Measurement Conversion Table

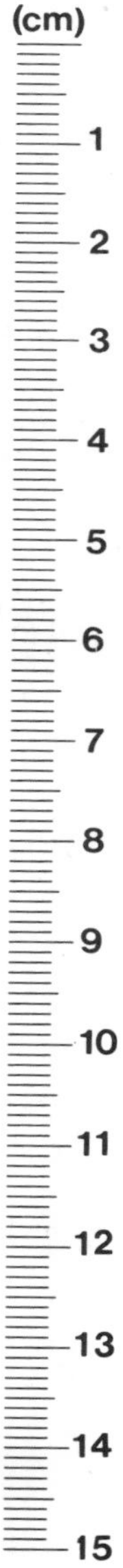

Metric System Equivalents

1 gram (g) = 1000 milligrams (mg)
1000 grams = 1 kilogram (kg)
.001 milligram = 1 microgram (mcg)
1 liter (L) = 1000 milliliters (ml)
1 milliliter = 1 cubic centimeter (cc)
1 meter = 100 centimeters (cm)
1 meter = 1000 millimeters (mm)

Conversion Equivalents

Volume

1 milliliter = 15 minims (M) = 15 drops (gtt)
5 milliliters = 1 fluidram (ʒ) = 1 teaspoon (tsp)
15 milliliters = 4 fluidrams = 1 tablespoon (T)
30 milliliters = 1 ounce (oz) = 2 tablespoons
500 milliliters = 1 pint (pt)
1000 milliliters = 1 quart (qt)

Weight

1 kilogram = 2.2 pound (lb)
1 gram (g) = 1000 milligrams = 15 grains (gr)
0.6 gram = 600 milligrams = 10 grains
0.5 gram = 500 milligrams = 7.5 grains
0.3 gram = 300 milligrams = 5 grains
0.06 gram = 60 milligrams = 1 grain

Length

2.5 centimeters = 1 inch

Centigrade/Fahrenheit Conversions

$C = (F - 32) \times 5/9$
$F = (C \times 9/5) + 32$

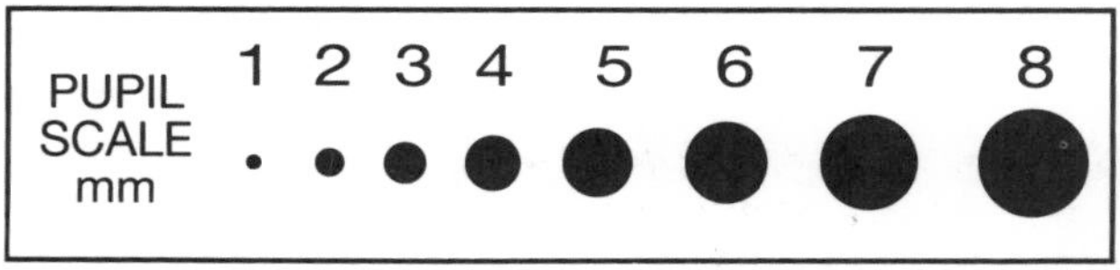

Davis's DRUG GUIDE for Nurses

Sixth Edition

JUDITH HOPFER DEGLIN, PharmD
Consultant Pharmacist
United Community Services, Inc.
Norwich
Connecticut

APRIL HAZARD VALLERAND, PhD, RN
University of Pennsylvania
School of Nursing
Philadelphia
Pennsylvania

F. A. DAVIS COMPANY • Philadelphia

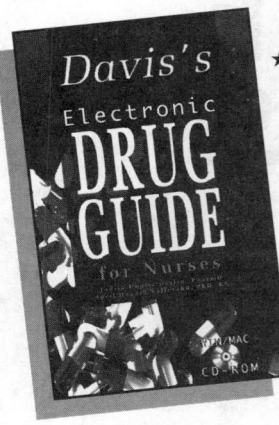

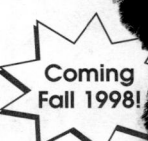

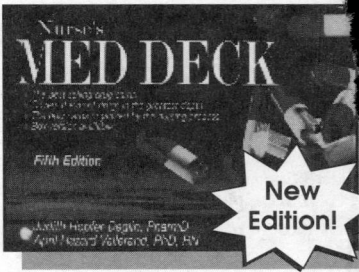

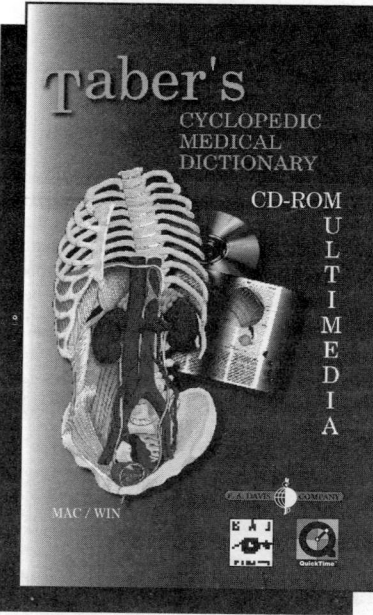

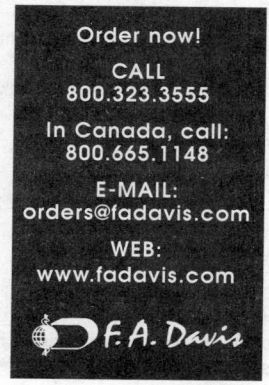

F. A. Davis Company
1915 Arch Street
Philadelphia, PA 19103

Printed in the United States of America

Last digit indicates print number 10 9 8 7 6 5 4 3 2 1

Publisher, Nursing: Robert Martone
Director of Production: Herbert J. Powell, Jr.
Senior Production Editor: Roberta Massey
Cover Designer: Louis J. Forgione

NOTE: As new scientific information becomes available through basic and clinical research, recommended treatments and drug therapies undergo changes. The authors and publisher have done everything possible to make this book accurate, up to date, and in accord with accepted standards at the time of publication. However, the reader is advised always to check product information (package inserts) for changes and new information regarding dose and contraindications before administering any drug. Caution is especially urged when using new or infrequently ordered drugs.

Library of Congress Cataloging-in-Publication Data

Deglin, Judith Hopfer, 1950 –
Davis's drug guide for nurses / Judith Hopfer Deglin, April Hazard Vallerand.—6th ed.
p. cm.
Includes bibliographical references and index.
0-8036-0365-7 (alk. paper)
1. Drugs—Handbooks, manuals, etc. 2. Nursing—Handbooks, manuals, etc. I. Vallerand, April Hazard. II. Title.
DNLM: 1. Drugs—handbooks. 2. Drugs—nurses' instruction.
RM301.12.D44 1998
615'.1'024613—dc21
DNLM/DLC
for Library of Congress

98-16214
CIP

In loving memory of my children, Samantha Ann and Randy Eli, both struck and killed by a drinking driver on January 9, 1997. They were the best part of us. Their lives were full of wonder and joy. Samantha taught us how to find the good in every person and Randy taught us how to make the smallest experience fun.

To my parents, Charlotte and Kurt Hopfer; my brothers, Sidney and Allen Hopfer; and my sister, Ricky Greenly; and their families for being there in the darkness.

To my husband, Stuart, for surviving with me through the deepest of despair.

To those numerous others who simply extended their love.

JHD

To my father, Keith, for teaching me the importance of doing my best.

To my other mom, Roberta, for always being there with support and understanding.

To Benjamin and Katharine, for their growing appreciation of what their Mom does.

To my husband, Warren, the best father, colleague, and friend I have ever known, for his unending support, encouragement, and love.

AHV

CONSULTANTS

Lizette A. Beltram, RPh
Coordinator of Pharmacy Operations
The William W. Backus Hospital
Norwich, Connecticut

Christine Bradway, MSN, RN, CS
Gerontologic Nurse Practitioner
University of Pennsylvania School of Nursing
Philadelphia, Pennsylvania

Regina S. Cunningham, RN, MA, AOCN
Chief Nursing Officer
Director of Ambulatory Services
The Cancer Institute of New Jersey
New Brunswick, New Jersey

Elizabeth A. Duthie, RN, MA
Director of Nursing Education and Patient Care Systems
New York University Medical Center
New York, New York

Corinne Impelliteri, BS, RPh
Staff Pharmacist
William W. Backus Hospital
Norwich, CT

Lenore H. Kurlowicz, PhD, RN, CS
Assistant Professor of Geropsychiatric Nursing
University of Pennsylvania School of Nursing
Psychiatric Consultation-Liaison Nurse
Hospital of the University of Pennsylvania
Philadelphia, Pennsylvania

Marie M. Lupo, RN, MSN, CNS, C, CDE
Clinical Nurse Specialist, Diabetes
Hackensack University Medical Center
Hackensack, New Jersey

Steven B. Meisel, PharmD
Assistant Director of Pharmacy
Fairview-Southdale Hospital
Edina, Minnesota

Lynda Nolan, MSN, MA, CRNP
High Risk Pregnancy Center
East Brunswick, New Jersey

Rosemary C. Polomano, PhD, RN, FAAN
Clinical Nurse Specialist, Pain Management
Hospital of the University of Pennsylvania
Philadelphia, Pennsylvania

Noel Dougherty Rosner, MSN, RN, ANP-C
Nurse Practitioner
Raritan Bay Medical Center
Department of Infectious Diseases
Perth Amboy, New Jersey

Mildred M. Russin, MSN, RN
University of Florida
Gainesville, Florida

Karen Sikorski, RN, MS
Clinical Nurse Specialist - Pain Management
OSF Center for Cancer Care
Rockford, Illinois
Elmhurst College
Elmhurst, Illinois

ACKNOWLEDGMENTS

We offer our thanks and gratitude to our families, whose support and patience with our endless computer time and phone calls gave us the time and strength to complete this manuscript.

To those at F. A. Davis, especially Bob Martone, Ruth De George, Herb Powell, John Morgan, Roberta Massey, and Jessica Howie Martin, who saw our projects through to completion.

Judi and April

NEW FEATURES AT A GLANCE

- **One hundred fifty drug monographs** have been added, along with 23 just-released FDA approvals highlighting use, dose, and Rx/OTC status.
  - Contains **Recent Drug Release Updates** for last-minute drug releases.
  - Free up-to-the-minute Drug Updates on the Web.
  - The new **Disk Version** of *Davis's Drug Guide for Nurses* offers access to more than 500 drugs by generic or trade name. Print entire monograph or parts—whatever you need to create customized med cards for quick clinical access.
- Many of the group monographs, in wide usage clinically, have been separated into individual monographs for easier use and user-friendliness.
- 100 full-color images of most commonly prescribed brand name drugs.
- It is the only nursing reference that thoroughly covers compatible drugs in syringe, Y-site, additive, and solution. This alerts the nurse to potential problems in the event the IV already in use is not compatible with another drug infusion.
- **Life span dosing considerations** for adult, geriatric, pediatric, and neonatal patients have been updated.
- Newly approved drug indications as well as new unlabeled uses are identified.
- Drugs with similar characteristics have been incorporated into **group monographs** that allow comparison among individual drugs in a group, a useful tool when switching from one agent in a group to another.
- All drugs include an **Availability** section identifying all available dosage forms with respective strengths, a handy addition for advanced practice nurses with prescriptive practice.
- A unique section, **Medication Misadventures: The Nurse's Role in Detecting, Preventing, and Documenting Adverse Drug Reactions and Medication Errors,** is included.
- **IV therapy** data have been completely updated, and **IV** rate information has been expanded to include the implications of drug administration at incorrect rates. This vital information is unique to *Davis's Drug Guide for Nurses, sixth edition.*
- 475 commonly used combination drugs have been completely rewritten and updated. This combination list now includes the amounts of each active ingredient.
- For quick clinical look-ups, a pull-out chart identifying **syringe compatibilities** and **equianalgesic doses** for **opioid analgesics.**
- All drug entries are labeled as Rx (prescription) or OTC (over-the-counter).
- "Use cautiously in" statements identify potentially dangerous additives in drugs such as alcohol, bisulfites, benzyl alcohol, or tartrazine should patients have a known intolerance to drug additives.
- "Do not confuse with" statements alert the nurse to drugs that sound alike, are spelled alike, or are commonly confused with other medications.
- Completely updated drug classifications for a total of 49.

WHAT'S NEW IN THE SIXTH EDITION

The sixth edition of *Davis's Drug Guide for Nurses* continues to set new standards for nursing drug references. While providing the most comprehensive, up-to-date, and practical information available to nurses, it also makes available the most relevant information required for the safe and effective administration and monitoring of drug therapy. Its consistent, easy-to-follow format ensures that, once the nurse is familiar with the layout of drug monographs, finding specific facts for individual drugs becomes a very efficient process.

The new Disk Version contains the most comprehensive drug coverage available. The floppy disk gives the user access to more than 500 drugs by generic or trade name with the option to print out an entire monograph or parts thereof.

In an effort to reflect the authors' commitment to providing the most up-to-date material available, 150 new drug monographs, 475 combination products, and 49 drug classifications are included. In an effort to continually update our users with the latest FDA releases, *free* up-to-the-minute *Drug Updates* are available on Davis's website at www.fadavis.com.

Existing monographs have been updated to include newly approved indications and unlabeled uses, as well as interactions with recently released drugs.

Situations in which a drug should be used with extreme caution are highlighted in a second color to increase awareness and hopefully prevent an adverse drug event.

Nursing implications have been streamlined to afford better accessibility to data, and IV administration information is more clearly delineated to facilitate rapid retrieval. In an effort to take a proactive role in the prevention of medication errors, we have included statements such as "do not confuse with . . . " that are highlighted in a second color to call attention to areas that may lead to life-threatening errors.

The dosage information includes the ranges recommended by manufacturers and approved by the Food and Drug Administration (FDA). Because special dosing considerations are usually required depending on the age, size, condition, and tolerance of the patient, more extensive **neonatal**, **pediatric**, and **geriatric** dosing information is provided in the sixth edition, as are more details on dosage modification in hepatic/renal disease. The book's information on contraindications, precautions, adverse reactions and side effects, and interactions is condensed to a level essential to responsible clinical practice.

This reference not only provides the pharmacologic profile of what each drug does and how it works, it also links essential nursing data—such as what parameters to assess in the patient taking the drug, how to administer the medication, and how to evaluate the drug's effectiveness—while it incorporates the nursing diagnoses applicable to its administration. In addition, the necessary information to provide appropriate patient and family teaching is presented.

The sixth edition of *Davis's Drug Guide for Nurses* fills the drug information needs of every student and practicing nurse and facilitates the safe and efficacious use of medications.

No other drug reference presents such depth of pharmacologic content within the framework of the nursing process and does it in such a convenient size and format.

From THE PUBLISHER

CONTENTS

HOW TO USE
DAVIS'S DRUG GUIDE FOR NURSES

The purpose of *Davis's Drug Guide for Nurses* is to provide readily accessible, easy-to-understand drug information for the most commonly used drugs for clinical use. The sections below describe the organization of the book and the information provided for each drug.

SPECIAL DOSING CONSIDERATIONS

In many clinical situations, the average dosing range can be inappropriate. This section presents general guidelines for conditions in which special considerations must be made to ensure optimal therapeutic outcome.

CLASSIFICATIONS

Brief summaries of the major therapeutic classifications are provided, along with a listing of those drugs included in *Davis's Drug Guide for Nurses* and the page numbers on which those monographs may be found.

DRUG MONOGRAPHS

The following information appears for each drug:

Generic/Trade Name: The generic name appears first, with a pronunciation key. This is followed by an alphabetical listing of trade names. The generic name is the official name of the drug assigned by the United States Adopted Names (USAN) Council in the United States and by the World Health Organization (WHO) in other countries. In many institutions, drugs are labeled generically. Canadian trade names appear in brackets. Common names, abbreviations, and selected foreign names are also included. For users who do not know the generic name, a color-coded Comprehensive Index, which contains entries for both trade names and generic names as well as classifications, provides this information quickly and easily.

Classification: Drugs may be classified by a variety of ways. For example, propranolol (Inderal) is classified first as an antianginal but is also used as an antiarrhythmic and an antihypertensive. For a better explanation of drug classifications, refer to the Classifications section of the book (pages C1–C75), which provides brief summaries of the classifications, lists the drugs contained in each classification, and identifies the page numbers on which the drugs can be found. The classifications are listed alphabetically.

Controlled Substance Schedule: If a drug is a controlled substance, its legal status or schedule is listed. This information alerts the reader to observe the necessary regulations when handling these drugs and should help instruct the patient regarding refill allotments. (See Appendix C for a description of the Schedule of Controlled Substances and a list of controlled substances included in *Davis's Drug Guide for Nurses*.)

Pregnancy Category: If the Food and Drug Administration (FDA) assigned pregnancy category is known, it is listed in this part of the monograph. A more detailed explanation of these categories (A, B, C, D, and X) is found in Appendix E. These categories allow for some assessment of risk to the fetus when a drug is used in the pregnant patient or in the patient who may be trying to conceive while receiving the drug.

Indications: The most common FDA uses of the drug are listed. Significant unlabeled uses are also included.

Action: This section contains a concise description of how a drug is known or believed to act in producing the desired therapeutic effect.

Pharmacokinetics: This information describes what happens to a drug following administration and includes an analysis of the absorption, distribution, metabolism, excretion, and half-life (amount of time for drug level to decrease by 50%).

Absorption: Absorption describes the process that follows drug administration and its subsequent delivery to systemic circulation. If only a small fraction is absorbed following oral administration (diminished bioavailability), then the oral dose will be much larger than the parenteral dose. Absorption into systemic circulation also follows other routes of administration such as topical, transdermal, intramuscular, subcutaneous, rectal, and ophthalmic routes. Drugs administered intravenously are usually 100% bioavailable.

Distribution: Following absorption, drugs are distributed, sometimes selectively, to various body tissues and fluids. These factors become important in choosing one drug over another, as in selecting antibiotics that may need to penetrate the central nervous system in the treatment of meningitis or avoiding drugs that cross the placenta in pregnancy or concentrate in breast milk during lactation. During distribution, many drugs interact with specific receptors and exert their pharmacologic effect.

Metabolism and Excretion: Following their intended action, drugs leave the body either by conversion by the liver to inactive compounds (metabolism or biotransformation), which are then excreted by the kidneys, or by renal elimination of unchanged drug. In addition, some drugs may be eliminated by other pathways such as biliary excretion, sweat, feces, and breath. If drugs are extensively liver metabolized, then patients with severe liver disease may require dosage reduction. If the kidney is the major organ of elimination, then dosage adjustment may be necessary in the face of renal impairment. For renally eliminated drugs, knowing creatinine clearance (CCr) provides a method of quantifying renal function and making dosage adjustments. Formulas may be used to estimate CCr and are helpful in adjusting dosage regimens (see Appendix F). The very young (premature infants and neonates) and the elderly (older than 60 years of age) have diminished renal excretory and hepatic metabolic capacity. These patients may require dosage reduction or increased dosing intervals.

Half-Life: The half-life of a drug is useful to know in planning effective regimens because it correlates roughly with the duration of action. Half-lives are given for patients with normal renal or hepatic function. Other conditions that may alter the half-life are noted.

Contraindications and Precautions: Situations in which drug use should be avoided or alternatives strongly considered are listed as contraindications. In general, most drugs are contraindicated in pregnancy or lactation, unless the potential benefits outweigh the possible risks to the mother or baby (e.g., anticonvulsants and antihypertensives). Contraindications may be absolute (i.e., the drug in question should be avoided completely) or relative, in which certain clinical situations may allow cautious use of the drug. The precautions portion includes disease states or clinical situations in which drug use involves particular risks or in which dosage modification may be necessary.

Adverse Reactions and Side Effects: To simplify long lists of possible reactions, a systems approach to side effects and adverse reactions has been taken. The order is such that these reactions have been listed in head-to-toe order for systems amenable to noting in this manner (CNS, EENT, Resp, CV, GI, GU). Other systems follow in alphabetical order (Endo, F and E, Hemat, Local, Metab, MS, Neuro), ending with a miscellaneous section. Although it is not possible to include all reported reactions, an effort has been made to include major side effects. Life-threatening adverse reactions or side effects are CAPITALIZED, while the most commonly encountered problems are underlined. Each group is alphabetized. In general, those underlined have an incidence of 10% or greater. Those not underlined occur in fewer than 10% but more than 1% of patients. Although life-threatening reactions may be rare (fewer than 1%), they are included because of their significance. The following abbreviations are used for body systems:

CNS: central nervous system
EENT: eye, ear, nose, and throat
Resp: respiratory
CV: cardiovascular
GI: gastrointestinal
GU: genitourinary
Derm: dermatologic
Endo: endocrinologic
F and E: fluid and electrolyte
Hemat: hematologic
Local: local
Metab: metabolic
MS: musculoskeletal
Neuro: neurologic
Misc: miscellaneous

Interactions: As the number of medications a patient receives increases, so does the likelihood of experiencing a drug-drug interaction. The most important drug-drug interactions and their results are explained. Significant drug-food interactions also are noted. Recommendations for avoiding or minimizing these interactions are also presented.

Route and Dosage: The usual routes of administration are grouped together and include recommended dosages for adults, children, and other more specific age groups (such as geriatric patients). Dosage units are given in the terms in which they will most likely be prescribed. For example, penicillin G dosage is given in units rather than in milligrams. Dosing intervals also are mentioned in the manner in which they are most likely to be ordered. Although antibiotics and antiarrhythmics should be given at regular intervals around the clock, it is neither necessary nor practical to give other medications, such as oral antihypertensives, in this manner. In situations in which dosage or interval is different from that commonly encountered, these indications are listed separately for clarification.

Availability: This section lists the strengths and concentrations of various dosage forms that are available. Such information is useful in planning more convenient regimens (fewer tablets/capsules, less injection volume) and in determining whether certain dosing forms are available (suppositories, oral concentrates, sustained or extended-release forms).

Time/Action Profile: This information is provided so that the onset of drug action, its peak effect, and its duration of activity can be anticipated and considered in planning administration schedules. The pharmacodynamics of each route of administration have been tabulated so that the reader may appreciate differences achieved by choosing one route over another. Durations of action of anti-infective agents generally have not been included. Most regimens for these agents are designed to avoid toxicity while ensuring high peak levels necessary for anti-infective action. Because of this, duration of action and blood level information are not necessarily comparable.

Nursing Implications: This section has been developed to help the nurse apply the nursing process to pharmacotherapeutics. It is divided into subsections that give the nurse a step-by-step guide to clinical assessment, implementation, and evaluation as they relate to medication administration.

Assessment: This subsection includes parameters for patient history and physical data that should be assessed before and monitored during drug therapy. The **General Info** section describes assessment that is pertinent to all patients taking the medication. Other sections also are identified to specify assessments based on the drug's various indications. **Lab Test Considerations** provide the nurse with information regarding which laboratory tests to monitor and how the results may be affected by the medication. **Toxicity and Overdose** discusses therapeutic serum drug levels and signs and symptoms of toxicity. The antidote and treatment for toxicity or overdose of appropriate medications also are included.

Potential Nursing Diagnoses: The nursing diagnoses approved by the North American Nursing Diagnoses Association (NANDA) are used. The three most pertinent diagnoses that apply to a patient receiving the medication are listed. Following each diagnosis, the location of the information from which the diagnosis has been developed is listed in parentheses to provide a reference for the nursing diagnosis—e.g., Infection, risk for (Indications, Side Effects). All of the NANDA diagnostic labels are listed in Appendix S.

Implementation: Guidelines specific for medication administration are discussed in this subsection. The information listed under the **General Info** heading applies to all routes of administration and includes timing of administration and details for patient care. Other headings in this section provide data regarding routes of administration. **PO** describes when and how to administer the drug, whether tablets may be crushed or capsules opened, and when to administer the medication in relation to food. **IV** provides details for reconstitution and dilution. **Direct IV** (IV Push), **Intermittent Infusion**, and **Continuous Infusion** specify amount and type of further dilution and stability information. **Rate** includes infusion time for each type of administration. **Syringe Compatibility/Incompatibility** identifies the medications each drug is compatible or incompatible with when mixed in a syringe. This type of compatibility is usually limited to 15 minutes after mixing. **Y-Site Compatibility/Incompatibility** identifies those medications that are compatible or incompatible with each drug when administered via Y-site injection or 3-way stopcock in IV tubing. **Additive Compatibility/Incompatibility** identifies those medications that are compatible or incompatible when admixed in solution. This type of compatibility is usually limited to 24 hours. **Solution Compatibility/Incompatibility** identifies solutions that are compatible or incompatible with the medication for dilution or administration purposes. Compatibility information is compiled from Trissel's *Handbook of Injectable Drugs*, ed 9. (See Bibliography, p. 1151.)

Patient/Family Teaching: This subsection includes material that should be taught to patients and/or families of patients. Side effects that should be reported, information on minimizing side effects, details on administration, and follow-up requirements are presented. The nurse also should refer to the **Adverse Reactions and Side Effects** and **Interactions** sections for additional data to complete the patient/family teaching plan. **Home Care Issues** discusses aspects to be considered for medications taken in the home setting.

Evaluation: Outcome criteria for determination of the effectiveness of the medication are provided.

SPECIAL DOSING CONSIDERATIONS

For almost every drug there is an average dosing range. There are many situations, however, when this average range can be either toxic or ineffective. The purpose of this section is to describe situations in which special dosing considerations must be made to ensure a successful therapeutic outcome. The guidelines presented are general but should lead to a finer appreciation of individual dosing parameters. When these clinical situations are encountered, the doses of drugs ordered should be reviewed and the necessary adjustments made. Many clinical situations change over time (renal/hepatic function, body size, age), requiring reassessment of dosing at regular intervals.

THE PEDIATRIC PATIENT

The most obvious reason for adjusting dosages in pediatric patients is size. Most drug dosages for this population are given on a mg/kg basis or even more specifically on the basis of body surface area (BSA). Body surface area is determined by using a Body Surface Area Nomogram (see Appendix G) or calculated by using formulas (Appendix F).

The neonate and the premature infant require additional adjustments besides those made on the basis of size. In this population, absorption following oral administration may be incomplete or altered because of changes in gastric pH or GI motility, distribution may be altered because of varying amounts of total body water, and metabolism and excretion may be delayed because liver and kidney function have not yet matured. Progressive hepatic and renal function maturation may necessitate frequent dosage adjustments during the course of therapy to reflect improved drug handling in the premature infant or neonate. Rapid weight changes in this age group require that additional frequent adjustments be made.

In addition to pharmacokinetic variables, other nursing considerations should be addressed. The route of administration chosen in pediatric patients often reflects the seriousness of the illness. The nurse should consider the child's developmental level and ability to understand the situation. Medications that must be administered intravenously or by intramuscular injection may seem frightening to a young child or may cause concern to the parents. The nurse should allay these fears by educating the parents and comforting the child. Intramuscular or subcutaneous injection sites should be carefully chosen in this age group to prevent possible nerve or tissue damage.

THE GERIATRIC PATIENT

In patients older than 55 to 60 years of age, the pharmacokinetic behavior of drugs changes. Drug absorption may be delayed secondary to diminished GI motility (from age or other drugs) or passive congestion of abdominal blood vessels, as seen in congestive heart failure. Distribution may be altered because of low plasma proteins, particularly in malnourished patients. Because plasma proteins are decreased, a larger proportion of free or unbound drug will result in an increase in drug action. The result may be a patient's becoming toxic while receiving a standard dose of a drug. Metabolism performed by the liver and excretion handled by the kidneys are both slowed as part of the aging process and may result in prolonged and exaggerated drug action. Body composition also changes with age. There is an increase in fatty tissue and a decrease in skeletal muscle and total body water. Height and weight usually decrease. A dosage of medication that was acceptable for the robust 50-year-old patient may be excessive in the same patient 20 years later.

An additional concern is that most elderly patients are receiving numerous drugs. With increasing numbers of drugs being used, there is an increased risk of one drug's negating, potentiating, or otherwise altering the effects of another drug (drug-drug interaction). In general, doses of most medications should be decreased in the geriatric population. Drugs to be specifically concerned about are the digitalis glycosides (digoxin and digitoxin), sedative/hypnotics, oral anticoagulants, nonsteroidal anti-inflammatory agents, and antihypertensives.

Dosing regimens should be kept simple in this patient population because many of these patients are taking multiple drugs. Doses should be scheduled so that the patient's day is not interrupted multiple times to take medications. The use of fixed-dose combination drugs may help to simplify dosing regimens. However, some of these combinations are more expensive than are the individual components.

In explaining medication regimens to elderly patients, the nurse should remember that hearing deficits are common in this group. Patients may find it embarrassing to disclose this information, and full compliance may be hindered. Verbal and written instructions should also be given in the language in which patients are fluent and at a level that they can understand.

THE OBSTETRIC PATIENT

During pregnancy, both the mother and the fetus must be considered. The placenta, once thought to be a protective barrier, is simply a membrane that is capable of protecting the fetus from only extremely large molecules. Transfer of drugs through the placenta to the fetus occurs by both passive and active processes. The fetus is particularly vulnerable during the first and the last trimesters of pregnancy. During the first trimester, the vital organs are being formed. Ingestion of drugs that cause harm (potential teratogens) during this stage of pregnancy may lead to fetal malformation or may cause miscarriage. Unfortunately, this is the time when a woman is least likely to know that she is pregnant. Therefore, it is wise to inform all patients of childbearing age of potential harm to an unborn child. In the third trimester, the major concern is that drugs administered to the mother and transferred to the fetus may not be safely metabolized and excreted by the fetus. This is especially true of drugs administered near term. After the infant is delivered, he or she no longer has the placenta to help with drug excretion. If drugs administered before delivery are allowed to accumulate, toxicity may result.

The possibility of medications altering sperm quality and quantity in potential fathers also is becoming an area of increasing concern. Male patients should be informed of this risk when taking any medications known to have this potential.

There are situations in which, for the sake of the mother's health and for protection of the fetus, drug administration is required throughout pregnancy. Two examples are the epileptic patient and the hypertensive patient. In these circumstances, the safest drug in the smallest effective dose is chosen. Because of changes in the behavior of drugs that may occur throughout pregnancy, dosage adjustments may be required during the progression of pregnancy and after delivery. A special situation related to drug behavior in pregnancy is the mother who abuses drugs. Infants born to mothers addicted to alcohol, sedatives (including benzodiazepines), heroin, and cocaine may be of low birth weight; may experience drug withdrawal after birth; and may display developmental delay. A careful history should alert the nurse to these possibilities.

RENAL DISEASE

The kidneys are the major organ of drug elimination. Some drugs are excreted only after being metabolized or biotransformed by the liver. Others may be eliminated unchanged by the kidneys. The premature infant has immature renal function. Elderly patients have an age-related decrease in renal function. To make dosage adjustments in patients with renal dysfunction, assessment must be made of the degree of renal impairment in the individual patient and the percentage of drug eliminated by the kidneys. The degree of renal function can be measured by laboratory testing, most commonly by the creatinine clearance (CCr or Ccr), which also can be approximated by calculation (Appendix F). The percentage of each drug excreted by the kidneys can be determined from references on pharmacokinetics. In addition, the dosage frequently can be optimized by measuring blood levels of the drug in the individual patient and making any further necessary changes. Two types of drugs for which this type of dosage adjustment are commonly used are digoxin and the aminoglycoside antibiotics (amikacin, gentamicin, and tobramycin).

LIVER DISEASE

The liver is the major organ for metabolism of drugs. For most drugs, this is an inactivation step. The inactive metabolites are subsequently excreted by the kidneys. The conversion process usually changes the drug from a relatively lipid or fat-soluble compound to a more water-soluble substance. Liver function is not as easily quantified as renal function; therefore, it is difficult to predict the correct dosage for a patient with liver dysfunction based on laboratory tests alone. In addition, it appears that only minimal liver function may be required for complete drug metabolism.

A patient who is severely jaundiced or who has very low serum proteins (particularly albumin) may be expected to have some problems metabolizing drugs. Chronic alcoholic patients are at risk for developing this type of situation. In advanced liver disease, drug absorption also may be impaired secondary to portal vascular congestion. Decreased levels of serum proteins also affect the amount of drug that may be bound. If less drug is bound to proteins, then more drug is unbound (free drug) and available to exert its pharmacologic effect. Examples of drugs that should be carefully dosed in patients with liver disease include theophylline, diuretics, and sedatives that are liver metabolized. Some drugs require the liver for activation (such as sulindac or cyclophosphamide) and should be avoided in patients with severely compromised liver function.

CONGESTIVE HEART FAILURE

Patients with congestive heart failure also require dosage modifications. In these patients, drug absorption may be impaired because of passive congestion of blood vessels feeding the GI tract. This same passive congestion slows drug delivery to the liver and delays metabolism. In addition, renal function may be compromised, leading to delayed elimination and prolonged drug action. Many patients who have congestive heart failure are already in a special dosing category because of their age. Dosages of drugs that are metabolized mainly by the liver or excreted mainly by the kidneys should be decreased in patients with apparent congestive heart failure.

BODY SIZE

In most situations, drug dosing is based on total body weight. Some drugs selectively penetrate fatty tissues. If the drug is known not to penetrate fatty tissues and if the patient is obese, dosage should be determined by ideal body weight or estimated lean body mass (e.g., digoxin, gentamicin). These quantities may be determined from tables of desirable weights or may be estimated using formulas for lean body mass when the patient's height and weight are known (see Appendix F). If this type of adjustment is not made, considerable toxicity may result.

Body size also should be appreciated in patients who are grossly underweight. Elderly patients, chronic alcoholics, patients with AIDS, and patients who are terminally ill from cancer or other chronic, debilitating illness may need careful attention to dosing, which may be based on the size of a normal adult (70 kg) patient. Patients who have had a limb amputated also need to have this change in body size taken into account.

DELIVERY TO SITES OF ACTION

To have a successful therapeutic outcome, the drug must reach its intended site of action. Under the most desirable of conditions, the drug will have only a minimal effect on other tissues or body systems. A good example is drugs that are applied topically for skin conditions and are only minimally absorbed. In many diseases, this arrangement is neither achievable nor practical. Often unusual routes of administration must be used to guarantee the presence of drug at the intended site of response. In patients with bacterial meningitis, parenteral administration of drugs may not produce high enough levels in the cerebrospinal fluid. Intrathecal administration may be required in addition to parenteral therapy, as is the case with the aminoglycoside antibiotics (amikacin, gentamicin, and tobramycin). The eye represents another barrier that is relatively impermeable to many drugs. To overcome this barrier, local instillation or injection may be required.

In some cases, local absorption may not occur, and the desired systemic effect will not happen. Drugs may not be absorbed into systemic circulation from subcutaneous sites in patients with shock or poor tissue perfusion due to other causes.

When considering the route of administration, identify the site at which the drug is intended to have its primary action. To achieve its maximal effect, it must be delivered to its intended site of action.

DRUG INTERACTIONS

The presence of additional drugs may also necessitate dosage adjustments. Drugs highly bound to plasma proteins, such as warfarin and phenytoin, may be displaced by other highly protein bound drugs. When this phenomenon occurs, the drug that has been displaced exhibits an increase in its activity because the free or unbound drug is active.

Some agents decrease the ability of the liver to metabolize other drugs. Drugs capable of doing this include cimetidine and chloramphenicol. Concurrently administered drugs that are highly metabolized by the liver may need to be administered in decreased dosages. Other agents such as phenobarbital, other barbiturates, and rifampin are capable of stimulating (inducing) the liver to metabolize drugs more rapidly, requiring larger doses to be administered.

Drugs that significantly alter urine pH can affect excretion of other drugs for which the excretory process is pH-dependent. Alkalinizing the urine will hasten the excretion of acidic drugs. Acidification of the urine will enhance reabsorption of acidic drugs, prolonging and enhancing drug action. In the reverse situation, drugs that acidify the urine will hasten the excretion of alkaline drugs. An example of this is administering sodium bicarbonate in cases of aspirin overdose. Alkalinizing the urine promotes renal excretion of aspirin.

Some drugs compete for enzyme systems with other drugs. Allopurinol inhibits the enzyme involved in uric acid production, but it also inhibits metabolism (inactivation) of 6-mercaptopurine, greatly increasing its toxicity. The dosage of mercaptopurine needs to be significantly reduced when coadministered with allopurinol.

DOSAGE FORMS

The nurse frequently encounters problems that relate to the dosage form itself. Some medications may not be commercially available in liquid or chewable dosage forms. The pharmacist may have to compound such dosage forms for an individual patient. It may be necessary to disguise the taste or appearance of a medication in food or a beverage for the patient to fully comply with a given regimen. Finally, some dosage forms, such as aerosol inhalers, may not be suitable for very young patients because use of the form requires cooperation beyond the patient's developmental level.

Before altering dosage forms (crushing tablets or opening capsules) or using them by routes for which they were not intended, check to be sure that the effect of the drug will not be altered and that patient safety will not be compromised by doing so. In general, neither extended nor sustained-release dosage forms should be crushed, nor should capsules containing beads of medication be opened. Altering these dosage forms may shorten and intensify their intended action. Others (sprinkle preparations) are designed to be opened. Enteric-coated tablets, which may appear to be sugar coated or candy coated, also should not be crushed. This coating may be designed to protect the stomach from the irritating effects of these drugs. Crushing the tablets will expose the stomach lining to these agents and increase GI irritation. If a dosage form needs to be crushed, it should be ingested right away. A glass of water should be taken before administration of powders or crushed tablets to wet the esophagus and prevent the material from sticking to upper GI mucosal surfaces.

ENVIRONMENTAL FACTORS

Cigarette smoke is capable of inducing liver enzymes to metabolize drugs more rapidly. Patients who smoke may need larger doses of liver-metabolized drugs to compensate for this. Patients who are passively exposed to cigarette smoke also may exhibit otherwise unexplained needs for larger doses of medications. The effect of cigarette smoke on drug metabolism may persist for months.

NUTRITIONAL FACTORS

Certain foods can alter the dosing requirement for some medications. Dietary calcium found in high concentrations in dairy products combines (chelates) with tetracycline and prevents its absorption. Many antibiotics are absorbed better if taken when the stomach is empty. Foods high in pyridoxine (vitamin B_6) can negate the anti-Parkinson effect of levodopa (this is counteracted with coadministration of carbidopa). Foods capable of altering urine pH may affect the excretion patterns of medications, enhancing or diminishing their effectiveness. There are no general guidelines for nutritional factors. It is prudent to check whether these problems exist or whether they may explain therapeutic failures and to make the necessary dosage adjustments.

SUMMARY

The average dosing range for drugs is intended for an average patient. However, every patient is an individual with specific drug-handling capabilities. Taking into account these special dosing considerations allows the planning of an individualized drug regimen that results in a desired therapeutic outcome while minimizing the risk of toxicity.

KEY TO COMMONLY USED ABBREVIATIONS

ABGs	arterial blood gases
ac	before meals
AD	right ear
ADHD	attention-deficit hyperactivity disorder
A-G ratio	albumin-globulin ratio
AIDS	acquired immunodeficiency syndrome
ALT	alanine aminotransferase
ANA	antinuclear antibodies
ANC	absolute neutrophil count
AS	left ear
AST	aspartate aminotransferase
AU	both ears
AV	atrioventricular
bid	two times a day
BP	blood pressure
BMI	body mass index
bpm	beats per minute
BUN	blood urea nitrogen
c̄	with
cap	capsule
CBC	complete blood count
CCr	creatinine clearance
CHF	congestive heart failure
CNS	central nervous system
COPD	chronic obstructive pulmonary disease
CPK	creatine phosphokinase
CR	controlled-release
CSF	colony-stimulating factor; cerebrospinal fluid
CV	cardiovascular
CVP	central venous pressure
D5/LR	5% dextrose and lactated Ringer's solution
D5/0.9% NaCl	5% dextrose and 0.9% NaCl; 5% dextrose and normal saline
D5/0.25% NaCl	5% dextrose and 0.25% NaCl; 5% dextrose and quarter normal saline
D5/0.45% NaCl	5% dextrose and 0.45% NaCl; 5% dextrose and half normal saline
D5W	5% dextrose in water
D10W	10% dextrose in water
Derm	dermatologic
dl	deciliter
DNA	deoxyribonucleic acid
ECG	electrocardiogram
EENT	eye, ear, nose, and throat
Endo	endocrine
ER	extended-release
F and E	fluid and electrolyte
g	gram(s)
GERD	gastroesophageal reflux disease
GFR	glomerular filtration rate

GI	gastrointestinal
gr	grain(s)
G6PD	glucose-6-phosphate dehydrogenase
gt(t)	drop(s)
GU	genitourinary
HDL	high-density lipoproteins
Hemat	hematologic
HIV	human immunodeficiency virus
hr(s)	hour(s)
HRT	hormone replacement therapy
hs	hour of sleep (bedtime)
IA	intra-articular
IL	intralesional
IM	intramuscular
in.	inch(es)
Inhaln	inhalation
IPPB	intermittent positive pressure breathing
IS	intrasynovial
IT	intrathecal
IU	international unit
IV	intravenous
K	potassium
KCl	potassium chloride
kg	kilogram
L	liter
LA	long-acting
LDH	lactic dehydrogenase
LDL	low-density lipoproteins
LR	lactated Ringer's solution
M	molar
MAO	monoamine oxidase
mcg	microgram(s)
mEq	milliequivalent
Metab	metabolic
mg	milligram(s)
min(s)	minute(s)
Misc	miscellaneous
ml	milliliter(s)
mo(s)	month(s)
MS	musculoskeletal; morphine sulfate
Na	sodium
NaCl	sodium chloride
0.9% NaCl	0.9% sodium chloride, normal saline
Neuro	neurologic
ng	nanogram(s)
NG	nasogastric
NPO	nothing by mouth
NS	sodium chloride, normal saline (0.9% NaCl)
NSAIDs/NSAIAs	nonsteroidal anti-inflammatory drugs/agents
OCD	obsessive-compulsive disorder
OD	right eye
Oint	ointment

Ophth .... ophthalmic
OS .... left eye
OTC .... over-the-counter
OU .... both eyes
oz .... ounce(s)
pc .... after meals
PCA .... patient-controlled analgesia
PO .... by mouth, orally
prn .... as needed
q .... every
qd .... every day
qh .... every hour
qid .... four times a day
qod .... every other day
q wk .... every week
q 2 h .... every 2 hours
q 3 h .... every 3 hours
q 4 h .... every 4 hours
RBC .... red blood cell count
Rect .... rectally or rectal
REM .... rapid eye movement
Resp .... respiratory
RNA .... ribonucleic acid
RTU .... ready to use
Rx .... prescription
s̄ .... without
SA .... sinoatrial
SC .... subcutaneous
sec(s) .... second(s)
SL .... sublingual
SR .... sustained-release
s̄s̄ .... one half
SSRI(s) .... selective serotonin reuptake inhibitor(s)
stat .... immediately
supp .... suppository
tab .... tablet
tbs .... tablespoon(s)
tid .... three times a day
Top .... topically or topical
tsp .... teaspoon(s)
U .... unit(s)
UK .... unknown
Vag .... vaginal
VLDL .... very low-density lipoproteins
WBC .... white blood cell count
wk(s) .... week(s)
yr(s) .... year(s)

MEDICATION MISADVENTURES: The Nurse's Role in Detecting, Preventing, and Documenting Adverse Drug Reactions and Medication Errors

Medication misadventures include all drug experiences that result in an unwanted or unintended response to drug therapy. The term includes both adverse drug reactions and medication errors.[1] The nurse should be familiar with the varied aspects of such experiences and be knowledgeable in how to detect, prevent (if possible), and document these events. Tantamount to this task and as the first step in this process, a detailed and accurate medication history should be obtained, and it should include questions about OTC (nonprescription) medications, dietary or social habits (smoking, alcohol, or drug abuse), and any previous reactions patients have had to medications (allergic and nonallergic).

ADVERSE DRUG REACTIONS

Unwanted or undesired drug effects fall into several categories. An appreciation of these categories can protect patients from subsequent misadventures when receiving the same drug or drugs in related chemical or pharmacologic categories. Before administering drugs, especially for the first time, it is wise to become familiar with the most commonly encountered adverse drug reactions (underlined in the **Adverse Reactions and Side Effects** section of each monograph). When they manifest, the nurse should know what measures should be taken and how to prioritize them. In addition to commonly encountered reactions, the nurse also should be aware of those rarely encountered but more disastrous reactions (CAPITALIZED in the **Adverse Reactions and Side Effects** section of each monograph). These may require immediate intervention at the time of the reaction or preparation prior to administering the drug in case they occur.

Adverse drug reactions should be suspected whenever there is a change in a patient's condition not interpreted as a therapeutic response to drugs being administered, particularly when a new drug has been introduced. Although intercurrent or progressive illness also may explain the appearance of new or worsening symptoms, adverse drug reactions and side effects should be strongly considered as a cause.

Recently, the term "adverse drug event" has been used to describe injury resulting from medical intervention related to a drug. This term is felt to be more comprehensive and clinically significant, while looking to preventability of such events.[2]

Dose-Related Reactions (Toxic Reactions): These reactions may mean several different things, but basically the dose prescribed for the patient is excessive. Some of the obvious reasons for this type of reaction include failure to take into account the patient's size (cachectic, elderly, or debilitated patients), failure to appreciate the distributive characteristics of the drug (some drugs do not enter fatty tissue well; basing dose on actual weight rather than ideal body weight may result in toxicity), failure to evaluate excretory/metabolic ability (renal or hepatic impairment from underlying disease or age), failure to determine the effect of other drugs being taken (displacement of drugs for protein binding sites), or increased sensitivity to a drug as a result of underlying illness (hypothyroid patients are very sensitive to the effects of digoxin). In any event, the clear course of action is to temporarily discontinue the drug and then to reduce the dose or increase the dosing interval, depending on the drug. In evaluating these reactions, the use of blood level monitoring may take the guesswork out of the situation. Patients should be taught that this type of reaction means that they may still receive the drug in question, despite the occurrence of the effect. They should not be under the misconception that they are "allergic" to the drug. Documentation of reactions as being dose related is important because it does not preclude use of the drug in question and may lend an appreciation for patient parameters that could determine doses of other drugs.

Side Effects: Side effects are usually considered to be symptoms that occur as a consequence of drug administration and are unrelated to the intended or desired action of the drug. Although they are undesirable and may be bothersome, they occur commonly enough at usual doses that patients should be aware of their occurrence and know how to deal with their presence. Certain side effects are so minimal that continued administration of the offending agent is allowed. An example of this type of situation is the headache that usually accompanies nitroglycerin administration. With chronic administration, this side effect dissipates and may be managed initially with acetaminophen. Other side effects require dosage alteration, the addition of another agent, or drug discontinuation, depending on patient response or severity of the reaction. Some antihypertensives may cause male impotence. If patients find this unacceptable, alternative agents should be sought. Opioid analgesics commonly cause constipation; however, the addition of a laxative to the medication regimen or simple dietary changes can eliminate or prevent this side effect. Appearance of neuroleptic malignant syndrome, a potentially life-threatening reaction that may occur as a consequence of phenothiazine therapy, precludes further use of the offending agent.

Documentation of side effects should identify the agent in question and time of occurrence, and it may help to avoid choosing the offending agent again if the side effect is serious or to serve as an aid to patient education if the drug is to be used again.

Idiosyncratic Reactions: These reactions occur without relation to dose. Their occurrence is unpredictable and sporadic. Reactions of this type may manifest in many different ways, including fever, blood dyscrasias, cardiovascular effects, or unwanted mental status changes. The time frame between the occurrence of a problem and initiation of therapy is sometimes the only clue linking drug to symptom. Several issues remain puzzling regarding these types of reactions. One is that this reaction may or may not recur when the patient is rechallenged with the same drug. The decision to proceed with rechallenge obviously depends on the necessity of continued therapy and choice of alternatives. Another issue is whether the same reaction will occur when similar drugs are given. Again, such decisions are made on an individual basis. Some idiosyncratic reactions may be explained by genetic differences in drug-metabolizing enzymes. Patient education is very important, as there must be clear understanding of the unpredictability of such events. Patients need to understand that the prescriber has taken into consideration the potential benefits of a particular drug and weighed them against any risks of therapy. When idiosyncratic reactions occur, they may not preclude further treatment with similar agents, but their occurrence should be documented so that the planning of future regimens may take them into account.

Hypersensitivity Reactions: Generally speaking, hypersensitivity reactions are usually allergic in nature and imply previous exposure to the agent. Manifestations of hypersensitivity reactions may range from mild rashes of all types, to nephritis, pneumonitis, or hemolytic anemia, to the potentially life-threatening manifestations of anaphylaxis. Drugs that are proteins (vaccines, enzymes) are more likely to induce hypersensitivity reactions on subsequent exposures. In many instances, antibody formation is involved in the process. In the case of these reactions, it is necessary to consider cross-sensitivity. The best example of this is hypersensitivity to penicillin. If a patient has a history of such a reaction to penicillin, then similar reactions may be expected with related anti-infectives (other penicillins and/or cephalospirins). Because of this, documenting hypersensitivity reactions is very important. Future regimens should avoid related agents or, if they are required, pretreatment (with antihistamines and/or glucocorticoids) or desensitization may be necessary.

Reactions That Occur as a Consequence of a Second (or Third or Fourth) Drug Being Added to the Regimen (Drug-Drug Interactions): Some adverse reactions or side effects may not manifest unless the presence of another drug initiates the process. Neither drug alone can be blamed for the problem, but nonetheless an adverse reaction has occurred. The management of these situations requires careful attention to which drug was started first, when the second agent was added, and how long it took for the reaction to manifest. An example is the interaction between digoxin and quinidine. When quinidine is added to the regimen of a patient who has been stabilized on an appropriate dose of digoxin, in the first several days many patients experience gastrointestinal complaints (nausea, vomiting). Initially, it would appear that, because the quinidine was just started, the quinidine is to blame. However, it has been documented that the presence of quinidine increases serum digoxin levels significantly within the first few days of therapy. In anticipation of this interaction, digoxin dosing may need to be decreased by as much as 50%, and then quinidine may be safely added to the regimen. If a drug-drug interaction occurs or is suspected, the continued need for both agents should be assessed and appropriate changes in agents or doses should be made. Documenting such events should help to prevent their recurrence. Certain classes of drugs are more likely to result in serious drug-drug interactions, and patients receiving these agents should be monitored carefully. In addition, it is useful to inform patients receiving these drugs to beware of the addition of new agents and to always check with a physician or pharmacist before taking any additional nonprescription drugs. Medications that may produce potentially serious drug-drug interactions are oral anticoagulants, oral hypoglycemic agents, nonsteroidal anti-inflammatory agents, theophylline, monoamine oxidase inhibitors, antihypertensives, anticonvulsants, cimetidine, lithium, and digitalis glycosides.

FOOD AND DRUG ADMINISTRATION MEDWATCH PROGRAM

Because of the demand for new drug entities, the time between development and marketing is becoming shorter. Consequently, there is a need to continuously survey the occurrence of adverse reactions after marketing has begun. In an effort to monitor and assess the occurrence of adverse reactions, the Food and Drug Administration (FDA) has launched MedWatch, a new program that gives health care practitioners the opportunity to report ***serious*** adverse reactions or product defects encountered from medications, medical devices, special nutritional products, or other FDA-regulated items. Through this reporting program, products may be withdrawn from the market if reporting is sufficient to warrant it. The FDA considers serious those reactions that may result in death, life-threatening illness or injury, hospitalization, disability, congenital anomaly, or those that may require medical/surgical intervention. In addition to reporting serious adverse reactions, health care providers should also report product problems including suspected contamination, questionable stability, defective components, or poor packaging/labeling. The FDA encourages all physicians, nurses, dentists, and pharmacists to become familiar with this program and to report serious adverse reactions or product problems, using the MedWatch reporting form. Reports should be submitted even if there is some uncertainty about the cause/effect relationship or if some details are missing. This form may be found in this edition of *Davis's Drug Guide for Nurses* and may be photocopied. Reports may also be faxed to the FDA (1-800-FDA-0178) or sent via computer modem (1-800-FDA-7737). If a reaction to a vaccine is suspected, it should be reported to the Vaccine Adverse Event Reporting System (VAERS; 1-800-822-7967). If a report is submitted, the FDA will hold the identity of the patient in strict confidence. Nurses, in addition to other health care providers, have the responsibility for reporting adverse reactions and are encouraged to participate in the MedWatch program.

MEDICATION ERRORS

Preventing Medication Errors: The most striking difference between adverse drug reactions and medication errors lies in the preventability of the latter. If the goal of optimal drug therapy is to provide the right drug, for the right patient, in the right dose, by the right route, at the right time, and for the right indication, then one can appreciate the many opportunities for potential errors in the process. There are also many checkpoints in the medication process, and the many people located along such checkpoints each play a role in detecting potential errors, preventing their occurrence, and documenting any effects that may occur as a consequence. Stages in the process are ordering (mainly done by physicians), transcribing (done by unit secretary or nurse), dispensing (by pharmacists), and administration (done by nurses). Because nurses are responsible for administering medications, they are often the last and probably the most important checkpoint in the system. Although errors may take place at this point, they can also be detected and ultimately prevented. The following additional recommendations for nurses have been suggested[3]:

- Become familiar with the institutional medication order process and administration system. Know where to obtain medications for a particular patient at a particular time. Is the time routinely floor stocked? Are initial or subsequent doses obtained from automated dispensing systems (such as Omnicell or Pyxis)? Does the institution use unit dose drug delivery? Many of these systems are designed to include additional checks and balances.
- Know where to go for drug information. Resources include physicians, pharmacists, libraries, and drug references. Lack of information has been identified as a common cause of adverse drug events. Much of this information is rapidly and readily available in electronic format or via the Internet.[2]
- Verify orders as much as possible. The transcription process is fraught with places for potential error.
- Use standard drug administration times. This helps to avoid confusion, particularly when lab test monitoring must be performed at a certain time following administration.
- When administering medications, inspect products for possible defects (cracks in capsules, cloudy injections, sediment in solutions). Report these as soon as possible. Verify the identity of the patient before administration. Keep medications clearly labeled as long as possible (leave in unit dose packaging right up to the bedside). Document administration in appropriate records. If a medication is unavailable for administration, resist the temptation to borrow from another patient's supply. Investigate why the drug is not there. There may be compelling reasons for the drug not to be administered pending confirmation of the order (potential interaction, history of previous reaction).
- Observe for any and all drug effects, including the presence of adverse reactions. It is just as important to document the desired therapeutic outcome as it is to report a rash.
- If any drug calculations are necessary, it is wise to check them with another person (physician, pharmacist, nurse, physician's assistant). The use of standard concentrations or infusion rate tables may be useful (see Appendix D).
- Be familiar with administration devices before using them and understand their benefits as well as potential disadvantages. The wide variety of high-technology delivery systems (infusion pumps, inhalers, transdermal patches) requires attention to their proper use.
- Teach patients as much as possible about their medications. Present this information in a format that the patient will understand. Determine reading and comprehension ability before teaching and clarify understanding during and following presentation of information. Use large print information, translators, pictures, or whatever it takes to produce an informed consumer. Initiate teaching with the first dose and reinforce the information with subsequent doses.
- If a medication is not given as ordered, for whatever reason, this must be documented.

Handling Medication Orders: In handling medication orders, care should be taken to avoid some of these common pitfalls, which may lead to medication errors:

Abbreviations: The use of abbreviations for names of drugs or directions for administration should be discouraged. For example, "AZT" could mean azathioprine, zidovudine, or aztreonam. Generic or brand names should be used. For confusing names, both the generic and brand name will add more clarity. Another example is the direction "qd" (every day), which could be misread as "qid" (four times a day) or "qod" (every other day). The use of standard names (generic/brand) should be encouraged.

Ambiguous Directions: Directions for medication administration should be clearly stated. Avoid "take as directed." Additional directions should be transcribed if they will alter the response to treatment or prevent an adverse reaction. This might include directions to take with food or on an empty stomach.

Dosage Problems: Write doses in strengths rather than dosage units (i.e., in mg, not in tablets or half tablets). Make sure to clearly write strengths that may be confused, such as milligrams and micrograms. Abbreviating these could also cause further confusion (mg; mcg). When the strength is specified in units, the word "units" should be spelled out. Using "U" as an abbreviation may be confused with the number "0."

Decimal Problems: Leading zeros should always appear in numbers less than 1 (such as 0.3), whereas terminal zeros to the right of the decimal point should not appear, as they may lead to tenfold dosage errors (misreading 5.0 as 50).

Which Measurement System? If at all possible, use the metric system. Older apothecary measurements are not only poorly standardized, their abbreviations are easily confused with other units of measurement.

What's in a Name? Many drugs have similar names. A few prominent examples of this phenomenon are vincristine and vinblastine, carboplatin and cisplatin, digoxin and digitoxin, ranitidine and rimantadine. When there may be doubt, the brand name and generic name may be written together to clarify the identity of the medication, and, of course, the dosage should be appropriate for the drug in question. Listing the indication may also be helpful.

Is What You See What You Get? Some drugs come in similar packaging. Fatalities have occurred when agents in such similar containers have been confused with each other. Avoid storing such drugs in close proximity and note the manufacturer's use of color coding and other devices to avoid confusion. None of these takes the place of close and repeated inspection.

Verbal Orders: Orders given verbally or over the phone should be put in writing as soon as possible. In doing so, the nurse should repeat the order clearly and make sure that numerical values are understood. This is especially problematic with numbers that end in "-teen" (fourteen may be easily confused with forty).

Hold Orders: Orders for temporarily stopping a medication should be clear as to what parameters should be observed in reinstituting therapy. Institutional hold policies should specify a certain period of time in order to avoid confusion. It may make more sense for many types of medication to be discontinued and therapy reinstituted at a later time.

Common Sense: Any order that just does not make sense, would result in a large number of tablets or large injection volume, or is geared toward a disease or problem the patient does not have should be confirmed. This includes administration by routes not necessary, as in an order for an intramuscular drug in a patient who is able to take solids.

Red Flags: Adverse drug events are more common in certain situations and more likely to occur with certain classes of drugs. Such problems are most liable to occur in Medical Intensive Care Units. In an area in which stress levels are already high and speed and precision often determine clinical outcome, extra vigilance may be warranted when dealing with medications. Among all agents used, *analgesics, anesthetics, sedatives, and antipsychotics* are most likely to be involved in adverse drug events. Situations arising during use of these drugs may include underdosing as well as overdosing and a lack of appreciation for individualizing regimens based on age, size, concurrent drug use, and intercurrent illness.[2]

WHAT IF AN ERROR DOES OCCUR?

If, after all preventive steps fail, a medication error occurs, it is vital that the incident be documented, even if no harm comes to the patient. Institutional reporting policies are designed to evaluate where the problem lies and to seek measures that should prevent its recurrence.

In an effort to compile data regarding the circumstances contributing to medication errors, the United States Pharmacopeial (USP) Convention, in cooperation with the Institute for Safe Medication Practices, has initiated a nationwide reporting system as part of its Practitioners' Reporting Network (USP PRN). The USP Medication Errors Reporting Program is designed to collect, analyze, and disseminate information that will hopefully aid in the design of systems to prevent the occurrence and recurrence of medication errors and their resultant morbidity and mortality. A copy of the report form is included as Appendix R. Nurses are strongly encouraged to participate in this unique program.

REFERENCES

1. Manasse, HR Jr: Medication use in an imperfect world: Drug misadventuring as an issue of public policy, Part 1. *Am J Hosp Pharm* 46:929–944, 1989.
2. Bates, DW, Cullen, DJ, Laird, N, et al: Incidence of adverse drug events and potential adverse drug events. *JAMA* 274:29–34, 1995.
3. ASHP Report: ASHP guidelines for preventing medication errors in hospitals. *Am J Hosp Pharm* 50:305–314, 1993.

CLASSIFICATIONS

▪ ANGIOTENSIN-CONVERTING ENZYME (ACE) INHIBITORS

See group monograph on page 60.

ACE Inhibitors Included in *Davis's Drug Guide for Nurses*:

benazepril 60
captopril 60
enalapril, enalaprilat 60
fosinopril 60
lisinopril 60
moexipril 60
quinapril 60
ramipril 60
trandolapril 60

▪ ANTIANEMICS

PHARMACOLOGIC PROFILE

General Use: Prevention and treatment of anemias.

General Action and Information: Iron (ferrous fumarate, ferrous gluconate, ferrous sulfate, iron dextran) is required for production of hemoglobin, which is necessary for oxygen transport to cells. Cyanocobalamin and hydroxocobalamin (vitamin B_{12}) and folic acid (vitamin B_9) are water-soluble vitamins that are required for red blood cell production. Epoetin stimulates production of red blood cells.

Contraindications: Undiagnosed anemias. Hemochromatosis, hemosiderosis, hemolytic anemia (iron). Uncontrolled hypertension (epoetin).

Precautions: Use parenteral iron cautiously in patients with a history of allergy or hypersensitivity reactions.

Interactions: Iron can decrease the absorption of tetracycline, fluoroquinolones, or penicillamine. Vitamin E may impair the therapeutic response to iron. Phenytoin and other anticonvulsants may decrease the absorption of folic acid. Response to vitamin B_{12} or folic acid may be delayed by chloramphenicol. Epoetin may increase the requirement for heparin during hemodialysis.

NURSING IMPLICATIONS

Assessment

- Assess patient's nutritional status and dietary history to determine possible cause of anemia and need for patient teaching.
- Monitor blood pressure prior to and throughout epoetin therapy. Inform physician if severe hypertension is present or if blood pressure begins to increase. Additional antihypertensive therapy may be required during initiation of therapy.
- **Lab Test Considerations:** Monitor hemoglobin, hematocrit, reticulocyte, and indices values before and periodically throughout therapy.
- See epoetin monograph for monitoring of specific lab indices.

Potential Nursing Diagnoses

- Activity intolerance (Indications).
- Nutrition, altered, less than body requirements (Indications).
- Knowledge deficit, related to medication regimen (Patient/Family Teaching).

Implementation

- Available in combination with many vitamins and minerals (see Appendix A).
- Transfusions are still required for severe symptomatic anemia. Supplemental iron should be initiated with epoetin and continued throughout therapy.

Patient/Family Teaching

- Encourage patients to comply with diet recommendations of health care professional. Explain that the best source of vitamins and minerals is a well-balanced diet with foods from the four basic food groups.
- Patients self-medicating with vitamin and mineral supplements should be cautioned not to exceed RDA (see Appendix L). The effectiveness of megadoses for treatment of various medical conditions is unproved and may cause side effects.

Evaluation

Clinical response is indicated by: ▪ Resolution of anemia.

Antianemics Included in *Davis's Drug Guide for Nurses*:

iron supplements
ferrous fumarate 537
ferrous gluconate 537
ferrous sulfate 537
iron dextran 537
polysaccharide-iron complex 537

hormone
epoetin 332

water-soluble vitamins
cyanocobalamin 1039
folic acid 409
hydroxocobalamin 1039

▪ ANTIANGINALS

PHARMACOLOGIC PROFILE

General Use: Nitrates are used to treat and prevent attacks of angina. Only nitrates (sublingual, lingual spray, or intravenous) may be used in the acute treatment of attacks of angina pectoris. Calcium channel blockers and beta-adrenergic blockers are used prophylactically in long-term management of angina.

General Action and Information: Several different groups of medications are used in the treatment of angina pectoris. The nitrates (isosorbide dinitrate, isosorbide mononitrate, and nitroglycerin) are available as a lingual spray, sublingual tablets, parenterals, transdermal systems, and sustained-release oral dosage forms. Nitrates dilate coronary arteries and cause systemic vasodilation (decreased preload). Calcium channel blockers dilate coronary arteries (some also slow heart rate). Beta-adrenergic blocking agents decrease myocardial oxygen consumption via a decrease in heart rate. Therapy may be combined if selection is designed to minimize side effects or adverse reactions.

Contraindications: Hypersensitivity. Avoid use of beta blockers or calcium channel blockers in advanced heart block, cardiogenic shock, or untreated congestive heart failure.

Precautions: Beta-adrenergic blockers should be used cautiously in patients with diabetes mellitus, pulmonary disease, or hypothyroidism.

Interactions: Nitrates, calcium channel blockers, and beta-adrenergic blockers may cause hypotension with other antihypertensive agents or acute ingestion of alcohol. Mibefradil, verapamil, diltiazem, and beta-adrenergic blockers may have additive myocardial depressant effects when used with other agents that affect cardiac function. Verapamil and mibefradil have a number of other significant drug-drug interactions.

NURSING IMPLICATIONS

Assessment

- Assess location, duration, intensity, and precipitating factors of patient's anginal pain.
- Monitor blood pressure and pulse periodically throughout therapy.

Potential Nursing Diagnoses

- Pain (Indications).
- Tissue perfusion, altered (Indications).
- Knowledge deficit, related to medication regimen (Patient/Family Teaching).

Implementation

- Available in various dose forms. See specific drugs for information on administration.

Patient/Family Teaching

- Instruct patient on concurrent nitrate therapy and prophylactic antianginal agents to continue taking both medications as ordered and to use SL nitroglycerin as needed for anginal attacks.
- Advise patient to contact health care professional immediately if chest pain does not improve; worsens after therapy; is accompanied by diaphoresis or shortness of breath; or if severe, persistent headache occurs.
- Caution patient to make position changes slowly to minimize orthostatic hypotension.
- Advise patient to avoid concurrent use of alcohol with these medications.

Evaluation

Effectiveness of therapy can be demonstrated by: ▪ Decrease in frequency and severity of anginal attacks ▪ Increase in activity tolerance.

Antianginals Included in *Davis's Drug Guide for Nurses*:

beta-adrenergic blocking agents
atenolol 82
metoprolol 647
nadolol 691
propranolol 863

calcium channel blockers
amlodipine 42
bepridil 98
diltiazem 284
mibefradil 656
nicardipine 719
nifedipine 723
verapamil 1026

nitrates and nitrites
amyl nitrite 1130
isosorbide dinitrate 543
isosorbide mononitrate 543
nitroglycerin 732

▪ ANTIARRHYTHMICS

PHARMACOLOGIC PROFILE

General Use: Suppression of cardiac arrhythmias.

General Action and Information: Correct cardiac arrhythmias by a variety of mechanisms, depending on the group used. The therapeutic goal is decreased symptomatology and increased hemodynamic performance. Choice of agent depends on etiology of arrhythmia and individual patient characteristics. Treatable causes of arrhythmias should be corrected before therapy is initiated (e.g., electrolyte disturbances). Major antiarrhythmics are generally classified by their effects on cardiac conduction tissue (see the following table). Adenosine, atropine, digitalis glycosides (digitoxin, digoxin), edrophonium, and isoproterenol are also used as antiarrhythmics.

MECHANISM OF ACTION OF MAJOR ANTIARRHYTHMIC DRUGS

GROUP	DRUGS	MECHANISM
I	moricizine	Shares properties of IA, IB, and IC agents
IA	quinidine, procainamide, disopyramide	Depress Na conductance, increase APD and ERP, decrease membrane responsiveness
IB	tocainide, lidocaine, phenytoin, mexiletine	Increase K conductance, decrease APD and ERP
IC	flecainide, propafenone	Profound slowing of conduction, markedly depress phase O
II	acebutolol, esmolol, propranolol	Interfere with Na conductance, depress cell membrane, decrease automaticity, and increase ERP of the AV node, block excess sympathetic activity
III	amiodarone, ibutilide, bretylium, sotalol	Interfere with norepinephrine, increase APD and ERP
IV	diltiazem, verapamil	Increase AV nodal ERP, Ca channel blocker

APD = action-potential duration; Ca = calcium; ERP = effective refractory period; K = potassium; Na = sodium.

Contraindications: Differ greatly among various agents. See individual drugs.

Precautions: Differ greatly among agents used. Appropriate dosage adjustments should be made in the elderly and those with renal or hepatic impairment, depending on agent chosen. Correctable causes (electrolyte abnormalities, drug toxicity) should be evaluated. See individual drugs.

Interactions: Differ greatly among agents used. See individual drugs.

NURSING IMPLICATIONS

Assessment

- Monitor ECG, pulse, and blood pressure continuously throughout IV administration and periodically throughout oral administration.

Potential Nursing Diagnoses

- Cardiac output, decreased (Indications).
- Knowledge deficit, related to medication regimen (Patient/Family Teaching).

Implementation

- Take apical pulse before administration of oral doses. Withhold dose and notify physician or other health care professional if heart rate is <50 bpm.
- Administer oral doses with a full glass of water. Most sustained-release preparations should be swallowed whole. Do not crush, break, or chew tablets or open capsules, unless specifically instructed.

Patient/Family Teaching

- Instruct patient to take oral doses around the clock, as directed, even if feeling better.
- Instruct patient or family member on how to take pulse. Advise patient to report changes in pulse rate or rhythm to health care professional.
- Caution patient to avoid taking OTC medications without consulting health care professional.
- Advise patient to carry identification describing disease process and medication regimen at all times.
- Emphasize the importance of follow-up exams to monitor progress.

Evaluation

Effectiveness of therapy can be demonstrated by: ▪ Resolution of cardiac arrhythmias without detrimental side effects.

Antiarrhythmics Included in *Davis's Drug Guide for Nurses*:

▪ ANTICHOLINERGICS

PHARMACOLOGIC PROFILE

General Use: Atropine—Bradyarrhythmias. **Scopolamine**—Nausea and vomiting related to motion sickness and vertigo. **Propantheline and glycopyrrolate**—Decreasing gastric secretory activity and increasing esophageal sphincter tone. **Dicyclomine and hyoscyamine**—Reducing GI motility and tone in the management of irritable bowel syndrome and other GI complaints. **Benztropine and trihexyphenidyl**—Management of dyskinesias, including parkinsonian syndrome. Atropine, scopolamine, and cyclopentolate are also used as ophthalmic mydriatics.

General Action and Information: Competitively inhibit the action of acetylcholine. In addition, atropine, glycopyrrolate, propantheline, and scopolamine are antimuscarinic in that they inhibit the action of acetylcholine at sites innervated by postganglionic cholinergic nerves.

Contraindications: Hypersensitivity, narrow-angle glaucoma, severe hemorrhage, tachycardia (due to thyrotoxicosis or cardiac insufficiency), or myasthenia gravis.

Precautions: Geriatric and pediatric patients are more susceptible to adverse effects. Use cautiously in patients with urinary tract pathology; those at risk for GI obstruction; and those with chronic renal, hepatic, pulmonary, or cardiac disease.

Interactions: Additive anticholinergic effects (dry mouth, dry eyes, blurred vision, constipation) with other agents possessing anticholinergic activity, including antihistamines, antidepressants, quinidine, and disopyramide. May alter GI absorption of other drugs by inhibiting GI motility and increasing transit time. Antacids may decrease absorption of anticholinergics.

NURSING IMPLICATIONS

Assessment

- Assess vital signs and ECG frequently during IV drug therapy. Report any significant changes in heart rate or blood pressure or increase in ventricular ectopy or angina promptly.
- Monitor intake and output ratios in elderly or surgical patients; may cause urinary retention.
- Assess patient regularly for abdominal distention and auscultate for bowel sounds. Constipation may become a problem. Increasing fluids and adding bulk to the diet may help alleviate constipation.

Potential Nursing Diagnoses

- Cardiac output, decreased (Indications).
- Oral mucous membrane, altered (Side Effects).
- Constipation (Side Effects).

Implementation

- **PO:** Administer oral doses of atropine, dicyclomine, glycopyrrolate, hyoscyamine, propantheline, or scopolamine 30 min before meals. Benztropine and trihexyphenidyl should be administered with or immediately after meals.
- Scopolamine transdermal patch should be applied at least 4 hr before travel.

Patient/Family Teaching

- **General Info:** Instruct patient that frequent rinses, sugarless gum or candy, and good oral hygiene may help relieve dry mouth.
- May cause drowsiness. Caution patient to avoid driving or other activities requiring alertness until response to medication is known.
- **Ophth:** Advise patients that ophthalmic preparations may temporarily blur vision and impair ability to judge distances. Dark glasses may be needed to protect eyes from bright light.

Evaluation

Effectiveness of therapy can be demonstrated by: ▪ Increase in heart rate ▪ Decrease in nausea and vomiting related to motion sickness or vertigo ▪ Dryness of mouth ▪ Dilation of pupils ▪ Decrease in GI motility ▪ Resolution of signs and symptoms of Parkinson's disease.

Anticholinergics Included in *Davis's Drug Guide for Nurses*:

▪ ANTICOAGULANTS/ANTIPLATELET AGENTS

PHARMACOLOGIC PROFILE

General Use: Prevention and treatment of thromboembolic disorders including deep vein thrombosis, pulmonary embolism, and atrial fibrillation with embolization. Antiplatelet agents, including aspirin, are used in a variety of settings to prevent thromboembolic events including stroke and myocardial infarction. Dipyridamole is commonly used after cardiac surgery.

General Action and Information: Anticoagulants are used to prevent clot extension and formation. They do not dissolve clots. The two types of anticoagulants in common use are parenteral heparins and oral warfarin. Therapy is usually initiated with heparin because of its rapid onset of action, while maintenance therapy consists of warfarin. Warfarin takes several days to produce therapeutic anticoagulation. In serious or severe thromboembolic events, heparin therapy may be preceded by thrombolytic therapy (alteplase, anistreplase, streptokinase, or urokinase). Low doses of heparin, low-molecular-weight heparins, and heparin-like compounds (ardeparin, danaparoid, dalteparin, enoxaparin) are used to prevent deep vein thrombosis after certain surgical procedures and in similar situations in which prolonged bed rest increases the risk of thromboembolism. Aspirin, clopidogrel, dipyridamole, and ticlopidine have antiplatelet activity and are used to prevent myocardial infarction or stroke. Abciximab, another antiplatelet agent, is used only with percutaneous coronary intervention (CPI).

Contraindications: Underlying coagulation disorders, ulcer disease, malignancy, recent surgery, or active bleeding.

Precautions: Anticoagulation should be undertaken cautiously in any patient with a potential site for bleeding. Pregnant or lactating patients should not receive warfarin. Heparin does not cross the placenta. Heparin and heparin-like agents should be used cautiously in patients receiving epidural analgesia.

Interactions: Warfarin is highly protein bound and may displace or be displaced by other highly protein-bound drugs. The resultant interactions depend on which drug is displaced. Bleeding may be potentiated by aspirin or large doses of penicillins or penicillin-like drugs, cefamandole, cefotetan, cefoperazone, plicamycin, valproic acid, or NSAIDs.

NURSING IMPLICATIONS

Assessment

- Assess patient taking anticoagulants for signs of bleeding and hemorrhage (bleeding gums; nosebleed; unusual bruising; tarry, black stools; hematuria; fall in hematocrit or blood pressure; guaiac-positive stools; urine; or nasogastric aspirate).
- Assess patient for evidence of additional or increased thrombosis. Symptoms will depend on area of involvement.
- Assess patient taking antiplatelet agents for symptoms of stroke, peripheral vascular disease, or myocardial infarction periodically throughout therapy.
- **Lab Test Considerations:** Monitor activated partial thromboplastin time (aPTT) or international normalized ratio (INR) with full-dose heparin therapy, prothrombin time (PT) with warfarin therapy, and hematocrit and other clotting factors frequently during therapy.
- Monitor bleeding time throughout antiplatelet therapy. Prolonged bleeding time, which is time- and dose-dependent, is expected.
- **Toxicity and Overdose:** If overdose occurs or anticoagulation needs to be immediately reversed, the antidote for heparins is protamine sulfate; for warfarin, the antidote is vitamin K (phytonadione [AquaMEPHYTON]). Administration of whole blood or plasma may also be required in severe bleeding due to warfarin because of the delayed onset of vitamin K.

Potential Nursing Diagnoses

- Tissue perfusion, altered (Indications).
- Injury, risk for (Side Effects).
- Knowledge deficit, related to medication regimen (Patient/Family Teaching).

Implementation

- Inform all personnel caring for patient of anticoagulant therapy. Venipunctures and injection sites require application of pressure to prevent bleeding or hematoma formation.
- Use an infusion pump with continuous infusions to ensure accurate dosage.

Patient/Family Teaching

- Caution patient to avoid activities leading to injury, to use a soft toothbrush and electric razor, and to report any symptoms of unusual bleeding or bruising to health care professional immediately.
- Instruct patient not to take OTC medications, especially those containing aspirin, NSAIDs, or alcohol, without advice of health care professional.
- Review foods high in vitamin K (see Appendix K) with patients on warfarin. Patient should have consistent limited intake of these foods, as vitamin K is the antidote for warfarin and greatly alternating intake of these foods will cause PT levels to fluctuate.
- Emphasize the importance of frequent lab tests to monitor coagulation factors.
- Instruct patient to carry identification describing medication regimen at all times and to inform all health care personnel caring for patient of anticoagulant therapy before laboratory tests, treatment, or surgery.

Evaluation

Clinical response can be evaluated by: ■ Prevention of undesired clotting and its sequelae without signs of hemorrhage ■ Prevention of stroke, myocardial infarction, and vascular death in patients at risk.

Anticoagulants/Antiplatelet Agents Included in *Davis's Drug Guide for Nurses*:

anticoagulants
ardeparin 473
dalteparin 473
danaparoid 473
enoxaparin 473
heparin 469
warfarin 1046

antiplatelet agents
abciximab 1129
aspirin 900
clopidogrel 216
dipyridamole 295
ticlopidine 982

■ ANTICONVULSANTS

PHARMACOLOGIC PROFILE

General Use: See the following table.

General Action and Information: Anticonvulsants include a variety of agents, all capable of depressing abnormal neuronal discharges in the CNS that may result in seizures. They may work by preventing the spread of seizure activity, depressing the motor cortex, raising seizure threshold, or altering levels of neurotransmitters, depending on the group. See individual drugs.

MAJOR ANTICONVULSANT CLASSES, DRUGS, AND MOST COMMON USES

CLASS	DRUGS	TYPE OF SEIZURE CONTROLLED
Barbiturates	amobarbital	Status epilepticus
	phenobarbital	Tonic-clonic and partial seizures, prophylaxis of febrile seizures
	primidone	Prophylaxis of partial seizures with complex symptomatology
Benzodiazepines	clonazepam	Absence seizures, akinetic seizures, myoclonic seizures
	clorazepate	Partial seizures
	diazepam (IV)	Status epilepticus, tonic-clonic seizures
	lorazepam (IV)	Status epilepticus
Hydantoins	fosphenytoin	Short-term parenteral management of seizures, treatment/prevention of seizures during neurosurgery
	phenytoin	Tonic-clonic and partial seizures with complex symptomatology
Succinimides	ethosuximide	Absence seizures

MAJOR ANTICONVULSANT CLASSES, DRUGS, AND MOST COMMON USES (CONTINUED)

CLASS	DRUGS	TYPE OF SEIZURE CONTROLLED
Miscellaneous	acetazolamide	Refractory seizures
	carbamazepine	Tonic-clonic seizures, complex partial seizures, mixed seizures
	felbamate	Partial seizures, Lennox-Gastaut syndrome
	gabapentin	Adjunctive treatment of partial seizures
	lamotrigine	Adjunctive treatment of partial seizures
	magnesium sulfate	Eclamptic seizures
	tiagabine	Adjunct treatment of partial seizures
	topiramate	Adjunctive therapy of partial-onset seizures
	valproates	Simple and complex partial seizures

Contraindications: Previous hypersensitivity.

Precautions: Use cautiously in patients with severe hepatic or renal disease; dosage adjustment may be required. Choose agents carefully in pregnant and lactating women. Fetal hydantoin syndrome may occur in offspring of patients who receive phenytoin during pregnancy. Felbamate is considered a second-line agent because of the risk of aplastic anemia and hepatic damage.

Interactions: Barbiturates stimulate the metabolism of other drugs that are metabolized by the liver, decreasing their effectiveness. Hydantoins are highly protein-bound and may displace or be displaced by other highly protein-bound drugs. Felbamate, lamotrigine, tiagabine, and topiramate are capable of interacting with several other anticonvulsants. For more specific interactions, see individual drugs. Many drugs are capable of lowering seizure threshold and may decrease the effectiveness of anticonvulsants, including tricyclic antidepressants and phenothiazines.

NURSING IMPLICATIONS

Assessment

- Assess location, duration, and characteristics of seizure activity.
- **Toxicity and Overdose:** Monitor serum drug levels routinely throughout anticonvulsant therapy, especially when adding or discontinuing other agents.

Potential Nursing Diagnoses

- Injury, risk for (Indications, Side Effects).
- Knowledge deficit, related to medication regimen (Patient/Family Teaching).

Implementation

- Administer anticonvulsants around the clock. Abrupt discontinuation may precipitate status epilepticus.
- Implement seizure precautions.

Patient/Family Teaching

- Instruct patient to take medication every day, exactly as directed.
- May cause drowsiness. Caution patient to avoid driving or other activities requiring alertness until response to medication is known. Do not resume driving until physician gives clearance based on control of seizures.
- Advise patient to avoid taking alcohol or other CNS depressants concurrently with these medications.
- Advise patient to carry identification describing disease process and medication regimen at all times.

Evaluation

Effectiveness of therapy can be demonstrated by: ▪ Decrease or cessation of seizures without excessive sedation.

Anticonvulsants Included in *Davis's Drug Guide for Nurses*:

▪ ANTIDEPRESSANTS

PHARMACOLOGIC PROFILE

General Use: Used in the treatment of various forms of endogenous depression, often in conjunction with psychotherapy. Other uses include: ▫ Treatment of anxiety (doxepin) ▫ Enuresis (imipramine) ▫ Chronic pain syndromes (amitriptyline, doxepin, imipramine, and nortriptyline). ▫ Smoking cessation (bupropion) ▫ Bulimia (fluoxetine) ▫ Obsessive-compulsive disorder (fluoxetine, sertraline).

General Action and Information: Antidepressant activity most likely due to preventing the reuptake of dopamine, norepinephrine, and serotonin by presynaptic neurons, resulting in accumulation of these neurotransmitters. The two major classes of antidepressants are the tricyclic antidepressants and the selective serotonin reuptake inhibitors (SSRIs). Most tricyclic agents possess significant anticholinergic and sedative properties, which explains many of their side effects (amitriptyline, amoxapine, doxepin, imipramine, nortriptyline). The SSRIs are more likely to cause insomnia (fluoxetine, fluvoxamine, paroxetine, sertraline).

Contraindications: Hypersensitivity. Should not be used in narrow-angle glaucoma. Should not be used in pregnancy or lactation or immediately after myocardial infarction.

Precautions: Use cautiously in older patients and those with pre-existing cardiovascular disease. Elderly men with prostatic enlargement may be more susceptible to urinary retention. Anticholinergic side effects (dry eyes, dry mouth, blurred vision, and constipation) may require dosage modification or drug discontinuation. Dosage requires slow titration; onset of therapeutic response may be 2–4 wk. May decrease seizure threshold, especially bupropion.

Interactions: Tricyclic antidepressants—May cause hypertension, tachycardia, and convulsions when used with monoamine oxidase (MAO) inhibitors. May prevent therapeutic response to some antihypertensives. Additive CNS depression with other CNS depressants. Sympathomimetic activity may be enhanced when used with other sympathomimetics. Additive anticholinergic effects with other drugs possessing anticholinergic properties. **MAO inhibitors**—Hypertensive crisis may occur with concurrent use of MAO inhibitors and amphetamines, methyldopa, levodopa, dopamine, epinephrine, norepinephrine, desipramine, imipramine, guanethidine, reserpine, vasoconstrictors, or ingestion of tyramine-containing foods. Hypertension or hypotension, coma, convulsions, and death may occur with meperidine or other opioid analgesics and MAO inhibitors. Additive hypotension with antihypertensives or spinal anesthesia and MAO inhibitors. Additive hypoglycemia with insulin or oral hypoglycemic agents and MAO inhibitors. **Fluoxetine, fluvoxamine, bupropion, paroxetine, sertraline,** or **venlafaxine** should not be used in combination with or within weeks of MAO inhibitors (see individual monographs). Risk of adverse reactions may be increased by **sumatriptan** or **zolmitriptan.**

NURSING IMPLICATIONS

Assessment

- Monitor mental status and affect. Assess for suicidal tendencies, especially during early therapy. Restrict amount of drug available to patient.
- **Toxicity and Overdose:** Concurrent ingestion of monamine oxidase inhibitors and tyramine-containing foods may lead to hypertensive crisis. Symptoms include chest pain, severe headache, nuchal rigidity, nausea and vomiting, photosensitivity, and enlarged pupils. Treatment includes IV phentolamine.

Potential Nursing Diagnoses

- Coping, ineffective individual (Indications).
- Injury, risk for (Side Effects).
- Knowledge deficit, related to medication regimen (Patient/Family Teaching).

Implementation

- Administer drugs that are sedating at bedtime to avoid excessive drowsiness during waking hours, and administer drugs that cause insomnia (fluoxetine, fluvoxamine, paroxetine, sertraline, monamine oxidase inhibitors) in the morning. Bupropion must be given in divided doses.

Patient/Family Teaching

- Caution patient to avoid alcohol and other CNS depressants. Patients receiving monamine oxidase inhibitors should also avoid OTC drugs and foods or beverages containing tyramine (see Appendix K for foods) during and for at least 2 wk after therapy has been discontinued, as they may precipitate a hypertensive crisis. Health care professional should be contacted immediately if symptoms of hypertensive crisis develop.
- Inform patient that dizziness or drowsiness may occur. Caution patient to avoid driving and other activities requiring alertness until response to the drug is known.
- Caution patient to make position changes slowly to minimize orthostatic hypotension.
- Advise patient to notify health care professional if dry mouth, urinary retention, or constipation occurs. Frequent rinses, good oral hygiene, and sugarless candy or gum may diminish dry mouth. An increase in fluid intake, fiber, and exercise may prevent constipation.
- Advise patient to notify health care professional of medication regimen before treatment or surgery. Monamine oxidase inhibitor therapy usually needs to be withdrawn at least 2 wk before use of anesthetic agents.
- Emphasize the importance of participation in psychotherapy and follow-up exams to evaluate progress.

Evaluation

Effectiveness of therapy can be demonstrated by: ■ Resolution of depression ■ Decrease in anxiety ■ Control of bedwetting in children over 6 yr of age ■ Management of chronic neurogenic pain.

Antidepressants Included in *Davis's Drug Guide for Nurses*:

tricyclic antidepressants

amitriptyline 40
amoxapine 44
desipramine 1134
doxepin 315
imipramine 511
nortriptyline 737

selective serotonin reuptake inhibitors

fluoxetine 398
fluvoxamine 407
paroxetine 766
sertraline 914

miscellaneous antidepressants

bupropion 133
maprotiline 601
mirtazapine 668
nefazodone 704
trazodone 1001
venlafaxine 1025

monoamine oxidase (MAO) inhibitors

phenelzine 676
tranylcypromine 676

monoamine oxidase (MAO) type B inhibitor

selegiline 911

▪ ANTIDIABETIC AGENTS

PHARMACOLOGIC PROFILE

General Use: Insulin is used in the management of insulin-dependent diabetes mellitus (IDDM, type I). It may also be used in non–insulin-dependent diabetes mellitus (NIDDM, type II) when diet and/or oral hypoglycemic therapy fails to adequately control blood sugar. The choice of insulin preparation (rapid-acting, intermediate-acting, long-acting) and source (beef, beef/pork, pork, semisynthetic, human recombinant DNA) depend on the degree of control desired, daily blood sugar fluctuations, and history of previous reactions. Oral hypoglycemics can be used only in non–insulin-dependent diabetes mellitus (NIDDM, type II). Oral agents are used when diet therapy alone fails to control blood sugar or symptoms or when patients are not amenable to using insulin. Some oral agents may be used with insulin. Newest among agents for management of hyperglycemia in non–insulin-dependent diabetics are the alpha-glucosidase inhibitors (acarbose and miglitol) and troglitazone (a thiazolidinedione).

General Action and Information: Insulin, a hormone produced by the pancreas, lowers blood glucose by increasing transport of glucose into cells and promotes the conversion of glucose to glycogen. It also promotes the conversion of amino acids to proteins in muscle, stimulates triglyceride formation, and inhibits the release of free fatty acids. The major types of oral hypoglycemic agents are the sulfonylureas, metformin, and acarbose. Sulfonylureas and metformin lower blood sugar by stimulating endogenous insulin secretion by beta cells of the pancreas and by increasing sensitivity to insulin at intracellular receptor sites. Intact pancreatic function is required. Acarbose and miglitol delay digestion of ingested carbohydrates, thus lowering blood sugar, especially after meals. They may be combined with sulfonylureas. Troglitazone improves sensitivity to insulin in muscle and adipose tissue and inhibits hepatic gluconeogenesis.

Contraindications: Insulin—Hypoglycemia. **Oral hypoglycemic agents**—Hypersensitivity (cross-sensitivity with other sulfonylureas and sulfonamides may exist). Hypoglycemia. Insulin-dependent diabetes mellitus (IDDM, type I). Avoid use in patients with severe kidney, liver, thyroid, and other endocrine dysfunction. Should not be used in pregnancy or lactation.

Precautions: Insulin—Infection, stress, or changes in diet may alter requirements. **Oral hypoglycemic agents**—Use cautiously in geriatric patients. Dosage reduction may be necessary. Infection, stress, or changes in diet may alter requirements. Use with sulfonylureas with caution in patients with a history of cardiovascular disease. Metformin may cause lactic acidosis. Troglitazone may cause hepatic damage.

Interactions: Insulin—Additive hypoglycemic effects with oral hypoglycemic agents. **Oral hypoglycemic agents**—Ingestion of alcohol may result in disulfiram-like reaction. Alcohol, glucocorticoids, rifampin, glucagon, and thiazide diuretics may decrease effectiveness. Anabolic steroids, chloramphenicol, clofibrate, MAO inhibitors, most NSAIDs, salicylates, sulfonamides, and warfarin may increase hypoglycemic effect. Beta-adrenergic blocking agents may produce hypoglycemia and mask signs and symptoms.

NURSING IMPLICATIONS

Assessment

- Observe patient for signs and symptoms of hypoglycemic reactions.
- Acarbose, miglitol, and troglitazone do not cause hypoglycemia when taken alone but may increase the hypoglycemic effect of other hypoglycemic agents.
- Patients who have been well controlled on metformin but develop illness or laboratory abnormalities should be assessed for ketoacidosis or lactic acidosis. Assess serum electrolytes, ketones, glucose, and, if indicated, blood pH, lactate, pyruvate, and metformin levels. If either form of acidosis is present, discontinue metformin immediately and treat acidosis.
- **Lab Test Considerations:** Serum glucose and glycosylated hemoglobin should be monitored periodically throughout therapy to evaluate effectiveness of treatment.

Potential Nursing Diagnoses

- Nutrition, altered, more than body requirements (Indications).
- Knowledge deficit, related to medication regimen (Patient/Family Teaching).
- Noncompliance (Patient/Family Teaching).

Implementation

- **General Info:** Patients stabilized on a diabetic regimen who are exposed to stress, fever, trauma, infection, or surgery may require sliding scale insulin. Withhold metformin and reinstitute after resolution of acute episode.
- Patients switching from daily insulin dose may require gradual conversion to oral hypoglycemics.
- **Insulin:** Available in different types and strengths and from different species. Check type, species' source, dose, and expiration date with another licensed nurse. Do not interchange insulins without physician's order. Use only insulin syringes to draw up dose. Use only U100 syringes to draw up insulin lispro dose.

Patient/Family Teaching

- **General Info:** Explain to patient that medication controls hyperglycemia but does not cure diabetes. Therapy is long-term.
- Review signs of hypoglycemia and hyperglycemia with patient. If hypoglycemia occurs, advise patient to take a glass of orange juice or 2–3 tsp of sugar, honey, or corn syrup dissolved in water (glucose, not table sugar, if taking acarbose or miglitol), and notify health care professional.
- Encourage patient to follow prescribed diet, medication, and exercise regimen to prevent hypoglycemic or hyperglycemic episodes.
- Instruct patient in proper testing of serum glucose and ketones.
- Advise patient to notify health care professional if nausea, vomiting, or fever develops; if unable to eat usual diet; or if blood sugar levels are not controlled.
- Advise patient to carry sugar or a form of glucose and identification describing medication regimen at all times.

- Insulin is the recommended method of controlling blood sugar during pregnancy. Counsel female patients to use a form of contraception other than oral contraceptives and to notify health care professional promptly if pregnancy is planned or suspected.
- **Insulin:** Instruct patient on proper technique for administration; include type of insulin, equipment (syringe and cartridge pens), storage, and syringe disposal. Discuss the importance of not changing brands of insulin or syringes, selection and rotation of injection sites, and compliance with therapeutic regimen.
- **Sulfonylureas:** Advise patient that concurrent use of alcohol may cause a disulfiram-like reaction (abdominal cramps, nausea, flushing, headache, and hypoglycemia).
- **Metformin:** Explain to patient the risk of lactic acidosis and the potential need for discontinuation of metformin therapy if a severe infection, dehydration, or severe or continuing diarrhea occurs or if medical tests or surgery is required.

Evaluation

Effectiveness of therapy can be demonstrated by: ▪ Control of blood glucose levels without the appearance of hypoglycemic or hyperglycemic episodes.

Antidiabetic Agents Included in *Davis's Drug Guide for Nurses*:

sulfonylureas
chlorpropamide 1132
glimepiride 498
glipizide 498
glyburide 498
tolazamide 1143
tolbutamide 1143

biguanide
metformin 627

alpha-glucosidase inhibitors
acarbose 1
miglitol 662

miscellaneous
troglitazone 1017

rapid-acting insulins
insulin lispro 521
regular insulin 521

intermediate-acting insulins
isophane suspension, NPH insulin 521
zinc suspension, lente insulin 521

long-acting insulin
extended zinc suspension, ultralente insulin 521

insulin mixture
regular plus NPH insulin 521

▪ ANTIDIARRHEALS

PHARMACOLOGIC PROFILE

General Use: For the control and symptomatic relief of acute and chronic nonspecific diarrhea.

General Action and Information: Diphenoxylate/atropine, difenoxin/atropine, and loperamide slow intestinal motility and propulsion. Attapulgite, kaolin/pectin, and bismuth subsalicylate affect fluid content of the stool. Polycarbophil acts as an antidiarrheal by taking on water within the bowel lumen to create a formed stool. Octreotide is used specifically for diarrhea associated with gastrointestinal endocrine tumors.

Contraindications: Previous hypersensitivity. Severe abdominal pain of unknown cause, especially when associated with fever.

Precautions: Use cautiously in patients with severe liver disease or inflammatory bowel disease. Safety in pregnancy and lactation not established (diphenoxylate/atropine and loperamide). Octreotide may aggravate gallbladder disease.

Interactions: Kaolin may decrease absorption of digoxin. Polycarbophil decreases the absorption of tetracycline. Octreotide may alter the response to insulin or oral hypoglycemic agents. Attapulgite may decrease absorption of medications administered orally within 3 hr before or 4 hr after.

NURSING IMPLICATIONS

Assessment

- Assess the frequency and consistency of stools and bowel sounds before and throughout therapy.
- Assess patient's fluid and electrolyte status and skin turgor for dehydration.

Potential Nursing Diagnoses

- Diarrhea (Indications).
- Constipation (Side Effects).
- Knowledge deficit, related to medication regimen (Patient/Family Teaching).

Implementation

- Shake liquid preparations before administration.

Patient/Family Teaching

- Instruct patient to notify health care professional if diarrhea persists; or if fever, abdominal pain, or palpitations occur.

Evaluation

Effectiveness of therapy can be demonstrated by: ▪ Decrease in diarrhea.

Antidiarrheals Included in *Davis's Drug Guide for Nurses*:

attapulgite 1131
bismuth subsalicylate 110
difenoxin/atropine 293
kaolin/pectin 549
loperamide 587
octreotide 740
polycarbophil 825

▪ ANTIDOTES

PHARMACOLOGIC PROFILE

General Use: See the following table.

General Action and Information: Antidotes are used in accidental and intentional overdoses of medications or toxic substances. The goal of antidotal therapy is to decrease systemic complications of the overdosage while supporting vital functions. Obtaining a precise history will determine aggressiveness of therapy, choice, and dose of agent. Some antidotes are designed to aid removal of the offending agent before systemic absorption occurs or to speed elimination (activated charcoal). Other agents are more specific and require more detailed history as to type and amount of agent ingested.

POISONS AND SPECIFIC ANTIDOTES

POISON	ANTIDOTE
acetaminophen	acetylcysteine
anticholinesterases	atropine, pralidoxime
benzodiazepines	flumazenil
cyanide	amyl nitrite, sodium nitrite, sodium thiosulfate
cyclophosphamide	mesna
digoxin, digitoxin	digoxin immune Fab
fluorouracil	leucovorin calcium
ethylene glycol (antifreeze)	fomepizole
heparin	protamine sulfate
iron	deferoxamine
lead	edetate calcium disodium, dimercaprol, succimer
methotrexate	leucovorin calcium
opioid analgesics, heroin	nalmefene, naloxone
tricyclic antidepressants	physostigmine
warfarin	phytonadione (vitamin K_1)

Contraindications: See individual drugs.

Precautions: See individual drugs.

Interactions: See individual drugs.

NURSING IMPLICATIONS

Assessment

- Inquire as to the type of drug or poison and time of ingestion.
- Consult reference, poison control center, or physician for symptoms of toxicity of ingested agent(s) and antidote. Monitor vital signs, affected systems, and serum levels closely.
- Monitor for suicidal ideation; institute suicide precautions as necessary.

Potential Nursing Diagnoses

- Coping, ineffective individual (Indications).
- Injury, risk for: poisoning (Patient/Family Teaching).
- Knowledge deficit, related to medication regimen (Patient/Family Teaching).

Implementation

- May be used in conjunction with induction of emesis or gastric aspiration and lavage, cathartics, agents to modify urine pH, and supportive measures for respiratory and cardiac effects of overdose or poisoning.

Patient/Family Teaching

- When counseling about poisoning in the home, discuss methods of prevention and the need to confer with poison control center, physician, or emergency department prior to administering syrup of ipecac and the need to bring ingested substance to the hospital for identification. Reinforce need to keep all medications and hazardous substances out of the reach of children.

Evaluation

Effectiveness of therapy is demonstrated by: ■ Prevention or resolution of toxic side effects of ingested agent.

Antidotes Included in *Davis's Drug Guide for Nurses*:

■ ANTIEMETICS

PHARMACOLOGIC PROFILE

General Use: Phenothiazines, benzquinamide, granisetron, metoclopramide, trimethobenzamide, and ondansetron are used to manage nausea and vomiting of many causes, including surgery, anesthesia, and antineoplastic and radiation therapy. Dimenhydrinate, scopolamine, and meclizine are used almost exclusively to prevent motion sickness. Dronabinol is used for short-term management of nausea and vomiting associated with antineoplastics and to stimulate appetite in patients with AIDS.

General Action and Information: Phenothiazines and benzquinamide act on the chemoreceptor trigger zone to inhibit nausea and vomiting. Dimenhydrinate, scopolamine, and meclizine act as antiemetics mainly by diminishing motion sickness. Metoclopramide decreases nausea and vomiting by its effects on gastric emptying. Dronabinol acts centrally to decrease nausea and vomiting. Dolasetron, granisetron, and ondansetron block the effects of serotonin.

Contraindications: Previous hypersensitivity.

Precautions: Use phenothiazines cautiously in children who may have viral illnesses. Choose agents carefully in pregnant patients (no agents are approved for safe use).

Interactions: Additive CNS depression with other CNS depressants including antidepressants, antihistamines, opioid analgesics, and sedative/hypnotics. Phenothiazines may produce hypotension when used with antihypertensives, nitrates, or acute ingestion of alcohol.

NURSING IMPLICATIONS

Assessment

- Assess nausea, vomiting, bowel sounds, and abdominal pain before and following administration.
- Monitor hydration status and intake and output. Patients with severe nausea and vomiting may require IV fluids in addition to antiemetics.

Potential Nursing Diagnoses

- Fluid volume deficit (Indications).
- Nutrition, altered, less than body requirements (Indications).
- Injury, risk for (Side Effects).

Implementation

- For prophylactic administration, follow directions for specific drugs so that peak effect corresponds to time of anticipated nausea.
- Phenothiazines should be discontinued 48 hr before and not resumed for 24 hr following myelography, as they lower seizure threshold.

Patient/Family Teaching

- Advise patient and family to use general measures to decrease nausea (begin with sips of liquids and small, nongreasy meals; provide oral hygiene; and remove noxious stimuli from environment).
- May cause drowsiness. Advise patient to call for assistance when ambulating and to avoid driving or other activities requiring alertness until response to medication is known.
- Advise patient to make position changes slowly to minimize orthostatic hypotension.

Evaluation

Effectiveness of therapy can be demonstrated by: ▪ Prevention of, or decrease in, nausea and vomiting.

Antiemetics Included in *Davis's Drug Guide for Nurses*:

▪ ANTIFUNGALS

PHARMACOLOGIC PROFILE

General Use: Treatment of fungal infections. Infections of skin or mucous membranes may be treated with topical or vaginal preparations. Deep-seated or systemic infections require oral or parenteral therapy. New parenteral formulations of amphotericin employ lipid encapsulation technology designed to decrease toxicity.

General Action and Information: Kill (fungicidal) or stop growth of (fungistatic) susceptible fungi by affecting the permeability of the fungal cell membrane or protein synthesis within the fungal cell itself.

Contraindications: Previous hypersensitivity.

Precautions: Because most systemic antifungals may have adverse effects on bone marrow function, use cautiously in patients with depressed bone marrow reserve. Amphotericin B commonly causes renal impairment. Flucytosine and fluconazole require dosage adjustment in the presence of renal impairment. Adverse reactions to fluconazole may be more severe in HIV-positive patients.

Interactions: Differ greatly among various agents. See individual drugs.

NURSING IMPLICATIONS

Assessment

- Assess patient for signs of infection and assess involved areas of skin and mucous membranes before and throughout therapy. Increased skin irritation may indicate need to discontinue medication.

Potential Nursing Diagnoses

- Infection, risk for (Indications).
- Skin integrity, impairment of (Indications).
- Knowledge deficit, related to medication regimen (Patient/Family Teaching).

Implementation

- **General Info:** Available in various dosage forms. Refer to specific drugs for directions for administration.
- **Topical:** Consult physician or other health care professional for cleansing technique before applying medication. Wear gloves during application. Do not use occlusive dressings unless specified by physician or other health care professional.

Patient/Family Teaching

- Instruct patient on proper use of medication form.
- Instruct patient to continue medication as directed for full course of therapy, even if feeling better.
- Advise patient to report increased skin irritation or lack of therapeutic response to health care professional.

Evaluation

Effectiveness of therapy can be demonstrated by: ▪ Resolution of signs and symptoms of infection. Length of time for complete resolution depends on organism and site of infection. Deep-seated fungal infections may require prolonged therapy (weeks–months). Recurrent fungal infections may be a sign of serious systemic illness.

Antifungals Included in *Davis's Drug Guide for Nurses*:

ophthalmic antifungal
natamycin 1115

systemic antifungals
amphotericin B 50
amphotericin B cholesteryl sulfate 50
amphotericin B lipid complex 50
amphotericin B liposome 50
dapsone 1133
fluconazole 382
flucytosine 385
griseofulvin 456
itraconazole 547
ketoconazole 550
miconazole 658
terbinafine 954

topical antifungals
amphotericin B 50
butenafine 69
ciclopirox 69
clotrimazole 69
econazole 69
haloprogin 69
ketoconazole 69
miconazole 69
naftifine 69
nystatin 69
oxiconazole 69
sulconazole 69
terbinafine 69
tolnaftate 69

vaginal antifungals
butoconazole 72
clotrimazole 72
miconazole 72
nystatin 72
terconazole 72
tioconazole 72

▪ ANTIGLAUCOMA AGENTS

PHARMACOLOGIC PROFILE

General Use: Management of glaucoma. Open-angle glaucoma is usually treated with medications. Other forms of glaucoma may require surgery.

General Action and Information: Agents used in the management of glaucoma decrease intraocular pressure by either decreasing the formation of aqueous humor or increasing the outflow of aqueous humor. Ophthalmic beta blockers and oral or ophthalmic carbonic anhydrase inhibitors decrease the production of aqueous humor. Direct-acting miotics, cholinesterase inhibitors, and sympathomimetics increase aqueous humor outflow.

Contraindications: Avoid use in patients with hypersensitivity to medications themselves, additives, or preservatives. Miotics should be avoided in patients with narrow-angle glaucoma.

Precautions: Use cautiously in patients with underlying cardiovascular disease, diabetes mellitus, or severe pulmonary disease.

Interactions: Beta blockers and carbonic anhydrase inhibitors have additive effects on intraocular pressure with other agents. Miotics and sympathomimetics also have additive effects and are frequently used together. Cholinesterase inhibitors may prolong the action of neuromuscular blocking agents.

NURSING IMPLICATIONS

Assessment

- Monitor patient for changes in vision, eye irritation, and persistent headache.
- Monitor patient for signs of systemic side effects. Notify physician or other health care professional if these signs occur.

Potential Nursing Diagnoses

- Sensory-perceptual alteration: visual (Indications, Side Effects).
- Knowledge deficit, related to medication regimen (Patient/Family Teaching).

Implementation

- When instilling eyedrops, have patient tilt head back, pull down on the lower lid, and instill drops into the conjunctival sac. Apply pressure to the inner canthus for 1 min following instillation to prevent systemic absorption.

Patient/Family Teaching

- Instruct patient to take as directed and not to discontinue without approval of health care professional. Lifelong therapy may be required.
- Instruct patient on correct technique for administration of ophthalmic medication. Emphasize the importance of not touching tip of container to eye, finger, or any other surface, and of preventing systemic absorption by placing pressure on the inner canthus.

- Explain to patient that temporary stinging and blurring of vision may occur. Health care professional should be notified if blurred vision or brow ache persists.
- Caution patient that night vision may be impaired. Advise patient not to drive at night until response to medication is known. To prevent injury at night, patient should use a night-light and keep environment uncluttered.
- Advise patient of the need for regular eye exams to monitor intraocular pressure and visual fields.

Evaluation

Effectiveness of therapy can be demonstrated by: ▪ Control of elevated intraocular pressure.

Antiglaucoma Agents Included in *Davis's Drug Guide for Nurses*:

beta blockers (ophthalmic)
betaxolol 1117
carteolol 1117
levobunolol 1117
metipranolol 1117
timolol 1117

carbonic anhydrase inhibitors
acetazolamide 152
dichlorphenamide 152
dorzolamide 1118
methazolamide 152

miotics (cholinesterase inhibitors)
demecarium 1118
isoflurophate 1119
physostigmine 1119

miotics (direct-acting)
carbachol 1118
pilocarpine 812, 1118

sympathomimetics
apraclonidine 1122
epinephrine 329, 1123

miscellaneous
glycerin 447, 1122

▪ ANTIGOUT AGENTS

PHARMACOLOGIC PROFILE

General Use: In the treatment of active gout (colchicine) and prevention of recurrent attacks (allopurinol, probenecid). Allopurinol and probenecid are also used to treat secondary hyperuricemia.

General Action and Information: Reduce the inflammatory response (colchicine) or lower serum uric acid by either enhancing its renal excretion (probenecid) or decreasing its production (allopurinol).

Contraindications: Hypersensitivity. Allopurinol should be avoided during acute attacks of gout.

Precautions: Akalinizing the urine enhances uricosuric effects. Rapid lowering of uric acid may cause precipitation of urate crystals in soft tissue.

Interactions: Probenecid promotes reabsorption and increases blood levels of many drugs including penicillins and cephalosporins. This interaction may be used to produce higher and more sustained blood levels of these drugs. Allopurinol increases toxicity from several antineoplastic agents (6-mercaptopurine, azathioprine). When allopurinol and ampicillin are used concurrently, the incidence of skin rash is greatly increased. Small doses of aspirin (<2 g/day) elevate serum uric acid and may interfere with the management of gout.

NURSING IMPLICATIONS

Assessment

- Assess for joint pain and swelling throughout therapy.
- Monitor intake and output ratios. Ensure that patient maintains adequate fluid intake (minimum 2500–3000 ml/day) to minimize risk of kidney stone formation.

Potential Nursing Diagnoses

- Pain (Indications).
- Knowledge deficit, related to medication regimen (Patient/Family Teaching).

Implementation

- Administer with or after meals to minimize gastric irritation.

Patient/Family Teaching

- Inform patient of the need for increased fluid intake.
- Advise patient to follow recommendations of health care professional regarding weight loss, diet, and alcohol consumption.

Evaluation

Effectiveness of therapy can be demonstrated by: ▪ Prevention or treatment of gout.

Antigout Agents Included in *Davis's Drug Guide for Nurses*:

allopurinol 22
colchicine 223
probenecid 841

▪ ANTIHISTAMINES

PHARMACOLOGIC PROFILE

General Use: Relief of symptoms associated with allergies, including rhinitis, urticaria, and angioedema, and as adjunctive therapy in anaphylactic reactions. Some antihistamines are used to treat motion sickness (dimenhydrinate and meclizine), insomnia (diphenhydramine), Parkinson-like reactions (diphenhydramine), and other nonallergic conditions.

General Action and Information: Antihistamines block the effects of histamine at the H_1 receptor. They do not block histamine release, antibody production, or antigen-antibody reactions. Most antihistamines have anticholinergic properties and may cause constipation, dry eyes, dry mouth, and blurred vision. In addition, many antihistamines cause sedation. Some phenothiazines have strong antihistaminic properties (hydroxyzine and promethazine).

Contraindications: Hypersensitivity and narrow-angle glaucoma. Should not be used in premature or newborn infants.

Precautions: Elderly patients may be more susceptible to adverse anticholinergic effects of antihistamines. Use cautiously in patients with pyloric obstruction, prostatic hypertrophy, hyperthyroidism, cardiovascular disease, or severe liver disease. Use cautiously in pregnancy and lactation.

Interactions: Additive sedation when used with other CNS depressants, including alcohol, antidepressants, opioid analgesics, and sedative/hypnotics. MAO inhibitors prolong and intensify the anticholinergic properties of antihistamines. Erythromycin, clarithromycin, ketoconazole, and itraconazole increase the risk of serious cardiac arrhythmias with astemizole.

NURSING IMPLICATIONS

Assessment

- **General Info:** Assess allergy symptoms (rhinitis, conjunctivitis, hives) before and periodically throughout therapy.
- Monitor pulse and blood pressure before initiating and throughout IV therapy.
- Assess lung sounds and character of bronchial secretions. Maintain fluid intake of 1500–2000 ml/day to decrease viscosity of secretions.
- **Nausea and Vomiting:** Assess degree of nausea and frequency and amount of emesis when administering for nausea and vomiting.
- **Anxiety:** Assess mental status, mood, and behavior when administering for anxiety.
- **Pruritus:** Observe the character, location, and size of affected area when administering for pruritic skin conditions.

Potential Nursing Diagnoses

- Airway clearance, ineffective (Indications).
- Injury, risk for (Adverse Reactions).
- Knowledge deficit, related to medication regimen (Patient/Family Teaching).

Implementation

- When used for prophylaxis of motion sickness, administer at least 30 min and preferably 1–2 hr before exposure to conditions that may precipitate motion sickness.
- When administering concurrently with opioid analgesics (hydroxyzine, promethazine), supervise ambulation closely to prevent injury secondary to increased sedation.

Patient/Family Teaching

- Inform patient that drowsiness may occur. Avoid driving or other activities requiring alertness until response to drug is known.
- Drowsiness is less likely to occur with astemizole and fexofenadine.
- Caution patient to avoid using concurrent alcohol or CNS depressants.
- Advise patient that good oral hygiene, frequent rinsing of mouth with water, and sugarless gum or candy may help relieve dryness of mouth.
- Instruct patient to contact health care professional if symptoms persist.

Evaluation

Effectiveness of therapy can be demonstrated by: ▪ Decrease in allergic symptoms ▪ Prevention or decreased severity of nausea and vomiting ▪ Decrease in anxiety ▪ Relief of pruritus ▪ Sedation when used as a sedative/hypnotic.

Antihistamines Included in *Davis's Drug Guide for Nurses*:

CLASSIFICATIONS

▪ ANTIHYPERTENSIVE AGENTS

PHARMACOLOGIC PROFILE

General Use: Treatment of hypertension of many causes, most commonly essential hypertension. Parenteral products are used in the treatment of hypertensive emergencies. Oral treatment should be initiated as soon as possible and individualized to ensure compliance for long-term therapy. Therapy is initiated with agents having minimal side effects. When such therapy fails, more potent drugs with different side effects are added in an effort to control blood pressure while causing minimal patient discomfort.

General Action and Information: As a group, the antihypertensives are used to lower blood pressure to a normal level (<90 mm Hg diastolic) or to the lowest level tolerated. The goal of antihypertensive therapy is prevention of end-organ damage. Antihypertensives are classified into groups according to their site of action. These include peripherally acting antiadrenergics; centrally acting alpha adrenergics; beta-adrenergic blockers; vasodilators; angiotensin-converting enzyme (ACE) inhibitors; angiotensin II antagonists; calcium channel blockers; diuretics; and indapamide, a diuretic with vasodilatory properties. Hypertensive emergencies may be managed with parenteral vasodilators such as diazoxide, nitroprusside, or enalaprilat.

Contraindications: Hypersensitivity to individual agents.

Precautions: Choose agents carefully in pregnancy, during lactation, or in patients receiving cardiac glycosides. ACE inhibitors and angiotensin II antagonists should be avoided during pregnancy. Alpha-adrenergic agonists and beta-adrenergic blockers should be used only in patients who will comply, because abrupt discontinuation of these agents may result in rapid and excessive rise in blood pressure (rebound phenomenon). Thiazide diuretics may increase the requirement for insulin, diet therapy, or oral hypoglycemic agents in diabetic patients. Vasodilators may cause tachycardia if used alone and are commonly used in combination with beta-adrenergic blocking agents. Most antihypertensives (except for beta-adrenergic blockers, angiotensin-converting enzyme [ACE] inhibitors, and calcium channel blockers) cause sodium and water retention and are usually combined with a diuretic.

Interactions: Many drugs can negate the therapeutic effectiveness of antihypertensives, including antihistamines, NSAIDs, sympathomimetic bronchodilators, decongestants, appetite suppressants, antidepressants, and MAO inhibitors. Hypokalemia from diuretics may increase the risk of cardiac glycoside toxicity. Potassium supplements and potassium-sparing diuretics may cause hyperkalemia when used with angiotensin-converting enzyme (ACE) inhibitors.

NURSING IMPLICATIONS

Assessment

- Monitor blood pressure and pulse frequently during dosage adjustment and periodically throughout therapy.
- Monitor intake and output ratios and daily weight.
- Monitor frequency of prescription refills to determine compliance.

Potential Nursing Diagnoses

- Tissue perfusion, altered (Indications).
- Knowledge deficit, related to medication regimen (Patient/Family Teaching).
- Noncompliance (Patient/Family Teaching).

Implementation

- Many antihypertensive agents are available as combination products to enhance compliance (see Appendix A).

Patient/Family Teaching

- Instruct patient to continue taking medication, even if feeling well. Abrupt withdrawal may cause rebound hypertension. Medication controls but does not cure hypertension.
- Encourage patient to comply with additional interventions for hypertension (weight reduction, low-sodium diet, regular exercise, discontinuation of smoking, moderation of alcohol consumption, and stress management).
- Instruct patient and family on proper technique for monitoring blood pressure. Advise them to check blood pressure weekly and report significant changes.
- Caution patient to make position changes slowly to minimize orthostatic hypotension. Advise patient that exercise or hot weather may enhance hypotensive effects.
- Advise patient to consult health care professional before taking any OTC medications, especially cold remedies.
- Advise patient to inform health care professional of medication regimen before treatment or surgery.
- Patients taking ACE inhibitors or angiotensin II antagonists should notify health care professional if pregnancy is planned or suspected.
- Emphasize the importance of follow-up exams to monitor progress.

Evaluation

Effectiveness of therapy can be demonstrated by: ▪ Decrease in blood pressure.

Antihypertensive Agents Included in *Davis's Drug Guide for Nurses*:

alpha-adrenergic blocking agent
phenoxybenzamine 1139

angiotensin-converting enzyme (ACE) inhibitors
benazepril 60
captopril 60
enalapril, enalaprilat 60
fosinopril 60
lisinopril 60
moexipril 60
quinapril 60
ramipril 60
trandolapril 60

angiotensin II antagonists
irbesartan 65
losartan 65
valsartan 65

beta-adrenergic blocking agents
acebutolol 2
atenolol 82
betaxolol 100
carteolol 160
carvedilol 163
labetalol 556
metoprolol 647
nadolol 691
penbutolol 771
pindolol 813
propranolol 863
timolol 985

calcium channel blockers
amlodipine 42
diltiazem 284
felodipine 366
isradipine 545
mibefradil 656
nicardipine 718
nifedipine 723
nisoldipine 729
verapamil 1026

centrally acting adrenergics
clonidine 213
guanabenz 462
guanfacine 465
methyldopa 638
methyldopate 638

diuretics
chlorothiazide 301
chlorthalidone 301
furosemide 414
hydrochlorothiazide 301
indapamide 516
methyclothiazide 1138
metolazone 645
torsemide 995
trichlormethiazide 1144

peripherally acting antiadrenergics
doxazosin 314
guanadrel 463
prazosin 837
terazosin 952

vasodilators
diazoxide 266
hydralazine 485
minoxidil 667
nitroprusside 735

▪ ANTI-INFECTIVES

PHARMACOLOGIC PROFILE

General Use: Treatment and prophylaxis of various bacterial infections. See specific drugs for spectrum and indications. Some infections may require additional surgical intervention and supportive therapy.

General Action and Information: Kill (bactericidal) or inhibit the growth of (bacteriostatic) susceptible pathogenic bacteria. Not active against viruses or fungi. Anti-infectives are subdivided into categories depending on chemical similarities and antimicrobial spectrum.

Contraindications: Known hypersensitivity to individual agents. Cross-sensitivity among related agents may occur.

Precautions: Culture and susceptibility testing are desirable to optimize therapy. Dosage modification may be required in patients with hepatic or renal insufficiency. Use cautiously in pregnant and lactating women. Prolonged inappropriate use of broad spectrum anti-infectives may lead to superinfection with fungi or resistant bacteria.

Interactions: Penicillins and aminoglycosides chemically inactivate each other and should not be physically admixed. Erythromycins may decrease hepatic metabolism of other drugs. Probenecid increases serum levels of penicillins and related compounds. Highly protein-bound anti-infectives such as sulfonamides may displace or be displaced by other highly bound drugs. See individual drugs. Extended-spectrum penicillins (mezlocillin, ticarcillin, piperacillin) and some cephalosporins (cefamandole, cefoperazone, cefotetan) may increase the risk of bleeding with anticoagulants, antiplatelet agents, or NSAIDs. Fluoroquinolone absorption is decreased by antacids, bismuth subsalicylate, iron salts, sucralfate, and zinc salts.

NURSING IMPLICATIONS

Assessment

- Assess patient for signs and symptoms of infection prior to and throughout therapy.
- Determine previous hypersensitivities in patients receiving penicillins or cephalosporins.
- Obtain specimens for culture and sensitivity prior to initiating therapy. First dose may be given before receiving results.

Potential Nursing Diagnoses

- Infection, risk for (Indications).
- Knowledge deficit, related to medication regimen (Patient/Family Teaching).
- Noncompliance (Patient/Family Teaching).

Implementation

- Most anti-infectives should be administered around the clock to maintain therapeutic serum drug levels.

Patient/Family Teaching

- Instruct patient to continue taking medication around the clock until finished completely, even if feeling better.
- Advise patient to report the signs of superinfection (black, furry overgrowth on the tongue; vaginal itching or discharge; loose or foul-smelling stools) and allergy to health care professional.
- Instruct patient to notify health care professional if fever and diarrhea develop, especially if stool contains pus, blood, or mucus. Advise patient not to treat diarrhea without consulting health care professional.
- Instruct patient to notify health care professional if symptoms do not improve.

Evaluation

Effectiveness of therapy can be demonstrated by: ▪ Resolution of the signs and symptoms of infection. Length of time for complete resolution depends on organism and site of infection.

Anti-infectives Included in *Davis's Drug Guide for Nurses*:

macrolides
azithromycin 91
clarithromycin 202
dirithromycin 1135
erythromycin 339

monobactam
aztreonam 93

penicillins
amoxicillin 46
amoxicillin/clavulanate 48
ampicillin 53
penicillin G benzathine 776
penicillin G potassium 776
penicillin G procaine 776
penicillin G sodium 776
penicillin V 776

penicillinase-resistant penicillins
cloxacillin 780
dicloxacillin 780
methicillin 780
nafcillin 780
oxacillin 780

sulfonamides
sulfacetamide 1116
sulfamethoxazole 937
sulfisoxazole 939
trimethoprim/sulfamethoxazole 1011

tetracyclines
demeclocycline 1134
doxycycline 961
minocycline 961
tetracycline 961

miscellaneous
bacitracin 1131
chloramphenicol 185
clindamycin 205
dapsone 1133
fosfomycin 413
metronidazole 650
nitrofurantoin 730
silver sulfadiazine 1142
spectinomycin 929
trimethoprim 1010
vancomycin 1022

■ ANTINEOPLASTICS

PHARMACOLOGIC PROFILE

General Use: Used in the treatment of various solid tumors, lymphomas, and leukemias. Also used in some autoimmune disorders such as rheumatoid arthritis (cyclophosphamide, methotrexate). Often used in combinations to minimize individual toxicities and increase response. Chemotherapy may be combined with other treatment modalities such as surgery and radiation therapy. Dosages vary greatly, depending on extent of disease, other agents used, and patient's condition. Some new formulations (daunorubicin, doxorubicin) encapsulated in a lipid membrane have less toxicity with greater efficacy.

General Action and Information: Act by many different mechanisms (see the following table). Most commonly affect DNA synthesis or function. Action may not be limited to neoplastic cells.

MECHANISM OF ACTION OF VARIOUS ANTINEOPLASTIC AGENTS

MECHANISM OF ACTION	AGENT	EFFECTS ON CELL CYCLE
ALKYLATING AGENTS Cause cross-linking of DNA	busulfan carboplatin chlorambucil cisplatin cyclophosphamide dacarbazine estramustine ifosfamide mechlorethamine melphalan procarbazine thiotepa	Cell cycle–nonspecific

MECHANISM OF ACTION OF VARIOUS ANTINEOPLASTIC AGENTS (CONTINUED)

MECHANISM OF ACTION	AGENT	EFFECTS ON CELL CYCLE
ANTHRACYCLINES	daunorubicin	Cell cycle–nonspecific
Interfere with DNA and RNA synthesis	doxorubicin	
	idarubicin	
ANTITUMOR ANTIBIOTICS	bleomycin	Cell cycle–nonspecific (except bleomycin)
Interfere with DNA and RNA synthesis	cladribine	
	dactinomycin	
	mitomycin	
	mitoxantrone	
	plicamycin	
	streptozocin	
ANTIMETABOLITES	cytarabine	Cell cycle–specific, work mostly in S phase (DNA synthesis)
Take the place of normal proteins	fludarabine	
	fluorouracil	
	hydroxyurea	
	mercaptopurine	
	methotrexate	
	thioguanine	
ENZYMES	asparaginase	Cell-cycle phase–specific
(Depletes asparagine)	pegaspargase	
ENZYME INHIBITORS	irinotecan	Cell-cycle phase–specific
Inhibit topoisomerase	topotecan	
HORMONAL AGENTS	bicalutamide	Unknown
Alter hormonal status in tumors that are sensitive	diethylstilbestrol (estrogens)	
	estramustine	
	flutamide	
	leuprolide	
	megestrol	
	nilutamide	
	tamoxifen	
	testosterone (androgens)	
Hormonal agents–aromatase inhibitors	anastrazole	Unknown
Inhibit enzyme responsible for activating estrogen	letrozole	
PODOPHYLLOTOXIN DERIVATIVES	etoposide	Cell-cycle phase–specific
(Damages DNA before mitosis)	teniposide	
TAXOIDS	docetaxel	Cell-cycle phase–specific
Interupt interphase and mitosis	paclitaxel	
VINCA ALKALOIDS	vinblastine	Cell cycle–specific, work during M phase (mitosis)
Interfere with mitosis	vincristine	
	vinorelbine	
ANTIPROLIFERATIVES	interferon alfa-2a	Unknown
	interferon alfa-2b	
ADRENAL SUPPRESSANT	mitotane	Unknown
IMMUNE MODULATORS	aldesleukin	Unknown
	BCG	Unknown
	levamisole	Unknown
MISCELLANEOUS	altretamine	Unknown
	masoprocol	Unknown
	pentostatin	Unknown
	porfimer	Unknown
	tretinoin (oral)	Unknown

Contraindications: Previous bone marrow depression or hypersensitivity. Contraindicated in pregnancy and lactation.

Precautions: Use cautiously in patients with active infections, decreased bone marrow reserve, radiation therapy, or other debilitating illnesses. Use cautiously in patients with childbearing potential.

Interactions: Allopurinol decreases metabolism of mercaptopurine. Toxicity from methotrexate may be increased by other nephrotoxic drugs or larger doses of aspirin or NSAIDs. Bone marrow depression is additive. See individual drugs.

NURSING IMPLICATIONS

Assessment

- Monitor for bone marrow depression. Assess for bleeding (bleeding gums, bruising, petechiae, guaiac stools, urine, and emesis) and avoid IM injections and rectal temperatures if platelet count is low. Apply pressure to venipuncture sites for 10 min. Assess for signs of infection during neutropenia. Anemia may occur. Monitor for increased fatigue, dyspnea, and orthostatic hypotension.
- Monitor intake and output ratios, appetite, and nutritional intake. Prophylactic antiemetics may be used. Adjusting diet as tolerated may help maintain fluid and electrolyte balance and nutritional status.
- Monitor IV site carefully and ensure patency. Discontinue infusion immediately if discomfort, erythema along vein, or infiltration occurs. Tissue ulceration and necrosis may result from infiltration.
- Monitor for symptoms of gout (increased uric acid, joint pain, and edema). Encourage patient to drink at least 2 liters of fluid each day. Allopurinol may be given to decrease uric acid levels. Alkalinization of urine may be ordered to increase excretion of uric acid.

Potential Nursing Diagnoses

- Infection, risk for (Side Effects).
- Nutrition, altered, less than body requirements (Adverse Reactions).
- Knowledge deficit, related to medication regimen (Patient/Family Teaching).

Implementation

- Solutions for injection should be prepared in a biologic cabinet. Wear gloves, gown, and mask while handling medication. Discard equipment in designated containers (see Appendix I for guidelines for safe handling).
- Check dose carefully. Fatalities have resulted from dosing errors.

Patient/Family Teaching

- Caution patient to avoid crowds and persons with known infections. Health care professional should be informed immediately if symptoms of infection occur.
- Instruct patient to report unusual bleeding. Advise patient of thrombocytopenia precautions.
- These drugs may cause gonadal suppression; however, patient should still use birth control, as most antineoplastics are teratogenic. Advise patient to inform health care professional immediately if pregnancy is suspected.
- Discuss with patient the possibility of hair loss. Explore methods of coping.
- Instruct patient to inspect oral mucosa for erythema and ulceration. If ulceration occurs, advise patient to use sponge brush and to rinse mouth with water after eating and drinking. Topical agents may be used if mouth pain interferes with eating. Stomatitis pain may require treatment with opioid analgesics.
- Instruct patient not to receive any vaccinations without advice of health care professional. Antineoplastics may decrease antibody response and increase risk of adverse reactions.
- Advise patient of need for medical follow-up and frequent lab tests.

Evaluation

Effectiveness of therapy can be demonstrated by: ▪ Decrease in size and spread of tumor ▪ Improvement in hematologic status in patients with leukemia.

Antineoplastics Included in *Davis's Drug Guide for Nurses*:

▪ ANTI-PARKINSON AGENTS

PHARMACOLOGIC PROFILE

General Use: Used in the treatment of parkinsonism of various causes: degenerative, toxic, infective, neoplastic, or drug-induced.

General Action and Information: Drugs used in the treatment of the parkinsonian syndrome and other dyskinesias are aimed at restoring the natural balance of two major neurotransmitters in the CNS: acetylcholine and dopamine. The imbalance is a deficiency in dopamine that results in excessive cholinergic activity. Drugs used are either anticholinergics (benztropine, biperiden, orphenadrine, and trihexyphenidyl) or dopaminergic agonists (amantadine, bromocriptine, levodopa, and pergolide). Pramipexole and ropinerole are two new nonergot dopamine agonists. Selegiline inhibits the enzyme that degrades dopamine, augmenting its effects.

Contraindications: Anticholinergics should be avoided in patients with narrow-angle glaucoma.

Precautions: Use cautiously in patients with severe cardiac disease, pyloric obstruction, or prostatic enlargement.

Interactions: Pyridoxine, MAO inhibitors, benzodiazepines, phenytoin, phenothiazines, and haloperidol may antagonize the effects of levodopa. Concurrent use of selegiline with opioid analgesics may result in two potentially fatal reactions (excitation, sweating, rigidity, and hypertension; or hypotension and coma). Doses of selegiline >10 mg/day may produce reactions with tyramine-containing foods. Agents that antagonize dopamine (phenothiazines, metoclopramide) may decrease effectiveness of dopamine agonists.

NURSING IMPLICATIONS

Assessment

- Assess parkinsonian and extrapyramidal symptoms (akinesia, rigidity, tremors, pill rolling, mask facies, shuffling gait, muscle spasms, twisting motions, and drooling) before and throughout course of therapy. On-off phenomenon may cause symptoms to appear or improve suddenly.
- Monitor blood pressure frequently during therapy. Instruct patient to remain supine during and for several hours after 1st dose of bromocriptine, as severe hypotension may occur.

Potential Nursing Diagnoses

- Physical mobility, impaired (Indications).
- Injury, risk for (Indications).
- Knowledge deficit, related to medication regimen (Patient/Family Teaching).

Implementation

- In the carbidopa/levodopa combination, the number following the drug name represents the milligram of each respective drug.

Patient/Family Teaching

- May cause drowsiness or dizziness. Advise patient to avoid driving or other activities that require alertness until response to medication is known.
- Caution patient to make position changes slowly to minimize orthostatic hypotension.
- Instruct patient that frequent rinsing of mouth, good oral hygiene, and sugarless gum or candy may decrease dry mouth. Patient should notify health care professional if dryness persists (saliva substitutes may be used). Also notify the dentist if dryness interferes with use of dentures.
- Advise patient to confer with health care professional before taking OTC medications, especially cold remedies, or drinking alcoholic beverages. Patients receiving levodopa should avoid multivitamins. Vitamin B_6 (pyridoxine) may interfere with levodopa's action.
- Caution patient that decreased perspiration may occur. Overheating may occur during hot weather. Patients should remain indoors in an air-conditioned environment during hot weather.
- Advise patient to increase activity, bulk, and fluid in diet to minimize constipating effects of medication.
- Advise patient to notify health care professional if confusion, rash, urinary retention, severe constipation, visual changes, or worsening of parkinsonian symptoms occur.

Evaluation

Effectiveness of therapy can be demonstrated by: ▪ Resolution of parkinsonian signs and symptoms ▪ Resolution of drug-induced extrapyramidal symptoms.

Anti-Parkinson Agents Included in *Davis's Drug Guide for Nurses*:

anticholinergics
benztropine 96
biperiden 107
trihexyphenidyl 1006

catechol-O-methyltransferase inhibitor
tolcapone 1126

dopamine agonists
amantadine 1129
bromocriptine 120
carbidopa/levodopa 572
levodopa 572
pergolide 792
pramipexole 836
ropinirole 898

monoamine oxidase (MAO) type B inhibitor
selegiline 911

▪ ANTIPSYCHOTIC AGENTS

PHARMACOLOGIC PROFILE

General Use: Treatment of acute and chronic psychoses, particularly when accompanied by increased psychomotor activity. Clomipramine is used only for obsessive-compulsive disorder (OCD). Use of clozapine is limited to schizophrenia unresponsive to conventional therapy. Selected agents are also used as antihistamines or antiemetics. Chlorpromazine is also used in the treatment of intractable hiccups.

General Action and Information: Block dopamine receptors in the brain; also alter dopamine release and turnover. Peripheral effects include anticholinergic properties and alpha-adrenergic blockade. Most antipsychotics are phenothiazines except for haloperidol, which is a butyrophenone; molindone, which resembles a phenothiazine in its action; clomipramine, which resembles tricyclic antidepressants; and loxapine and clozapine, which are miscellaneous compounds. Newer agents such as olanzapine, quetiapine, and risperidone may have fewer adverse reactions. Phenothiazines differ in their ability to produce sedation (greatest with chlorpromazine, promazine, thioridazine, and thiothixene), extrapyramidal reactions (greatest with fluphenazine, perphenazine, prochlorperazine, and trifluoperazine), and anticholinergic effects (greatest with chlorpromazine and promazine).

Contraindications: Hypersensitivity. Cross-sensitivity may exist among phenothiazines. Should not be used in narrow-angle glaucoma. Should not be used in patients who have CNS depression.

Precautions: Safety in pregnancy and lactation not established. Use cautiously in patients with symptomatic cardiac disease. Avoid exposure to extremes in temperature. Use cautiously in severely ill or debilitated patients, diabetics, and patients with respiratory insufficiency, prostatic hypertrophy, or intestinal obstruction. May lower seizure threshold. Clozapine may cause agranulocytosis. Most agents are capable of causing neuroleptic malignant syndrome.

Interactions: Additive hypotension with acute ingestion of alcohol, antihypertensives, or nitrates. Antacids may decrease absorption. Phenobarbital may increase metabolism and decrease effectiveness. Additive CNS depression with other CNS depressants, including alcohol, antihistamines, antidepressants, opioid analgesics, or sedative/hypnotics. Lithium may decrease blood levels and effectiveness of phenothiazines. May decrease the therapeutic response to levodopa. May increase the risk of agranulocytosis with antithyroid agents.

NURSING IMPLICATIONS

Assessment

- Assess patient's mental status (orientation, mood, behavior) before and periodically throughout therapy.
- Monitor blood pressure (sitting, standing, lying), pulse, and respiratory rate before and frequently during the period of dosage adjustment.
- Observe patient carefully when administering medication to ensure medication is actually taken and not hoarded.
- Monitor patient for onset of akathisia (restlessness or desire to keep moving) and extrapyramidal side effects(*parkinsonian*—difficulty speaking or swallowing, loss of balance control, pill rolling, mask-like face, shuffling gait, rigidity, tremors; and *dystonic*—muscle spasms, twisting motions, twitching, inability to move eyes, weakness of arms or legs) every 2 mo during therapy and 8–12 wk after therapy has been discontinued. Parkinsonian effects are more common in geriatric patients and dystonias are more common in younger patients. Notify health care professional if these symptoms occur, as reduction in dosage or discontinuation of medication may be necessary. Trihexyphenidyl or diphenhydramine may be used to control these symptoms.
- Monitor for tardive dyskinesia (uncontrolled rhythmic movement of mouth, face, and extremities; lip smacking or puckering; puffing of cheeks; uncontrolled chewing; rapid or worm-like movements of tongue). Notify health care professional immediately if these symptoms occur; these side effects may be irreversible.
- Monitor for development of neuroleptic malignant syndrome (fever, respiratory distress, tachycardia, convulsions, diaphoresis, hypertension or hypotension, pallor, tiredness, severe muscle stiffness, loss of bladder control). Notify health care professional immediately if these symptoms occur.

Potential Nursing Diagnoses

- Thought processes, altered (Indications).
- Knowledge deficit, related to medication regimen (Patient/Family Teaching).
- Noncompliance (Patient/Family Teaching).

Implementation

- **General Info:** Keep patient recumbent for at least 30 min following parenteral administration to minimize hypotensive effects.
- To prevent contact dermatitis, avoid getting solution on hands.
- Phenothiazines should be discontinued 48 hr before and not resumed for 24 hr following myelography, as they lower the seizure threshold.
- **PO:** Administer with food, milk, or a full glass of water to minimize gastric irritation.
- Dilute most concentrates in 120 ml of distilled or acidified tap water or fruit juice just before administration.

Patient/Family Teaching

- Advise patient to take medication exactly as directed and not to skip doses or double up on missed doses. Abrupt withdrawal may lead to gastritis, nausea, vomiting, dizziness, headache, tachycardia, and insomnia.
- Advise patient to make position changes slowly to minimize orthostatic hypotension.
- Medication may cause drowsiness. Caution patient to avoid driving or other activities requiring alertness until response to the medication is known.
- Caution patient to avoid taking alcohol or other CNS depressants concurrently with this medication.
- Advise patient to use sunscreen and protective clothing when exposed to the sun to prevent

photosensitivity reactions. Extremes of temperature should also be avoided, as these drugs impair body temperature regulation.

- Advise patient that increasing activity, bulk, and fluids in the diet helps minimize the constipating effects of this medication.
- Instruct patient to use frequent mouth rinses, good oral hygiene, and sugarless gum or candy to minimize dry mouth.
- Advise patient to notify health care professional of medication regimen before treatment or surgery.
- Emphasize the importance of routine follow-up examinations and continued participation in psychotherapy as indicated.

Evaluation

Effectiveness of therapy can be demonstrated by: ▪ Decrease in excitable, paranoic, or withdrawn behavior ▪ Relief of nausea and vomiting ▪ Relief of intractable hiccups.

Antipsychotic Agents Included in *Davis's Drug Guide for Nurses*:

phenothiazines
chlorpromazine 193
fluphenazine 400
mesoridazine 622
perphenazine 795
prochlorperazine 847
promazine 851
thioridazine 967
thiothixene 1143
trifluoperazine 1004

butyrophenone
haloperidol 467

miscellaneous
clomipramine 209
clozapine 219
loxapine 591
olanzapine 742
pimozide 1140
quetiapine 878
risperidone 892

▪ ANTIPYRETICS

PHARMACOLOGIC PROFILE

General Use: Used to lower fever of many causes (infection, inflammation, and neoplasms).

General Action and Information: Antipyretics lower fever by affecting thermoregulation in the CNS and by inhibiting the action of prostaglandins peripherally. Aspirin has the most profound effect on platelet function as compared with other salicylates, ibuprofen, ketoprofen, or naproxen.

Contraindications: Avoid aspirin, ibuprofen, ketoprofen, or naproxen in patients with bleeding disorders (risk of bleeding is less with other salicylates). Aspirin and other salicylates should be avoided in children and adolescents.

Precautions: Use aspirin, ibuprofen, ketoprofen, or naproxen cautiously in patients with ulcer disease. Avoid chronic use of large doses of acetaminophen.

Interactions: Large doses of aspirin may displace other highly protein-bound drugs. Additive GI irritation with aspirin, ibuprofen, ketoprofen, naproxen, and other NSAIDs or glucocorticoids. Aspirin, ibuprofen, ketoprofen, or naproxen may increase the risk of bleeding with other agents affecting hemostasis (anticoagulants, thrombolytics, antineoplastics, and certain anti-infectives).

NURSING IMPLICATIONS

Assessment

- Assess fever; note presence of associated symptoms (diaphoresis, tachycardia, and malaise).

Potential Nursing Diagnoses

- Body temperature, altered, risk for (Indications).
- Knowledge deficit, related to medication regimen (Patient/Family Teaching).

Implementation

- Administration with food or antacids may minimize GI irritation (aspirin, ibuprofen, ketoprofen, naproxen).
- Available in oral and rectal dosage forms and in combination with other drugs.

Patient/Family Teaching

- Advise patient to consult health care professional if fever is not relieved by routine doses or if greater than 39.5°C (103°F) or lasts longer than 3 days.
- Centers for Disease Control warns against giving aspirin to children or adolescents with varicella (chickenpox) or influenza-like or viral illnesses because of a possible association with Reye's syndrome.

Evaluation

Effectiveness of therapy can be demonstrated by: ▪ Reduction of fever.

Antipyretics Included in *Davis's Drug Guide for Nurses*:

acetaminophen 4
aspirin 900
choline and magnesium salicylates 900
choline salicylate 900
ibuprofen 501
ketoprofen 551
naproxen 702
salsalate 900

▪ ANTIRETROVIRALS

PHARMACOLOGIC PROFILE

General Use: The goal of antiretroviral therapy in the management of HIV infection is to improve CD4 cell counts and decrease viral load. If accomplished, this generally results in slowed progession of the disease, improved quality of life, and decreased opportunistic infections. Perinatal use of agents also prevents transmission of the virus to the fetus. Postexposure prophylaxis with antiretrovirals is also recommended.

General Action and Information: Because of the rapid emergence of resistance and toxicities of individual agents, HIV infection is almost always managed by a combination of agents. Selections and doses are based on individual toxicities, underlying organ system disease, concurrent drug therapy, and severity of illness. Various combination are used; up to 4 agents may be used simultaneously. More than 100 agents are currently being tested in addition to those already approved by the FDA.

Contraindications: Hypersensitivity. Because of highly varying toxicities among agents, see individual monographs for more specific information.

Precautions Many agents require modification for renal impairment. Protease inhibitors may cause hyperglycemia and should be used cautiously in patients with diabetes. Hemophiliacs may also be at risk of bleeding when taking protease inhibitors. See individual monographs for specific information.

Interactions: There are many signficant interactions among the antiretrovirals. They are affected by drugs that alter metabolism; some agents themselves affect metabolism. See individual agents.

NURSING IMPLICATIONS

Assessment

- Assess patient for change in severity of symptoms of HIV and for symptoms of opportunistic infections throughout therapy.
- **Lab Test Considerations:** Monitor viral load and CD4 counts prior to and periodically during therapy.

Potential Nursing Diagnoses

- Infection, risk for (Indications).
- Knowledge deficit, related to medication regimen (Patient/Family Teaching).
- Noncompliance (Patient/Family Teaching).

Implementation

- Administer doses around the clock.

Patient/Family Teaching

- Instruct patient to take medication exactly as directed, around the clock, even if sleep is interrupted. Emphasize the importance of complying with therapy, not taking more than prescribed amount, and not discontinuing without consulting health care professional. Missed doses should be taken as soon as remembered unless almost time for next dose; patient should not double doses. Inform patient that long-term effects are unknown at this time.
- Instruct patient that antiretrovirals should not be shared with others.
- Inform patient that antiretroviral therapy does not cure HIV and does not reduce the risk of transmission of HIV to others through sexual contact or blood contamination. Caution patient to use a condom during sexual contact and to avoid sharing needles or donating blood to prevent spreading the AIDS virus to others.
- Advise patient to avoid taking any Rx or OTC medications without consulting health care professional.
- Emphasize the importance of regular follow-up exams and blood counts to determine progress and monitor for side effects.

Evaluation

Effectiveness of therapy can be demonstrated by: ▪ Decrease in viral load and increase in CD4 counts in patients with HIV.

Antiretrovirals Included in *Davis's Drug Guide for Nurses*:

non-nucleoside reverse transcriptase inhibitors
delavirdine 1134
nevirapine 714

nucleoside reverse transcriptase inhibitors
didanosine 270
lamivudine 560
stavudine 931
zalcitabine 1049
zidovudine 1051

protease inhibitors
indinavir 517
nelfinavir 706a
ritonavir 894
saquinavir 905

■ ANTITHYROID AGENTS

PHARMACOLOGIC PROFILE

General Use: Used in the treatment of hyperthyroidism of various causes (Graves' disease, multinodular goiter, thyroiditis, and thyrotoxic crisis) in children, pregnant women, and other patients in whom hyperthyroidism is not expected to be permanent. These agents are also used to prepare patients for thyroidectomy or for patients in whom thyroidectomy is contraindicated. Beta-adrenergic blockers (propranolol) are sometimes used in conjunction with antithyroid agents to control symptoms (tachycardia and tremor) but have no effect on thyroid status. Iodine and iodides are also used as radiation protectants.

General Action and Information: Inhibit thyroid hormone formation (iodine) or inhibit oxidation of iodine (methimazole and propylthiouracil).

Contraindications: Hypersensitivity. Previous bone marrow depression.

Precautions: Use methimazole cautiously in patients with decreased bone marrow reserve.

Interactions: Lithium may cause thyroid abnormalities and interfere with the response to antithyroid therapy. Phenothiazines may increase the risk of agranulocytosis.

NURSING IMPLICATIONS

Assessment

- **General Info:** Monitor response of symptoms of hyperthyroidism or thyrotoxicosis (tachycardia, palpitations, nervousness, insomnia, fever, diaphoresis, heat intolerance, tremors, weight loss, diarrhea).
- Assess patient for development of hypothyroidism (intolerance to cold, constipation, dry skin, headache, listlessness, tiredness, or weakness). Dosage adjustment may be required.
- Assess patient for skin rash or swelling of cervical lymph nodes. Treatment may be discontinued if this occurs.
- Monitor thyroid function studies before and periodically throughout therapy.
- **Iodides:** Assess for signs and symptoms of iodism (metallic taste, stomatitis, skin lesions, cold symptoms, severe GI upset) or anaphylaxis. Report these symptoms promptly to physician or other health care provider.

Potential Nursing Diagnoses

- Knowledge deficit, related to medication regimen (Patient/Family Teaching).

Implementation

- Mix iodide solutions in a full glass of fruit juice, water, or milk. Administer after meals to minimize GI irritation.

Patient/Family Teaching

- Instruct patient to take medication exactly as directed. Missing doses may precipitate hyperthyroidism.
- Advise patient to consult health care professional regarding dietary sources of iodine (iodized salt, shellfish, cabbage, kale, turnips).
- Advise patient to carry identification describing medication regimen at all times and to notify health care professional of medical regimen before treatment or surgery.
- Emphasize the importance of routine exams to monitor progress and check for side effects.

Evaluation

Effectiveness of therapy can be demonstrated by: ▪ Decrease in severity of symptoms of hyperthyroidism ▪ Decrease in vascularity and friability of the thyroid gland before preparation for surgery ▪ Protection of the thyroid gland during radiation emergencies.

Antithyroid Agents Included in *Davis's Drug Guide for Nurses*:

methimazole 631
potassium iodide 530
propylthiouracil 867
strong iodine solution 530

▪ ANTITUBERCULARS/ANTIMYCOBACTERIALS

PHARMACOLOGIC PROFILE

General Use: Used in the treatment and prevention of tuberculosis and diseases caused by other mycobacteria, including *Mycobacterium avium* complex (MAC), seen mostly in HIV patients. Combinations are used in the treatment of active disease tuberculosis to rapidly decrease the infectious state and delay or prevent the emergence of resistant strains. In selected situations, intermittent (twice weekly) regimens may be employed. Streptomycin is also used as an antitubercular. Azithromycin and clarithromycin are useful in the prevention and management of MAC disease. Rifampin is used in the prevention of meningococcal meningitis and *Haemophilus influenzae* type b disease.

General Action and Information: Kill (tuberculocidal) or inhibit the growth of (tuberculostatic) mycobacteria responsible for causing tuberculosis. Combination therapy with two or more agents is required, unless used as prophylaxis (isoniazid alone).

Contraindications: Hypersensitivity. Severe liver disease.

Precautions: Use cautiously in patients with a history of liver disease or in elderly or debilitated patients. Ethambutol requires ophthalmologic follow-up. Safety in pregnancy and lactation not established, although selected agents have been used without adverse effects on the fetus. Compliance is required for optimal response.

Interactions: Isoniazid inhibits the metabolism of phenytoin. Rifampin and rifabutin stimulate hepatic drug-metabolizing enzymes and may decrease the effects of drugs that are metabolized by the liver. Rifampin and rifabutin significantly decrease saquinavir levels (combination should be avoided).

NURSING IMPLICATIONS

Assessment

- Mycobacterial studies and susceptibility tests should be performed prior to and periodically throughout therapy to detect possible resistance.
- Assess lung sounds and character and amount of sputum periodically throughout therapy.

Potential Nursing Diagnoses

- Infection, risk for (Indications).
- Knowledge deficit, related to medication regimen (Patient/Family Teaching).
- Noncompliance (Patient/Family Teaching).

Implementation

- Most medications can be administered with food or antacids if GI irritation occurs.

Patient/Family Teaching
- Advise patient of the importance of continuing therapy even after symptoms have subsided.
- Emphasize the importance of regular follow-up examinations to monitor progress and check for side effects.
- Inform patients taking *rifabutin* or *rifampin* that saliva, sputum, sweat, tears, urine, and feces may become red-orange to red-brown and that soft contact lenses may become permanently discolored.

Evaluation
Effectiveness of therapy can be demonstrated by: ▪ Resolution of the signs and symptoms of tuberculosis ▪ Negative sputum cultures.

Antituberculars/antimycobacterials Included in *Davis's Drug Guide for Nurses*:

azithromycin 91
clarithromycin 202
ethambutol 353
isoniazid 541
pyrazinamide 1141
rifabutin 889
rifampin 890
streptomycin 32

▪ ANTITUSSIVES/EXPECTORANTS

PHARMACOLOGIC PROFILE
General Use: Used for the symptomatic relief of cough due to various causes, including viral upper respiratory infections. Not intended for chronic use.

General Action and Information: Antitussives (codeine, dextromethorphan, diphenhydramine, hydrocodone, and hydromorphone) suppress cough by central mechanisms. Expectorants (acetylcysteine and guaifenesin) aid in mobilizing pulmonary secretions. Benzonatate decreases cough by a local anesthetic action. Productive cough should not be suppressed unless it interferes with sleeping or other activities of daily living. Increasing fluid intake probably serves as the best expectorant, decreasing the viscosity of secretions so that they may be more easily mobilized.

Contraindications: Hypersensitivity.

Precautions: Use cautiously in children. Should not be used for prolonged periods unless under the advice of a physician or other health care professional.

Interactions: Centrally acting antitussives may have additive CNS depression with other CNS depressants.

NURSING IMPLICATIONS
Assessment
- Assess frequency and nature of cough, lung sounds, and amount and type of sputum produced.

Potential Nursing Diagnoses
- Airway clearance, ineffective (Indications).
- Knowledge deficit, related to medication regimen (Patient/Family Teaching).

Implementation
- Unless contraindicated, maintain fluid intake of 1500–2000 ml to decrease viscosity of bronchial secretions.

Patient/Family Teaching

- Instruct patient to cough effectively, sit upright, and take several deep breaths before attempting to cough.
- Advise patient to minimize cough by avoiding irritants (cigarette smoke, fumes, dust). Humidification of environmental air, frequent sips of water, and sugarless hard candy may also decrease the frequency of dry, irritating cough.
- Caution patient to avoid taking concurrent alcohol or CNS depressants.
- May cause dizziness or drowsiness. Caution patient to avoid driving or other activities requiring alertness until response to medication is known.
- Advise patient that any cough lasting over 1 wk or accompanied by fever, chest pain, persistent headache, or skin rash warrants medical attention.

Evaluation

Effectiveness of therapy can be demonstrated by: ▪ Decrease in frequency and intensity of cough without eliminating patient's cough reflex.

Antitussives Included in *Davis's Drug Guide for Nurses*:

benzonatate 1131
codeine 221
dextromethorphan 258
diphenhydramine 291
hydrocodone 487
hydromorphone 490

Expectorants Included in *Davis's Drug Guide for Nurses*:

acetylcysteine 6
guaifenesin 460

▪ ANTIULCER AGENTS

PHARMACOLOGIC PROFILE

General Use: Treatment and prophylaxis of peptic ulcer and gastric hypersecretory conditions such as Zollinger-Ellison syndrome. Histamine H_2-receptor antagonists and omeprazole are also used in the management of gastroesophageal reflux disease (GERD).

General Action and Information: Because a great majority of peptic ulcer disease may be traced to gastrointestinal infection with the organism *Helicobacter pylori*, eradication of the organism decreases symptomatology and recurrence. Anti-infectives with significant activity against the organism include amoxicillin, clarithromycin, metronidazole, and tetracycline. Bismuth also has anti-infective activity against *H. pylori*. Regimens may include 2 anti-infectives plus a gastric acid–pump inhibitor (lansoprazole, omeprazole) or 3 anti-infectives or 3 anti-infectives plus a gastric acid–pump inhibitor.

REGIMENS FOR ERADICATING *H. PYLORI*

Regimen	Dosing
omeprazole clarithromycin	40 mg once daily on 1st day, then 20 mg once daily for 2 wk 500 mg 3 times daily for 2 wk
ranitidine bismuth citrate clarithromycin	400 mg twice daily for 4 wk 500 mg 3 times daily for 2 wk

REGIMENS FOR ERADICATING *H. PYLORI* (CONTINUED)

Regimen	Dosing
metronidazole tetracycline bismuth subsalicylate	250 mg 4 times daily (at meals and bedtime) for 2 wk 500 mg 4 times daily (at meals and bedtime) for 2 wk 525 mg 4 times daily (at meals and bedtime) for 2 wk
lansoprazole clarithromycin amoxicillin	30 mg daily for 2 wk 500 mg twice daily for 2 wk 1 g twice daily for for 2 wk
lansoprazole amoxicillin	30 mg daily for 2 wk 1 g 3 times daily for for 2 wk

Other medications used in the management of gastric/duodenal ulcer disease are aimed at neutralizing gastric acid (antacids), decreasing acid secretion (histamine H_2 antagonists, lansoprazole, misoprostol, omeprazole), or protecting the ulcer surface from further damage (misoprostol, sucralfate). Histamine H_2-receptor antagonists (blockers) competitively inhibit the action of histamine at the H_2 receptor, located primarily in gastric parietal cells, resulting in inhibition of gastric acid secretion. Misoprostol decreases gastric acid secretion and increases production of protective mucus. Omeprazole and lansoprazole prevent the transport of hydrogen ions into the gastric lumen.

Contraindications: Hypersensitivity.

Precautions: Most histamine H_2 antagonists require dosage reduction in renal impairment and in the elderly. Magnesium-containing antacids should be used cautiously in patients with renal impairment. Misoprostol should be used cautiously in women with childbearing potential.

Interactions: Calcium and magnesium-containing antacids decrease the absorption of tetracycline and fluoroquinolones. Cimetidine inhibits the ability of the liver to metabolize several drugs, increasing the risk of toxicity from warfarin, tricyclic antidepressants, theophylline, metoprolol, phenytoin, propranolol, and lidocaine. Omeprazole decreases metabolism of phenytoin, diazepam, and warfarin. All agents that increase gastric pH will decrease the absorption of ketoconazole.

NURSING IMPLICATIONS

Assessment

- **General Info:** Assess patient routinely for epigastric or abdominal pain and frank or occult blood in the stool, emesis, or gastric aspirate.
- **Antacids:** Assess for heartburn and indigestion as well as the location, duration, character, and precipitating factors of gastric pain.
- **Histamine H_2 Antagonists:** Assess elderly and severely ill patients for confusion routinely. Notify physician or other health care professional promptly should this occur.
- **Misoprostol:** Assess women of childbearing age for pregnancy. Medication is usually begun on 2nd or 3rd day of menstrual period following a negative serum pregnancy test within 2 wk of beginning therapy.
- **Lab Test Considerations:** *Histamine H_2 antagonists* antagonize the effects of pentagastrin and histamine during gastric acid secretion test. Avoid administration during the 24 hr preceding the test.
- May cause false-negative results in skin tests using allergen extracts. These drugs should be discontinued 24 hr prior to the test.

Potential Nursing Diagnoses

- Pain (Indications).
- Knowledge deficit, related to medication regimen (Patient/Family Teaching).

Implementation

- **Antacids:** Antacids cause premature dissolution and absorption of enteric-coated tablets and may interfere with absorption of other oral medications. Separate administration of antacids and other oral medications by at least 1 hr.
- Shake liquid preparations well before pouring. Follow administration with water to ensure passage to stomach. Liquid and powder dosage forms are considered to be more effective than chewable tablets.
- Chewable tablets must be chewed thoroughly before swallowing. Follow with half a glass of water.
- Administer 1 and 3 hr after meals and at bedtime for maximum antacid effect.
- **Misoprostol:** Administer with meals and at bedtime to reduce the severity of diarrhea.
- **Omeprazole and Lansoprazole:** Administer before meals, preferably in the morning. Capsules should be swallowed whole; do not open, crush, or chew.
- □ May be administered concurrently with antacids.
- **Sucralfate:** Administer on an empty stomach 1 hr before meals and at bedtime. Do not crush or chew tablets. Shake suspension well prior to administration. If nasogastric administration is required, consult pharmacist, as protein-binding properties of sucralfate have resulted in formation of a bezoar when administered with enteral feedings and other medications.

Patient/Family Teaching

- **General Info:** Instruct patient to take medication as directed for the full course of therapy, even if feeling better. If a dose is missed, it should be taken as soon as remembered but not if almost time for next dose. Do not double doses.
- Advise patient to avoid alcohol, products containing aspirin, NSAIDs, and foods that may cause an increase in GI irritation.
- Advise patient to report onset of black, tarry stools to the physician or other health care professional promptly.
- Inform patient that cessation of smoking may help prevent the recurrence of duodenal ulcers.
- **Antacids:** Caution patient to consult health care professional before taking antacids for more than 2 wk or if problem is recurring. Advise patient to consult health care professional if relief is not obtained or if symptoms of gastric bleeding (black, tarry stools; coffee-ground emesis) occur.
- **Misoprostol:** Emphasize that sharing of this medication may be dangerous.
- □ Inform patient that misoprostol may cause spontaneous abortion. Women of childbearing age must be informed of this effect through verbal and written information and must use contraception throughout therapy. If pregnancy is suspected, the woman should stop taking misoprostol and immediately notify her health care professional.
- **Sucralfate:** Advise patient to continue with course of therapy for 4–8 wk, even if feeling better, to ensure ulcer healing.
- Advise patient that an increase in fluid intake, dietary bulk, and exercise may prevent drug-induced constipation.

Evaluation

Effectiveness of therapy can be demonstrated by: ▪ Decrease in GI pain and irritation ▪ Prevention of gastric irritation and bleeding. Healing of duodenal ulcers can be seen by x rays or endoscopy. Therapy with histamine H_2 antagonists is continued for at least 6 wk after initial episode ▪ Decreased symptoms of gastroesophageal reflux disease ▪ Increase in the pH of gastric secretions (antacids) ▪ Prevention of gastric ulcers in patients receiving chronic NSAID therapy (misoprostol only).

Antiulcer Agents Included in *Davis's Drug Guide for Nurses*:

antacids
aluminum hydroxide 27, 594
calcium carbonate 144
magaldrate 594
magnesium hydroxide 596
magnesium hydroxide/aluminum hydroxide 594
sodium bicarbonate 918

anti-infectives
amoxicillin 46
bismuth subsalicylate 110
clarithromycin 202
metronidazole 650
tetracycline 961

gastric acid–pump inhibitors
lansoprazole 563
omeprazole 744

histamine H_2-receptor antagonists
cimetidine 477
famotidine 477
nizatidine 477
ranitidine 477

miscellaneous
misoprostol 670
sucralfate 936

■ ANTIVIRALS

PHARMACOLOGIC PROFILE

General Use: Acyclovir, famciclovir, and valacyclovir are used in the management of herpesvirus infections. Acyclovir also is used in the management of chickenpox. Amantadine and rimantadine are used primarily in the prevention of influenza A viral infections. Trifluridine is used for ophthalmic viral infections. Cidofovir, ganciclovir, and foscarnet are used in the treatment of cytomegalovirus (CMV) retinitis.

General Action and Information: Most agents inhibit viral replication. Amantadine and rimantadine prevent penetration of the virus into host cells.

Contraindications: Previous hypersensitivity.

Precautions: All require dosage adjustment in renal impairment. Acyclovir may cause renal impairment. Acyclovir and amantadine may cause CNS toxicity. Vidarabine commonly causes GI adverse reactions. Foscarnet increases risk of seizures.

Interactions: Acyclovir may have additive CNS and nephrotoxicity with drugs causing similar adverse reactions. Amantadine may have additive anticholinergic properties with other drugs, causing anticholinergic side effects. Adverse reactions to vidarabine may be potentiated by concurrent allopurinol.

NURSING IMPLICATIONS

Assessment

- **General Info:** Assess patient for signs and symptoms of infection before and throughout therapy.
- **Ophth:** Assess eye lesions before and daily during therapy.
- **Topical:** Assess lesions before and daily during therapy.

Potential Nursing Diagnoses

- Infection, risk for (Indications).
- Skin integrity, impairment of (Indications).
- Knowledge deficit, related to medication regimen (Patient/Family Teaching).

Implementation

- Most systemic antiviral agents should be administered around the clock to maintain therapeutic serum drug levels.

Patient/Family Teaching

- Instruct patient to continue taking medication around the clock for full course of therapy, even if feeling better.
- Advise patient that antivirals and antiretrovirals do not prevent transmission to others. Precautions should be taken to prevent spread of virus.
- Instruct patient in correct technique for topical or ophthalmic preparations.
- Instruct patient to notify health care professional if symptoms do not improve.

Evaluation

Effectiveness of therapy can be demonstrated by: ▪ Prevention or resolution of the signs and symptoms of viral infection. Length of time for complete resolution depends on organism and site of infection.

Antivirals Included in *Davis's Drug Guide for Nurses*:

acyclovir 9
amantadine 1129
cidofovir 196
foscarnet 411
ganciclovir 419
rimantadine 1141
trifluridine 1116
vidarabine 1144

▪ BETA-ADRENERGIC BLOCKING AGENTS

PHARMACOLOGIC PROFILE

General Use: Used in the management of hypertension, angina pectoris, tachyarrhythmias, hypertrophic subaortic stenosis, migraine headache (prophylaxis), myocardial infarction (prevention), glaucoma (betaxolol, levobunolol, metipranolol, and timolol), pheochromocytoma, tremors (propranolol only), congestive heart failure (carvedilol only), and hyperthyroidism (management of symptoms only).

General Action and Information: Beta-adrenergic receptor blocking agents compete with adrenergic (sympathetic) neurotransmitters (epinephrine and norepinephrine) for beta-adrenergic receptor sites. Beta-adrenergic receptor sites are located chiefly in the heart, where stimulation results in increased heart rate, contractility, and AV conduction. Beta$_2$-adrenergic receptors are found mainly in bronchial and vascular smooth muscle and the uterus. Stimulation of beta$_2$-adrenergic receptors produces vasodilation, bronchodilation, and uterine relaxation. Blockade of these receptors antagonizes the effect of the neurotransmitters. Beta blockers may be relatively *selective* for beta$_1$-adrenergic receptors (acebutolol, atenolol, betaxolol, esmolol, and metoprolol) or *nonselective* (carteolol, carvedilol, labetalol, levobunolol, nadolol, penbutolol, pindolol, propranolol, sotalol, and timolol), blocking both beta$_1$- and beta$_2$-adrenergic receptors. Carvedilol and labetalol have additional alpha-adrenergic blocking action. Acebutolol, carteolol, penbutolol, and pindolol possess *intrinsic sympathomimetic action (ISA)*, which may result in less bradycardia than other agents. Ophthalmic beta blockers decrease production of aqueous humor.

Contraindications: Uncompensated congestive heart failure, acute bronchospasm, some forms of valvular heart disease, bradyarrhythmias, and heart block.

Precautions: Use cautiously in pregnant and lactating women (may cause fetal bradycardia and hypoglycemia). Use cautiously in any form of lung disease, bradyarrhythmias, or underlying compensated congestive heart failure. Use cautiously in diabetics and patients with severe liver disease. Beta-adrenergic blockers should not be discontinued abruptly in patients with cardiovascular disease.

Interactions: May cause additive myocardial depression and bradycardia when used with other agents having this effect (cardiac glycosides and selected antiarrhythmics). May antagonize the therapeutic effect of bronchodilators. May alter insulin dosage requirements. Cimetidine may decrease metabolism and increase the effect of certain beta blockers.

NURSING IMPLICATIONS

Assessment

- **General Info:** Monitor blood pressure and pulse frequently during dosage adjustment and periodically throughout therapy.
- Monitor intake and output ratios and daily weight. Assess patient routinely for signs and symptoms of congestive heart failure (dyspnea, rales/crackles, weight gain, peripheral edema, and jugular venous distention).
- **Angina:** Assess frequency and severity of episodes of chest pain periodically throughout therapy.
- **Migraine Prophylaxis:** Assess frequency and severity of migraine headaches periodically throughout therapy.

Potential Nursing Diagnoses

- Tissue perfusion, altered (Indications).
- Knowledge deficit, related to medication regimen (Patient/Family Teaching).
- Noncompliance (Patient/Family Teaching).

Implementation

- Take apical pulse before administration. If heart rate is <50 bpm or if arrhythmias occur, hold medication and notify physician or other health care professional.
- Many beta-adrenergic blockers are available as combination products to enhance compliance (see Appendix A).

Patient/Family Teaching

- **General Info:** Instruct patient to continue taking medication, even if feeling well. Abrupt withdrawal may cause life-threatening arrhythmias, hypertension, or myocardial ischemia. Medication controls but does not cure hypertension.
- Encourage patient to comply with additional interventions for hypertension (weight reduction, low-sodium diet, regular exercise, discontinuation of smoking, moderation of alcohol consumption, and stress management).
- Instruct patient and family on proper technique for monitoring blood pressure. Advise them to check blood pressure weekly and report significant changes.
- Caution patient to make position changes slowly to minimize orthostatic hypotension. Advise patient that exercising or hot weather may enhance hypotensive effects.
- Advise patient to consult health care professional before taking any OTC medication, especially cold remedies.
- Caution patient that these medications may cause increased sensitivity to cold.
- Diabetics should monitor blood sugar closely, especially if weakness, malaise, irritability, or fatigue occurs. May mask tachycardia and increased blood pressure as signs of hypoglycemia, but dizziness and sweating may still occur.
- Advise patient to inform health care professional of medication regimen before treatment or surgery.

- Advise patient to carry identification describing disease process and medication regimen at all times.
- Emphasize the importance of follow-up exams to monitor progress.
- **Ophth:** Instruct patient in correct technique for administration of ophthalmic preparations.

Evaluation

Effectiveness of therapy can be demonstrated by: ▪ Decrease in blood pressure ▪ Decrease in frequency and severity of anginal attacks ▪ Control of arrhythmias ▪ Prevention of myocardial infarction ▪ Prevention of migraine headaches ▪ Decrease in tremors ▪ Lowering of intraocular pressure.

Beta-Adrenergic Blocking Agents Included in *Davis's Drug Guide for Nurses*:

nonselective beta-adrenergic blocking agents

carteolol 160
carvedilol 163
labetalol 556
levobunolol (ophth only) 1117
metipranolol (ophth only) 1117
nadolol 691
penbutolol 771
pindolol 813
propranolol 863
sotalol 927
timolol 985

selective beta-adrenergic blocking agents

acebutolol 2
atenolol 82
betaxolol 100
esmolol 342
metoprolol 647

ophthalmic beta-adrenergic blocking agents

betaxolol 1117
carteolol 1117
levobunolol 1117
metipranolol 1117
timolol 1117

▪ BRONCHODILATORS

PHARMACOLOGIC PROFILE

General Use: Used in the treatment of reversible airway obstruction due to asthma or COPD. Recently revised recommendations for management of asthma recommend that rapid-acting inhaled beta-agonist bronchodilators (not salmeterol) be reserved as acute relievers of bronchospasm; repeated or chronic use indicates the need for additional long-term contol agents including inhaled glucocorticoids, mast cell stabilizers, and long-acting bronchodilators (oral theophylline or beta agonists). The place of the new agents zafirlukast and zileuton has not yet been established.*

General Action and Information: Beta-adrenergic agonists (albuterol, epinephrine, isoproterenol, metaproterenol, pirbuterol, and terbutaline) produce bronchodilation by stimulating the production of cyclic adenosine monophosphate (cAMP). Newer agents (albuterol, bitolterol, metaproterenol, pirbuterol, and terbutaline) are relatively selective for pulmonary ($beta_2$) receptors, whereas older agents produce cardiac stimulation ($beta_1$-adrenergic effects) in addition to bronchodilation. Onset of action allows use in management of acute attacks except for salmeterol, which has delayed onset. Phosphodiesterase inhibitors (aminophylline, dyphylline, oxtriphylline, and theophylline) inhibit the breakdown of cAMP. Ipratropium is an anticholinergic compound that produces bronchodilation by blocking the action of acetylcholine in the respi-

*Highlights of the Expert Panel Report 2: Guidelines for the diagnosis and management of asthma. NIH Publication No. 97-4051A. May 1997.

CLASSIFICATIONS

ratory tract. Zafirlukast and zileuton are leukotriene modifiers. Leukotrienes are components of slow-reacting substance of anaphylaxis A (SRS-A), which may be a cause of bronchospasm.

Contraindications: Hypersensitivity to agents, preservatives (bisulfites), or propellants used in their formulation. Avoid use in uncontrolled cardiac arrhythmias.

Precautions: Use cautiously in patients with diabetes, cardiovascular disease, or hyperthyroidism.

Interactions: Therapeutic effectiveness may be antagonized by concurrent use of beta-adrenergic blocking agents. Additive sympathomimetic effects with other adrenergic (sympathetic) drugs, including vasopressors and decongestants. Cardiovascular effects may be potentiated by antidepressants and MAO inhibitors.

NURSING IMPLICATIONS

Assessment

- Assess blood pressure, pulse, respiration, lung sounds, and character of secretions before and throughout therapy.
- Patients with a history of cardiovascular problems should be monitored for ECG changes and chest pain.

Potential Nursing Diagnoses

- Airway clearance, ineffective (Indications).
- Activity intolerance (Indications).
- Knowledge deficit, related to medication regimen (Patient/Family Teaching).

Implementation

- Administer around the clock to maintain therapeutic plasma levels.

Patient/Family Teaching

- Emphasize the importance of taking only the prescribed dose at the prescribed time intervals.
- Encourage the patient to drink adequate liquids (2000 ml/day minimum) to decrease the viscosity of the airway secretions.
- Advise patient to avoid OTC cough, cold, or breathing preparations without consulting health care professional and to minimize intake of xanthine-containing foods or beverages (colas, coffee, and chocolate), as these may increase side effects and cause arrhythmias.
- Caution patient to avoid smoking and other respiratory irritants.
- Instruct patient on proper use of metered-dose inhaler (see Appendix H).
- Advise patient to contact health care professional promptly if the usual dose of medication fails to produce the desired results, symptoms worsen after treatment, or toxic effects occur.
- Patients using other inhalation medications and bronchodilators should be advised to use bronchodilator first and allow 5 min to elapse before administering the other medication, unless otherwise directed by health care professional.

Evaluation

Effectiveness of therapy can be demonstrated by: ▪ Decreased bronchospasm ▪ Increased ease of breathing.

Bronchodilators Included in *Davis's Drug Guide for Nurses*:

beta-adrenergic agonists
albuterol 16
bitolterol 113
epinephrine 329
isoproterenol 1137
metaproterenol 625
pirbuterol 818
salmeterol 903
terbutaline 955

leukotriene antagonists
zafirlukast 1048
zileuton 1053

phosphodiesterase inhibitors (xanthines)
aminophylline 124
dyphylline 124
oxtriphylline 124
theophylline 124

anticholinergic agent
ipratropium 533

▪ CALCIUM CHANNEL BLOCKERS

PHARMACOLOGIC PROFILE

General Use: Used in the treatment of hypertension (amlodipine, diltiazem, felodipine, isradipine, nicardipine, nifedipine, nisoldipine, verapamil) or in the treatment and prophylaxis of angina pectoris or coronary artery spasm (amlodipine, bepridil, diltiazem, nicardipine, verapamil). Verapamil and diltiazem are also used for control of arrhythmias. Nimodipine is used to prevent neurologic damage due to certain types of cerebral vasospasm.

General Action and Information: Block calcium entry into cells of vascular smooth muscle and myocardium. Dilate coronary arteries in both normal and ischemic myocardium and inhibit coronary artery spasm. Decrease AV conduction (bepridil, mibefradil, verapamil, and diltiazem). Nimodipine appears to have a relatively selective effect on cerebral blood vessels.

Contraindications: Hypersensitivity. Contraindicated in bradycardia, 2nd- and 3rd- degree heart block, or uncompensated congestive heart failure (bepridil, mibefradil, verapamil).

Precautions: Safety in pregnancy and lactation not established. Use cautiously in patients with liver disease or uncontrolled arrhythmias. Bepridil has been associated with serious arrhythmias and agranulocytosis.

Interactions: Additive myocardial depression with beta-adrenergic blocking agents and disopyramide (verapamil and diltiazem). Effectiveness may be decreased by phenobarbital or phenytoin and increased by propranolol or cimetidine. Verapamil and diltiazem may increase serum digoxin levels and cause toxicity. Mibefradil has a number of serious interactions; consult individual monograph.

NURSING IMPLICATIONS

Assessment

- **General Info:** Monitor blood pressure and pulse before and periodically during therapy.
- Monitor intake and output ratios and daily weight. Assess patient routinely for signs and symptoms of congestive heart failure (dyspnea, rales/crackles, weight gain, peripheral edema, jugular venous distention).
- Patients receiving digitalis glycosides concurrently with calcium channel blockers should have routine serum digitalis glycoside levels and be monitored for signs and symptoms of digitalis glycoside toxicity.

- **Angina:** Assess frequency and severity of episodes of chest pain periodically throughout therapy.
- **Arrhythmias:** ECG should be monitored continuously during IV therapy and periodically during long-term therapy with verapamil.
- **Cerebral Vasospasm:** Assess patient's neurologic status (level of consciousness, movement) before and periodically during therapy with nimodipine.
- **Lab Test Considerations:** Total serum calcium concentrations are not affected by calcium channel blockers.

Potential Nursing Diagnoses

- Tissue perfusion, altered (Indications).
- Pain (Indications).
- Knowledge deficit, related to medication regimen (Patient/Family Teaching).

Implementation

- May be administered without regard to meals. May be administered with meals if GI irritation becomes a problem. Administer bepridil and verapamil with meals or milk to minimize gastric irritation.
- Do not open, crush, break, or chew sustained-release capsules or tablets, except for Verelan (verapamil) capsules, which may be opened and sprinkled in liquids or on soft foods. Empty tablets that appear in stool are not significant. Crush and mix diltiazem with food or fluids for patients having difficulty swallowing.
- Sublingual nifedipine may be administered by puncturing the capsule with a sterile needle and squeezing to administer the liquid into the buccal pouch. The dose used is the same as the oral dose. Chewing or puncturing and swallowing capsule has shown similar effectiveness as SL route for hypertensive emergencies.

Patient/Family Teaching

- **General Info:** Advise patient to take medication exactly as directed, even if feeling well.
- Instruct patient on correct technique for monitoring pulse. Instruct patient to contact health care professional if heart rate is <50 bpm.
- Caution patient to make position changes slowly to minimize orthostatic hypotension.
- May cause dizziness or drowsiness. Caution patient to avoid driving or other activities requiring alertness until response to medication is known.
- Instruct patient on importance of maintaining good dental hygiene and seeing dentist frequently for teeth cleaning to prevent tenderness, bleeding, and gingival hyperplasia (gum enlargement).
- Instruct patient to avoid concurrent use of alcohol or OTC medications, especially cold preparations, without consulting health care professional.
- Advise patient to inform health care professional of medication regimen before treatment or surgery.
- Advise patient to carry identification describing disease process and medication regimen at all times.
- Emphasize the importance of follow-up exams to monitor progress.
- **Angina:** Instruct patients on concurrent nitrate therapy to continue taking both medications as ordered and to use SL nitroglycerin as needed for anginal attacks.
- Advise patient to contact health care professional if chest pain worsens, does not improve after therapy, or is accompanied by diaphoresis or shortness of breath; or if severe, persistent headache occurs.
- Caution patient to discuss exercise restrictions with health care professional prior to exertion.
- **Hypertension:** Encourage patient to comply with additional interventions for hypertension (weight reduction, low-sodium diet, regular exercise, discontinuation of smoking, moderation

of alcohol consumption, stress management). Medication controls but does not cure hypertension.

- Instruct patient and family on proper technique for monitoring blood pressure. Advise them to check blood pressure weekly and report significant changes.

Evaluation

Effectiveness of therapy can be demonstrated by: ▪ Decrease in blood pressure ▪ Decrease in frequency and severity of anginal attacks ▪ Decrease in need for nitrate therapy ▪ Increase in activity tolerance and sense of well-being ▪ Suppression and prevention of supraventricular tachyarrhythmias ▪ Improvement in neurologic deficits due to vasospasm following subarachnoid hemorrhage.

Calcium Channel Blockers Included in *Davis's Drug Guide for Nurses*:

▪ CHOLINERGICS

PHARMACOLOGIC PROFILE

General Use: Used in the treatment of nonobstructive urinary retention (bethanechol) and in the diagnosis (edrophonium) and treatment (neostigmine and pyridostigmine) of myasthenia gravis. Physostigmine is used in the diagnosis and management of cholinergic excess, which occurs following antidepressant overdosage. Cholinesterase inhibitors may be used to reverse nondepolarizing neuromuscular blocking agents. Edrophonium has been used in the treatment of supraventricular tachyarrhythmias. Acetylcholine is administered as an eyedrop to produce miosis during ophthalmic surgery.

General Action and Information: Cholinergics intensify and prolong the action of acetylcholine by either mimicking its effects at cholinergic receptor sites (bethanechol) or preventing the breakdown of acetylcholine by inhibiting cholinesterases (edrophonium, neostigmine, physostigmine, and pyridostigmine). Effects include increased tone in GU and skeletal muscle, decreased intraocular pressure, increased secretions, and decreased bladder capacity.

Contraindications: Hypersensitivity. Avoid use in patients with possible obstruction of the GI or GU tract.

Precautions: Use with extreme caution in patients with a history of asthma, peptic ulcer disease, cardiovascular disease, epilepsy, or hyperthyroidism. Safety in pregnancy and lactation not established. Atropine should be available to treat excessive dosage.

Interactions: Additive cholinergic effects. Do not use with depolarizing neuromuscular blocking agents. Use with ganglionic blocking agents may result in severe hypotension.

NURSING IMPLICATIONS

Assessment

- **General Info:** Monitor pulse, respiratory rate, and blood pressure frequently throughout parenteral administration.

CLASSIFICATIONS

- **Myasthenia Gravis:** Assess neuromuscular status (ptosis, diplopia, vital capacity, ability to swallow, and extremity strength) before and at time of peak effect.
- Assess patient for overdosage and underdosage or resistance. Both have similar symptoms (muscle weakness, dyspnea, and dysphagia), but symptoms of overdosage usually occur within 1 hr of administration, while underdosage symptoms occur 3 hr or more after administration. A Tensilon test (edrophonium chloride) may be used to distinguish between overdosage and underdosage.
- **Antidote to Nondepolarizing Neuromuscular Blocking Agents:** Monitor reversal of effects of neuromuscular blocking agents with a peripheral nerve stimulator.
- **Urinary Retention:** Monitor intake and output ratios. Palpate abdomen for bladder distention. Catheterization may be done to assess postvoid residual.
- **Glaucoma:** Monitor patient for changes in vision, eye irritation, and persistent headache.
- **Toxicity and Overdose:** Atropine is the specific antidote.

Potential Nursing Diagnoses

- Urinary elimination, altered (Indications).
- Breathing pattern, ineffective (Indications).
- Knowledge deficit, related to medication regimen (Patient/Family Teaching).

Implementation

- **Myasthenia Gravis:** For patients who have difficulty chewing, medication may be administered 30 min before meals.

Patient/Family Teaching

- **General Info:** Instruct patients with myasthenia gravis to take medication exactly as ordered. Taking the dose late may result in myasthenic crisis. Taking the dose early may result in a cholinergic crisis. This regimen must be continued as a lifelong therapy.
- **Ophth:** Instruct patient on correct method of application of drops or ointment (see Appendix H).
- Explain to patient that pupil constriction and temporary stinging and blurring of vision are expected. Notify health care professional if blurred vision and brow ache persist.
- Caution patient that night vision may be impaired.
- Advise patient of the need for regular eye exams to monitor intraocular pressure and visual fields.

Evaluation

Effectiveness of therapy can be demonstrated by: ▪ Reversal of CNS symptoms secondary to anticholinergic excess resulting from drug overdosage or ingestion of poisonous plants ▪ Control of elevated intraocular pressure ▪ Increase in bladder function and tone ▪ Decrease in abdominal distention ▪ Relief of myasthenic symptoms ▪ Differentiation of myasthenic from cholinergic crisis ▪ Reversal of paralysis after anesthesia ▪ Resolution of supraventricular tachycardia.

Cholinergics Included in *Davis's Drug Guide for Nurses*:

cholinomimetic
bethanechol 102

cholinesterase inhibitors
demecarium 1118
echothiophate 1118
edrophonium 325
neostigmine 706
physostigmine 1119
pyridostigmine 873

■ DIURETICS

PHARMACOLOGIC PROFILE

General Use: Thiazide and loop diuretics are used alone or in combination in the treatment of hypertension or edema due to congestive heart failure or other causes. Potassium-sparing diuretics have weak diuretic and antihypertensive properties and are used mainly to conserve potassium in patients receiving thiazide or loop diuretics. Osmotic diuretics are often used in the management of cerebral edema.

General Action and Information: Enhance the selective excretion of various electrolytes and water by affecting renal mechanisms for tubular secretion and reabsorption. Groups commonly used are thiazide diuretics and thiazide-like diuretics (chlorthalidone, hydrochlorothiazide, indapamide, and metolazone), loop diuretics (bumetanide, ethacrynic acid, and furosemide), potassium-sparing diuretics (amiloride, spironolactone, and triamterene), and osmotic diuretics (mannitol). Mechanisms vary, depending on agent.

Contraindications: Hypersensitivity. Thiazide diuretics may exhibit cross-sensitivity with other sulfonamides.

Precautions: Use with caution in patients with renal or hepatic disease. Safety in pregnancy and lactation not established.

Interactions: Additive hypokalemia with glucocorticoids, amphotericin B, mezlocillin, piperacillin, or ticarcillin. Hypokalemia enhances digitalis glycoside toxicity. Potassium-losing diuretics decrease lithium excretion and may cause toxicity. Additive hypotension with other antihypertensives or nitrates. Potassium-sparing diuretics may cause hyperkalemia when used with potassium supplements or ACE inhibitors.

NURSING IMPLICATIONS

Assessment

- **General Info:** Assess fluid status throughout therapy. Monitor daily weight, intake and output ratios, amount and location of edema, lung sounds, skin turgor, and mucous membranes.
- Assess patient for anorexia, muscle weakness, numbness, tingling, paresthesia, confusion, and excessive thirst. Notify physician or other health care professional promptly if these signs of electrolyte imbalance occur.
- **Hypertension:** Monitor blood pressure and pulse before and during administration. Monitor frequency of prescription refills to determine compliance in patients treated for hypertension.
- **Increased Intracranial Pressure:** Monitor neurologic status and intracranial pressure readings in patients receiving osmotic diuretics to decrease cerebral edema.
- **Increased Intraocular Pressure:** Monitor for persistent or increased eye pain or decreased visual acuity.
- **Lab Test Considerations:** Monitor electrolytes (especially potassium), blood glucose, BUN, and serum uric acid levels before and periodically throughout course of therapy.
- Thiazide diuretics may cause increased serum cholesterol, low-density lipoprotein (LDL), and triglyceride concentrations.

Potential Nursing Diagnoses

- Fluid volume excess (Indications).
- Knowledge deficit, related to medication regimen (Patient/Family Teaching).

Implementation

- Administer oral diuretics in the morning to prevent disruption of sleep cycle.
- Many diuretics are available in combination with antihypertensives or potassium-sparing diuretics.

Patient/Family Teaching

- **General Info:** Instruct patient to take medication exactly as directed. Advise patients on antihypertensive regimen to continue taking medication, even if feeling better. Medication controls but does not cure hypertension.
- Caution patient to make position changes slowly to minimize orthostatic hypotension. Caution patient that the use of alcohol, exercise during hot weather, or standing for long periods during therapy may enhance orthostatic hypotension.
- Instruct patient to consult health care professional regarding dietary potassium guidelines.
- Instruct patient to monitor weight weekly and report significant changes.
- Caution patient to use sunscreen and protective clothing to prevent photosensitivity reactions.
- Advise patient to consult health care professional before taking OTC medication concurrently with this therapy.
- Instruct patient to notify health care professional of medication regimen before treatment or surgery.
- Advise patient to contact health care professional immediately if muscle weakness, cramps, nausea, dizziness, or numbness or tingling of extremities occurs.
- Emphasize the importance of routine follow-up.
- **Hypertension:** Reinforce the need to continue additional therapies for hypertension (weight loss, regular exercise, restricted sodium intake, stress reduction, moderation of alcohol consumption, and cessation of smoking).
- Instruct patients with hypertension in the correct technique for monitoring weekly blood pressure.

Evaluation

Effectiveness of therapy can be demonstrated by: ▪ Decreased blood pressure ▪ Increased urine output ▪ Decreased edema ▪ Reduced intracranial pressure ▪ Prevention of hypokalemia in patients taking diuretics ▪ Treatment of hyperaldosteronism.

Diuretics Included in *Davis's Drug Guide for Nurses*:

loop diuretics
bumetanide 128
furosemide 414
torsemide 995

osmotic diuretic
mannitol 599

potassium-sparing diuretics
amiloride 298
spironolactone 298
triamterene 298

thiazide and thiazide-like diuretics
chlorothiazide 301
chlorthalidone 301
hydrochlorothiazide 301
indapamide 516
metolazone 645

▪ ELECTROLYTES/ELECTROLYTE MODIFIERS

PHARMACOLOGIC PROFILE

General Use: Used to prevent or treat deficiencies or excesses of electrolytes. Acidifiers and alkalinizers are used to increase solubility and promote renal excretion of substances that accumulate in certain disease states (kidney stones and uric acid).

General Action and Information: Electrolytes are essential for homeostasis. Maintenance of electrolyte levels within normal levels is required for many physiologic processes such as cardiac, nerve, and muscle function; bone growth and stability; and other processes. Electrolytes may also serve as catalysts in many enzymatic reactions.

Contraindications: Contraindicated in situations in which replacement would cause excess or when risk factors for retention are present.

Precautions: Use cautiously in disease states in which electrolyte imbalances are common, such as hepatic or renal disease, adrenal disorders, pituitary disorders, and diabetes mellitus.

Interactions: Depend on individual agents. Akalinizers and acidifiers can alter excretion of drugs whose renal elimination is pH-dependent. See specific entries.

NURSING IMPLICATIONS

Assessment

- Observe patient carefully for evidence of electrolyte excess or insufficiency. Monitor lab values before and periodically throughout therapy.

Potential Nursing Diagnoses

- Nutrition, altered, less than body requirements (Indications).
- Knowledge deficit, related to medication and dietary regimens (Patient/Family Teaching).

Implementation

- **Potassium chloride:** Do not administer parenteral potassium chloride undiluted.

Patient/Family Teaching

- Review diet modifications with patients with chronic electrolyte disturbances.

Evaluation

Effectiveness of therapy can be demonstrated by: ▪ Return to normal serum electrolyte concentrations and resolution of clinical symptoms of electrolyte imbalance ▪ Changes in pH or composition of urine, which prevent formation of renal calculi.

Electrolytes/Electrolyte Modifiers Included in *Davis's Drug Guide for Nurses*:

phosphates
monobasic potassium and sodium phosphates 828
potassium and sodium phosphates 828
potassium phosphate 830

potassium exchange resin
sodium polystyrene sulfonate 926

potassium salts
potassium acetate 832
potassium bicarbonate/potassium chloride 832
potassium bicarbonate/potassium citrate 832
potassium chloride 832
potassium chloride/potassium bicarbonate/potassium citrate 832
potassium gluconate 832
potassium gluconate/potassium chloride 832
potassium gluconate/potassium citrate 832
trikates 832

replacement solution
sodium chloride 921

urinary acidifiers
monobasic potassium and sodium phosphates 828
potassium and sodium phosphates 828

urinary alkalinizer
sodium citrate and citric acid 923

■ GLUCOCORTICOIDS

PHARMACOLOGIC PROFILE

General Use: Used in replacement doses (20 mg of hydrocortisone or equivalent) to treat adrenocortical insufficiency. Larger doses are usually used for their anti-inflammatory, immunosuppressive, or antineoplastic activity. Used adjunctively in many other situations including hypercalcemia and autoimmune diseases. Topical glucocorticoids are used in a variety of inflammatory and allergic conditions. Inhalant glucocorticoids are used in the chronic management of reversible airway disease (asthma); intranasal and ophthalmic glucocorticoids are used in the management of chronic allergic/inflammatory conditions.

General Action and Information: Produce profound and varied metabolic effects in addition to modifying the normal immune response and suppressing inflammation. Available in a variety of dosage forms including oral, injectable, topical, and inhalation. Prolonged use of large amounts of topical or inhaled agents may result in systemic absorption and/or adrenal suppression.

Contraindications: Serious infections (except for certain forms of meningitis). Do not administer live vaccines to patients on larger doses.

Precautions: Chronic treatment will result in adrenal suppression. Do not discontinue abruptly. Additional doses may be needed during stress (surgery and infection). Safety in pregnancy and lactation not established. Chronic use in children will result in decreased growth. May mask signs of infection. Use lowest dose possible for shortest time possible. Alternate-day therapy is preferable during chronic treatment.

Interactions: Additive hypokalemia with amphotericin B, potassium-losing diuretics, mezlocillin, piperacillin, and ticarcillin. Hypokalemia may increase the risk of cardiac glycoside toxicity. May increase requirements for insulin or oral hypoglycemic agents. Phenytoin, phenobarbital, and rifampin stimulate metabolism and may decrease effectiveness. Oral contraceptives may block metabolism. Cholestyramine and colestipol may decrease absorption.

NURSING IMPLICATIONS

Assessment

- These drugs are indicated for many conditions. Assess involved systems before and periodically throughout course of therapy.

- Assess patient for signs of adrenal insufficiency (hypotension, weight loss, weakness, nausea, vomiting, anorexia, lethargy, confusion, restlessness) prior to and periodically throughout course of therapy.
- Children should have periodic evaluations of growth.

Potential Nursing Diagnoses

- Infection, risk for (Side Effects).
- Knowledge deficit, related to medication regimen (Patient/Family Teaching).
- Body image disturbance (Side Effects).

Implementation

- **General Info:** If dose is ordered daily or every other day, administer in the morning to coincide with the body's normal secretion of cortisol.
- **PO:** Administer with meals to minimize gastric irritation.

Patient/Family Teaching

- Emphasize need to take medication exactly as directed. Review symptoms of adrenal insufficiency that may occur when stopping the medication and that may be life-threatening.
- Encourage patients on long-term therapy to eat a diet high in protein, calcium, and potassium and low in sodium and carbohydrates.
- These drugs cause immunosuppression and may mask symptoms of infection. Instruct patient to avoid people with known contagious illnesses and to report possible infections. Advise patient to consult health care professional before receiving any vaccinations.
- Discuss possible effects on body image. Explore coping mechanisms.
- Advise patient to carry identification in the event of an emergency in which patient cannot relate medical history.

Evaluation

Effectiveness of therapy can be demonstrated by: ▪ Suppression of the inflammatory and immune responses in autoimmune disorders, allergic reactions, and organ transplants ▪ Replacement therapy in adrenal insufficiency ▪ Resolution of skin inflammation, pruritus, or other dermatologic conditions.

Glucocorticoids Included in *Davis's Drug Guide for Nurses*:

systemic glucocorticoids (short-acting)

systemic glucocorticoids (intermediate-acting)

systemic glucocorticoids (long-acting)

topical glucocorticoids

CLASSIFICATIONS

inhalant/intranasal glucocorticoids
beclomethasone 430, 433
budesonide 430, 433
flunisolide 430, 433
fluticasone 430, 433
triamcinolone 430, 433

ophthalmic glucocorticoids
dexamethasone 1120
fluorometholone 1120
prednisolone 1120
rimexolone 1120

▪ HORMONES

PHARMACOLOGIC PROFILE

General Use: Used in the treatment of deficiency states including diabetes (insulin), diabetes insipidus (desmopressin), hypothyroidism (thyroid hormone), and menopause (estrogens). Combinations of hormones (estrogens and progestins) are used as oral contraceptive agents. Hormones may be used for treatment of hormonally sensitive tumors (androgens and estrogens) and in other selected situations. Estrogens are commonly used to replace hormones in menopausal women as part of hormone replacment therapy (HRT) to minimize vasomotor symptoms and prevent osteoporosis. See individual drugs.

General Action and Information: Natural or synthetic substances that have a specific effect on target tissue. Differ greatly in their effects, depending on individual agent and function of target tissue.

Contraindications: Differ greatly among agents. See individual entries.

Precautions: Use cautiously in patients with severe cardiac, hepatic, or renal disease. When used in deficiency states, appropriate laboratory monitoring is necessary to adjust dosages and monitor progress.

Interactions: Differ greatly among agents. See individual entries.

NURSING IMPLICATIONS

Assessment

- **General Info:** Monitor patient for symptoms of hormonal excess or insufficiency.
- **Sex Hormones:** Blood pressure and hepatic function tests should be monitored periodically throughout therapy.
- **Epoetin:** Monitor blood pressure, hematocrit, hemoglobin, reticulocyte count, and RBC, as well as symptoms of anemia, throughout therapy. Uncontrolled hypertension is contraindicated.

Potential Nursing Diagnoses

- Sexual dysfunction (Indications).
- Body image disturbance (Indications, Side Effects).
- Knowledge deficit, related to medication regimen (Patient/Family Teaching).

Implementation

- **Sex Hormones:** Continue to administer according to schedule prior to hospitalization.

Patient/Family Teaching

- **General Info:** Explain dosage schedule (and withdrawal bleeding with female sex hormones).
- Emphasize importance of follow-up examinations to monitor effectiveness of therapy and to ensure proper development of children and early detection of possible side effects.

- **Female Sex Hormones:** Advise patient to report signs and symptoms of fluid retention, thromboembolic disorders, mental depression, or hepatic dysfunction to health care professional.

Evaluation

Effectiveness of therapy can be demonstrated by: ▪ Resolution of clinical symptoms of hormone imbalance including menopausal symptoms and effective contraception ▪ Correction of fluid and electrolyte imbalances ▪ Control of the spread of advanced metastatic breast or prostate cancer ▪ Slowed progression of postmenopausal osteoporosis ▪ Increase in hematocrit (epoetin) ▪ Induction of ovulation in women with primary hypothalamic amenorrhea (gonadorelin) ▪ Resolution of the signs of precocious puberty (histrelin, nafarelin).

Hormones Included in *Davis's Drug Guide for Nurses*:

contraceptives, hormonal
monophasic oral contraceptives 225
biphasic oral contraceptives 225
triphasic oral contraceptives 225
progestin-only oral contraceptives 225
contraceptive implant 225
injectable contraceptive 225

adrenocorticotropic hormones
corticotropin 1133
cosyntropin 1133

androgenic hormones
danazol 243
testosterone 958

antidiuretic hormones
desmopressin 252
vasopressin 1144

estrogenic hormones
dienestrol 1134
diethylstilbestrol 272
estrogens, conjugated 348
estropipate 351

gastrointestinal hormone
octreotide 740

gonadotropin-releasing hormones
goserelin 453
histrelin 1137
nafarelin 694

gonadotropins
gonadotropin, chorionic 1137
menotropins 1138

growth hormones
somatrem 458
somatropin 458

ovulation inducer
clomiphene 208

oxytocic hormone
oxytocin 758

progestins
medroxyprogesterone 611
progesterone 1140, 1141

thyroid hormones
levothyroxine 975
liothyronine 975
liotrix 975
thyroid 975

miscellaneous
calcitonin 142
epoetin 332
glucagon 428
insulins 521

▪ IMMUNOSUPPRESSANTS

PHARMACOLOGIC PROFILE

General Use: Azathioprine, cyclosporine, daclizumab, mycophenolate, and tacrolimus are used with glucocorticoids in the prevention of transplantation rejection reactions. Muromonab-CD3 is used to manage rejection reactions not controlled by other agents. Azathioprine, cyclophosphamide, and methotrexate are used in the management of selected autoimmune diseases (nephrotic syndrome of childhood and severe rheumatoid arthritis).

General Action and Information: Inhibit cell-mediated immune responses by different mechanisms. In addition to azathioprine and cyclosporine, which are used primarily for their immunomodulating properties, cyclophosphamide and methotrexate are used to suppress the immune responses in certain disease states (nephrotic syndrome of childhood and severe rheumatoid arthritis). Muromonab-CD3 is a recombinant immunoglobulin antibody that alters T-cell function. Daclizumab is a monoclonal antibody.

Contraindications: Hypersensitivity to drug or vehicle.

Precautions: Use cautiously in patients with infections. Safety in pregnancy and lactation not established.

Interactions: Allopurinol inhibits the metabolism of azathioprine. Drugs that alter liver metabolizing processes may change the effect of cyclosporine. The risk of toxicity of methotrexate may be increased by other nephrotoxic drugs, large doses of aspirin, or NSAIDs. Muromonab-CD3 has additive immunosuppressive properties; concurrent immunosuppressive doses should be decreased or eliminated.

NURSING IMPLICATIONS

Assessment

- **General Info:** Monitor for infection (vital signs, sputum, urine, stool, WBC). Notify physician or other health care professional immediately if symptoms occur.
- **Organ Transplant:** Assess for symptoms of organ rejection throughout therapy.
- **Lab Test Considerations:** Monitor CBC and differential throughout therapy.

Potential Nursing Diagnoses

- Infection, risk for (Side Effects).
- Knowledge deficit, related to medication regimen (Patient/Family Teaching).

Implementation

- Protect transplant patients from staff and visitors who may carry infection.
- Maintain protective isolation as indicated.

Patient/Family Teaching

- Reinforce the need for lifelong therapy to prevent transplant rejection. Review symptoms of rejection for transplanted organ and stress need to notify health care professional immediately if they occur.
- Advise patient to avoid contact with contagious persons and those who have recently taken oral poliovirus vaccine. Patients should not receive vaccinations without first consulting with health care professional.
- Emphasize the importance of follow-up exams and lab tests.

Evaluation

Effectiveness of therapy can be demonstrated by: ▪ Prevention or reversal of rejection of organ transplants or decrease in symptoms of autoimmune disorders.

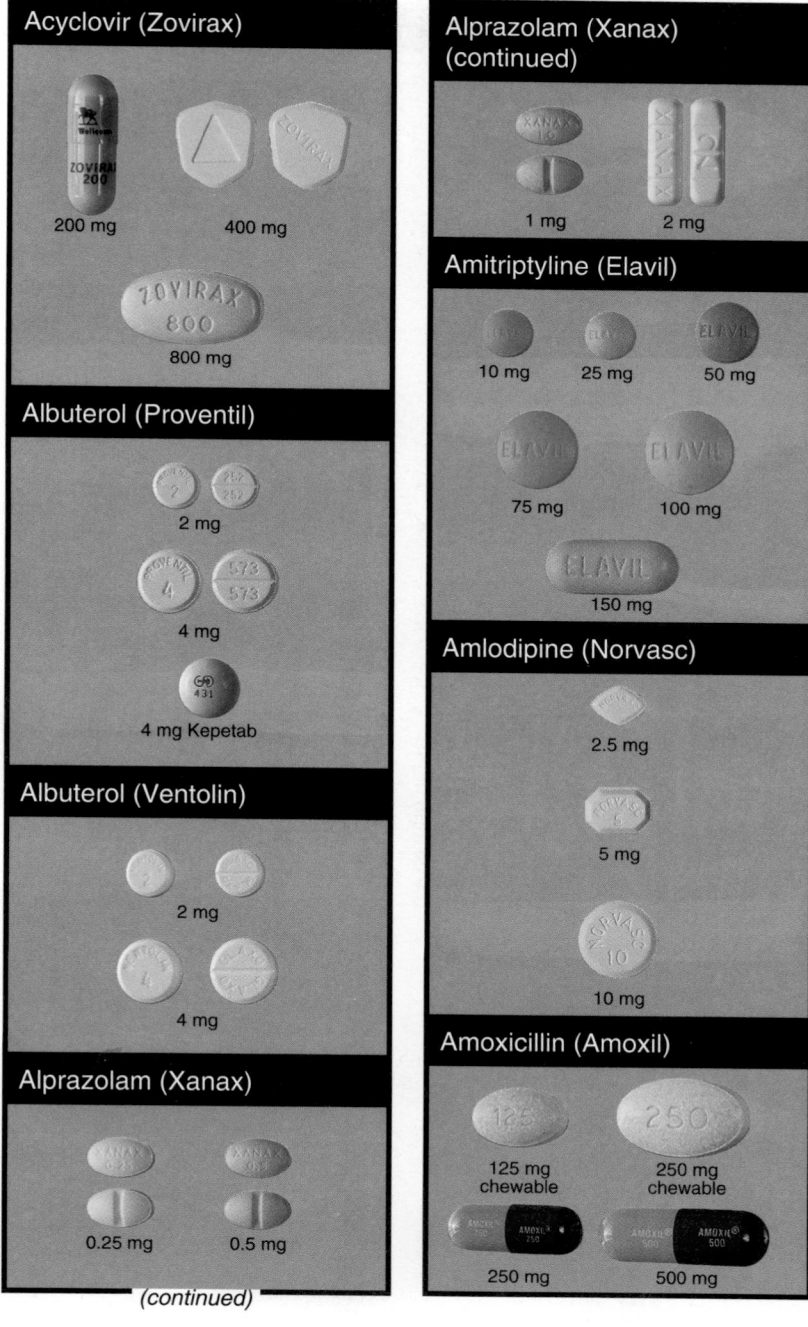

Acyclovir (Zovirax)

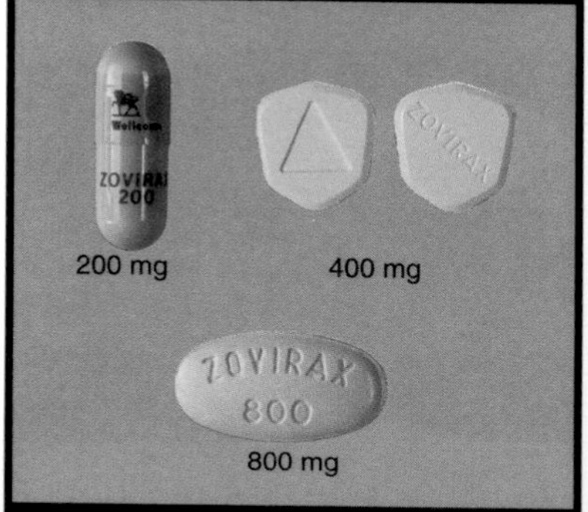

200 mg 400 mg

800 mg

Albuterol (Proventil)

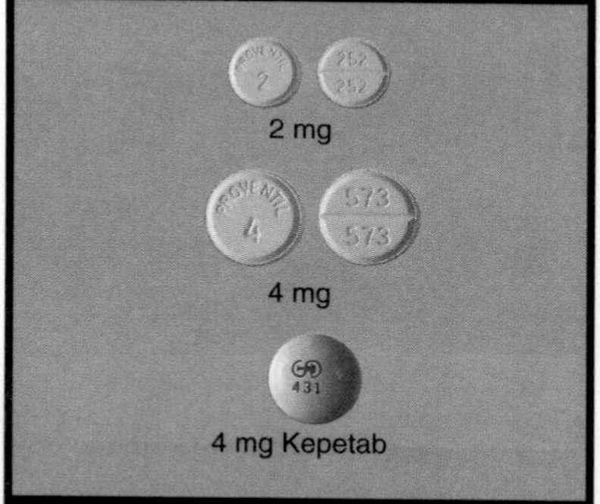

2 mg

4 mg

4 mg Kepetab

Albuterol (Ventolin)

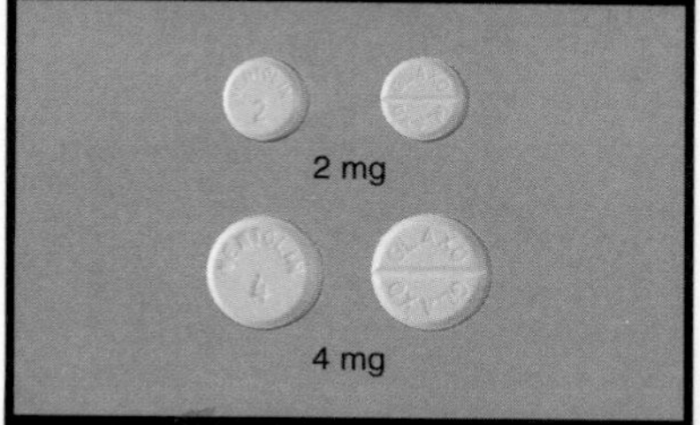

2 mg

4 mg

Alprazolam (Xanax)

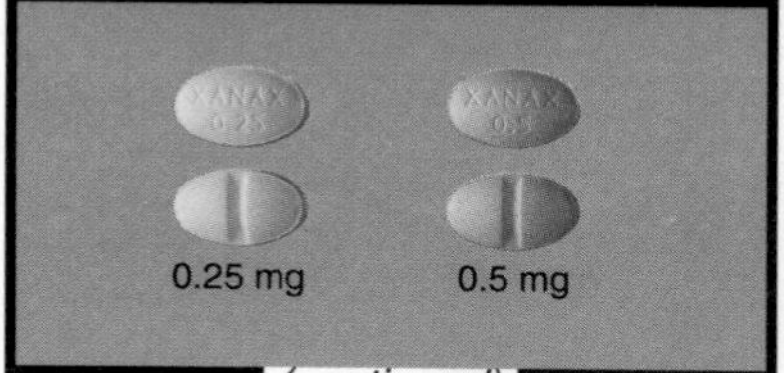

0.25 mg 0.5 mg

(continued)

Alprazolam (Xanax) (continued)

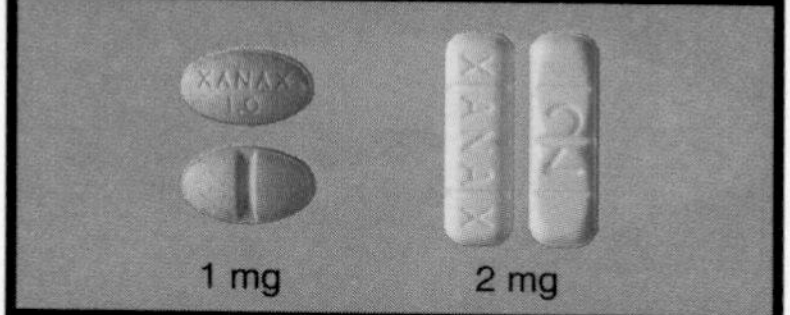

1 mg 2 mg

Amitriptyline (Elavil)

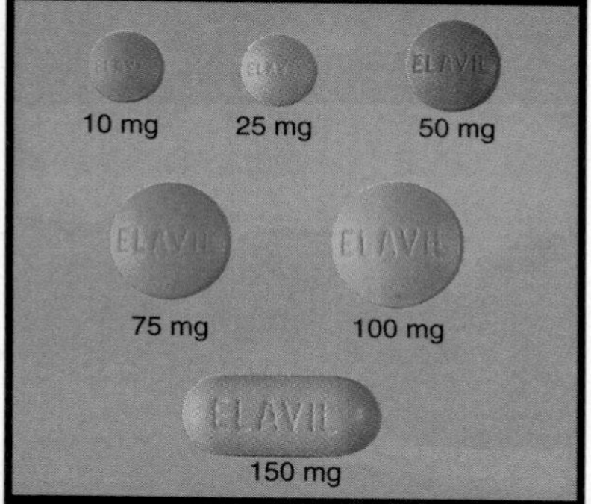

10 mg 25 mg 50 mg

75 mg 100 mg

150 mg

Amlodipine (Norvasc)

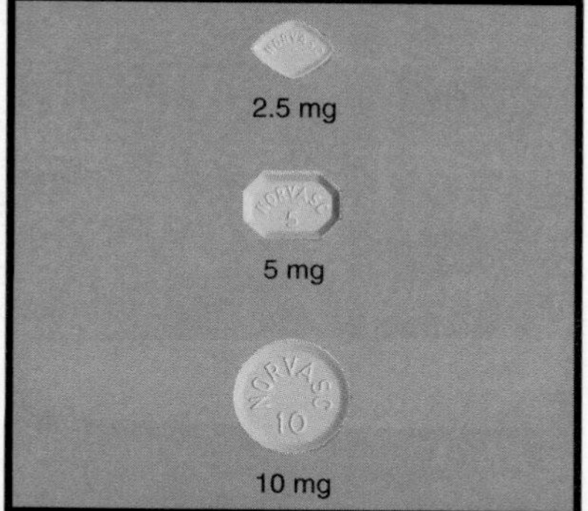

2.5 mg

5 mg

10 mg

Amoxicillin (Amoxil)

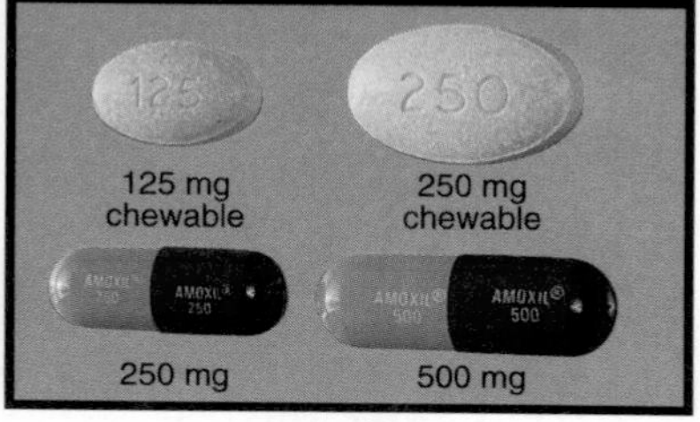

125 mg chewable 250 mg chewable

250 mg 500 mg

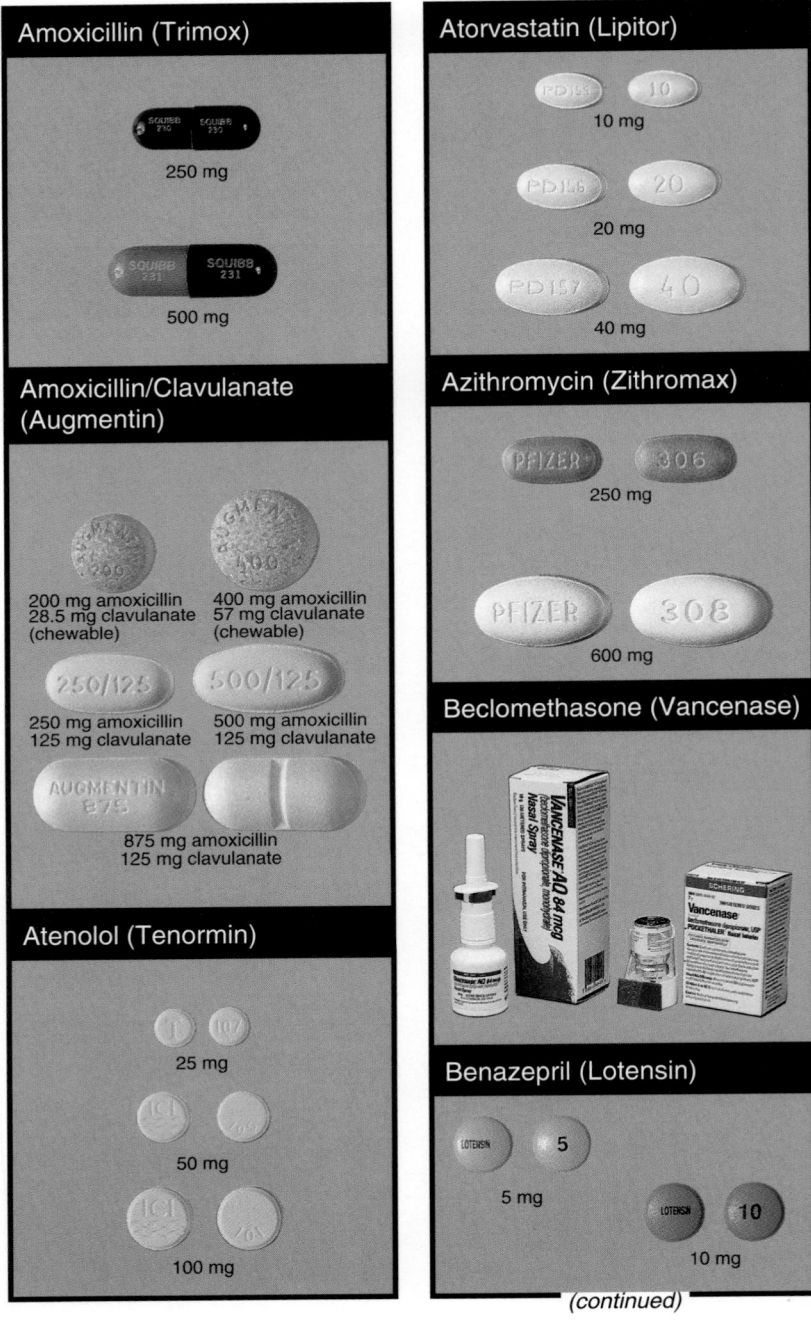

Amoxicillin (Trimox)

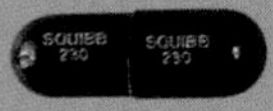

250 mg

500 mg

Amoxicillin/Clavulanate (Augmentin)

200 mg amoxicillin
28.5 mg clavulanate
(chewable)

400 mg amoxicillin
57 mg clavulanate
(chewable)

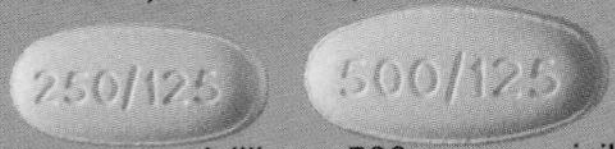

250 mg amoxicillin
125 mg clavulanate

500 mg amoxicillin
125 mg clavulanate

875 mg amoxicillin
125 mg clavulanate

Atenolol (Tenormin)

25 mg

50 mg

100 mg

Atorvastatin (Lipitor)

10 mg

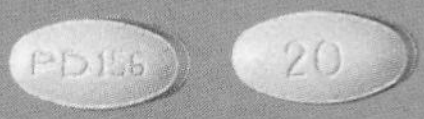

20 mg

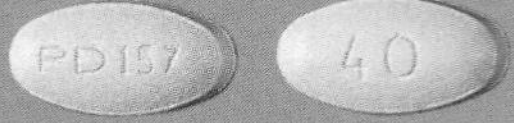

40 mg

Azithromycin (Zithromax)

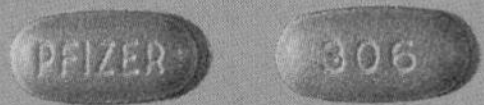

250 mg

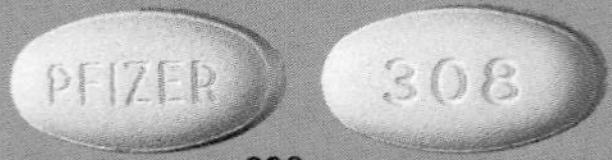

600 mg

Beclomethasone (Vancenase)

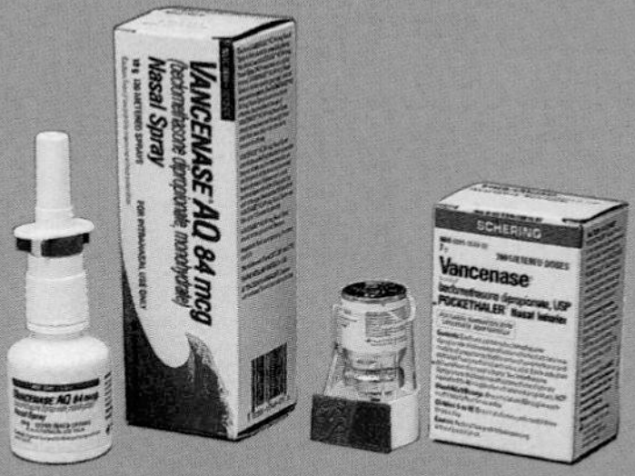

Benazepril (Lotensin)

5 mg

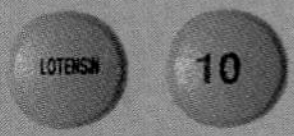

10 mg

(continued)

Benazepril (Lotensin) (continued)

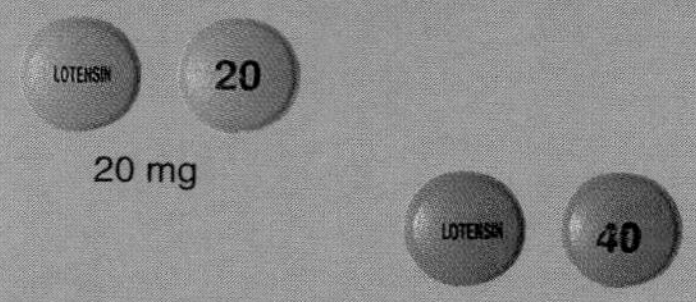

20 mg

40 mg

Buspirone (Buspar)

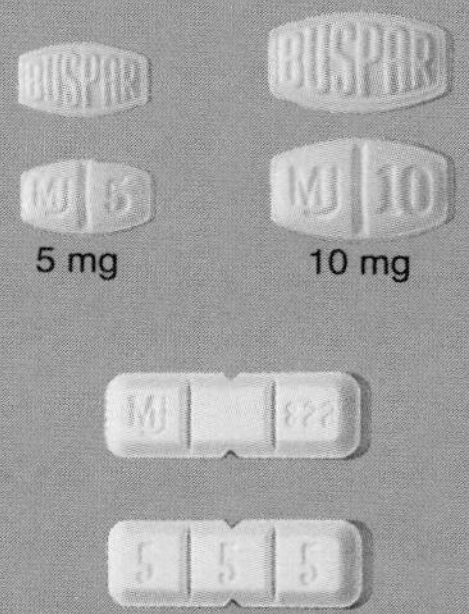

5 mg

10 mg

15 mg

Cefaclor (Ceclor)

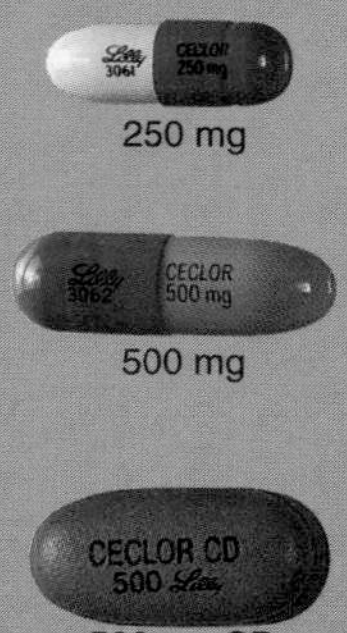

250 mg

500 mg

500 mg CD

Cefprozil (Cefzil)

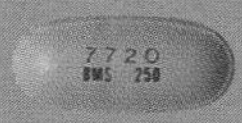

250 mg

(continued)

Cefprozil (Cefzil) (continued)

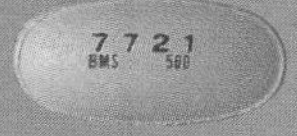

500 mg

Cefuroxime (Ceftin)

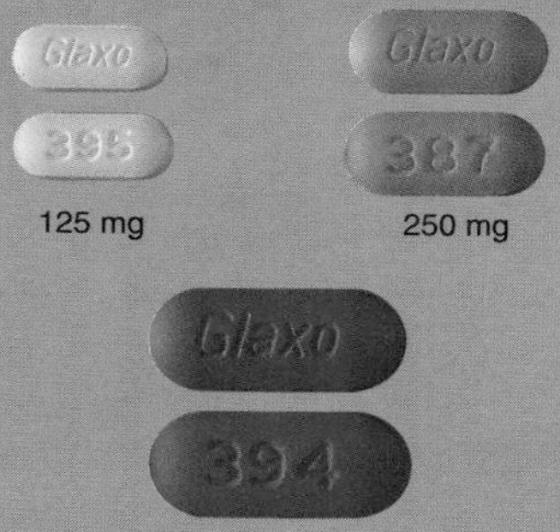

125 mg

250 mg

500 mg

Cephalexin (Keflex)

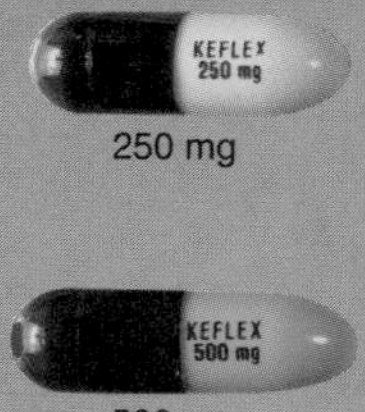

250 mg

500 mg

Cimetidine (Tagamet)

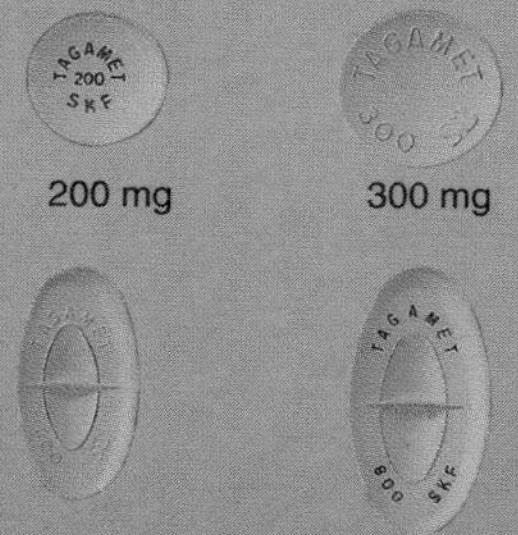

200 mg

300 mg

400 mg Tiltab

800 mg Tiltab

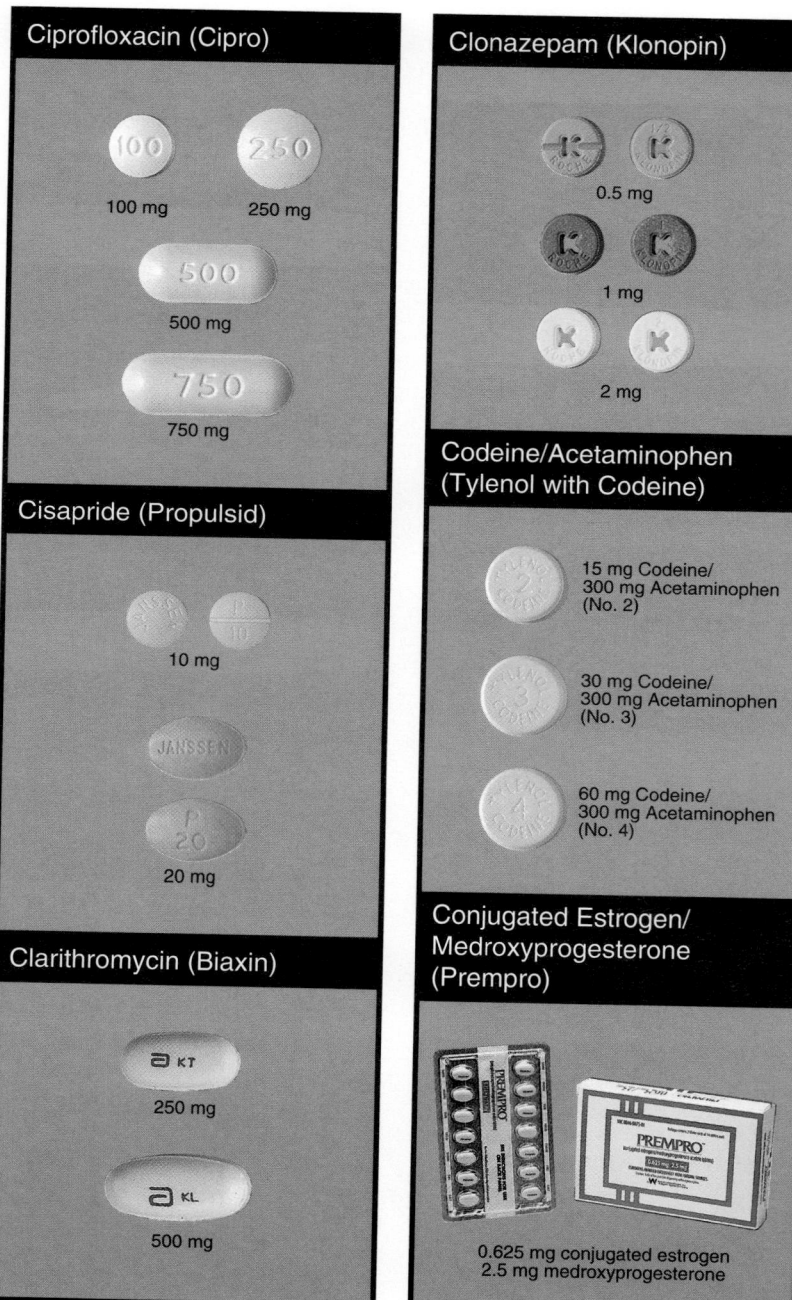

Ciprofloxacin (Cipro)

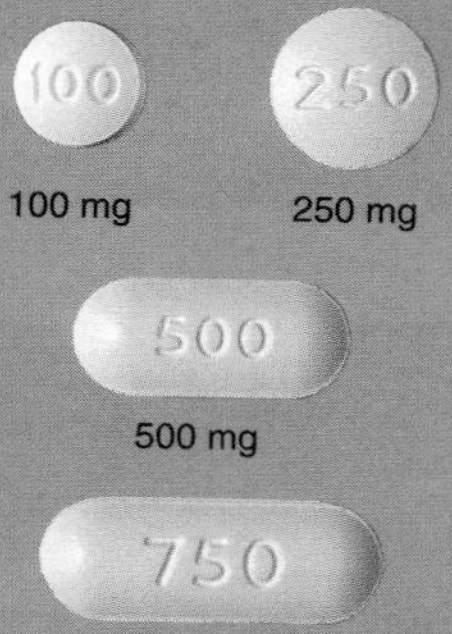

100 mg 250 mg

500 mg

750 mg

Cisapride (Propulsid)

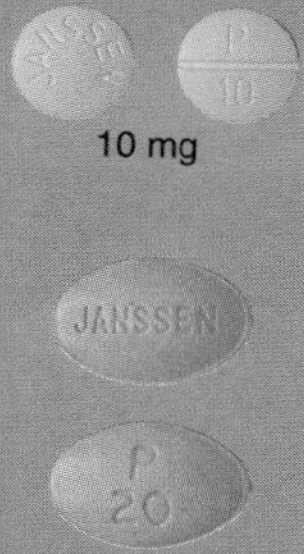

10 mg

20 mg

Clarithromycin (Biaxin)

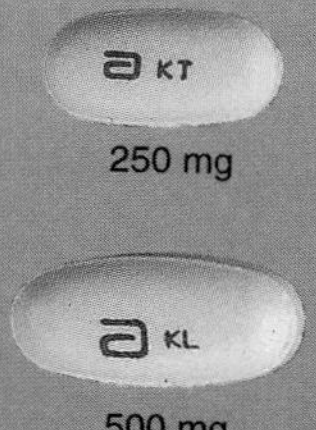

250 mg

500 mg

Clonazepam (Klonopin)

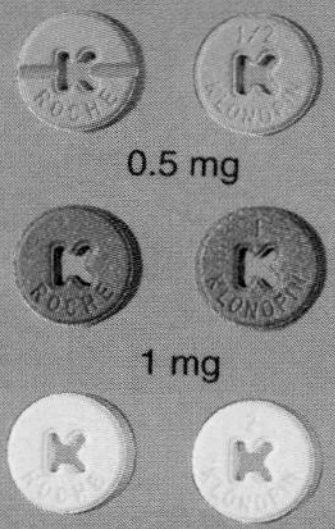

0.5 mg

1 mg

2 mg

Codeine/Acetaminophen (Tylenol with Codeine)

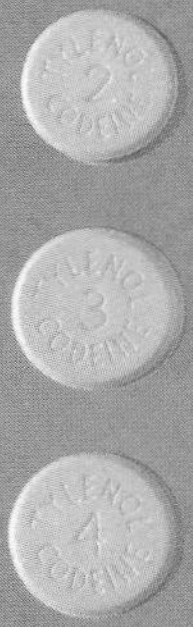

15 mg Codeine/
300 mg Acetaminophen
(No. 2)

30 mg Codeine/
300 mg Acetaminophen
(No. 3)

60 mg Codeine/
300 mg Acetaminophen
(No. 4)

Conjugated Estrogen/ Medroxyprogesterone (Prempro)

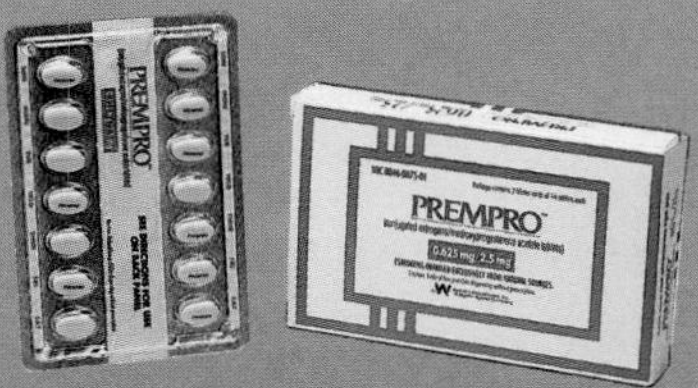

0.625 mg conjugated estrogen
2.5 mg medroxyprogesterone

Conjugated Estrogens (Premarin)

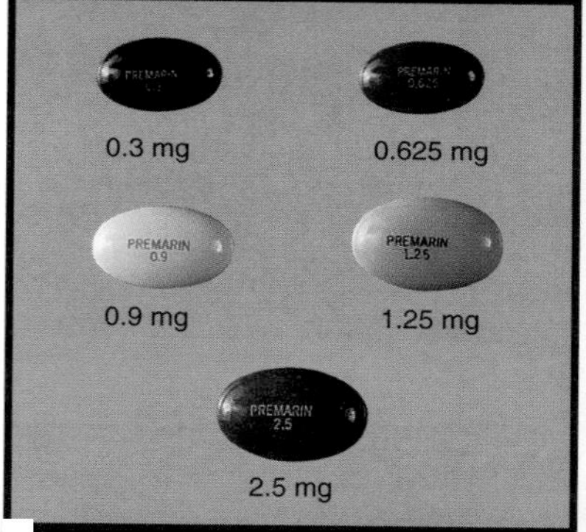

0.3 mg | 0.625 mg | 0.9 mg | 1.25 mg | 2.5 mg

Cyclobenzaprine (Flexeril)

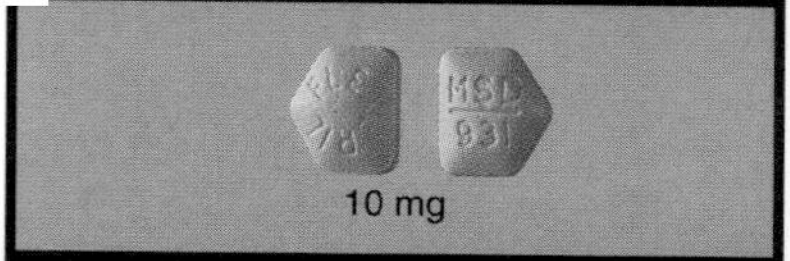

10 mg

Diazepam (Valium)

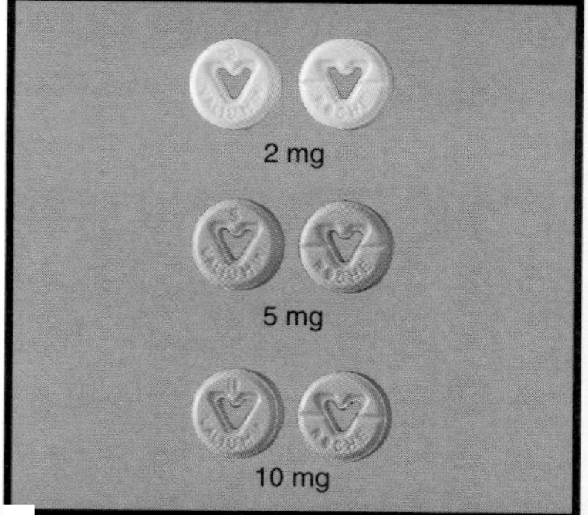

2 mg | 5 mg | 10 mg

Digoxin (Lanoxin)

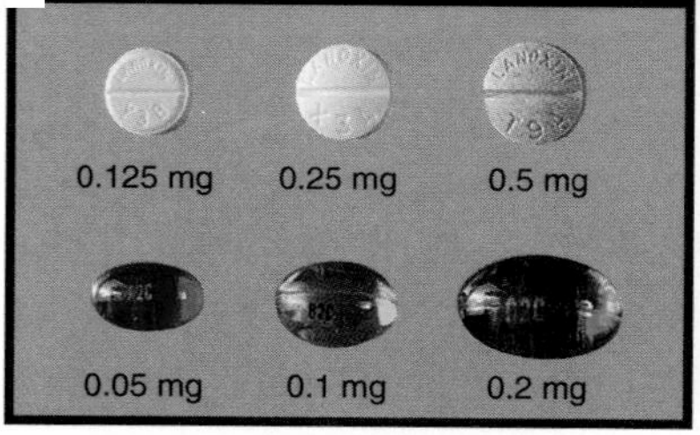

0.125 mg | 0.25 mg | 0.5 mg | 0.05 mg | 0.1 mg | 0.2 mg

Diltiazem (Cardizem)

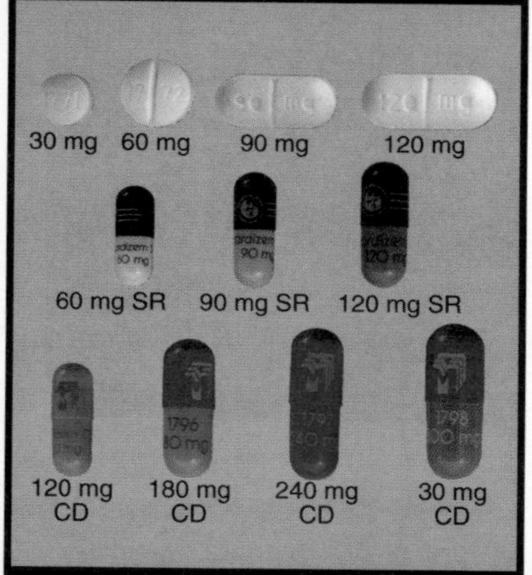

30 mg | 60 mg | 90 mg | 120 mg | 60 mg SR | 90 mg SR | 120 mg SR | 120 mg CD | 180 mg CD | 240 mg CD | 30 mg CD

Divalproex (Depakote)

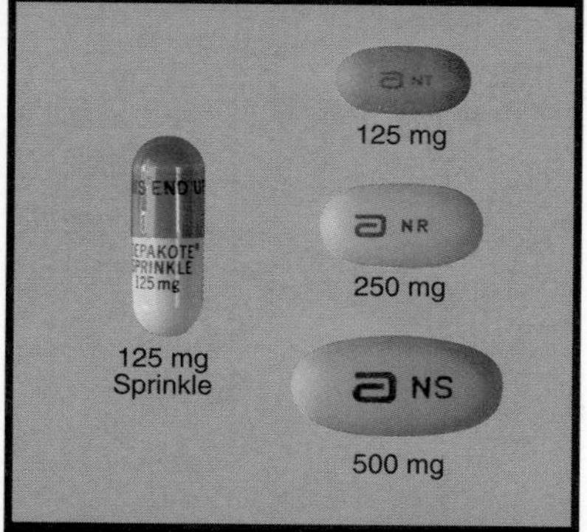

125 mg | 250 mg | 125 mg Sprinkle | 500 mg

Doxazosin (Cardura)

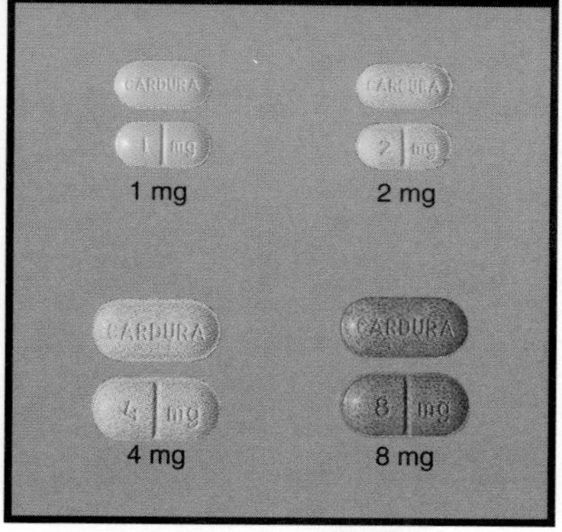

1 mg | 2 mg | 4 mg | 8 mg

Enalapril (Vasotec)

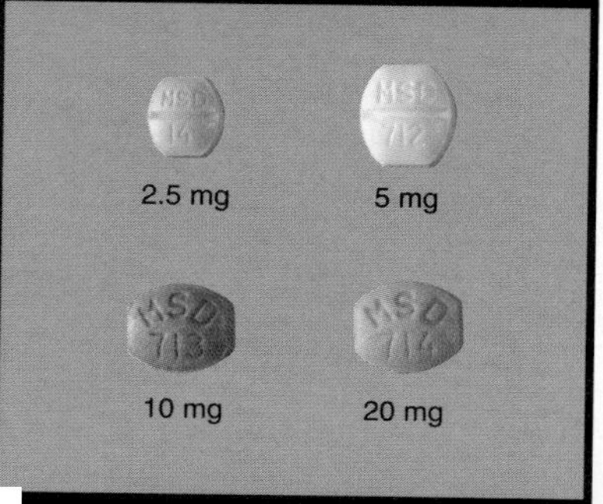

Erythromycin

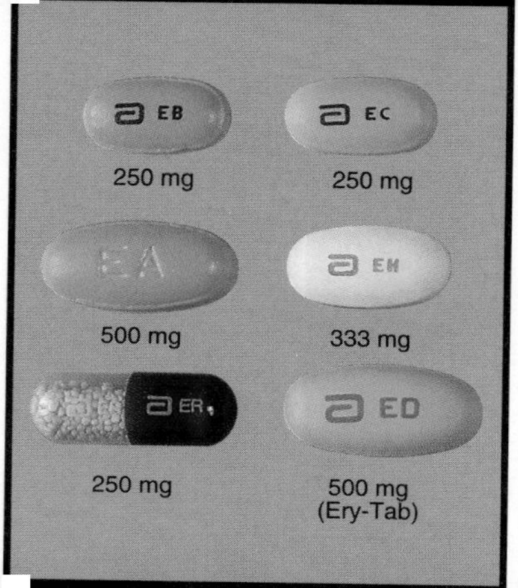

Estradiol (Estrace)

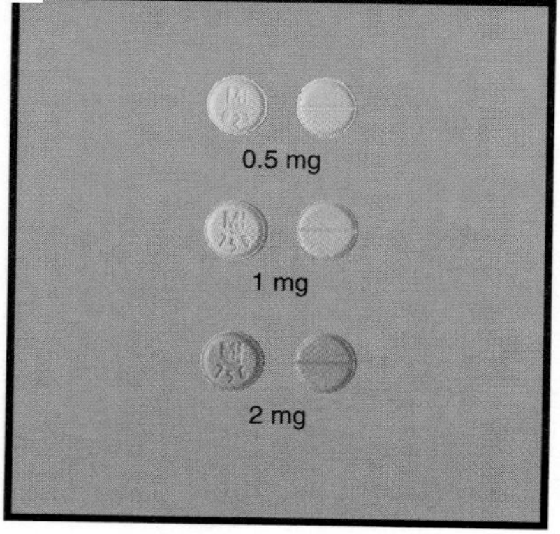

Estradiol (Estraderm)

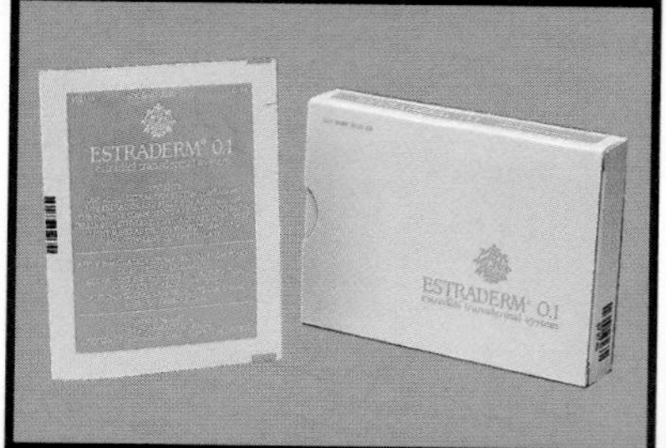

Etodolac (Lodine)

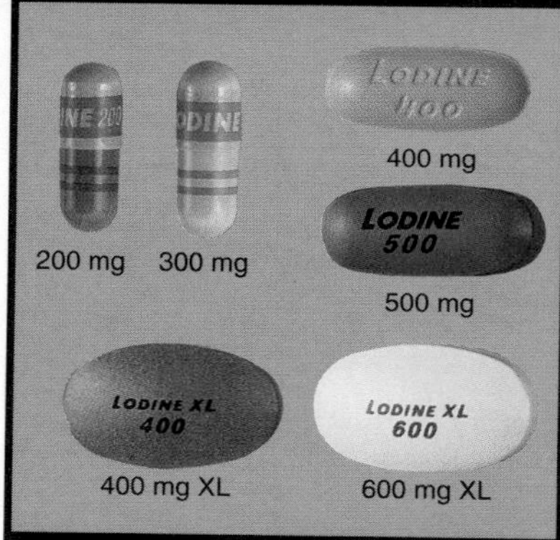

Famotidine (Pepcid)

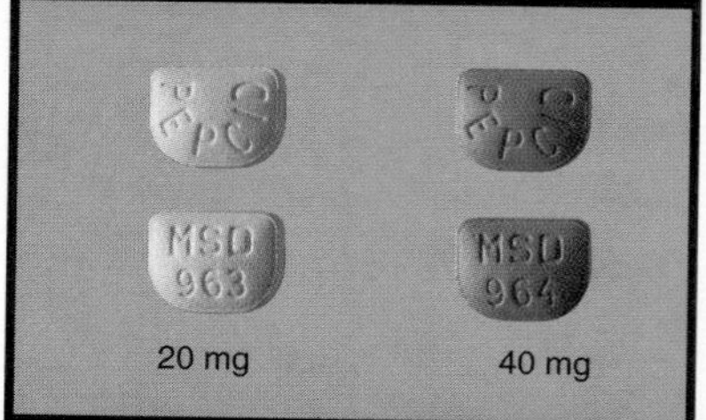

Fexofenadine (Allegra)

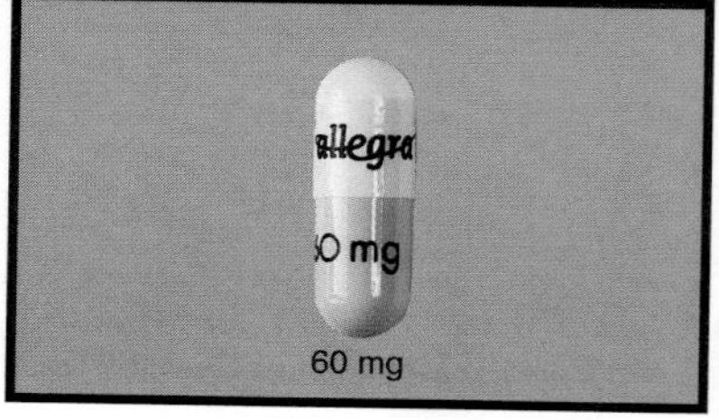

Fluconazole (Diflucan)

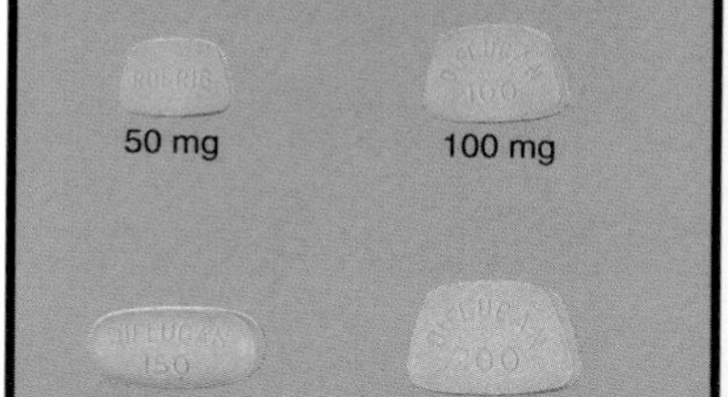

50 mg

100 mg

150 mg

200 mg

Fluoxetine (Prozac)

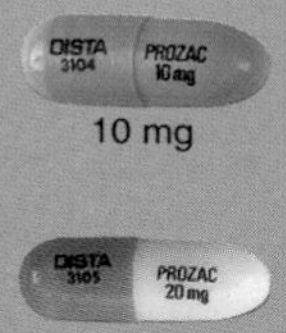

10 mg

20 mg

Fluticasone (Flonase)

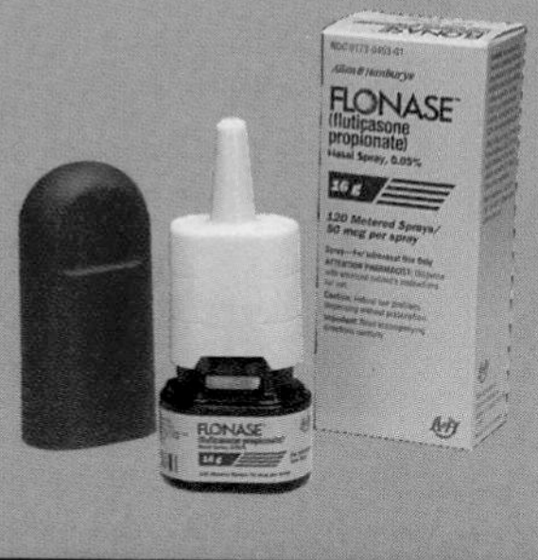

Fluvastatin (Lescol)

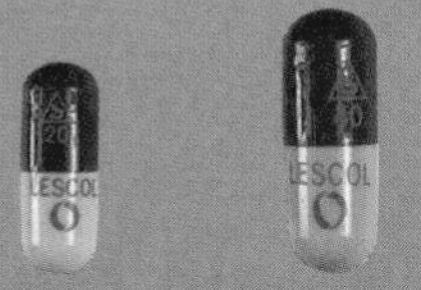

20 mg

40 mg

Furosemide (Lasix)

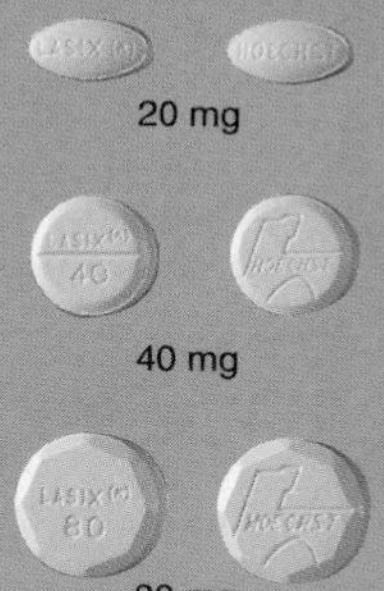

20 mg

40 mg

80 mg

Gemfibrozil (Lopid)

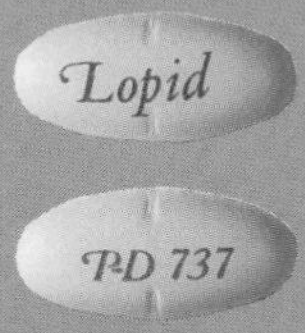

600 mg

Glipizide (Glucotrol)

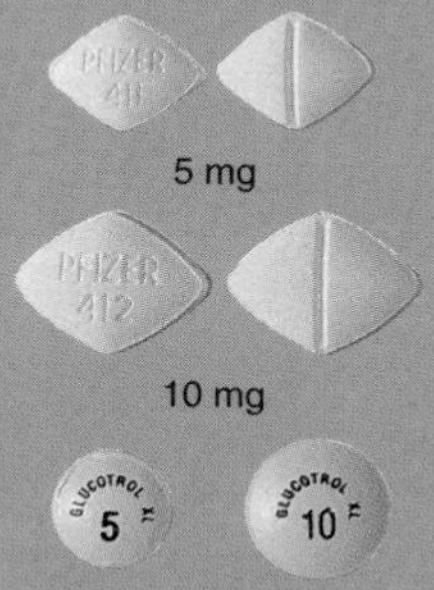

5 mg

10 mg

5 mg 10 mg
Extended Release

Glyburide (DiaBeta)

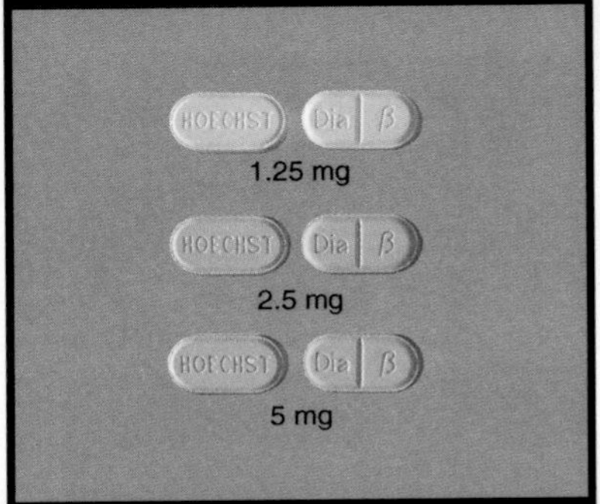

Haloperidol (Haldol)

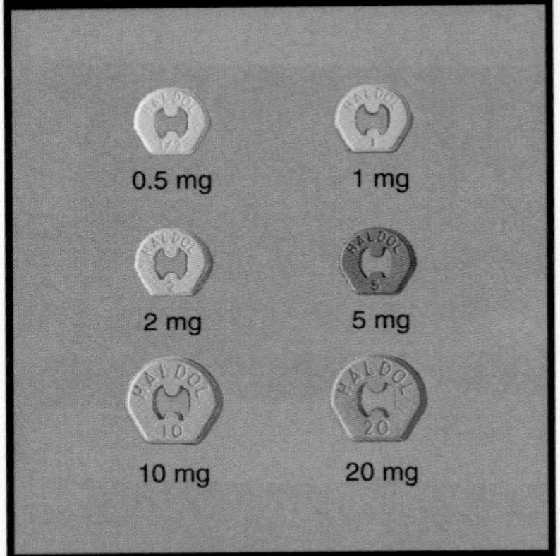

Hydrochlorothiazide (Hydrodiuril)

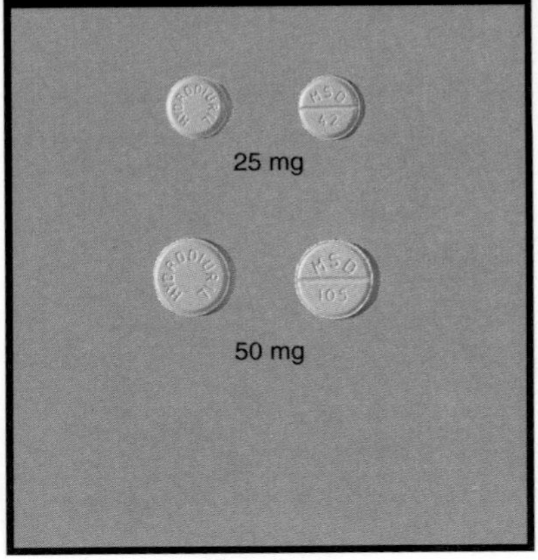

Hydrocodone/Acetaminophen (Lortab)

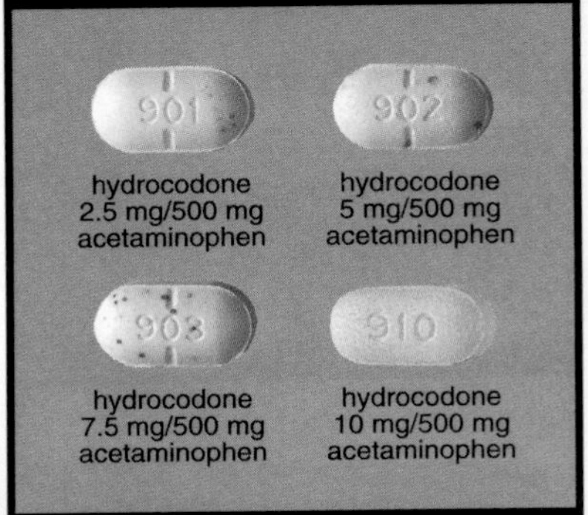

Ibuprofen (Motrin)

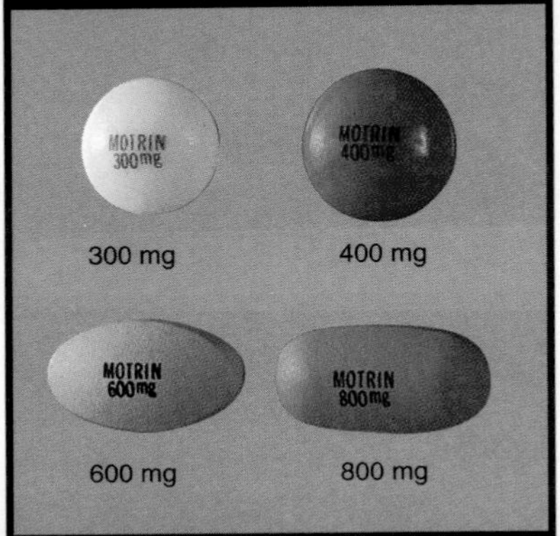

Ipratropium (Atrovent)

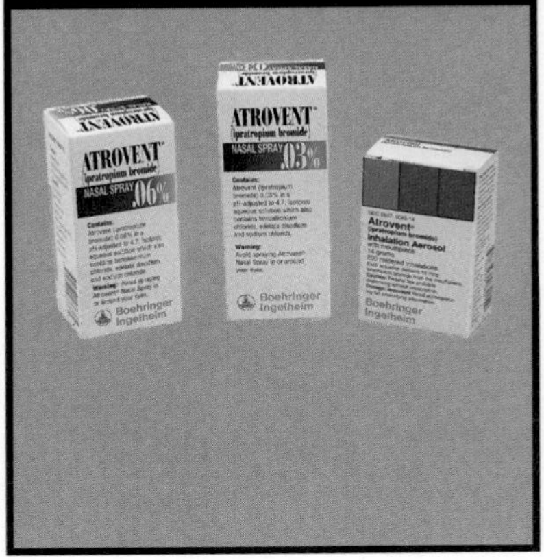

Isosorbide Mononitrate (Imdur)

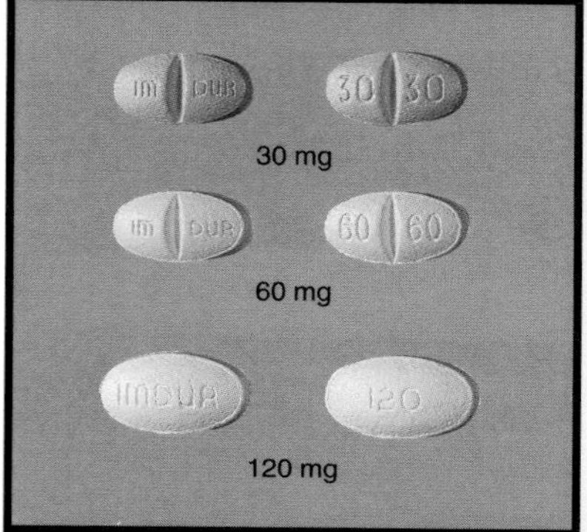

30 mg

60 mg

120 mg

Levothyroxine (Synthroid)

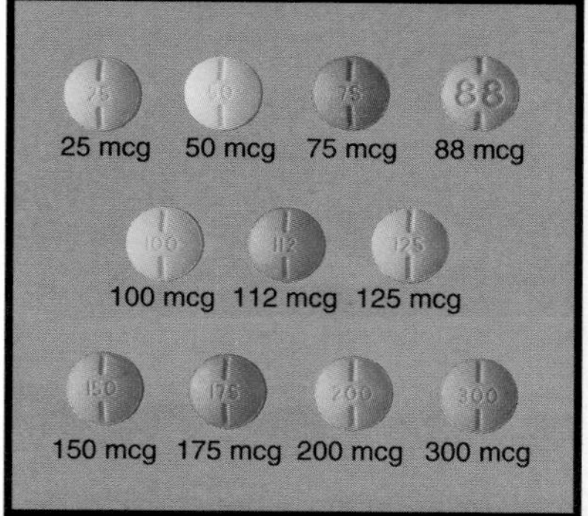

25 mcg 50 mcg 75 mcg 88 mcg

100 mcg 112 mcg 125 mcg

150 mcg 175 mcg 200 mcg 300 mcg

Lisinopril (Prinivil)

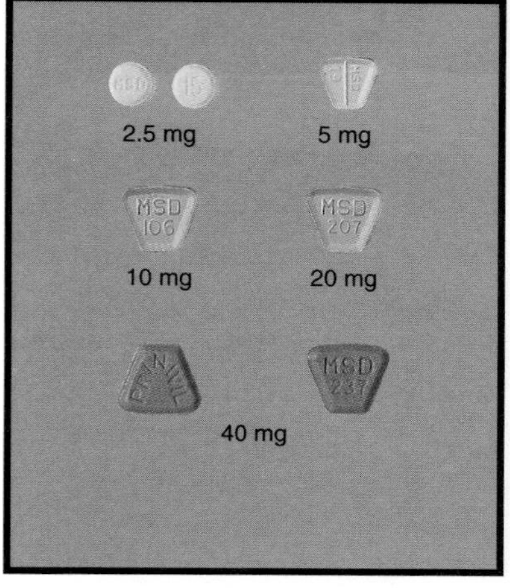

2.5 mg 5 mg

10 mg 20 mg

40 mg

Lisinopril (Zestril)

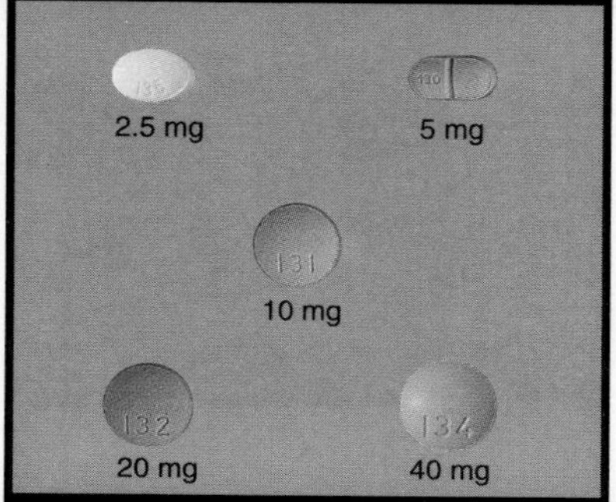

2.5 mg 5 mg

10 mg

20 mg 40 mg

Loracarbef (Lorabid)

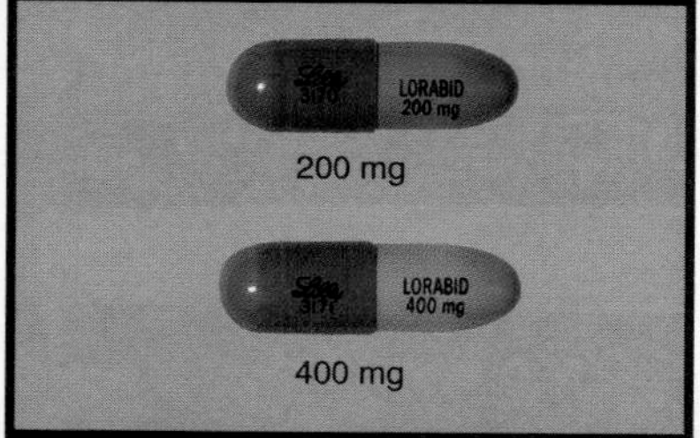

200 mg

400 mg

Loratadine (Claritin)

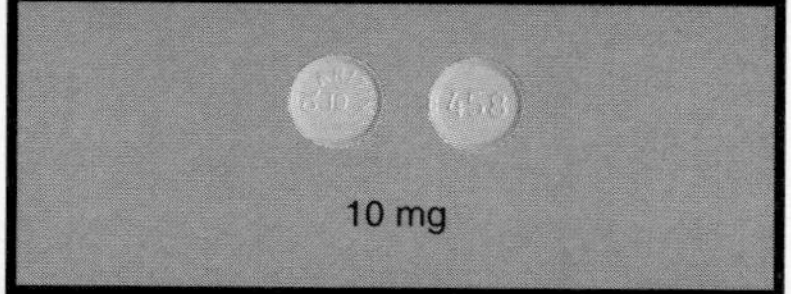

10 mg

Loratadine/Pseudoephedrine (Claritin-D)

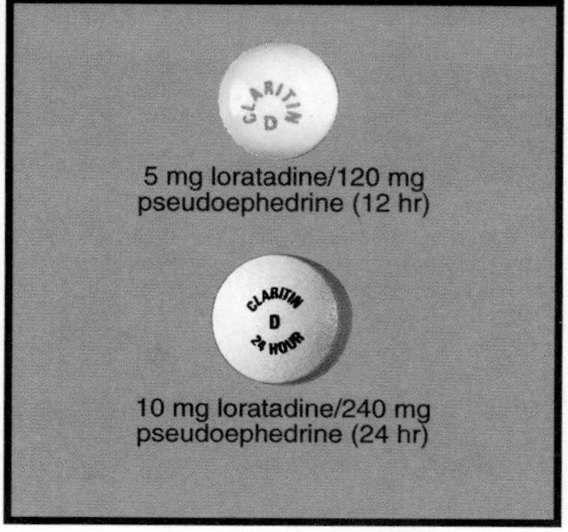

5 mg loratadine/120 mg pseudoephedrine (12 hr)

10 mg loratadine/240 mg pseudoephedrine (24 hr)

Lorazepam (Ativan)

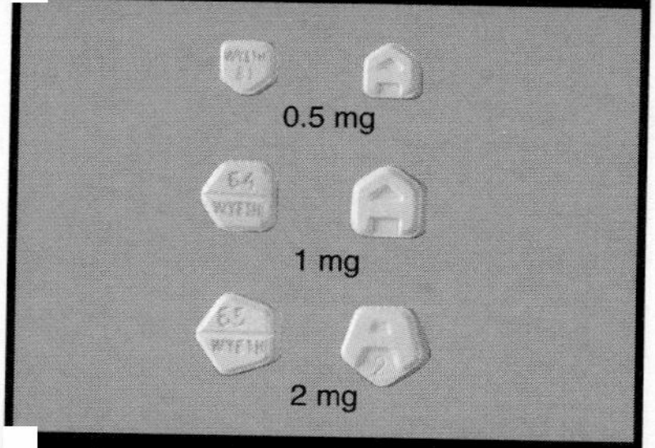

0.5 mg

1 mg

2 mg

Losartan (Cozaar)

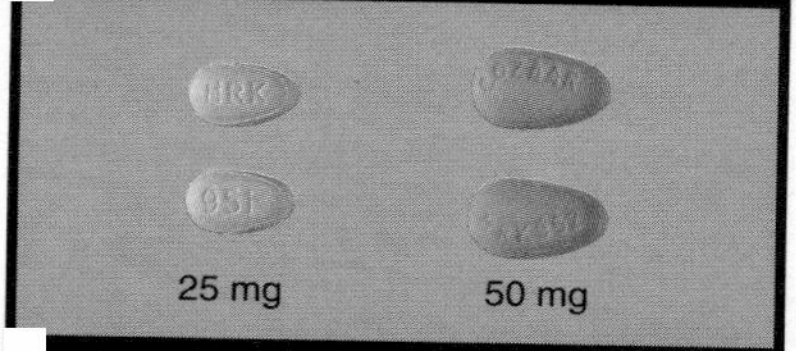

25 mg

50 mg

Lovastatin (Mevacor)

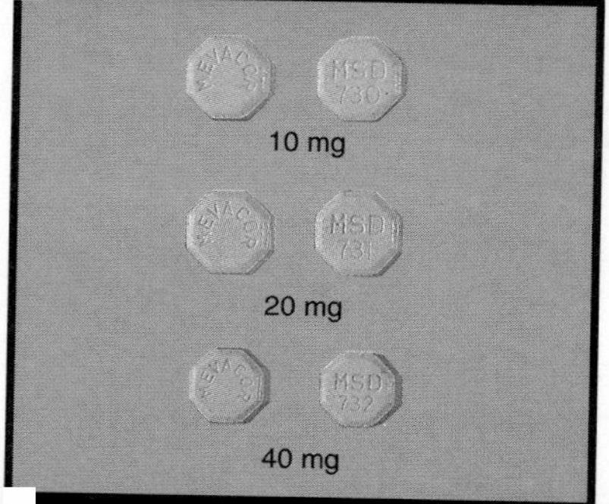

10 mg

20 mg

40 mg

Medroxyprogesterone (Cycrin)

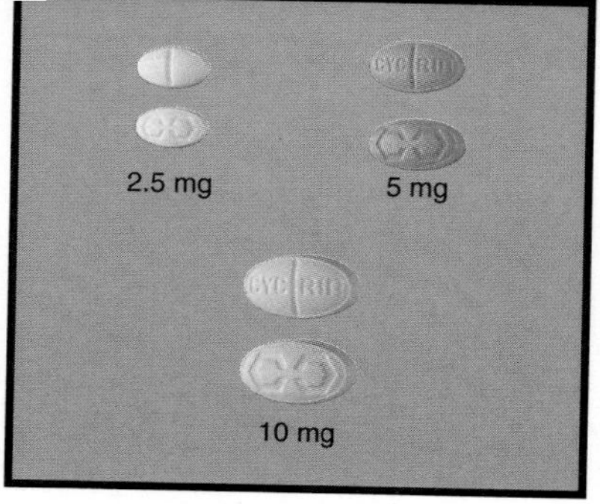

2.5 mg

5 mg

10 mg

Metformin (Glucophage)

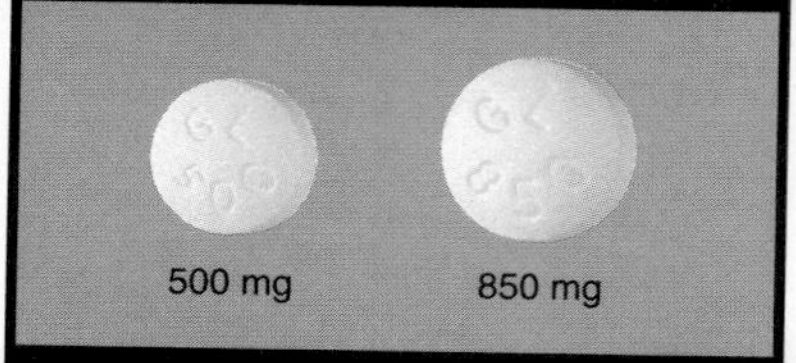

500 mg

850 mg

Methylphenidate (Ritalin)

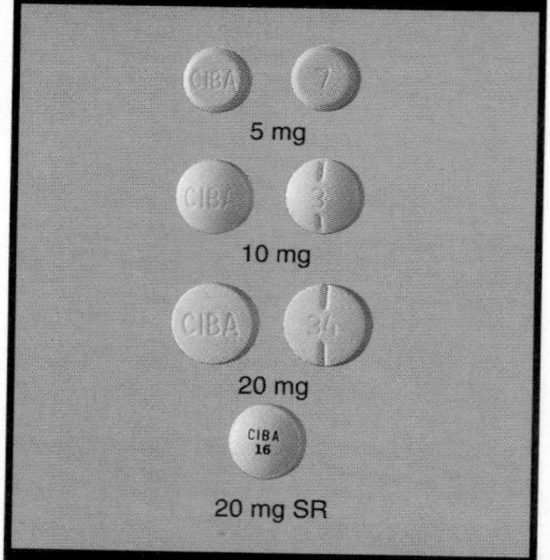

5 mg

10 mg

20 mg

20 mg SR

Metoprolol (Lopressor)

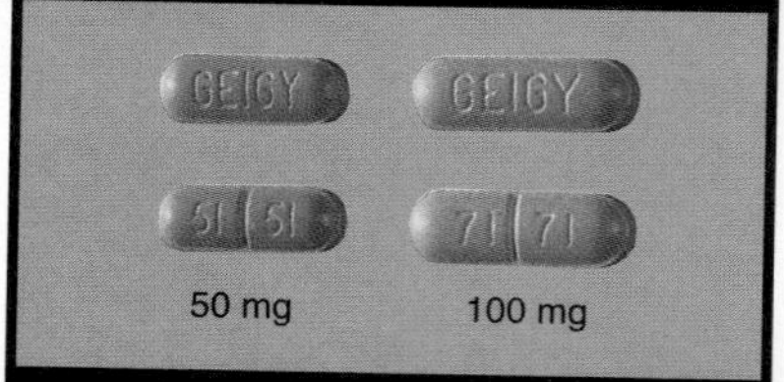

50 mg

100 mg

Metoprolol (Toprol XL)

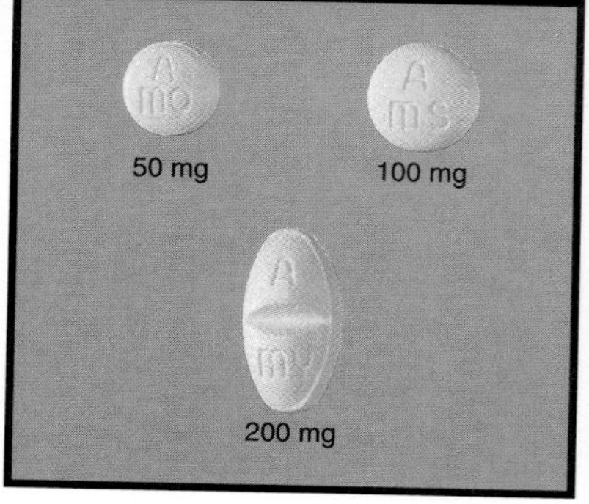

50 mg

100 mg

200 mg

Nabumetone (Relafen)

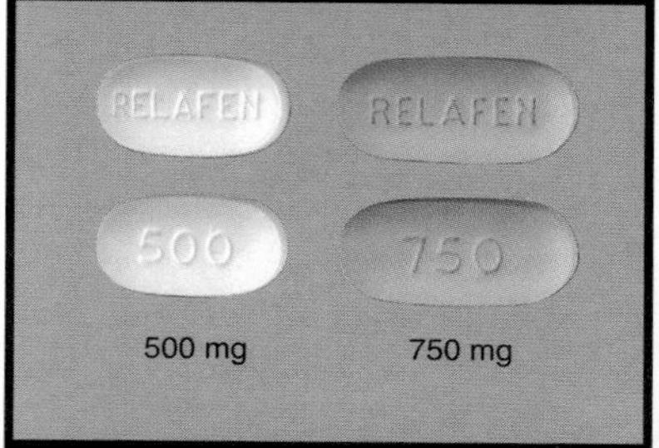

500 mg 750 mg

Naproxen (Naprosyn)

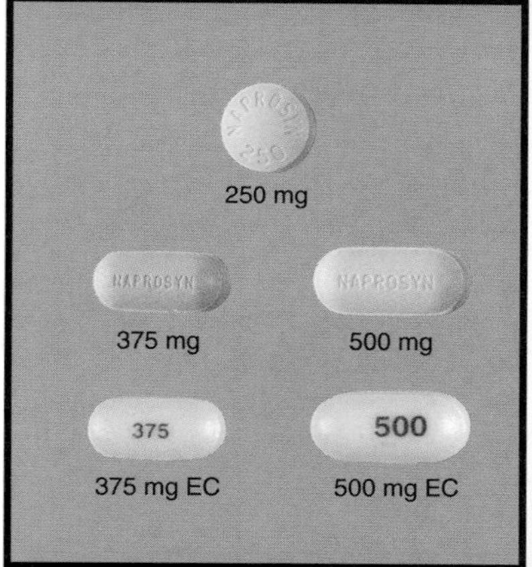

250 mg
375 mg 500 mg
375 mg EC 500 mg EC

Nifedipine (Adalat)

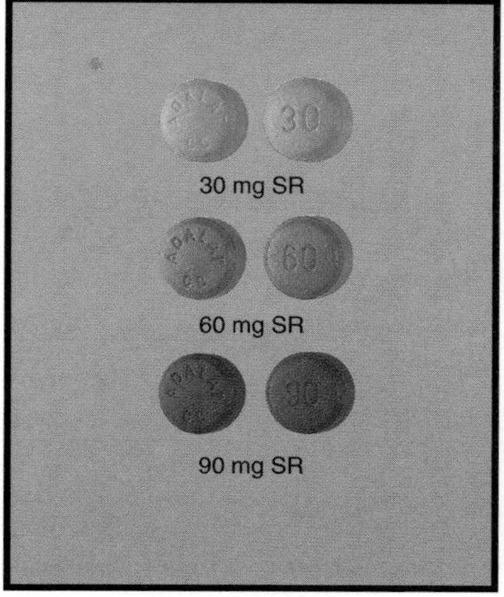

30 mg SR
60 mg SR
90 mg SR

Nifedipine (Procardia)

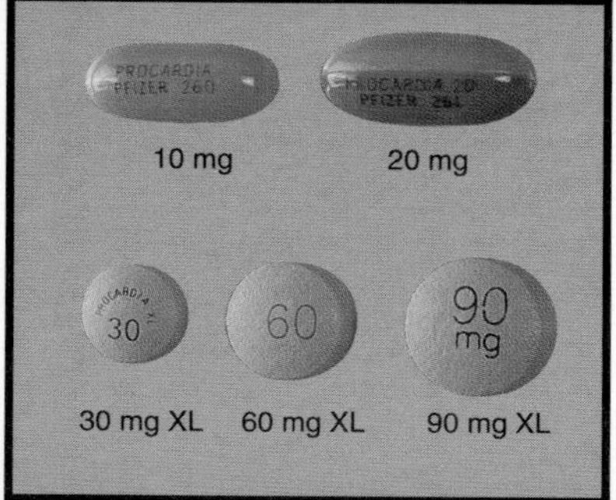

10 mg 20 mg
30 mg XL 60 mg XL 90 mg XL

Nitroglycerin (Nitrostat)

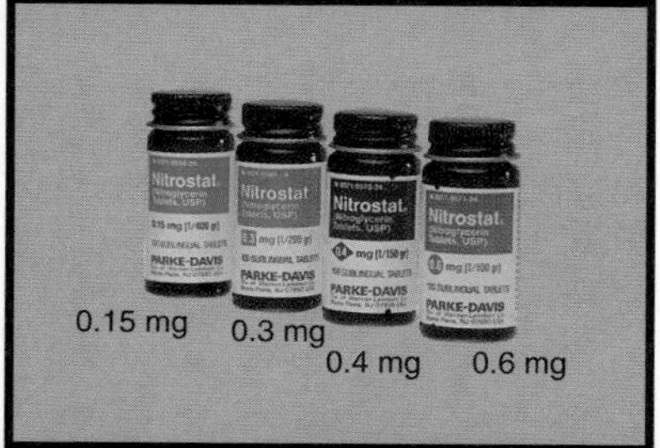

0.15 mg 0.3 mg 0.4 mg 0.6 mg

Nizatidine (Axid)

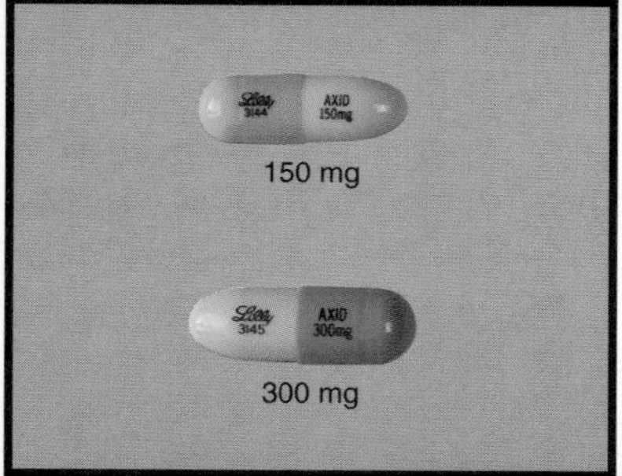

150 mg
300 mg

Omeprazole (Prilosec)

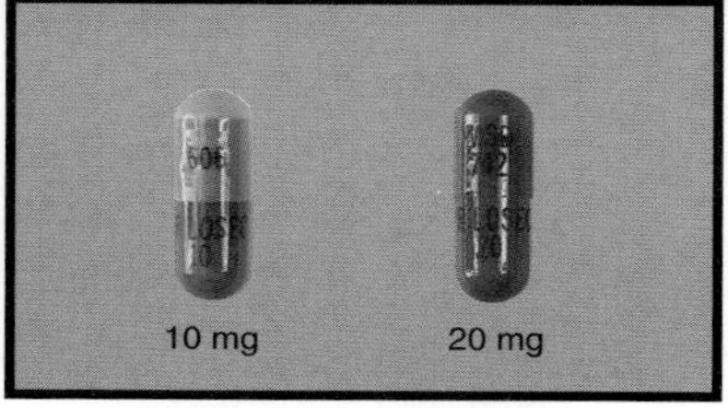
10 mg 20 mg

Oxaprozin (Daypro)

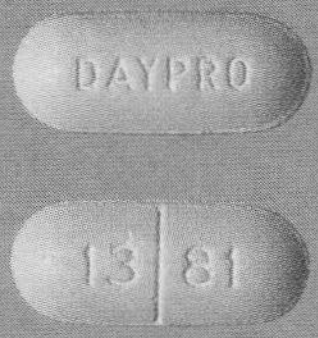

600 mg

Oxycodone/Acetaminophen (Percocet)

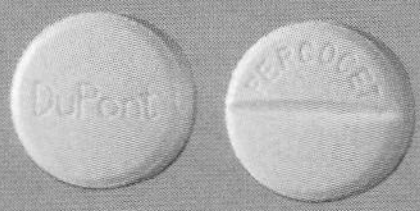

5 mg oxycodone/
325 mg acetaminophen

Paroxetine (Paxil)

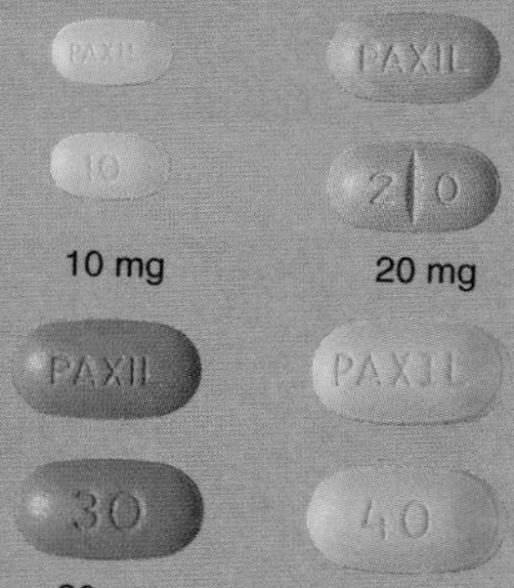

10 mg 20 mg

30 mg 40 mg

Penicillin V Potassium (Veetids)

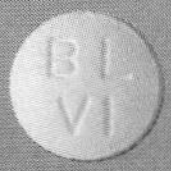

250 mg

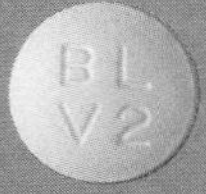

500 mg

Pentoxifylline (Trental)

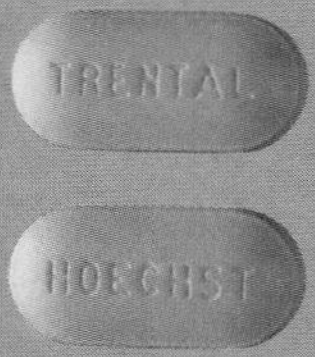

400 mg

Phenytoin extended (Dilantin Kapseals)

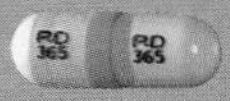

30 mg

100 mg

Potassium Chloride (K-Dur)

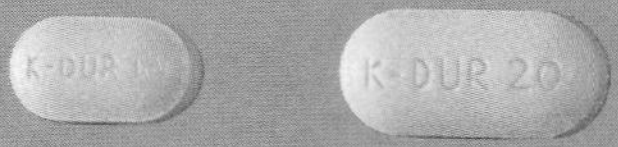

10 mEq 20 mEq

Potassium Chloride (Klor-Con)

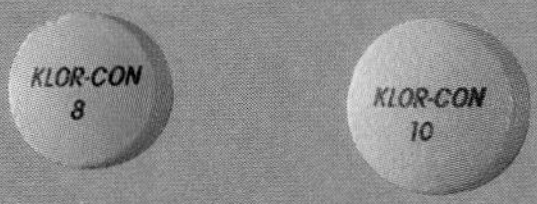

600 mg
(8 mEq)

750 mg
(10 mEq) ER

Pravastatin (Pravachol)

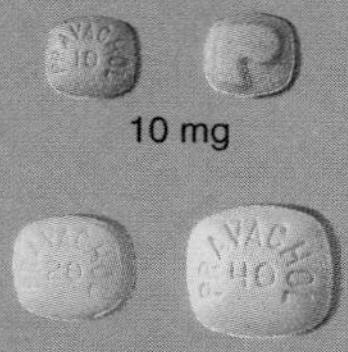

10 mg

20 mg 40 mg

Prednisone (Deltasone)

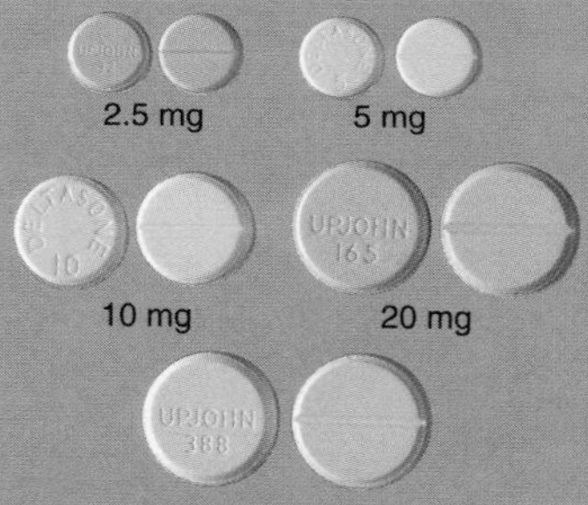

2.5 mg 5 mg

10 mg 20 mg

50 mg

Propoxyphene/ Acetaminophen (Darvocet-N)

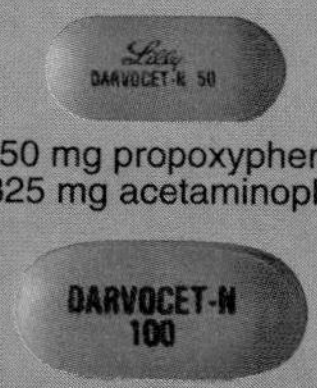

50 mg propoxyphene/
325 mg acetaminophen

100 mg propoxyphene/
325 mg acetaminophen

Provera (Medroxyprogesterone)

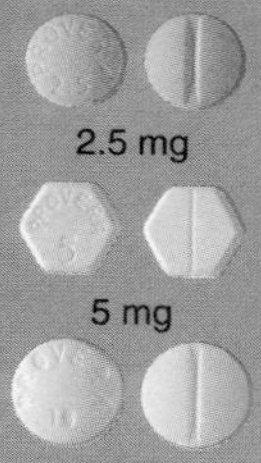

2.5 mg

5 mg

10 mg

Quinapril (Accupril)

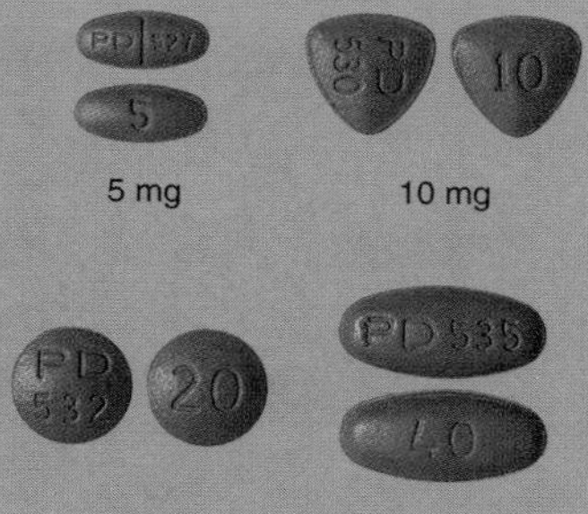

5 mg 10 mg

20 mg 40 mg

Ranitidine (Zantac)

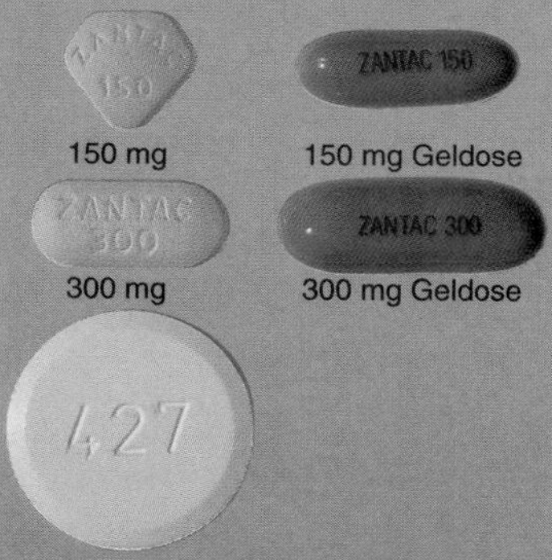

150 mg 150 mg Geldose

300 mg 300 mg Geldose

150 mg Efferdose

Risperidone (Risperdal)

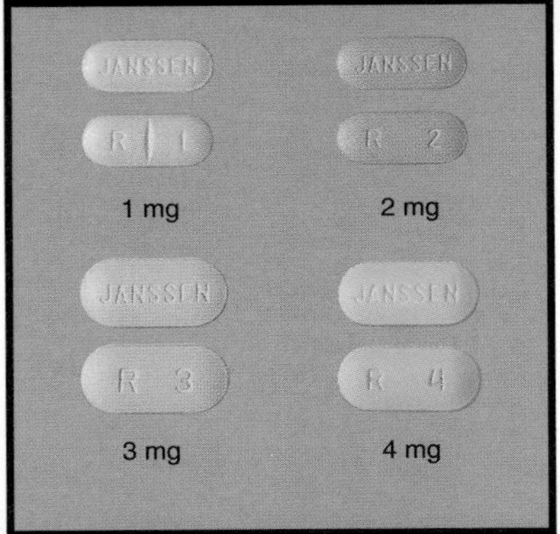

1 mg 2 mg

3 mg 4 mg

Salmeterol (Serevent)

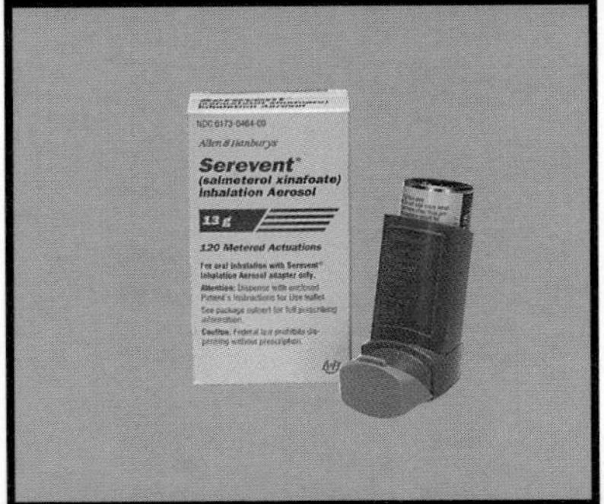

Sertraline (Zoloft)

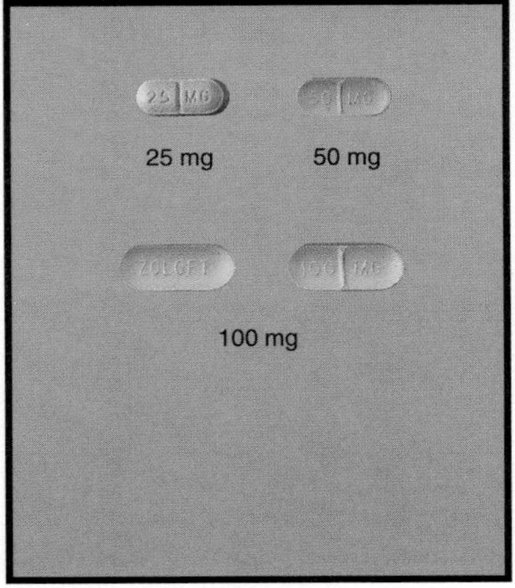

25 mg 50 mg

100 mg

Simvastatin (Zocor)

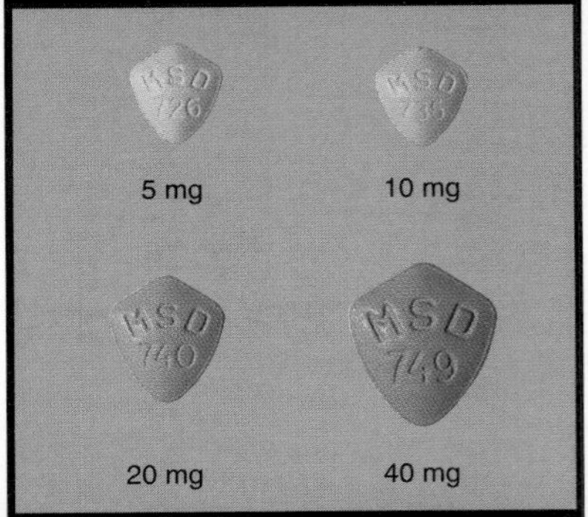

5 mg 10 mg

20 mg 40 mg

Sumatriptan (Imitrex)

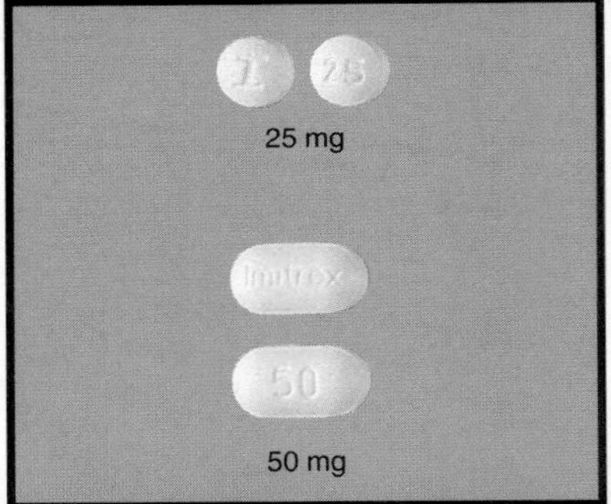

25 mg

50 mg

Terazosin (Hytrim)

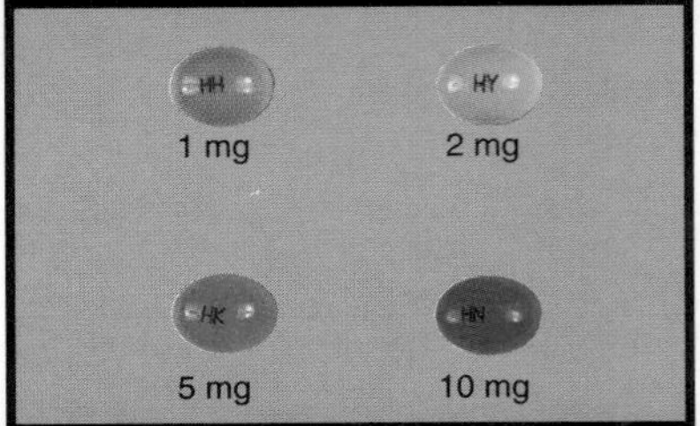

1 mg 2 mg

5 mg 10 mg

Tramadol (Ultram)

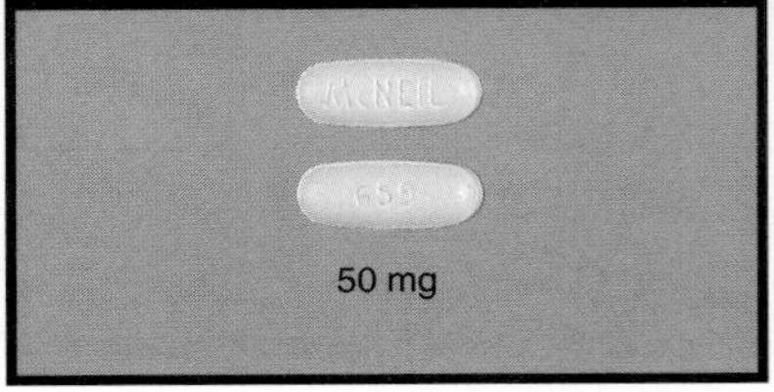

50 mg

Triamcinolone (Azmacort)

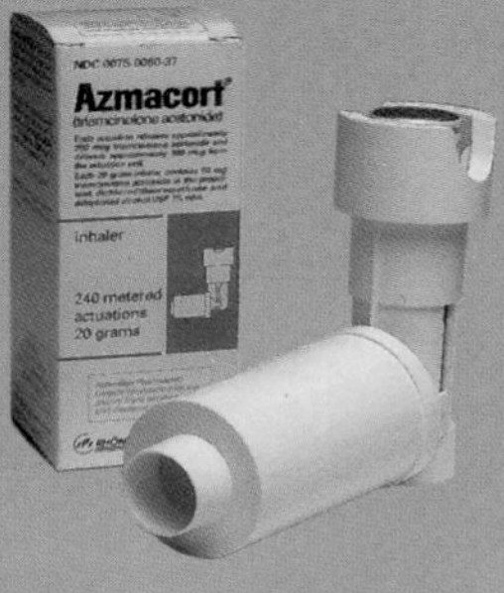

Triamterene/ Hydrochlorothiazide (Dyazide)

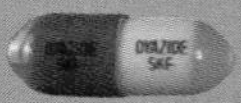

37.5 mg triamterene/
25 mg hydrochlorothiazide

Trimethoprim/ Sulfamethoxazole (Bactrim)

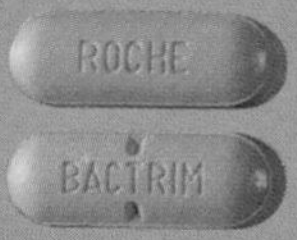

80 mg trimethoprim/
400 mg sulfamethoxazole

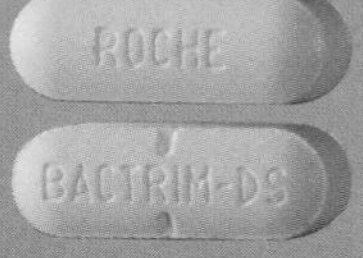

160 mg trimethoprim/
800 mg sulfamethoxazole (D)

Troglitazone (Rezulin)

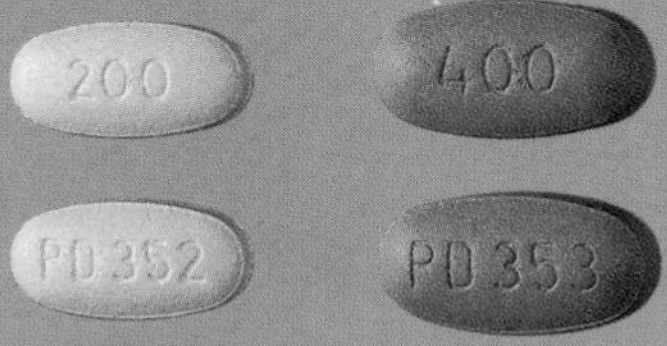

200 mg 400 mg

Venlafaxine (Effexor)

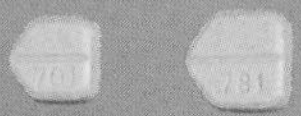

25 mg 37.5 mg

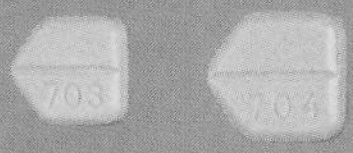

50 mg 75 mg

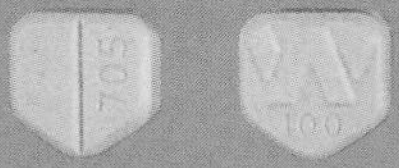

100 mg

Verapamil (Calan)

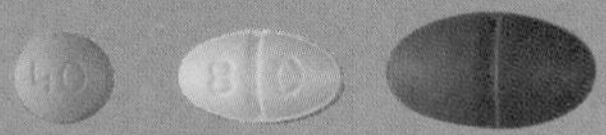

40 mg 80 mg 120 mg

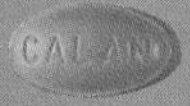

120 mg SR

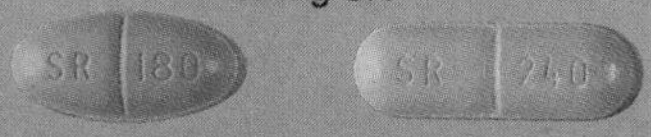

180 mg SR 240 mg SR

Verapamil (Isoptin)

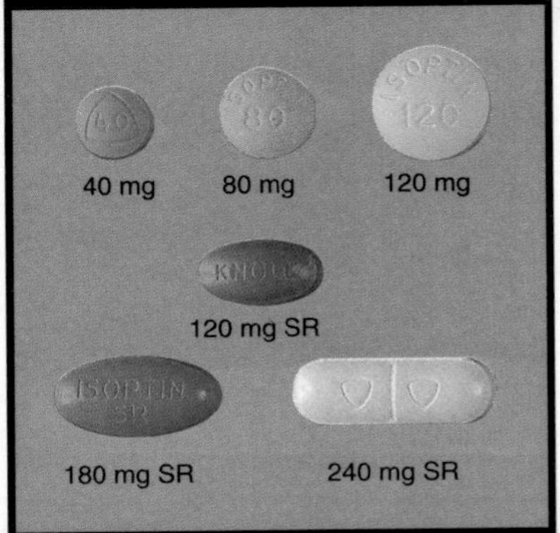

Verapamil (Verelan)

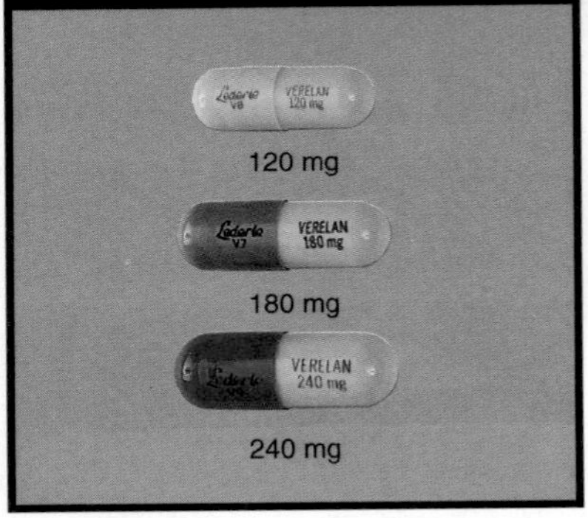

Warfarin (Coumadin)

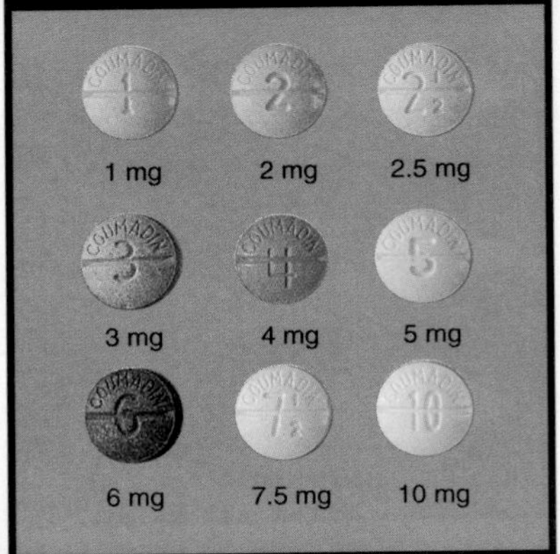

Zolpidem (Ambien)

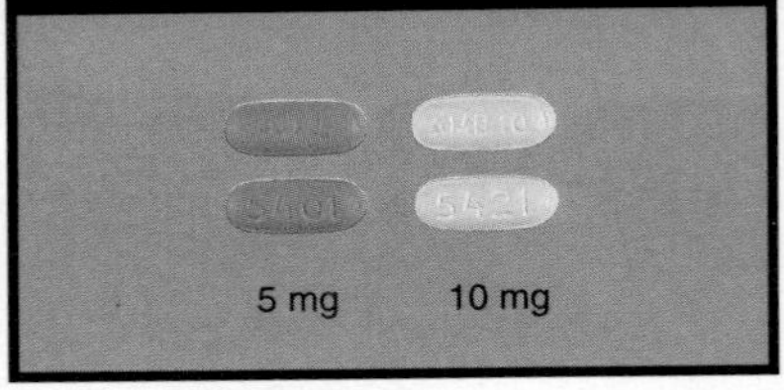

Immunosuppressants Included in *Davis's Drug Guide for Nurses*:

▪ INOTROPIC AGENTS

PHARMACOLOGIC PROFILE

General Use: Management of congestive heart failure or cardiac decompensation unresponsive to conventional therapy with cardiac glycosides, diuretics, or vasodilators. Also used during cardiac surgery.

General Action and Information: Increase cardiac output mainly by direct myocardial effects and some peripheral vascular effects. Digitalis glycosides (digoxin and digitoxin) act by direct effects on the myocardium.

Contraindications: Hypersensitivity. Avoid use in patients with hypertrophic cardiomyopathy.

Precautions: Safety in pregnancy and lactation not established.

Interactions: Beta-adrenergic blockers may negate the effects of dobutamine or dopamine. Several drugs may increase the arrhythmogenic and hypertensive effects of dobutamine or dopamine. Amrinone may produce excessive hypotension when given with disopyramide. Agents that cause hypokalemia, hypomagnesemia, or hypercalcemia increase the risk of cardiac glycoside toxicity. Bradycardia from beta blockers may be additive with digitalis glycosides. Quinidine increases serum digoxin levels.

NURSING IMPLICATIONS

Assessment

- Monitor pulse, blood pressure, ECG, and hemodynamic parameters frequently during parenteral administration and periodically throughout oral administration.
- Monitor intake and output ratios and daily weights. Assess patient for signs and symptoms of congestive heart failure (peripheral edema, rales/crackles, dyspnea, weight gain, and jugular venous distention) throughout therapy.
- Before administering initial loading dose, determine if patient has taken any cardiac glycoside preparations in the preceding 2–3 wk.
- **Lab Test Considerations:** Serum electrolyte levels, especially potassium, magnesium, and calcium, and renal and hepatic function should be evaluated periodically during therapy.
- **Toxicity and Overdose:** Patients taking digitalis glycosides should have serum levels measured regularly.

Potential Nursing Diagnoses

- Cardiac output, decreased (Indications).
- Knowledge deficit, related to medication regimen (Patient/Family Teaching).

Implementation

- Hypokalemia should be corrected before administration of amrinone, milrinone, digoxin, or digitoxin.
- Hypovolemia should be corrected with volume expanders before administration.

CLASSIFICATIONS

Patient/Family Teaching

- Advise patient to notify health care professional if symptoms are not relieved or worsen.
- Instruct patient to notify nurse immediately if pain or discomfort at the insertion site occurs during IV administration.

Evaluation

Effectiveness of therapy can be demonstrated by: ▪ Increased cardiac output ▪ Decrease in severity of congestive heart failure ▪ Increased urine output.

Inotropic Agents Included in *Davis's Drug Guide for Nurses*:

▪ LAXATIVES

PHARMACOLOGIC PROFILE

General Use: Used to treat or prevent constipation or to prepare the bowel for radiologic or endoscopic procedures.

General Action and Information: Induce one or more bowel movements per day. Groups include stimulants (bisacodyl, cascara and its derivatives, senna), saline laxatives (magnesium salts and phosphates), stool softeners (docusate), bulk-forming agents (polycarbophil and psyllium), lubricants (mineral oil), and osmotic cathartics (glycerin, lactulose, polyethylene glycol/electrolyte). Increasing fluid intake, exercising, and adding more dietary fiber are also useful in the management of chronic constipation.

Contraindications: Hypersensitivity. Contraindicated in persistent abdominal pain, nausea, or vomiting of unknown cause, especially if accompanied by fever or other signs of an acute abdomen.

Precautions: Excessive or prolonged use may lead to dependence. Should not be used in children unless advised by a physician or other health care professional.

Interactions: Theoretically may decrease the absorption of other orally administered drugs by decreasing transit time.

NURSING IMPLICATIONS

Assessment

- Assess patient for abdominal distention, presence of bowel sounds, and usual pattern of bowel function.
- Assess color, consistency, and amount of stool produced.

Potential Nursing Diagnoses

- Constipation (Indications).
- Knowledge deficit, related to medication regimen (Patient/Family Teaching).

Implementation

- Many laxatives may be administered at bedtime for morning results.
- Taking oral doses on an empty stomach will usually produce more rapid results.

- Do not crush or chew enteric-coated tablets. Take with a full glass of water or juice.
- Stool softeners and bulk laxatives may take several days for results.

Patient/Family Teaching

- Advise patients, other than those with spinal cord injuries, that laxatives should be used only for short-term therapy. Long-term therapy may cause electrolyte imbalance and dependence.
- Advise patient to increase fluid intake to a minimum of 1500–2000 ml/day during therapy to prevent dehydration.
- Encourage patients to use other forms of bowel regulation: increasing bulk in the diet, increasing fluid intake, and increasing mobility. Normal bowel habits are individualized and may vary from 3 times/day to 3 times/wk.
- Instruct patients with cardiac disease to avoid straining during bowel movements (Valsalva maneuver).
- Advise patient that laxatives should not be used when constipation is accompanied by abdominal pain, fever, nausea, or vomiting.

Evaluation

Effectiveness of therapy can be demonstrated by: ▪ A soft, formed bowel movement ▪ Evacuation of the colon.

Laxatives Included in *Davis's Drug Guide for Nurses*:

bulk-forming agents
polycarbophil 825
psyllium 872

lubricant
mineral oil 665

osmotic agents
glycerin 447
lactulose 558
polyethylene glycol/electrolyte 827

saline laxatives
magnesium citrate 596
magnesium hydroxide 596
magnesium sulfate 596
phosphate/biphosphate 809

stimulants
bisacodyl 108
casanthranol 165
cascara sagrada 165
senna 913

stool softener
docusate 307

▪ LIPID-LOWERING AGENTS

PHARMACOLOGIC PROFILE

General Use: Used as a part of a total plan including diet and exercise to reduce blood lipids in an effort to reduce the morbidity and mortality of atherosclerotic cardiovascular disease and its sequelae.

General Action and Information: HMG-CoA reductase inhibitors (fluvastatin, lovastatin, simvastatin, pravastatin) inhibit an enzyme involved in cholesterol synthesis. Bile acid sequestrants (cholestyramine, colestipol) bind cholesterol in the GI tract. Niacin and gemfibrozil act by other mechanisms (see individual monographs).

Contraindications: Hypersensitivity.

Precautions: Safety in pregnancy, lactation, and children not established. See individual drugs. Dietary therapy should be given a 2–3 mo trial before drug therapy is initiated.

CLASSIFICATIONS

Interactions: Bile acid sequestrants (cholestyramine and colestipol) may bind lipid-soluble vitamins (A, D, E, and K) and other concurrently administered drugs in the GI tract. The risk of myopathy from HMG-CoA reductase inhibitors is increased by niacin, erythromycin, gemfibrozil, mibefradil (not all agents), and cyclosporine.

NURSING IMPLICATIONS

Assessment

- Obtain a diet history, especially in regard to fat and alcohol consumption.
- **Lab Test Considerations:** Serum cholesterol and triglyceride levels should be evaluated before initiating and periodically throughout therapy. Medication should be discontinued if paradoxical increase in cholesterol level occurs.
- Liver function tests should be assessed before and periodically throughout therapy. May cause an increase in levels.

Potential Nursing Diagnoses

- Knowledge deficit, related to medication regimen (Patient/Family Teaching).
- Noncompliance (Patient/Family Teaching).

Implementation

- See specific medications to determine timing of doses in relation to meals.

Patient/Family Teaching

- Advise patient that these medications should be used in conjunction with diet restrictions (fat, cholesterol, carbohydrates, and alcohol), exercise, and cessation of smoking.

Evaluation

Effectiveness of therapy can be demonstrated by: ▪ Decreased serum triglyceride and low-density lipoprotein (LDL) cholesterol levels and improved high-density lipoprotein (HDL) cholesterol ratios. Therapy is usually discontinued if the clinical response is not evident after 3 mo of therapy.

Lipid-Lowering Agents Included in *Davis's Drug Guide for Nurses*:

▪ NEUROMUSCULAR BLOCKING AGENTS

Nondepolarizing, see page 708. Succinylcholine, see page 934.

■ NONOPIOID ANALGESICS/NONSTEROIDAL ANTI-INFLAMMATORY AGENTS

PHARMACOLOGIC PROFILE

General Use: Most agents in this group are used to control mild to moderate pain, fever, and various inflammatory conditions, such as rheumatoid arthritis and osteoarthritis. Acetaminophen has analgesic and antipyretic properties but is not effective as an anti-inflammatory agent. Phenazopyridine is used as a urinary tract analgesic only.

General Action and Information: The largest group of nonopioid analgesics is the nonsteroidal anti-inflammatory agents (NSAIDs). Although not labeled for all actions, NSAIDs and salicylates have analgesic, antipyretic, and anti-inflammatory properties. The mechanism for analgesia is probably due to inhibition of prostaglandin synthesis. Antipyretic action is due to prostaglandin synthesis inhibition in the CNS and vasodilation. Prostaglandin synthesis inhibition also explains the ability to suppress inflammation. Acetaminophen possesses antipyretic and analgesic action but has no anti-inflammatory properties.

Contraindications: Hypersensitivity to aspirin is a contraindication for the whole class of NSAIDs. Only acetaminophen is safe for occasional use in pregnancy or lactation.

Precautions: Use NSAIDs cautiously in patients with a history of bleeding disorders or gastrointestinal bleeding (effect may be less with nonaspirin salicylates) and in severe hepatic, renal, or cardiovascular disease. Safety of NSAIDs in pregnancy is not established and in general should be avoided, especially in large doses or in the 3rd trimester.

Interactions: NSAIDs prolong bleeding time and potentiate the effect of anticoagulants, thrombolytic agents, plicamycin, some cephalosporins, and valproic acid. Chronic use of NSAIDs with aspirin may result in increased GI side effects and decreased effectiveness. NSAIDs may decrease the response to diuretics or antihypertensive therapy. Chronic use of acetaminophen with NSAIDs may increase the risk of adverse renal reactions. Methotrimeprazine will produce additive hypotension with other agents that lower blood pressure.

NURSING IMPLICATIONS

Assessment

- **General Info:** Patients who have asthma, aspirin-induced allergy, and nasal polyps are at increased risk for developing hypersensitivity reactions. Assess for rhinitis, asthma, and urticaria.
- Assess amount, frequency, and type of drugs taken in patients self-medicating, especially with OTC drugs. Prolonged use of acetaminophen and salicylates or NSAIDs increases the risk of renal adverse effects. For short-term use, combined doses of acetaminophen and salicylates should not exceed the recommended dose of either drug given alone.
- **Arthritis:** Assess pain and range of motion before and 1–2 hr following administration.
- **Pain:** Assess pain (note type, location, and intensity) before and 1–2 hr following administration.
- **Fever:** Monitor temperature; note signs associated with fever (diaphoresis, tachycardia, and malaise).
- **Lab Test Considerations:** May cause prolonged bleeding time, which may persist following discontinuation of therapy.

CLASSIFICATIONS

Potential Nursing Diagnoses

- Pain (Indications).
- Physical mobility, impaired (Indications).
- Knowledge deficit, related to medication regimen (Patient/Family Teaching).

Implementation

- **General Info:** Administration in higher than recommended doses does not provide increased effectiveness but may cause increased side effects.
- Coadministration with opioid analgesics may have additive analgesic effects and may permit lower opioid doses.
- **PO:** For rapid initial effect, administer 30 min before or 2 hr after meals. May be administered with food, milk, or antacids to decrease GI irritation. Food slows but does not reduce the extent of absorption.
- **Dysmenorrhea:** Administer as soon as possible after the onset of menses. Prophylactic treatment has not been shown to be effective.

Patient/Family Teaching

- Advise patient to take medication exactly as directed and not to take more than the recommended amount. Severe and permanent liver damage may result from prolonged use or high doses of acetaminophen. Renal damage may occur with prolonged use of acetaminophen and salicylates or NSAIDs. Adults should not take acetaminophen longer than 10 days and children not longer than 5 days unless directed by health care professional. Short-term doses of acetaminophen with salicylates or NSAIDs should not exceed the recommended daily dose of either drug alone. Caution patient that drinking 3 or more glasses of alcohol/day may increase the risk of liver damage with acetaminophen or GI bleeding with aspirin or NSAIDs.
- Advise patients to take these medications with a full glass of water and to remain in an upright position for 15–30 min after administration.
- These medications may occasionally cause drowsiness or dizziness. Advise patient to avoid driving or other activities requiring alertness until response to medication is known.
- Caution patient to avoid the concurrent use of alcohol, aspirin, acetaminophen, or other OTC medications without consultation with health care professional.
- Instruct patients not to take OTC preparations for more than 3 days for fever and to consult health care professional if symptoms persist or worsen.
- Advise patient to inform health care professional of medication regimen before treatment or surgery.

Evaluation

Effectiveness of therapy can be demonstrated by: ▪ Improved joint mobility ▪ Decrease in severity of pain. Patients who do not respond to one NSAID may respond to another ▪ Reduction in fever.

Nonopioid Analgesics/Nonsteroidal Anti-inflammatory Agents Included in *Davis's Drug Guide for Nurses*:

nonsteroidal anti-inflammatory agents
aspirin 900
choline and magnesium salicylates 900
choline salicylate 900
diclofenac 268
etodolac 356
fenoprofen 368
flurbiprofen 404
ibuprofen 501
indomethacin 519
ketoprofen 551
ketorolac 554
meclofenamate 610
nabumetone 690
naproxen 702

oxaprozin 749
piroxicam 820
salsalate 900
sulindac 941
tolmetin 990

nonopioid analgesics
acetaminophen 4
bromfenac 119
etodolac 356
fenoprofen 368
ibuprofen 501
ketoprofen 551
ketorolac 554
meclofenamate 610
naproxen 702
phenazopyridine 798

salicylates
aspirin 900
choline and magnesium salicylates 900
choline salicylate 900
salsalate 900

▪ OPIOID ANALGESICS

PHARMACOLOGIC PROFILE

General Use: Management of moderate to severe pain. Some agents used as general anesthetic adjuncts (alfentanil, fentanyl, remifentanil, and sufentanil).

General Action and Information: Opioids bind to opiate receptors in the CNS, where they act as agonists of endogenously occurring opioid peptides (eukephalins and endorphins). The result is alteration to the perception of and response to pain.

Contraindications: Hypersensitivity to individual agents.

Precautions: Use cautiously in patients with undiagnosed abdominal pain, head trauma or pathology, liver disease, or history of addiction to opioids. Use smaller doses initially in the elderly and those with respiratory diseases. Chronic use may result in tolerance and the need for larger doses to relieve pain. Psychological or physical dependence may occur.

Interactions: Increases the CNS depressant properties of other drugs, including alcohol, antihistamines, antidepressants, sedative/hypnotics, phenothiazines, and MAO inhibitors. Use of partial-antagonist opioid analgesics (buprenorphine, butorphanol, dezocine, nalbuphine, and pentazocine) may precipitate opioid withdrawal in physically dependent patients. Use with MAO inhibitors or procarbazine may result in severe paradoxical reactions (especially with meperidine). Nalbuphine or pentazocine may decrease the analgesic effects of other concurrently administered opioid analgesics.

NURSING IMPLICATIONS

Assessment

- Assess type, location, and intensity of pain prior to and at peak following administration. When titrating opioid doses, increases of 25–50% should be administered until there is either a 50% reduction in the patient's pain rating on a numerical or visual analogue scale or the patient reports satisfactory pain relief. A repeat dose can be safely administered at the time of the peak if previous dose is ineffective and side effects are minimal. Patients requiring higher doses of opioid agonist-antagonists should be converted to an opioid agonist. Opioid agonist-antagonists are not recommended for prolonged use or as first-line therapy for acute or cancer pain.
- An equianalgesic chart (see Appendix B) should be used when changing routes or when changing from one opioid to another.

- Assess blood pressure, pulse, and respirations before and periodically during administration. If respiratory rate is <10/min, assess level of sedation. Physical stimulation may be sufficient to prevent significant hypoventilation. Dose may need to be decreased by 25–50%. Initial drowsiness will diminish with continued use.
- Assess prior analgesic history. Antagonistic properties of agonist-antagonists may induce withdrawal symptoms (vomiting, restlessness, abdominal cramps, and increased blood pressure and temperature) in patients physically dependent on opioids.
- Prolonged use may lead to physical and psychological dependence and tolerance. This should not prevent patient from receiving adequate analgesia. Most patients who receive opioid analgesics for pain do not develop psychological dependence. Progressively higher doses may be required to relieve pain with long-term therapy.
- Assess bowel function routinely. Prevention of constipation should be instituted with increased intake of fluids and bulk, stool softeners, and laxatives to minimize constipating effects. Stimulant laxatives should be administered routinely if opioid use exceeds 2–3 days, unless contraindicated.
- Monitor intake and output ratios. If significant discrepancies occur, assess for urinary retention and inform physician or other health care professional.
- **Toxicity and Overdose:** If an opioid antagonist is required to reverse respiratory depression or coma, naloxone (Narcan) is the antidote. Dilute the 0.4-mg ampule of naloxone in 10 ml of 0.9% NaCl and administer 0.5 ml (0.02 mg) by direct IV push every 2 min. For children and patients weighing <40 kg, dilute 0.1 mg of naloxone in 10 ml of 0.9% NaCl for a concentration of 10 mcg/ml and administer 0.5 mcg/kg every 1–2 min. Titrate dose to avoid withdrawal, seizures, and severe pain.

Potential Nursing Diagnoses

- Pain (Indications).
- Sensory-perceptual alteration: visual, auditory (Side Effects).
- Injury, risk for (Side Effects).
- Knowledge deficit, related to medication regimen (Patient/Family Teaching).

Implementation

- Do not confuse morphine with hydromorphone or meperidine; errors have resulted in fatalities.
- Explain therapeutic value of medication before administration to enhance the analgesic effect.
- Regularly administered doses may be more effective than prn administration. Analgesic is more effective if given before pain becomes severe.
- Coadministration with nonopioid analgesics may have additive analgesic effects and may permit lower doses.
- Medication should be discontinued gradually after long-term use to prevent withdrawal symptoms.

Patient/Family Teaching

- Instruct patient on how and when to ask for pain medication.
- Medication may cause drowsiness or dizziness. Caution patient to call for assistance when ambulating or smoking and to avoid driving or other activities requiring alertness until response to medication is known.
- Advise patient to make position changes slowly to minimize orthostatic hypotension.
- Caution patient to avoid concurrent use of alcohol or other CNS depressants with this medication.
- Encourage patient to turn, cough, and breathe deeply every 2 hr to prevent atelectasis.

Evaluation

Effectiveness of therapy can be demonstrated by: ▪ Decreased severity of pain without a significant alteration in level of consciousness or respiratory status.

Opioid Analgesics Included in *Davis's Drug Guide for Nurses*:

▪ SEDATIVE/HYPNOTICS

PHARMACOLOGIC PROFILE

General Use: Sedatives are used to treat various anxiety states and to provide sedation before procedures. Hypnotics are used to treat insomnia. Selected agents are useful as anticonvulsants (clorazepate, diazepam, and phenobarbital), as skeletal muscle relaxants (diazepam), as adjuncts in the treatment of alcohol withdrawal syndrome (chlordiazepoxide, clorazepate, diazepam, and oxazepam), and as general anesthetic adjuncts or amnestics. Some phenothiazines are also used as sedatives.

General Action and Information: Cause generalized CNS depression. May produce tolerance with chronic use and have potential for psychological or physical dependence. These agents have no analgesic properties.

Contraindications: Hypersensitivity. Should not be used in comatose patients or in those with pre-existing CNS depression. Should not be used in patients with uncontrolled severe pain. Avoid use during pregnancy or lactation.

Precautions: Use cautiously in patients with hepatic dysfunction, severe renal impairment, or severe underlying pulmonary disease. Use with caution in patients who may be suicidal or who may have been addicted to drugs previously. Hypnotic use should be short-term. Geriatric patients may be more sensitive to CNS depressant effects (initial dosage reduction may be required).

Interactions: Additive CNS depression with alcohol, antihistamines, antidepressants, opioid analgesics, or phenothiazines. Barbiturates induce hepatic drug-metabolizing enzymes and can decrease the effectiveness of drugs metabolized by the liver. Should not be used with MAO inhibitors.

NURSING IMPLICATIONS

Assessment

- **General Info:** Monitor blood pressure, pulse, and respiratory status frequently throughout IV administration.

- Prolonged high-dose therapy may lead to psychological or physical dependence. Restrict the amount of drug available to patient, especially if patient is depressed, suicidal, or has a history of addiction.
- **Insomnia:** Assess sleep patterns before and periodically throughout therapy.
- **Anxiety:** Assess degree of anxiety and level of sedation (ataxia, dizziness, and slurred speech) before and periodically throughout therapy.
- **Seizures:** Observe and record intensity, duration, and characteristics of seizure activity. Institute seizure precautions.
- **Muscle Spasms:** Assess muscle spasms, associated pain, and limitation of movement before and throughout therapy.
- **Alcohol Withdrawal:** Assess patient experiencing alcohol withdrawal for tremors, agitation, delirium, and hallucinations. Protect patient from injury.

Potential Nursing Diagnoses

- Sleep pattern disturbance (Indications).
- Injury, risk for (Side Effects).
- Knowledge deficit, related to medication regimen (Patient/Family Teaching).

Implementation

- Supervise ambulation and transfer of patients following administration of hypnotic doses. Remove cigarettes. Side rails should be raised and call bell within reach at all times. Keep bed in low position.

Patient/Family Teaching

- Discuss the importance of preparing environment for sleep (dark room, quiet, avoidance of nicotine and caffeine). If less effective after a few weeks, consult health care professional; do not increase dose. Gradual withdrawal may be required to prevent reactions following prolonged therapy.
- May cause daytime drowsiness. Caution patient to avoid driving or other activities requiring alertness until response to medication is known.
- Advise patient to avoid the use of alcohol and other CNS depressants concurrently with these medications.
- Advise patient to inform health care professional if pregnancy is planned or suspected.

Evaluation

Effectiveness of therapy can be demonstrated by: ▪ Improvement in sleep patterns ▪ Decrease in anxiety level ▪ Control of seizures ▪ Decrease in muscle spasm ▪ Decrease in tremulousness ▪ More rational ideation when used for alcohol withdrawal.

Sedative/Hypnotics Included in *Davis's Drug Guide for Nurses*:

antihistamines
diphenhydramine 291
hydroxyzine 496
promethazine 853

barbiturates
butalbital compound 137
pentobarbital 789
phenobarbital 799
thiopental 1143

benzodiazepines
alprazolam 23
chlordiazepoxide 187
diazepam 263
flurazepam 403
lorazepam 589
midazolam 660
oxazepam 750
quazepam 1141
temazepam 951
triazolam 1002

miscellaneous
buspirone 134
chloral hydrate 181
zolpidem 1056

▪ SKELETAL MUSCLE RELAXANTS

PHARMACOLOGIC PROFILE

General Use: Two major uses are spasticity associated with spinal cord diseases or lesions (baclofen and dantrolene) or adjunctive therapy in the symptomatic relief of acute painful musculoskeletal conditions (cyclobenzaprine, diazepam, and methocarbamol). IV dantrolene is also used to treat and prevent malignant hyperthermia.

General Action and Information: Act either centrally (baclofen, carisoprodol, cyclobenzaprine, diazepam, and methocarbamol) or directly (dantrolene).

Contraindications: Baclofen and oral dantrolene should not be used in patients in whom spasticity is used to maintain posture and balance.

Precautions: Safety in pregnancy and lactation not established. Use cautiously in patients with a previous history of liver disease.

Interactions: Additive CNS depression with other CNS depressants, including alcohol, antihistamines, antidepressants, opioid analgesics, and sedative/hypnotics.

NURSING IMPLICATIONS

Assessment

- Assess patient for pain, muscle stiffness, and range of motion before and periodically throughout therapy.

Potential Nursing Diagnoses

- Pain (Indications).
- Physical mobility, impaired (Indications).
- Injury, risk for (Side Effects).

Implementation

- Provide safety measures as indicated. Supervise ambulation and transfer of patients.

Patient/Family Teaching

- Encourage patient to comply with additional therapies prescribed for muscle spasm (rest, physical therapy, heat).
- Medication may cause drowsiness. Caution patient to avoid driving or other activities requiring alertness until response to drug is known.
- Advise patient to avoid concurrent use of alcohol or other CNS depressants with these medications.

Evaluation

Effectiveness of therapy can be demonstrated by: ▪ Decreased musculoskeletal pain ▪ Decreased muscle spasticity ▪ Increased range of motion ▪ Prevention or decrease in temperature and skeletal rigidity in malignant hyperthermia.

Skeletal Muscle Relaxants Included in *Davis's Drug Guide for Nurses*:

centrally acting
baclofen 95
carisoprodol 157
chlorzoxazone 1133
cyclobenzaprine 229
diazepam 263
methocarbamol 633
orphenadrine 1139

direct-acting
dantrolene 245

▪ THROMBOLYTIC AGENTS

See group monograph on page 970.

Thrombolytic Agents Included in *Davis's Drug Guide for Nurses*:

alteplase 970
anistreplase 970
reteplase 970
streptokinase 970
urokinase 970

▪ VASCULAR HEADACHE SUPPRESSANTS

PHARMACOLOGIC PROFILE

General Use: Used for acute treatment of vascular headaches (migraine, cluster headaches, migraine variants). Other agents such as some beta-adrenergic blockers and some calcum channel blockers are used for suppression of frequently occurring vascular headaches.

General action and information: Ergot derivative agents (ergotamine, dihydroergotamine) directly stimulate alpha-adrenergic and serotonergic receptors, producing vascular smooth muscle vasoconstriction. Sumatriptan and zolmitriptan produce vasoconstriction by acting as serotonin agonists.

Contraindications: Avoid using these agents in patients with ischemic cardiovascular disease.

Precautions: Use cautiously in patients with a history of or risk for cardiovascular disease.

Interactions: Avoid concurrent use of ergot derivative agents with serotonin agonist agents; see also individual agents.

NURSING IMPLICATIONS

Assessment

- Assess pain location, intensity, duration, and associated symptoms (photophobia, phonophobia, nausea, vomiting) during migraine attack.

Potential Nursing Diagnoses

- Pain (Indications).
- Knowledge deficit, related to medication regimen (Patient/Family Teaching).

Implementation

- Medication should be administered at the first sign of a headache.

Patient/Family Teaching

- Inform patient that medication should be used only during a migraine attack. It is meant to be used for relief of migraine attacks but not to prevent or reduce the number of attacks.
- Advise patient that lying down in a darkened room following medication administration may further help relieve headache.
- May cause dizziness or drowsiness. Caution patient to avoid driving or other activities requiring alertness until response to medication is known.
- Advise patient to avoid alcohol, which aggravates headaches.

Evaluation

Effectiveness of therapy can be demonstrated by: ▪ Relief of migraine attack.

Vascular Headache Suppressants Included in *Davis's Drug Guide for Nurses*:

ergot derivatives
dihydroergotamine 336
ergotamine 336

serotonin agonists
sumatriptan 942
zolmitriptan 1056a

▪ VASOPRESSORS

PHARMACOLOGIC PROFILE

General Use: Used to correct the hemodynamic imbalances that may persist despite adequate fluid replacement in the treatment of shock. Phenylephrine is also used as a topical decongestant and mydriatic.

General Action and Information: Stimulate adrenergic receptors, resulting in vasoconstriction (alpha-adrenergic effects) and/or myocardial stimulation (beta-adrenergic effects).

Contraindications: Contraindicated in occlusive vascular diseases, uncorrected arrhythmias, or hypotension secondary to fluid deficit.

Precautions: Use cautiously in patients with underlying cardiovascular disease. Safety in pregnancy and lactation not established.

Interactions: Use with MAO inhibitors may result in severe hypertension. Beta-adrenergic blockers may block therapeutic effectiveness.

NURSING IMPLICATIONS

Assessment

- Monitor blood pressure, pulse, respiration, ECG, and hemodynamic parameters every 5–15 min during and after administration. Notify physician if significant changes in vital signs or arrhythmias occur. Consult physician for parameters for pulse, blood pressure, or ECG changes for adjusting dosage or discontinuing medication.
- Monitor urine output frequently throughout administration. Notify physician promptly if urine output decreases.
- Assess IV site frequently throughout infusion. Administer into a large vein to minimize the risk of extravasation. Extravasation of dopamine, norepinephrine, or phenylephrine may cause severe irritation, necrosis, and sloughing of tissue. If extravasation occurs, affected area should be infiltrated with 10–15 ml of 0.9% NaCl containing 5–10 mg of phentolamine.

Potential Nursing Diagnoses

- Cardiac output, decreased (Indications).
- Tissue perfusion, altered (Indications).

Implementation

- Hypovolemia should be corrected before administration of vasopressors.
- Infusions must be administered via infusion pump to ensure precise amount delivered. Rate of administration is titrated according to patient response (blood pressure, heart rate, urine flow, peripheral perfusion, presence of ectopic activity, and cardiac output).

Patient/Family Teaching

- Instruct patient to inform nurse immediately if chest pain, dyspnea, or pain at infusion site occurs.

Evaluation

Effectiveness of therapy can be demonstrated by: ▪ Increase in blood pressure ▪ Increase in peripheral circulation ▪ Increase in urine output.

Vasopressors Included in *Davis's Drug Guide for Nurses*:

▪ VITAMINS

PHARMACOLOGIC PROFILE

General Use: Used in the prevention and treatment of vitamin deficiencies and as supplements in various metabolic disorders.

General Action and Information: Serve as components of enzyme systems that catalyze numerous varied metabolic reactions. Necessary for homeostasis. Water-soluble vitamins (B-vitamins, vitamin C, and pantothenic acid) rarely cause toxicity. Fat-soluble vitamins (vitamins A, D, E, and K) may accumulate and cause toxicity.

Contraindications: Hypersensitivity to additives, preservatives, or colorants.

Precautions: Dosage should be adjusted to avoid toxicity, especially for fat-soluble vitamins.

Interactions: Pyridoxine in large amounts may interfere with the effectiveness of levodopa. Cholestyramine, colestipol, and mineral oil decrease absorption of fat-soluble vitamins.

NURSING IMPLICATIONS

Assessment

- Assess patient for signs of vitamin deficiency before and periodically throughout therapy.
- Assess nutritional status through 24-hr diet recall. Determine frequency of consumption of vitamin-rich foods.

Potential Nursing Diagnoses

- Nutrition, altered, less than body requirements (Indications).
- Knowledge deficit, related to medication regimen (Patient/Family Teaching).

Implementation

- Because of infrequency of single vitamin deficiencies, combinations are commonly administered.

Patient/Family Teaching

- Encourage patients to comply with diet recommendations of physician or other health care professional. Explain that the best source of vitamins is a well-balanced diet with foods from the four basic food groups.
- Patients self-medicating with vitamin supplements should be cautioned not to exceed RDA (see Appendix L). The effectiveness of megadoses for treatment of various medical conditions is unproved and may cause side effects and toxicity.

Evaluation

Effectiveness of therapy may be demonstrated by: ▪ Prevention of or decrease in the symptoms of vitamin deficiencies.

Vitamins Included in *Davis's Drug Guide for Nurses*:

fat-soluble vitamins
calcitriol 1042
dihydrotachysterol 1042
ergocalciferol 1042
vitamin A 1036
vitamin D analogues 1042
vitamin E (alpha tocopherol) 1045
vitamin K (phytonadione) 810

water-soluble vitamins
folic acid (vitamin B_6) 409
hydroxocobalamin (vitamin B_{12}) 1039
niacin, niacinamide (vitamin B_3) 716
pyridoxine (vitamin B_5) 875
riboflavin (vitamin B_2) 888
thiamine (vitamin B_1) 964
vitamin B cyanocobalamin (vitamin B_{12}) 1039
vitamin C (ascorbic acid) 76

miscellaneous
multiple vitamins (oral and parenteral) 683
vitamin B complex with C (oral and parenteral) 1038

A

ACARBOSE

(aye-**kar**-bose)
Precose

CLASSIFICATION(S):
Oral hypoglycemic agent (alpha-glucosidase inhibitor)

Pregnancy Category B

INDICATIONS

▪ Management of non–insulin-dependent diabetes mellitus (NIDDM) in conjunction with dietary therapy; may be used with sulfonylurea oral hypoglycemic agents.

ACTION

▪ Lowers blood sugar by inhibiting the enzyme alpha-glucosidase in the GI tract. Result is delayed glucose absorption. **Therapeutic Effects:** ▪ Lowering of blood sugar in diabetic patients, especially postprandial hyperglycemia.

PHARMACOKINETICS

Absorption: <2% systemically absorbed; action is primarily local (in the GI tract).
Distribution: UK.
Metabolism and Excretion: Minimal amounts absorbed are excreted by the kidneys.
Half-life: 2 hr.

CONTRAINDICATIONS AND PRECAUTIONS

Contraindicated in: ▪ Hypersensitivity ▪ Diabetic ketoacidosis ▪ Cirrhosis ▪ Patients with renal impairment (not recommended if serum creatinine >2 mg/dl) ▪ Pregnancy, lactation, or children.
Use Cautiously in: ▪ Patients with □ Fever □ Infection □ Trauma □ Stress (may cause hyperglycemia requiring alternative therapy).

ADVERSE REACTIONS AND SIDE EFFECTS*

GI: abdominal pain, diarrhea, flatulence, elevated transaminases.

INTERACTIONS

Drug-Drug: ▪ **Thiazide** and **loop diuretics**, **glucocorticoids**, **phenothiazines**, **thyroid preparations**, **estrogens**, **oral contraceptives**, **phenytoin**, **nicotinic acid**, **sympathomimetics**, **calcium channel blockers**, and **isoniazid** may increase glucose levels in diabetic patients and lead to loss of control of blood sugar ▪ Effects are decreased by concurrent use of **intestinal adsorbents including charcoal** and **digestive enzyme preparations (amylase, pancreatin)**; concurrent use should be avoided ▪ Potentiates the effects of **sulfonylurea oral hypoglycemic agents**.

ROUTE AND DOSAGE

▪ **PO (Adults):** 25 mg 3 times daily; may be increased q 4–8 wk as needed and tolerated (range 50–100 mg 3 times daily; not to exceed 50 mg 3 times daily in patients ≤60 kg or 100 mg 3 times daily in patients >60 kg).

AVAILABILITY

▪ ***Tablets:*** 50 mg[Rx], 100 mg[Rx].

TIME/ACTION PROFILE (effect on blood sugar)

	ONSET	PEAK	DURATION
PO	UK	1 hr	UK

NURSING IMPLICATIONS

ASSESSMENT

□ Observe patient for signs and symptoms of hypoglycemic reactions (sweating, hunger, weakness, dizziness, tremor, tachycardia, anxiety), especially when taking concurrently with other oral hypoglycemic agents.
▪ ***Lab Test Considerations:*** Serum glucose and glycosylated hemoglobin should be monitored periodically throughout therapy to evaluate effectiveness of treatment.
□ Monitor AST and ALT every 3 mo for the 1st yr and then periodically. Elevated levels may require dosage reduction or discontinuation of acarbose.
▪ ***Toxicity and Overdose:*** Symptoms of overdose are transient increase in flatulence, diarrhea, and abdominal discomfort. Acarbose alone does not cause hypoglycemia;

*CAPITALS indicate life-threatening; underlines indicate most frequent.

however, other concurrently administered hypoglycemic agents may produce hypoglycemia requiring treatment. Mild hypoglycemia may be treated with administration of oral glucose. Severe hypoglycemia should be treated with IV D5W or glucagon, followed by continuous IV infusion of more dilute dextrose solution at a rate sufficient to keep serum glucose at approximately 100 mg/dl.

POTENTIAL NURSING DIAGNOSES

- Nutrition, altered, more than body requirements (Indications).
- Knowledge deficit, related to medication regimen (Patient/Family Teaching).
- Noncompliance.

IMPLEMENTATION

- **General Info:** Patients stabilized on a diabetic regimen who are exposed to stress, fever, trauma, infection, or surgery may require administration of insulin.
- □ Does not cause hypoglycemia when taken while fasting but may increase hypoglycemic effect of other hypoglycemic agents.
- **PO:** Administer with 1st bite of each meal 3 times/day.

PATIENT/FAMILY TEACHING

- □ Instruct patient to take medication at same time each day. If a dose is missed and the meal is completed without taking the dose, skip missed dose and take next dose with the next meal. Do not double doses.
- □ Explain to patient that this medication controls hyperglycemia but does not cure diabetes. Therapy is long-term.
- □ Review signs of hypoglycemia and hyperglycemia with patient. If hypoglycemia occurs, advise patient to take a form of oral glucose rather than sugar (absorption of sugar is blocked by acarbose) and notify health care professional.
- □ Encourage patient to follow prescribed diet, medication, and exercise regimen to prevent hypoglycemic or hyperglycemic episodes.
- □ Instruct patient in proper testing of serum glucose and urine ketones. Monitor closely during periods of stress or illness. Notify health care professional if significant changes occur.
- □ Caution patient to avoid other medications while on this therapy without consulting health care professional.
- □ Advise patient to inform health care professional of medication regimen prior to treatment or surgery.
- □ Advise patient to carry a form of oral glucose and identification describing disease process and medication regimen at all times.
- □ Emphasize the importance of routine follow-up examinations.

EVALUATION

Effectiveness of therapy can be demonstrated by: ▪ Control of blood glucose levels without the appearance of hypoglycemic or hyperglycemic episodes.

ACEBUTOLOL

(a-se-**byoo**-toe-lole)
{Monitan}, Sectral

CLASSIFICATION(S):
Antiarrhythmic (group II), Antihypertensive agent, Beta-adrenergic blocking agent (selective)

Pregnancy Category B

INDICATIONS

▪ Treatment of hypertension (single agent or with other antihypertensives) ▪ Treatment of ventricular tachyarrhythmias. **Unlabeled Uses:** ▪ Prophylaxis of myocardial infarction, treatment of angina pectoris, management of anxiety, tremors, thyrotoxicosis, mitral valve prolapse, idiopathic hypertrophic subaortic stenosis.

ACTION

▪ Blocks stimulation of $beta_1$(myocardial) -adrenergic receptors. Does not usually affect $beta_2$ (pulmonary, vascular, or uterine) receptor sites ▪ Mild intrinsic sympathomimetic activity (ISA). **Therapeutic Effects:** ▪ Decreased heart rate ▪ Decreased AV conduction ▪ Decreased blood pressure.

PHARMACOKINETICS

Absorption: Well absorbed following oral administration but rapidly undergoes metabolism. **Distribution:** Minimal penetration of the CNS.

Crosses the placenta and enters breast milk in small amounts.
Metabolism and Excretion: Mostly metabolized to diacetolol, which is also a beta blocker.
Half-life: 3–4 hr (8–13 hr for diacetolol).

CONTRAINDICATIONS AND PRECAUTIONS

Contraindicated in: ▪ Uncompensated congestive heart failure ▪ Pulmonary edema ▪ Cardiogenic shock ▪ Bradycardia or heart block.
Use Cautiously in: ▪ Renal or hepatic impairment (dosage reduction recommended if CCr <50 ml/min/1.73 m^2) ▪ Geriatric patients (increased sensitivity) ▪ Thyrotoxicosis (may mask symptoms) ▪ Diabetes mellitus (may mask symptoms of hypoglycemia) ▪ Pregnancy, lactation, or children (safety not established; neonatal bradycardia, hypotension, hypoglycemia, and respiratory depression may occur rarely) ▪ History of severe allergic reactions (intensity of reactions may be increased).

ADVERSE REACTIONS AND SIDE EFFECTS*

CNS: <u>fatigue</u>, <u>weakness</u>, anxiety, depression, dizziness, drowsiness, insomnia, memory loss, nervousness, nightmares.
EENT: blurred vision, stuffy nose.
Resp: bronchospasm, wheezing.
CV: BRADYCARDIA, CONGESTIVE HEART FAILURE, PULMONARY EDEMA, hypotension, peripheral vasoconstriction.
GI: constipation, diarrhea, nausea, vomiting.
GU: <u>impotence</u>, diminished libido, urinary frequency.
Derm: rashes.
Endo: hyperglycemia, hypoglycemia.
MS: arthralgia, joint pain.

INTERACTIONS

Drug-Drug: ▪ **General anesthesia, IV phenytoin,** and **verapamil** may cause additive myocardial depression ▪ Concurrent use with **digitalis glycosides** may increase bradycardia ▪ **Antihypertensive agents,** acute ingestion of **alcohol,** or **nitrates** may cause additive hypotension ▪ Use with **epinephrine** may result in unopposed alpha-adrenergic stimulation ▪ Concurrent **thyroid** use may decrease effectiveness ▪ Concurrent use with **insulin** may result in prolonged hypoglycemia ▪ May decrease effectiveness of **theophylline.**

ROUTE AND DOSAGE

- **PO (Adults):** 400–800 mg/day—single dose or twice daily (up to 1200 mg/day or 800 mg/day in geriatric patients).

AVAILABILITY

▪ ***Capsules:*** 200 mg[Rx], 400 mg[Rx] ▪ ***Tablets:*** 200mg[Rx], 400 mg[Rx].

TIME/ACTION PROFILE

	ONSET	PEAK	DURATION
PO (effect on BP)	1–1.5 hr	2–8 hr	12–24 hr
PO (antiarrhythmic)	1 hr	4–6 hr	up to 10 hr

NURSING IMPLICATIONS

ASSESSMENT

- □ Monitor blood pressure, ECG, and pulse frequently during dosage adjustment period and periodically throughout therapy.
- □ Monitor intake and output ratios and daily weights. Assess routinely for signs and symptoms of congestive heart failure (dyspnea, rales/crackles, weight gain, peripheral edema, jugular venous distention).
- ▪ ***Lab Test Considerations:*** May cause increased BUN, serum lipoprotein, potassium, triglyceride, and uric acid levels.
- □ May cause increased serum alkaline phosphatase, LDH, AST, and ALT levels.
- □ May cause increased ANA titers.
- □ May cause increase in blood glucose levels.

POTENTIAL NURSING DIAGNOSES

- Cardiac output, decreased (Side Effects).
- Knowledge deficit, related to medication regimen (Patient/Family Teaching).
- Noncompliance, related to medication regimen (Patient/Family Teaching).

IMPLEMENTATION

- **PO:** Take apical pulse prior to administering. If <50 bpm or if arrhythmia occurs, withhold medication and notify physician or other health care professional.

***CAPITALS indicate life-threatening; <u>underlines</u> indicate most frequent.**

□ May be administered with food or on an empty stomach.

PATIENT/FAMILY TEACHING

■ **General Info:** Instruct patient to take medication exactly as directed, at the same time each day, even if feeling well; do not skip or double up on missed doses. If a dose is missed, it should be taken as soon as possible up to 4 hr before next dose. Abrupt withdrawal may precipitate life-threatening arrhythmias, hypertension, or myocardial ischemia.

□ Teach patient and family how to check pulse and blood pressure. Instruct them to check pulse daily and blood pressure biweekly and to report significant changes to health care professional.

□ May cause drowsiness or dizziness. Caution patients to avoid driving or other activities that require alertness until response to the drug is known.

□ Caution patient that this medication may increase sensitivity to cold.

□ Instruct patient to consult health care professional before taking any OTC medications, especially cold preparations, concurrently with this medication.

□ Diabetics should closely monitor blood sugar, especially if weakness, malaise, irritability, or fatigue occurs.

□ Advise patient to notify health care professional if slow pulse, difficulty breathing, wheezing, cold hands and feet, dizziness, lightheadedness, confusion, depression, rash, fever, sore throat, unusual bleeding, or bruising occurs.

□ Instruct patient to inform health care professional of medication regimen prior to treatment or surgery.

□ Advise patient to carry identification describing disease process and medication regimen at all times.

■ **Hypertension:** Reinforce the need to continue additional therapies for hypertension (weight loss, sodium restriction, stress reduction, regular exercise, moderation of alcohol consumption, and smoking cessation). Acebutolol controls but does not cure hypertension.

EVALUATION

Effectiveness of therapy can be demonstrated by: ■ Decrease in blood pressure ■ Control of arrhythmias without appearance of detrimental side effects.

ACETAMINOPHEN

(a-seat-a-**min**-oh-fen)

{Abenol}, Acephen, Aceta, Actamin, {Actimol}, Aminofen, Apacet, APAP, {Apo-Acetaminophen}, Arthritis Foundation Pain Reliever Aspirin-Free, Aspirin Free Anacin, Aspirin Free Pain Relief, Atasol, Banesin, Dapa, Dapacin, Datril, {Exdol}, Fem-Etts, Feverall, Genapap, Genebs, Halenol, Liquiprin, Mapap, Maranox, Meda, Neopap, Panadol, paracetamol, Redutemp, {Robigesic}, {Rounox}, Silapap, Snaplets-FR, St. Joseph's Aspirin-Free, Tapanol, Tempra, Tylenol, Uni-Ace, Valorin

CLASSIFICATION(S):
Antipyretic, Nonopioid analgesic

Pregnancy Category B

INDICATIONS

■ Mild to moderate pain ■ Fever.

ACTION

■ Inhibits the synthesis of prostaglandins that may serve as mediators of pain and fever. **Therapeutic Effects:** ■ Analgesia ■ Antipyresis ■ No significant anti-inflammatory properties.

PHARMACOKINETICS

Absorption: Well absorbed following oral administration. Rectal absorption is variable.
Distribution: Widely distributed. Crosses the placenta; enters breast milk.
Protein Binding: Low at therapeutic doses; 20–50% at toxic levels.
Metabolism and Excretion: 85–95% metabolized by the liver. Metabolites may be toxic in overdose situation. Metabolites excreted by the kidneys.
Half-life: 1–4 hr.

A

CONTRAINDICATIONS AND PRECAUTIONS

Contraindicated in: ▪ Previous hypersensitivity ▪ Products containing alcohol, aspartame, saccharin, sugar, or tartrazine (FDC yellow dye #5) should be avoided in patients who have hypersensitivity or intolerance to these compounds.

Use Cautiously in: ▪ Severe hepatic disease ▪ Renal disease ▪ Chronic alcohol use/abuse ▪ Malnutrition.

ADVERSE REACTIONS AND SIDE EFFECTS*

GI: HEPATIC NECROSIS (overdose).
Derm: rash, urticaria.

INTERACTIONS

Drug-Drug: ▪ Chronic concurrent use with **NSAIDs,** including **aspirin,** may increase the risk of adverse renal reactions ▪ **Diflunisal** increases acetaminophen blood levels and may increase the risk of hepatotoxicity with chronic concurrent use ▪ Chronic high-dose acetaminophen (>2 g/day) may increase the risk of bleeding with **warfarin** ▪ Hepatotoxicity may be additive with other **hepatotoxic substances,** including **alcohol.**

ROUTE AND DOSAGE

Children ≤12 yr should not receive >5 doses/24 hr without notifying physician or other health care professional.

- **PO (Adults):** 325–650 mg q 4–6 hr or 1 g 3–4 times daily (not to exceed 4 g/day).
- **PO (Children):** 10–15 mg/kg q 4 hr.
- **Rect (Adults and Children >12 yr):** 650 mg q 4–6 hr.
- **Rect (Children 6–12 yr):** 325 mg q 4–6 hr (not to exceed 2.6 g/24 hr).
- **Rect (Children 3–6 yr):** 125 mg q 4–6 hr (not to exceed 720 mg/24 hr).
- **Rect (Children 1–3 yr):** 80 mg q 4 hr.
- **Rect (Children 3–11 mo):** 80 mg q 6 hr.

AVAILABILITY

▪ ***Chewable tablets:*** 80 mg^{OTC}, 120 mg^{OTC}, 160 mg^{OTC} ▪ ***Granules:*** 80 mg/packet^{OTC} ▪ ***Oral powder (capsule for sprinkle):*** 80 mg^{OTC}, 160 mg^{OTC} ▪ ***Tablets:*** 120 mg^{OTC}, 160 mg^{OTC}, 325 mg^{OTC}, 500 mg^{OTC}, 650 mg^{OTC} ▪ ***Extended-release tablets:*** 650 mg^{OTC} ▪ ***Capsules:*** 325 mg^{OTC}, 500 mg^{OTC} ▪ ***Solution:*** {80 mg/ml^{OTC}}, 100 mg/ml^{OTC}, 80 mg/1.66 ml^{OTC}, 80 mg/5 ml^{OTC}, 120 mg/5 ml^{OTC}, 130 mg/5 ml^{OTC}, 160 mg/5 ml^{OTC} ▪ ***Liquid:*** 160 mg/5 ml^{OTC}, 500 mg/15 ml^{OTC} ▪ ***Elixir:*** 80 mg/2.5 ml^{OTC}, 80 mg/5 ml^{OTC}, 120 mg/5 ml^{OTC}, 160 mg/5 ml^{OTC} ▪ ***Suspension:*** 32 mg/ml^{OTC}, 48 mg/ml^{OTC}, 80 mg/ml^{OTC}, 100 mg/ml^{OTC}, {80 mg/5 ml^{OTC}}, 160 mg/5 ml^{OTC} ▪ ***Syrup:*** 16 mg/ml^{OTC} ▪ ***Suppositories:*** 80 mg^{OTC}, 120 mg^{OTC}, 300 mg^{OTC}, 325 mg^{OTC}, 650 mg^{OTC} ▪ ***In combination with:*** many other medications. See Appendix A.

TIME/ACTION PROFILE (analgesia and antipyresis)

	ONSET	PEAK	DURATION
PO	0.5–1 hr	1–3 hr	3–4 hr
PO-ER	UK	UK	up to 8 hr
Rect	0.5–1 hr	1–3 hr	3–4 hr

NURSING IMPLICATIONS

ASSESSMENT

- **General Info:** Assess overall health status and alcohol usage before administering acetaminophen. Malnourished patients or chronic alcohol abusers are at higher risk of developing hepatotoxicity with chronic use of usual doses of this drug.
- □ Assess amount, frequency, and type of drugs taken in patients self-medicating, especially with OTC drugs. Prolonged use of acetaminophen and salicylates or NSAIDs increases the risk of renal adverse effects. For short-term use, combined doses of acetaminophen and salicylates should not exceed the recommended dose of either drug given alone.
- **Pain:** Assess type, location, and intensity prior to and 30–60 min following administration.
- **Fever:** Assess fever; note presence of associated signs (diaphoresis, tachycardia, and malaise).
- ***Lab Test Considerations:*** Hepatic, hematologic, and renal function should be evaluated periodically throughout prolonged, high-dose therapy.
- □ May alter results of blood glucose monitoring. May cause falsely decreased values when measured with glucose oxidase/peroxidase method, but probably not with hexokinase/

*CAPITALS indicate life-threatening; underlines indicate most frequent.

glucose-6-phosphate dehydrogenase (G6PD) method. May also cause falsely increased values with certain instruments; see manufacturer's instruction manual.

- □ Increased serum bilirubin, LDH, AST, ALT, and prothrombin time may indicate hepatotoxicity.
- ■ ***Toxicity and Overdose:*** If overdose occurs, acetylcysteine (Mucomyst) is the antidote.

POTENTIAL NURSING DIAGNOSES

- ■ Pain (Indications).
- ■ Body temperature, altered, risk for (Indications).
- ■ Knowledge deficit, related to medication regimen (Patient/Family Teaching).

IMPLEMENTATION

- ■ **General Info:** When combined with opioids do not exceed the maximum recommended daily dose of acetaminophen.
- ■ **PO:** Administer with a full glass of water.
- □ May be taken with food or on an empty stomach.

PATIENT/FAMILY TEACHING

- □ Advise patient to take medication exactly as directed and not to take more than the recommended amount. Severe and permanent liver damage may result from prolonged use or high doses of acetaminophen. Renal damage may occur with prolonged use of acetaminophen and salicylates or NSAIDs. Adults should not take acetaminophen longer than 10 days and children not longer than 5 days unless directed by health care professional. Short-term doses of acetaminophen with salicylates or NSAIDs should not exceed the recommended daily dose of either drug alone.
- □ Advise patient to avoid alcohol (3 or more glasses per day increase the risk of liver damage) if taking more than an occasional 1–2 doses and to avoid taking concurrently with salicylates or NSAIDs for more than a few days, unless directed by health care professional.
- □ Advise parents to check concentrations of liquid preparations. Errors have resulted in serious liver damage.
- □ Inform patients with diabetes that acetaminophen may alter results of blood glucose monitoring. Advise patient to notify health care professional if changes are noted.
- □ Advise patient to consult the health care professional if discomfort or fever is not relieved by routine doses of this drug or if fever is greater than 39.5°C (103°F) or lasts longer than 3 days.

EVALUATION

Effectiveness of therapy can be demonstrated by: ■ Relief of mild to moderate pain ■ Reduction of fever.

ACETYLCYSTEINE

(a-se-teel-**sis**-teen)

Mucomyst, Mucosil

CLASSIFICATION(S):

Antidote (acetaminophen), Mucolytic

Pregnancy Category B

INDICATIONS

■ **PO:** Overdosage of acetaminophen ■ **Inhalation:** Mucolytic.

ACTION

■ **PO:** Decreases the buildup of a hepatotoxic metabolite in acetaminophen overdosage ■ **Inhalation:** Degrades mucus, allowing easier mobilization and expectoration. **Therapeutic Effects:** ■ **PO:** Prevention of liver damage following acetaminophen overdose by decreasing the buildup of a hepatotoxic metabolite ■ **Inhalation:** Lowers the viscosity of mucus.

PHARMACOKINETICS

Absorption: Absorbed from the GI tract following oral administration. Action is local following inhalation; remainder may be absorbed from pulmonary epithelium.

Distribution: UK.

Protein Binding: UK.

Metabolism and Excretion: Metabolized by the liver.

Half-life: UK.

CONTRAINDICATIONS AND PRECAUTIONS

Contraindicated in: ■ Hypersensitivity.

Use Cautiously in: ■ Severe respiratory insufficiency or asthma ■ Geriatric or debilitated patients ▪ History of GI bleeding (oral only) ▪ Pregnancy or lactation (safety not established).

ADVERSE REACTIONS AND SIDE EFFECTS*

CNS: drowsiness.
EENT: rhinorrhea, stomatitis.
Resp: increased secretions.
GI: nausea, vomiting.
Derm: urticaria.
Misc: chills, fever.

INTERACTIONS

Drug-Drug: ▪ **Activated charcoal** may adsorb acetylcysteine and decrease its effectiveness as an antidote.

ROUTE AND DOSAGE

❑ Acetaminophen Overdose

▪ **PO (Adults and Children):** 140 mg/kg initially, followed by 70 mg/kg q 4 hr for 17 additional doses.

❑ Mucolytic

▪ **Inhalation (Adults and Children):** *Nebulization via face mask:* 1–10 ml of 20% solution or 2–20 ml of 10% solution q 2–6 hr; *nebulization via tent or croupette:* amount of 10–20% solution required to produce heavy mist; *direct instillation:* 1–2 ml of 10–20% solution q 1–4 hr.

AVAILABILITY

▪ ***Solution:*** 10%[Rx], 20%[Rx].

TIME/ACTION PROFILE

	ONSET	PEAK	DURATION
PO (antidote)	UK	UK	4 hr
Inhaln (mucolytic)	1 min	5–10 min	short

NURSING IMPLICATIONS

ASSESSMENT

▪ **Antidote in Acetaminophen Overdose:** Assess type, amount, and time of acetaminophen ingestion. Assess plasma acetaminophen levels. Initial levels are drawn at least 4 hr after ingestion of acetaminophen. Plasma level determinations may be difficult to interpret following ingestion of extended-release preparations. Do not wait for results to administer dose.

☐ Monitor AST, ALT, and bilirubin levels along with prothrombin time every 24 hr for 96 hr in patients with plasma acetaminophen levels, which indicate potential hepatotoxicity.

☐ Monitor cardiac and renal function (creatinine, BUN), serum glucose, and electrolytes. Maintain fluid and electrolyte balance, correct hypoglycemia, and administer vitamin K_1 or fresh frozen plasma or clotting factor concentrate if prothrombin time ratio exceeds 1.5 or 3, respectively.

☐ Assess patient for nausea, vomiting, and urticaria. Notify physician if these occur.

▪ **Mucolytic:** Assess respiratory function (lung sounds, dyspnea) and color, amount, and consistency of secretions before and immediately following treatment to determine effectiveness of therapy.

POTENTIAL NURSING DIAGNOSES

▪ Violence, risk for, directed at self (Indications).
▪ Airway clearance, ineffective (Indications).
▪ Knowledge deficit, related to medication regimen (Patient/Family Teaching).

IMPLEMENTATION

▪ **General Info:** After opening, may turn light purple; does not alter potency. Refrigerate open vials and discard after 96 hr.

☐ Drug reacts with rubber and metals (iron, nickel, copper); avoid contact with these substances.

▪ **PO: Acetaminophen Overdose**—First empty stomach contents by inducing emesis or lavage. Dilute 20% solution with cola, water, or juice to a final concentration of 1 : 3 for patients weighing up to 20 kg or with enough diluent to make a 5% solution for patients weighing more than 20 kg, to increase palatability. May be administered by duodenal tube if patient is unable to swallow. If patient vomits loading dose or maintenance doses within 1 hr of administration, readminister dose.

▪ **Inhalation: Mucolytic**—Encourage adequate fluid intake (2000–3000 ml/day) to decrease viscosity of secretions.

☐ For nebulization, the 20% solution may be di-

*CAPITALS indicate life-threatening; underlines indicate most frequent.

luted with 0.9% NaCl for injection or inhalation or sterile water for injection or inhalation. May use 10% solution undiluted. May be administered by nebulization, or 1–2 ml may be instilled directly into airway. During administration, when 25% of medication remains in nebulizer, dilute with equal amount of 0.9% NaCl or sterile water.

- □ An increased volume of liquefied bronchial secretions may occur following administration. Have suction equipment available for patients unable to effectively clear airways.
- □ If bronchospasm occurs during treatment, discontinue and consult health care professional regarding possible addition of bronchodilator to therapy. Patients with asthma or hyperactive airway disease should be given a bronchodilator prior to acetylcysteine to prevent bronchospasm.
- □ Rinse patient's mouth and wash face following treatment, as drug leaves a sticky residue.

PATIENT/FAMILY TEACHING

- ▪ **Inhalation:** Instruct patient to clear airway by coughing deeply before taking aerosol treatment.
- □ Inform patient that unpleasant odor of this drug becomes less noticeable as treatment progresses.

EVALUATION

Effectiveness of therapy can be demonstrated by: ▪ Decreased acetaminophen levels □ No further increase in hepatic damage during acetaminophen overdose therapy ▪ Decreased dyspnea and clearing of lung sounds when used as a mucolytic.

ACTIVATED CHARCOAL

Acta-Char Liquid-A, Actidose-Aqua, {Aqueous Charcodote}, {Charac-50}, CharcoAid 2000, {Charcodote}, Insta-Char, Insta-Char Aqueous Suspension, Liqui-Char, SuperChar Aqueous

CLASSIFICATION(S):
Antidote (adsorbent)

Pregnancy Category C

INDICATIONS

▪ Acute management of many oral poisonings following emesis/lavage.

ACTION

▪ Binds drugs and chemicals within the GI tract. **Therapeutic Effects:** ▪ Decreased intestinal absorption of drugs or chemicals in the overdose situation, thereby preventing toxicity.

PHARMACOKINETICS

Absorption: None.
Distribution: None.
Metabolism and Excretion: Excreted unchanged in the feces.
Half-life: UK.

CONTRAINDICATIONS AND PRECAUTIONS

Contraindicated in: ▪ No known contraindications.
Use Cautiously in: ▪ Poisonings due to cyanide, corrosives, ethanol, methanol, petroleum distillates, organic solvents, mineral acids, or iron ▪ Endoscopic examination (observation will be obscured).

ADVERSE REACTIONS AND SIDE EFFECTS*

GI: black stools, constipation, diarrhea, vomiting.

INTERACTIONS

Drug-Drug: ▪ **Other drugs** including **ipecac** and **laxatives** will be adsorbed by charcoal and as a result will not be systemically absorbed from the GI tract.
Drug-Food: ▪ **Milk**, **ice cream**, and **sherbet** will decrease the ability of charcoal to absorb other agents.

ROUTE AND DOSAGE

□ **Antidote**

- ▪ **PO (Adults):** 25–100 g (may be repeated q 4–6 hr).
- ▪ **PO (Children 1–12 yr):** 25–50 g (may be repeated q 4–6 hr).

{} = Available in Canada only.
***CAPITALS indicate life-threatening; underlines indicate most frequent.**

- **PO (Children < 1 yr):** 1 g/kg (may be repeated q 4–6 hr).

AVAILABILITY

- ***Powder:*** 15-, {25-}, 30-, 40-, 120-, 125-, 240-g[OTC] containers - ***Oral suspension:*** 12.5 g/60 ml[OTC], 15 g/72 ml[OTC], 15 g/120 ml[OTC], 25 g/120 ml[OTC], 30 g/120 ml[OTC], 50 g/240 ml[OTC], 15 g/120 ml[OTC], 25 g/125 ml[OTC], 50 g/225 ml[OTC], 50 g/250 ml[OTC] - ***In combination with:*** sorbitol (Actidose with Sorbitol, Charcoaid, {Pediatric Charcodote}, {Charac-tol}, {Charcodote TFS})[OTC].

TIME/ACTION PROFILE (antidote)

	ONSET	PEAK	DURATION
PO	within min	UK	4–12 hr

NURSING IMPLICATIONS

ASSESSMENT

- Assess neurologic status; administer only if patient is alert (unless airway is protected).
- Inquire as to the type of drug or poison and time of ingestion.
- Consult reference, poison control center, or physician for symptoms of toxicity of ingested agent(s).
- Monitor blood pressure, pulse, respiratory and neurologic status, and urine output as indicated by toxicity of agent(s). Notify physician if symptoms persist or worsen.
- ***Lab Test Considerations:*** Chronic use may impair absorption of essential nutrients. This may result in decreased mineral or electrolyte levels.

POTENTIAL NURSING DIAGNOSES

- Violence, risk for, directed at self (Indications).
- Injury, risk for (Indications).

IMPLEMENTATION

- **Treatment of Poisoning:** Activated charcoal is most effective if administered within 30 min of ingestion of drug or poison. Dosage may be repeated for drugs subjected to enterohepatic elimination to minimize further absorption.
- Administer syrup of ipecac first and wait until emesis occurs before administering activated charcoal.
- Tablets and capsules should not be used in the treatment of poisoning.
- **PO:** Mix dose in 6–8 oz water; administer as a slurry (unless using suspension with or without sorbitol). Do not administer with milk products (milk, ice cream, or sherbet). May need to be diluted with additional water to be thin enough to administer through a nasogastric tube.
- Shake oral suspension well before administration.
- Rapid ingestion may cause vomiting. If vomiting occurs shortly after administering dose, confer with physician about repeating dose.
- Do not administer other oral drugs for 2 hr before or after administering activated charcoal.
- Slurry is constipating; physician may order a laxative to speed removal of the drug. Sorbitol or magnesium citrate is commonly used for this purpose and may cause diarrhea. Some products contain sorbitol.

PATIENT/FAMILY TEACHING

- **General Info:** Inform patient that stools will turn black.
- **Poisoning:** When counseling, discuss methods of prevention, need to confer with poison control center, physician, or emergency department prior to administering, and need to bring ingested substance to emergency room for identification.

EVALUATION

Effectiveness of therapy can be demonstrated by: - Prevention or resolution of toxic effects of ingested agent.

ACYCLOVIR

(ay-**sye**-kloe-veer)
{Avirax}, Zovirax

CLASSIFICATION(S):
Antiviral

Pregnancy Category C

INDICATIONS

▪ **PO:** Treatment and prophylaxis of recurrent genital herpes infections. Treatment of localized cutaneous herpes zoster infections (shingles) and chickenpox (varicella) ▪ **IV:** Treatment of severe initial episodes of genital herpes in non-immunosuppressed patients. Management of mucosal or cutaneous herpes simplex infections or herpes zoster infections (shingles) in immunosuppressed patients. Treatment of herpes simplex encephalitis in patients>6 mo ▪ **Topical:** Treatment of herpes genitalis infections.

ACTION

▪ Interferes with viral DNA synthesis. **Therapeutic Effects:** ▪ Inhibition of viral replication, decreased viral shedding, and reduced time to healing of lesions.

PHARMACOKINETICS

Absorption: Oral absorption is poor (15–30%), although therapeutic blood levels are achieved.
Distribution: Widely distributed. CSF concentrations are 50% of plasma. Crosses the placenta.
Metabolism and Excretion: >90% eliminated unchanged by the kidneys; remainder metabolized by the liver.
Half-life: 2.1–3.5 hr (increased in renal failure).

CONTRAINDICATIONS AND PRECAUTIONS

Contraindicated in: ▪ Hypersensitivity.
Use Cautiously in: ▪ Pre-existing serious neurologic, hepatic, pulmonary, or fluid and electrolyte abnormalities ▪ Renal impairment (dosage alteration recommended if CCr <50 ml/min) ▪ Obese patients (dose should be based on ideal body weight) ▪ Pregnancy and lactation (safety not established).

ADVERSE REACTIONS AND SIDE EFFECTS*

CNS: SEIZURES, dizziness, headache, hallucinations, trembling.
GI: diarrhea, nausea, vomiting, abdominal pain, anorexia.
GU: RENAL FAILURE, crystalluria, hematuria.
Derm: acne, hives, skin rashes, unusual sweating.
Endo: changes in menstrual cycle.
Local: pain, phlebitis.
MS: joint pain.
Misc: polydipsia.

INTERACTIONS

Drug-Drug: ▪ **Probenecid** increases blood levels of acyclovir ▪ Concurrent use of other **nephrotoxic drugs** increases the risk of adverse renal effects ▪ **Zidovudine** and intrathecal **methotrexate** may increase the risk of CNS side effects.

ROUTE AND DOSAGE

❑ Initial Genital Herpes

- **PO (Adults):** 200 mg q 4 hr while awake (5 times a day) for 10 days.
- **IV (Adults):** 5 mg/kg q 8 hr for 5 days.

❑ Chronic Suppressive Therapy for Recurrent Genital Herpes

- **PO (Adults):** 400 mg twice daily or 200 mg 3–5 times daily for up to 12 mo.

❑ Intermittent Therapy for Recurrent Genital Herpes

- **PO (Adults):** 200 mg q 4 hr while awake (5 times a day) for 5 days, initiated at first sign of symptoms.

❑ Acute Treatment of Herpes Zoster

- **PO (Adults):** 800 mg q 4 hr while awake (5 times a day) for 7–10 days.

❑ Chickenpox

- **PO (Adults and Children):** 20 mg/kg (not to exceed 800 mg/dose) qid for 5 days.

❑ Mucosal and Cutaneous Herpes Simplex Infections in Immunosuppressed Patients

- **IV (Adults and Children >12 yr):** 5–10 mg/kg q 8 hr for 7–10 days.
- **IV (Children <12 yr):** 250 mg/m² q 8 hr for 7 days.
- **Topical (Adults):** ½-in. ribbon of 5% ointment for every 4-square-in. area q 3 hr 6 times/day for 7 days.

***CAPITALS indicate life-threatening; underlines indicate most frequent.**

Herpes Simplex Encephalitis

- **IV (Adults):** 10 mg/kg q 8 hr for 10 days.
- **IV (Children <12 yr):** 500 mg/m^2 q 8 hr for 10 days.

Varicella Zoster Infections in Immunosuppressed Patients

- **IV (Adults):** 10 mg/kg q 8 hr for 7 days.
- **IV (Children <12 yr):** 500 mg/m^2 q 8 hr for 7 days.

AVAILABILITY

▪ ***Capsules:*** 200 mg[Rx] ▪ ***Tablets:*** 200 mg[Rx], 400 mg[Rx], 800 mg[Rx] ▪ ***Suspension:*** 200 mg/5 ml[Rx] ▪ ***Injection:*** 500-mg vials[Rx], 1000-mg vials[Rx].

TIME/ACTION PROFILE (antiviral blood levels)

	ONSET	PEAK	DURATION
PO	UK	1.5–2.5 hr	4 hr
IV	prompt	end of infusion	8 hr

NURSING IMPLICATIONS

ASSESSMENT

- Assess lesions before and daily during therapy.
- Monitor neurologic status in patients with herpes encephalitis.
- ***Lab Test Considerations:*** Monitor BUN, serum creatinine, and CCr before and during therapy. Increased BUN and serum creatinine levels or decreased CCr may indicate renal failure.

POTENTIAL NURSING DIAGNOSES

- Skin integrity, impaired (Indications, Patient/Family Teaching).
- Knowledge deficit, related to medication regimen (Patient/Family Teaching).

IMPLEMENTATION

- **General Info:** Acyclovir treatment should be started as soon as possible after herpes simplex symptoms appear and within 24 hr of herpes zoster outbreak.
- **PO:** Acyclovir may be administered with food or on an empty stomach, with a full glass of water.
- Shake oral suspension well before administration.
- **IV:** Maintain adequate hydration (2000–3000 ml/day), especially during first 2 hr following IV infusion, to prevent crystalluria.
- Observe infusion site for phlebitis. Rotate infusion site to prevent phlebitis.
- Acyclovir sodium should not be administered topically, IM, SC, PO, or in the eye.
- **Intermittent Infusion:** Reconstitute 500-mg or 1-g vial with 10 ml or 20 ml, respectively, of sterile water for injection for a concentration of 50 mg/ml. Do not reconstitute with bacteriostatic water with benzyl alcohol or parabens. Shake well to dissolve completely. Dilute in at least 100 ml of D5W, D5/0.25% NaCl, D5/0.45% NaCl, D5/0.9% NaCl, 0.9% NaCl, or LR for a concentration not to exceed 7 mg/ml. Use reconstituted solution within 12 hr. Once diluted for infusion, should be used within 24 hr. Refrigeration results in precipitation, which dissolves at room temperature.
- ***Rate:*** Administer via infusion pump over at least 1 hr to minimize renal tubular damage.
- **Y-Site Compatibility:** ▪ allopurinol ▪ amikacin ▪ ampicillin ▪ cefamandole ▪ cefazolin ▪ cefonicid ▪ cefoperazone ▪ cefotaxime ▪ cefoxitin ▪ ceftazidime ▪ ceftizoxime ▪ ceftriaxone ▪ cefuroxime ▪ cephapirin ▪ chloramphenicol ▪ cimetidine ▪ clindamycin ▪ dexamethasone sodium phosphate ▪ dimenhydrinate ▪ diphenhydramine ▪ doxycycline ▪ erythromycin lactobionate ▪ filgrastim ▪ fluconazole ▪ gallium nitrate ▪ gentamicin ▪ heparin ▪ hydrocortisone sodium succinate ▪ hydromorphone ▪ imipenem/cilastatin ▪ lorazepam ▪ magnesium sulfate ▪ melphalan ▪ methylprednisolone sodium succinate ▪ metoclopramide ▪ metronidazole ▪ multivitamin infusion ▪ nafcillin ▪ oxacillin ▪ paclitaxel ▪ penicillin G potassium ▪ pentobarbital ▪ perphenazine ▪ piperacillin ▪ potassium chloride ▪ ranitidine ▪ sodium bicarbonate ▪ tacrolimus ▪ teniposide ▪ theophylline ▪ thiotepa ▪ ticarcillin ▪ tobramycin ▪ trimethoprim-sulfamethoxazole ▪ vancomycin ▪ zidovudine.
- **Y-Site Incompatibility:** ▪ amifostine ▪ aztreonam ▪ dobutamine ▪ dopamine ▪ fludarabine ▪ foscarnet ▪ idarubicin ▪ ondansetron ▪ piperacillin/tazobactam ▪ sargramostim ▪ vinorelbine.
- **Additive Compatibility:** ▪ fluconazole.
- **Additive Incompatibility:** ▪ blood products ▪ protein-containing solutions.

- **Topical:** Apply to skin lesions only; do not use in the eye.

PATIENT/FAMILY TEACHING

- **General Info:** Advise patient to take medication exactly as directed for the full course of therapy. If a dose is missed, take as soon as possible but not just before next dose is due; do not double doses. Acyclovir should not be used more frequently or longer than prescribed.
- □ Advise patients that the additional use of OTC creams, lotions, and ointments may delay healing and may cause spreading of lesions.
- □ Inform patient that acyclovir is not a cure, as the virus lies dormant in the ganglia, and it will not prevent the spread of infection to others.
- □ Advise patient that condoms should be used during sexual contact and that no sexual contact should be made while lesions are present.
- □ Patient should consult health care professional if symptoms are not relieved following 7 days of topical therapy or if oral acyclovir does not decrease the frequency and severity of recurrences.
- □ Instruct women with genital herpes to have yearly PAP smears because they may be more likely to develop cervical cancer.
- **Topical:** Instruct patient to apply ointment in sufficient quantity to cover all lesions every 3 hr, 6 times/day for 7 days. One ½-in. ribbon of ointment covers approximately 4 square in. Use a finger cot or glove when applying to prevent inoculation of other areas or spread to other people. Keep affected areas clean and dry. Loose-fitting clothing should be worn to prevent irritation.
- □ Avoid drug contact in or around eyes. Report any unexplained eye symptoms to health care professional immediately, as ocular herpetic infection can lead to blindness.

EVALUATION

Effectiveness of therapy can be demonstrated by: ▪ Crusting over and healing of skin lesions ▪ Decrease in frequency and severity of recurrences ▪ Shortening of time to complete healing and cessation of pain in herpes zoster ▪ Decrease in intensity of chickenpox.

ADENOSINE

(a-**den**-oh-seen)

Adenocard, Adenoscan

CLASSIFICATION(S):

Antiarrhythmic

Pregnancy Category C

INDICATIONS

▪ Conversion of paroxysmal supraventricular tachycardia (PSVT) to normal sinus rhythm when vagal maneuvers are unsuccessful ▪ As a diagnostic agent (with noninvasive techniques) to assess myocardial perfusion defects occurring as a consequence of coronary artery disease.

ACTION

▪ Restores normal sinus rhythm by interrupting re-entrant pathways in the AV node ▪ Slows conduction time through the AV node ▪ Also produces coronary artery vasodilation. **Therapeutic Effects:** ▪ Restoration of normal sinus rhythm.

PHARMACOKINETICS

Absorption: Following IV administration, absorption is complete.
Distribution: Taken up by erythrocytes and vascular endothelium.
Metabolism and Excretion: Rapidly converted to inosine and adenosine monophosphate.
Half-life: <10 sec.

CONTRAINDICATIONS AND PRECAUTIONS

Contraindicated in: ▪ Hypersensitivity ▪ 2nd- or 3rd-degree AV block or sick sinus syndrome, unless a functional artificial pacemaker is present.
Use Cautiously in: ▪ Patients with a history of asthma (may induce bronchospasm) ▪ Unstable angina ▪ Pregnancy, lactation, or children (safety not established).

ADVERSE REACTIONS AND SIDE EFFECTS*

CNS: apprehension, dizziness, headache, head pressure, light-headedness.

*CAPITALS indicate life-threatening; underlines indicate most frequent.

EENT: blurred vision, throat tightness.
Resp: shortness of breath, chest pressure, hyperventilation.
CV: facial flushing, transient arrhythmias, chest pain, hypotension, palpitations.
GI: metallic taste, nausea.
Derm: burning sensation, facial flushing, sweating.
MS: neck and back pain.
Neuro: numbness, tingling.
Misc: heaviness in arms, pressure sensation in groin.

INTERACTIONS

Drug-Drug: ▪ **Carbamazepine** may increase the risk of progressive heart block ▪ **Dipyridamole** potentiates the effects of adenosine (dosage reduction of adenosine recommended) ▪ Effects of adenosine may be decreased by **theophylline** or **caffeine** (larger doses of adenosine may be required) ▪ Concurrent use with digitalis glycosides may increase the risk of ventricular fibrillation.

ROUTE AND DOSAGE

- **IV (Adults):** *Antiarrhythmic*—6 mg by rapid IV bolus; if no results, repeat 1–2 min later as 12-mg rapid bolus. This dose may be repeated (single dose not to exceed 12 mg). *Diagnostic use*—140 mcg/kg/min for 6 min (0.84 mg/kg total).

AVAILABILITY

- ***Injection:*** 6 mg/2-ml vial[Rx] (Adenocard), 3 mg/1 ml in 30-ml vial[Rx] (Adenoscan).

TIME/ACTION PROFILE (antiarrhythmic effect)

	ONSET	PEAK	DURATION
IV	immediate	UK	1–2 min

NURSING IMPLICATIONS

ASSESSMENT

- □ Monitor heart rate frequently (every 15–30 sec) and ECG continuously throughout therapy. Once conversion to normal sinus rhythm is achieved, transient arrhythmias (premature ventricular contractions, atrial premature contractions, sinus tachycardia, sinus bradycardia, skipped beats, AV nodal block) may occur, but generally last a few seconds.
- □ Monitor blood pressure during therapy.
- □ Assess respiratory status (breath sounds, rate) following administration. Patients with history of asthma may experience bronchospasm.

POTENTIAL NURSING DIAGNOSES

- ▪ Cardiac output, decreased (Indications).
- ▪ Knowledge deficit, related to medication regimen (Patient/Family Teaching).

IMPLEMENTATION

- ▪ **General Info:** Do not confuse adenosine (Adenocard) with ***adenosine phosphate***.
- □ Crystals may occur if adenosine is refrigerated. Warm to room temperature to dissolve crystals. Solution must be clear before use. Discard unused portions.
- ▪ **Direct IV:** Administer undiluted.
- ▪ ***Rate:*** Administer over 1–2 sec via direct IV or into proximal IV line. Follow with rapid saline flush to ensure injection reaches systemic circulation. Slow administration may cause increased heart rate in response to vasodilation.
- ▪ **Continuous Infusion:** Administer 30-ml vial undiluted as a peripheral infusion. Do not administer solutions that are discolored or contain particulate matter. Discard unused portion.
- ▪ ***Rate:*** Administer at a rate of 140 mcg/kg/min over 6 min for a total dose of 0.84 mg/kg. Thallium-201 should be injected as close to the venous access as possible at the midpoint (after 3 min) of the infusion.
- ▪ **Y-Site Compatibility:** ▪ ▪ Thallium-201.

PATIENT/FAMILY TEACHING

- □ Caution patient to make position changes slowly to minimize orthostatic hypotension. Doses >12 mg decrease blood pressure by decreasing peripheral vascular resistance.
- □ Instruct patient to report facial flushing, shortness of breath, or dizziness.

EVALUATION

Effectiveness of therapy can be demonstrated by: ▪ Conversion of supraventricular tachycardia to normal sinus rhythm ▪ Diagnosis of myocardial perfusion defects.

ALBUMIN, Human
(al-**byoo**-min)
Albuminar, Albutein, Buminate, normal human serum albumin, Plasbumin

CLASSIFICATION(S):
Volume expander

Pregnancy Category C

INDICATIONS

▪ Expansion of plasma volume and maintenance of cardiac output in situations associated with fluid volume deficit including shock, hemorrhage, and burns ▪ Temporary replacement of albumin in diseases associated with low levels of plasma proteins such as nephrotic syndrome or end-stage liver disease, resulting in relief or reduction of associated edema.

ACTION

▪ Provides colloidal oncotic pressure, which serves to mobilize fluid from extravascular tissues back into the intravascular space. **Therapeutic Effects:** ▪ Increase in intravascular fluid volume.

PHARMACOKINETICS

Absorption: Following IV administration, absorption is essentially complete.
Distribution: Confined to the intravascular space, unless capillary permeability is increased.
Metabolism and Excretion: Probably degraded by the liver.
Half-life: 2–3 wk.

CONTRAINDICATIONS AND PRECAUTIONS

Contraindicated in: ▪ Allergic reactions to albumin ▪ Severe anemia ▪ Congestive heart failure ▪ Normal or increased intravascular volume.
Use Cautiously in: ▪ Severe hepatic or renal disease ▪ Dehydration (additional fluids may be required).

ADVERSE REACTIONS AND SIDE EFFECTS*

CNS: headache.
CV: PULMONARY EDEMA, fluid overload, hypertension, hypotension, tachycardia.
GI: increased salivation, nausea, vomiting.
Derm: rash, urticaria.
MS: back pain.
Misc: chills, fever, flushing.

INTERACTIONS

Drug-Drug: ▪ None significant.

ROUTE AND DOSAGE

Dose is highly individualized and depends on condition being treated.

❑ **5% Albumin**

❑ ***Shock***

- **IV (Adults):** 500 ml, may be repeated within 30 min.
- **IV (Children):** 50 ml.
- **IV (Infants and Neonates):** 10–20 ml/kg as a 5% solution.

❑ **25% Albumin**

❑ ***Hypoproteinemia***

- **IV (Adults):** 50–75 g
- **IV (Children):** 25 g

❑ ***Acute Nephrosis***

- **IV (Adults):** 100 ml given daily with a loop diuretic for 7–10 days (until response to glucocorticoids occurs).

AVAILABILITY

▪ ***Injection:*** 5%[Rx], 25%[Rx].

TIME/ACTION PROFILE (oncotic effect)

	ONSET	PEAK	DURATION
IV	15–30 min	UK	UK

NURSING IMPLICATIONS

ASSESSMENT

▪ **General Info:** Monitor vital signs, CVP, and intake and output prior to and frequently throughout therapy. If fever, tachycardia, or hypotension occurs, stop infusion and notify physician immediately. Antihistamines may be

*CAPITALS indicate life-threatening; underlines indicate most frequent.

required to suppress this hypersensitivity response. Hypotension may also result from infusing too rapidly. May be given without regard to patient's blood group.

- □ Assess for signs of vascular overload (elevated CVP, rales/crackles, dyspnea, hypertension, jugular venous distention) during and following administration.
- ▪ **Surgical Patients:** Assess for increased bleeding following administration caused by increased blood pressure and circulating blood volume. Albumin does not contain clotting factors.
- ▪ ***Lab Test Considerations:*** Serum albumin levels should increase with albumin therapy.
- □ Monitor serum sodium levels; may cause increased concentrations.
- □ Infusions of normal serum albumin may cause false elevation of alkaline phosphatase levels.
- ▪ **Hemorrhage:** Monitor hemoglobin and hematocrit levels. These values may decrease because of hemodilution.

POTENTIAL NURSING DIAGNOSES

- ▪ Cardiac output, decreased (Indications).
- ▪ Fluid volume deficit, active loss (Indications).
- ▪ Fluid volume excess (Side Effects).

IMPLEMENTATION

- ▪ **General Info:** Follow manufacturer's recommendations for administration. Administer through a large-gauge (at least 20-gauge) needle or catheter. Following administration, record lot number in patient record.
- □ Solution should be clear amber; 25% albumin solution is equal to 5 times the osmotic value of plasma. Do not administer solutions that are discolored or contain particulate matter. Each liter of normal serum albumin contains 130–160 mEq of sodium and is thus no longer labeled "salt-poor" albumin.
- □ Administration of large quantities of normal serum albumin may need to be supplemented with whole blood to prevent anemia. If more than 1000 ml of 5% normal serum albumin are given or if hemorrhage has occurred, the administration of whole blood or packed red blood cells may be needed. Hydration status should be monitored and maintained with additional fluids.
- ▪ **Continuous Infusion:** Administer 5% normal serum albumin undiluted. Normal serum albumin 25% may be administered undiluted or diluted in 0.9% NaCl, D5W, or sodium lactate injection. Infusion must be completed within 4 hr.
- ▪ ***Rate:*** Rate of administration is determined by concentration of solution, blood volume, indication, and patient response. In patients with normal blood volume, administer at 1–2 ml/min. The rate for children is usually ¼ to ½ the adult rate.
- □ *Hypovolemia:* 5% or 25% normal serum albumin may be administered as rapidly as tolerated and repeated in 15–30 min if necessary.
- □ *Burns:* Rate after the first 24 hr should be set to maintain a plasma albumin level of 2.5 g/100 ml or a total serum protein level of 5.2 g/100 ml.
- □ *Hypoproteinemia:* Normal serum albumin 25% is the preferred solution because of the increased concentration of protein. The rate should not exceed 3 ml/min of 25% or 5–10 ml/min of 5% solution to prevent circulatory overload and pulmonary edema. This treatment provides a temporary rise in plasma protein until the hypoproteinemia is corrected.
- ▪ **Y-Site Compatibility:** ▪ diltiazem.
- ▪ **Y-Site Incompatibility:** ▪ vancomycin ▪ verapamil.
- ▪ **Solution Compatibility:** ▪ Normal serum albumin is compatible with 0.9% NaCl, D5W, D5/0.9% NaCl, D5/0.45% NaCl, sodium lactate ⅙ M, D5/LR, and lactated Ringer's solution.

PATIENT/FAMILY TEACHING

- □ Explain the purpose of this solution to the patient.
- □ Instruct patient to report signs and symptoms of hypersensitivity reaction.

EVALUATION

Effectiveness of therapy can be demonstrated by: ▪ Increase in blood pressure and blood volume when used to treat shock and burns ▪ Increased urinary output reflects the mobilization of fluid from extravascular tissues ▪ Elevated serum plasma protein in patients with hypoproteinemia.

ALBUTEROL

(al-**byoo**-ter-ole)

Airet, {Gen-Salbutamol}, {Novo-Salmol}, Proventil, salbutamol, Ventodisk, Ventolin, Volmax

CLASSIFICATION(S):

Bronchodilator (beta-adrenergic agonist)

Pregnancy Category C

INDICATIONS

▪ Used as a bronchodilator in the management of reversible airway obstruction due to asthma or COPD ▪ **Inhalation:** Used as a quick-relief agent for acute bronchospasm and for prevention of exercise-induced bronchospasm ▪ **PO:** Used as a long-term control agent in patients with chronic/persistent bronchospasm.

ACTION

▪ Results in the accumulation of cyclic adenosine monophosphate (cAMP) at beta-adrenergic receptors ▪ Produces bronchodilation ▪ Relatively selective for beta$_2$ (pulmonary) receptors. **Therapeutic Effects:** ▪ Bronchodilation.

PHARMACOKINETICS

Absorption: Well absorbed following oral administration but rapidly undergoes extensive metabolism.
Distribution: Small amounts appear in breast milk.
Metabolism and Excretion: Extensively metabolized by the liver and other tissues.
Half-life: 3.8 hr.

CONTRAINDICATIONS AND PRECAUTIONS

Contraindicated in: ▪ Hypersensitivity to adrenergic amines ▪ Hypersensitivity to fluorocarbons (inhaler).
Use Cautiously in: ▪ Cardiac disease ▪ Hypertension ▪ Hyperthyroidism ▪ Diabetes ▪ Glaucoma ▪ Elderly patients (more susceptible to adverse reactions; may require dosage reduction) ▪ Pregnancy (near term), lactation, and children <2 yr (safety not established) ▪ Excessive use may lead to tolerance and paradoxical bronchospasm (inhaler).

ADVERSE REACTIONS AND SIDE EFFECTS*

CNS: nervousness, restlessness, tremor, headache, insomnia.
CV: angina, arrhythmias, hypertension.
GI: nausea, vomiting.
Endo: hyperglycemia.

INTERACTIONS

Drug-Drug: ▪ Concurrent use with other **adrenergic (sympathomimetic) agents** will have additive adrenergic side effects ▪ Use with **MAO inhibitors** may lead to hypertensive crisis ▪ **Beta-adrenergic blockers** may negate therapeutic effect.

ROUTE AND DOSAGE

- **PO (Adults and Children ≥14 yr):** 2–6 mg 3–4 times daily (not to exceed 32 mg/day) or 4–8 mg of extended-release tablets (Proventil Repetabs) twice daily.
- **PO (Children 6–14 yr):** 2 mg 3–4 times daily or 0.3–0.6 mg/kg/day in 2 divided doses as extended-release product. May be carefully increased as needed (not to exceed 24 mg/day).
- **PO (Children 2–6 yr):** 0.1 mg/kg 3 times daily (not to exceed 2 mg 3 times daily initially); may be carefully increased to 0.2 mg/kg 3 times daily (not to exceed 4 mg 3 times daily).
- **Inhalation (Adults and Children ≥12 yr):** *Via metered-dose inhaler*—2 inhalations q 4–6 hr or 2 inhalations 15 min prior to exercise (90 mcg/spray).
- **Inhalation (Adults and Children >12 yr):** *Via nebulization or IPPB*—1.25–5 mg 3–4 times daily.
- **Inhalation (Adults and Children ≥12 yr):** *Via Rotahaler inhalation device*—200 mcg (as Ventolin Rotacaps) q 4–6 hr (up to 400 mcg q 4–6 hr). May also be given 15 min prior to exercise.

AVAILABILITY

▪ ***Tablets:*** 2 mg[Rx], 4 mg[Rx] ▪ ***Extended-release tablets:*** 4 mg[Rx] ▪ ***Oral solution:*** 2 mg/5

{} = Available in Canada only.
*CAPITALS indicate life-threatening; underlines indicate most frequent.

ml[Rx] ▪ ***Metered-dose aerosol:*** 90 mcg/spray[Rx], {100 mcg/spray[Rx]}, {80 inhalations/canister[Rx]}, {200 inhalations/canister[Rx]} ▪ ***Inhalation solution:*** 0.83 mg/ml[Rx], {1 mg/ml[Rx]}, {2 mg/ml[Rx]}, 5 mg/ml[Rx] ▪ ***Capsules for inhalation (Rotacaps):*** 200 mcg[Rx], 400 mcg[Rx] ▪ ***In combination with:*** ipratropium (Combivent). See Appendix A.

TIME/ACTION PROFILE (bronchodilation)

	ONSET	PEAK	DURATION
PO	15–30 min	2–3 hr	8 hr or more
PO–ER	30 min	2–3 hr	12 hr
Inhaln	5–15 min	60–90 min	3–6 hr

NURSING IMPLICATIONS

ASSESSMENT

- Assess lung sounds, pulse, and blood pressure before administration and during peak of medication. Note amount, color, and character of sputum produced.
- Monitor pulmonary function tests before initiating therapy and periodically throughout course to determine effectiveness of medication.
- Observe for paradoxical bronchospasm (wheezing). If condition occurs, withhold medication and notify physician or other health care professional immediately.
- ***Lab Test Considerations:*** May cause transient decrease in serum potassium concentrations with nebulization or higher than recommended doses.

POTENTIAL NURSING DIAGNOSES

- Airway clearance, ineffective (Indications).
- Knowledge deficit, related to medication regimen (Patient/Family Teaching).

IMPLEMENTATION

- **PO:**
- Administer oral medication with meals to minimize gastric irritation.
- Extended-release tablets should be swallowed whole; do not break, crush, or chew.
- **Inhalation:** Allow at least 1 min between inhalations of aerosol medication.
- For nebulization or intermittent positive pressure breathing (IPPB), the 0.83 mg/ml solution does not require dilution prior to administration. The 5 mg/ml solution must be diluted with 2–5 or more ml of 0.9% NaCl or sterile water for inhalation. Diluted solutions are stable for 24 hr at room temperature or 48 hr if refrigerated.
- For nebulizer, compressed air or oxygen flow should be 6–10 L/min; a single treatment of 3 ml lasts about 10 min.
- IPPB usually lasts 5–20 min.

PATIENT/FAMILY TEACHING

- **General Info:** Instruct patient to take albuterol exactly as directed. If on a scheduled dosing regimen, take a missed dose as soon as remembered, spacing remaining doses at regular intervals. Do not double doses. Caution patient not to exceed recommended dose; may cause adverse effects, paradoxical bronchospasm, or loss of effectiveness of medication. Advise patient that all agents should not be used for acute attacks.
- Instruct patient to contact physician or other health care professional immediately if shortness of breath is not relieved by medication or is accompanied by diaphoresis, dizziness, palpitations, or chest pain.
- Advise patient to consult health care professional before taking any OTC medications or alcohol concurrently with this therapy. Caution patient to also avoid smoking and other respiratory irritants.
- Inform patient that albuterol may cause an unusual or bad taste.
- **Inhalation:** Instruct patient in the proper use of the metered-dose inhaler or Rotahaler (see Appendix H).
- Advise patients to use albuterol first if using other inhalation medications, and allow 5 min to elapse before administering other inhalant medications unless otherwise directed.
- Advise patient to rinse mouth with water after each inhalation dose to minimize dry mouth.
- Instruct patient to notify health care professional if no response to the usual dose of albuterol or if contents of one canister are used in less than 2 wk.

EVALUATION

Effectiveness of therapy can be demonstrated by: ▪ Prevention or relief of bronchospasm.

ALDESLEUKIN
(al-dess-**loo**-kin)
interleukin-2, IL-2, Proleukin

CLASSIFICATION(S):
Antineoplastic (modified recombinant interleukin)

Pregnancy Category C

INDICATIONS

■ Management of metastatic renal cell carcinoma.

ACTION

■ Increases cellular immunity (noted as lymphocytosis and eosinophilia), increases the production of cytokines (including tumor necrosis factor, interleukin-1, and gamma interferon), and inhibits tumor growth. **Therapeutic Effects:** ■ Regression of renal cell carcinoma.

PHARMACOKINETICS

Absorption: IV administration results in complete bioavailability.
Distribution: Rapidly distributes to intravascular, extracellular space. 70% is taken up by the liver, kidneys, and lungs.
Metabolism and Excretion: Metabolized to amino acids by renal tubular cells.
Half-life: 85 min.

CONTRAINDICATIONS AND PRECAUTIONS

Contraindicated in: ■ Hypersensitivity to aldesleukin or mannitol ■ Cross-sensitivity to *E. coli*–derived proteins may occur ■ Patients with any history of cardiac or pulmonary disease as assessed by abnormal thallium stress testing or abnormal pulmonary function testing ■ Patients who have experienced any of the following toxicities during previous courses of aldesleukin—sustained ventricular tachycardia (≥5 beats), angina pectoris or myocardial infarction as indicated by ECG changes, respiratory problems requiring more than 72 hr of intubation, pericardial tamponade, renal toxicity requiring more than 72 hr of dialysis, CNS dysfunction consisting of more than 48 hr of coma or psychosis, intractable seizures, bowel perforation or ischemia, GI bleeding requiring surgical intervention ■ Patients who have had allograft organ transplantation (increased risk of rejection).
Use Cautiously in: ■ Patients with a history of cardiovascular, respiratory, hepatic, or renal disease ■ Patients with a history of seizures or suspected CNS metastases (symptoms may be exaggerated and seizures may occur) ■ Patients with childbearing potential ■ Pregnancy, lactation, or children <18 yr (safety not established).

ADVERSE REACTIONS AND SIDE EFFECTS*

Resp: APNEA, RESPIRATORY FAILURE, dyspnea, pulmonary congestion, pulmonary edema, hemoptysis, pleural effusion, pneumothorax, tachypnea, wheezing.
CV: CARDIAC ARREST, CONGESTIVE HEART FAILURE, MYOCARDIAL INFARCTION, STROKE, arrhythmias, hypotension, tachycardia, myocardial ischemia, pericardial effusion, thrombosis.
GI: BOWEL PERFORATION, diarrhea, jaundice, nausea, stomatitis, vomiting, ascites, hepatomegaly.
GU: oliguria/anuria, proteinuria, dysuria, hematuria, renal failure.
Derm: EXFOLIATATIVE DERMATITIS, pruritus.
F and E: acidosis, hypocalcemia, hypokalemia, hypomagnesemia, hypophosphatemia, alkalosis, hyperkalemia, hyperuricemia, hyponatremia.
Hemat: anemia, coagulation disorders, leukopenia, thrombocytopenia, eosinophilia, leukocytosis.
Misc: CAPILLARY LEAK SYNDROME, chills, fever, weight gain, weight loss.

INTERACTIONS

Drug-Drug: ■ **Glucocorticoids** decrease antineoplastic effectiveness. Avoid concurrent use ■ Additive hypotension may occur with **antihypertensives** ■ Concurrent **cardiotoxic, hepatotoxic, myelotoxic,** or **nephrotoxic drug therapy** increases the risk of toxicity in these organs.

ROUTE AND DOSAGE

■ **IV (Adults):** 600,000 IU/kg (0.037 mg/kg) every 8 hr for 14 doses. Cycle is repeated once

*CAPITALS indicate life-threatening; underlines indicate most frequent.

after a 9-day rest period to a total of 28 doses. After a rest period of 7 wk, patients who have had a beneficial response may be evaluated for additional courses.

AVAILABILITY

- ***Vials:*** containing 22 million IU[Rx].

TIME/ACTION PROFILE (tumor regression after completion of first course)

	ONSET	PEAK	DURATION
IV	4 wk	UK	12 mo

NURSING IMPLICATIONS

ASSESSMENT

- □ Monitor ECG continuously during infusion. Cardiac function, including thallium stress testing, should be determined prior to initiation of therapy. Supraventricular arrhythmias may respond to digoxin or verapamil and usually resolve after completion of therapy.
- □ Monitor vital signs at least daily throughout therapy. Fever, chills, rigors, and malaise usually occur within hours of administration. Acetaminophen and an NSAID, such as indomethacin, should be administered prior to initiation of aldesleukin therapy to reduce fever. Meperidine may be given to control rigors associated with fever.
- □ Assess patient for the development of capillary leak syndrome (hypotension, hypovolemia, edema, ascites, pleural effusions). This initially manifests as a drop in arterial blood pressure beginning 2–12 hr from start of administration. If blood pressure decreases to <90 mm Hg, constant ECG monitoring, hourly vital signs, and CVP monitoring are recommended.
- □ Monitor respiratory status and pulse oximetry frequently. Pulmonary function tests, including arterial blood gases, and chest x ray should be monitored prior to and periodically throughout therapy. Pulmonary toxicity (respiratory failure, tachypnea, wheezing) and pulmonary infiltration may become apparent by the 4th day of therapy and usually resolve within a few weeks after therapy. Respiratory failure may require intubation.
- □ Monitor weight daily. Weight gain during therapy may be more than 10% of pretreatment weight. Reversal of weight gain, via diuresis of fluid, may take up to 1–2 wk after therapy.
- □ Monitor for changes in mental status. Hold administration if patient develops moderate-to-severe lethargy or somnolence. Low doses of haloperidol have been used for debilitating mental status changes.
- □ Assess frequently for signs of infection, particularly sepsis and bacterial endocarditis. Antibiotic prophylaxis directed against *Staphylococcus aureus* may be used for patients with central lines. Any intercurrent infections should be managed aggressively. Aldesleukin impairs the function of white blood cells.
- □ Assess for signs of anemia (increased fatigue, dyspnea, orthostatic hypotension) and bleeding (bleeding gums, bruising, petechiae, guaiac stools, urine, and emesis). Ranitidine or cimetidine may be given for prophylaxis of GI irritation and bleeding. Transfusions of red blood cells and/or platelets may be required.
- □ Assess nutrition and bowel status. Stomatitis may require a liquid diet. Nausea, vomiting, and diarrhea occur in most patients and may lead to hypokalemia and acidosis. Antiemetics and antidiarrheals may be given as needed and are usually discontinued 12 hr after last dose.
- □ Assess skin daily for rash or blisters on skin. Notify physician if these occur; exfoliative dermatitis may be fatal.
- ***Lab Test Considerations:*** Monitor CBC, differential, platelet count, blood chemistries including electrolytes, and renal and hepatic function prior to and daily throughout therapy. May cause elevated bilirubin, BUN, serum creatinine, transaminase, and alkaline phosphatase levels. May cause anemia, thrombocytopenia, hypomagnesemia, acidosis, hypocalcemia, hypophosphatemia, hypokalemia, hyperuricemia, hypoalbuminemia, and hypoproteinemia.
- □ Monitor thyroid function periodically during therapy.

POTENTIAL NURSING DIAGNOSES

- Infection, risk for (Side Effects).
- Knowledge deficit, related to medication regimen (Patient/Family Teaching).

IMPLEMENTATION

- **General Info:** Aldesleukin should be administered only in a hospital setting with intensive care facilities.
- **Intermittent Infusion:** Reconstitute each vial with 1.2 ml of sterile water for injection for a concentration of 18 million IU (1.1 mg)/ml. Direct the sterile water at the side of the vial during reconstitution and swirl contents gently to prevent excessive foaming. Do not shake. Solution should be clear and colorless to slightly yellow. Administer within 48 hr of reconstitution. Discard unused portion.
  - Dilute reconstituted dose in 50 ml of D5W. Do not reconstitute or dilute with bacteriostatic water for injection, 0.9% NaCl, or albumin.
  - Do not use an in-line filter during administration of aldesleukin.
- ***Rate:*** Infuse each dose over 15 min.
- **Y-Site Compatibility:** ▪ amphotericin B ▪ calcium gluconate ▪ diphenhydramine ▪ dopamine ▪ fluconazole ▪ foscarnet ▪ heparin ▪ magnesium sulfate ▪ metoclopramide ▪ ondansetron ▪ potassium chloride ▪ ranitidine ▪ thiethylperazine ▪ trimethoprim/sulfamethoxazole
- **Y-Site Incompatibility:** ▪ ganciclovir ▪ lorazepam ▪ pentamidine ▪ prochlorperazine ▪ promethazine
- **Additive Incompatibility:** ▪ Do not mix with other drugs.

PATIENT/FAMILY TEACHING

- Instruct patient to notify health care professional if dyspnea, sore throat, fever, chills, yellow skin, unusual bleeding or bruising, or fatigue occurs. Caution patient to avoid crowds and persons with known infections. Instruct patient to use a soft toothbrush and electric razor and to be especially careful to avoid falls. Patients should be cautioned not to drink alcohol or take medication containing aspirin or NSAIDs, as these may precipitate gastric bleeding.
- Inform patient that visual problems usually begin shortly after aldesleukin administration and may persist for several weeks but are reversible.
- Advise patient to use a nonhormonal method of contraception throughout therapy.

EVALUATION

Effectiveness of therapy can be demonstrated by: ▪ Decrease in size or spread of renal cell carcinoma.

ALENDRONATE

(a-**len**-drone-ate)
Fosamax

CLASSIFICATION(S):
Bone resorption inhibitor (biphosphonate)

Pregnancy Category C

INDICATIONS

▪ Treatment and prevention of osteoporosis in postmenopausal women ▪ Prevention of fractures in women with osteoporosis ▪ Treatment of Paget's disease of the bone.

ACTION

▪ Inhibits resorption of bone by inhibiting osteoclast activity. **Therapeutic Effects:** ▪ Reversal of the progression of osteoporosis ▪ Decreased progression of Paget's disease.

PHARMACOKINETICS

Absorption: Poorly absorbed following oral administration.
Distribution: Transiently distributes to soft tissue, then distributes to bone.
Metabolism and Excretion: Excreted in urine.
Half-life: 10 yr (reflects release of drug from skeleton).

CONTRAINDICATIONS AND PRECAUTIONS

Contraindicated in: ▪ Renal insufficiency (CCr <35 ml/min) ▪ Pregnancy or lactation.
Use Cautiously in: ▪ Patients with active GI pathology (dysphagia, esophageal disease, gastritis, duodenitis, ulcers) ▪ Pre-existing hypocalcemia or vitamin D deficiency.

ADVERSE REACTIONS AND SIDE EFFECTS

CNS: headache.
GI: abdominal distention, abdominal pain, acid regurgitation, constipation, diarrhea, dyspepsia, dysphagia, esophageal ulcer, flatulence, gastritis, nausea, taste perversion, vomiting.
Derm: erythema, rash.
MS: musculoskeletal pain.

INTERACTIONS

Drug-Drug: ▪ **Calcium supplements, antacids**, and **other oral medications** decrease the absorption of alendronate ▪ Doses >10 mg/day increase the risk of adverse GI events when used with **NSAIDs.**
Drug-Food: ▪ Food significantly decreases absorption. Caffeine (coffee, tea, cola), mineral water, and orange juice also decrease absorption.

ROUTE AND DOSAGE

- **PO (Adults):** *Treatment of osteoporosis*—10 mg once daily. *Prevention of osteoporosis*—5 mg once daily. *Paget's disease*—40 mg once daily for 6 mo. Re-treatment may be considered for patients who relapse.

AVAILABILITY

- ***Tablets:*** 10 mg[Rx].

TIME/ACTION PROFILE (inhibition of bone resorption)

	ONSET	PEAK	DURATION
PO	1 mo	3–6 mo	3 wk–7 mo*

*Following discontinuation of alendronate.

NURSING IMPLICATIONS

ASSESSMENT

- **Osteoporosis:** Assess patients for low bone mass prior to and periodically during therapy.
- **Paget's disease:** Assess for symptoms of Paget's disease (bone pain, headache, decreased visual and auditory acuity, increased skull size).
- ***Lab Test Considerations:***
  - *Osteoporosis:* Assess serum calcium prior to and periodically during therapy. Hypocalcemia and vitamin D deficiency should be treated prior to initiating alendronate therapy. May cause mild, transient elevations of calcium and phosphate.
  - *Paget's Disease:* Monitor alkaline phosphatase prior to and periodically during therapy. Alendronate is indicated for patients with alkaline phosphatase two times the upper limit of normal.

POTENTIAL NURSING DIAGNOSES

- Injury, risk for (Indications).
- Knowledge deficit, related to diet and medication regimen (Patient/Family Teaching).

IMPLEMENTATION

- **PO:** Administer first thing in the morning with 6–8 oz plain water 30 min prior to other medications, beverages, or food.

PATIENT/FAMILY TEACHING

- Instruct patient on the importance of taking exactly as directed, first thing in the morning, 30 min prior to other medications, beverages, or food. Waiting longer than 30 min will improve absorption. Alendronate should be taken with 6–8 oz plain water (mineral water, orange juice, coffee, and other beverages decrease absorption). If a dose is missed, skip dose and resume the next morning; do not double doses or take later in the day. Do not discontinue without consulting health care professional.
- Caution patient to remain upright for 30 min following dose to facilitate passage to stomach and minimize risk of esophageal irritation.
- Advise patient to eat a balanced diet and consult health care professional about the need for supplemental calcium and vitamin D.
- Encourage patient to participate in regular exercise and to modify behaviors that increase the risk of osteoporosis (stop smoking, reduce alcohol consumption).
- Advise female patient to notify health care professional if pregnancy is planned or suspected or if she is nursing.

EVALUATION

Effectiveness of therapy can be demonstrated by: ▪ Prevention of or decrease in the progression of osteoporosis in postmenopausal women ▪ Decrease in the progression of Paget's disease.

ALLOPURINOL
(al-oh-**pure**-i-nole)
{Apo-Allopurinol}, Lopurin, {Purinol}, Zyloprim

CLASSIFICATION(S):
Antigout agent (xanthine oxidase inhibitor)

Pregnancy Category C

INDICATIONS

■ Prevention of attack of gouty arthritis and nephropathy ■ Treatment of secondary hyperuricemia, which may occur during treatment of tumors or leukemias.

ACTION

■ Inhibits the production of uric acid. **Therapeutic Effects:** ■ Lowering of serum uric acid levels.

PHARMACOKINETICS

Absorption: Well absorbed (80%) following oral administration.
Distribution: Widely distributed in tissue water.
Metabolism and Excretion: Metabolized to oxypurinol, an active compound with a long half-life. Both allopurinol and oxypurinol are excreted mainly by the kidneys.
Half-life: 2–3 hr (oxypurinol 24 hr).

CONTRAINDICATIONS AND PRECAUTIONS

Contraindicated in: ■ Hypersensitivity ■ Pregnancy or lactation.
Use Cautiously in: ■ Acute attacks of gout ■ Renal insufficiency (dosage reduction required if CCr <20 ml/min) ■ Dehydration (adequate hydration necessary).

ADVERSE REACTIONS AND SIDE EFFECTS*

CNS: drowsiness.
GI: diarrhea, hepatitis, nausea, vomiting.
GU: renal failure.
Derm: rash, urticaria.
Hemat: bone marrow depression.
Misc: hypersensitivity reactions.

INTERACTIONS

Drug-Drug: ■ Use with **mercaptopurine** and **azathioprine** increases bone marrow depressant properties—dosages of these drugs should be reduced ■ Use with **ampicillin** or **amoxicillin** increases the risk of rash ■ Use with **oral hypoglycemics** and **warfarin** increases the effects of these drugs ■ Use with **thiazide diuretics** or **captopril** increases the risk of hypersensitivity reactions ■ Large doses of allopurinol may increase the risk of **theophylline** toxicity.

ROUTE AND DOSAGE

❑ **Management of Gout**

- **PO (Adults):** *Initially*—100 mg/day; increase at weekly intervals based on serum uric acid (not to exceed 800 mg/day). Doses >300 mg/day should be given in divided doses. *Maintenance dose*—100–200 mg 2–3 times daily. Doses of <300 mg may be given as a single daily dose.

❑ **Management of Secondary Hyperuricemia**

- **PO (Adults):** 600–800 mg/day in divided doses starting 12 hr–3 days prior to chemotherapy or radiation.
- **PO (Children 6–10 yr):** 100 mg 3 times daily or 300 mg as a single dose.
- **PO (Children <6 yr):** <50 mg 3 times daily.

AVAILABILITY

■ ***Tablets:*** 100 mg[Rx], {200 mg[Rx]}, 300 mg[Rx].

TIME/ACTION PROFILE (hypouricemic effect)

ONSET	PEAK	DURATION†
2–3 days	1–3 wk	1–2 wk

†Duration after discontinuation of allopurinol.

NURSING IMPLICATIONS

ASSESSMENT

❑ Monitor for joint pain and swelling. Addition of colchicine or NSAIDs may be necessary for acute attacks. Prophylactic doses of colchicine or an NSAID should be administered concurrently during the first 3–6 mo of therapy be-

{} = Available in Canada only.
*CAPITALS indicate life-threatening; underlines indicate most frequent.

cause of an increased frequency of acute attacks of gouty arthritis during early therapy.

- Monitor intake and output ratios. Decreased kidney function can cause drug accumulation and toxic effects. Ensure that patient maintains adequate fluid intake (minimum 2500–3000 ml/day) to minimize risk of kidney stone formation.
- Assess patient for rash or more severe hypersensitivity reactions. Discontinue allopurinol immediately if rash occurs. Therapy should be discontinued permanently if reaction is severe. Therapy may be reinstated after a mild reaction has subsided, at a lower dose (50 mg/day with very gradual titration). If skin rash recurs, discontinue permanently.
- ***Lab Test Considerations:*** Serum and urine uric acid levels usually begin to decrease 2–3 days after initiation of therapy.
- Monitor blood glucose in patients receiving oral hypoglycemic agents. May cause hypoglycemia.
- Hematologic, renal, and liver function tests should be monitored prior to and periodically throughout therapy, especially during the first few months. May cause elevation of serum alkaline phosphatase, bilirubin, AST, and ALT levels. Decreased CBC and platelets may indicate bone marrow depression. Elevated BUN, serum creatinine, and CCr may indicate nephrotoxicity. These are usually reversed with discontinuation of therapy.

POTENTIAL NURSING DIAGNOSES

- Pain (Indications).
- Knowledge deficit, related to medication regimen (Patient/Family Teaching).

IMPLEMENTATION

- **PO:** May be administered with milk or meals to minimize gastric irritation. May be crushed and given with fluid or mixed with food for patients who have difficulty swallowing.

PATIENT/FAMILY TEACHING

- Instruct patient to take allopurinol exactly as directed. If a dose is missed, take as soon as remembered. If dosing schedule is once daily, do not take if remembered the next day. If dosing schedule is more than once a day, take up to 300 mg for the next dose.
- Instruct patient to continue taking allopurinol along with an NSAID or colchicine during an acute attack of gout. Allopurinol helps prevent but does not relieve acute gout attacks.
- Alkaline diet may be ordered. Urinary acidification with large doses of vitamin C or other acids may increase kidney stone formation (see Appendix K). Advise patient of need for increased fluid intake.
- May occasionally cause drowsiness. Caution patient to avoid driving or other activities requiring alertness until response to drug is known.
- Instruct patient to report skin rash or influenza symptoms (chills, fever, muscle aches and pains, nausea, or vomiting) occurring with or shortly after skin rash to health care professional immediately; may indicate hypersensitivity.
- Advise patient that large amounts of alcohol increase uric acid concentrations and may decrease the effectiveness of allopurinol.
- Emphasize the importance of follow-up exams to monitor effectiveness and side effects.

EVALUATION

Effectiveness of therapy can be demonstrated by: ▪ Decreased serum and urinary uric acid levels. May take 2–6 wk to observe clinical improvement in patients treated for gout.

ALPRAZOLAM

(al-**pray**-zoe-lam)

{Apo-Alpraz}, {Novo-Alprazol}, {Nu-Alpraz}, Xanax

CLASSIFICATION(S):

Sedative/hypnotic (benzodiazepine)

Schedule IV

Pregnancy Category D

INDICATIONS

▪ Treatment of anxiety ▪ Management of panic attacks. **Unlabeled Uses:** ▪ Management of symptoms of premenstrual syndrome (PMS).

ACTION

▪ Acts at many levels in the CNS to produce anxiolytic effect ▪ May produce CNS depression

{} = **Available in Canada only.**

▪ Effects may be mediated by gamma-aminobutyric acid (GABA), an inhibitory neurotransmitter. **Therapeutic Effects:** ▪ Relief of anxiety.

PHARMACOKINETICS

Absorption: Slowly but completely absorbed from the GI tract.
Distribution: Widely distributed, crosses blood-brain barrier. Probably crosses the placenta and enters breast milk. Accumulation is minimal.
Metabolism and Excretion: Metabolized by the liver to an active compound that is subsequently rapidly metabolized.
Half-life: 12–15 hr.

CONTRAINDICATIONS AND PRECAUTIONS

Contraindicated in: ▪ Hypersensitivity ▪ Cross-sensitivity with other benzodiazepines may exist ▪ Patients with pre-existing CNS depression ▪ Severe uncontrolled pain ▪ Narrow-angle glaucoma ▪ Pregnancy and lactation.
Use Cautiously in: ▪ Hepatic dysfunction (dosage reduction required) ▪ History of suicide attempt or drug dependence ▪ Elderly or debilitated patients (dosage reduction required).

ADVERSE REACTIONS AND SIDE EFFECTS*

CNS: dizziness, drowsiness, lethargy, confusion, hangover, headache, mental depression, paradoxical excitation.
EENT: blurred vision.
GI: constipation, diarrhea, nausea, vomiting.
Derm: rashes.
Misc: physical dependence, psychological dependence, tolerance.

INTERACTIONS

Drug-Drug: ▪ **Alcohol, antidepressants, other benzodiazepines, antihistamines,** and **opioid analgesics**—concurrent use results in additive CNS depression ▪ **Cimetidine, oral contraceptives, disulfiram, erythromycin, fluoxetine, isoniazid, ketoconazole, metoprolol, propoxyphene, propranolol,** or **valproic acid** may decrease the metabolism of alprazolam, enhancing its actions ▪ May decrease efficacy of **levodopa** ▪ **Rifampin** or **barbiturates** may increase metabolism and decrease effectiveness of alprazolam ▪ Sedative effects may be decreased by **theophylline.**
Drug-Food: ▪ Concurrent ingestion of **grapefruit juice** increases blood levels.

ROUTE AND DOSAGE

❑ **Anxiety**

▪ **PO (Adults):** 0.25–0.5 mg 2–3 times daily (not >4 mg/day; begin with 0.25 mg 2–3 times daily in geriatric/debilitated patients).

❑ **Panic Attacks**

▪ **PO (Adults):** 0.5 mg 3 times daily; may be increased as needed (not >10 mg/day).

AVAILABILITY

▪ ***Tablets:*** 0.25 mg^{Rx}, 0.5 mg^{Rx}, 1 mg^{Rx}, 2 mg^{Rx}
▪ ***Oral solution:*** 0.1 mg/ml^{Rx}, 1 mg/ml ^{Rx}.

TIME/ACTION PROFILE (sedation)

	ONSET	PEAK	DURATION
PO	1–2 hr	1–2 hr	up to 24 hr

NURSING IMPLICATIONS

ASSESSMENT

- ❑ Assess degree and manifestations of anxiety and mental status prior to and periodically during therapy.
- ❑ Assess patient for drowsiness, light-headedness, and dizziness. These symptoms usually disappear as therapy progresses. Dosage should be reduced if these symptoms persist.
- ❑ Prolonged high-dose therapy may lead to psychological or physical dependence. Risk is greater in patients taking >4 mg/day. Restrict the amount of drug available to patient.
- ▪ ***Lab Test Considerations:*** Monitor CBC and liver and renal function periodically during long-term therapy. May cause decreased hematocrit and neutropenia.

POTENTIAL NURSING DIAGNOSES

- ▪ Anxiety (Indications).
- ▪ Injury, risk for (Side Effects).
- ▪ Knowledge deficit, related to medication regimen (Patient/Family Teaching).

***CAPITALS indicate life-threatening; underlines indicate most frequent.**

IMPLEMENTATION

- **General Info:** If early morning anxiety or anxiety between doses occurs, the same total daily dose should be divided into more frequent intervals.
- **PO:** May be administered with food if GI upset occurs.
- □ Tablets may be crushed and taken with food or fluids if patient has difficulty swallowing.

PATIENT/FAMILY TEACHING

- □ Instruct patient to take medication exactly as directed; do not skip or double up on missed doses. If a dose is missed, take within 1 hr; otherwise, skip the dose and return to regular schedule. If medication is less effective after a few weeks, check with health care professional; do not increase dose. Abrupt withdrawal may cause sweating, vomiting, muscle cramps, tremors, and convulsions.
- □ May cause drowsiness or dizziness. Caution patient to avoid driving and other activities requiring alertness until response to the medication is known.
- □ Advise patient to avoid the use of alcohol or other CNS depressants concurrently with alprazolam. Instruct patient to consult health care professional before taking OTC medications concurrently with this medication.

EVALUATION

Effectiveness of therapy can be demonstrated by: ▪ Decreased sense of anxiety □ Increased ability to cope ▪ Decreased frequency and severity of panic attacks. Treatment with this medication should not exceed 4 mo without re-evaluation of the patient's need for the drug ▪ Decreased symptoms of premenstrual syndrome.

ALTRETAMINE

(al-**tret**-a-meen)

Hexalen, hexamethylmelamine, {Hexastat}

CLASSIFICATION(S):

Antineoplastic

Pregnancy Category D

INDICATIONS

▪ Management of ovarian cancer unresponsive to treatment with other agents.

ACTION

▪ Mechanism unknown, but may disrupt DNA and RNA synthesis. **Therapeutic Effects:** ▪ Death of rapidly replicating cells, particularly malignant ones.

PHARMACOKINETICS

Absorption: Well absorbed following oral administration. Requires metabolism for conversion to antineoplastic compounds.

Distribution: Reaches high concentrations in liver, kidney, and small intestine. Poor penetration into brain.

Metabolism and Excretion: Mostly metabolized by the liver to compounds with antineoplastic activity.

Half-life: 4.7–10.2 hr.

CONTRAINDICATIONS AND PRECAUTIONS

Contraindicated in: ▪ Hypersensitivity ▪ Pregnancy or lactation.

Use Cautiously in: ▪ Pre-existing neurologic diseases ▪ Patients with childbearing potential ▪ Infections ▪ Decreased bone marrow reserve ▪ Other chronic debilitating illnesses ▪ Children (safety not established).

ADVERSE REACTIONS AND SIDE EFFECTS*

CNS: SEIZURES, fatigue.

GI: <u>nausea</u>, <u>vomiting</u>, anorexia, hepatic toxicity.

GU: gonadal suppression, renal toxicity.

Derm: alopecia (<1%), pruritus, skin rash.

Endo: gonadal suppression.

Hemat: <u>anemia</u>, leukopenia, thrombocytopenia.

Neuro: <u>peripheral neuropathy</u>.

INTERACTIONS

Drug-Drug: ▪ Concurrent use with **MAO inhibitors** may produce orthostatic hypotension ▪ May decrease antibody response and increase risk of adverse reactions from **live virus vaccines** ▪ Additive bone marrow depression may occur with other **antineoplastic agents** or **ra-**

{} = Available in Canada only.

***CAPITALS indicate life-threatening; <u>underlines</u> indicate most frequent.**

diation therapy ▪ **Cimetidine** increases blood levels and risk of toxicity.

ROUTE AND DOSAGE

- **PO (Adults):** 65 mg/m² 4 times daily (after meals and at bedtime) for 14 or 21 days of each 28-day cycle. Dosage reduction to 50 mg/m² 4 times daily (after meals and at bedtime) recommended after 14 or more days' rest for any of the following: GI intolerance, severe bone marrow depression, or progressive neurologic toxicity.

AVAILABILITY

- ***Capsules:*** 50 mg^Rx^, {100 mg^Rx^}.

TIME/ACTION PROFILE (effects on blood counts)

	ONSET	PEAK	DURATION
PO	UK	3–4 wk	6 wk

NURSING IMPLICATIONS

ASSESSMENT

- Nausea and vomiting of gradual onset frequently occur. Tolerance may develop after several weeks of therapy. Treatment includes antiemetics or dosage reduction and, rarely, discontinuation. Monitor amount of emesis and notify physician if emesis exceeds guidelines to prevent dehydration.
- Monitor for bone marrow depression throughout therapy. Although the patient is often asymptomatic, symptoms include anemia (unusual tiredness), leukopenia (fever, chills, sore throat, cough or hoarseness, lower back or side pain, painful or difficult urination), and thrombocytopenia (bleeding gums, bruising, petechiae, guaiac stools, urine, and emesis). Notify physician if these symptoms occur.
- Avoid IM injections and rectal temperatures. Apply pressure to venipuncture sites for 10 min.
- Assess patient for signs of neurotoxicity including CNS effects (anxiety, clumsiness, confusion, dizziness, mental depression, weakness, seizures) and peripheral neuropathy (numbness, tingling, paresthesia) prior to initiation of each course and routinely throughout therapy. Pyridoxine may minimize peripheral neuropathy; usually reversible on discontinuation of altretamine. If neurotoxicity continues after dosage reduction, discontinue therapy.
- ***Lab Test Considerations:*** Monitor CBC and platelets prior to each course of therapy, monthly, and as clinically indicated. The nadir of leukopenia and thrombocytopenia occurs in 3–4 wk with 21-day therapy and recovers in 6 wk with intermittent dosing; with continuous dosing the nadir occurs in 6–8 wk. Dose should be held for 14 or more days and resumed at 50 mg/m²/day 4 times daily for any of the following: GI intolerance unresponsive to conventional therapy, WBC <2000 mm³, granulocytes <1000 mm³, platelet count <75,000 mm³, or progressive neurologic toxicity.

POTENTIAL NURSING DIAGNOSES

- Infection, risk for (Adverse Reactions).
- Injury, risk for (Side Effects).
- Knowledge deficit, related to medication regimen (Patient/Family Teaching).

IMPLEMENTATION

- **PO:** Administer doses after meals and at bedtime to reduce nausea and vomiting.

PATIENT/FAMILY TEACHING

- Instruct patient to notify health care professional promptly if fever; sore throat; signs of infection; bleeding gums; bruising; petechiae; blood in stools, urine, or emesis; increased fatigue, dyspnea, or orthostatic hypotension occurs. Caution patient to avoid crowds and persons with known infections. Instruct patient to use soft toothbrush and electric razor and to avoid falls. Caution patient not to drink alcoholic beverages or take medications containing aspirin or NSAIDs; may precipitate GI bleeding.
- Instruct patient to report promptly any numbness or tingling in extremities.
- Instruct patient not to receive any vaccinations without advice of health care professional.
- Advise patient of the need for contraception.
- Emphasize the need for periodic lab tests to monitor for side effects.

EVALUATION

Effectiveness of therapy can be demonstrated by: ▪ Decrease in size or spread of malignancy.

A

ALUMINUM HYDROXIDE

AlternaGEL, Alu-Cap, {Alugel}, Aluminet, Alu-Tab, Amphojel, Basalgel, Dialume

CLASSIFICATION(S):

Antacid, Electrolyte modifier (hypophosphatemic)

Pregnancy Category UK

INDICATIONS

▪ Lowering of phosphate levels in patients with chronic renal failure ▪ Adjunctive therapy in the treatment of peptic, duodenal, and gastric ulcers ▪ Hyperacidity, indigestion, reflux esophagitis.

ACTION

▪ Binds phosphate in the GI tract ▪ Neutralizes gastric acid and inactivates pepsin. **Therapeutic Effects:** ▪ Lowering of serum phosphate levels ▪ Healing of ulcers and decreased pain associated with ulcers or gastric hyperacidity ▪ Constipation limits use alone in the treatment of ulcer disease ▪ Frequently found in combination with magnesium-containing compounds.

PHARMACOKINETICS

Absorption: With chronic use, small amounts of aluminum are systemically absorbed.
Distribution: If absorbed, aluminum distributes widely, crosses the placenta, and enters breast milk. Concentrates in the CNS with chronic use.
Metabolism and Excretion: Mostly excreted in feces. Small amounts absorbed are excreted by the kidneys.
Half-life: UK.

CONTRAINDICATIONS AND PRECAUTIONS

Contraindicated in: ▪ Severe abdominal pain of unknown cause.
Use Cautiously in: ▪ Hypercalcemia ▪ Hypophosphatemia ▪ Pregnancy (generally considered safe; chronic high-dose therapy should be avoided).

ADVERSE REACTIONS AND SIDE EFFECTS*

GI: constipation.
F and E: hypophosphatemia.

INTERACTIONS

Drug-Drug: ▪ Absorption of **tetracyclines, chlorpromazine, iron salts, isoniazid, digoxin,** or **fluoroquinolones** may be decreased ▪ **Salicylate** blood levels may be decreased ▪ **Quinidine, mexiletine,** and **amphetamine** levels may be increased if enough antacid is ingested such that urine pH is increased.

ROUTE AND DOSAGE

❑ **Hypophosphatemic**

▪ **PO (Adults):** 1.9–4.8 g (30–40 ml of regular suspension or 15–20 ml of concentrated suspension) 3–4 times daily.
▪ **PO (Children):** 50–150 mg/kg/24 hr in 4–6 divided doses; titrate to normal serum phosphate levels.

❑ **Antacid**

▪ **PO (Adults):** 500–1500 mg (5–30 ml) 3–6 times daily.

AVAILABILITY

▪ ***Capsules:*** 475 mg[OTC], 500 mg[OTC] ▪ ***Tablets:*** 300 mg[OTC], 600 mg[OTC] ▪ ***Suspension:*** 320 mg/5 ml[OTC], 450 mg/5 ml[OTC], 600 mg/5 ml[OTC], 675 mg/5 ml[OTC] ▪ ***In combination with:*** magnesium carbonate, calcium carbonate, simethicone, and mineral oil. See Appendix A.

TIME/ACTION PROFILE

	ONSET	PEAK	DURATION
PO†	hr–days	days–wk	days
PO‡	15–30 min	30 min	30 min–3 hr

†Hypophosphatemic effect.
‡Antacid effect.

NURSING IMPLICATIONS

ASSESSMENT

❑ Assess location, duration, character, and precipitating factors of gastric pain.
▪ ***Lab Test Considerations:*** Monitor serum

{} = Available in Canada only.
*CAPITALS indicate life-threatening; underlines indicate most frequent.

phosphate and calcium levels periodically during chronic use of aluminum hydroxide.
- □ May cause increased serum gastrin and decreased serum phosphate concentrations.
- □ In treatment of severe ulcer disease, guaiac stools and emesis and monitoring pH of gastric secretions.

POTENTIAL NURSING DIAGNOSES

- ▪ Pain (Indications).
- ▪ Constipation (Side Effects).
- ▪ Knowledge deficit, related to medication regimen (Patient/Family Teaching).

IMPLEMENTATION

- ▪ **General Info:** Antacids cause premature dissolution and absorption of enteric-coated tablets and may interfere with absorption of other oral medications. Separate administration of aluminum hydroxide and oral medications by at least 1–2 hr.
- □ Tablets must be chewed thoroughly before swallowing to prevent entering small intestine in undissolved form. Follow with a glass of water.
- □ Shake liquid preparations well before pouring. Follow administration with water to ensure passage into stomach.
- □ Liquid dosage forms are considered to be more effective than tablets.
- ▪ **Hypophosphatemic:** For phosphate lowering, follow dose with full glass of water or fruit juice.
- ▪ **Antacid:** May be given in conjunction with magnesium-containing antacids to minimize constipation, except in patients with renal failure. Administer 1 and 3 hr after meals and at bedtime for maximum antacid effect.
- □ For treatment of peptic ulcer, aluminum hydroxide may be administered every 1–2 hr while awake or diluted with 2–3 parts water and administered intragastrically every 30 min for 12 or more hr per day. Physician may order nasogastric tube clamped following administration.
- □ For reflux esophagitis, administer 15 ml 20–40 min after meals and at bedtime.

PATIENT/FAMILY TEACHING

- ▪ **General Info:** Instruct patient to take aluminum hydroxide exactly as directed. If on a regular dosing schedule and a dose is missed, take as soon as remembered if not almost time for next dose; do not double doses.
- □ Advise patient not to take aluminum hydroxide within 1–2 hr of other medications without consulting health care professional.
- □ Advise patients to check label for sodium content. Patients with congestive heart failure, hypertension, or those on sodium restriction should use low-sodium preparations.
- □ Inform patients of potential for constipation from aluminum hydroxide.
- ▪ **Hypophosphatemic:** Patients taking aluminum hydroxide for hyperphosphatemia should be taught the importance of a low-phosphate diet.
- ▪ **Antacid:** Caution patient to consult health care professional before taking antacids for more than 2 wk if problem is recurring, if taking other medications, if relief is not obtained, or if symptoms of gastric bleeding (black tarry stools, coffee-ground emesis) occur.

EVALUATION

Effectiveness of therapy can be demonstrated by: ▪ Decrease in serum phosphate levels ▪ Decrease in GI pain and irritation □ Increase in the pH of gastric secretions. In treatment of peptic ulcer, antacid therapy should be continued for at least 4–6 wk after symptoms have disappeared because there is no correlation between disappearance of symptoms and healing of ulcers.

AMIFOSTINE

(a-mi-**foss**-teen)
Ethyol

CLASSIFICATION(S):
Cytoprotective agent (for cisplatin)

Pregnancy Category C

INDICATIONS

▪ Reduces renal toxicity from cisplatin in patients being treated for ovarian cancer.

ACTION

▪ Converted in tissue to a compound that binds and detoxifies damaging metabolites of cisplatin ▪ May also act as a scavenger of compounds generated following exposure to cisplatin. **Ther-**

apeutic Effects: ▪ Decreased renal damage from cisplatin.

PHARMACOKINETICS

Absorption: IV administration results in complete bioavailability.
Distribution: UK.
Metabolism and Excretion: Rapidly metabolized in plasma.
Half-life: 8 min.

CONTRAINDICATIONS AND PRECAUTIONS

Contraindicated in: ▪ Known sensitivity to aminothiol compounds or mannitol ▪ Hypotension or dehydration ▪ Lactation.
Use Cautiously in: ▪ Elderly patients or patients with cardiovascular disease (risk of adverse reactions may be increased) ▪ Pregnancy or children (safety not established).

ADVERSE REACTIONS AND SIDE EFFECTS*

CNS: dizziness, somnolence.
EENT: sneezing.
CV: hypotension.
GI: nausea, vomiting, hiccups.
Derm: flushing.
F and E: hypocalcemia.
Misc: allergic reactions, chills.

INTERACTIONS

Drug-Drug: ▪ Concurrent use of **antihypertensives** may increase the risk of hypotension.

ROUTE AND DOSAGE

- **IV (Adults):** 910 mg/m² once daily, within 30 min before chemotherapy.

AVAILABILITY

- ***Powder for injection:*** 500 mg/vial (with 500 mg mannitol)Rx.

TIME/ACTION PROFILE

	ONSET	PEAK	DURATION
IV	UK	UK	UK

NURSING IMPLICATIONS

ASSESSMENT

- Monitor blood pressure prior to and every 5 min during infusion. If significant hypotension requiring interruption of therapy occurs, place patient in Trendelenburg position and administer an infusion of 0.9% NaCl using a separate IV line. If blood pressure returns to normal in 5 min and patient is asymptomatic, infusion may be resumed.
- Assess fluid status prior to administration. Correct dehydration prior to instituting therapy. Nausea and vomiting are frequent and may be severe. Prophylactic antiemetic agents including dexamethasone 20 mg IV and a serotonin antagonist antiemetic (dolasetron, ondansetron, granisetron) should be administered prior to and during infusion. Monitor fluid status closely.
- ***Lab Test Considerations:*** Monitor serum calcium concentrations prior to and periodically during therapy. May cause hypocalcemia. Calcium supplements may be necessary.

POTENTIAL NURSING DIAGNOSES

- Injury, risk for (Indications).
- Knowledge deficit, related to medication regimen (Patient/Family Teaching).

IMPLEMENTATION

- **Intermittent Infusion:** Reconstitute with 9.5 ml of sterile 0.9% NaCl. Dilute further with 0.9% NaCl for a concentration of 5–40 mg/ml. Do not administer solutions that are discolored or contain particulate matter. Solution is stable for 5 hr at room temperature or 24 hr if refrigerated.
- ***Rate:*** Administer over 15 min within 30 min of chemotherapy administration. Longer infusion times are not as well tolerated.
- **Y-Site Compatibility:** ▪ amikacin ▪ aminophylline ▪ ampicillin ▪ ampicillin/sulbactam ▪ aztreonam ▪ bleomycin ▪ bumetanide ▪ buprenorphine ▪ butorphanol ▪ calcium gluconate ▪ carboplatin ▪ carmustine ▪ cefazolin ▪ cefonicid ▪ cefotaxime ▪ cefotetan ▪ cefoxitin ▪ ceftazidime ▪ ceftizoxime ▪ ceftriaxone ▪ cefuroxime ▪ cimetidine ▪ ciprofloxacin ▪ clindamycin ▪ cyclophosphamide ▪ cytarabine ▪ dacarbazine ▪ dactinomycin ▪ daunorubicin

*CAPITALS indicate life-threatening; underlines indicate most frequent.

▪ dexamethasone ▪ diphenhydramine ▪ dobutamine ▪ dopamine ▪ doxorubicin ▪ doxycycline ▪ droperidol ▪ enalaprilat ▪ etoposide ▪ famotidine ▪ floxuridine ▪ fluconazole ▪ fludarabine ▪ fluorouracil ▪ furosemide ▪ gallium nitrate ▪ gentamicin ▪ haloperidol ▪ heparin ▪ hydrocortisone ▪ hydromorphone ▪ idarubicin ▪ ifosfamide ▪ imipenem/cilastatin ▪ leucovorin ▪ lorazepam ▪ magnesium sulfate ▪ mannitol ▪ mechlorethamine ▪ meperidine ▪ mesna ▪ methotrexate ▪ methylprednisolone ▪ metoclopramide ▪ metronidazole ▪ mezlocillin ▪ mitomycin ▪ mitoxantrone ▪ morphine ▪ nalbuphine ▪ netilmicin ▪ ondansetron ▪ piperacillin ▪ plicamycin ▪ potassium chloride ▪ promethazine ▪ ranitidine ▪ sodium bicarbonate ▪ streptozocin ▪ teniposide ▪ thiotepa ▪ ticarcillin ▪ ticarcillin/clavulanate ▪ tobramycin ▪ trimethoprim/sulfamethoxazole ▪ trimetrexate ▪ vancomycin ▪ vinblastine ▪ vincristine ▪ zidovudine.

- **Y-Site Incompatibility:** ▪ amphotericin B ▪ cefoperazone ▪ cisplatin ▪ miconazole ▪ minocycline ▪ prochlorperazine.
- **Additive Incompatibility:** ▪ ▪ Do not mix with other solutions or medications.

PATIENT/FAMILY TEACHING

- Explain the purpose of amifostine infusion to patient.
- Inform patient that amifostine may cause hypotension, nausea, vomiting, flushing, chills, dizziness, somnolence, hiccups, and sneezing.

EVALUATION

Effectiveness of therapy can be demonstrated by: ▪ Prevention of renal toxicity associated with repeated administration of cisplatin in patients with ovarian cancer.

AMINO ACIDS

Aminees, Aminosyn, BranchAmin, FreAmine, HepatAmine, NeprAmine, Novamine, ProcalAmine, RenAmin, Travasol, Trophamine

CLASSIFICATION(S):
Caloric agent (protein source)

Pregnancy Category C

INDICATIONS

▪ Provides protein to patients who are unable to ingest enough protein by mouth to maintain positive nitrogen balance □ Used perioperatively in patients who are unable to ingest protein (GI disorders), as an extra source of protein in patients with large requirements who are unable to ingest enough (extensive burns, severe trauma, overwhelming sepsis) □ Usually used with a carbohydrate source (dextrose) and a fat source (fat emulsion) as part of a total parenteral nutrition (TPN, hyperalimentation) program or protein-sparing regimen. Electrolytes, minerals, trace elements, and vitamins are also included. **Treatment must be individualized for each patient. Initiation of therapy requires facilities and personnel skilled in its use.**

ACTION

▪ Promotes protein synthesis by acting as a protein calorie source; decreases rate of protein breakdown (catabolism). **Therapeutic Effects:** ▪ Maintenance of positive nitrogen balance.

PHARMACOKINETICS

Absorption: Following IV administration, absorption is essentially complete.
Distribution: Widely distributed.
Metabolism and Excretion: Metabolized as part of anabolic processes, then excreted in urine as urea nitrogen.
Half-life: UK.

CONTRAINDICATIONS AND PRECAUTIONS

Contraindicated in: ▪ No known contraindications.
Use Cautiously in: ▪ Uncontrolled sepsis ▪ Advanced cardiac, renal, and hepatic disease (specific formulations may be required) ▪ Pregnancy, lactation, children, infants, burn patients, trauma patients, transplant patients (specific formulations may be required).

ADVERSE REACTIONS AND SIDE EFFECTS

CNS: confusion, headache.
CV: congestive heart failure, hypertension, hypotension.

F and E: electrolyte disturbances, hypervolemia, hypovolemia.
Metab: azotemia, fatty acid deficiency, hyperammonemia, hyperglycemia, hypoglycemia.

INTERACTIONS

Drug-Drug: ▪ **Glucocorticoids, diuretics,** or **tetracyclines** may exaggerate negative nitrogen balance.

ROUTE AND DOSAGE

Doses must be individualized to meet metabolic needs. If amino acids are part of total parenteral nutrition (hyperalimentation), then additional calories (dextrose and lipid emulsions) must be provided with electrolytes, vitamins, trace minerals, and other micronutrients.

- **IV (Adults):** 1–2 g protein/kg/day.
- **IV (Children):** 2–4 g protein/kg/day.
- **IV (Neonates):** 2–3 g protein/kg/day.

AVAILABILITY

- ***Injection:*** 2.75%Rx, 3%Rx, 3.5%Rx, 4%Rx, 4.25%Rx, 5%Rx, 5.2%Rx, 5.4%Rx, 5.5%Rx, 6%Rx, 6.5%Rx, 7%Rx, 8%Rx, 8.5%Rx, 10%Rx, 11.4%Rx, 15%Rx amino acids.

TIME/ACTION PROFILE

	ONSET	PEAK	DURATION
IV	UK	UK	UK

NURSING IMPLICATIONS

ASSESSMENT

- □ Nutritional status must be assessed prior to and periodically throughout therapy because amino acids are most commonly used as a component of total parenteral nutrition. Parameters to assess include height, weight, skinfold thickness, arm circumference, total protein, serum albumin, CBC, electrolytes, nitrogen balance, function of gastrointestinal tract, and caloric need. Special formulas available for patients with cardiac, hepatic, or renal dysfunction; patients under extreme stress (trauma, sepsis); and children.
- □ Monitor intake and output; assess for fluid overload (rales/crackles, dyspnea, peripheral edema).
- □ Monitor for infection (fever, chills, diaphoresis). If sepsis occurs, physician may order changing site, culturing catheter tip, hanging new solution and tubing, and obtaining blood cultures. Because of the risk of infection associated with hyperalimentation, patients with uncontrolled sepsis should be treated before therapy is initiated.
- □ Monitor vital signs, fluid and electrolyte status, glucose, weight, and nitrogen balance. Patients on long-term therapy require monitoring of trace elements.
- ▪ ***Lab Test Considerations:*** May cause increased BUN. A 10–15% increase for 3 consecutive days may necessitate discontinuing therapy or altering formulation.
- □ May cause increased ammonia and ketone levels.

POTENTIAL NURSING DIAGNOSES

- ▪ Nutrition, altered, less than body requirements (Indications).
- ▪ Infection, risk for (Side Effects).
- ▪ Knowledge deficit, related to medication regimen (Patient/Family Teaching).

IMPLEMENTATION

- ▪ **General Info:** Component of total parenteral nutrition. Usually given in conjunction with hypertonic dextrose and lipids. Trace elements, vitamins, electrolytes, and insulin are usually incorporated into formulation. May also be administered as a part of multicomponent admixtures, all-in-one, 3-in-1, or triple mix, which combine amino acids, dextrose, and lipids in one container.
- ▪ **Continuous Infusion:**
- □ Solution should be clear. Do not administer if precipitates have formed. Addition of multivitamins will result in bright yellow color.
- □ If administered peripherally, change peripheral site every 48–72 hr or according to institutional policy. Monitor for thrombophlebitis. Avoid infiltration; may cause tissue necrosis.
- □ Peripheral line may be used to administer protein-sparing regimen using dilute amino acid solution (3.5%) with or without D5W or D10W and fat emulsion. Central line must be used to administer more concentrated solution when mixed with hypertonic glucose.
- □ Fat emulsion may be piggybacked with amino acids. Fat emulsion container should be hung at a higher level than amino acid container.
- □ Use aseptic technique with central line.

Change dressing every 48 hr or according to institutional policy. Auscultate breath sounds and assess site for erythema, edema, and leakage.

- *Rate:* Infuse through 0.22-micron filter unless mixed with dextrose and fat emulsion in a 3-in-1 admixture. Control rate with pump or controller.
- **Y-Site Compatibility:** ▪ aminophylline ▪ ascorbic acid ▪ calcium gluconate ▪ cefamandole ▪ cefazolin ▪ cefoperazone ▪ cefotaxime ▪ cefoxitin ▪ ceftazidime ▪ ceftriaxone ▪ cephalothin ▪ cephapirin ▪ chloramphenicol ▪ cimetidine ▪ ciprofloxacin ▪ clindamycin ▪ diazepam ▪ digoxin ▪ dobutamine ▪ dopamine ▪ doxycycline ▪ erythromycin lactobionate ▪ fat emulsion ▪ fluconazole ▪ folic acid ▪ foscarnet ▪ furosemide ▪ gentamicin ▪ haloperidol ▪ heparin ▪ hydrocortisone sodium succinate ▪ idarubicin ▪ isoproterenol ▪ kanamycin ▪ lidocaine ▪ meperidine ▪ methicillin ▪ metronidazole ▪ mezlocillin ▪ miconazole ▪ morphine ▪ nafcillin ▪ netilmicin ▪ norepinephrine ▪ oxacillin ▪ penicillin G potassium ▪ piperacillin ▪ potassium chloride ▪ ranitidine ▪ sargramostim ▪ ticarcillin ▪ ticarcillin/clavulanate ▪ tobramycin ▪ urokinase ▪ vancomycin.
- **Y-Site Incompatibility:** ▪ indomethacin ▪ midazolam ▪ phenytoin ▪ trace elements.
- **Additive Incompatibility:** ▪ Do not add anything to solution without conferring with pharmacist. Total parenteral nutrition solutions should be prepared aseptically in a biologic cabinet.

PATIENT/FAMILY TEACHING

- □ If used as a component of total parenteral nutrition, assure patient that solution is capable of fulfilling all nutritional needs.
- □ Instruct patient to report fever, chills, swelling and pain, or leakage at infusion site immediately.
- ▪ **Home Care Issues:** Patients receiving total parenteral nutrition at home may receive infusion only at night. Prior to discharge the patient and family must understand rationale for therapy, procedures, and symptoms to report to physician. Patients must correctly demonstrate aseptic technique in caring for site, spiking bag, priming tubing, and regulating infusion pump. Discharge planning should be coordinated with home care agency that will provide equipment, solutions, and professional support to the patient and family.

EVALUATION

Effectiveness of therapy can be demonstrated by: ▪ Increased weight □ Improvement of nutritional parameters □ Improved healing.

AMINOGLYCOSIDES (oral, parenteral)*

amikacin
(am-i-**kay**-sin)
Amikin

gentamicin
(jen-ta-**mye**-sin)
{Alcomicin}, {Cidomycin}, Garamycin, Genoptic, Gentacidin, Gentafair, Gentak, Gentamar, Gentrasul, G-Mycin, G-Myticin, Ocu-Mycin, Jenamicin, Spectro-Genta

kanamycin
(kan-a-**mye**-sin)
Kantrex

neomycin
(neo-oh-**mye**-sin)
Mycifradin, Myciguent

netilmicin
(ne-til-**mye**-sin)
Netromycin

streptomycin
(strep-toe-**mye**-sin)

tobramycin
(toe-bra-**mye**-sin)
Nebcin, Tobrex

CLASSIFICATION(S):
Anti-infectives

Pregnancy Category C (kanamycin, topical use of others), D (amikacin, gentamicin, netilmicin, streptomycin, tobramycin)

*See Appendix O for ophthalmic use.

INDICATIONS

▪ **Amikacin, gentamicin, kanamycin, netilmicin, and tobramycin:** Treatment of serious gram-negative bacillary infections and infections caused by staphylococci when penicillins or other less toxic drugs are contraindicated ▪ **Streptomycin:** In combination with other agents in the management of active tuberculosis ▪ **Neomycin:** Used orally to prepare the GI tract for surgery, to decrease the number of ammonia-producing bacteria in the gut as part of the management of hepatic encephalopathy, and to treat some forms of infectious diarrhea ▪ **Gentamicin, streptomycin:** In combination with other agents in the management of serious interococcal infections ▪ **Topical and ophthalmic gentamicin, neomycin, and tobramycin:** Treatment of localized infections due to susceptible organisms ▪ **Gentamicin IM, IV:** Part of endocarditis prophylaxis (see Appendix N). **Unlabeled Uses:** ▪ **Amikacin:** In combination with other agents in the management of *Mycobacterium avium* complex infections.

ACTION

▪ Inhibits protein synthesis in bacteria at level of 30S ribosome. **Therapeutic Effects:** ▪ Bactericidal action. **Spectrum:** ▪ Most aminoglycosides notable for activity against: ▫ *Pseudomonas aeruginosa* ▫ *Klebsiella pneumoniae* ▫ *Escherichia coli* ▫ *Proteus* ▫ *Serratia* ▫ *Acinetobacter* ▫ *Staphylococcus aureus* ▪ In treatment of enterococcal infections, synergy with a penicillin is required ▪ Streptomycin and amikacin also active against *Mycobacterium.*

PHARMACOKINETICS

Absorption: Well absorbed after IM administration. IV administration results in complete bioavailability. Some absorption follows administration by other routes.
Distribution: Widely distributed throughout extracellular fluid; crosses the placenta; small amounts enter breast milk. Poor penetration into CSF.
Metabolism and Excretion: Excretion is >90% renal.
Half-life: 2–4 hr (↑ in renal impairment).

CONTRAINDICATIONS AND PRECAUTIONS

Contraindicated in: ▪ Hypersensitivity ▪ Most parenteral products contain bisulfites and should be avoided in patients with known intolerance ▪ Products containing benzyl alcohol should be avoided in neonates ▪ Cross-sensitivity among aminoglycosides may occur.
Use Cautiously in: ▪ Renal impairment (dosage adjustments necessary; blood level monitoring useful in preventing ototoxicity and nephrotoxicity) ▪ Hearing impairment ▪ Geriatric patients and premature infants (difficulty in assessing auditory and vestibular function; age-related renal impairment) ▪ Neonates (increased risk of neuromuscular blockade; difficulty in assessing auditory and vestibular function; immature renal function) ▪ Neuromuscular diseases such as myasthenia gravis ▪ Obese patients (dosage should be based on ideal body weight) ▪ Pregnancy (tobramycin and streptomycin may cause congenital deafness) ▪ Lactation, infants, and neonates (safety not established).

ADVERSE REACTIONS AND SIDE EFFECTS*

EENT: ototoxicity (vestibular and cochlear).
GU: nephrotoxicity.
F and E: hypomagnesemia.
MS: muscle paralysis (high parenteral doses).
Misc: hypersensitivity reactions.

INTERACTIONS

Drug-Drug: ▪ Inactivated by **penicillins** and **cephalosporins** when coadministered to patients with renal insufficiency ▪ Possible respiratory paralysis after **inhalation anesthetics** or **neuromuscular blockers** ▪ Increased incidence of ototoxicity with **loop diuretics** ▪ Increased incidence of nephrotoxicity with other **nephrotoxic drugs.**

ROUTE AND DOSAGE

All parenteral doses should be adjusted on the basis of serum levels and renal function.

▫ Amikacin

- **IM, IV (Adults and Children):** *Most infections*—5 mg/kg q 8 hr *or* 7 mg/kg q 12 hr (not to exceed 1.5 g/day for >10 days). *Urinary tract infections in adults*—250 mg q 12 hr. *Once-daily dosing*—15–20 mg/kg q 24 hr (unlabeled).
- **IM, IV (Infants):** 10 mg/kg initially; 7.5 mg/kg every 12 hr.
- **IM, IV (Infants—premature):** 10 mg/kg initially; 7.5 mg/kg every 18–24 hr.

*CAPITALS indicate life-threatening; underlines indicate most frequent.

❑ **Gentamicin**

- **IM, IV (Adults):** *Most infections*—1–2 mg/kg q 8 hr (up to 8 mg/kg/day for life-threatening infections or 15 mg/kg/day for intraocular infections). *Uncomplicated urinary tract infections in adults* ≥*60 kg*—160 mg once daily or 80 mg q 12 hr. *Uncomplicated urinary tract infections in adults* <*60 kg*—3 mg/kg once daily or 1.5 mg/kg q 12 hr. *Once-daily dosing*—4–7 mg/kg q 24 hr (unlabeled).
- **IM, IV (Children):** 2–2.5 mg/kg q 8 hr.
- **IM, IV (Infants and Neonates >7 days):** 2.5 mg/kg q 8–16 hr (dosing interval may vary from q 4 hr to q 24 hr, depending on clinical situation).
- **IM, IV (Neonates—full term or premature <7 days):** 2.5 mg/kg q 12–24 hr.
- **IT (Adults):** 4–8 mg once daily.
- **IT (Children ≥3 mo):** 1–2 mg once daily (up to 8 mg/day in children with functioning ventricular shunts).
- **Topical (Adults and Children):** Apply cream/ointment 3–4 times daily.

❑ **Kanamycin**

- **IM, IV (Adults, Children, and Infants):** 3.75 mg/kg q 6 hr, 5 mg/kg q 8 hr, or 7.5 mg/kg q 12 hr (not to exceed 1.5 g/day in adults or 30 mg/kg/day in children).
- **PO (Adults):** *Preoperative intestinal antisepsis*—1 g q hr for 4 doses, then 1 g q 6 hr for 36–72 hr; *hepatic encephalopathy*—2–3 g q 6 hr.

❑ **Neomycin**

- **PO (Adults):** *Preoperative intestinal antisepsis*—1 g q hr for 4 doses, then 1 g q 4 hr for 24 hr *or* 1 g 19 hr, 18 hr, and 9 hr before surgery; *hepatic encephalopathy*—1–3 g q 6 hr for 5–6 days.
- **PO (Children):** *Preoperative intestinal antisepsis*—14.7 mg/kg (417 mg/m^2) q 4 hr for 3 days; *hepatic encephalopathy*—625 mg–1.75 g/m^2 q 6 hr for 5–6 days.
- **Topical (Adults and Children):** Apply cream or ointment 1–5 times daily.

❑ **Netilmicin**

- **IM, IV (Adults):** *Most infections*—1.3–2.2 mg/kg q 8 hr or 2–3.25 mg/kg q 12 hr (up to 7 mg/kg/day or 12 mg/kg/day in cystic fibrosis patients); *complicated urinary tract infections*—1.2–2 mg/kg q 12 hr. *Once-daily dosing*—4–8 mg/kg q 24 hr (unlabeled).
- **IM, IV (Infants and Children 6 wk–12 yr):** 1.83–2.67 mg/kg q 8 hr or 2.75–4 mg/kg q 12 hr.
- **IM, IV (Infants <6 wk):** 2–3.25 mg/kg q 12 hr.

❑ **Streptomycin**

- **IM (Adults):** *Tuberculosis*—1 g/day initially, decreased to 1 g 2–3 times weekly; *other infections*—250 mg–1 g q 6 hr or 500 mg–2 g q 12 hr.
- **IM (Children):** *Tuberculosis*—20 mg/kg/day (not to exceed 1 g/day); *other infections*—5–10 mg/kg q 6 hr or 10–20 mg/kg q 12 hr.

❑ **Tobramycin**

- **IM, IV (Adults):** 0.75–1.25 mg/kg q 6 hr or 1–2 mg/kg q 8 hr (up to 10 mg/kg/day in cystic fibrosis patients).
- **IM, IV (Children and Older Infants):** 1.5–1.9 mg/kg q 6 hr or 2–2.5 mg/kg q 8–16 hr, up to 10 mg/kg/day in cystic fibrosis patients (dosing interval may vary from q 4 hr–q 24 hr, depending on clinical situation).
- **IM, IV (Infants <1 wk):** Up to 2 mg/kg q 12–24 hr.

AVAILABILITY

❑ **Amikacin**

▪ ***Injection:*** 50 mg/ml^{Rx}, 250 mg/ml^{Rx}.

❑ **Gentamicin**

▪ ***Injection:*** 10 mg/ml^{Rx}, 40 mg/ml^{Rx} ▪ ***Premixed injection:*** 40 mg/50 ml^{Rx}, 40 mg/100 ml^{Rx}, 60 mg/50 ml^{Rx}, 60 mg/100 ml^{Rx}, 70 mg/50 ml^{Rx}, 80 mg/50 ml^{Rx}, 80 mg/100 ml^{Rx}, 90 mg/100 ml^{Rx}, 100 mg/50 ml^{Rx}, 100 mg/100 ml^{Rx}, 120 mg/100 ml^{Rx}, 160 mg/100 ml^{Rx}, 180 mg/100 ml^{Rx} ▪ ***Intrathecal injection:*** 2 mg/ml^{Rx} ▪ ***Topical cream:*** 0.1%^{Rx} ▪ ***Topical ointment:*** 0.1%^{Rx}.

❑ **Kanamycin**

▪ ***Injection:*** 37.5 mg/ml^{Rx}, 250 mg/ml^{Rx}, 333.3 mg/ml^{Rx}.

❑ **Neomycin**

▪ ***Oral solution:*** 125 mg/5 ml^{Rx} ▪ ***Tablets:*** 500 mg^{Rx} ▪ ***Cream:*** 0.5%^{OTC} ▪ ***Ointment:*** 0.5%^{Rx,OTC} ▪ ***In combination with:*** other topical antibiotics or anti-inflammatory agents for skin, ear, and eye infections. See Appendix A.

❑ **Netilmicin**

▪ ***Injection:*** 25 mg/ml[Rx], 50 mg/ml[Rx], 100 mg/ml[Rx].

❑ **Streptomycin**

▪ {500 mg/ml[Rx]}, 1 g[Rx].

❑ **Tobramycin**

▪ ***Injection:*** 10 mg/ml[Rx], 40 mg/ml[Rx], 1.2-g vial[Rx].

TIME/ACTION PROFILE (blood levels*)

	ONSET	PEAK	DURATION
IM	rapid	30–90 min	N/A
IV	rapid	15–30 min†	N/A

*All parenterally administered aminoglycosides.
†Postdistribution peak occurs 30 min after the end of a 30-min infusion and 15 min after the end of a 1-hr infusion.

NURSING IMPLICATIONS

ASSESSMENT

▪ **General Info:** Assess patient for infection (vital signs, wound appearance, sputum, urine, stool, WBC) at beginning of and throughout therapy.

□ Obtain specimens for culture and sensitivity prior to initiating therapy. First dose may be given before receiving results.

□ Evaluate eighth cranial nerve function by audiometry prior to and throughout therapy. Hearing loss is usually in the high-frequency range. Prompt recognition and intervention are essential in preventing permanent damage. Also monitor for vestibular dysfunction (vertigo, ataxia, nausea, vomiting). Eighth cranial nerve dysfunction is associated with persistently elevated peak aminoglycoside levels. Aminoglycosides should be discontinued if tinnitus or subjective hearing loss occurs.

□ Monitor intake and output and daily weight to assess hydration status and renal function.

□ Assess patient for signs of superinfection (fever, upper respiratory infection, vaginal itching or discharge, increasing malaise, diarrhea). Report to physician or other health care professional.

▪ **Hepatic Encephalopathy:** Monitor neurologic status. Prior to administering oral medication, assess patient's ability to swallow.

▪ ***Lab Test Considerations:*** Monitor renal function by urinalysis, specific gravity, BUN, creatinine, and CCr prior to and throughout therapy.

□ May cause increased BUN, AST, ALT, serum alkaline phosphatase, bilirubin, creatinine, and LDH concentrations.

□ May cause decreased serum calcium, magnesium, potassium, and sodium concentrations.

▪ ***Toxicity and Overdose:*** Blood levels should be monitored periodically during therapy. Timing of blood levels is important in interpreting results. Draw blood for peak levels 1 hr after IM injection and 30 min after a 30-min IV infusion is completed. Trough levels should be drawn just prior to next dose. Peak level for **amikacin** and **kanamycin** should not exceed 35 mcg/ml; trough level should not exceed 5 mcg/ml. Peak level for **gentamicin** and **tobramycin** should not exceed 10 mcg/ml; trough level should not exceed 2 mcg/ml. Peak level for **netilmicin** should not exceed 16 mcg/ml; trough level should not exceed 2 mcg/ml. Peak level for **streptomycin** should not exceed 25 mcg/ml.

POTENTIAL NURSING DIAGNOSES

▪ Infection, risk for (Indications).

▪ Sensory-perceptual alterations: auditory (Side Effects).

▪ Knowledge deficit, related to medication regimen (Patient/Family Teaching).

IMPLEMENTATION

▪ **General Info:** Keep patient well hydrated (1500–2000 ml/day) during therapy.

▪ **Preoperative Bowel Prep:** Neomycin is usually used in conjunction with erythromycin, a low-residue diet, and a cathartic or enema.

▪ **PO:** May be administered without regard to meals.

▪ **IM:** IM administration should be deep into a well-developed muscle. Alternate injection sites.

❑ **Amikacin**

▪ **Intermittent Infusion:** Dilute 500 mg of amikacin in 100–200 ml of D5W, D10W, 0.9% NaCl, D5/0.9% NaCl, D5/0.45% NaCl, D5/0.25% NaCl, or lactated Ringer's solution. Solution may be pale yellow without decreased potency. Stable for 24 hr at room temperature.

- *Rate:* Infuse over 30–60 min (over 1–2 hr for infants).
- **Syringe Incompatibility:** ▪ heparin.
- **Y-Site Compatibility:** ▪ acyclovir ▪ amifostine ▪ amiodarone ▪ aztreonam ▪ cyclophosphamide ▪ diltiazem ▪ enalaprilat ▪ esmolol ▪ filgrastim ▪ fluconazole ▪ fludarabine ▪ foscarnet ▪ furosemide ▪ idarubicin ▪ labetalol ▪ lorazepam ▪ magnesium sulfate ▪ melphalan ▪ midazolam ▪ morphine ▪ ondansetron ▪ paclitaxel ▪ perphenazine ▪ sargramostim ▪ teniposide ▪ thiotepa ▪ vinorelbine ▪ zidovudine.
- **Y-Site Incompatibility:** ▪ hetastarch.
- **Additive Incompatibility:** ▪ Manufacturer does not recommend admixing.

❑ Gentamicin

- **Intermittent Infusion:** Dilute each dose in 50–200 ml of D5W, 0.9% NaCl, or lactated Ringer's solution to provide a concentration not to exceed 1 mg/ml. Also available in commercially mixed piggyback injections. Do not use solutions that are discolored or that contain a precipitate.
- *Rate:* Infuse slowly over 30 min–2 hr. For pediatric patients, the volume of diluent may be reduced but should be sufficient to permit infusion over 30 min–2 hr.
- **Syringe Incompatibility:** ▪ ampicillin ▪ cefamandole ▪ heparin.
- **Y-Site Compatibility:** ▪ acyclovir ▪ amifostine ▪ amiodarone ▪ atracurium ▪ aztreonam ▪ ciprofloxacin ▪ cyclophosphamide ▪ diltiazem ▪ enalaprilat ▪ esmolol ▪ famotidine ▪ filgrastim ▪ fluconazole ▪ fludarabine ▪ foscarnet ▪ granisetron ▪ hydromorphone ▪ insulin ▪ labetalol ▪ lorazepam ▪ magnesium sulfate ▪ melphalan ▪ meperidine ▪ midazolam ▪ morphine ▪ multivitamins ▪ ondansetron ▪ paclitaxel ▪ pancuronium ▪ perphenazine ▪ sargramostim ▪ tacrolimus ▪ teniposide ▪ thiotepa ▪ tolazoline ▪ vecuronium ▪ vinorelbine ▪ vitamin B complex with C ▪ zidovudine.
- **Y-Site Incompatibility:** ▪ furosemide ▪ heparin ▪ hetastarch ▪ idarubicin ▪ indomethacin.
- **Additive Compatibility:** ▪ atracurium ▪ aztreonam ▪ bleomycin ▪ cimetidine ▪ ciprofloxacin ▪ metronidazole ▪ ofloxacin ▪ ranitidine.
- **Additive Incompatibility:** ▪ amphotericin B ▪ heparin.

❑ Kanamycin

- **Intermittent Infusion:** Dilute each 500 mg in 100–200 ml or each 1 g in 200–400 ml of D5W, D10W, D5/0.9% NaCl, 0.9% NaCl, or lactated Ringer's solution. Dilute in a proportionately smaller volume for pediatric patients. Darkening of solution does not alter potency.
- *Rate:* Infuse slowly over 30–60 min.
- **Syringe Incompatibility:** ▪ heparin.
- **Y-Site Compatibility:** ▪ cyclophosphamide ▪ furosemide ▪ hydromorphone ▪ magnesium sulfate ▪ meperidine ▪ morphine ▪ perphenazine ▪ potassium chloride ▪ vitamin B complex with C.
- **Additive Incompatibility:** ▪ Manufacturer does not recommend admixing with other antibacterial agents.

❑ Netilmicin

- **Intermittent Infusion:** Dilute each dose in 50–200 ml of D5/LR, D5/0.9% NaCl, D5W, D10W, Ringer's or lactated Ringer's solution, 0.9% NaCl, 3% NaCl, or 5% NaCl. Dilute in a proportionately smaller volume for pediatric doses. Solution clear and colorless to pale yellow. Stable 72 hours at room temperature.
- *Rate:* Infuse slowly over 30 min–2 hr.
- **Syringe Incompatibility:** ▪ heparin.
- **Y-Site Compatibility:** ▪ amifostine ▪ aminophylline ▪ aztreonam ▪ calcium gluconate ▪ filgrastim ▪ fludarabine ▪ melphalan ▪ sargramostim ▪ teniposide ▪ thiotepa ▪ vinorelbine.
- **Y-Site Incompatibility:** ▪ furosemide ▪ heparin.
- **Additive Compatibility:** ▪ aminocaproic acid ▪ atropine ▪ clindamycin ▪ dexamethasone sodium phosphate ▪ edetate calcium disodium ▪ fibrinolysin and deoxyribonuclease ▪ hydrocortisone sodium succinate ▪ metronidazole ▪ multivitamins ▪ potassium chloride ▪ teniposide ▪ vitamin B complex with C.

❑ Streptomycin

- **IM:** Reconstitute by adding 4.2–4.5 ml of 0.9% NaCl or sterile water for injection to each 1-g vial for a concentration of 200 mg/ml, or add 3.2–3.5 ml of diluent for a concentration of 250 mg/ml. Add 17 ml of diluent to each 5-g vial for a concentration of 250 mg/ml, or add 6.5 ml for a concentration of 500 mg/ml. Do not administer concentrations

>500 mg/ml. Solution is stable for 2–28 days at room temperature or for 14 days if refrigerated, depending on manufacturer.

- **IV:** Flush IV line with D5W or 0.9% NaCl following administration.
- If aminoglycosides and penicillins or cephalosporins must be administered concurrently, administer in separate sites, at least 1 hr apart.

Tobramycin

- **Intermittent Infusion:** Dilute each dose of tobramycin in 50–100 ml of D5W, D10W, D5/0.9% NaCl, 0.9% NaCl, Ringer's or lactated Ringer's solution to provide a concentration not >1 mg/ml. Pediatric doses may be diluted in proportionately smaller amounts. Stable for 24 hr at room temperature, 96 hr if refrigerated. Also available in commercially mixed piggyback injections.
- ***Rate:*** Infuse slowly over 30–60 min in both adult and pediatric patients.
- **Syringe Incompatibility:** ▪ cefamandole ▪ clindamycin ▪ heparin.
- **Y-Site Compatibility:** ▪ acyclovir ▪ amifostine ▪ amiodarone ▪ aztreonam ▪ ciprofloxacin ▪ cyclophosphamide ▪ diltiazem ▪ enalaprilat ▪ esmolol ▪ filgrastim ▪ fluconazole ▪ fludarabine ▪ foscarnet ▪ furosemide ▪ hydromorphone ▪ insulin ▪ labetalol ▪ magnesium sulfate ▪ melphalan ▪ meperidine ▪ midazolam ▪ morphine ▪ perphenazine ▪ tacrolimus ▪ teniposide ▪ thiotepa ▪ tolazoline ▪ vinorelbine ▪ zidovudine.
- **Y-Site Incompatibility:** ▪ heparin ▪ hetastarch ▪ indomethacin ▪ sargramostim.
- **Additive Incompatibility:** ▪ Manufacturer recommends administering separately; do not admix.
- **Topical:** Cleanse skin prior to application. Wear gloves during application.

PATIENT/FAMILY TEACHING

- **General Info:** Instruct patient to report signs of hypersensitivity, tinnitus, vertigo, hearing loss, rash, dizziness, or difficulty urinating.
- Advise patient of the importance of drinking plenty of liquids.
- Teach patients with a history of rheumatic heart disease or valve replacement the importance of using antimicrobial prophylaxis before invasive medical or dental procedures.
- **PO:** Instruct patient to take as directed for full course of therapy. Missed doses should be taken as soon as possible if not almost time for next dose; do not double doses.
- Caution patient that medication may cause nausea, vomiting, or diarrhea.
- **Topical:** Instruct patient to wash affected skin gently and pat dry. Apply a thin film of ointment. Apply occlusive dressing only if ordered by physician. Patient should assess skin and inform health care professional if skin irritation develops or infection worsens.

EVALUATION

Clinical response to therapy can be evaluated by: ▪ Resolution of the signs and symptoms of infection. If no response is seen within 3–5 days, new cultures should be taken ▪ Prevention of infection in intestinal surgery ▪ Improved neurologic status in hepatic encephalopathy ▪ Endocarditis prophylaxis.

AMIODARONE

(am-ee-**oh**-da-rone)
Cordarone

CLASSIFICATION(S):
Antiarrhythmic (group III)

Pregnancy Category D

INDICATIONS

▪ Management/prophylaxis of life-threatening ventricular arrhythmias unresponsive to less toxic agents. **Unlabeled Uses:** ▪ **PO:** Management of supraventricular tachyarrhythmias.

ACTION

▪ Prolongs action potential and refractory period ▪ Inhibits adrenergic stimulation ▪ Slows the sinus rate, increases PR and QT intervals, and decreases peripheral vascular resistance (vasodilation). **Therapeutic Effects:** ▪ Suppression of arrhythmias.

PHARMACOKINETICS

Absorption: IV administration results in complete bioavailability. Slowly and variably absorbed from the GI tract (35–65%).
Distribution: Distributed to and accumulates slowly in body tissues. Reaches high levels in fat, muscle, liver, lungs, and spleen. Crosses the placenta and enters breast milk.

Metabolism and Excretion: Metabolized by the liver, excreted into bile. Minimal renal excretion. One metabolite has antiarrhythmic activity.
Half-life: 13–107 days.

CONTRAINDICATIONS AND PRECAUTIONS

Contraindicated in: ▪ Severe sinus node dysfunction ▪ 2nd- and 3rd-degree AV block ▪ Bradycardia (has caused syncope unless a pacemaker is in place) ▪ Pregnancy and lactation.
Use Cautiously in: ▪ History of congestive heart failure ▪ Thyroid disorders ▪ Severe pulmonary or liver disease ▪ Children (safety not established).

ADVERSE REACTIONS AND SIDE EFFECTS*

CNS: dizziness, fatigue, malaise, headache, insomnia.
EENT: corneal microdeposits, abnormal smell, dry eyes, optic neuritis, optic neuropathy, photophobia.
Resp: ADULT RESPIRATORY DISTRESS SYNDROME, PULMONARY FIBROSIS.
CV: CONGESTIVE HEART FAILURE, WORSENING OF ARRHYTHMIAS, bradycardia, hypotension.
GI: LIVER FUNCTION ABNORMALITIES, anorexia, constipation, nausea, vomiting, abdominal pain, abnormal taste.
GU: decreased libido, epididymitis.
Derm: photosensitivity, blue discoloration.
Endo: hypothyroidism, hyperthyroidism.
Neuro: ataxia, involuntary movement, paresthesia, peripheral neuropathy, poor coordination, tremor.

INTERACTIONS

Drug-Drug: ▪ Increases blood levels and may lead to toxicity from **digoxin** (decrease dose of digoxin by 50%) ▪ Increases blood levels and may lead to toxicity from other **group I antiarrhythmics (quinidine, procainamide, mexiletine, lidocaine,** or **flecainide**—decrease doses of other drugs by 30–50%) ▪ Increases blood levels of **cyclosporine, dextromethorphan, methotrexate, phenytoin,** and **theophylline** ▪ **Phenytoin** decreases amiodarone blood levels ▪ Increases the activity of **warfarin** (decrease dose of warfarin by 33–50%) ▪ Increased risk of bradyarrhythmias, sinus arrest, or AV heart block with **beta blockers** or **calcium channel blockers** ▪ **Cholestyramine** may decrease amiodarone blood levels ▪ **Cimetidine** increases amiodarone blood levels.

ROUTE AND DOSAGE

- **PO (Adults):** 800–1600 mg/day in 1–2 doses for 1–3 wk, then 600–800 mg/day in 1–2 doses for 1 mo, then 400 mg/day maintenance dose.
- **PO (Children):** 10 mg/kg/day (800 mg/1.72 m^2/day) for 10 days or until response or adverse reaction occurs, then 5 mg/kg/day (400 mg/1.72 m^2/day) for several weeks, then decreased to 2.5 mg/kg/day (200 mg/1.72 m^2/day) or lowest effective dose.
- **IV (Adults):** 150 mg over 10 min, followed by 360 mg over the next 6 hr and then 540 mg over the next 18 hr. Continue infusion at 0.5 mg/min until oral therapy is initiated. If arrhythmia recurs, a small loading infusion of 150 mg over 10 min should be given; in addition, the rate of the maintenance infusion may be increased. ***Conversion to initial oral therapy***—If duration of IV infusion was <1 wk, oral dose should be 800–1000 mg/day; if IV infusion was 1–3 wk, oral dose should be 600–800 mg/day; if IV infusion was >3 wk, oral dose should be 400 mg/day.

AVAILABILITY

▪ ***Tablets:*** 200 mg[Rx] ▪ ***Injection:*** 50 mg/ml in 3-ml ampules[Rx].

TIME/ACTION PROFILE (suppression of ventricular arrhythmias)

	ONSET	PEAK	DURATION
PO	1–3 wk	UK	wks–mos
IV	2 hr	UK	UK

NURSING IMPLICATIONS

ASSESSMENT

- **General Info:** ECG should be monitored continuously during IV therapy or initiation of oral therapy. Monitor heart rate and rhythm

*CAPITALS indicate life-threatening; underlines indicate most frequent.

throughout therapy; PR prolongation, slight QRS widening, T-wave amplitude reduction with T-wave widening and bifurcation, and U waves may occur. QT prolongation may be associated with worsening of arrhythmias and should be monitored closely during IV therapy. Report bradycardia or increase in arrhythmias promptly; patients receiving IV therapy may require slowing rate, discontinuing infusion, or inserting a temporary pacemaker.

- Assess patient for signs of pulmonary toxicity (rales/crackles, decreased breath sounds, pleuritic friction rub, fatigue, dyspnea, cough, pleuritic pain, fever). Chest x ray and pulmonary function tests are recommended prior to therapy. Monitor chest x ray every 3–6 mo during therapy to detect diffuse interstitial changes or alveolar infiltrates. Usually reversible after withdrawal but may be fatal.
- **IV:** Assess patient for signs and symptoms of adult respiratory distress syndrome (ARDS) throughout therapy. Report dyspnea, tachypnea, or rales/crackles promptly. Bilateral, diffuse pulmonary infiltrates are seen on chest x ray.
- Monitor blood pressure frequently. Hypotension usually occurs during first several hours of therapy and is related to rate of infusion. If hypotension occurs, slow rate.
- **PO:** Ophthalmic exams should be performed prior to and regularly throughout therapy and if visual changes (photophobia, halos around lights, decreased acuity) occur. May cause permanent loss of vision.
- Assess patient for signs of thyroid dysfunction, especially during initial therapy. Lethargy; weight gain; edema of the hands, feet, and periorbital region; and cool, pale skin suggest hypothyroidism and may require decrease in dosage or discontinuation of therapy and thyroid supplementation. Tachycardia; weight loss; nervousness; sensitivity to heat; insomnia; and warm, flushed, moist skin suggest hyperthyroidism and may require discontinuation of therapy and treatment with antithyroid agents.
- ***Lab Test Considerations:*** Monitor liver and thyroid functions prior to and periodically throughout therapy. Drug effects persist long after discontinuation. Thyroid function abnormalities are common, but clinical thyroid dysfunction is uncommon.
- May cause increased AST, ALT, and serum alkaline phosphatase concentrations.
- May cause asymptomatic elevations in antinuclear antibody (ANA) titer concentrations.

POTENTIAL NURSING DIAGNOSES

- Cardiac output, decreased (Indications).
- Gas exchange, impaired (Side Effects).
- Knowledge deficit, related to medication regimen (Patient/Family Teaching).

IMPLEMENTATION

- **General Info:** Patients should be hospitalized and monitored closely during IV therapy and initiation of oral therapy. IV therapy should be administered only by physicians experienced in treating life-threatening arrhythmias.
- Do not confuse amiodarone with amrinone (written orders should include brand names).
- Hypokalemia and hypomagnesemia may decrease effectiveness or cause additional arrhythmias; correct prior to therapy.
- Assist patient during ambulation to prevent falls. Neurotoxicity (ataxia, proximal muscle weakness, tingling or numbness in fingers or toes, uncontrolled movements, tremors) is common during initial therapy, but may occur within 1 wk to several months of initiation of therapy and may persist for more than 1 yr after withdrawal. Dosage reduction is recommended.
- Monitor closely when converting from IV to oral therapy, especially in elderly patients.
- **PO:** May be administered with meals and in divided doses if GI intolerance occurs.
- **IV:** Administer via volumetric pump; drop size may be reduced, causing altered dosing with drop counter infusion sets.
- Infusions longer than 1 hr should not exceed 2 mg/ml unless administered through a central venous catheter.
- Administer through an in-line filter.
- Infusions exceeding 2 hr must be administered in glass or polyolefin bottles to prevent adsorption. However, polyvinyl chloride (PVC) tubing must be used during administration as concentrations and infusion rate recommendations have been based on PVC tubing.
- **Intermittent Infusion:** Recommended starting dose of about 1000 mg over 24 hr is administered during loading and maintenance infusions.

Initial loading dose

- Add 3 ml (150 mg) of amiodarone to 100 ml D5W for a concentration of 1.5 mg/ml.
- ***Rate:*** Administer rapidly over 10 min (see Appendix D).

Loading infusion

- Add 18 ml (900 mg) of amiodarone to 500 ml of D5W for a concentration of 1.8 mg/ml.
- ***Rate:*** Administer slowly, 360 mg over next 6 hr at a rate of 1 mg/min.

Maintenance infusion

- Administer remainder of loading infusion.
- ***Rate:*** Administer 540 mg over the remaining 18 hr at a rate of 0.5 mg/min.
- **Continuous Infusion:** After initial 24 hr, infusion may continue using a concentration of 1–6 mg/ml. Administer concentrations of >2 mg/ml via central venous catheter.
- ***Rate:*** Administer at maintenance infusion rate of 0.5 mg/min (720 mg/24 hr). May be increased to achieve effective arrhythmia suppression but should not exceed 30 mg/min.
- **Supplemental Infusions:** If breakthrough episodes of ventricular fibrillation or hemodynamically unstable ventricular tachycardia occur, dilute 150 mg of amiodarone in 100 ml of D5W.
- ***Rate:*** Administer over 10 min to minimize hypotension.
- **Y-Site Compatibility:** ▪ amikacin ▪ bretylium ▪ clindamycin ▪ dobutamine ▪ dopamine ▪ doxycycline ▪ erythromycin lactobionate ▪ esmolol ▪ gentamicin ▪ insulin ▪ isoproterenol ▪ labetalol ▪ metaraminol ▪ metronidazole ▪ midazolum ▪ morphine ▪ norepinephrine ▪ penicillin G potassium ▪ phentolamine ▪ phenylephrine ▪ potassium chloride ▪ procainamide ▪ tobramycin ▪ vancomycin.
- **Y-Site Incompatibility:** ▪ aminophylline ▪ cefamandole ▪ cefazolin ▪ heparin ▪ mezlocillin ▪ sodium bicarbonate.
- **Additive Incompatibility:** ▪ aminophylline ▪ cefamandole ▪ cefazolin ▪ heparin ▪ mezlocillin ▪ sodium bicarbonate.

PATIENT/FAMILY TEACHING

- Instruct patient to take this medication exactly as directed. If a dose is missed, do not take at all. Consult health care professional if more than two doses are missed.
- Inform patient that side effects may not appear until several days, weeks, or years after initiation of therapy and may persist for several months after withdrawal.
- Teach patients to monitor pulse daily and report abnormalities.
- Advise patients that photosensitivity reactions may occur through window glass, thin clothing, and sunscreens. Protective clothing and sunblock are recommended during and for 4 mo following therapy. If photosensitivity occurs, dosage reduction may be useful.
- Inform patients that bluish discoloration of the face, neck, and arms is a possible side effect of this drug following prolonged use. This is usually reversible and will fade over several months. Notify health care professional if this occurs.
- Instruct male patients to notify health care professional if signs of epididymitis (pain and swelling in scrotum) occur. May require reduction in dose.
- Instruct patient to notify health care professional of medication regimen prior to treatment or surgery.
- Emphasize the importance of follow-up exams, including chest x ray and pulmonary function tests every 3–6 mo and ophthalmic exams after 6 mo of therapy, and then annually.

EVALUATION

Effectiveness of therapy can be demonstrated by: ▪ Cessation of life-threatening ventricular arrhythmias. Adverse effects may take up to 4 mo to resolve.

AMITRIPTYLINE

(a-mee-**trip**-ti-leen)
{Apo-Amitriptyline}, Elavil, Endep, Enovil, {Levate}, {Novotriptyn}

CLASSIFICATION(S):
Antidepressant (tricyclic)

Pregnancy Category C

INDICATIONS

▪ Treatment of depression, often in conjunction with psychotherapy. **Unlabeled Uses:** ▪ Chronic pain syndromes.

ACTION

▪ Potentiates the effect of serotonin and norepinephrine in the CNS ▪ Has significant anticholinergic properties. **Therapeutic Effects:** ▪ Antidepressant action.

PHARMACOKINETICS

Absorption: Well absorbed from the GI tract.
Distribution: Widely distributed.
Metabolism and Excretion: Extensively metabolized by the liver. Some metabolites are pharmacologically active. Undergoes enterohepatic recirculation and secretion into gastric juices. Probably crosses the placenta and enters breast milk.
Half-life: 10–50 hr.

CONTRAINDICATIONS AND PRECAUTIONS

Contraindicated in: ▪ Narrow-angle glaucoma ▪ Pregnancy and lactation.
Use Cautiously in: ▪ Elderly patients ▪ Patients with pre-existing cardiovascular disease ▪ Prostatic hypertrophy (increased risk of urinary retention) ▪ History of seizures (threshold may be lowered).

ADVERSE REACTIONS AND SIDE EFFECTS*

CNS: lethargy, sedation.
EENT: blurred vision, dry eyes, dry mouth.
CV: ARRHYTHMIAS, hypotension, ECG changes.
GI: constipation, hepatitis, paralytic ileus.
GU: urinary retention.
Derm: photosensitivity.
Endo: changes in blood glucose, gynecomastia.
Hemat: blood dyscrasias.
Misc: increased appetite, weight gain.

INTERACTIONS

Drug-Drug: ▪ May cause hypotension, tachycardia, and potentially fatal reactions when used with **MAO inhibitors** (avoid concurrent use—discontinue 2 wk prior to amitriptyline) ▪ May prevent the therapeutic response to **clonidine, guanedrel**, and **guanethidine** ▪ Additive CNS depression with other **CNS depressants** including **alcohol, antihistamines, clonidine, opioid analgesics**, and **sedative/hypnotics** ▪ **Adrenergic** and **anticholinergic** side effects may be additive with other **agents having these properties** ▪ **Cimetidine, fluoxetine, phenothiazines,** or **oral contraceptives** increase levels and may cause toxicity ▪ Increased risk of agranulocytosis with **antithyroid drugs.**

ROUTE AND DOSAGE

- **PO (Adults):** 50–100 mg/day single bedtime dose or divided doses. Dose may be gradually increased up to 150–300 mg/day.
- **PO (Children >12 yr):** 10 mg tid and 20 mg at hs. May be slowly increased to 100 mg/day as a single bedtime dose or divided doses.
- **PO (Children 6–12 yr):** 10–30 mg/day (1–5 mg/kg/day) in 2 divided doses.
- **PO (Geriatric Patients):** 25 mg at hs. May be slowly increased up to 10 mg tid and 20 mg at hs (daily dose not to exceed 100 mg).
- **IM (Adults):** 20–30 mg 4 times daily.

AVAILABILITY

▪ ***Tablets:*** 10 mg[Rx], 25 mg[Rx], 50 mg[Rx], 75 mg[Rx], 100 mg[Rx], 150 mg[Rx] ▪ ***Syrup:*** 10 mg/5 ml[Rx] ▪ ***Injection:*** 10 mg/ml[Rx].

TIME/ACTION PROFILE (antidepressant effect)

	ONSET	PEAK	DURATION
PO	2–3 wk	2–6 wk	days–wks
IM	2–3 wk	2–6 wk	days–wks

NURSING IMPLICATIONS

ASSESSMENT

- Monitor mental status and affect. Assess for suicidal tendencies, especially during early therapy. Restrict amount of drug available to patient.
- Monitor blood pressure and pulse prior to and during initial therapy. Notify physician or other health care professional of decreases in blood pressure (10–20 mm Hg) or sudden increase in pulse rate. Patients taking high doses or with a history of cardiovascular disease should have ECG monitored prior to and periodically throughout therapy.

▪ ***Lab Test Considerations:*** Assess leukocyte and differential blood counts, liver function, and serum glucose periodically. May cause an elevated serum bilirubin and alkaline phosphatase. May cause bone marrow de-

***CAPITALS indicate life-threatening; underlines indicate most frequent.**

pression. Serum glucose may be increased or decreased.

POTENTIAL NURSING DIAGNOSES

- Coping, ineffective, individual (Indications).
- Injury, risk for (Side Effects).
- Knowledge deficit, related to medication regimen (Patient/Family Teaching).

IMPLEMENTATION

- **General Info:** Dose increases should be made at bedtime because of sedation. Dose titration is a slow process; may take weeks to months. May give entire dose at bedtime.
- **PO:** Administer medication with or immediately after a meal to minimize gastric upset. Tablet may be crushed and given with food or fluids.
- **IM:** For short-term IM administration only. Do not administer IV.

PATIENT/FAMILY TEACHING

- □ Instruct patient to take medication exactly as directed. If a dose is missed, take as soon as possible unless almost time for next dose; if regimen is a single dose at bedtime, do not take in the morning because of side effects. Advise patient that drug effects may not be noticed for at least 2 wk. Abrupt discontinuation may cause nausea, vomiting, diarrhea, headache, trouble sleeping with vivid dreams, and irritability.
- □ May cause drowsiness and blurred vision. Caution patient to avoid driving and other activities requiring alertness until response to drug is known.
- □ Orthostatic hypotension, sedation, and confusion are common during early therapy, especially in the elderly. Protect patient from falls and advise patient to make position changes slowly.
- □ Advise patient to avoid alcohol or other CNS depressant drugs during and for 3–7 days after therapy has been discontinued.
- □ Instruct patient to notify health care professional if urinary retention occurs or if dry mouth or constipation persists. Sugarless candy or gum may diminish dry mouth, and an increase in fluid intake or bulk may prevent constipation. If symptoms persist, dose reduction or discontinuation may be necessary. Consult health care professional if dry mouth persists for more than 2 wk.
- □ Caution patient to use sunscreen and protective clothing to prevent photosensitivity reactions.
- □ Inform patient of need to monitor dietary intake. Increase in appetite may lead to undesired weight gain.
- □ Advise patient to notify health care professional of medication regimen prior to treatment or surgery.
- □ Therapy for depression is usually prolonged. Emphasize the importance of follow-up exams to monitor effectiveness and side effects.

EVALUATION

Effectiveness of therapy can be demonstrated by: ▪ Increased sense of well-being □ Renewed interest in surroundings □ Increased appetite □ Improved energy level □ Improved sleep ▪ Decrease in chronic pain symptoms ▪ Full therapeutic effects may be seen 2–6 wk after initiating therapy.

AMLODIPINE

(am-**loe**-di-peen)

Norvasc

CLASSIFICATION(S):

Calcium channel blocker (antihypertensive agent)

Pregnancy Category C

INDICATIONS

▪ Alone or with other agents in the management of hypertension, angina pectoris, and vasospastic (Prinzmetal's) angina.

ACTION

▪ Inhibits the transport of calcium into myocardial and vascular smooth muscle cells, resulting in inhibition of excitation-contraction coupling and subsequent contraction. **Therapeutic Effects:** ▪ Systemic vasodilation resulting in decreased blood pressure ▪ Coronary vasodilation resulting in decreased frequency and severity of attacks of angina.

PHARMACOKINETICS

Absorption: Well absorbed following oral administration (64–90%).

Distribution: Probably crosses the placenta.
Protein Binding: 95–98%.
Metabolism and Excretion: Mostly metabolized by the liver.
Half-life: 30–50 hr.

CONTRAINDICATIONS AND PRECAUTIONS

Contraindicated in: ▪ Hypersensitivity ▪ Sick sinus syndrome ▪ 2nd- or 3rd-degree AV block (unless an artificial pacemaker is in place) ▪ Blood pressure <90 mm Hg.
Use Cautiously in: ▪ Severe hepatic impairment (dosage reduction recommended) ▪ Geriatric patients (dosage reduction recommended; increased risk of hypotension) ▪ History of serious ventricular arrhythmias or congestive heart failure ▪ Pregnancy, lactation, or children (safety not established).

ADVERSE REACTIONS AND SIDE EFFECTS*

CNS: abnormal dreams, anxiety, confusion, dizziness/light-headedness, drowsiness, headache, jitteriness, nervousness, psychiatric disturbances, shakiness, weakness.
EENT: blurred vision, disturbed equilibrium, tinnitus.
Resp: congestion, cough, dyspnea, epistaxis, shortness of breath.
CV: ARRHYTHMIAS, CONGESTIVE HEART FAILURE, peripheral edema, bradycardia, chest pain, hypotension, palpitations, syncope, tachycardia.
GI: abnormal liver function studies, anorexia, constipation, diarrhea, dry mouth, dysgeusia, dyspepsia, nausea, vomiting.
GU: dysuria, nocturia, polyuria, sexual dysfunction, urinary frequency.
Derm: STEVENS-JOHNSON SYNDROME, dermatitis/rash, erythema multiforme, flushing, increased sweating, photosensitivity, pruritus/urticaria, rash.
Endo: gynecomastia, hyperglycemia.
Hemat: anemia, leukopenia, thrombocytopenia.
Metab: weight gain.
MS: joint stiffness, muscle cramps.
Neuro: paresthesia, tremor.
Misc: gingival hyperplasia.

INTERACTIONS

Drug-Drug: ▪ Additive hypotension may occur when used concurrently with **fentanyl, other antihypertensives, nitrates,** acute ingestion of **alcohol**, or **quinidine** ▪ Antihypertensive effects may be decreased by concurrent use of **NSAIDs.**
Drug-Food: ▪ Blood levels are increased by concurrent ingestion of **grapefruit juice.**

ROUTE AND DOSAGE

- **PO (Adults):** 5–10 mg as a single dose (range 2.5–10 mg). Initiate therapy with 2.5 mg/day in geriatric or small patients or patients with hepatic insufficiency.

AVAILABILITY

▪ ***Tablets:*** 2.5 mg[Rx], 5 mg[Rx], 10 mg[Rx] ▪ ***In combination with:*** benazepril (Lotrel)[Rx]. See Appendix A.

TIME/ACTION PROFILE (cardiovascular effects)

	ONSET	PEAK	DURATION
PO	UK	6–9	24 hr

NURSING IMPLICATIONS

ASSESSMENT

- **General Info:** Monitor blood pressure and pulse prior to therapy, during dosage titration, and periodically during therapy. Monitor ECG periodically during prolonged therapy.
- Monitor intake and output ratios and daily weight. Assess for signs of congestive heart failure (peripheral edema, rales/crackles, dyspnea, weight gain, jugular venous distention).
- **Angina:** Assess location, duration, intensity, and precipitating factors of patient's anginal pain.
- ***Lab Test Considerations:*** Total serum calcium concentrations are not affected by calcium channel blockers.

POTENTIAL NURSING DIAGNOSES

- Tissue perfusion, altered (Indications).
- Pain (Indications).
- Knowledge deficit, related to medication regimen (Patient/Family Teaching).

*CAPITALS indicate life-threatening; underlines indicate most frequent.

IMPLEMENTATION

- **PO:** May be administered without regard to meals.

PATIENT/FAMILY TEACHING

- **General Info:** Advise patient to take medication exactly as directed, even if feeling well. If a dose is missed, take as soon as possible unless almost time for next dose; do not double doses. May need to be discontinued gradually.
- Instruct patient on correct technique for monitoring pulse. Instruct patient to contact health care professional if heart rate is <50 bpm.
- Caution patient to change positions slowly to minimize orthostatic hypotension.
- May cause drowsiness or dizziness. Advise patient to avoid driving or other activities requiring alertness until response to the medication is known.
- Instruct patient on importance of maintaining good dental hygiene and seeing dentist frequently for teeth cleaning to prevent tenderness, bleeding, and gingival hyperplasia (gum enlargement).
- Instruct patient to avoid concurrent use of alcohol or OTC medications, especially cold preparations, without consulting health care professional.
- Advise patient to notify health care professional if irregular heartbeats, dyspnea, swelling of hands and feet, pronounced dizziness, nausea, constipation, or hypotension occurs or if headache is severe or persistent.
- Caution patient to wear protective clothing and use sunscreen to prevent photosensitivity reactions.
- Advise patient to inform health care professional of medication regimen before treatment or surgery.
- **Angina:** Instruct patient on concurrent nitrate or beta-blocker therapy to continue taking both medications as directed and to use SL nitroglycerin as needed for anginal attacks.
- Advise patient to contact health care professional if chest pain does not improve or worsens after therapy, occurs with diaphoresis, shortness of breath occurs, or if severe, persistent headache occurs.
- Caution patient to discuss exercise restrictions with health care professional prior to exertion.
- **Hypertension:** Encourage patient to comply with other interventions for hypertension (weight reduction, low-sodium diet, smoking cessation, moderation of alcohol consumption, regular exercise, and stress management). Medication controls but does not cure hypertension.
- Instruct patient and family in proper technique for monitoring blood pressure. Advise patient to take blood pressure weekly and to report significant changes to health care professional.

EVALUATION

Effectiveness of therapy can be demonstrated by: ▪ Decrease in blood pressure ▪ Decrease in frequency and severity of anginal attacks ▫ Decrease in need for nitrate therapy ▫ Increase in activity tolerance and sense of well-being.

AMOXAPINE

(a-**mox**-a-peen)

Asendin

CLASSIFICATION(S):

Antidepressant (tricyclic)

Pregnancy Category C

INDICATIONS

- Treatment of depression accompanied by anxiety, often used in conjunction with psychotherapy.

ACTION

▪ Potentiates the effects of serotonin and norepinephrine in the CNS ▪ Has significant anticholinergic properties ▪ Also has antianxiety effect related to sedative properties. **Therapeutic Effects:** ▪ Antidepressant and antianxiety action.

PHARMACOKINETICS

Absorption: Well absorbed following oral administration.

Distribution: Widely distributed. Enters breast milk.

Metabolism and Excretion: Extensively metabolized by the liver.

Half-life: 8 hr.

CONTRAINDICATIONS AND PRECAUTIONS

Contraindicated in: ▪ Narrow-angle glaucoma ▪ Pregnancy and lactation.

Use Cautiously in: ▪ Elderly patients (dosage reduction required) ▪ History of cardiovascular disease ▪ Elderly men (increased susceptibility to urinary retention) ▪ History of seizures (threshold may be lowered) ▪ Children <16 yr (safety not established).

ADVERSE REACTIONS AND SIDE EFFECTS*

CNS: NEUROLEPTIC MALIGNANT SYNDROME, fatigue, sedation, extrapyramidal reactions, tardive dyskinesia.

EENT: blurred vision, dry eyes, dry mouth.

CV: ARRHYTHMIAS, hypotension, ECG changes.

GI: constipation, increased appetite, paralytic ileus.

GU: urinary retention, testicular swelling.

Derm: photosensitivity, rash.

Endo: gynecomastia, sexual dysfunction.

Hemat: blood dyscrasias.

Misc: fever, weight gain.

INTERACTIONS

Drug-Drug: ▪ May cause hypotension, tachycardia, and potentially fatal reactions when used with **MAO inhibitors** (avoid concurrent use—discontinue 2 wk prior to amoxapine) ▪ May prevent the therapeutic response to **clonidine, guanadrel**, and **guanethidine** ▪ Additive CNS depression with other **CNS depressants** including **alcohol, clonidine, antihistamines, opioid analgesics**, and **sedative/hypnotics** ▪ **Adrenergic** and **anticholinergic** side effects may be additive with other **agents having these properties** ▪ **Cimetidine, fluoxetine, phenothiazines**, or **oral contraceptives** increase levels and may cause toxicity ▪ Increased risk of agranulocytosis with **antithyroid drugs.** ▪ Increased risk of extrapyramidal reactions with other **drugs causing extrapyramidal reactions (phenothiazines).**

ROUTE AND DOSAGE

- **PO (Adults):** 50 mg 2–3 times daily, increase to 100 mg 2–3 times daily by end of 1 week (not to exceed 300 mg daily in outpatients, 600 mg daily in divided doses in hospitalized patients). Once optimal dose is achieved, may be given as a single bedtime dose; no single dose to exceed 300 mg.
- **PO (Geriatric Patients):** 25 mg 2–3 times daily, may be increased to 50 mg 2–3 times daily (not >300 mg/day).

AVAILABILITY

- ***Tablets:*** 25 mg[Rx], 50 mg[Rx], 100 mg[Rx], 150 mg[Rx].

TIME/ACTION PROFILE (antidepressant effect)

	ONSET	PEAK	DURATION
PO	1–2 wk	2–6 wk	days–wks

NURSING IMPLICATIONS

ASSESSMENT

- Monitor mental status and affect. Assess for suicidal tendencies, especially during early therapy. Restrict amount of drug available to patient.
- Monitor blood pressure and pulse prior to and during initial therapy. Notify physician or other health care professional of decreases in blood pressure (10–20 mm Hg) or sudden increase in pulse rate. Patients taking high doses or with a history of cardiovascular disease should have ECG monitored prior to and periodically throughout therapy.
- Observe for onset of extrapyramidal side effects (akathisia—restlessness; dystonia—muscle spasms and twisting motions; pseudoparkinsonism—mask facies, rigidity, tremors, drooling, shuffling gait, dysphagia, pill-rolling motions). Dosage reduction or discontinuation may be necessary. Trihexyphenidyl or diphenhydramine may be used to control these symptoms.
- Monitor for tardive dyskinesia (lip smacking or puckering, puffing of cheeks, rhythmic chewing or worm-like movement of tongue and mouth, uncontrolled movements of extremities). Notify physician or other health care professional immediately if these symptoms occur, as they may be irreversible.
- Monitor for development of neuroleptic malignant syndrome (fever, respiratory distress, tachycardia, convulsions, diaphoresis, hyper-

*CAPITALS indicate life-threatening; underlines indicate most frequent.

tension or hypotension, pallor, tiredness, severe muscle stiffness, loss of bladder control). Notify physician or other health care professional immediately if these symptoms occur.

- ***Lab Test Considerations:*** May cause elevated serum prolactin levels.
  - □ Monitor CBC and differential during chronic therapy. May rarely cause bone marrow suppression.
  - □ In chronic therapy periodically monitor hepatic and renal function. Serum glucose may be increased or decreased.

POTENTIAL NURSING DIAGNOSES

- Coping, ineffective, individual (Indications).
- Injury, risk for (Side Effects).
- Knowledge deficit, related to medication regimen (Patient/Family Teaching).

IMPLEMENTATION

- **General Info:** Dose increases should be made at bedtime because of sedation. Dosage titration is a slow process; may take weeks to months. May give entire dose (if <300 mg) at bedtime, when dose is stabilized.
- **PO:** Administer medication with or immediately following a meal to minimize gastric irritation.

PATIENT/FAMILY TEACHING

- □ Instruct patient to take medication exactly as directed. Abrupt discontinuation may cause nausea, headache, and malaise.
- □ May cause drowsiness and blurred vision. Caution patient to avoid driving and other activities requiring alertness until response to drug is known.
- □ Orthostatic hypotension, sedation, and confusion are common during early therapy, especially in the elderly. Protect patient from falls and advise patient to make position changes slowly.
- □ Advise patient to avoid alcohol or other CNS depressant drugs during and for 3–7 days after therapy.
- □ Instruct patient to notify health care professional if dry mouth or constipation persists or if urinary retention, uncontrolled movements, or rigidity occurs. Sugarless candy or gum may diminish dry mouth, and an increase in fluid intake or bulk may prevent constipation. If these symptoms persist, dosage reduction or discontinuation may be necessary. Consult health care professional if dry mouth persists for more than 2 wk.
- □ Advise patient to inform health care professional if breast enlargement or sexual dysfunction occurs.
- □ Caution patient to use sunscreen and protective clothing to prevent photosensitivity reactions.
- □ Inform patient to monitor dietary intake. Increased appetite may lead to undesired weight gain.
- □ Advise patient to notify health care professional of medication regimen prior to treatment or surgery.
- □ Therapy for depression is usually prolonged. Emphasize the importance of follow-up exams to monitor effectiveness and side effects.

EVALUATION

Effectiveness of therapy can be demonstrated by: ▪ Increased sense of well-being □ Renewed interest in surroundings □ Increased appetite □ Improved energy level □ Improved sleep □ Decreased anxiety. Initial response may be noted in 4–7 days in some patients. Most patients respond within 2 wk.

AMOXICILLIN

(a-mox-i-**sill**-in)

Amoxil, {Apo-Amoxi}, {Novamoxin}, {Nu-Amoxi}, Polymox, Trimox, Wymox

CLASSIFICATION(S):
Anti-infective (aminopenicillin)

Pregnancy Category B

INDICATIONS

▪ Treatment of the following infections: □ Skin and skin structure infections □ Otitis media □ Sinusitis □ Respiratory infections □ Genitourinary infections □ Meningitis □ Septicemia ▪ Endocarditis prophylaxis ▪ Management of ulcer disease due to *Helicobacter pylori*. **Unlabeled Uses:** ▪ Lyme disease.

ACTION

▪ Binds to bacterial cell wall, causing cell death. **Therapeutic Effects:** ▪ Bactericidal action; spectrum is broader than penicillin. **Spectrum:** ▪ Active against: ▫ Streptococci ▫ Pneumococci ▫ Enterococci ▫ *Haemophilus influenzae* ▫ *Escherichia coli* ▫ *Proteus mirabilis* ▫ *Neisseria meningitidis* ▫ *Shigella* ▫ *Salmonella* ▫ *Borrelia burgdorferi*. ▫ *H. pylori*.

PHARMACOKINETICS

Absorption: Well absorbed from the duodenum (75–90%). More resistant to acid inactivation than other penicillins.
Distribution: Diffuses readily into most body tissues and fluids. CSF penetration is increased when meninges are inflamed. Crosses the placenta; enters breast milk in small amounts.
Metabolism and Excretion: 70% excreted unchanged in the urine. 30% metabolized by the liver.
Half-life: 1–1.3 hr.

CONTRAINDICATIONS AND PRECAUTIONS

Contraindicated in: ▪ Hypersensitivity to penicillins.
Use Cautiously in: ▪ Severe renal insufficiency (dosage reduction necessary) ▪ Has been used safely during pregnancy and lactation ▪ Infectious mononucleosis (increased incidence of rash).

ADVERSE REACTIONS AND SIDE EFFECTS*

CNS: SEIZURES (high doses).
GI: PSEUDOMEMBRANOUS COLITIS, diarrhea, nausea, vomiting.
Derm: rashes, urticaria.
Hemat: blood dyscrasias.
Misc: allergic reactions including ANAPHYLAXIS and SERUM SICKNESS, superinfection.

INTERACTIONS

Drug-Drug: ▪ **Probenecid** decreases renal excretion and increases blood levels of amoxicillin—therapy may be combined for this purpose ▪ May potentiate the effect of **warfarin** ▪ May decrease the effectiveness of **oral contraceptives.**

ROUTE AND DOSAGE

▫ Most Infections

- **PO (Adults and Children >20 kg):** 250–500 mg q 8 hr.
- **PO (Children 8–20 kg):** 6.7–13.3 mg/kg q 8 hr.
- **PO (Children 6–8 kg):** 50–100 mg q 8 hr.
- **PO (Children <6 kg):** 25–50 mg q 8 hr.

▫ *Helicobacter Pylori*

- **PO (Adults):** 500 mg 4 times daily or 750 mg 3 times daily (unlabeled).

▫ Endocarditis Prophylaxis

- **PO (Adults):** 2 g 1 hr prior to procedure.
- **PO (Children):** 50 mg/kg 1 hr prior to procedure.

AVAILABILITY

▪ ***Chewable tablets:*** 125 mg[Rx], 250 mg[Rx] ▪ ***Capsules:*** 250 mg[Rx], 500 mg[Rx] ▪ ***Suspension:*** 50 mg/ml[Rx], 125 mg/5 ml[Rx], 250 mg/5 ml[Rx] ▪ ***In combination with:*** clarithromycin and lansoprazole in a compliance package (Prevpac). See Appendix A.

TIME/ACTION PROFILE (blood levels)

	ONSET	PEAK	DURATION
PO	30 min	1–2 hr	8 hr

NURSING IMPLICATIONS

ASSESSMENT

▫ Assess patient for infection (vital signs; appearance of wound, sputum, urine, and stool; WBC) at beginning of and throughout therapy.
▫ Obtain a history before initiating therapy to determine previous use of and reactions to penicillins or cephalosporins. Persons with a negative history of penicillin sensitivity may still have an allergic response.
▫ Observe for signs and symptoms of anaphylaxis (rash, pruritus, laryngeal edema, wheezing). Notify the physician or other health care professional immediately if these occur.
▫ Obtain specimens for culture and sensitivity

*CAPITALS indicate life-threatening; underlines indicate most frequent.

prior to therapy. First dose may be given before receiving results.

- *Lab Test Considerations:* May cause increased serum alkaline phosphatase, LDH, AST, and ALT concentrations.
- May cause false-positive direct Coombs' test result.

POTENTIAL NURSING DIAGNOSES

- Infection, risk for (Indications, Side Effects).
- Knowledge deficit, related to medication regimen (Patient/Family Teaching).
- Noncompliance, related to medication regimen (Patient/Family Teaching).

IMPLEMENTATION

- **PO:** Administer around the clock. May be given without regard to meals. May be given with meals to decrease GI side effects. Capsule contents may be emptied and swallowed with liquids. Chewable tablets should be crushed or chewed before swallowing with liquids.
- Shake oral suspension before administering. Suspension may be given straight or mixed in formula, milk, fruit juice, water, or ginger ale. Administer immediately after mixing. Discard refrigerated reconstituted suspension after 10 days.

PATIENT/FAMILY TEACHING

- Instruct patients to take medication around the clock and to finish the drug completely as directed, even if feeling better. Advise patients that sharing of this medication may be dangerous.
- Instruct female patients taking oral contraceptives to use an alternate or additional nonhormonal method of contraception during therapy with amoxicillin and until next menstrual period.
- Advise patient to report the signs of superinfection (furry overgrowth on the tongue, vaginal itching or discharge, loose or foul-smelling stools) and allergy.
- Instruct the patient to notify health care professional if symptoms do not improve or if nausea or diarrhea persists when drug is administered with food.
- Teach patients with a history of rheumatic heart disease or valve replacement the importance of using antimicrobial prophylaxis before invasive medical or dental procedures (see Appendix N).

EVALUATION

Clinical response to therapy can be evaluated by: ▪ Resolution of the signs and symptoms of infection. Length of time for complete resolution depends on the organism and site of infection ▪ Endocarditis prophylaxis.

AMOXICILLIN/CLAVULANATE

(a-mox-i-**sill**-in/klav-yoo-**lan**-ate)

Augmentin, {Clavulin}

CLASSIFICATION(S):

Anti-infective (aminopenicillin/beta-lactamase inhibitor)

Pregnancy Category B

INDICATIONS

▪ Treatment of a variety of infections including: ▫ Skin and skin structure infections ▫ Otitis media ▫ Sinusitis ▫ Respiratory tract infections ▫ Genitourinary tract infections ▫ Meningitis ▫ Septicemia.

ACTION

▪ Binds to bacterial cell wall, causing cell death; spectrum of amoxicillin is broader than penicillin. Clavulanate resists action of beta-lactamase, an enzyme produced by bacteria that is capable of inactivating some penicillins. **Therapeutic Effects:** ▪ Bactericidal action against susceptible bacteria. **Spectrum:** ▪ Active against: ▫ Streptococci ▫ Pneumococci ▫ Enterococci ▫ *Haemophilus influenzae* ▫ *Escherichia coli* ▫ *Proteus mirabilis* ▫ *Neisseria menigitidis* ▫ *Shigella* ▫ *Salmonella* ▫ *Moraxella catarrhalis.*

PHARMACOKINETICS

Absorption: Well absorbed from the duodenum (75–90%). More resistant to acid inactivation than other penicillins.

Distribution: Diffuses readily into most body tissues and fluids. CSF penetration is increased

in the presence of inflamed meninges. Crosses the placenta and enters breast milk in small amounts.
Metabolism and Excretion: 70% excreted unchanged in the urine; 30% metabolized by the liver.
Half-life: 1–1.3 hr.

CONTRAINDICATIONS AND PRECAUTIONS

Contraindicated in: ▪ Hypersensitivity to penicillins ▪ Hypersensitivity to clavulanate ▪ Suspension and chewable tablets contain aspartame and should be avoided in phenylketonurics.
Use Cautiously in: ▪ Severe renal insufficiency (dosage reduction necessary) ▪ Infectious mononucleosis (increased incidence of rash).

ADVERSE REACTIONS AND SIDE EFFECTS*

CNS: SEIZURES (high doses).
GI: PSEUDOMEMBRANOUS COLITIS, diarrhea, nausea, vomiting.
Derm: rashes, urticaria.
Hemat: blood dyscrasias.
Misc: allergic reactions including ANAPHYLAXIS and SERUM SICKNESS, superinfection.

INTERACTIONS

Drug-Drug: ▪ **Probenecid** decreases renal excretion and increases blood levels of amoxicillin—therapy may be combined for this purpose ▪ May potentiate the effect of **warfarin** ▪ Concurrent **allopurinol** therapy increases risk of rash ▪ May decrease the effectiveness of **oral contraceptives.**

ROUTE AND DOSAGE

❑ Most Infections

- **PO (Adults and Children >40 kg): Tablets:** 1–500 mg tablet q 12 hr or 1–250 mg tablet q 8 hr. **Suspension:** 500 mg q 12 hr as 125 mg/5 ml or 250 mg/5 ml suspension.
- **PO (Children ≥3 mo):** 12.5 mg/kg q 12 hr (as 200 mg/5ml or 400 mg/5 ml suspension) or 6.6 mg/kg q 8 hr (as 125 mg/5 ml or 250 mg/5 ml suspension).

❑ Severe Infections, Respiratory Tract Infections, or Otitis Media

- **PO (Adults):** 875 mg (1 tablet) q 12 hr or 500 mg (1 tablet) q 8 hr.
- **PO (Children ≥3 mo):** 22.5 mg/kg q 12 hr (as 200 mg/5ml or 400 mg/5 ml suspension) or 13.3 mg/kg q 8 hr (as 125 mg/5 ml or 250 mg/5 ml suspension).

AVAILABILITY

▪ ***Tablets:*** 250 mg amoxicillin with 125 mg clavulanic acid^Rx^, 500 mg amoxicillin with 125 mg clavulanate^Rx^, 875 mg amoxicillin with 125 mg clavulanate^Rx^ ▪ ***Chewable tablets:*** 125 mg amoxicillin with 31.25 mg clavulanate^Rx^, 200 mg amoxicillin with 28.5 mg clavulanate^Rx^, 250 mg amoxicillin with 62.5 mg clavulanate^Rx^, 400 mg amoxicillin with 57 mg clavulanate^Rx^ ▪ ***Suspension:*** 125 mg amoxicillin with 31.25 mg clavulanic acid/5 ml^Rx^, 200 mg amoxicillin with 28.5 mg clavulanic acid/5 ml^Rx^, 250 mg amoxicillin with 62.5 mg clavulanate/5 ml^Rx^, 400 mg amoxicillin with 57 mg clavulanic acid/5 ml^Rx^.

TIME/ACTION PROFILE (peak blood levels)

	ONSET	PEAK	DURATION
PO	30 min	1–2 hr	8 hr

NURSING IMPLICATIONS

ASSESSMENT

- ❑ Assess patient for infection (vital signs; appearance of wound, sputum, urine, and stool; WBC) at beginning of and throughout therapy.
- ❑ Obtain a history before initiating therapy to determine previous use of and reactions to penicillins or cephalosporins. Persons with a negative history of penicillin sensitivity may still have an allergic response.
- ❑ Observe for signs and symptoms of anaphylaxis (rash, pruritus, laryngeal edema, wheezing). Notify the physician or other health care professional immediately if these occur.
- ❑ Obtain specimens for culture and sensitivity prior to therapy. First dose may be given before receiving results.
- ▪ ***Lab Test Considerations:*** May cause increased serum alkaline phosphatase, LDH, AST, and ALT concentrations.

*CAPITALS indicate life-threatening; underlines indicate most frequent.

□ May cause false-positive direct Coombs' test result.

POTENTIAL NURSING DIAGNOSES

- Infection, risk for (Indications, Side Effects).
- Knowledge deficit, related to medication regimen (Patient/Family Teaching).
- Noncompliance, related to medication regimen (Patient/Family Teaching).

IMPLEMENTATION

- **PO:** Administer around the clock. May be given without regard to meals. May be given with meals to decrease GI side effects. Capsule contents may be emptied and swallowed with liquids. Chewable tablets should be crushed or chewed before swallowing with liquids. Shake oral suspension before administering. Refrigerated reconstituted suspension should be discarded after 10 days.

□ Two 250-mg tablets are not bioequivalent to one 500-mg tablet. 250-mg tablets and 250-mg chewable tablets are also not interchangeable.

PATIENT/FAMILY TEACHING

□ Instruct patients to take medication around the clock and to finish the drug completely as directed, even if feeling better. Advise patients that sharing of this medication may be dangerous.

□ Instruct female patients taking oral contraceptives to use an alternate or additional method of contraception during therapy and until next menstrual period.

□ Advise patient to report the signs of superinfection (furry overgrowth on the tongue, vaginal itching or discharge, loose or foul-smelling stools) and allergy.

□ Instruct the patient to notify health care professional if symptoms do not improve or if nausea or diarrhea persists when drug is administered with food.

EVALUATION

Clinical response to therapy can be evaluated by: ▪ Resolution of the signs and symptoms of infection. Length of time for complete resolution depends on the organism and site of infection.

AMPHOTERICIN B DEOXYCHOLATE
(am-foe-**ter**-i-sin)
Fungizone

AMPHOTERICIN B CHOLESTERYL SULFATE
Amphotec

AMPHOTERICIN B LIPID COMPLEX
Abelcet

AMPHOTERICIN B LIPOSOME
AmBisome

CLASSIFICATION(S):
Antifungals

Pregnancy Category B

INDICATIONS

▪ **IV:** Treatment of active, progressive, potentially fatal fungal infections ▪ **Amphotericin B liposome:** Management of suspected fungal infections in febrile neutropenic patients □ Treatment of visceral leishmaniasis ▪ **PO:** Treatment of oral candidiasis ▪ **Topical:** Treatment of superficial fungal infections.

ACTION

▪ Binds to fungal cell membrane, allowing leakage of cellular contents ▪ Toxicity (especially acute infusion reactions and nephrotoxicity) is less with lipid formulations. **Therapeutic Effects:** ▪ Fungistatic action. **Spectrum:** ▪ Active against: □ Aspergillosis □ Blastomycosis □ *Candida* □ Coccidioidomycosis □ Cryptococcosis □ Histoplasmosis □ Leishmaniasis □ Mucormycosis.

PHARMACOKINETICS

Absorption: Not absorbed orally. Topical and oral preparations are not significantly absorbed.
Distribution: Following administration, distributed to body tissues and fluids. Poor penetration into CSF. *Cholesteryl*—taken up by liver, spleen, and bone marrow, then slowly released.
Metabolism and Excretion: Elimination is very prolonged. Detectable in urine up to 7 wk after discontinuation.

Half-life: Biphasic—initial phase, 24–48 hr; terminal phase, 15 days. *Cholesteryl*—28 hr. *Liposomal*—174 hr.

CONTRAINDICATIONS AND PRECAUTIONS

Contraindicated in: ▪ Hypersensitivity ▪ Lactation.

Use Cautiously in: ▪ Renal impairment or electrolyte abnormalities (decrease dose or temporarily discontinue if BUN ≥40 mg/100 ml or serum creatinine ≥3 mg/100 ml ▪ Patients receiving concurrent leucocyte transfusions (increased risk of pulmonary toxicity with lipid complex formulation only) ▪ Pregnancy (safety not established).

ADVERSE REACTIONS AND SIDE EFFECTS*

CNS: headache, dizziness, tremor.
Resp: dyspnea, hypoxia, wheezing.
CV: hypotension, arrhythmias.
GI: diarrhea, nausea, vomiting, abdominal pain, enlarged abdomen.
GU: nephrotoxicity, hematuria.
F and E: hypokalemia, hypocalcemia (cholesteryl only), hypomagnesemia.
Hemat: anemia, dyscrasias.
Local: phlebitis.
MS: arthralgia, myalgia.
Neuro: peripheral neuropathy.
Misc: HYPERSENSITIVITY REACTIONS, chills, fever, acute infusion reactions.

INTERACTIONS

Drug-Drug: ▪ Increased risk of nephrotoxicity with other **nephrotoxic agents** ▪ **Diuretics, glucocorticoids, mezlocillin, piperacillin,** or **ticarcillin** may potentiate hypokalemia ▪ **Diuretics** may potentiate hypomagnesemia.

ROUTE AND DOSAGE

❑ **Amphotericin Deoxycholate (Fungizone)**

- **IV (Adults):** Give test dose of 1 mg, then initial dose of 0.25 mg/kg; increase daily doses slowly to 0.5 mg/kg (can give up to 1 mg/kg/day or 1.5 mg/kg every other day).
- **IV (Children):** 0.25 mg/kg infused initially; increase by 0.25 mg/kg every other day to maximum of 1 mg/kg/day.
- **Topical (Adults and Children):** Apply 2–4 times daily.
- **PO (Adults and Children):** 1 ml 4 times daily.

❑ **Amphotericin B Cholesteryl Sulfate (Amphotec)**

- **IV (Adults and Children):** 3–4 mg/kg/day (up to 6 mg/kg/day).

❑ **Amphotericin B Lipid Complex (Abelcet)**

- **IV (Adults and Children):** 5 mg/kg/day.

❑ **Amphotericin B Liposome (AmBisome)**

- **IV (Adults and Children):** *Suspected fungal infections*—3 mg/kg q 24 hr; *documented fungal infections*—3–5 mg/kg q 24 hr; *visceral leishmaniasis (immunocompetent patients)*—3 mg/kg q 24 hr on days 1–5, then 3 mg/kg on days 14 and 21; *visceral leishmaniasis (immunosuppressed patients)*—4 mg/kg q 24 hr on days 1–5, then 4 mg/kg on days 10, 17, 24, 31, and 38.

AVAILABILITY

❑ **Amphotericin Deoxycholate**

▪ ***Injection:*** 50-mg vial[Rx] ▪ ***Cream, lotion, ointment:*** 3%[Rx] ▪ ***Oral suspension:*** 100 mg/ml in 24-ml bottles[Rx].

❑ **Amphotericin B Cholesteryl Sulfate**

▪ ***Powder for injection:*** 50 mg in 20-ml vial[Rx], 100 mg in 50-ml vial[Rx].

❑ **Amphotericin B Lipid Complex**

▪ ***Suspension for injection:*** 100 mg/20-ml vial[Rx].

TIME/ACTION PROFILE (blood levels)

	ONSET	PEAK	DURATION
IV	rapid	end of infusion	24 hr

NURSING IMPLICATIONS

ASSESSMENT

❑ Monitor patient closely during test dose and the first 1–2 hr of each dose for fever, chills,

*CAPITALS indicate life-threatening; underlines indicate most frequent.

headache, anorexia, nausea, or vomiting. Premedicating with antipyretics, corticosteroids, antihistamines, meperidine, and antiemetics and maintaining sodium balance may decrease these reactions. Febrile reaction usually subsides within 4 hr after the infusion is completed.

- Assess injection site frequently for thrombophlebitis or leakage. Drug is very irritating to tissues. Adding heparin to IV solution may decrease the likelihood of thrombophlebitis.
- Monitor vital signs every 15–30 min during test dose and every 30 min for 2–4 hr after administration. Meperidine and dantrolene have been used to prevent and treat rigors. Assess respiratory status (lung sounds, dyspnea) daily. Notify physician of changes. If respiratory distress occurs, discontinue infusion immediately; anaphylaxis may occur. Equipment for cardiopulmonary resuscitation should be readily available.
- Monitor intake and output and weigh daily. Adequate hydration (2000–3000 ml/day) may minimize nephrotoxicity.
- ***Lab Test Considerations:*** Monitor CBC and platelet counts weekly, BUN and serum creatinine every other day while increasing dose and then twice weekly, and potassium and magnesium levels biweekly. Life-threatening hypokalemia may occur following each dose. If BUN exceeds 40 mg/100 ml or serum creatinine exceeds 3 mg/100 ml, dosage should be decreased or discontinued until renal function improves. May cause decreased hemoglobin, hematocrit, and magnesium levels.

POTENTIAL NURSING DIAGNOSES

- Infection, risk for (Indications).
- Knowledge deficit, related to medication regimen (Patient/Family Teaching).

IMPLEMENTATION

- **General Info:** Do not confuse amphotericin B cholesteryl (Amphotec) with amphotericin deoxycholate (Fungizone) or amphotericin B lipid complex (Abelcet); they are not interchangeable.
- This drug should be administered IV only to hospitalized patients or those under close supervision. Diagnosis should be confirmed prior to administration.

Amphotericin B Deoxycholate

- **IV:** Reconstitute 50-mg vial with 10 ml of sterile water for injection without bacteriostatic agent. Concentration equals 5 mg/ml. Shake until clear. Further dilute each 1 mg with at least 10 ml of D5W (pH >4.2) for a concentration of 100 mcg (0.1 mg)/ml. Do not use other diluents. Avoid use of precipitated solution. Use 20-gauge needle; change for each step of dilution. Wear gloves while handling.
- Store in dark area. Reconstituted solution is stable for 24 hr at room temperature and 1 wk if refrigerated.
- **Test Dose:** Administer 1 mg in 20 ml of D5W over 10–30 min to determine patient tolerance. If medication is withheld for 7 days, restart at lowest dose level. In severe, life-threatening infections, test dose may be omitted.
- **Intermittent Infusion:** Administer preferably through central line. If peripheral site is used, change site with each dose to prevent phlebitis. If an in-line filter is used, the mean pore diameter should be no less than 1 micron. Short-term exposure to light (8 hr) does not alter potency.
- ***Rate:*** Administer slowly via infusion pump over 2–6 hr.
- **Syringe Compatibility:** ▪ heparin.
- **Y-Site Compatibility:** ▪ aldesleukin ▪ diltiazem ▪ tacrolimus ▪ teniposide ▪ thiotepa ▪ zidovudine.
- **Y-Site Incompatibility:** ▪ allopurinol sodium ▪ amifostine ▪ enalaprilat ▪ filgrastim ▪ fluconazole ▪ fludarabine ▪ foscarnet ▪ melphalan ▪ ondansetron ▪ paclitaxel ▪ piperacillin/tazobactam ▪ vinorelbine.
- **Additive Compatibility:** ▪ heparin ▪ hydrocortisone ▪ sodium bicarbonate.
- **Additive Incompatibility:** ▪ calcium chloride ▪ calcium gluconate ▪ cimetidine ▪ diphenhydramine ▪ potassium chloride ▪ ranitidine.
- **Solution Incompatibility:** ▪ lactated Ringer's injection ▪ saline solutions.

Amphotericin B Cholesteryl

- **IV:** Reconstitute 50-mg vial with 10 ml and 100-mg vial with 20 ml of sterile water for injection. Concentration equals 5 mg/ml. Shake gently until solids have dissolved. Solution may be opalescent. Further dilute with

D5W for a concentration of 0.6 mg/ml. Do not use other diluents. Avoid use of precipitated solution. Use 20-gauge needle; change for each step of dilution. Wear gloves while handling.

□ Refrigerate after reconstitution and further dilution; use within 24 hr.

- **Test Dose:** Administer 10 ml of the final preparation (containing 1.6–8.3 mg) over 15–30 min to determine patient tolerance. Observe patient closely for next 30 min. If medication is withheld for 7 days, restart at lowest dose level. In severe, life-threatening infections, test dose may be omitted.
- **Intermittent Infusion:** Do not filter or use an in-line filter.
- ***Rate:*** Administer at a rate of 1 mg/kg/hr via infusion pump. If patient tolerates infusion without adverse reactions, infusion time may be shortened to a minimum of 2 hr. If reactions occur or patient cannot tolerate volume, infusion time may be extended. Rapid infusions may cause hypotension, hypokalemia, arrhythmias, and shock.
- **Additive Compatibility:** ▪ heparin.
- **Additive Incompatibility:** ▪ electrolytes.
- **Solution Incompatibility:** ▪ saline solutions.

□ Amphotericin B Lipid Complex

- **IV:** Prepare imediately before use. Shake vial gently until yellow sediment at bottom has dissolved. Withdraw dose from required number of vials with 18-gauge needle. Replace needle from syringe filled with amphotericin B lipid complex with 5-micron filter needle. Each filter needle may be used to filter the contents of no more than 4 vials. Insert filter needle of syringe into IV bag of D5W and empty contents of syringe into bag for a concentration of 1 mg/ml (2mg/ml in pediatric patients or patients who cannot tolerate large volumes of fluid). Do not use admixtures containing foreign matter. Vials are for single use only; discard unused material.

□ Refrigerate after dilution. May be stored in refrigerator for up to 48 hr and an additional 6 hr at room temperature.

- **Intermittent Infusion:** Do not use an in-line filter.
- ***Rate:*** Administer at a rate of 2.5 mg/kg/hr via infusion pump. If infusion exceeds 2 hr, mix contents by shaking infusion bag every 2 hr.
- **Y-Site Incompatibility:** ▪ Flush IV line with D5W prior to infusion or use a separate line.
- **Additive Incompatibility:** ▪ electrolytes.
- **Solution Incompatibility:** ▪ saline solutions.
- **Topical:** While wearing gloves, apply topical preparations liberally and rub in well. Shake lotion before applying. Do not use occlusive dressings. Discontinue if lesions worsen or signs of hypersensitivity develop.

PATIENT/FAMILY TEACHING

- **General Info:** Explain need for long duration of IV or topical therapy.
- **PO:** Instruct patient to swish medication around in mouth as long as possible before swallowing.
- **IV:** Inform patient of potential side effects and discomfort at IV site. Advise patient to notify health care professional if side effects occur.
- **Home Care Issue:** Instruct family or caregiver on dilution, rate, and administration of drug and proper care of IV equipment.
- **Topical:** Advise patient that topical preparations may stain clothing. Cream or lotion may be removed with soap and warm water; ointment may be removed with cleaning fluid.

EVALUATION

Effectiveness of therapy can be demonstrated by: ▪ Resolution of signs and symptoms of infection. Several weeks to months of therapy may be required to prevent relapse.

AMPICILLIN

(am-pi-**sill**-in)

{Ampicin}, {Apo-Ampi}, {Nu-Ampi}, {Novo-Ampicillin}, Omnipen, Penbritin, Principen, Polycillin, Totacillin

CLASSIFICATION(S):

Anti-infective (aminopenicillin)

Pregnancy Category B

INDICATIONS

▪ Treatment of the following infections: □ Skin and skin structure infections, soft tissue infections ▫ Otitis media ▫ Sinusitis ▫ Respiratory infections ▫ Genitourinary infections ▫ Meningitis ▫ Septicemia ▪ Endocarditis prophylaxis.

ACTION

▪ Binds to bacterial cell wall, resulting in cell death. **Therapeutic Effects:** ▪ Bactericidal action; spectrum is broader than penicillin. **Spectrum:** ▪ Active against: ▫ Streptococci ▫ Pneumococci ▫ Enterococci ▫ *Haemophilus influenzae* ▫ *Escherichia coli* ▫ *Proteus mirabilis* ▫ *Neisseria meningitidis* ▫ *Neisseria gonorrhoeae* ▫ *Shigella* ▫ *Salmonella*.

PHARMACOKINETICS

Absorption: Moderately absorbed from the duodenum (30–50%).
Distribution: Diffuses readily into body tissues and fluids. CSF penetration is increased in the presence of inflamed meninges. Crosses the placenta; enters breast milk in small amounts.
Metabolism and Excretion: Variably metabolized by the liver (12–50%). Renal excretion is variable (25–60% after oral dosing; 50–85% following IM administration).
Half-life: 1–1.5 hr.

CONTRAINDICATIONS AND PRECAUTIONS

Contraindicated in: ▪ Hypersensitivity to penicillins.
Use Cautiously in: ▪ Severe renal insufficiency (dosage reduction required if CCr <10 ml/min). ▪ Infectious mononucleosis (increased incidence of rash) ▪ Has been used during pregnancy and lactation.

ADVERSE REACTIONS AND SIDE EFFECTS*

CNS: SEIZURES (high doses).
GI: diarrhea, nausea, vomiting.
Derm: rashes, urticaria.
Hemat: blood dyscrasias.
Misc: allergic reactions including ANAPHYLAXIS and SERUM SICKNESS, superinfection.

INTERACTIONS

Drug-Drug: ▪ **Probenecid** decreases renal excretion and increases blood levels of ampicillin—therapy may be combined for this purpose ▪ May potentiate the effect of **warfarin** ▪ Incidence of rash increases with concurrent **allopurinol** therapy ▪ May decrease the effectiveness of **oral contraceptives.**

ROUTE AND DOSAGE

- **PO (Adults and Children ≥20 kg):** 250–500 mg q 6 hr (up to 4 g/day).
- **PO (Children <20 kg):** 12.5–25 mg/kg q 6 hr *or* 16.7–33.3 mg/kg q 8 hr.
- **IM, IV (Adults and Children ≥20 kg):** 250–500 mg q 6 hr up to 1–2 g q 6 hr for serious infections (not to exceed 14 g/day).
- **IM, IV (Children <20 kg):** *Most infections*—12.5 mg/kg q 6 hr.
- **IM, IV (Neonates ≥2 kg):** *Bacterial meningitis*—50 mg/kg q 8 hr for 1st week of life, then q 6 hr.
- **IM, IV (Neonates <2 kg):** *Bacterial meningitis*—25–50 mg/kg for 1st week of life, then q 50 mg/kg q 8 hr.

AVAILABILITY

▪ ***Capsules:*** 250 mg[Rx], 500 mg[Rx] ▪ ***Suspension:*** 100 mg/ml[Rx], 125 mg/5 ml[Rx], 250 mg/5 ml[Rx], 500 mg/5 ml[Rx] ▪ ***In combination with:*** probenecid (Polycillin-PRB, Probampacin). See Appendix A. ▪ ***Injection:*** 125 mg[Rx], 250 mg[Rx], 1-, 2-, 10-g vials[Rx].

TIME/ACTION PROFILE (blood levels)

	ONSET	PEAK	DURATION
PO	rapid	1.5–2 hr	4–6 hr
IM	rapid	1 hr	4–6 hr
IV	rapid	end of infusion	4–6 hr

NURSING IMPLICATIONS

ASSESSMENT

▫ Assess patient for infection (vital signs, wound appearance, sputum, urine, stool, and WBC) at beginning of and throughout therapy.

▫ Obtain a history before initiating therapy to determine previous use and reactions to penicillins or cephalosporins. Persons with a negative history of penicillin sensitivity may still have an allergic response.

▫ Obtain specimens for culture and sensitivity prior to therapy. First dose may be given before receiving results.

*CAPITALS indicate life-threatening; underlines indicate most frequent.

- Observe patient for signs and symptoms of anaphylaxis (rash, pruritus, laryngeal edema, wheezing). Discontinue the drug and notify the physician or other health care professional immediately if these occur. Keep epinephrine, an antihistamine, and resuscitation equipment close by in the event of an anaphylactic reaction.
- Assess skin for "ampicillin rash," a nonallergic, dull red, macular or maculopapular, mildly pruritic rash.
- ***Lab Test Considerations:*** May cause increased AST and ALT.
- May cause transient decreases in estradiol, total conjugated estriol, estriol-glucuronide, or conjugated estrone in pregnant women.
- May cause a false-positive direct Coombs' test result.

POTENTIAL NURSING DIAGNOSES

- Infection, risk for (Indications, Side Effects).
- Knowledge deficit, related to medication regimen (Patient/Family Teaching).
- Noncompliance, related to medication regimen (Patient/Family Teaching).

IMPLEMENTATION

- **PO:** Administer around the clock on an empty stomach at least 1 hr before or 2 hr after meals with a full glass of water. Capsules may be opened and mixed with water. Reconstituted oral suspensions retain potency for 7 days at room temperature and 14 days if refrigerated. Combination with probenecid should be used immediately after reconstitution.
- **IM:** Reconstitute for IM or IV use by adding sterile water for injection 0.9–1.2 ml to the 125-mg vial, 0.9–1.9 ml to the 250-mg vial, 1.2–1.8 ml to the 500-mg vial, 2.4–7.4 ml to the 1-g vial, and 6.8 ml to the 2-g vial.
- **Direct IV:** Add 5 ml of sterile or bacteriostatic water for injection to each 125-, 250-, or 500-mg vial or at least 7.4–10 ml of diluent to each 1- or 2-g vial.
- ***Rate:*** Doses of 125–500 mg may be given over 3–5 min within 1 hr of reconstitution. Rapid administration may cause seizures.
- **Intermittent Infusion:** Dilute in 50 ml or more of 0.9% NaCl, D5W, D5/0.45% NaCl, or lactated Ringer's solution for a concentration of no more than 30 mg/ml; administer within 4 hr (more stable in NaCl).
- ***Rate:*** Administer (1–2 g) doses over 10–15 min.
- **Syringe Compatibility:** ▪ chloramphenicol ▪ heparin ▪ procaine.
- **Syringe Incompatibility:** ▪ erythromycin lactobionate ▪ gentamicin ▪ kanamycin ▪ metoclopramide.
- **Y-Site Compatibility:** ▪ acyclovir ▪ allopurinol sodium ▪ amifostine ▪ cyclophosphamide ▪ enalaprilat ▪ esmolol ▪ famotidine ▪ filgrastim ▪ fludarabine ▪ foscarnet ▪ heparin ▪ insulin, regular ▪ labetalol ▪ magnesium sulfate ▪ melphalan ▪ meperidine ▪ morphine ▪ multivitamins ▪ ofloxacin ▪ perphenazine ▪ phytonadione ▪ potassium chloride ▪ tacrolimus ▪ teniposide ▪ theophylline ▪ thiotepa ▪ tolazoline ▪ vitamin B complex with C.
- **Y-Site Incompatibility:** ▪ epinephrine ▪ fluconazole ▪ hydralazine ▪ midazolam ▪ ondansetron ▪ sargramostim ▪ verapamil ▪ vinorelbine. If aminoglycosides and penicillins must be administered concurrently, administer in separate sites at least 1 hr apart.
- **Additive Incompatibility:** ▪ amikacin ▪ gentamicin ▪ kanamycin ▪ tobramycin.

PATIENT/FAMILY TEACHING

- Instruct patient to take medication around the clock and to finish the drug completely as directed, even if feeling better. Advise patients that sharing of this medication can be dangerous.
- Advise patient to report the signs of superinfection (furry overgrowth on the tongue, vaginal itching or discharge, loose or foul-smelling stools) and allergy.
- Advise patients taking oral contraceptives to use an alternate or additional nonhormonal method of contraception while taking ampicillin and until next menstrual period.
- Instruct the patient to notify health care professional if symptoms do not improve.
- Patients with a history of rheumatic heart disease or valve replacement need to be taught the importance of using antimicrobial prophylaxis before invasive medical or dental procedures (see Appendix N).

EVALUATION

Clinical response to therapy can be evaluated by: ▪ Resolution of the signs and symptoms of infection. Length of time for complete resolution depends on the organism and site of infection ▪ Endocarditis prophylaxis.

AMPICILLIN/SULBACTAM

(am-pi-**sill**-in/sul-**bak**-tam)

Unasyn

CLASSIFICATION(S):

Anti-infective (aminopenicillin/beta-lactamase inhibitor)

Pregnancy Category B (Ampicillin)

INDICATIONS

▪ Treatment of the following infections: ▫ Skin and skin structure infections, soft tissue infections ▫ Otitis media ▫ Sinusitis ▫ Respiratory infections ▫ Genitourinary infections ▫ Meningitis ▫ Septicemia.

ACTION

▪ Binds to bacterial cell wall, resulting in cell death; spectrum is broader than penicillin. Addition of sulbactam increases resistance to beta-lactamases, enzymes produced by bacteria that may inactivate ampicillin. **Therapeutic Effects:** ▪ Bactericidal action. **Spectrum:** ▪ Active against: ▫ Streptococci ▫ Pneumococci ▫ Enterococci ▫ *Haemophilus influenzae* ▫ *Escherichia coli* ▫ *Proteus mirabilis* ▫ *Neisseria meningitidis* ▫ *Neisseria gonorrhoeae* ▫ *Shigella* ▫ *Salmonella* ▫ *Bacteroides fragilis* ▫ *Moraxella catarrhalis* ▪ Use should be reserved for infections caused by beta-lactamase–producing strains.

PHARMACOKINETICS

Absorption: Well absorbed from IM sites.
Distribution: Ampicillin diffuses readily into body tissues and fluids. CSF penetration is increased when meninges are inflamed. Crosses the placenta; enters breast milk in small amounts.
Metabolism and Excretion: Ampicillin is variably metabolized by the liver (12–50%). Renal excretion is also variable. Sulbactam is eliminated unchanged in urine.
Half-life: *Ampicillin*—1–1.5 hr; *sulbactam*—1–1.4 hr.

CONTRAINDICATIONS AND PRECAUTIONS

Contraindicated in: ▪ Hypersensitivity to penicillins or sulbactam.
Use Cautiously in: ▪ Severe renal insufficiency (dosage reduction required if CCr <30 ml/min) ▪ Infectious mononucleosis (increased incidence of rash) ▪ Has been used during pregnancy and lactation (ampicillin).

ADVERSE REACTIONS AND SIDE EFFECTS*

CNS: SEIZURES (high doses).
GI: PSEUDOMEMBRANOUS COLITIS, diarrhea, nausea, vomiting.
Derm: rashes, urticaria.
Hemat: blood dyscrasias.
Local: pain at IM site, pain at IV site.
Misc: allergic reactions including ANAPHYLAXIS and SERUM SICKNESS, superinfection.

INTERACTIONS

Drug-Drug: ▪ **Probenecid** decreases renal excretion and increases blood levels of ampicillin—therapy may be combined for this purpose ▪ May potentiate the effect of **warfarin** ▪ Concurrent **allopurinol** therapy (increased incidence of rash) ▪ May decrease the effectiveness of **oral contraceptives.**

ROUTE AND DOSAGE

- **IM, IV (Adults and Children ≥40 kg):** 1.5–3 g (1 g ampicillin plus 0.5 g sulbactam–2 g ampicillin plus 1 g sulbactam) q 6–8 hr (not to exceed 4 g sulbactam/day).
- **IV (Children ≥ 1 yr):** 75 mg (50 mg ampicillin/25 mg sulbactam)/kg q 6 hr.

AVAILABILITY

▪ ***Injection:*** 1 g ampicillin with 500 mg sulbactam[Rx], 2 g ampicillin with 1 g sulbactam[Rx].

TIME/ACTION PROFILE (blood levels)

	ONSET	PEAK	DURATION
IM	rapid	1 hr	6–8 hr
IV	immediate	end of infusion	6–8 hr

***CAPITALS indicate life-threatening; underlines indicate most frequent.**

NURSING IMPLICATIONS

ASSESSMENT

- Assess patient for infection (vital signs, wound appearance, sputum, urine, stool, WBC) at beginning and throughout therapy.
- Obtain a history before initiating therapy to determine previous use of and reactions to penicillins or cephalosporins. Persons with a negative history of penicillin sensitivity may still have an allergic response.
- Obtain specimens for culture and sensitivity prior to therapy. First dose may be given before receiving results.
- Observe patient for signs and symptoms of anaphylaxis (rash, pruritus, laryngeal edema, wheezing). Discontinue the drug and notify the physician or other health care professional immediately if these occur. Keep epinephrine, an antihistamine, and resuscitation equipment close by in the event of an anaphylactic reaction.
- ***Lab Test Considerations:*** May cause increased AST, ALT, LDH, bilirubin, alkaline phosphatase, BUN, and creatinine.
- May cause decreased hemoglobin, hematocrit, RBC, WBC, neutrophils, and lymphocytes.
- May cause transient decreases in estradiol, total conjugated estriol, estriol-glucuronide, or conjugated estrone in pregnant women.
- May cause a false-positive Coombs' test result.

POTENTIAL NURSING DIAGNOSES

- Infection, risk for (Indications, Side Effects).
- Knowledge deficit, related to medication regimen (Patient/Family Teaching).

IMPLEMENTATION

- **IM:** Reconstitute for IM use by adding 3.2 ml of sterile water or 0.5% or 2% lidocaine HCl to the 1.5-g vial or 6.4 ml to the 3-g vial. Administer within 1 hr of preparation, deep IM into well-developed muscle.
- **IV:** For IV use, add 3.2 ml of sterile water for injection to each 1.5-g vial and 6.4 ml to each 3-g vial for a concentration of 250 mg ampicillin/ml and 125 mg sulbactam/ml. Foaming should dissipate upon standing. Administer only clear solutions.
- **Direct IV:** May be administered over 10–15 min (1–2 g) within 1 hr of reconstitution. More rapid administration may cause seizures.
- **Intermittent Infusion:** Dilute immediately for infusion in 50–100 ml or more of 0.9% NaCl, D5W, D5/0.45% NaCl, or lactated Ringer's solution. Stability of solution varies from 2–8 hr at room temperature or 3–72 hr if refrigerated, depending on concentration and diluent.
- ***Rate:*** Administer over 15–30 min.
- **Y-Site Compatibility:** ▪ amifostine ▪ enalaprilat ▪ famotidine ▪ filgrastim ▪ fluconazole ▪ fludarabine ▪ gallium nitrate ▪ heparin ▪ insulin ▪ meperidine ▪ morphine ▪ paclitaxel ▪ tacrolimus ▪ teniposide ▪ theophylline ▪ thiotepa.
- **Y-Site Incompatibility:** ▪ ciprofloxacin ▪ idarubicin ▪ ondansetron ▪ sargramostim. If aminoglycosides and penicillins must be given concurrently, administer in separate sites at least 1 hr apart.
- **Additive Compatibility:** ▪ aztreonam.

PATIENT/FAMILY TEACHING

- Advise patient to report signs of superinfection (furry overgrowth on the tongue, vaginal itching or discharge, loose or foul-smelling stools) and allergy.
- Advise patients taking oral contraceptives to use an alternative or additional nonhormonal method of contraception while taking ampicillin/sulbactam and until next menstrual period.
- Instruct the patient to notify health care professional if symptoms do not improve.

EVALUATION

Clinical response to therapy can be evaluated by: ▪ Resolution of signs and symptoms of infection. Length of time for complete resolution depends on the organism and site of infection.

AMRINONE

(**am**-ri-none)

Inocor

CLASSIFICATION(S):

Inotropic agent

Pregnancy Category C

INDICATIONS

▪ Short-term treatment of congestive heart failure unresponsive to digitalis glycosides, diuretics, and vasodilators.

ACTION

▪ Increases myocardial contractility ▪ Decreases preload and afterload by a direct dilating effect on vascular smooth muscle. **Therapeutic Effects:** ▪ Increased cardiac output (inotropic effect).

PHARMACOKINETICS

Absorption: IV administration results in complete bioavailability.
Distribution: UK.
Metabolism and Excretion: 50% metabolized by the liver; 10–40% excreted unchanged by the kidneys.
Half-life: 3.6–5.8 hr (increased in congestive heart failure).

CONTRAINDICATIONS AND PRECAUTIONS

Contraindicated in: ▪ Hypersensitivity to amrinone or bisulfites ▪ Idiopathic hypertrophic subaortic stenosis.
Use Cautiously in: ▪ Atrial fibrillation or flutter (may increase ventricular response; pretreatment with cardiac glycosides may be necessary) ▪ Recent aggressive diuretic therapy (correct fluid and electrolyte disorders prior to administering amrinone) ▪ Thrombocytopenia (platelets $<100{,}000/mm^3$ ▪ Pregnancy, lactation, or children (safety not established).

ADVERSE REACTIONS AND SIDE EFFECTS*

Resp: dyspnea.
CV: arrhythmias, hypotension.
GI: diarrhea, hepatotoxicity, nausea, vomiting.
F and E: hypokalemia.
Hemat: thrombocytopenia.
Misc: tachyphylaxis, fever, hypersensitivity reactions.

INTERACTIONS

Drug-Drug: ▪ Inotropic effects may be additive with **digitalis glycosides** ▪ Hypotension may be exaggerated by **disopyramide.**

ROUTE AND DOSAGE

See infusion rate chart in Appendix D.

▪ **IV (Adults):** 0.75 mg/kg loading dose; may be repeated in 30 min if necessary, then 5–10 mcg/kg/min infusion (total daily dose should not exceed 10 mg/kg).

AVAILABILITY

▪ ***Injection:*** 5 mg/ml[Rx].

TIME/ACTION PROFILE (inotropic effect)

	ONSET	PEAK	DURATION†
IV	2–5 min	10 min	0.5–2 hr

†After infusion is discontinued.

NURSING IMPLICATIONS

ASSESSMENT

□ Monitor blood pressure, pulse, ECG, respiratory rate, cardiac index, pulmonary capillary wedge pressure, and central venous pressure frequently during administration. Notify physician promptly if hypotension occurs. Tachyphylaxis (rapid development of tolerance) commonly develops within the first 72 hr.

□ Monitor intake and output and weigh daily. Assess for resolution of signs of congestive heart failure (peripheral edema, dyspnea, rales/crackles, weight gain). Fluid intake may need to be increased cautiously to ensure adequate cardiac filling pressure.

▪ ***Lab Test Considerations:*** Platelet counts, serum electrolytes, liver enzymes, and renal function should be evaluated periodically throughout therapy. If platelet count is $<150{,}000/mm^3$ notify physician promptly; may require dose reduction. Increased liver enzymes may indicate hepatotoxicity. May cause decreased potassium levels.

POTENTIAL NURSING DIAGNOSES

▪ Cardiac output, decreased (Indications).
▪ Activity intolerance (Indications).
▪ Fluid volume excess (Indications).

IMPLEMENTATION

▪ **General Info:** Hypokalemia should be corrected prior to administration.

***CAPITALS indicate life-threatening; underlines indicate most frequent.**

- Patients with atrial fibrillation/flutter may require digitalis glycoside therapy prior to treatment; amrinone enhances atrioventricular conduction.
- **Direct IV:** May be administered undiluted.
- *Rate:* Administer loading dose over 2–3 min.
- **Continuous Infusion:** Dilute amrinone with 0.9% NaCl or 0.45% NaCl only, for a concentration of 1–3 mg/ml. Dilution with dextrose products may lead to decomposition of amrinone, but may be administered through Y-tubing or directly into tubing of a running dextrose solution. Administer via infusion pump to ensure accurate dosage. Change tubing whenever concentration of solution is changed. Solution should be clear yellow. Use reconstituted solution within 24 hr of preparation.
- *Rate:* Rate is titrated according to patient response.
- **Syringe Compatibility:** ▪ propranolol ▪ verapamil.
- **Y-Site Compatibility:** ▪ amifostine ▪ aminophylline ▪ atropine ▪ bretylium ▪ calcium chloride ▪ cimetidine ▪ digoxin ▪ dobutamine ▪ dopamine ▪ epinephrine ▪ famotidine ▪ hydrocortisone sodium succinate ▪ isoproterenol ▪ lidocaine ▪ metaraminol bitartrate ▪ methylprednisolone sodium succinate ▪ nitroglycerin ▪ nitroprusside ▪ norepinephrine ▪ phenylephrine ▪ potassium chloride ▪ propranolol ▪ thiotepa ▪ verapamil.
- **Y-Site Incompatibility:** ▪ furosemide ▪ sodium bicarbonate.

PATIENT/FAMILY TEACHING

- □ Advise patient to report an increase in dyspnea or chest pain, or the onset of hypersensitivity reactions promptly.
- □ Advise patient to change positions slowly to minimize any drug-induced postural hypotension.

EVALUATION

Effectiveness of therapy can be demonstrated by: ▪ Increase in cardiac index and diuresis □ Decrease in pulmonary capillary wedge pressure, dyspnea, and edema.

ANASTRAZOLE

(a-**nass**-stra-zole)
Arimidex

CLASSIFICATION(S):
Antineoplastic (aromatase inhibitor)

Pregnancy Category D

INDICATIONS

▪ Treatment of advanced breast cancer in postmenopausal patients with disease progression despite tamoxifen therapy.

ACTION

▪ Inhibits the enzyme aromatase, which is partially responsible for conversion of precursors to estrogen. **Therapeutic Effects:** ▪ Lowers levels of circulating estrogen, which may halt progression of estrogen-sensitive breast cancer.

PHARMACOKINETICS

Absorption: 83–85% absorbed following oral administration.
Distribution: UK.
Metabolism and Excretion: 85% metabolized by the liver; 11% excreted renally.
Half-life: 50 hr.

CONTRAINDICATIONS AND PRECAUTIONS

Contraindicated in: ▪ Pregnancy.
Use Cautiously in: ▪ Women with childbearing potential ▪ Lactation or children (safety not established).

ADVERSE REACTIONS AND SIDE EFFECTS*

CNS: headache, weakness, dizziness.
EENT: pharyngitis.
Resp: dyspnea, increased cough.
CV: peripheral edema.
GI: nausea, abdominal pain, anorexia, constipation, diarrhea, dry mouth, vomiting.
GU: pelvic pain, vaginal bleeding, vaginal dryness.
Derm: rash, sweating.

***CAPITALS indicate life-threatening; underlines indicate most frequent.**

Metab: weight gain.
MS: back pain, bone pain.
Neuro: paresthesia.
Misc: hot flashes, pain.

INTERACTIONS

Drug-Drug: ▪ None significant.

ROUTE AND DOSAGE

- **PO (Adults):** 1 mg daily.

AVAILABILITY

- ***Tablets:*** 1 mg[Rx].

TIME/ACTION PROFILE (lowering of serum estradiol)

	ONSET	PEAK	DURATION
PO	within 24 hr	14 days	6 days*

*Following cessation of therapy.

NURSING IMPLICATIONS

ASSESSMENT

- □ Assess patient for pain and other side effects periodically throughout therapy.
- ▪ ***Lab Test Considerations:*** May cause elevated GTT, AST, ALT, alkaline phosphatase, total cholesterol and LDL cholesterol levels.

POTENTIAL NURSING DIAGNOSES

- Pain (Side Effects).
- Knowledge deficit, related to medication regimen (Patient/Family Teaching).

IMPLEMENTATION

- Take medication consistently with regard to food.

PATIENT/FAMILY TEACHING

- □ Instruct patient to take medication as directed.
- □ Inform patient of potential for adverse reactions and advise her to notify health care professional if side effects are problematic.
- □ Advise patient that vaginal bleeding may occur during first few weeks after changing over from other hormonal therapy. Continued bleeding should be evaluated.

EVALUATION

Effectiveness of therapy can be demonstrated by: ▪ Slowing of disease progression in women with advanced breast cancer.

ANGIOTENSIN-CONVERTING ENZYME (ACE) INHIBITORS

benazepril
(ben-**aye**-ze-pril)
Lotensin

captopril
(**kap**-toe-pril)
Capoten

enalapril, enalaprilat
(e-**nal**-a-pril, e-**nal**-a-pril-at)

fosinopril
(foe-**sin**-oh-pril)

lisinopril
(lyse-**in**-oh-pril)

moexipril
(moe-**eks**-i-pril)
Univasc

quinapril
(**kwin**-a-pril)

ramipril
(ra-**mi**-pril)
Altace

trandolapril
(tran-**doe**-la-pril)
Mavik

CLASSIFICATION(S):
Antihypertensive agents

Pregnancy Category C (first trimester), D (second and third trimesters)

INDICATIONS

▪ Alone or with other agents in the management of hypertension ▪ **Captopril, enalapril, fosinopril, lisinopril, quinapril, ramipril, trandolapril:** Management of congestive heart failure ▪ **Captopril, lisinopril, ramipril:** Reduction of risk of death or development of congestive heart failure following myocardial infarction ▪ **Captopril:** Decreased progression of diabetic nephropathy.

ACTION

▪ Prevents the production of angiotensin II, a potent vasoconstrictor that stimulates the production of aldosterone by blocking its conversion to the active form—result is systemic vasodilation. **Therapeutic Effects:** ▪ Lowering of blood pressure in hypertensive patients ▪ Decreased preload and afterload in patients with congestive heart failure ▪ Decreased development of overt heart failure in patients surviving myocardial infarction ▪ Decreased progression of diabetic nephropathy.

PHARMACOKINETICS

Absorption: *Benazepril:* 37% absorbed following oral administration. *Captopril:* 75% following oral administration (decreased by food). *Enalapril:* 60% absorbed following oral administration. *Enalaprilat:* IV administration results in complete bioavailability. *Fosinopril:* 36% absorbed following oral administration. *Lisinopril:* 25% absorbed following oral administration (much variability). *Moexipril:* Converted to moexiprilat (the active form) following oral administration; absorption is variable (decreased by food), resulting in 13% bioavailability as moexiprilat. *Quinapril:* 60% absorbed following oral administration (high-fat meal may decrease absorption). *Ramipril:* 50–60% absorbed following oral administration. *Trandolapril:* Converted to trandolaprilat (the active form) following oral administration; bioavailability of trandolapril is 10%, 70% for trandolaprilat.

Distribution: All ACE inhibitors cross the placenta. *Benazepril, benazeprilat, captopril,* and *fosinoprilat:* Enter breast milk in small amounts. *Ramipril:* Probably does not enter breast milk. *Enalapril* and *enalaprilat:* Small amounts cross the blood-brain barrier. *Trandolapril:* UK.

Metabolism and Excretion: *Benazepril:* Converted by the liver to benazeprilat, the active metabolite. Eliminated by the kidneys. *Captopril:* 50% metabolized by the liver to inactive compounds, 50% excreted unchanged by the kidneys. *Fosinopril:* Converted by the liver and GI mucosa to fosinoprilat, the active metabolite: 50% eliminated by the kidneys; 50% fecal elimination. *Lisinopril:* 100% eliminated by the kidneys. *Moexipril:* 7% excreted in urine, 53% in feces. *Quinapril:* Converted by the liver, GI mucosa, and tissue to quinaprilat, the active metabolite: 61% eliminated by the kidneys; 37% fecal elimination. *Ramipril:* Metabolized by the liver to ramiprilat, the active metabolite: 60% eliminated by the kidneys; 40% fecal elimination. *Trandolapril:* Converted by liver to trandolaprilat; 33% excreted in urine as trandolaprilat, 66% in feces.

Half-life: *Benazeprilat:* 10–11 hr. *Captopril:* <3 hr (increased in renal impairment). *Enalapril* and *enalaprilat:* 11 hr (increased in renal impairment). *Fosinoprilat:* 11.5 hr. *Lisinopril:* 12 hr (increased in renal impairment). *Moexiprilat:* 12 hr. *Quinapril:* 1–2 hr. *Ramiprilat:* 13–17 hr (increased in renal impairment). *Trandolaprilat:* 10 hr.

CONTRAINDICATIONS AND PRECAUTIONS

Contraindicated in: ▪ Hypersensitivity ▪ Cross-sensitivity among ACE inhibitors may occur ▪ Pregnancy.

Use Cautiously in: ▪ Renal impairment, hepatic impairment, hypovolemia, hyponatremia, elderly patients, concurrent diuretic therapy (initial dosage reduction recommended for *benazepril, enalapril, lisinopril, trandolapril* if CCr <30 ml/min; *quinapril* if CCr <30–60 ml/min; *ramipril* if CCr <40 ml/min) ▪ Aortic stenosis ▪ Cerebrovascular or cardiac insufficiency ▪ Lactation or children (safety not established; most agents) ▪ Surgery/anesthesia (hypotension may be exaggerated).

Use Extreme Caution in: ▪ Family history of angioedema.

ADVERSE REACTIONS AND SIDE EFFECTS*

CNS: dizziness, fatigue, headache, insomnia, weakness.

Resp: <u>cough</u>.

CV: <u>hypotension</u>, angina pectoris, tachycardia.

GI: <u>loss of taste perception</u>, anorexia, diarrhea, nausea.

GU: <u>proteinuria</u>, impotence, renal failure.

Derm: rashes.

F and E: hyperkalemia.

***CAPITALS indicate life-threatening; <u>underlines</u> indicate most frequent.**

Hemat: AGRANULOCYTOSIS, NEUTROPENIA.
Misc: ANGIOEDEMA, fever.

INTERACTIONS

Drug-Drug: ▪ Excessive hypotension may occur with concurrent use of **diuretics** ▪ Additive hypotension with other **antihypertensives, nitrates, phenothiazines,** and acute ingestion of **alcohol** ▪ Hyperkalemia may result from concurrent use of **potassium supplements, potassium-sparing diuretics,** or **cyclosporine** ▪ Antihypertensive response may be blunted by **NSAIDs** ▪ Absorption may be decreased by **antacids** ▪ Increases levels and may increase the risk of **lithium** or **digoxin** toxicity ▪ **Probenecid** decreases elimination and increases levels of captopril ▪ Risk of hypersensitivity reactions increased by concurrent **allopurinol** ▪ **Capsaicin** may increase the incidence of cough ▪ **Rifampin** may decrease the effectiveness of enalapril ▪ **Tetracycline** absorption is decreased by quinapril (because of magnesium in tablets).

ROUTE AND DOSAGE

❑ Benazepril

- **PO (Adults):** 5–10 mg once daily, increased gradually to maintenance dose of 20–40 mg/day as single dose or 2 divided doses (begin with 5 mg/day in patients receiving diuretics).

❑ Captopril

- **PO (Adults):** *Hypertension*—12.5–25 mg 2–3 times daily, may be increased at 1–2 wk intervals up to 150 mg 3 times daily (usual dose 50 mg 3 times daily; begin with 6.25–12.5 mg 2–3 times daily in patients receiving diuretics). *Congestive heart failure*—12.5 mg 2–3 times daily, may be increased up to 50–100 mg 3 times daily (range 12.5–450 mg/day). *Postmyocardial infarction*—6.25-mg test dose, followed by 12.5 mg 3 times daily, may be increased up to 50 mg 3 times daily. *Diabetic nephropathy*—25 mg 3 times daily.
- **PO (Children):** 300 mcg (0.3 mg)/kg 3 times daily, may be increased by 300 mcg (0.3 mg)/kg q 8–24 hr (initiate therapy at 150 mcg [0.15 mg]/kg in patients receiving diuretics or patients with renal impairment).
- **PO (Neonates):** 10 mcg (0.01 mg)/kg 2–3 times daily, may be increased as needed.

❑ Enalapril/Enalaprilat

- **PO (Adults):** *Hypertension*—5 mg/day, increased as required by response (usual range 10–40 mg/day in 1–2 divided doses; initiate therapy at 2.5 mg/day in patients receiving diuretics). *Congestive heart failure*—2.5 mg 1–2 times daily, then 5 mg/day, increased as required by response (usual range 5–20 mg/day in 1–2 divided doses).
- **IV (Adults):** 0.625–1.25 mg (0.625 mg if receiving diuretics) q 6 hr.

❑ Fosinopril

- **PO (Adults):** *Hypertension*—10 mg once daily, may be increased as required (range 20–40 mg once daily). *Congestive heart failure*—10 mg once daily (5 mg in patients who have moderate to severe renal impairment or who have been vigorously diuresed), may be increased over several weeks up to 40 mg/day (usual range 20–40 mg/day).

❑ Lisinopril

- **PO (Adults):** *Hypertension*—10 mg once daily, can be increased up to 20–40 mg/day (initiate therapy at 5 mg/day in patients receiving diuretics). *Congestive heart failure*—2.5–5 mg once daily, can be increased up to 50 mg/day. *Improved survival after myocardial infarction*—5 mg once daily for 2 days, then 10 mg daily for 6 wk.

❑ Moexipril

- **PO (Adults):** 7.5 mg once daily, may be increased as needed (usual range is 7.5–30 mg/day in 1–2 divided doses; begin with 3.75 mg in patients receiving diuretics).

❑ Quinapril

- **PO (Adults):** Initial dose 5–10 mg/day, may be increased at 2-wk intervals (range 20–80 mg/day in 1–2 divided doses; initiate therapy at 5 mg/day in patients receiving diuretics).

❑ Ramipril

- **PO (Adults):** *Hypertension*—2.5 mg once daily, slowly may be increased up to 20 mg/day in 1–2 divided doses (initiate therapy at 1.25 mg/day in patients receiving diuretics). *Congestive heart failure following MI*—1.25–2.5 mg twice daily initially, may be increased up to 5 mg twice daily.

❑ **Trandolapril**

▪ **PO (Adults):** *Non-black patients:*—1 mg once daily; *black patients:*—2 mg once daily. May be increased weekly up to 4 mg once daily; twice daily dosing may be necessary in some patients (begin with 0.5 mg/day in patients with reduced renal function, hepatic cirrhosis, or those receiving diuretics).

AVAILABILITY

❑ **Benazepril**

▪ ***Tablets:*** 5 mg^{Rx}, 10 mg^{Rx}, 20 mg^{Rx}, 40 mg^{Rx} ▪ ***In combination with:*** amlodipine (Lotrel^{Rx}). See Appendix A.

❑ **Captopril**

▪ ***Tablets:*** 12.5 mg^{Rx}, 25 mg^{Rx}, 50 mg^{Rx}, 100 mg^{Rx} ▪ ***In combination with:*** hydrochlorothiazide (Capozide^{Rx}). See Appendix A.

❑ **Enalapril**

▪ ***Tablets:*** 2.5 mg^{Rx}, 5 mg^{Rx}, 10 mg^{Rx}, 20 mg^{Rx} ▪ ***In combination with:*** diltiazem (Teczem^{Rx}), felodipine (Lexxel^{Rx}), hydrochlorothiazide (Vaseretic^{Rx}). See Appendix A.

❑ **Enalaprilat**

▪ ***Injection:*** 1.25 mg/ml^{Rx}.

❑ **Fosinopril**

▪ ***Tablets:*** 10 mg^{Rx}, 20 mg^{Rx}.

❑ **Lisinopril**

▪ ***Tablets:*** 2.5 mg^{Rx}, 5 mg^{Rx}, 10 mg ^{Rx}, 20 mg^{Rx}, 40 mg^{Rx} ▪ ***In combination with:*** hydrochlorothiazide (Prinzide^{Rx}, Zestoretic^{Rx}). See Appendix A.

❑ **Moexipril**

▪ ***Tablets:*** 7.5 mg^{Rx}, 15 mg^{Rx}.

❑ **Quinapril**

▪ ***Tablets:*** 5 mg^{Rx}, 10 mg^{Rx}, 20 mg^{Rx}, 40 mg^{Rx}.

❑ **Ramipril**

▪ ***Capsules:*** 1.25 mg^{Rx}, 2.5 mg^{Rx}, 5 mg^{Rx}, 10 mg^{Rx}.

❑ **Trandolapril**

▪ ***Tablets:*** 1 mg^{Rx}, 2 mg^{Rx}, 4 mg^{Rx} ▪ ***In combination with:*** verapamil (Tarka^{Rx}). See Appendix A.

TIME/ACTION PROFILE (effect on blood pressure—single dose*)

	ONSET	PEAK	DURATION
Benazepril	within 1 hr	2–4 hr	24 hr
Captopril	15–60 min	60–90 min	6–12 hr
Enalapril PO	1 hr	4–6 hr	24 hr
Enalapril IV	15 min	1–4 hr	6 hr
Fosinopril	within 1 hr	2–6 hr	24 hr
Lisinopril	1 hr	6 hr	24 hr
Moexipril	within 1 hr	3–6 hr	up to 24 hr
Quinapril	within 1 hr	2–4 hr	up to 24 hr
Ramipril	within 1–2 hr	4–6.5 hr	24 hr
Trandolapril	within 1 hr	4–10 hr	up to 24 hr

*Full effects may not be noted for several weeks.

NURSING IMPLICATIONS

ASSESSMENT

▪ **Hypertension:** Monitor blood pressure and pulse frequently during initial dosage adjustment and periodically throughout therapy. Notify physician or other health care professional of significant changes.

❑ Monitor frequency of prescription refills to determine compliance.

▪ **Congestive Heart Failure:** Monitor weight and assess patient routinely for resolution of fluid overload (peripheral edema, rales/crackles, dyspnea, weight gain, jugular venous distention).

▪ ***Lab Test Considerations:*** Monitor BUN, creatinine, and electrolyte levels periodically. Serum potassium may be increased, and BUN and creatinine transiently increased while sodium levels may be decreased. If elevated BUN or serum creatinine concentrations occur, dosage reduction or withdrawal may be required.

❑ Monitor CBC periodically during therapy. May rarely cause slight decrease in hemoglobin and hematocrit.

❑ May cause elevated AST, ALT, alkaline phosphatase, serum bilirubin, uric acid, and glucose.

❑ Assess urine protein prior to and periodically during therapy for up to 1 yr in patients with renal impairment or those receiving >150 mg/day of captopril. If excessive or increasing proteinuria occurs, re-evaluate ACE inhibitor therapy.

❑ May cause positive antinuclear antibody (ANA) titer.

- WBC with differential should be monitored prior to initiation of therapy, monthly for the first 3–6 mo, and periodically thereafter for up to 1 yr in patients at risk for neutropenia (patients with renal impairment, collagen-vascular disease, or those receiving high doses) or at first sign of infection. Discontinue therapy if neutrophil count is $<1000/mm^3$.
- *Captopril:* May cause false-positive test results for urine acetone.

POTENTIAL NURSING DIAGNOSES

- Cardiac output, altered, decreased (Indications, Side Effects).
- Knowledge deficit, related to medication regimen (Patient/Family Teaching).
- Noncompliance (Patient/Family Teaching).

IMPLEMENTATION

- **PO:** Precipitous drop in blood pressure during first 1–3 hr following first dose may require volume expansion with normal saline but is not normally considered an indication for stopping therapy. Discontinuing diuretic therapy or increasing salt intake 1 wk prior to initiation may decrease risk of hypotension. Monitor closely for at least 1 hr after blood pressure has stabilized. Resume diuretics if blood pressure is not controlled.

Captopril

- Administer 1 hr before or 2 hr after meals. May be crushed if patient has difficulty swallowing. Tablets may have a sulfurous odor.
- An oral solution may be prepared by crushing a 25-mg tablet and dissolving it in 25–100 ml of water. Shake for at least 5 min and administer within 30 min.

Enaprilat

- **Direct IV:** May be administered undiluted.
- ***Rate:*** Administer over at least 5 min.
- **Intermittent Infusion:** Dilute in up to 50 ml of D5W, 0.9% NaCl, D5/0.9% NaCl, or D5/LR. Diluted solution is stable for 24 hr.
- ***Rate:*** Administer as a slow infusion.
- **Y-Site Compatibility:** ▪ amikacin ▪ aminophylline ▪ ampicillin ▪ ampicillin/sulbactam ▪ aztreonam ▪ butorphanol ▪ calcium gluconate ▪ cefazolin ▪ cefoperazone ▪ ceftazidime ▪ ceftizoxime ▪ chloramphenicol ▪ cimetidine ▪ clindamycin ▪ dextran 40 ▪ dobutamine ▪ dopamine ▪ erythromycin lactobionate ▪ esmolol ▪ famotidine ▪ fentanyl ▪ filgrastim ▪ ganciclovir ▪ gentamicin ▪ heparin ▪ hetastarch ▪ hydrocortisone sodium succinate ▪ labetalol ▪ lidocaine ▪ magnesium sulfate ▪ melphalan ▪ methylprednisolone sodium succinate ▪ metronidazole ▪ morphine ▪ nafcillin ▪ nicardipine ▪ nitroprusside ▪ penicillin G potassium ▪ phenobarbital ▪ piperacillin ▪ piperacillin/tazobactam ▪ potassium chloride ▪ potassium phosphate ▪ ranitidine ▪ sodium acetate ▪ teniposide ▪ tobramycin ▪ trimethoprim/sulfamethoxazole ▪ vancomycin ▪ vinorelbine.
- **Y-Site Incompatibility:** ▪ amphotericin B ▪ cefepime ▪ phenytoin.
- **Additive Compatibility:** ▪ dobutamine ▪ dopamine ▪ heparin ▪ nitroglycerin ▪ nitroprusside ▪ potassium chloride.

Moexipril

- **PO:** Administer captopril and moexipril on an empty stomach, 1 hr prior to a meal.

Ramipril

- **PO:** Capsules may be opened and sprinkled on applesauce, added to apple juice, or dissolved in 4 oz water for patients with difficulty swallowing. Effectiveness is same as capsule.

PATIENT/FAMILY TEACHING

- **General Info:** Instruct patient to take medication exactly as directed at the same time each day, even if feeling well. Missed doses should be taken as soon as possible but not if almost time for next dose. Do not double doses. Warn patient not to discontinue ACE inhibitor therapy unless directed by health care professional.
- Caution patient to avoid salt substitutes or foods containing high levels of potassium or sodium unless directed by health care professional (see Appendix K).
- Caution patient to change positions slowly to minimize hypotension, particularly after initial dose. Patients should also be advised that exercising in hot weather may increase hypotensive effects.
- Advise patient to consult health care professional before taking any OTC medications, especially cold remedies.

- □ May cause dizziness. Caution patient to avoid driving and other activities requiring alertness until response to medication is known.
- □ Advise patient to inform health care professional of medication regimen prior to treatment or surgery.
- □ Advise patient that medication may cause impairment of taste that generally resolves within 8–12 wk, even with continued therapy.
- □ Instruct patient to notify health care professional if rash; mouth sores; sore throat; fever; swelling of hands or feet; irregular heart beat; chest pain; dry cough; hoarseness; swelling of face, eyes, lips, or tongue; difficulty swallowing or breathing occurs; or if taste impairment or skin rash persists. Persistent dry cough may occur and may not subside until medication is discontinued. Consult health care professional if cough becomes bothersome. Also notify health care professional if nausea, vomiting, or diarrhea occurs and continues.
- □ Emphasize the importance of follow-up examinations to monitor progress.
- ■ **Hypertension:** Encourage patient to comply with additional interventions for hypertension (weight reduction, discontinuation of smoking, moderation of alcohol consumption, regular exercise, and stress management). Medication controls but does not cure hypertension.
- □ Instruct patient and family on correct technique for monitoring blood pressure. Advise them to check blood pressure at least weekly and to report significant changes to health care professional.

EVALUATION

Effectiveness of therapy can be demonstrated by: ▪ Decrease in blood pressure without appearance of side effects ▪ Decrease in signs and symptoms of congestive heart failure ▪ Reduction of risk of death or development of congestive heart failure following myocardial infarction ▪ Decrease in progression of diabetic nephropathy.

ANGIOTENSIN II RECEPTOR ANTAGONISTS

irbesartan
(ir-be-**sar**-tan)
Avapro

losartan
(loe-**sar**-tan)
Cozaar

valsartan
(val-**sar**-tan)
Diovan

CLASSIFICATION(S):
Antihypertensive agents

Pregnancy Category C (first trimester); D (second and third trimesters)

INDICATIONS

▪ Alone or with other agents in the management of hypertension.

ACTION

▪ Blocks the vasoconstrictor and aldosterone-producing effects of angiotensin II at various receptor sites, including vascular smooth muscle and the adrenal glands. **Therapeutic Effects:** ▪ Lowering of blood pressure.

PHARMACOKINETICS

Absorption: *Irbesartan*—60–80% absorbed; *losartan*—well absorbed but undergoes extensive first-pass hepatic metabolism, resulting in 33% bioavailability; *valsartan*—25% absorbed following oral administration.

Distribution: UK.

Metabolism and Excretion: *Irbesartan*—Some hepatic metabolism, some biliary excretion, some elimination as unchanged drug in urine; *losartan*—undergoes extensive first-pass hepatic metabolism; 14% is converted to an active metabolite. 4% of losartan is excreted unchanged by the kidneys; although 6% of the active metabolite is excreted unchanged by the kidneys, some biliary elimination also occurs; *valsartan*—20% metabolized by the liver; mostly excreted in feces via bile.

Half-life: *Irbesartan*—11–15 hr; *losartan*—2 hr (6–9 hr for metabolite); *valsartan*—6 hr.

CONTRAINDICATIONS AND PRECAUTIONS

Contraindicated in: ▪ Hypersensitivity ▪ Pregnancy or lactation.

Use Cautiously in: ▪ Volume- or salt-depleted patients or patients receiving high doses of diuretics (correct deficits before initiating therapy or initiate at lower doses) ▪ Black patients (losartan may not be as effective as monotherapy; additional agents may be required) ▪ Impaired renal function due to primary renal disease or congestive heart failure (may worsen renal function) ▪ Hepatic impairment (lower initial doses of losartan or valsartan recommended) ▪ Patients with childbearing potential ▪ Children <18 yr (safety not established).

ADVERSE REACTIONS AND SIDE EFFECTS

CNS: dizziness, fatigue, headache.
CV: hypotension.
GI: diarrhea, drug-induced hepatitis.
GU: impaired renal function.
F and E: hyperkalemia.

INTERACTIONS

Drug-Drug: ▪ **Cimetidine** may increase the effects of losartan ▪ **NSAIDs** and **phenobarbital** may decrease antihypertensive effects ▪ Additive antihypertensive effects with other **antihypertensives** and **diuretics.** Risk of hypotension is increased by concurrent **diuretic** therapy (use lower initial doses).

ROUTE AND DOSAGE

❑ **Irbesartan**

- **PO (Adults):** 150 mg once daily; may be increased to 300 mg once daily. *Patients receiving diuretics, who are volume depleted, or who are being hemodialyzed*—initiate with 75 mg/day.

❑ **Losartan**

- **PO (Adults):** 50 mg/day initially (range 25–100 mg/day as a single daily dose or 2 divided doses). *Patients receiving diuretics, who are volume depleted, or who have impaired hepatic function*—25 mg/day initially; may be increased as tolerated.

❑ **Valsartan**

- **PO (Adults):** 80 mg/day as a single dose initially in patients who are not receiving diuretics or other antihypertensives; may be increased to 160–320 mg/day.

AVAILABILITY

❑ **Irbesartan**

- ***Tablets:*** 75 mg[Rx], 150 mg[Rx], 300 mg[Rx].

❑ **Losartan**

- ***Tablets:*** 25 mg[Rx], 50 mg[Rx] ▪ ***In combination with:*** hydrochlorothiazide (Hyzaar[Rx]; see Appendix A).

❑ **Valsartan**

- ***Capsules:*** 80 mg[Rx], 160 mg[Rx].

TIME/ACTION PROFILE (antihypertensive effect*)

	ONSET	PEAK	DURATION
Irbesartan	within 24 hr	2 wk	1 wk†
Losartan	1 wk	6 hr	24 hr
Valsartan	within 2 wk	4 wk	24 hr

*Onset of antihypertensive effect with chronic dosing.
†Following discontinuation.

NURSING IMPLICATIONS

ASSESSMENT

- ❑ Assess blood pressure (lying, sitting, standing) and pulse periodically throughout therapy.
- ▪ ***Lab Test Considerations:*** May rarely cause elevations in BUN and serum creatinine.
- ❑ May cause elevated serum bilirubin.
- ❑ May occasionally cause hyperkalemia.

POTENTIAL NURSING DIAGNOSES

- Injury, risk for (Adverse Reactions).
- Knowledge deficit, related to medication regimen (Patient/Family Teaching).
- Noncompliance (Patient/Family Teaching).

IMPLEMENTATION

- **General Info:** Volume depletion should be corrected, if possible, prior to initiation of therapy.
- **PO:** May be administered without regard to meals.

PATIENT/FAMILY TEACHING

- ❑ Emphasize the importance of continuing to take as directed, even if feeling well. Take missed doses as soon as remembered if not almost time for next dose; do not double doses. Medication controls but does not cure hypertension. Instruct patient to take medication at the same time each day.
- ❑ Encourage patient to comply with additional interventions for hypertension (weight reduction, low-sodium diet, discontinuation of

smoking, moderation of alcohol consumption, regular exercise, stress management).

- Instruct patient and family on proper technique for monitoring blood pressure. Advise them to check blood pressure at least weekly and to report significant changes.
- Caution patient to avoid sudden changes in position to decrease orthostatic hypotension. Use of alcohol, standing for long periods, exercising, and hot weather may increase orthostatic hypotension.
- Advise women of childbearing age to use contraception and notify health care professional if pregnancy is suspected or planned.
- Advise patient to consult health care professional before taking any OTC cough, cold, or allergy remedies or other medications.
- Instruct patient to notify health care professional of medication regimen prior to treatment or surgery.
- Emphasize the importance of follow-up exams to evaluate effectiveness of medication.

EVALUATION

Effectiveness of therapy can be demonstrated by: ▪ Decrease in blood pressure without appearance of excessive side effects.

ANILERIDINE

(a-ni-**lerr**-i-deen)

{Leritine}

CLASSIFICATION(S):

Opioid analgesic (agonist)

Pregnancy Category UK

INDICATIONS

▪ Moderate to severe pain ▪ Relief of apprehension in congestive heart failure (CHF) ▪ Anesthesia adjunct ▪ Analgesic during labor ▪ Preoperative sedation.

ACTION

▪ Binds to opiate receptors in the CNS. Alters the perception of and response to painful stimuli, while producing generalized CNS depression. **Therapeutic Effects:** ▪ Decrease in severity of pain/apprehension.

PHARMACOKINETICS

Absorption: Well absorbed following oral, IM, or SC administration.

Distribution: UK.

Metabolism and Excretion: Mostly metabolized by the liver; minimal renal excretion.

Half-life: UK.

CONTRAINDICATIONS AND PRECAUTIONS

Contraindicated in: ▪ Hypersensitivity ▪ Some products contain bisulfites and should be avoided in patients with known intolerance.

Use Cautiously in: ▪ Head trauma ▪ Increased intracranial pressure ▪ Severe renal, hepatic, or pulmonary disease ▪ Hypothyroidism ▪ Adrenal insufficiency ▪ Alcoholism ▪ Geriatric or debilitated patients (dosage reduction suggested) ▪ Undiagnosed abdominal pain ▪ Prostatic hypertrophy ▪ Pregnancy or lactation (avoid chronic use; has been used during labor but may cause respiratory depression in the newborn) ▪ Children <12 yr (safety not established).

ADVERSE REACTIONS AND SIDE EFFECTS*

CNS: dizziness, euphoria, excitement, nervousness, restlessness.

EENT: disturbed vision.

Resp: RESPIRATORY DEPRESSION.

GI: constipation, dry mouth, nausea, vomiting.

Derm: flushing, itching, sweating.

Misc: physical dependence, psychological dependence, tolerance.

INTERACTIONS

Drug-Drug: ▪ Use with **extreme caution** in patients receiving **MAO inhibitors** (may result in unpredictable, severe reactions—decrease initial dose to 25% of usual dose) ▪ Additive CNS depression with **alcohol, sedative/hypnotics,** and **antihistamines** ▪ Administration of **partial-antagonist opioid analgesics** may precipitate opioid withdrawal in physically dependent patients ▪ **Buprenorphine, dezocine, nalbuphine,** or **pentazocine** may decrease analgesia.

{} = Available in Canada only.

***CAPITALS indicate life-threatening; underlines indicate most frequent.**

ROUTE AND DOSAGE

Larger doses may be required during chronic therapy.

❑ Analgesia/Preoperative Use/Supplement to Anesthesia

- **PO (Adults):** 25–50 mg q 6 hr; if pain is extremely severe, initial dose may be 50 mg or more frequent intervals may be used but should be reserved for nonambulatory patients.
- **SC, IM (Adults):** *Analgesia*—25–50 mg q 4–6 hr; for more severe pain, 75–100 mg and smaller, more frequent doses used (not to exceed 200 mg/24 hr). *Preoperative use*—50–75 mg.
- **IV (Adults):** *Supplement to anesthesia*—5–10 mg followed by 0.6 mg/min.

❑ Analgesia during Labor

- **IV, IM, SC (Adults):** 50 mg IM or SC; may be repeated in 3–4 hr (not to exceed 100–200 mg total dose) or 40 mg IM or SC given concurrently with 10 mg IV.

AVAILABILITY

- ***Tablets:*** 25 mg[Rx] ▪ ***Injection:*** 25 mg/ml[Rx].

TIME/ACTION PROFILE

	ONSET	PEAK	DURATION
PO, IM, IV, SC	within 15 min	UK	2–3 hr

NURSING IMPLICATIONS

ASSESSMENT

- ❑ Assess type, location, and intensity of pain prior to and 1 hr following IV administration. When titrating opioid doses, increases of 25–50% should be administered until there is either a 50% reduction in the patient's pain rating on a numerical or visual analogue scale or the patient reports satisfactory pain relief. A repeat dose can be safely administered at the time of the peak if previous dose is ineffective and side effects are minimal.
- ❑ Assess blood pressure, pulse, and respirations before and periodically during administration. If respiratory rate is <10/min, assess level of sedation. Physical stimulation may be sufficient to prevent significant hypoventilation. Subsequent doses may need to be decreased by 25–50%. Initial drowsiness will diminish with continued use.
- ❑ Prolonged use may lead to physical and psychological dependence and tolerance. This should not prevent patient from receiving adequate analgesia. Most patients who receive anileridine for pain do not develop psychological dependence. Progressively higher doses may be required to relieve pain with long-term therapy.
- ❑ Assess bowel function routinely. Prevention of constipation should be instituted with increased intake of fluids and bulk, and laxatives to minimize constipating effects. Stimulant laxatives should be administered routinely if opioid use exceeds 2–3 days, unless contraindicated.
- ***Toxicity and Overdose:*** If an opioid antagonist is required to reverse respiratory depression or coma, naloxone (Narcan) is the antidote. Dilute the 0.4-mg ampule of naloxone in 10 ml of 0.9% NaCl and administer 0.5 ml (0.02 mg) by direct IV push every 2 min. For children and adults weighing <40 kg, dilute 0.1 mg of naloxone in 10 ml of 0.9% NaCl for a concentration of 10 mcg/ml and administer 0.5 mcg/kg every 1–2 min. Titrate dose to avoid withdrawal, seizures, and severe pain.

POTENTIAL NURSING DIAGNOSES

- Pain (Indications).
- Sensory-perceptual alterations: visual, auditory (Side Effects).
- Injury, risk for (Side Effects).
- Knowledge deficit, related to medication regimen (Patient/Family Teaching).

IMPLEMENTATION

- **General Info:** Explain therapeutic value of medication prior to administration to enhance the analgesic effect.
- ❑ Regularly administered doses may be more effective than prn administration. Analgesic is more effective if given before pain becomes severe.
- ❑ Coadministration with nonopioid analgesics may have additive analgesic effects and may permit lower doses.
- ❑ Anileridine should be discontinued gradually after long-term use to prevent withdrawal symptoms.

- **PO:** Doses may be administered with food or milk to minimize GI irritation.
- **IV:** Solution is clear and colorless; do not administer discolored solution.
- **Direct IV:** Dilute 5–10 mg with at least 10 ml of 0.9% NaCl for injection. Do not administer undiluted.
- ***Rate:*** Administer slowly. Rapid administration may lead to increased respiratory depression, hypotension, and circulatory collapse.
- **Continuous Infusion:** Dilute 50–100 mg in 500 ml of D5W for continuous infusion as an anesthesia adjunct.
- ***Rate:*** Administer via infusion pump at a rate of approximately 0.6 mg/min. Dose should be titrated to ensure adequate pain relief without excessive sedation, respiratory depression, or hypotension.

PATIENT/FAMILY TEACHING

- Instruct patient how and when to ask for pain medication.
- May cause sedation and dizziness. Caution patient to call for assistance when ambulating or smoking and to avoid driving or other activities requiring alertness until response to medication is known.
- Advise patient to change positions slowly to minimize orthostatic hypotension.
- Caution patient to avoid concurrent use of alcohol or other CNS depressants with this medication.
- Encourage patient to turn, cough, and breathe deeply every 2 hr to prevent atelectasis.

EVALUATION

Effectiveness of therapy can be demonstrated by: ▪ Decrease in severity of pain without a significant alteration in level of consciousness or respiratory status.

ANTIFUNGALS (topical)

butenafine
(byoo-**ten**-a-feen)
Mentax

ciclopirox
(sye-kloe-**peer**-ox)
Loprox

clotrimazole
(kloe-**trye**-ma-zole)
{Canesten}, {Clotrimaderm}, Lotrimin, Mycelex, Mycelex OTC, {Myclo}, {Neo-Zol}

econazole
(ee-**kon**-a-zole)
Spectazole

haloprogin
(hal-oh-**proe**-jin)
Halotex

ketoconazole
(kee-toe-**kon**-a-zole)
Nizoral

miconazole
(mye-**kon**-a-zole)
Lotrimin AF, Micatin, Monistat-Derm, Zeasorb-AF

naftifine
(**naff**-ti-feen)
Naftin

nystatin
(nye-**stat**-in)
Mycostatin, {Nadostine}, Nilstat, {Nyaderm}, Nystex

oxiconazole
(ox-i-**kon**-a-zole)
Oxistat

sulconazole
(sul-**kon**-a-zole)
Exelderm

terbinafine
(ter-**bin**-a-feen)
Lamisil

tolnaftate
(tol-**naff**-tate)
Aftate, Dr. Scholl's Athlete's Foot, NP·27, Tinactin, Ting

CLASSIFICATION(S):
Antifungals (topical)

{} = Available in Canada only.

Pregnancy Category B (butenafine, ciclopirox, clotrimazole, haloprogin, naftifine, oxiconazole, terbinafine), C (econazole, sulconazole), UK (ketoconazole, miconazole, nystatin, tolnaftate)

INDICATIONS

▪ Treatment of a variety of cutaneous fungal infections, including cutaneous candidiasis, tinea pedis (athlete's foot), tinea cruris (jock itch), tinea corporis (ringworm), and tinea versicolor.

ACTION

▪ Butenafine, nystatin, clotrimazole, econazole, ketoconazole, miconazole, and oxiconazole affect the synthesis of the fungal cell wall, allowing leakage of cellular contents. **Therapeutic Effects:** ▪ Fungistatic or fungicidal action depending on agent and concentration, with resultant decrease in symptoms of fungal infection.

PHARMACOKINETICS

Absorption: Most agents are minimally, if at all, absorbed through intact skin.
Distribution: Distribution following topical administration not known. Action is primarily local.
Metabolism and Excretion: Metabolism and excretion not known following local application.
Half-life: *Ciclopirox*—1.7 hr; *miconazole*—24.1 hr (terminal).

CONTRAINDICATIONS AND PRECAUTIONS

Contraindicated in: ▪ Hypersensitivity to active ingredients, additives, preservatives, or bases ▪ Some products contain alcohol or bisulfites and should be avoided in patients with known intolerance.
Use Cautiously in: ▪ Nail and scalp infections (may require additional systemic therapy) ▪ Pregnancy or lactation (safety not established).

ADVERSE REACTIONS AND SIDE EFFECTS

Local: burning, itching, local hypersensitivity reactions, redness, stinging.

INTERACTIONS

Drug-Drug: ▪ If sufficient ketoconazole is absorbed through skin, it may increase the cardiotoxicity of **astemizole** or the nephrotoxicity of **cyclosporine.**

ROUTE AND DOSAGE

❑ **Butenafine**

▪ **Topical (Adults):** Apply once daily for 4 wk.

❑ **Ciclopirox**

▪ **Topical (Adults):** Apply cream or lotion twice daily for 2 wk.

❑ **Clotrimazole**

▪ **Topical (Adults):** Apply cream, solution, or lotion twice daily for 1–4 wk.

❑ **Econazole**

▪ **Topical (Adults):** Apply cream once daily for tinea pedis, tinea cruris, or tinea versicolor. Apply twice daily for cutaneous candidiasis. Use for 2–4 wk.

❑ **Haloprogin**

▪ **Topical (Adults):** Apply daily for 2–4 wk.

❑ **Ketoconazole**

▪ **Topical (Adults):** Apply cream once daily for cutaneous candidiasis or twice daily for seborrheic dermatitis. For dandruff, use shampoo twice weekly (wait 3 days between treatments) for 4 wk, then intermittently.

❑ **Miconazole**

▪ **Topical (Adults):** Apply cream, powder, or spray twice daily (once daily for tinea versicolor) for up to 1 mo.

❑ **Naftifine**

▪ **Topical (Adults):** Apply cream once daily or gel twice daily.

❑ **Nystatin**

▪ **Topical (Adults and Children):** Apply cream, ointment, or powder 2–3 times daily until healing is complete.

❑ **Oxiconazole**

▪ **Topical (Adults and Children):** Apply cream or lotion 1–2 times daily for 2 wk–1 mo.

❑ **Sulconazole**

▪ **Topical (Adults):** Apply 1–2 times daily (twice daily for tinea pedis).

❑ **Terbinafine**

▪ **Topical (Adults):** Apply twice daily for tinea pedis (athlete's foot) or 1–2 times daily for tinea cruris (jock itch) or tinea corporis (ringworm) for 1–4 wk.

❑ **Tolnaftate**

▪ **Topical (Adults):** Apply twice daily for 2–3 wk.

AVAILABILITY

❑ **Butenafine**

▪ ***Cream:*** 1%[Rx].

❑ **Ciclopirox**

▪ ***Cream:*** 1%[Rx] ▪ ***Lotion:*** 1%[Rx] ▪ ***Ointment:*** 3%[OTC].

❑ **Clotrimazole**

▪ ***Cream:*** {1%[Rx,OTC]} ▪ ***Solution:*** 1%[Rx,OTC] ▪ ***Lotion:*** 1%[Rx,OTC] ▪ ***In combination with:*** betamethasone (Lotrisone)[Rx]. See Appendix A.

❑ **Econazole**

▪ ***Cream:*** 1%[Rx].

❑ **Haloprogin**

▪ ***Cream:*** 1%[Rx] ▪ ***Solution:*** 1%[Rx].

❑ **Ketoconazole**

▪ ***Cream:*** 2%[Rx] ▪ ***Shampoo:*** 2%[Rx,OTC].

❑ **Miconazole**

▪ ***Cream:*** {2%[Rx,OTC]} ▪ ***Lotion:*** 2%[Rx] ▪ ***Powder:*** 2%[OTC] ▪ ***Aerosol powder:*** 2%[OTC] ▪ ***Spray:*** 2%[OTC].

❑ **Naftifine**

▪ ***Cream:*** {1%[Rx,OTC]} ▪ ***Gel:*** 1%[Rx,OTC].

❑ **Nystatin**

▪ ***Cream:*** {100,000 units/g[Rx,OTC]} ▪ ***Ointment:*** {100,000 units/g[Rx,OTC]} ▪ ***Powder:*** {100,000 units/g[Rx,OTC]} ▪ ***In combination with:*** triamcinolone (Mycogen II, Mycolog II, Myci-Triacet II, Mytrex)[Rx]. See Appendix A.

❑ **Oxiconazole**

▪ ***Cream:*** 1%[Rx] ▪ ***Lotion:*** 1%[Rx].

❑ **Sulconazole**

▪ ***Cream:*** 1%[Rx] ▪ ***Solution:*** 1%[Rx].

❑ **Terbinafine**

▪ ***Cream:*** 1%[Rx].

❑ **Tolnaftate**

▪ ***Cream:*** 1%[OTC] ▪ ***Solution:*** 1%[OTC] ▪ ***Gel:*** 1%[OTC] ▪ ***Powder:*** 1%[OTC] ▪ ***Spray powder:*** 1%[OTC] ▪ ***Spray liquid:*** 1%[OTC].

TIME/ACTION PROFILE (resolution of symptoms/lesions)

	ONSET	PEAK	DURATION
Butenafine	UK	up to 4 wk	UK
Ciclopirox	within 1st wk	UK	12 hr
Clotrimazole	within 1st wk	UK	12 hr
Miconazole	2–3 days	2 wk	12–24 hr

NURSING IMPLICATIONS

ASSESSMENT

▫ Inspect involved areas of skin and mucous membranes prior to and frequently during therapy. Increased skin irritation may indicate need to discontinue medication.

POTENTIAL NURSING DIAGNOSES

▪ Skin integrity, impaired (Indications).
▪ Infection, risk for (Indications).
▪ Knowledge deficit, related to medication regimen (Patient/Family Teaching).

IMPLEMENTATION

▪ **General Info:** Consult physician or other health care professional for proper cleansing technique prior to applying medication.

▫ Choice of vehicle is based on use. Ointments, creams, and liquids are used as primary therapy. Lotion is usually preferred in intertriginous areas; if cream is used, apply sparingly to avoid maceration. Powders are usually used as adjunctive therapy but may be used as primary therapy for mild conditions.

▪ **Topical:** Apply small amount to cover affected area completely. Avoid the use of occlusive wrappings or dressings unless directed by physician or other health care professional.

▪ **Ketoconazole shampoo:** Moisten hair and scalp thoroughly with water. Apply sufficient shampoo to produce enough lather to wash scalp and hair and gently massage it over the entire scalp area for approximately 1 min. Rinse hair thoroughly with warm water. Repeat process, leaving shampoo on hair for an additional 3 min. After the 2nd shampoo, rinse and dry hair with towel or warm air flow. Shampoo twice a week for 4 wk with at least 3 days between each shampooing and then intermittently as needed to maintain control.

- **Triacetin:** For spray products, shake well. Dry affected areas prior to spraying. Spray onto affected nails, holding actuator down 1–2 sec.

PATIENT/FAMILY TEACHING

- Instruct patient to apply medication as directed for full course of therapy, even if feeling better. Emphasize the importance of avoiding the eyes.
- Caution patient that some products may stain fabric, skin, or hair. Check label information. Fabrics stained from cream or lotion can usually be cleaned by handwashing with soap and warm water; stains from ointments can usually be removed with standard cleaning fluids.
- Patients with athlete's foot should be taught to wear well-fitting, ventilated shoes and to change shoes and socks at least once a day.
- Advise patient to report increased skin irritation or lack of response to therapy to health care professional.

EVALUATION

Effectiveness of therapy can be demonstrated by: ▪ Decrease in skin irritation and resolution of infection. Early relief of symptoms may be seen in 2–3 days. For *Candida,* tinea cruris, and tinea corporis, 2 wk are needed, and for tinea pedis, therapeutic response may take 3–4 wk. Recurrent fungal infections may be a sign of systemic illness.

ANTIFUNGALS (vaginal)

butoconazole
(**byoo**-toe-kon-a-zole)
Femstat

clotrimazole
(kloe-**trye**-ma-zole)
{Canesten}, {Clotrimaderm}, Gyne-Lotrimin, FemCare, Femizole, Mycelex, {Myclo-Gyne}

miconazole
(mye-**kon**-a-zole)
Miconazole, Monistat

nystatin
(nye-**stat**-in)
Mycostatin, Nilstat

terconazole
(ter-**kon**-a-zole)
Terazol

tioconazole
(tye-oh-**kon**-a-zole)
{Gyne-Trosyd}, Vagistat

CLASSIFICATION(S):
Antifungals (vaginal)

Pregnancy Category A (nystatin), B (clotrimazole, miconazole), C (butoconazole, terconazole), UK (tioconazole)

INDICATIONS

- Treatment of vulvovaginal candidiasis.

ACTION

- Damage fungal cell membrane, allowing leakage of cellular contents. Not active against bacteria. **Therapeutic Effects:** ▪ Inhibited growth/death of susceptible *Candida* with decrease in accompanying symptoms of vulvovaginitis (vaginal burning, itching, discharge).

PHARMACOKINETICS

Absorption: *Nystatin, miconazole, and tioconazole* are minimally absorbed; 5.5% of *butoconazole* is absorbed, 3–10% of *clotrimazole,* 5–15% of *terconazole* following intravaginal administration.
Distribution: UK. Action is primarily local.
Metabolism and Excretion: Small amounts of *clotrimazole* absorbed are rapidly metabolized.
Half-life: *Miconazole*—20–25 hr (following parenteral administration).

CONTRAINDICATIONS AND PRECAUTIONS

Contraindicated in: ▪ Hypersensitivity to active ingredients, additives, or preservatives ▪ Buto-

conazole is contraindicated in the first trimester of pregnancy ▪ Lactation (except terconazole).
Use Cautiously in: ▪ Patients with recurrent vulvovaginal yeast infections ▪ Lactation (safe use not established for terconazole).

ADVERSE REACTIONS AND SIDE EFFECTS*

CNS: *terconazole*—headache.
Local: irritation, sensitization, vulvovaginal burning.
Misc: hypersensitivity reactions; *terconazole*—body pain.

INTERACTIONS

Drug-Drug: ▪ None significant.

ROUTE AND DOSAGE

❑ **Butoconazole**

- **Vag (Adults and Adolescents):** *Vaginal cream*—1 applicatorful (5 g) at bedtime for 3–6 days.

❑ **Clotrimazole**

- **Vag (Adults and Adolescents):** *Vaginal tablets*—100 mg at bedtime for 7 nights (preferred regimen for pregnancy) *or* 200 mg at bedtime for 3 nights *or* 500 mg (one 500-mg vaginal tablet) as a single bedtime dose. *Vaginal cream*—1 applicatorful (5 g) at bedtime for 7–14 days.

❑ **Miconazole**

- **Vag (Adults and Adolescents):** *Vaginal suppositories*— one 200-mg or one 400-mg suppository at bedtime for 3 days or one 100-mg suppository at bedtime for 7 days. *Vaginal cream*—1 applicatorful at bedtime for 7 days.

❑ **Nystatin**

- **Vag (Adults and Adolescents):** *Vaginal tablets*—100,000 U (1 tablet) daily for 2 wk.

❑ **Terconazole**

- **Vag (Adults and Adolescents):** *Vaginal cream*—1 applicatorful (5 g) of 0.4% cream at bedtime for 7 days or 1 applicatorful (5 g) of 0.8% cream at bedtime for 3 days. *Vaginal suppositories*—1 suppository (80 mg) at bedtime for 3 days.

❑ **Tioconazole**

- **Vag (Adults and Adolescents):** *Vaginal ointment*—1 applicatorful (4.6 g) at bedtime as a single dose.

AVAILABILITY

❑ **Butoconazole**

- ***Vaginal cream:*** 2%^OTC^.

❑ **Clotrimazole**

- ***Vaginal tablets:*** 100 mg^OTC^, {200 mg^Rx^}, 500 mg^Rx,OTC^ ▪ ***Vaginal cream:*** 1%^OTC^, {2%^Rx^}.

❑ **Miconazole**

- ***Vaginal cream:*** 2%^OTC^ ▪ ***Vaginal suppositories:*** 100 mg^OTC^, 200 mg^Rx,OTC^, {400 mg^OTC^}.

❑ **Nystatin**

- ***Vaginal tablets:*** 100,000 units^Rx^.

❑ **Terconazole**

- ***Vaginal cream:*** 0.4%^Rx^, 0.8%^Rx^ ▪ ***Vaginal suppositories:*** 80 mg^Rx^.

❑ **Tioconazole**

- ***Vaginal ointment:*** 6.5%^OTC^.

TIME/ACTION PROFILE

	ONSET	PEAK	DURATION
All agents	rapid	UK	24 hr

NURSING IMPLICATIONS

ASSESSMENT

- ❑ Inspect involved areas of skin and mucous membranes prior to and frequently throughout therapy. Increased skin irritation may indicate need to discontinue medication.

POTENTIAL NURSING DIAGNOSES

- Infection, risk for (Indications).
- Skin integrity, impaired (Indications).
- Knowledge deficit, related to medication regimen (Patient/Family Teaching).

IMPLEMENTATION

- **General Info:** Consult physician or other health care professional for proper cleansing

*CAPITALS indicate life-threatening; underlines indicate most frequent.

technique prior to applying medication. Sitz baths and vaginal douches may be ordered concurrently with this therapy.
- **Vag:** Applicators are supplied for vaginal administration.

PATIENT/FAMILY TEACHING

- Instruct patient to apply medication as directed for full course of therapy, even if feeling better. Therapy should be continued during menstrual period.
- Instruct patient on proper use of vaginal applicator. Medication should be inserted high into the vagina at bedtime. Instruct patient to remain recumbent for at least 30 min following insertion. Advise use of sanitary napkins to prevent staining of clothing or bedding.
- Advise patient to consult health care professional regarding douching and intercourse during therapy. Vaginal medication may cause minor skin irritation in sexual partner. Advise patient to refrain from sexual contact during therapy or have male partner wear a condom. Some products may weaken latex contraceptive devices.
- Advise patient to report to health care professional increased skin irritation or lack of response to therapy. A second course may be necessary if symptoms persist.

EVALUATION

Clinical response to therapy can be evaluated by: ▪ Decrease in skin irritation and vaginal discomfort. Therapeutic response is usually seen after 1 wk. Diagnosis should be reconfirmed with smears or cultures prior to a second course of therapy to rule out other pathogens associated with vulvovaginitis. Recurrent vaginal infections may be a sign of systemic illness.

ANTIHEMOPHILIC FACTOR

Alphanate, Bioclate, Helixate, HYATE:C, Humate-P, Koate-HP, Kogenate, Monoclate-P, Profilate HP, Recombinate

CLASSIFICATION(S):
Hemostatic

Pregnancy Category C

INDICATIONS

▪ Management of hemophilia A associated with a deficiency of factor VIII ▪ Antihemophilic factor (porcine, HYATE:C) is used in patients with antibodies to factor VIII.

ACTION

▪ An essential clotting factor required for the conversion of prothrombin to thrombin. **Therapeutic Effects:** ▪ Correction of deficiency states with resultant decreased bleeding.

PHARMACOKINETICS

Absorption: Following IV administration absorption is complete.
Distribution: Rapidly cleared from plasma; does not cross the placenta.
Metabolism and Excretion: Used up in the clotting process.
Half-life: 8.4–19.3 hr (reduced in the presence of inhibitor antibodies and during active bleeding).

CONTRAINDICATIONS AND PRECAUTIONS

Contraindicated in: ▪ Hypersensitivity to hamster, mouse, or bovine proteins (in recombinant and monoclonal antibody products); hypersensivity to porcine products (HYATE:C only).
Use Cautiously in: ▪ Hypersensitivity to antihemophilic factor ▪ Pregnancy (safety not established).

ADVERSE REACTIONS AND SIDE EFFECTS

CNS: headache, lethargy, loss of consciousness, sedation.
EENT: visual disturbances.
CV: chest tightness, hypotension, tachycardia.
GI: nausea, vomiting.
Derm: flushing, urticaria.
Hemat: intravascular hemolysis.
MS: back pain.
Neuro: paresthesia.
Misc: allergic reactions, hepatitis B, C, D, or HIV virus infection (small risk from frequent use of large amounts), jaundice, rigor.

INTERACTIONS

Drug-Drug: ▪ None significant.

A

ROUTE AND DOSAGE

Consult individual product information for more specific dosing information. Dosage may be calculated using the following formula: Dose AHF (units) = body weight (kg) × desired AHF increase (% normal) × 0.5. Each unit of AHF/kg may be expected to produce a 2% rise in factor VIII activity.

❑ **Prevention of Spontaneous Hemorrhage**

- **IV (Adults and Children):** 10 AHF units/kg (or amount necessary to increase plasma factor VIII levels by 5–30% of normal, depending on situation).

❑ **Treatment of Minor Hemorrhage**

- **IV (Adults and Children):** A single infusion of the amount necessary to increase plasma factor VIII levels by ≥20% of normal.

❑ **Treatment of Moderate Hemorrhage/ Minor Surgery**

- **IV (Adults and Children):** 15–25 units/kg (or amount necessary to increase plasma factor VIII levels by 30–50% of normal); may require additional doses of 10–15 IU/kg q 12–24 hr.

❑ **Treatment of Severe Hemorrhage**

- **IV (Adults and Children):** 40–50 units/kg (or amount needed to increase plasma factor VIII levels by 60–100% of normal) initially, then 20–25 units/kg 8–12 hr as needed.

❑ **Management of Perioperative Hemostasis—Major Surgery**

- **IV (Adults and Children):** Amount necessary to raise plasma factor VIII levels to 80–100% of normal given 1 hr prior to procedure, then amount necessary to maintain plasma factor VIII levels of at least 30% of normal for 10–14 days postoperatively.

❑ **Management of Perioperative Hemostasis—Tooth Extraction**

- **IV (Adults and Children):** Amount necessary to raise plasma factor VIII levels to 50% given prior to surgery.

❑ **Prevention of Bleeding in Patients with Factor VIII Antibodies (HYATE:C)**

- **IV (Adults and Children >50 kg):** 100–150 porcine units/kg (may be increased as needed).

AVAILABILITY

- ***Injection:*** 250-unit, 500-unit, 750-unit, 1000-unit, 1500-unit vials[Rx].

TIME/ACTION PROFILE (levels of factor VIII)

	ONSET	PEAK	DURATION
IV	rapid	1–2 hr	8–12 hr

NURSING IMPLICATIONS

ASSESSMENT

- □ Monitor blood pressure, pulse, and respirations. If tachycardia occurs, slow or stop infusion rate and notify physician.
- □ Obtain history of current trauma; estimate amount of blood loss.
- □ Monitor for renewed bleeding every 15–30 min. Immobilize and apply ice to affected joints.
- □ Monitor intake and output ratios; note color of urine. Notify physician of significant discrepancy or if urine becomes red or orange. Patients with types A, B, and AB blood are particularly at risk for hemolytic reaction.
- □ Assess for allergic reaction (wheezing, tachycardia, urticaria, hives, chest tightness, stinging at IV site, nausea and vomiting, lethargy). Diphenhydramine (Benadryl) may be used as a premedication to prevent acute reactions. Stop infusion, notify physician.
- ***Lab Test Considerations:*** Monitor plasma factor VIII levels. To prevent spontaneous bleeding, at least 5% of the normal factor VIII level must be present.
- □ Obtain baseline and periodic CBC, platelet count, direct Coombs' test, urinalysis, partial thromboplastin time (PTT), thromboplastin generation test, and prothrombin generation test. Decreased hematocrit and increased Coombs' test may indicate hemolytic anemia.
- □ Monitor coagulation studies before, during, and after therapy to assess effectiveness of therapy.
- □ Patients with increased inhibitor levels may not respond or may require increased doses.

POTENTIAL NURSING DIAGNOSES

- Tissue perfusion, altered (Indications).
- Injury, risk for (Indications).
- Knowledge deficit, related to medication regimen (Patient/Family Teaching).

IMPLEMENTATION

- **General Info:** Inform all personnel of bleeding tendency. Apply pressure to venipuncture sites for at least 5 min; avoid all IM injections.
- □ Dosage varies with degree of clotting factor deficit, desired level of clotting factors, and weight.
- □ Obtain type and crossmatch of blood in case a transfusion is necessary.
- □ The first dose of antihemophilic factor is given 1 hr before surgery.
- **Direct IV:** Administer IV only. Refrigerate concentrate until just prior to reconstitution. Warm concentrate and diluent (provided by manufacturer) to room temperature before reconstituting. Use plastic syringe for preparation and administration. Use an additional needle as an air vent to the vial when reconstituting. After adding diluent, rotate vial gently until completely dissolved. Solution may vary in color from light yellow to clear with a bluish tint. Do not refrigerate after reconstitution; use within 3 hr. Preparations should be filtered prior to administration.
- ***Rate:*** Rate is based on patient's response. Administer at a rate of 2 ml/min. May be given over up to 10 min.
- **Y-site/Additive Incompatibility:** Do not admix or administer in the same line with any other medication or solution.

PATIENT/FAMILY TEACHING

- □ Instruct patient to notify nurse immediately if bleeding recurs. Advise patient to observe for bleeding of gums, skin, urine, stool, or emesis.
- □ Advise patient to carry identification describing disease process at all times.
- □ Caution patient to avoid products containing aspirin or NSAIDs, as they may further impair clotting.
- □ Review prevention of bleeding with patient (use soft toothbrush, avoid IM and SC injections, avoid potentially traumatic activities).
- □ Inform newly diagnosed hemophilia patients of the need for hepatitis B vaccine. Advise patient that the risk of hepatitis or AIDS transmission may be diminished by the use of heat-treated, pasteurized, solvent/detergent-treated, or monoclonal antibody preparations. Screening programs should also decrease the risk.

EVALUATION

Effectiveness of therapy can be demonstrated by: ▪ Prevention of spontaneous bleeding ▪ Cessation of bleeding.

ASCORBIC ACID

(as-**kor**-bik **as**-id)

{Apo-C}, Ascorbicap, Cebid, Cecon, Cecore-500, Cemill, Cenolate, Cetane, Cevalin, Cevi-Bid, Flavorcee, Mega-C/A Plus, Ortho/CS, Sunkist

CLASSIFICATION(S):
Vitamin (water-soluble)

Pregnancy Category C

INDICATIONS

▪ Treatment/prevention of vitamin C deficiency (scurvy) with dietary supplementation ▪ Supplemental therapy in some GI diseases, during long-term parenteral nutrition or chronic hemodialysis ▪ States of increased requirements such as: □ Pregnancy □ Lactation □ Stress □ Hyperthyroidism □ Trauma □ Burns □ Infancy. **Unlabeled Uses:** ▪ Prevention of the common cold.

ACTION

▪ Necessary for collagen formation and tissue repair ▪ Involved in oxidation reduction reactions; tyrosine, folic acid, iron, and carbohydrate metabolism; lipid and protein synthesis; cellular respiration; and resistance to infection. **Therapeutic Effects:** ▪ Replacement in deficiency states ▪ Supplementation during increased requirements.

PHARMACOKINETICS

Absorption: Actively absorbed following oral administration by a saturable process.
Distribution: Widely distributed. Crosses the placenta; enters breast milk.
Metabolism and Excretion: Converted to compounds that are excreted by the kidneys.
Half-life: UK.

CONTRAINDICATIONS AND PRECAUTIONS

Contraindicated in: ▪ Tartrazine hypersensitivity (some products contain tartrazine—FDC yellow dye #5).
Use Cautiously in: ▪ Recurrent kidney stones ▪ Avoid chronic use of large doses in pregnant women.

ADVERSE REACTIONS AND SIDE EFFECTS

CNS: drowsiness, fatigue, headache, insomnia.
GI: cramps, diarrhea, heartburn, nausea, vomiting.
GU: kidney stones.
Derm: flushing.
Hemat: deep vein thrombosis, hemolysis (in G6PD deficiency), sickle cell crisis.
Local: pain at SC or IM sites.

INTERACTIONS

Drug-Drug: ▪ If urinary acidification occurs, may increase excretion and decrease effects of **mexiletine, amphetamines,** or **tricyclic antidepressants** ▪ Large doses (>10 g/day) may decrease response to **warfarin** ▪ Increases iron toxicity when given concurrently with **deferoxamine.**

ROUTE AND DOSAGE

- **PO (Adults):** *Scurvy*—500 mg/day for at least 14 days. *Prevention of deficiency*—50–100 mg/day.
- **PO (Children):** *Scurvy*—100–300 mg/day for at least 14 days. *Prevention of deficiency*—30–45 mg/day.
- **IM (Adults):** *Scurvy*—100–500 mg/day for at least 14 days.
- **IM (Children):** *Scurvy*—100–300 mg/day for at least 14 days.
- **IV (Adults and Children):** *Prevention of deficiency*—determined by need.

AVAILABILITY

▪ ***Tablets:*** 25 mg^{OTC}, 50 mg^{OTC}, 100 mg^{OTC}, 125 mg^{OTC}, 250 mg^{OTC}, 500 mg^{OTC}, 1 g^{OTC}, 1.5 g^{OTC} ▪ ***Chewable tablets:*** 60 mg^{OTC}, 100 mg^{OTC}, 250 mg^{OTC}, 500 mg^{OTC}, 1 g^{OTC} ▪ ***Extended-release tablets:*** 500 mg^{OTC}, 1 g^{OTC}, 1.5 g^{OTC} ▪ ***Extended-release capsules:*** 500 mg^{OTC} ▪ ***Solution:*** {50 mg/0.6 ml^{OTC}}, 100 mg/ml^{OTC} ▪ ***Syrup:*** 250 mg/5 ml^{OTC} ▪ ***Injection:*** {222 mg/ml^{Rx}}, 250 mg/ml^{Rx}, {500 mg/ml^{OTC}} ▪ ***In combination with:*** other vitamins and minerals in multivitamin preparations.

TIME/ACTION PROFILE (response to skeletal and hemorrhagic changes in scurvy)

	ONSET	PEAK	DURATION
PO, IM, IV, SC	2 days–3 wk	UK	UK

NURSING IMPLICATIONS

ASSESSMENT

- **Vitamin C Deficiency:** Assess for signs of vitamin C deficiency (faulty bone and tooth development, gingivitis, bleeding gums, loosened teeth) before and during therapy.
- ***Lab Test Considerations:*** Megadoses of ascorbic acid (>10 times the RDA requirement) may cause false-negative results for occult blood in the stool.
- □ May cause decreased serum bilirubin and increased urine oxalate, urate, and cysteine levels.

POTENTIAL NURSING DIAGNOSES

- Nutrition, altered, less than body requirements (Indications).
- Knowledge deficit, related to medication regimen (Patient/Family Teaching).

IMPLEMENTATION

- **General Info:** Often ordered as a part of multivitamin supplementation, because inadequate diet often results in multiple-vitamin deficiency.
- □ Pressure in ampules may be increased at room temperature; wrap with protective cover before breaking.
- **PO:** Extended-release tablets and capsules should be swallowed whole without crushing, breaking, or chewing; contents of capsules may be mixed with jelly or jam. Chewable tablets should be chewed well or crushed before swallowing. Oral solution may be taken di-

rectly by mouth or mixed with fruit juice, cereal, or other food.
- **Direct IV:** Ascorbic acid may be administered IV undiluted.
- ***Rate:*** Administer at a rate of 100 mg over at least 1 min. Rapid IV administration may result in temporary dizziness and fainting.
- **Intermittent Infusion:** Dilute with D5W, D10W, 0.9% NaCl, 0.45% NaCl, lactated Ringer's or Ringer's solution, dextrose/saline or dextrose/Ringer's combinations.
- **Syringe Compatibility:** ▪ metoclopramide.
- **Syringe Incompatibility:** ▪ cefazolin ▪ doxapram.
- **Additive Compatibility:** ▪ amikacin ▪ calcium chloride ▪ calcium gluceptate ▪ calcium gluconate ▪ cephalothin ▪ chloramphenicol ▪ chlorpromazine ▪ colistimethate ▪ cyanocobalamin ▪ diphenhydramine ▪ heparin ▪ kanamycin ▪ methicillin ▪ methyldopate ▪ penicillin G potassium ▪ polymyxin B ▪ prednisolone ▪ procaine ▪ prochlorperazine ▪ promethazine ▪ verapamil.
- **Additive Incompatibility:** ▪ bleomycin ▪ cephapirin ▪ nafcillin ▪ sodium bicarbonate ▪ warfarin.

PATIENT/FAMILY TEACHING

- **General Info:** Advise patient to take this medication as directed and not to exceed dose prescribed. Excess doses may lead to diarrhea and urinary stone formation. If a dose is missed, skip dose and return to dosage schedule.
- **Vitamin C Deficiency:** Encourage patient to comply with diet recommendations of health care professional. Explain that the best source of vitamins is a well-balanced diet.
- □ Foods high in ascorbic acid include citrus fruits, tomatoes, strawberries, cantaloupe, and raw peppers. Gradual loss of ascorbic acid occurs when fresh food is stored, but not when frozen. Rapid loss is caused by drying, salting, and cooking.
- □ Patients self-medicating with vitamin supplements should be cautioned not to exceed RDA (see Appendix L). The effectiveness of megadoses of vitamins for treatment of various medical conditions is unproven and may cause side effects. Abrupt withdrawal of megadoses of ascorbic acid may cause rebound deficiency.

EVALUATION

Effectiveness of therapy can be demonstrated by: ▪ Decrease in the symptoms of ascorbic acid deficiency.

ASPARAGINASE

(a-**spare**-a-gin-ase)
Elspar, {Kidrolase}

CLASSIFICATION(S):
Antineoplastic (enzyme)

Pregnancy Category C

INDICATIONS

▪ Part of combination chemotherapy in the treatment of acute lymphocytic leukemia (ALL).

ACTION

▪ Catalyst in the conversion of asparagine (an amino acid) to aspartic acid and ammonia ▪ Depletes asparagine in leukemic cells. **Therapeutic Effects:** ▪ Death of leukemic cells.

PHARMACOKINETICS

Absorption: Is absorbed from IM sites.
Distribution: Remains in the intravascular space. Poor penetration into the CSF.
Metabolism and Excretion: Slowly sequestered in the reticuloendothelial system.
Half-life: IV: 8–30 hr; IM: 39–49 hr.

CONTRAINDICATIONS AND PRECAUTIONS

Contraindicated in: ▪ Previous hypersensitivity ▪ Pregnancy or lactation.
Use Cautiously in: ▪ History of hypersensitivity reactions ▪ Severe liver disease ▪ Renal or pancreatic disease ▪ CNS depression ▪ Clotting abnormalities ▪ Chronic debilitating illnesses ▪ Patients with childbearing potential.

A

ADVERSE REACTIONS AND SIDE EFFECTS*

CNS: SEIZURES, agitation, coma, confusion, depression, dizziness, fatigue, hallucinations, headache, irritability, somnolence.
GI: <u>nausea</u>, <u>vomiting</u>, anorexia, cramps, hepatotoxicity, pancreatitis, weight loss.
Derm: rashes, urticaria.
Endo: hyperglycemia.
Hemat: coagulation abnormalities, transient bone marrow depression.
Metab: hyperammonemia, hyperuricemia.
Misc: hypersensitivity reactions including ANAPHYLAXIS.

INTERACTIONS

Drug-Drug: ▪ May negate the antineoplastic activity of **methotrexate** ▪ May enhance the hepatotoxicity of other **hepatotoxic drugs** ▪ Concurrent IV use with or immediately preceding **vincristine** and **prednisone** may result in increased neurotoxicity and hyperglycemia ▪ May alter the response to **live vaccines** (decreased antibody response, increased risk of adverse reactions).

ROUTE AND DOSAGE

Various other regimens may be used.

❑ **Multiple-Agent Induction Regimen (in combination with vincristine and prednisone)**

- **IV (Children):** 1000 IU/kg/day for 10 successive days beginning on day 22 of regimen.
- **IM (Children):** 6000 IU/m² on days 4, 7, 10, 13, 16, 19, 22, 25, 28.

❑ **Single-Agent Therapy for Acute Lymphocytic Leukemia**

- **IV (Adults and Children):** 200 IU/kg daily for 28 days.

❑ **Desensitization Regimen**

- **IV (Adults and Children):** Administer 1 IU, then double dose every 10 min until total dose for that day has been given or reaction occurs.

❑ **Test Dose**

- **Intradermal (Adults and Children):** 2 IU.

AVAILABILITY

▪ ***Injection:*** 10,000 IU-vial (with mannitol)[Rx].

TIME/ACTION PROFILE (depletion of asparagine)

	ONSET	PEAK†	DURATION
IM	immediate	14–24 hr	23–33 days
IV	immediate	UK	23–33 days

†Plasma levels of asparaginase.

NURSING IMPLICATIONS

ASSESSMENT

- ◻ Monitor vital signs prior to and frequently during therapy. Inform physician if fever or chills occur.
- ◻ Monitor intake and output. Notify physician of significant discrepancies. Encourage patient to drink 2000–3000 ml/day to promote excretion of uric acid. Allopurinol and alkalinization of the urine may be used to prevent urate stone formation.
- ◻ Monitor for hypersensitivity reaction (urticaria, diaphoresis, facial swelling, joint pain, hypotension, bronchospasm). Epinephrine and resuscitation equipment should be readily available. Reaction may occur up to 2 hr after administration. If patient requires continued therapy, pegaspargase (p.768) is an alternative.
- ◻ Assess nausea, vomiting, and appetite. Weigh weekly. An antiemetic may be given prior to administration.
- ◻ Monitor affect and neurologic status. Notify physician if depression, drowsiness, or hallucinations occur. Symptoms usually resolve 2–3 days after drug is discontinued.
- ▪ ***Lab Test Considerations:*** Monitor CBC prior to and periodically throughout therapy. May alter coagulation studies. Platelets, PT, PTT, and thrombin time may be increased. May cause elevated BUN.
- ◻ Hepatotoxicity may be manifested by increased AST, ALT, alkaline phosphatase, bilirubin, or cholesterol. Liver function tests usually return to normal after therapy. May cause pancreatitis; monitor frequently for elevated amylase or glucose.
- ◻ Monitor blood glucose during therapy. May

***CAPITALS indicate life-threatening; <u>underlines</u> indicate most frequent.**

cause hyperglycemia treatable with fluids and insulin. May be fatal.

- ▫ May cause elevated serum and urine uric acid concentrations.
- ▫ May interfere with thyroid function tests.

POTENTIAL NURSING DIAGNOSES

- ▪ Injury, risk for (Side Effects).
- ▪ Infection, risk for (Side Effects).
- ▪ Knowledge deficit, related to medication regimen (Patient/Family Teaching).

IMPLEMENTATION

- ▪ **General Info:** Solution should be prepared in a biologic cabinet. Wear gloves, gown, and mask while handling medication. Discard equipment in specially designated containers (see Appendix I).
- ▫ If coagulopathy develops, apply pressure to venipuncture sites; avoid IM injections.
- ▪ **Test Dose:** Intradermal test dose must be performed prior to initial dose, and doses must be separated by more than 1 wk. Reconstitute vial with 5 ml of sterile water for injection or 0.9% NaCl for injection (without preservatives). Add 0.1 ml of this 2000-IU/ml solution to 9.9 ml additional diluent to yield a 20-IU/ml solution. Inject 0.1 ml (2 IU) intradermally. Observe site for 1 hr for formation of wheal. Wheal is indicative of a positive reaction.
- ▪ **Desensitization Therapy:** Begin by administering 1 IU intravenously. Double dose every 10 min if hypersensitivity does not occur until full daily dose is administered.
- ▪ **IM:** Prepare for IM dose by adding 2 ml of 0.9% NaCl for injection (without preservatives) to the 10,000-IU vial. Shake vial gently. Administer no more than 2 ml per injection site.
- ▪ **Direct IV:** Prepare IV dose by diluting 10,000-IU vial with 5 ml of sterile water for injection or 0.9% NaCl (without preservatives). If gelatinous fibers are present, administration through a 5-micron filter will not alter potency. Administration through a 0.2-micron filter may cause loss of potency. Solution should be clear after reconstitution. Discard if cloudy. Stable for 8 hr if refrigerated.
- ▪ ***Rate:*** Administer through Y-site of rapidly flowing IV of D5W or 0.9% NaCl over at least 30 min. Maintain IV infusion for 2 hr after dose.
- ▪ **Y-Site Compatibility:** ▪ methotrexate ▪ sodium bicarbonate.
- ▪ **Additive Incompatibility:** ▪ Information unavailable. Do not admix with other drugs.

PATIENT/FAMILY TEACHING

- ▫ Instruct patient to notify health care professional if abdominal pain, severe nausea and vomiting, jaundice, fever, chills, sore throat, bleeding or bruising, excess thirst or urination, or mouth sores occur. Caution patient to avoid crowds and persons with known infections. Instruct patient to use soft toothbrush, electric razor, and to be especially careful to avoid falls. Patients should also be cautioned not to drink alcoholic beverages or take medication containing aspirin or NSAIDs because these may precipitate gastric bleeding.
- ▫ Advise patient of the need for contraception because of teratogenic effects of asparaginase.
- ▫ Instruct patient not to receive any vaccinations without advice of health care professional. Advise parents that this may alter immunization schedule.
- ▫ Emphasize need for periodic lab test to monitor for side effects.

EVALUATION

Effectiveness of therapy can be demonstrated by: ▪ Improvement of hematologic status in patients with leukemia.

ASTEMIZOLE

(a-**stem**-mi-zole)

Hismanal

CLASSIFICATION(S):

Antihistamine

Pregnancy Category C

INDICATIONS

▪ Symptomatic relief of allergic symptoms (rhinitis, urticaria) caused by histamine release ▪ May cause less sedation and fewer anticholinergic effects than other antihistamines.

ACTION

▪ Antagonizes the effects of histamine at H_1-receptor sites; does not bind to or inactivate histamine. **Therapeutic Effects:** ▪ Decreased symptoms of histamine excess (sneezing, rhinorrhea, nasal and ocular pruritus, ocular tearing, and redness).

PHARMACOKINETICS

Absorption: Well absorbed following oral administration.
Distribution: UK.
Metabolism and Excretion: Highly metabolized by the liver, partially converted to desmethylastemizole, an active metabolite.
Half-life: 100 hr—astemizole; 12–19 days—desmethylastemizole.

CONTRAINDICATIONS AND PRECAUTIONS

Contraindicated in: ▪ Hypersensitivity ▪ Acute attacks of asthma ▪ Lactation ▪ Significant hepatic dysfunction or concurrent ketoconazole, itraconazole, erythromycin, other macrolide anti-infectives, ibutilide, fluvoxamine, nefazodone, indinavir, ritonavir, or nelfinavir (increased risk of arrhythmias) ▪ History of syncope during previous astemizole therapy.
Use Cautiously in: ▪ Narrow-angle glaucoma ▪ Liver disease ▪ Elderly patients (more susceptible to adverse reactions) ▪ Underlying cardiovascular disease ▪ Pregnancy or children <12 yr (safety not established).

ADVERSE REACTIONS AND SIDE EFFECTS*

CNS: ataxia, dizziness, drowsiness, fatigue, headache, inability to concentrate, stimulation, syncope.
EENT: conjunctivitis, pharyngitis.
Resp: cough.
CV: ARRHYTHMIAS.
GI: abdominal pain, diarrhea, dry mouth, flatulence, nausea.
Derm: eczema, rash.
MS: joint pain.
Misc: increased appetite, weight gain.

INTERACTIONS

Drug-Drug: ▪ Concurrent **ketoconazole, itraconazole, indinavir, nelfinavir, ritonavir, clarithromycin, fluconazole, fluvoxamine, ibutilide, mibefradil, nefazodone,** or **erythromycin** increases the risk of cardiac arrhythmias ▪ Additive CNS depression with other **CNS depressants** including **alcohol, opioid analgesics,** and **sedative/hypnotics** ▪ **MAO inhibitors** intensify and prolong the anticholinergic effects and sedation.
Drug-Food: ▪ **Food** decreases the absorption of astemizole ▪ Concurrent ingestion of **grapefruit juice** increases absorption.

ROUTE AND DOSAGE

- **PO (Adults and Children >12 yr):** 10 mg/day.
- **PO (Children 6–12 yr):** 5 mg once daily (unlabeled).
- **PO (Children <6 yr):** 2 mg/10 kg once daily (unlabeled).

AVAILABILITY

▪ ***Tablets:*** 10 mg[Rx] ▪ ***Suspension:*** {2 mg/ml[OTC]}.

TIME/ACTION PROFILE (antihistaminic effects)

	ONSET	PEAK	DURATION
PO	<1–3 days	9–12 days	up to several wk

NURSING IMPLICATIONS

ASSESSMENT

- □ Assess allergy symptoms (rhinitis, conjunctivitis, hives) prior to and periodically throughout therapy.
- □ Assess lung sounds and character of bronchial secretions. Maintain fluid intake of 1500–2000 ml/day to decrease viscosity of secretions.
- ▪ ***Lab Test Considerations:*** May cause false-negative allergy skin testing.

POTENTIAL NURSING DIAGNOSES

- ▪ Airway clearance, ineffective (Indications).
- ▪ Injury, risk for (Adverse Reactions).
- ▪ Knowledge deficit, related to medication regimen (Patient/Family Teaching).

IMPLEMENTATION

- ▪ **PO:** Administer on an empty stomach.

***CAPITALS indicate life-threatening; underlines indicate most frequent.**

PATIENT/FAMILY TEACHING

- □ Instruct patient to take medication at least 1 hr before or 2 hr after eating.
- □ May cause drowsiness. Caution patient to avoid driving or other activities requiring alertness until response to medication is known.
- □ Discuss possibility of increased appetite. Patients on chronic therapy may need to limit caloric intake and increase activity to avoid undesired weight gain.
- □ Advise patient to avoid taking alcohol or other CNS depressants concurrently with this drug.
- □ Advise patient that good oral hygiene, frequent rinsing of mouth with water, and sugarless gum or candy may minimize dry mouth. Patient should notify dentist if dry mouth persists >2 wk.
- □ Instruct patient to contact health care professional immediately if dizziness, fainting, or fast or irregular heartbeat occurs, or if symptoms persist.

EVALUATION

Effectiveness of therapy can be demonstrated by: ▪ Decrease in allergic symptoms.

ATENOLOL

(a-**ten**-oh-lole)

{Apo-Atenolol}, {Novo-Atenolol}, Tenormin

CLASSIFICATION(S):

Antianginal, Antihypertensive agent, Beta-adrenergic blocking agent (selective)

Pregnancy Category D

INDICATIONS

▪ Management of hypertension ▪ Management of angina pectoris ▪ Prevention of myocardial infarction.

ACTION

▪ Blocks stimulation of $beta_1$ (myocardial) -adrenergic receptors. Does not usually affect $beta_2$ (pulmonary, vascular, uterine) -receptor sites. **Therapeutic Effects:** ▪ Decreased blood pressure and heart rate ▪ Decreased frequency of attacks of angina pectoris ▪ Prevention of myocardial infarction.

PHARMACOKINETICS

Absorption: 50–60% absorbed following oral administration.

Distribution: Minimal penetration of CNS. Crosses the placenta and enters breast milk.

Metabolism and Excretion: 40–50% excreted unchanged by the kidneys; remainder excreted in feces as unabsorbed drug.

Half-life: 6–9 hr.

CONTRAINDICATIONS AND PRECAUTIONS

Contraindicated in: ▪ Uncompensated congestive heart failure ▪ Pulmonary edema ▪ Cardiogenic shock ▪ Bradycardia or heart block.

Use Cautiously in: ▪ Renal impairment (dosage reduction recommended if CCr ≤35 ml/min) ▪ Hepatic impairment ▪ Geriatric patients (increased sensitivity to beta-adrenergic blockers; initial dosage reduction recommended) ▪ Pulmonary disease (including asthma; $beta_1$ selectivity may be lost at higher doses) ▪ Diabetes mellitus (may mask signs of hypoglycemia) ▪ Thyrotoxicosis (may mask symptoms) ▪ Patients with a history of severe allergic reactions (intensity of reactions may be increased) ▪ Pregnancy, lactation, or children (safety not established; all agents cross the placenta and may cause fetal/neonatal bradycardia, hypotension, hypoglycemia, or respiratory depression).

ADVERSE REACTIONS AND SIDE EFFECTS*

CNS: <u>fatigue</u>, <u>weakness</u>, anxiety, depression, dizziness, drowsiness, insomnia, memory loss, mental status changes, nervousness, nightmares.

EENT: blurred vision, stuffy nose.

Resp: bronchospasm, wheezing.

CV: BRADYCARDIA, CONGESTIVE HEART FAILURE, PULMONARY EDEMA, hypotension, peripheral vasoconstriction.

GI: constipation, diarrhea, liver function abnormalities, nausea, vomiting.

GU: <u>impotence</u>, decreased libido, urinary frequency.

{} = Available in Canada only.

***CAPITALS indicate life-threatening; <u>underlines</u> indicate most frequent.**

Derm: rashes.
Endo: hyperglycemia, hypoglycemia.
MS: arthralgia, back pain, joint pain.

INTERACTIONS

Drug-Drug: ▪ **General anesthesia, IV phenytoin, mibefradil,** and **verapamil** may cause additive myocardial depression ▪ Additive bradycardia may occur with **digitalis glycosides** ▪ Additive hypotension may occur with other **antihypertensives,** acute ingestion of **alcohol,** or **nitrates** ▪ Concurrent use with **amphetamines, cocaine, ephedrine, epinephrine, norepinephrine, phenylephrine,** or **pseudoephedrine** may result in unopposed alpha-adrenergic stimulation (excessive hypertension, bradycardia) ▪ Concurrent **thyroid** administration may decrease effectiveness ▪ May alter the effectiveness of **insulin** or **oral hypoglycemic agents** (dosage adjustments may be necessary) ▪ May decrease the effectiveness of **theophylline** ▪ May decrease the beneficial $beta_1$-cardiovascular effects of **dopamine** or **dobutamine** ▪ Use cautiously within 14 days of **MAO inhibitor** therapy (may result in hypertension).

ROUTE AND DOSAGE

- **PO (Adults):** *Antianginal*—50 mg once daily; may be increased after 1 wk to 100 mg/day (up to 200 mg/day). *Antihypertensive*—25–50 mg once daily; may be increased after 2 wk to 50–100 mg once daily. *Myocardial infarction*—50 mg (given 10 min following last IV dose), then 50 mg 12 hr later, then 100 mg/day as a single dose or in 2 divided doses for 6–9 days or until hospital discharge.
- **IV (Adults):** *Myocardial infarction*—5 mg, followed by another 5 mg after 10 min; after 10 more min follow with oral dosing.

AVAILABILITY

▪ ***Tablets:*** 25 mg[Rx], 50 mg[Rx], 100 mg[Rx] ▪ ***Injection:*** 500 mcg (0.5 mg)/ml[Rx] ▪ ***In combination with:*** chlorthalidone (Tenoretic)[Rx]. See Appendix A.

TIME/ACTION PROFILE (cardiovascular effects)

	ONSET	PEAK	DURATION
PO	1 hr	2–4 hr	24 hr
IV	rapid	5 min	UK

NURSING IMPLICATIONS

ASSESSMENT

- ▫ Monitor blood pressure, ECG, and pulse frequently during dosage adjustment period and periodically throughout therapy.
- ▫ Monitor intake and output ratios and daily weights. Assess routinely for congestive heart failure (dyspnea, rales/crackles, weight gain, peripheral edema, jugular venous distention).
- ▪ **Angina:** Assess frequency and characteristics of angina periodically throughout therapy.
- ▪ ***Lab Test Considerations:*** May cause increased BUN, serum lipoprotein, potassium, triglyceride, and uric acid levels.
- ▫ May cause increased ANA titers.
- ▫ May cause increase in blood glucose levels.
- ▪ ***Toxicity and Overdose:*** Monitor patients receiving beta-adrenergic blocking agents for signs of overdose (bradycardia, severe dizziness or fainting, severe drowsiness, dyspnea, bluish fingernails or palms, seizures). Notify physician immediately if these signs occur.

POTENTIAL NURSING DIAGNOSES

- ▪ Cardiac output, decreased (Side Effects).
- ▪ Knowledge deficit, related to medication regimen (Patient/Family Teaching).
- ▪ Noncompliance, related to medication regimen (Patient/Family Teaching).

IMPLEMENTATION

- ▪ **PO:** Take apical pulse prior to administering drug. If <50 bpm or if arrhythmia occurs, withhold medication and notify physician or other health care professional.
- ▪ **Direct IV:** IV therapy for acute myocardial infarction should be initiated as soon as possible after patient arrives at the hospital.
- ▫ May be diluted in D5W, 0.9% NaCl, or D5/0.9% NaCl. Stable for 48 hr.
- ▪ ***Rate:*** Administer 5 mg over 5 min, followed by another 5 mg 10 min later.
- ▪ **Y-Site Compatibility:** ▪ meperidine ▪ morphine.

PATIENT/FAMILY TEACHING

- ▪ **General Info:** Instruct patient to take atenolol as directed at the same time each day, even if feeling well; do not skip or double up on missed doses. If a dose is missed, it should be taken as soon as possible up to 8 hr before next dose. Abrupt withdrawal may cause life-threatening arrhythmias, hypertension, or myocardial ischemia.

- Advise patient to make sure enough medication is available for weekends, holidays, and vacations. A written prescription may be kept in wallet in case of emergency.
- Teach patient and family how to check pulse and blood pressure. Instruct them to check pulse daily and blood pressure biweekly and to report significant changes.
- May cause drowsiness or dizziness. Caution patients to avoid driving or other activities that require alertness until response to the drug is known.
- Advise patients to change positions slowly to minimize orthostatic hypotension.
- Caution patient that atenolol may increase sensitivity to cold.
- Instruct patient to consult health care professional before taking any OTC medications, especially cold preparations, concurrently with this medication.
- Diabetics should closely monitor blood sugar, especially if weakness, malaise, irritability, or fatigue occurs. Medication does not block sweating as a sign of hypoglycemia.
- Advise patient to notify health care professional if slow pulse, difficulty breathing, wheezing, cold hands and feet, dizziness, lightheadedness, confusion, depression, rash, fever, sore throat, unusual bleeding, or bruising occurs.
- Instruct patient to inform health care professional of medication regimen prior to treatment or surgery.
- Advise patient to carry identification describing disease process and medication regimen at all times.
- **Hypertension:** Reinforce the need to continue additional therapies for hypertension (weight loss, sodium restriction, stress reduction, regular exercise, moderation of alcohol consumption, and smoking cessation). Medication controls but does not cure hypertension.

EVALUATION

Effectiveness of therapy can be demonstrated by: ▪ Decrease in blood pressure ▪ Reduction in frequency of angina ▫ Increase in activity tolerance ▪ Prevention of myocardial infarction.

ATOVAQUONE

(a-**toe**-va-kwone)

Mepron

CLASSIFICATION(S):

Antiprotozoal

Pregnancy Category C

INDICATIONS

▪ Treatment of mild to moderate *Pneumocystis carinii* pneumonia (PCP) in patients who are unable to tolerate trimethoprim/sulfamethoxazole.

ACTION

▪ Inhibits the action of enzymes necessary to nucleic acid and ATP synthesis in protozoa. **Therapeutic Effects:** ▪ Antiprotozoal action against *Pneumocystis carinii*.

PHARMACOKINETICS

Absorption: Absorption is poor but is increased by food, particularly fat.

Distribution: Enters CSF in very low concentrations (less than 1% of plasma levels).

Metabolism and Excretion: Undergoes enterohepatic recycling; elimination occurs in feces.

Half-life: 2.2–2.9 days.

CONTRAINDICATIONS AND PRECAUTIONS

Contraindicated in: ▪ Hypersensitivity.

Use Cautiously in: ▪ Decreased hepatic, renal, or cardiac function (dosage modification may be necessary) ▪ GI disorders (absorption may be limited) ▪ Pregnancy, lactation, or children (safety not established).

ADVERSE REACTIONS AND SIDE EFFECTS*

CNS: headache, insomnia.

Resp: cough.

GI: diarrhea, nausea, vomiting.

Derm: rash.

Misc: fever.

*CAPITALS indicate life-threatening; underlines indicate most frequent.

INTERACTIONS

Drug-Drug: ▪ May interact with **drugs that are highly bound to plasma proteins** (does not appear to interact with phenytoin).
Drug-Food: ▪ **Food** enhances absorption.

ROUTE AND DOSAGE

▪ **PO (Adults):** 750 mg twice daily for 21 days.

AVAILABILITY

▪ ***Suspension:*** 750 mg/5 ml[Rx].

TIME/ACTION PROFILE (blood levels)

	ONSET	PEAK	DURATION
PO	UK	1–8 hr; 24–96 hr*	12 hr

*Two peaks are due to enterohepatic recycling.

NURSING IMPLICATIONS

ASSESSMENT

□ Assess patient for signs of *Pneumocystis carinii* pneumonia (vital signs, lung sounds, sputum, WBC) at beginning of and throughout therapy.
□ Obtain specimens prior to initiating therapy. First dose may be given before receiving results.
▪ ***Lab Test Considerations:*** Monitor hematologic and hepatic functions. May cause mild, transient anemia and neutropenia. May also cause elevated serum amylase, AST, ALT, and alkaline phosphatase.
□ Monitor electrolytes. May cause hyponatremia.

POTENTIAL NURSING DIAGNOSES

▪ Infection, risk for (Indications, Side Effects).
▪ Knowledge deficit, related to medication regimen (Patient/Family Teaching).

IMPLEMENTATION

▪ **PO:** Administer with food twice daily for 21 days.

PATIENT/FAMILY TEACHING

□ Instruct patient to take atovaquone exactly as directed around the clock for the full course of therapy, even if feeling better. Emphasize the importance of taking atovaquone with food, especially foods high in fat; taking without food may decrease plasma concentrations and effectiveness.
□ Advise patient to notify health care professional if rash occurs.

EVALUATION

Clinical response to therapy can be evaluated by: ▪ Resolution of the signs and symptoms of *Pneumocystis carinii* pneumonia.

ATROPINE

(**at**-ro-peen)
Atro-Pen

CLASSIFICATION(S):
Antiarrhythmic, Anticholinergic (antimuscarinic)

Pregnancy Category C

INDICATIONS

▪ **IM:** Given preoperatively to decrease oral and respiratory secretions ▪ **IV:** Treatment of sinus bradycardia and heart block ▪ **PO:** Adjunctive therapy in the management of peptic ulcer and irritable bowel syndrome ▪ **IV:** Reversal of adverse muscarinic effects of anticholinesterase agents (neostigmine, physostigmine, or pyridostigmine) ▪ **IM, IV:** Treatment of anticholinesterase (organophosphate pesticide) poisoning.

ACTION

▪ Inhibits the action of acetylcholine at postganglionic sites located in: □ Smooth muscle □ Secretory glands □ CNS (antimuscarinic activity) ▪ Low doses decrease: □ Sweating □ Salivation □ Respiratory secretions ▪ Intermediate doses result in: □ Mydriasis (pupillary dilation) □ Cycloplegia (loss of visual accommodation) □ Increased heart rate ▪ GI and GU tract motility are decreased at larger doses. **Therapeutic Effects:** ▪ Increased heart rate ▪ Decreased GI and respiratory secretions ▪ Reversal of muscarinic effects ▪ May have a spasmolytic action on the biliary and genitourinary tracts.

PHARMACOKINETICS

Absorption: Well absorbed following oral, SC, or IM administration.
Distribution: Readily crosses the blood-brain

barrier. Crosses the placenta and enters breast milk.
Metabolism and Excretion: Mostly metabolized by the liver; 30–50% excreted unchanged by the kidneys.
Half-life: 13–38 hr.

CONTRAINDICATIONS AND PRECAUTIONS

Contraindicated in: ▪ Hypersensitivity ▪ Narrow-angle glaucoma ▪ Acute hemorrhage ▪ Tachycardia secondary to cardiac insufficiency or thyrotoxicosis.
Use Cautiously in: ▪ Elderly and the very young (increased susceptibility to adverse reactions) ▪ Intra-abdominal infections ▪ Prostatic hypertrophy ▪ Chronic renal, hepatic, pulmonary, or cardiac disease ▪ Pregnancy and lactation (safety not established; IV administration may produce fetal tachycardia).

ADVERSE REACTIONS AND SIDE EFFECTS*

CNS: drowsiness, confusion.
EENT: blurred vision, cycloplegia, dry eyes, mydriasis.
CV: tachycardia, palpitations.
GI: dry mouth, constipation.
GU: urinary hesitancy, retention.
Misc: decreased sweating.

INTERACTIONS

Drug-Drug: ▪ Additive anticholinergic effects with other **anticholinergic compounds**, including **antihistamines, tricyclic antidepressants, quinidine,** and **disopyramide** ▪ Anticholinergics may alter the absorption of other **orally administered drugs** by slowing motility of the GI tract ▪ **Antacids** decrease the absorption of anticholinergics ▪ May increase GI mucosal lesions in patients taking **oral potassium chloride tablets.**

ROUTE AND DOSAGE

❑ Preanesthesia (To Decrease Saliva-tion/Secretions)

- **PO (Adults):** 2 mg.
- **IM, IV, SC (Adults):** 0.2–0.6 mg 30–60 min preop.
- **IM, SC (Children ≥20 kg):** 0.4 mg (range 0.2–1 mg) 30–60 min preop.
- **IM, SC (Children 12–16 kg):** 0.3 mg 30–60 min preop.
- **IM, SC (Children 7–9 kg):** 0.2 mg 30–60 min preop.
- **IM, SC (Children <3 kg):** 0.1 mg 30–60 min preop.

❑ Bradycardia

- **IV (Adults):** 0.5–1.0 mg; may repeat as needed q 5 min or 0.4–1 mg q 1–2 hr to a total of 3 mg or 0.04 mg/kg (total vagolytic dose).
- **IV (Children):** 0.02 mg/kg (range is 0.1–0.5 mg in children or up to 1 mg in adolescents); may repeat q 5 min up to a total dose of 1 mg in children (2 mg in adolescents).

❑ Reversal of Adverse Muscarinic Effects of Anticholinesterases

- **IV (Adults):** 0.6–1.2 mg for each 0.5–2.5 mg of neostigmine methylsulfate or 10–20 mg of pyridostigmine bromide concurrently with anticholinesterase.

❑ Organophosphate Poisoning

- **IM, IV (Adults):** 1–2 mg initially, then 2 mg q 5–60 min as needed. *Severe cases*—2–6 mg initially and repeated every 5–60 min as needed. May be followed by oral therapy. Pralidoxime may be given concurrently.
- **IM, IV (Children):** 0.05 mg/kg q 10–30 min as needed. Pralidoxime may be given concurrently.

❑ Anticholinergic Effects

- **PO (Adults):** 400 mcg (0.4 mg)–600 mcg (0.6 mg) q 4–6 hr.
- **PO (Children):** 0.01 mg/kg (not to exceed 0.4 mg or 0.3 mg/m²/dose) q 4–6 hr.

AVAILABILITY

▪ ***Tablets:*** 0.4 mg Rx ▪ ***In combination with:*** phenobarbital oral solution (Antrocol) Rx. See Appendix A ▪ ***Injection:*** 0.05 mg/ml Rx, 0.1 mg/ml Rx, 0.3 mg/ml Rx, 0.4 mg/ml Rx, 0.5 mg/ml Rx, 0.8 mg/ml Rx, 1 mg/ml Rx, 2 mg/0.7 ml Auto-injector Rx ▪ ***In combination with:*** meperidine Rx, neostigmine Rx.

*CAPITALS indicate life-threatening; underlines indicate most frequent.

TIME/ACTION PROFILE (inhibition of salivation)

	ONSET	PEAK	DURATION
PO	30 min	30–60 min	4–6 hr
IM, SC	rapid	15–50 min	4–6 hr
IV	immediate	2–4 min	4–6 hr

NURSING IMPLICATIONS

ASSESSMENT

- □ Assess vital signs and ECG tracings frequently during IV drug therapy. Report any significant changes in heart rate or blood pressure, or increased ventricular ectopy or angina to physician promptly.
- □ Monitor intake and output ratios in elderly or surgical patients because atropine may cause urinary retention.
- □ Assess patients routinely for abdominal distention and auscultate for bowel sounds. If constipation becomes a problem, increasing fluids and adding bulk to the diet may help alleviate constipation.
- ▪ ***Toxicity and Overdose:*** If overdose occurs, physostigmine is the antidote.

POTENTIAL NURSING DIAGNOSES

- ▪ Cardiac output, decreased (Indications).
- ▪ Oral mucous membrane, altered (Side Effects).
- ▪ Constipation (Side Effects).

IMPLEMENTATION

- ▪ **PO:** Oral doses of atropine are usually given 30 min before meals.
- ▪ **IM:** Intense flushing of the face and trunk may occur 15–20 min following IM administration. In children, this response is called "atropine flush" and is not harmful.
- ▪ **Direct IV:** Give IV undiluted or dilute in 10 ml of sterile water.
- ▪ ***Rate:*** Administer at a rate of 0.6 mg over 1 min. Do not add to IV solution. Inject through Y-tubing or 3-way stopcock. When given IV in doses less than 0.4 mg or over more than 1 min, atropine may cause paradoxical bradycardia, which usually resolves in approximately 2 min.
- ▪ **Syringe Compatibility:** ▪ benzquinamide ▪ butorphanol ▪ chlorpromazine ▪ cimetidine ▪ dimenhydrinate ▪ diphenhydramine ▪ droperidol ▪ fentanyl ▪ glycopyrrolate ▪ heparin ▪ hydromorphone ▪ hydroxyzine ▪ meperidine ▪ metoclopramide ▪ midazolam ▪ milrinone ▪ morphine ▪ nalbuphine ▪ pentazocine ▪ perphenazine ▪ prochlorperazine ▪ promazine ▪ promethazine ▪ propiomazine ▪ ranitidine ▪ scopolamine ▪ sufentanil.
- ▪ **Y-Site Compatibility:** ▪ amrinone ▪ famotidine ▪ heparin ▪ hydrocortisone sodium succinate ▪ nafcillin ▪ potassium chloride ▪ sufentanil ▪ vitamin B complex with C.

PATIENT/FAMILY TEACHING

- □ Instruct patient to take exactly as directed. If a dose is missed, take as soon as remembered unless almost time for next dose. Do not double doses.
- □ May cause drowsiness. Caution patients to avoid driving or other activities requiring alertness until response to medication is known.
- □ Instruct patient that oral rinses, sugarless gum or candy, and frequent oral hygiene may help relieve dry mouth.
- □ Caution patients that atropine impairs heat regulation. Strenuous activity in a hot environment may cause heat stroke.
- □ Instruct patient to consult health care professional before taking any OTC medications concurrently with atropine.
- □ Inform male patients with benign prostatic hypertrophy that atropine may cause urinary hesitancy and retention. Changes in urinary stream should be reported to health care professional.

EVALUATION

Effectiveness of therapy can be demonstrated by: ▪ Increase in heart rate ▪ Dryness of mouth ▪ Reversal of muscarinic effects.

AZATADINE

(a-**za**-ta-deen)

Optimine

CLASSIFICATION(S):

Antihistamine

Pregnancy Category B

INDICATIONS

▪ Symptomatic relief of allergic symptoms (rhinitis, urticaria) caused by histamine release.

ACTION

▪ Antagonizes the effects of histamine at H_1-receptor sites; does not bind to or inactivate histamine. **Therapeutic Effects:** ▪ Decreased symptoms of histamine excess (sneezing, rhinorrhea, nasal and ocular pruritus, ocular tearing and redness).

PHARMACOKINETICS

Absorption: Well absorbed following oral administration.
Distribution: Probably crosses the placenta.
Metabolism and Excretion: Extensively metabolized by the liver; 20% excreted unchanged by the kidneys.
Half-life: 12 hr.

CONTRAINDICATIONS AND PRECAUTIONS

Contraindicated in: ▪ Hypersensitivity ▪ Acute attacks of asthma ▪ Lactation (avoid use).
Use Cautiously in: ▪ Narrow-angle glaucoma ▪ Liver disease ▪ Geriatric patients (more susceptible to adverse reactions) ▪ Hyperthyroidism ▪ Hypertension ▪ Pregnancy or children <12 yr (safety not established).

ADVERSE REACTIONS AND SIDE EFFECTS*

CNS: dizziness, sedation, excitation, headache, seizures.
EENT: tinnitus, blurred vision, nasal stuffiness.
Resp: thickened bronchial secretions, wheezing.
CV: hypertension, arrhythmias, chest tightness, hypotension, palpitations, tachycardia.
GI: epigastric distress, anorexia, constipation, diarrhea, dry mouth, vomiting.
GU: early menses, urinary hesitancy, urinary retention.
Derm: sweating.
Hemat: AGRANULOCYTOSIS, anemia, thrombocytopenia.

INTERACTIONS

Drug-Drug: ▪ Additive CNS depression with other **CNS depressants** including **alcohol, opioid analgesics,** and **sedative/hypnotics** ▪ **MAO inhibitors** intensify and prolong the anticholinergic effects of antihistamines.

ROUTE AND DOSAGE

▪ **PO (Adults and Children >12 yr):** 1–2 mg q 8–12 hr as needed.
▪ **PO (Children >12 yr):** 0.5–1 mg twice daily as needed.

AVAILABILITY

▪ ***Tablets:*** 1 mg[Rx] ▪ ***In combination with:*** pseudoephedrine (Trinalin)[Rx]. See Appendix A.

TIME/ACTION PROFILE (antihistaminic effects)

	ONSET	PEAK	DURATION
PO	15–60 min	4 hr	12 hr

NURSING IMPLICATIONS

ASSESSMENT

- Assess allergy symptoms (rhinitis, conjunctivitis, hives) prior to and periodically throughout therapy.
- Assess lung sounds and character of bronchial secretions. Maintain fluid intake of 1500–2000 ml/day to decrease viscosity of secretions.
- ***Lab Test Considerations:*** May cause false-negative allergy skin testing. Discontinue antihistamines at least 72 hr before testing.

POTENTIAL NURSING DIAGNOSES

- Airway clearance, ineffective (Indications).
- Injury, risk for (Adverse Reactions).
- Knowledge deficit, related to medication regimen (Patient/Family Teaching).

IMPLEMENTATION

- **PO:** Administer oral doses with food or milk to decrease GI irritation.

PATIENT/FAMILY TEACHING

- Instruct patient to take azatadine exactly as directed.
- May cause drowsiness. Caution patient to avoid driving or other activities requiring alertness until effects of the medication are known.
- Advise patient to avoid taking alcohol or other CNS depressants concurrently with this drug.
- Advise patient that good oral hygiene, frequent rinsing of mouth, and sugarless gum or candy

*CAPITALS indicate life-threatening; underlines indicate most frequent.

A

may help relieve dry mouth. Patient should notify dentist if dry mouth persists >2 wk.

- Elderly patients are at risk for orthostatic hypotension. Advise patient to make position changes slowly.
- Instruct patient to contact health care professional if symptoms persist.

EVALUATION

Effectiveness of therapy can be demonstrated by: ▪ Decrease in allergic symptoms.

AZATHIOPRINE

(ay-za-**thye**-oh-preen)
Imuran

CLASSIFICATION(S):
Immunosuppressant
Pregnancy Category D

INDICATIONS

▪ Prevention of renal transplant rejection (with corticosteroids, local radiation, or other cytotoxic agents) ▪ Treatment of severe, active, erosive rheumatoid arthritis unresponsive to more conventional therapy. **Unlabeled Uses:** ▪ Management of Crohn's disease.

ACTION

▪ Antagonizes purine metabolism with subsequent inhibition of DNA and RNA synthesis. **Therapeutic Effects:** ▪ Suppression of cell-mediated immunity and altered antibody formation.

PHARMACOKINETICS

Absorption: Readily absorbed following oral administration.
Distribution: Crosses the placenta. Enters breast milk in low concentrations.
Metabolism and Excretion: Metabolized to mercaptopurine, which is further metabolized. Minimal renal excretion of unchanged drug.
Half-life: 3 hr.

CONTRAINDICATIONS AND PRECAUTIONS

Contraindicated in: ▪ Hypersensitivity ▪ Concurrent use of mycophenolate ▪ Pregnancy or lactation.
Use Cautiously in: ▪ Infections ▪ Malignancies ▪ Decreased bone marrow reserve ▪ Previous or concurrent radiation therapy ▪ Other chronic debilitating illnesses ▪ Patients with childbearing potential.

ADVERSE REACTIONS AND SIDE EFFECTS*

EENT: retinopathy.
Resp: pulmonary edema.
GI: anorexia, hepatotoxicity, nausea, vomiting, diarrhea, mucositis, pancreatitis.
Derm: alopecia, rash.
Hemat: anemia, leukopenia, pancytopenia, thrombocytopenia.
MS: arthralgia.
Misc: SERUM SICKNESS, chills, fever, Raynaud's phenomenon, retinopathy.

INTERACTIONS

Drug-Drug: ▪ Additive myelosuppression with **antineoplastics, cyclosporine,** and **myelosuppressive agents** ▪ **Allopurinol** inhibits the metabolism of azathioprine, increasing toxicity. Dosage of azathioprine should be decreased by 25–33% with concurrent allopurinol ▪ May decrease antibody response to **live virus vaccines** and increase the risk of adverse reactions.

ROUTE AND DOSAGE

Renal Allograft Rejection Prevention

- **PO, IV (Adults and Children):** 3–5 mg/kg/day initially; maintenance dose 1–3 mg/kg/day.

Rheumatoid Arthritis

- **PO (Adults and Children):** 1 mg/kg/day for 6–8 wk, increase by 0.5 mg/kg/day q 4 wk until response or up to 2.5 mg/kg/day, then decrease by 0.5 mg/kg/day q 4–8 wk to minimal effective dose.

AVAILABILITY

▪ ***Tablets:*** 50 mg[Rx] ▪ ***Injection:*** 100-mg vial[Rx].

TIME/ACTION PROFILE

	ONSET	PEAK	DURATION
PO (anti-inflammatory)	6–8 wk	12 wk	UK
IV (immunosuppression)	days–wks	UK	days–wks

*CAPITALS indicate life-threatening; underlines indicate most frequent.

NURSING IMPLICATIONS

ASSESSMENT

- **General Info:** Assess for infection (vital signs, sputum, urine, stool, WBC) throughout therapy.
- Monitor intake and output and daily weight. Decreased urine output may lead to toxicity with this medication.
- **Rheumatoid Arthritis:** Assess range of motion; degree of swelling, pain, and strength in affected joints; and ability to perform activities of daily living prior to and periodically throughout therapy.
- ***Lab Test Considerations:*** Monitor renal, hepatic, and hematologic functions prior to beginning therapy, weekly during the 1st mo, bimonthly for the next 2–3 mo, and monthly thereafter.
- Notify physician if leukocyte count is <3000 or platelet count is <100,000/mm^3; may necessitate a reduction in dosage or temporary discontinuation of therapy.
- A decrease in hemoglobin may indicate bone marrow suppression.
- Hepatotoxicity may be manifested by increased alkaline phosphatase, bilirubin, AST, ALT, and amylase concentrations. Usually occurs within 6 mo of transplant, rarely with rheumatoid arthritis, and is reversible upon discontinuation of azathioprine.
- May decrease serum and urine uric acid and plasma albumin.

POTENTIAL NURSING DIAGNOSES

- Infection, risk for (Indications).
- Knowledge deficit, related to medication regimen (Patient/Family Teaching).

IMPLEMENTATION

- **General Info:** Protect transplant patients from staff and visitors who may carry infection. Maintain protective isolation as indicated.
- **PO:** May be administered with or after meals or in divided dose to minimize nausea.
- **IV:** Reconstitute 100 mg with 10 ml of sterile water for injection. Swirl vial gently until completely dissolved. Reconstituted solution may be administered up to 24 hr after preparation.
- Solution should be prepared in a biologic cabinet. Wear gloves, gown, and mask while handling medication. Discard equipment in specially designated containers (see Appendix I).
- **Intermittent Infusion:** Solution may be further diluted in 50 ml of 0.9% NaCl, 0.45% NaCl, or D5W. Do not admix.
- ***Rate:*** Usually infused over 30–60 min; may range from 5 min–8 hr.

PATIENT/FAMILY TEACHING

- **General Info:** Instruct patient to take azathioprine exactly as directed. If a dose is missed on a once-daily regimen, omit dose; if on several-times-a-day dosing, take as soon as possible or double next dose. Consult health care professional if more than 1 dose is missed or if vomiting occurs shortly after dose is taken. Do not discontinue without consulting health care professional.
- Advise patient to report unusual tiredness or weakness; cough or hoarseness; fever or chills; lower back or side pain; painful or difficult urination; severe diarrhea; black, tarry stools; blood in urine; or transplant rejection to health care professional immediately.
- Reinforce the need for lifelong therapy to prevent transplant rejection.
- Instruct the patient to consult health care professional before taking any OTC medications or receiving any vaccinations while taking this medication.
- Advise patient to avoid contact with persons with contagious diseases and persons who have recently taken oral poliovirus vaccine.
- This drug may have teratogenic properties. Advise patient to use contraception during and for at least 4 mo after therapy is completed.
- Emphasize the importance of follow-up exams and lab tests.
- **Rheumatoid Arthritis:** Concurrent therapy with salicylates, NSAIDs, or glucocorticoids may be necessary. Patient should continue physical therapy and adequate rest. Explain that joint damage will not be reversed; goal is to slow or stop disease process.

EVALUATION

Effectiveness of therapy can be demonstrated by: ▪ Prevention of transplant rejection ▪ Decreased stiffness, pain, and swelling in affected joints in 6–8 wk in rheumatoid arthritis. Therapy is discontinued if no improvement in 12 wk.

A

AZITHROMYCIN
(aye-**zith**-row-my-sin)
Zithromax

CLASSIFICATION(S):
Anti-infective (macrolide)

Pregnancy Category B

INDICATIONS

▪ Treatment of the following infections due to susceptible organisms: ▫ Upper respiratory tract infections, including streptococcal pharyngitis and tonsillitis ▫ Lower respiratory tract infections, including bronchitis and pneumonia ▫ Skin and skin structure infections ▫ Nongonococcal urethritis, cervicitis, gonorrhea, and chancroid ▪ Prevention of disseminated *Mycobacterium avium* complex (MAC) infection in patients with advanced HIV infection. **Unlabeled Uses:** ▪ Prevention of bacterial endocarditis.

ACTION

▪ Inhibits protein synthesis at the level of the 50S bacterial ribosome. **Therapeutic Effects:** ▪ Bacteriostatic action against susceptible bacteria. **Spectrum:** ▪ Active against the following gram-positive aerobic bacteria: ▫ *Staphylococcus aureus* ▫ *Streptococcus pneumoniae* ▫ *Streptococcus pyogenes* (group A strep) ▪ Active against these gram-negative aerobic bacteria: ▫ *Haemophilus influenzae* ▫ *Moraxella catarrhalis* ▫ *Neisseria gonorrhoeae* ▪ Also active against: ▫ *Mycoplasma* ▫ *Legionella* ▫ *Chlamydia trachomatis* ▫ *Ureaplasma urealyticum* ▫ *Borrelia burgdorferi* ▫ *Mycobacterium avium* ▪ Not active against methicillin-resistant *Staphylococcus aureus*.

PHARMACOKINETICS

Absorption: Rapidly absorbed (40%) following oral administration. IV administration results in complete bioavailability.
Distribution: Widely distributed to body tissues and fluids. Intracellular and tissue levels exceed those in serum; low CSF levels.
Metabolism and Excretion: Mostly excreted unchanged in bile; 4.5% excreted unchanged in urine.
Half-life: 11–14 hr after single dose; 68 hr after several doses.

CONTRAINDICATIONS AND PRECAUTIONS

Contraindicated in: ▪ Hypersensitivity to azithromycin, erythromycin, or other macrolide anti-infectives.
Use Cautiously in: ▪ Severe liver impairment (dosage adjustment may be required) ▪ Pregnancy, lactation, and children <2 yr (safety not established).

ADVERSE REACTIONS AND SIDE EFFECTS*

CNS: dizziness, drowsiness, fatigue, headache.
CV: chest pain, palpitations.
GI: abdominal pain, diarrhea, nausea, cholestatic jaundice, dyspepsia, flatulence, melena.
GU: nephritis, vaginitis.
Derm: photosensitivity, rashes.
Endo: hyperglycemia.
F and E: hyperkalemia.
Misc: ANGIOEDEMA.

INTERACTIONS

Drug-Drug: ▪ **Aluminum-** and **magnesium-containing antacids** decrease peak serum levels of azithromycin ▪ May increase serum levels and the risk of toxicity from **pimozide** or **carbamazepine** ▪ May increase the effect of **warfarin.**
Drug-Food: ▪ **Food** decreases absorption.

ROUTE AND DOSAGE

▫ Most Respiratory and Skin Infections

- **PO (Adults):** 500 mg on 1st day, then 250 mg/day for 4 more days (total dose of 1.5 g).
- **PO (Children 2–15 yr):** 10 mg/kg (not >500 mg/dose) on 1st day, then 5 mg/kg (not >250 mg/dose) for 4 more days.

▫ Community-Acquired Pneumonia

- **IV, PO (Adults):** 500 mg IV q 24 hr for at least 2 doses, then 500 mg PO q 24 hr for a total of 7–10 days.

▫ Pelvic Inflammatory Disease

- **IV, PO (Adults):** 500 mg IV q 24 hr for 1–2 days, then 250 mg PO q 24 hr for a total of 7 days.

***CAPITALS indicate life-threatening; underlines indicate most frequent.**

❑ **Endocarditis Prophylaxis**

- **PO (Adults):** 500 mg 1 hr before procedure.
- **PO (Children):** 15 mg/kg 1 hr before procedure.

❑ **Nongonococcal Urethritis, Cervicitis, Chancroid, Chlamydia**

- **PO (Adults):** Single 1-g dose.

❑ **Gonorrhea**

- **PO (Adults):** Single 2-g dose.

❑ **Prevention of Disseminated MAC Infection**

- **PO (Adults):** 1.2 g once weekly (alone or with rifabutin).

AVAILABILITY

▪ ***Capsules:*** 250 mg[Rx] ▪ ***Tablets:*** 250 mg[Rx], 600 mg[Rx] ▪ ***Powder for oral suspension:*** 1 g/pkt[Rx] ▪ ***Oral suspension:*** 100 mg/5 ml in 15-ml bottles[Rx], 200 mg/5 ml in 15- and 22.5-ml bottles[Rx].

TIME/ACTION PROFILE (serum levels)

	ONSET	PEAK	DURATION
PO	rapid	2.5–3.2 hr	24 hr
IV	rapid	end of infusion	24 hr

NURSING IMPLICATIONS

ASSESSMENT

- ❑ Assess patient for infection (vital signs; appearance of wound, sputum, urine, and stool; WBC) at beginning of and throughout therapy.
- ❑ Obtain specimens for culture and sensitivity prior to initiating therapy. First dose may be given before receiving results.
- ▪ ***Lab Test Considerations:*** May cause increased serum bilirubin, AST, ALT, LDH, and alkaline phosphatase concentrations.
- ❑ May cause elevated creatine phosphokinase, potassium, prothrombin time, BUN, serum creatinine, and blood glucose concentrations.
- ❑ May occasionally cause decreased WBC and platelet count.

POTENTIAL NURSING DIAGNOSES

- Infection, risk for (Indications, Side Effects).
- Knowledge deficit, related to medication regimen (Patient/Family Teaching).
- Noncompliance, related to medication regimen (Patient/Family Teaching).

IMPLEMENTATION

- **PO:** Administer 1 hr before or 2 hr after meals.
- **Intermittent Infusion:** Reconstitute by adding 4.8 ml of sterile water for injection to the 500-mg vial and shake until dissolved, for a concentration of 100 mg/ml. Do not administer solution containing particulate matter. Dilute further by transferring 5 ml of the 100 mg/ml solution to 250 ml or 500 ml of 0.9% NaCl, 0.45% NaCl, D5W, LR, D5/0.45% NaCl, or D5/LR for a concentration of 2 mg/ml or 1 mg/ml, respectively. Solution is stable for 24 hr at room temperature or for 7 days if refrigerated.
- ***Rate:*** Administer the 1 mg/ml solution over 3 hr or the 2 mg/ml solution over 1 hr. Do not administer as a bolus.

PATIENT/FAMILY TEACHING

- ❑ Instruct patients to take medication as directed and to finish the drug completely, even if they are feeling better. Missed doses should be taken as soon as possible unless almost time for next dose; do not double doses. Advise patients that sharing of this medication may be dangerous.
- ❑ Instruct patient not to take azithromycin with food or antacids.
- ❑ May cause drowsiness and dizziness. Caution patient to avoid driving or other activities requiring alertness until response to medication is known.
- ❑ Advise patient to use sunscreen and protective clothing to prevent photosensitivity reactions.
- ❑ Advise patient to report the signs of superinfection (black, furry overgrowth on the tongue; vaginal itching or discharge; loose or foul-smelling stools).
- ❑ Instruct patient to notify health care professional if fever and diarrhea develop, especially if stool contains blood, pus, or mucus.
- ❑ Advise patient to notify health care professional if pregnancy is planned or suspected.
- ❑ Advise patients being treated for nongonococcal urethritis or cervicitis that sexual partners should also be treated.
- ❑ Instruct patient to notify health care professional if symptoms do not improve.

EVALUATION

Clinical response to therapy can be evaluated by: ▪ Resolution of the signs and symptoms of infection. Length of time for complete resolution depends on the organism and site of infection.

AZTREONAM

(az-**tree**-oh-nam)

Azactam

CLASSIFICATION(S):

Anti-infective (monobactam)

Pregnancy Category B

INDICATIONS

▪ Treatment of serious gram-negative infections including: ▫ Bone and joint infections ▫ Septicemia ▫ Skin and skin structure infections ▫ Intra-abdominal infections ▫ Gynecologic infections ▫ Respiratory tract infections ▫ Urinary tract infections.

ACTION

▪ Binds to the bacterial cell wall membrane, causing cell death. **Therapeutic Effects:** ▪ Bactericidal action against susceptible bacteria. **Spectrum:** ▪ Displays significant activity against gram-negative aerobic organisms only: ▫ *Escherichia coli* ▫ *Serratia* ▫ *Klebsiella* ▫ *Enterobacter* ▫ *Shigella* ▫ *Providencia* ▫ *Salmonella* ▫ *Neisseria gonorrhoeae* ▫ *Haemophilus influenzae* ▪ Has good activity against *Pseudomonas aeruginosa*, including strains resistant to other drugs ▪ Not active against: ▫ *Staphylococcus aureus* ▫ *Enterococcus* ▫ *Bacteroides fragilis* ▫ Streptococci.

PHARMACOKINETICS

Absorption: Well absorbed following IM administration.

Distribution: Widely distributed. Crosses the placenta and enters breast milk in low concentrations.

Metabolism and Excretion: 65–75% excreted unchanged by the kidneys. Small amounts metabolized by the liver.

Half-life: 1.5–2.2 hr (increased in renal impairment).

CONTRAINDICATIONS AND PRECAUTIONS

Contraindicated in: ▪ Hypersensitivity ▪ Cross-sensitivity with penicillins or cephalosporins may occur rarely.

Use Cautiously in: ▪ Renal impairment (dosage reduction required if CCr <30 ml/min/1.73 m^2) ▪ Pregnancy, lactation, and young children (safety not established).

ADVERSE REACTIONS AND SIDE EFFECTS*

CNS: SEIZURES.

GI: altered taste (IV only), diarrhea, nausea, vomiting.

Derm: rashes.

Local: pain at IM site, phlebitis at IV site.

Misc: allergic reactions including ANAPHYLAXIS, superinfection.

INTERACTIONS

Drug-Drug: ▪ Serum levels may be increased by **furosemide** or **probenecid.**

ROUTE AND DOSAGE

- **IM, IV (Adults):** *Most infections*—0.5–2 g q 6–12 hr; *life-threatening infections*—2 g q 6–8 hr; *urinary tract infections*—0.5–1 g q 8–12 hr.
- **IM, IV (Children):** *Most infections*—30 mg/kg q 6–8 hr; *serious infections*—50 mg/kg q 4–6 hr.

AVAILABILITY

▪ ***Injection:*** 0.5-g[Rx], 1-g[Rx], 2-g vials and infusion bottles[Rx].

TIME/ACTION PROFILE (blood levels)

	ONSET	PEAK	DURATION
IM	rapid	60 min	6–8 hr
IV	rapid	end of infusion	6–8 hr

NURSING IMPLICATIONS

ASSESSMENT

- **General Info:** Assess patient for infection (vital signs; wound appearance, sputum, urine, and stool; WBC) at beginning of and throughout therapy.

▫ Obtain a history before initiating therapy to determine previous use of and reactions to

*CAPITALS indicate life-threatening; underlines indicate most frequent.

penicillins and cephalosporins. Patients allergic to these drugs may exhibit hypersensitivity reactions to aztreonam.

- Obtain specimens for culture and sensitivity prior to initiating therapy. First dose may be given before receiving results.
- ***Lab Test Considerations:*** May cause elevations in AST, ALT, alkaline phosphatase, LDH, and serum creatinine. May cause increased prothrombin and partial thromboplastin times, and positive Coombs' test.

POTENTIAL NURSING DIAGNOSES

- Infection, risk for (Indications).
- Knowledge deficit, related to medication regimen (Patient/Family Teaching).

IMPLEMENTATION

- **General Info:** After adding diluent to vial, shake immediately and vigorously. Not for multidose use; discard unused solution.
- **IM:** Use 15-ml vial and dilute each g of aztreonam with at least 3 ml of 0.9% NaCl, or sterile or bacteriostatic water for injection. Stable at room temperature for 48 hr or 7 days if refrigerated.
- Administer into large, well-developed muscle.
- **Direct IV:** For direct IV use, add 6–10 ml of sterile water for injection to each 15- or 30-ml vial.
- ***Rate:*** Administer slowly over 3–5 min by direct injection or into tubing of a compatible solution.
- **Intermittent Infusion:** Constitute the 100-ml vial with at least 50 ml/g and dilute further with 50–100 ml of 0.9% NaCl, Ringer's or lactated Ringer's solution, D5W, D10W, D5/0.9% NaCl, D5/0.45% NaCl, D5/0.25% NaCl, sodium lactate, 5% or 10% mannitol. Final concentration should not exceed 20 mg/ml. Solution is stable for 48 hr at room temperature and 7 days if refrigerated. Solutions range from colorless to light, straw yellow or may develop a pink tint upon standing; this does not affect potency.
- ***Rate:*** Infuse over 20–60 min.
- **Syringe Compatibility:** ▪ clindamycin.
- **Y-Site Compatibility:** ▪ amikacin ▪ aminophylline ▪ ampicillin ▪ ampicillin/sulbactam ▪ bleomycin ▪ bumetanide ▪ buprenorphine ▪ butorphanol ▪ calcium gluconate ▪ carboplatin ▪ carmustine ▪ cefazolin ▪ cefepime ▪ cefonicid ▪ cefoperazone ▪ cefotaxime ▪ cefotetan ▪ cefoxitin ▪ ceftazidime ▪ ceftizoxime ▪ ceftriaxone ▪ cimetidine ▪ ciprofloxacin ▪ cisplatin ▪ clindamycin ▪ cyclophosphamide ▪ cytarabine ▪ dacarbazine ▪ dactinomycin ▪ dexamethasone sodium phosphate ▪ diltiazem ▪ diphenhydramine ▪ dobutamine ▪ dopamine ▪ droperidol ▪ enalaprilat ▪ etoposide ▪ famotidine ▪ filgrastim ▪ floxuridine ▪ fluconazole ▪ fludarabine ▪ fluorouracil ▪ foscarnet ▪ furosemide ▪ gallium nitrate ▪ gentamicin ▪ haloperidol ▪ heparin ▪ hydrocortisone ▪ hydromorphone ▪ idarubicin ▪ ifosfamide ▪ imipenem/cilastatin ▪ regular insulin ▪ leucovorin ▪ magnesium sulfate ▪ mannitol ▪ mechlorethamine ▪ melphalan ▪ meperidine ▪ mesna ▪ methotrexate ▪ methylprednisolone sodium succinate ▪ metoclopramide ▪ mezlocillin ▪ morphine ▪ nalbuphine ▪ netilmicin ▪ ondansetron ▪ piperacillin ▪ piperacillin/tazobactam ▪ plicamycin ▪ potassium chloride ▪ promethazine ▪ ranitidine ▪ sargramostim ▪ sodium bicarbonate ▪ teniposide ▪ thiotepa ▪ ticarcillin ▪ ticarcillin/clavulanate ▪ tobramycin ▪ trimethoprim/sulfamethoxazole ▪ vinblastine ▪ vincristine ▪ vinorelbine ▪ zidovudine.
- **Y-Site Incompatibility:** ▪ acyclovir ▪ amphotericin B ▪ chlorpromazine ▪ daunorubicin ▪ ganciclovir ▪ lorazepam ▪ metronidazole ▪ miconazole ▪ mitomycin ▪ mitoxantrone ▪ prochlorperazine ▪ streptozocin.
- **Additive Compatibility:** ▪ ampicillin/sulbactam ▪ cefazolin ▪ ciprofloxacin ▪ clindamycin ▪ gentamicin ▪ tobramycin ▪ May be admixed with ampicillin in 0.9% NaCl; stable for 24 hr at room temperature and 48 hr if refrigerated.
- **Additive Incompatibility:** ▪ nafcillin ▪ metronidazole.

PATIENT/FAMILY TEACHING

- **General Info:** Advise patient to report the signs of superinfection (furry overgrowth on the tongue, vaginal itching or discharge, loose or foul-smelling stools) and allergy.
- **IV:** Warn patient that IV infusion may cause mild taste alteration.

EVALUATION

Effectiveness of therapy can be demonstrated by: ▪ Resolution of signs and symptoms of infection. Length of time for complete resolution depends on the organism and site of infection.

B

BACLOFEN
(**bak**-loe-fen)
Lioresal

CLASSIFICATION(S):
Skeletal muscle relaxant (centrally acting)

Pregnancy Category C

INDICATIONS

▪ **PO:** Treatment of reversible spasticity associated with multiple sclerosis or spinal cord lesions ▪ **IT:** Treatment of severe spasticity originating in the spinal cord. **Unlabeled Uses:** ▪ Management of pain in trigeminal neuralgia.

ACTION

▪ Inhibits reflexes at the spinal level. **Therapeutic Effects:** ▪ Relief of muscle spasticity; bowel and bladder function may also be improved.

PHARMACOKINETICS

Absorption: Well absorbed following oral administration.
Distribution: Widely distributed; crosses the placenta.
Metabolism and Excretion: 70–80% eliminated unchanged by the kidneys.
Half-life: 2.5–4 hr.

CONTRAINDICATIONS AND PRECAUTIONS

Contraindicated in: ▪ Hypersensitivity.
Use Cautiously in: ▪ Patients in whom spasticity is used to maintain posture and balance ▪ Epileptics (may lower seizure threshold) ▪ Elderly (increased susceptibility to CNS side effects) ▪ Renal impairment (dosage reduction may be required) ▪ Pregnancy, lactation, and children (safety not established).

ADVERSE REACTIONS AND SIDE EFFECTS*

CNS: SEIZURES (IT), dizziness, drowsiness, fatigue, weakness, confusion, depression, headache, insomnia.
EENT: nasal congestion, tinnitus.
CV: edema, hypotension.
GI: nausea, constipation.
GU: frequency.
Derm: pruritus, rash.
Metab: hyperglycemia, weight gain.
Neuro: ataxia.
Misc: hypersensitivity reactions, sweating.

INTERACTIONS

Drug-Drug: ▪ Additive CNS depression with other **CNS depressants** including **alcohol, antihistamines, opioid analgesics,** and **sedative/hypnotics** ▪ Use with **MAO inhibitors** may lead to increased CNS depression or hypotension.

ROUTE AND DOSAGE

- **PO (Adults):** 5 mg 3 times daily. May increase q 3 days by 5 mg/dose to maximum of 80 mg/day (total daily dose may also be given in divided doses 4 times daily).
- **IT (Adults):** 100–800 mcg/day infusion; dose is determined by response during screening phase.
- **IT (Children):** 25–1200 mcg/day infusion (average 275 mcg/day); dose is determined by response during screening phase.

AVAILABILITY

▪ ***Tablets:*** 10 mg[Rx], 20 mg[Rx] ▪ ***Intrathecal injection:*** 10 mg/20 ml (500 mcg/ml)[Rx], 10 mg/5 ml (2000 mcg/ml)[Rx].

TIME/ACTION PROFILE (effects on spasticity)

	ONSET	PEAK	DURATION
PO	hrs–wks	UK	UK
IT	0.5–1 hr	4 hr	4–8 hr

NURSING IMPLICATIONS

ASSESSMENT

- **General Info:** Assess muscle spasticity prior to and periodically throughout therapy.
- Observe patient for drowsiness, dizziness, or ataxia. A change in dose may alleviate these problems.
- **IT:** Monitor patient closely during test dose and titration. Resuscitative equipment should be immediately available for life-threatening or intolerable side effects.
- ***Lab Test Considerations:*** May cause in-

*CAPITALS indicate life-threatening; underlines indicate most frequent.

crease in serum glucose, alkaline phosphatase, AST, and ALT levels.

POTENTIAL NURSING DIAGNOSES

- Physical mobility, impaired (Indications).
- Injury, risk for (Adverse Reactions).
- Knowledge deficit, related to medication regimen (Patient/Family Teaching).

IMPLEMENTATION

- **PO:** May be administered with milk or food to minimize gastric irritation.
- **IT:** For *screening phase,* dilute for a concentration of 50 mcg/ml with sterile preservative-free NaCl for injection. Test dose should be administered over at least 1 min. Patient should be observed for a significant decrease in muscle tone or frequency or severity of spasm. If response is inadequate, 2 additional test doses, each 24 hr apart, 75 mcg/1.5 ml and 100 mcg/2 ml respectively, may be administered. Patients with an inadequate response should not receive chronic IT therapy.
- □ Dose titration for implantable IT pumps is based on patient response. If no substantive response after dose increase, check pump function and catheter patency.

PATIENT/FAMILY TEACHING

- □ Instruct patient to take baclofen as directed. Take a missed dose within 1 hr; do not double doses. Caution patient to avoid abrupt withdrawal of this medication as it may precipitate an acute withdrawal reaction (hallucinations, increased spasticity, seizures, mental changes, restlessness). Baclofen should be discontinued gradually over 2 wk or more.
- □ May cause dizziness and drowsiness. Advise patient to avoid driving or other activities requiring alertness until response to drug is known.
- □ Instruct patient to change positions slowly to minimize orthostatic hypotension.
- □ Advise patient to avoid concurrent use of alcohol or other CNS depressants while taking this medication.
- □ Instruct patient to notify health care professional if frequent urge to urinate or painful urination, constipation, nausea, headache, insomnia, tinnitus, depression, or confusion persists. Advise patient to report signs and symptoms of hypersensitivity (rash, itching) promptly.

EVALUATION

Effectiveness of therapy can be demonstrated by: ▪ Decrease in muscle spasticity and associated musculoskeletal pain with an increased ability to perform activities of daily living ▪ Decreased pain in patients with trigeminal neuralgia. May take weeks to obtain optimal effect.

BENZTROPINE

(**benz**-troe-peen)

{Apo-Benztropine}, Cogentin

CLASSIFICATION(S):

Anti-Parkinson agent (anticholinergic)

Pregnancy Category C

INDICATIONS

▪ Adjunctive treatment of all forms of Parkinson's disease, including drug-induced extrapyramidal effects and acute dystonic reactions.

ACTION

▪ Blocks cholinergic activity in the CNS, which is partially responsible for the symptoms of Parkinson's disease ▪ Restores the natural balance of neurotransmitters in the CNS. **Therapeutic Effects:** ▪ Reduction of rigidity and tremors.

PHARMACOKINETICS

Absorption: Well absorbed following PO and IM administration.
Distribution: UK.
Metabolism and Excretion: UK.
Half-life: UK.

CONTRAINDICATIONS AND PRECAUTIONS

Contraindicated in: ▪ Hypersensitivity ▪ Children <3 yr ▪ Narrow-angle glaucoma ▪ Tardive dyskinesia.
Use Cautiously in: ▪ Geriatric patients (increased risk of adverse reactions) ▪ Prostatic hypertension ▪ Seizure disorders ▪ Cardiac arrhythmias ▪ Pregnancy and lactation (safety not established).

ADVERSE REACTIONS AND SIDE EFFECTS*

CNS: confusion, depression, dizziness, hallucinations, headache, sedation, weakness.
EENT: blurred vision, dry eyes, mydriasis.
CV: arrhythmias, hypotension, palpitations, tachycardia.
GI: constipation, dry mouth, ileus, nausea.
GU: hesitancy, urinary retention.
Misc: decreased sweating.

INTERACTIONS

Drug-Drug: ▪ Additive anticholinergic effects with **drugs sharing anticholinergic properties**, such as **antihistamines, phenothiazines, quinidine, disopyramide**, and **tricyclic antidepressants** ▪ Counteracts the cholinergic effects of **bethanechol** ▪ **Antacids** and **antidiarrheals** may decrease absorption.

ROUTE AND DOSAGE

❑ Parkinsonism

- **PO (Adults):** 1–2 mg/day in 1–2 divided doses (range 0.5–6 mg/day).

❑ Acute Dystonic Reactions

- **IM, IV (Adults):** 1–2 mg, then 1–2 mg PO twice daily.

❑ Drug-Induced Extrapyramidal Reactions

- **PO, IM, IV (Adults):** 1–4 mg given once or twice daily (1–2 mg 2–3 times daily may also be used PO).

AVAILABILITY

▪ ***Tablets:*** 0.5 mg[Rx], 1 mg[Rx], 2 mg[Rx] ▪ ***Injection:*** 1 mg/ml[Rx].

TIME/ACTION PROFILE (antidyskinetic activity)

	ONSET	PEAK	DURATION
PO	1–2 hr	several days	24 hr
IM, IV	within min	UK	24 hr

NURSING IMPLICATIONS

ASSESSMENT

- **General Info:** Assess parkinsonian and extrapyramidal symptoms (restlessness or desire to keep moving, rigidity, tremors, pill rolling, mask-like face, shuffling gait, muscle spasms, twisting motions, difficulty speaking or swallowing, loss of balance control) prior to and throughout therapy.
- ❑ Assess bowel function daily. Monitor for constipation, abdominal pain, distention, or absence of bowel sounds.
- ❑ Monitor intake and output ratios and assess patient for urinary retention (dysuria, distended abdomen, infrequent voiding of small amounts, overflow incontinence).
- ❑ Patients with mental illness are at risk of developing exaggerated symptoms of their disorder during early therapy with benztropine. Withhold drug and notify physician or other health care professional if significant behavioral changes occur.
- **IM/IV:** Monitor pulse and blood pressure closely and maintain bed rest for 1 hr after administration. Advise patients to change positions slowly to minimize orthostatic hypotension.

POTENTIAL NURSING DIAGNOSES

- Physical mobility, impaired (Indications).
- Injury, risk for (Indications).
- Knowledge deficit, related to medication regimen (Patient/Family Teaching).

IMPLEMENTATION

- **PO:** Administer with food or immediately after meals to minimize gastric irritation. May be crushed and administered with food if patient has difficulty swallowing.
- **IM:** Parenteral route is used only for dystonic reactions.
- **Direct IV:** IV route is rarely used because onset is same as with IM route.
- ***Rate:*** Administer at a rate of 1 mg over 1 min.
- **Syringe Compatibility:** ▪ metoclopramide.
- **Y-Site Compatibility:** ▪ fluconazole ▪ tacrolimus.

PATIENT/FAMILY TEACHING

- ❑ Encourage patient to take benztropine as directed. Missed doses should be taken as soon as possible, up to 2 hr before the next dose. Taper gradually when discontinuing or a withdrawal reaction may occur (anxiety, tachycar-

***CAPITALS indicate life-threatening; underlines indicate most frequent.**

dia, insomnia, return of parkinsonian or extrapyramidal symptoms).

- May cause drowsiness or dizziness. Advise patient to avoid driving or other activities that require alertness until response to the drug is known.
- Instruct patient that frequent rinsing of mouth, good oral hygiene, and sugarless gum or candy may decrease dry mouth. Patient should notify health care professional if dryness persists (saliva substitutes may be used). Also, notify the dentist if dryness interferes with use of dentures.
- Caution patient to change positions slowly to minimize orthostatic hypotension.
- Instruct patient to notify health care professional if difficulty with urination, constipation, abdominal discomfort, rapid or pounding heartbeat, confusion, eye pain, or rash occurs.
- Advise patient to confer with health care professional prior to taking OTC medications, especially cold remedies, or drinking alcoholic beverages.
- Caution patient that this medication decreases perspiration. Overheating may occur during hot weather. Patient should notify health care professional if unable to remain indoors in an air-conditioned environment during hot weather.
- Advise patient to avoid taking antacids or antidiarrheals within 1–2 hr of this medication.
- Emphasize the importance of routine follow-up exams.

EVALUATION

Effectiveness of therapy can be demonstrated by: ▪ Decrease in tremors and rigidity and an improvement in gait and balance. Therapeutic effects are usually seen 2–3 days after the initiation of therapy.

BEPRIDIL

(**be**-pri-dil)

Bepadin, Vascor

CLASSIFICATION(S):

Antianginal, Calcium channel blocker

Pregnancy Category C

INDICATIONS

▪ Management of angina pectoris.

ACTION

▪ Inhibits the transport of calcium into myocardial and vascular smooth muscle cells, resulting in inhibition of excitation-contraction coupling and subsequent contraction ▪ Inhibits fast sodium inward current in myocardial and vascular smooth muscles ▪ Also has effects on conduction that may result in onset of new serious arrhythmias (proarrhythmic action). **Therapeutic Effects:** ▪ Coronary vasodilation resulting in decreased frequency and severity of attacks of angina.

PHARMACOKINETICS

Absorption: Well absorbed following oral administration.

Distribution: Crosses the placenta and enters breast milk.

Metabolism and Excretion: Mostly metabolized by the liver; inactive metabolites excreted by the kidneys.

Half-life: 42 hr (following cessation of multiple dosing).

CONTRAINDICATIONS AND PRECAUTIONS

Contraindicated in: ▪ Hypersensitivity ▪ Sick sinus syndrome ▪ 2nd- or 3rd-degree AV block (unless an artificial pacemaker is in place) ▪ Blood pressure <90 mm Hg ▪ Serious ventricular arrhythmias, severe cardiac insufficiency, prolonged QT interval.

Use Cautiously in: ▪ Severe hepatic impairment (dosage reduction recommended) ▪ Geriatric patients (dosage reduction recommended; increased risk of hypotension) ▪ Severe renal impairment (dosage reduction necessary) ▪ History of serious ventricular arrhythmias or congestive heart failure ▪ Pregnancy, lactation, or children (safety not established).

ADVERSE REACTIONS AND SIDE EFFECTS*

CNS: dizziness, headache, nervousness, abnormal dreams, anxiety, confusion, psychiatric disturbances, sedation, shakiness, weakness.

***CAPITALS indicate life-threatening; underlines indicate most frequent.**

EENT: blurred vision, disturbed equilibrium, epistaxis, tinnitus.
Resp: congestion, cough, dyspnea, shortness of breath.
CV: ARRHYTHMIAS, CONGESTIVE HEART FAILURE, peripheral edema, bradycardia, chest pain, hypotension, palpitations, syncope, tachycardia.
GI: nausea, abnormal liver function studies, anorexia, constipation, diarrhea, dry mouth, dysgeusia, dyspepsia, vomiting.
GU: dysuria, nocturia, polyuria, sexual dysfunction, urinary frequency.
Derm: dermatitis/rash, erythema multiforme, increased sweating, photosensitivity, pruritus/urticaria.
Endo: gynecomastia, hyperglycemia.
Hemat: anemia, leukopenia, thrombocytopenia.
Metab: weight gain.
MS: joint stiffness, muscle cramps.
Neuro: paresthesia, tremor.
Misc: STEVENS-JOHNSON SYNDROME, gingival hyperplasia.

INTERACTIONS

Drug-Drug: ▪ Additive hypotension may occur when used concurrently with **fentanyl** ▪ Concurrent use with **antiarrhythmics (quinidine, procainamide), tricyclic antidepressants,** or **digitalis glycosides** increases the risk of ventricular arrhythmias.

ROUTE AND DOSAGE

- **PO (Adults):** 200 mg once daily, may increase after 10 days to 300 mg/day (not to exceed 400 mg/day).

AVAILABILITY

- ***Tablets:*** 200 mg[Rx], 300 mg[Rx], 400 mg[Rx].

TIME/ACTION PROFILE

	ONSET	PEAK	DURATION
PO	8 days*	UK	24 hr

*Onset of steady-state antianginal effect with chronic dosing.

NURSING IMPLICATIONS

ASSESSMENT

- **General Info:** Monitor blood pressure and pulse prior to therapy, during dosage titration, and periodically throughout therapy. Monitor ECG periodically during prolonged therapy. Bepridil may cause increased QT interval and altered T-wave morphology.
- □ Monitor intake and output ratios and daily weight. Assess for signs of congestive heart failure (peripheral edema, rales/crackles, dyspnea, weight gain, jugular venous distention).
- **Angina:** Assess location, duration, intensity, and precipitating factors of patient's anginal pain.
- ***Lab Test Considerations:*** Total serum calcium concentrations are not affected by calcium channel blockers.
- □ Monitor serum potassium periodically. Hypokalemia increases the risk of arrhythmias and should be corrected.
- □ Monitor renal and hepatic functions periodically during long-term therapy. May cause increase in hepatic enzymes after several days of therapy, which return to normal upon discontinuation of therapy.

POTENTIAL NURSING DIAGNOSES

- Tissue perfusion, altered (Indications).
- Pain (Indications).
- Knowledge deficit, related to medication regimen (Patient/Family Teaching).

IMPLEMENTATION

- **PO:** Administer bepridil with meals or milk to minimize gastric irritation.

PATIENT/FAMILY TEACHING

- **General Info:** Advise patient to take medication exactly as directed, even if feeling well. If a dose is missed, take as soon as possible unless almost time for next dose; do not double doses. May need to be discontinued gradually.
- □ Instruct patient on correct technique for monitoring pulse. Instruct patient to contact health care professional if heart rate is <50 bpm.
- □ Caution patient to change positions slowly to minimize orthostatic hypotension.
- □ May cause drowsiness or dizziness. Advise patient to avoid driving or other activities requiring alertness until response to the medication is known.
- □ Instruct patient on importance of maintaining good dental hygiene and seeing dentist frequently for teeth cleaning to prevent tender-

ness, bleeding, and gingival hyperplasia (gum enlargement).

□ Instruct patient to avoid concurrent use of alcohol or OTC medications, especially cold preparations, without consulting health care professional.

□ Advise patient to notify health care professional if irregular heart beats, dyspnea, swelling of hands and feet, pronounced dizziness, nausea, constipation, or hypotension occurs or if headache is severe or persistent.

□ Advise patient to inform health care professional of medication regimen before treatment or surgery.

■ **Angina:** Instruct patient on concurrent nitrate or beta-blocker therapy to continue taking both medications as directed and use SL nitroglycerin as needed for anginal attacks.

□ Advise patient to contact physician if chest pain does not improve or worsens after therapy or occurs with diaphoresis; if shortness of breath occurs; or if severe, persistent headache occurs.

□ Caution patient to discuss exercise restrictions with health care professional prior to exertion.

EVALUATION

Effectiveness of therapy can be demonstrated by: ■ Decrease in frequency and severity of anginal attacks □ Decrease in need for nitrate therapy □ Increase in activity tolerance and sense of well-being.

BETAXOLOL†

(be-**tax**-oh-lol)

Kerlone

CLASSIFICATION(S):

Antihypertensive agent, Beta-adrenergic blocking agent (selective)

Pregnancy Category C

†See Appendix O for ophthalmic use.

INDICATIONS

■ Management of hypertension.

ACTION

■ Blocks stimulation of $beta_1$ (myocardial) -adrenergic receptors. Does not usually affect $beta_2$ (pulmonary, vascular, uterine) -receptor sites. **Therapeutic Effects:** ■ Decreased blood pressure and heart rate.

PHARMACOKINETICS

Absorption: Well absorbed following oral administration.

Distribution: Widely distributed.

Metabolism and Excretion: Mostly metabolized by the liver, 20% excreted unchanged by the kidneys.

Half-life: 15–20 hr.

CONTRAINDICATIONS AND PRECAUTIONS

Contraindicated in: ■ Uncompensated congestive heart failure ■ Pulmonary edema ■ Cardiogenic shock ■ Bradycardia or heart block.

Use Cautiously in: ■ Renal or hepatic impairment ■ Geriatric patients (increased sensitivity to beta-adrenergic blockers; initial dosage reduction recommended) ■ Pulmonary disease (including asthma; $beta_1$ selectivity may be lost at higher doses) ■ Diabetes mellitus ■ Thyrotoxicosis ■ Patients with a history of severe allergic reactions (intensity of reactions may be increased) ■ Pregnancy, lactation, or children (safety not established; all agents cross the placenta and may cause fetal/neonatal bradycardia, hypotension, hypoglycemia, or respiratory depression).

ADVERSE REACTIONS AND SIDE EFFECTS*

CNS: fatigue, weakness, anxiety, depression, dizziness, drowsiness, insomnia, memory loss, mental status changes, nightmares.

EENT: blurred vision, stuffy nose.

Resp: bronchospasm, wheezing.

CV: BRADYCARDIA, CONGESTIVE HEART FAILURE, PULMONARY EDEMA, hypotension, peripheral vasoconstriction.

GI: constipation, diarrhea, liver function abnormalities, nausea, vomiting.

GU: impotence, decreased libido, urinary frequency.

***CAPITALS indicate life-threatening; underlines indicate most frequent.**

Derm: rashes.
Endo: hyperglycemia, hypoglycemia.
MS: arthralgia, back pain, joint pain.

INTERACTIONS

Drug-Drug: ▪ **General anesthesia, IV phenytoin,** and **verapamil** may cause additive myocardial depression ▪ Additive bradycardia may occur with **digitalis glycosides** ▪ Additive hypotension may occur with other **antihypertensives,** acute ingestion of **alcohol,** or **nitrates** ▪ Concurrent use with **amphetamines, cocaine, ephedrine, epinephrine, norepinephrine, phenylephrine,** or **pseudoephedrine** may result in unopposed alpha-adrenergic stimulation (excessive hypertension, bradycardia) ▪ Concurrent **thyroid** administration may decrease effectiveness ▪ May alter the effectiveness of **insulin** or **oral hypoglycemic agents** (dosage adjustments may be necessary) ▪ May decrease the effectiveness of **theophylline** ▪ May decrease the beneficial beta_1-cardiovascular effects of **dopamine** or **dobutamine** ▪ Use cautiously within 14 days of **MAO inhibitor** therapy (may result in hypertension).

ROUTE AND DOSAGE

- **PO (Adults):** 10 mg once daily, may be increased to 20 mg after 7 days; start with 5 mg in geriatric patients or patients with renal impairment.

AVAILABILITY

- ***Tablets:*** 10 mg[Rx], 20 mg[Rx].

TIME/ACTION PROFILE (antihypertensive effect)

	ONSET	PEAK	DURATION
PO	3–4 hr	3–4 hr	24 hr

NURSING IMPLICATIONS

ASSESSMENT

- Monitor blood pressure, ECG, and pulse frequently during dose adjustment and periodically during therapy.
- Monitor intake and output ratios and daily weights. Assess routinely for signs and symptoms of congestive heart failure (dyspnea, rales/crackles, weight gain, peripheral edema, jugular venous distention).
- **Angina:** Assess frequency and characteristics of angina periodically during therapy.
- ***Lab Test Considerations:*** May cause increased BUN, serum lipoprotein, potassium, triglyceride, and uric acid levels.
- May cause increased ANA titers.
- May cause increase in blood glucose levels.
- ***Toxicity and Overdose:*** Monitor patients receiving beta-adrenergic blocking agents for signs of overdose (bradycardia, severe dizziness or fainting, severe drowsiness, dyspnea, bluish fingernails or palms, seizures). Notify physician or health care professional immediately if these signs occur.
- Glucagon has been used to treat bradycardia and hypotension.

POTENTIAL NURSING DIAGNOSES

- Cardiac output, decreased (Side Effects).
- Knowledge deficit, related to medication regimen (Patient/Family Teaching).
- Noncompliance, related to medication regimen (Patient/Family Teaching).

IMPLEMENTATION

- **PO:** Take apical pulse prior to administering. If <50 bpm or if arrhythmia occurs, withhold medication and notify physician or other health care professional.
- May be administered without regard to food.

PATIENT/FAMILY TEACHING

- **General Info:** Instruct patient to take medication exactly as directed, at the same time each day, even if feeling well; do not skip or double up on missed doses. Take missed doses as soon as possible up to 4 hr before next dose. Abrupt withdrawal may precipitate life-threatening arrhythmias, hypertension, or myocardial ischemia.
- Advise patient to make sure enough medication is available for weekends, holidays, and vacations. A written prescription may be kept in wallet in case of emergency.
- Teach patient and family how to check pulse and blood pressure. Instruct them to check pulse daily and blood pressure biweekly and to report significant changes.
- May cause drowsiness or dizziness. Caution patients to avoid driving or other activities that require alertness until response to the drug is known.
- Advise patients to change positions slowly to minimize orthostatic hypotension.

B

□ Caution patient that this medication may increase sensitivity to cold.
□ Instruct patient to consult health care professional before taking any OTC medications, especially cold preparations, concurrently with this medication.
□ Diabetics should closely monitor blood sugar, especially if weakness, malaise, irritability, or fatigue occurs. Betaxolol may mask some signs of hypoglycemia, but sweating and dizziness may occur.
□ Advise patient to notify health care professional if slow pulse, difficulty breathing, wheezing, cold hands and feet, dizziness, confusion, depression, rash, fever, sore throat, unusual bleeding, or bruising occurs.
□ Instruct patient to inform health care professional of medication regimen prior to treatment or surgery.
□ Advise patient to carry identification describing disease process and medication regimen at all times.

▪ **Hypertension:** Reinforce the need to continue additional therapies for hypertension (weight loss, sodium restriction, stress reduction, regular exercise, moderation of alcohol consumption, and smoking cessation). Medication controls but does not cure hypertension.

EVALUATION

Effectiveness of therapy can be demonstrated by: ▪ Decrease in blood pressure without appearance of detrimental side effects.

BETHANECHOL

(be-**than**-e-kole)
Duvoid, Urebeth, Urecholine

CLASSIFICATION(S):
Cholinergic (direct-acting)

Pregnancy Category C

INDICATIONS

▪ Postpartum and postoperative nonobstructive urinary retention or urinary retention due to neurogenic bladder.

ACTION

▪ Stimulates cholinergic receptors. Effects include: □ Contraction of the urinary bladder □ Decreased bladder capacity □ Increased frequency of ureteral peristaltic waves □ Increased tone and peristalsis in the GI tract □ Increased pressure in the lower esophageal sphincter □ Increased gastric secretions. **Therapeutic Effects:** ▪ Bladder emptying.

PHARMACOKINETICS

Absorption: Poorly absorbed following oral administration, requiring larger doses by mouth than subcutaneously.
Distribution: Does not cross the blood-brain barrier.
Metabolism and Excretion: UK.
Half-life: UK.

CONTRAINDICATIONS AND PRECAUTIONS

Contraindicated in: ▪ Hypersensitivity ▪ Mechanical obstruction of the GI or GU tract.
Use Cautiously in: ▪ History of asthma ▪ Ulcer disease ▪ Cardiovascular disease ▪ Epilepsy ▪ Hyperthyroidism ▪ Sensitivity to cholinergic agents or effects ▪ Children, pregnancy, and lactation (safety not established).

ADVERSE REACTIONS AND SIDE EFFECTS*

CNS: headache, malaise.
EENT: lacrimation, miosis.
Resp: bronchospasm.
CV: HEART BLOCK, SYNCOPE/CARDIAC ARREST, bradycardia, hypotension.
GI: abdominal discomfort, diarrhea, nausea, salivation, vomiting.
GU: urgency.
Misc: flushing, sweating, hypothermia.

INTERACTIONS

Drug-Drug: ▪ **Quinidine** and **procainamide** may antagonize cholinergic effects ▪ Additive cholinergic effects with **cholinesterase inhibitors** ▪ Use with **ganglionic blocking agents** may result in severe hypotension ▪ Do not use with **depolarizing neuromuscular blocking agents** ▪ Effectiveness will be decreased by **anticholinergic agents.**

***CAPITALS indicate life-threatening; underlines indicate most frequent.**

ROUTE AND DOSAGE

- **PO (Adults):** 25–50 mg 3 times daily. Dose may be determined by administering 5–10 mg q 1–2 hr until response is obtained or total of 50 mg administered *or* by starting with 10 mg, giving 25 mg 6 hr later, then, if needed, 50 mg 6 hr later.
- **PO (Children):** 0.2 mg/kg 3 times daily or 0.15 mg/kg 4 times daily.
- **SC (Adults):** 5 mg 3–4 times daily. Dose may be determined by administering 2.5 mg q 15–30 min until response is obtained or total of 4 doses administered.
- **SC (Children):** 0.06 mg/kg 3 times daily or 0.15 mg/kg 4 times daily.

AVAILABILITY

- ***Tablets:*** 5 mg[Rx], 10 mg[Rx], 25 mg[Rx], 50 mg[Rx]
- ***Injection:*** 5 mg/ml[Rx].

TIME/ACTION PROFILE (response on bladder muscle)

	ONSET	PEAK	DURATION
PO	30–90 min	1 hr	6 hr
SC	5–15 min	15–30 min	2 hr

NURSING IMPLICATIONS

ASSESSMENT

- Monitor blood pressure, pulse, and respirations before administering and for at least 1 hr following SC administration.
- Monitor intake and output ratios. Palpate abdomen for bladder distention. Notify physician or other health care professional if drug fails to relieve condition for which it was prescribed. Catheterization may be ordered to assess postvoid residual.
- ***Lab Test Considerations:*** May cause an increase in serum AST, amylase, and lipase concentrations.
- ***Toxicity and Overdose:*** Observe patient for drug toxicity (sweating, flushing, abdominal cramps, nausea, salivation). If overdosage occurs, treatment includes atropine sulfate (specific antidote).

POTENTIAL NURSING DIAGNOSES

- Urinary elimination, altered patterns of (Indications).
- Knowledge deficit, related to medication regimen (Patient/Family Teaching).

IMPLEMENTATION

- **General Info:** A test dose is usually used prior to maintenance to determine minimum effective dose.
- Oral and SC doses are *not* interchangeable.
- **PO:** Administer medication on an empty stomach, 1 hr before or 2 hr after meals, to prevent nausea and vomiting.
- **SC:** Parenteral solution is intended only for subcutaneous administration. Do not give IM or IV. Inadvertent IM or IV administration may cause cholinergic overstimulation (circulatory collapse, drop in blood pressure, abdominal cramps, bloody diarrhea, shock, and cardiac arrest).
- Do not use if solution is discolored or contains a precipitate.

PATIENT/FAMILY TEACHING

- Instruct patient to take medication exactly as directed. Missed doses should be taken as soon as possible within 2 hr; otherwise, return to regular dosing schedule. Do not double doses.
- Caution patient to change positions slowly to minimize orthostatic hypotension.
- Advise patient to report abdominal discomfort, salivation, sweating, or flushing to health care professional.

EVALUATION

Effectiveness of therapy can be demonstrated by: ▪ Increase in bladder function and tone.

BICALUTAMIDE

(bye-ka-**loot**-a-mide)
Casodex

CLASSIFICATION(S):
Antineoplastic (hormone)

Pregnancy Category X

INDICATIONS

- Treatment of metastatic prostate carcinoma in conjunction with luteinizing hormone-releasing hormone (LHRH) analogues (goserelin, leuprolide).

ACTION

- Antagonizes the effects of androgen at the cellular level. **Therapeutic Effects:** - Decreased spread of prostate carcinoma.

PHARMACOKINETICS

Absorption: Well absorbed following oral administration.
Distribution: UK.
Metabolism and Excretion: Mostly metabolized by the liver.
Half-life: 5.8 days.

CONTRAINDICATIONS AND PRECAUTIONS

Contraindicated in: - Hypersensitivity - Pregnancy.
Use Cautiously in: - Moderate to severe liver impairment - Patients with childbearing potential - Lactation and children (safety not established).

ADVERSE REACTIONS AND SIDE EFFECTS*

CNS: weakness, dizziness, headache, insomnia.
Resp: dyspnea.
CV: chest pain, hypertension, peripheral edema.
GI: constipation, diarrhea, nausea, abdominal pain, increased liver enzymes, vomiting.
GU: hematuria, impotence, incontinence, nocturia, urinary tract infections.
Derm: alopecia, rashes, sweating.
Endo: breast pain, gynecomastia.
Hemat: anemia.
Metab: hyperglycemia, weight loss.
MS: back pain, pelvic pain, bone pain.
Neuro: paresthesia.
Misc: generalized pain, hot flashes, flu-like syndrome, infection.

INTERACTIONS

Drug-Drug: - May increase the effect of **warfarin.**

ROUTE AND DOSAGE

- **PO (Adults):** 50 mg once daily (must be given concurrently with LHRH analogue).

AVAILABILITY

- ***Tablets:*** 50 mg[Rx].

TIME/ACTION PROFILE (blood levels)

	ONSET	PEAK	DURATION
PO	UK	31.3 hr	UK

NURSING IMPLICATIONS

ASSESSMENT

- □ Assess patient for GI adverse effects. Diarrhea is the most common cause of discontinuation of therapy.
- ***Lab Test Considerations:*** Monitor serum prostate-specific antigen (PSA) periodically to determine response to therapy. If levels rise, assess patient for disease progression. May require periodic LHRH analogue administration without bicalutamide.
- □ Monitor liver function tests prior to and periodically during therapy. May cause elevated serum alkaline phosphatase, AST, ALT, and bilirubin concentrations. If transaminases increase >2 times normal, bicalutamide should be discontinued; levels usually return to normal after discontinuation.
- □ May cause increased BUN and serum creatinine, and decreased hemoglobin and white blood cell counts.

POTENTIAL NURSING DIAGNOSES

- Diarrhea (Adverse Reactions).
- Knowledge deficit, related to medication regimen (Patient/Family Teaching).

IMPLEMENTATION

- **General Info:** Start treatment with bicalutamide at the same time as LHRH analogue.
- **PO:** May be administered in the morning or evening, without regard to food.

PATIENT/FAMILY TEACHING

- □ Instruct patient to take bicalutamide exactly as directed at the same time each day. Do not discontinue without consulting health care professional.
- □ Advise patient not to take other medications without consulting health care professional.
- □ Instruct patient to report diarrhea that is severe or persistent.
- □ Discuss with patient the possibility of hair loss. Explore methods of coping.

*CAPITALS indicate life-threatening; underlines indicate most frequent.

- Emphasize the importance of regular follow-up exams and blood tests to determine progress, and monitor for side effects.

EVALUATION

Effectiveness of therapy can be demonstrated by: ▪ Decreased spread of prostate carcinoma.

BILE ACID SEQUESTRANTS

cholestyramine
(koe-less-**tear**-a-meen)
Prevalite, Questran, Questran Light

colestipol
(koe-**les**-ti-pole)
Colestid

CLASSIFICATION(S):
Lipid-lowering agents

Pregnancy Category UK

INDICATIONS

▪ Management of primary hypercholesterolemia ▪ Pruritus associated with elevated levels of bile acids. **Unlabeled Uses:** ▪ Diarrhea associated with excess bile acids.

ACTION

▪ Bind bile acids in the GI tract, forming an insoluble complex. Result is increased clearance of cholesterol. **Therapeutic Effects:** ▪ Decreased plasma cholesterol and low-density lipoproteins ▪ Decreased pruritus.

PHARMACOKINETICS

Absorption: Action takes place in the GI tract. No absorption occurs.
Distribution: No distribution.
Metabolism and Excretion: After binding bile acids, insoluble complex is eliminated in the feces.
Half-life: UK.

CONTRAINDICATIONS AND PRECAUTIONS

Contraindicated in: ▪ Hypersensitivity ▪ Complete biliary obstruction ▪ Some products contain aspartame and should be avoided in patients with phenylketonuria.
Use Cautiously in: ▪ History of constipation.
Use with Extreme Caution in: ▪ Children (may cause intestinal obstruction; deaths have occurred).

ADVERSE REACTIONS AND SIDE EFFECTS*

EENT: irritation of the tongue.
GI: abdominal discomfort, constipation, flatulence, nausea, hemorrhoids, impaction, perianal irritation, steatorrhea, vomiting.
Derm: irritation, rashes.
F and E: hyperchloremic acidosis.
Metab: vitamin A, D, and K deficiency.

INTERACTIONS

Drug-Drug: ▪ May decrease absorption/effects of orally administered **acetaminophen, amiodarone, clindamycin, clofibrate, digitalis glycosides, diuretics, gemfibrozil, glipizide, glucocorticoids, imipramine, mycophenolate, methotrexate, methyldopa, niacin, NSAIDs, penicillin, phenytoin, phosphates, propranolol, tetracyclines, tolbutamide, thyroid, ursodiol, warfarin,** and **fat-soluble vitamins (A, D, E, and K)** ▪ May decrease absorption of other **orally administered medications.**

ROUTE AND DOSAGE

Cholestyramine

- **PO (Adults):** 4 g 1–2 times daily (may be divided up and given 6 times daily).
- **PO (Children):** 240 mg/kg/day in 2–3 divided doses (not >8 g/day).

Colestipol

- **PO (Adults):** *Granules*—5 g 1–2 times daily, may be increased q 1–2 mo up to 30 g/day in 1–2 doses. *Tablets*—2 g 1–2 times daily, may be increased q 1–2 mo up to 16 g/day in 1–2 doses.

AVAILABILITY

Cholestyramine

Questran Light ▪ ***Powder for suspension (with aspartame and sucrose):*** 5-g packets or bulk container with 5-g scoop (contains 4 g cholestyramine/5 g powder)[Rx]

***CAPITALS** indicate life-threatening; **underlines** indicate most frequent.

Questran ▪ ***Powder for suspension:*** 9-g packets or bulk container with 9-g scoop (contains 4 g cholestyramine/9 g powder)Rx.

❑ Colestipol

▪ ***Granules for suspension:*** 5-g packets or bulk container with 5-g scoopRx ▪ ***Flavored granules for suspension (with aspartame):*** 7.5-g packets or bulk container with 7.5-g scoop (contains 5 g colestipol/7.5 g granules); orange flavoredRx ▪ ***Tablets:*** 1 gRx.

TIME/ACTION PROFILE (hypocholesterolemic effects)

	ONSET	PEAK	DURATION
Cholestyramine	24–48 hr	1–3 wk	2–4 wk
Colestipol	24–48 hr	1 mo	1 mo

NURSING IMPLICATIONS

ASSESSMENT

- **Hypercholesterolemia:** Obtain a diet history, especially in regard to fat consumption.
- **Pruritus:** Assess severity of itching and skin integrity. Dose may be decreased when relief of pruritus occurs.
- **Diarrhea:** Assess frequency, amount, and consistency of stools.
- ***Lab Test Considerations:*** Serum cholesterol and triglyceride levels should be evaluated before initiating, frequently during first few months and periodically throughout therapy. Discontinue medication if paradoxical increase in cholesterol level occurs.
  - ❑ May cause an increase in AST, ALT, phosphorus, chloride, and alkaline phosphatase and a decrease in serum calcium, sodium, and potassium levels.
  - ❑ May also cause prolonged prothrombin time (PT).

POTENTIAL NURSING DIAGNOSES

- Constipation (Side Effects).
- Knowledge deficit, related to medication regimen (Patient/Family Teaching).
- Noncompliance (Patient/Family Teaching).

IMPLEMENTATION

- **General Info:** Parenteral or water-miscible forms of fat-soluble vitamins (A, D, K) and folic acid may be ordered for patients on chronic therapy.
- **PO:** Administer before meals.
  - ❑ Administer other medications 1 hr before or 4–6 hr after the administration of this medication.
  - ❑ Colestipol tablets should be swallowed whole; do not cut, crush, or chew.

PATIENT/FAMILY TEACHING

- ❑ Instruct patient to take medication exactly as directed; do not skip doses or double up on missed doses.
- ❑ Instruct patient to take medication before meals. Mix cholestyramine with 4–6 oz water, milk, fruit juice, or other noncarbonated beverages. Shake vigorously. Colestipol can be mixed with water, juice, or carbonated beverages. Slowly stir in a large glass. Rinse glass with small amount of additional beverage to ensure all medication is taken. May also mix with highly fluid soups, cereals, or pulpy fruits (applesauce, crushed pineapple). Allow powder to sit on fluid and hydrate for 1–2 min prior to mixing. Do not take dry. Variations in the color of cholestyramine do not alter stability.
- ❑ Advise patient that this medication should be used in conjunction with diet restrictions (fat, cholesterol, carbohydrates, alcohol), exercise, and cessation of smoking.
- ❑ Explain that constipation may occur. Increase in fluids and bulk in diet, exercise, stool softeners, and laxatives may be required to minimize the constipating effects. Instruct patient to notify health care professional if constipation, nausea, flatulence, and heartburn persist or if stools become frothy and foul smelling.
- ❑ Advise patient to notify health care professional if unusual bleeding or bruising; petechiae; or black, tarry stools occur. Treatment with vitamin K may be necessary.

EVALUATION

Effectiveness of therapy can be demonstrated by: ▪ Decrease in serum low-density lipoprotein (LDL) cholesterol levels. Therapy is usually discontinued if the clinical response remains poor after 3 mo of therapy ▪ Decrease in severity of pruritus. Relief usually occurs 1–3 wk after therapy is initiated ▪ Decrease in frequency and severity of diarrhea.

B

BIPERIDEN
(by-**per**-i-den)
Akineton

CLASSIFICATION(S):
Anti-Parkinson agent (anticholinergic)

Pregnancy Category C

INDICATIONS
▪ Adjunctive treatment of all forms of Parkinson's disease, including drug-induced extrapyramidal effects and acute dystonic reactions.

ACTION
▪ Blocks cholinergic activity in the CNS, which is partially responsible for the symptoms of Parkinson's disease ▪ Restores the natural balance of neurotransmitters in the CNS. **Therapeutic Effects:** ▪ Reduction of rigidity and tremors.

PHARMACOKINETICS
Absorption: Well absorbed following oral or IM administration.
Distribution: UK.
Metabolism and Excretion: UK.
Half-life: UK.

CONTRAINDICATIONS AND PRECAUTIONS
Contraindicated in: ▪ Hypersensitivity ▪ Narrow-angle glaucoma ▪ Bowel obstruction ▪ Megacolon ▪ Tardive dyskinesia.
Use Cautiously in: ▪ Geriatric patients (increased risk of adverse reactions; lower doses may be necessary) ▪ Prostatic enlargement ▪ Seizure disorders ▪ Cardiac arrhythmias ▪ Pregnancy and lactation (safety not established).

ADVERSE REACTIONS AND SIDE EFFECTS*
CNS: confusion, depression, dizziness, hallucinations, headache, sedation, weakness.
EENT: blurred vision, dry eyes, mydriasis.
CV: arrhythmias, hypotension, palpitations, tachycardia.
GI: constipation, dry mouth, ileus, nausea.
GU: hesitancy, urinary retention.
Misc: decreased sweating.

INTERACTIONS
Drug-Drug: ▪ Additive anticholinergic effects with **drugs sharing anticholinergic properties** such as **antihistamines, phenothiazines, quinidine, disopyramide**, and **tricyclic antidepressants** ▪ Counteracts the cholinergic effects of **bethanechol** ▪ **Antacids** or **antidiarrheals** may decrease absorption.

ROUTE AND DOSAGE
❑ **Parkinsonism**
- **PO (Adults):** 2 mg 3–4 times daily initially (not to exceed 16 mg/day).

❑ **Extrapyramidal Reactions**
- **PO (Adults):** 2 mg 1–3 times daily.
- **IM, IV (Adults):** 2 mg, may repeat q 30 min (not to exceed 8 mg or 4 doses/24 hr).
- **IM (Children):** 40 mcg (0.04 mg)/kg or 1.2 mg/m², may repeat q 30 min (not to exceed 4 doses/24 hr).

AVAILABILITY
▪ ***Tablets:*** 2 mg[Rx] ▪ ***Injection:*** 5 mg/ml[Rx].

TIME/ACTION PROFILE (relief of symptoms)

	ONSET	PEAK	DURATION
PO	UK	UK	UK
IM	10–30 min	UK	UK
IV	UK	UK	1–8 hr

NURSING IMPLICATIONS

ASSESSMENT
- **General Info:** Assess parkinsonian and extrapyramidal symptoms (restlessness or desire to keep moving, rigidity, tremors, pill rolling, mask-like face, shuffling gait, muscle spasms, twisting motions, difficulty speaking or swallowing, loss of balance control) prior to and throughout therapy.
- ❑ Assess bowel function daily. Monitor for constipation, abdominal pain, distention, or the absence of bowel sounds.
- ❑ Monitor intake and output ratios and assess patient for urinary retention (dysuria, distended abdomen, infrequent voiding of small amounts, overflow incontinence).

*CAPITALS indicate life-threatening; underlines indicate most frequent.

□ After parenteral administration, monitor pulse and blood pressure closely and maintain bed rest for 1 hr. Advise patients to change positions slowly to minimize orthostatic hypotension.
□ Patients with mental illness are at risk of developing exaggerated symptoms of their disorder during early therapy with this medication. Withhold drug and notify physician or other health care professional if significant behavioral changes occur.

POTENTIAL NURSING DIAGNOSES

- Physical mobility, impaired (Indications).
- Knowledge deficit, related to medication regimen (Patient/Family Teaching).

IMPLEMENTATION

- **PO:** Administer with food or immediately after meals to minimize gastric irritation.
- **Direct IV:** Administer each dose over at least 1 min to minimize hypotension and mild bradycardia.

PATIENT/FAMILY TEACHING

□ Advise patient to take medication exactly as directed. Missed doses should be taken as soon as possible up to 2 hr before the next dose. Drug should be tapered gradually when discontinuing or a withdrawal reaction may occur (anxiety, tachycardia, insomnia, return of parkinsonian or extrapyramidal symptoms).
□ May cause drowsiness, dizziness, or blurred vision. Advise patient to avoid driving or other activities that require alertness until response to the drug is known.
□ Caution patient to change positions slowly to minimize orthostatic hypotension.
□ Advise patient that frequent mouth rinses, good oral hygiene, and sugarless gum or candy may decrease dry mouth. Patient should notify health care professional if dry mouth persists (saliva substitutes may be used). Also notify the dentist if dry mouth interferes with use of dentures.
□ Instruct patient to notify health care professional if difficulty with urination, constipation, abdominal discomfort, rapid or pounding heartbeat, confusion, eye pain, or rash occurs.
□ Advise patient to confer with health care professional prior to taking OTC medications, especially cold remedies, or drinking alcoholic beverages.
□ Caution patient that this medication decreases perspiration. Overheating may occur during hot weather. Patients should notify health care professional if they cannot remain indoors in an air-conditioned environment during hot weather.
□ Advise patient to avoid antacids or antidiarrheals within 1–2 hr of this medication.
□ Emphasize the importance of routine follow-up exams.

EVALUATION

Effectiveness of therapy can be demonstrated by: ▪ Decrease in tremors and rigidity and an improvement in gait and balance in Parkinson's disease ▪ Resolution of drug-induced extrapyramidal reactions.

BISACODYL

(bis-a-**koe**-dill)

{Bisac-Evac}, {Bisaco-Lax}, {Bisacolax}, Carter's Little Pills, Dacodyl, Deficol, Dulcagen, Dulcolax, Fleet Bisacodyl, {Laxit}, Theralax

CLASSIFICATION(S):
Laxative (stimulant)

Pregnancy Category UK

INDICATIONS

▪ Treatment of constipation ▪ Evacuation of the bowel prior to radiologic studies or surgery ▪ Part of a bowel regimen in spinal cord injury patients.

ACTION

▪ Stimulates peristalsis ▪ Alters fluid and electrolyte transport, producing fluid accumulation in the colon. **Therapeutic Effects:** ▪ Evacuation of the colon.

PHARMACOKINETICS

Absorption: Variable absorption follows oral administration; rectal absorption is minimal; action is local in the colon.

Distribution: Small amounts of metabolites excreted in breast milk.
Metabolism and Excretion: Small amounts absorbed are metabolized by the liver.
Half-life: UK.

CONTRAINDICATIONS AND PRECAUTIONS

Contraindicated in: ▪ Hypersensitivity ▪ Abdominal pain ▪ Obstruction ▪ Nausea or vomiting (especially with fever or other signs of an acute abdomen).
Use Cautiously in: ▪ Severe cardiovascular disease ▪ Anal or rectal fissures ▪ Excess or prolonged use (may result in dependence) ▪ Products containing tannic acid (Clysodrast) should not be used as multiple enemas (increased risk of hepatotoxicity) ▪ May be used during pregnancy and lactation.

ADVERSE REACTIONS AND SIDE EFFECTS*

GI: abdominal cramps, nausea, diarrhea, rectal burning.
F and E: hypokalemia (with chronic use).
MS: muscle weakness (with chronic use).
Misc: protein-losing enteropathy, tetany (with chronic use).

INTERACTIONS

Drug-Drug: ▪ **Antacids, histamine H_2-receptor agonists,** and **gastric acid–pump inhibitors** may remove enteric coating of tablets ▪ May decrease the absorption of other **orally administered drugs** because of increased motility and decreased transit time.

ROUTE AND DOSAGE

- **PO (Adults and Children ≥ 12 yr):** 5–15 mg (up to 30 mg/day) as a single dose.
- **PO (Children > 3 yr):** 5–10 mg (0.3 mg/kg) as a single dose.
- **Rect (Adults and Children ≥ 12 yr):** 10 mg single dose.
- **Rect (Children 2–11 yr):** 5–10 mg single dose.
- **Rect (Children <2 yr):** 5 mg single dose.

AVAILABILITY

▪ ***Enteric-coated tablets:*** 5 mg[OTC] ▪ ***Suppositories:*** 5 mg[OTC], 10 mg[OTC] ▪ ***Rectal solution:*** 10 mg/37 ml[OTC] ▪ ***In combination with:*** tannic acid (Clysodrast)[OTC], docusate (Dulcodos)[OTC], hydroxypropyl methylcellulose (Fleet Bisacodyl Prep)[OTC]. See Appendix A.

TIME/ACTION PROFILE (evacuation of bowel)

	ONSET	PEAK	DURATION
PO	6–12 hr	UK	UK
Rect	15–60 min	UK	UK

NURSING IMPLICATIONS

ASSESSMENT

▪ **General Info:** Assess patient for abdominal distention, presence of bowel sounds, and usual pattern of bowel function.
□ Assess color, consistency, and amount of stool produced.

POTENTIAL NURSING DIAGNOSES

▪ Constipation (Indications).
▪ Knowledge deficit, related to medication regimen (Patient/Family Teaching).

IMPLEMENTATION

▪ **General Info:** May be administered at bedtime for morning results.
▪ **PO:** Taking on an empty stomach will produce more rapid results.
□ Do not crush or chew enteric-coated tablets. Take with a full glass of water or juice.
□ Do not administer oral doses within 1 hr of milk or antacids; this may lead to premature dissolution of tablet and gastric or duodenal irritation.
▪ **Rect:** Suppository or enema can be given at the time a bowel movement is desired. Lubricate suppositories with water or water-soluble lubricant prior to insertion. Encourage patient to retain the suppository or enema 15–30 min before expelling.

PATIENT/FAMILY TEACHING

□ Advise patients, other than those with spinal cord injuries, that laxatives should be used only for short-term therapy. Prolonged therapy may cause electrolyte imbalance and dependence.
□ Advise patient to increase fluid intake to at

*CAPITALS indicate life-threatening; underlines indicate most frequent.

least 1500–2000 ml/day during therapy to prevent dehydration.

- □ Encourage patients to use other forms of bowel regulation (increasing bulk in the diet, increasing fluid intake, or increasing mobility). Normal bowel habits may vary from 3 times/day to 3 times/wk.
- □ Instruct patients with cardiac disease to avoid straining during bowel movements (Valsalva maneuver).
- □ Advise patient that bisacodyl should not be used when constipation is accompanied by abdominal pain, fever, nausea, or vomiting.

EVALUATION

Effectiveness of therapy can be demonstrated by: ▪ The patient's having a soft, formed bowel movement when used for constipation ▪ Evacuation of colon before surgery or radiologic studies, or for patients with spinal cord injury.

BISMUTH SUBSALICYLATE

(**bis**-muth sub-sa-**li**-si-late)

Bismatrol, Bismed, Pepto-Bismol, Pink Bismuth, {PMS-Bismuth Subsalicylate}

CLASSIFICATION(S):
Antidiarrheal

Pregnancy Category C

INDICATIONS

▪ Adjunctive therapy in the treatment of mild to moderate diarrhea ▪ Treatment of nausea, abdominal cramping, heartburn, and indigestion that may accompany diarrheal illnesses ▪ Used with anti-infectives in the treatment of ulcer disease associated with *Helicobacter pylori*. **Unlabeled Uses:** ▪ Treatment and prevention of traveler's (enterotoxigenic *Escherichia coli*) diarrhea.

ACTION

▪ Promotes intestinal adsorption of fluids and electrolytes ▪ Decreases synthesis of intestinal prostaglandins. **Therapeutic Effects:** ▪ Relief of diarrhea.

PHARMACOKINETICS

Absorption: Bismuth is not absorbed; salicylate split from parent compound is >90% absorbed from the small intestine. Salicylate is highly bound to albumin.

Distribution: Salicylate crosses the placenta and enters breast milk.

Metabolism and Excretion: Bismuth is excreted unchanged in the feces. Salicylate undergoes extensive hepatic metabolism.

Half-life: Salicylate—2–3 hr for low doses; 15–30 hr with larger doses.

CONTRAINDICATIONS AND PRECAUTIONS

Contraindicated in: ▪ Elderly patients who may be impacted ▪ Children or teenagers during or after recovery from chickenpox or flu-like illness (contains salicylate) ▪ Aspirin hypersensitivity; cross-sensitivity with NSAIDs or oil of wintergreen may occur.

Use Cautiously in: ▪ Infants, elderly, or debilitated patients (impaction may occur) ▪ Patients undergoing radiologic examination of the GI tract (bismuth is radiopaque) ▪ Pregnancy or lactation (safety not established; avoid chronic use of large doses) ▪ Diabetes mellitus ▪ Gout.

ADVERSE REACTIONS AND SIDE EFFECTS

GI: constipation, gray-black stools, impaction.

INTERACTIONS

Drug-Drug: ▪ If taken with **aspirin,** may potentiate signs of salicylate toxicity ▪ May decrease the absorption of **tetracycline** or **enoxacin** (chewable tablets only) ▪ May decrease the effectiveness of **probenecid** (large doses).

ROUTE AND DOSAGE

- **PO (Adults):** *Antidiarrheal*—524 mg q 30 min or 1048 or 1056 mg q 60 min as needed (not to exceed 4.2 g/24 hr). *Antiulcer*—524 mg 4 times daily.
- **PO (Children 9–12 yr):** 262 or 264 mg q 30–60 min (not to exceed 2.1 g/24 hr).
- **PO (Children 6–9 yr):** 174.6 or 176 mg q 30–60 min (not to exceed 1.4 g/24 hr).

- **PO (Children 3–6 yr):** 88 mg q 30–60 min (not to exceed 704 mg/24 hr).
- **PO (Children <3 yr weighing >13 kg):** 88 mg, may repeat q 4 hr (not to exceed 6 doses/24 hr).
- **PO (Children <3 yr weighing 6.4–8 kg):** 44 mg, may repeat q 4 hr (not to exceed 6 doses/24 hr).

AVAILABILITY

▪ ***Tablets:*** 262 mg[OTC] ▪ ***Chewable tablets:*** 262 mg (contain calcium carbonate)[OTC], {300 mg[OTC]} ▪ ***Liquid:*** 262 mg/15 ml[OTC], {264 mg/15 ml[OTC]}, 525 mg/15 ml[OTC] ▪ ***In combination with:*** kaolin/pectin (Kaodene Non-Narcotic)[OTC]. See Appendix A.

TIME/ACTION PROFILE (relief of diarrhea and other GI symptoms)

	ONSET	PEAK	DURATION
PO	within 24 hr	UK	UK

NURSING IMPLICATIONS

ASSESSMENT

- **Diarrhea:** Assess the frequency and consistency of stools, presence of nausea and indigestion, and bowel sounds prior to and throughout therapy.
- □ Assess patient's fluid and electrolyte balance and skin turgor for dehydration if diarrhea is prolonged.
- **Ulcers:** Assess patient for epigastric or abdominal pain and frank or occult blood in the stool, emesis, or gastric aspirate.
- ***Lab Test Considerations:*** Chronic high doses may cause falsely increased uric acid levels with colorimetric assay. May also cause increased or decreased urine vanillylmandelic acid (VMA) concentrations.
- □ May interfere with radiologic examination of the GI tract.
- □ May cause abnormal results with alkaline phosphatase, AST, and ALT tests.
- □ May cause decreased potassium levels and serum T_3 and T_4 concentrations.
- □ Large doses of salicylates may also cause prolonged prothrombin time (PT).
- □ For additional lab test considerations related to salicylate content, see salicylates, page 900.

POTENTIAL NURSING DIAGNOSES

- Diarrhea (Indications).
- Constipation (Side Effects).
- Knowledge deficit, related to medication regimen (Patient/Family Teaching).

IMPLEMENTATION

- **PO:** Shake liquid before using. Chewable tablets may be chewed or allowed to dissolve before swallowing.

PATIENT/FAMILY TEACHING

- **General Info:** Instruct patient to take medication exactly as directed.
- □ Inform patient that medication may temporarily cause stools and tongue to appear gray-black.
- □ Advise patient taking concurrent aspirin products that bismuth subsalicylate should be discontinued if ringing in the ears occurs.
- **Diarrhea:** Instruct patient to notify health care professional if diarrhea persists for more than 2 days or if accompanied by a high fever.
- □ Centers for Disease Control and Prevention warns against giving salicylates to children or adolescents with varicella (chickenpox) or influenza-like or viral illnesses because of a possible association with Reye's syndrome.
- **Ulcers:** Advise patient to consult health care professional prior to taking other OTC ulcer remedies concurrently with bismuth subsalicylate.

EVALUATION

Effectiveness of therapy can be demonstrated by: ▪ Decrease in diarrhea ▪ Decrease in symptoms of indigestion ▪ Prevention of traveler's diarrhea ▪ Treatment of ulcers.

BISOPROLOL

(bis-**oh**-pro-lole)
Zebeta

CLASSIFICATION(S):
Antihypertensive agent, Beta-adrenergic blocking agent (selective)

Pregnancy Category C

INDICATIONS

- Management of hypertension.

ACTION

▪ Blocks stimulation of $beta_1$ (myocardial) -adrenergic receptors. Does not usually affect $beta_2$ (pulmonary, vascular, uterine) -receptor sites. **Therapeutic Effects:** ▪ Decreased blood pressure and heart rate.

PHARMACOKINETICS

Absorption: Well absorbed following oral administration, but 20% undergoes first-pass hepatic metabolism.
Distribution: UK.
Metabolism and Excretion: 50% excreted unchanged by the kidneys; remainder renally excreted as metabolites; 2% excreted in feces.
Half-life: 9–12 hr.

CONTRAINDICATIONS AND PRECAUTIONS

Contraindicated in: ▪ Uncompensated congestive heart failure ▪ Pulmonary edema ▪ Cardiogenic shock ▪ Bradycardia or heart block.
Use Cautiously in: ▪ Renal impairment (dosage reduction recommended if CCr <40 ml/min) ▪ Hepatic impairment (dosage reduction recommended) ▪ Geriatric patients (increased sensitivity to beta-adrenergic blockers; initial dosage reduction recommended) ▪ Pulmonary disease (including asthma; $beta_1$ selectivity may be lost at higher doses) ▪ Diabetes mellitus (may mask signs of hypoglycemia) ▪ Thyrotoxicosis (may mask symptoms) ▪ Patients with a history of severe allergic reactions (intensity of reactions may be increased) ▪ Pregnancy, lactation, or children (safety not established; all agents cross the placenta and may cause fetal/neonatal bradycardia, hypotension, hypoglycemia, or respiratory depression).

ADVERSE REACTIONS AND SIDE EFFECTS*

CNS: fatigue, weakness, anxiety, depression, dizziness, drowsiness, insomnia, memory loss, mental status changes, nervousness, nightmares.
EENT: blurred vision, stuffy nose.
Resp: bronchospasm, wheezing.
CV: BRADYCARDIA, CONGESTIVE HEART FAILURE, PULMONARY EDEMA, hypotension, peripheral vasoconstriction.
GI: constipation, diarrhea, liver function abnormalities, nausea, vomiting.
GU: impotence, decreased libido, urinary frequency.
Derm: rashes.
Endo: hyperglycemia, hypoglycemia.
MS: arthralgia, back pain, joint pain.

INTERACTIONS

Drug-Drug: ▪ **General anesthesia, IV phenytoin,** and **verapamil** may cause additive myocardial depression ▪ Additive bradycardia may occur with **digitalis glycosides** ▪ Additive hypotension may occur with other **antihypertensives**, acute ingestion of **alcohol,** or **nitrates** ▪ Concurrent use with **amphetamines, cocaine, ephedrine, epinephrine, norepinephrine, phenylephrine,** or **pseudoephedrine** may result in unopposed alpha-adrenergic stimulation (excessive hypertension, bradycardia) ▪ Concurrent **thyroid** administration may decrease effectiveness ▪ May alter the effectiveness of **insulin** or **oral hypoglycemic agents** (dosage adjustments may be necessary) ▪ May decrease the effectiveness of **theophylline** ▪ May decrease the beneficial $beta_1$-cardiovascular effects of **dopamine** or **dobutamine** ▪ Use cautiously within 14 days of **MAO inhibitor** therapy (may result in hypertension).

ROUTE AND DOSAGE

- **PO (Adults):** 5 mg once daily, may be increased to 10 mg once daily (range 2.5–20 mg/day); start with 2.5 mg/day in patients with bronchospasm.

AVAILABILITY

▪ ***Tablets:*** 5 mg[Rx], 10 mg[Rx] ▪ ***In combination with:*** hydrochlorothiazide (Ziac)[Rx]. See Appendix A.

TIME/ACTION PROFILE (antihypertensive effect)

	ONSET	PEAK	DURATION
PO	UK	1–4 hr	24 hr

NURSING IMPLICATIONS

ASSESSMENT

- ▫ Monitor blood pressure, ECG, and pulse frequently during dosage adjustment period and periodically throughout therapy.
- ▫ Monitor intake and output ratios and daily

*CAPITALS indicate life-threatening; underlines indicate most frequent.

weights. Assess routinely for signs and symptoms of congestive heart failure (dyspnea, rales/crackles, weight gain, peripheral edema, jugular venous distention).
- Monitor frequency of prescription refills to determine compliance.
- ***Lab Test Considerations:*** May cause increased BUN, serum lipoprotein, potassium, triglyceride, and uric acid levels.
- May cause increased ANA titers.
- May cause increase in blood glucose levels.

POTENTIAL NURSING DIAGNOSES

- Cardiac output, decreased (Side Effects).
- Knowledge deficit, related to medication regimen (Patient/Family Teaching).
- Noncompliance, related to medication regimen (Patient/Family Teaching).

IMPLEMENTATION

- **PO:** Take apical pulse prior to administering. If <50 bpm or if arrhythmia occurs, withhold medication and notify physician or other health care professional.
- May be administered without regard to meals.

PATIENT/FAMILY TEACHING

- **General Info:** Instruct patient to take medication exactly as directed, at the same time each day, even if feeling well; do not skip or double up on missed doses. If a dose is missed, it should be taken as soon as possible up to 4 hr before next dose. Abrupt withdrawal may precipitate life-threatening arrhythmias, hypertension, or myocardial ischemia.
- Teach patient and family how to check pulse and blood pressure. Instruct them to check pulse daily and blood pressure biweekly and to report significant changes to health care professional.
- May cause drowsiness. Caution patients to avoid driving or other activities that require alertness until response to the drug is known.
- Advise patients to change positions slowly to minimize orthostatic hypotension.
- Caution patient that this medication may increase sensitivity to cold.
- Instruct patient to consult health care professional before taking any OTC medications, especially cold preparations, concurrently with this medication. Patients on antihypertensive therapy should also avoid excessive amounts of coffee, tea, and cola.
- Diabetics should closely monitor blood sugar, especially if weakness, malaise, irritability, or fatigue occurs. Medication does not block dizziness or sweating as signs of hypoglycemia.
- Advise patient to notify health care professional if slow pulse, difficulty breathing, wheezing, cold hands and feet, dizziness, lightheadedness, confusion, depression, rash, fever, sore throat, unusual bleeding, or bruising occurs.
- Instruct patient to inform health care professional of medication regimen prior to treatment or surgery.
- Advise patient to carry identification describing disease process and medication regimen at all times.
- **Hypertension:** Reinforce the need to continue additional therapies for hypertension (weight loss, sodium restriction, stress reduction, regular exercise, moderation of alcohol consumption, and smoking cessation). Medication controls but does not cure hypertension.

EVALUATION

Effectiveness of therapy can be demonstrated by: ■ Decrease in blood pressure.

BITOLTEROL
(bye-**tole**-ter-ole)
Tornalate

CLASSIFICATION(S):
Bronchodilator (adrenergic agonist)

Pregnancy Category C

INDICATIONS

■ Used as a quick-relief agent in the management of reversible airway disease due to asthma or COPD.

ACTION

■ Results in the accumulation of cyclic adenosine monophosphate (cAMP) at beta-adrenergic receptors ■ Produces bronchodilation ■ Inhibits the release of mediators of immediate hypersensitivity reactions from mast cells ■ Relatively selective for $beta_2$-adrenergic (pulmonary) receptor sites with less effect on $beta_1$ (cardiac)

-adrenergic receptors. **Therapeutic Effects:** ▪ Bronchodilation.

PHARMACOKINETICS

Absorption: Some absorption occurs following inhalation.
Distribution: Action is primarily local.
Metabolism and Excretion: Converted in the lungs to colterol, the active compound.
Half-life: UK.

CONTRAINDICATIONS AND PRECAUTIONS

Contraindicated in: ▪ Hypersensitivity to adrenergic amines ▪ Known hypersensitivity or intolerance to alcohol.
Use Cautiously in: ▪ Cardiac disease ▪ Hypertension ▪ Hyperthyroidism ▪ Diabetes ▪ Glaucoma ▪ Elderly patients (more susceptible to adverse reactions; may require dosage reduction) ▪ Excessive use may lead to tolerance and paradoxical bronchospasm ▪ Pregnancy (near term), lactation, and children <2 yr (safety not established).

ADVERSE REACTIONS AND SIDE EFFECTS*

CNS: nervousness, restlessness, tremor, headache, insomnia.
Resp: PARADOXICAL BRONCHOSPASM.
CV: angina, arrhythmias, hypertension, tachycardia.
GI: nausea, vomiting.
Endo: hyperglycemia.

INTERACTIONS

Drug-Drug: ▪ Concurrent use with other **adrenergic (sympathomimetic) agents** will have additive adrenergic side effects ▪ Use with **MAO inhibitors** may lead to hypertensive crisis ▪ **Beta-adrenergic blockers** may negate therapeutic effect.

ROUTE AND DOSAGE

- **Inhalation (Adults and Children ≥12 yr):** *Treatment*—2 inhalations (1–3 min apart), followed by an additional inhalation if needed (not to exceed 2 inhalations q 4 hr or 3 inhalations q 6 hr). *Prophylaxis*—2 inhalations q 8 hr (370 mcg/spray).

AVAILABILITY

- ***Metered-dose aerosol:*** 370 mcg/spray (≥300 inhalations/15-ml container)[Rx].

TIME/ACTION PROFILE (bronchodilation)

	ONSET	PEAK	DURATION
Inhaln	3–4 min	30–60 min	5–8 hr

NURSING IMPLICATIONS

ASSESSMENT

- □ Assess lung sounds, respiratory pattern, pulse, and blood pressure before administration and during peak of medication. Note amount, color, and character of sputum produced. Report abnormal findings.
- □ Monitor pulmonary function tests before initiating therapy and periodically throughout course to determine effectiveness of medication.
- □ Observe for paradoxical bronchospasm (wheezing). If condition occurs, withhold medication and notify physician or other health care professional immediately.
- □ Observe patient for drug tolerance and rebound bronchospasm. Patients requiring more than 3 inhalation treatments in 24 hr should be under close supervision. If minimal or no relief is seen after 3–5 inhalation treatments within 6–12 hr, further treatment with aerosol alone is not recommended.
- ▪ ***Lab Test Considerations:*** May cause decreased serum potassium concentrations, which are usually transient and dose related; rarely occurs at recommended doses and is more pronounced with frequent use of high doses.
- ▪ ***Toxicity and Overdose:*** Symptoms of overdose include persistent agitation, chest pain or discomfort, decreased blood pressure, dizziness, hyperglycemia, hypokalemia, seizures, tachyarrhythmias, persistent trembling, and vomiting.
- □ Treatment includes discontinuing beta-adrenergic agonists and symptomatic, supportive therapy. Cardioselective beta-adrenergic

*CAPITALS indicate life-threatening; underlines indicate most frequent.

blocking agents are used cautiously, as they may induce bronchospasm.

POTENTIAL NURSING DIAGNOSES

- Airway clearance, ineffective (Indications).
- Knowledge deficit, related to medication regimen (Patient/Family Teaching).

IMPLEMENTATION

- **Inhalation:** See Appendix H for use of the metered-dose inhaler.

PATIENT/FAMILY TEACHING

- Instruct patient to take medication exactly as directed. If on a scheduled dosing regimen, take a missed dose as soon as possible; space remaining doses at regular intervals. Do not double doses. Caution patient not to exceed recommended dose; may cause adverse effects, paradoxical bronchospasm, or loss of effectiveness of medication.
- Review correct administration technique with patient. See Appendix H for administration with metered-dose inhaler. Wait 1–5 min before administering next dose. Mouthpiece should be washed after each use. Do not spray inhaler near eyes.
- Instruct patient to use bronchodilator first if using other inhalation medications, and allow 5 min to elapse between administering other inhalation medications, unless otherwise directed.
- Advise patient to rinse mouth with water after each inhalation dose to minimize dry mouth.
- Instruct patient to maintain adequate fluid intake (2000–3000 ml/day) to help liquefy tenacious secretions.
- Advise patient to consult health care professional if respiratory symptoms are not relieved or worsen after treatment or if chest pain, headache, severe dizziness, palpitations, nervousness, or weakness occurs.
- Instruct patient to notify health care professional if contents of one canister are used up in less than 2 wk.
- Advise patient to save inhaler; refill canisters may be available.
- Advise patient to consult health care professional before taking any OTC medications or alcoholic beverages concurrently with this therapy. Caution patient also to avoid smoking and other respiratory irritants.

EVALUATION

Effectiveness of therapy can be demonstrated by: ▪ Relief of bronchospasm ▪ Increase in ease of breathing.

BLEOMYCIN

(blee-oh-**mye**-sin)

Blenoxane

CLASSIFICATION(S):

Antineoplastic (antitumor antibiotic)

Pregnancy Category D

INDICATIONS

▪ Treatment of: □ Lymphomas □ Squamous cell carcinoma □ Testicular embryonal cell carcinoma □ Choriocarcinoma □ Teratocarcinoma ▪ Intrapleural administration to prevent the reaccumulation of malignant effusions.

ACTION

▪ Inhibits DNA and RNA synthesis. **Therapeutic Effects:** ▪ Death of rapidly replicating cells, particularly malignant ones.

PHARMACOKINETICS

Absorption: Well absorbed from IM and SC sites. Absorption follows intrapleural and intraperitoneal administration.

Distribution: Widely distributed, concentrates in skin, lungs, peritoneum, kidneys, and lymphatics.

Metabolism and Excretion: 60–70% excreted unchanged by the kidneys.

Half-life: 2 hr (↑ in renal impairment).

CONTRAINDICATIONS AND PRECAUTIONS

Contraindicated in: ▪ Hypersensitivity ▪ Pregnancy or lactation.

Use Cautiously in: ▪ Renal impairment (dosage reduction required if CCr <35 ml/min) ▪ Pulmonary impairment ▪ Patients with childbearing potential ▪ Nonmalignant chronic debilitating illness ▪ Elderly patients (increased risk of pulmonary toxicity).

ADVERSE REACTIONS AND SIDE EFFECTS*

CNS: aggressive behavior, disorientation, weakness.
Resp: PULMONARY FIBROSIS, pneumonitis.
CV: hypotension, peripheral vasoconstriction.
GI: anorexia, nausea, stomatitis, vomiting.
Derm: hyperpigmentation, mucocutaneous toxicity, alopecia, erythema, rashes, urticaria, vesiculation.
Hemat: LEUKOPENIA, anemia, thrombocytopenia.
Local: pain at tumor site, phlebitis at IV site.
Metab: weight loss.
Misc: ANAPHYLACTOID REACTIONS, chills, fever.

INTERACTIONS

Drug-Drug: ▪ Hematologic toxicity increased with concurrent use of **radiation therapy** and other **antineoplastic agents** ▪ Concurrent use with **cisplatin** decreases elimination of bleomycin and may increase toxicity ▪ Increased risk of pulmonary toxicity with other **antineoplastic agents** or thoracic **radiation** ▪ **General anesthesia** increases the risk of pulmonary toxicity ▪ Increased risk of Raynaud's syndrome when used with **vinblastine.**

ROUTE AND DOSAGE

Lymphoma patients should receive initial test doses of 2 units or less for the first 2 doses.

- **IV, IM, SC (Adults and Children):** 0.25–0.5 unit/kg (10–20 units/m²) weekly or twice weekly initially. If favorable response, lower maintenance doses given (1 unit/day or 5 units/wk IM or IV). May also be given as continuous IV infusion at 0.25 unit/kg or 15 units/m²/day for 4–5 days.
- **Intrapleural (Adults):** 60 units instilled for 4 hr, then removed.

AVAILABILITY

- ***Injection:*** 15 units/vial[Rx].

TIME/ACTION PROFILE (tumor response)

	ONSET	PEAK	DURATION
IV, IM, SC	2–3 wk	UK	UK

NURSING IMPLICATIONS

ASSESSMENT

- □ Monitor vital signs prior to and frequently during therapy.
- □ Assess for fever and chills. May occur 3–6 hr after administration and last 4–12 hr.
- □ Monitor for anaphylactic (fever, chills, hypotension, wheezing) and idiosyncratic (confusion, hypotension, fever, chills, wheezing) reactions. Keep resuscitation equipment and medications on hand. Lymphoma patients are at particular risk for idiosyncratic reactions that may occur immediately or several hours after therapy, usually after the first or second dose.
- □ Assess respiratory status for dyspnea and rales/crackles. Chest x ray should be monitored prior to and periodically during therapy. Pulmonary toxicity occurs primarily in elderly patients (age 70 or older) who have received 400 or more units or at lower doses in patients having received other antineoplastics or thoracic radiation. May occur 4–10 wk after therapy. Discontinue and do not resume bleomycin if pulmonary toxicity occurs.
- □ Assess nausea, vomiting, and appetite. Weigh weekly. Modify diet as tolerated. Antiemetics may be given prior to administration.
- ▪ ***Lab Test Considerations:*** Monitor CBC prior to and periodically throughout therapy. May cause mild thrombocytopenia and leukopenia (nadir occurs in 2 wk).
- □ Monitor baseline and periodic renal and hepatic function.

POTENTIAL NURSING DIAGNOSES

- Injury, risk for (Side Effects).
- Body image disturbance (Side Effects).
- Knowledge deficit, related to medication regimen (Patient/Family Teaching).

IMPLEMENTATION

- ▪ **General Info:** Solution should be prepared in a biologic cabinet. Wear gloves, gown, and mask while handling medication. Discard equipment in specially designated containers (see Appendix I).
- □ Lymphoma patients should receive a 1- or 2-

***CAPITALS indicate life-threatening; underlines indicate most frequent.**

unit test dose 2–4 hrs prior to initiation of therapy. Monitor closely for anaphylactic reaction. May not detect reactors.

- □ Premedication with acetaminophen, steroids, and diphenhydramine may reduce drug fever and risk of anaphylaxis
- □ Reconstituted solution is stable for 24 hr at room temperature and for 14 days if refrigerated.
- ■ **IM, SC:** Reconstitute vial with 1–5 ml of sterile water for injection, 0.9% NaCl, or bacteriostatic water for injection. Do not reconstitute with diluents containing benzyl alcohol when used for neonates.
- ■ **Direct IV:** Prepare IV doses by diluting 15-unit vial with at least 5 ml of 0.9% NaCl.
- ■ ***Rate:*** Administer slowly over 10 min.
- ■ **Syringe Compatibility:** ■ cisplatin ■ cyclophosphamide ■ doxorubicin ■ droperidol ■ fluorouracil ■ furosemide ■ heparin ■ leucovorin calcium ■ methotrexate ■ metoclopramide ■ mitomycin ■ vinblastine ■ vincristine.
- ■ **Y-Site Compatibility:** ■ amifostine ■ aztreonam ■ cefepime ■ cisplatin ■ cyclophosphamide ■ doxorubicin ■ droperidol ■ filgrastim ■ fludarabine ■ fluorouracil ■ heparin ■ leucovorin calcium ■ melphalan ■ methotrexate ■ metoclopramide ■ mitomycin ■ ondansetron ■ paclitaxel ■ piperacillin/tazobactam ■ sargramostim ■ teniposide ■ thiotepa ■ vinblastine ■ vincristine ■ vinorelbine.
- ■ **Intrapleural:** Dissolve 60 units in 50–100 ml of 0.9% NaCl.
- □ May be administered through thoracostomy tube by physician. Position patient as directed.

PATIENT/FAMILY TEACHING

- □ Instruct patient to notify health care professional if fever, chills, wheezing, faintness, diaphoresis, shortness of breath, prolonged nausea and vomiting, or mouth sores occur.
- □ Encourage patient not to smoke, as this may worsen pulmonary toxicity.
- □ Explain to the patient that skin toxicity may manifest itself as skin sensitivity, hyperpigmentation (especially at skin folds and points of skin irritation), and skin rashes and thickening.
- □ Instruct patient to inspect oral mucosa for erythema and ulceration. If ulceration occurs, advise patient to use sponge brush and rinse mouth with water after eating and drinking. Opioid analgesics may be required if pain interferes with eating.
- □ Discuss with patient the possibility of hair loss. Explore coping strategies.
- □ Advise patient of the need for contraception.
- □ Instruct patient not to receive any vaccinations without advice of health care professional.
- □ Emphasize need for periodic lab tests to monitor for side effects.

EVALUATION

Effectiveness of therapy can be demonstrated by: ■ Decrease in tumor size without evidence of hypersensitivity or pulmonary toxicity.

B

BRETYLIUM

(bre-**till**-ee-yum)

{Bretylate}, Bretylol

CLASSIFICATION(S):

Antiarrhythmic (group III)

Pregnancy Category C

INDICATIONS

■ Treatment of ventricular tachycardia ■ Prophylaxis against ventricular fibrillation ■ Treatment of other serious ventricular arrhythmias resistant to lidocaine.

ACTION

■ Initially releases norepinephrine, then blocks its release ■ Also has positive inotropic effects. **Therapeutic Effects:** ■ Suppression of ventricular tachycardia and fibrillation.

PHARMACOKINETICS

Absorption: Well absorbed following IM administration.

Distribution: Reaches high concentration in areas of adrenergic innervation.

Metabolism and Excretion: Eliminated entirely unchanged by the kidneys.

Half-life: 5–10 hr (↑ in renal impairment).

CONTRAINDICATIONS AND PRECAUTIONS

Contraindicated in: ■ No significant contraindications.

{} = Available in Canada only.

Use Cautiously in: ▪ Suspected digitalis glycoside toxicity (increased risk of arrhythmias) ▪ Patients with fixed cardiac output (may produce severe hypotension requiring supportive therapy) ▪ Renal insufficiency (increased dosing interval recommended) ▪ Pregnancy, lactation, and children (safety not established).

ADVERSE REACTIONS AND SIDE EFFECTS*

CNS: dizziness, faintness.
EENT: nasal stuffiness.
CV: postural hypotension, angina, bradycardia, transient hypertension.
GI: nausea, vomiting, diarrhea.

INTERACTIONS

Drug-Drug: ▪ Combination with other **antiarrhythmics** may be additive or antagonistic ▪ Avoid using in suspected **digitalis glycoside** toxicity (initial release of norepinephrine may aggravate arrhythmias) ▪ Enhances actions of **adrenergic vasopressors** (dopamine, norepinephrine).

ROUTE AND DOSAGE

See infusion rate table in Appendix D.

❑ Ventricular Fibrillation/Ventricular Tachycardia

- **IV (Adults):** 5 mg/kg bolus over 15–30 sec initially; if no response, increase to 10 mg/kg, repeat as necessary (not to exceed 30 mg/kg/24 hr). For maintenance: 5–10 mg/kg q 6 hr or 1–2 mg/min continuous infusion.

❑ Other Ventricular Arrhythmias

- **IV (Adults):** 5–10 mg/kg q 1–2 hr; then q 6 hr as maintenance; may also be given as a continuous infusion at 1–2 mg/min.
- **IM (Adults):** 5–10 mg/kg, repeat q 1–2 hr if arrhythmia persists, then q 6–8 hr.

AVAILABILITY

▪ ***Injection:*** 50 mg/ml[Rx] ▪ ***Premixed injection in D5W:*** 1 mg/ml[Rx], 2 mg/ml[Rx], 4 mg/ml[Rx].

TIME/ACTION PROFILE (suppression of arrhythmias)

	ONSET	PEAK	DURATION
IM (VFib)	20–60 min	UK	6–24 hr
IM (VT, PVCs)	20 min–2 hr	6–9 hr	UK
IV (VFib)	5–10 min	end of infusion	6–24 hr
IV (VT, PVCs)	20 min–2 hr	UK	UK

NURSING IMPLICATIONS

ASSESSMENT

- ☐ Patients receiving this medication should be hospitalized in a unit where ECG and blood pressure can be constantly monitored. Assess patient for arrhythmias and changes in blood pressure frequently. A transient increase in arrhythmias and hypertension may occur within 1 hr after initial administration; may be decreased by slowing rate of administration.
- ☐ Assess patient frequently for orthostatic hypotension, keep supine until tolerance to hypotension develops (usually within several days). Instruct patient to change positions slowly; assist with ambulation. If systolic blood pressure <75 mm Hg or patient is symptomatic, notify physician. Dopamine, dobutamine, or norepinephrine, and volume replacement may be necessary.

POTENTIAL NURSING DIAGNOSES

- Cardiac output, decreased (Indications).
- Injury, risk for (Adverse Reactions).

IMPLEMENTATION

- **General Info:** Dosage should be reduced gradually and discontinued over 3–5 days with close ECG monitoring. Maintenance with an oral antiarrhythmic may be initiated.
- **IM:** Administer IM undiluted. Rotate injection sites frequently during IM injection to prevent atrophy and necrosis of muscle tissue caused by repeated injections. May repeat injection at 1–2 hr intervals if arrhythmia persists.
- **Direct IV:** For ventricular fibrillation, give IV undiluted; arrhythmia usually resolves within minutes. Employ usual resuscitative procedures, including CPR and electrical cardioversion, prior to and following injection.
- ***Rate:*** Administer over 15–30 sec.
- **Intermittent Infusion:** Dilute 500 mg in at least 50 ml of D5W, 0.9% NaCl, D5/0.45%

*CAPITALS indicate life-threatening; underlines indicate most frequent.

NaCl, D5/0.9% NaCl, D5/LR, ⅙ M sodium lactate, or lactated Ringer's solution.

- *Rate:* Administer over more than 8 min. More rapid infusion in the alert patient may cause nausea and vomiting.
- **Continuous Infusion:** Bretylium can be diluted in any amount of solution (1 g in 1000 ml equals 1 mg/ml).
- *Rate:* Infuse at 1–2 mg of diluted solution/min. Administer via infusion pump to ensure accurate dosage. (See Appendix D for Infusion Rate Table.)
- **Y-Site Compatibility:** ▪ amiodarone ▪ amrinone ▪ diltiazem ▪ dobutamine ▪ famotidine ▪ isoproterenol ▪ ranitidine.

PATIENT/FAMILY TEACHING

- ☐ Instruct patient to change positions slowly to minimize orthostatic hypotension.

EVALUATION

Clinical response to therapy can be evaluated by: ▪ Suppression of existing ventricular arrhythmias ▪ Prevention of additional arrhythmias.

BROMFENAC

(**brom**-fe-nak)

Duract

CLASSIFICATION(S):

Nonopioid analgesic/Nonsteroidal anti-inflammatory agent

Pregnancy Category C

INDICATIONS

▪ Short-term management of pain (not to exceed 10 days).

ACTION

▪ Inhibits prostaglandin synthesis, producing peripherally mediated analgesia ▪ Also has antipyretic and anti-inflammatory properties. **Therapeutic Effects:** ▪ Decreased pain.

PHARMACOKINETICS

Absorption: 67% absorbed following oral administration.

Distribution: UK.

Metabolism and Excretion: Entirely metabolized by the liver.

Half-life: 1.3 hr (increased in geriatric patients and severe hepatic impairment).

CONTRAINDICATIONS AND PRECAUTIONS

Contraindicated in: ▪ Hypersensitivity ▪ Cross-sensitivity with other NSAIDs may occur ▪ Lactation.

Use Cautiously in: ▪ History of GI bleeding ▪ Volume depletion, impaired renal or hepatic function, heart failure, geriatric patients, and patients receiving diuretics (increased risk of adverse renal reactions) ▪ History of asthma ▪ Coagulation disorders ▪ Pregnancy and children (use not recommended during 2nd half of pregnancy).

ADVERSE REACTIONS AND SIDE EFFECTS*

CNS: dizziness, drowsiness, headache, weakness.

CV: edema.

GI: GI BLEEDING, dyspepsia, abdominal pain, constipation, diarrhea, drug-induced hepatitis, eructation, flatulence, nausea, vomiting.

Hemat: anemia.

INTERACTIONS

Drug-Drug: ▪ Blood levels are increased by **cimetidine** ▪ May increase serum levels and risk of toxicity from **lithium** ▪ May increase the risk of bleeding with **warfarin** ▪ May decrease the effectiveness of **diuretics** or **antihypertensive** therapy.

Drug-Food: ▪ Concurrent administration with a **high-fat meal** decreases absorption.

ROUTE AND DOSAGE

- **PO (Adults):** 25 mg q 6–8 hr; may require 50 mg if taken with a high-fat meal (not to exceed 150 mg/day).

AVAILABILITY

- ***Capsules:*** 25 mg[Rx].

TIME/ACTION PROFILE (analgesic effect)

	ONSET	PEAK	DURATION
PO	within 30 min	2–3 hr	6–7 hr

*CAPITALS indicate life-threatening; underlines indicate most frequent.

NURSING IMPLICATIONS

ASSESSMENT

- □ Assess pain and limitation of movement; note type, location, and intensity prior to and 30–60 min following administration.
- □ Patients who have asthma, aspirin-induced allergy, and nasal polyps are at increased risk for developing hypersensitivity reactions.
- ▪ ***Lab Test Considerations:*** Bromfenac may prolong bleeding time and inhibit platelet aggregation for 24 hr after administration.
- □ May cause anemia.
- □ May cause elevated liver function tests.

POTENTIAL NURSING DIAGNOSES

- ▪ Pain (Indications).
- ▪ Knowledge deficit, related to medication regimen (Patient/Family Teaching).

IMPLEMENTATION

- ▪ **General Info:** Dose and frequency are determined by decrease in pain intensity following first dose and time to return of pain necessitating next dose.
- □ Administration in higher than recommended doses does not provide increased effectiveness but may increase side effects.
- ▪ **PO:** If bromfenac is administered with a high-fat meal, 50-mg dose may be needed.

PATIENT/FAMILY TEACHING

- □ Instruct patient to take bromfenac with a full glass of water and to remain in an upright position for 15–30 min after administration. Discuss need for dose modifications based on diet with patient.
- □ Caution patient to avoid concurrent use of alcohol, aspirin, acetaminophen, other NSAIDs, or other OTC medications without consulting health care professional.
- □ May cause drowsiness or dizziness. Caution patient to avoid driving or other activities requiring alertness until response to medication is known.
- □ Advise patient to consult health care professional if rash, itching, black stools, or influenza-like syndrome (chills, fever, muscle aches, pain) occurs.

EVALUATION

Effectiveness of therapy can be demonstrated by: ▪ Decrease in severity of mild to moderate pain.

BROMOCRIPTINE

(broe-moe-**krip**-teen)

Parlodel

CLASSIFICATION(S):

Anti-Parkinson agent (dopamine agonist)

Pregnancy Category UK

INDICATIONS

▪ Adjunct to levodopa in the treatment of parkinsonism ▪ Treatment of hyperprolactinemia (amenorrhea/galactorrhea), including associated female infertility ▪ Treatment of acromegaly. **Unlabeled Uses:** ▪ Management of pituitary prolactinomas ▪ Management of neuroleptic malignant syndrome.

ACTION

▪ Activates dopamine receptors in the CNS ▪ Decreases prolactin secretion. **Therapeutic Effects:** ▪ Relief of rigidity and tremor in parkinsonism ▪ Restoration of fertility in hyperprolactinemia ▪ Decreased growth hormone in acromegaly.

PHARMACOKINETICS

Absorption: Poorly absorbed (30%) from the GI tract.

Distribution: UK.

Metabolism and Excretion: Completely metabolized by the liver.

Half-life: Biphasic—initial phase 4–4.5 hr, terminal phase 45–50 hr.

CONTRAINDICATIONS AND PRECAUTIONS

Contraindicated in: ▪ Hypersensitivity to bromocriptine, ergot alkaloids, or bisulfites (capsules only) ▪ Severe cardiovascular disease or peripheral vascular disease ▪ Children <15 yr ▪ Lactation.

Use Cautiously in: ▪ Cardiac disease ▪ Mental disturbances ▪ May restore fertility (additional contraception may be required if pregnancy is undesirable) ▪ Severe liver impairment (dosage reduction required) ▪ Pregnancy (safety not established).

ADVERSE REACTIONS AND SIDE EFFECTS*

CNS: dizziness, confusion, drowsiness, hallucinations, headache, insomnia, nightmares.
EENT: burning eyes, nasal stuffiness, visual disturbances.
Resp: effusions, pulmonary infiltrates.
CV: MYOCARDIAL INFARCTION, hypotension.
GI: nausea, abdominal pain, anorexia, dry mouth, metallic taste, vomiting.
Derm: urticaria.
MS: leg cramps.
Misc: digital vasospasm (acromegaly only).

INTERACTIONS

Drug-Drug: ▪ Additive hypotension with **antihypertensives** ▪ Additive CNS depression with **antihistamines, alcohol, opioid analgesics,** and **sedative/hypnotics** ▪ Additive neurologic effects with **levodopa** ▪ Effective on prolactin levels, may be antagonized by **phenothiazines, haloperidol, methyldopa, tricyclic antidepressants,** and **reserpine.**

ROUTE AND DOSAGE

❑ Parkinsonism

- **PO (Adults):** 1.25 mg 1–2 times daily, increased by 2.5 mg/day in 2–4 wk intervals (range is 2.5–100 mg/day in divided doses; up to 40 mg/day have been used).

❑ Hyperprolactinemia

- **PO (Adults):** 1.25–2.5 mg/day initially, may be gradually increased q 3–7 days up to 2.5 mg 2–3 times daily.

❑ Acromegaly

- **PO (Adults):** 1.25–2.5 mg/day for 3 days, increase by 1.25–2.5 mg q 3–7 days until optimal response is obtained (usual range 10–30 mg/day; up to 100 mg/day).

❑ Pituitary Adenomas

- **PO (Adults):** 1.25 mg 2–3 times daily, may be increased over several weeks (range 2.5–20 mg/day).

❑ Neuroleptic Malignant Syndrome (Unlabeled)

- **PO (Adults):** 5 mg once daily initially, dosage increased as required up to 20 mg/day.

AVAILABILITY

▪ *Tablets:* 2.5 mg[Rx], 5 mg[Rx] ▪ *Capsules:* 5 mg[Rx].

TIME/ACTION PROFILE (suppression of various parameters)

	ONSET	PEAK	DURATION
PO†	30–90 min	1–2 hr	8–12 hr
PO‡	2 hr	8 hr	24 hr
PO§	1–2 hr	4–8 wk¶	4–8 hr

†Effect on parkinsonian symptoms.
‡Effect on serum prolactin levels.
§Effect on growth hormone.
¶During chronic therapy.

NURSING IMPLICATIONS

ASSESSMENT

- **General Info:** Assess patient for allergy to ergot derivatives.
- ❑ Monitor blood pressure prior to and frequently during drug therapy. Instruct patient to remain supine during and for several hours after 1st dose; severe hypotension may occur. Supervise ambulation and transfer during initial dosing to prevent injury from hypotension.
- **Parkinson's Disease:** Assess symptoms (restlessness or desire to keep moving, rigidity, tremors, pill rolling, mask-like face, shuffling gait, muscle spasms, twisting motions, difficulty speaking or swallowing, loss of balance control) prior to and throughout therapy.
- **Acromegaly:** Physical examination including ring size, heel pad thickness, and soft tissue volume should be assessed throughout therapy.
- **Hyperprolactinemia:** Sella turcica should be evaluated prior to therapy and yearly with computerized axial tomography (CAT) scan or magnetic resonance imaging (MRI) scan.
- **Neuroleptic Malignant Syndrome:** Monitor symptoms (fever, respiratory distress, tachycardia, convulsions, diaphoresis, hypertension, hypotension, pallor, tiredness) for improvement.

*CAPITALS indicate life-threatening; underlines indicate most frequent.

- *Lab Test Considerations:* May cause elevated serum BUN, AST, ALT, CPK, alkaline phosphatase, and uric acid levels; usually transient and clinically insignificant.
- *Female infertility:* Serum prolactin concentrations and anterior pituitary function should be measured prior to therapy. Ovulation should be monitored during therapy.
- *Acromegaly:* Serum growth hormone and insulin-like growth factor (IGF-I) concentrations should be monitored periodically during therapy.
- *Hyperprolactinemia:* Serum prolactin concentrations should be measured monthly during initial therapy and twice yearly during maintenance therapy to determine effectiveness of therapy.

POTENTIAL NURSING DIAGNOSES

- Physical mobility, impaired (Indications).
- Injury, risk for (Indications, Side Effects).
- Knowledge deficit, related to medication regimen (Patient/Family Teaching).

IMPLEMENTATION

- **General Info:** This medication is often given concurrently with levodopa or a levodopa-carbidopa combination in the treatment of Parkinson's disease.
- **PO:** Administer with food or milk to minimize gastric distress. Tablets may be crushed if patient has difficulty swallowing. Taking at bedtime may decrease nausea.

PATIENT/FAMILY TEACHING

- **General Info:** Instruct patient to take medication exactly as directed. If a dose is missed it should be taken within 4 hr of the scheduled dose or omitted. Do not double doses.
- May cause drowsiness and dizziness. Caution patients to avoid driving and other activities requiring alertness until response to medication is known.
- Caution patient to avoid concurrent use of alcohol during the course of therapy.
- Instruct patient to inform health care professional if increasing shortness of breath is noted; pulmonary infiltrates and pleural effusions may occur with long-term therapy.
- Advise women to consult with health care professional regarding a nonhormonal method of birth control. Women should contact health care professional promptly if pregnancy is suspected.
- Emphasize the importance of regular follow-up examinations to determine effectiveness and monitor side effects.
- **Infertility:** Instruct women treated for infertility to obtain daily basal body temperatures to determine when ovulation occurs.
- **Pituitary Tumors:** Instruct patients taking bromocriptine for pituitary tumors to inform health care professional immediately if signs of tumor enlargement (blurred vision, sudden headache, severe nausea, and vomiting) occur.

EVALUATION

Effectiveness of therapy can be demonstrated by: ■ Decrease in tremor, rigidity, and bradykinesia □ Improvement in balance and gait in patients with Parkinson's disease ■ Decrease in galactorrhea in patients with hyperprolactinemia ■ Resumption of normal ovulatory menstrual cycles with restoration of fertility (in patients with amenorrhea and galactorrhea, menses usually resume within 6–8 wk, and galactorrhea subsides within 8–12 wk) ■ Decreased serum levels of growth hormone in patients with acromegaly ■ Decrease in the symptoms of neuroleptic malignant syndrome.

BROMPHENIRAMINE

(brome-fen-**eer**-a-meen)

Bromphen, Chlorphed, Codimal-A, Conjec-B, Cophene-B, Dehist, Dimetane, Dimetapp Allergy Liqui-Gels, Histaject Modified, Nasahist B, ND Stat Revised, Oraminic II, Veltane

CLASSIFICATION(S):
Antihistamine

Pregnancy Category B

INDICATIONS

■ Symptomatic relief of allergic symptoms (rhinitis, urticaria) caused by histamine release ■ Severe allergic or hypersensitivity reactions, including anaphylaxis and transfusion reactions.

ACTION

■ Antagonizes the effects of histamine at H_1-receptor sites; does not bind to or inactivate histamine. **Therapeutic Effects:** ▪ Decreased symptoms of histamine excess (sneezing, rhinorrhea, nasal and ocular pruritus, ocular tearing and redness).

PHARMACOKINETICS

Absorption: Well absorbed following PO/IM administration.
Distribution: Widely distributed; minimal amounts excreted in breast milk; crosses the blood-brain barrier.
Metabolism and Excretion: Extensively metabolized by the liver.
Half-life: 12–35 hr.

CONTRAINDICATIONS AND PRECAUTIONS

Contraindicated in: ▪ Hypersensitivity ▪ Acute attacks of asthma ▪ Lactation (avoid use) ▪ Known alcohol intolerance (some elixirs).
Use Cautiously in: ▪ Narrow-angle glaucoma ▪ Liver disease ▪ Geriatric patients (more susceptible to adverse reactions; use lower initial dose) ▪ Pregnancy (safety not established).

ADVERSE REACTIONS AND SIDE EFFECTS*

CNS: drowsiness, sedation, dizziness, excitation (in children).
EENT: blurred vision.
CV: hypertension, arrhythmias, hypotension, palpitations.
GI: dry mouth, constipation, obstruction.
GU: retention, urinary hesitancy.
Derm: sweating.
Misc: hypersensitivity reaction (IV use).

INTERACTIONS

Drug-Drug: ▪ Additive CNS depression with other **CNS depressants** including **alcohol, opioids**, and **sedative/hypnotics** ▪ **MAO inhibitors** intensify and prolong the anticholinergic effects of antihistamines.

ROUTE AND DOSAGE

- **PO (Adults):** 4 mg q 4–6 hr daily as needed (not to exceed 24 mg/day), or 8 mg q 8–12 hr of extended-release tablets or 12 mg q 12 hr of extended-release tablets.
- **PO (Children 6–12 yr):** 2 mg q 4–6 hr as needed (not to exceed 12 mg/day) or 8–12 mg as extended-release tablets q 12 hr.
- **PO (Children 2–6 yr):** 1 mg q 4–6 hr as needed (not to exceed 6 mg/day).
- **SC, IM, IV (Adults):** 10 mg q 8–12 hr as needed (not to exceed 40 mg/day).
- **SC, IM, IV (Children):** 125 mcg (0.125 mg)/kg or 3.75 mg/m² 3–4 times daily as needed.

AVAILABILITY

▪ ***Tablets:*** 4 mg[Rx,OTC] ▪ ***Extended-release tablets:*** 8 mg[Rx,OTC], 12 mg[Rx,OTC] ▪ ***Capsules:*** 4 mg[Rx] ▪ ***Elixir:*** 2 mg/5 ml[Rx,OTC] ▪ ***Injection:*** 10 mg/ml[Rx].

TIME/ACTION PROFILE (relief of allergic symptoms)

	ONSET	PEAK	DURATION
PO	15–30 min	1–2 hr	6–8 hr†
SC, IM	20–30 min	UK	8–12 hr
IV	rapid	UK	8–12 hr

†Duration is longer (8–12 hr) for sustained-release oral preparations.

NURSING IMPLICATIONS

ASSESSMENT

- **Allergy:** Assess allergy symptoms (rhinitis, conjunctivitis, hives) prior to and periodically during therapy.
- ▫ Assess lung sounds and character of bronchial secretions. Maintain fluid intake of 1500–2000 ml/day to decrease viscosity of secretions.
- **Transfusion Reaction or Anaphylaxis:** Monitor for resolution of symptoms of allergic transfusion reaction or anaphylaxis (urticaria, wheezing, bronchospasm, hypotension). Monitor pulse and blood pressure prior to and throughout therapy.
- **IV:** Observe patient for sweating, hypotension, dizziness, drowsiness, or hypersensitivity reactions when administering medication intravenously. Elderly patients are more susceptible to side effects with this medication.
- ***Lab Test Considerations:*** May cause false negatives in allergy skin testing. Discontinue antihistamines at least 72 hr before testing.

*CAPITALS indicate life-threatening; underlines indicate most frequent.

POTENTIAL NURSING DIAGNOSES

- Airway clearance, ineffective (Indications).
- Injury, risk for (Adverse Reactions).
- Knowledge deficit, related to medication regimen (Patient/Family Teaching).

IMPLEMENTATION

- **PO:** Administer oral doses with food or milk to decrease GI irritation. Extended-release tablets should be swallowed whole; do not crush, break, or chew.
- **Direct IV:** May be given IV undiluted, but further dilution of each ml of 10 mg/ml solution with 10 ml of 0.9% NaCl for injection is recommended to reduce side effects.
- ***Rate:*** Administer each single dose slowly over at least 1 min.
- **Intermittent Infusion:** May be further diluted in 0.9% NaCl or D5W for IV infusion. The 100 mg/ml concentration is not recommended for IV use.

PATIENT/FAMILY TEACHING

- Instruct patient to take medication as directed; do not double doses.
- Commonly causes drowsiness. Caution patient to avoid driving or other activities requiring alertness until response to the medication is known.
- Advise patient to avoid taking alcohol or other CNS depressants concurrently with this drug.
- Frequent oral rinses, good oral hygiene, and sugarless gum or candy may help relieve dry mouth.
- Instruct patient to contact health care professional if symptoms persist.

EVALUATION

Effectiveness of therapy can be demonstrated by: ▪ Decrease in allergic symptoms.

BRONCHODILATORS (xanthines)

aminophylline
(am-in-**off**-i-lin)
Phyllocontin, Truphylline

dyphylline
(**dye**-fi-lin)
Dilor, Lufyllin, Dyflex-200, Neothylline

oxtriphylline
(ox-**trye**-fi-lin)
Choledyl, Choledyl SA

theophylline
(thee-**off**-i-lin)
Aerolate, {Apo-Theo LA}, Asmalix, Elixophyllin, Quibron-T, Respbid, Slo-Phyllin, Theochron, Theoclear, Theo-24, Theo-Dur, Theolair, Theo-Time, Theovent, Theo-X, T-Phyl, Uniphyl

CLASSIFICATION(S):
Bronchodilators

Pregnancy Category B

INDICATIONS

▪ Used as a bronchodilator in long-term control of reversible airway obstruction due to asthma or COPD. **Unlabeled Uses:** ▪ Respiratory and myocardial stimulant in apnea of infancy.

ACTION

▪ Inhibits phosphodiesterase, producing increased tissue concentrations of cyclic adenosine monophosphate (cAMP). Increased levels of cAMP result in: ▫ Bronchodilation ▫ CNS stimulation ▫ Positive inotropic and chronotropic effects ▫ Diuresis ▫ Gastric acid secretion. Aminophylline is a salt of theophylline and releases free theophylline following administration. **Therapeutic Effects:** ▪ Bronchodilation.

PHARMACOKINETICS

Absorption: Aminophylline and oxtriphylline release theophylline following administration. *Aminophylline*—well absorbed from oral dosage forms; absorption from extended-release dosage forms is slow but complete. *Dyphylline*—well absorbed (75%) following oral administration. *Oxtriphylline*—well absorbed following oral administration; absorption of enteric-coated and sustained-release forms may be delayed and unreliable. *Theophylline*—well

absorbed from PO dosage forms; absorption from extended-release dosage forms is slow but complete.
Distribution: *Aminophylline* and *oxtriphylline*—widely distributed as theophylline; cross the placenta; breast milk concentrations are 70% of plasma levels; not distributed into adipose tissue. *Dyphylline*—achieves high concentrations in breast milk. *Theophylline*—widely distributed; crosses the placenta; breast milk concentrations are 70% of plasma levels; does not distribute into adipose tissue.
Metabolism and Excretion: *Aminophylline, oxtriphylline,* and *theophylline*—aminophylline and oxytriphylline are converted to theophylline; theophylline is metabolized by the liver (90%) to caffeine, which may accumulate in neonates; metabolites are renally excreted; 10% excreted unchanged by the kidneys. *Dyphylline*—85% excreted unchanged by the kidneys.
Half-life: *Theophylline*—3–13 hr (increased in patients >60 yr, neonates, patients with congestive heart failure [CHF] or liver disease; decreased in cigarette smokers and children). *Dyphylline*—1.8–2.1 hr (increased in renal impairment).

CONTRAINDICATIONS AND PRECAUTIONS

Contraindicated in: ▪ Uncontrolled arrhythmias ▪ Hyperthyroidism.
Use Cautiously in: ▪ Elderly patients (>60 yr), CHF, or liver disease (dosage reduction required) ▪ Obese patients (dose should be based on ideal body weight) ▪ Has been used safely in pregnancy.

ADVERSE REACTIONS AND SIDE EFFECTS*

CNS: SEIZURES, anxiety, headache, insomnia.
CV: ARRHYTHMIAS, tachycardia, angina, palpitations.
GI: nausea, vomiting, anorexia, cramps.
Neuro: tremor.

INTERACTIONS

Drug-Drug: ▪ Additive CV and CNS side effects with **adrenergic (sympathomimetic) agents** ▪ May decrease the therapeutic effect of **lithium** ▪ **Nicotine (cigarettes, gum, transdermal patches), adrenergic agents, barbiturates, phenytoin, ketoconazole,** and **rifampin** may increase metabolism and may decrease effectiveness ▪ **Erythromycin, beta blockers, clarithromycin, cimetidine, influenza vaccination, oral contraceptives, glucocorticoids, disulfiram, fluvoxamine, interferon, mexiletine, thiabendazole, some fluoroquinolones,** and large doses of **allopurinol** decrease metabolism and may lead to toxicity ▪ Increased risk of arrhythmias with **halothane** ▪ **Isoniazid, carbamazepine,** and **loop diuretics** may increase or decrease theophylline levels.
Drug-Food: ▪ Excessive regular intake of **charcoal-broiled foods** may decrease effectiveness ▪ Excessive intake of **xanthine-containing foods** or **beverages (colas, coffee, chocolate)** may increase the risk of CV and CNS side effects.

ROUTE AND DOSAGE

Dose should be determined by theophylline serum level monitoring (not dyphylline). Loading dose should be decreased or eliminated if theophylline preparation has been used in preceding 24 hr. Aminophylline is 79–86% theophylline; oxtriphylline is 64% theophylline. Dyphylline is not a salt of theophylline. Extended-release (sustained-release) products may be given q 8–24 hr.

❑ Aminophylline/Theophylline

- **PO (Adults):** *Loading dose*—6 mg/kg, then 3 mg/kg q 6 hr for 2 doses, then 3 mg/kg q 8 hr maintenance dose (up to 13 mg/kg or 900 mg/day).
- **PO (Adults with CHF or Liver Disease):** *Loading dose*—6 mg/kg, then 2 mg/kg q 8 hr for 2 doses, then 1–2 mg/kg q 12 hr maintenance dose.
- **PO (Geriatric Patients and Patients with Cor Pulmonale):** 6 mg/kg loading dose, then 2 mg/kg q 6 hr for 2 doses, then 2 mg/kg q 8 hr maintenance dose.
- **PO (Children 9–16 yr or Young Adult Smokers):** *Loading dose*—6 mg/kg, then 3 mg/kg q 4 hr for 3 doses, then 3 mg/kg q 6 hr maintenance dose (up to 20 mg/kg/day in children 9–12 yr or 18 mg/kg/day in children 12–16 yr).
- **PO (Children 6 mo–9 yr):** *Loading*

***CAPITALS indicate life-threatening; underlines indicate most frequent.**

dose—4 mg/kg q 4 hr for 3 doses, then 4 mg/kg q 6 hr maintenance dose (up to 24 mg/kg/day).

- **PO, IV (Premature Neonates up to 40 wk postconception age):** 1 mg/kg q 12 hr.
- **PO, IV (Neonates at birth or 40 week postconception):** *Up to 4 wk postnatal age*—1–2 mg/kg q 12 hr; *4–8 wk postnatal age*—1–2 mg/kg q 8 hr; *over 8 wk postnatal age*—1–3 mg/kg q 6 hr.
- **IV (Adults):** *Loading dose*—4.7 mg/kg, then 0.55 mg/kg/hr for 12 hr, then 0.36 mg/kg/hr maintenance infusion rate.
- **IV (Adults with CHF or Liver Disease):** *Loading dose*—4.7 mg/kg, then 0.39 mg/kg/hr for 12 hr, then 0.08–0.16 mg/kg/hr maintenance infusion rate.
- **IV (Geriatric Patients and Patients with Cor Pulmonale)):** *Loading dose*—4.7 mg/kg, then 0.47 mg/kg/hr for 12 hr, then 0.24 mg/kg/hr maintenance infusion rate.
- **IV (Children 9–16 yr or Young Adult Smokers):** 4.7 mg/kg, then 0.79 mg/kg/hr for 12 hr, then 0.63 mg/kg/hr maintenance infusion rate.
- **IV (Children 6 mo–9 yr):** 4.7 mg/kg, then 0.95 mg/kg/hr for 12 hr, then 0.79 mg/kg/hr maintenance infusion rate.

❑ **Dyphylline**

- **PO (Adults):** Up to 15 mg/kg q 6 hr.
- **IM (Adults):** 250–500 mg q 6 hr (not to exceed 15 mg/kg/dose).

❑ **Oxtriphylline**

Daily dose may be divided and given as sustained-release (SA tablets) q 12 hr.

- **PO (Adults—Nonsmokers):** 4.7 mg/kg q 8 hr.
- **PO (Children 9–16 yr and Adult Smokers):** 4.7 mg/kg q 6 hr.
- **PO (Children 1–9 yr):** 6.2 mg/kg q 6 hr.

AVAILABILITY

❑ **Aminophylline**

▪ ***Tablets:*** 100 mgRx, 200 mgRx ▪ ***Enteric-coated tablets:*** 100 mgRx, 200 mgRx ▪ ***Extended-release tablets:*** 225 mgRx, {350 mgRx} ▪ ***Oral solution:*** 105 mg/5 mlRx ▪ ***Suppositories:*** 250 mgRx, 500 mgRx ▪ ***Injection:*** 250 mg/10 mlRx.

❑ **Dyphylline**

▪ ***Tablets:*** 200 mgRx, 400 mgRx ▪ ***Elixir:*** 33.3 mg/5 mlRx, 53.3 mg/5 mlRx ▪ ***Injection:*** 250 mg/mlRx.

❑ **Oxtriphylline**

▪ ***Tablets:*** 100 mgRx, 200 mgRx ▪ ***Sustained-release tablets:*** {400 mgRx}, {600 mgRx} ▪ ***Syrup:*** 50 mg/5 mlRx ▪ ***Elixir:*** 100 mg/5 mlRx.

❑ **Theophylline**

▪ ***Immediate-release tablets:*** 100 mgRx, 125 mgRx, 200 mgRx, 250 mgRx, 300 mgRx ▪ ***Timed-release tablets (8–12 hr):*** 100 mgRx, 200 mgRx, 250 mgRx, 300 mgRx, 500 mgRx ▪ ***Timed-release tablets (8–24 hr):*** 100 mgRx, 200 mgRx, 300 mgRx, 450 mgRx ▪ ***Timed-release tablets (12–24 hr):*** 100 mgRx, 200 mgRx, 300 mgRx ▪ ***Timed-release tablets (24 hr):*** 400 mgRx ▪ ***Immediate-release capsules:*** 100 mgRx, 200 mgRx ▪ ***Timed-release capsules (8–12 hr):*** 50 mgRx, 60 mgRx, 65 mgRx, 75 mgRx, 100 mgRx, 125 mgRx, 130 mgRx, 200 mgRx, 250 mgRx, 260 mgRx ▪ ***Timed-release capsules (12 hr):*** 50 mgRx, 125 mgRx, 130 mgRx, 250 mgRx, 260 mgRx ▪ ***Timed-release capsules (24 hr):*** 100 mgRx, 200 mgRx, 300 mgRx ▪ ***Syrup:*** 80 mg/15 mgRx, 150 mg/15 mlRx ▪ ***Elixir:*** 80 mg/15 mlRx ▪ ***Solution:*** 80 mg/15 mlRx, 150 mg/15 mlRx ▪ ***Injection (with dextrose):*** 0.4 mg/mlRx, 0.8 mg/mlRx, 1.6 mg/mlRx, 2 mg/mlRx, 3.2 mg/mlRx, 4 mg/mlRx.

TIME/ACTION PROFILE (bronchodilation)

	ONSET*	PEAK	DURATION
Aminophylline PO	15–60 min	1–2 hr	6–8 hr
Aminophylline PO–ER	UK	4–7 hr	8–12 hr
Aminophylline IV	rapid	end of infusion	6–8 hr
Dyphylline PO	UK	1 hr	6 hr
Dyphylline IM	UK	UK	UK
Oxtriphylline PO–liquid	UK	1 hr	UK
Oxtriphylline PO–tablet	15–60 min	5 hr	6–8 hr
Oxtriphylline PO–SA tablet	UK	4–7 hr	12 hr
Theophylline PO	rapid	1–2 hr	6 hr
Theophylline PO–ER	delayed	4–8 hr	8–24 hr
Theophylline IV	rapid	end of infusion	6–8 hr

*Provided a loading dose has been given and steady-state blood levels exist.

B

NURSING IMPLICATIONS

ASSESSMENT

- **General Info:** Assess blood pressure, pulse, respiratory status (rate, lung sounds, use of accessory muscles) prior to and throughout therapy. Ensure that oxygen therapy is correctly instituted during acute asthma attacks.
- □ Monitor intake and output ratios for an increase in diuresis or fluid overload.
- □ Patients with a history of cardiovascular problems should be monitored for chest pain and ECG changes (PACs, supraventricular tachycardia, PVCs, ventricular tachycardia). Resuscitative equipment should be readily available.
- □ Monitor pulmonary function tests before and periodically during therapy to determine therapeutic efficacy in patients with chronic bronchitis or emphysema.
- ***Lab Test Considerations:*** Monitor ABGs, acid-base, and fluid and electrolyte balance in patients receiving parenteral therapy or whenever required by patient's condition.
- ***Toxicity and Overdose:*** Monitor drug levels routinely, especially in patients requiring high doses or during prolonged intensive therapy. Serum sample should be obtained at time of peak absorption. Peak levels should be evaluated 15–30 min after IV loading dose, 1–2 hr after rapid-acting forms, and 4–12 hr after extended-release forms. Therapeutic plasma levels range from 5–15 mcg/ml. Drug levels in excess of 20 mcg/ml are associated with toxicity. Caffeine ingestion may falsely elevate drug concentration levels.
- □ Standard theophylline assays do not measure dyphylline concentrations.
- □ Observe patient for symptoms of drug toxicity (anorexia, nausea, vomiting, stomach cramps, diarrhea, confusion, headache, restlessness, flushing, increased urination, insomnia, tachycardia, arrhythmias, seizures). Notify physician or other health care professional immediately if these occur. Tachycardia, ventricular arrhythmias, or seizures may be the first sign of toxicity.

POTENTIAL NURSING DIAGNOSES

- Airway clearance, ineffective (Indications).
- Activity intolerance (Indications).
- Knowledge deficit, related to medication regimen (Patient/Family Teaching).

IMPLEMENTATION

- **General Info:** Administer around the clock to maintain therapeutic plasma levels. Once-a-day doses should be administered in the morning.
- □ Do not refrigerate elixirs, solutions, syrups, or suspensions, as crystals may form. Crystals should dissolve when liquid is warmed to room temperature.
- □ Wait at least 4–6 hr after stopping IV therapy to begin immediate-release oral dosage; for extended-release oral dosage form, give first oral dose at time of IV discontinuation.
- **PO:** Administer oral preparations with food or a full glass of water to minimize GI irritation. Food slows but does not reduce the extent of absorption. May be administered 1 hr before or 2 hr after meals for more rapid absorption. Use calibrated measuring device to ensure accurate dose of liquid preparations. Swallow tablets whole; do not crush, break, or chew enteric-coated or extended-release tablets (extended-release may be broken if scored).
- **IM:** Do not use if precipitate is present. May be caused by exposure to cold.
- □ Inject slowly; avoid IV administration.

□ **Aminophylline**

- **IV:** May be diluted in D5W, D10W, D20W, 0.9% NaCl, 0.45% NaCl, D5/0.9% NaCl, D5/0.45% NaCl, D5/0.25% NaCl, or lactated Ringer's solution. Mixture is stable for 24 hr if refrigerated.
- □ Do not administer discolored or precipitated solution. Flush main IV line prior to administration.
- □ If extravasation occurs, local injection of 1% procaine and application of heat may relieve pain and promote vasodilation.
- **Loading Dose:** Administer over 20–30 min.
- ***Rate:*** Do not exceed 20–25 mg/min. Administer via infusion pump to ensure accurate dosage. Rapid administration may cause chest pain, dizziness, hypotension, tachypnea, flushing, arrhythmias, or a reaction to the solution or administration technique (chills; fever; redness, pain, or swelling at injection site).
- **Continuous Infusion:** Usually given as a loading dose in a small volume followed by continuous infusion in larger volume.
- ***Rate:*** See Route and Dosage section for rates.

- **Syringe Compatibility:** ▪ heparin ▪ metoclopramide.
- **Syringe Incompatibility:** ▪ doxapram.
- **Y-Site Compatibility:** ▪ amifostine ▪ amrinone ▪ aztreonam ▪ cimetidine ▪ enalaprilat ▪ esmolol ▪ famotidine ▪ filgrastim ▪ fluconazole ▪ fludarabine ▪ foscarnet ▪ gallium nitrate ▪ labetalol ▪ melphalan ▪ morphine ▪ netilmicin ▪ paclitaxel ▪ pancuronium ▪ piperacillin/tazobactam ▪ potassium chloride ▪ ranitidine ▪ sargramostim ▪ tacrolimus ▪ teniposide ▪ thiotepa ▪ tolazoline ▪ vecuronium ▪ vitamin B complex with vitamin C.
- **Y-Site Incompatibility:** ▪ amiodarone ▪ ciprofloxacin ▪ diltiazem ▪ dobutamine ▪ hydralazine ▪ ondansetron ▪ vinorelbine.
- **Additive Incompatibility:** ▪ Admixing is not recommended because of dose titration and incompatibilities.

❑ Theophylline

- **Continuous Infusion:** IV theophylline and 5% dextrose are packed in a moisture-barrier overwrap. Remove immediately before administration and squeeze bag to check for leaks. Discard if solution is not clear.
- **Loading Dose:** ▪ Administer over 20–30 min. If patient has had another form of theophylline prior to loading dose, serum theophylline level should be obtained and loading dose proportionately reduced.
- ***Rate:*** Do not exceed 20–25 mg/min. Rapid administration may cause chest pain, dizziness, hypotension, tachypnea, flushing, arrhythmias, or a reaction to the solution or administration technique (chills; fever; redness, pain, or swelling at injection site). Infusion rate may be increased after 12 hr. Administer via infusion pump to ensure accurate dosage. Monitor ECG continuously, as tachyarrhythmias may occur.
- **Y-Site Compatibility:** ▪ acyclovir ▪ ampicillin ▪ ampicillin/sulbactam ▪ aztreonam ▪ cefazolin ▪ cefotetan ▪ ceftazidime ▪ cimetidine ▪ clindamycin ▪ dexamethasone ▪ diltiazem ▪ dobutamine ▪ dopamine ▪ doxycycline ▪ erythromycin lactobionate ▪ famotidine ▪ fluconazole ▪ gentamicin ▪ haloperidol ▪ heparin ▪ hydrocortisone sodium succinate ▪ lidocaine ▪ methyldopate ▪ methylprednisolone sodium succinate ▪ metronidazole ▪ nafcillin ▪ nitroglycerin ▪ nitroprusside ▪ penicillin G potassium ▪ piperacillin ▪ potassium chloride ▪ ranitidine ▪ ticarcillin ▪ ticarcillin/clavulanate ▪ tobramycin ▪ vancomycin.
- **Y-Site Incompatibility:** ▪ hetastarch ▪ phenytoin.
- **Additive Incompatibility:** ▪ Admixing is not recommended because of dose titration and incompatibilities.

PATIENT/FAMILY TEACHING

- □ Emphasize the importance of taking only the prescribed dose at the prescribed time intervals. Missed doses should be taken as soon as possible or omitted if close to next dose.
- □ Encourage the patient to drink adequate liquids (2000 ml/day minimum) to decrease the viscosity of the airway secretions.
- □ Advise patient to avoid OTC cough, cold, or breathing preparations without consulting health care professional. These medications may increase side effects and cause arrhythmias.
- □ Encourage patients not to smoke. A change in smoking habits may necessitate a change in dosage.
- □ Advise patient to minimize intake of xanthine-containing foods or beverages (colas, coffee, chocolate) and not to eat charcoal-broiled foods daily.
- □ Instruct patient not to change brands without consulting health care professional.
- □ Advise patient to contact health care professional promptly if the usual dose of medication fails to produce the desired results, symptoms worsen after treatment, or toxic effects occur.
- □ Emphasize the importance of having serum levels routinely tested every 6–12 mo.

EVALUATION

Effectiveness of therapy can be demonstrated by: ▪ Increased ease in breathing □ Clearing of lung fields on auscultation ▪ Respiratory and myocardial stimulation in apnea of infancy.

BUMETANIDE

(byoo-**met**-a-nide)
Bumex

CLASSIFICATION(S):
Diuretic (loop)

Pregnancy Category C

INDICATIONS

▪ Management of: ▫ Edema secondary to congestive heart failure ▫ Hepatic or renal disease. ▪ **Unlabeled Uses:** ▪ Treatment of hypertension.

ACTION

▪ Inhibits the reabsorption of sodium and chloride from the loop of Henle and distal renal tubule ▪ Increases renal excretion of water, sodium, chloride, magnesium, hydrogen, and calcium ▪ May have renal and peripheral vasodilatory effects ▪ Effectiveness persists in impaired renal function. **Therapeutic Effects:** ▪ Diuresis and subsequent mobilization of excess fluid (edema, pleural effusions) ▪ Lowering of blood pressure.

PHARMACOKINETICS

Absorption: Rapidly and completely absorbed after oral or IM administration.
Distribution: UK.
Metabolism and Excretion: Partially metabolized by the liver; 50% eliminated unchanged by the kidneys and 20% excreted in feces.
Half-life: 60–90 min.

CONTRAINDICATIONS AND PRECAUTIONS

Contraindicated in: ▪ Hypersensitivity ▪ Cross-sensitivity with thiazides and sulfonamides may exist ▪ Pre-existing uncorrected electrolyte imbalance, hepatic coma, or anuria.
Use Cautiously in: ▪ Severe liver disease accompanied by cirrhosis or ascites (may precipitate hepatic coma; concurrent use with potassium-sparing diuretics may be necessary) ▪ Electrolyte depletion ▪ Geriatric patients (difficulty assessing hearing status; increased risk of hypotension) ▪ Diabetes mellitus ▪ Increasing azotemia ▪ Pregnancy, lactation, or children (safety not established).

ADVERSE REACTIONS AND SIDE EFFECTS*

CNS: dizziness, encephalopathy, headache.
EENT: hearing loss, tinnitus.
CV: hypotension.
GI: constipation, diarrhea, dry mouth, dyspepsia, nausea, vomiting.
GU: excessive urination.
Derm: photosensitivity, rashes.
Endo: hyperglycemia.
F and E: dehydration, hypochloremia, hypokalemia, hypomagnesemia, hyponatremia, hypovolemia, metabolic alkalosis.
Metab: hyperglycemia, hyperuricemia.
MS: muscle cramps.
Misc: increased BUN.

INTERACTIONS

Drug-Drug: ▪ Additive hypotension with **antihypertensives** or **nitrates** ▪ Additive hypokalemia with other **diuretics, mezlocillin, piperacillin, amphotericin B,** and **glucocorticoids** ▪ Hypokalemia may increase **digitalis glycoside** toxicity ▪ Decreases **lithium** excretion, may cause toxicity ▪ Increased risk of ototoxicity with **aminoglycosides** ▪ May increase the effectiveness of **warfarin, thrombolytics** ▪ May increase the risk of hypomagnesemia with **amphotericin B.**

ROUTE AND DOSAGE

- **PO (Adults):** 0.5–2 mg/day as a single dose. Up to 2 additional doses may be given during the day q 4–5 hr (up to 10 mg/day). Alternate day or q 2–3 day regimens may also be used.
- **IM, IV (Adults):** 0.5–1 mg, may be repeated q 2–3 hr as needed (up to 10 mg/day).

AVAILABILITY

▪ ***Tablets:*** 0.5 mg[Rx], 1 mg[Rx], 2 mg[Rx] ▪ ***Injection:*** 0.25 mg/ml[Rx].

TIME/ACTION PROFILE

	ONSET	PEAK	DURATION
PO	30–60 min	1–2 hr	3–6 hr
IM	40 min	1–2 hr	4–6 hr
IV	within min	15–45 min	3–6 hr

NURSING IMPLICATIONS

ASSESSMENT

▫ Assess fluid status throughout therapy. Monitor daily weight, intake and output ratios, amount and location of edema, lung sounds,

*CAPITALS indicate life-threatening; underlines indicate most frequent.

skin turgor, and mucous membranes. Notify physician or other health care professional if thirst, dry mouth, lethargy, weakness, hypotension, or oliguria occurs.

- Monitor blood pressure and pulse before and during administration. Monitor frequency of prescription refills to determine compliance in patients treated for hypertension.
- Assess patients receiving digitalis glycosides for anorexia, nausea, vomiting, muscle cramps, paresthesia, and confusion. Patients taking digitalis glycosides are at increased risk of digitalis toxicity because of the potassium-depleting effect of the diuretic. Potassium supplements or potassium-sparing diuretics may be used concurrently to prevent hypokalemia.
- Assess patient for tinnitus and hearing loss. Audiometry is recommended for patients receiving prolonged high-dose IV therapy. Hearing loss is most common following rapid or high-dose IV administration in patients with decreased renal function or in those taking other ototoxic drugs.
- Assess for allergy to sulfonamides.
- ***Lab Test Considerations:*** Monitor electrolytes, renal and hepatic function, serum glucose and uric acid levels prior to and periodically throughout therapy. May cause decreased serum potassium, calcium, and magnesium concentrations. May also cause increased BUN, serum glucose, creatinine, and uric acid levels.
- May cause an increase in urinary phosphate concentrations.

POTENTIAL NURSING DIAGNOSES

- Fluid volume excess (Indications).
- Fluid volume deficit (Side Effects).
- Knowledge deficit, related to medication regimen (Patient/Family Teaching).

IMPLEMENTATION

- **General Info:** Administer medication in the morning to prevent disruption of sleep cycle.
- IV is preferred over IM for parenteral administration.
- **PO:** Administer orally with food or milk to minimize gastric irritation.
- **Direct IV:** Administer undiluted.
- ***Rate:*** Administer slowly over 2 min.
- **Intermittent Infusion:** Dilute in D5W, 0.9% NaCl, or lactated Ringer's solution, and administer through Y-tubing or 3-way stopcock. Use reconstituted solution within 24 hr.
- ***Rate:*** May be administered over 12 hr for patients with renal impairment.
- **Y-Site Compatibility:** ▪ amifostine ▪ aztreonam ▪ cefepime ▪ diltiazem ▪ filgrastim ▪ lorazepam ▪ melphalan ▪ meperidine ▪ morphine ▪ piperacillin/tazobactam ▪ teniposide ▪ thiotepa ▪ vinorelbine.

PATIENT/FAMILY TEACHING

- **General Info:** Instruct patient to take bumetanide exactly as directed. Missed doses should be taken as soon as possible; do not double doses.
- Caution patient to make position changes slowly to minimize orthostatic hypotension. Caution patient that the use of alcohol, exercise during hot weather, or standing for long periods may enhance orthostatic hypotension.
- Instruct patient to consult health care professional regarding a diet high in potassium (see Appendix K).
- Advise patient to consult health care professional before taking OTC medication concurrently with this therapy.
- Instruct patient to notify health care professional of medication regimen prior to treatment or surgery.
- Caution patient to use sunscreen and protective clothing to prevent photosensitivity reactions.
- Advise patient to contact health care professional immediately if muscle weakness, cramps, nausea, dizziness, numbness or tingling of extremities occurs.
- Emphasize the importance of routine follow-up exams.
- **Hypertension:** Advise patients on antihypertensive regimen to continue taking medication even if feeling better. Bumetanide controls but does not cure hypertension.
- Reinforce the need to continue additional therapies for hypertension (weight loss, exercise, restricted sodium intake, stress reduction, regular exercise, moderation of alcohol consumption, cessation of smoking).

EVALUATION

Effectiveness of therapy can be demonstrated by: ▪ Decrease in edema ▫ Increase in urinary output ▪ Decrease in blood pressure.

BUPRENORPHINE
(byoo-pre-**nor**-feen)
Buprenex

CLASSIFICATION(S):
Opioid analgesic (agonist/antagonist)

Schedule V
Pregnancy Category C

INDICATIONS

▪ Management of moderate to severe acute pain.

ACTION

▪ Binds to opiate receptors in the CNS ▪ Alters the perception of and response to painful stimuli, while producing generalized CNS depression ▪ Has partial antagonist properties that may result in opioid withdrawal in physically dependent patients. **Therapeutic Effects:** ▪ Decreased severity of pain.

PHARMACOKINETICS

Absorption: Well absorbed from IM sites.
Distribution: Crosses the placenta and enters breast milk. CNS concentration is 15–25% of plasma levels.
Metabolism and Excretion: Mostly metabolized by the liver.
Half-life: 2–3 hr.

CONTRAINDICATIONS AND PRECAUTIONS

Contraindicated in: ▪ Hypersensitivity.
Use Cautiously in: ▪ Increased intracranial pressure ▪ Severe renal, hepatic, or pulmonary disease ▪ Hypothyroidism ▪ Adrenal insufficiency ▪ Alcoholism ▪ Elderly or debilitated patients (dosage reduction required) ▪ Undiagnosed abdominal pain ▪ Prostatic hypertrophy ▪ Pregnancy, labor, lactation, or children <13 yr (safety not established).

ADVERSE REACTIONS AND SIDE EFFECTS*

CNS: confusion, dysphoria, hallucinations, sedation, dizziness, euphoria, floating feeling, headache, unusual dreams.
EENT: blurred vision, diplopia, miosis (high doses).
Resp: respiratory depression.
CV: hypertension, hypotension, palpitations.
GI: nausea, constipation, dry mouth, ileus, vomiting.
GU: urinary retention.
Derm: sweating, clammy feeling.
Misc: physical dependence, psychological dependence, tolerance.

INTERACTIONS

Drug-Drug: ▪ Use with extreme caution in patients receiving **MAO inhibitors** (increased CNS and respiratory depression and hypotension—decrease buprenorphine dose by 50%; may need to decrease MAO inhibitor dose) ▪ Additive CNS depression with **alcohol, antihistamines, antidepressants,** and **sedative/hypnotics** ▪ May decrease effectiveness of other **opioid analgesics.**

ROUTE AND DOSAGE

- **IM, IV (Adults):** 0.3 mg q 4–6 hr as needed. May repeat initial dose after 30 min (up to 0.3 mg q 4 hr or 0.6 mg q 6 hr); 0.6-mg doses should be given only IM.
- **IM, IV (Children 2–12 yr):** 2–6 mcg (0.002–0.006 mg)/kg q 4–6 hr.

AVAILABILITY

▪ ***Injection:*** 300 mcg (0.3 mg)/ml[Rx].

TIME/ACTION PROFILE (analgesia)

	ONSET	PEAK	DURATION
IM	15 min	60 min	6 hr†
IV	rapid	less than 60 min	6 hr†

†4–5 hr in children.

NURSING IMPLICATIONS

ASSESSMENT

□ Assess type, location, and intensity of pain prior to and 1 hr following IM and 5 min (peak) following IV administration. When titrating opioid doses, increases of 25–50% should be administered until there is either a 50% reduction in the patient's pain rating on a numerical or visual analogue scale or the

*CAPITALS indicate life-threatening; underlines indicate most frequent.

patient reports satisfactory pain relief. A repeat dose can be safely administered at the time of the peak if previous dose is ineffective and side effects are minimal. Single doses of 600 mcg (0.6 mg) should be administered IM. Patients requiring doses higher than 600 mcg (0.6 mg) should be converted to an opioid agonist. Buprenorphine is not recommended for prolonged use or as first-line therapy for acute or cancer pain.

- An equianalgesic chart (see Appendix B) should be used when changing routes or when changing from one opioid to another.
- Assess blood pressure, pulse, and respirations before and periodically during administration. If respiratory rate is <10/min, assess level of sedation. Dose may need to be decreased by 25–50%. Buprenorphine 0.3–0.4 mg has approximately equal analgesic and respiratory depressant effects to morphine 10 mg.
- Assess prior analgesic history. Antagonistic properties may induce withdrawal symptoms (vomiting, restlessness, abdominal cramps, increased blood pressure and temperature) in patients who are physically dependent on opioid agonists. Symptoms may occur up to 15 days after discontinuation and persist for 1–2 wk.
- Buprenorphine has a lower potential for dependence than other opioids; however, prolonged use may lead to physical and psychological dependence and tolerance. This should not prevent patient from receiving adequate analgesia. Most patients receiving buprenorphine for pain do not develop psychological dependence. If tolerance develops, changing to an opioid agonist may be required to relieve pain.
- ***Lab Test Considerations:*** May cause elevated serum amylase and lipase levels.
- ***Toxicity and Overdose:*** If an opioid antagonist is required to reverse respiratory depression or coma, naloxone (Narcan) is the antidote. Dilute the 0.4-mg ampule of naloxone in 10 ml of 0.9% NaCl and administer 0.5 ml (0.02 mg) by direct IV push every 2 min. For children and patients weighing <40 kg, dilute 0.1 mg of naloxone in 10 ml of 0.9% NaCl for a concentration of 10 mcg/ml and administer 0.5 mcg/kg every 1–2 min. Titrate dose to avoid withdrawal, seizures, and severe pain.

POTENTIAL NURSING DIAGNOSES

- Pain (Indications).
- Injury, risk for (Side Effects).

IMPLEMENTATION

- **General Info:** Explain therapeutic value of medication prior to administration to enhance the analgesic effect.
- Regularly administered doses may be more effective than prn administration. Analgesic is more effective if given before pain becomes severe.
- Coadministration with nonopioid analgesics has additive effects and may permit lower opioid doses.
- **IM:** Administer IM injections deep into well-developed muscle. Rotate sites of injections.
- **Direct IV:** May give IV undiluted. Administer slowly. Rapid administration may cause respiratory depression, hypotension, and cardiac arrest.
- **Syringe Compatibility:** ▪ midazolam.
- **Y-Site Compatibility:** ▪ amifostine ▪ filgrastim ▪ melphalan ▪ piperacillin/tazobactam ▪ teniposide ▪ thiotepa ▪ vinorelbine.
- **Solution Compatibility:** ▪ 0.9% NaCl ▪ D5W ▪ D5/0.9% NaCl ▪ lactated Ringer's injection ▪ Ringer's injection.

PATIENT/FAMILY TEACHING

- Instruct patient on how and when to ask for pain medication.
- Medication may cause drowsiness or dizziness. Advise patient to call for assistance when ambulating and to avoid driving or other activities requiring alertness until response to medication is known.
- Encourage patient to turn, cough, and deep breathe every 2 hr to prevent atelectasis.
- Instruct patient to change positions slowly to minimize orthostatic hypotension.
- Advise patient to avoid concurrent use of alcohol or other CNS depressants.
- Advise patient that good oral hygiene, frequent mouth rinses, and sugarless gum or candy may decrease dry mouth.

EVALUATION

Effectiveness of therapy can be demonstrated by: ▪ Decrease in severity of pain without a significant alteration in level of consciousness or respiratory status.

BUPROPION
(byoo-**proe**-pee-on)
Wellbutrin, Zyban

CLASSIFICATION(S):
Antidepressant, Smoking deterrent

Pregnancy Category B

INDICATIONS

▪ Treatment of depression, often in conjunction with psychotherapy (Wellbutrin) ▪ Smoking cessation (Zyban).

ACTION

▪ Decreases neuronal reuptake of dopamine in the CNS ▪ Diminished neuronal uptake of serotonin and norepinephrine (less than tricyclic antidepressants). **Therapeutic Effects:** ▪ Diminished depression ▪ Decreased craving for cigarettes.

PHARMACOKINETICS

Absorption: Although well absorbed, rapidy and extensively metabolized by the liver.
Distribution: UK.
Metabolism and Excretion: Extensively metabolized by the liver. Some conversion to active metabolites.
Half-life: 14 hr (active metabolites may have longer half-lives).

CONTRAINDICATIONS AND PRECAUTIONS

Contraindicated in: ▪ Hypersensitivity ▪ History of seizures, bulimia, and anorexia nervosa ▪ Concurrent MAO inhibitor therapy.
Use Cautiously in: ▪ History of cranial trauma ▪ Renal or hepatic impairment (dosage reduction recommended) ▪ Recent history of myocardial infarction ▪ Unstable cardiovascular status ▪ Pregnancy, lactation, or children (safety not established).

ADVERSE REACTIONS AND SIDE EFFECTS*

CNS: SEIZURES, agitation, headache, insomnia, mania, psychoses.
GI: dry mouth, nausea, vomiting, change in appetite, weight gain, weight loss.
Neuro: tremor.

INTERACTIONS

Drug-Drug: ▪ Increased risk of adverse reactions when used with **levodopa** or **MAO inhibitors** ▪ Increased risk of seizures with **phenothiazines, antidepressants,** cessation of **benzodiazepines,** or cessation of **alcohol.**

ROUTE AND DOSAGE

▪ **PO (Adults):** *Depression*—100 mg twice daily (morning and evening) initially; after 3 days may be increased to 100 mg 3 times daily; after 4 wk of therapy, may increase to a maximum daily dose of 450 mg/day in divided doses (no single dose to exceed 150 mg; wait at least 6 hr between doses at the 300 mg/day dose or at least 4 hr between doses at the 450 mg/day dose). *Smoking cessation*—150 mg once daily for 3 days, then 150 mg twice daily for 7–12 wk (doses should be at least 8 hr apart).

AVAILABILITY

▪ ***Tablets:*** 75 mg[Rx], 100 mg[Rx] ▪ ***Sustained-release tablets:*** 50 mg[Rx], 100 mg[Rx], 150 mg[Rx].

TIME/ACTION PROFILE (antidepressant effect)

	ONSET	PEAK	DURATION
PO	1–3 wk	UK	UK

NURSING IMPLICATIONS

ASSESSMENT

- Monitor mood changes. Inform physician or other health care professional if patient demonstrates significant increase in anxiety, nervousness, or insomnia.
- Assess for suicidal tendencies, especially during early therapy. Restrict amount of drug available to patient.
- ***Lab Test Considerations:*** Monitor hepatic and renal function closely in patients with kidney or liver impairment to prevent elevated serum and tissue bupropion concentrations.

*CAPITALS indicate life-threatening; underlines indicate most frequent.

POTENTIAL NURSING DIAGNOSES

- Coping, ineffective individual (Indications).
- Knowledge deficit, related to medication regimen (Patient/Family Teaching).

IMPLEMENTATION

- **General Info:** Administer doses in equally spaced time increments throughout day to minimize the risk of seizures.
  - May be initially administered concurrently with sedatives to minimize agitation. This is not usually required after the 1st wk of therapy.
  - Insomnia may be decreased by avoiding bedtime doses.
  - May be administered with food to lessen GI irritation.
  - Nicotine patches may be used concurrently with bupropion.
- **PO:** Tablets should be swallowed whole; do not break, crush, or chew.

PATIENT/FAMILY TEACHING

- Instruct patient to take bupropion exactly as directed. If a dose taken for depression is missed, take as soon as possible and space day's remaining doses evenly at not less than 4-hr intervals. Missed doses for smoking cessation should be omitted. Do not double doses or take more than prescribed. May require 4 wk or longer for full effects. Do not discontinue without consulting health care professional. May require gradual reduction prior to discontinuation.
- Bupropion may impair judgment or motor and cognitive skills. Caution patient to avoid driving and other activities requiring alertness until response to medication is known.
- Advise patient to avoid alcohol during therapy and to consult with health care professional before taking other medications with bupropion.
- Inform patient that frequent mouth rinses, good oral hygiene, and sugarless gum or candy may minimize dry mouth. If dry mouth persists for more than 2 wk, consult health care professional regarding use of saliva substitute.
- Advise patient to notify health care professional if rash or other troublesome side effects occur.
- Instruct female patients to inform health care professional if pregnancy is planned or suspected.
- Emphasize the importance of follow-up exams to monitor progress. Encourage patient participation in psychotherapy.
- **Smoking Cessation:** Smoking should be stopped during the 2nd week of therapy to allow for the onset of buproprion and to maximize the chances of quitting.

EVALUATION

Effectiveness of therapy can be demonstrated by: ▪ Increased sense of well-being ▫ Renewed interest in surroundings. Acute episodes of depression may require several months of treatment ▪ Cessation of smoking.

BUSPIRONE
(byoo-**spye**-rone)
BuSpar

CLASSIFICATION(S):
Antianxiety agent

Pregnancy Category B

INDICATIONS

- Management of anxiety.

ACTION

▪ Binds to serotonin and dopamine receptors in the brain ▪ Increases norepinephrine metabolism in the brain. **Therapeutic Effects:** ▪ Relief of anxiety.

PHARMACOKINETICS

Absorption: Rapidly absorbed.
Distribution: UK.
Metabolism and Excretion: Extensively metabolized by the liver; 20–40% excreted in feces.
Half-life: 2–3 hr.

CONTRAINDICATIONS AND PRECAUTIONS

Contraindicated in: ▪ Hypersensitivity.
Use Cautiously in: ▪ Patients receiving other antianxiety agents (other agents should be slowly withdrawn to prevent withdrawal or rebound phenomenon) ▪ Severe liver disease ▪ Patients

receiving other psychoactive drugs ▪ Pregnancy, lactation, and children (safety not established).

ADVERSE REACTIONS AND SIDE EFFECTS*

CNS: dizziness, drowsiness, excitement, fatigue, headache, insomnia, nervousness, weakness, personality changes.
EENT: blurred vision, nasal congestion, sore throat, tinnitus, altered taste or smell, conjunctivitis.
Resp: chest congestion, hyperventilation, shortness of breath.
CV: chest pain, palpitations, tachycardia, hypertension, hypotension, syncope.
GI: nausea, abdominal pain, constipation, diarrhea, dry mouth, vomiting.
GU: changes in libido, dysuria, urinary frequency, urinary hesitancy.
Derm: rashes, alopecia, blisters, dry skin, easy bruising, edema, flushing, pruritus.
Endo: irregular menses.
MS: myalgia.
Neuro: incoordination, numbness, paresthesia, tremor.
Misc: clamminess, sweating, fever.

INTERACTIONS

Drug-Drug: ▪ Use with **MAO inhibitors** may result in hypertension ▪ May increase the risk of hepatic effects from **trazadone** ▪ Avoid concurrent use with **alcohol.**

ROUTE AND DOSAGE

- **PO (Adults):** 5 mg 3 times daily, increase by 5 mg/day q 2–3 days as needed (not to exceed 60 mg/day). Usual dose is 20–30 mg/day.

AVAILABILITY

- ***Tablets:*** 5 mg[Rx], 10 mg[Rx].

TIME/ACTION PROFILE (relief of anxiety)

	ONSET	PEAK	DURATION
PO	7–10 days	3–4 wk	UK

NURSING IMPLICATIONS

ASSESSMENT

- **General Info:** Assess degree and manifestations of anxiety prior to and periodically throughout therapy.
- □ Buspirone does not appear to cause physical or psychological dependence or tolerance. However, patients with a history of drug abuse should be assessed for tolerance or dependence, and the amount of drug available to these patients should be restricted.

POTENTIAL NURSING DIAGNOSES

- Anxiety (Indications).
- Injury, risk for (Side Effects).
- Knowledge deficit, related to medication regimen (Patient/Family Teaching).

IMPLEMENTATION

- **General Info:** Patients changing from other antianxiety agents should receive gradually decreasing doses. Buspirone will not prevent withdrawal symptoms.
- **PO:** May be administered with food to minimize gastric irritation. Food slows but does not alter extent of absorption.

PATIENT/FAMILY TEACHING

- □ Instruct patient to take buspirone exactly as directed. If a dose is missed, take as soon as possible if not just before next dose; do not double doses. Do not take more than amount prescribed.
- □ May cause dizziness or drowsiness. Caution patient to avoid driving or other activities requiring alertness until response to the medication is known.
- □ Advise patient to avoid concurrent use of alcohol or other CNS depressants with this medication.
- □ Advise patient to consult health care professional before taking OTC medications with this drug.
- □ Instruct patient to notify health care professional if any chronic abnormal movements occur (dystonia, motor restlessness, involuntary movements of facial or cervical muscles) or if pregnancy is suspected.

*CAPITALS indicate life-threatening; underlines indicate most frequent.

□ Emphasize the importance of follow-up exams to determine effectiveness of medication.

EVALUATION

Effectiveness of therapy can be demonstrated by: ■ Increase in sense of well-being □ Decrease in subjective feelings of anxiety. Some improvement may be seen in 7–10 days. Optimal results take 3–4 wk of therapy. Buspirone is usually used for short-term therapy (3–4 wk). If prescribed for long-term therapy, efficacy should be periodically assessed.

BUSULFAN

(byoo-**sul**-fan)

Myleran

CLASSIFICATION(S):

Antineoplastic (alkylating agent)

Pregnancy Category D

INDICATIONS

■ Treatment of chronic myelogenous leukemia and bone marrow disorders.

ACTION

■ Disrupts nucleic acid function and protein synthesis (cell-cycle phase–nonspecific). **Therapeutic Effects:** ■ Death of rapidly growing cells, especially malignant ones.

PHARMACOKINETICS

Absorption: Rapidly absorbed from the GI tract.

Distribution: UK.

Metabolism and Excretion: Extensively metabolized by the liver.

Half-life: 2.5 hr.

CONTRAINDICATIONS AND PRECAUTIONS

Contraindicated in: ■ Hypersensitivity ■ Failure to respond to previous courses ■ Pregnancy or lactation.

Use Cautiously in: ■ Active infections ■ Decreased bone marrow reserve ■ Other chronic debilitating diseases ■ Patients with childbearing potential.

ADVERSE REACTIONS AND SIDE EFFECTS*

Resp: PULMONARY FIBROSIS.

GI: hepatitis, nausea, vomiting.

Derm: alopecia.

Endo: gonadal suppression, gynecomastia.

Hemat: <u>bone marrow depression.</u>

Metab: hyperuricemia.

INTERACTIONS

Drug-Drug: ■ Additive bone marrow suppression with other **antineoplastic agents** or **radiation therapy** ■ May decrease the antibody response to and risk of adverse reactions from **live virus vaccines.**

ROUTE AND DOSAGE

- **PO (Adults):** *Induction*—1.8 mg/m²/day or 60 mcg (0.06 mg)/kg/day until WBCs <15,000/mm³. Usual dose is 4–8 mg/day (range 1–12 mg/day). *Maintenance*—1–3 mg/day.
- **PO (Children):** 0.06–0.12 mg/kg/day or 1.8–4.6 mg/m²/day initially. Titrate dose to maintain WBC of approximately 20,000/mm³.

AVAILABILITY

■ ***Tablets:*** 2 mg[Rx].

TIME/ACTION PROFILE (effects on blood counts)

	ONSET	PEAK	DURATION
PO	1–2 wk	wks	up to 1 mo†

†Complete recovery may take up to 20 mo.

NURSING IMPLICATIONS

ASSESSMENT

□ Assess for signs of infection (fever, chills, sore throat, cough, hoarseness, lower back or side pain, difficult or painful urination). Notify physician if these symptoms occur.

□ Assess for bleeding (bleeding gums, bruising, petechiae, guaiac stools, urine, emesis). Avoid IM injections and rectal temperatures. Hold pressure on all venipuncture sites for at least 10 min.

□ Monitor intake and output ratios and daily weights. Report significant changes in totals.

*CAPITALS indicate life-threatening; <u>underlines</u> indicate most frequent.

- ▫ Monitor for symptoms of gout (increased uric acid, joint pain, lower back or side pain, swelling of feet or lower legs). Encourage patient to drink at least 2 liters of fluid each day. Allopurinol may be given to decrease uric acid levels. Alkalinization of urine may be ordered to increase excretion of uric acid.
- ▫ Anemia may occur. Monitor for increased fatigue, dyspnea, and orthostatic hypotension.
- ▫ Assess for pulmonary fibrosis (fever, cough, shortness of breath) periodically during and following therapy. Discontinue therapy at the first sign of pulmonary fibrosis. Usually occurs 8 mo–10 yr (average 4 yr) after initiation of therapy.
- ***Lab Test Considerations:*** Monitor CBC with differential and platelet count prior to and weekly during course of therapy. The nadir of leukopenia occurs within 10–15 days and nadir of white cell count at 11–30 days. Recovery usually occurs within 12–20 wk. Notify physician if WBC is <15,000 mm³ or if a precipitous drop occurs. Institute thrombocytopenia precautions if platelet count is <150,000/mm³. Bone marrow depression may be severe and progressive, with recovery taking 1 mo–2 yr after discontinuation of therapy.
- ▫ Monitor serum ALT, bilirubin, alkaline phosphatase, and uric acid prior to and periodically during therapy. May cause elevated uric acid levels.
- ▫ May cause false-positive cytology results of breast, bladder, cervix, and lung tissues.

POTENTIAL NURSING DIAGNOSES

- Body image disturbance (Side Effects).
- Injury, risk for (Side Effects).
- Infection, risk for (Side Effects).

IMPLEMENTATION

- **PO:** Administer at the same time each day. Administer on an empty stomach to decrease nausea and vomiting.

PATIENT/FAMILY TEACHING

- ▫ Instruct patient to take medication exactly as directed, at the same time each day, even if nausea and vomiting are a problem. Consult health care professional if vomiting occurs shortly after dose is taken. If a dose is missed, do not take at all; do not double doses.
- ▫ Advise patient to notify health care professional if fever; chills; dyspnea; persistent cough; sore throat; signs of infection; bleeding gums; bruising; petechiae; or blood in urine, stool, or emesis occurs. Caution patient to avoid crowds and persons with known infections. Instruct patient to use soft toothbrush and electric razor. Caution patient not to drink alcoholic beverages or take products containing aspirin or NSAIDs.
- ▫ Caution patient to avoid crowds and persons with known infections. Health care professional should be informed immediately if symptoms of infection occur.
- ▫ Discuss with patient the possibility of hair loss. Explore methods of coping.
- ▫ Review with patient the need for contraception during therapy. Women need to use contraception even if amenorrhea occurs.
- ▫ Instruct patient not to receive any vaccinations without advice of health care professional.
- ▫ Advise patient to notify health care professional if unusual bleeding; bruising; or flank, stomach, or joint pain occurs. Advise patients on long-term therapy to notify health care professional immediately if cough, shortness of breath, and fever occur or if darkening of skin, diarrhea, dizziness, fatigue, anorexia, confusion, or nausea and vomiting become pronounced.

EVALUATION

Effectiveness of therapy can be demonstrated by: ▪ Decrease in leukocyte count to within normal limits ▫ Decreased night sweats ▫ Increase in appetite ▫ Increased sense of well-being. Therapy is resumed when leukocyte count reaches 50,000/mm³.

BUTALBITAL COMPOUND
(byoo-**tal**-bi-tal)

butalbital, acetaminophen†
Bancap, Conten, Phrenilin, Phrenilin Forte, Sedapap, Tencon, Triaprin

butalbital, acetaminophen, caffeine†
Amaphen, Anolor-300, Anoquan, Arcet, Butace, Dolmar, Endolor, Esgic, Esgic-Plus, Ezol, Femcet, Fioricet, Isocet, Isopap, Medigesic,

Pacaps, Pharmagesic, Repan, Tencet, Triad, Two-Dyne

butalbital, aspirin‡
Axotal

butalbital, aspirin, caffeine‡
Butalgen, Fiorgen, Fiorinal, Fiormor, Fortabs, Isobutal, Isobutyl, Isollyl, Isolin, Lanorinal, Laniroif, Marnal, {Tecnal}, Vibutal

CLASSIFICATION(S):
Nonopioid analgesics with barbiturates

Schedule III
Pregnancy Category C

†For information on acetaminophen component of this formulation, see acetaminophen monograph on page 4.
‡For information on aspirin component of this formulation, see salicylates monograph on page 900.

INDICATIONS

▪ Management of mild to moderate pain.

ACTION

▪ Contain an analgesic (aspirin or acetaminophen) for relief of pain, a barbiturate (butalbital) for its sedative effect, and some contain caffeine, which may be of benefit in vascular headaches. **Therapeutic Effects:** ▪ Decreased severity of pain with some sedation.

PHARMACOKINETICS

Absorption: Well absorbed.
Distribution: Widely distributed; cross the placenta and enter breast milk.
Metabolism and Excretion: Mostly metabolized by the liver.
Half-life: 35 hr.

CONTRAINDICATIONS AND PRECAUTIONS

Contraindicated in: ▪ Hypersensitivity to individual components ▪ Cross-sensitivity may occur ▪ Comatose patients or those with pre-existing CNS depression ▪ Uncontrolled severe pain ▪ Pregnancy or lactation ▪ Aspirin should be avoided in patients with bleeding disorders or thrombocytopenia ▪ Acetaminophen should be avoided in patients with severe hepatic or renal disease ▪ Caffeine should be avoided in patients with severe cardiovascular disease.
Use Cautiously in: ▪ History of suicide attempt or drug addiction ▪ Chronic alcohol use/abuse (for aspirin and acetaminophen content) ▪ Geriatric patients (dosage reduction required) ▪ Use should be short-term only ▪ Children (safety not established).

ADVERSE REACTIONS AND SIDE EFFECTS*

CNS: *caffeine*—drowsiness, hangover, delirium, depression, excitation, headache (with chronic use), insomnia, irritability, lethargy, nervousness, vertigo.
Resp: respiratory depression.
CV: *caffeine*—palpitations, tachycardia.
GI: *caffeine*—constipation, diarrhea, epigastric distress, heartburn, nausea, vomiting.
Derm: dermatitis, rash.
Misc: hypersensitivity reactions including ANGIOEDEMA and SERUM SICKNESS, physical dependence, psychological dependence, tolerance.

INTERACTIONS

Drug-Drug: ▪ Additive CNS depression with other **CNS depressants**, including **alcohol, antihistamines, antidepressants, opioid analgesics,** and **sedative/hypnotics** ▪ May increase the liver metabolism and decrease the effectiveness of other drugs including **oral contraceptives, chloramphenicol, acebutolol, propranolol, metoprolol, timolol, doxycycline, glucocorticoids, tricyclic antidepressants, phenothiazines, phenylbutazone,** and **quinidine** ▪ **MAO inhibitors, primidone,** and **valproic acid** may prevent metabolism and increase the effectiveness of butalbital ▪ May enhance the hematologic toxicity of **cyclophosphamide.**

ROUTE AND DOSAGE

▪ **PO (Adults):** 1–2 capsules or tablets (50–100 mg butalbital) every 4 hr as needed for pain (not to exceed 4 g acetaminophen or aspirin/24 hr).

{} = Available in Canada only.
***CAPITALS indicate life-threatening; underlines indicate most frequent.**

AVAILABILITY

▪ ***Tablets and capsules***Rx: In combination with aspirin, acetaminophen, caffeine, and codeineRx. See Appendix A.

TIME/ACTION PROFILE

	ONSET	PEAK	DURATION
PO	15–30 min	1–2 hr	2–6 hr

NURSING IMPLICATIONS

ASSESSMENT

□ Assess type, location, and intensity of pain prior to and 60 min following administration.
□ Prolonged use may lead to physical and psychological dependence and tolerance. This should not prevent patient from receiving adequate analgesia. Most patients who receive butalbital compound for pain do not develop psychological dependence.
□ Assess frequency of use. Frequent, chronic use may lead to daily headaches in headache-prone individuals because of physical dependence on caffeine and other components. Chronic headaches from overmedication are difficult to treat and may require hospitalization for treatment and prophylaxis.

POTENTIAL NURSING DIAGNOSES

▪ Pain (Indications).
▪ Injury, risk for (Side Effects).

IMPLEMENTATION

▪ **General Info:** Explain therapeutic value of medication prior to administration to enhance the analgesic effect.
□ Regularly administered doses may be more effective than prn administration. Analgesic is more effective if given before pain becomes severe.
□ Medication should be discontinued gradually after long-term use to prevent withdrawal symptoms.
▪ **PO:** Oral doses should be administered with food, milk, or a full glass of water to minimize GI irritation.

PATIENT/FAMILY TEACHING

□ Instruct patient to take medication exactly as directed. Do not increase dose because of the habit-forming potential of butalbital. If medication appears less effective after a few weeks, consult health care professional. Severe and permanent liver damage may result from prolonged use or high doses of acetaminophen. Renal damage may occur with prolonged use of acetaminophen or aspirin. Doses of acetaminophen or aspirin should not exceed the maximum recommended daily dose.
□ Advise patients with vascular headaches to take medication at first sign of headache. Lying down in a quiet, dark room may also be helpful. Medications taken for prophylaxis should be continued.
□ Instruct patient on how and when to ask for pain medication.
□ May cause drowsiness or dizziness. Advise patient to avoid driving and other activities requiring alertness until response to medication is known.
□ Caution patient to avoid concurrent use of alcohol or other CNS depressants.
□ Advise patient to use an additional nonhormonal method of contraception while taking butalbital compound.

EVALUATION

Effectiveness of therapy can be demonstrated by: ▪ Decrease in severity of pain without a significant alteration in level of consciousness.

BUTORPHANOL

(byoo-**tor**-fa-nole)
Stadol, Stadol NS

CLASSIFICATION(S):
Opioid analgesic (agonist/antagonist)

Pregnancy Category C

INDICATIONS

▪ Management of moderate to severe pain ▪ Analgesia during labor ▪ Sedation prior to surgery ▪ Supplement in balanced anesthesia.

ACTION

▪ Binds to opiate receptors in the CNS ▪ Alters the perception of and response to painful stimuli, while producing generalized CNS depression ▪ Has partial antagonist properties that may result in opioid withdrawal in physically dependent patients. **Therapeutic Effects:** ▪ Decreased severity of pain.

PHARMACOKINETICS

Absorption: Well absorbed from IM sites and nasal mucosa.
Distribution: Crosses the placenta and enters breast milk.
Metabolism and Excretion: Mostly metabolized by the liver; 11–14% excreted in the feces. Minimal renal excretion.
Half-life: 3–4 hr.

CONTRAINDICATIONS AND PRECAUTIONS

Contraindicated in: ▪ Hypersensitivity ▪ Patients physically dependent on opioids who have not been detoxified (may precipitate withdrawal).
Use Cautiously in: ▪ Head trauma ▪ Increased intracranial pressure ▪ Severe renal, hepatic, or pulmonary disease (increase interval to q 6–8 hr initially in hepatic/renal impairment) ▪ Hypothyroidism ▪ Adrenal insufficiency ▪ Alcoholism ▪ Geriatric or debilitated patients (in geriatric patients, decrease usual dose by 50%; given at twice the usual interval initially) ▪ Undiagnosed abdominal pain ▪ Prostatic hypertrophy ▪ Pregnancy, lactation, or children <18 yr (safety not established but has been used during labor—may cause respiratory depression in the newborn).

ADVERSE REACTIONS AND SIDE EFFECTS*

CNS: confusion, dysphoria, hallucinations, sedation, euphoria, floating feeling, headache, unusual dreams.
EENT: blurred vision, diplopia, miosis (high doses).
Resp: respiratory depression.
CV: hypertension, hypotension, palpitations.
GI: nausea, constipation, dry mouth, ileus, vomiting.
GU: urinary retention.
Derm: sweating, clammy feeling.
Misc: physical dependence, psychological dependence, tolerance.

INTERACTIONS

Drug-Drug: ▪ Use with extreme caution in patients receiving **MAO inhibitors** (may produce severe, potentially fatal reactions—reduce initial dose of butorphanol to 25% of usual dose) ▪ Additive CNS depression with **alcohol, antihistamines, antidepressants,** and **sedative/hypnotics** ▪ May precipitate withdrawal in patients who are physically dependent on **opioids** and have not been detoxified ▪ May decrease effects of concurrently administered **opioid analgesics.**

ROUTE AND DOSAGE

- **IM (Adults):** 2 mg q 3–4 hr as needed (range 1–4 mg).
- **IV (Adults):** 1 mg q 3–4 hr as needed (range 0.5–2 mg).
- **IM, IV (Geriatric Patients):** 1 mg q 4–6 hr, increased as necessary.
- **Intranasal (Adults):** 1 mg (1 spray in one nostril) initially. An additional dose may be given 60–90 min later. This sequence may be repeated in 3–4 hr. If pain is severe, an initial dose of 2 mg (1 spray in each nostril) may be given. May be repeated in 3–4 hr.
- **Intranasal (Geriatric Patients):** 1 mg (1 spray in one nostril) initially. An additional dose may be given 90–120 min later. This sequence may be repeated in 3–4 hr.

AVAILABILITY

▪ ***Injection:*** 1 mg/ml^Rx, 2 mg/ml^Rx ▪ ***Intranasal solution:*** 10 mg/ml, in 2.5-ml metered-dose spray pump (14–15 doses; 1 mg/spray)^Rx.

TIME/ACTION PROFILE (analgesia)

	ONSET	PEAK	DURATION
IM	1–30 min	30–60 min	3–4 hr
IV	1 min	4–5 min	2–4 hr
Intranasal	within 15 min	1–2 hr	4–5 hr

NURSING IMPLICATIONS

ASSESSMENT

- ☐ Assess type, location, and intensity of pain prior to and 30–60 min following IM, 5 min following IV, and 60–90 min following intra-

*CAPITALS indicate life-threatening; underlines indicate most frequent.

nasal administration. When titrating opioid doses, increases of 25–50% should be administered until there is either a 50% reduction in the patient's pain rating on a numerical or visual analogue scale or the patient reports satisfactory pain relief. A repeat dose can be safely administered at the time of the peak if previous dose is ineffective and side effects are minimal. Patients requiring doses higher than 4 mg should be converted to an opioid agonist. Butorphanol is not recommended for prolonged use or as first-line therapy for acute or cancer pain.

- An equianalgesic chart (see Appendix B) should be used when changing routes or when changing from one opioid to another.
- Assess blood pressure, pulse, and respirations before and periodically during administration. If respiratory rate is <10/min, assess level of sedation. Dose may need to be decreased by 25–50%. Respiratory depression does not increase in severity, only in duration, with increased dosage.
- Assess prior analgesic history. Antagonistic properties may induce withdrawal symptoms (vomiting, restlessness, abdominal cramps, increased blood pressure and temperature) in patients who are physically dependent on opioid agonists.
- Butorphanol has a lower potential for dependence than other opioids; however, prolonged use may lead to physical and psychological dependence and tolerance. This should not prevent the patient from receiving adequate analgesia. Most patients receiving butorphanol for pain do not develop psychological dependence. If tolerance develops, changing to an opioid agonist may be required to relieve pain.
- ***Lab Test Considerations:*** May cause elevated serum amylase and lipase levels.
- ***Toxicity and Overdose:*** If an opioid antagonist is required to reverse respiratory depression or coma, naloxone (Narcan) is the antidote. Dilute the 0.4-mg ampule of naloxone in 10 ml of 0.9% NaCl and administer 0.5 ml (0.02 mg) by direct IV push every 2 min. For children and patients weighing <40 kg, dilute 0.1 mg of naloxone in 10 ml of 0.9% NaCl for a concentration of 10 mcg/ml and administer 0.5 mcg/kg every 1–2 min. Titrate dose to avoid withdrawal, seizures, and severe pain.

POTENTIAL NURSING DIAGNOSES

- Pain (Indications).
- Injury, risk for (Side Effects).
- Sensory-perceptual alterations: visual, auditory (Side Effects).
- Knowledge deficit, related to medication regimen (Patient/Family Teaching).

IMPLEMENTATION

- **General Info:** Explain therapeutic value of medication prior to administration to enhance the analgesic effect.
- Regularly administered doses may be more effective than prn administration. Analgesic is more effective if given before pain becomes severe.
- Coadministration with nonopioid analgesics may have additive analgesic effects and permit lower opioid doses.
- **IM:** Administer IM injections deep into well-developed muscle. Rotate sites of injections.
- **Direct IV:** May give IV undiluted.
- ***Rate:*** Administer over 3–5 min. Rapid administration may cause respiratory depression, hypotension, and cardiac arrest.
- **Syringe Compatibility:** ▪ atropine ▪ chlorpromazine ▪ cimetidine ▪ diphenhydramine ▪ droperidol ▪ fentanyl ▪ hydroxyzine ▪ meperidine ▪ methotrimeprazine ▪ metoclopramide ▪ midazolam ▪ morphine ▪ pentazocine ▪ perphenazine ▪ prochlorperazine ▪ promethazine ▪ scopolamine ▪ thiethylperazine.
- **Syringe Incompatibility:** ▪ dimenhydrinate ▪ pentobarbital.
- **Y-Site Compatibility:** ▪ allopurinol sodium ▪ amifostine ▪ aztreonam ▪ cefepime ▪ enalaprilat ▪ esmolol ▪ filgrastim ▪ fludarabine ▪ labetalol ▪ melphalan ▪ paclitaxel ▪ piperacillin/tazobactam ▪ sargramostim ▪ teniposide ▪ thiotepa ▪ vinorelbine.
- **Intranasal:** Administer 1 spray in nostril.

PATIENT/FAMILY TEACHING

- Instruct patient on how and when to ask for pain medication.
- Medication may cause drowsiness or dizziness. Advise patient to call for assistance when ambulating and to avoid driving or other activities requiring alertness until response to the medication is known.
- Encourage patient to turn, cough, and breathe deeply every 2 hr to prevent atelectasis.

- Instruct patient to change positions slowly to minimize orthostatic hypotension.
- Caution patient to avoid concurrent use of alcohol or other CNS depressants with this medication.
- Advise patient that good oral hygiene, frequent mouth rinses, and sugarless gum or candy may decrease dry mouth.
- **Intranasal:** Instruct patient on proper use of nasal spray. See package insert for detailed instructions. Instruct patient to replace protective clip and clear cover following use and to store the unit in the child-resistant container. Caution patient that medication should not be used by anyone other than for whom it was prescribed. Excess medication should be disposed of as soon as it is no longer needed. To dispose of, unscrew cap, rinse bottle and pump with water, and dispose of in waste can.
- If 2-mg dose is prescribed, administer additional spray in other nostril. May cause dizziness and dysphoria. Patient should remain recumbent following administration of 2-mg dose until response to medication is known.

EVALUATION

Effectiveness of therapy can be demonstrated by: ▪ Decrease in severity of pain without a significant alteration in level of consciousness or respiratory status.

CALCITONIN, human
(kal-si-**toe**-nin)
Cibacalcin

CALCITONIN, salmon
Calcimar, Miacalcin, Osteocalcin, Salmonine

CLASSIFICATION(S):
Electrolyte modifier (hypocalcemic), Hormone

Pregnancy Category C

INDICATIONS

▪ Treatment of Paget's disease of bone ▪ Adjunctive therapy for hypercalcemia ▪ Management of postmenopausal osteoporosis.

ACTION

▪ Decreases serum calcium by a direct effect on bone, kidney, and GI tract ▪ Promotes renal excretion of calcium. **Therapeutic Effects:** ▪ Decreased rate of bone turnover ▪ Lowering of serum calcium.

PHARMACOKINETICS

Absorption: Completely absorbed from IM and SC sites. Rapidly absorbed from nasal mucosa; absorption is 3% compared with parenteral administration.
Distribution: UK.
Metabolism and Excretion: Rapidly metabolized in kidneys, blood, and tissues.
Half-life: 70–90 min.

CONTRAINDICATIONS AND PRECAUTIONS

Contraindicated in: ▪ Hypersensitivity to salmon protein or gelatin diluent ▪ Pregnancy or lactation (use not recommended).
Use Cautiously in: ▪ Children (safety not established).

ADVERSE REACTIONS AND SIDE EFFECTS*

CNS: headaches.
EENT: *nasal only*—epistaxis, nasal irritation, rhinitis.
GI: *IM, SC*—nausea, vomiting, altered taste, diarrhea.
GU: *IM, SC*—urinary frequency.
Derm: rashes.
Local: injection site reactions.
MS: *nasal*—arthralgia, back pain.
Misc: allergic reactions including ANAPHYLAXIS, facial flushing, swelling, tingling, and tenderness in the hands.

INTERACTIONS

Drug-Drug: ▪ **Vitamin D** and **calcium supplements** will antagonize the calcium-lowering effect of calcitonin.

ROUTE AND DOSAGE

- **Calcitonin—Human**
- **SC (Adults):** *Paget's disease*—250–500 mcg/day; some patients may require 500 mcg only 2–3 times weekly.

*CAPITALS indicate life-threatening; underlines indicate most frequent.

❑ **Calcitonin—Salmon**

Precede therapy with 1-IU intradermal skin test.

- **IM, SC (Adults):** *Hypercalcemia*—4 IU/kg q 12 hr initially, can increase up to 8 IU/kg q 6 hr. *Osteoporosis*—100 IU/day. *Paget's disease*—100 IU/day initially, then may decrease to 50 IU q 2 days as maintenance dose.
- **Intranasal (Adults):** *Osteoporosis*—1 spray (200 IU) in alternating nostrils daily.

AVAILABILITY

❑ **Calcitonin—Human**

- ***Powder for injection:*** 500 mcg/vial[Rx].

❑ **Calcitonin—Salmon**

- ***Injection:*** 100 IU/ml[Rx], 200 IU/ml[Rx] ▪ ***Nasal spray:*** 200 IU/0.09 ml spray in 2-ml bottles[Rx].

TIME/ACTION PROFILE

	ONSET	PEAK	DURATION
IM, SC*	UK	2 hr	6–8 hr
Intranasal†	rapid	31–39 min	UK

*Effects on serum calcium.
†Serum levels of administered calcitonin.

NURSING IMPLICATIONS

ASSESSMENT

- ❑ Observe patient for signs of hypersensitivity (skin rash, fever, hives, anaphylaxis, serum sickness). Keep epinephrine, antihistamines, and oxygen nearby in the event of a reaction.
- ❑ Assess patient for signs of hypocalcemic tetany (nervousness, irritability, paresthesia, muscle twitching, tetanic spasms, convulsions) during the first several doses of calcitonin. Parenteral calcium, such as calcium gluconate, should be available in case of this event.
- ***Lab Test Considerations:*** Serum calcium and alkaline phosphatase should be monitored periodically throughout therapy. These levels should normalize within a few months of initiation of therapy.
- ❑ Urine hydroxyproline (24 hr) may be monitored periodically in patients with Paget's disease.

POTENTIAL NURSING DIAGNOSES

- Pain (Indications).
- Injury, risk for (Indications, Side Effects).
- Knowledge deficit, related to medication regimen (Patient/Family Teaching).

IMPLEMENTATION

- **General Info:** Assess for sensitivity to calcitonin-salmon by administering an intradermal test dose on the inner aspect of the forearm prior to initiating therapy. Test dose is prepared in a dilution of 10 IU/ml by withdrawing 0.05 ml in a tuberculin syringe and filling to 1 ml with 0.9% NaCl for injection. Mix well and discard 0.9 ml. Administer 0.1 ml and observe site for 15 min. More than mild erythema or wheal constitutes positive response.
- ❑ Store solution in refrigerator.
- **IM, SC:** Inspect injection site for the appearance of redness, swelling, or pain. Rotate injection sites. SC is the preferred route. Use IM route if dose exceeds 2 ml in volume. Use multiple sites to minimize inflammatory reaction.
- ❑ Do not administer solutions that are discolored or contain particulate matter.

PATIENT/FAMILY TEACHING

- **General Info:** Advise patient to take medication exactly as directed. If dose is missed and medication is scheduled for twice a day, take only if possible within 2 hr of correct time. If scheduled for daily dose, take only if remembered that day. If scheduled for every other day, take when remembered and restart alternate day schedule. If taking 1 dose 3 times weekly (Mon, Wed, Fri), take missed dose the next day and set each injection back 1 day; resume regular schedule the following week. Do not double doses.
- ❑ Instruct patient in the proper method of self-injection.
- ❑ Advise patient to report signs of hypercalcemic relapse (deep bone or flank pain, renal calculi, anorexia, nausea, vomiting, thirst, lethargy) or allergic response promptly.
- ❑ Reassure patient that flushing and warmth following injection are transient and usually last about 1 hr.
- ❑ Explain that nausea following injection tends to decrease even with continued therapy.
- ❑ Instruct patient to follow low-calcium diet if recommended by health care professional (see Appendix K). Women with postmenopausal osteoporosis should adhere to a diet high in calcium and vitamin D.
- **Osteoporosis:** Advise patients receiving calcitonin for the treatment of osteoporosis that

exercise has been found to arrest and reverse bone loss. The patient should discuss any exercise limitations with health care professional before beginning program.

- **Intranasal:** Instruct patient on correct use of nasal spray. Before first use, activate pump by holding upright and depressing white side arms down toward bottle 6 times until a fine spray is emitted. Following activation, place nozzle firmly in nostril with head in an upright position and depress the pump toward the bottle.
- □ Advise patient to notify health care professional if significant nasal irritation occurs.

EVALUATION

Effectiveness of therapy can be demonstrated by: ▪ Lowered serum calcium levels ▪ Decreased bone pain ▪ Slowed progression of postmenopausal osteoporosis. Significant increases in bone marrow density may be seen as early as a month after initiation of therapy.

CALCIUM SALTS

calcium acetate, 25% Ca or 12.6 mEq/g
(**kal**-see-um **ass**-e-tate)
Calphron, PhosLo

calcium carbonate, 40% Ca or 20 mEq/g
(**kal**-see-um **kar**-bo-nate)
Alka-Mints, Amitone, {Apo-Cal}, BioCal, Calcarb, Calci-Chew, Calciday, Calcilac, Calci-Mix, {Calcite}, {Calglycine}, Cal-Plus, {Calsan}, Caltrate, Chooz, Dicarbosil, Equilet, Gencalc, Liqui-Cal, Liquid Cal-600, Maalox Antacid Caplets, Mallamint, {Mylanta Lozenges}, Nephro-Calci, {Nu-Cal}, Os-Cal, Oysco, Oyst-Cal, Oystercal, Rolaids Calcium Rich, Titralac, Tums, Tums E-X

calcium chloride, 27% Ca or 13.6 mEq/g
(**kal**-see-um **kloh**-ride)

calcium citrate, 21% Ca or 12 mEq/g
(**kal**-see-um **si**-trate)
Citrical, Citrical Liquitab

calcium glubionate, 6.4% Ca or 3.2 mEq/g
(**kal**-see-um gloo-**bye**-oh-nate)
{Calcium-Sandoz}, Neo-Calglucon

calcium gluceptate, 8.2% Ca or 4.1 mEq/g
(**kal**-see-um **gloo**-sep-tate)

calcium gluconate, 9% Ca or 4.5 mEq/g
(**kal**-see-um **gloo**-koh-nate)
Kalcinate

calcium lactate, 13% Ca or 6.5 mEq/g
(**kal**-see-um **lak**-tate)

tricalcium phosphate, 39% Ca or 19.5 mEq/g
Posture

CLASSIFICATION(S):
Electrolytes

Pregnancy Category C, UK

INDICATIONS

▪ **PO, IV:** Treatment and prevention of hypocalcemia ▪ **PO:** Adjunct in the prevention of postmenopausal osteoporosis ▪ **IV:** Emergency treatment of hyperkalemia and hypermagnesemia and adjunct in cardiac arrest (calcium chloride, calcium gluconate, calcium glubionate) ▪ **Calcium carbonate:** May be used as an antacid ▪ **Calcium acetate:** Control of hyperphosphatemia in end-stage renal disease.

ACTION

▪ Essential for nervous, muscular, and skeletal systems ▪ Maintain cell membrane and capillary permeability ▪ Act as an activator in the transmission of nerve impulses and contraction of cardiac, skeletal, and smooth muscle ▪ Essential for bone formation and blood coagulation. **Therapeutic Effects:** ▪ Replacement of calcium

{} = Available in Canada only.

in deficiency states. Control of hyperphosphatemia in end-stage renal disease without promoting aluminum absorption (calcium acetate).

PHARMACOKINETICS

Absorption: Absorption from the GI tract requires vitamin D. IV administration results in complete bioavailability.
Distribution: Readily enters extracellular fluid. Crosses the placenta and enters breast milk.
Metabolism and Excretion: Excreted mostly in the feces; 20% eliminated by the kidneys.
Half-life: UK.

CONTRAINDICATIONS AND PRECAUTIONS

Contraindicated in: ▪ Hypercalcemia ▪ Renal calculi ▪ Ventricular fibrillation.
Use Cautiously in: ▪ Patients receiving digitalis glycosides ▪ Severe respiratory insufficiency ▪ Renal disease ▪ Cardiac disease.

ADVERSE REACTIONS AND SIDE EFFECTS*

CNS: syncope (IV only), tingling.
CV: CARDIAC ARREST (IV only), arrhythmias, bradycardia.
GI: constipation, nausea, vomiting.
GU: calculi, hypercalcuria.
Local: phlebitis (IV only).

INTERACTIONS

Drug-Drug: ▪ Hypercalcemia increases the risk of **digitalis glycoside** toxicity ▪ Chronic use with **antacids** in renal insufficiency may lead to milk-alkali syndrome ▪ Ingestion by mouth decreases the absorption of orally administered **tetracycline, fluoroquinolones, phenytoin,** and **iron salts** ▪ Excessive amounts may decrease the effects of **calcium channel blocking agents** ▪ May decrease the effectiveness of **atenolol** ▪ Concurrent use with **thiazide diuretics** may result in hypercalcemia ▪ May decrease the ability of **sodium polystyrene sulfonate** to decrease serum potassium.
Drug-Food: ▪ **Cereals, spinach,** or **rhubarb** may decrease the absorption of calcium supplements ▪ Calcium acetate should not be given concurrently with other calcium supplements.

ROUTE AND DOSAGE

Doses are expressed in mg, g, or mEq of calcium.

- **PO (Adults):** *Prevention of hypocalcemia, treatment of depletion, osteoporosis*—1–2 g/day. *Antacid*—0.5–1.5 g as needed (calcium carbonate only). *Hyperphosphatemia in end-stage renal disease (calcium acetate only)*—Amount necessary to control serum phosphate and calcium.
- **PO (Children):** *Supplementation*—45–65 mg/kg/day.
- **PO (Infants):** *Neonatal hypocalcemia*—50–150 mg/kg (not to exceed 1 g).
- **IV (Adults):** *Emergency treatment of hypocalcemia, cardiac standstill*—7–14 mEq. *Hypocalcemic tetany*—4.5–16 mEq; repeat until symptoms are controlled. *Hyperkalemia with cardiac toxicity*—2.25–14 mEq; may repeat in 1–2 min. *Hypermagnesemia*—7 mEq.
- **IV (Children):** *Emergency treatment of hypocalcemia*—1–7 mEq. *Hypocalcemic tetany*—0.5–0.7 mEq/kg 3–4 times daily.
- **IV (Infants):** *Emergency treatment of hypocalcemia*—<1 mEq. *Hypocalcemic tetany*—2.4 mEq/kg/day in divided doses.

AVAILABILITY

❑ Calcium Acetate

▪ ***Tablets:*** 250 mg (65 mg Ca)OTC, 667 mg (169 mg Ca)OTC, 668 mg (169 mg Ca)OTC, 1 g (250 mg Ca)OTC ▪ ***Capsules:*** 500 mg (125 mg Ca)OTC.

❑ Calcium Carbonate

▪ ***Tablets:*** 500 mg (200 mg Ca)OTC, 600 mg (240 mg Ca)OTC, 650 mg (260 mg Ca)OTC, 667 mg (266.8 mg Ca)OTC, 1 g (400 mg Ca)OTC, 1.25 g (500 mg Ca)OTC, 1.5 g (600 mg Ca)OTC ▪ ***Chewable tablets:*** 350 mg (300 mg Ca)OTC, 420 mg (168 mg Ca)OTC, 500 mg (200 mg Ca)OTC, 750 mg (300 mg Ca)OTC, 1 g (400 mg Ca)OTC, 1.25 g (500 mg Ca)OTC ▪ ***Gum tablets:*** 500 mg (200 mg Ca)OTC ▪ ***Capsules:*** 1.25 g (500 mg Ca)OTC ▪ ***Lozenges:*** 600 mg (240 mg Ca)OTC ▪ ***Oral suspension:*** 1.25 g (500 mg Ca)/5 mlOTC ▪ ***Powder:*** 6.5 g (2400 mg Ca)/packetOTC.

❑ Calcium Chloride

▪ ***Injection:*** 10% (1.36 mEq/ml)Rx.

*CAPITALS indicate life-threatening; underlines indicate most frequent.

▫ **Calcium Glubionate**

- ***Syrup:*** 1.8 g (115 mg Ca)/5 ml[OTC].

▫ **Calcium Gluceptate**

- ***Injection:*** 22% (0.9 mEq/ml)[Rx].

▫ **Calcium Gluconate**

- ***Tablets:*** 500 mg (45 mg Ca)[OTC], 650 mg (58.5 mg Ca)[OTC], 975 mg (87.75 mg Ca)[OTC], 1 g (90 mg Ca)[OTC] ▪ ***Injection:*** 10% (0.45 mEq/ml)[Rx].

▫ **Calcium Lactate**

- ***Tablets:*** 325 mg (42.45 mg Ca)[OTC], 650 mg (84.5 mg Ca)[OTC].

TIME/ACTION PROFILE (effects on serum calcium)

	ONSET	PEAK	DURATION
PO	UK	UK	UK
IV	immediate	immediate	0.5–2 hr

NURSING IMPLICATIONS

ASSESSMENT

- **Calcium Supplement/Replacement:** Observe patient closely for symptoms of hypocalcemia (paresthesia, muscle twitching, laryngospasm, colic, cardiac arrhythmias, Chvostek's or Trousseau's sign). Notify physician or other health care professional if these occur. Protect symptomatic patients by elevating and padding side rails and keeping bed in low position.
- ▫ Monitor blood pressure, pulse, and ECG frequently throughout parenteral therapy. May cause vasodilation with resulting hypotension, bradycardia, arrhythmias, and cardiac arrest. Transient increases in blood pressure may occur during IV administration, especially in the elderly or in patients with hypertension.
- ▫ Assess IV site for patency. Extravasation may cause cellulitis, necrosis, and sloughing.
- ▫ Monitor patient on digitalis glycosides for signs of toxicity.
- **Antacid:** When used as an antacid, assess for heartburn, indigestion, and abdominal pain. Inspect abdomen; auscultate bowel sounds.
- ***Lab Test Considerations:*** Monitor serum calcium or ionized calcium, chloride, sodium, potassium, magnesium, albumin, and parathyroid hormone (PTH) concentrations prior to and periodically throughout therapy for treatment of hypocalcemia.
- ▫ May cause decreased serum phosphate concentrations with excessive and prolonged use. When used to treat hyperphosphatemia in renal failure patients, monitor phosphate levels.
- ***Toxicity and Overdose:*** Observe patient for appearance of nausea, vomiting, anorexia, thirst, severe constipation, paralytic ileus, and bradycardia. Contact physician or other health care professional immediately if these signs of hypercalcemia occur.

POTENTIAL NURSING DIAGNOSES

- Nutrition, altered, less than body requirements (Indications).
- Injury, risk for, related to osteoporosis or electrolyte imbalance (Indications).
- Knowledge deficit, related to diet and medication regimen (Patient/Family Teaching).

IMPLEMENTATION

- **General Info:** Milligram doses of calcium chloride, calcium gluconate, and calcium gluceptate are not equal; do not confuse. Chloride and gluconate forms are stocked on most hospital crash carts. Physician should specify form of calcium desired. Doses should be expressed in mEq.
- ▫ In arrest situations, the use of calcium chloride is now limited to patients with hyperkalemia, hypocalcemia, and calcium channel blocker toxicity.
- **PO:** Administer calcium carbonate or phosphate 1–1.5 hr after meals and at bedtime. Chewable tablets should be well chewed before swallowing. Dissolve effervescent tablets in glass of water. Follow oral doses with a full glass of water, except when using calcium carbonate as a phosphate binder in renal dialysis. Administer calcium glubionate syrup before meals; may dilute in water or fruit juice for infants or children. Administer with meals for patients with hyperphosphatemia.
- **IM:** IM administration of calcium gluconate and calcium gluceptate may be tolerated in an emergency if IV administration is not feasible. For child, administer only in thigh. For adult, administer only in gluteal region. Do not administer calcium chloride IM.
- **IV:** IV solution should be warmed to body temperature and given through a small-bore needle in a large vein to minimize phlebitis. Do not administer through a scalp vein. May

cause cutaneous burning sensation, peripheral vasodilation, and drop in blood pressure. Patient should remain recumbent for 30–60 min following IV administration. Administer slowly. High concentrations may cause cardiac arrest.

- If infiltration occurs, discontinue IV. May be treated with application of heat, elevation, and local infiltration of normal saline, 1% procaine HCl, or hyaluronidase.
- Rapid administration may cause tingling, sensation of warmth, and a metallic taste. Halt infusion if these symptoms occur, and resume infusion at a slower rate when they subside.
- Do not administer solutions that are not clear or that contain a precipitate.

Calcium Chloride

- **Direct IV:** May be administered undiluted by IV push.
- **Intermittent/Continuous Infusion:** May be diluted with D5W, D10W, 0.9% NaCl, D5/0.25% NaCl, D5/0.45% NaCl, D5/0.9% NaCl, or D5/LR.
- ***Rate:*** Maximum rate for adults is 0.7–1.4 mEq/min (0.5–1 ml of 10% solution); for children, 0.5 ml/min.
- **Syringe Compatibility:** ▪ milrinone.
- **Y-Site Compatibility:** ▪ amrinone ▪ dobutamine ▪ epinephrine ▪ esmolol ▪ morphine ▪ paclitaxel.
- **Y-Site Incompatibility:** ▪ sodium bicarbonate.

Calcium Gluceptate

- **Direct IV:** May be administered undiluted.
- ***Rate:*** Administer at a rate not to exceed 2 ml (1.8 mEq)/min for adults, 0.5 ml (0.45 mEq)/min for children. In exchange transfusion for neonates, 0.5 ml (0.45 mEq) is given after each 100 ml of citrated blood.
- **Intermittent Infusion:** May be further diluted in D5W, D10W, 0.9% NaCl, 0.45% NaCl, D5/LR, or lactated Ringer's solution. Solution should be clear; do not use if crystals are present.
- ***Rate:*** Do not exceed 200 mg/min.

Calcium Gluconate

- **Direct IV:** Administer slowly by direct IV push.
- ***Rate:*** Maximum administration rate for adults is 1.5–2 ml/min.
- **Continuous Infusion:** May be further diluted in 1000 ml of D5W, D10W, D20W, D5/0.9% NaCl, 0.9% NaCl, D5/LR, or lactated Ringer's solution.
- ***Rate:*** Administer at a rate not to exceed 200 mg/min over 12–24 hr.
- **Syringe Incompatibility:** ▪ metoclopramide.
- **Y-Site Compatibility:** ▪ aldesleukin ▪ allopurinol sodium ▪ amifostine ▪ aztreonam ▪ cefazolin ▪ cefepime ▪ ciprofloxacin ▪ dobutamine ▪ enalaprilat ▪ epinephrine ▪ famotidine ▪ filgrastim ▪ labetalol ▪ melphalan ▪ midazolam ▪ netilmicin ▪ piperacillin/tazobactam ▪ potassium chloride ▪ sargramostim ▪ tacrolimus ▪ teniposide ▪ thiotepa ▪ tolazoline ▪ vinorelbine ▪ vitamin B complex with C.
- **Y-Site Incompatibility:** ▪ fluconazole ▪ indomethacin.

PATIENT/FAMILY TEACHING

- **General Info:** Instruct patient not to take enteric-coated tablets within 1 hr of calcium carbonate as this will result in premature dissolution of the tablets.
- Do not administer concurrently with foods containing large amounts of oxalic acid (spinach, rhubarb), phytic acid (brans, cereals), or phosphorus (milk or dairy products). Administration with milk products may lead to milk-alkali syndrome (nausea, vomiting, confusion, headache). Do not take within 1–2 hr of other medications if possible.
- Instruct patients on a regular schedule to take missed doses as soon as possible, then go back to regular schedule.
- Advise patient that calcium carbonate may cause constipation. Review methods of preventing constipation (increasing bulk in diet, increasing fluid intake, increasing mobility) and using laxatives. Severe constipation may indicate toxicity.
- Advise patient to avoid excessive use of beverages containing alcohol or caffeine or tobacco.
- **Calcium Supplement:** Encourage patients to maintain a diet adequate in vitamin D (see Appendix K).
- **Osteoporosis:** Advise patients that exercise has been found to arrest and reverse bone loss. Patient should discuss any exercise limitations with health care professional before beginning program.

C

EVALUATION

Effectiveness of therapy can be demonstrated by: ▪ Increase in serum calcium levels ▪ Decrease in the signs and symptoms of hypocalcemia ▪ Resolution of indigestion ▪ Control of hyperphosphatemia in patients with renal failure (calcium acetate only).

CAPSAICIN

(cap-**say**-sin)

{Axsam}, Capsin, Capzasin•P, Dolorac, No Pain-HP, Pain Doctor, Pain-X, R-Gel, Zostrix, Zostrix-HP

CLASSIFICATION(S):
Analgesic (topical)

Pregnancy Category UK

INDICATIONS

▪ Temporary management of pain due to rheumatoid arthritis and osteoarthritis ▪ Treatment of pain associated with postherpetic neuralgia or diabetic neuropathy. **Unlabeled Uses:** ▪ Treatment of postmastectomy pain syndrome ▪ Treatment of reflex sympathetic dystrophy syndrome.

ACTION

▪ May deplete and prevent the reaccumulation of a chemical (substance P) responsible for transmitting painful impulses from peripheral sites to the central nervous system. **Therapeutic Effects:** ▪ Relief of discomfort associated with peripheral painful syndromes.

PHARMACOKINETICS

Absorption: UK.
Distribution: UK.
Metabolism and Excretion: UK.
Half-life: UK.

CONTRAINDICATIONS AND PRECAUTIONS

Contraindicated in: ▪ Hypersensitivity to capsaicin or hot peppers ▪ Not for use near eyes or on open or broken skin.
Use Cautiously in: ▪ Pregnancy, lactation, or children <2 yr (safety not established).

ADVERSE REACTIONS AND SIDE EFFECTS

Resp: cough.
Derm: transient burning.

INTERACTIONS

Drug-Drug: ▪ None significant.

ROUTE AND DOSAGE

▪ **Topical (Adults and Children ≥2 yr):** Apply to affected areas 3–4 times daily.

AVAILABILITY

▪ ***Cream:*** 0.025%^{OTC}, 0.075%^{OTC} ▪ ***Gel:*** 0.05%^{OTC} ▪ ***Lotion:*** 0.025%^{OTC} ▪ ***Roll-on:*** 0.075%^{OTC}.

TIME/ACTION PROFILE

	ONSET	PEAK	DURATION
Top	1–2 wk	2–4 wk*	UK

*May take up to 6 wk for head and neck neuralgias.

NURSING IMPLICATIONS

ASSESSMENT

□ Assess pain intensity and location prior to and periodically throughout therapy.

POTENTIAL NURSING DIAGNOSES

▪ Pain, chronic (Indications).
▪ Knowledge deficit, related to medication regimen (Patient/Family Teaching).

IMPLEMENTATION

▪ **Topical:** Apply to affected area not more than 3–4 times daily. Avoid getting medication into eyes or on broken or irritated skin. Do not bandage tightly.
□ Topical lidocaine may be applied during the first 1–2 wk of treatment to reduce initial discomfort.

PATIENT/FAMILY TEACHING

□ Instruct patient on the correct method for application of capsaicin. Rub cream into affected area well so that little or no cream is left on the surface. Gloves should be worn during application or hands should be washed immediately after application. If application is to

hands for arthritis, do not wash hands for at least 30 min following application.
- □ Advise patient to apply missed doses as soon as possible unless almost time for next dose. Pain relief lasts only as long as capsaicin is used regularly.
- □ Advise patient that transient burning may occur with application, especially if applied fewer than 3–4 times daily. Burning usually disappears after the first few days but may continue for 2–4 wk or longer. Burning is increased by heat, sweating, bathing in warm water, humidity, and clothing. Burning usually decreases in frequency and intensity the longer capsaicin is used. Decreasing number of daily doses will not lessen burning but may decrease amount of pain relief and may prolong period of burning.
- □ Caution patient to flush with water if capsaicin gets into eyes and to wash with warm, but not hot, soapy water if capsaicin gets on other sensitive areas of the body.
- □ Instruct patient with herpes zoster (shingles) not to apply capsaicin cream until lesions have healed completely.
- □ Advise patient to discontinue use and notify health care professional if pain persists longer than 1 month, worsens, or if signs of infection are present.

EVALUATION

Effectiveness of therapy can be demonstrated by: ▪ Decrease in discomfort associated with: □ Postherpetic neuropathy □ Diabetic neuropathy □ Rheumatoid arthritis □ Osteoarthritis. Pain relief usually begins within 1–2 wk with arthritis, 2–4 wk with neuralgias, and 4–6 wk with neuralgias of the head and neck.

CARBAMAZEPINE

(kar-ba-**maz**-e-peen)

{Apo-Carbamazepine}, Atretol, Carbatrol, Epitol, {Novo-Carbamaz}, Tegretol, {Tegretol CR}, Tegretol-XR

CLASSIFICATION(S):
Anticonvulsant

Pregnancy Category C

INDICATIONS

▪ Prophylaxis of tonic-clonic, mixed, and complex-partial seizures ▪ Management of pain in trigeminal neuralgia. **Unlabeled Uses:** ▪ Other forms of neurogenic pain.

ACTION

▪ Decreases synaptic transmission in the CNS by affecting sodium channels in neurons. **Therapeutic Effects:** ▪ Prevention of seizures ▪ Relief of pain in trigeminal neuralgia.

PHARMACOKINETICS

Absorption: Absorption is slow but complete. Suspension produces earlier, higher peak and lower trough levels.
Distribution: Widely distributed. Crosses the blood-brain barrier. Crosses the placenta and enters breast milk in high concentrations.
Metabolism and Excretion: Extensively metabolized by the liver; epoxide metabolite has anticonvulsant and antineuralgic activity.
Half-life: *Carbamazapine*—single dose—25–65 hr, chronic dosing—8–29 hr; *epoxide*—5–8 hr.

CONTRAINDICATIONS AND PRECAUTIONS

Contraindicated in: ▪ Hypersensitivity ▪ Bone marrow depression.
Use Cautiously in: ▪ Cardiac disease ▪ Hepatic disease ▪ Elderly men with prostatic hypertrophy ▪ Increased intraocular pressure ▪ Pregnancy and lactation (safety not established).

ADVERSE REACTIONS AND SIDE EFFECTS*

CNS: <u>ataxia</u>, <u>drowsiness</u>, fatigue, psychosis, vertigo.
EENT: blurred vision, corneal opacities.
Resp: pneumonitis.
CV: congestive heart failure, hypertension, hypotension, syncope.
GI: hepatitis.
GU: hesitancy, urinary retention.
Derm: photosensitivity, rashes, urticaria.
Endo: syndrome of inappropriate antidiuretic hormone (SIADH).

{} = Available in Canada only.
***CAPITALS indicate life-threatening; <u>underlines</u> indicate most frequent.**

Hemat: AGRANULOCYTOSIS, APLASTIC ANEMIA, THROMBOCYTOPENIA, eosinophilia, leukopenia.
Misc: chills, fever, lymphadenopathy.

INTERACTIONS

Drug-Drug: ▪ May decrease effectiveness of **glucocorticoids, doxycycline, felbamate, quinidine, warfarin, oral contraceptives, barbiturates, benzodiazepines, theophylline,** and other **anticonvulsants** ▪ Concurrent use (within 2 wk) of **MAO inhibitors** may result in hyperpyrexia, hypertension, seizures, and death ▪ **Verapamil, diltiazem, propoxyphene, erythromycin,** or **cimetidine** increases levels and may cause toxicity ▪ May increase risk of hepatotoxicity from **isoniazid** ▪ **Felbamate** decreases carbamazepine levels but increases levels of active metabolite.

ROUTE AND DOSAGE

- **PO (Adults):** *Anticonvulsant*—200 mg twice daily (tablets) or 100 mg 4 times daily (suspension); increase by 200 mg/day q 7 days until therapeutic levels are achieved (range is 600–1200 mg/day in divided doses q 6–8 hr; not to exceed 1 g/day in 12–15-yr-olds. Extended-release tablets are given 1–2 times daily (XR, CR). *Antineuralgic*—100 mg twice daily (tablets) or 50 mg 4 times daily (suspension); increase by up to 200 mg/day until pain is relieved, then maintenance dose of 200–1200 mg/day in divided doses (usual range, 400–800 mg/day).
- **PO (Children 6–12 yr):** 100 mg twice daily (tablets) or 50 mg 4 times daily (suspension) increased by 100 mg weekly until therapeutic levels are obtained (usual range 400–800 mg/day; not to exceed 1 g/day). Extended-release tablets (XR, CR) are given 1–2 times daily.
- **PO (Children <6 yr):** 10–20 mg/kg/day in 2–3 divided doses; may be increased by 100 mg/day at weekly intervals. Usual maintenance dose is 250–350 mg/day (not to exceed 400 mg/day).

AVAILABILITY

▪ ***Tablets:*** 200 mg[Rx] ▪ ***Chewable tablets:*** 100 mg[Rx], {200 mg[Rx]} ▪ ***Extended-release tablets:*** 100 mg[Rx], {200 mg[Rx]}, 400 mg[Rx] ▪ ***Oral suspension:*** 100 mg/5 ml[Rx].

TIME/ACTION PROFILE (anticonvulsant activity)

	ONSET	PEAK	DURATION
PO	2–4 days*	2–12 hr†	UK

*Onset of antineuralgic activity is 8–72 hr.
†Listed for tablets; peak level occurs 1.5 hr after a chronic dose of suspension.

NURSING IMPLICATIONS

ASSESSMENT

- **Seizures:** Assess frequency, location, duration, and characteristics of seizure activity.
- **Trigeminal Neuralgia:** Assess for facial pain (location, intensity, duration). Ask patient to identify stimuli that may precipitate facial pain (hot or cold foods, bedclothes, touching face).
- ***Lab Test Considerations:*** Monitor CBC, including platelet count, reticulocyte count, and serum iron, weekly during the first 3 mo and monthly thereafter for evidence of potentially fatal blood cell abnormalities. Medication should be discontinued if bone marrow depression occurs.
  - Liver function tests, urinalysis, and BUN should be routinely performed. May cause elevated AST, ALT, serum alkaline phosphatase, bilirubin, BUN, urine protein, and urine glucose levels.
  - Monitor serum ionized calcium levels every 6 mo or if seizure frequency increases. Thyroid function tests and ionized serum calcium concentrations may be decreased; hypocalcemia decreases seizure threshold.
  - Monitor ECG and serum electrolytes prior to and periodically during therapy. May cause hyponatremia.
  - May occasionally cause increased serum cholesterol, high-density lipoprotein, and triglyceride concentrations.
  - May cause false-negative pregnancy test results with tests that determine human chorionic gonadotropin.
- ***Toxicity and Overdose:*** Serum blood levels should be routinely monitored throughout course of therapy. Therapeutic levels range from 6–12 mcg/ml.

POTENTIAL NURSING DIAGNOSES

- Injury, risk for (Indications, Side Effects).
- Pain, chronic (Indications).

- Knowledge deficit, related to medication regimen (Patient/Family Teaching).

IMPLEMENTATION

- **General Info:** Implement seizure precautions as indicated.
- **PO:** Administer medication with food to minimize gastric irritation. Tablets may be crushed if patient has difficulty swallowing. Do not crush or chew extended-release tablets. If suspension is administered via nasogastric tube, mix with an equal volume of diluent prior to administration.

PATIENT/FAMILY TEACHING

- **General Info:** Instruct patient to take carbamazepine around the clock, exactly as directed. If a dose is missed, take as soon as possible but not just before next dose; do not double doses. Notify health care professional if more than one dose is missed. Medication should be gradually discontinued to prevent seizures.
  - May cause dizziness or drowsiness. Advise patients to avoid driving or other activities requiring alertness until response to medication is known.
  - Instruct patients that fever, sore throat, mouth ulcers, easy bruising, petechiae, unusual bleeding, abdominal pain, chills, pale stools, dark urine, or jaundice be reported to health care professional immediately.
  - Advise patient not to take alcohol or other CNS depressants concurrently with this medication.
  - Caution patients to use sunscreen and protective clothing to prevent photosensitivity reactions.
  - Inform patient that frequent mouth rinses, good oral hygiene, and sugarless gum or candy may help reduce dry mouth. Saliva substitute may be used. Consult dentist if dry mouth persists >2 wk.
  - Advise female patients to use a nonhormonal form of contraception while taking carbamazepine.
  - Instruct patient to notify health care professional of medication regimen prior to treatment or surgery.
  - Emphasize the importance of follow-up lab tests and eye exams to monitor for side effects.
- **Seizures:** Advise patients to carry identification describing disease and medication regimen at all times.

EVALUATION

Effectiveness of therapy can be demonstrated by: ▪ Absence or reduction of seizure activity ▪ Decrease in trigeminal neuralgia pain. Patients with trigeminal neuralgia who are painfree should be re-evaluated every 3 mo to determine minimum effective dose.

CARBENICILLIN

(kar-ben-i-**sill**-in)

Geocillin, {Pyopen}

CLASSIFICATION(S):

Anti-infective (extended-spectrum penicillin)

Pregnancy Category B

INDICATIONS

- Treatment of urinary tract infections or prostatitis due to susceptible organisms.

ACTION

- Binds to bacterial cell wall membrane, causing cell death. **Therapeutic Effects:** ▪ Bactericidal against susceptible bacteria. Spectrum is broader than other penicillins. **Spectrum:** ▪ Active against: □ *Pseudomonas aeruginosa* □ *Escherichia coli* □ *Proteus mirabilis* □ *Proteus vulgaris* □ *Morganella morganii* □ *Enterobacter* □ enterococci ▪ Not active against penicillinase-producing staphylococci.

PHARMACOKINETICS

Absorption: Oral form is rapidly but incompletely absorbed.
Distribution: Widely distributed. Enters CSF well when meninges are inflamed. Crosses the placenta; enters breast milk in low concentrations.
Metabolism and Excretion: 36% excreted unchanged by the kidneys.
Half-life: 0.8–1 hr (increased in renal impairment).

CONTRAINDICATIONS AND PRECAUTIONS

Contraindicated in: ▪ Hypersensitivity to penicillins or cephalosporins.
Use Cautiously in: ▪ Severe renal impairment (if CCr <10 ml/min, therapeutic concentrations will not be achieved in urine) ▪ Severe liver disease ▪ Pregnancy or lactation (safety not established).

ADVERSE REACTIONS AND SIDE EFFECTS*

GI: diarrhea, nausea.
Derm: rashes, urticaria.
Hemat: blood dyscrasias.
Misc: hypersensitivity reactions including ANAPHYLAXIS and SERUM SICKNESS, superinfection.

INTERACTIONS

Drug-Drug: ▪ **Probenecid** decreases renal excretion and increases blood levels.

ROUTE AND DOSAGE

- **PO (Adults):** 382–764 mg (1–2 tablets) every 6 hr.

AVAILABILITY

- ***Tablets:*** 500 mg (contains 382 mg carbenicillin)Rx.

TIME/ACTION PROFILE (blood levels)

	ONSET	PEAK	DURATION
PO	30 min	30–120 min	6 hr

NURSING IMPLICATIONS

ASSESSMENT

- □ Assess patient for infection (vital signs; WBC; appearance of urine; dysuria; urgency; frequency; perineal, sacral, or suprapubic pain) at beginning of and throughout therapy.
- □ Obtain a history before initiating therapy to determine previous use of and reactions to penicillins or cephalosporins. Persons with a negative history of penicillin sensitivity may still have an allergic response.
- □ Obtain specimens for culture and sensitivity prior to initiating therapy. First dose may be given before receiving results.
- □ Observe patient for signs and symptoms of anaphylaxis (rash, pruritus, laryngeal edema, wheezing). Discontinue the drug and notify the physician or other health care professional immediately if these occur. Keep epinephrine, an antihistamine, and resuscitation equipment close by in the event of an anaphylactic reaction.

POTENTIAL NURSING DIAGNOSES

- Infection, risk for (Indications, Side Effects).
- Knowledge deficit, related to medication regimen (Patient/Family Teaching).
- Noncompliance, related to medication regimen (Patient/Family Teaching).

IMPLEMENTATION

- **PO:** Administer around the clock on an empty stomach at least 1 hr before or 2 hr after meals, with a full glass of water.

PATIENT/FAMILY TEACHING

- □ Instruct patient to take medication around the clock and to finish the drug completely as directed, even if feeling better. Advise patient that sharing of this medication may be dangerous.
- □ Advise patient to report the signs of superinfection (furry overgrowth on the tongue, vaginal itching or discharge, loose or foul-smelling stools) and allergy.
- □ Instruct the patient to notify health care professional if symptoms do not improve.

EVALUATION

Clinical response to therapy can be evaluated by: ▪ Resolution of the signs and symptoms of infection. Length of time for complete resolution depends on the organism and site of infection.

CARBONIC ANHYDRASE INHIBITORS (oral)†

acetazolamide

(a-set-a-**zole**-a-mide)
{Acetazolam}, AK-Zol, {Apo-Acetazolamide}, Dazamide, Diamox, Diamox Sequels, Storzolamide

*CAPITALS indicate life-threatening; underlines indicate most frequent.
{} = Available in Canada only.

dichlorphenamide
(dye-klor-**fen**-a-mide)
Daranide

methazolamide
(meth-a-**zole**-a-mide)
Neptazane

CLASSIFICATION(S):
Antiglaucoma agents

Pregnancy Category C

†See Appendix O for ophthalmic use.

INDICATIONS

▪ Lowering of intraocular pressure in the treatment of glaucoma ▪ **Acetazolamide:** ▫ Adjunct treatment ▫ Acute altitude sickness. **Unlabeled Uses:** ▪ **Acetazolamide:** Prevention of renal calculi composed of uric acid or cystine.

ACTION

▪ Inhibition of carbonic anhydrase in the eye results in decreased secretion of aqueous humor ▪ Inhibit renal carbonic anhydrase, resulting in self-limiting urinary excretion of sodium, potassium, bicarbonate, and water ▪ CNS inhibition of carbonic anhydrase and resultant diuresis may decrease abnormal neuronal firing ▪ Alkaline diuresis prevents precipitation of uric acid or cystine in the urinary tract. **Therapeutic Effects:** ▪ Lowering of intraocular pressure ▪ Control of some types of seizures ▪ Prevention and treatment of acute altitude sickness ▪ Prevention of uric acid or cystine renal calculi.

PHARMACOKINETICS

Absorption: Well absorbed following oral administration. IV administration results in complete bioavailability.

Distribution: Cross the placenta. Acetazolamide enters breast milk.

Metabolism and Excretion: *Acetazolamide*—excreted mostly unchanged in urine. *Methazolamide*—15–30% excreted unchanged in urine; 2.4–5.8 hr excreted mostly unchanged in urine.

Half-life: *Acetazolamide*—2.4–5.8 hr. *Methazolamide*—14 hr.

CONTRAINDICATIONS AND PRECAUTIONS

Contraindicated in: ▪ Hypersensitivity or cross-sensitivity with sulfonamides may occur ▪ Avoid during first trimester of pregnancy. Concurrent use of oral and ophthalmic carbonic anhydrase inhibitors (dorzolamide) is not recommended.

Use Cautiously in: ▪ Chronic respiratory disease ▪ Electrolyte abnormalities ▪ Renal or hepatic disease ▪ Diabetes mellitus ▪ Second or third trimester of pregnancy or lactation (safety not established).

ADVERSE REACTIONS AND SIDE EFFECTS*

CNS: <u>depression</u>, <u>tiredness</u>, <u>weakness</u>, drowsiness.

EENT: transient nearsightedness.

GI: <u>anorexia</u>, <u>metallic taste</u>, nausea, vomiting.

GU: crystalluria, renal calculi.

Derm: rashes.

Endo: hyperglycemia.

F and E: <u>hyperchloremic acidosis</u>, hypokalemia.

Hemat: APLASTIC ANEMIA, HEMOLYTIC ANEMIA, LEUKOPENIA.

Metab: <u>weight loss</u>, hyperuricemia.

Neuro: <u>paresthesias</u>.

Misc: allergic reactions.

INTERACTIONS

Drug-Drug: ▪ Excretion of **barbiturates, aspirin,** and **lithium** is decreased and may lead to decreased effectiveness ▪ Excretion of **amphetamines, quinidine, procainamide,** and possibly **tricyclic antidepressants** is decreased and may lead to toxicity.

ROUTE AND DOSAGE

▫ **Acetazolamide**

- **PO (Adults):** *Glaucoma*—250–1000 mg/day in 1–4 divided doses (up to 250 mg q 4 hr) or 500 mg extended-release capsules twice daily. *Epilepsy*—4–30 mg/kg/day in 1–4 divided doses (range 375 mg–1g/day). *Altitude sickness*—250 mg 2–4 times daily started 24–48 hr before ascent, continued for 48 hr or longer to control symptoms. *Antiurolithic*—250 mg at bedtime.
- **PO (Children):** *Glaucoma*—8–30 mg/kg

*CAPITALS indicate life-threatening; <u>underlines</u> indicate most frequent.

(300–900 mg/m^2)/day in divided doses (usual range 10–15 mg/kg/day). *Epilepsy*—4–30 mg/kg/day in 1–4 divided doses.

- **IM, IV (Adults):** 250–500 mg, may repeat in 2–4 hr.
- **IM, IV (Children):** 5–10 mg/kg q 6 hr.

❑ **Dichlorphenamide**

- **PO (Adults):** 100–200 mg followed by 100 mg q 12 hr initially, then maintenance dose of 25–50 mg 1–3 times daily.

❑ **Methazolamide**

- **PO (Adults):** 50–100 mg 2–3 times daily.

AVAILABILITY

❑ **Acetazolamide**

- ***Tablets:*** 125 mg^{Rx}, 250 mg^{Rx} ▪ ***Extended-release capsules:*** 500 mg^{Rx} ▪ ***Injection:*** 500 mg/vial^{Rx}.

❑ **Dichlorphenamide**

- ***Tablets:*** 25 mg^{Rx}, 50 mg^{Rx}.

❑ **Methazolamide**

- ***Tablets:*** 25 mg^{Rx}, 50 mg^{Rx}.

TIME/ACTION PROFILE (lowering of intraocular pressure)

	ONSET	PEAK	DURATION
Acetazolamide PO	1 hr	2–4 hr	8–12 hr
Acetazolamide PO-ER	2 hr	8–18 hr	18–24 hr
Acetazolamide IV	2 min	15 min	4–5 hr
Dichlorphenamide PO	0.5–1 hr	2–4 hr	6–12 hr
Methazolamide PO	2–4 hr	6–8 hr	10–18 hr

NURSING IMPLICATIONS

ASSESSMENT

- **General Info:** Observe patient for signs of hypokalemia (muscle weakness, malaise, fatigue, ECG changes, vomiting).
- ▫ Assess for allergy to sulfonamides.
- **Intraocular Pressure:** Assess for eye discomfort or decrease in visual acuity.
- **Seizures:** Monitor neurologic status in patients receiving acetazolamide for seizures. Initiate seizure precautions.
- **Altitude Sickness:** Monitor for decrease in severity of symptoms (headache, nausea, vomiting, fatigue, dizziness, drowsiness, shortness of breath). Notify physician or other health care professional immediately if neurologic symptoms worsen or patient becomes more dyspneic and rales or crackles develop.
- ***Lab Test Considerations:*** Serum electrolytes, complete blood counts, and platelet counts should be evaluated initially and periodically throughout prolonged therapy. May cause decreased potassium, bicarbonate, WBCs, and RBCs. May cause increased serum chloride.
- ▫ May cause increase in serum and urine glucose; monitor serum and urine glucose carefully in diabetic patients.
- ▫ May cause false-positive results for urine protein and 17-hydroxysteroid tests.
- ▫ May cause increased blood ammonia, bilirubin, uric acid, urine urobilinogen, and calcium. May decrease urine citrate.

POTENTIAL NURSING DIAGNOSES

- Sensory-perceptual alterations: visual (Indications).
- Knowledge deficit, related to medication regimen (Patient/Family Teaching).

IMPLEMENTATION

- **General Info:** Encourage fluids to 2000–3000 ml/day, unless contraindicated, to prevent crystalluria and stone formation.
- ▫ A potassium supplement without chloride should be administered concurrently with carbonic anhydrase inhibitors.
- **PO:** Give with food to minimize GI irritation. Tablets may be crushed and mixed with fruit-flavored syrup to minimize bitter taste for patients with difficulty swallowing. Long-acting capsules may be opened and sprinkled on soft food, but do not crush, chew, or swallow contents dry.
- **IM:** Extremely painful; avoid if possible.
- **Direct IV:** Dilute 500 mg of acetazolamide in at least 5 ml of sterile water for injection. Use reconstituted solution within 24 hr.
- ***Rate:*** Administer over at least 1 min.
- **Intermittent Infusion:** Further dilute in D5W, D10W, 0.45% NaCl, 0.9% NaCl, Ringer's or lactated Ringer's solution, or combinations of dextrose and saline or dextrose and Ringer's solution.
- ***Rate:*** Infuse over 4–8 hr.

- **Additive Compatibility:** ▪ cimetidine ▪ ranitidine.
- **Additive Incompatibility:** ▪ multiple vitamins.

PATIENT/FAMILY TEACHING

- **General Info:** Instruct patient to take exactly as directed. If a dose is missed, take as soon as possible unless almost time for next dose. Do not double doses. Patients on anticonvulsant therapy may need to gradually withdraw medication.
- Advise patient to report numbness or tingling of extremities, weakness, rash, sore throat, unusual bleeding or bruising, or fever to health care professional. If hematopoietic reactions, fever, rash, or renal problems occur, carbonic anhydrase inhibitor therapy should be discontinued.
- May occasionally cause drowsiness. Caution patient to avoid driving and other activities that require alertness until response to the drug is known.
- Caution patient to use sunscreen and wear protective clothing to prevent photosensitivity reactions.
- **Intraocular Pressure:** Advise patient of the need for periodic ophthalmologic exams; loss of vision may be gradual and painless.

EVALUATION

Effectiveness of therapy can be demonstrated by: ▪ Decrease in intraocular pressure when used for glaucoma. If therapy is not effective or patient is unable to tolerate one carbonic anhydrase inhibitor, using another may be effective and more tolerable ▪ Decrease in the frequency of seizures ▪ Prevention of altitude sickness ▪ Prevention of uric acid or cystine stones in the urinary tract.

CARBOPLATIN

(kar-boe-**pla**-tin)

Paraplatin, {Paraplatin-AQ}

CLASSIFICATION(S):

Antineoplastic (alkylating agent)

Pregnancy Category D

INDICATIONS

▪ In combination with other agents as initial treatment of advanced ovarian carcinoma ▪ Palliative treatment of ovarian carcinoma unresponsive to other chemotherapeutic modalities.

ACTION

▪ Inhibits DNA synthesis by producing cross-linking of parent DNA strands (cell-cycle phase–nonspecific). **Therapeutic Effects:** ▪ Death of rapidly replicating cells, particularly malignant ones.

PHARMACOKINETICS

Absorption: IV administration results in complete bioavailability.
Distribution: UK.
Metabolism and Excretion: Excreted mostly by the kidneys.
Half-life: 2.6–5.9 hr (increased in renal impairment).

CONTRAINDICATIONS AND PRECAUTIONS

Contraindicated in: ▪ Hypersensitivity to carboplatin, cisplatin, or mannitol ▪ Pregnancy or lactation.

Use Cautiously in: ▪ Hearing loss ▪ Electrolyte abnormalities ▪ Renal impairment (dosage reduction recommended if creatinine <60 ml/min) ▪ Active infections ▪ Diminished bone marrow reserve (dosage reduction recommended) ▪ Other chronic debilitating illnesses ▪ Patients with childbearing potential.

ADVERSE REACTIONS AND SIDE EFFECTS*

CNS: weakness.
EENT: ototoxicity.
GI: abdominal pain, nausea, vomiting, constipation, diarrhea, hepatitis, stomatitis.
GU: gonadal suppression, nephrotoxicity.
Derm: alopecia, rash.
F and E: hypocalcemia, hypokalemia, hypomagnesemia, hyponatremia.
Hemat: ANEMIA, LEUKOPENIA, THROMBOCYTOPENIA.

{} = Available in Canada only.
***CAPITALS indicate life-threatening; underlines indicate most frequent.**

Neuro: peripheral neuropathy.
Misc: hypersensitivity reactions including ANAPHYLACTIC-LIKE REACTIONS.

INTERACTIONS

Drug-Drug: ▪ Additive nephrotoxicity and ototoxicity with other **nephrotoxic** and **ototoxic drugs (aminoglycosides, loop diuretics)** ▪ Additive bone marrow depression with other **bone marrow–depressing drugs** or **radiation therapy** ▪ May decrease the antibody response to **live virus vaccines** and increase the risk of adverse reactions.

ROUTE AND DOSAGE

Other dosing formulas are used.

- **IV (Adults):** *Initial treatment*—300 mg/m^2 with cyclophosphamide at 4-wk intervals. *Treatment of refractory tumors*—360 mg/m^2 as a single dose; may be repeated at 4-wk intervals, depending on response.

AVAILABILITY

- ***Injection:*** 50-mg vials[Rx], 150-mg vials[Rx], 450-mg vials[Rx].

TIME/ACTION PROFILE (effects on blood counts)

	ONSET	PEAK	DURATION
IV	UK	21 days	28 days

NURSING IMPLICATIONS

ASSESSMENT

- □ Assess for nausea and vomiting; often occurs 6–12 hr after therapy and may persist for 24 hr. Prophylactic antiemetics may be used. Adjust diet as tolerated to maintain fluid and electrolyte balance and ensure adequate nutritional intake.
- □ Monitor for bone marrow depression. Assess for bleeding (bleeding gums, bruising, petechiae, guaiac stools, urine, and emesis) and avoid IM injections and rectal temperatures if platelet count is low. Apply pressure to venipuncture sites for 10 min. Assess for signs of infection during neutropenia. Anemia may occur and may be cumulative; transfusions are frequently required. Monitor for increased fatigue, dyspnea, and orthostatic hypotension.
- □ Monitor for signs of anaphylaxis (rash, urticaria, pruritus, wheezing, tachycardia, hypotension). Discontinue medication immediately and notify physician if these occur. Epinephrine and resuscitation equipment should be readily available.
- □ Audiometry is recommended prior to initiation of therapy and if ototoxicity is suspected during therapy.
- ▪ ***Lab Test Considerations:*** CBC, differential, and clotting studies should be monitored prior to and routinely throughout therapy. The nadirs of thrombocytopenia and leukopenia occur after 21 days and recover by 30 days after a dose. Nadir of granulocyte counts usually occurs after 21–28 days and recovers by day 35. Withhold subsequent doses until neutrophil count is >2000/mm^3 and platelet count is >100,000/mm^3.
- □ Monitor renal function prior to initiation of therapy and before each course of carboplatin. May cause elevated BUN and serum creatinine concentrations and decreased CCr.
- □ Monitor hepatic function prior to and periodically throughout therapy. May cause elevated serum bilirubin, alkaline phosphatase, and AST concentrations.
- □ May cause decreased serum potassium, calcium, magnesium, and sodium concentrations.

POTENTIAL NURSING DIAGNOSES

- ▪ Infection, risk for (Adverse Reactions).
- ▪ Injury, risk for (Side Effects).
- ▪ Knowledge deficit, related to medication regimen (Patient/Family Teaching).

IMPLEMENTATION

- ▪ **General Info:** Do not confuse with cisplatin.
- □ Do not use aluminum needles or equipment during preparation or administration, because aluminum reacts with the drug.
- □ Solution should be prepared in a biologic cabinet. Wear gloves, gown, and mask while handling medication. Discard equipment in specially designated containers (see Appendix I).
- ▪ **Intermittent Infusion:** Reconstitute to a concentration of 10 mg/ml with sterile water for injection, D5W, or 0.9% NaCl for injection. May be further diluted in D5W or 0.9% NaCl to a concentration of 0.5 mg/ml. Stable for 8 hr at room temperature.
- □ May also be administered over 24 hr or by dividing total dose into 5 consecutive pulse doses; may decrease nausea and vomiting but

does not decrease nephrotoxicity or ototoxicity.

- *Rate:* Administer over 15–60 min.
- **Y-Site Compatibility:** ▪ amifostine ▪ aztreonam ▪ cefepime ▪ filgrastim ▪ fludarabine ▪ granisetron ▪ melphalan ▪ ondansetron ▪ paclitaxel ▪ piperacillin/tazobactam ▪ sargramostim ▪ teniposide ▪ thiotepa ▪ vinorelbine.

PATIENT/FAMILY TEACHING

- ☐ Instruct patient to notify health care professional promptly if fever; chills; sore throat; signs of infection; lower back or side pain; difficult or painful urination; bleeding gums; bruising; petechiae; blood in stools, urine, or emesis; increased fatigue, dyspnea, or orthostatic hypotension occurs. Caution patient to avoid crowds and persons with known infections. Instruct patient to use soft toothbrush and electric razor and to avoid falls. Patients should be cautioned not to drink alcoholic beverages or take medication containing aspirin or NSAIDs because they may precipitate gastric bleeding.
- ☐ Instruct patient to promptly report any numbness or tingling in extremities or face, decreased coordination, difficulty with hearing or ringing in the ears, unusual swelling, or weight gain to health care professional. The risks of ototoxicity, neurotoxicity, and nephrotoxicity are less than with cisplatin.
- ☐ Instruct patient not to receive any vaccinations without advice of health care professional.
- ☐ Advise patient of the need for contraception (if patient is not infertile as a result of surgical or radiation therapy).
- ☐ Instruct patient to inspect oral mucosa for erythema and ulceration. If ulceration occurs, advise patient to notify health care professional, rinse mouth with water after eating, and use sponge brush. Mouth pain may require treatment with opioids.
- ☐ Discuss with patient the possibility of hair loss. Explore methods of coping.
- ☐ Emphasize the need for periodic lab tests to monitor for side effects.

EVALUATION

Effectiveness of therapy can be demonstrated by: ▪ Decrease in size or spread of ovarian carcinoma.

CARISOPRODOL

(kar-i-soe-**proe**-dole)
Soma, Vanadom

CLASSIFICATION(S):
Skeletal muscle relaxant (centrally acting)

Pregnancy Category UK

C

INDICATIONS

▪ Adjunct to rest and physical therapy in the treatment of muscle spasm associated with acute painful musculoskeletal conditions.

ACTION

▪ Skeletal muscle relaxation, probably due to CNS depression. **Therapeutic Effects:** ▪ Skeletal muscle relaxation.

PHARMACOKINETICS

Absorption: Well absorbed following oral administration.
Distribution: Crosses the placenta; high concentrations in breast milk.
Metabolism and Excretion: Mostly metabolized by the liver.
Half-life: 8 hr.

CONTRAINDICATIONS AND PRECAUTIONS

Contraindicated in: ▪ Hypersensitivity to carisoprodol or to meprobamate ▪ Porphyria or suspected porphyria.
Use Cautiously in: ▪ Severe liver or kidney disease ▪ Pregnancy, lactation, or children <12 yr (safety not established).

ADVERSE REACTIONS AND SIDE EFFECTS*

CNS: dizziness, drowsiness, agitation, ataxia, depression, headache, insomnia, irritability, syncope.
Resp: asthmatic attacks.
CV: hypotension, tachycardia.
GI: epigastric distress, hiccups, nausea, vomiting.
Derm: flushing, rashes.
Hemat: eosinophilia, leukopenia.

***CAPITALS indicate life-threatening; underlines indicate most frequent.**

Misc: ANAPHYLACTIC SHOCK, fever, psychological dependence, severe idiosyncratic reaction.

INTERACTIONS

Drug-Drug: ▪ Additive CNS depression with other **CNS depressants** including **alcohol, antihistamines, opioid analgesics,** and **sedative/hypnotics.**

ROUTE AND DOSAGE

- **PO (Adults):** 350 mg 4 times daily.
- **PO (Children 5–12 yr):** 6.25 mg/kg 4 times daily.

AVAILABILITY

▪ ***Tablets:*** 350 mg[Rx] ▪ ***In combination with:*** aspirin (Soma compound) and codeine[Rx]. See Appendix A.

TIME/ACTION PROFILE (skeletal muscle relaxation)

	ONSET	PEAK	DURATION
PO	30 min	UK	4–6 hr

NURSING IMPLICATIONS

ASSESSMENT

- Assess patient for pain, muscle stiffness, and range of motion prior to and periodically throughout therapy.
- Observe patient for idiosyncratic symptoms that may appear within minutes or hours of administration during the first dose. Symptoms include extreme weakness, quadriplegia, dizziness, ataxia, dysarthria, visual disturbances, agitation, euphoria, confusion, and disorientation. Usually subsides over several hours.

POTENTIAL NURSING DIAGNOSES

- Pain (Indications).
- Physical mobility, impaired (Indications).
- Injury, risk for (Side Effects).

IMPLEMENTATION

- **General Info:** Provide safety measures as indicated. Supervise ambulation and transfer of patients.
- **PO:** Administer with food to minimize GI irritation. Last dose should be given at bedtime.

PATIENT/FAMILY TEACHING

- Instruct patient to take medication exactly as directed. Missed doses should be taken within 1 hr; if not, omit and return to regular dosing schedule. Do not double doses.
- Encourage patient to comply with additional therapies prescribed for muscle spasm (rest, physical therapy, heat, etc.).
- May cause dizziness or drowsiness. Advise patient to avoid driving or other activities requiring alertness until response to drug is known.
- Instruct patient to change positions slowly to minimize orthostatic hypotension.
- Advise patient to avoid concurrent use of alcohol and other CNS depressants while taking this medication.
- Instruct patient to notify health care professional if signs of allergy (rash, hives, swelling of tongue or lips, dyspnea) or idiosyncratic reaction occur.

EVALUATION

Effectiveness of therapy can be demonstrated by: ▪ Decreased musculoskeletal pain and muscle spasticity ▫ Increased range of motion.

CARMUSTINE

(kar-**mus**-teen)

BCNU, BiCNU, Gliadel

CLASSIFICATION(S):
Antineoplastic (alkylating agent)

Pregnancy Category D

INDICATIONS

▪ Alone or in combination with other treatment modalities (surgery, radiation) in the treatment of: ▫ Brain tumors ▫ Multiple myeloma ▫ Hodgkin's disease ▫ Other lymphomas.

ACTION

▪ Inhibits DNA and RNA synthesis (cell-cycle phase–nonspecific). **Therapeutic Effects:** ▪ Death of rapidly replicating cells, especially malignant ones.

PHARMACOKINETICS

Absorption: Following IV administration, absorption is complete. Following implantation, action is primarily local.
Distribution: Highly lipid-soluble, readily penetrates CSF. Enters breast milk.
Metabolism and Excretion: Rapidly metabolized. Some metabolites have antineoplastic activity.
Half-life: *Biologic*—15–30 min; *chemical*—5 min.

CONTRAINDICATIONS AND PRECAUTIONS

Contraindicated in: ▪ Hypersensitivity ▪ Pregnancy or lactation.
Use Cautiously in: ▪ Infections ▪ Depressed bone marrow reserve ▪ Other chronic debilitating illnesses ▪ Patients with childbearing potential.

ADVERSE REACTIONS AND SIDE EFFECTS*

Resp: PULMONARY FIBROSIS, pulmonary infiltrates.
GI: hepatotoxicity, nausea, vomiting, anorexia, diarrhea, esophagitis.
GU: renal failure.
Derm: alopecia.
Hemat: LEUKOPENIA, THROMBOCYTOPENIA, anemia.
Local: pain at IV site.

INTERACTIONS

Drug-Drug: ▪ Additive bone marrow depression with other **antineoplastics** or **radiation therapy** ▪ **Smoking** increases the risk of pulmonary toxicity ▪ May decrease the antibody response to **live virus vaccines** and increase the risk of adverse reactions ▪ Myelosuppression may be potentiated by **cimetidine.**

ROUTE AND DOSAGE

- **IV (Adults and Children):** 150–200 mg/m² single dose every 6–8 wk *or* 75–100 mg/m²/day for 2 days q 6 wk *or* 40 mg/m²/day for 5 days q 6 wk.
- **Intracavitary (Adults):** Up to 61.6 mg (8 implants) placed in cavity created during surgical resection of brain tumor.

AVAILABILITY

▪ ***Injection:*** 100-mg vial^Rx^ ▪ ***Intracavitary wafer:*** 7.7 mg^Rx^.

TIME/ACTION PROFILE (effect on platelet counts)

	ONSET	PEAK	DURATION
IV	days	4–5 wk	6 wk

NURSING IMPLICATIONS

ASSESSMENT

- □ Monitor vital signs prior to and frequently during therapy.
- □ Monitor for bone marrow depression. Assess for bleeding (bleeding gums, bruising, petechiae, guaiac stools, urine, and emesis) and avoid IM injections and rectal temperatures if platelet count is low. Apply pressure to venipuncture sites for 10 min. Assess for signs of infection during neutropenia. Anemia may occur; monitor for increased fatigue, dyspnea, and orthostatic hypotension.
- □ Assess respiratory status for dyspnea or cough. Pulmonary toxicity usually occurs after high cumulative doses or several courses of therapy but may also occur following 1–2 courses of low doses. Symptoms may be rapid or gradual in onset; damage may be reversible or irreversible. Delayed pulmonary fibrosis may occur years after therapy. Notify physician promptly if symptoms occur.
- □ Monitor IV site closely. Carmustine is an irritant. Instruct patient to notify nurse immediately if discomfort occurs at IV site. Discontinue IV immediately if infiltration occurs. Ice may be applied to site. May cause hyperpigmentation of skin along vein.
- □ Monitor intake and output, appetite, and nutritional intake. Assess for nausea and vomiting, which occurs within 2 hr of administration and persists for 4–6 hr. Administration of an antiemetic prior to and during therapy and adjusting diet as tolerated may help maintain fluid and electrolyte balance and nutritional status.
- ***Lab Test Considerations:*** Monitor CBC with differential and platelet count prior to and throughout therapy. The nadir of thrombocytopenia occurs in 4–5 wk; the nadir of leukopenia, in 5–6 wk. Recovery usually occurs

***CAPITALS indicate life-threatening; underlines indicate most frequent.**

in 6–7 wk but may take 10–12 wk after prolonged therapy. Withhold dose and notify physician if platelet count is $<100,000/mm^3$ or leukocyte count is $<4000/mm^3$. Anemia is usually mild.

□ Monitor serum bilirubin, AST, ALT, and LDH prior to and periodically throughout therapy. May cause mild, reversible increase in AST, alkaline phosphatase, and bilirubin.

□ Monitor BUN, serum creatinine, and uric acid prior to and periodically during therapy. Notify physician if BUN is elevated.

POTENTIAL NURSING DIAGNOSES

- Injury, risk for (Side Effects).
- Body image disturbance (Side Effects).
- Knowledge deficit, related to medication regimen (Patient/Family Teaching).

IMPLEMENTATION

- **General Info:** Solution should be prepared in a biologic cabinet. Wear gloves, gown, and mask while handling medication. Discard equipment in designated containers. Contact with skin may cause transient hyperpigmentation (see Appendix I).
- **Intermittent Infusion:** Dilute contents of each 100-mg vial with 3 ml of absolute ethyl alcohol provided as a diluent. Dilute this solution with 27 ml of sterile water for injection for a concentration of 3.3 mg/ml. Further dilute with 500 ml of D5W or 0.9% NaCl in a glass container.

□ Solution is clear and colorless. Do not use vials that contain an oily film, which indicates decomposition. Reconstituted solution is stable for 24 hr when refrigerated and protected from light. Solution contains no preservatives; do not use as a multi-dose vial.

□ IV lines may be flushed with 5–10 ml of 0.9% NaCl prior to and following carmustine infusion to minimize irritation at the injection site.

- ***Rate:*** Administer dose over 1–2 hr. Rapid infusion rate may cause local pain, burning at site, and flushing. Facial flushing occurs within 2 hr and may persist for 4 hr.
- **Y-Site Compatibility:** ▪ amifostine ▪ aztreonam ▪ cefepime ▪ filgrastim ▪ fludarabine ▪ melphalan ▪ ondansetron ▪ piperacillin/tazobactam ▪ sargramostim ▪ teniposide ▪ thiotepa ▪ vinorelbine.
- **Additive Incompatibility:** ▪ sodium bicarbonate.

PATIENT/FAMILY TEACHING

□ Instruct patient to notify health care professional if fever; chills; sore throat; signs of infection; lower back or side pain; difficult or painful urination; bleeding gums; bruising; petechiae; or blood in urine, stool, or emesis occurs. Caution patient to avoid crowds and persons with known infections. Instruct patient to use soft toothbrush and electric razor. Patients should be cautioned not to drink alcoholic beverages or take products containing aspirin or NSAIDs.

□ Instruct patient to notify health care professional if shortness of breath or increased cough occurs. Encourage patient not to smoke, because smokers are at greater risk for pulmonary toxicity.

□ Instruct patient to inspect oral mucosa for redness and ulceration. If mouth sores occur, advise patient to use sponge brush and rinse mouth with water after eating and drinking. Stomatitis may require treatment with opioid analgesics.

□ Discuss with patient the possibility of hair loss. Explore coping strategies.

□ Advise patient of the need for contraception.

□ Instruct patient not to receive any vaccinations without advice of health care professional.

□ Emphasize need for periodic lab tests to monitor for side effects.

EVALUATION

Effectiveness of therapy can be demonstrated by: ▪ Decrease in size and spread of tumor □ Improvement in hematologic parameters in nonsolid cancers.

CARTEOLOL

(**kar**-tee-oh-lole)

Cartrol

CLASSIFICATION(S):

Antihypertensive agent, Beta-adrenergic blocking agent (nonselective)

Pregnancy Category C

INDICATIONS

▪ Management of hypertension. **Unlabeled Uses:** ▪ Management of angina pectoris.

ACTION

▪ Blocks stimulation of $beta_1$ (myocardial) and $beta_2$ (pulmonary, vascular, and uterine) -adrenergic receptor sites ▪ Also has intrinsic sympathomimetic activity (ISA), which may produce less bradycardia. **Therapeutic Effects:** ▪ Decreased heart rate and blood pressure.

PHARMACOKINETICS

Absorption: 85% absorbed following oral administration.
Distribution: UK.
Metabolism and Excretion: Some metabolism by the liver, with conversion to at least one active compound (8-hydroxycarteolol); 50–70% excreted unchanged by the kidneys.
Half-life: 6–8 hr (8–12 hr for 8-hydroxycarteolol; both are increased in renal impairment).

CONTRAINDICATIONS AND PRECAUTIONS

Contraindicated in: ▪ Uncompensated congestive heart failure ▪ Pulmonary edema ▪ Cardiogenic shock ▪ Bradycardia or heart block.
Use Cautiously in: ▪ Renal impairment ▪ Hepatic impairment ▪ Geriatric patients (increased sensitivity to beta-adrenergic blockers; initial dosage reduction recommended) ▪ Pulmonary disease (including asthma; $beta_1$ selectivity may be lost at higher doses) ▪ Diabetes mellitus (may mask signs of hypoglycemia) ▪ Thyrotoxicosis (may mask symptoms) ▪ Patients with a history of severe allergic reactions (intensity of reactions may be increased) ▪ Pregnancy, lactation, or children (safety not established; all agents cross the placenta and may cause fetal/neonatal bradycardia, hypotension, hypoglycemia, or respiratory depression).

ADVERSE REACTIONS AND SIDE EFFECTS*

CNS: fatigue, weakness, anxiety, depression, dizziness, drowsiness, insomnia, memory loss, mental status changes, nightmares.
EENT: blurred vision, dry eyes, nasal stuffiness.
Resp: bronchospasm, wheezing.
CV: BRADYCARDIA, CONGESTIVE HEART FAILURE, PULMONARY EDEMA, orthostatic hypotension, peripheral vasoconstriction.
GI: constipation, diarrhea, nausea.
GU: impotence, decreased libido.
Derm: itching, rashes.
Endo: hyperglycemia, hypoglycemia.
MS: arthralgia, back pain, muscle cramps.
Neuro: paresthesia.

INTERACTIONS

Drug-Drug: ▪ **General anesthesia, IV phenytoin, mibefradil,** and **verapamil** may cause additive myocardial depression ▪ Additive bradycardia may occur with **digitalis glycosides** ▪ Additive hypotension may occur with other **antihypertensives,** acute ingestion of **alcohol,** or **nitrates** ▪ Concurrent use with **amphetamines, cocaine, ephedrine, epinephrine, norepinephrine, phenylephrine,** or **pseudoephedrine** may result in unopposed alpha-adrenergic stimulation (excessive hypertension, bradycardia) ▪ Concurrent **thyroid** administration may decrease effectiveness ▪ May alter the effectiveness of **insulin** or **oral hypoglycemic agents** (dosage adjustments may be necessary) ▪ May decrease the effectiveness of **beta-adrenergic bronchodilators** and **theophylline** ▪ May decrease the beneficial $beta_1$ cardiovascular effects of **dopamine** or **dobutamine** ▪ Use cautiously within 14 days of **MAO inhibitor** therapy (may result in hypertension) ▪ Concurrent use with **clonidine** increases hypotension and bradycardia ▪ May exaggerate withdrawal phenomenon from clonidine ▪ Concurrent **NSAIDs** may decrease antihypertensive action.

ROUTE AND DOSAGE

- **PO (Adults):** 2.5 mg once daily, may be increased up to 10 mg/day.

AVAILABILITY

▪ ***Tablets:*** 2.5 mg[Rx], 5 mg[Rx].

TIME/ACTION PROFILE

	ONSET	PEAK	DURATION
PO	UK	1–3 hr	≥24 hr

NURSING IMPLICATIONS

ASSESSMENT

- **General Info:** Monitor blood pressure and pulse frequently during dosage adjustment period and periodically throughout therapy. As-

*CAPITALS indicate life-threatening; underlines indicate most frequent.

sess for orthostatic hypotension when assisting patient up from supine position.

□ Monitor intake and output ratios and daily weight. Assess patient routinely for evidence of fluid overload (peripheral edema, dyspnea, rales/crackles, fatigue, weight gain, jugular venous distention).

▪ **Hypertension:** Check frequency of refills to determine compliance.

▪ **Angina:** Assess frequency and characteristics of angina periodically during therapy.

▪ ***Lab Test Considerations:*** May cause increased BUN, serum lipoprotein, potassium, triglyceride, and uric acid levels.

□ May cause increased ANA titers.

□ May cause increase in blood glucose levels.

▪ ***Toxicity and Overdose:*** Monitor patients receiving beta-adrenergic blocking agents for signs of overdose (bradycardia, severe dizziness or fainting, severe drowsiness, dyspnea, bluish fingernails or palms, seizures). Notify physician or other health care professional immediately if these signs occur.

POTENTIAL NURSING DIAGNOSES

▪ Cardiac output, decreased (Side Effects).

▪ Knowledge deficit, related to medication regimen (Patient/Family Teaching).

▪ Noncompliance, related to medication regimen (Patient/Family Teaching).

IMPLEMENTATION

▪ **General Info:** Discontinuation of concurrent clonidine should be gradual, with beta blocker discontinued first; then, after several days, discontinue clonidine.

▪ **PO:** Take apical pulse prior to administering. If <50 bpm or if arrhythmia occurs, withhold medication and notify physician or other health care professional.

□ Administer without regard to food.

PATIENT/FAMILY TEACHING

▪ **General Info:** Instruct patient to take medication exactly as directed, at the same time each day, even if feeling well; do not skip or double up on missed doses. If a dose is missed, it should be taken as soon as possible up to 4 hr before next dose. Abrupt withdrawal may precipitate life-threatening arrhythmias, hypertension, or myocardial ischemia.

□ Advise patient to make sure enough medication is available for weekends, holidays, and vacations. A written prescription may be kept in wallet in case of emergency.

□ Teach patient and family how to check pulse and blood pressure. Instruct them to check pulse daily and blood pressure biweekly. Advise patient to hold dose and contact health care professional if pulse is <50 bpm or blood pressure changes significantly.

□ May cause drowsiness or dizziness. Caution patients to avoid driving or other activities that require alertness until response to the drug is known.

□ Advise patient to change positions slowly to minimize orthostatic hypotension, especially during initiation of therapy or when dose is increased.

□ Caution patient that this medication may increase sensitivity to cold.

□ Instruct patient to consult health care professional before taking any OTC medications, especially cold preparations, concurrently with this medication.

□ Diabetics should closely monitor blood sugar, especially if weakness, malaise, irritability, or fatigue occurs. Medication may mask some signs of hypoglycemia, but dizziness and sweating may still occur.

□ Advise patient to notify health care professional if slow pulse, difficulty breathing, wheezing, cold hands and feet, dizziness, confusion, depression, rash, fever, sore throat, unusual bleeding, or bruising occurs.

□ Instruct patient to inform health care professional of medication regimen prior to treatment or surgery.

□ Advise patient to carry identification describing disease process and medication regimen at all times.

▪ **Hypertension:** Reinforce the need to continue additional therapies for hypertension (weight loss, sodium restriction, stress reduction, regular exercise, moderation of alcohol consumption, and smoking cessation). Medication controls but does not cure hypertension.

▪ **Angina:** Caution patient to avoid overexertion with decrease in chest pain.

EVALUATION

Effectiveness of therapy can be demonstrated by: ▪ Decrease in blood pressure without appearance of detrimental side effects ▪ Reduction in frequency of anginal attacks ▫ Increase in activity tolerance.

CARVEDILOL
(kar-**ve**-di-lole)
Coreg

CLASSIFICATION(S):
Antihypertensive agent, Beta-adrenergic blocking agent (nonselective)

Pregnancy Category C

INDICATIONS

▪ Management of hypertension ▪ Management of mild to moderate congestive heart failure (due to ischemia or cardiomyopathy) with digitalis glycosides, diuretics, and ACE inhibitors.

ACTION

▪ Blocks stimulation of $beta_1$ (myocardial) and $beta_2$ (pulmonary, vascular, and uterine) -adrenergic receptor sites ▪ Also has $alpha_1$-adrenergic blocking activity, which may result in orthostatic hypotension. **Therapeutic Effects:** ▪ Decreased heart rate and blood pressure ▪ Slowing of the progression of congestive heart failure.

PHARMACOKINETICS

Absorption: Well absorbed but rapidly undergoes extensive first-pass hepatic metabolism, resulting in 25–35% bioavailability.
Distribution: UK.
Metabolism and Excretion: Extensively metabolized, excreted in feces via bile, <2% excreted unchanged in urine.
Half-life: 7–10 hr.

CONTRAINDICATIONS AND PRECAUTIONS

Contraindicated in: ▪ Uncompensated congestive heart failure ▪ Pulmonary edema ▪ Cardiogenic shock ▪ Bradycardia or heart block ▪ Severe hepatic impairment or bronchial asthma/bronchospasm.
Use Cautiously in: ▪ Renal impairment ▪ Hepatic impairment ▪ Geriatric patients (increased sensitivity to beta-adrenergic blockers; initial dosage reduction recommended) ▪ Pulmonary disease (including asthma) ▪ Diabetes mellitus (may mask signs of hypoglycemia) ▪ Thyrotoxicosis (may mask symptoms) ▪ Peripheral vascular disease ▪ Patients with a history of severe allergic reactions (intensity of reactions may be increased) ▪ Pregnancy, lactation, or children (safety not established; all agents cross the placenta and may cause fetal/neonatal bradycardia, hypotension, hypoglycemia, or respiratory depression).

ADVERSE REACTIONS AND SIDE EFFECTS*

CNS: <u>dizziness</u>, <u>fatigue</u>, <u>weakness</u>, anxiety, depression, drowsiness, insomnia, memory loss, mental status changes, nervousness, nightmares.
EENT: blurred vision, dry eyes, nasal stuffiness.
Resp: bronchospasm, wheezing.
CV: BRADYCARDIA, CONGESTIVE HEART FAILURE, PULMONARY EDEMA, <u>orthostatic hypotension</u>, peripheral vasoconstriction.
GI: <u>diarrhea</u>, constipation, nausea.
GU: <u>impotence</u>, decreased libido.
Derm: itching, rashes.
Endo: <u>hyperglycemia</u>, hypoglycemia.
MS: arthralgia, back pain, muscle cramps.
Neuro: paresthesia.

INTERACTIONS

Drug-Drug: ▪ **General anesthesia, IV phenytoin, diltiaziem,** and **verapamil** may cause additive myocardial depression ▪ Additive bradycardia may occur with **digitalis glycosides** ▪ Additive hypotension may occur with other **antihypertensives,** acute ingestion of **alcohol,** or **nitrates** ▪ Concurrent use with **clonidine** increases hypotension and bradycardia ▪ May exaggerate withdrawal phenomenon from **clonidine** ▪ Concurrent **thyroid** administration may decrease effectiveness ▪ May alter the effectiveness of **insulin** or **oral hypoglycemic agents** (dosage adjustments may be necessary) ▪ May decrease the effectiveness of **theophylline** ▪ May decrease the beneficial $beta_1$ cardiovascular effects of **dopamine** or **dobutamine** ▪ Use cautiously within 14 days of **MAO inhibitor** therapy (may result in hypertension) ▪ **Cimetidine** may increase toxicity from carvedilol, labetalol, timolol, or propranolol ▪ Concurrent **NSAIDs** may decrease antihyper-

***CAPITALS indicate life-threatening; <u>underlines</u> indicate most frequent.**

C

tensive action ▪ Effectiveness may be decreased by **rifampin** ▪ May increase serum **digoxin** levels.

ROUTE AND DOSAGE

- **PO (Adults):** *Hypertension*—6.25 mg twice daily, may be increased q 7–14 days up to 25 mg twice daily; *congestive heart failure*—3.125 mg twice daily for 2 wk; may be increased to 6.25 mg twice daily. Dose may be doubled q 2 wk as tolerated (not to exceed 25 mg twice daily in patients <85 kg or 50 mg twice daily in patients >85 kg).

AVAILABILITY

- ***Tablets:*** 3.125 mg[Rx], 6.25 mg[Rx], 12.5 mg[Rx], 25 mg[Rx].

TIME/ACTION PROFILE (cardiovascular effects)

	ONSET	PEAK	DURATION
PO	within 1 hr	1–2 hr	12 hr

NURSING IMPLICATIONS

ASSESSMENT

- **General Info:** Monitor blood pressure and pulse frequently during dosage adjustment period and periodically throughout therapy. Assess for orthostatic hypotension when assisting patient up from supine position.
- □ Monitor intake and output ratios and daily weight. Assess patient routinely for evidence of fluid overload (peripheral edema, dyspnea, rales/crackles, fatigue, weight gain, jugular venous distention). Patients may experience worsening of symptoms during initiation of therapy for congestive heart failure.
- **Hypertension:** Check frequency of refills to determine compliance.
- ***Lab Test Considerations:*** May cause increased BUN, serum lipoprotein, potassium, triglyceride, and uric acid levels.
- □ May cause increased ANA titers.
- □ May cause increase in blood glucose levels.
- ***Toxicity and Overdose:*** Monitor patients receiving beta-adrenergic blocking agents for signs of overdose (bradycardia, severe dizziness or fainting, severe drowsiness, dyspnea, bluish fingernails or palms, seizures). Notify physician or other health care professional immediately if these signs occur.

POTENTIAL NURSING DIAGNOSES

- Cardiac output, decreased (Side Effects).
- Knowledge deficit, related to medication regimen (Patient/Family Teaching).
- Noncompliance, related to medication regimen (Patient/Family Teaching).

IMPLEMENTATION

- **General Info:** Discontinuation of concurrent clonidine should be gradual, with beta blocker discontinued first; then, after several days, discontinue clonidine.
- **PO:** Take apical pulse prior to administering. If <50 bpm or if arrhythmia occurs, withhold medication and notify physician or other health care professional.
- □ Administer without regard to food.

PATIENT/FAMILY TEACHING

- **General Info:** Instruct patient to take medication exactly as directed, at the same time each day, even if feeling well; do not skip or double up on missed doses. If a dose is missed, it should be taken as soon as possible up to 4 hr before next dose. Abrupt withdrawal may precipitate life-threatening arrhythmias, hypertension, or myocardial ischemia.
- □ Advise patient to make sure enough medication is available for weekends, holidays, and vacations. A written prescription may be kept in wallet in case of emergency.
- □ Teach patient and family how to check pulse and blood pressure. Instruct them to check pulse daily and blood pressure biweekly. Advise patient to hold dose and contact health care professional if pulse is <50 bpm or blood pressure changes significantly.
- □ May cause drowsiness or dizziness. Caution patients to avoid driving or other activities that require alertness until response to the drug is known.
- □ Advise patient to change positions slowly to minimize orthostatic hypotension, especially during initiation of therapy or when dose is increased.
- □ Caution patient that this medication may increase sensitivity to cold.
- □ Instruct patient to consult health care professional before taking any OTC medications, especially cold preparations, concurrently with this medication.
- □ Diabetics should closely monitor blood sugar,

especially if weakness, malaise, irritability, or fatigue occurs. Medication may mask some signs of hypoglycemia, but dizziness and sweating may still occur.

- Advise patient to notify health care professional if slow pulse, difficulty breathing, wheezing, cold hands and feet, dizziness, confusion, depression, rash, fever, sore throat, unusual bleeding, or bruising occurs.
- Instruct patient to inform health care professional of medication regimen prior to treatment or surgery.
- Advise patient to carry identification describing disease process and medication regimen at all times.
- **Hypertension:** Reinforce the need to continue additional therapies for hypertension (weight loss, sodium restriction, stress reduction, regular exercise, moderation of alcohol consumption, and smoking cessation). Medication controls but does not cure hypertension.

EVALUATION

Effectiveness of therapy can be demonstrated by: ▪ Decrease in blood pressure without appearance of detrimental side effects ▪ Decrease in severity of congestive heart failure.

CASCARA DERIVATIVES

casanthranol
(ka-**san**-thra-nole)

cascara sagrada
(kas-**kar**-a sa-**grad**-a)

CLASSIFICATION(S):
Laxative (stimulant)

Pregnancy Category C

INDICATIONS

▪ Treatment of constipation. Particularly useful when constipation is secondary to prolonged bed rest or constipating drugs. Casanthranol is available only in combination with other laxatives.

ACTION

▪ Stimulates peristalsis ▪ Alters fluid and electrolyte transport, producing fluid accumulation in the colon. **Therapeutic Effects:** ▪ Evacuation of the colon. Cascara is another name for cascara sagrada, which is naturally derived from the bark of the buckthorn tree. Casanthranol is the active ingredient that has been extracted from cascara.

PHARMACOKINETICS

Absorption: Minimally absorbed. Converted in the colon to active drug.
Distribution: UK.
Metabolism and Excretion: Small amounts absorbed are metabolized by the liver.
Half-life: UK.

CONTRAINDICATIONS AND PRECAUTIONS

Contraindicated in: ▪ Hypersensitivity ▪ Abdominal pain, obstruction, nausea, or vomiting, especially when associated with fever or other signs of acute abdomen ▪ Aromatic cascara sagrada fluid extract contains alcohol and should be avoided in patients with known intolerance ▪ Pregnancy or lactation.
Use Cautiously in: ▪ Severe cardiovascular disease ▪ Anal or rectal fissures ▪ Excessive or prolonged use may lead to dependence.

ADVERSE REACTIONS AND SIDE EFFECTS*

GI: abdominal cramps, nausea, diarrhea.
GU: discoloration of urine.
F and E: hypokalemia (with chronic use).

INTERACTIONS

Drug-Drug: ▪ May decrease the absorption of concurrently administered **oral medications** because of increased motility and decreased transit time.

ROUTE AND DOSAGE

Casanthranol

- **PO (Adults):** 30–90 mg once daily.
- **PO (Children 2–11 yr):** 15–45 mg once daily.
- **PO (Children <2 yr):** 7.5–22.5 mg once daily.

Cascara Sagrada

- **PO (Adults):** 300 mg–1 g once daily.
- **PO (Children 2–11 yr):** 150–500 mg once daily.

*CAPITALS indicate life-threatening; underlines indicate most frequent.

- **PO (Children <2 yr):** 75–250 mg once daily.

❑ Cascara Sagrada Extract

- **PO (Adults):** 200–400 mg once daily.
- **PO (Children 2–11 yr):** 100–200 mg once daily.
- **PO (Children <2 yr):** 50–100 mg once daily.

❑ Cascara Sagrada Fluid Extract

- **PO (Adults):** 0.5–1.5 ml once daily.
- **PO (Children 2–11 yr):** 0.25 ml–0.75 ml once daily.
- **PO (Children <2 yr):** 0.12–0.38 ml once daily.

❑ Aromatic Cascara Fluid Extract

- **PO (Adults):** 2–6 ml once daily.
- **PO (Children 2–11 yr):** 1–3 ml once daily.
- **PO (Children <2 yr):** 0.5–1.5 ml once daily.

AVAILABILITY

❑ Casanthranol

- ***Tablets and liquid:*** in combination with docusate, milk of magnesia.[OTC] See Appendix A.

❑ Cascara Sagrada

- ***Powder, extract tablets, fluid extract, and aromatic fluid extract:*** alone and in combination with docusate, aloe, milk of magnesia.[OTC] See Appendix A.

TIME/ACTION PROFILE (evacuation of colon)

	ONSET	PEAK	DURATION
PO	6–12 hr	UK	UK

NURSING IMPLICATIONS

ASSESSMENT

- ❑ Assess patient for abdominal distention, presence of bowel sounds, and usual pattern of bowel function.
- ❑ Assess color, consistency, and amount of stool produced.
- ***Lab Test Considerations:*** May cause increased serum glucose and decreased serum potassium with prolonged use.

POTENTIAL NURSING DIAGNOSES

- Constipation (Indications).
- Diarrhea (Side Effects).
- Knowledge deficit, related to medication regimen (Patient/Family Teaching).

IMPLEMENTATION

- **PO:** Administer with full glass of water. Administer at bedtime for evacuation 6–12 hr later. Administer on an empty stomach for more rapid results.
- ❑ Do not administer within 2 hr of other medications.

PATIENT/FAMILY TEACHING

- ❑ Advise patients that laxatives should be used only for short-term (not longer than 1 wk without approval of health care professional) therapy. Long-term therapy may cause electrolyte imbalance and dependence.
- ❑ Encourage patients to use other forms of bowel regulation such as increasing bulk in the diet, increasing fluid intake (6–8 glasses of fluid/day), and increasing mobility. Normal bowel habits are individualized and may vary from 3 times/day to 3 times/wk.
- ❑ Inform patients that this medication may cause a change in urine color to a pink, red, violet, or brown.
- ❑ Instruct patients with cardiac disease to avoid straining during bowel movements (Valsalva maneuver).
- ❑ Advise patients not to use laxatives when abdominal pain, nausea, vomiting, or fever is present.

EVALUATION

Effectiveness of therapy can be demonstrated by: ▪ The patient's having a soft, formed bowel movement.

CEPHALOSPORINS—FIRST GENERATION

cefadroxil

(sef-a-**drox**-ill)

Duricef, Ultracef

cefazolin
(sef-**a**-zoe-lin)
Ancef, {Gen-Cefazolin}, Kefzol, Zolicef

cephalexin
(sef-a-**lex**-in)
{Apo-Cephalex}, Cefanex, C-Lexin, Keflex, Keftab, {Novo-Lexin}, {Nu-Cephalex}

cephalothin
(sef-**a**-loe-thin)
Keflin

cephapirin
(sef-a-**pye**-rin)
Cefadyl

cephradine
(**sef**-re-deen)
Velosef

CLASSIFICATION(S):
Anti-infectives (first-generation cephalosporins)
Pregnancy Category B

INDICATIONS

▪ Treatment of: ▫ Skin and skin structure infections (including burn wounds) ▫ Pneumonia ▫ Otitis media ▫ Urinary tract infections ▫ Bone and joint infections ▫ Septicemia (including endocarditis) due to susceptible organisms ▪ **Cefazolin, cephalothin, cephapirin, cephradine:** Perioperative prophylaxis ▪ Not suitable for the treatment of meningitis.

ACTION

▪ Bind to bacterial cell wall membrane, causing cell death. **Therapeutic Effects:** ▪ Bactericidal action against susceptible bacteria. **Spectrum:** ▪ Active against many gram-positive cocci including: ▫ *Streptococcus pneumoniae* ▫ Group A beta-hemolytic streptococci ▫ Penicillinase-producing staphylococci ▪ Not active against: ▫ Methicillin-resistant staphylococci ▫ *Bacteroides fragilis* ▫ *Enterococcus* ▪ Limited activity against some gram-negative rods including: ▫ *Klebsiella pneumoniae* ▫ *Proteus mirabilis* ▫ *Escherichia coli*.

PHARMACOKINETICS

Absorption: *Cefadroxil, cephalexin,* and *cephradine* are well absorbed following oral administration. *Cefazolin, cephalothin, cephapirin,* and *cephradine* are well absorbed following IM administration.
Distribution: Widely distributed. All cross the placenta and enter breast milk in low concentrations. Minimal CSF penetration
Protein Binding: *Cefadroxil*—20%; *cefazolin*—80–86%; *cephalexin*—10%; *cephalothin*—70%; *cephapirin*—54%; *cephradine*—8–17%.
Metabolism and Excretion: Excreted almost entirely unchanged by the kidneys.
Half-life: *Cefadroxil*—78–96 min; *cefazolin*—90–120 min; *cephalexin*—50–80 min; *cephalothin*—30–50 min; *cephapirin*—24–36 min; *cephradine*—48–80 min (all are increased in renal impairment).

CONTRAINDICATIONS AND PRECAUTIONS

Contraindicated in: ▪ Hypersensitivity to cephalosporins ▪ Serious hypersensitivity to penicillins.
Use Cautiously in: ▪ Renal impairment (dosage reduction and/or increased dosing interval recommended for: *cefadroxil* if CCr ≤50 ml/min, *cephradine* and *cephapirin* if CCr ≤20 ml/min, *cephalothin* if CCr ≤50 ml/min, *cefazolin* if CCr <55 ml/min) ▪ Patients >50 yr (increased risk of nephrotoxicity from *cephalothin*) ▪ Pregnancy or lactation (half-life is shorter and blood levels lower during pregnancy; have been used safely).

ADVERSE REACTIONS AND SIDE EFFECTS*

CNS: SEIZURES (high doses).
GI: PSEUDOMEMBRANOUS COLITIS, diarrhea, nausea, vomiting, cramps.
GU: nephrotoxicity (*cephalothin* only), interstitial nephritis (*cefadroxil* only).
Derm: rashes, urticaria.
Hemat: blood dyscrasias, hemolytic anemia.
Local: pain at IM site, phlebitis at IV site.
Misc: allergic reactions including ANAPHYLAXIS and SERUM SICKNESS, superinfection.

{} = Available in Canada only.
***CAPITALS indicate life-threatening; underlines indicate most frequent.**

INTERACTIONS

Drug-Drug: ▪ **Probenecid** decreases excretion and increases blood levels of renally excreted cephalosporins ▪ Increased risk of nephrotoxicity when **aminoglycosides** are used with cephalothin.

ROUTE AND DOSAGE

❑ Cefadroxil

- **PO (Adults):** *Group A beta-hemolytic streptococcal pharyngitis*—500 mg q 12 hr or 1 g q 24 hr for 10 days. *Skin and soft tissue infections*—500 mg q 12 hr or 1 g q 24 hr. *Urinary tract infections*—500 mg–1 g q 12 hr or 1–2 g q 24 hr.
- **PO (Children):** *Group A beta-hemolytic streptococcal pharyngitis*—15 mg/kg q 12 hr or 30 mg/kg q 24 hr for 10 days. *Skin and soft tissue infections*—15 mg/kg q 12 hr or 30 mg/kg q 24 hr. *Urinary tract infections*—500 mg or 15 mg/kg q 12 hr.

❑ Cefazolin

- **IM, IV (Adults):** *Most infections*—250 mg–1.5 g q 6–8 hr. *Perioperative prophylaxis*—1 g within 60 min of incision, then q 8 hr for up to 24 hr.
- **IM, IV (Children and Infants >1 mo):** 6.25–25 mg/kg q 6 hr or 8.3–33.3 mg/kg q 8 hr.

❑ Cephalexin

- **PO (Adults):** *Most infections*—250–500 mg q 6 hr. *Cystitis, skin and soft tissue infections, streptococcal pharyngitis*—500 mg q 12 hr.
- **PO (Children):** *Most infections*—6.25–25 mg/kg q 6 hr. *Skin and soft tissue infections, streptococcal pharyngitis*—12.5–50 mg/kg q 12 hr.

❑ Cephalothin

- **IM, IV (Adults):** *Most infections*—0.5–2 g q 4–6 hr.
- **IM, IV (Children):** *Most infections*—13.3–26.6 mg/kg q 4 hr or 20–40 mg/kg q 6 hr.

❑ Cephapirin

- **IM, IV (Adults):** *Most infections*—0.5–1 g q 4–6 hr.
- **IM, IV (Children >3 mo):** *Most infections*—10–20 mg/kg q 6 hr.

❑ Cephradine

- **PO (Adults):** *Most infections*—250–500 mg q 6 hr or 500–1000 mg q 12 hr.
- **PO (Children >9 mo):** *Most infections*—6.25–25 mg/kg q 6 hr.
- **IM, IV (Adults):** *Most infections*—500 mg–1 g q 6 hr.
- **IM, IV (Children >1 yr):** *Most infections*—12.5–25 mg/kg q 6 hr (up to 300 mg/kg/day).

AVAILABILITY

❑ Cefadroxil

▪ ***Capsules:*** 500 mg[Rx] ▪ ***Tablets:*** 1 g[Rx] ▪ ***Oral suspension:*** 125 mg/5 ml[Rx], 250 mg/5 ml[Rx], 500 mg/5 ml[Rx].

❑ Cefazolin

▪ ***Powder for injection:*** 250 mg[Rx], 500 mg[Rx], 1 g[Rx], 5 g[Rx], 10 g[Rx], 20 g[Rx] ▪ ***Premixed containers:*** 500 mg/50 ml D5W[Rx], 1 g/50 ml D5W[Rx].

❑ Cephalexin

▪ ***Capsules:*** 250 mg[Rx], 500 mg[Rx] ▪ ***Tablets:*** 250 mg[Rx], 500 mg[Rx] ▪ ***Oral suspension:*** 100 mg/ml[Rx], 125 mg/5 ml[Rx], 250 mg/5 ml[Rx].

❑ Cephalothin

▪ ***Powder for injection:*** 1 g[Rx], 2 g[Rx], 20 g[Rx] ▪ ***Premixed containers:*** 1 g/50 ml D5W[Rx], 2 g/50 ml D5W[Rx].

❑ Cephapirin

▪ ***Powder for injection:*** 500 mg[Rx], 1 g[Rx], 2 g[Rx], 4 g[Rx], 20 g[Rx].

❑ Cephradine

▪ ***Capsules:*** 250 mg[Rx], 500 mg[Rx] ▪ ***Oral suspension:*** 125 mg/5 ml[Rx], 250 mg/5 ml[Rx] ▪ ***Powder for injection:*** 250 mg[Rx], 500 mg[Rx], 1 g[Rx], 2 g[Rx].

TIME/ACTION PROFILE (blood levels)

	ONSET	PEAK	DURATION
Cefadroxil PO	rapid	1.5–2 hr	12–24 hr
Cefazolin IM	rapid	1–2 hr	6–12 hr
Cefazolin IV	rapid	end of infusion	6–12 hr
Cephalexin PO	rapid	1 hr	6–12 hr
Cephalothin IM	rapid	0.5 hr	4–6 hr
Cephalothin IV	rapid	end of infusion	4–6 hr
Cephapirin IM	rapid	0.5 hr	4–6 hr
Cephapirin IV	rapid	end of infusion	4–6 hr
Cephradine PO	rapid	1–2 hr	6–12 hr
Cephradine IM	rapid	1–2 hr	6–12 hr
Cephradine IV	rapid	end of infusion	6–12 hr

NURSING IMPLICATIONS

ASSESSMENT

- Assess patient for infection (vital signs; appearance of wound, sputum, urine, and stool; WBC) at beginning of and throughout therapy.
- Before initiating therapy, obtain a history to determine previous use of and reactions to penicillins or cephalosporins. Persons with a negative history of penicillin sensitivity may still have an allergic response.
- Obtain specimens for culture and sensitivity before initiating therapy. First dose may be given before receiving results.
- Observe patient for signs and symptoms of anaphylaxis (rash, pruritus, laryngeal edema, wheezing). Discontinue drug and notify physician or other health care professional immediately if these problems occur. Keep epinephrine, an antihistamine, and resuscitation equipment close by in case of an anaphylactic reaction.
- Monitor intake and output ratios and daily weight in patients taking *cephalothin*. Patients with impaired renal function, older than age 50, or receiving other nephrotoxic drugs are at risk for developing nephrotoxicity with high-dose therapy.
- ***Lab Test Considerations:*** May cause positive results for Coombs' test in patients receiving high doses or in neonates whose mothers were given cephalosporins prior to delivery.
- May cause increased AST, ALT, serum alkaline phosphatase, bilirubin, LDH, BUN, creatinine.
- *Cephalothin* may cause falsely elevated test results for serum and urine creatinine; do not obtain serum samples within 2 hr of administration.
- May rarely cause leukopenia, neutropenia, agranulocytosis, thrombocytopenia, eosinophilia, lymphocytosis, and thrombocytosis.

POTENTIAL NURSING DIAGNOSES

- Infection, risk for (Indications, Side Effects).
- Diarrhea (Adverse Reactions).
- Knowledge deficit, related to medication regimen (Patient/Family Teaching).

IMPLEMENTATION

- **PO:** Administer around the clock. May be administered on full or empty stomach. Administration with food may minimize GI irritation. Shake oral suspension well before administering. Refrigerate oral suspensions.
- **IM:** Reconstitute IM doses with sterile or bacteriostatic water for injection or 0.9% NaCl for injection. May be diluted with lidocaine to minimize injection discomfort.
- Inject deep into a well-developed muscle mass; massage well.
- **IV:** Monitor site frequently for thrombophlebitis (pain, redness, swelling). Change sites every 48–72 hr to prevent phlebitis.
- Do not use solutions that are cloudy or contain a precipitate.
- If aminoglycosides are administered concurrently, administer in separate sites, if possible, at least 1 hr apart. If second site is unavailable, flush line between medications.
- **Direct IV:** Dilute in at least 1 g/10 ml of sterile water for injection. Do not use preparations containing benzyl alcohol for neonates.
- ***Rate:*** Administer slowly over 3–5 min.

Cefazolin

- **Intermittent Infusion:** Reconstituted 500-mg or 1-g solution may be diluted in 50–100 ml of 0.9% NaCl, D5W, D10W, D5/0.25% NaCl, D5/0.45% NaCl, D5/09% NaCl, D5/LR, or lactated Ringer's solution. Solution is stable for 24 hr at room temperature and 96 hr if refrigerated.
- ***Rate:*** Administer over 30–60 min.
- **Syringe Compatibility:** ▪ heparin ▪ vitamin B complex.
- **Syringe Incompatibility:** ▪ ascorbic acid injection ▪ cimetidine ▪ lidocaine.
- **Y-Site Compatibility:** ▪ acyclovir ▪ amifostine ▪ atracurium ▪ aztreonam ▪ calcium gluconate ▪ cyclophosphamide ▪ diltiazem ▪ enalaprilat ▪ esmolol ▪ famotidine ▪ filgrastim ▪ fluconazole ▪ fludarabine ▪ foscarnet ▪ gallium nitrate ▪ heparin ▪ insulin ▪ labetalol ▪ lidocaine ▪ magnesium sulfate ▪ melphalan ▪ meperidine ▪ midazolam ▪ morphine ▪ multivitamins ▪ ondansetron ▪ pancuronium ▪ perphenazine ▪ sargramostim ▪ tacrolimus ▪ teniposide ▪ theophylline ▪ thiotepa ▪ vecuronium ▪ vitamin B complex with C.
- **Y-Site Incompatibility:** ▪ idarubicin ▪ pentamidine ▪ vinorelbine.

Cephalothin

- **Intermittent Infusion:** Reconstituted 1-mg or 2-g solution may be diluted in 50 ml of

D5W, D10W, D5/09% NaCl, D5/LR, lactated Ringer's solution, or 0.5% NaCl for intermittent infusion. Stable for 24 hr at room temperature and 96 hr if refrigerated. Solution may darken but this change will not alter potency.

- *Rate:* Administer each gram over 15–30 min.
- **Continuous Infusion:** May also be diluted in 500–1000 ml for continuous infusion.
- **Syringe Compatibility:** ▪ cimetidine.
- **Syringe Incompatibility:** ▪ metoclopramide.
- **Y-Site Compatibility:** ▪ Discontinue other IV solutions during IV administration of cephalothin.
- **Additive Compatibility:** ▪ hydrocortisone sodium succinate.

❑ Cephapirin

- **Intermittent Infusion:** Reconstituted solutions may be further diluted in 50–100 ml of 0.9% NaCl, D5W, D10W, D20W, D5/0.25% NaCl, D5/0.45% NaCl, D5/0.9% NaCl, or D5/LR. Stable for 24 hr at room temperature and 10 days if refrigerated.
- *Rate:* Administer over at least 15–20 min.
- **Continuous Infusion:** Solution may also be diluted in 500–1000 ml for continuous infusion.
- **Y-Site Compatibility:** ▪ acyclovir ▪ cyclophosphamide ▪ famotidine ▪ heparin ▪ hydrocortisone sodium succinate ▪ hydromorphone ▪ magnesium sulfate ▪ meperidine ▪ morphine ▪ multivitamins ▪ perphenazine ▪ potassium chloride ▪ vitamin B complex with C.

❑ Cephradine

- **Intermittent Infusion:** Dilute each gram in at least 10 ml of D5W, D10W, 0.9% NaCl, or D5/0.9% NaCl. May vary in color from light straw to yellow; color changes do not alter potency. Stable for 10 hr at room temperature or 48 hr if refrigerated.
- *Rate:* Administer over 30–60 min.
- **Solution Incompatibility:** ▪ lactated Ringer's injection ▪ Ringer's injection.

PATIENT/FAMILY TEACHING

- ❑ Instruct patient to take medication around the clock at evenly spaced times and to finish the medication completely as directed, even if feeling better. Missed doses should be taken as soon as possible unless almost time for next dose; do not double doses. Instruct patient to use calibrated measuring device with liquid preparations. Advise patient that sharing this medication may be dangerous.
- ❑ Advise patient to report signs of superinfection (furry overgrowth on the tongue, vaginal itching or discharge, loose or foul-smelling stools) and allergy.
- ❑ Instruct patient to notify health care professional if fever and diarrhea develop, especially if diarrhea contains blood, mucus, or pus. Advise patient not to treat diarrhea without consulting health care professional.

EVALUATION

Clinical response to therapy can be evaluated by: ▪ Resolution of signs and symptoms of infection. Length of time for complete resolution depends on the organism and site of infection ▪ Decreased incidence of infection when used for prophylaxis.

CEPHALOSPORINS—SECOND GENERATION

cefaclor
(**sef**-a-klor)
Ceclor

cefamandole
(sef-a-**man**-dole)
Mandol

cefmetazole
(sef-**met**-a-zole)
Zefazone

cefonicid
(se-**fon**-i-sid)
Monocid

cefotetan
(sef-oh-**tee**-tan)
Cefotan

cefoxitin
(se-**fox**-i-tin)
Mefoxin

cefprozil
(sef-**proe**-zil)
Cefzil

cefuroxime
(se-fyoor-**ox**-eem)
Ceftin, Kefurox, Zinacef

loracarbef
(lore-a-**kar**-beff)
Lorabid

CLASSIFICATION(S):
Anti-infectives (second-generation cephalosporins)

Pregnancy Category B

INDICATIONS

▪ Treatment of the following infections: ▫ Respiratory tract infections ▫ Skin and skin structure infections ▫ Bone and joint infections (not cefmetazole, cefprozil, or loracarbef) ▫ Urinary tract and gynecologic infection (not cefprozil) ▫ Septicemia (not cefmetazole, cefprozil, or loracarbef) ▪ **Cefamandole, cefotetan:** Intra-abdominal, gynecologic, and biliary tract infections ▪ **Cefuroxime:** Meningitis ▪ **Cefaclor, cefprozil, cefuroxime:** Otitis media ▪ **Cefamandole, cefmetazole, cefonicid, ceforanide, cefotetan, cefoxitin, cefuroxime:** Perioperative prophylaxis.

ACTION

▪ Bind to bacterial cell wall membrane, causing cell death. **Therapeutic Effects:** ▪ Bactericidal action against susceptible bacteria. **Spectrum:** ▪ Similar to that of first-generation cephalosporins but have increased activity against several other gram-negative pathogens including: ▫ *Haemophilus influenzae* ▫ *Escherichia coli* ▫ *Klebsiella pneumoniae* ▫ *Neisseria gonorrhoeae* (including penicillinase-producing strains) ▫ *Proteus* ▫ *Moraxella catarrhalis* ▪ Cefamandole, cefotetan, and cefoxitin have activity against *Bacteroides fragilis* ▪ Not active against methicillin-resistant staphylococci or enterococci.

PHARMACOKINETICS

Absorption: Well absorbed following IM administration. *Cefaclor, cefprozil, cefuroxime,* and *loracarbef*—well absorbed following PO administration.

Distribution: Widely distributed. Penetration into CSF is poor, but adequate for cefuroxime to be used in treating meningitis. All cross the placenta and enter breast milk in low concentrations.

Metabolism and Excretion: Excreted primarily unchanged by the kidneys.

Half-life: *Cefaclor*—35–54 min; *cefamandole*—30–60 min; *cefmetazole*—72 min; *cefonicid*—270 min; *cefotetan*—3–4.6 hr; *cefoxitin*—40–60 min; *cefmetazole*—72 min; *cefprozil*—90 min; *cefuroxime*—80 min; *loracarbef*—1 hr (all are increased in renal impairment).

CONTRAINDICATIONS AND PRECAUTIONS

Contraindicated in: ▪ Hypersensitivity to cephalosporins ▪ Serious hypersensitivity to penicillins.

Use Cautiously in: ▪ Renal impairment (dosage reduction/increased dosing interval recommended for: *cefamandole* if CCr ≤80 ml/min, *cefmetazole* if CCr ≤90 ml/min, *cefonicid* if CCr <80 ml/min, *cefotetan* if CCr ≤30 ml/min, *cefoxitin* if CCr ≤50 ml/min, *cefprozil* if CCr <30 ml/min, *cefuroxime* if CCr ≤20 ml/min, *loracarbef* if CCr <50 ml/min) ▪ Elderly, debilitated, or emaciated patients (may need supplemental vitamin K to prevent bleeding) ▪ Pregnancy and lactation (have been used safely).

ADVERSE REACTIONS AND SIDE EFFECTS*

CNS: SEIZURES (high doses).
GI: PSEUDOMEMBRANOUS COLITIS, <u>diarrhea</u>, <u>nausea</u>, <u>vomiting</u>, cramps.
Derm: <u>rashes</u>, urticaria.
Hemat: bleeding (↑ with cefamandole, cefmetazole, cefotetan), blood dyscrasias, hemolytic anemia.
Local: <u>pain</u> at IM site, <u>phlebitis</u> at IV site.
Misc: allergic reactions including ANAPHYLAXIS and SERUM SICKNESS, superinfection.

INTERACTIONS

Drug-Drug: ▪ **Probenecid** decreases excretion and increases blood levels ▪ If **alcohol** is ingested within 48–72 hr of cefamandole, cefmetazole, or cefotetan, a disulfiram-like reaction may occur ▪ Cefamandole, cefmetazole, and cefotetan may potentiate the effects of **anticoagu-**

***CAPITALS indicate life-threatening; <u>underlines</u> indicate most frequent.**

lants and increase the risk of bleeding with **antiplatelet agents, thrombolytic agents, NSAIDs, plicamycin,** or **valproic acid.**

ROUTE AND DOSAGE

❑ Cefaclor

- **PO (Adults):** 250–500 mg q 8 hr or 375–500 mg q 12 hr as extended-release tablets.
- **PO (Children >1 mo):** 6.7–13.4 mg/kg q 8 hr or 10–20 mg/kg q 12 hr (up to 60 mg/kg/day or 1.5 g/day have been used).

❑ Cefamandole

- **IM, IV (Adults):** *Most infections*—0.5–2 g q 4–6 hr. *Urinary tract infections*—500 mg–1 g q 8 hr. *Perioperative prophylaxis*—1 g within 60 min of incision, then q 6 hr for 24 hr.
- **IM, IV (Children >1 mo):** 8.3–16.7 mg/kg q 4 hr or 12.5–25 mg/kg q 6 hr or 16.7–33.3 mg/kg q 8 hr.

❑ Cefmetazole

- **IV (Adults):** *Most infections*—2 g q 6–12 hr. *Gonorrhea*—1 g IM given with or 30 min after 1 g probenecid PO.

❑ Cefonicid

- **IM, IV (Adults):** *Most infections*—0.5–1 g q 24 hr. *Severe/life-threatening infections*—2 g q 24 hr.

❑ Cefotetan

- **IM, IV (Adults):** *Most infections*—1–2 g q 12 hr. *Severe/life-threatening infections*—2–3 g q 12 hr. *Urinary tract infections*—500 mg–1 g q 12 hr or 1–2 g q 24 hr.

❑ Cefoxitin

- **IM, IV (Adults):** *Most infections*—1 g q 6–8 hr. *Severe infections*—1 g q 4 hr or 2 g q 6–8 hr. *Life-threatening infections*—2 g q 4 hr or 3 g q 6 hr. *Perioperative prophylaxis*—1–2 g within 60 min of incision, then q 6 hr for up to 24 hr.
- **IM, IV (Children and Infants >3 mo):** *Most infections*—13.3–26.7 mg/kg q 4 hr or 20–40 mg/kg q 6 hr.

❑ Cefprozil

- **PO (Adults):** *Most infections*—250–500 mg q 12 hr or 500 mg q 24 hr.
- **PO (Children 6 mo–12 yr):** *Otitis media*—15 mg/kg q 12 hr.
- **PO (Children 2–12 yr):** *Pharyngitis/tonsillitis*—7.5 mg/kg q 12 hr.

❑ Cefuroxime

- **PO (Adults and Children >12 yr):** *Most infections*—250–500 mg q 12 hr. *Urinary tract infections*—125–250 mg q 12 hr. *Gonorrhea*—1 g single dose.
- **PO (Children <12 yr):** *Most infections*—125 mg q 12 hr as tablets. *Otitis media*—250 mg q 12 hr as tablets.
- **PO (Children 3 mo–12 yr):** *Otitis media, impetigo*—15 mg/kg q 12 hr as oral suspension. *Pharyngitis/tonsillitis*—10 mg/kg q 12 hr as oral suspension.
- **IM, IV (Adults):** *Most infections*—750 mg–1.5 g q 8 hr. *Bacterial meningitis*—up to 3 g q 8 hr. *Gonorrhea*—1.5 g IM (750 mg in two sites) with 1 g probenecid PO.
- **IM, IV (Children and Infants >3 mo):** *Most infections*—16.7–33.3 mg/kg q 8 hr or 15–50 mg/kg q 12 hr. *Bone infections*—50 mg/kg q 8 hr. *Bacterial meningitis*—50–60 mg/kg q 6 hr or 66.7–80 mg/kg q 8 hr.
- **IM, IV (Neonates):** *Most infections*—10–33.3 mg/kg q 8 hr or 15–50 mg/kg q 12 hr. *Bacterial meningitis*—33.3 mg/kg q 8 hr or 50 mg/kg q 12 hr.

❑ Loracarbef

- **PO (Adults):** *Most infections*—200–400 mg q 12 hr. *Cystitis*—200 mg q 24 hr.
- **PO (Children 6 mo–12 yr):** *Pharyngitis/skin and soft tissue infections*—7.5 mg q 12 hr. *Otitis media*—15 mg/kg q 12 hr.

AVAILABILITY

❑ Cefaclor

▪ ***Capsules:*** 250 mg^Rx^, 500 mg^Rx^ ▪ ***Extended-release tablets (CD):*** 375 mg^Rx^, 500 mg^Rx^ ▪ ***Oral suspension:*** 125 mg/5 ml^Rx^, 187 mg/5 ml^Rx^, 250 mg/5 ml^Rx^, 375 mg/5 ml^Rx^.

❑ Cefamandole

▪ ***Powder for injection:*** 1 g^Rx^, 2 g^Rx^, 10 g^Rx^ ▪ ***Premixed containers:*** 1 g/50 ml D5W^Rx^, 2 g/50 ml D5W^Rx^.

❑ Cefmetazole

▪ ***Powder for injection:*** 1 g^Rx^, 2 g^Rx^.

❑ Cefonicid

▪ ***Powder for injection:*** 500 mg^Rx^, 1 g^Rx^, 10 g^Rx^.

❑ **Cefotetan**

▪ ***Powder for injection:*** 1 g[Rx], 2 g[Rx], 10 g[Rx].

❑ **Cefoxitin**

▪ ***Powder for injection:*** 1 g[Rx], 2 g[Rx], 10 g[Rx] ▪ ***Premixed containers:*** 1 g/50 ml D5W[Rx], 2 g/50 ml D5W[Rx].

❑ **Cefprozil**

▪ ***Tablets:*** 250 mg[Rx], 500 mg[Rx] ▪ ***Oral suspension:*** 125 mg/5 ml[Rx], 250 mg/5 ml[Rx].

❑ **Cefuroxime**

▪ ***Tablets:*** 125 mg[Rx], 250 mg[Rx], 500 mg[Rx] ▪ ***Oral suspension:*** 125 mg/5 ml[Rx] ▪ ***Powder for injection:*** 750 mg[Rx], 1.5 g[Rx], 7.5 g[Rx] ▪ ***Premixed containers:*** 750 mg/50 ml[Rx], 1.5 g/50 ml[Rx].

❑ **Loracarbef**

▪ ***Capsules:*** 200 mg[Rx] ▪ ***Oral suspension:*** 100 mg/5 ml[Rx].

TIME/ACTION PROFILE

	ONSET	PEAK	DURATION
Cefaclor PO	rapid	30–60 min	6–12 hr
Cefaclor PO-CD	UK	UK	12 hr
Cefamandole IM	rapid	30–120 min	4–8 hr
Cefamandole IV	rapid	end of infusion	4–8 hr
Cefmetazole IV	rapid	end of infusion	6–12 hr
Cefonicid IM	rapid	60 min	12–24 hr
Cefotetan IM	rapid	1–3 hr	12 hr
Cefotetan IV	rapid	end of infusion	12 hr
Cefoxitin IM	rapid	30 min	4–8 hr
Cefoxitin IV	rapid	end of infusion	4–8 hr
Cefprozil PO	UK	1–2 hr	12–24 hr
Cefuroxime PO	UK	2 hr	8–12 hr
Cefuroxime IM	rapid	15–60 min	6–12 hr
Cefuroxime IV	rapid	end of infusion	6–12 hr
Loracarbef PO	rapid	0.5–1.2 hr	12 hr

NURSING IMPLICATIONS

ASSESSMENT

- Assess patient for infection (vital signs; appearance of wound, sputum, urine, and stool; WBC) at beginning of and throughout therapy.
- Before initiating therapy, obtain a history to determine previous use of and reactions to penicillins or cephalosporins. Persons with a negative history of penicillin sensitivity may still have an allergic response.
- Obtain specimens for culture and sensitivity before initiating therapy. First dose may be given before receiving results.
- Observe patient for signs and symptoms of anaphylaxis (rash, pruritus, laryngeal edema, wheezing). Discontinue the drug and notify the physician or other health care professional immediately if these symptoms occur. Keep epinephrine, an antihistamine, and resuscitation equipment close by in the event of an anaphylactic reaction.

▪ ***Lab Test Considerations:*** May cause positive results for Coombs' test in patients receiving high doses or in neonates whose mothers were given cephalosporins prior to delivery.

- Monitor prothrombin time and assess patient for bleeding (guaiac stools; check for hematuria, bleeding gums, ecchymosis) daily in high-risk patients or those receiving *cefamandole, cefmetazole,* or *cefotetan;* may cause hypoprothrombinemia.
- *Cefuroxime* may also cause false-negative blood glucose results with ferricyanide tests. Use glucose enzymatic or hexokinase tests to determine blood glucose.
- May cause increased AST, ALT, serum alkaline phosphatase, bilirubin, LDH, BUN, and creatinine.
- *Cefotetan, cephalothin,* and *cefoxitin* may cause falsely elevated test results for serum and urine creatinine; do not obtain serum samples within 2 hr of administration.
- *Cefamandole* may cause false-positive test results for urine protein with acid and denaturization-precipitation tests.
- May rarely cause leukopenia, neutropenia, agranulocytosis, thrombocytopenia, eosinophilia, lymphocytosis, and thrombocytosis.

POTENTIAL NURSING DIAGNOSES

- Infection, risk for (Indications, Side Effects).
- Diarrhea (Adverse Reactions).
- Knowledge deficit, related to medication regimen (Patient/Family Teaching).

IMPLEMENTATION

▪ **PO:** Administer around the clock. May be administered on full or empty stomach. Administration with food may minimize GI irritation. Shake oral suspension well before administering.

- Administer *cefaclor* extended-release tablets with food; do not crush, break, or chew.
- *Cefuroxime* tablets should be swallowed whole, not crushed; crushed tablets have a

strong, persistent bitter taste. Tablets may be taken without regard to meals. Suspension must be taken with food. Shake well each time before using. Tablets and suspension are not interchangeable.

- **IM:** Reconstitute IM doses with sterile or bacteriostatic water for injection or 0.9% NaCl for injection. May be diluted with lidocaine to minimize injection discomfort.
  - Inject deep into a well-developed muscle mass; massage well.
  - When administering 2-g dose of *cefonicid*, divide in half and inject into two large muscle mass sites.
- **IV:** Change sites every 48–72 hr to prevent phlebitis. Monitor site frequently for thrombophlebitis (pain, redness, swelling).
  - If aminoglycosides are administered concurrently, administer in separate sites if possible, at least 1 hr apart. If second site is unavailable, flush line between medications.
- **Direct IV:** Dilute in at least 1 g/10 ml. Do not use preparations containing benzyl alcohol for neonates.
- ***Rate:*** Administer slowly over 3–5 min.

Cefamandole

- **Intermittent Infusion:** Reconstituted solution may be diluted in 100 ml of 0.9% NaCl, D5W, D10W, D5/0.25% NaCl, D5/0.9% NaCl, or D5/LR. Solution ranges in color from light yellow to amber. Do not use if solution is a different color or contains a precipitate. Solution is stable for 24 hr at room temperature and 96 hr if refrigerated.
  - Reconstitution causes gas to form. Vial can be vented prior to withdrawal, or use gas to assist in withdrawal of the solution by inverting the vial over the syringe needle, allowing the solution to flow into the needle.
  - Powder is difficult to dissolve. Reconstitute by keeping powder at stopper end of vial and adding diluent to other end of vial. Shake vigorously to dissolve.
- ***Rate:*** Administer over 15–30 min.
- **Continuous Infusion:** May be diluted in up to 1000 ml for continuous infusion.
- **Syringe Compatibility:** ▪ heparin.
- **Syringe Incompatibility:** ▪ cimetidine.
- **Y-Site Compatibility:** ▪ acyclovir ▪ cyclophosphamide ▪ hydromorphone ▪ magnesium sulfate ▪ meperidine ▪ morphine ▪ perphenazine.
- **Y-Site Incompatibility:** ▪ amiodarone ▪ hetastarch.
- **Solution Incompatibility:** ▪ lactated Ringer's solution ▪ Ringer's solution.

Cefmetazole

- **Intermittent Infusion:** Reconstituted solution may be further diluted in 50–100 ml of 0.9% NaCl, D5W, or lactated Ringer's solution for a concentration of 1–20 mg/ml. Solution is stable for 24 hr at room temperature and 7 days if refrigerated.
- ***Rate:*** Administer over 30–60 min.

Cefonicid

- **Intermittent Infusion:** Reconstituted solution may be further diluted in 50–100 ml of D5W, D10W, D5/LR, Ringer's or lactated Ringer's solution, D5/0.25% NaCl, D5/0.45% NaCl, D5/0.9% NaCl, or 0.9% NaCl. Solution may be colorless to light amber. Stable for 24 hr at room temperature and 72 hr if refrigerated.
- ***Rate:*** Administer over 20–30 min.
- **Y-Site Compatibility:** ▪ acyclovir ▪ amifostine ▪ aztreonam ▪ teniposide ▪ thiotepa.
- **Y-Site Incompatibility:** ▪ filgrastim ▪ sargramostim.

Cefotetan

- **Intermittent Infusion:** Reconstituted solution may be further diluted in 50–100 ml of D5W or 0.9% NaCl. Solution may be colorless or yellow. Solution is stable for 24 hr at room temperature or 96 hr if refrigerated.
- ***Rate:*** Administer over 20–30 min.
- **Y-Site Compatibility:** ▪ amifostine ▪ aztreonam ▪ diltiazem ▪ famotidine ▪ filgrastim ▪ fluconazole ▪ fludarabine ▪ insulin ▪ melphalan ▪ meperidine ▪ morphine ▪ paclitaxel ▪ sargramostim ▪ tacrolimus ▪ teniposide ▪ theophylline ▪ thiotepa.
- **Y-Site Incompatibility:** ▪ vinorelbine.

Cefoxitin

- **Intermittent Infusion:** Reconstituted solution may be further diluted in 50–100 ml of D5W, D10W, 0.9% NaCl, D5/0.45% NaCl, D5/0.25% NaCl, D5/0.9% NaCl, D5/LR, Ringer's or lactated Ringer's solution. Stable for 24 hr at room temperature and 1 wk if refrigerated. Darkening of powder does not alter potency.
- ***Rate:*** Administer over 15–30 min.

- **Continuous Infusion:** May be diluted in 500–1000 ml for continuous infusion.
- **Syringe Compatibility:** ▪ heparin.
- **Y-Site Incompatibility:** ▪ Manufacturer recommends stopping other medications during infusion.

❑ Cefuroxime

- **Intermittent Infusion:** Solution may be further diluted in 100 ml of 0.9% NaCl, D5W, D10W, D5/0.45% NaCl, or D5/0.9% NaCl. Stable for 24 hr at room temperature and 1 wk if refrigerated.
- *Rate:* Administer over 15–60 min.
- **Continuous Infusion:** May also be diluted in 500–1000 ml for continuous infusion.
- **Y-Site Compatibility:** ▪ acyclovir ▪ amifostine ▪ atracurium ▪ aztreonam ▪ cyclophosphamide ▪ diltiazem ▪ famotidine ▪ fludarabine ▪ foscarnet ▪ hydromorphone ▪ melphalan ▪ meperidine ▪ morphine ▪ ondansetron ▪ pancuronium ▪ perphenazine ▪ sargramostim ▪ tacrolimus ▪ teniposide ▪ thiotepa ▪ vecuronium.
- **Y-Site Incompatibility:** ▪ filgrastim ▪ fluconazole ▪ midazolam ▪ vinorelbine.

PATIENT/FAMILY TEACHING

- ❑ Instruct patient to take medication around the clock at evenly spaced times and to finish the medication completely, even if feeling better. Missed doses should be taken as soon as possible unless almost time for next dose; do not double doses. Advise patient that sharing of this medication may be dangerous.
- ❑ Advise patient to report signs of superinfection (furry overgrowth on the tongue, vaginal itching or discharge, loose or foul-smelling stools) and allergy.
- ❑ Caution patients that concurrent use of alcohol with *cefamandole, cefmetazole,* or *cefotetan* may cause a disulfiram-like reaction (abdominal cramps, nausea, vomiting, headache, hypotension, palpitations, dyspnea, tachycardia, sweating, flushing). Alcohol and alcohol-containing medications should be avoided during and for several days after therapy.
- ❑ Instruct patient to notify health care professional if fever and diarrhea develop, especially if stool contains blood, pus, or mucus. Advise patient not to treat diarrhea without consulting health care professional.

EVALUATION

Clinical response to therapy can be evaluated by: ▪ Resolution of signs and symptoms of infection. Length of time for complete resolution depends on the organism and site of infection ▪ Decreased incidence of infection when used for prophylaxis.

C

CEPHALOSPORINS—THIRD GENERATION

cefepime
(**seff**-e-peem)
Maxipime

cefixime
(se-**fix**-eem)
Suprax

cefoperazone
(sef-oh-**per**-a-zone)
Cefobid

cefotaxime
(sef-oh-**taks**-eem)
Claforan

cefpodoxime
(sef-poe-**dox**-eem)
Vantin

ceftazidime
(sef-**tay**-zi-deem)
Ceptaz, Fortaz, Tazicef, Tazidime

ceftibuten
(sef-tye-**byoo**-ten)
Cedax

ceftizoxime
(sef-ti-**zox**-eem)
Cefizox

ceftriaxone
(sef-try-**ax**-one)
Rocephin

CLASSIFICATION(S):
Anti-infectives (third-generation cephalosporins)

Pregnancy Category B

INDICATIONS

■ Treatment of □ Skin and skin structure infections □ Bone and joint infections □ Urinary and gynecologic infections including gonorrhea □ Respiratory tract infections □ Intra-abdominal infections □ Septicemia ■ **Cefotaxime, ceftazidime, ceftizoxime, ceftriaxone:** Meningitis ■ **Ceftriaxone:** Perioperative prophylaxis ■ **Cefepime:** Empiric treatment of febrile neutropenic patients ■ **Ceftriaxone:** Single-dose treatment of acute bacterial otitis media ■ **Cefotaxime, ceftriaxone:** Lyme disease.

ACTION

■ Bind to the bacterial cell wall membrane, causing cell death. **Therapeutic Effects:** ■ Bactericidal action against susceptible bacteria. **Spectrum:** ■ Similar to that of second-generation cephalosporins, but activity against staphylococci is less, while activity against gram-negative pathogens is greater, even for organisms resistant to first- and second-generation agents ■ Notable is increased action against: □ *Enterobacter* □ *Haemophilus influenzae* □ *Escherichia coli* □ *Klebsiella pneumoniae* □ *Neisseria* □ *Proteus* □ *Providencia* □ *Serratia* □ *Moraxella catarrhalis* □ *Borrelia burgdorferi* ■ Some agents have enhanced activity against: □ *Pseudomonas aeruginosa* (ceftazidime, cefoperazone) ■ All except cefixime, ceftibuten, and cefpodoxime have some activity against anaerobes, including *Bacteroides fragilis.*

PHARMACOKINETICS

Absorption: Well absorbed following IM administration. *Cefixime, ceftibuten,* and *cefpodoxime* are well absorbed following oral administration (cefixime suspension produces higher blood levels than tablets).

Distribution: Widely distributed. Cross the placenta; enter breast milk in low concentrations. CSF penetration better than with first- and second-generation agents.

Metabolism and Excretion: *Cefepime, cefixime, ceftazidime, cefpodoxime,* and *ceftizoxime*—>85% excreted in urine. *Cefoperazone*—excreted in the bile. *Ceftibuten, ceftriaxone,* and *cefotaxime*—partly metabolized and partly excreted in the urine.

Half-life: *Cefepime*—120 min; *cefixime*—180–240 min; *cefoperazone*—102–156 min; *cefotaxime*—60 min; *cefpodoxime*—120–180 min; *ceftazidime*—114–120 min; *ceftibuten*—120–144 min; *ceftizoxime*—84–114 min; *ceftriaxone*—348–522 min (all except *cefoperazone* and *ceftriaxone* are increased in renal impairment).

CONTRAINDICATIONS AND PRECAUTIONS

Contraindicated in: ■ Hypersensitivity to cephalosporins ■ Serious hypersensitivity to penicillins ■ Hypersensitivity to L-arginine (Ceptaz formulation only).

Use Cautiously in: ■ Renal impairment (decreased dosing/increased dosing interval recommended for: *cefepime* and *cefixime* if CCr ≤60 ml/min, *cefotaxime* if CCr <20 ml/min, *cefpodoxime* if CCr <30 ml/min, *ceftazidime* if CCr ≤50 ml/min, *ceftibuten* if CCr <50 ml/min, *ceftizoxime* if CCr ≤80 ml/min) ■ Severe hepatic/biliary impairment (dosage reduction/increased dosing interval recommended for *cefoperazone*) ■ Combined severe hepatic and renal impairment (dosage reduction/increased dosing interval recommended for *cefoperazone* and *ceftriaxone*) ■ Diabetes (*ceftibuten* suspension contains 1 g sucrose/5 ml) ■ Pregnancy and lactation (have been used safely).

ADVERSE REACTIONS AND SIDE EFFECTS*

CNS: SEIZURES (high doses).
GI: PSEUDOMEMBRANOUS COLITIS, diarrhea, nausea, vomiting, cramps, pseudolithiasis (ceftriaxone).
Derm: rashes, urticaria.
Hemat: bleeding (↑ with cefoperazone), blood dyscrasias, hemolytic anemia.
Local: pain at IM site, phlebitis at IV site.
Misc: allergic reactions including ANAPHYLAXIS and SERUM SICKNESS, superinfection.

INTERACTIONS

Drug-Drug: ■ **Probenecid** decreases excretion and increases serum levels (cefixime, cefotaxime, cefpodoxime, ceftizoxime) ■ Ingestion of **alcohol** within 48–72 hr of cefoperazone may result in a disulfiram-like reaction ■ Cefoperazone may potentiate the effects of **anticoagu-**

***CAPITALS indicate life-threatening; underlines indicate most frequent.**

lants and increase the risk of bleeding with **antiplatelet agents, thrombolytic agents, NSAIDs, plicamycin,** or **valproic acid.**

ROUTE AND DOSAGE

❑ **Cefepime**

- **IM (Adults):** 0.5–1 g q 12 hr.
- **IV (Adults):** 0.5–2 g q 12 hr.

❑ **Cefixime**

- **PO (Adults and Children >12 yr or >50 kg):** *Most infections*—400 mg q 24 hr or 200 mg q 12 hr. *Gonorrhea*—400 mg single dose.
- **PO (Children):** 8 mg/kg q 24 hr or 4 mg/kg q 12 hr (when treating otitis media, use suspension only).

❑ **Cefoperazone**

- **IM, IV (Adults):** *Mild to moderate infections*—1–2 g q 12 hr. *Severe infections*—2–4 g q 8 hr or 3–6 g q 12 hr.

❑ **Cefotaxime**

- **IM, IV (Adults):** *Most infections*—1 g q 12 hr. *Moderate or severe infections*—1–2 g q 6–8 hr. *Life-threatening infections*—2 g q 4 hr.
- **IM, IV (Children >1 mo):** 8.3–30 mg/kg q 4 hr or 12.5–45 mg/kg q 6 hr.
- **IV (Neonates 1–4 wk):** 50 mg/kg q 8 hr.
- **IV (Neonates ≤1 wk):** 50 mg/kg q 12 hr.

❑ **Cefpodoxime**

- **PO (Adults):** *Most infections*—200 mg q 12 hr. *Skin and soft tissue infections*—400 mg q 12 hr. *Urinary tract infections/pharyngitis*—100 mg q 12 hr. *Gonorrhea*—200 mg single dose.
- **PO (Children 6 mo–12 yr):** *Pharyngitis/tonsillitis/otitis media*—5 mg/kg q 12 hr; may be given as 10 mg/kg once daily for otitis media (not to exceed 200 mg/day for pharyngitis/tonsillitis or 400 mg/day for otitis media).

❑ **Ceftazidime**

- **IM, IV (Adults):** *Most infections*—500 mg–2 g q 8–12 hr. *Pneumonia/skin structure infections*—0.5–1 g q 8–12 hr. *Bone and joint infections*—2 g q 12 hr. *Severe/life-threatening infections*—2 g q 8 hr. *Complicated urinary tract infections*—500 mg q 8–12 hr. *Uncomplicated urinary tract infections*—250 mg q 12 hr.
- **IM, IV (Children 1 mo–12 yr):** 30–50 mg/kg q 8 hr.
- **IV (Neonates ≤4 wk):** 30 mg/kg q 12 hr.

❑ **Ceftibuten**

- **PO (Adults and Children ≥12 yr):** 400 mg q 24 hr for 10 days.
- **PO (Children 6 mo–12 yr):** 9 mg/kg/day for 10 days (up to 400 mg/day).

❑ **Ceftizoxime**

- **IM, IV (Adults):** *Severe infections*—1–2 g q 8–12 hr. *Life-threatening infections*—3–4 g q 8 hr. *Mild/moderate infections*—1 g q 8–12 hr. *Uncomplicated urinary tract infections*—500 mg q 12 hr.
- **IM, IV (Children >6 mo):** 50 mg/kg q 6–8 hr (not to exceed 200 mg/kg/day).

❑ **Ceftriaxone**

- **IM, IV (Adults):** *Most infections*—0.5–1 g q 12 hr or 1–2 g q 24 hr. *Gonorrhea*—250 mg IM. *Meningitis*—2 g q 12 hr.
- **IM, IV (Children):** *Most infections*—25–37.5 mg/kg q 12 hr. *Meningitis*—100 mg/kg q 24 hr or 50 mg/kg q 12 hr. *Skin/soft tissue infections*—50–75 mg/kg q 24 hr. *Acute otitis media*—50 mg/kg IM single dose.

AVAILABILITY

❑ **Cefepime**

- ***Powder for injection:*** 500-mg, 1-g, 2-g vials^Rx^, 1-g, 2-g piggyback bottles^Rx^.

❑ **Cefixime**

- ***Tablets:*** 200 mg^Rx^, 400 mg^Rx^ ▪ ***Oral suspension:*** 100 mg/5 ml^Rx^.

❑ **Cefoperazone**

- ***Powder for injection:*** 1 g^Rx^, 2 g^Rx^ ▪ ***Premixed containers:*** 1 g/50 ml^Rx^, 2 g/50 ml^Rx^.

❑ **Cefotaxime**

- ***Powder for injection:*** 1 g^Rx^, 2 g^Rx^, 10 g^Rx^ ▪ ***Premixed containers:*** 1 g/50 ml^Rx^, 2 g/50 ml^Rx^.

❑ **Cefpodoxime**

- ***Tablets:*** 100 mg^Rx^, 200 mg^Rx^ ▪ ***Oral suspension:*** 50 mg/5 ml^Rx^, 100 mg/5 ml^Rx^.

□ **Ceftazidime**

▪ ***Powder for injection:*** 500 mg[Rx], 1 g[Rx], 2 g[Rx], 6 g[Rx], 10 g[Rx] ▪ ***Premixed containers:*** 1 g/50 ml[Rx], 2 g/50 ml[Rx].

□ **Ceftibuten**

▪ ***Capsules:*** 400 mg[Rx] ▪ ***Oral suspension:*** 90 mg/5 ml[Rx], 180 mg/5 ml[Rx].

□ **Ceftizoxime**

▪ ***Powder for injection:*** 500 mg[Rx], 1 g[Rx], 2 g[Rx], 10 g[Rx] ▪ ***Premixed containers:*** 1 g/50 ml[Rx], 2 g/50 ml[Rx].

□ **Ceftriaxone**

▪ ***Powder for injection:*** 250 mg[Rx], 500 mg[Rx], 1 g[Rx], 2 g[Rx], 10 g[Rx] ▪ ***Premixed containers:*** 1 g/50 ml[Rx], 2 g/50 ml[Rx].

TIME/ACTION PROFILE

	ONSET	PEAK	DURATION
Cefepime IM	rapid	1–2 hr	12 hr
Cefepime IV	rapid	end of infusion	12 hr
Cefixime PO	rapid	2–6 hr	24 hr
Cefoperazone IM	rapid	1–2 hr	12 hr
Cefoperazone IV	rapid	end of infusion	12 hr
Cefotaxime IM	rapid	0.5 hr	4–12 hr
Cefotaxime IV	rapid	end of infusion	4–12 hr
Cefpodoxime PO	UK	2–3 hr	12 hr
Ceftazidime IM	rapid	1 hr	6–12 hr
Ceftazidime IV	rapid	end of infusion	6–12 hr
Ceftizoxime IM	rapid	0.5–1.5 hr	6–12 hr
Ceftizoxime IV	rapid	end of infusion	6–12 hr
Ceftriaxone IM	rapid	1–2 hr	12–24 hr
Ceftriaxone IV	rapid	end of infusion	12–24 hr

NURSING IMPLICATIONS

ASSESSMENT

- □ Assess patient for infection (vital signs; appearance of wound, sputum, urine, and stool; WBC) at beginning of and throughout therapy.
- □ Before initiating therapy, obtain a history to determine previous use of and reactions to penicillins or cephalosporins. Persons with a negative history of penicillin sensitivity may still have an allergic response.
- □ Obtain specimens for culture and sensitivity before initiating therapy. First dose may be given before receiving results.
- □ Observe patient for signs and symptoms of anaphylaxis (rash, pruritus, laryngeal edema, wheezing). Discontinue the drug and notify the physician or other health care professional immediately if these symptoms occur. Keep epinephrine, an antihistamine, and resuscitation equipment close by in the event of an anaphylactic reaction.
- ▪ ***Lab Test Considerations:*** May cause positive results for Coombs' test in patients receiving high doses or in neonates whose mothers were given cephalosporins prior to delivery.
- □ Monitor prothrombin time and assess patient for bleeding (guaiac stools; check for hematuria, bleeding gums, ecchymosis) daily in patients receiving *cefoperazone,* as this agent may cause hypoprothrombinemia.
- □ May cause increased AST, ALT, serum alkaline phosphatase, bilirubin, LDH, BUN, and creatinine.
- □ May rarely cause leukopenia, neutropenia, agranulocytosis, thrombocytopenia, eosinophilia, lymphocytosis, and thrombocytosis.

POTENTIAL NURSING DIAGNOSES

- ▪ Infection, risk for (Indications, Side Effects).
- ▪ Diarrhea (Adverse Reactions).
- ▪ Knowledge deficit, related to medication regimen (Patient/Family Teaching).

IMPLEMENTATION

- ▪ **PO:** Administer around the clock. May be administered on full or empty stomach. Administration with food may minimize GI irritation. Shake oral suspension well before administering. *Cefixime* tablets may be crushed and dissolved in water. Swirl glass with additional water to ensure all medication is received. Tablets are not bioequivalent with suspension.
- ▪ **IM:** Reconstitute IM doses with sterile or bacteriostatic water for injection or 0.9% NaCl for injection. May be diluted with lidocaine to minimize injection discomfort.
- □ Inject deep into a well-developed muscle mass; massage well.
- ▪ **IV:** Monitor injection site frequently for thrombophlebitis (pain, redness, swelling). Change sites every 48–72 hr to prevent phlebitis.
- □ If aminoglycosides are administered concurrently, administer in separate sites, if possible, at least 1 hr apart. If second site is unavailable, flush lines between medications.
- ▪ **Direct IV:** Dilute in at least 1 g/10 ml. Avoid direct IV administration of *cefoperazone* and

ceftriaxone. Do not use preparations containing benzyl alcohol for neonates.
- *Rate:* Administer slowly over 3–5 min.

❑ Cefepime

- **Intermittent Infusion:** Dilute in 50–100 ml for a concentration of 1–40 mg/ml with D5W, 0.9% NaCl, D10W, M/6 sodium lactate injection, D5/0.9% NaCl, D5/LR, D5/Normosol-R, or D5/Normosol-M injection.
  - Solution is stable for 24 hr at room temperature and 7 days if refrigerated.
- *Rate:* Administer over 30 min.
- **Y-Site Compatibility:** ▪ amikacin ▪ clindamycin ▪ heparin ▪ potassium chloride ▪ theophylline.

❑ Cefoperazone

- **Intermittent Infusion:** Reconstitute each gram with at least 2.8 ml of sterile or bacteriostatic water for injection or 0.9% NaCl. Shake vigorously and allow to stand for visualization and clarity. Solution may be colorless to straw-colored. Each gram in solution should be further diluted in 20–40 ml of 0.9% NaCl, D5W, D10W, D5/0.25% NaCl, D5/0.9% NaCl, D5/LR, or lactated Ringer's solution. Solution is stable for 24 hr at room temperature and 5 days if refrigerated.
- *Rate:* Administer over 15–30 min.
- **Continuous Infusion:** For continuous infusion, concentration should be 2–25 mg/ml.
- **Syringe Compatibility:** ▪ heparin.
- **Y-Site Compatibility:** ▪ acyclovir ▪ aztreonam ▪ cyclophosphamide ▪ enalaprilat ▪ esmolol ▪ famotidine ▪ fludarabine ▪ foscarnet ▪ hydromorphone ▪ magnesium sulfate ▪ melphalan ▪ morphine ▪ teniposide ▪ thiotepa.
- **Y-Site Incompatibility:** ▪ amifostine ▪ filgrastim ▪ hetastarch ▪ labetalol ▪ meperidine ▪ ondansetron ▪ pentamidine ▪ perphenazine ▪ promethazine ▪ sargramostim ▪ vinorelbine.

❑ Cefotaxime

- **Intermittent Infusion:** Reconstituted solution may be further diluted in 50–100 ml of D5W, D10W, lactated Ringer's solution, D5/0.25% NaCl, D5/0.45% NaCl, D5/0.9% NaCl, or 0.9% NaCl. Solution may appear light yellow to amber. Solution is stable for 24 hr at room temperature and 5 days if refrigerated.
- *Rate:* Administer over 20–30 min.
- **Syringe Compatibility:** ▪ heparin ▪ ofloxacin.
- **Y-Site Compatibility:** ▪ acyclovir ▪ amifostine ▪ aztreonam ▪ cyclophosphamide ▪ diltiazem ▪ famotidine ▪ fludarabine ▪ hydromorphone ▪ lorazepam ▪ magnesium sulfate ▪ melphalan ▪ meperidine ▪ midazolam ▪ morphine ▪ ondansetron ▪ perphenazine ▪ sargramostim ▪ teniposide ▪ thiotepa ▪ tolazoline ▪ vinorelbine.
- **Y-Site Incompatibility:** ▪ filgrastim ▪ fluconazole ▪ hetastarch ▪ pentamidine.

❑ Ceftazidime

- **Intermittent Infusion:** Reconstituted solution may be further diluted in at least 1 g/10 ml of 0.9% NaCl, D5W, D10W, D5/0.25% NaCl, D5/0.45% NaCl, D5/0.9% NaCl, or lactated Ringer's solution. Dilution causes carbon dioxide to form inside vial, resulting in positive pressure; vial may require venting after dissolution to preserve sterility of vial. Not required with L-arginine formulation (Ceptaz). Solution may appear yellow to amber; darkening does not alter potency. Solution is stable for 18 hr at room temperature and 7 days if refrigerated.
- *Rate:* Administer over 15–30 min.
- **Y-Site Compatibility:** ▪ acyclovir ▪ amifostine ▪ aztreonam ▪ ciprofloxacin ▪ diltiazem ▪ enalaprilat ▪ esmolol ▪ famotidine ▪ filgrastim ▪ fludarabine ▪ foscarnet ▪ gallium nitrate ▪ granisetron ▪ heparin ▪ hydromorphone ▪ labetalol ▪ melphalan ▪ meperidine ▪ morphine ▪ ondansetron ▪ paclitaxel ▪ ranitidine ▪ tacrolimus ▪ teniposide ▪ thiotepa ▪ vinorelbine ▪ zidovudine.
- **Y-Site Incompatibility:** ▪ fluconazole ▪ idarubicin ▪ midazolam ▪ pentamidine.

❑ Ceftizoxime

- **Intermittent Infusion:** Reconstituted solution may be further diluted in 50–100 ml of D5W, D10W, 0.9% NaCl, D5/0.25% NaCl, D5/0.45% NaCl, D5/0.9% NaCl, or lactated Ringer's solution. Solution is stable for 8 hr at room temperature and 48 hr if refrigerated.
- *Rate:* Administer over 15–30 min.
- **Y-Site Compatibility:** ▪ acyclovir ▪ amifostine ▪ aztreonam ▪ enalaprilat ▪ esmolol ▪ famotidine ▪ fludarabine ▪ foscarnet ▪ hydromorphone ▪ labetalol ▪ melphalan ▪ meperidine

▪ morphine ▪ ondansetron ▪ sargramostim ▪ teniposide ▪ thiotepa ▪ vinorelbine.

▪ **Y-Site Incompatibility:** ▪ filgrastim.

❑ Ceftriaxone

▪ **Intermittent Infusion:** Reconstitute each 250-mg vial with 2.4 ml, each 500-mg vial with 4.8 ml, each 1-g vial with 9.6 ml, and each 2-g vial with 19.2 ml of sterile water for injection, 0.9% NaCl, or D5W for a concentration of 100 mg/ml. Solution may be further diluted in 50–100 ml of 0.9% NaCl, D5W, D10W, D5/0.45% NaCl, or lactated Ringer's solution. Solution may appear light yellow to amber. Solution is stable for 3 days at room temperature.

▪ ***Rate:*** Administer over 15–30 min in adults and 10–30 min in newborns or children.

▪ **Y-Site Compatibility:** ▪ acyclovir ▪ amifostine ▪ aztreonam ▪ diltiazem ▪ fludarabine ▪ foscarnet ▪ gallium nitrate ▪ heparin ▪ melphalan ▪ meperidine ▪ methotrexate ▪ morphine ▪ paclitaxel ▪ sargramostim ▪ tacrolimus ▪ teniposide ▪ theophylline ▪ thiotepa ▪ zidovudine.

▪ **Y-Site Incompatibility:** ▪ filgrastim ▪ fluconazole ▪ pentamidine ▪ vancomycin ▪ vinorelbine.

PATIENT/FAMILY TEACHING

□ Instruct patient to take medication at evenly spaced times and to finish the medication completely, even if feeling better. Missed doses should be taken as soon as possible unless almost time for next dose; do not double doses. Advise patient that sharing of this medication may be dangerous.

□ Advise patient to report signs of superinfection (furry overgrowth on the tongue, vaginal itching or discharge, loose or foul-smelling stools) and allergy.

□ Caution patients that concurrent use of alcohol with *cefoperazone* may cause a disulfiram-like reaction (abdominal cramps, nausea, vomiting, headache, hypotension, palpitations, dyspnea, tachycardia, sweating, flushing). Alcohol and alcohol-containing medications should be avoided during and for several days after therapy.

□ Instruct patient to notify health care professional if fever and diarrhea develop, especially if stool contains blood, pus, or mucus. Advise patient not to treat diarrhea without consulting health care professional.

EVALUATION

Clinical response to therapy can be evaluated by: ▪ Resolution of the signs and symptoms of infection. Length of time for complete resolution depends on the organism and site of infection ▪ Decreased incidence of infection when used for prophylaxis.

CETIRIZINE

(se-**ti**-ri-zeen)

Zyrtec

CLASSIFICATION(S):

Antihistamine

Pregnancy Category B

INDICATIONS

▪ Relief of allergic symptoms caused by histamine release including: □ Seasonal and perennial allergic rhinitis □ Chronic urticaria.

ACTION

▪ Antagonizes the effects of histamine at H_1-receptor sites; does not bind to or inactivate histamine ▪ Anticholinergic effects are minimal and sedation is dose related. **Therapeutic Effects:** ▪ Decreased symptoms of histamine excess (sneezing, rhinorrhea, nasal and ocular pruritus, ocular tearing and redness).

PHARMACOKINETICS

Absorption: Well absorbed following oral administration.

Distribution: UK.

Metabolism and Excretion: Excreted primarily unchanged by the kidneys.

Half-life: 8 hr (decreased in children, increased in renal impairment).

CONTRAINDICATIONS AND PRECAUTIONS

Contraindicated in: ▪ Hypersensitivity ▪ Acute attacks of asthma ▪ Not recommended for use during lactation.

Use Cautiously in: ▪ Patients with hepatic or renal impairment (dosage reduction recommended if CCr <30 ml/min or hepatic function is impaired) ▪ Pregnancy or children <6 yr (safety not established).

ADVERSE REACTIONS AND SIDE EFFECTS

CNS: dizziness, drowsiness, fatigue.
EENT: pharyngitis.
GI: dry mouth.

INTERACTIONS

Drug-Drug: ▪ Additive CNS depression may occur with **alchohol, opioids,** or **sedative/hypnotics.**

ROUTE AND DOSAGE

▪ **PO (Adults):** 5–10 mg once daily.
▪ **PO (Children 6–11 yr):** 5–10 mg daily.

AVAILABILITY

▪ ***Tablets:*** 5 mg[Rx], 10 mg[Rx] ▪ ***Syrup:*** 5 mg/5 ml[Rx].

TIME/ACTION PROFILE (antihistaminic effects)

	ONSET	PEAK	DURATION
PO	30 min	4–8 hr	24 hr

NURSING IMPLICATIONS

ASSESSMENT

□ Assess allergy symptoms (rhinitis, conjunctivitis, hives) prior to and periodically throughout therapy.
□ Assess lung sounds and character of bronchial secretions. Maintain fluid intake of 1500–2000 ml/day to decrease viscosity of secretions.
▪ ***Lab Test Considerations:*** May cause false-negative allergy skin testing.

POTENTIAL NURSING DIAGNOSES

▪ Airway clearance, ineffective (Indications).
▪ Injury, risk for (Adverse Reactions).
▪ Knowledge deficit, related to medication regimen (Patient/Family Teaching).

IMPLEMENTATION

▪ **PO:** Administer once daily without regard to food.

PATIENT/FAMILY TEACHING

□ Instruct patient to take medication as directed.
□ May cause dizziness and drowsiness. Caution patient to avoid driving or other activities requiring alertness until response to medication is known.
□ Advise patient to avoid taking alcohol or other CNS depressants concurrently with this drug.
□ Advise patient that good oral hygiene, frequent rinsing of mouth with water, and sugarless gum or candy may minimize dry mouth. Patient should notify dentist if dry mouth persists >2 wk.
□ Instruct patient to contact health care professional if dizziness occurs or if symptoms persist.

EVALUATION

Effectiveness of therapy can be demonstrated by: ▪ Decrease in allergic symptoms.

CHLORAL HYDRATE

(**klor**-al **hye**-drate)
Aquachloral, {Novo-Chlorhydrate}, {PMS-Chloral Hydrate}

CLASSIFICATION(S):
Sedative/hypnotic

Schedule IV
Pregnancy Category C

INDICATIONS

▪ Short-term sedative and hypnotic (effectiveness decreases after 2 wk of use) ▪ Sedation or reduction of anxiety preoperatively (anesthetic adjunct).

ACTION

▪ Converted to trichloroethanol, which is the active drug. Has generalized CNS depressant properties. **Therapeutic Effects:** ▪ Sedation or induction of sleep.

PHARMACOKINETICS

Absorption: Well absorbed following oral or rectal administration.
Distribution: Widely distributed. Crosses the

placenta and enters breast milk in low concentrations.
Metabolism and Excretion: Converted by liver to trichloroethanol, which is active. Trichloroethanol is, in turn, metabolized by the liver and kidneys to inactive compounds.
Half-life: *Trichloroethanol*—8–10 hr.

CONTRAINDICATIONS AND PRECAUTIONS

Contraindicated in: ▪ Hypersensitivity ▪ Coma or pre-existing CNS depression ▪ Uncontrolled severe pain ▪ Pregnancy and lactation ▪ Esophagitis, gastritis, or ulcer disease ▪ Proctitis (rectal use) ▪ Tartrazine hypersensitivity (some rectal products).
Use Cautiously in: ▪ Hepatic dysfunction ▪ Severe renal impairment ▪ Patients who may be suicidal or who may have been addicted to drugs previously ▪ Geriatric patients (dosage reduction recommended).

ADVERSE REACTIONS AND SIDE EFFECTS*

CNS: excess sedation, disorientation, dizziness, hangover, headache, incoordination, irritability.
Resp: respiratory depression.
GI: diarrhea, nausea, vomiting, flatulence.
Derm: rashes.
Misc: tolerance, physical dependence, psychological dependence.

INTERACTIONS

Drug-Drug: ▪ Additive CNS depression with other **CNS depressants** including **alcohol, antihistamines, antidepressants, sedative/hypnotics,** and **opioid analgesics** ▪ May potentiate **warfarin** ▪ When given within 24 hr of IV **furosemide,** may cause diaphoresis, changes in blood pressure, and flushing.

ROUTE AND DOSAGE

- **PO (Adults):** *Hypnotic*—500–1000 mg 15–30 min before bedtime. *Preoperative sedation*—500 mg–1 g 30 min before surgery. *Daytime sedation*—250 mg 3 times daily.
- **PO (Geriatric Patients):** *Hypnotic*—250 mg 15–30 min before bedtime.
- **Rect (Adults):** *Sedation*—325 mg 3 times daily. *Hypnotic*—500–1000 mg.
- **PO, Rect (Children):** *Pre-EEG sedation*—25 mg/kg. *Sedation prior to dental/medical procedures*—50 mg/kg (up to 1 g; range 25–100 mg/kg; cumulative dose should not exceed 100 mg/kg or 2 g).

AVAILABILITY

- ***Capsules:*** 250 mg[Rx], 500 mg[Rx], 650 mg[Rx]
- ***Syrup:*** 250 mg/5 ml[Rx], 500 mg/5 ml[Rx]
- ***Suppositories:*** 325 mg[Rx], 500 mg[Rx].

TIME/ACTION PROFILE (sedation)

	ONSET	PEAK	DURATION
PO	30 min	1 hr	4–8 hr
Rect	0.5–1 hr	UK	4–8 hr

NURSING IMPLICATIONS

ASSESSMENT

- □ Assess mental status, sleep patterns, and potential for abuse prior to administering this medication. Prolonged use may lead to physical and psychological dependence. Limit amount of drug available to the patient.
- □ Assess level of consciousness at time of peak effect. Notify physician or other health care professional if desired sedation does not occur or if paradoxical reaction occurs.
- ▪ ***Lab Test Considerations:*** Interferes with tests for urinary 17-hydroxycorticosteroids and urinary catecholamines.

POTENTIAL NURSING DIAGNOSES

- Sleep pattern disturbance (Indications).
- Anxiety (Indications).
- Injury, risk for (Side Effects).

IMPLEMENTATION

- ▪ **General Info:** Before administering, reduce external stimuli and provide comfort measures to increase effectiveness of medication.
- □ Protect patient from injury. Place bed side rails up. Assist with ambulation. Remove cigarettes from patients receiving hypnotic dose.
- □ When administered before outpatient procedures for sedation in children, dose should be administered at the facility where procedure is to be performed, and monitoring must continue until level of consciousness is safe for discharge.

*CAPITALS indicate life-threatening; underlines indicate most frequent.

- **PO:** Capsules should be swallowed whole with a full glass of water or juice to minimize gastric irritation; do not chew. Dilute syrup in a half glass of water or juice.
- **Rect:** If suppository is too soft for insertion, chill in refrigerator for 30 min or run under cold water before removing foil wrapper.

PATIENT/FAMILY TEACHING

- □ Instruct patient to take chloral hydrate exactly as directed. Missed doses should be omitted; do not double doses. If used for 2 wk or longer, abrupt withdrawal may result in CNS excitement, tremor, anxiety, hallucinations, and delirium.
- □ Chloral hydrate causes drowsiness and dizziness. Caution patient to avoid driving or other activities requiring alertness until response to medication is known.
- □ Caution patient that concurrent alcohol use may create an additive effect that results in tachycardia, vasodilation, flushing, headache, hypotension, and pronounced CNS depression. Alcohol and other CNS depressants should be avoided while taking chloral hydrate.
- □ Advise patient to discontinue use and notify health care professional if skin rash, dizziness, irritability, impaired thought processes, headache, or motor incoordination occurs.

EVALUATION

Effectiveness of therapy can be demonstrated by: ▪ Sedation ▪ Improvement in sleep pattern.

CHLORAMBUCIL

(klor-**am**-byoo-sill)
Leukeran

CLASSIFICATION(S):
Antineoplastic (alkylating agent), Immunosuppressant

Pregnancy Category D

INDICATIONS

▪ Management of chronic lymphocytic leukemia, malignant lymphoma, and Hodgkin's disease (alone and in combination with other agents).

ACTION

▪ An alkylating agent that interferes with cellular protein synthesis (cell-cycle phase–nonspecific). **Therapeutic Effects:** ▪ Death of rapidly replicating cells, particularly malignant ones.

PHARMACOKINETICS

Absorption: Rapidly and completely absorbed from the GI tract.
Distribution: Crosses the placenta.
Metabolism and Excretion: Extensively metabolized by the liver.
Half-life: 1.5 hr.

CONTRAINDICATIONS AND PRECAUTIONS

Contraindicated in: ▪ Hypersensitivity ▪ Previous resistance ▪ Pregnancy or lactation.
Use Cautiously in: ▪ Patients with childbearing potential ▪ Infection ▪ Other chronic debilitating diseases ▪ Geriatric patients (more sensitive to immunosuppressants).

ADVERSE REACTIONS AND SIDE EFFECTS*

Resp: pulmonary fibrosis.
GI: nausea, stomatitis (rare), vomiting.
GU: decreased sperm count, infertility.
Derm: alopecia (rare), dermatitis, rash.
Hemat: LEUKOPENIA, anemia, thrombocytopenia.
Metab: <u>hyperuricemia</u>.
Misc: allergic reactions, risk of second malignancy.

INTERACTIONS

Drug-Drug: ▪ Additive bone marrow depression with other **bone marrow depressants (antineoplastics)** or **immunosuppressants** ▪ May decrease antibody response to **live virus vaccines** and increase the risk of adverse reactions.

ROUTE AND DOSAGE

- **PO (Adults):** 0.1–0.2 mg/kg/day (3–6 mg/m^2/day) (usual range 4–10 mg/day as a single dose or in divided doses), then adjust dose on basis of blood counts; *or* 0.4 mg/kg (12 mg/m^2) twice weekly, increased by 0.1 mg/kg (3 mg/m^2) q 2 wk, then adjusted as necessary.
- **PO (Geriatric Patients):** Initial dose should not be more than 2–4 mg/day.

***CAPITALS indicate life-threatening; <u>underlines</u> indicate most frequent.**

- **PO (Children):** 0.1–0.2 mg/kg/day (4.5 mg/m^2/day) single dose or in divided doses.

AVAILABILITY
- ***Tablets:*** 2 mg[Rx].

TIME/ACTION PROFILE (effects on white blood cell counts)

	ONSET	PEAK	DURATION
PO	7–14 days	7–14 days	14–28 days

NURSING IMPLICATIONS

ASSESSMENT
- Monitor for bone marrow depression. Assess for bleeding (bleeding gums, bruising, petechiae, guaiac stools, urine, and emesis) and avoid IM injections and rectal temperatures if platelet count is low. Apply pressure to venipuncture sites for 10 min. Assess for signs of infection during neutropenia. Anemia may occur. Monitor for increased fatigue, dyspnea, and orthostatic hypotension.
- Monitor intake and output ratios and daily weights. Report significant changes in totals.
- Monitor for symptoms of gout (increased uric acid, joint pain, edema). Encourage patient to drink at least 2 liters of fluid/day. Allopurinol may be given to decrease uric acid levels. Alkalinization of urine may be ordered to increase excretion of uric acid.
- ***Lab Test Considerations:*** Monitor CBC and differential prior to and weekly during course of therapy. Report significant drops in granulocyte count. Leukopenia usually occurs around the 3rd week of therapy and persists for 1–2 wk following a short course of therapy. The nadir of leukopenia occurs in 7–14 days after a single high dose, with recovery in 2–3 wk. The neutrophil count may decrease for 10 days after last dose. Monitor platelet count throughout therapy. Thrombocytopenia usually occurs around 3rd week of therapy and persists for 1–2 wk following a short course of therapy. The nadir of thrombocytopenia occurs in 1–2 wk after a single dose, with recovery in 2–3 wk. Institute thrombocytopenia precautions if platelet count is $<150,000/mm^3$.
- Monitor liver function tests, BUN, serum creatinine, and uric acid prior to and periodically during course of therapy. May cause elevated ALT and alkaline phosphatase, which may reflect hepatotoxicity.

POTENTIAL NURSING DIAGNOSES
- Injury, risk for (Side Effects).
- Infection, risk for (Side Effects).
- Knowledge deficit, related to medication regimen (Patient/Family Teaching).

IMPLEMENTATION
- **PO:** Administer oral medication either 1 hr before or 2 hr after meals. Can be compounded into a suspension by pharmacist for patients who have difficulty swallowing.

PATIENT/FAMILY TEACHING
- Instruct patient to take medication exactly as directed, even if nausea or vomiting is a problem. Consult health care professional if vomiting occurs shortly after dose is taken. If a dose is missed and the medication is ordered daily, take when remembered that day. If ordered more frequently, take as soon as possible unless almost time for next dose. Do not double doses.
- Instruct patient to report unusual bleeding or bruising. Advise patient of thrombocytopenia precautions (use soft toothbrush, electric razor, and avoid falls; do not drink alcoholic beverages or take medication containing aspirin or NSAIDs because they may precipitate gastric bleeding).
- Caution patient to avoid crowds and persons with known infections. Health care professional should be informed immediately if symptoms of infection (fever, sore throat, chills, cough, hoarseness, lower back or side pain, difficult or painful urination) or rash occurs.
- Instruct patient to inspect oral mucosa for redness and ulceration. If mouth sores occur, advise patient to use sponge brush and rinse mouth with water after eating and drinking. Stomatitis may require treatment with opioid analgesics.
- Advise patients on long-term therapy to notify health care professional immediately if cough, shortness of breath, and fever occur.
- Instruct patient to inform health care professional if nausea and vomiting persist. Antiemetics may be used, although these side ef-

fects usually last less than 1 day and tend to decrease with continued therapy.
- □ Discuss with patient the possibility of hair loss. Explore methods of coping.
- □ This drug may cause irreversible gonadal suppression; however, patient should still use birth control. Instruct patient to inform health care professional if pregnancy is suspected.
- □ Instruct patient not to receive any vaccinations without advice of health care professional.

EVALUATION

Effectiveness of therapy can be demonstrated by: ▪ Improvement of hematopoietic values in leukemia ▪ Decrease in size and spread of the tumor. Therapeutic effects are usually seen by the 3rd week of therapy.

CHLORAMPHENICOL†
(klor-am-**fen**-i-kole)
AK-Chlor, Chloracol, Chlorofair, Chloromycetin, Chloroptic, Econochlor, {Fenicol}, I-Chlor, {Novochlorocap}, Ocu-Chlor, Ophthochlor, {Ophtho-Chloram}, {Pentamycetin}, {Sopamycetin}, Spectro-Chlor

CLASSIFICATION(S):
Anti-infective (miscellaneous)

Pregnancy Category UK

†See Appendix O for ophthalmic use.

INDICATIONS

▪ **PO, IV: :** Management of the following serious infections when less toxic agents cannot be used: □ Skin and soft tissue infections □ Intra-abdominal infections □ CNS infections (including meningitis) □ Bacteremia ▪ **Ophth:** Management of local infections.

ACTION

▪ Inhibits protein synthesis in susceptible bacteria at the level of the 50S ribosome. **Therapeutic Effects:** ▪ Bacteriostatic action. **Spectrum:** ▪ Wide variety of gram-positive aerobic organisms including: □ *Streptococcus pneumoniae* and other streptococci ▪ Gram-negative pathogens: □ *Haemophilus influenzae* □ *Neisseria meningitidis* □ *Salmonella* □ *Shigella* □ Some Enterococci ▪ Anaerobes: □ *Bacteroides fragilis* □ *Bacteroides melaninogenicus* ▪ Other organisms inhibited: □ *Rickettsia* □ *Chlamydia* □ *Mycoplasma.*

PHARMACOKINETICS

Absorption: Well absorbed following oral administration. Some systemic and intraocular absorption follows ophthalmic administration.
Distribution: Widely distributed. Crosses the blood-brain barrier with CSF levels 60% of serum values. Crosses the placenta; enters breast milk.
Metabolism and Excretion: Mostly metabolized by the liver; <10% excreted unchanged by the kidneys.
Half-life: 1.5–3.5 hr.

CONTRAINDICATIONS AND PRECAUTIONS

Contraindicated in: ▪ Hypersensitivity ▪ Previous toxic reaction to chloramphenicol.
Use Cautiously in: ▪ Newborns, patients with severe hepatic or renal disease, geriatric patients (increased risk of reactions due to inability to metabolize and excrete chloramphenicol) ▪ Pregnancy or lactation (safety not established).

ADVERSE REACTIONS AND SIDE EFFECTS*

CNS: confusion, depression, headache.
EENT: blurred vision, optic neuritis.
GI: bitter taste (IV only), diarrhea, nausea, vomiting.
Derm: rashes.
Hemat: APLASTIC ANEMIA, <u>bone marrow depression</u>.
Neuro: peripheral neuritis.
Misc: GRAY SYNDROME in newborns, fever.

INTERACTIONS

Drug-Drug: ▪ May increase effects of the following drugs: **oral hypoglycemic agents, warfarin,** and **phenytoin** ▪ **Phenobarbital** or **rifampin** may decrease chloramphenicol blood levels ▪ May delay response to **vitamin B_{12}** or **folic acid** therapy ▪ Bone marrow depression may be additive with **bone marrow–depress-**

{} = Available in Canada only.
***CAPITALS indicate life-threatening; <u>underlines</u> indicate most frequent.**

ing agents (antineoplastics) ▪ Chronic high-dose **acetaminophen** may increase toxicity.

ROUTE AND DOSAGE

- **PO, IV (Adults):** 12.5 mg/kg q 6 hr (up to 4 g/day).
- **PO, IV (Infants >2 wk and Children):** *Most infections*—12 mg/kg q 6 hr or 25 mg/kg q 12 hr. *Bacteremia/meningitis*—up to 75–100 mg/kg/day.
- **PO, IV (Infants, Premature and Full Term, <2 wk):** *Most infections*—6.25 mg/kg q 6 hr. *Bacteremia/meningitis*—up to 75–100 mg/kg/day.

AVAILABILITY

▪ ***Capsules:*** 250 mg[Rx] ▪ ***Powder for injection:*** 1-g vials[Rx].

TIME/ACTION PROFILE (blood levels)

	ONSET	PEAK	DURATION
PO	rapid	1–3 hr	6–12 hr
IV	rapid	end of infusion	6–12 hr

NURSING IMPLICATIONS

ASSESSMENT

- **General Info:** Assess patient for infection (vital signs, wound appearance, sputum, urine, stool, and WBC) at beginning of and throughout therapy.
- □ This drug should be administered systemically only to hospitalized patients or those under close medical supervision. Diagnosis should be confirmed with cultures prior to administration.
- □ Assess patients daily for signs of bone marrow depression (petechiae, sore throat, fatigue, unusual bleeding, bruising). Patients who have impaired liver or renal function, infants, children, and the elderly are at the greatest risk of developing adverse effects.
- **Premature Infants and Neonates:** Assess for gray syndrome (abdominal distention, blue-gray skin coloring, uneven breathing, unresponsiveness, low body temperature, cyanosis, hypotension, and respiratory distress).
- ***Lab Test Considerations:*** CBC and platelet count should be monitored every 2 days throughout therapy. The drug should be stopped if anemia, reticulocytopenia, leukopenia, or thrombocytopenia develops.
- ***Toxicity and Overdose:*** Monitor serum levels weekly, especially in low-birth-weight infants, patients with impaired or immature metabolic function, or patients receiving other medications metabolized by the liver. Therapeutic levels: peak, 10–25 mcg/ml. Concentrations exceeding 25 mcg/ml increase the risk of reversible bone marrow depression and gray syndrome.

POTENTIAL NURSING DIAGNOSES

- Infection, risk for (Indications, Adverse Reactions).
- Knowledge deficit, related to medication regimen (Patient/Family Teaching).

IMPLEMENTATION

- **General Info:** Medication should be administered around the clock.
- **PO:** Give oral doses with a full glass of water 1 hr before or 2 hr after meals.
- **Direct IV:** Reconstitute to a 10% solution by adding 10 ml of sterile water for injection or D5W to each 1 g for a concentration of not greater than 100 mg/ml. Do not use preparations containing benzyl alcohol in neonates.
- ***Rate:*** Inject slowly over at least 1 min.
- **Intermittent Infusion:** May be further diluted in 50–100 ml of D5W, D10W, D5/0.9% NaCl, D5/0.45% NaCl, D5/0.25% NaCl, D5/LR, 0.45% NaCl, 0.9% NaCl, or lactated Ringer's solution. Solution may form crystals at low temperatures. Shake well to dissolve crystals. Do not administer cloudy solutions.
- ***Rate:*** Administer over 30–60 min.
- **Y-Site Compatibility:** ▪ acyclovir ▪ cyclophosphamide ▪ enalaprilat ▪ esmolol ▪ foscarnet ▪ hydromorphone ▪ labetalol ▪ magnesium sulfate ▪ meperidine ▪ morphine ▪ perphenazine ▪ tacrolimus.
- **Y-Site Incompatibility:** ▪ fluconazole.

PATIENT/FAMILY TEACHING

- **General Info:** Instruct patient to take medication exactly as directed and to finish prescription, even if feeling better. Missed doses should be taken as soon as possible unless almost time for next dose. Do not double doses. Caution patient that sharing of this medication may be dangerous.
- □ Advise patient to contact health care professional immediately if signs of unusual bleed-

ing; bruising; fever; sore throat; nausea; vomiting; diarrhea; numbness, tingling, or burning pain or weakness in hands or feet occurs. Medication should be discontinued with the onset of these symptoms.
- Instruct patient to report signs of superinfection (stomatitis, perianal itching, vaginal discharge, fever).
- Emphasize the importance of follow-up exams. Bone marrow depression may develop weeks to months after drug therapy has been discontinued.
- **IV:** Reassure patient that bitter taste 15–20 sec following injection is limited to 2–3 min.

EVALUATION

Clinical response to therapy can be evaluated by: ▪ Resolution of the signs and symptoms of infection. Length of time for complete resolution depends on the organism and site of infection.

CHLORDIAZEPOXIDE

(klor-dye-az-e-**pox**-ide)
{Apo-Chlordiazepoxide}, Libritabs, Librium, {Novopoxide}, {Solium}

CLASSIFICATION(S):
Sedative/hypnotic (benzodiazepine)

Schedule IV
Pregnancy Category D

INDICATIONS

▪ Adjunct management of anxiety ▪ Treatment of alcohol withdrawal.

ACTION

▪ Acts at many levels of the CNS to produce anxiolytic effect ▪ Depresses the CNS, probably by potentiating gamma-aminobutyric acid (GABA), an inhibitory neurotransmitter. **Therapeutic Effects:** ▪ Sedation ▪ Relief of anxiety.

PHARMACOKINETICS

Absorption: Well absorbed from the GI tract. IM absorption may be slow and unpredictable.
Distribution: Widely distributed. Crosses the blood-brain barrier. Crosses the placenta; enters breast milk.
Metabolism and Excretion: Highly metabolized by the liver. Some products of metabolism are active as CNS depressants.
Half-life: 5–30 hr.

CONTRAINDICATIONS AND PRECAUTIONS

Contraindicated in: ▪ Hypersensitivity ▪ Some products contain tartrazine and should be avoided in patients with known intolerance ▪ Cross-sensitivity with other benzodiazepines may occur ▪ Comatose patients or those with pre-existing CNS depression ▪ Uncontrolled severe pain ▪ Narrow-angle glaucoma ▪ Pregnancy and lactation ▪ Children ≤6 yr ▪ Porphyria.
Use Cautiously in: ▪ Hepatic dysfunction ▪ Severe renal impairment ▪ Patients who may be suicidal or who may have been addicted to drugs previously ▪ Geriatric or debilitated patients (initial dosage reduction required).

ADVERSE REACTIONS AND SIDE EFFECTS*

CNS: <u>dizziness</u>, <u>drowsiness</u>, hangover, headache, mental depression, paradoxical excitation.
EENT: blurred vision.
GI: constipation, diarrhea, nausea, vomiting.
Derm: rashes.
Local: <u>pain at IM site</u>.
Misc: physical dependence, psychological dependence, tolerance.

INTERACTIONS

Drug-Drug: ▪ **Alcohol, antidepressants, antihistamines,** and **opioids**—concurrent use results in additive CNS depression ▪ **Cimetidine, oral contraceptives, disulfiram, fluoxetine, isoniazid, ketoconazole, metoprolol, propoxyphene, propranolol,** or **valproic acid** may enhance its actions ▪ May decrease efficacy of **levodopa** ▪ **Rifampin** or **barbiturates** may decrease effectiveness of chlordiazepoxide ▪ Sedative effects may be decreased by **theophylline.**

ROUTE AND DOSAGE

- **PO (Adults):** *Alcohol withdrawal*—50–100 mg, repeated until agitation is controlled (up to 400 mg/day). *Anxiety*—5–25 mg 3–4 times daily.

- **PO (Geriatric Patients or Debilitated Patients):** *Anxiety*—5 mg 2–4 times daily initially, increased as needed.
- **PO (Children >6 yr):** *Anxiety*—5 mg 2–4 times daily, up to 10 mg 2–3 times daily.
- **IM, IV (Adults):** *Alcohol withdrawal*—50–100 mg initially; may be repeated in 2–4 hr. *Anxiety*—50–100 mg initially, then 25–50 mg 3–4 times daily as required (25–50 mg initially in elderly patients). *Preoperative sedation*—50–100 mg 1 hr preop.
- **IM, IV (Geriatric Patients or Debilitated Patients):** *Anxiety/sedation*—25–50 mg/dose.
- **IM, IV (Children >12 yr):** *Anxiety/sedation*—25–50 mg/dose.

AVAILABILITY

■ ***Capsules:*** 5 mg[Rx], 10 mg[Rx], 25 mg[Rx] ■ ***Tablets:*** 5 mg[Rx], 10 mg[Rx], 25 mg[Rx] ■ ***Injection:*** 100-mg ampule[Rx] ■ ***In combination with:*** amitriptyline (Limbitrol), clidinium[Rx]. See Appendix A.

TIME/ACTION PROFILE (sedation)

	ONSET	PEAK	DURATION
PO	1–2 hr	0.5–4 hr	up to 24 hr
IM	15–30 min	UK	UK
IV	1–5 min	UK	0.25–1 hr

NURSING IMPLICATIONS

ASSESSMENT

- **General Info:** Assess patient for anxiety and level of sedation (ataxia, dizziness, slurred speech) periodically throughout therapy.
- □ Monitor blood pressure, heart rate, and respiratory rate frequently when administering parenterally. Report significant changes immediately.
- □ Prolonged high-dose therapy may lead to psychological or physical dependence. Restrict the amount of drug available to patient.
- **Alcohol Withdrawal:** Assess patient for tremors, agitation, delirium, and hallucinations. Protect patient from injury.
- ***Lab Test Considerations:*** Patients on prolonged therapy should have CBC and liver function tests evaluated periodically. May cause an increase in serum bilirubin, AST, and ALT.
- □ May alter results of urine 17-ketosteroids and 17-ketogenic steroids. May cause decreased response on metyrapone tests and decreased thyroidal uptake of ^{123}I and ^{131}I.

POTENTIAL NURSING DIAGNOSES

- Anxiety (Indications).
- Injury, risk for (Side Effects).
- Knowledge deficit, related to medication regimen (Patient/Family Teaching).

IMPLEMENTATION

- **General Info:** IV administration is usually the preferred route for parenteral administration because of the slow, erratic absorption following IM administration.
- □ Following parenteral administration, have patient remain recumbent, and observe for 3–8 hr or longer, depending on patient response.
- □ Equipment to maintain a patent airway should be immediately available when chlordiazepoxide is administered intravenously.
- □ Use parenteral solution immediately after reconstitution and discard any unused portion.
- **PO:** Administer after meals or with milk to minimize GI irritation. Tablets may be crushed and taken with food or fluids if patient has difficulty swallowing.
- **IM:** Reconstitute with 2 ml of diluent provided by manufacturer only. Do not use solution if opalescent or hazy. Agitate gently to minimize bubbling. Administer slowly, deep into a well-developed muscle mass to minimize pain at injection site. Solution reconstituted with IM diluent should not be given IV.
- **Direct IV:** Reconstitute 100 mg in 5 ml of 0.9% NaCl or sterile water for injection. Do not use IM diluent.
- ***Rate:*** Administer prescribed dose slowly over at least 1 min. Rapid administration may cause apnea, hypotension, bradycardia, or cardiac arrest.
- **Syringe Incompatibility:** ■ benzquinamide.
- **Y-Site Compatibility:** ■ heparin ■ hydrocortisone sodium succinate ■ potassium chloride ■ vitamin B complex with C.

PATIENT/FAMILY TEACHING

- □ Instruct patient to take chlordiazepoxide exactly as directed. If medication is less effective after a few weeks, check with health care professional; do not increase dose. Medication should be tapered at the completion of long-term therapy. Sudden cessation of medication may lead to withdrawal (insomnia, irritability, nervousness, tremors).

- May cause drowsiness or dizziness. Caution patient to avoid driving or other activities requiring alertness until response to medication is known.
- Advise patient to avoid the use of alcohol and other CNS depressants concurrently with this medication.
- Instruct patient to consult health care professional before taking OTC medications.
- Instruct patient to notify health care professional if pregnancy is planned or suspected.

EVALUATION

Effectiveness of therapy can be demonstrated by: ▪ Decreased sense of anxiety ▫ Increased ability to cope ▪ Decreased tremulousness and more rational ideation when used for alcohol withdrawal.

C

CHLOROQUINE

(**klor**-oh-kwin)

Aralen

CLASSIFICATION(S):

Antimalarial

Pregnancy Category UK

INDICATIONS

▪ Prophylaxis and treatment of malaria ▪ Treatment of amebic liver abscess. **Unlabeled Uses:** ▪ Treatment of severe rheumatoid arthritis.

ACTION

▪ Inhibits protein synthesis in susceptible organisms by inhibiting DNA and RNA polymerase. **Therapeutic Effects:** ▪ Death of plasmodia responsible for causing malaria ▪ Improvement in inflammatory arthritis.

PHARMACOKINETICS

Absorption: Well absorbed following oral administration.

Distribution: Widely distributed; high tissue concentrations achieved. Crosses the placenta, enters breast milk.

Metabolism and Excretion: 30% metabolized by the liver. Metabolite also has antiplasmodial activity; 70% excreted unchanged by the kidneys.

Half-life: 72–120 hr.

CONTRAINDICATIONS AND PRECAUTIONS

Contraindicated in: ▪ Hypersensitivity ▪ Hypersensitivity to other 4-aminoquinolones (hydroxychloroquine) ▪ Visual damage caused by chloroquine or other 4-aminoquinolones.

Use Cautiously in: ▪ Liver disease ▪ Alcoholism ▪ Patients receiving hepatotoxic drugs ▪ Psoriasis ▪ G6PD deficiency ▪ Bone marrow depression ▪ Pregnancy (although safety not established, has been used) ▪ Children (extremely sensitive to chloroquine effects).

ADVERSE REACTIONS AND SIDE EFFECTS*

CNS: SEIZURES, anxiety, confusion, dizziness, fatigue, headache, irritability, personality changes.

EENT: keratopathy, ototoxicity, retinopathy, visual disturbances.

CV: ECG changes, hypotension.

GI: abdominal cramps, anorexia, diarrhea, epigastric discomfort, nausea, vomiting.

GU: rusty yellow or brown discoloration of urine.

Derm: alopecia, dermatoses, photosensitivity, pigmentary changes, pruritus, skin eruptions.

Hemat: AGRANULOCYTOSIS, APLASTIC ANEMIA, LEUKOPENIA, thrombocytopenia.

Neuro: neuromyopathy, peripheral neuritis.

INTERACTIONS

Drug-Drug: ▪ May increase the risk of hepatotoxicity when administered with other **hepatotoxic agents** ▪ **Penicillamine** increases the risk of hematologic toxicity ▪ Increased risk of dermatologic toxicity when given with other **agents having dermatologic toxicity** ▪ May decrease rabies antibody titers when given concurrently with human diploid cell **rabies vaccine** ▪ **Urinary acidifiers** may increase renal excretion and decrease effectiveness.

Drug-Food: ▪ **Foods that acidify urine** (see

*CAPITALS indicate life-threatening; underlines indicate most frequent.

Appendix K) may increase excretion and decrease effectiveness.

ROUTE AND DOSAGE

Doses expressed as chloroquine base: 1 mg of chloroquine base = 1.67 mg chloroquine phosphate or 1.25 mg chloroquine hydrochloride.

Malaria

- **PO (Adults):** *Suppression/chemoprophylaxis*—300 mg once weekly, starting 1–2 wk prior to entering malarious areas and for 4 wk afterward. *Treatment*—600 mg initially, then 300 mg at 6–8 hr, 24 hr, and 48 hr after initial dose (not to exceed 1 g/24 hr).
- **PO (Children):** *Suppression/chemoprophylaxis*—5 mg/kg once weekly, starting 1–2 wk prior to entering malarious areas and for 4 wk afterward (not to exceed 300 mg/day). *Treatment*—10 mg/kg initially, 5 mg/kg at 6 hr, 24 hr, and 48 hr after initial dose (not to exceed 12.5 mg/kg/24 hr).
- **IM (Adults):** 160–200 mg, may repeat in 6 hr (not to exceed 800 mg/24 hr).
- **IM, SC (Children):** 3.5 mg/kg, may repeat in 6 hr (not to exceed 10 mg/kg/24 hr).
- **IV (Children):** 13.3 mg/kg initially, then 6.6 mg/kg q 6–8 hr.

Amebic Liver Abscess

- **PO (Adults):** 150 mg 4 times daily for 2 days, then 150 mg twice daily for 2–3 wk (in combination with other antiprotozoals).
- **PO (Children):** 6 mg/kg (up to 300 mg)/day for 3 wk.
- **IM (Adults):** 160–200 mg/day for 10–12 days.
- **IM (Children):** 6 mg/kg/day for 10–12 days.

Rheumatoid Arthritis

- **PO (Adults):** Up to 2.4 mg/kg/day (based on ideal body weight).

AVAILABILITY

Chloroquine Phosphate

- ***Tablets:*** 250 mg (150-mg base)Rx, 500 mg (300-mg base)Rx.

Chloroquine Hydrochloride

- ***Injection:*** 50 mg (40-mg base)/mlRx ▪ ***In combination with:*** primaquine (Aralen phosphate with primaquine phosphate)Rx.

TIME/ACTION PROFILE (antimalarial activity)

	ONSET	PEAK	DURATION
PO	rapid	1–2 hr	days–wks
IM	rapid	UK	days–wks

NURSING IMPLICATIONS

ASSESSMENT

- **General Info:** Determine baseline for future reference that includes current symptoms of disease prior to administration.
- Assess deep tendon reflexes periodically to determine muscle weakness. Therapy may be discontinued should this occur.
- **Malaria:** Assess patient for improvement in signs and symptoms of condition daily throughout therapy.
- **Rheumatoid Arthritis:** Assess degree of joint pain and limitation of motion monthly.
- ***Lab Test Considerations:*** Monitor CBC and platelet count periodically throughout therapy. May cause decreased WBC and platelet counts.

POTENTIAL NURSING DIAGNOSES

- Infection, risk for (Indications).
- Pain, chronic (Indications).
- Knowledge deficit, related to medication regimen (Patient/Family Teaching).

IMPLEMENTATION

- **General Info:** For malaria prophylaxis, chloroquine therapy should be started 2 wk prior to potential exposures and continued for 6 wk after leaving the area.
- **PO:** Administer with milk or meals to minimize GI distress.
- IM: Parenteral administration may cause severe reaction (seizures, respiratory distress, shock, and cardiovascular collapse) or sudden death in children. Avoid if possible.
- Avoid intravenous injection; aspirate to ensure needle placement in muscle. Rotate sites. IM dose may be repeated in 6 hr if necessary. Change to oral route as soon as possible.
- **Intermittent Infusion:** Dilute in 0.9% NaCl for injection in quantity sufficient to infuse slowly.
- ***Rate:*** Administer initial dose over 8 hr. Subsequent doses should infuse over 4 hr.

PATIENT/FAMILY TEACHING

- □ Instruct patient to take medication exactly as directed and continue full course of therapy, even if feeling better. Missed doses should be taken as soon as remembered, except with regimens requiring doses more than once a day, for which missed doses should be taken within 1 hr or omitted. Do not double doses.
- □ Review methods of minimizing exposure to mosquitoes with patients receiving chloroquine prophylactically (use repellent, wear long-sleeved shirt and long trousers, use screen or netting).
- □ Chloroquine may cause dizziness. Caution patient to avoid driving or other activities requiring alertness until response to medication is known.
- □ Advise patients to avoid use of alcohol while taking chloroquine.
- □ Caution patient to keep chloroquine out of the reach of children; fatalities have occurred with ingestion of 3 or 4 tablets.
- □ Explain need for periodic ophthalmic exams for patients on prolonged high-dose therapy. Advise patient that the risk of ocular damage may be decreased by the use of dark glasses in bright light. Protective clothing and sunscreen should also be used to reduce risk of dermatoses.
- □ Inform patient that chloroquine may cause rusty yellow or brown discoloration of the urine.
- □ Advise patient to notify health care professional promptly if sore throat, fever, unusual bleeding or bruising, blurred vision, difficulty reading, visual changes, ringing in the ears, difficulty hearing, mental changes, or muscle weakness occurs or if diarrhea, anorexia, nausea, stomach pain, vomiting, or rash becomes pronounced or bothersome. Most adverse reactions are dose related.
- ▪ **Rheumatoid Arthritis:** Instruct patient to contact health care professional if no improvement is noticed within a few days. Treatment may require up to 6 mo for full benefit.

EVALUATION

Effectiveness of therapy can be demonstrated by: ▪ Prevention of or improvement in signs and symptoms of malaria ▪ Regression of amebic liver abscess ▪ Decrease in the symptoms and progression of rheumatoid arthritis.

CHLORPHENIRAMINE

(klor-fen-**eer**-a-meen)

Aller-Chlor, Chlo-Amine, Chlorate, Chlor-Niramine, Chlor-Pro, Chlor-Trimeton, {Chlor-Tripolon}, Chlorspan, Chlortab, Clortab, Clor-100, Gen-Allerate, {Novo-Pheniram}, PediaCare Allergy Formula, Pfeiffer's Allergy, Phenetron, Telachlor, Teldrin, Trymegen

CLASSIFICATION(S):

Antihistamine

Pregnancy Category B

INDICATIONS

▪ Relief of allergic symptoms caused by histamine release, including: □ Nasal allergies □ Allergic dermatoses ▪ Management of severe allergic or hypersensitivity reactions, including anaphylaxis and transfusion reactions.

ACTION

▪ Antagonizes the effects of histamine at H_1-receptor sites; does not bind to or inactivate histamine. **Therapeutic Effects:** ▪ Decreased symptoms of histamine excess (sneezing, rhinorrhea, nasal and ocular pruritus, ocular tearing and redness).

PHARMACOKINETICS

Absorption: Well absorbed following oral and parenteral administration.

Distribution: Widely distributed. Minimal amounts excreted in breast milk. Crosses the blood-brain barrier.

Metabolism and Excretion: Extensively metabolized by the liver.

Half-life: 12–15 hr.

CONTRAINDICATIONS AND PRECAUTIONS

Contraindicated in: ▪ Hypersensitivity ▪ Acute attacks of asthma ▪ Lactation (avoid use) ▪ Known alcohol intolerance (some liquid forms).

Use Cautiously in: ▪ Narrow-angle glaucoma

▪ Liver disease ▪ Geriatric patients (more susceptible to adverse reactions) ▪ Pregnancy (safety not established).

ADVERSE REACTIONS AND SIDE EFFECTS*

CNS: drowsiness, dizziness, excitation (in children).
EENT: blurred vision.
CV: hypertension, arrhythmias, hypotension, palpitations.
GI: dry mouth, constipation, obstruction.
GU: retention, urinary hesitancy.

INTERACTIONS

Drug-Drug: ▪ Additive CNS depression with other **CNS depressants** including **alcohol, opioids**, and **sedative/hypnotics** ▪ **MAO inhibitors** intensify and prolong anticholinergic effects of antihistamines ▪ Additive anticholinergic effects with other **drugs possessing anticholinergic properties** including **antidepressants, atropine, haloperidol, phenothiazines, quinidine**, and **disopyramide**.

ROUTE AND DOSAGE

- **PO (Adults):** 4 mg q 4–6 hr *or* 8–12 mg of extended-release formulation q 8–12 hr (not to exceed 24 mg/day).
- **PO (Geriatric Patients):** 4 mg twice daily or 8 mg of extended-release formulation at bedtime.
- **PO (Children 6–12 yr):** 2 mg 3–4 times daily (not to exceed 12 mg/day).
- **SC, IM, IV (Adults):** 5–40 mg single dose (not to exceed 40 mg/day).
- **SC (Children):** 87.5 mcg (0.0875 mg)/kg or 2.5 mg/m^2 q 6 hr as needed.

AVAILABILITY

▪ ***Tablets:*** 4 mg^{Rx,OTC}, 8 mg^{Rx,OTC}, 12 mg^{Rx,OTC} ▪ ***Chewable tablets:*** 2 mg^{Rx,OTC} ▪ ***Timed-release tablets:*** 8 mg^{Rx,OTC}, 12 mg^{Rx,OTC} ▪ ***Timed-release capsules:*** 8 mg^{Rx,OTC}, 12 mg^{Rx,OTC} ▪ ***Syrup:*** 1 mg/5 ml^{Rx,OTC}, 2 mg/5 ml^{Rx,OTC}, {2.5 mg/5 ml^{Rx,OTC}} ▪ ***Injection:*** 10 mg/ml^{Rx}, 100 mg/ml^{Rx} ▪ ***In combination with:*** decongestants^{Rx,OTC}. See Appendix A.

TIME/ACTION PROFILE (antihistaminic effects)

	ONSET	PEAK	DURATION
PO	15–30 min	6 hr	4–12 hr
PO–ER	UK	UK	8–24 hr
SC	UK	UK	4–12 hr
IM	UK	UK	4–12 hr
IV	rapid	UK	4–12 hr

NURSING IMPLICATIONS

ASSESSMENT

- □ Assess allergy symptoms (rhinitis, conjunctivitis, hives) prior to and periodically throughout therapy.
- □ Monitor pulse and blood pressure before initiating and throughout IV therapy.
- □ Assess lung sounds and character of bronchial secretions. Maintain fluid intake of 1500–2000 ml/day to decrease viscosity of secretions.
- ▪ ***Lab Test Considerations:*** May cause false-negative reactions on allergy skin tests; discontinue 4 days prior to testing.

POTENTIAL NURSING DIAGNOSES

- ▪ Airway clearance, ineffective (Indications).
- ▪ Injury, risk for (Adverse Reactions).
- ▪ Knowledge deficit, related to medication regimen (Patient/Family Teaching).

IMPLEMENTATION

- ▪ **PO:** Administer oral doses with food or milk to decrease GI irritation. Extended-release tablets and capsules should be swallowed whole; do not crush, break, or chew. Chewable tablets should not be swallowed whole; chew well before swallowing.
- ▪ **IM, SC:** The 100 mg/ml solution is recommended for IM or SC routes only. The 10 mg/ml solution may be used for IM, SC, or IV.
- ▪ **Direct IV:** May be given undiluted. Use only the 10 mg/ml strength for IV administration.
- ▪ ***Rate:*** Administer each 10 mg dose over at least 1 min.

PATIENT/FAMILY TEACHING

- □ Instruct patient to take chlorpheniramine exactly as directed.
- □ May cause drowsiness. Caution patient to

***CAPITALS** indicate life-threatening; underlines indicate most frequent.**

avoid driving or other activities requiring alertness until response to drug is known.
- Caution patient to avoid using alcohol or other CNS depressants concurrently with this drug.
- Advise patient that good oral hygiene, frequent rinsing of mouth with water, and sugarless gum or candy may help relieve dryness of mouth.
- Instruct patient to contact health care professional if symptoms persist.

EVALUATION

Effectiveness of therapy can be demonstrated by: ▪ Decrease in allergic symptoms.

CHLORPROMAZINE

(klor-**proe**-ma-zeen)
{Chlorpromanyl}, {Largactil}, {Novo-Chlorpromazine}, Thorazine, Thor-Prom

CLASSIFICATION(S):
Antiemetic, Antipsychotic agent (phenothiazine)

Pregnancy Category UK

INDICATIONS

▪ Acute and chronic psychoses, particularly when accompanied by increased psychomotor activity ▪ Nausea and vomiting ▪ Intractable hiccups ▪ Preoperative sedation ▪ Treatment of acute intermittent porphyria. **Unlabeled Uses:** ▪ Vascular headache.

ACTION

▪ Alters the effects of dopamine in the CNS ▪ Has significant anticholinergic/alpha-adrenergic blocking activity. **Therapeutic Effects:** ▪ Diminished signs/symptoms of psychosis ▪ Relief of nausea/vomiting/intractable hiccups ▪ Decreased symptoms of porphyria.

PHARMACOKINETICS

Absorption: Variable absorption from tablets/suppositories; better with oral liquid formulations. Well absorbed following IM administration.
Distribution: Widely distributed; high CNS concentrations. Crosses the placenta; enters breast milk.
Metabolism and Excretion: Highly metabolized by the liver and GI mucosa. Some metabolites are active.
Half-life: 30 hr.

CONTRAINDICATIONS AND PRECAUTIONS

Contraindicated in: ▪ Hypersensitivity ▪ Hypersensitivity to sulfites (injectable) or benzyl alcohol (sustained-release capsules) ▪ Cross-sensitivity with other phenothiazines may occur ▪ Narrow-angle glaucoma ▪ Bone marrow depression ▪ Severe liver/cardiovascular disease.
Use Cautiously in: ▪ Geriatric/debilitated patients (decrease initial dose) ▪ Diabetes ▪ Respiratory disease ▪ Prostatic hypertrophy ▪ CNS tumors ▪ Epilepsy ▪ Intestinal obstruction ▪ Pregnancy or lactation (safety not established).

ADVERSE REACTIONS AND SIDE EFFECTS*

CNS: NEUROLEPTIC MALIGNANT SYNDROME, <u>sedation</u>, extrapyramidal reactions, tardive dyskinesia.
EENT: <u>blurred vision</u>, <u>dry eyes</u>, lens opacities.
CV: <u>hypotension</u> (↑ with IM, IV), tachycardia.
GI: <u>constipation</u>, <u>dry mouth</u>, anorexia, hepatitis, ileus.
GU: urinary retention.
Derm: <u>photosensitivity</u>, pigment changes, rashes.
Endo: galactorrhea.
Hemat: AGRANULOCYTOSIS, leukopenia.
Metab: hyperthermia.
Misc: allergic reactions.

INTERACTIONS

Drug-Drug: ▪ Additive hypotension with **antihypertensives** ▪ Additive CNS depression with **alcohol, antidepressants, antihistamines, MAO inhibitors, opioids, sedative/hypnotics**, or **general anesthetics** ▪ **Phenobarbital** may decrease effectiveness ▪ Concurrent use with **lithium** may produce acute encephalopathy, decreased chlorpromazine absorption, increased lithium excretion, increased risk of extrapyramidal reactions, or masking of **lithium** toxicity ▪ **Antacids** or **adsorbent antidiarrheals** may

{} = Available in Canada only.
***CAPITALS indicate life-threatening; <u>underlines</u> indicate most frequent.**

decrease adsorption ▪ Increased risk of agranulocytosis with **antithyroid drugs** ▪ May decrease anti-Parkinson activity of **levodopa** and **bromocriptine** ▪ Decreases vasopressor response to **epinephrine** and **norepinephrine** ▪ Decreases antihypertensive effect of **guanethidine** ▪ Concurrent use with **beta blockers** may produce an increased response ▪ Increased risk of anticholinergic effects with **antihistamines, tricyclic antidepressants, quinidine**, or **disopyramide.**

ROUTE AND DOSAGE

- **PO (Adults):** *Psychoses*—10–25 mg 2–4 times daily; may increase every 3–4 days (usual dose is 200 mg/day; up to 1 g/day) or 30–300 mg 1–3 times daily as extended-release capsules. *Nausea and vomiting*—10–25 mg q 4 hr as needed. *Preoperative sedation*—25–50 mg 2–3 hr before surgery. *Hiccups/porphyria*—25–50 mg 3–4 times daily.
- **PO (Children):** *Psychoses/nausea and vomiting*—0.55 mg/kg (15 mg/m^2) q 4–6 hr as needed. *Preoperative sedation*—0.55 mg/kg (15 mg/m^2) 2–3 hr before surgery.
- **Rect (Adults):** *Nausea/vomiting*—50–100 mg q 6–8 hr as needed.
- **Rect (Children >6 mo):** 1 mg/kg q 6–8 hr as needed.
- **IM (Adults):** *Severe psychoses*—25–50 mg initially, may be repeated in 1 hr; increase to maximum of 400 mg q 3–12 hr if needed (up to 1 g/day). *Nausea/vomiting*—25 mg initially, may repeat with 25–50 mg q 3–4 hr as needed. *Nausea/vomiting during surgery*—12.5 mg, may be repeated in 30 min as needed. *Preoperative sedation*—12.5–25 mg 1–2 hr prior to surgery. *Hiccups/tetanus*—25–50 mg 3–4 times daily. *Porphyria*—25 mg q 6–8 hr until patient can take PO.
- **IM (Children >6 mo):** *Psychoses/nausea and vomiting*—0.55 mg/kg (15 mg/m^2) q 6–8 hr (not to exceed 40 mg/day in children 6 mo–5 yr, or 75 mg/day in children 5–12 yr). *Nausea/vomiting during surgery*—0.275 mg/kg, may repeat in 30 min as needed. *Preoperative sedation*—0.55 mg/kg 1–2 hr prior to surgery. *Tetanus*—0.55 mg/kg q 6–8 hr.
- **IV (Adults):** *Nausea/vomiting during surgery*—up to 25 mg. *Hiccups/tetanus*—25–50 mg.
- **IV (Children):** *Nausea/vomiting during surgery*—0.275 mg/kg. *Tetanus*—0.55 mg/kg.

AVAILABILITY

▪ ***Tablets:*** 10 mg^{Rx}, 25 mg^{Rx}, 50 mg^{Rx}, 100 mg^{Rx}, 200 mg^{Rx} ▪ ***Sustained-release capsules:*** 30 mg^{Rx}, 75 mg^{Rx}, 150 mg^{Rx}, 200 mg^{Rx}, 300 mg^{Rx} ▪ ***Syrup:*** 10 mg/5 ml^{Rx}, {25 mg/5 ml^{Rx}}, {100 mg/5 ml^{Rx}} ▪ ***Oral concentrate:*** 30 mg/ml^{Rx}, {40 mg/ml^{Rx}}, 100 mg/ml^{Rx} ▪ ***Suppositories:*** 25 mg^{Rx}, 100 mg^{Rx} ▪ ***Injection:*** 25 mg/ml^{Rx}.

TIME/ACTION PROFILE (antipsychotic activity, antiemetic activity, sedation)

	ONSET	PEAK	DURATION
PO	30–60 min	UK	4–6 hr
PO–ER	30–60 min	UK	10–12 hr
Rect	1–2 hr	UK	3–4 hr
IM	UK	UK	4–8 hr
IV	rapid	UK	UK

NURSING IMPLICATIONS

ASSESSMENT

- **General Info:** Assess patient's mental status (orientation, mood, behavior) prior to and periodically throughout therapy.
- □ Monitor blood pressure (sitting, standing, lying), pulse, and respiratory rate prior to and frequently during the period of dosage adjustment.
- □ Observe patient carefully when administering medication to ensure medication is actually taken and not hoarded.
- □ Assess fluid intake and bowel function. Increased bulk and fluids in the diet may help minimize constipation.
- □ Monitor patient for onset of akathisia (restlessness or desire to keep moving) and extrapyramidal side effects (*parkinsonian*—difficulty speaking or swallowing, loss of balance control, pill rolling, mask-like face, shuffling gait, rigidity, tremors; and *dystonic*—muscle spasms, twisting motions, twitching, inability to move eyes, weakness of arms or legs) every 2 mo during therapy and 8–12 wk after therapy has been discontinued. Notify physician or other health care professional if these symptoms occur; reduction in dose or discontin-

uation may be necessary. Trihexyphenidyl or diphenhydramine may be used to control these symptoms.

- Monitor for tardive dyskinesia (uncontrolled rhythmic movement of mouth, face, and extremities; lip smacking or puckering; puffing of cheeks; uncontrolled chewing; rapid or worm-like movements of tongue). Report these symptoms immediately; may be irreversible.
- Monitor for development of neuroleptic malignant syndrome (fever, respiratory distress, tachycardia, convulsions, diaphoresis, hypertension or hypotension, pallor, tiredness, severe muscle stiffness, loss of bladder control). Report these symptoms immediately.
- **Preoperative Sedation:** Assess level of anxiety prior to and following administration.
- **Vascular Headache:** Assess type, location, intensity, and duration of pain and accompanying symptoms.
- ***Lab Test Considerations:*** Monitor CBC, liver function tests, and ocular exams periodically throughout therapy. May cause decreased hematocrit, hemoglobin, leukocytes, granulocytes, platelets. May cause elevated bilirubin, AST, ALT, and alkaline phosphatase. Agranulocytosis occurs 4–10 wk after initiation of therapy with recovery 1–2 wk following discontinuation. May recur if medication is restarted. Liver function abnormalities may require discontinuation of therapy. May cause false-positive or false-negative pregnancy tests and false-positive urine bilirubin test results.

POTENTIAL NURSING DIAGNOSES

- Thought processes, altered (Indications).
- Knowledge deficit, related to medication regimen (Patient/Family Teaching).
- Noncompliance (Patient/Family Teaching).

IMPLEMENTATION

- Keep patient recumbent for at least 30 min following parenteral administration to minimize hypotensive effects.
- To prevent contact dermatitis, avoid getting solution on hands.
- Phenothiazines should be discontinued 48 hr before and not resumed for 24 hr following myelography, because they lower the seizure threshold.
- **Hiccups:** Initial treatment is with oral doses. If hiccups persist 2–3 days, IM injection may be used, followed by IV infusion.
- **PO:** Administer oral doses with food, milk, or a full glass of water to minimize gastric irritation. Tablets may be crushed. Do not open capsules; swallow whole. Sustained-release capsules may be opened but contents should not be chewed. Dilute concentrate just prior to administration in 120 ml of coffee, tea, tomato or fruit juice, milk, water, soup, or carbonated beverages.
- **Rect:** If suppository is too soft for insertion, chill in refrigerator for 30 min or run under cold water before removing foil wrapper.
- **IM:** Do not inject SC. Inject slowly into deep, well-developed muscle. May be diluted with 0.9% NaCl or 2% procaine. Lemon-yellow color does not alter potency of solution. Do not administer solution that is markedly discolored or contains a precipitate.
- **Direct IV:** Dilute with 0.9% NaCl for a concentration not to exceed 1 mg/ml.
- ***Rate:*** Inject slowly at a rate of at least 1 mg/min for adults and 0.5 mg/min for children.
- **Continuous Infusion:** May dilute 25–50 mg in 500–1000 ml of D5W, D10W, 0.45% NaCl, 0.9% NaCl, Ringer's or lactated Ringer's injection, dextrose/Ringer's or dextrose/lactated Ringer's combinations.
- **Syringe Compatibility:** ▪ atropine ▪ benztropine ▪ butorphanol ▪ diphenhydramine ▪ doxapram ▪ droperidol ▪ fentanyl ▪ glycopyrrolate ▪ hydromorphone ▪ hydroxyzine ▪ meperidine ▪ metoclopramide ▪ midazolam ▪ morphine ▪ pentazocine ▪ scopolamine.
- **Syringe Incompatibility:** ▪ cimetidine ▪ dimenhydrinate ▪ heparin ▪ pentobarbital ▪ thiopental.
- **Y-Site Compatibility:** ▪ cisplatin ▪ cyclophosphamide ▪ cytarabine ▪ doxorubicin ▪ filgrastim ▪ fluconazole ▪ heparin ▪ hydrocortisone sodium succinate ▪ ondansetron ▪ potassium chloride ▪ teniposide ▪ thiotepa ▪ vinorelbine ▪ vitamin B complex with C.
- **Y-Site Incompatibility:** ▪ amifostine ▪ aztreonam ▪ cefepime ▪ fludarabine ▪ melphalan ▪ methotrexate ▪ paclitaxel ▪ piperacillin/tazobactam ▪ sargramostim.

PATIENT/FAMILY TEACHING

- Advise patient to take medication exactly as directed and not to skip doses or double up on missed doses. If a dose is missed, take within 1 hr or omit dose and return to regular schedule. Abrupt withdrawal may lead to gastritis, nausea, vomiting, dizziness, headache, tachycardia, and insomnia.

- Inform patient of possibility of extrapyramidal symptoms and tardive dyskinesia. Instruct patient to report these symptoms immediately to health care professional.
- Advise patient to change positions slowly to minimize orthostatic hypotension.
- Medication may cause drowsiness. Caution patient to avoid driving or other activities requiring alertness until response to the medication is known.
- Caution patient to avoid taking alcohol or other CNS depressants concurrently with this medication.
- Advise patient to use sunscreen and protective clothing when exposed to the sun. Exposed surfaces may develop a temporary pigment change (ranging from yellow-brown to grayish purple). Extremes of temperature (exercise, hot weather, hot baths or showers) should also be avoided, because this drug impairs body temperature regulation.
- Instruct patient to use frequent mouth rinses, good oral hygiene, and sugarless gum or candy to minimize dry mouth. Consult health care professional if dry mouth continues for >2 wk.
- Advise patient not to take chlorpromazine within 2 hr of antacids or antidiarrheal medication.
- Inform patient that this medication may turn urine a pink-to-reddish-brown color.
- Advise patient to notify health care professional of medication regimen prior to treatment or surgery.
- Instruct patient to notify health care professional promptly if sore throat, fever, unusual bleeding or bruising, rash, weakness, tremors, visual disturbances, dark-colored urine, or clay-colored stools occur.
- Emphasize the importance of routine follow-up exams and continued participation in psychotherapy as indicated.

EVALUATION

Effectiveness of therapy can be demonstrated by: ▪ Decrease in excitable, paranoid, or withdrawn behavior. Therapeutic effects may not be seen for 7–8 wk ▪ Relief of nausea and vomiting ▪ Relief of hiccups ▪ Preoperative sedation ▪ Management of porphyria ▪ Relief of vascular headache.

CIDOFOVIR

(sye-doe-**foe**-veer)
Vistide

CLASSIFICATION(S):
Antiviral

Pregnancy Category C

INDICATIONS

▪ Management of cytomegalovirus (CMV) retinitis in HIV-infected patients.

ACTION

▪ Suppresses replication of the CMV by inhibiting viral DNA synthesis. **Therapeutic Effects:** ▪ Slows progression of CMV retinitis; may not be curative.

PHARMACOKINETICS

Absorption: IV administration results in complete bioavailability.
Distribution: UK.
Metabolism and Excretion: Excreted mostly unchanged by the kidneys.
Half-life: UK.

CONTRAINDICATIONS AND PRECAUTIONS

Contraindicated in: ▪ Hypersensitivity to cidofovir, probenecid, or sulfonamides ▪ Serum creatinine >1.5 mg/dl, CCr ≤55 ml/min, or urine protein ≥100 mg/dl (≥2+ proteinuria) ▪ Concurrent use of foscarnet, amphotericin B, aminoglycoside anti-infectives, NSAIDs, or IV pentamidine.

Use Cautiously in: ▪ Pregnancy or children (safety not established); breast-feeding is not recommended in HIV-positive patients.

Use with Extreme Caution in: ▪ Any condition that increases the risk of dehydration.

ADVERSE REACTIONS AND SIDE EFFECTS*

CNS: headache, weakness.
EENT: ocular hypotony.
Resp: dyspnea, pneumonia.
GI: abdominal pain, nausea, vomiting, anorexia, diarrhea.
GU: FANCONI'S SYNDROME, proteinuria, renal toxicity.
Derm: alopecia, rash.
F and E: decreased serum bicarbonate.
Hemat: anemia, neutropenia.
Misc: chills, fever, infection.

INTERACTIONS

Drug-Drug: ▪ Risk of nephrotoxicity is increased by concurrent **aminoglycosides, amphotericin B, foscarnet,** and **pentamidine** and should be avoided ▪ **Probenecid,** which is required concurrently, may interact with **acetaminophen, acyclovir, ACE inhibitors, barbiturates, benzodiazepines, bumetanide, methotrexate, famotidine, furosemide, NSAIDs, theophylline,** and **zidovudine.**

ROUTE AND DOSAGE

- **IV (Adults):** 5 mg/kg once weekly for 2 wk, followed by 5 mg/kg every 2 wk (must be given with probenecid).

AVAILABILITY

▪ ***Solution for injection:*** 75 mg/ml in 5-ml ampules[Rx].

TIME/ACTION PROFILE

	ONSET	PEAK	DURATION
IV	rapid	end of infusion	UK

NURSING IMPLICATIONS

ASSESSMENT

- ▫ Monitor vision for progression of CMV retinitis. Monitor ocular symptoms, intraocular pressure, and visual acuity periodically.
- ▫ Antiemetics and administration after a meal may minimize nausea and vomiting associated with probenecid. If allergic reactions occur in association with probenecid, pretreatment with antihistamines or acetaminophen should be considered.
- ▫ Monitor vital signs periodically. May cause fever, hypotension, and tachycardia. Monitor patients for early signs and symptoms of infection.
- ▪ ***Lab Test Considerations:*** Renal function, measured by serum creatinine and urine protein, must be monitored within 48 hr prior to each dose and throughout cidofovir therapy. In patients with proteinuria, administer IV hydration and repeat urine protein test. If renal function deteriorates, dose modification or temporary discontinuation should be considered.
- ▫ Monitor white blood count prior to each dose. Granulocytopenia may occur.
- ▫ May cause hyperglycemia, hyperlipemia, hypocalcemia, hypokalemia, and elevated alkaline phosphatase, AST, and ALT.

POTENTIAL NURSING DIAGNOSES

- Infection, risk for (Indications).
- Knowledge deficit, related to medication regimen (Patient/Family Teaching).

IMPLEMENTATION

- ▪ Probenecid and saline prehydration must be given with cidofovir to minimize renal toxicity. *Probenecid* must be administered 2 g orally given 3 hr before, then 1 g given 2 hr and 8 hr following completion of cidofovir infusion. *Saline prehydration* with 1 liter of 0.9% NaCl must be given over 1–2 hr prior to cidofovir. A second liter over 1–3 hr is recommended concurrently with or following cidofovir.
- ▫ Patients receiving foscarnet, amphotericin B, aminoglycoside, NSAIDs, or IV pentamidine should wait at least 7 days following these agents to begin cidofovir.
- ▪ **Intermittent Infusion:** Dilute in 100 ml of 0.9% NaCl. Solution is stable for 24 hr if refrigerated. Allow refrigerated solution to return to room temperature prior to administration.
- ▪ ***Rate:*** Administer over 1 hr.
- ▪ **Additive Incompatibility:** ▪ Information unavailable. Do not admix with other solutions or medications.

PATIENT/FAMILY TEACHING

- ▫ Inform patient that cidofovir is not a cure for CMV retinitis and that retinitis may continue to progress during and after therapy.

***CAPITALS indicate life-threatening; underlines indicate most frequent.**

- □ Inform patient that concurrent antiretroviral therapy may be continued. However, zidovudine therapy should be temporarily discontinued or decreased by 50% on the days of cidofovir therapy because of the effects of probenicid on zidovudine.
- □ Advise patient of the possibility of renal toxicity from cidofovir. Emphasize the importance of routine lab tests to monitor renal function.
- □ Inform patient that cidofovir may have teratogenic effects. Women should use contraception during and for 1 mo following therapy. Men should use barrier contraception during and for 3 mo following therapy.
- □ Discuss with patient the possibility of hair loss. Explore coping strategies.
- □ Advise patients to have routine ophthalmologic exams following cidofovir therapy.

EVALUATION

Effectiveness of therapy can be demonstrated by: ▪ Decrease in symptoms and arrest of progression of CMV retinitis in HIV-infected patients.

CISAPRIDE
(**sis**-a-pride)
{Prepulsid}, Propulsid

CLASSIFICATION(S):
Gastrointestinal (prokinetic agent)

Pregnancy Category C

INDICATIONS

▪ Management of nocturnal symptoms (heartburn) associated with gastroesophageal reflux disease (GERD). **Unlabeled Uses:** ▪ Management of gastroparesis due to diabetes, pseudo-obstruction, or other causes.

ACTION

▪ Enhances the release of acetylcholine at the myenteric plexus. Increases the strength of esophageal peristalsis and increases lower esophageal sphincter pressure. Also acts as a serotonin-4 agonist. **Therapeutic Effects:** ▪ Reduced nocturnal symptoms of GERD.

PHARMACOKINETICS

Absorption: Rapidly absorbed following oral administration, although bioavailability is low (35–40%).
Distribution: Enters breast milk in low concentrations.
Metabolism and Excretion: Extensively metabolized by the liver (>90%).
Half-life: 8–10 hr.

CONTRAINDICATIONS AND PRECAUTIONS

Contraindicated in: ▪ Hypersensitivity ▪ Situations in which increased GI motility may be harmful (GI hemorrhage, mechanical obstruction, or perforation).
Use Cautiously in: ▪ Pregnancy or lactation (safety not established).

ADVERSE REACTIONS AND SIDE EFFECTS

CNS: dizziness, fatigue, headache.
Resp: pharyngitis, rhinitis.
CV: chest pain.
GI: abdominal pain, constipation, diarrhea, dyspepsia, flatulence, vomiting.
F and E: dehydration.
MS: back pain, myalgia.

INTERACTIONS

Drug-Drug: ▪ **Anticholinergics** may decrease the effects of cisapride ▪ May accelerate the sedative effects of **benzodiazepines** or **alcohol** ▪ May increase the effects of **warfarin** ▪ May alter the effects of **drugs with narrow therapeutic margins** (digoxin, anticonvulsants; blood level monitoring recommended) ▪ **Cimetidine** increases plasma levels of cisapride ▪ GI absorption of **cimetidine** and **ranitidine** is accelerated ▪ **Delavirdine, ketoconazole, itraconazole, miconazole, fluconazole, troleandomycin (TAO), erythromycin, dirithromycin,** and **clarithromycin** decrease metabolism and increase levels of cisapride; may result in serious arrhythmias (avoid concurrent use).

{} = Available in Canada only.

ROUTE AND DOSAGE

- **PO (Adults):** *Treatment*—5–10 mg 3–4 times daily. *Prevention*—10 mg twice daily or 20 mg once daily at bedtime.
- **PO (Children):** 0.15–0.3 mg/kg 3–4 times daily.

AVAILABILITY

- ***Tablets:*** {5 mg Rx}, 10 mgRx, 20 mgRx ▪ ***Oral suspension:*** 1 mg/mlRx.

TIME/ACTION PROFILE (effects on lower esophageal sphincter pressure)

	ONSET	PEAK	DURATION
PO	30–60 min	70 min	UK

NURSING IMPLICATIONS

ASSESSMENT

- Assess patient for nocturnal symptoms (heartburn) associated with GERD.

POTENTIAL NURSING DIAGNOSES

- Pain (Indications).
- Knowledge deficit, related to medication regimen (Patient/Family Teaching).

IMPLEMENTATION

- **PO:** Administer 15 min before each meal and at bedtime.

PATIENT/FAMILY TEACHING

- Instruct patient to take cisapride as directed, even if feeling better. If a dose is missed, take as soon as possible unless almost time for next dose.
- Cisapride may cause drowsiness; caution patient to avoid driving or other activities requiring alertness until response to medication is known.
- Advise patient to consult health care professional before taking OTC medications while taking cisapride.
- Advise patient to avoid alcohol or other depressants while taking cisapride; cisapride may enhance the sedative effects of these products.

EVALUATION

Effectiveness of therapy can be demonstrated by: ▪ Decrease in nocturnal symptoms of GERD. Treatment may continue for up to 8 wk.

CISPLATIN

(sis-**pla**-tin)

Platinol-AQ

CLASSIFICATION(S):

Antineoplastic (alkylating agent)

Pregnancy Category UK

INDICATIONS

- Alone or in combination (with other antineoplastics, surgery, or radiation) in the management of: ▫ Metastatic testicular and ovarian carcinoma ▫ Advanced bladder cancer ▫ Head and neck cancer ▫ Cervical cancer ▫ Lung cancer ▫ Other tumors.

ACTION

- Inhibits DNA synthesis by producing cross-linking of parent DNA strands (cell-cycle phase–nonspecific). **Therapeutic Effects:** ▪ Death of rapidly replicating cells, particularly malignant ones.

PHARMACOKINETICS

Absorption: Following IV administration, absorption is essentially complete.
Distribution: Widely distributed; accumulates for months after administration.
Metabolism and Excretion: Excreted mainly by the kidneys.
Half-life: 30–100 hr.

CONTRAINDICATIONS AND PRECAUTIONS

Contraindicated in: ▪ Hypersensitivity ▪ Pregnancy or lactation.
Use Cautiously in: ▪ Hearing loss ▪ Renal impairment (dosage reduction recommended) ▪ Electrolyte abnormalities ▪ Active infections ▪ Bone marrow depression ▪ Chronic debilitating illnesses ▪ Patients with childbearing potential.

C

ADVERSE REACTIONS AND SIDE EFFECTS*

CNS: SEIZURES.
EENT: ototoxicity, tinnitus.
GI: severe nausea, vomiting, diarrhea, hepatotoxicity.
GU: infertility, nephrotoxicity.
F and E: hypocalcemia, hypokalemia, hypomagnesemia.
Hemat: LEUKOPENIA, THROMBOCYTOPENIA, anemia.
Local: phlebitis at IV site.
Metab: hyperuricemia.
Neuro: peripheral neuropathy.
Misc: anaphylactoid reactions.

INTERACTIONS

Drug-Drug: ▪ Additive nephrotoxicity and ototoxicity with other **nephrotoxic** and **ototoxic drugs (aminoglycosides, loop diuretics)** ▪ Increased risk of hypokalemia and hypomagnesemia with **loop diuretics** and **amphotericin B** ▪ May decrease **phenytoin** levels ▪ Additive bone marrow depression with other **antineoplastic agents** or **radiation therapy** ▪ May decrease the antibody response to **live virus vaccines** and increase the risk of adverse reactions.

ROUTE AND DOSAGE

Other regimens are used.

- **IV (Adults):** *Metastatic testicular tumors*—20 mg/m² daily for 5 days. *Metastatic ovarian cancer*—50 mg/m², repeat q 3 wk in combination with other agents or 100 mg/m² q 4 wk if used as a single agent. *Advanced bladder cancer*—50–70 mg/m² q 3–4 wk as a single agent.

AVAILABILITY

- ***Powder for injection:*** 10-mg, 50-mg vials[Rx]
- ***Injection:*** 1 mg/ml in 50- and 100-mg vials[Rx].

TIME/ACTION PROFILE (effects on blood counts)

	ONSET	PEAK	DURATION
IV	UK	18–23 days	39 days

NURSING IMPLICATIONS

ASSESSMENT

- □ Monitor blood pressure, pulse, respiratory rate, and temperature frequently during administration. Report significant changes.
- □ Monitor intake and output and specific gravity frequently throughout therapy. Report discrepancies immediately. To reduce the risk of nephrotoxicity, a urinary output of at least 100 ml/hr should be maintained for 4 hr before initiating and for at least 24 hr after administration.
- □ Encourage patient to drink 2000–3000 ml/day to promote excretion of uric acid. Allopurinol and alkalinization of the urine may be used to help prevent uric acid nephropathy.
- □ Assess patency of IV site frequently during therapy. Cisplatin may cause severe irritation and necrosis of tissue if extravasation occurs. If a large amount of highly concentrated cisplatin solution extravasates, mix 4 ml of 10% sodium thiosulfate with 6 ml of sterile water or 1.6 ml of 25% sodium thiosulfate with 8.4 ml of sterile water and inject 1–4 ml (1 ml for each ml extravasated) through existing line or cannula. Inject SC if needle has been removed. Sodium thiosulfate inactivates cisplatin.
- □ Severe and protracted nausea and vomiting usually occur 1–4 hr after a dose; vomiting may last for 24 hr. Parenteral antiemetic agents should be administered 30–45 min prior to therapy and routinely around the clock for the next 24 hr. Monitor amount of emesis and notify physician or other health care professional if emesis exceeds guidelines to prevent dehydration. Nausea and anorexia may persist for up to 1 wk.
- □ Monitor for bone marrow depression. Assess for bleeding (bleeding gums, bruising, petechiae, guaiac stools, urine, and emesis) and avoid IM injections and rectal temperatures if platelet count is low. Apply pressure to venipuncture sites for 10 min. Assess for signs of infection during neutropenia. Anemia may occur. Monitor for increased fatigue, dyspnea, and orthostatic hypotension.
- □ Monitor for signs of anaphylaxis (facial edema, wheezing, dizziness, fainting, tachy-

*CAPITALS indicate life-threatening; underlines indicate most frequent.

cardia, hypotension). Discontinue medication immediately and report symptoms. Epinephrine and resuscitation equipment should be readily available.

- Medication may cause ototoxicity and neurotoxicity. Assess patient frequently for dizziness, tinnitus, hearing loss, loss of coordination, loss of taste, or numbness and tingling of extremities; may be irreversible. Notify physician or other health care professional promptly if these occur. Audiometry should be performed prior to initiation and periodically throughout therapy. Hearing loss usually occurs first with high frequencies and may be unilateral or bilateral.

- ***Lab Test Considerations:*** Monitor CBC with differential and platelet count prior to and routinely throughout course of therapy. The nadir of leukopenia, thrombocytopenia, and anemia occurs within 18–23 days and recovery 39 days after a dose. Withhold further doses until WBC is $>4000/mm^3$ and platelet count is $>100,000/mm^3$.
- Monitor BUN, serum creatinine, and CCr prior to initiation of therapy and before each course of cisplatin to detect nephrotoxicity. May cause increased BUN and creatinine and decreased calcium, magnesium, phosphate, sodium, and potassium levels that usually occur the 2nd wk after a dose. Do not administer additional doses until BUN is <25 mg/100 ml and serum creatinine is <1.5 mg/100 ml. May cause increased uric acid level, which usually peaks 3–5 days after a dose.
- May cause transiently increased serum bilirubin and AST concentrations.
- May cause positive Coombs' test.

POTENTIAL NURSING DIAGNOSES

- Infection, risk for (Adverse Reactions).
- Injury, risk for (Side Effects).
- Knowledge deficit, related to medication regimen (Patient/Family Teaching).

IMPLEMENTATION

- **General Info:** Do not confuse with carboplatin. To prevent confusion, orders should include generic and brand names.
- Hydrate patient with at least 1–2 liters of IV fluid 8–12 hr before initiating therapy with cisplatin. Amifostine (p. 28) may be administered to minimize nephrotoxicity.
- Do not use aluminum needles or equipment during preparation or administration. Aluminum reacts with the drug, forms a black or brown precipitate, and renders it ineffective.
- Unopened vials of powder and constituted solution must not be refrigerated.
- Solution should be prepared in a biologic cabinet. Wear gloves, gown, and mask while handling medication. Discard equipment in specially designated containers (see Appendix I).
- **Intermittent Infusion:** Reconstitute 10-mg vials with 10 ml of sterile water for injection and 50-mg vial with 50 ml. Stable for 20 hr if reconstituted with sterile water, for 72 hr with bacteriostatic water. Do not refrigerate, as crystals will form. Solution should be clear and colorless; discard if turbid or if it contains precipitates.
- Dilution in 2 liters of 5% dextrose in 0.3% or 0.45% NaCl containing 37.5 g of mannitol is recommended.
- ***Rate:*** Infuse over 6–8 hr.
- **Continuous Infusion:** Has been administered as continuous infusion over 24 hr to 5 days with resultant decrease in nausea and vomiting. Clarify dose to ensure cumulative dosage is not confused with daily dose; errors may be fatal.
- **Syringe Compatibility:** ▪ bleomycin ▪ cyclophosphamide ▪ doxapram ▪ doxorubicin ▪ droperidol ▪ fluorouracil ▪ furosemide ▪ heparin ▪ leucovorin calcium ▪ methotrexate ▪ metoclopramide ▪ mitomycin ▪ vinblastine ▪ vincristine.
- **Y-Site Compatibility:** ▪ aztreonam ▪ bleomycin ▪ chlorpromazine ▪ cimetidine ▪ cyclophosphamide ▪ dexamethasone ▪ diphenhydramine ▪ doxorubicin ▪ droperidol ▪ famotidine ▪ filgrastim ▪ fludarabine ▪ fluorouracil ▪ furosemide ▪ ganciclovir ▪ granisetron ▪ heparin ▪ hydromorphone ▪ leucovorin calcium ▪ lorazepam ▪ melphalan ▪ methotrexate ▪ methylprednisolone ▪ metoclopromide ▪ mitomycin ▪ morphine ▪ ondansetron ▪ paclitaxel ▪ prochlorperazine edisylate ▪ promethazine ▪ ranitidine ▪ sargramostim ▪ teniposide ▪ vinblastine ▪ vincristine ▪ vinorelbine.
- **Y-Site Incompatibility:** ▪ amifostine ▪ cefepime ▪ gallium nitrate ▪ piperacillin/tazobactam ▪ thiotepa.
- **Additive Compatibility:** ▪ etoposide ▪ floxuridine ▪ ifosfamide ▪ leucovorin calcium

C

▪ magnesium sulfate ▪ mannitol ▪ ondansetron ▪ 0.9% NaCl ▪ D5/0.9% NaCl.

▪ **Additive Incompatibility:** ▪ fluorouracil ▪ mesna ▪ sodium bicarbonate ▪ thiotepa.

PATIENT/FAMILY TEACHING

□ Instruct patient to report pain at injection site immediately.

□ Instruct patient to notify health care professional promptly if fever; chills; cough; hoarseness; sore throat; signs of infection; lower back or side pain; painful or difficult urination; bleeding gums; bruising; petechiae; blood in stools, urine, or emesis; increased fatigue; dyspnea; or orthostatic hypotension occurs. Caution patient to avoid crowds and persons with known infections. Instruct patient to use soft toothbrush and electric razor and to avoid falls. Caution patient not to drink alcoholic beverages or take medication containing aspirin or NSAIDS; may precipitate gastric bleeding.

□ Instruct patient to report promptly any numbness or tingling in extremities or face, difficulty with hearing or tinnitus, unusual swelling, or joint pain.

□ Instruct patient not to receive any vaccinations without advice of health care professional.

□ Advise patient of the need for contraception, although cisplatin may cause infertility.

□ Emphasize the need for periodic lab tests to monitor for side effects.

EVALUATION

Effectiveness of therapy can be demonstrated by: ▪ Decrease in size or spread of malignancies. Therapy should not be administered more frequently than every 3–4 wk, and only if lab values are within acceptable parameters and patient is not exhibiting signs of ototoxicity or other serious adverse effects.

CLARITHROMYCIN

(klare-**ith**-row-my-sin)

Biaxin

CLASSIFICATION(S):

Anti-infective (macrolide)

Pregnancy Category C

INDICATIONS

▪ Treatment of the following infections: □ Upper respiratory tract infections including streptococcal pharyngitis and sinusitis □ Lower respiratory tract infections including bronchitis and pneumonia ▪ Treatment (with ethambutol) and prevention of disseminated *Mycobacterium avium* complex (MAC) ▪ Treatment of the following infections in children: □ Otitis media □ Sinusitis □ Pharyngitis □ Skin and skin structure infections ▪ Part of a combination regimen (with a gastric acid–pump inhibitor and amoxicillin or with ranitidine bismuth citrate) for ulcer disease due to *Helicobacter pylori* ▪ Endocarditis prophylaxis.

ACTION

▪ Inhibits protein synthesis at the level of the 50S bacterial ribosome. **Therapeutic Effects:** ▪ Bacteriostatic action against susceptible bacteria. **Spectrum:** ▪ Active against the following gram-positive aerobic bacteria: □ *Staphylococcus aureus* □ *Streptococcus pneumoniae* □ *Streptococcus pyogenes* (group A strep) ▪ Active against these gram-negative aerobic bacteria: □ *Haemophilus influenzae* □ *Moraxella catarrhalis* ▪ Also active against: □ *Mycoplasma* □ *Legionella* □ *Helicobacter pylori* □ *Mycobacterium avium* ▪ Not active against methicillin-resistant *Staphylococcus aureus*.

PHARMACOKINETICS

Absorption: Rapidly absorbed (50%) following oral administration.

Distribution: Widely distributed to body tissues and fluids; tissue levels may exceed those in serum.

Metabolism and Excretion: 10–15% conversion by the liver to 14-hydroxyclarithromycin, which has anti-infective activity; 20–30% excreted unchanged in urine.

Half-life: 250-mg dose—3–4 hr; 500-mg dose—5–7 hr.

CONTRAINDICATIONS AND PRECAUTIONS

Contraindicated in: ▪ Hypersensitivity to clarithromycin, erythromycin, or other macrolide anti-infectives ▪ Pregnancy and lactation (avoid use during pregnancy unless no alternatives available).

Use Cautiously in: ▪ Severe liver and/or renal

impairment (dosage adjustment required if CCr <30 ml/min).

ADVERSE REACTIONS AND SIDE EFFECTS*

CNS: headache.
GI: PSEUDOMEMBRANOUS COLITIS, abdominal pain/discomfort, abnormal taste, diarrhea, dyspepsia, nausea.

INTERACTIONS

Drug-Drug: ▪ May increase serum levels and the risk of toxicity from **carbamazepine, digoxin,** or **theophylline** ▪ May increase the effect of **warfarin** ▪ May decrease effects of **zidovudine** ▪ May increase risk of arrhythmias with **astemizole, cisapride,** or **pimozide** ▪ Blood levels are increased by **delavirdine.**

ROUTE AND DOSAGE

- **PO (Adults):** *Bronchitis (not* H. influenzae*)/pneumonia/skin and soft tissue infections*—250 mg q 12 hr. *Bronchitis* (H. influenzae)*/sinusitus/disseminated* MAC/H. pylori—500 mg q 12 hr. *Endocarditis prophylaxis*—500 mg 1 hr before procedure.
- **PO (Children):** *Most infections*—7.5 mg/kg q 12 hr (up to 500 mg/dose for MAC). *Endocarditis prophylaxis*—15 mg/kg 1 hr before procedure.

AVAILABILITY

▪ ***Tablets:*** 250 mg[Rx], 500 mg[Rx] ▪ ***Oral suspension:*** 125 mg/5 ml[Rx], 250 mg/5 ml[Rx] ▪ ***In combination with:*** amoxicillin and lansoprozole as part of a compliance package (Prevpac). See Appendix A..

TIME/ACTION PROFILE (serum levels)

	ONSET	PEAK	DURATION
PO	UK	2 hr	12 hr

NURSING IMPLICATIONS

ASSESSMENT

- ▫ Assess patient for infection (vital signs; appearance of wound, sputum, urine, and stool; WBC) at beginning of and throughout therapy.
- ▫ Obtain specimens for culture and sensitivity prior to initiating therapy. First dose may be given before receiving results.
- ▪ ***Lab Test Considerations:*** May rarely cause increased serum AST and ALT concentrations.
- ▫ May rarely cause elevated BUN.

POTENTIAL NURSING DIAGNOSES

- ▪ Infection, risk for (Indications, Side Effects).
- ▪ Knowledge deficit, related to medication regimen (Patient/Family Teaching).
- ▪ Noncompliance, related to medication regimen (Patient/Family Teaching).

IMPLEMENTATION

- ▪ **PO:** Administer around the clock, without regard to meals. Food slows but does not decrease the extent of absorption.
- ▫ Shake suspension well before administration.
- ▫ Do not administer within 4 hr of zidovudine.

PATIENT/FAMILY TEACHING

- ▫ Instruct patient to take medication around the clock and to finish the drug completely as directed, even if feeling better. Missed doses should be taken as soon as possible, unless almost time for next dose. Do not double doses. Advise patient that sharing of this medication may be dangerous.
- ▫ Advise patient to report the signs of superinfection (black, furry overgrowth on the tongue, vaginal itching or discharge, loose or foul-smelling stools).
- ▫ Instruct patient to notify health care professional if fever and diarrhea develop, especially if stool contains blood, pus, or mucus. Advise patient not to treat diarrhea without consulting health care professional.
- ▫ Caution patients taking zidovudine that clarithromycin and zidovudine must be taken at least 4 hr apart.
- ▫ Advise patient to notify health care professional if pregnancy is planned or suspected.
- ▫ Instruct the patient to notify health care professional if symptoms do not improve within a few days.

EVALUATION

Clinical response to therapy can be evaluated by: ▪ Resolution of the signs and symptoms of infection. Length of time for complete resolution depends on the organism and site of infection.

*CAPITALS indicate life-threatening; underlines indicate most frequent.

CLEMASTINE
(**klem**-as-teen)
Contac Allergy 12 Hour, Tavist

CLASSIFICATION(S):
Antihistamine

Pregnancy Category B

INDICATIONS

▪ Relief of allergic symptoms caused by histamine release including: □ Allergic rhinitis □ Urticaria.

ACTION

Antagonizes the effects of histamine at H_1-receptor sites; does not bind to or inactivate histamine. **Therapeutic Effects:** ▪ Decreased symptoms of histamine excess (sneezing, rhinorrhea, nasal and ocular pruritus, ocular tearing and redness).

PHARMACOKINETICS

Absorption: Well absorbed following oral administration.
Distribution: Enters breast milk in high concentrations.
Metabolism and Excretion: Extensively metabolized by the liver.
Half-life: UK.

CONTRAINDICATIONS AND PRECAUTIONS

Contraindicated in: ▪ Hypersensitivity ▪ Acute attacks of asthma ▪ Lactation (avoid use) ▪ Known alcohol intolerance (liquid form).
Use Cautiously in: ▪ Narrow-angle glaucoma ▪ Liver disease ▪ Geriatric patients (more susceptible to adverse reactions) ▪ Pregnancy or children <6 yr (safety not established).

ADVERSE REACTIONS AND SIDE EFFECTS*

CNS: drowsiness, confusion, dizziness, paradoxical excitation (children).
EENT: blurred vision.
CV: hypertension, arrhythmias, hypotension, palpitations.
GI: dry mouth, constipation, obstruction.
GU: retention, urinary hesitancy.
Derm: sweating.

INTERACTIONS

Drug-Drug: ▪ Additive CNS depression with other **CNS depressants**, including **alcohol, opioids,** and **sedative/hypnotics** ▪ **MAO inhibitors** intensify and prolong the anticholinergic effects of antihistamines.

ROUTE AND DOSAGE

- **PO (Adults):** *Most allergic conditions*—1.34 mg twice daily. *Allergic dermatoses*—2.68 mg 1–3 times daily.
- **PO (Children 6–12 yr):** *Most allergic conditions*—0.67 mg twice daily. *Allergic dermatoses*—1.34 mg twice daily (not to exceed 4.02 mg/day).

AVAILABILITY

▪ ***Tablets:*** {1 mg[OTC]}, 1.34 mg[OTC], 2.68 mg[Rx] ▪ ***Syrup:*** {0.67 mg/ml[Rx,OTC]} ▪ ***In combination with:*** phenylpropanolamine (Tavist-D)[OTC]. See Appendix A.

TIME/ACTION PROFILE (antihistaminic effects)

	ONSET	PEAK	DURATION
PO	15–60 min	1–2 hr	12 hr

NURSING IMPLICATIONS

ASSESSMENT

□ Assess allergy symptoms (rhinitis, conjunctivitis, hives, urticaria) prior to and periodically throughout therapy.
□ Assess lung sounds and character of bronchial secretions. Maintain fluid intake of 1500–2000 ml/day to decrease viscosity of secretions.
▪ ***Lab Test Considerations:*** May cause false-negative reactions on allergy skin tests; discontinue 3 days prior to testing.
▪ ***Toxicity and Overdose:*** Symptoms of toxicity in children include excitement, hyperreflexia, hallucinations, tremors, ataxia, fever, seizures, fixed dilated pupils, dry mouth, and facial flushing. The dose that causes seizures approximates the lethal dose. Adults are more likely to experience severe drowsiness.

***CAPITALS indicate life-threatening; underlines indicate most frequent.**

POTENTIAL NURSING DIAGNOSES

- Airway clearance, ineffective (Indications).
- Injury, risk for (Adverse Reactions).
- Knowledge deficit, related to medication regimen (Patient/Family Teaching).

IMPLEMENTATION

- **PO:** Administer with food or milk to decrease GI irritation.

PATIENT/FAMILY TEACHING

- Instruct patient to take medication as directed. Do not take more than recommended amount. Missed doses should be taken as soon as possible unless almost time for next dose. Do not double doses.
- May cause drowsiness. Caution patient to avoid driving or other activities requiring alertness until response to drug is known.
- Caution patient to avoid using alcohol or other CNS depressants concurrently with this drug.
- Advise patient that good oral hygiene, frequent rinsing of mouth with water, and sugarless gum or candy may help relieve dry mouth. Patient should notify dentist if dry mouth persists for >2 wk.
- Geriatric patients are at risk for orthostatic hypotension. Advise patient to change positions slowly.
- Instruct patient to contact health care professional if symptoms persist or if difficulty with urination; changes in vision; confusion; severe dry mouth, nose, and throat; or dizziness occurs. May be more common in geriatric patients. Parents should notify health care professional if their child has difficulty sleeping, becomes unusually excited or irritable, or develops shortness of breath or facial flushing.

EVALUATION

Effectiveness of therapy can be demonstrated by: ▪ Decrease in allergic symptoms.

CLINDAMYCIN

(klin-da-**mye**-sin)

Cleocin, Cleocin T, Clinda-Derm, C/T/S, {Dalacin C}, {Dalacin T}

CLASSIFICATION(S):
Anti-infective (miscellaneous)

Pregnancy Category B

INDICATIONS

▪ **PO, IM, IV:** Treatment of: ▫ Skin and skin structure infections ▫ Respiratory tract infections ▫ Septicemia ▫ Intra-abdominal infections ▫ Gynecologic infections ▫ Osteomyelitis ▪ Endocarditis prophylaxis ▪ **Topical:** Severe acne ▪ **Vag:** Bacterial vaginosis. **Unlabeled Uses:** ▪ **PO, IM, IV:** : Treatment of *Pneumocystis carinii* pneumonia, CNS toxoplasmosis, and babesiosis.

ACTION

▪ Inhibits protein synthesis in susceptible bacteria at the level of the 50S ribosome. **Therapeutic Effects:** ▪ Bactericidal or bacteriostatic, depending on susceptibility and concentration. **Spectrum:** ▪ Active against most gram-positive aerobic cocci, including: ▫ Staphylococci ▫ *Streptococcus pneumoniae* ▫ Other streptococci, but not enterococci ▪ Has good activity against those anaerobic bacteria that cause bacterial vaginosis, including *Bacteroides fragilis, Gardnerella vaginalis, Mobiluncus* spp, *Mycoplasma hominis,* and *Corynebacterium* ▪ Also active against *Pneumocystis carinii* and *Toxoplasma gondii*.

PHARMACOKINETICS

Absorption: Well absorbed following PO/IM administration. Minimal absorption following topical/vaginal use.
Distribution: Widely distributed. Does not significantly cross blood-brain barrier. Crosses the placenta; enters breast milk.
Metabolism and Excretion: Mostly metabolized by the liver.
Half-life: 2–3 hr.

CONTRAINDICATIONS AND PRECAUTIONS

Contraindicated in: ▪ Hypersensitivity ▪ Previous pseudomembranous colitis ▪ Severe liver impairment ▪ Diarrhea ▪ Known alcohol intolerance (topical solution, suspension).

{} = **Available in Canada only.**

Use Cautiously in: ▪ Pregnancy or lactation (safety not established).

ADVERSE REACTIONS AND SIDE EFFECTS*

CNS: dizziness, headache, vertigo.
CV: arrhythmias, hypotension.
GI: PSEUDOMEMBRANOUS COLITIS, diarrhea, bitter taste (IV only), nausea, vomiting.
Derm: rashes.
Local: phlebitis at IV site.

INTERACTIONS

Drug-Drug: ▪ **Kaolin** may decrease GI absorption ▪ May enhance the neuromuscular blocking action of other **neuromuscular blocking agents** ▪ **Topical:** Concurrent use with **irritants, abrasives,** or **desquamating agents** may result in additive irritation.

ROUTE AND DOSAGE

- **PO (Adults):** *Most infections*—150–300 mg q 6 hr. P. carinii *pneumonia*—1200–1800 mg/day in divided doses with 15–30 mg primaquine/day (unlabeled). *CNS toxoplasmosis*—1200–2400 mg/day in divided doses with pyrimethamine 50–100 mg/day (unlabeled).
- **PO (Children >1 mo):** 2–5 mg/kg q 6 hr or 2.7–6.7 mg/kg q 8 hr. (Children ≤10 kg should receive at least 37.5 mg q 8 hr.)
- **IM, IV (Adults):** *Most infections*—300–600 mg q 6–8 hr or 900 mg q 8 hr (up to 4.8 g/day IV has been used; single IM doses of >600 mg are not recommended). P. carinii *pneumonia*—2400–2700 mg/day in divided doses with primaquine (unlabeled). *Toxoplasmosis*—1200–4800 mg/day in divided doses with pyrimethamine.
- **IM, IV (Children >1 mo):** 3.75–10 mg/kg (87.5–112.5 mg/m^2) q 6 hr or 5–13.3 mg/kg (116.7–150 mg/m^2) q 8 hr (300 mg/day minimum; up to 7.5 mg/kg q 6 hr for bone infections).
- **IM, IV (Infants <1 mo):** 3.75–5 mg q 6 hr or 5–6.7 mg/kg q 8 hr.
- **Vag (Adults and Adolescents):** 1 applicatorful (5 g) hs for 7 days.
- **Topical (Adults and Adolescents):** *Solution*—1% solution/suspension applied twice daily (range 1– 4 times daily). *Gel*—1% gel applied twice daily.

AVAILABILITY

▪ ***Capsules:*** 75 mg^Rx^, 150 mg^Rx^, 300 mg^Rx^ ▪ ***Oral suspension:*** 75 mg/5 ml^Rx^ ▪ ***Injection:*** 150 mg/ml^Rx^ ▪ ***Topical:*** 1% lotion, gel, solution, suspension^Rx^ ▪ ***Vaginal:*** 2% cream^Rx^.

TIME/ACTION PROFILE (blood levels)

	ONSET	PEAK	DURATION
PO	rapid	45 min	6–8 hr
IM	rapid	1.3 hr	6–8 hr
IV	rapid	end of infusion	6–8 hr

NURSING IMPLICATIONS

ASSESSMENT

- □ Assess patient for infection (vital signs; appearance of wound, sputum, urine, and stool; WBC) at beginning of and throughout therapy.
- □ Obtain specimens for culture and sensitivity prior to initiating therapy. First dose may be given before receiving results.
- □ Monitor bowel elimination. Diarrhea, abdominal cramping, fever, and bloody stools should be reported to health care professional promptly as a sign of pseudomembranous colitis. This may begin up to several weeks following the cessation of therapy.
- □ Assess patient for hypersensitivity (skin rash, urticaria).
- ▪ ***Lab Test Considerations:*** Monitor CBC; may cause transient decrease in leukocytes, eosinophils, and platelets.
- □ May cause elevated alkaline phosphatase, bilirubin, CPK, AST, and ALT concentrations.

POTENTIAL NURSING DIAGNOSES

- Infection, risk for (Indications, Side Effects).
- Diarrhea (Side Effects).
- Knowledge deficit, related to medication regimen (Patient/Family Teaching).

IMPLEMENTATION

- **PO:** Administer with a full glass of water. May be given with meals. Shake liquid preparations

*CAPITALS indicate life-threatening; underlines indicate most frequent.

well. Do not refrigerate. Stable for 14 days at room temperature.

- **IM:** Do not administer >600 mg in a single IM injection.
- **Intermittent Infusion:** Do not administer as an undiluted IV bolus. Dilute each 300 or 600 mg for IV administration with at least 50 ml and 900 or 1200 mg with at least 100 ml of D5W, D10W, D5/0.45% NaCl, D5/0.9% NaCl, D5/Ringer's injection, 0.9% NaCl, or lactated Ringer's solution for injection. Stable for 24 hr at room temperature. Crystals may occur if refrigerated, but dissolve when warmed to room temperature. Do not administer solution with undissolved crystals.
- ***Rate:*** Administer each 300 mg over a minimum of 10 min. Do not give more than 1200 mg in a single 1-hr infusion.
- **Continuous Infusion:** May also be initially administered as a single rapid infusion, followed by continuous IV infusion.
- ***Rate:*** May also administer at an infusion rate of 10–20 mg/min for 30 min, followed by a continuous infusion rate of 0.75–1.25 mg/min.
- **Syringe Compatibility:** ▪ amikacin ▪ aztreonam ▪ gentamicin ▪ heparin.
- **Syringe Incompatibility:** ▪ tobramycin.
- **Y-Site Compatibility:** ▪ amiodarone ▪ aztreonam ▪ cyclophosphamide ▪ diltiazem ▪ enalaprilat ▪ esmolol ▪ fludarabine ▪ foscarnet ▪ heparin ▪ hydromorphone ▪ labetalol ▪ magnesium sulfate ▪ melphalan ▪ meperidine ▪ morphine ▪ multivitamins ▪ ondansetron ▪ perphenazine ▪ piperacillin/tazobactam ▪ sargramostim ▪ tacrolimus ▪ teniposide ▪ theophylline ▪ vinorelbine ▪ vitamin B complex with C ▪ zidovudine.
- **Y-Site Incompatibility:** ▪ filgrastim ▪ fluconazole ▪ idarubicin.
- **Vag:** Applicators are supplied for vaginal administration. When treating bacterial vaginosis, concurrent treatment of male partner is not usually necessary.
- **Topical:** Contact with eyes, mucous membranes, and open cuts should be avoided during topical application. If accidental contact occurs, rinse with copious amounts of cool water.
- □ Wash affected areas with warm water and soap, rinse, and pat dry prior to application. Apply to entire affected area.

PATIENT/FAMILY TEACHING

- **General Info:** Instruct patient to take medication around the clock at evenly spaced times and to finish the drug completely as directed, even if feeling better. If a dose is missed, take as soon as possible unless almost time for next dose. Do not double doses. Advise patient that sharing of this medication may be dangerous.
- □ Instruct patient to notify health care professional immediately if diarrhea, abdominal cramping, fever, or bloody stools occur and not to treat with antidiarrheals without consulting health care professional.
- □ Advise patient to report signs of superinfection (furry overgrowth on the tongue, vaginal or anal itching or discharge).
- □ Notify health care professional if no improvement within a few days.
- □ Patients with a history of rheumatic heart disease or valve replacement need to be taught the importance of antimicrobial prophylaxis before invasive medical or dental procedures (see Appendix N).
- **IV:** Inform patient that bitter taste occurring with IV administration is not significant.
- **Vag:** Instruct patient on proper use of vaginal applicator. Insert high into vagina at bedtime. Instruct patient to remain recumbent for at least 30 min following insertion. Advise patient to use sanitary napkin to prevent staining of clothing or bedding. Continue therapy during menstrual period.
- □ Advise patient to refrain from vaginal sexual intercourse during treatment.
- □ Caution patient that mineral oil in clindamycin cream may weaken latex or rubber contraceptive devices. Such products should not be used within 72 hr of vaginal cream.
- **Topical:** Caution patient applying topical clindamycin that solution is flammable (vehicle is isopropyl alcohol). Avoid application while smoking or near heat or flame.
- □ Advise patient to notify health care professional if excessive drying of skin occurs.
- □ Advise patient to wait 30 min after washing or shaving area before applying.

EVALUATION

Clinical response to therapy can be evaluated by: ▪ Resolution of the signs and symptoms of infection. Length of time for complete resolution depends on the organism and site of infection ▪ Endocarditis prophylaxis ▪ Improvement in acne vulgaris lesions. Improvement should be seen in 6 wk but may take 8–12 wk for maximum benefit.

CLOMIPHENE

(**kloe**-mi-feen)
Clomid, Milophene, Serophene

CLASSIFICATION(S):
Hormone (ovulation inducer)

Pregnancy Category X

INDICATIONS

▪ Induces ovulation in anovulatory women who desire pregnancy. Requires intact anterior pituitary, thyroid, and adrenal function. **Unlabeled Uses:** ▪ Male infertility due to oligospermia.

ACTION

▪ Stimulates release of pituitary gonadotropins, follicle-stimulating hormone, and luteinizing hormone, resulting in ovulation and the development of the corpus luteum. **Therapeutic Effects:** ▪ Induction of ovulation.

PHARMACOKINETICS

Absorption: Well absorbed following oral administration.
Distribution: UK.
Metabolism and Excretion: Apparently metabolized by the liver, with enterohepatic recirculation and biliary elimination. Excreted in feces.
Half-life: 5 days.

CONTRAINDICATIONS AND PRECAUTIONS

Contraindicated in: ▪ Liver disease ▪ Ovarian cysts ▪ Pregnancy.
Use Cautiously in: ▪ Known sensitivity to pituitary gonadotropins ▪ Polycystic ovary syndrome.

ADVERSE REACTIONS AND SIDE EFFECTS*

CNS: fatigue, headache, insomnia, light-headedness, nervousness, restlessness.
EENT: blurred vision, photophobia, scotoma, visual disturbances.
CV: hot flashes, flushing.
GI: abdominal pain, bloating, distention, increased appetite, nausea, vomiting.
GU: increased urine volume, urinary frequency.
Derm: allergic dermatitis, rashes, reversible hair loss, urticaria.
Endo: cyst formation, ovarian enlargement, breast discomfort, multiple births.
Metab: weight gain.

INTERACTIONS

Drug-Drug: ▪ None significant.

ROUTE AND DOSAGE

▪ **PO (Adults):** 25–50 mg/day for 5 days; if ovulation does not occur, a second course of 100 mg/day for 5 days may be given 30 days after the initial course. A maximum of 3 courses may be administered. Some patients require up to 250 mg/day.

AVAILABILITY

▪ ***Tablets:*** 50 mg[Rx].

TIME/ACTION PROFILE (ovulation)

	ONSET	PEAK	DURATION
PO	5–14 days	UK	UK

NURSING IMPLICATIONS

ASSESSMENT

□ A pelvic examination to determine ovarian size should be completed prior to therapy.
□ An endometrial biopsy is recommended in older patients prior to clomiphene therapy to rule out the presence of endometrial carcinoma.
□ Assess patient for abdominal pain throughout therapy. Occurrence requires immediate pelvic examination to determine ovarian enlargement or cyst formation. If these occur, discontinue therapy until ovaries have returned to pretreatment size, usually within a few days to weeks. Dose and duration of next course should be decreased.
▪ ***Lab Test Considerations:*** Estrogen excretion determinations, histological studies of the luteal phase endometrium, serum progester-

*CAPITALS indicate life-threatening; underlines indicate most frequent.

one, and urinary excretion of pregnanediol may be used to determine whether ovulation has occurred following a course of clomiphene.

- □ Liver function tests should be performed prior to course of therapy.
- □ Immunologic assay for human chorionic gonadotropin (HCG) should be used to determine pregnancy if menses does not occur prior to next dose of clomiphene and should be measured 10 days or more after exogenous HCG is administered.

POTENTIAL NURSING DIAGNOSES

- ▪ Knowledge deficit, related to medication regimen (Patient/Family Teaching).

IMPLEMENTATION

- ▪ **General Info:** Clomiphene therapy is usually begun on the 5th day of the menstrual cycle.

PATIENT/FAMILY TEACHING

- □ Instruct patient to take clomiphene exactly as directed at the same time each day. Missed doses should be taken as soon as remembered and the dose doubled if not remembered until the time of the next dose. Notify health care professional if more than one dose is missed.
- □ Advise patient that conception should be attempted with intercourse every other day starting 48 hr prior to ovulation. Ovulation usually occurs 7 days (range 5–10) after last dose of clomiphene.
- □ Instruct patient in the correct method for measuring basal body temperature. A record of the daily basal body temperature should be maintained prior to and throughout course of therapy. Emphasize the importance of compliance with all aspects of therapy.
- □ Prior to therapy, patient should be informed of the potential for multiple births.
- □ Medication may cause visual disturbances or dizziness. Caution patient to avoid driving until the response to the medication is known.
- □ Instruct patient to notify health care professional immediately if pregnancy is suspected; clomiphene should not be taken during pregnancy.
- □ Advise patient that ophthalmologic exams should be performed to evaluate the possibility of ocular toxicity if treatment is continued for more than 1 yr.
- □ Advise patient to notify health care professional promptly if bloating, stomach or pelvic pain, blurred vision, jaundice, persistent hot flashes, breast discomfort, headache, or nausea and vomiting occur.
- □ Emphasize the importance of close monitoring by health care professional throughout therapy.

EVALUATION

Effectiveness of therapy can be demonstrated by: ▪ Occurrence of ovulation measured by estrogen excretion, biphasic body temperature curve, urinary excretion of pregnanediol at postovulatory levels, and endometrial histologic changes. If conception is not achieved after 3–4 courses of clomiphene, diagnosis should be re-evaluated.

CLOMIPRAMINE

(kloe-**mip**-ra-meen)
Anafranil

CLASSIFICATION(S):
Antidepressant (antiobsessive agent)

Pregnancy Category C

INDICATIONS

▪ Management of obsessive-compulsive disorder (OCD). **Unlabeled Uses:** ▪ Treatment of depression.

ACTION

▪ Potentiates the effect of serotonin (antiobsessional effect) and norepinephrine in the CNS. Has moderate anticholinergic effects. **Therapeutic Effects:** ▪ Diminished obsessive-compulsive behavior.

PHARMACOKINETICS

Absorption: Well absorbed from the GI tract.
Distribution: Widely distributed.
Metabolism and Excretion: Extensively metabolized by the liver. Some conversion to a pharmacologically active metabolite (desmethylclomipramine). Undergoes enterohepatic recirculation and secretion into gastric juices.
Half-life: 21–31 hr.

CONTRAINDICATIONS AND PRECAUTIONS

Contraindicated in: ▪ Hypersensitivity ▪ Narrow-angle glaucoma ▪ Recent myocardial infarction ▪ Concurrent MAO inhibitor or clonidine use (avoid if possible) ▪ Pregnancy or lactation.
Use Cautiously in: ▪ History of seizures (threshold may be lowered) ▪ Geriatric patients ▪ Patients with pre-existing cardiovascular disease ▪ Elderly men with prostatic hypertrophy (may be more susceptible to urinary retention) ▪ Hyperthyroidism (increased risk of arrhythmias) ▪ Children <10 yr (safety not established).

ADVERSE REACTIONS AND SIDE EFFECTS*

CNS: SEIZURES, lethargy, sedation, weakness, aggressive behavior.
EENT: blurred vision, dry eyes, dry mouth, vestibular disorder.
CV: ARRHYTHMIAS, ECG changes, orthostatic hypotension.
GI: constipation, nausea, vomiting, eructation.
GU: male sexual dysfunction, urinary retention.
Derm: dry skin, photosensitivity.
Endo: gynecomastia.
Hemat: anemia.
MS: muscle weakness.
Neuro: extrapyramidal reactions.
Misc: hyperthermia, weight gain.

INTERACTIONS

Drug-Drug: ▪ May cause hypotension and tachycardia when used with **MAO inhibitors** (concurrent use not recommended) ▪ May prevent the therapeutic response to **antihypertensives** ▪ Use with **clonidine** may result in hypertensive crisis (avoid concurrent use) ▪ Additive CNS depression with other **CNS depressants** including **alcohol, antihistamines, opioids**, and **sedative/hypnotics** ▪ Adrenergic and anticholinergic side effects may be additive with other **agents having adrenergic/anticholinergic properties** ▪ Effects and toxicity may be increased by concurrent **SSRI antidepressants, phenothiazines, cimetidine**, or **oral contraceptives** ▪ **Nicotine** may increase metabolism and decrease effectiveness ▪ Transient delirium may occur with **disulfiram.**

ROUTE AND DOSAGE

- **PO (Adults):** *Antiobsessive*—25 mg/day, increased over 2-wk period to 100 mg/day in divided doses. May be further increased over several weeks up to 250–300 mg/day in divided doses. Once stabilizing dose is reached, entire daily dose may be given at bedtime. *Antidepressant*—25 mg 3 times daily, may be increased as needed (unlabeled).
- **PO (Geriatric Patients):** 20–30 mg/day initially, may be increased as needed.
- **PO (Children >10 yr and Adolescents):** 25 mg/day initially, increased over 2-wk period to 3 mg/kg/day or 100 mg/day (whichever is smaller) in divided doses. May be further increased to 3 mg/kg/day or 200 mg/day (whichever is smaller) in divided doses. Once stabilizing dose is reached, entire daily dose may be given at bedtime.

AVAILABILITY

- ***Capsules:*** 10 mg[Rx], 25 mg[Rx], 50 mg[Rx], 75 mg[Rx].

TIME/ACTION PROFILE

	ONSET	PEAK	DURATION
PO	1–6 wk	UK	UK

NURSING IMPLICATIONS

ASSESSMENT

- ☐ Monitor mental status and affect. Assess patient for frequency of obsessive-compulsive behaviors. Note degree to which these thoughts and behaviors interfere with daily functioning.
- ☐ Monitor blood pressure and pulse prior to and during initial therapy. Notify physician or other health care professional of decreases in blood pressure (10–20 mm Hg) or sudden increase in pulse rate. Patients taking high doses or with a history of cardiovascular disease should have ECG monitored prior to and periodically throughout therapy.
- ☐ Observe for onset of extrapyramidal parkin-

*CAPITALS indicate life-threatening; underlines indicate most frequent.

sonian side effects (difficulty speaking or swallowing, loss of balance control, pill rolling, mask-like face, shuffling gait, rigidity, tremors). Notify physician or other health care professional if these symptoms occur, as reduction in dose or discontinuation of medication may be necessary. Trihexyphenidyl or diphenhydramine may be used to control these symptoms.

- ***Lab Test Considerations:*** Serum glucose may be increased or decreased.
- □ Monitor CBC and differential during chronic therapy. May rarely cause bone marrow suppression.
- □ In chronic therapy, periodically monitor hepatic and renal function.

POTENTIAL NURSING DIAGNOSES

- Coping, ineffective individual (obsessive-compulsive behaviors), related to repressed anxiety (Indications).
- Injury, risk for (Side Effects).
- Knowledge deficit, related to medication regimen (Patient/Family Teaching).

IMPLEMENTATION

- **PO:** Administer medication with or immediately following a meal to minimize gastric irritation. After titration of dose, total daily dose may be given at bedtime.

PATIENT/FAMILY TEACHING

- □ Instruct patient to take medication exactly as directed. Abrupt discontinuation may cause nausea, headache, and malaise.
- □ May cause drowsiness and blurred vision. Caution patient to avoid driving and other activities requiring alertness until response to drug is known.
- □ Orthostatic hypotension, sedation, and confusion are common during early therapy, especially in geriatric patients. Protect patient from falls and advise patient to change positions slowly.
- □ Advise patient to avoid alcohol or other CNS depressant drugs during course of therapy and for 3–7 days after cessation of therapy.
- □ Instruct patient to notify health care professional if dry mouth or constipation persists or if urinary retention, uncontrolled movements, or rigidity occurs. Sugarless candy or gum may diminish dry mouth, and an increase in fluid intake or bulk may prevent constipation. If these symptoms persist, dosage reduction or discontinuation may be necessary. Consult health care professional if dry mouth persists for more than 2 wk.
- □ Advise patient to inform health care professional if sexual dysfunction occurs.
- □ Caution patient to use sunscreen and protective clothing to prevent photosensitivity reactions.
- □ Inform patient of need to monitor dietary intake, as possible increase in appetite may lead to undesired weight gain.
- □ Advise patient to notify health care professional of medication regimen prior to treatment or surgery.
- □ Emphasize the importance of follow-up exams to monitor effectiveness and side effects.

EVALUATION

Effectiveness of therapy can be demonstrated by: ▪ Diminished obsessive-compulsive behavior.

CLONAZEPAM

(kloe-**na**-ze-pam)
Klonopin, {Rivotril}, {Syn-Clonazepam}

CLASSIFICATION(S):
Anticonvulsant (benzodiazepine)

Schedule IV
Pregnancy Category C

INDICATIONS

▪ Prophylaxis of: □ Petit mal □ Petit mal variant □ Akinetic □ Myoclonic seizures ▪ Management of panic disorder. **Unlabeled Uses:** ▪ Uncontrolled leg movements during sleep ▪ Neuralgias ▪ Sedation.

ACTION

▪ Anticonvulsant effects may be due to presynaptic inhibition ▪ Produces sedative effects in the CNS, probably by stimulating inhibitory GABA re-

{} = **Available in Canada only.**

ceptors. **Therapeutic Effects:** ▪ Prevention of seizures.

PHARMACOKINETICS

Absorption: Well absorbed from the GI tract.
Distribution: Probably crosses the blood-brain barrier and the placenta.
Metabolism and Excretion: Mostly metabolized by the liver.
Half-life: 18–50 hr.

CONTRAINDICATIONS AND PRECAUTIONS

Contraindicated in: ▪ Hypersensitivity to clonazepam or other benzodiazepines ▪ Severe liver disease.
Use Cautiously in: ▪ Narrow-angle glaucoma ▪ Chronic respiratory disease ▪ Do not discontinue abruptly ▪ Pregnancy, lactation, or children (safety not established; chronic use during pregnancy may result in withdrawal in the neonate).

ADVERSE REACTIONS AND SIDE EFFECTS*

CNS: behavioral changes, drowsiness.
EENT: abnormal eye movements, diplopia, nystagmus.
Resp: increased secretions.
CV: palpitations.
GI: constipation, diarrhea, hepatitis.
GU: dysuria, nocturia, urinary retention.
Hemat: anemia, eosinophilia, leukopenia, thrombocytopenia.
Neuro: ataxia, hypotonia.
Misc: fever, physical dependence, psychological dependence, tolerance.

INTERACTIONS

Drug-Drug: ▪ **Alcohol, antidepressants, antihistamines,** other **benzodiazepines,** and **opioids**—concurrent use results in additive CNS depression ▪ **Cimetidine, oral contraceptives, disulfiram, fluoxetine, isoniazid, ketoconazole, metoprolol, propoxyphene, propranolol,** or **valproic acid** may decrease the metabolism of clonazepam, enhancing its actions ▪ May decrease efficacy of **levodopa** ▪ **Rifampin** or **barbiturates** may increase the metabolism and decrease effectiveness of clonazepam ▪ Sedative effects may be decreased by **theophylline** ▪ May increase serum **phenytoin** levels ▪ **Phenytoin** may decrease serum clonazepam levels.

ROUTE AND DOSAGE

- **PO (Adults):** 0.5 mg 3 times daily; may increase by 0.5–1 mg q 3rd day. Total daily maintenance dose not to exceed 20 mg. *Panic disorder*—0.125 mg twice daily; increase after 3 days toward target dose of 1 mg/day (some patients may require up to 4 mg/day).
- **PO (Children <10 yr or 30 kg):** Initial daily dose 0.01–0.03 mg/kg/day (not to exceed 0.05 mg/kg/day) given in 2–3 equally divided doses; increase by no more than 0.25–0.5 mg q 3rd day until therapeutic blood levels are reached (not to exceed 0.2 mg/kg/day).

AVAILABILITY

- ***Tablets:*** 0.5 mg[Rx], 1 mg[Rx], 2 mg[Rx].

TIME/ACTION PROFILE (anticonvulsant activity)

	ONSET	PEAK	DURATION
PO	20–60 min	1–2 hr	6–12 hr

NURSING IMPLICATIONS

ASSESSMENT

- ☐ Observe and record intensity, duration, and location of seizure activity.
- ☐ Assess degree and manifestations of anxiety and mental status prior to and periodically during therapy.
- ☐ Assess patient for drowsiness, unsteadiness, and clumsiness. These symptoms are dose related and most severe during initial therapy; may decrease in severity or disappear with continued or long-term therapy.
- ▪ ***Lab Test Considerations:*** Patients on prolonged therapy should have CBC and liver function tests evaluated periodically. May cause an increase in serum bilirubin, AST, and ALT.
- ☐ May cause decreased thyroidal uptake of sodium iodide ^{123}I and ^{131}I.
- ▪ ***Toxicity and Overdose:*** Therapeutic serum concentrations are 20–80 ng/ml.

***CAPITALS indicate life-threatening; underlines indicate most frequent.**

POTENTIAL NURSING DIAGNOSES

- Injury, risk for (Indications, Side Effects).
- Knowledge deficit, related to medication regimen (Patient/Family Teaching).

IMPLEMENTATION

- **General Info:** Institute seizure precautions for patients on initial therapy or undergoing dose manipulations.
- **PO:** Administer with food to minimize gastric irritation. Tablets may be crushed if patient has difficulty swallowing.

PATIENT/FAMILY TEACHING

- Instruct patient to take medication exactly as directed. Missed doses should be taken within 1 hr or omitted; do not double doses. Abrupt withdrawal of clonazepam may cause status epilepticus, tremors, nausea, vomiting, and abdominal and muscle cramps.
- Medication may cause drowsiness or dizziness. Advise patient to avoid driving or other activities requiring alertness until response to drug is known.
- Caution patient to avoid taking alcohol or other CNS depressants concurrently with this medication.
- Advise patient to notify health care professional of medication regimen prior to treatment or surgery.
- Instruct patient and family to notify health care professional of unusual tiredness, bleeding, sore throat, fever, clay-colored stools, yellowing of skin, or behavioral changes.
- Patient on anticonvulsant therapy should carry identification describing disease process and medication regimen at all times.
- Emphasize the importance of follow-up exams to determine effectiveness of the medication.

EVALUATION

Effectiveness of therapy can be demonstrated by: ▪ Decrease or cessation of seizure activity without undue sedation. Dosage adjustments may be required after several months of therapy ▪ Decrease in frequency and severity of panic attacks ▪ Relief of leg movements during sleep ▪ Decrease in pain from neuralgia.

CLONIDINE

(klon-i-deen)

Catapres, Catapres-TTS, {Dixarit}, Duraclon

CLASSIFICATION(S):

Analgesic (centrally acting), Antihypertensive agent (centrally acting adrenergic)

Pregnancy Category C

C

INDICATIONS

▪ **PO, Transdermal:** Management of mild to moderate hypertension ▪ **Epidural:** Management of cancer pain unresponsive to opioids alone. **Unlabeled Uses:** ▪ Management of opioid withdrawal.

ACTION

▪ Stimulates alpha-adrenergic receptors in the CNS; result is inhibition of cardioacceleration and vasoconstriction center ▪ Prevents pain signal transmission to the CNS by stimulating alpha$_2$-adrenergic receptors in the spinal cord. **Therapeutic Effects:** ▪ Decreased blood pressure ▪ Decreased pain.

PHARMACOKINETICS

Absorption: Well absorbed from the GI tract and skin. Enters systemic circulation following epidural use. Some absorption follows sublingual administration.

Distribution: Widely distributed; enters CNS. Crosses the placenta readily; enters breast milk in high concentrations.

Metabolism and Excretion: Mostly metabolized by the liver; 40–50% eliminated unchanged in urine.

Half-life: *Plasma*—12–22 hr; *CNS*—1.3 hr.

CONTRAINDICATIONS AND PRECAUTIONS

Contraindicated in: ▪ Hypersensitivity ▪ *Epidural*—injection site infection, anticoagulant therapy, or bleeding problems.

Use Cautiously in: ▪ Serious cardiac or cerebrovascular disease ▪ Renal insufficiency

▪ Geriatric patients (dosage reduction may be required) ▪ Pregnancy or lactation (safety not established).

ADVERSE REACTIONS AND SIDE EFFECTS*

CNS: drowsiness, depression, dizziness, nervousness, nightmares.
CV: bradycardia, hypotension (↑ with epidural), palpitations.
GI: dry mouth, constipation, nausea, vomiting.
GU: impotence.
Derm: rash, sweating.
F and E: sodium retention.
Metab: weight gain.
Misc: withdrawal phenomenon.

INTERACTIONS

Drug-Drug: ▪ Additive sedation with **CNS depressants** including **alcohol, antihistamines, opioids**, and **sedative/hypnotics** ▪ Additive hypotension with other **antihypertensive agents** and **nitrates** ▪ Additive bradycardia with **myocardial depressants**, including **beta-adrenergic blockers** ▪ **MAO inhibitors, amphetamines, beta blockers, prazosin**, or **tricyclic antidepressants** may decrease antihypertensive effect ▪ Withdrawal phenomenon may be increased by discontinuation of **beta blockers** ▪ Epidural clonidine prolongs the effects of epidurally administered **local anesthetics** ▪ May decrease effectiveness of **levodopa** ▪ Increased risk of adverse cardiovascular reactions with **verapamil.**

ROUTE AND DOSAGE

- **PO (Adults):** *Hypertension—Initial dose*—100 mcg (0.1 mg) bid, increase by 100–200 mcg (0.1–0.2 mg)/day q 2–4 days. *Usual maintenance dose* is 200–600 mcg (0.2–0.6 mg)/day in 2–3 divided doses (up to 2.4 mg/day). *Urgent treatment*—200 mcg (0.2 mg) loading dose, then 100 mcg (0.1 mg) q hr until blood pressure is controlled or 800 mcg (0.8 mg) total has been administered; follow with maintenance dosing. *Opioid withdrawal*—300 mcg (0.3 mg)–1.2 mg/day, may be decreased by 50%/day for 3 days, then discontinued or decreased by 100–200 mcg (0.1–0.2 mg)/day.
- **PO (Geriatric Patients):** 100 mcg (0.1 mg) at bedtime initially, increased as needed.
- **PO (Children):** 50–400 mcg (0.05–0.4 mg) twice daily.
- **Transdermal (Adults):** *Hypertension*—Transdermal system delivering 100–300 mcg (0.1–0.3 mg)/24 hr applied every 7 days. Initiate with 100 mcg (0.1 mg)/24 hr system; dosage increments may be made q 1–2 wk when system is changed.
- **Epidural (Adults):** 30 mcg/hr initially; titrated according to need.
- **Epidural (Children):** 0.5 mcg/kg/hr initially; titrated according to need.

AVAILABILITY

▪ ***Tablets:*** {25 mcg (0.025 mg)[Rx]}, 100 mcg (0.1 mg)[Rx], 200 mcg (0.2 mg)[Rx], 300 mcg (0.3 mg)[Rx] ▪ ***Transdermal systems:*** Catapres-TTS 1[Rx] contains 2.5 mg total clonidine content, releases 0.1 mg/24 hr, Catapres-TTS 2[Rx] contains 5 mg total clonidine content, releases 0.2 mg/24 hr, Catapres-TTS 3[Rx] contains 7.5 mg total clonidine content, releases 0.3 mg/24 hr ▪ ***Solution for epidural injection*** : 100 mcg/ml in 10-ml vials[Rx] ▪ ***In combination with:*** chlorthalidone (Combipres).[Rx] See Appendix A.

TIME/ACTION PROFILE (PO, TD = antihypertensive effect; epidural = analgesia)

	ONSET	PEAK	DURATION
PO	30–60 min	2–4 hr	8–12 hr
TD	2–3 days	UK	7 days†
Epidural	UK	UK	UK

†8 hr following removal of patch.

NURSING IMPLICATIONS

ASSESSMENT

- **General Info:** Monitor intake and output ratios and daily weight, and assess for edema daily, especially at beginning of therapy.
- □ Monitor blood pressure and pulse frequently during initial dosage adjustment and periodically throughout therapy. Report significant changes.
- **Pain:** Assess location, character, and intensity of pain prior to, frequently during first few days, and routinely throughout administration.

*CAPITALS indicate life-threatening; underlines indicate most frequent.

- Monitor for fever as potential sign of catheter infection.
- **Opioid Withdrawal:** Monitor patient for signs and symptoms of opioid withdrawal (tachycardia, fever, runny nose, diarrhea, sweating, nausea, vomiting, irritability, stomach cramps, shivering, unusually large pupils, weakness, difficulty sleeping, gooseflesh).
- ***Lab Test Considerations:*** May cause transient increase in blood glucose levels.
- May cause decreased urinary catecholamine and vanillylmandelic acid (VMA) concentrations; these may increase upon abrupt withdrawal.
- May cause weakly positive Coombs' test.

POTENTIAL NURSING DIAGNOSES

- Pain (Indications).
- Injury, risk for (Side Effects).
- Knowledge deficit, related to medication regimen (Patient/Family Teaching).

IMPLEMENTATION

- **General Info:** In the perioperative setting, continue clonidine up to 4 hr prior to surgery and resume as soon as possible thereafter. Do not interrupt *transdermal clonidine* during surgery. Monitor blood pressure carefully.
- **PO:** Administer last dose of the day at bedtime.
- **Transdermal:** Transdermal system should be applied once every 7 days. May be applied to any hairless site; avoid cuts or calluses. Absorption is greater when placed on chest or upper arm and decreased when placed on thigh. Rotate sites. Wash area with soap and water; dry thoroughly before application. Apply firm pressure over patch to ensure contact with skin, especially around edges. Remove old system and discard. System includes a protective adhesive overlay to be applied over medication patch to ensure adhesion, should medication patch loosen.

PATIENT/FAMILY TEACHING

- **General Info:** Instruct patient to take clonidine at the same time each day, even if feeling well. If a dose is missed, take as soon as remembered. If more than 1 oral dose in a row is missed or if transdermal system is late in being changed by 3 or more days, consult health care professional. All routes of clonidine should be gradually discontinued over 2–4 days to prevent rebound hypertension.
- Advise patient to make sure enough medication is available for weekends, holidays, and vacations. A written prescription may be kept in wallet in case of emergency.
- Clonidine may cause drowsiness, which usually diminishes with continued use. Advise patient to avoid driving or other activities requiring alertness until response to medication is known.
- Caution patient to avoid sudden changes in position to decrease orthostatic hypotension. Use of alcohol, standing for long periods, exercising, and hot weather may increase orthostatic hypotension.
- If dry mouth occurs, frequent mouth rinses, good oral hygiene, and sugarless gum or candy may decrease effect. If dry mouth continues for more than 2 wk, consult health care professional.
- Caution patient to avoid concurrent use of alcohol or other CNS depressants with this medication.
- Advise patient to consult health care professional before taking any OTC cough, cold, or allergy remedies.
- Advise patient to notify health care professional of medication regimen prior to treatment or surgery.
- Advise patient to notify health care professional if itching or redness of skin (with transdermal patch), mental depression, swelling of feet and lower legs, paleness or cold feeling in fingertips or toes, or vivid dreams or nightmares occur. May require discontinuation of therapy, especially with depression.
- **Hypertension:** Encourage patient to comply with additional interventions for hypertension (weight reduction, low-sodium diet, discontinuation of smoking, moderation of alcohol consumption, regular exercise, and stress management). Medication helps control but does not cure hypertension.
- Instruct patient and family on proper technique for blood pressure monitoring. Advise them to check blood pressure at least weekly and report significant changes.
- **Transdermal:** Instruct patient on proper application of transdermal system. Do not cut or trim unit. Transdermal system can remain in place during bathing or swimming.

EVALUATION

Effectiveness of therapy can be demonstrated by: ▪ Decrease in blood pressure ▪ Decrease in severity of pain ▪ Decrease in the signs and symptoms of opioid withdrawal.

CLOPIDOGREL

(kloe-**pi**-doe-grel)

Plavix

CLASSIFICATION(S):

Platelet aggregation inhibitor

Pregnancy Category B

INDICATIONS

▪ Reduction of atherosclerotic events (myocardial infarction, stroke, vascular death) in patients at risk for such events (recent myocardial infarction, stroke, or peripheral vascular disease).

ACTION

▪ Inhibits platelet aggregation by irreversibly inhibiting the binding of adenosine triphosphate (ATP) to platelet receptors. **Therapeutic Effects:** ▪ Decreased occurrence of atherosclerotic events in patients at risk.

PHARMACOKINETICS

Absorption: Well absorbed following oral administration but rapidly metabolized to an active antiplatelet compound. Parent drug has no antiplatelet activity.
Distribution: UK.
Metabolism and Excretion: Rapidly and extensively converted by the liver to its active metabolite, which is then eliminated 50% in urine and 45% in feces.
Half-life: 8 hr (active metabolite).

CONTRAINDICATIONS AND PRECAUTIONS

Contraindicated in: ▪ Hypersensitivity ▪ Pathologic bleeding (peptic ulcer, intracranial hemorrhage) ▪ Lactation.
Use Cautiously in: ▪ Patients at risk for bleeding (trauma, surgery, or other pathologic conditions) ▪ History of GI bleeding or ulcer disease ▪ Severe hepatic impairment ▪ Pregnancy or children (safety not established; use in pregnancy only if clearly indicated).

ADVERSE REACTIONS AND SIDE EFFECTS*

Incidence of adverse reactions similar to aspirin.
CNS: depression, dizziness, fatigue, headache.
EENT: epistaxis.
Resp: cough, dyspnea.
CV: chest pain, edema, hypertension.
GI: GI BLEEDING, abdominal pain, diarrhea, dyspepsia, gastritis.
Derm: pruritus, purpura, rash.
Hemat: BLEEDING, NEUTROPENIA.
Metab: hypercholesterolemia.
MS: arthralgia, back pain.

INTERACTIONS

Drug-Drug: ▪ Concurrent **abciximab, aspirin, NSAIDs, heparin, thrombolytic agents, ticlopidine**, or **warfarin** may increase the risk of bleeding ▪ May inhibit the metabolism and increase the effects of **phenytoin, tolbutamide, tamoxifen, warfarin, torsemide, fluvastatin**, and many **NSAIDs.**

ROUTE AND DOSAGE

▪ **PO (Adults):** 75 mg once daily.

AVAILABILITY

▪ ***Tablets:*** 75 mg[Rx].

TIME/ACTION PROFILE (effects on platelet function)

	ONSET	PEAK	DURATION
PO	within 24 hr	3–7 days	5 days†

†Following discontinuation.

NURSING IMPLICATIONS

ASSESSMENT

□ Assess patient for symptoms of stroke, peripheral vascular disease, or myocardial infarction periodically throughout therapy.
▪ ***Lab Test Considerations:*** Monitor bleeding time throughout therapy. Prolonged bleeding time, which is time- and dose-dependent, is expected.
□ Monitor CBC with differential and platelet count periodically during therapy. Neutropenia may rarely occur.

***CAPITALS indicate life-threatening; underlines indicate most frequent.**

POTENTIAL NURSING DIAGNOSES

- Injury, risk for (Indications, Side Effects).
- Knowledge deficit, related to medication regimen (Patient/Family Teaching).

IMPLEMENTATION

- **PO:** Administer once daily without regard to food.

PATIENT/FAMILY TEACHING

- Instruct patient to take medication exactly as directed. Missed doses should be taken as soon as possible unless almost time for next dose; do not double doses.
- Advise patient to notify health care professional promptly if fever, chills, sore throat, or unusual bleeding or bruising occurs.
- Advise patient to notify health care professional of medication regimen prior to treatment or surgery.
- Instruct patient to avoid taking OTC medications containing aspirin or NSAIDs without consulting health care professional.

EVALUATION

Effectiveness of therapy can be demonstrated by: ▪ Prevention of stroke, myocardial infarction, and vascular death in patients at risk.

CLORAZEPATE

(klor-**az**-e-pate)

{Apo-Clorazepate}, Gen-XENE, {Novo-Clopate}, Tranxene, Tranxene-SD

CLASSIFICATION(S):

Antianxiety agent, Anticonvulsant, Sedative/hypnotic (benzodiazepine)

Schedule IV

Pregnancy Category UK

INDICATIONS

▪ Treatment of anxiety ▪ Management of alcohol withdrawal ▪ Management of simple partial seizures.

ACTION

▪ Acts at many levels in the CNS to produce anxiolytic effect and CNS depression (by stimulating inhibitory GABA receptors) ▪ Produces skeletal muscle relaxation (by inhibiting spinal polysynaptic afferent pathways) ▪ Also has anticonvulsant effect (enhances presynaptic inhibition). **Therapeutic Effects:** ▪ Relief of anxiety ▪ Sedation ▪ Prevention of seizures.

PHARMACOKINETICS

Absorption: Well absorbed from the GI tract as desmethyldiazepam.
Distribution: Widely distributed. Crosses the placenta; enters breast milk.
Metabolism and Excretion: Metabolized by the liver; some conversion to active compounds.
Half-life: 48 hr.

CONTRAINDICATIONS AND PRECAUTIONS

Contraindicated in: ▪ Hypersensitivity ▪ Cross-sensitivity with other benzodiazepines may occur ▪ Pre-existing CNS depression ▪ Severe uncontrolled pain ▪ Narrow-angle glaucoma ▪ Pregnancy or lactation.
Use Cautiously in: ▪ Pre-existing hepatic dysfunction ▪ Patients who may be suicidal or have been addicted to drugs in the past ▪ Geriatric or debilitated patients (dosage reduction required) ▪ Severe pulmonary disease.

ADVERSE REACTIONS AND SIDE EFFECTS*

CNS: dizziness, drowsiness, lethargy, hangover, headache, mental depression, paradoxical excitation.
EENT: blurred vision.
Resp: respiratory depression.
GI: constipation, diarrhea, nausea, vomiting.
Derm: rashes.
Misc: physical dependence, psychological dependence, tolerance.

INTERACTIONS

Drug-Drug: ▪ **Alcohol, antidepressants, antihistamines,** and **opioids**—concurrent use results in additive CNS depression ▪ **Cimetidine, oral contraceptives, disulfiram, fluoxetine,**

{} = Available in Canada only.
*CAPITALS indicate life-threatening; underlines indicate most frequent.

isoniazid, ketoconazole, metoprolol, propoxyphene, propranolol, or **valproic acid** may decrease the metabolism of clorazepate, enhancing its actions ▪ May decrease efficacy of **levodopa** ▪ **Rifampin** or **barbiturates** may increase the metabolism and decrease effectiveness of clorazepate ▪ Sedative effects may be decreased by **theophylline.**

ROUTE AND DOSAGE

- **PO (Adults):** *Anxiety*—7.5–15 mg 2–4 times daily or 15 mg at bedtime initially. May also be given in a single dose of 11.25–22.5 mg at bedtime. *Alcohol withdrawal*—30 mg initially, then 15 mg 2–4 times daily on 1st day, then gradually decreased over subsequent days. *Anticonvulsant*—7.5 mg 3 times daily; can increase by no more than 7.5 mg/day at weekly intervals (daily dose not to exceed 90 mg).
- **PO (Geriatric Patients or Debilitated Patients):** *Anxiety*—3.73–15 mg/day, may be increased.
- **PO (Children 9–12 yr):** 7.5 mg twice daily initially, may increase by 7.5 mg/wk (not to exceed 60 mg/day).

AVAILABILITY

▪ ***Tablets:*** 3.75 mg^{Rx}, 7.5 mg^{Rx}, 11.25 mg^{Rx}, 15 mg^{Rx}, 22.5 mg^{Rx} ▪ ***Capsules:*** 3.75 mg^{Rx}, 7.5 mg^{Rx}, 15 mg^{Rx}.

TIME/ACTION PROFILE (sedation)

	ONSET	PEAK	DURATION
PO	1–2 hr	1–2 hr	up to 24 hr

NURSING IMPLICATIONS

ASSESSMENT

- **General Info:** Assess patient for drowsiness, unsteadiness, and clumsiness. These symptoms are dose related and most severe during initial therapy; may decrease in severity or disappear with continued or long-term therapy.
- □ Prolonged high-dose therapy may lead to psychological or physical dependence. Restrict amount of drug available to patient.
- **Anxiety:** Assess degree and manifestations of anxiety prior to and periodically throughout therapy.
- **Alcohol Withdrawal:** Assess patient experiencing alcohol withdrawal for tremors, agitation, delirium, and hallucinations. Protect from injury.
- **Seizures:** Observe and record intensity, duration, and location of seizure activity.
- ***Lab Test Considerations:*** Patients on prolonged therapy should have CBC and liver function tests evaluated periodically. May cause an increase in serum bilirubin, AST, and ALT.
- □ May cause decreased thyroidal uptake of sodium iodide ^{123}I and ^{131}I.

POTENTIAL NURSING DIAGNOSES

- Anxiety (Indications).
- Injury, risk for (Indications, Side Effects).
- Knowledge deficit, related to medication regimen (Patient/Family Teaching).

IMPLEMENTATION

- **PO:** If gastric irritation is a problem, may be administered with food or fluids. Capsule should be swallowed whole; do not open.
- □ Avoid administration of antacids within 1 hr of medication, as absorption of clorazepate may be delayed.

PATIENT/FAMILY TEACHING

- **General Info:** Instruct patient to take medication exactly as directed, not to skip or double up on missed doses. Abrupt withdrawal of clorazepate may cause status epilepticus, tremors, nausea, vomiting, and abdominal and muscle cramps.
- □ Medication may cause drowsiness or dizziness. Advise patient to avoid driving or other activities requiring alertness until response to drug is known.
- □ Caution patient to avoid taking alcohol or other CNS depressants concurrently with this medication.
- □ Instruct patient to contact health care professional immediately if pregnancy is suspected.
- □ Advise patient to notify health care professional of medication regimen prior to treatment or surgery.
- □ Instruct patient and family to notify health care professional of unusual tiredness, bleeding, sore throat, fever, clay-colored stools, yellowing of skin, or behavioral changes.
- □ Emphasize the importance of follow-up exams to determine effectiveness of the medication.
- **Seizures:** Patients on anticonvulsant therapy

should carry identification describing disease process and medication regimen at all times.

EVALUATION

Effectiveness of therapy can be demonstrated by: ▪ Increase in sense of well-being ▫ Decrease in subjective feelings of anxiety ▪ Control of acute alcohol withdrawal ▪ Decrease or cessation of seizure activity without undue sedation.

CLOZAPINE
(**cloz**-a-peen)
Clozaril

CLASSIFICATION(S):
Antipsychotic agent

Pregnancy Category B

INDICATIONS

▪ Treatment of schizophrenic patients unresponsive to or intolerant of standard therapy with other antipsychotics.

ACTION

▪ Binds to dopamine receptors in the CNS ▪ Also has anticholinergic and alpha-adrenergic blocking activity ▪ Produces fewer extrapyramidal reactions and less tardive dyskinesia than standard antipsychotics but carries high risk of hematologic abnormalities. **Therapeutic Effects:** ▪ Diminished schizophrenic behavior.

PHARMACOKINETICS

Absorption: Well absorbed following oral administration.
Distribution: Rapid and extensive distribution; crosses blood-brain barrier and placenta.
Metabolism and Excretion: Mostly metabolized on first pass through the liver.
Half-life: 8–12 hr.

CONTRAINDICATIONS AND PRECAUTIONS

Contraindicated in: ▪ Hypersensitivity ▪ Bone marrow depression ▪ Lactation ▪ Severe CNS depression/coma.
Use Cautiously in: ▪ Prostatic enlargement ▪ Narrow-angle glaucoma ▪ Malnourished patients or patients with cardiovascular, hepatic, or renal disease (use lower initial dose, titrate more slowly) ▪ Diabetes ▪ Seizure disorder ▪ Children <16 yr (safety not established).

ADVERSE REACTIONS AND SIDE EFFECTS*

CNS: NEUROLEPTIC MALIGNANT SYNDROME, SEIZURES, dizziness, sedation.
EENT: visual disturbances.
CV: hypotension, tachycardia, ECG changes, hypertension.
GI: constipation, abdominal discomfort, dry mouth, increased salivation, nausea, vomiting.
Derm: rash, sweating.
Endo: hyperglycemia.
Hemat: AGRANULOCYTOSIS, LEUKOPENIA.
Neuro: extrapyramidal reactions.
Misc: fever, weight gain.

INTERACTIONS

Drug-Drug: ▪ Additive anticholinergic effects with other **agents having anticholinergic properties** including **antihistamines, quinidine, disopyramide,** and **antidepressants** ▪ Additive CNS depression with **alcohol, antidepressants, antihistamines, opioids,** or **sedative/hypnotics** ▪ Additive hypotension with **nitrates,** acute ingestion of **alcohol,** or **antihypertensives** ▪ Increased risk of bone marrow suppression with **antineoplastic agents** or **radiation therapy** ▪ Use with **lithium** increases the risk of adverse CNS reactions, including seizures.

ROUTE AND DOSAGE

▪ **PO (Adults):** 25 mg 1–2 times daily initially; increase by 25–50 mg/day over a period of 2 wk up to target dose of 300–450 mg/day. May increase by up to 100 mg/day once or twice weekly (not to exceed 900 mg/day).

AVAILABILITY

▪ ***Tablets:*** 25 mg[Rx], 100 mg[Rx].

TIME/ACTION PROFILE (antipsychotic effect)

	ONSET	PEAK	DURATION
PO	UK	wks	4–12 hr

***CAPITALS indicate life-threatening; underlines indicate most frequent.**

NURSING IMPLICATIONS

ASSESSMENT

- Monitor patient's mental status (delusions, hallucinations, and behavior) prior to and periodically throughout therapy.
- Monitor blood pressure (sitting, standing, lying) and pulse rate prior to and frequently during initial dosage titration.
- Observe patient carefully when administering medication to ensure medication is actually taken and not hoarded.
- Monitor patient for onset of akathisia (restlessness or desire to keep moving) and extrapyramidal side effects (*parkinsonian*—difficulty speaking or swallowing, loss of balance control, pill rolling, mask-like face, shuffling gait, rigidity, tremors and dystonic muscle spasms, twisting motions, twitching, inability to move eyes, weakness of arms or legs) every 2 mo during therapy and 8–12 wk after therapy has been discontinued. Notify physician or other health care professional if these symptoms occur, as reduction in dose or discontinuation of medication may be necessary. Trihexyphenidyl or diphenhydramine may be used to control these symptoms.
- Although not yet reported for clozapine, monitor for possible tardive dyskinesia (uncontrolled rhythmic movement of mouth, face, and extremities, lip smacking or puckering, puffing of cheeks, uncontrolled chewing, rapid or worm-like movements of tongue). Report these symptoms immediately; may be irreversible.
- Monitor frequency and consistency of bowel movements. Increasing bulk and fluids in the diet may help to minimize constipation.
- Clozapine lowers the seizure threshold. Institute seizure precautions for patients with history of seizure disorder.
- Transient fevers may occur, especially during first 3 wk of therapy. Fever is usually self-limiting but may require discontinuation of medication. Also, monitor for development of neuroleptic malignant syndrome (fever, respiratory distress, tachycardia, convulsions, diaphoresis, hypertension or hypotension, pallor, tiredness). Notify physician immediately if these symptoms occur.
- ***Lab Test Considerations:*** Monitor WBC and differential count prior to initiation of therapy and WBC count weekly during therapy and for 4 wk after discontinuation of clozapine. Because of the risk of agranulocytosis, clozapine is available only in a 1-wk supply through the *Clozaril Patient Management System,* which combines WBC testing, patient monitoring, and controlled distribution through participating pharmacies. If WBC is <3000 mm^3 or granulocyte count is <1500 mm^3, withhold clozapine and monitor patient for signs and symptoms of infection.
- ***Toxicity and Overdose:*** Overdose is treated with activated charcoal and supportive therapy. Monitor patient for several days because of risk of delayed effects.
- Avoid use of epinephrine and its derivatives when treating hypotension, and avoid quinidine and procainamide when treating arrhythmias.

POTENTIAL NURSING DIAGNOSES

- Violence, risk for, directed at others (Indications).
- Thought processes, altered, related to panic anxiety (Indications).
- Injury, risk for (Side Effects).

IMPLEMENTATION

- **PO:** Administer capsules with food or milk to decrease gastric irritation.

PATIENT/FAMILY TEACHING

- Instruct patient to take medication exactly as directed. Patients on long-term therapy may need to discontinue gradually over 1–2 wk.
- Inform patient of possibility of extrapyramidal symptoms. Instruct patient to report these symptoms immediately.
- Advise patient to change positions slowly to minimize orthostatic hypotension.
- May cause seizures and drowsiness. Caution patient to avoid driving or other activities requiring alertness while taking clozapine.
- Caution patient to avoid concurrent use of alcohol, other CNS depressants, and OTC medications without consulting health care professional.
- Instruct patient to use frequent mouth rinses, good oral hygiene, and sugarless gum or candy to minimize dry mouth.
- Advise patient to notify health care profes-

sional of medication regimen prior to treatment or surgery.

- □ Instruct patient to notify health care professional promptly if sore throat, fever, lethargy, weakness, malaise, or flu-like symptoms occur or if pregnancy is planned or suspected.
- □ Advise patient of need for continued medical follow-up for psychotherapy, eye exams, and laboratory tests.

EVALUATION

Effectiveness of therapy can be demonstrated by: ▪ Diminished schizophrenic behavior.

CODEINE

(koe-**deen**)

{Paveral}

CLASSIFICATION(S):

Antitussive, Opioid analgesic (agonist)

Schedule II, III, IV, V (depends on content)

INDICATIONS

▪ Management of mild to moderate pain ▪ Antitussive (in smaller doses). **Unlabeled Uses:** ▪ Management of diarrhea.

ACTION

▪ Binds to opiate receptors in the CNS. Alters the perception of and response to painful stimuli, while producing generalized CNS depression ▪ Decreases cough reflex ▪ Decreases GI motility. **Therapeutic Effects:** ▪ Decreased severity of pain ▪ Suppression of the cough reflex ▪ Relief of diarrhea.

PHARMACOKINETICS

Absorption: 50% absorbed from the GI tract. Completely absorbed from IM sites. Oral and parenteral doses are not equal.

Distribution: Widely distributed. Crosses the placenta; enters breast milk.

Metabolism and Excretion: Mostly metabolized by the liver; 10% converted to morphine, 5–15% excreted unchanged in urine.

Half-life: 2.5–4 hr.

CONTRAINDICATIONS AND PRECAUTIONS

Contraindicated in: ▪ Hypersensitivity.

Use Cautiously in: ▪ Head trauma ▪ Increased intracranial pressure ▪ Severe renal, hepatic, or pulmonary disease ▪ Hypothyroidism ▪ Adrenal insufficiency ▪ Alcoholism ▪ Geriatric or debilitated patients (dosage reduction required; more susceptible to CNS depression, constipation) ▪ Undiagnosed abdominal pain ▪ Prostatic hypertrophy ▪ Has been used during labor; respiratory depression may occur in the newborn ▪ Pregnancy or lactation (avoid chronic use).

ADVERSE REACTIONS AND SIDE EFFECTS*

CNS: <u>confusion</u>, <u>sedation</u>, dysphoria, euphoria, floating feeling, hallucinations, headache, unusual dreams.

EENT: blurred vision, diplopia, miosis.

Resp: respiratory depression.

CV: <u>hypotension</u>, bradycardia.

GI: <u>constipation</u>, <u>nausea</u>, <u>vomiting</u>.

GU: urinary retention.

Derm: flushing, sweating.

Misc: physical dependence, psychological dependence, tolerance.

INTERACTIONS

Drug-Drug: ▪ Use with extreme caution in patients receiving **MAO inhibitors** (reduce initial dosage to 25% of usual dose) ▪ Additive CNS depression with **alcohol, antidepressants, antihistamines,** and **sedative/hypnotics** ▪ Administration of **partial antagonists (buprenorphine, butorphanol, nalbuphine,** or **pentazocine)** may precipitate opioid withdrawal in physically dependent patients ▪ **Nalbuphine** or **pentazocine** may decrease analgesia.

ROUTE AND DOSAGE

- **PO (Adults):** *Analgesic*—15–60 mg q 3–6 hr as needed. *Antitussive*—10–20 mg q 4–6 hr as needed (not to exceed 120 mg/day). *Antidiarrheal*—30 mg up to 4 times daily.
- **PO (Children 6–12 yr):** *Analgesic*—0.5

{} = Available in Canada only.

***CAPITALS indicate life-threatening; <u>underlines</u> indicate most frequent.**

mg/kg (15 mg/m^2) q 4–6 hr (up to 4 times daily) as needed. *Antitussive*—5–10 mg q 4–6 hr as needed (not to exceed 60 mg/day). *Antidiarrheal*—0.5 mg/kg up to 4 times daily.

- **PO (Children 2–5 yr):** *Analgesic*—0.5 mg/kg (15 mg/m^2) q 4–6 hr (up to 4 times daily) as needed. *Antitussive*—0.25 mg/kg up to 4 times daily. *Antidiarrheal*—0.5 mg/kg up to 4 times daily.
- **IM, IV, SC (Adults):** *Analgesic*—15–60 mg q 4–6 hr as needed.
- **IM, IV, SC (Infants and Children):** *Analgesic*—0.5 mg/kg (15 mg/m^2) q 4–6 hr as needed.

AVAILABILITY

▪ ***Tablets:*** 15 mg^{Rx}, 30 mg^{Rx}, 60 mg^{Rx} ▪ ***Oral solution:*** {10 mg/5 ml^{Rx}}, 15 mg/5 ml^{Rx} ▪ ***Injection:*** 30 mg/ml^{Rx}, 60 mg/ml^{Rx} ▪ ***In combination with:*** antihistamines, decongestants, antipyretics, caffeine, butalbital, and nonopioid analgesics^{Rx}. See Appendix A.

TIME/ACTION PROFILE (analgesia)

	ONSET	PEAK	DURATION
PO	30–45 min	60–120 min	4 hr
IM	10–30 min	30–60 min	4 hr
SC	10–30 min	UK	4 hr

NURSING IMPLICATIONS

ASSESSMENT

- **General Info:** Assess blood pressure, pulse, and respirations before and periodically during administration. If respiratory rate is <10/min, assess level of sedation. Physical stimulation may be sufficient to prevent significant hypoventilation. Dose may need to be decreased by 25–50%. Initial drowsiness will diminish with continued use.
- □ Assess bowel function routinely. Prevention of constipation should be instituted with increased intake of fluids, bulk, and laxatives to minimize constipating effects. Stimulant laxatives should be administered routinely if opioid use exceeds 2–3 days, unless contraindicated.
- **Pain:** Assess type, location, and intensity of pain prior to and 1 hr (peak) following administration. When titrating opioid doses, increases of 25–50% should be administered until there is either a 50% reduction in the patient's pain rating on a numerical or visual analogue scale or the patient reports satisfactory pain relief. A repeat dose can be safely administered at the time of the peak if previous dose is ineffective and side effects are minimal.
- □ An equianalgesic chart (see Appendix B) should be used when changing routes or when changing from one opioid to another.
- □ Prolonged use may lead to physical and psychological dependence and tolerance. This should not prevent patient from receiving adequate analgesia. Most patients who receive codeine for pain do not develop psychological dependence. If progressively higher doses are required, consider conversion to a stronger opioid.
- **Cough:** Assess cough and lung sounds during antitussive use.
- ***Lab Test Considerations:*** May cause increased plasma amylase and lipase concentrations.
- ***Toxicity and Overdose:*** If an opioid antagonist is required to reverse respiratory depression or coma, naloxone (Narcan) is the antidote. Dilute the 0.4-mg ampule of naloxone in 10 ml of 0.9% NaCl and administer 0.5 ml (0.02 mg) by direct IV push every 2 min. For children and patients weighing <40 kg, dilute 0.1 mg of naloxone in 10 ml of 0.9% NaCl for a concentration of 10 mcg/ml and administer 0.5 mcg/kg every 1–2 min. Titrate dose to avoid withdrawal, seizures, and severe pain.

POTENTIAL NURSING DIAGNOSES

- Pain (Indications).
- Sensory-perceptual alterations: visual, auditory (Side Effects).
- Injury, risk for (Side Effects).

IMPLEMENTATION

- **General Info:** Explain therapeutic value of medication prior to administration to enhance the analgesic effect.
- □ Regularly administered doses may be more effective than prn administration. Analgesic is more effective if given before pain becomes severe.

- Coadministration with nonopioid analgesics may have additive analgesic effects and permit lower doses.
- Medications should be discontinued gradually after long-term use to prevent withdrawal symptoms.
- When combined with nonopioid analgesics (aspirin, acetaminophen) #2 = 15 mg, #3 = 30 mg, #4 = 60 mg codeine. Codeine as an individual drug is a Schedule II substance. In combination with other drugs, tablet form is Schedule III, liquid is Schedule IV, and elixir or cough suppressant is Schedule V (see Appendix C).

- **PO:** Oral doses may be administered with food or milk to minimize GI irritation.
- **IM, SC:** Do not administer solution that is more than slightly discolored or contains a precipitate.
- **Direct IV:** Codeine is usually administered IM or SC, but slow IV injection has been used.
- **Syringe Compatibility:** ▪ glycopyrrolate ▪ hydroxyzine.

PATIENT/FAMILY TEACHING

- Instruct patient on how and when to ask for pain medication.
- Codeine may cause drowsiness or dizziness. Advise patient to call for assistance when ambulating or smoking. Caution ambulatory patient to avoid driving or other activities requiring alertness until response to medication is known.
- Advise patient to change positions slowly to minimize orthostatic hypotension.
- Caution patient to avoid concurrent use of alcohol or other CNS depressants with this medication.
- Encourage patient to turn, cough, and breathe deeply every 2 hr to prevent atelectasis.
- Advise patient that good oral hygiene, frequent mouth rinses, and sugarless gum or candy may decrease dry mouth.

EVALUATION

Effectiveness of therapy can be demonstrated by: ▪ Decrease in severity of pain without a significant alteration in level of consciousness or respiratory status ▪ Suppression of cough ▪ Control of diarrhea.

COLCHICINE

(**kol**-chi-seen)

CLASSIFICATION(S):
Antigout agent

Pregnancy Category C

INDICATIONS

▪ Acute attacks of gouty arthritis (larger doses) ▪ Prevention of recurrences of gout (smaller doses). **Unlabeled Uses:** ▪ Treatment of hepatic cirrhosis and familial Mediterranean fever.

ACTION

▪ Interferes with the functions of white blood cells in initiating and perpetuating the inflammatory response to monosodium urate crystals. **Therapeutic Effects:** ▪ Decreased pain and inflammation in acute attacks of gout ▪ Prevention of recurrent attacks of gout.

PHARMACOKINETICS

Absorption: Absorbed from the GI tract, then re-enters GI tract from biliary secretions, when more absorption may occur.
Distribution: Concentrates in white blood cells.
Metabolism and Excretion: Partially metabolized by the liver. Secreted in bile back into GI tract; eliminated in the feces. Small amount excreted in the urine.
Half-life: 20 min (plasma), 60 hr (white blood cells).

CONTRAINDICATIONS AND PRECAUTIONS

Contraindicated in: ▪ Hypersensitivity ▪ Pregnancy ▪ Severe renal (CCr <10 ml/min) or GI disease.
Use Cautiously in: ▪ Elderly or debilitated patients (toxicity may be cumulative) ▪ Renal impairment (dosage reduction suggested if CCr <50 ml/min; total IV dose not >2 mg) ▪ Lactation or children (safety not established).

ADVERSE REACTIONS AND SIDE EFFECTS*

GI: diarrhea, nausea, vomiting, abdominal pain.
GU: anuria, hematuria, renal damage.

*CAPITALS indicate life-threatening; underlines indicate most frequent.

Derm: alopecia.
Hemat: AGRANULOCYTOSIS, APLASTIC ANEMIA, leukopenia, thrombocytopenia.
Local: phlebitis at IV site.
Neuro: peripheral neuritis.

INTERACTIONS

Drug-Drug: ▪ Additive bone marrow depression may occur with **bone marrow depressants** or **radiation therapy** ▪ Additive adverse GI effects with **NSAIDs** ▪ May cause reversible malabsorption of **vitamin B_{12}**.

ROUTE AND DOSAGE

- **PO (Adults):** *Treatment of acute attacks*—0.5–1.2 mg, then 0.5–0.6 mg q 1–2 hr or 1–1.2 mg q 2 hr until relief, GI side effects, or a total cumulative dose of 6 mg is achieved. *Prophylaxis*—0.5–0.6 mg daily (may be used up to 3 times daily or as little as 1–4 times weekly). If surgery is planned, give 3 times daily for 3 days before and 3 days after procedure.
- **IV (Adults):** *Treatment of acute attack*—2 mg initially, then 0.5 mg q 6 hr or 1 mg q 6–12 hr, until relief or cumulative dose of 4 mg has been given. Other regimens may use lower doses. *Prophylaxis*—0.5–1 mg 1–2 times daily. Other regimens may use lower doses.

AVAILABILITY

▪ ***Tablets:*** 0.5 mg[Rx], 0.6 mg[Rx], {1 mg[Rx]} ▪ ***Injection:*** 0.5 mg/ml in 2-ml ampules[Rx] ▪ ***In combination with:*** probenecid (ColBenemid, Co-Prebenecid, Proben-C)[Rx]. See Appendix A.

TIME/ACTION PROFILE (anti-inflammatory activity)

	ONSET	PEAK	DURATION
PO	12 hr	24–72 hr	UK
IV	within 6–12 hr	UK	UK

NURSING IMPLICATIONS

ASSESSMENT

- Assess involved joints for pain, mobility, and edema throughout therapy. During initiation of therapy, monitor for drug response every 1–2 hr.
- Monitor intake and output ratios. Fluids should be encouraged to promote a urinary output of at least 2000 ml/day.
- ***Lab Test Considerations:*** In patients receiving prolonged therapy, monitor baseline and periodic CBC; report significant decrease in values. May cause decreased platelet count.
- May cause an increase in AST and alkaline phosphatase.
- May cause false-positive results for urine hemoglobin.
- May interfere with results of urinary 17-hydroxycorticosteroid concentrations.
- ***Toxicity and Overdose:*** Assess patient for toxicity (weakness, abdominal discomfort, nausea, vomiting, diarrhea). If these symptoms occur, discontinue medication and notify physician or other health care professional. Opioids may be needed to treat diarrhea.

POTENTIAL NURSING DIAGNOSES

- Pain (Indications).
- Physical mobility, impaired (Indications).
- Knowledge deficit, related to medication regimen (Patient/Family Teaching).

IMPLEMENTATION

- **General Info:** Intermittent therapy with 3 days between courses may be used to decrease risk of toxicity.
- **PO:** Administer oral doses with food to minimize gastric irritation.
- **IV:** Avoid extravasation; may cause necrosis of skin and soft tissue.
- Do not administer oral and IV colchicine concurrently or sequentially. Do not administer additional colchicine for 3 days after oral therapy or at least 7 days (21 days for geriatric patients) after IV therapy.
- **Direct IV:** May be administered undiluted. If a lower concentration is desired, may dilute to a volume of 10–20 ml with sterile water or 0.9% NaCl for injection. Do not administer solutions that are turbid.
- ***Rate:*** Administer slowly over 2–10 min. Rapid administration may cause cardiac arrhythmias.
- **Y-Site Incompatibility:** ▪ Do not dilute colchicine with or inject into IV tubing containing D5W, solutions containing a bacteriostatic agent, or any other solution that might change the pH of the colchicine solution because precipitation will occur.

PATIENT/FAMILY TEACHING

- Review medication administration schedule. If dose is missed, take as soon as remembered unless almost time for next dose. Do not double doses.
- Instruct patients taking prophylactic doses not to increase to therapeutic doses during an acute attack to prevent toxicity. An NSAID or glucocorticoid, preferably via intrasynovial injection, should be used to treat acute attacks.
- Advise patient to follow recommendations of health care professional regarding weight loss, diet, and alcohol consumption.
- Instruct patient to report nausea, vomiting, abdominal pain, diarrhea, unusual bleeding, bruising, sore throat, fatigue, malaise, or rash promptly. Medication should be withheld if gastric symptoms, indicative of toxicity, occur.
- Surgery may precipitate an acute attack of gout. Advise patient to confer with health care professional regarding dose 3 days before surgical or dental procedures.

EVALUATION

Effectiveness of therapy can be demonstrated by: ▪ Decrease in pain and swelling in affected joints within 12 hr □ Relief of symptoms within 24–48 hr ▪ Prevention of acute gout attacks.

CONTRACEPTIVES, HORMONAL

MONOPHASIC ORAL CONTRACEPTIVES

mestranol/norethindrone
(**mes**-tre-nole/nor-eth-**in**-drone)
Genora 1/50, Nelova 1/50M, Norethin 1/50M, Norinyl 1+50, Ortho-Novum 1/50

ethinyl estradiol/norethindrone
(**eth**-in-il ess-tra-**dye**-ole/nor-eth-**in**-drone)
Brevicon, Genora 0.5/35, Genora 1/35, Loestrin 21 1.5/30, Loestrin 21 1/20, Modicon, N.E.E. 1/35, Nelova 0.5/35E, Nelova 1/35E, Norcept-E 1/35, Norethin 1/35E, Norinyl 1+35, Norlestrin 1/50, Norlestrin 2.5/50, Ortho-Novum 1/35, Ovcon 35, Ovcon 50

ethinyl estradiol/ethynodiol
(**eth**-in-il ess-tra-**dye**-ole/e-thye-noe-**dye**-ole)
Demulen, Demulen 1/35

ethinyl estradiol/norgestrel
(**eth**-in-il ess-tra-**dye**-ole/nor-**jess**-trel)
Lo/Ovral, Ovral

ethinyl estradiol/levonorgestrel
(**eth**-in-il ess-tra-**dye**-ole/lee-voe-nor-**jess**-trel)
Alesse, Levlen, Nordette

desogestrel/ethinyl estradiol
(dess-oh-**jess**-trel/**eth**-in-il ess-tra-**dye**-ole)
Desogen

BIPHASIC ORAL CONTRACEPTIVES

ethinyl estradiol/norethindrone
Nelova 10/11, Ortho-Novum 10/11

TRIPHASIC ORAL CONTRACEPTIVES

ethinyl estradiol/norethindrone
Ortho-Novum 7/7/7, Tri-Norinyl

ethinyl estradiol/norgestrel
Tri-Levlen, Triphasil

norgestimate/ethinyl estradiol
Ortho Tri-Cyclen

PROGESTIN-ONLY ORAL CONTRACEPTIVES

norethindrone
Micronor, Nor-Q D

PROGRESSIVE ESTROGEN ORAL CONTRACEPTIVES

Estrostep, Estrostep Fe

norgestrel
Ovrette

CONTRACEPTIVE IMPLANT

levonorgestrel
Norplant

INJECTABLE CONTRACEPTIVE

medroxyprogesterone
(me-**drox**-ee-proe-jess-te-rone)
Depo-Provera

CLASSIFICATION(S):
Hormones (estrogens, progestins, contraceptives)

Pregnancy Category X

INDICATIONS

▪ Prevention of pregnancy ▪ Regulation of menstrual cycle ▪ Emergency contraception (some products) ▪ Management of acne in women >14 yr who desire contraception, have no health problems, and have failed topical treatment.

ACTION

▪ **Monophasic Oral Contraceptives:** Provide a fixed dosage of estrogen/progestin over a 21-day cycle. Ovulation is inhibited by suppression of follicle-stimulating hormone (FSH) and luteinizing hormone (LH). May alter cervical mucus and the endometrial environment, preventing penetration by sperm and implantation of the egg ▪ **Biphasic Oral Contraceptives:** Ovulation is inhibited by suppression of FSH and LH. May alter cervical mucus and the endometrial environment, preventing penetration by sperm and implantation of the egg. In addition, smaller dose of progestin in phase 1 allows for proliferation of endometrium. Larger amount in phase 2 allows for adequate secretory development ▪ **Triphasic Oral Contraceptives:** Ovulation is inhibited by suppression of FSH and LH. May alter cervical mucus and the endometrial environment, preventing penetration by sperm and implantation of the egg. Varying doses of estrogen/progestin may more closely mimic natural hormonal fluctuations ▪ **Progressive Estrogen:** Contains constant amount of progestin with 3 progressive doses of estrogen ▪ **Progestin-Only Contraceptives and Contraceptive Implant:** Mechanism not clearly known. May alter cervical mucus and the endometrial environment, preventing penetration by sperm and implantation of the egg. Ovulation may also be suppressed ▪ **Medroxyprogesterone Injection:** Inhibits gonadotropin secretion, follicle maturation, and ovulation. Also produces endometrial thinning.
Therapeutic Effects: ▪ Prevention of pregnancy.

PHARMACOKINETICS

Absorption: Well absorbed following oral administration. Slowly absorbed from implant or IM injection.
Distribution: UK.
Metabolism and Excretion: Mostly metabolized by the liver.
Half-life: UK.

CONTRAINDICATIONS AND PRECAUTIONS

Contraindicated in: ▪ History of thromboembolic disorders, cardiovascular disease, cerebrovascular disease, liver tumors, or gallbladder disease ▪ Lactation (avoid use) ▪ Hypersensitivity to parabens (injectable only).
Use Cautiously in: ▪ Surgical procedures (depending on procedure, may want to discontinue 2–4 wk prior to surgery) ▪ History of cigarette smoking or age >30–35 yr (increased risk of cardiovascular or thromboembolic phenomenon) ▪ Presence of other cardiovascular risk factors (obesity, hyperglycemia, elevated lipids, hypertension) ▪ History of diabetes mellitus, bleeding disorders, or headaches ▪ Some products increase risk of breast or liver cancer in high-risk patients.
Use with Extreme Caution in: ▪ Products containing >50 mcg estrogen (increased risk of thromboembolic disorders and other vascular problems).

ADVERSE REACTIONS AND SIDE EFFECTS*

CNS: depression, migraine headache.
EENT: contact lens intolerance, optic neuritis, retinal thrombosis.
CV: CEREBRAL HEMORRHAGE, CEREBRAL THROMBOSIS, CORONARY THROMBOSIS, PULMONARY EMBOLISM, edema, hypertension, Raynaud's disease, thromboembolic phenomena, thrombophlebitis.
GI: abdominal cramps, bloating, cholestatic jaundice, gallbladder disease, liver tumors, nausea, vomiting.

***CAPITALS indicate life-threatening; underlines indicate most frequent.**

GU: amenorrhea, breakthrough bleeding, dysmenorrhea, spotting.
Derm: melasma, rash.
Endo: hyperglycemia.
Misc: weight change.

INTERACTIONS

Drug-Drug: ▪ Oral contraceptive efficacy may be decreased by **penicillins, chloramphenicol, dihydroergotamine, mineral oil, oral neomycin, sulfonamides, barbiturates, chronic alcohol use, carbamazepine, glucocorticoids (systemic), griseofulvin, phenylbutazone, phenytoin, primidone, rifampin,** or **tetracyclines** ▪ May increase the effects/risk of toxicity from **tricyclic antidepressants, benzodiazepines, beta-adrenergic blocking agents, caffeine, glucocorticoids,** and **theophylline** ▪ Increased risk of hepatic toxicity with **dantrolene** (estrogen only) ▪ **Carbamazepine** or **phenytoin** may decrease the efficacy of contraceptive implants ▪ **Smoking** increases the risk of thromboembolic phenomena (estrogen only) ▪ May interfere with the effectiveness of **bromocriptine.**

ROUTE AND DOSAGE

❑ Monophasic Oral Contraceptives

▪ **PO (Adults):** On 21-day regimen, take first tablet on first Sunday after menses begin (take on Sunday if menses begin on Sunday) for 21 days, then skip 7 days and begin again. Regimen may also be started on first day of menses, continue for 21 days, then skip 7 days and begin again. Some regimens contain 7 placebo tablets, so that 1 tablet is taken every day for 28 days.

❑ Biphasic Oral Contraceptives

▪ **PO (Adults):** Given in 2 phases. First phase is 10 days of smaller amount of progestin. Second phase is larger amount of progestin. Amount of estrogen remains constant for same length of time (total of 21 days), then skip 7 days and begin again. Some regimens contain 7 placebo tablets for 28-day regimen.

❑ Triphasic Oral Contraceptives

▪ **PO (Adults):** Progestin amount varies throughout a 21-day cycle. Estrogen component stays the same or may vary. Some regimens contain 7 placebo tablets for 28-day regimen.

❑ Progressive Estrogen Oral Contraceptives

▪ **PO (Adults):** Estrogen amount increases q 7 days throughout a 21-day cycle. Progestin component stays the same. Some regimens contain 7 placebo tablets for 28-day regimen.

❑ Progestin-Only Oral Contraceptives

▪ **PO (Adults):** Start on first day of menses. Taken daily and continuously.

❑ Contraceptive Implant

▪ **Subdermal: (Adults):** 6 capsules implanted subdermally during first 7 days of menses; replaced q 5 yr.

❑ Injectable Contraceptive

▪ **IM (Adults):** 150 mg within first 5 days of menses or within 5 days postpartum, if not breast-feeding. If breast-feeding, give 6 wk postpartum; repeat q 3 mo.

❑ Emergency Contraception

▪ **PO (Adults and Adolescents):** Given within 72 hr of unprotected intercourse and repeated 12 hr later. *Ovral*—2 white tablets; *Lo/Ovral*—4 white tablets; *Levlen, Nordette*—4 light orange tablets; *Triphasil, Tri-Levlen*—4 yellow tablets.

❑ Acne

▪ **PO (Adults):** Ortho Tri-Cyclen only, taken daily for 21 days, off for 7 days.

AVAILABILITY

Tablets: Usually in monthly packs with enough (21) active tablets to complete a 28-day cycle. Some contain 7 inert tablets to complete the cycle[Rx].

❑ Levonorgestrel

▪ ***Implant:*** Package of 6 implantable capsules containing 36 mg of levonorgestrel each[Rx].

❑ Medroxyprogesterone

▪ ***Injectable:*** 150 mg/ml[Rx].

TIME/ACTION PROFILE (prevention of pregnancy)

	ONSET	PEAK	DURATION
PO	1 mo	1 mo	1 mo*
Implant	1 mo	1 mo	5 yr
IM	1 mo	1 mo	3 mo

*Only during month of taking contraceptive.

NURSING IMPLICATIONS

ASSESSMENT

- Assess blood pressure prior to and periodically throughout therapy.
- ***Lab Test Considerations:*** Monitor hepatic function periodically throughout therapy.
- *Estrogens only*—May cause increased serum glucose, sodium, triglyceride, very high-density lipoprotein (VHDL), total cholesterol, prothrombin, and factors VII, VIII, IX, and X levels. May cause decreased low-density lipoptotein (LDL) and antithrombin III levels.
- May cause false interpretations of thyroid function tests, false increases in norepinephrine platelet-induced aggregability, and false decreases in metyrapone tests.
- *Progestins only*—May cause increased LDL concentrations. May cause decreased serum alkaline phosphatase and high-density lipoprotein (HDL) concentrations.

POTENTIAL NURSING DIAGNOSES

- Knowledge deficit, related to medication regimen (Patient/Family Teaching).
- Noncompliance (Patient/Family Teaching).

IMPLEMENTATION

- **PO:** Oral doses may be administered with or immediately after food to reduce nausea.
- **Levonorgestrel Implant:** ▪ 6-capsule implant is inserted subdermally in midportion of upper arm about 8–10 cm above the elbow crease.
- **IM:** Shake vial vigorously just before use to ensure uniform suspension. Administer deep IM into gluteal or deltoid muscle. If period between injections is >14 wk, determine that patient is not pregnant before administering the drug.

PATIENT/FAMILY TEACHING

- Instruct patient to take oral medication as directed at the same time each day. Pills should be taken in proper sequence and kept in the original container.
- *If single daily dose is missed:* Take as soon as remembered; if not until next day, take 2 tablets and continue on regular dosing schedule. *If 2 days in a row are missed:* Take 2 tablets a day for the next 2 days and continue on regular dosing schedule, using a second method of birth control for the remaining cycle. *If 3 days in a row are missed:* Discontinue medication and use another form of birth control until period begins or pregnancy is ruled out; then begin a new cycle of tablets. *For 28-day dosing schedule:* If schedule is followed for first 21 days and 1 dose is missed of the last 7 tablets, it is important to take the 1st tablet of next month's cycle on the regularly scheduled day.
- Advise patient of the need to use another form of contraception for the first 3 wk when beginning to use oral contraceptives.
- Advise patient that a second method of birth control should also be used during each cycle in which any of the following are used: *Oral contraceptives*—ampicillin, adrenocorticoids, bacampicillin, barbiturates, carbamazepine, chloramphenicol, dihydroergotamine, glucocorticoids (systemic), griseofulvin, mineral oil, oral neomycin, penicillin V, phenylbutazone, primidone, rifampin, sulfonamides, tetracyclines, or valproic acid. *Levonorgestrel implant*—carbamazepine or phenytoin.
- Explain dosage schedule and maintenance routine. Discontinuing medication suddenly may cause withdrawal bleeding.
- If nausea becomes a problem, advise patient that eating solid food often provides relief.
- Advise patient to report signs and symptoms of fluid retention (swelling of ankles and feet, weight gain), thromboembolic disorders (pain, swelling, tenderness in extremities, headache, chest pain, blurred vision), mental depression, hepatic dysfunction (yellowed skin or eyes, pruritus, dark urine, light-colored stools), or abnormal vaginal bleeding.
- Instruct patient to stop taking medication and notify health care professional if pregnancy is suspected.
- Caution patient that cigarette smoking during estrogen therapy may increase risk of serious side effects, especially for women over age 35.
- Caution patients to use sunscreen and protective clothing to prevent increased pigmentation.
- Caution patient that oral contraceptives do not protect against HIV or other sexually transmitted diseases.
- Advise patient to notify health care professional of medication regimen prior to treatment or surgery.

- Emphasize the importance of routine follow-up physical exams including blood pressure; breast, abdomen, and pelvic examinations; and PAP smears every 6–12 mo.

EVALUATION

Effectiveness of therapy can be demonstrated by: ▪ Prevention of pregnancy ▪ Regulation of the menstral cycle ▪ Decrease in acne.

CYCLOBENZAPRINE

(sye-kloe-**ben**-za-preen)
Cycloflex, Flexeril

CLASSIFICATION(S):
Skeletal muscle relaxant (centrally acting)

Pregnancy Category B

INDICATIONS

▪ Management of acute painful musculoskeletal conditions associated with muscle spasm. **Unlabeled Uses:** ▪ Management of fibromyalgia.

ACTION

▪ Reduces tonic somatic muscle activity at the level of the brain stem. Structurally similar to tricyclic antidepressants. **Therapeutic Effects:** ▪ Reduction in muscle spasm and hyperactivity without loss of function.

PHARMACOKINETICS

Absorption: Well absorbed from the GI tract.
Distribution: UK.
Metabolism and Excretion: Mostly metabolized by the liver.
Half-life: 1–3 days.

CONTRAINDICATIONS AND PRECAUTIONS

Contraindicated in: ▪ Hypersensitivity ▪ Should not be used within 14 days of MAO inhibitor therapy ▪ Immediate period after myocardial infarction ▪ Severe or symptomatic cardiovascular disease ▪ Cardiac conduction disturbances ▪ Hyperthyroidism.
Use Cautiously in: ▪ Cardiovascular disease ▪ Pregnancy, lactation, and children <15 yr (safety not established).

ADVERSE REACTIONS AND SIDE EFFECTS*

CNS: dizziness, drowsiness, confusion, fatigue, headache, nervousness.
EENT: dry mouth, blurred vision.
CV: arrhythmias.
GI: constipation, dyspepsia, nausea, unpleasant taste.
GU: urinary retention.

INTERACTIONS

Drug-Drug: ▪ Additive CNS depression with other **CNS depressants,** including **alcohol, antihistamines, opioids,** and **sedative/hypnotics** ▪ Additive anticholinergic effects with **drugs possessing anticholinergic properties,** including **antihistamines, antidepressants, atropine, disopyramide, haloperidol,** and **phenothiazines** ▪ Avoid use within 14 days of **MAO inhibitor** therapy (hyperpyretic crisis, convulsions, and death may occur) ▪ May blunt the response to **guanadrel** or **guanethidine.**

ROUTE AND DOSAGE

- **PO (Adults):** *Acute painful musculoskeletal conditions*—10 mg 3 times daily (range 20–40 mg/day in 2–4 divided doses; not to exceed 60 mg/day). *Fibromyalgia*—5–40 mg at bedtime (unlabeled).

AVAILABILITY

▪ ***Tablets:*** 10 mg[Rx].

TIME/ACTION PROFILE (skeletal muscle relaxation)

	ONSET	PEAK†	DURATION
PO	1 hr	4–6 hr	12–24 hr

†Full effects may not occur for 1–2 wk.

NURSING IMPLICATIONS

ASSESSMENT

- Assess patient for pain, muscle stiffness, and range of motion prior to and periodically throughout therapy.

POTENTIAL NURSING DIAGNOSES

- Pain (Indications).
- Physical mobility, impaired (Indications).
- Injury, risk for (Side Effects).

*CAPITALS indicate life-threatening; underlines indicate most frequent.

IMPLEMENTATION

- **PO:** May be administered with meals to minimize gastric irritation.

PATIENT/FAMILY TEACHING

- Instruct patient to take medication exactly as directed; do not take more than the prescribed amount. Missed doses should be taken within 1 hr of time ordered; otherwise, return to normal dosage schedule. Do not double doses.
- Medication may cause drowsiness, dizziness, and blurred vision. Caution patient to avoid driving or other activities requiring alertness until response to drug is known.
- Advise patient to avoid concurrent use of alcohol or other CNS depressants with this medication.
- If constipation becomes a problem, advise patient that increasing fluid intake and bulk in diet and stool softeners may alleviate this condition.
- Advise patient to notify health care professional if symptoms of urinary retention (distended abdomen, feeling of fullness, overflow incontinence, voiding small amounts) occur.
- Inform patient that good oral hygiene, frequent mouth rinses, and sugarless gum or candy may help relieve dry mouth.

EVALUATION

Effectiveness of therapy can be demonstrated by: ▪ Relief of muscular spasm in acute skeletal muscle conditions. Maximum effects may not be evident for 1–2 wk. Use is usually limited to 2–3 wk; however, has been effective for at least 12 wk in the management of fibromyalgia.

CYCLOPHOSPHAMIDE

(sye-kloe-**foss**-fa-mide)
Cytoxan, Neosar, {Procytox}

CLASSIFICATION(S):
Antineoplastic (alkylating agent), Immunosuppressant

Pregnancy Category C

INDICATIONS

▪ Alone or with other modalities (other chemotherapeutic agents, radiation therapy, surgery) in the management of: ▫ Hodgkin's disease ▫ Malignant lymphomas ▫ Multiple myeloma ▫ Leukemias ▫ Mycosis fungoides ▫ Neuroblastoma ▫ Ovarian carcinoma ▫ Breast carcinoma and a variety of other tumors ▪ Minimal change nephrotic syndrome in children. **Unlabeled Uses:** ▪ Severe active rheumatoid arthritis or Wegener's granulomatosis.

ACTION

▪ Interferes with DNA replication and RNA transcription, ultimately disrupting protein synthesis (cell-cycle phase–nonspecific). **Therapeutic Effects:** ▪ Death of rapidly replicating cells, particularly malignant ones ▪ Also has immunosuppressant action in smaller doses.

PHARMACOKINETICS

Absorption: Inactive parent drug is well absorbed from the GI tract. Converted to active drug by the liver.
Distribution: Widely distributed. Limited penetration of the blood-brain barrier. Crosses the placenta; enters breast milk.
Metabolism and Excretion: Converted to active drug by the liver; 30% eliminated unchanged by the kidneys.
Half-life: 4–6.5 hr.

CONTRAINDICATIONS AND PRECAUTIONS

Contraindicated in: ▪ Hypersensitivity ▪ Pregnancy or lactation.
Use Cautiously in: ▪ Active infections ▪ Bone marrow depression ▪ Other chronic debilitating illnesses ▪ Patients with childbearing potential.

ADVERSE REACTIONS AND SIDE EFFECTS*

Resp: PULMONARY FIBROSIS.
CV: MYOCARDIAL FIBROSIS, hypotension.
GI: anorexia, nausea, vomiting.
GU: HEMORRHAGIC CYSTITIS, hematuria.
Derm: alopecia.
Endo: gonadal suppression, syndrome of inap-

{} = Available in Canada only.
*CAPITALS indicate life-threatening; underlines indicate most frequent.

propriate antidiuretic hormone (SIADH).
Hemat: LEUKOPENIA, thrombocytopenia, anemia.
Metab: hyperuricemia.
Misc: secondary neoplasms.

INTERACTIONS

Drug-Drug: ▪ **Phenobarbital** or **rifampin** may increase the toxicity of cyclophosphamide ▪ Concurrent **allopurinol** or **thiazide diuretics** may exaggerate bone marrow depression ▪ May prolong neuromuscular blockade from **succinylcholine** ▪ Cardiotoxicity may be additive with other **cardiotoxic agents (cytarabine, daunorubicin, doxorubicin)** ▪ May decrease serum **digoxin** levels ▪ Additive bone marrow depression with other **antineoplastics** or **radiation therapy** ▪ May potentiate the effects of **warfarin** ▪ May decrease antibody response to **live virus vaccines** and increase the risk of adverse reactions ▪ Prolongs the effects of **cocaine.**

ROUTE AND DOSAGE

Many regimens are used.

- **PO (Adults):** 1–5 mg/kg/day.
- **PO (Children):** *Induction*—2–8 mg/kg/day (60–250 mg/m²/day) in divided doses for 6 days or longer. *Maintenance*—2–5 mg/kg (50–150 mg/m²) twice weekly.
- **IV (Adults):** 40–50 mg/kg in divided doses over 2–5 days *or* 10–15 mg/kg q 7–10 days *or* 3–5 mg/kg twice weekly *or* 1.5–3 mg/kg/day. Other regimens may use larger doses.
- **IV (Children):** *Induction*—2–8 mg/kg/day (60–250 mg/m²/day) in divided doses for 6 days or longer. Total dose for 7 days may be given as a single weekly dose. *Maintenance*—10–15 mg/kg every 7–10 days or 30 mg/kg q 3–4 wk.

AVAILABILITY

▪ ***Tablets:*** 25 mg^Rx^, 50 mg^Rx^ ▪ ***Injection:*** 100 mg^Rx^, 200 mg^Rx^, 500 mg^Rx^, {750 mg^Rx^}, 1 g^Rx^, 2 g^Rx^.

TIME/ACTION PROFILE (effects on blood counts)

	ONSET	PEAK	DURATION
PO, IV	7 days	7–15 days	21 days

NURSING IMPLICATIONS

ASSESSMENT

- ☐ Monitor blood pressure, pulse, respiratory rate, and temperature frequently during administration. Report significant changes.
- ☐ Monitor urinary output frequently throughout therapy. To reduce the risk of hemorrhagic cystitis, fluid intake should be at least 3000 ml/day for adults and 1000–2000 ml/day for children. May be administered with mesna (see p. 621).
- ☐ Monitor for bone marrow depression. Assess for bleeding (bleeding gums, bruising, petechiae, guaiac stools, urine, and emesis) and avoid IM injections and rectal temperatures if platelet count is low. Apply pressure to venipuncture sites for 10 min. Assess for signs of infection during neutropenia. Anemia may occur. Monitor for increased fatigue, dyspnea, and orthostatic hypotension.
- ☐ Assess nausea, vomiting, and appetite. Weigh weekly. Antiemetics may be given 30 min prior to administration of medication to minimize GI effects. Anorexia and weight loss can be minimized by feeding frequent light meals.
- ☐ Encourage patient to drink 2000–3000 ml/day to promote excretion of uric acid. Alkalinization of the urine may be used to help prevent uric acid nephropathy.
- ☐ Assess cardiac and respiratory status for dyspnea, rales/crackles, weight gain, edema. Pulmonary toxicity may occur after prolonged therapy. Cardiotoxicity may occur early in therapy and is characterized by symptoms of congestive heart failure.
- ▪ ***Lab Test Considerations:*** Monitor CBC with differential and platelet count prior to and periodically throughout therapy. The nadir of leukopenia occurs in 7–12 days (recovery in 17–21 days). Leukocytes should be maintained at 2500–4000/mm³. May also cause thrombocytopenia (nadir 10–15 days), and rarely causes anemia.
- ☐ Monitor BUN, creatinine, and uric acid prior to and frequently during therapy to detect nephrotoxicity.
- ☐ Monitor ALT, AST, LDH, and serum bilirubin prior to and frequently during therapy to detect hepatotoxicity.
- ☐ Urinalysis should be evaluated before initiating therapy and frequently during course of ther-

C

apy to detect hematuria or change in specific gravity indicative of SIADH.

- May suppress positive reactions to skin tests for *Candida,* mumps, *Trichophyton,* and tuberculin purified protein derivative (PPD). May also produce false-positive results in PAP smears.

POTENTIAL NURSING DIAGNOSES

- Infection, risk for (Side Effects).
- Body image disturbance (Side Effects).
- Knowledge deficit, related to medication regimen (Patient/Family Teaching).

IMPLEMENTATION

- **General Info:** Clarify dose to ensure cumulative dose is not confused with daily dose; errors may be fatal.
- **PO:** Administer medication on an empty stomach. If severe gastric irritation develops, medication may be given with food.
- Oral solution can be formed by diluting powder for injection in aromatic elixir to a concentration of 1–5 mg of cyclophosphamide/ml. Reconstituted preparations should be refrigerated and used within 2 wk.
- **IV:** Solution for IV administration should be prepared in a biologic cabinet. Wear gloves, gown, and mask while handling IV medication. Discard IV equipment in specially designated containers (see Appendix I).
- Prepare IV solution by diluting each 100 mg with 5 ml of sterile water or bacteriostatic water for injection containing parabens. Shake solution gently and allow to stand until clear. Use solution without bacteriostatic water within 6 hr. Solution prepared with bacteriostatic water is stable for 24 hr at room temperature, 6 days if refrigerated.
- **Direct IV:** Administer reconstituted solution directly.
- ***Rate:*** Administer at a rate of 100 mg over 1 min.
- **Intermittent Infusion:** May be further diluted in up to 250 ml of D5W, 0.9% NaCl, D5/0.9% NaCl, 0.45% NaCl, lactated Ringer's solution, or dextrose/Ringer's solution.
- **Syringe Compatibility:** ▪ bleomycin ▪ cisplatin ▪ doxapram ▪ doxorubicin ▪ droperidol ▪ fluorouracil ▪ furosemide ▪ heparin ▪ leucovorin calcium ▪ methotrexate ▪ metoclopramide ▪ mitomycin ▪ vinblastine ▪ vincristine.
- **Y-Site Compatibility:** ▪ amifostine ▪ amikacin ▪ ampicillin ▪ aztreonam ▪ bleomycin ▪ cefamandole ▪ cefazolin ▪ cefepime ▪ cefoperazone ▪ cefotaxime ▪ cefoxitin ▪ cefuroxime ▪ cephalothin ▪ cephapirin ▪ chloramphenicol ▪ chlorpromazine ▪ cimetidine ▪ cisplatin ▪ clindamycin ▪ dexamethasone ▪ diphenhydramine ▪ doxorubicin ▪ doxycycline ▪ droperidol ▪ erythromycin lactobionate ▪ famotidine ▪ filgrastim ▪ fludarabine ▪ fluorouracil ▪ furosemide ▪ gallium nitrate ▪ ganciclovir ▪ gentamicin ▪ granisetron ▪ heparin ▪ hydromorphone ▪ idarubicin ▪ kanamycin ▪ leucovorin calcium ▪ lorazepam ▪ melphalan ▪ methotrexate ▪ methylprednisolone ▪ metoclopramide ▪ metronidazole ▪ mezlocillin ▪ minocycline ▪ mitomycin ▪ morphine ▪ nafcillin ▪ ondansetron ▪ oxacillin ▪ paclitaxel ▪ penicillin G potassium ▪ piperacillin ▪ piperacillin/tazobactam ▪ prochlorperazine ▪ promethazine ▪ ranitidine ▪ sargramostim ▪ teniposide ▪ thiotepa ▪ ticarcillin ▪ ticarcillin/clavulanate ▪ tobramycin ▪ trimethoprim/sulfamethoxazole ▪ vancomycin ▪ vinblastine ▪ vincristine ▪ vinorelbine.
- **Additive Compatibility:** ▪ fluorouracil ▪ methotrexate ▪ mitoxantrone ▪ ondansetron.

PATIENT/FAMILY TEACHING

- Instruct patient to take dose in early morning. Emphasize need for adequate fluid intake for 72 hr after therapy. Patient should void frequently to decrease bladder irritation from metabolites excreted by the kidneys. Report hematuria immediately. If a dose is missed, health care professional should be contacted.
- Instruct patient to notify health care professional promptly if fever; sore throat; signs of infection; lower back or side pain; difficult or painful urination; sores in the mouth or on the lips; yellow discoloration of skin or eyes; bleeding gums; bruising; petechiae; blood in urine, stool, or emesis; unusual swelling; joint pain; shortness of breath; or confusion occurs. Caution patient to avoid crowds and persons with known infections. Instruct patient to use soft toothbrush and electric razor and to avoid falls. Patient should also be cautioned not to drink alcoholic beverages or to take products containing aspirin or NSAIDs; may precipitate GI hemorrhage.
- Advise patient that this medication may cause

sterility and menstrual irregularities or cessation of menses. This drug is also teratogenic, and contraceptive measures should continue for at least 4 mo after completion of therapy.

- □ Discuss with patient the possibility of hair loss. Explore methods of coping. May also cause darkening of skin and fingernails.
- □ Instruct patient not to receive any vaccinations without advice of health care professional.

EVALUATION

Effectiveness of therapy can be demonstrated by: ▪ Decrease in size or spread of malignant tumors ▪ Improvement of hematologic status in patients with leukemia. Maintenance therapy is instituted if leukocyte count remains between 2500 and 4000/mm^3 and if patient does not demonstrate serious side effects ▪ Management of minimal change nephrotic syndrome in children.

CYCLOSPORINE

(**sye**-kloe-spor-een)
Neoral, Sandimmune

CLASSIFICATION(S):
Immunosuppressant

Pregnancy Category C

INDICATIONS

▪ **PO, IV:** Prevention and treatment of rejection in renal, cardiac, and hepatic transplantation (with glucocorticoids) ▪ **PO:** Treatment of severe active rheumatoid arthritis ▪ Treatment of severe recalcitrant psoriasis in adult nonimmunocompromised patients. **Unlabeled Uses:** ▪ Management of recalcitrant ulcerative colitis.

ACTION

▪ Inhibits normal immune responses (cellular and humoral) by inhibiting interleukin-2, a factor necessary for initiation of T-cell activity. **Therapeutic Effects:** ▪ Prevention of rejection reactions ▪ Slowed progression of rheumatoid arthritis or psoriasis.

PHARMACOKINETICS

Absorption: Erratically absorbed (range 10–60%) after oral administration, with significant first-pass metabolism by the liver. Microemulsion (Neoral) has better bioavailability.
Distribution: Widely distributed, mainly into extracellular fluid and blood cells. Crosses the placenta; enters breast milk.
Metabolism and Excretion: Extensively metabolized by the liver; excreted in bile, small amounts excreted unchanged in urine.
Half-life: Children—7 hr; adults—19 hr.

CONTRAINDICATIONS AND PRECAUTIONS

Contraindicated in: ▪ Hypersensitivity to cyclosporine or polyoxethylated castor oil (vehicle for IV form) ▪ Should not be given to pregnant or lactating women unless benefits outweigh risks ▪ Disulfiram therapy or known alcohol intolerance (IV and oral liquid dosage forms contain alcohol).
Use Cautiously in: ▪ Severe hepatic impairment (dosage reduction recommended) ▪ Renal impairment (frequent dosage changes may be necessary) ▪ Active infection ▪ Children (larger or more frequent doses may be required).

ADVERSE REACTIONS AND SIDE EFFECTS*

CNS: SEIZURES, <u>tremor</u>, confusion, flushing, headache, psychiatric problems.
CV: <u>hypertension</u>.
GI: <u>diarrhea</u>, <u>hepatotoxicity</u>, <u>nausea</u>, <u>vomiting</u>, abdominal discomfort, anorexia.
GU: <u>nephrotoxicity</u>.
Derm: <u>hirsutism</u>, acne.
F and E: hyperkalemia, hypomagnesemia.
Hemat: LEUKOPENIA, anemia, thrombocytopenia.
Metab: hyperlipidemia, hyperuricemia.
Neuro: hyperesthesia, paresthesia.
Misc: <u>gingival hyperplasia</u>, <u>hypersensitivity reactions</u>, <u>infections</u>.

INTERACTIONS

Drug-Drug: ▪ Increased blood levels and/or risk of toxicity with **amphotericin B, aminoglycosides, amiodarone, anabolic steroids,** some **calcium channel blockers, cimetidine, danazol, erythromycin, fluconazole, fluoroquinolones, ketoconazole, metoclopramide, miconazole, NSAIDs, melphalan,** or **oral contraceptives** ▪ Additive immunosup-

***CAPITALS indicate life-threatening; <u>underlines</u> indicate most frequent.**

pression with other **immunosuppressants (cyclophosphamide, azathioprine, glucocorticoids)** ▪ **Barbiturates, phenytoin, rifampin, carbamazepine,** or **sulfonamides** may decrease the effect of cyclosporine ▪ Additive hyperkalemia may occur with **potassium-sparing diuretics, potassium supplements,** or **ACE inhibitors** ▪ Increases serum levels and risk of toxicity from **digoxin** (decrease digoxin dose by 50%) ▪ Prolongs the action of **neuromuscular blocking agents** ▪ Increased risk of seizures with **imipenem/cilastatin** ▪ May decrease antibody response to **live virus vaccines** and increase the risk of adverse reactions ▪ Increased risk of rhabdomyolysis with **lovastatin** ▪ Concurrent use with **tacrolimus** should be avoided.
Drug-Food: ▪ Concurrent ingestion of **grapefruit juice** increases absorption ▪ **Food** decreases absorption of microemulsion products (Neoral).

ROUTE AND DOSAGE

Doses are adjusted on the basis of serum level monitoring.

❑ Prevention of Transplant Rejection

- **PO (Adults and Children):** 12–15 mg/kg/day (first dose before transplant) for 1–2 wk, taper by 5% weekly to maintenance dose of 5–10 mg/kg/day. Children may require larger or more frequent dosing because of faster clearance.
- **IV (Adults and Children):** 2–6 mg/kg/day (⅓ PO dose) initially, change to PO as soon as possible. Children may require larger or more frequent dosing because of faster clearance.

❑ Rheumatoid Arthritis

- **PO (Adults):** 2.5 mg/kg/day given in 2 divided doses; may increase by 0.5–0.75 mg/kg/day after 8 and 12 weeks; up to 4 mg/kg/day. Decrease dose by 25–50% if adverse reactions occur.

❑ Severe Psoriasis

- **PO (Adults):** 2.5 mg/kg/day given in 2 divided doses, for at least 4 wk; then may increase by 0.5 mg/kg/day q 2 wk, up to 4 mg/kg/day. Decrease dose by 25–50% if adverse reactions occur.

AVAILABILITY

▪ ***Microemulsion soft gelatin capsules (Neoral):*** 25 mg[Rx], 100 mg[Rx] ▪ ***Microemulsion oral solution (Neoral):*** 100 mg/ml[Rx] ▪ ***Soft gelatin capsules:*** 25 mg[Rx], 100 mg[Rx] ▪ ***Oral solution:*** 100 mg/ml[Rx] ▪ ***Injection:*** 50 mg/ml in 5-ml ampules[Rx].

TIME/ACTION PROFILE (blood levels)

	ONSET	PEAK	DURATION
PO	UK*	3.5 hr	UK
IV	UK	end of infusion	UK

*Onset of action in rheumatoid arthritis is 4–8 wk and may last 4 wk after discontinuation; for psoriasis, onset is 2–6 wk and lasts 6 wk following discontinuation.

NURSING IMPLICATIONS

ASSESSMENT

- **General Info:** Monitor intake and output ratios, daily weight, and blood pressure throughout therapy. Report significant changes.
- **Prevention of Transplant Rejection:** Assess for symptoms of organ rejection throughout therapy.
- **IV:** Monitor patient for signs and symptoms of hypersensitivity (wheezing, dyspnea, flushing of face or neck) continuously during at least the first 30 min of each treatment and frequently thereafter. Oxygen, epinephrine, and equipment for treatment of anaphylaxis should be available with each IV dose.
- **Arthritis:** Assess pain and limitation of movement prior to and during administration.
  - ❑ Prior to initiating therapy, perform a physical exam including blood pressure on 2 occasions to determine baseline. Monitor blood pressure every 2 wk during initial 3 mo, then monthly if stable. If hypertension occurs, dose should be reduced.
- **Psoriasis:** Assess skin lesions prior to and during therapy.
- ***Lab Test Considerations:*** Serum creatinine, BUN, CBC, magnesium, potassium, uric acid, and lipids should be measured at baseline, every 2 wk during initial therapy, and then monthly if stable. Nephrotoxicity may occur; report significant increases.
  - ❑ May cause hepatotoxicity; monitor for elevated AST, ALT, alkaline phosphatase, amylase, and bilirubin.
  - ❑ May cause increased serum potassium and

uric acid levels and decreased serum magnesium levels.

□ Serum lipid levels may be elevated.

■ ***Toxicity and Overdose:*** Serum cyclosporine levels should be evaluated periodically during therapy. Dose may be adjusted daily, in response to levels, during initiation of therapy. Guidelines for desired serum levels will vary among institutions.

POTENTIAL NURSING DIAGNOSES

■ Infection, risk for (Side Effects).
■ Pain (Indications).
■ Knowledge deficit, related to medication regimen (Patient/Family Teaching).

IMPLEMENTATION

■ **General Info:** Given with other immunosuppressive agents. Protect transplant patients from staff and visitors who may carry infection. Maintain protective isolation as indicated.

□ Microemulsion products (Neoral) and other products (Sandimmune) are not interchangeable.

■ **PO:** Draw up oral solution in the pipette provided with the medication. Mix oral solution with milk, chocolate milk, or orange juice, preferably at room temperature. Stir well and drink at once. Use a glass container and rinse with more diluent to ensure that total dose is taken. Administer oral doses with meals. Wipe pipette dry; do not wash after use.

■ **Intermittent Infusion:** Dilute each 1 ml (50 mg) of IV concentrate immediately before use with 20–100 ml of D5W or 0.9% NaCl for injection. Solution is stable for 24 hr in D5W. In 0.9% NaCl, it is stable for 6 hr in a polyvinylchloride container and 12 hr in a glass container at room temperature.

■ ***Rate:*** Infuse slowly over 2–6 hr via infusion pump.

■ **Continuous Infusion:** May be administered over 24 hr.

■ **Y-Site Compatibility:** ■ sargramostim.

■ **Additive Incompatibility:** ■ magnesium sulfate.

PATIENT/FAMILY TEACHING

□ Instruct patient to take medication at the same time each day and with regard to food, as directed. Do not skip doses or double up on missed doses. Take missed doses as soon as remembered within 12 hr. Do not discontinue medication without advice of health care professional.

□ Reinforce the need for lifelong therapy to prevent transplant rejection. Review symptoms of rejection for transplanted organ, and stress need to notify health care professional immediately if they occur.

□ Instruct patient to avoid grapefruit and grapefruit juice to prevent interaction with cyclosporine.

□ Advise patient of common side effects (nephrotoxicity, increased blood pressure, hand tremors, increased facial hair, gingival hyperplasia).

□ Teach patient the correct method for monitoring blood pressure. Instruct patient to notify health care professional of significant changes in blood pressure or if hematuria, increased frequency, cloudy urine, decreased urine output, fever, sore throat, tiredness, or unusual bruising occurs.

□ Instruct patient on proper oral hygiene. Meticulous oral hygiene and dental examinations for teeth cleaning and plaque control every 3 mo will help decrease gingival inflammation and hyperplasia.

□ Instruct patient to consult health care professional before taking any OTC medications or receiving any vaccinations while taking this medication.

□ Advise patient to notify health care professional if pregnancy is planned or suspected.

□ Emphasize the importance of follow-up exams and lab tests.

EVALUATION

Effectiveness of therapy can be demonstrated by: ■ Prevention of rejection of transplanted tissues ■ Decrease in severity of pain □ Increased ease of joint movement ■ Decrease in progression of psoriasis.

CYPROHEPTADINE

(si-proe-**hep**-ta-deen)
Periactin

CLASSIFICATION(S):
Antihistamine

Pregnancy Category B

C

INDICATIONS

▪ Relief of allergic symptoms caused by histamine release including: □ Seasonal and perennial allergic rhinitis □ Chronic urticaria □ Cold urticaria. **Unlabeled Uses:** ▪ Stimulation of appetite.

ACTION

▪ Antagonizes the effects of histamine at H_1-receptor sites; does not bind to or inactivate histamine ▪ Also blocks the effects of serotonin, which may result in increased appetite. **Therapeutic Effects:** ▪ Decreased symptoms of histamine excess (sneezing, rhinorrhea, nasal and ocular pruritus, ocular tearing and redness) ▪ Decreased cold urticaria.

PHARMACOKINETICS

Absorption: Apparently well absorbed after oral dosing.
Distribution: UK.
Metabolism and Excretion: Mostly metabolized by the liver.
Half-life: UK.

CONTRAINDICATIONS AND PRECAUTIONS

Contraindicated in: ▪ Hypersensitivity ▪ Acute attacks of asthma ▪ Lactation ▪ Known alcohol intolerance (syrup only).
Use Cautiously in: ▪ Geriatric patients ▪ Narrow-angle glaucoma ▪ Liver disease ▪ Pregnancy (safety not established).

ADVERSE REACTIONS AND SIDE EFFECTS*

CNS: drowsiness, excitation (↑ in children).
EENT: blurred vision.
CV: arrhythmias, hypotension, palpitations.
GI: dry mouth, constipation.
GU: hesitancy, retention.
Derm: photosensitivity, rashes.
Misc: weight gain.

INTERACTIONS

Drug-Drug: ▪ Additive CNS depression with other **CNS depressants**, including **alcohol, opioids**, and **sedative/hypnotics** ▪ **MAO inhibitors** may intensify and prolong the anticholinergic effects of antihistamines.

ROUTE AND DOSAGE

▪ **PO (Adults):** 4 mg q 8 hr (range 4–20 mg/day in 3 divided doses; up to 32 mg/day).
▪ **PO (Children 6–14 yr):** 2–4 mg q 8–12 hr (not to exceed 16 mg/day).
▪ **PO (Children 2–6 yr):** 2 mg q 8–12 hr (not to exceed 12 mg/day).

AVAILABILITY

▪ ***Tablets:*** 4 mg[Rx,OTC] ▪ ***Syrup:*** 2 mg/5 ml[Rx,OTC].

TIME/ACTION PROFILE (antihistaminic effects)

	ONSET	PEAK	DURATION
PO	15–60 min	1–2 hr	8 hr

NURSING IMPLICATIONS

ASSESSMENT

▪ **Allergy:** Assess symptoms (rhinitis, conjunctivitis, hives) prior to and periodically throughout therapy.
□ Assess lung sounds and respiratory function prior to and periodically throughout therapy. May cause thickening of bronchial secretions. Maintain fluid intake of 1500–2000 ml/day to decrease viscosity of secretions.
▪ **Appetite Stimulant:** Monitor food intake and weight routinely.
▪ ***Lab Test Considerations:*** May cause false-negative reactions on allergy skin tests; discontinue 72 hr prior to testing.
□ Increased serum amylase and prolactin concentrations may occur when cyproheptadine is administered with a thyrotropin-releasing hormone.

POTENTIAL NURSING DIAGNOSES

▪ Airway clearance, ineffective (Indications).
▪ Injury, risk for (Side Effects).
▪ Knowledge deficit, related to medication regimen (Patient/Family Teaching).

IMPLEMENTATION

▪ **PO:** Administer with food, water, or milk to minimize gastric irritation.

PATIENT/FAMILY TEACHING

□ Instruct patient to take cyproheptadine exactly as directed. Missed dose should be taken as soon as remembered. Do not double doses.

*CAPITALS indicate life-threatening; underlines indicate most frequent.

Syrup should be accurately measured using calibrated medication cup or measuring device.

□ Medication may cause drowsiness. Advise patient to avoid driving or other activities requiring alertness until response to the drug is known.
□ Advise patient to use sunscreen and protective clothing to prevent a photosensitivity reaction.
□ Caution patient to avoid concurrent use of alcohol and other CNS depressants.
□ Advise patient that frequent mouth rinses, good oral hygiene, and sugarless gum or candy may decrease dry mouth. Patient should notify dentist if dry mouth persists for >2 wk.

EVALUATION

Effectiveness of therapy can be demonstrated by: ▪ Alleviation of allergic symptoms □ Alleviation of cold urticaria ▪ Improvement of appetite.

CYTARABINE

(sye-**tare**-a-been)

Ara-C, cytosine arabinoside, {Cytosar}, Cytosar-U

CLASSIFICATION(S):

Antineoplastic (antimetabolite)

Pregnancy Category D

INDICATIONS

▪ **IV:** Used mainly in combination chemotherapeutic regimens for the treatment of leukemias and non-Hodgkin's lymphomas ▪ **IT:** Treatment of meningeal leukemia.

ACTION

▪ Inhibits DNA synthesis by inhibiting DNA polymerase (cell-cycle S phase–specific). **Therapeutic Effects:** ▪ Death of rapidly replicating cells, particularly malignant ones.

PHARMACOKINETICS

Absorption: Absorption occurs from SC sites, but blood levels are less than with IV administration.
Distribution: Widely distributed. Crosses the blood-brain barrier but not in sufficient quantities. Crosses the placenta.
Metabolism and Excretion: Metabolized mostly by the liver; <10% excreted unchanged by the kidneys.
Half-life: 1–3 hr.

CONTRAINDICATIONS AND PRECAUTIONS

Contraindicated in: ▪ Hypersensitivity ▪ Pregnancy or lactation.
Use Cautiously in: ▪ Active infections ▪ Decreased bone marrow reserve ▪ Renal/hepatic disease ▪ Other chronic debilitating illnesses ▪ Patients with childbearing potential.

ADVERSE REACTIONS AND SIDE EFFECTS*

CNS: CNS dysfunction (high dose), headache.
EENT: corneal toxicity (high dose), hemorrhagic conjunctivitis (high dose).
Resp: PULMONARY EDEMA (high dose).
GI: <u>nausea</u>, <u>vomiting</u>, hepatitis, hepatotoxicity, severe GI ulceration (high dose), stomatitis.
Derm: alopecia, rash.
Endo: gonadal suppression.
Hemat: <u>anemia</u>, <u>leukopenia</u>, <u>thrombocytopenia</u>.
Metab: hyperuricemia.
Misc: cytarabine syndrome, fever.

INTERACTIONS

Drug-Drug: ▪ Additive bone marrow depression with other **antineoplastics** or **radiation therapy** ▪ Increased risk of cardiomyopathy when used in high-dose regimens with **cyclophosphamide** ▪ May decrease antibody response to **live virus vaccines** and increase the risk of adverse reactions.

ROUTE AND DOSAGE

Dosage regimens vary widely.

▪ **IV (Adults):** *Induction dose*—200 mg/m²/day for 5 days q 2 wk as a single agent or 2–6 mg/kg/day (100–200 mg/m²/day) as a single daily dose or in 2–3 divided doses for 5–10 days or until remission occurs as part of combination chemotherapy. *Maintenance*—70–200 mg/m²/day for 2–5 days monthly. *High-dose regimen*—2–3 g/m² q 12 hr for up to 12 doses.

{} = Available in Canada only.
***CAPITALS indicate life-threatening; <u>underlines</u> indicate most frequent.**

- **SC (Adults):** *Maintenance*—1 mg/kg 1–2 times weekly.
- **IT (Adults):** 5–75 mg/m² or 30–100 mg q 2–7 days or daily for 4–5 days; may also be given as 30 mg/m² once every 4 days until CSF is normal, followed by an additional dose.

AVAILABILITY

- ***Powder for injection:*** 100 mg[Rx], 500 mg[Rx], 1g[Rx], 2 g[Rx].

TIME/ACTION PROFILE (effects on white blood cell counts)

	ONSET	PEAK	DURATION
SC, IV (1st phase)	24 hr	7–9 days	12 days
SC, IV (2nd phase)	15–24 days	15–24 days	25–34 days

NURSING IMPLICATIONS

ASSESSMENT

- Monitor for bone marrow depression. Assess for bleeding (bleeding gums, bruising, petechiae, guaiac stools, urine, and emesis) and avoid IM injections and rectal temperatures if platelet count is low. Apply pressure to venipuncture sites for 10 min. Assess for signs of infection during neutropenia. Anemia may occur. Monitor for increased fatigue, dyspnea, and orthostatic hypotension.
- Monitor intake and output ratios and daily weights. Report significant changes in totals.
- Monitor for symptoms of gout (increased uric acid, joint pain, edema). Encourage patient to drink at least 2 liters of fluid each day. Allopurinol may decrease uric acid levels. Alkalinization of urine may increase excretion of uric acid.
- Assess nutritional status. Nausea and vomiting may occur within 1 hr of administration, especially if IV dose is administered rapidly. Administering an antiemetic prior to and periodically throughout therapy and adjusting diet as tolerated may help maintain fluid and electrolyte balance and nutritional status.
- Monitor patient for development of *cytarabine or ara-C syndrome* (fever, myalgia, bone pain, chest pain, maculopapular rash, conjunctivitis, malaise), which usually occurs 6–12 hr following administration. Glucocorticoids may be used for treatment or prevention. If patient responds to glucocorticoids, continue cytarabine and glucocorticoids.
- ***Lab Test Considerations:*** Monitor CBC with differential and platelet count prior to and frequently throughout therapy. Leukocyte counts begin to drop within 24 hr of administration. The initial nadir occurs in 7–9 days. After a small rise in the count, the second, deeper nadir occurs 15–24 days after administration. Platelet counts begin to fall 5 days after a dose, with a nadir at 12–15 days. Leukocyte and thrombocyte counts usually begin to rise 10 days after the nadirs. Therapy is usually withdrawn if leukocyte count is <1000/mm³ or platelet count is <50,000/mm³. Bone marrow aspirations are recommended every 2 wk until remission occurs.
- Renal (BUN and creatinine) and hepatic function (AST, ALT, bilirubin, alkaline phosphatase, and LDH) should be monitored prior to and routinely throughout therapy.
- May cause increased uric acid concentrations.

POTENTIAL NURSING DIAGNOSES

- Infection, risk for (Adverse Reactions).
- Injury, risk for (Side Effects).
- Knowledge deficit, related to medication regimen (Patient/Family Teaching).

IMPLEMENTATION

- **General Info:** Solution should be prepared in a biologic cabinet. Wear gloves, gown, and mask while handling IV medication. Discard IV equipment in specially designated containers (see Appendix I).
- May be given SC, direct IV, intermittent IV, continuous IV, or IT.
- Do not confuse high-dose and regular therapy. Fatalities have occurred with high-dose therapy.
- **SC, IV:** Reconstitute 100-mg vials with 5 ml of bacteriostatic water for injection with benzyl alcohol 0.9% for a concentration of 20 mg/ml. Reconstitute 500-mg vials with 10 ml for a concentration of 50 mg/ml, 1-g vials with 10 ml, and 2-g vials with 20 ml for a concentration of 100 mg/ml. Reconstituted solution is stable for 48 hr. Do not administer a cloudy solution.
- **Direct IV:** Administer each 100 mg direct IV push over 1–3 min.
- **Intermittent Infusion:** May be further di-

luted in 100 ml of 0.9% NaCl or D5W. May also be diluted in D10W, D5/0.9% NaCl, Ringer's solution, lactated Ringer's solution, or D5/LR.

- ***Rate:*** Infuse over 30 min.
- **Continuous Infusion:** Rate and concentration for IV infusion are ordered individually by physician.
- **Syringe Compatibility:** ▪ metoclopramide.
- **Y-Site Compatibility:** ▪ amifostine ▪ aztreonam ▪ cefepime ▪ chlorpromazine ▪ dexamethasone ▪ diphenhydramine ▪ droperidol ▪ famotidine ▪ filgrastim ▪ fludarabine ▪ furosemide ▪ granisetron ▪ heparin ▪ hydromorphone ▪ idarubicin ▪ lorazepam ▪ melphalan ▪ methotrexate ▪ methylprednisolone ▪ metoclopramide ▪ morphine ▪ ondansetron ▪ paclitaxel ▪ piperacillin/tazobactam ▪ prochlorperazine ▪ promethazine ▪ ranitidine ▪ sargramostim ▪ teniposide ▪ thiotepa ▪ vinorelbine.
- **Y-Site Incompatibility:** ▪ gallium nitrate ▪ ganciclovir.
- **Additive Compatibility:** ▪ etoposide ▪ methotrexate ▪ mitoxantrone ▪ potassium chloride ▪ prednisolone sodium phosphate ▪ sodium bicarbonate ▪ vincristine.
- **Additive Incompatibility:** ▪ fluorouracil ▪ heparin ▪ regular insulin ▪ nafcillin ▪ oxacillin ▪ penicillin G sodium.
- **IT:** Reconstitute with preservative-free 0.9% NaCl or other suitable diluent. Use immediately to prevent bacterial contamination.

PATIENT/FAMILY TEACHING

- □ Caution patient to avoid crowds and persons with known infections. Report symptoms of infection (fever; chills; cough; hoarseness; sore throat; lower back or side pain; painful or difficult urination) immediately.
- □ Instruct patient to report unusual bleeding. Advise patient of thrombocytopenia precautions (use soft toothbrush and electric razor; avoid falls; do not drink alcoholic beverages or take medication containing aspirin or NSAIDs; may precipitate gastric bleeding).
- □ Instruct patient to inspect oral mucosa for redness and ulceration. If mouth sores occur, advise patient to use sponge brush and rinse mouth with water after eating and drinking. Stomatitis may require treatment with opioid analgesics.
- □ Advise patient that this medication may have teratogenic effects. Contraception should be used during therapy and for at least 4 mo after therapy is concluded.
- □ Instruct patient not to receive any vaccinations without advice of health care professional.
- □ Emphasize the need for periodic lab tests to monitor for side effects.

EVALUATION

Effectiveness of therapy can be demonstrated by: ▪ Improvement of hematopoietic values in leukemias ▪ Decrease in size and spread of the tumor in non-Hodgkin's lymphomas. Therapy is continued every 2 wk until patient is in complete remission or thrombocyte count or leukocyte count falls below acceptable levels.

D

DACARBAZINE

(da-**kar**-ba-zeen)

{DTIC}, DTIC-Dome

CLASSIFICATION(S):

Antineoplastic (alkylating agent)

Pregnancy Category C

INDICATIONS

▪ Treatment of metastatic malignant melanoma (single agent) ▪ Treatment of advanced Hodgkin's disease (with other agents).

ACTION

▪ Disrupts DNA and RNA synthesis (cell-cycle phase–nonspecific). **Therapeutic Effects:** ▪ Death of rapidly growing tissue cells, especially malignant ones.

PHARMACOKINETICS

Absorption: IV administration results in complete bioavailability.

Distribution: Large volume of distribution; probably concentrates in liver; some CNS penetration.

Metabolism and Excretion: 50% metabolized

by the liver, 50% excreted unchanged by the kidneys.
Half-life: 5 hr (increased in renal disease).

CONTRAINDICATIONS AND PRECAUTIONS

Contraindicated in: ▪ Hypersensitivity ▪ Pregnancy or lactation ▪ Concurrent radiation therapy.
Use Cautiously in: ▪ Active infections ▪ Decreased bone marrow reserve ▪ Other chronic debilitating diseases ▪ Children (safety not established) ▪ Renal disease ▪ Patients with childbearing potential.

ADVERSE REACTIONS AND SIDE EFFECTS*

GI: HEPATIC NECROSIS, anorexia, nausea, vomiting, diarrhea, hepatic vein thrombosis.
Derm: alopecia, facial flushing, photosensitivity.
Endo: gonadal suppression.
Hemat: bone marrow depression.
Local: pain at IV site, phlebitis at IV site, tissue necrosis.
MS: myalgia.
Neuro: facial paresthesia.
Misc: ANAPHYLAXIS, facial flushing, fever, flu-like syndrome, malaise.

INTERACTIONS

Drug-Drug: ▪ Additive bone marrow depression with other **antineoplastic agents** ▪ Additive hepatotoxicity with other **hepatotoxic drugs** ▪ **Phenytoin** or **phenobarbital** may increase metabolism and decrease effectiveness ▪ May decrease antibody response to **live virus vaccines** and increase the risk of adverse reactions.

ROUTE AND DOSAGE

Other regimens are used.
- **IV (Adults):** *Malignant melanoma*—2–4.5 mg/kg/day for 10 days q 4 wk or 250 mg/m²/day for 5 days q 3 wk. *Hodgkin's disease*—150 mg/m²/day for 5 days (in combination with other agents) q 4 wk or 375 mg/m² (with other agents) q 15 days.

AVAILABILITY

- ***Powder for injection:*** 100 mg[Rx], 200 mg[Rx].

TIME/ACTION PROFILE (effects on blood counts)

	ONSET	PEAK	DURATION
IV (WBCs)	16–20 days	21–25 days	3–5 days
IV (platelets)	UK	16 days	3–5 days

NURSING IMPLICATIONS

ASSESSMENT

- Monitor vital signs prior to and frequently during therapy.
- Monitor for bone marrow depression. Assess for bleeding (bleeding gums, bruising, petechiae, guaiac stools, urine, and emesis) and avoid IM injections and rectal temperatures if platelet count is low. Apply pressure to venipuncture sites for 10 min. Assess for signs of infection during neutropenia. Anemia may occur. Monitor for increased fatigue, dyspnea, and orthostatic hypotension.
- Monitor IV site closely. Dacarbazine is an irritant. Instruct patient to notify nurse immediately if discomfort at IV site occurs. Discontinue IV immediately if infiltration occurs. Applications of hot packs may relieve pain, burning sensation, and irritation at injection site.
- Monitor intake and output, appetite, and nutritional intake. Assess for nausea and vomiting, which may be severe and last 1–12 hr. Administration of an antiemetic prior to and periodically during therapy, restricting oral intake for 4–6 hr prior to administration, and adjusting diet as tolerated may help maintain fluid and electrolyte balance and nutritional status. Nausea usually decreases on subsequent doses.
- ***Lab Test Considerations:*** Monitor CBC and differential prior to and periodically throughout therapy. The nadir of thrombocytopenia occurs in 16 days. The nadir of leukopenia occurs in 3–4 wk. Recovery begins in 5 days. Withhold dose and notify physician if platelet count is $<100,000/mm^3$ or leukocyte count is $<4000/mm^3$.
- Monitor for increased AST, ALT, uric acid, and BUN.

POTENTIAL NURSING DIAGNOSES

- Infection, risk for (Side Effects).
- Injury, risk for (Side Effects).

*CAPITALS indicate life-threatening; underlines indicate most frequent.

- Knowledge deficit, related to medication regimen (Patient/Family Teaching).

IMPLEMENTATION

- **General Info:** Reconstitute each 100-mg vial with 9.9 ml and each 200-mg vial with 19.7 ml of sterile water for injection for a concentration of 10 mg/ml. Solution is colorless or clear yellow. Do not use solution that has turned pink. Solution is stable for 8 hr at room temperature and for 72 hr if refrigerated.
  - Solution should be prepared in a biologic cabinet. Wear gloves, gown, and mask while handling medication. Discard equipment in designated containers (see Appendix I).
- **Direct IV:** Administer over 1 min into a free-flowing IV infusion.
- **Intermittent Infusion:** Further dilute with up to 250 ml of D5W or 0.9% NaCl. Stable for 24 hr if refrigerated or 8 hr at room temperature.
- ***Rate:*** Administer over 15–30 min.
- **Y-Site Compatibility:** ▪ amifostine ▪ aztreonam ▪ filgrastim ▪ fludarabine ▪ granisetron ▪ melphalan ▪ ondansetron ▪ paclitaxel ▪ sargramostim ▪ teniposide ▪ thiotepa ▪ vinorelbine.
- **Y-Site Incompatibility:** ▪ cefepime ▪ piperacillin/tazobactam.
- **Additive Compatibility:** ▪ bleomycin ▪ carmustine ▪ cyclophosphamide ▪ cytarabine ▪ dactinomycin ▪ doxorubicin ▪ fluorouracil ▪ mercaptopurine ▪ methotrexate ▪ ondansetron ▪ vinblastine.
- **Additive Incompatibility:** ▪ hydrocortisone sodium succinate.

PATIENT/FAMILY TEACHING

- Instruct patient to notify health care professional if fever; chills; sore throat; signs of infection; bleeding gums; bruising; petechiae; or blood in urine, stool, or emesis occurs. Caution patient to avoid crowds and persons with known infections. Instruct patient to use soft toothbrush and electric razor. Patients should be cautioned not to drink alcoholic beverages or take products containing aspirin or NSAIDs; may increase GI irritation.
- May cause photosensitivity. Instruct patient to avoid sunlight or wear protective clothing and use sunscreen for 2 days after therapy.
- Instruct patient to inform health care professional if flu-like syndrome occurs. Symptoms include fever, myalgia, and general malaise. May occur after several courses of therapy. Usually occurs 1 wk after administration. May persist for 1–3 wk. Acetaminophen may be used for relief of symptoms.
- Discuss with patient the possibility of hair loss. Explore coping strategies.
- Advise patient of the need for a nonhormonal method of contraception.
- Instruct patient not to receive any vaccinations without advice of health care professional.

EVALUATION

Effectiveness of therapy can be demonstrated by: ▪ Decrease in size and spread of malignant melanoma or Hodgkin's lymphoma.

D

DACTINOMYCIN

(dak-ti-noe-**mye**-sin)

actinomycin-D, Cosmegen

CLASSIFICATION(S):

Antineoplastic (antibiotic)

Pregnancy Category C

INDICATIONS

▪ Used alone and in combination with other treatment modalities (other antineoplastic agents, radiation therapy, or surgery) in the management of: □ Wilms' tumor □ Rhabdomyosarcoma □ Ewing's sarcoma □ Trophoblastic neoplasms □ Testicular carcinoma □ Other malignancies.

ACTION

▪ Inhibits RNA synthesis by forming a complex with DNA (cell-cycle phase–nonspecific). **Therapeutic Effects:** ▪ Death of rapidly replicating cells, particularly malignant ones ▪ Also has immunosuppressive properties.

PHARMACOKINETICS

Absorption: IV administration results in complete bioavailability.

Distribution: Widely distributed, with extensive tissue binding; does not cross the blood-brain barrier. Crosses the placenta.

Metabolism and Excretion: Excreted in bile and subsequently in the feces as unchanged drug (50%); small amounts excreted unchanged by the kidneys.
Half-life: 36 hr.

CONTRAINDICATIONS AND PRECAUTIONS

Contraindicated in: ▪ Hypersensitivity ▪ Pregnant or lactating women.
Use Cautiously in: ▪ Active infections ▪ Decreased bone marrow reserve ▪ Concurrent radiation therapy ▪ Other chronic debilitating illnesses ▪ Obese or edematous patients (dose should be based on body surface area) ▪ Patients with childbearing potential.

ADVERSE REACTIONS AND SIDE EFFECTS*

CNS: lethargy, malaise.
GI: nausea, stomatitis, vomiting, hepatotoxicity, ulceration.
Derm: alopecia, photosensitivity, radiation recall, rashes.
Endo: gonadal suppression.
Hemat: anemia, leukopenia, thrombocytopenia.
Local: phlebitis at IV site.
Misc: fever.

INTERACTIONS

Drug-Drug: ▪ Additive bone marrow depression with other **antineoplastics** or **radiation therapy** ▪ May increase the risk of cardiotoxicity with **doxorubicin** ▪ May decrease antibody response to **live virus vaccines** and increase risk of adverse reactions.

ROUTE AND DOSAGE

- **IV (Adults):** 10–15 mcg/kg/day for up to 5 days q 4–6 wk or 500 mcg/m^2 (up to 2 mg) weekly for 3 wk.
- **IV (Children >6 mo):** 15 mcg/kg (450–500 mcg/m^2) daily for up to 5 days *or* 2.5 mg/m^2 total dose divided into 7 daily doses; may be repeated in 4–6 wk.

AVAILABILITY

- ***Powder for injection:*** 0.5-mg vials[Rx].

TIME/ACTION PROFILE (effects on blood counts)

	ONSET	PEAK	DURATION
IV	7 days	14 days	21–28 days

NURSING IMPLICATIONS

ASSESSMENT

- □ Monitor vital signs prior to and frequently during therapy.
- □ Monitor for bone marrow depression. Assess for bleeding (bleeding gums, bruising, petechiae, guaiac stools, urine, and emesis) and avoid IM injections and rectal temperatures if platelet count is low. Apply pressure to venipuncture sites for 10 min. Assess for signs of infection during neutropenia. Anemia may occur. Monitor for increased fatigue, dyspnea, and orthostatic hypotension.
- □ Assess IV site frequently for inflammation or infiltration. Dactinomycin is a vesicant. Patient should notify nurse if pain or irritation at injection site occurs. If extravasation occurs, infusion must be stopped and restarted in another vein to avoid damage to SC tissue. Standard treatments include local injections of steroids and application of ice compresses. Saline may be infused through the line into infiltrated area to dilute the drug.
- □ Monitor intake and output, appetite, and nutritional intake. Assess for nausea and vomiting; usually begin a few hours after administration and persist for up to 20 hr. Administration of an antiemetic prior to and periodically during therapy and adjustment of diet as tolerated may help maintain fluid and electrolyte balance and nutritional status. IV fluids and allopurinol may be given to decrease uric acid levels in patients unable to maintain satisfactory oral intake.
- ▪ ***Lab Test Considerations:*** May cause increased uric acid levels.
- □ Monitor CBC and differential prior to and periodically throughout therapy. Platelets and leukocyte counts begin to drop 7–10 days after beginning therapy. The nadirs of thrombocytopenia and leukopenia occur in 3 wk. Recovery occurs 3 wk later.
- □ Monitor for hepatotoxicity (increased AST, ALT, LDH, and serum bilirubin).

***CAPITALS indicate life-threatening; underlines indicate most frequent.**

POTENTIAL NURSING DIAGNOSES

- Infection, risk for (Adverse Reactions).
- Oral mucous membrane, altered (Side Effects).
- Knowledge deficit, related to medication regimen (Patient/Family Teaching).

IMPLEMENTATION

- **General Info:** Avoid contact with skin. If spillage occurs, irrigate skin with copious amount of water for 15 min. If splashed into eye, irrigate with water and consult ophthalmologist.
- □ Solution for IV administration should be prepared in a biologic cabinet. Wear gloves, gown, and mask while handling IV medication. Discard IV equipment in specially designated containers (see Appendix I).
- **IV:** Reconstitute each 0.5-mg vial with 1.1 ml of sterile water for injection without preservatives for a concentration of 0.5 mg/ml. Use of 0.9% NaCl or preservatives, benzyl alcohol, or parabens for reconstitution causes precipitation. Solution color is gold. Discard any unused solution.
- **Direct IV:** Change needle between reconstitution and direct IV administration.
- ***Rate:*** May be injected into Y-site of free-flowing infusions of 0.9% NaCl or D5W at a rate of 0.5 mg/min.
- **Intermittent Infusion:** May be further diluted in 50 ml of 0.9% NaCl or D5W.
- ***Rate:*** Infuse over 10–15 min.
- **Y-Site Compatibility:** ▪ amifostine ▪ aztreonam ▪ cefepime ▪ fludarabine ▪ melphalan ▪ ondansetron ▪ sargramostim ▪ teniposide ▪ thiotepa ▪ vinorelbine.
- **Y-Site Incompatibility:** ▪ filgrastim.

PATIENT/FAMILY TEACHING

- □ Instruct patient to notify health care professional if fever; chills; sore throat; signs of infection; bleeding gums; bruising; petechiae; or blood in urine, stool, or emesis occurs. Caution patient to avoid crowds and persons with known infections. Instruct patient to use soft toothbrush and electric razor. Patients should be cautioned not to drink alcoholic beverages or take products containing aspirin or NSAIDs; may increase GI irritation.
- □ Instruct patient to inspect oral mucosa for erythema and ulceration. If ulceration occurs, advise patient to use sponge brush and rinse mouth with water after eating and drinking. Stomatitis may require treatment with opioid analgesics.
- □ Inform patient that this medication may cause irreversible gonadal suppression. Advise patient that this medication may have teratogenic effects. A nonhormonal method of contraception should be used during therapy and for at least 4 mo after therapy is concluded.
- □ Discuss with patient the possibility of hair loss, which usually occurs 7–10 days after administration. Explore coping strategies.
- □ Instruct patient not to receive any vaccinations without advice of health care professional.
- □ Emphasize the need for periodic lab tests to monitor for side effects.

EVALUATION

Effectiveness of therapy can be demonstrated by: ▪ Decrease in size or spread of malignancy.

D

DANAZOL

(**da**-na-zole)

{Cyclomen}, Danocrine

CLASSIFICATION(S):

Hormone (androgen)

Pregnancy Category X

INDICATIONS

▪ Treatment of moderate endometriosis unresponsive to conventional therapy ▪ Palliative therapy of fibrocystic breast disease ▪ Prophylaxis of hereditary angioedema.

ACTION

▪ Inhibits pituitary output of gonadotropins, resulting in suppression of ovarian function. Has weak androgenic-anabolic activity. **Therapeutic Effects:** ▪ Atrophy of ectopic endometrial tissue in endometriosis ▪ Decreased pain and nodularity in fibrocystic breast disease ▪ Correction of biochemical abnormalities in hereditary angioedema.

PHARMACOKINETICS

Absorption: Absorbed from the GI tract.
Distribution: UK.
Metabolism and Excretion: Metabolized by the liver.
Half-life: 4.5 hr.

TIME/ACTION PROFILE (disease response)

	ONSET	PEAK	DURATION
PO (endometriosis)	UK	6–8 wk	60–90 days
PO (fibrocystic disease)	1 mo	2–6 mo	1 yr
PO (angioedema)	UK	1–3 mo	UK

CONTRAINDICATIONS AND PRECAUTIONS

Contraindicated in: ▪ Hypersensitivity ▪ Male patients with breast or prostate cancer ▪ Hypercalcemia ▪ Severe hepatic, renal, or cardiac disease ▪ Pregnancy or lactation.
Use Cautiously in: ▪ Previous history of liver disease ▪ Coronary artery disease ▪ Prepubertal males.

ADVERSE REACTIONS AND SIDE EFFECTS*

CNS: emotional lability.
EENT: deepening of voice.
CV: edema.
GI: hepatitis (cholestatic jaundice).
GU: amenorrhea, clitoral enlargement, testicular atrophy.
Derm: acne, hirsutism, oiliness.
Endo: amenorrhea, anovulation, decreased breast size (females), decreased libido.
Metab: weight gain.

INTERACTIONS

Drug-Drug: ▪ May potentiate **warfarin, oral hypoglycemic agents, insulin,** or **glucocorticoids** ▪ May increase **cyclosporine** levels and risk of toxicity.

ROUTE AND DOSAGE

- **PO (Adults and Adolescents):** *Endometriosis*—400 mg twice daily (for milder cases may initiate therapy with 100–200 mg twice daily) for 3–6 mo (up to 9 mo). *Fibrocystic breast disease*—50–200 mg twice daily. *Hereditary angioedema*—200 mg 2–3 times daily. Attempt to decrease dosage by 50% or less q 1–3 mo. If acute attack occurs, increase dose by up to 200 mg/day.

AVAILABILITY

- ***Capsules:*** 50 mg[Rx], 100 mg[Rx], 200 mg[Rx].

NURSING IMPLICATIONS

ASSESSMENT

- **Endometriosis:** Assess patient for endometrial pain prior to and periodically throughout therapy.
- **Fibrocystic Breast Disease:** Assess patient for breast pain, tenderness, and nodules prior to and monthly throughout therapy. To rule out carcinoma, mammography or cyst biopsy is recommended prior to therapy and during treatment if nodules persist or enlarge.
- **Hereditary Angioedema:** Monitor patient for edematous attacks throughout therapy, especially during dosage adjustments.
- ***Lab Test Considerations:*** Liver function tests should be monitored periodically throughout therapy.
  - □ Semen volume and viscosity, sperm count, and motility determinations are recommended every 3–4 mo during treatment for hereditary angioedema, especially in adolescents.
  - □ May alter results of glucose tolerance or thyroid function tests. May also cause serum glucose and low-density lipoprotein concentrations and decreased high-density lipoprotein concentrations.

POTENTIAL NURSING DIAGNOSES

- Sexual dysfunction (Side Effects).
- Body image disturbance (Side Effects).
- Knowledge deficit, related to medication regimen (Patient/Family Teaching).

IMPLEMENTATION

- **General Info:** In patients with endometriosis or fibrocystic breast disease, therapy should be started during menstruation or preceded by a pregnancy test. Advise patient to notify physician immediately if pregnancy is suspected.

*CAPITALS indicate life-threatening; underlines indicate most frequent.

- **PO:** Medication may be administered with meals to minimize GI irritation.

PATIENT/FAMILY TEACHING

- **General Info:** Instruct patient to take medication exactly as directed. Missed doses should be taken as soon as remembered, if not almost time for next dose; do not double doses.
  - Advise patient to use a nonhormonal form of contraception during therapy. Inform patient that amenorrhea is expected with higher doses. Instruct patient to notify health care professional if regular menstruation does not occur within 60–90 days after discontinuation of therapy or if pregnancy is suspected.
  - Advise patient to notify health care professional if masculinizing effects occur (abnormal growth of facial hair or other body hair, deepening of the voice).
  - Advise patient to use sunscreen and protective clothing to prevent photosensitivity reactions.
  - Emphasize the importance of routine visits to health care professional to check progress during therapy.
- **Fibrocystic Breast Disease:** Teach patient the correct technique for monthly breast self-exam. Instruct patient to report increase in size of nodules to health care professional promptly.

EVALUATION

Effectiveness of therapy can be demonstrated by: ▪ Decrease in symptoms of endometriosis. Therapy for endometriosis usually requires 3–6 mo and may extend to 9 mo to decrease symptoms ▪ Relief of pain and tenderness in fibrocystic breast disease, which is usually relieved by the first month and eliminated in 2–3 mo. Elimination of nodularity usually requires 4–6 mo ▪ Resolutions of signs and symptoms of hereditary angioedema. Initial response in hereditary angioedema may require 1–3 mo of therapy; efforts should be made to decrease dosage at 1–3-mo intervals.

DANTROLENE

(**dan**-troe-leen)
Dantrium

CLASSIFICATION(S):
Skeletal muscle relaxant (direct-acting)

Pregnancy Category C

INDICATIONS

▪ **PO:** Treatment of spasticity associated with: □ Spinal cord injury □ Stroke □ Cerebral palsy □ Multiple sclerosis ▪ Prophylaxis of malignant hyperthermia ▪ **IV:** Emergency treatment of malignant hyperthermia. **Unlabeled Uses:** ▪ Management of neuroleptic malignant syndrome.

ACTION

▪ Acts directly on skeletal muscle, causing relaxation by decreasing calcium release from sarcoplasmic reticulum in muscle cells ▪ Prevents intense catabolic process associated with malignant hyperthermia. **Therapeutic Effects:** ▪ Reduction of muscle spasticity ▪ Prevention of malignant hyperthermia.

PHARMACOKINETICS

Absorption: 35% absorbed after oral administration.
Distribution: UK.
Metabolism and Excretion: Almost entirely metabolized by the liver.
Half-life: 8.7 hr.

CONTRAINDICATIONS AND PRECAUTIONS

Contraindicated in: ▪ No contraindications to IV form in treatment of hyperthermia ▪ Pregnancy and lactation ▪ Situations in which spasticity is used to maintain posture or balance.
Use Cautiously in: ▪ Cardiac, pulmonary, or previous liver disease ▪ Females, patients >35 yr (increased risk of hepatotoxicity).

ADVERSE REACTIONS AND SIDE EFFECTS*

CNS: drowsiness, muscle weakness, confusion, dizziness, headache, insomnia, malaise, nervousness.
EENT: excessive lacrimation, visual disturbances.
Resp: pleural effusions.

*CAPITALS indicate life-threatening; underlines indicate most frequent.

D

CV: changes in BP, tachycardia.
GI: HEPATOTOXICITY, diarrhea, anorexia, cramps, dysphagia, GI bleeding, vomiting.
GU: crystalluria, dysuria, frequency, impotence, incontinence, nocturia.
Derm: pruritus, sweating, urticaria.
Hemat: eosinophilia.
Local: irritation at IV site, phlebitis.
MS: myalgia.
Misc: chills, drooling, fever.

INTERACTIONS

Drug-Drug: ▪ Additive CNS depression with **CNS depressants,** including **alcohol, antihistamines, opioids, sedative/hypnotics,** and **parenteral magnesium sulfate** ▪ Increased risk of hepatotoxicity with other **hepatotoxic agents** or **estrogens** ▪ Increased risk of arrhythmias with **verapamil.**

ROUTE AND DOSAGE

- **PO (Adults):** *Spasticity*—25 mg/day initially; increase by 25 mg/day q 4–7 days until desired response or total of 100 mg 4 times daily is reached. *Prevention of malignant hyperthermia*—4–8 mg/kg/day in 3–4 divided doses for 1–2 days prior to procedure, last dose 3–4 hr preop. *Post-hyperthermic crisis follow-up*—4–8 mg/kg/day in 3–4 divided doses for 1–3 days following IV treatment.
- **PO (Children >5 yr):** *Spasticity*—0.5 mg/kg twice daily; increase by 0.5 mg/kg/day q 4–7 days until desired response is obtained or dosage of 3 mg/kg 4 times daily is reached (not to exceed 400 mg/day). *Prevention of malignant hyperthermia*—4–8 mg/kg/day in 3–4 divided doses for 1–2 days prior to procedure, last dose 3–4 hr preop. *Post-hyperthermic crisis follow-up*—4–8 mg/kg/day in 3–4 divided doses for 1–3 days following IV treatment.
- **IV (Adults and Children):** *Treatment of malignant hyperthermia*—at least 1 mg/kg (up to 3 mg/kg), continued until symptoms decrease or a cumulative dose of 10 mg/kg has been given. If symptoms reappear, dosage may be repeated. *Prevention of malignant hyperthermia*—2.5 mg/kg prior to anesthesia.

AVAILABILITY

- ***Capsules:*** 25 mg[Rx], 50 mg[Rx], 100 mg[Rx]
- ***Powder for injection:*** 20 mg/vial[Rx].

TIME/ACTION PROFILE (effects on spasticity)

	ONSET	PEAK	DURATION
PO	1 wk	UK	6–12 hr
IV	rapid	rapid	UK

NURSING IMPLICATIONS

ASSESSMENT

- **General Info:** Assess bowel function periodically. Persistent diarrhea may warrant discontinuation of therapy.
- **Muscle Spasticity:** Assess neuromuscular status and muscle spasticity before initiating therapy and periodically during its course to determine response to therapy.
- **Malignant Hyperthermia:** Assess previous anesthesia history of all surgical patients. Also assess for family history of reactions to anesthesia (malignant hyperthermia or perioperative death).
  - □ Monitor ECG, vital signs, electrolytes, and urine output continuously when administering IV for malignant hyperthermia.
  - □ Monitor patient for difficulty swallowing and choking during meals on the day of administration.
- ***Lab Test Considerations:*** Monitor liver function frequently during therapy. Liver function abnormalities (elevated AST, ALT, alkaline phosphatase, bilirubin, GGTP) may require discontinuation of therapy.
  - □ Renal function and CBC should be evaluated prior to and periodically during therapy in patients receiving prolonged therapy.

POTENTIAL NURSING DIAGNOSES

- Physical mobility, impaired (Indications).
- Pain (Indications).
- Injury, risk for (Side Effects).

IMPLEMENTATION

- **PO:** If gastric irritation becomes a problem, may be administered with food. Oral suspensions may be made by opening capsules and adding them to fruit juices or other liquid. Drink immediately after mixing.

- Oral dose for spasticity should be divided into 4 doses/day.
- **Direct IV:** Reconstitute each 20 mg with 60 ml of sterile water for injection without a bacteriostatic agent for a concentration of 333 mcg/ml. Shake until solution is clear. Solution must be used within 6 hr. Protect diluted solution from direct light.
- ***Rate:*** Administer each single dose by rapid continuous IV push through Y-tubing or 3-way stopcock. Follow immediately with subsequent doses as indicated. Medication is very irritating to tissues; observe infusion site frequently to avoid extravasation.
- **Intermittent Infusion:** Prophylactic dose has been administered as an infusion.
- ***Rate:*** Administer over 1 hr prior to anesthesia.

PATIENT/FAMILY TEACHING

- **General Info:** Advise patient not to take more medication than the amount prescribed to minimize risk of hepatotoxicity and other side effects. If a dose is missed, do not take unless remembered within 1 hr. Do not double doses.
- May cause dizziness, drowsiness, visual disturbances, and muscle weakness. Advise patient to avoid driving and other activities requiring alertness until response to drug is known. Following IV dose for surgery, patients may experience decreased grip strength, leg weakness, light-headedness, and difficulty swallowing for up to 48 hr. Caution patients to avoid activities requiring alertness and to use caution when walking down stairs and eating during this period.
- Advise patient to avoid taking alcohol or other CNS depressants concurrently with this medication.
- Instruct patient to notify health care professional if rash; itching; yellow eyes or skin; dark urine; or clay-colored, bloody, or black, tarry stools occur or if nausea, weakness, malaise, fatigue, or diarrhea persists. May require discontinuation of therapy.
- Advise patient to wear sunscreen and protective clothing to prevent photosensitivity reactions.
- Emphasize the importance of follow-up exams to check progress in long-term therapy and blood tests to monitor for side effects.
- **Malignant Hyperthermia:** Patients with malignant hyperthemia should carry identification describing disease process at all times.

EVALUATION

Effectiveness of therapy can be demonstrated by: ▪ Relief of muscle spasm in musculoskeletal conditions. One wk or more may be required to see improvement; if there is no observed improvement in 45 days, the medication is usually discontinued ▪ Prevention of or decrease in temperature and skeletal rigidity in malignant hyperthermia.

DAUNORUBICIN HYDROCHLORIDE

(daw-noe-**roo**-bi-sin)
Cerubidine

DAUNORUBICIN CITRATE LIPOSOME

(daw-noe-**roo**-bi-sin **lye**-poe-sohm)
DaunoXome

CLASSIFICATION(S):
Antineoplastics (antibiotic)

Pregnancy Category D

INDICATIONS

▪ **Daunorubicin HCl (Cerubidine):** Used in combination with other antineoplastic agents in the treatment of leukemias ▪ **Daunorubicin Citrate Liposome (DaunoXome):** Management of advanced Kaposi's sarcoma in HIV-infected patients.

ACTION

▪ Forms a complex with DNA, which subsequently inhibits DNA and RNA synthesis (cell-cycle phase–nonspecific) ▪ Encapsulation in a liposome (DaunoXome) increases uptake by tumor and decreases systemic toxicity. **Therapeutic Effects:** ▪ Death of rapidly replicating cells, particularly malignant ones. Also has immunosuppressive properties.

PHARMACOKINETICS

Absorption: Administered IV only, resulting in complete bioavailability. DaunoXome is released from the liposome following uptake by tumor.
Distribution: Widely distributed. Crosses the placenta.

Metabolism and Excretion: Extensively metabolized by the liver. Converted partially to a compound that also has antineoplastic activity (daunorubicinol); 40% eliminated by biliary excretion.
Half-life: *Daunorubicin HCl*—18.5 hr. *Daunorubicinol*—26.7 hr. *Daunorubicin citrate liposome*—55.4 hr.

CONTRAINDICATIONS AND PRECAUTIONS

Contraindicated in: ▪ Hypersensitivity to daunorubucin or any other components in the formulation ▪ Symptomatic congestive heart failure (for Cerubidine) ▪ Arrhythmias (for Cerubidine) ▪ Pregnant or lactating women.
Use Cautiously in: ▪ Patients with childbearing potential ▪ Active infections or decreased bone marrow reserve ▪ Geriatric patients or patients with other chronic debilitating illnesses (dosage reduction recommended for patients ≥60 yr for Cerubidine) ▪ May reactivate skin lesions produced by previous radiation therapy ▪ Children (safety not established for DaunoXome) ▪ Hepatic or renal impairment (dosage reduction recommended if serum creatinine >3 mg/dl or serum bilirubin >1.2 mg/dl) ▪ Patients who have received previous anthracycline therapy or who have underlying cardiovascular disease (increased risk of cardiotoxicity).

ADVERSE REACTIONS AND SIDE EFFECTS*

CNS: *DaunoXome*—fatigue, headache, depression, dizziness, insomnia, malaise.
EENT: rhinitis, abnormal vision, sinusitis.
CV: CARDIOTOXICITY; *Cerubidine*—arrhythmias; *DaunoXome*—chest pain, edema.
GI: nausea, vomiting; *Cerubidine*—esophagitis, stomatitis; *DaunoXome*—abdominal pain, anorexia, constipation, diarrhea, stomatitis, tenesmus.
GU: red urine, gonadal suppression.
Derm: alopecia; *DaunoXome*—increased sweating, pruritus.
Hemat: anemia, leukopenia, thrombocytopenia.
Local: phlebitis at IV site.
Metab: hyperuricemia.
MS: *DaunoXome*—back pain, arthralgia, myalgia.
Neuro: *DaunoXome*—neuropathy.
Misc: chills, fever; *DaunoXome*—allergic reactions, chills, fever, triad of back pain, flushing and chest tightness, influenza-like symptoms.

INTERACTIONS

Drug-Drug: ▪ Additive myelosuppression with other **antineoplastic agents** ▪ May decrease antibody response to **live virus vaccines** and increase risk of adverse reactions ▪ **Cyclophosphamide** increases the risk of cardiotoxicity.

ROUTE AND DOSAGE

❑ Daunorubicin Hydrochloride (Cerubidine)

Other dose regimens are used. In adults, cumulative dose should not exceed 550 mg/m² (450 mg/m² if previous chest radiation).

- **IV (Adults <60 yr):** 45 mg/m²/day for 3 days in first course, then for 2 days of second course (as part of combination regimen).
- **IV (Adults ≥60 yr):** 30 mg/m²/day for 3 days in first course, then for 2 days of second course (as part of combination regimen).
- **IV (Children >2 yr):** 25 mg/m² once weekly (as part of combination regimen). In children <2 yr or <0.5 m², dosage should be determined on a mg/kg basis.

❑ Daunorubicin Citrate Liposome (DaunoXome)

- **IV (Adults):** 40 mg/m²q 2 wk.

AVAILABILITY

❑ Daunorubicin Hydrochloride (Cerubidine)

- ***Powder for injection:*** 20 mg/vial[Rx].

❑ Daunorubicin Citrate Liposome (DaunoXome)

- ***Liposomal dispersion for injection:*** 2 mg/ml in 25-ml vial[Rx].

TIME/ACTION PROFILE (effects on blood counts)

	ONSET	PEAK	DURATION
IV (Cerubidine)	7–10 days	10–14 days	21 days
IV (Daunorubicin)	UK	UK	UK

*CAPITALS indicate life-threatening; underlines indicate most frequent.

NURSING IMPLICATIONS

ASSESSMENT

- ☐ Monitor vital signs prior to and frequently during therapy.
- ☐ Monitor for bone marrow depression. Assess for bleeding (bleeding gums, bruising, petechiae, guaiac stools, urine, and emesis) and avoid IM injections and rectal temperatures if platelet count is low. Apply pressure to venipuncture sites for 10 min. Assess for signs of infection during neutropenia. Anemia may occur. Monitor for increased fatigue, dyspnea, and orthostatic hypotension.
- ☐ Assess IV site frequently for inflammation or infiltration. Instruct patient to notify nurse immediately if pain or irritation at injection site occurs. If extravasation occurs, infusion must be stopped and restarted in another vein to avoid damage to SC tissue. Notify physician immediately. *Daunorubicin hydrocholride (Cerubidine)* is a vesicant. Standard treatments include local injections of steroids and application of ice compresses.
- ☐ Monitor intake and output, appetite, and nutritional intake. Assess for nausea and vomiting, which, although mild, may persist for 24–48 hr. Administration of an antiemetic prior to and periodically during therapy and adjusting diet as tolerated may help maintain fluid and electrolyte balance and nutritional status. Encourage fluid intake of 2000–3000 ml/day. Allopurinol and alkalinization of the urine may be used to help prevent urate stone formation.
- ☐ Assess patient for evidence of cardiotoxicity, which manifests as congestive heart failure (peripheral edema, dyspnea, rales/crackles, weight gain, jugular venous distention) and usually occurs 1–6 mo after initiation of therapy. Chest x ray, echocardiography, ECGs, and radionuclide angiography determination of ejection fraction may be ordered prior to and periodically throughout therapy. A 30% decrease in QRS voltage and decrease in systolic ejection fraction are early signs of cardiotoxicity. Patients who receive total cumulative doses >550/mm², who have a history of cardiac disease, or who have received mediastinal radiation are at greater risk of developing cardiotoxicity. May be irreversible and fatal, but usually responds to early treatment.
- ▪ **Daunorubicin Citrate Liposome:** Assess patient for back pain, flushing, and chest tightness. Usually occurs during first 5 min of infusion and subsides with interruption of therapy. Symptoms do not usually recur when infusion is restarted at a slower rate.
- ▪ ***Lab Test Considerations:*** Monitor uric acid levels.
- ☐ *Daunorubicin hydrochloride:* Monitor CBC and differential prior to and periodically throughout therapy. The leukocyte count nadir occurs 10–14 days after administration. Recovery usually occurs within 21 days after administration of daunorubicin.
- ☐ Monitor AST, ALT, LDH, and serum bilirubin. May cause transiently elevated serum alkaline phosphatase, bilirubin, and AST concentrations.
- ☐ *Daunorubicin citrate liposome:* Monitor CBC and differential prior to each course of therapy. May cause severe bone marrow depression, especially granulocytopenia. Repeat blood counts prior to each dose and do not administer if absolute granulocyte count is <750 cells/mm³.
- ☐ Monitor hepatic and renal function prior to each dose.

POTENTIAL NURSING DIAGNOSES

- ▪ Infection, risk for (Adverse Reactions).
- ▪ Cardiac output, decreased (Side Effects).
- ▪ Knowledge deficit, related to medication regimen (Patient/Family Teaching).

IMPLEMENTATION

- ▪ **General Info:** Do not confuse daunorubicin hydrochloride (Cerubidine) with daunorubicin citrate liposome (DaunoXome) or with doxorubicin (Adriamycin, Rubex). To prevent confusion, orders should include generic and brand name.
- ☐ Solution should be prepared in a biologic cabinet. Wear gloves, gown, and mask while handling IV medication. Discard IV equipment in specially designated containers (see Appendix I).

☐ Daunorubicin Hydrochloride (Cerubidine)

- ▪ **IV:** Reconstitute each 20 mg with 4 ml of sterile water for injection for a concentration of 5 mg/ml. Shake gently to dissolve. Reconstituted medication is stable for 24 hr at room

D

temperature, 48 hr if refrigerated. Protect from sunlight.

□ Do not use aluminum needles when reconstituting or injecting daunorubicin, as aluminum darkens the solution.

- **Direct IV:** Dilute further in 10–15 ml of 0.9% NaCl. Administer direct IV push through Y-site into free-flowing infusion of 0.9% NaCl or D5W.
- ***Rate:*** Administer over at least 2–3 min. Rapid administration rate may cause facial flushing or erythema along the vein.
- **Intermittent Infusion:** Has also been diluted in 50 or 100 ml of 0.9% NaCl.
- ***Rate:*** Administer 50 ml over 10–15 min or 100 ml over 30–45 min.
- **Y-Site Compatibility:** ▪ amifostine ▪ filgrastim ▪ melphalan ▪ methotrexate ▪ ondansetron ▪ sodium bicarbonate ▪ teniposide ▪ thiotepa ▪ vinorelbine.
- **Y-Site Incompatibility:** ▪ aztreonam ▪ cefepime ▪ fludarabine ▪ piperacillin/tazobactam.
- **Additive Incompatibility:** ▪ Manufacturer does not recommend admixing daunorubicin hydrochloride.

□ Daunorubicin Citrate Liposome (DaunoXome)

- **Intermittent Infusion:** Dilute with D5W for a concentration of 1 mg/ml. Do not use an in-line filter for infusion. Reconstituted infusion may be stored for up to 6 hr in refrigerator.
- ***Rate:*** Administer dose over 1 hr.
- **Additive Incompatibility:** ▪ Information unavailable. Do not admix with other solutions or medications.

PATIENT/FAMILY TEACHING

□ Instruct patient to notify health care professional if fever; chills; sore throat; signs of infection; bleeding gums; bruising; petechiae; or blood in urine, stool, or emesis occurs. Caution patient to avoid crowds and persons with known infections. Instruct patient to use soft toothbrush and electric razor. Patient should be cautioned not to drink alcoholic beverages or take products containing aspirin or NSAIDs.

□ Instruct patient to inspect oral mucosa for erythema and ulceration. If ulceration occurs, advise patient to use sponge brush and rinse mouth with water after eating and drinking. Stomatitis pain may require management with opioid analgesics. Period of highest risk is 3–7 days after administration of dose.

□ Instruct patient to notify health care professional immediately if irregular heartbeat, shortness of breath, or swelling of lower extremities occurs.

□ Discuss with patient possibility of hair loss. Explore methods of coping. Regrowth of hair usually begins within 5 wk after discontinuing therapy.

□ Inform patient that medication may turn urine reddish color for 1–2 days following administration.

□ Inform patient that this medication may cause irreversible gonadal suppression. Advise patient that this medication may have teratogenic effects. Contraception should be used during therapy and for at least 4 mo after therapy is concluded.

□ Instruct patient not to receive any vaccinations without advice of health care professional.

□ Emphasize the need for periodic lab tests to monitor for side effects.

EVALUATION

Effectiveness of therapy can be demonstrated by: ▪ Improvement of hematologic status in patients with leukemia ▪ Arrested progression of Kaposi's sarcoma in patients with HIV infection. Therapy is continued until there is evidence of progression (new visceral sites of involvement, progression of visceral disease, development of 10 or more new cutaneous lesions or 25% increase in the number of lesions at baseline, change in character of >25% of lesions from flat to raised, increase in surface area of lesions) or until complications of HIV disease preclude continuation of therapy.

DEFEROXAMINE

(de-fer-**ox**-a-meen)
Desferal

CLASSIFICATION(S):
Antidote (heavy metal antagonist)

Pregnancy Category C

INDICATIONS

- Management of acute toxic iron ingestion
- Management of secondary iron overload syn-

dromes associated with multiple transfusion therapy.

ACTION

▪ Chelates unbound iron, forming a water-soluble complex (ferrioxamine) in plasma that is easily excreted by the kidneys. **Therapeutic Effects:** ▪ Removal of excess iron. Also chelates aluminum.

PHARMACOKINETICS

Absorption: Poorly absorbed following oral administration. Well absorbed following IM administration and SC administration.
Distribution: Appears to be widely distributed.
Metabolism and Excretion: Metabolized by tissues and plasma enzymes. Unchanged drug and chelated form excreted by the kidneys; 33% of iron removed is eliminated in the feces via biliary excretion.
Half-life: 1 hr.

CONTRAINDICATIONS AND PRECAUTIONS

Contraindicated in: ▪ Early pregnancy or childbearing potential (however, may be used safely in pregnant patients with moderate to severe acute iron intoxication) ▪ Severe renal disease ▪ Anuria.
Use Cautiously in: ▪ Children <3 yr (safety not established).

ADVERSE REACTIONS AND SIDE EFFECTS*

EENT: blurred vision, cataracts, ototoxicity.
CV: hypotension, tachycardia.
GI: abdominal pain, diarrhea.
GU: red urine.
Derm: erythema, flushing, urticaria.
Local: induration at injection site, pain at injection site.
MS: leg cramps.
Misc: allergic reactions, fever, shock following rapid IV administration.

INTERACTIONS

Drug-Drug: ▪ **Ascorbic acid** may increase the effectiveness of deferoxamine but may also increase cardiac iron toxicity.

ROUTE AND DOSAGE

❑ Acute Iron Ingestion

- **IM, IV (Adults and Children ≥3 yr):** 1 g (20 mg/kg or 600 mg/m^2), then 500 mg (10 mg/kg or 300 mg/m^2) q 4 hr for 2 doses. Additional doses of 500 mg (10 mg/kg or 300 mg/m^2) q 4–12 hr may be needed (not to exceed 6 g/24 hr).

❑ Chronic Iron Overload

- **IM, IV (Adults and Children ≥3 yr):** 500 mg–1 g daily; additional doses of 2 g should be given IV for each unit of blood transfused.
- **SC (Adults and Children ≥3 yr):** 1–2 g/day (20–40 mg/kg/day) infused over 8–24 hr.

AVAILABILITY

▪ ***Injection:*** 500 mg/vial^{Rx}.

TIME/ACTION PROFILE (effects on hematologic parameters)

	ONSET	PEAK	DURATION
IV	rapid	UK	UK
IM	UK	UK	UK
SC	UK	UK	UK

NURSING IMPLICATIONS

ASSESSMENT

- ❑ In acute poisoning, assess time, amount, and type of iron preparation ingested.
- ❑ Monitor signs of iron toxicity: early acute (abdominal pain, bloody diarrhea, emesis), late acute (decreased level of consciousness, shock, metabolic acidosis).
- ❑ Monitor vital signs closely, especially during IV administration. Report hypotension, erythema, urticaria, or signs of allergic reaction. Keep epinephrine, an antihistamine, and resuscitation equipment close by in the event of an anaphylactic reaction.
- ❑ May cause oculotoxicity or ototoxicity. Report decreased visual acuity or hearing loss. Audiovisual exams should be performed every 3 mo in patients with chronic iron overload.
- ❑ Monitor intake and output and urine color. Inform physician or other health care professional if patient is anuric. Chelated iron is ex-

*CAPITALS indicate life-threatening; underlines indicate most frequent.

creted primarily by the kidneys; urine may turn red.

- *Lab Test Considerations:* Monitor serum iron, total iron binding capacity (TIBC), ferritin levels, and urinary iron excretion prior to and periodically throughout therapy.
- □ Monitor liver function studies to assess damage from iron poisoning.

POTENTIAL NURSING DIAGNOSES

- Injury, risk for poisoning (Patient/Family Teaching).
- Knowledge deficit, related to medication regimen (Patient/Family Teaching).

IMPLEMENTATION

- **General Info:** Reconstitute 500-mg vial with 2 ml of sterile water for injection. Dissolve powder completely prior to administration. Solution is stable for 1 wk after reconstitution if protected from light.
- □ Used in conjunction with induction of emesis or gastric aspiration and lavage with sodium bicarbonate, and supportive measures for shock and metabolic acidosis in acute poisoning.
- **Trial Dose:** May be administered between 2–4 hr after ingestion of iron and after GI tract has been cleaned out. Monitor urine for color change (orange-rose color indicates significant iron ingestion) until serum iron and total iron binding capacity results are available.
- □ May be administered IM or by IV infusion over 4 hr.
- **IM:** Administer deep IM and massage well. Rotate sites. IM administration may cause transient severe pain.
- **SC:** SC route is used to treat chronically elevated iron levels.
- □ Therapy is administered into abdominal subcutaneous tissue via infusion pump for 8–24 hr per treatment.
- **IV:** Reconstitute, then further dilute in D5W, 0.9% NaCl, or lactated Ringer's solution.
- ***Rate:*** Maximum infusion rate is 15 mg/kg/hr. Rapid infusion rate may cause hypotension, erythema, urticaria, wheezing, convulsions, tachycardia, or shock.
- □ May be administered at the same time as blood transfusion in persons with chronically elevated serum iron levels. Use separate site for administration.

PATIENT/FAMILY TEACHING

- □ Reinforce need to keep iron preparations, all medications, and hazardous substances out of the reach of children.
- □ Reassure patient that red coloration of urine is expected and reflects excretion of excess iron.
- □ Advise patient not to take vitamin C preparations without consulting health care professional, as tissue toxicity may increase.
- □ Encourage patients requiring chronic therapy to keep follow-up appointments for lab tests. Eye and hearing exams may be monitored every 3 mo.

EVALUATION

Effectiveness of therapy can be demonstrated by: ▪ Return of serum iron concentrations to a normal level (50–150 mcg/100 ml).

DESMOPRESSIN

(des-moe-**press**-in)
DDAVP, DDAVP Rhinal Tube, DDAVP Rhinyle Drops, Stimate

CLASSIFICATION(S):
Hormone (antidiuretic)

Pregnancy Category B

INDICATIONS

▪ **Intranasal:** Management of primary nocturnal enuresis unresponsive to other treatment modalities ▪ **PO, SC, IV, Intranasal:** Treatment of diabetes insipidus caused by a deficiency of vasopressin ▪ **Intranasal:** Controls bleeding in certain types of hemophilia and von Willebrand's disease.

ACTION

▪ An analogue of naturally occurring vasopressin (antidiuretic hormone). Primary action is enhanced reabsorption of water in the kidneys. **Therapeutic Effects:** ▪ Prevention of nocturnal enuresis ▪ Maintenance of appropriate body water content in diabetes insipidus ▪ Control of bleeding in certain types of hemophilia or von Willebrand's disease.

PHARMACOKINETICS

Absorption: 5% absorbed following oral administration; some 10–20% absorbed from nasal mucosa.
Distribution: Distribution not fully known. Enters breast milk.
Metabolism and Excretion: UK.
Half-life: 75 min.

CONTRAINDICATIONS AND PRECAUTIONS

Contraindicated in: ▪ Hypersensitivity ▪ Hypersensitivity to chlorobutanol ▪ Patients with type IIB or platelet-type (pseudo) von Willebrand's disease.
Use Cautiously in: ▪ Angina pectoris ▪ Hypertension ▪ Pregnancy or lactation (safety not established).

ADVERSE REACTIONS AND SIDE EFFECTS

CNS: drowsiness, headache, listlessness.
EENT: *intranasal*—nasal congestion, rhinitis.
Resp: dyspnea.
CV: hypertension, hypotension, tachycardia (large IV doses only).
GI: mild abdominal cramps, nausea.
GU: vulval pain.
Derm: flushing.
F and E: water intoxication/hyponatremia.
Local: phlebitis at IV site.

INTERACTIONS

Drug-Drug: ▪ **Chlorpropamide, clofibrate,** or **carbamazepine** may enhance the antidiuretic response to desmopressin ▪ **Demeclocycline, lithium,** or **norepinephrine** may diminish the antidiuretic response to desmopressin ▪ Large doses may enhance the effects of vasopressors.

ROUTE AND DOSAGE

❑ **Primary Nocturnal Enuresis**

- **Intranasal (Adults and Children ≥6 yr):** 20 mcg (10 mcg in each nostril) at bedtime (range 10–40 mcg).

❑ **Diabetes Insipidus**

- **PO (Adults):** 0.05 mg twice daily; adjusted as needed (usual range 0.1–1.2 mg/day in 2–3 divided doses).
- **PO (Children):** 0.05 mg daily initially; adjusted as needed.
- **Intranasal (Adults):** *Using nasal tube delivery system or spray pump (0.1 mg/ml)*—0.1–0.4 ml/day as a single dose or 2–3 divided doses.
- **Intranasal (Children 3 mo–12 yr):** *Using nasal tube delivery system or spray pump (0.1 mg/ml)*—0.05–0.3 ml/day as a single dose or 2 divided doses.
- **SC, IV (Adults):** 2–4 mcg/day in 2 divided doses.

❑ **Antihemorrhagic**

- **IV (Adults and Children >3 mo):** 0.3 mcg/kg repeated as needed.
- **Intranasal (Adults and Children ≥50 kg):** 1 spray (150 mcg) in each nostril.
- **Intranasal (Adults and Children <50 kg):** 1 spray in one nostril (150 mcg).

D

AVAILABILITY

▪ ***Tablets:*** 0.1 mg Rx, 0.2 mg Rx ▪ ***Nasal spray pump:*** 10 mcg/spray–5-ml bottle (0.1 mg/ml) contains 50 doses (DDAVP) Rx ▪ ***Rhinal tube delivery system-nasal solution:*** 2.5-ml vials with applicator tubes (0.1 mg/ml) Rx ▪ ***Nasal solution:*** 1.5 mg/ml (150 mcg/dose) in 2.5-ml bottle (contains 25 doses) Rx ▪ ***Injection:*** 4 mcg/ml Rx, 15 mcg/ml Rx.

TIME/ACTION PROFILE (PO, intranasal = antidiuretic effect; IV = effect on factor VIII activity)

	ONSET	PEAK	DURATION
PO	1 hr	4–7 hr	UK
Intranasal	1 hr	1–5 hr	8–20 hr
IV	within min	15–30 min	3 hr*

*4–24 hr in mild hemophilia A.

NURSING IMPLICATIONS

ASSESSMENT

- **General Info:** Chronic intranasal use may cause tolerance or if administered more frequently than every 24–48 hr IV tachyphylaxis (short-term tolerance) may develop.
- **Nocturnal Enuresis:** Monitor frequency of enuresis throughout therapy.
- **Diabetes Insipidus:** Monitor urine and plasma osmolality and urine volume frequently. Assess patient for symptoms of dehydration (excessive thirst, dry skin and mucous membranes, tachycardia, poor skin

turgor). Weigh patient daily and assess for edema.

- **Hemophilia:** Monitor plasma factor VIII coagulant, factor VIII antigen, and ristocetin cofactor. May also assess activated partial thromboplastin time (aPTT) for hemophilia A and skin bleeding time for von Willebrand's disease. Assess patient for signs of bleeding.
- □ Monitor blood pressure and pulse during IV infusion.
- □ Monitor intake and output and adjust fluid intake (especially in children and elderly) to avoid overhydration in patients receiving desmopressin for hemophilia.
- ***Toxicity and Overdose:*** Signs and symptoms of water intoxication include confusion, drowsiness, headache, weight gain, difficulty urinating, seizures, and coma.
- □ Treatment of overdose includes decreasing dosage and, if symptoms are severe, administration of furosemide.

POTENTIAL NURSING DIAGNOSES

- Fluid volume deficit (Indications).
- Fluid volume excess (Adverse Reactions).
- Knowledge deficit, related to medication regimen (Patient/Family Teaching).

IMPLEMENTATION

- **General Info:** IV desmopressin has 10 times the antidiuretic effect of intranasal desmopressin.
- **PO:** Begin oral doses 12 hr after last intranasal dose. Monitor response closely.
- **Diabetes Insipidus:** Parenteral dose for antidiuretic effect is administered direct IV or SC.
- **Hemophilia:** Parenteral dose for control of bleeding is administered via IV infusion. If used preoperatively, administer 30 min prior to procedure.
- **Direct IV:** Administer each dose over 1 min for diabetes insipidus.
- **Intermittent Infusion:** Dilute each dose in 50 ml of 0.9% NaCl for adults and children >10 kg and in 10 ml in children weighing <10 kg.
- ***Rate:*** Infuse slowly over 15–30 min for hemophilia.
- **Intranasal:** If intranasal dose is used preoperatively, administer 2 hr before procedure.

PATIENT/FAMILY TEACHING

- **General Info:** Advise patient to notify health care professional if bleeding is not controlled or if headache, dyspnea, heartburn, nausea, abdominal cramps, vulval pain, or severe nasal congestion or irritation occurs.
- □ Caution patient to avoid concurrent use of alcohol with this medication.
- **Diabetes Insipidus:** Instruct patient on intranasal administration. Medication is supplied with a flexible calibrated catheter (rhinyle). Draw solution into rhinyle. Insert one end of tube into nostril, blow on the other end to deposit solution deep into nasal cavity. An air-filled syringe may be attached to the plastic catheter for children, infants, or obtunded patients. Tube should be rinsed under water after each use.
- □ If nasal spray is used, prime pump prior to first use by pressing down 4 times. Caution patient that nasal spray should not be used beyond the labeled number of sprays; subsequent sprays may not deliver accurate dose. Do not attempt to transfer remaining solution to another bottle.
- □ If a dose is missed, instruct patient to take it as soon as remembered but not if it is almost time for the next dose. Do not double doses.
- □ Advise patient that rhinitis or upper respiratory infection may decrease effectiveness of this therapy. If increased urine output occurs, patient should contact health care professional for dosage adjustment.
- □ Patients with diabetes insipidus should carry identification describing disease process and medication regimen at all times.

EVALUATION

Effectiveness of therapy can be demonstrated by: ■ Decreased frequency of nocturnal enuresis ■ Decrease in urine volume □ Relief of polydipsia □ Increased urine osmolality ■ Control of bleeding in hemophilia.

DEXRAZOXANE

(dex-ra-**zox**-ane)

Zinecard

CLASSIFICATION(S):
Cardioprotective agent

Pregnancy Category C

INDICATIONS

▪ Reducing incidence and severity of cardiomyopathy from doxorubicin in women with metastatic breast cancer who have already received a cumulative dose of doxorubicin >300 mg/m².

ACTION

▪ Acts as an intracellular chelating agent. **Therapeutic Effects:** ▪ Diminishes the cardiotoxic effects of doxorubicin.

PHARMACOKINETICS

Absorption: IV administration results in complete bioavailability.
Distribution: UK.
Metabolism and Excretion: Some metabolism occurs; 42% eliminated in urine.
Half-life: 2.1–2.5 hr.

CONTRAINDICATIONS AND PRECAUTIONS

Contraindicated in: ▪ Any other type of chemotherapy except other anthracyclines (doxorubicin-like agents).
Use Cautiously in: ▪ Pregnancy, lactation, or children (safety not established).

ADVERSE REACTIONS AND SIDE EFFECTS

Hemat: myelosuppression.
Local: pain at injection site.

INTERACTIONS

Drug-Drug: ▪ Myelosuppression may be additive with **antineoplastic agents** or **radiation therapy.** Antitumor effects of concurrent combination chemotherapy with **fluorouracil** and **cyclophosphamide** may be diminished by dexrazoxane.

ROUTE AND DOSAGE

▪ **IV (Adults):** 10 mg of dexrazoxane/1 mg doxorubicin.

AVAILABILITY

▪ ***Injection:*** 250-mg vial^Rx^, 500-mg vial^Rx^.

TIME/ACTION PROFILE (cardioprotective effect)

	ONSET	PEAK	DURATION
IV	rapid	UK	UK

NURSING IMPLICATIONS

ASSESSMENT

□ Assess extent of cardiomyopathy (cardiomegaly on x ray, basilar rales, S_3 gallop, dyspnea, decline in left ventricular ejection fraction) prior to and periodically throughout therapy.
▪ ***Lab Test Considerations:*** Monitor CBC and platelet count frequently throughout therapy. Thrombocytopenia, leukopenia, and granulocytopenia from chemotherapy may be more severe at nadir with dexrazoxane therapy.

POTENTIAL NURSING DIAGNOSES

▪ Cardiac output, decreased (Indications).
▪ Pain, acute (Side Effects).
▪ Knowledge deficit, related to medication regimen (Patient/Family Teaching).

IMPLEMENTATION

▪ **General Info:** Doxorubicin should be administered within 30 min following dexrazoxane administration.
□ Solution should be prepared in a biologic cabinet. Wear gloves, gown, and mask while handling IV medication. Discard IV equipment in specially designated containers (see Appendix I).
□ Do not administer solutions that are discolored or contain particulate matter. Reconstituted solution and diluted solution are stable in an IV bag for 6 hr at room temperature or if refrigerated. Discard unused solutions.
▪ **Direct IV:** Reconstitute dexrazoxane with 0.167 molar (M/6) sodium lactate injection for a concentration of 10 mg/ml.
▪ ***Rate:*** Administer via slow IV push.
▪ **Intermittent Infusion:** Reconstituted solution may also be diluted with 0.9% NaCl or D5W for a concentration of 1.3– 5.0 mg/ml. Solution is stable for 6 hr at room temperature or refrigerated.
▪ ***Rate:*** May also be administered via rapid IV infusion.
▪ **Additive Incompatibility:** ▪ Do not mix with other medications.

PATIENT/FAMILY TEACHING

□ Explain the purpose of the medication to the patient.

D

- Emphasize the need for continued monitoring of cardiac function.

EVALUATION

Effectiveness of therapy can be demonstrated by: ▪ Reduction of incidence and severity of cardiomyopathy associated with doxorubicin administration in women with metastatic breast cancer.

DEXTROAMPHETAMINE

(dex-troe-am-**fet**-a-meen)
Dexedrine, Dextrostat

CLASSIFICATION(S):
CNS stimulant

Schedule II
Pregnancy Category C

INDICATIONS

▪ Treatment of narcolepsy ▪ Adjunct in the management of attention-deficit hyperactivity disorder (ADHD).

ACTION

▪ Produces CNS stimulation by releasing norepinephrine from nerve endings. Pharmacologic effects: ▫ CNS and respiratory stimulation ▫ Vasoconstriction ▫ Mydriasis (pupillary dilation) ▫ Contraction of the urinary bladder sphincter. **Therapeutic Effects:** ▪ Increased motor activity and mental alertness and decreased fatigue in narcoleptic patients ▪ Increased attention span in ADHD.

PHARMACOKINETICS

Absorption: Well absorbed following oral administration.
Distribution: Widely distributed with high concentrations in the brain and CSF. Crosses the placenta; enters breast milk; potentially embryotoxic.
Metabolism and Excretion: Some metabolism by the liver. Urinary excretion is pH-dependent. Alkaline urine promotes reabsorption and prolongs action.
Half-life: 10–12 hr (6.8 hr in children).

CONTRAINDICATIONS AND PRECAUTIONS

Contraindicated in: ▪ Pregnancy or lactation ▪ Hyperexcitable states, including hyperthyroidism ▪ Psychotic personalities ▪ Suicidal or homicidal tendencies ▪ Chemical dependence ▪ Glaucoma ▪ Some products contain tartrazine and should be avoided in patients with known hypersensitivity.
Use Cautiously in: ▪ Cardiovascular disease ▪ Hypertension ▪ Diabetes mellitus ▪ Elderly or debilitated patients ▪ Continual use (may result in psychological dependence or physical addiction).

ADVERSE REACTIONS AND SIDE EFFECTS*

CNS: hyperactivity, insomnia, restlessness, tremor, depression, dizziness, headache, irritability.
CV: palpitations, tachycardia, arrhythmias, hypertension, hypotension.
GI: anorexia, constipation, cramps, diarrhea, dry mouth, metallic taste, nausea, vomiting.
GU: impotence, increased libido.
Derm: urticaria.
Misc: physical dependence, psychological dependence.

INTERACTIONS

Drug-Drug: ▪ Additive adrenergic effects with other **adrenergic agents** ▪ Use with **MAO inhibitors** can result in hypertensive crisis ▪ Alkalinizing the urine **(sodium bicarbonate, acetazolamide)** prolongs effect ▪ Acidification of urine **(ammonium chloride,** large doses of **ascorbic acid)** decreases effect ▪ **Phenothiazines** may decrease the effect of dextroamphetamine ▪ May antagonize the response to **antihypertensives** ▪ Increased risk of cardiovascular side effects with **beta blockers** or **tricyclic antidepressants.**

ROUTE AND DOSAGE

▫ Attention-Deficit Hyperactivity Disorder

- **PO (Adults):** 5–60 mg/day in divided doses. Sustained-release capsules should not be used as initial therapy.
- **PO (Children ≥6 yr):** 5 mg 1–2 times

***CAPITALS indicate life-threatening; underlines indicate most frequent.**

daily, increase by 5 mg at weekly intervals. Sustained-release capsules should not be used as initial therapy.

- **PO (Children 3–5 yr):** 2.5 mg/day, increase by 2.5 mg at weekly intervals.

□ **Narcolepsy**

- **PO (Adults):** 5–60 mg/day single dose or in divided doses. Sustained-release capsules should not be used as initial therapy.
- **PO (Children ≥12 yr):** 10 mg/day, increase by 10 mg/day at weekly intervals until response is obtained or adult dose is reached.
- **PO (Children 6–12 yr):** 5 mg/day, increase by 5 mg/day at weekly intervals until response is obtained or adult dose is reached.

AVAILABILITY

■ ***Tablets:*** 5 mg[Rx], 10 mg[Rx] ■ ***Sustained-release capsules:*** 5 mg[Rx], 10 mg[Rx], 15 mg[Rx] ■ ***In combination with:*** amphetamine (Adderall)[Rx]. See Appendix A.

TIME/ACTION PROFILE (CNS stimulation)

	ONSET	PEAK	DURATION
PO	1–2 hr	UK	2–10 hr
PO-ER	UK	UK	up to 24 hr

NURSING IMPLICATIONS

ASSESSMENT

- **General Info:** Monitor blood pressure, pulse, and respiration before administering and periodically throughout therapy.
- **Attention-Deficit Hyperactivity Disorder:** Monitor weight biweekly and inform physician of significant loss. Monitor height periodically in children; report growth inhibition.
- □ Assess attention span, impulse control, motor and vocal tics, and interactions with others in patients with ADHD.
- **Narcolepsy:** Observe and document frequency of narcoleptic episodes.
- □ May produce a false sense of euphoria and well-being. Provide frequent rest periods and observe patient for rebound depression after the effects of the medication have worn off.
- □ Has high dependence and abuse potential. Tolerance to medication occurs rapidly; do not increase dose.
- ***Lab Test Considerations:*** May interfere with urinary steroid determinations.
- □ May cause increased plasma corticosteroid concentrations; greatest in evening.

POTENTIAL NURSING DIAGNOSES

- Thought processes, altered (Side Effects).
- Knowledge deficit, related to medication regimen (Patient/Family Teaching).

IMPLEMENTATION

- **General Info:** Therapy should utilize the lowest effective dose.
- **PO:** Sustained-release capsules should be swallowed whole; do not break, crush, or chew.
- **Attention-Deficit Hyperactivity Disorder:** When symptoms are controlled, dose reduction or interruption of therapy may be possible during summer months or may be given on each of the 5 school days with medication-free weekends and holidays.

D

PATIENT/FAMILY TEACHING

- **General Info:** Instruct patient to take medication at least 6 hr before bedtime to avoid sleep disturbances. Missed doses should be taken as soon as remembered up to 6 hr before bedtime. Do not double doses. Instruct patient not to alter dosage without consulting health care professional. Abrupt cessation of high doses may cause extreme fatigue and mental depression.
- □ Inform patient that the effects of drug-induced dry mouth can be minimized by rinsing frequently with water or chewing sugarless gum or candies.
- □ Advise patient to avoid the intake of large amounts of caffeine.
- □ Medication may impair judgment. Advise patients to use caution when driving or during other activities requiring alertness.
- □ Advise patient to notify health care professional if nervousness, restlessness, insomnia, dizziness, anorexia, or dry mouth becomes severe.
- □ Inform patient that periodic holiday from the drug may be ordered to assess progress and decrease dependence.

EVALUATION

Effectiveness of therapy can be demonstrated by: ■ Improved attention span. Therapy should be interrupted and need reassessed periodically ■ Decrease in narcoleptic symptoms.

DEXTROMETHORPHAN

(dex-troe-meth-**or**-fan)

{Balminil DM}, Benylin Adult, Benylin Pediatric, {Broncho-Grippol-DM}, {Calmylin #1}, Children's Hold, Creo-Terpin, Delsym, {DM Syrup}, Drix-oral Liquid Cough Caps, Hold, {Kof-fex}, Mediquell, {Neo-DM}, {Or-nex·DM}, Pertussin Cough Suppressant, Pertussin CS, Pertus-sin ES, {Robidex}, Robitussin Cough Calmers, Robitussin Maximum Strength Cough Suppressant, Robi-tussin Pediatric, {Sedatuss}, Sucrets Cough Control Formula, Vicks For-mula 44 Pediatric Formula

CLASSIFICATION(S):
Antitussive

Pregnancy Category UK

INDICATIONS

▪ Symptomatic relief of coughs caused by minor viral upper respiratory tract infections or inhaled irritants ▪ Most effective for chronic nonproductive cough ▪ A common ingredient in nonprescription cough and cold preparations.

ACTION

▪ Suppresses the cough reflex by a direct effect on the cough center in the medulla. Related to opioids structurally but has no analgesic properties. **Therapeutic Effects:** ▪ Relief of irritating nonproductive cough.

PHARMACOKINETICS

Absorption: Rapidly absorbed from the GI tract. Extended-release product is slowly absorbed.
Distribution: Distribution not known. Probably crosses the placenta and enters breast milk.
Metabolism and Excretion: Metabolized to dextrorphan, an active metabolite. Dextromethorphan and dextrorphan are renally excreted.
Half-life: UK.

CONTRAINDICATIONS AND PRECAUTIONS

Contraindicated in: ▪ Hypersensitivity ▪ Patients taking MAO inhibitors or selective serotonin reuptake inhibitors (SSRIs) ▪ Should not be used for chronic productive coughs ▪ Some products contain alcohol and should be avoided in patients with known intolerance.
Use Cautiously in: ▪ Cough that lasts more than 1 wk or is accompanied by fever, rash, or headache—health care professional should be consulted ▪ Diabetes (some products contain sucrose) ▪ Pregnancy (has been used safely) ▪ Lactation or children <2 yr (safety not established).

ADVERSE REACTIONS AND SIDE EFFECTS

CNS: *high dose:* dizziness, sedation.
GI: nausea.

INTERACTIONS

Drug-Drug: ▪ Use with **MAO inhibitors** or **SSRIs** may result in serotonin syndrome (nausea, confusion, changes in blood pressure). Concurrent use should be avoided; may result in excitation, hypotension, and hyperpyrexia ▪ Additive CNS depression with **antihistamines, alcohol, antidepressants, sedative/hypnotics,** or **opioids** ▪ **Quinidine** may increase blood levels and side effects of dextromethorphan.

ROUTE AND DOSAGE

- **PO (Adults and Children >12 yr):** 10–20 mg q 4 hr or 30 mg q 6–8 hr or 60 mg of extended-release preparation bid (not to exceed 120 mg/day).
- **PO (Children 6–12 yr):** 5–10 mg q 4 hr or 15 mg q 6–8 hr or 30 mg of extended-release preparation q 12 hr (not to exceed 60 mg/day).
- **PO (Children 2–6 yr):** 2.5–5 mg q 4 hr or 7.5 mg q 6–8 hr or 15 mg of extended-release preparation q 12 hr (not to exceed 30 mg/day).

AVAILABILITY

▪ ***Lozenges:*** 2.5 mg^{OTC}, 5 mg^{OTC} ▪ ***Liquid:*** 3.5 mg/5 ml^{OTC}, 7.5 mg/5 ml^{OTC}, 15 mg/5 ml^{OTC}

▪ ***Syrup:*** 15 mg/15 ml[OTC], 10 mg/5 ml[OTC] ▪ ***Extended-release suspension:*** 30 mg/5 ml[OTC] ▪ ***In combination with:*** antihistamines, decongestants, and expectorants in cough and cold preparations. See Appendix A.

TIME/ACTION PROFILE (cough suppression)

	ONSET	PEAK	DURATION
PO	15–30 min	UK	3–6 hr
PO-ER	UK	UK	9–12 hr

NURSING IMPLICATIONS

ASSESSMENT

- **General Info:** Assess frequency and nature of cough, lung sounds, and amount and type of sputum produced. Unless contraindicated, maintain fluid intake of 1500–2000 ml to decrease viscosity of bronchial secretions.

POTENTIAL NURSING DIAGNOSES

- Airway clearance, ineffective (Indications).
- Knowledge deficit, related to medication regimen (Patient/Family Teaching).

IMPLEMENTATION

- **General Info:** Dextromethorphan 15–30 mg is equivalent in cough suppression to codeine 8–15 mg.
- **PO:** Do not give fluids immediately after administering to prevent dilution of vehicle. Shake oral suspension well before administration.

PATIENT/FAMILY TEACHING

- □ Instruct patient to cough effectively: Sit upright and take several deep breaths before attempting to cough.
- □ Advise patient to minimize cough by avoiding irritants, such as cigarette smoke, fumes, and dust. Humidification of environmental air, frequent sips of water, and sugarless hard candy may also decrease the frequency of dry, irritating cough.
- □ Caution patient to avoid taking alcohol or other CNS depressants concurrently with this medication.
- □ May occasionally cause dizziness. Caution patient to avoid driving or other activities requiring alertness until response to the medication is known.
- □ Advise patient that any cough lasting over 1 wk or accompanied by fever, chest pain, persistent headache, or skin rash warrants medical attention.

EVALUATION

Effectiveness of therapy can be demonstrated by: ▪ Decrease in frequency and intensity of cough without eliminating patient's cough reflex.

DEXTROSE

glucose, Glutose, Insta-glucose, Insulin Reaction

CLASSIFICATION(S):
Caloric agent (carbohydrate)

Pregnancy Category C

INDICATIONS

▪ **IV:** Lower-concentration (2.5–11.5%) injection provides hydration and calories ▪ Higher concentrations (up to 70%) treat hypoglycemia and in combination with amino acids provide calories for parenteral nutrition ▪ **PO:** Corrects hypoglycemia in conscious patients.

ACTION

▪ Provides calories. **Therapeutic Effects:** ▪ Provision of calories ▪ Prevention and treatment of hypoglycemia.

PHARMACOKINETICS

Absorption: Well absorbed following oral administration.
Distribution: Widely distributed and rapidly utilized.
Metabolism and Excretion: Metabolized to carbon dioxide and water. When renal threshold is exceeded, dextrose is excreted unchanged by the kidneys.
Half-life: UK.

CONTRAINDICATIONS AND PRECAUTIONS

Contraindicated in: ▪ Allergy to corn or corn products ▪ Hypertonic solution (>5%) should not be given to patients with CNS bleeding or anuria or who are at risk of dehydration.
Use Cautiously in: ▪ Known diabetic patients (frequent lab assessment necessary to quantitate appropriate doses) ▪ Chronic alcoholics or se-

D

verely malnourished patients (administration requires initial pretreatment with thiamine).

ADVERSE REACTIONS AND SIDE EFFECTS

Endo: inappropriate insulin secretion (long-term use).
F and E: fluid overload, hypokalemia, hypomagnesemia, hypophosphatemia.
Local: local pain and irritation at IV site (hypertonic solution).
Metab: glycosuria, hyperglycemia.

INTERACTIONS

Drug-Drug: ▪ Will alter requirements for **insulin** or **oral hypoglycemic agents** in diabetic patients.

ROUTE AND DOSAGE

❑ Hydration (as 5% solution)

- **IV (Adults and Children):** 0.5–0.8 g/kg/hr.

❑ Hypoglycemia

- **PO (Adults and Children):** *Conscious patients*—10–20 g, may repeat in 10–20 min.
- **IV (Adults):** 20–50 ml of 50% solution infused slowly (3 ml/min).
- **IV (Infants and Neonates):** 250–500 mg/kg/dose (as 25% dextrose); repeated doses of 10–12 ml of 25% dextrose may be required.

AVAILABILITY

▪ ***Oral gel:*** 40% in 25-g and 30-g tubes and 80-g bottle[OTC] ▪ ***Chewable tablets:*** 5 g[OTC] ▪ ***Solution for injection:*** 2.5%[Rx], 5%[Rx], 10%[Rx], 20%[Rx], 25%[Rx], 30%[Rx], 40%[Rx], 50%[Rx], 60%[Rx], 70%[Rx] ▪ ***In combination with:*** sodium chloride, other electrolytes, and amino acids.

TIME/ACTION PROFILE (effects on blood sugar in diabetic patients)

	ONSET	PEAK	DURATION
PO	rapid	rapid	brief
IV	rapid	rapid	brief

NURSING IMPLICATIONS

ASSESSMENT

- ❑ Assess the hydration status of patients receiving IV dextrose. Monitor intake and output and electrolyte concentrations. Assess patient for dehydration or edema.
- ❑ Assess nutritional status, function of gastrointestinal tract, and caloric needs of patient.
- ❑ Diabetics and patients receiving hypertonic dextrose solution (>5%) should have serum glucose monitored regularly.
- ❑ Monitor IV site frequently for phlebitis and infection.
- ▪ ***Lab Test Considerations:*** May cause an elevated serum glucose level.

POTENTIAL NURSING DIAGNOSES

- Fluid volume deficit (Indications).
- Nutrition, altered, less than body requirements (Indications).
- Fluid volume excess (Adverse Reactions).

IMPLEMENTATION

- ▪ **General Info:** Dextrose solution alone does not contain enough calories to sustain an individual for a prolonged period. Dextrose contains 3.4 kcal/g. D5W contains 170 cal/liter and D10W contains 340 cal/liter.
- ▪ **PO:** Concentrated dextrose gels and chewable tablets may be used in the treatment of hypoglycemia in conscious patients. The dose should be repeated if symptoms persist and serum glucose has not increased by at least 20 mg/100 ml within 20 min. May be followed by more complex carbohydrates.
- ▪ **IV:** Hypertonic dextrose solution (>10%) should be administered IV into a central vein. For emergency treatment of hypoglycemia, administer slowly into a large peripheral vein to prevent phlebitis or sclerosis of the vein. Assess IV site frequently. Rapid infusions may cause hyperglycemia or fluid shifts. When hypertonic solution is discontinued, taper solution and administer D5W or D10W to prevent rebound hypoglycemia.
- ❑ Patients requiring prolonged infusions of dextrose should have electrolytes added to the dextrose solution to prevent water intoxication and maintain fluid and electrolyte balance.
- ▪ **Additive Incompatibility:** ▪ whole blood.

PATIENT/FAMILY TEACHING

- ❑ Explain the purpose of dextrose administration to patient.
- ❑ Instruct diabetic patient on the correct method for self–blood glucose monitoring.

□ Advise patient on when and how to administer dextrose products for hypoglycemia.

EVALUATION

Effectiveness of therapy can be demonstrated by: ▪ Correction and maintenance of adequate hydration status and normal serum glucose levels ▪ Maintenance of adequate caloric intake.

DEZOCINE

(**dez**-oh-seen)
Dalgan

CLASSIFICATION(S):
Opioid analgesic (agonist/antagonist)

Pregnancy Category C

INDICATIONS

▪ Short-term management of moderate to severe pain.

ACTION

▪ Binds to opiate receptors in the CNS ▪ Alters the perception of and the response to painful stimuli, while causing generalized CNS depression ▪ Has partial antagonist properties, which may result in opioid withdrawal in physically dependent patients. **Therapeutic Effects:** ▪ Relief of moderate to severe pain.

PHARMACOKINETICS

Absorption: Rapidly and completely absorbed following IM administration.
Distribution: UK.
Metabolism and Excretion: Mostly metabolized by the liver; <1% excreted unchanged by the kidneys.
Half-life: 2.4 hr (range 1.2–7.4 hr).

CONTRAINDICATIONS AND PRECAUTIONS

Contraindicated in: ▪ Hypersensitivity to dezocine or bisulfites.
Use Cautiously in: ▪ Head trauma ▪ Increased intracranial pressure ▪ Severe renal, hepatic, or pulmonary disease (dosage reduction recommended) ▪ Undiagnosed abdominal pain ▪ Geriatric or debilitated patients (initial dosage reduction recommended) ▪ Patients who are physically dependent on opioid analgesic agonists (may precipitate withdrawal) or who have recently received systemic opioids ▪ Pregnancy, labor, lactation, or children <18 yr (safety not established).

ADVERSE REACTIONS AND SIDE EFFECTS*

CNS: sedation, anxiety, confusion, crying, dizziness, slurred speech.
EENT: blurred vision, double vision, miosis.
Resp: respiratory depression.
CV: orthostatic hypotension.
GI: abdominal pain, constipation, dry mouth, nausea, vomiting.
GU: hesitancy, retention, urinary frequency.
Derm: flushing or redness of skin.
Misc: physical dependence, psychological dependence, tolerance.

INTERACTIONS

Drug-Drug: ▪ Use with caution in patients receiving **MAO inhibitors** (may result in unpredictable reactions) ▪ Additive CNS depression with **alcohol, antihistamines**, and **sedative/hypnotics** ▪ May precipitate withdrawal in patients who are dependent on **opioid analgesic agonists** ▪ May diminish the analgesic effects of other **opioid analgesics.**

ROUTE AND DOSAGE

- **IM (Adults):** 10 mg initially every 3–6 hr (range 5–20 mg) as needed (not to exceed 120 mg/day).
- **IV (Adults):** 5 mg initially every 2–4 hr (range 2.5–10 mg) as needed (not to exceed 120 mg/day).

AVAILABILITY

▪ ***Injection:*** 5 mg/ml[Rx], 10 mg/ml[Rx], 15 mg/ml[Rx].

TIME/ACTION PROFILE (analgesic)

	ONSET	PEAK	DURATION
IM	within 30 min	1–2 hr	3–6 hr
IV	within 15 min	UK	2–4 hr

*CAPITALS indicate life-threatening; underlines indicate most frequent.

D

NURSING IMPLICATIONS

ASSESSMENT

- □ Assess type, location, and intensity of pain prior to and 1–2 hr following IM or 15 min following IV administration. When titrating opioid doses, increases of 25–50% should be administered until there is either a 50% reduction in the patient's pain rating on a numerical or visual analogue scale or the patient reports satisfactory pain relief. A repeat dose can be safely administered at the time of the peak if previous dose is ineffective and side effects are minimal. Patients requiring doses higher than 15–20 mg should be converted to an opioid agonist. Dezocine is not recommended for prolonged use or as first-line therapy for acute or cancer pain.
- □ An equianalgesic chart (see Appendix B) should be used when changing routes or when changing from one opioid to another. Dezocine is equianalgesic mg per mg with morphine.
- □ Assess blood pressure, pulse, and respirations before and periodically during administration. If respiratory rate is <10/min, assess level of sedation. Dose may need to be decreased by 25–50%. Respiratory depression occurs more rapidly and is more pronounced for the first 1–2 hr than that of morphine but persists for the same duration as an equianalgesic dose of morphine.
- □ Assess prior analgesic history. Antagonistic properties may induce withdrawal symptoms (vomiting, restlessness, abdominal cramps, and increased blood pressure and temperature) in patients physically dependent on opioids.
- □ Although this drug has a low potential for dependence, prolonged use may lead to physical and psychological dependence and tolerance. This should not prevent patient from receiving adequate analgesia. Most patients who receive dezocine for pain do not develop psychological dependence. If tolerance develops, changing to an opioid agonist may be required to relieve pain.
- ■ ***Lab Test Considerations:*** May cause elevated serum alkaline phosphatase and AST levels and decreased hemoglobin concentrations.
- ■ ***Toxicity and Overdose:*** If an opioid antagonist is required to reverse respiratory depression or coma, naloxone (Narcan) is the antidote. Dilute the 0.4-mg ampule of naloxone in 10 ml of 0.9% NaCl and administer 0.5 ml (0.02 mg) by direct IV push every 2 min. For children and patients weighing <40 kg, dilute 0.1 mg of naloxone in 10 ml of 0.9% NaCl for a concentration of 10 mcg/ml and administer 0.5 mcg/kg every 1–2 min. Titrate dose to avoid withdrawal, seizures, and severe pain.

POTENTIAL NURSING DIAGNOSES

- ■ Pain (Indications).
- ■ Injury, risk for (Side Effects).
- ■ Sensory-perceptual alterations: visual, auditory (Side Effects).

IMPLEMENTATION

- ■ **General Info:** Explain therapeutic value of medication prior to administration to enhance the analgesic effect.
- □ Regularly administered doses may be more effective than prn administration. Analgesic is more effective if given before pain becomes severe.
- □ Coadministration with nonopioid analgesics may have additive effects and permit lower opioid doses.
- ■ **IM:** Administer IM injections deep into well-developed muscle. Rotate sites of injections. Avoid SC injections.
- ■ **Direct IV:** May give IV undiluted.
- ■ ***Rate:*** Administer slowly, each 5 mg over 3–5 min.

PATIENT/FAMILY TEACHING

- □ Instruct patient on how and when to ask for pain medication.
- □ Dezocine may cause drowsiness or dizziness. Advise patient to call for assistance when ambulating and to avoid driving or other activities requiring alertness until response to the medication is known.
- □ Caution patient to change positions slowly to minimize orthostatic hypotension.
- □ Advise patient that frequent mouth rinses, good oral hygiene, and sugarless gum or candy may decrease dry mouth.
- □ Encourage patient to turn, cough, and breathe deeply every 2 hr to prevent atelectasis.
- □ Advise patient to avoid concurrent use of al-

cohol or other CNS depressants with this medication.

EVALUATION

Effectiveness of therapy can be demonstrated by: ▪ Decrease in severity of pain without a significant alteration in level of consciousness or respiratory status.

DIAZEPAM

(dye-**az**-e-pam)

{Apo-Diazepam}, Diastat, {Diazemuls}, {Dizac}, D-Val, {Novodipam}, {PMS-Diazepam}, Valium, Valrelease, {Vivol}

CLASSIFICATION(S):

Anticonvulsant (benzodiazepine), Sedative/hypnotic (benzodiazepine), Skeletal muscle relaxant (centrally acting)

Schedule IV

Pregnancy Category D

INDICATIONS

▪ Adjunct in the management of: ▫ Anxiety ▫ Preoperative sedation ▫ Conscious sedation ▪ Provides light anesthesia and anterograde amnesia ▪ Treatment of status epilepticus/uncontrolled seizures ▪ Skeletal muscle relaxant ▪ Management of the symptoms of alcohol withdrawal.

ACTION

▪ Depresses the CNS, probably by potentiating gamma-aminobutyric acid (GABA), an inhibitory neurotransmitter ▪ Produces skeletal muscle relaxation by inhibiting spinal polysynaptic afferent pathways ▪ Has anticonvulsant properties due to enhanced presynaptic inhibition. **Therapeutic Effects:** ▪ Relief of anxiety ▪ Sedation ▪ Amnesia ▪ Skeletal muscle relaxation ▪ Decreased seizure activity.

PHARMACOKINETICS

Absorption: Rapidly absorbed from the GI tract. Absorption from IM sites may be slow and unpredictable. Well absorbed (90%) from rectal mucosa.

Distribution: Widely distributed. Crosses the blood-brain barrier. Crosses the placenta; enters breast milk.

Metabolism and Excretion: Highly metabolized by the liver. Some products of metabolism are active as CNS depressants.

Half-life: 20–70 hr (up to 200 hr for metabolites).

CONTRAINDICATIONS AND PRECAUTIONS

Contraindicated in: ▪ Hypersensitivity ▪ Cross-sensitivity with other benzodiazepines may occur ▪ Comatose patients ▪ Pre-existing CNS depression ▪ Uncontrolled severe pain ▪ Narrow-angle glaucoma ▪ Pregnancy or lactation ▪ Some products contain alcohol, propylene glycol, or tartrazine and should be avoided in patients with known hypersensitivity or intolerance.

Use Cautiously in: ▪ Hepatic dysfunction ▪ Severe renal impairment ▪ History of suicide attempt or drug dependence ▪ Geriatric or debilitated patients (dosage reduction required) ▪ Children (dosage should not exceed 0.25 mg/kg).

ADVERSE REACTIONS AND SIDE EFFECTS*

CNS: <u>dizziness</u>, <u>drowsiness</u>, <u>lethargy</u>, depression, hangover, headache, paradoxical excitation.

EENT: blurred vision.

Resp: respiratory depression.

CV: hypotension (IV only).

GI: constipation, diarrhea, nausea, vomiting.

Derm: rashes.

Local: pain (IM), phlebitis (IV), venous thrombosis.

Misc: physical dependence, psychological dependence, tolerance.

INTERACTIONS

Drug-Drug: ▪ **Alcohol, antidepressants, antihistamines,** and **opioids**—concurrent use results in additive CNS depression ▪ **Cimetidine, oral contraceptives, disulfiram, fluoxetine, isoniazid, ketoconazole, metoprolol, propoxyphene, propranolol,** or **valproic acid** may decrease the metabolism of diazepam, en-

{} = Available in Canada only.

***CAPITALS indicate life-threatening; <u>underlines</u> indicate most frequent.**

hancing its actions ▪ May decrease the efficacy of **levodopa** ▪ **Rifampin** or **barbiturates** may increase the metabolism and decrease effectiveness of diazepam ▪ Sedative effects may be decreased by **theophylline.**

ROUTE AND DOSAGE

❑ Antianxiety/Anticonvulsant

- **PO (Adults):** 2–10 mg 2–4 times daily or 15–30 mg of extended-release form once daily.
- **PO (Children >6 mo):** 1–2.5 mg 3–4 times daily; may be increased.

❑ Precardioversion

- **IV (Adults):** 5–15 mg 5–10 min precardioversion.

❑ Pre-endoscopy

- **IV (Adults):** 2.5–20 mg.
- **IM (Adults):** 5–10 mg 30 min pre-endoscopy.

❑ Status Epilepticus/Acute Seizure Activity

- **IV (Adults):** 5–10 mg, may repeat q 10–15 min to a total of 30 mg, may repeat regimen again in 2–4 hr (IM route may be used if IV route unavailable); larger doses may be required.
- **IM, IV (Children ≥5 yr):** 1 mg q 2–5 min to a total of 10 mg, repeat q 2–4 hr.
- **IM, IV (Children 1 mo–5 yr):** 0.2–0.5 mg q 2–5 min to maximum of 5 mg.
- **Rect (Adults):** 0.2 mg/kg; may repeat 4–12 hr later.
- **Rect (Children 6–11 yr):** 0.3 mg/kg; may repeat 4–12 hr later.
- **Rect (Children 2–5 yr):** 0.5 mg/kg; may repeat 4–12 hr later.

❑ Skeletal Muscle Relaxation

- **PO (Adults):** 2–10 mg 3–4 times daily or 15–30 mg of extended-release form once daily.
- **PO (Geriatric Patients or Debilitated Patients):** 2–2.5 mg 1–2 times daily initially.
- **PO (Children):** 1–2.5 mg 3–4 times daily.
- **IM, IV (Adults):** 5–10 mg; may repeat in 2–4 hr (larger doses may be required for tetanus).
- **IM, IV (Geriatric Patients or Debilitated Patients):** 2–5 mg; may repeat in 2–4 hr (larger doses may be required for tetanus).
- **IM, IV (Children ≥5 yr):** *Tetanus*—5–10 mg q 3–4 hr.
- **IM, IV (Children > 1 mo):** *Tetanus*—1–2 mg q 3–4 hr.

❑ Alcohol Withdrawal

- **PO (Adults):** 10 mg 3–4 times in first 24 hr, decrease to 5 mg 3–4 times daily.
- **IM, IV (Adults):** 10 mg initially, then 5–10 mg in 3–4 hr as needed; larger or more frequent doses have been used.

❑ Psychoneurotic Reactions

- **IM, IV (Adults):** 2–10 mg, may be repeated in 3–4 hr.

AVAILABILITY

▪ ***Tablets:*** 2 mg[Rx], 5 mg[Rx], 10 mg[Rx] ▪ ***Sustained-release capsules:*** 15 mg[Rx] ▪ ***Oral solution:*** 5 mg/ml (Intensol)[Rx], 5 mg/5 ml[Rx] ▪ ***Injection:*** 5 mg/ml (contains 10% alcohol and 40% propylene glycol)[Rx] ▪ ***Rectal gel delivery system:*** 2.5 mg[Rx], 10 mg[Rx], 15 mg[Rx], 20 mg[Rx] ▪ ***Sterile emulsion for injection:*** 5 mg/ml (contains egg phospholipids and soybean oil)[Rx].

TIME/ACTION PROFILE (sedation)

	ONSET	PEAK	DURATION
PO	30–60 min	1–2 hr	up to 24 hr
PO-ER	UK	UK	24 hr
IM	within 20 min	0.5–1.5 hr	UK
IV	1–5 min	15–30 min	15–60 min*
Rect	UK	1–2 hr	4–12 hr

*In status epilepticus, anticonvulsant duration is 15–20 min.

NURSING IMPLICATIONS

ASSESSMENT

- **General Info:** Monitor blood pressure, pulse, and respiratory rate prior to and periodically throughout therapy and frequently during IV therapy.
  - ☐ Assess IV site frequently during administration; diazepam may cause phlebitis and venous thrombosis.
  - ☐ Prolonged high-dose therapy may lead to psychological or physical dependence. Restrict amount of drug available to patient. Observe depressed patients closely for suicidal tendencies.
- **Anxiety:** Assess degree of anxiety and level of sedation (ataxia, dizziness, slurred speech) prior to and periodically throughout therapy.

- **Seizures:** Observe and record intensity, duration, and location of seizure activity. The initial dose of diazepam offers seizure control for 15–20 min after administration. Institute seizure precautions.
- **Muscle Spasms:** Assess muscle spasm, associated pain, and limitation of movement prior to and throughout therapy.
- **Alcohol Withdrawal:** Assess patient experiencing alcohol withdrawal for tremors, agitation, delirium, and hallucinations. Protect patient from injury.
- ***Lab Test Considerations:*** Hepatic and renal function and CBC should be evaluated periodically throughout course of prolonged therapy.

POTENTIAL NURSING DIAGNOSES

- Anxiety (Indications).
- Physical mobility, impaired (Indications).
- Injury, risk for (Side Effects).

IMPLEMENTATION

- **General Info:** Patient should be kept on bed rest and observed for at least 3 hr following parenteral administration.
- □ Sterile emulsion for injection (Dizac) is for IV use only.
- □ If opioids are used concurrently with parenteral diazepam, decrease opioid dose by ⅓ and titrate dose to effect.
- **PO:** Tablets may be crushed and taken with food or water if patient has difficulty swallowing. Swallow sustained-release capsules whole; do not crush, break, or chew.
- □ Mix Intensol preparation with liquid or semisolid food such as water, juices, soda, applesauce, or pudding. Administer entire amount immediately. Do not store.
- **IM:** IM injections are painful and erratically absorbed. If IM route is used, inject deeply into deltoid muscle for maximum absorption.
- **IV:** Resuscitation equipment should be available when diazepam is administered IV.
- **Direct IV:** For IV administration do not dilute or mix with any other drug. If direct IV push is not feasible, administer IV push into tubing as close to insertion site as possible. Continuous infusion is not recommended because of precipitation in IV fluids and absorption of diazepam into infusion bags and tubing. Injection may cause burning and venous irritation; avoid small veins.
- ***Rate:*** Administer slowly at a rate of 5 mg over at least 1 min. Infants and children should receive total dose over a minimum of 3–5 min. Rapid injection may cause apnea, hypotension, bradycardia, or cardiac arrest.
- **Syringe Compatibility:** ▪ cimetidine.
- **Syringe Incompatibility:** ▪ heparin ▪ sufentanil.
- **Y-Site Compatibility:** ▪ dobutamine ▪ nafcillin ▪ sufentanil.
- **Y-Site Incompatibility:** ▪ atracurium ▪ cefepime ▪ diltiazem ▪ fluconazole ▪ foscarnet ▪ heparin ▪ hydromorphone ▪ pancuronium ▪ potassium chloride ▪ vecuronium ▪ vitamin B complex with C.
- **Rect:** Do not repeat *Diastat* rectal dose more than 5 times/mo or 1 episode every 5 days. Round dose up to next available dose unit.
- □ Diazepam injection has been used for rectal administration. Instill via catheter or cannula fitted to the syringe or directly from a 1-ml syringe inserted 4–5 cm into the rectum. A dilution of diazepam injection with propylene glycol containing 1 mg/ml has also been used.
- □ Do not dilute with other solutions, IV fluids, or medications.

PATIENT/FAMILY TEACHING

- **General Info:** Instruct patient to take medication exactly as directed and not to take more than prescribed or increase dose if less effective after a few weeks without checking with health care professional. Abrupt withdrawal of diazepam may cause insomnia, unusual irritability or nervousness, and seizures. Advise patient that sharing of this medication may be dangerous.
- □ Medication may cause drowsiness, clumsiness, or unsteadiness. Advise patient to avoid driving or other activities requiring alertness until response to medication is known.
- □ Caution patient to avoid taking alcohol or other CNS depressants concurrently with this medication.
- □ Advise patient to notify health care professional if pregnancy is suspected or planned.
- □ Emphasize the importance of follow-up examinations to determine effectiveness of the medication.
- **Seizures:** Patients on anticonvulsant therapy should carry identification describing disease process and medication regimen at all times.

- Carefully review patient/caregiver package insert for Diastat rectal gel with caregiver prior to administration.

EVALUATION

Effectiveness of therapy can be demonstrated by: ▪ Decrease in anxiety level. Full therapeutic antianxiety effects occur after 1–2 wk of therapy ▪ Decreased recall of surgical or diagnostic procedures ▪ Control of seizures ▪ Decrease in muscle spasms ▪ Decreased tremulousness and more rational ideation when used for alcohol withdrawal.

DIAZOXIDE

(dye-az-**ox**-ide)

Hyperstat, Proglycem

CLASSIFICATION(S):

Antihypertensive agent (vasodilator), Hyperglycemic

Pregnancy Category C

INDICATIONS

▪ **IV:** Emergency treatment of hypertension ▪ **PO:** Treatment of hypoglycemia associated with hyperinsulinism or other causes.

ACTION

▪ Directly relaxes vascular smooth muscle in peripheral arterioles. Produces reflex tachycardia and increased cardiac output ▪ Inhibits insulin release from the pancreas and decreases peripheral utilization of glucose. **Therapeutic Effects:** ▪ Lowering of blood pressure ▪ Increased blood glucose.

PHARMACOKINETICS

Absorption: Well absorbed following oral administration.
Distribution: Crosses the blood-brain barrier and placenta.
Metabolism and Excretion: 50% metabolized by the liver; 50% excreted unchanged by the kidneys.
Half-life: 21–45 hr.

CONTRAINDICATIONS AND PRECAUTIONS

Contraindicated in: ▪ Hypersensitivity ▪ Hypersensitivity to bisulfites (IV only). Cross-sensitivity with sulfonamides may occur.
Use Cautiously in: ▪ Diabetics (hyperglycemia accompanies use) ▪ Cardiovascular disease ▪ Uremia ▪ Pregnancy and lactation (safety not established; may inhibit labor).

ADVERSE REACTIONS AND SIDE EFFECTS*

CV: CONGESTIVE HEART FAILURE, hypotension, tachycardia, angina, arrhythmias, edema, flushing.
Derm: hirsutism.
Endo: hyperglycemia.
F and E: sodium and water retention.
Local: phlebitis at IV site.

INTERACTIONS

Drug-Drug: ▪ Concurrent **diuretic** therapy may potentiate hyperglycemic, hyperuricemic, and hypotensive effects ▪ May increase the metabolism and decrease the effectiveness of **phenytoin** ▪ **Phenytoin, corticosteroids,** and **estrogen/progesterone** may increase hyperglycemia ▪ May increase the effects of **warfarin** ▪ May alter the effects of **insulin** or **oral hypoglycemic agents.**

ROUTE AND DOSAGE

Hypertension

- **IV (Adults and Children):** 1–3 mg/kg (not to exceed 150 mg/dose) every 5–15 min until blood pressure is lowered to desired level (not to exceed 1.2 g/day in adults).

Hypoglycemia

- **PO (Adults and Children):** 1 mg/kg q 8 hr initially, further adjustments made on the basis of response. Usual maintenance dose is 3–8 mg/kg/day given in divided doses every 8–12 hr.
- **PO (Infants and Newborns):** 3.3 mg/kg q 8 hr initially, further adjustments made on the basis of response. Usual maintenance dose is 8–15 mg/kg/day in divided doses every 8–12 hr.

***CAPITALS indicate life-threatening; underlines indicate most frequent.**

AVAILABILITY

▪ ***Capsules:*** 50 mg[Rx], {100 mg[Rx]} ▪ ***Oral suspension:*** 50 mg/ml[Rx] ▪ ***Injection:*** 15 mg/ml[Rx], 300 mg/20 ml[Rx].

TIME/ACTION PROFILE

	ONSET	PEAK	DURATION
PO*	1 hr	8–12 hr	8 hr
IV†	immediate	5 min	3–12 hr

*Blood sugar.
†Blood pressure.

NURSING IMPLICATIONS

ASSESSMENT

▪ **General Info:** Assess for allergy to sulfonamide drugs.
□ Assess patient routinely for signs and symptoms of congestive heart failure (peripheral edema, dyspnea, rales/crackles, fatigue, weight gain, jugular venous distention). Notify physician if these occur.
▪ **Hypertension:** Monitor blood pressure and pulse every 5 min until stable and then hourly. Report significant changes immediately.
▪ **Hypoglycemia:** Assess patient for signs of hyperglycemia (drowsiness, fruity breath, increased urination, unusual thirst). Monitor blood glucose on diabetic patients requiring frequent doses.
▪ ***Lab Test Considerations:*** May cause increased serum glucose, BUN, alkaline phosphatase, AST, sodium, and uric acid levels.
□ Monitor blood glucose in diabetic patients requiring frequent parenteral doses.
□ May cause decreased CCr, hematocrit, and hemoglobin.
▪ ***Toxicity and Overdose:*** If severe hypotension occurs, treatment includes Trendelenburg position, volume infusion, and sympathomimetics (norepinephrine).
□ Patients who develop marked hyperglycemia must be monitored for 7 days while blood glucose concentrations stabilize.

POTENTIAL NURSING DIAGNOSES

▪ Cardiac output, decreased (Side Effects).
▪ Knowledge deficit, related to medication regimen (Patient/Family Teaching).

IMPLEMENTATION

▪ **General Info:** Loop diuretics are commonly given concurrently with this medication to prevent sodium and water retention.
□ Oral and injectable solution must be protected from light. Do not administer darkened solution.
▪ **PO:** Shake oral suspension well before use.
▪ **Direct IV:** Do not administer SC or IM. Injection may cause warmth and pain along injected vein. Monitor IV site closely; extravasation causes cellulitis and pain. Cold packs may be applied if extravasation occurs.
▪ ***Rate:*** Administer undiluted over 30 sec or less only into a peripheral vein to prevent cardiac arrhythmias. May be repeated every 5–15 min as indicated.
□ Have patient remain recumbent for at least 1 hr following IV administration. Take blood pressure standing prior to ambulation.
▪ **Syringe Compatibility:** ▪ heparin.
▪ **Y-Site Incompatibility:** ▪ hydralazine ▪ propranolol.

PATIENT/FAMILY TEACHING

▪ **Hypoglycemia:** Instruct patient to take medication as directed, at the same time each day.
□ Encourage patient to follow prescribed diet, medication, and exercise regimen to prevent hypoglycemic or hyperglycemic episodes.
□ Review signs of hypoglycemia and hyperglycemia with patient.
□ Advise patient not to switch from capsule to oral suspension form without consulting health care professional, as oral suspension produces higher blood concentrations.
□ Advise patient to inform health care professional of medication regimen prior to treatment or surgery.
▪ **Hypertension:** Instruct patient to change positions slowly to minimize orthostatic hypotension.
□ Caution patient to avoid taking other medications, especially OTC cold medicine, without consulting health care professional.
□ Emphasize the importance of routine follow-up exams, especially during the first few weeks of therapy.

EVALUATION

Effectiveness of therapy can be demonstrated by: ▪ Decrease in blood pressure with-

D

out the appearance of side effects. This drug is utilized in short-term treatment of hypertension. Oral antihypertensives should be introduced as soon as the hypertensive crisis is controlled ▪ Management of hypoglycemia and return to normal serum glucose concentrations. If diazoxide is not effective within 2–3 wk, therapy should be re-evaluated.

DICLOFENAC

(dye-**kloe**-fen-ak)

diclofenac potassium

Cataflam, {Voltaren Rapide}

diclofenac sodium

{Apo-Diclo}, {Novo-Difenac}, Nu-Diclo, Voltaren, {Voltaren-SR}

CLASSIFICATION(S):

Analgesic (nonopioid), Nonsteroidal anti-inflammatory agent

Pregnancy Category B (first trimester)

INDICATIONS

▪ Management of inflammatory disorders including: ▫ Rheumatoid arthritis ▫ Osteoarthritis ▫ Ankylosing spondylitis ▪ Relief of mild to moderate pain or dysmenorrhea.

ACTION

▪ Inhibits prostaglandin synthesis. **Therapeutic Effects:** ▪ Suppression of pain and inflammation.

PHARMACOKINETICS

Absorption: Well absorbed following oral administration. Diclofenac sodium is a delayed-release dosage form. Diclofenac potassium is an immediate-release dosage form.

Distribution: Crosses the placenta; enters breast milk.

Metabolism and Excretion: ≥50% metabolized on first pass through the liver.

Half-life: 1.2–2 hr.

CONTRAINDICATIONS AND PRECAUTIONS

Contraindicated in: ▪ Hypersensitivity ▪ Cross-sensitivity may occur with other NSAIDs including aspirin ▪ Active GI bleeding/ulcer disease.

Use Cautiously in: ▪ Severe cardiovascular/renal/hepatic disease ▪ History of ulcer disease ▪ Elderly patients (dosage reduction recommended; more susceptible to adverse reactions) ▪ Bleeding tendency or concurrent anticoagulant therapy ▪ Pregnancy, lactation, and children (safety not established; not recommended for use during second half of pregnancy).

ADVERSE REACTIONS AND SIDE EFFECTS*

CV: dizziness, drowsiness, headache, hypertension.

GI: GI BLEEDING, <u>abdominal pain</u>, <u>dyspepsia</u>, <u>heartburn</u>, diarrhea, hepatotoxicity.

GU: acute renal failure, dysuria, frequency, hematuria, nephritis, proteinuria.

Derm: eczema, photosensitivity, rashes.

F and E: edema.

Hemat: prolonged bleeding time.

Misc: allergic reactions including ANAPHYLAXIS.

INTERACTIONS

Drug-Drug: ▪ Concurrent use with **aspirin** may decrease effectiveness ▪ Additive adverse GI effects with **aspirin**, other **NSAIDs, colchicine, glucocorticoids**, or **alcohol** ▪ Chronic use with **acetaminophen** may increase the risk of adverse renal reactions ▪ May decrease the effectiveness of **diuretics, antihypertensives, insulin**, or **hypoglycemic agents** ▪ Increases serum **digoxin** levels (dosage adjustment may be necessary) ▪ May increase levels and increase the risk of toxicity from **cyclosporine, lithium**, or **methotrexate** ▪ **Probenecid** increases risk of toxicity from diclofenac ▪ Increased risk of bleeding with **some cephalosporins, plicamycin, thrombolytic agents, valproic acid**, or **anticoagulants** ▪ Increased risk of adverse hematologic reactions with **antineoplastic agents** or **radiation therapy.** Concurrent use with **potassium-sparing diuretics** increases the risk of hyperkalemia ▪ Concurrent use with

{} = Available in Canada only.

***CAPITALS indicate life-threatening; <u>underlines</u> indicate most frequent.**

gold compounds may increase the risk of adverse renal reactions.

ROUTE AND DOSAGE

❑ **Osteoarthritis**

- **PO (Adults):** *Diclofenac sodium or potassium*—50 mg 2–3 times daily. *Diclofenac sodium*—75 mg twice daily.

❑ **Rheumatoid Arthritis**

- **PO (Adults):** *Diclofenac sodium or potassium*—50 mg 3–4 times daily. *Diclofenac sodium*—75 mg twice daily.

❑ **Ankylosing Spondylitis**

- **PO (Adults):** *Diclofenac sodium*—25 mg 4 times daily; an additional 25 mg is given at bedtime.

❑ **Analgesia/Dysmenorrhea**

- **PO (Adults):** *Diclofenac potassium*—50 mg 3 times daily; initial dose may be 100 mg (not to exceed 200 mg during the first 24 hr or 150 mg/day on subsequent days).

AVAILABILITY

▪ ***Diclofenac potassium immediate-release tablets:*** 25 mg[Rx], 50 mg[Rx], 75 mg[Rx] ▪ {***Diclofenac sodium delayed-release (enteric-coated) tablets:*** 25 mg[Rx], 50 mg[Rx], 75 mg[Rx]} ▪ ***Diclofenac sodium extended-release tablets:*** {75 mg[Rx]}, {100 mg[Rx]} ▪ ***Suppositories:*** {50 mg[Rx]}, {100 mg[Rx]} ▪ ***In combination with:*** 200 mcg misoprostol (Arthrotec[Rx]). See Appendix A.

TIME/ACTION PROFILE

	ONSET	PEAK	DURATION
PO (inflammation)	few days–1 wk	2 wk or more	UK
PO (pain)	30 min	UK	up to 8 hr

NURSING IMPLICATIONS

ASSESSMENT

- **General Info:** Patients who have asthma, aspirin-induced allergy, and nasal polyps are at increased risk for developing hypersensitivity reactions.
- **Pain:** Assess pain and limitation of movement; note type, location, and intensity prior to and 30–60 min following administration.
- **Arthritis:** Assess arthritic pain (note type, location, intensity) and limitation of movement prior to and periodically during therapy.
- ***Lab Test Considerations:*** Diclofenac has minimal effect on bleeding time and platelet aggregation.
  - ❑ May cause decreased hemoglobin, hematocrit, leukocyte, and platelet counts.
  - ❑ Monitor liver function tests within 8 wk of initiating diclofenac therapy and periodically during therapy. May cause elevated serum alkaline phosphatase, LDH, AST, and ALT concentrations.
  - ❑ Monitor BUN, serum creatinine, and electrolytes periodically during therapy. May cause increased BUN, serum creatinine, and electrolyte concentrations and decreased urine electrolyte concentrations.
  - ❑ May cause decreased serum and increased urine uric acid concentrations.

D

POTENTIAL NURSING DIAGNOSES

- Pain (Indications).
- Physical mobility, impaired (Indications).
- Knowledge deficit, related to medication regimen (Patient/Family Teaching).

IMPLEMENTATION

- **General Info:** Administration in higher than recommended doses does not provide increased effectiveness but may cause increased side effects.
- **PO:** Administer after meals, with food, or with an antacid containing aluminum or magnesium to minimize gastric irritation. May take first 1–2 doses on an empty stomach for more rapid onset. Do not crush or chew enteric-coated or sustained-release tablets.
- **Dysmenorrhea:** Administer as soon as possible after the onset of menses. Prophylactic treatment has not been shown to be effective.

PATIENT/FAMILY TEACHING

- **PO:** Instruct patient to take diclofenac with a full glass of water and to remain in an upright position for 15–30 min after administration. If a dose is missed, take as soon as possible within 1–2 hr if taking once or twice/day or unless almost time for next dose if taking more than twice/day. Do not double doses.
  - ❑ Caution patient to avoid concurrent use of alcohol, aspirin, acetaminophen, other NSAIDs,

or other OTC medications without consulting health care professional.

- May cause drowsiness or dizziness. Caution patient to avoid driving or other activities requiring alertness until response to medication is known.
- Instruct patient to notify health care professional of medication regimen prior to treatment or surgery.
- Caution patient to wear sunscreen and protective clothing to prevent photosensitivity reactions.
- Advise patient to consult health care professional if rash, itching, visual disturbances, tinnitus, weight gain, edema, black stools, persistent headache, or influenza-like syndrome (chills, fever, muscle aches, pain) occurs.

EVALUATION

Effectiveness of therapy can be demonstrated by: ▪ Decrease in severity of mild to moderate pain ▫ Increased ease of joint movement. Patients who do not respond to one NSAID may respond to another. May require 2 wk or more for maximum effects.

DIDANOSINE

(dye-**dan**-oh-seen)
ddI, dideoxyinosine, Videx

CLASSIFICATION(S):
Antiretroviral (nucleoside reverse transcriptase inhibitor)

Pregnancy Category B

INDICATIONS

▪ Treatment of HIV infection in patients who are intolerant to zidovudine therapy or who have had previous zidovudine therapy.

ACTION

▪ Inhibits viral replication by interfering with viral RNA-directed DNA polymerase (reverse transcriptase). Must be converted intracellularly by the phosphorylation process to its active form. **Therapeutic Effects:** ▪ Increase in CD4 cell counts and decreased viral load, which may result in decreased incidence of opportunistic infections and slowed progression in HIV-infected patients.

PHARMACOKINETICS

Absorption: Rapidly degrades at gastric pH. Buffers in formulation neutralize gastric acid and allow for maximal absorption (33–37%).
Distribution: CSF levels are 21% of plasma levels in adults.
Metabolism and Excretion: 55% eliminated by the kidneys (urinary excretion appears to be less in children).
Half-life: 1.6 hr (0.8 hr in children).

CONTRAINDICATIONS AND PRECAUTIONS

Contraindicated in: ▪ Hypersensitivity ▪ Lactation ▪ Phenylketonuria (tablets contain phenylalanine).
Use Cautiously in: ▪ History of gout ▪ Patients on sodium-restricted diets (tablets contain 264.5 mg sodium) ▪ Renal impairment (dosage modification required if CCr <60 ml/min) ▪ History of seizures ▪ Diabetes mellitus.

ADVERSE REACTIONS AND SIDE EFFECTS*

CNS: SEIZURES, <u>headache</u>, dizziness, insomnia, lethargy, pain, weakness.
EENT: <u>rhinitis</u>, ear pain, epistaxis, photophobia, retinal depigmentation (children only).
Resp: <u>cough</u>, asthma.
CV: arrhythmias, edema, hypertension, vasodilation.
GI: PANCREATITIS, <u>LIVER FAILURE</u>, <u>anorexia</u>, <u>diarrhea</u>, <u>liver function abnormalities</u>, <u>nausea</u>, <u>vomiting</u>, abdominal pain, constipation, dry mouth, stomatitis.
GU: urinary frequency.
Derm: alopecia, ecchymoses, rash.
Endo: hyperglycemia.
Hemat: <u>granulocytopenia</u>, anemia, bleeding, leukopenia.
Metab: hyperlipidemia, hyperuricemia, weight loss.
MS: arthritis, myalgia.
Neuro: <u>peripheral neuropathy</u>, poor coordination.
Misc: <u>chills</u>, <u>fever</u>.

***CAPITALS indicate life-threatening; <u>underlines</u> indicate most frequent.**

INTERACTIONS

Drug-Drug: ▪ Presence of buffers in didanosine will decrease absorption of **ketoconazole, itraconazole, dapsone, tetracyclines, fluoroquinolones** ▪ Increased risk of peripheral neuropathy with other **drugs causing peripheral neuropathy** (isoniazid, phenytoin, zalcitabine, stavudine, ethambutol, chloramphenicol, and others) ▪ Increased risk of pancreatitis with other **drugs causing pancreatitis** (alcohol, thiazide diuretics, IV pentamidine, tetracyclines, and others) ▪ Increased risk of bone marrow depression with other **drugs causing bone marrow depression.**

Drug-Food: ▪ Administration of didanosine with **food** decreases absorption by 50%.

ROUTE AND DOSAGE

When tablets are used, adults and children >1 yr should receive 2 tablets/dose to ensure adequate buffering. Children <1 yr may receive 1 tablet. Tablets and buffered powder are not interchangeable because of differences in bioavailabilty.

- **PO (Adults ≥60 kg):** *Tablets*—200 mg bid; *buffered powder packets*—250 mg bid.
- **PO (Adults <60 kg):** *Tablets*—125 mg bid; *buffered powder packets*—167 mg q 12 hr.
- **PO (Children):** *Tablets*—90–120 mg/m² q 12 hr; *buffered powder packets*—112.5–150 mg/m² q 12 hr.
- **PO (Children with BSA 1.1–1.4 m²):** *Tablets*—100 mg q 8–12 hr; *reconstituted pediatric powder*—125 mg q 8–12 hr.
- **PO (Children with BSA 0.8–1 m²):** *Tablets*—75 mg q 8–12 hr; *reconstituted pediatric powder*—94 mg q 8–12 hr.
- **PO (Children with BSA 0.5–0.7 m²):** *Tablets*—50 mg q 8–12 hr; *reconstituted pediatric powder*—62 mg q 8–12 hr.
- **PO (Children with BSA <0.4 m²):** *Tablets*—25 mg q 8–12 hr; *reconstituted pediatric powder*—31 mg q 8–12 hr.

AVAILABILITY

▪ ***Chewable/dispersible buffered tablets:*** 25 mg^Rx^, 50 mg^Rx^, 100 mg^Rx^, 150 mg^Rx^ ▪ ***Buffered powder packets for oral solution:*** 100 mg^Rx^, 167 mg^Rx^, 250 mg^Rx^, 375 mg^Rx^ ▪ ***Pediatric powder for oral solution (requires reconstitution):*** 10 mg/ml^Rx^, 20 mg/ml^Rx^.

TIME/ACTION PROFILE (retroviral plasma levels)

	ONSET	PEAK	DURATION
PO	UK	0.5–1 hr	8–12 hr

NURSING IMPLICATIONS

ASSESSMENT

- □ Monitor patient for symptoms of opportunistic infection prior to and throughout therapy.
- □ Monitor patient for peripheral neuropathy (distal numbness, tingling, or pain in feet or hands) throughout therapy. Dose may need to be decreased.
- □ Monitor patient for symptoms of pancreatitis (abdominal pain, nausea, vomiting, increased amylase, lipase, or triglyceride concentrations). If amylase is elevated 1.5–2 times the normal limit and/or the patient has symptoms of pancreatitis, didanosine should be discontinued. Pancreatitis may be fatal.
- ▪ ***Lab Test Considerations:*** Monitor viral load and CD4 count prior to and routinely during therapy to determine response.
- □ Monitor CBC, hepatic function, and uric acid concentrations throughout therapy. May cause leukopenia, granulocytopenia, thrombocytopenia, and anemia. May cause elevated AST, ALT, alkaline phosphatase, bilirubin, uric acid, amylase, lipase, and triglyceride concentrations.
- □ May cause hyperglycemia.
- □ Monitor serum potassium concentrations routinely. Diarrhea from buffer may cause a decrease in serum potassium concentrations.

POTENTIAL NURSING DIAGNOSES

- ▪ Infection, risk for (Indications, Side Effects).
- ▪ Injury, risk for (Side Effects).
- ▪ Knowledge deficit, related to medication regimen (Patient/Family Teaching).

IMPLEMENTATION

- ▪ **General Info:** Commonly identified by abbreviation "ddI," but generic and brand name should be used when ordering to prevent errors.
- □ If diarrhea develops in patients taking buffered powder for oral solution, chewable/dis-

persible buffered tablets may cause less diarrhea.

- □ If solution or powder spills or leaks, a wet mop or damp sponge should be used for cleaning to avoid generation of dust. Clean surface with soap and water as needed.
- ▪ **PO:** Administer every 12 hr on an empty stomach, 1 hr before or 2 hr after meals. Do not administer ketoconazole, dapsone, tetracyclines, or fluoroquinolones within 2 hr of didanosine.
- □ Tablets should be chewed thoroughly, manually crushed, or dispersed in at least 1 oz water prior to administration. To disperse, add 1 or 2 tablets to at least 1 oz water and stir until a uniform dispersion forms. Dispersion should be taken immediately.
- □ Buffered powder for oral solution should be mixed in at least 4 oz water; do not mix with fruit juice or other acid-containing liquid. Stir 2–3 min until the powder dissolves completely. Solution should be taken immediately.
- □ Solution for pediatric use is mixed by pharmacist and is stable for 30 days if refrigerated. Shake admixture immediately before administering.

PATIENT/FAMILY TEACHING

- □ Instruct patient on the importance of taking didanosine exactly as directed, even if feeling better. Caution patient not to share or trade this medication with others.
- □ May cause dizziness. Caution patient to avoid driving or other activities requiring alertness until response to medication is known.
- □ Inform patient that didanosine may cause hyperglycemia. Advise patient to notify health care professional if increased thirst or hunger; unexplained weight loss; increased urination; fatigue; or dry, itchy skin occurs.
- □ Advise patient to consult health care professional before taking other medications concurrently with didanosine.
- □ Caution patient to avoid crowds and persons with known infections.
- □ Advise patient to notify health care professional immediately if numbness or tingling of the hands or feet, stomach pain, nausea, or vomiting occurs.
- □ Caution patient to use a condom to prevent transmission of HIV and not to share needles with anyone.
- □ Children should have dilated retinal exams every 3–6 mo or if there is a change in vision throughout therapy.
- □ Emphasize the importance of regular exams to monitor for side effects.

EVALUATION

Effectiveness of therapy can be demonstrated by: ▪ Decreased incidence of opportunistic infection and slowed progression of HIV infection.

DIETHYLSTILBESTROL

(dye-eth-il-stil-**bess**-trole)

DES, {Honvol}, Stilphostrol

CLASSIFICATION(S):

Antineoplastic (hormone), Hormone (estrogen)

Pregnancy Category X

INDICATIONS

▪ Palliatively in advanced, inoperable metastatic prostate carcinoma and postmenopausal breast carcinoma (Stilphostrol used for prostate carcinoma only).

ACTION

▪ Promotes the growth and development of female sex organs and the maintenance of secondary sex characteristics in women ▪ Metabolic effects include reduced blood cholesterol, protein synthesis, and sodium and water retention ▪ Competes for androgen binding sites in prostate cancer. **Therapeutic Effects:** ▪ Decreased tumor spread in androgen-sensitive tumors.

PHARMACOKINETICS

Absorption: Well absorbed from the GI tract.
Distribution: Widely distributed. Crosses the placenta; probably enters breast milk.
Metabolism and Excretion: Metabolized by the liver.
Half-life: UK.

CONTRAINDICATIONS AND PRECAUTIONS

Contraindicated in: ▪ Thromboembolic disease ▪ Undiagnosed vaginal bleeding ▪ Pregnancy (use may result in harm to the fetus) ▪ Lactation.
Use Cautiously in: ▪ Underlying cardiovascular disease ▪ Severe hepatic or renal disease ▪ May increase the risk of endometrial carcinoma.

ADVERSE REACTIONS AND SIDE EFFECTS*

CNS: headache, dizziness, lethargy.
EENT: intolerance to contact lenses, worsening of myopia or astigmatism.
CV: MYOCARDIAL INFARCTION, THROMBOEMBOLISM, edema, hypertension.
GI: nausea, anorexia, increased appetite, jaundice, vomiting.
GU: *women*—amenorrhea, breakthrough bleeding, dysmenorrhea, cervical erosions, loss of libido, vaginal candidiasis; *men*—impotence, testicular atrophy.
Derm: acne, oily skin, photosensitivity, pigmentation, urticaria.
Endo: gynecomastia (men), hyperglycemia.
F and E: hypercalcemia, sodium and water retention.
Metab: weight changes.
MS: leg cramps.
Misc: breast tenderness.

INTERACTIONS

Drug-Drug: ▪ May alter requirement for **warfarin, oral hypoglycemic agents,** or **insulin** ▪ **Barbiturates** or **rifampin** may decrease effectiveness ▪ May interfere with the desired effects of **bromocriptine** ▪ May increase the risk of hepatotoxicity from **dantrolene** ▪ May increase blood levels and risk of toxicity from **cyclosporine.**

ROUTE AND DOSAGE

❑ **Postmenopausal Breast Carcinoma**

▪ **PO (Adults):** 15 mg/day.

❑ **Prostate Carcinoma**

▪ **PO (Adults):** *Diethylstilbestrol*—1–3 mg/day initially, then decrease to 1 mg/day. *Diethylstilbestrol diphosphate*—50–200 mg 3 times daily.

▪ **IV (Adults):** 500 mg—1 g/day initially until response is obtained (5 or more days), then 250–500 mg 1–2 times weekly.

AVAILABILITY

❑ **Diethylstilbestrol**

▪ ***Tablets:*** 1 mg[Rx], 5 mg[Rx] ▪ ***Tablets (enteric-coated):*** 1 mg[Rx], 5 mg[Rx].

❑ **Diethylstilbestrol Diphosphate**

▪ ***Tablets:*** 50 mg[Rx], {83 mg[Rx]} ▪ ***Injection:*** 50 mg/ml[Rx].

TIME/ACTION PROFILE (antineoplastic effect)†

	ONSET	PEAK	DURATION
PO	up to 4–8 wk	UK	UK

†Onset of response for carcinomas may take 4–8 wk.

NURSING IMPLICATIONS

ASSESSMENT

□ Assess blood pressure prior to and periodically throughout therapy.
□ Monitor intake and output ratios and weekly weight. Report significant discrepancies or steady weight gain.
▪ ***Lab Test Considerations:*** May cause increased serum glucose, sodium, triglyceride, phospholipid, cortisol, prolactin, prothrombin, and factor VII, VIII, IX, and X levels. May decrease serum folate, pyridoxine, antithrombin III, and pregnanediol excretion concentrations.
□ May alter thyroid hormone assays.
□ May cause hypercalcemia in patients with metastatic bone lesions.

POTENTIAL NURSING DIAGNOSES

▪ Knowledge deficit, related to medication regimen (Patient/Family Teaching).

IMPLEMENTATION

▪ **PO:** Administer oral doses with or immediately after food to reduce nausea.
□ Do not break, crush, or chew enteric-coated tablets.
▪ **IV:** Dilute solution in 250–500 ml of D5W or 0.9% NaCl.
▪ ***Rate:*** Infuse at a rate of 1–2 ml/min for the first 10–15 min. If infusion is tolerated, adjust

*CAPITALS indicate life-threatening; underlines indicate most frequent.

the rate so that the entire dose has infused within 1 hr.

PATIENT/FAMILY TEACHING

- Instruct patient to take oral medication as directed. If a dose is missed, take as soon as remembered as long as it is not just before next dose. Do not double doses.
- If nausea becomes a problem, advise patient that eating solid food often provides relief.
- Advise patient to report signs and symptoms of fluid retention (swelling of ankles and feet, weight gain), thromboembolic disorders (pain, swelling, tenderness in extremities, headache, chest pain, blurred vision), mental depression, or hepatic dysfunction (yellowed skin or eyes, pruritus, dark urine, light-colored stools) to health care professional.
- Instruct patient to stop taking medication and notify health care professional if pregnancy is suspected. Caution patient of the increase in cervical and vaginal carcinoma in female offspring and in testicular tumors in male offspring if this drug is taken during pregnancy.
- Caution patient that cigarette smoking during estrogen therapy may increase risk of serious side effects, especially for women over age 35.
- Advise patient to notify health care professional of medication regimen prior to treatment or surgery.
- Caution patient to use sunscreen and protective clothing to prevent photosensitivity reactions.
- Emphasize the importance of routine follow-up physical exams including blood pressure; breast, abdomen, and pelvic exams; and PAP smears every 6–12 mo.

EVALUATION

Effectiveness of therapy can be demonstrated by: ▪ Control of the spread of advanced metastatic breast or prostatic cancer.

DIFLUNISAL

(dye-**floo**-ni-sal)
{Apo-Diflunisal}, Dolobid, Novo-Diflunisal

CLASSIFICATION(S):
Analgesic (nonopioid), Nonsteroidal anti-inflammatory agent

Pregnancy Category C (first trimester)

INDICATIONS

▪ Inflammatory disorders including: ▫ Rheumatoid arthritis ▫ Osteoarthritis ▪ Treatment of mild to moderate pain.

ACTION

▪ Inhibits prostaglandin synthesis ▪ Diflunisal is an NSAID chemically related to aspirin. **Therapeutic Effects:** ▪ Suppression of pain and inflammation.

PHARMACOKINETICS

Absorption: Well absorbed from the GI tract.
Distribution: Crosses the placenta; enters breast milk.
Metabolism and Excretion: Metabolized by the liver.
Half-life: 8–12 hr.

CONTRAINDICATIONS AND PRECAUTIONS

Contraindicated in: ▪ Hypersensitivity ▪ Cross-sensitivity may exist with other NSAIDs, including aspirin ▪ Active GI bleeding or ulcer disease.
Use Cautiously in: ▪ Severe cardiovascular, renal, or hepatic disease ▪ History of ulcer disease ▪ Adolescents (may increase the risk of Reye's syndrome if used during viral illness) ▪ Pregnancy (not recommended for use during second half of pregnancy) ▪ Lactation or children (safety not established).

ADVERSE REACTIONS AND SIDE EFFECTS*

CNS: dizziness, drowsiness, headache, psychic disturbances.
EENT: blurred vision, rhinitis, tinnitus.
CV: arrhythmias, changes in blood pressure, edema.
GI: GI BLEEDING, discomfort, nausea, constipation, diarrhea, vomiting.
GU: renal failure.

{} = Available in Canada only.
*CAPITALS indicate life-threatening; underlines indicate most frequent.

Derm: rashes.
Hemat: blood dyscrasias, prolonged bleeding time.
MS: muscle aches.
Misc: allergic reactions including ANAPHYLAXIS, chills.

INTERACTIONS

Drug-Drug: ▪ Concurrent use with **aspirin** may decrease effectiveness ▪ Additive adverse GI effects with **aspirin**, other **NSAIDs, colchicine, glucocorticoids**, or **alcohol** ▪ Chronic use with **acetaminophen** may increase the risk of adverse renal and hepatic reactions ▪ May decrease the effectiveness of **diuretics** or **antihypertensive therapy** ▪ May increase the hypoglycemic effects of **insulin** or **oral hypoglycemic agents** ▪ May increase serum **lithium** levels and increase the risk of toxicity ▪ Increases the risk of toxicity from **methotrexate** ▪ **Probenecid** increases risk of toxicity from diflunisal ▪ Increased risk of bleeding with **some cephalosporins, plicamycin, valproic acid, thrombolytic agents**, or **anticoagulants** ▪ May increase levels and increase the risk of toxicity from **cyclosporine, lithium**, or **methotrexate** ▪ Increased risk of adverse hematologic reactions with **antineoplastic agents** or **radiation therapy** ▪ Administration with **antacids** decreases absorption of diflunisal ▪ May increase the risk of adverse renal reactions when used with **gold compounds.**

ROUTE AND DOSAGE

- **PO (Adults):** *Anti-inflammatory*—250–500 mg twice daily. *Analgesic*—500 mg–1 g initially, then 250–500 mg q 8–12 hr.

AVAILABILITY

- ***Tablets:*** 250 mg[Rx], 500 mg[Rx].

TIME/ACTION PROFILE

	ONSET	PEAK	DURATION
PO (analgesic)	1 hr	2–3 hr	8–12 hr
PO (anti-inflammatory)	few days–1 wk	2 wk	UK

NURSING IMPLICATIONS

ASSESSMENT

- **General Info:** Patients who have asthma, aspirin-induced allergy, and nasal polyps are at increased risk for developing hypersensitivity reactions.
- **Arthritis:** Assess pain and range of motion prior to and periodically during therapy.
- **Pain:** Assess pain (type, location, and intensity) prior to and 1–2 hr following administration.
- ***Lab Test Considerations:*** BUN, serum creatinine, CBC, and liver function tests should be evaluated periodically in patients receiving prolonged course of therapy.
  - ☐ Serum potassium, creatinine, AST, ALT, and LDH may show increased levels. Serum uric acid levels may be decreased.
  - ☐ May cause minimally prolonged bleeding time, which may persist for less than 1 day following discontinuation of therapy.

POTENTIAL NURSING DIAGNOSES

- Pain (Indications).
- Physical mobility, impaired (Indications).
- Knowledge deficit, related to medication regimen (Patient/Family Teaching).

D

IMPLEMENTATION

- **General Info:** Coadministration with opioid analgesics may have additive analgesic effects and may permit lower opioid doses.
- **PO:** For rapid initial effect, administer 30 min before or 2 hr after meals. May be administered with food, milk, or antacids to decrease GI irritation. Capsules should be swallowed whole; do not crush or chew.

PATIENT/FAMILY TEACHING

- ☐ Advise patient to take diflunisal with a full glass of water and to remain in an upright position for 15–30 min after administration.
- ☐ Instruct patient to take diflunisal exactly as directed. If a dose is missed, it should be taken as soon as remembered but not if almost time for the next dose. Do not double doses.
- ☐ May cause drowsiness or dizziness. Advise patient to avoid driving or other activities requiring alertness until response to the medication is known.
- ☐ Caution patient to avoid concurrent use of alcohol, aspirin, NSAIDs, acetaminophen, or other OTC medications without consulting health care professional.
- ☐ Instruct patient to notify health care profes-

sional of medication regimen prior to treatment or surgery.
- Caution patient to wear sunscreen and protective clothing to prevent photosensitivity reactions.
- Advise patient to consult health care professional if rash, itching, visual disturbances, tinnitus, weight gain, edema, black stools, persistent headache, or influenza-like syndrome (chills, fever, muscle aches, pain) occurs.
- Centers for Disease Control and Prevention warns against giving aspirin or salicylates to children or adolescents with varicella (chickenpox) or influenza-like or viral illnesses because of a possible association with Reye's syndrome.

EVALUATION

Effectiveness of therapy can be demonstrated by: ▪ Decrease in severity of mild to moderate pain ▪ Improved joint mobility. Partial arthritic relief is usually seen within 1–2 wk, with maximum effectiveness seen in several weeks. Patients who do not respond to one NSAID may respond to another.

DIGITOXIN

(di-ji-**tox**-in)

Crystodigin, {Digitaline}

CLASSIFICATION(S):

Antiarrhythmic, Inotropic agent

Pregnancy Category C

INDICATIONS

▪ Treatment of congestive heart failure ▪ Tachyarrhythmias ▫ Atrial fibrillation and atrial flutter (slows ventricular rate) ▫ Paroxysmal atrial tachycardia.

ACTION

▪ Increases the force of myocardial contraction ▪ Prolongs refractory period of the AV node ▪ Decreases conduction through the SA and AV nodes. **Therapeutic Effects:** ▪ Increased cardiac output (positive inotropic effect) and slowing of the heart rate (negative chronotropic effect).

PHARMACOKINETICS

Absorption: Completely absorbed following oral administration.
Distribution: Widely distributed.
Metabolism and Excretion: Primarily metabolized by the liver; some metabolites have cardiac activity.
Half-life: 118–216 hr.

CONTRAINDICATIONS AND PRECAUTIONS

Contraindicated in: ▪ Hypersensitivity ▪ Uncontrolled ventricular arrhythmias ▪ AV block ▪ Idiopathic hypertrophic subaortic stenosis ▪ Constrictive pericarditis.
Use Cautiously in: ▪ Electrolyte abnormalities (hypokalemia, hypercalcemia, and hypomagnesemia may predispose to toxicity) ▪ Geriatric patients (very sensitive to toxic effects) ▪ Myocardial infarction ▪ Renal impairment (dosage reduction of digoxin required) ▪ Pregnancy and lactation (safety not established).

ADVERSE REACTIONS AND SIDE EFFECTS*

CNS: fatigue, headache, weakness.
EENT: blurred vision, yellow vision.
CV: ARRHYTHMIAS, bradycardia, ECG changes.
GI: anorexia, nausea, vomiting, diarrhea.
Endo: gynecomastia.
Hemat: thrombocytopenia.

INTERACTIONS

Drug-Drug: ▪ Concurrent use with **phenobarbital, phenytoin,** or **rifampin** may result in decreased effectiveness of digitoxin ▪ Use of digitoxin with **succinylcholine** may increase cardiac irritability ▪ **Thiazide** and **loop diuretics, mezlocillin, piperacillin, ticarcillin, amphotericin B,** and **glucocorticoids,** which cause hypokalemia, may increase the risk of toxicity ▪ **Quinidine, cyclosporine, amiodarone, verapamil, diltiazem, propofenone,** and **diclofenac** increase serum levels and may lead to toxicity (serum level monitoring/dosage reduction recommended) ▪ Additive bradycardia may occur with **beta-adrenergic blocking agents** and other **antiarrhythmic agents (quinidine, disopyramide)** ▪ Absorption is

{} = Available in Canada only.
***CAPITALS indicate life-threatening; underlines indicate most frequent.**

decreased by concurrent **antacids, kaolin-pectin, cholestyramine,** or **colestipol** ▪ **Thyroid hormones** may decrease therapeutic effects.

Drug-Food: ▪ Concurrent ingestion of a **high-fiber meal** may decrease absorption.

ROUTE AND DOSAGE

For rapid effect, a larger initial loading/digitalizing dose should be given in several divided doses over 12–24 hr. All dosing must be evaluated by individual response. In general, doses required for atrial arrhythmias are higher than those for inotropic effect.

- **PO (Adults and Children >12 yr):** *Rapid digitalization*—600 mcg (0.6 mg) initially, then 400 mcg (0.4 mg) 4–6 hr later, then 200 mcg (0.2 mg) 4–6 hr after that, followed by maintenance dose. *Slow digitalization*—200 mcg (0.2 mg) twice daily for 4 days, followed by maintenance dose. *Maintenance dose*—50–300 mcg (0.05–0.3 mg)/day.
- **PO (Children >2 yr):** *Digitalizing dose*—0.03 mg/kg (0.75 mg/m^2) given in 3–4 divided doses at least 6 hr apart, followed by maintenance dose. *Maintenance dose*—10% of the digitalizing dose.
- **PO (Children 1–2 yr):** *Digitalizing dose*—0.04 mg/kg given in 3–4 divided doses at least 6 hr apart, followed by maintenance dose. *Maintenance dose*—10% of the digitalizing dose.
- **PO (Children < 1 yr):** *Digitalizing dose*—0.045 mg/kg given in 3–4 divided doses at least 6 hr apart, followed by maintenance dose. *Maintenance dose*—10% of the digitalizing dose.

AVAILABILITY

- ***Tablets:*** 100 mcg[Rx], 200 mcg[Rx].

TIME/ACTION PROFILE (antiarrhythmic or inotropic effects, provided that a loading dose has been given)

	ONSET	PEAK	DURATION
Digitoxin–PO	60 –240 min	8–12 hr	2–3 wk*

*Duration listed is that for normal renal function; in impaired renal function, duration will be longer.

NURSING IMPLICATIONS

ASSESSMENT

- ▫ Monitor apical pulse for 1 full min prior to administering. Withhold dose and notify physician if pulse rate is <60 bpm in an adult, <70 bpm in a child, or <90 bpm in an infant. Also notify physician or health care professional promptly of any significant changes in rate, rhythm, or quality of pulse.
- ▫ Monitor ECG periodically during therapy. Notify physician or health care professional if bradycardia or new arrhythmias occur.
- ▫ Monitor intake and output ratios and daily weights. Assess for peripheral edema, and auscultate lungs for rales/crackles throughout therapy.
- ▫ Before administering initial loading dose, determine if patient has taken any digitalis preparations in the preceding 2–3 wk.
- ▪ ***Lab Test Considerations:*** Serum electrolyte levels (especially potassium, magnesium, and calcium) and renal and hepatic functions should be evaluated periodically during course of therapy. Notify physician or other health care professional prior to giving dose if patient is hypokalemic. Hypokalemia, hypomagnesemia, or hypercalcemia may make the patient more susceptible to digitalis toxicity.
- ▪ ***Toxicity and Overdose:*** Therapeutic serum digitoxin levels range from 20 to 35 ng/ml. Serum levels may be drawn 4–10 hr after a dose is administered, although they are usually drawn immediately prior to the next dose.
- ▫ Observe patient for signs and symptoms of toxicity. In adults and older children, the first signs of toxicity usually include abdominal pain, anorexia, nausea, vomiting, visual disturbances, bradycardia, and other arrhythmias. In infants and small children, the first symptoms of overdose are usually cardiac arrhythmias. If these appear, withhold drug and notify physician or health care professional immediately.
- ▫ If signs of toxicity occur and are not severe, discontinuation of digitalis glycoside may be all that is required.
- ▫ If hypokalemia is present and renal function is adequate, potassium salts may be administered. Do not administer if hyperkalemia or heart block exists.
- ▫ Correction of arrhythmias due to digitalis toxicity may be attempted with lidocaine, procainamide, quinidine, propranolol, or phenytoin. Temporary ventricular pacing may be useful in advanced heart block.

D

□ Treatment of life-threatening arrhythmias may include administration of digoxin immune Fab (Digibind, see p. 282), which binds to the digitalis glycoside molecule in the blood and is excreted by the kidneys.

POTENTIAL NURSING DIAGNOSES

- Cardiac output, decreased (Indications).
- Knowledge deficit, related to medication regimen (Patient/Family Teaching).

IMPLEMENTATION

- **General Info:** For rapid digitalization, the initial dose is higher than the maintenance dose; ¼–½ of the total digitalizing dose is given initially. The remainder of the dose will be administered in ¼ increments at 4–8 hr intervals.
- **PO:** Oral preparations can be administered without regard to meals. Tablets can be crushed and administered with food or fluids if patient has difficulty swallowing.

PATIENT/FAMILY TEACHING

□ Instruct patient to take medication exactly as directed, at the same time each day. Missed doses should be taken within 12 hr of scheduled dose or not taken at all. Do not double doses. Consult health care professional if doses for 2 or more days are missed. Do not discontinue medication without consulting health care professional.

□ Teach patient to take pulse and to contact health care professional before taking medication if pulse rate is <60 or >100.

□ Review signs and symptoms of digitalis toxicity with patient and family. Advise patient to notify health care professional immediately if these or symptoms of congestive heart failure occur. Inform patient that these symptoms may be mistaken for those of colds or flu.

□ Advise patient that sharing of this medication can be dangerous.

□ Caution patient to avoid concurrent use of OTC medications without consulting health care professional. Advise patient to avoid antacids or antidiarrheals within 2 hr of digitoxin.

□ Advise patient to notify health care professional of this medication regimen prior to treatment.

□ Patients taking digitoxin should carry identification describing disease process and medication regimen at all times.

□ Emphasize the importance of routine follow-up exams to determine effectiveness and to monitor for toxicity.

EVALUATION

Effectiveness of therapy can be demonstrated by: ▪ Decrease in severity of congestive heart failure ▪ Increase in cardiac output ▪ Decrease in ventricular response in atrial tachyarrhythmias ▪ Termination of paroxysmal atrial tachycardia.

DIGOXIN

(di-**jox**-in)

Lanoxicaps, Lanoxin

CLASSIFICATION(S):

Antiarrhythmic, Inotropic agent

Pregnancy Category C

INDICATIONS

▪ Treatment of congestive heart failure ▪ Tachyarrhythmias □ Atrial fibrillation and atrial flutter (slows ventricular rate) □ Paroxysmal atrial tachycardia.

ACTION

▪ Increases the force of myocardial contraction ▪ Prolongs refractory period of the AV node ▪ Decreases conduction through the SA and AV node. **Therapeutic Effects:** ▪ Increased cardiac output (positive inotropic effect) and slowing of the heart rate (negative chronotropic effect).

PHARMACOKINETICS

Absorption: 60–85% absorbed following oral administration of tablets; 75–80% absorbed following administration of elixir. Absorption from liquid-filled capsules is 90–100%; 80% absorbed from IM sites, but this route is not recommended because of extreme pain and irritation.

Distribution: Widely distributed; crosses the placenta and enters breast milk.

Metabolism and Excretion: Excreted almost entirely unchanged by the kidneys.

Half-life: 36–48 hr (increased in renal impairment).

CONTRAINDICATIONS AND PRECAUTIONS

Contraindicated in: ▪ Hypersensitivity ▪ Uncontrolled ventricular arrhythmias ▪ AV block ▪ Idiopathic hypertrophic subaortic stenosis ▪ Constrictive pericarditis ▪ Known alcohol intolerance (elixir only).

Use Cautiously in: ▪ Electrolyte abnormalities (hypokalemia, hypercalcemia, and hypomagnesemia may predispose to toxicity) ▪ Geriatric patients (very sensitive to toxic effects) ▪ Myocardial infarction ▪ Renal impairment (dosage reduction of digoxin required) ▪ Obese patients (dose should be based on ideal body weight) ▪ Pregnancy and lactation (although safety has not been established, has been used during pregnancy without adverse effects on the fetus).

ADVERSE REACTIONS AND SIDE EFFECTS*

CNS: <u>fatigue</u>, headache, weakness.
EENT: blurred vision, yellow vision.
CV: ARRHYTHMIAS, <u>bradycardia</u>, ECG changes.
GI: <u>anorexia</u>, <u>nausea</u>, <u>vomiting</u>, diarrhea.
Endo: gynecomastia.
Hemat: thrombocytopenia.

INTERACTIONS

Drug-Drug: ▪ **Thiazide** and **loop diuretics, mezlocillin, piperacillin, ticarcillin, amphotericin B,** and **glucocorticoids,** which cause hypokalemia, may increase the risk of toxicity ▪ **Quinidine, cyclosporine, amiodarone, verapamil, diltiazem, propofenone,** and **diclofenac** increase serum levels and may lead to toxicity (serum level monitoring/dosage reduction recommended) ▪ **Spironolactone** increases half-life (reduced dosage/increased dosing interval may be required) ▪ Additive bradycardia may occur with **beta-adrenergic blocking agents** and other **antiarrhythmic agents (quinidine, disopyramide)** ▪ Absorption is decreased by concurrent **antacids, kaolin-pectin, cholestyramine,** or **colestipol** ▪ **Thyroid hormones** may decrease therapeutic effects.

Drug-Food: ▪ Concurrent ingestion of a **high-fiber meal** may decrease absorption.

ROUTE AND DOSAGE

For rapid effect, a larger initial loading/digitalizing dose should be given in several divided doses over 12–24 hr. Maintenance doses are determined for digoxin by renal function. All dosing must be evaluated by individual response. In general, doses required for atrial arrhythmias are higher than those for inotropic effect. When determining dosage, consider that bioavailability of gelatin capsules (Lanoxicaps) is greater than that of tablets.

- **IV (Adults):** *Digitalizing dose*—0.6–1.0 mg (10–15 mcg/kg) given as 50% of the dose initially and additional fractions given at 4–8 hr intervals.
- **IV (Children >10 yr):** *Digitalizing dose*—8–12 mcg/kg given as 50% of the dose initially and additional fractions given at 4–8 hr intervals.
- **IV (Children 5–10 yr):** *Digitalizing dose*—15–30 mcg/kg given as 50% of the dose initially and additional fractions given at 4–8 hr intervals.
- **IV (Children 2–5 yr):** *Digitalizing dose*—25–35 mcg/kg given as 50% of the dose initially and additional fractions given at 4–8 hr intervals.
- **IV (Children 1–24 mo):** *Digitalizing dose*—30–50 mcg/kg given as 50% of the dose initially and additional fractions given at 4–8 hr intervals.
- **IV (Infants—full term):** *Digitalizing dose*—20–30 mcg/kg given as 50% of the dose initially and additional fractions given at 4–8 hr intervals.
- **IV (Infants—premature):** *Digitalizing dose*—15–25 mcg/kg given as 50% of the dose initially and additional fractions given at 4–8 hr intervals.
- **PO (Adults):** *Digitalizing dose*—0.75–1.25 mg (10–15 mg/kg) given as 50% of the dose initially and additional fractions given at 4–8 hr intervals. *Maintenance dose*—0.063–0.5 mg/day as tablets or 0.350–0.5 mg/day as gelatin capsules, depending on patient's lean body weight, renal function, and serum level.

*CAPITALS indicate life-threatening; <u>underlines</u> indicate most frequent.

D

- **PO (Children >10 yr):** *Digitalizing dose*—10–15 mcg/kg given as 50% of the dose initially and additional fractions given at 6–8 hr intervals. *Maintenance dose*—25–35% of the loading dose given daily as a single dose.
- **PO (Children 5–10 yr):** *Digitalizing dose*—20–35 mcg/kg given as 50% of the dose initially and additional fractions given at 6–8 hr intervals. *Maintenance dose*—25–35% of the loading dose given daily in 2 divided doses.
- **PO (Children 2–5 yr):** *Digitalizing dose*—30–40 mcg/kg given as 50% of the dose initially and additional fractions given at 6–8 hr intervals. *Maintenance dose*—25–35% of the loading dose given daily in 2 divided doses.
- **PO (Children 1–24 mo):** *Digitalizing dose*—35–60 mcg/kg given as 50% of the dose initially and additional fractions given at 6–8 hr intervals. *Maintenance dose*—25–35% of the loading dose given daily in 2 divided doses.
- **PO (Infants—full term):** *Digitalizing dose*—25–35 mcg/kg given as 50% of the dose initially and additional fractions given at 6–8 hr intervals. *Maintenance dose*—25–35% of the loading dose given daily in 2 divided doses.
- **PO (Infants—premature):** *Digitalizing dose*—20–30 mcg/kg given as 50% of the dose initially and additional fractions given at 6–8 hr intervals. *Maintenance dose*—20–30% of the loading dose given daily in 2 divided doses.

AVAILABILITY

- ***Tablets:*** 0.125 mg[Rx], 0.25 mg[Rx], 0.5 mg[Rx]
- ***Capsules:*** 0.05 mg[Rx], 0.1 mg[Rx], 0.2 mg[Rx]
- ***Pediatric elixir:*** 0.05 mg/ml[Rx] ▪ ***Injection:*** 0.25 mg/ml[Rx] ▪ ***Pediatric injection:*** 0.1 mg/ml[Rx].

TIME/ACTION PROFILE (antiarrhythmic or inotropic effects, provided that a loading dose has been given)

	ONSET	PEAK	DURATION
Digoxin–PO	30–120 min	2–6 hr	2–4 days*
Digoxin–IM	30 min	4–6 hr	2–4 days*
Digoxin–IV	5–30 min	1–5 hr	2–4 days*

*Duration listed is that for normal renal function; in impaired renal function, duration will be longer.

NURSING IMPLICATIONS

ASSESSMENT

- Monitor apical pulse for 1 full min prior to administering. Withhold dose and notify physician if pulse rate is <60 bpm in an adult, <70 bpm in a child, or <90 bpm in an infant. Also notify physician or health care professional promptly of any significant changes in rate, rhythm, or quality of pulse.
- Monitor blood pressure periodically in patients receiving IV digoxin.
- Monitor ECG throughout IV administration and periodically during therapy. Notify physician or health care professional if bradycardia or new arrhythmias occur.
- Observe IV site for redness or infiltration; extravasation can lead to tissue irritation and sloughing.
- Monitor intake and output ratios and daily weights. Assess for peripheral edema, and auscultate lungs for rales/crackles throughout therapy.
- Before administering initial loading dose, determine if patient has taken any digitalis preparations in the preceding 2–3 wk.
- ***Lab Test Considerations:*** Serum electrolyte levels (especially potassium, magnesium, and calcium) and renal and hepatic functions should be evaluated periodically during therapy. Notify physician or other health care professional prior to giving dose if patient is hypokalemic. Hypokalemia, hypomagnesemia, or hypercalcemia may make the patient more susceptible to digitalis toxicity.
- ***Toxicity and Overdose:*** Therapeutic serum digoxin levels range from 0.5 to 2 ng/ml. Serum levels may be drawn 4–10 hr after a dose is administered, although they are usually drawn immediately prior to the next dose.
- Observe patient for signs and symptoms of toxicity. In adults and older children, the first signs of toxicity usually include abdominal pain, anorexia, nausea, vomiting, visual disturbances, bradycardia, and other arrhythmias. In infants and small children, the first symptoms of overdose are usually cardiac arrhythmias. If these appear, withhold drug and notify physician or health care professional immediately.
- If signs of toxicity occur and are not severe,

discontinuation of digitalis glycoside may be all that is required.
- ▫ If hypokalemia is present and renal function is adequate, potassium salts may be administered. Do not administer if hyperkalemia or heart block exists.
- ▫ Correction of arrhythmias due to digitalis toxicity may be attempted with lidocaine, procainamide, quinidine, propranolol, or phenytoin. Temporary ventricular pacing may be useful in advanced heart block.
- ▫ Treatment of life-threatening arrhythmias may include administration of digoxin immune Fab (Digibind, see p. 282), which binds to the digitalis glycoside molecule in the blood and is excreted by the kidneys.

POTENTIAL NURSING DIAGNOSES

- Cardiac output, decreased (Indications).
- Knowledge deficit, related to medication regimen (Patient/Family Teaching).

IMPLEMENTATION

- **General Info:** For rapid digitalization, the initial dose is higher than the maintenance dose; ¼–½ of the total digitalizing dose is given initially. The remainder of the dose will be administered in ¼ increments at 4–8 hr intervals.
- ▫ When changing from parenteral to oral dosage forms, dosage adjustments may be necessary because of pharmacokinetic variations in percentage of digoxin absorbed. 100 mcg (0.1 mg) digoxin injection or 100 mcg (0.1 mg) liquid-filled capsule = 125 mcg (0.125 mg) tablet or 125 mcg (0.125 mg) of elixir.
- **PO:** Oral preparations can be administered without regard to meals. Tablets can be crushed and administered with food or fluids if patient has difficulty swallowing. Use calibrated measuring device for liquid preparations. Do not alternate between dosage forms; bioavailability of capsules is not equal to tablets or elixir.
- **IM:** Administer deep into gluteal muscle and massage well to reduce painful local reactions. Do not administer more than 2 ml of digoxin in each IM site. IM administration is not generally recommended.
- **Direct IV:** IV doses may be given undiluted or each 1 ml may be diluted in 4 ml of sterile water, 0.9% NaCl, D5W, or lactated Ringer's solution for injection. Less diluent will cause precipitation. Use diluted solution immediately. Do not use solution that is discolored or contains precipitate.
- ***Rate:*** Administer each dose through Y-site injection over a minimum of 5 min.
- **Syringe Compatibility:** ▪ heparin ▪ milrinone.
- **Y-Site Compatibility:** ▪ amrinone ▪ ciprofloxacin ▪ diltiazem ▪ famotidine ▪ meperidine ▪ milrinone ▪ morphine ▪ potassium chloride ▪ tacrolimus ▪ vitamin B complex with C.
- **Y-Site Incompatibility:** ▪ fluconazole ▪ foscarnet.
- **Additive Incompatibility:** ▪ Manufacturer recommends that digoxin not be admixed with other drugs.

PATIENT/FAMILY TEACHING

- ▫ Instruct patient to take medication exactly as directed, at the same time each day. Missed doses should be taken within 12 hr of scheduled dose or not taken at all. Do not double doses. Consult health care professional if doses for 2 or more days are missed. Do not discontinue medication without consulting health care professional.
- ▫ Teach patient to take pulse and to contact health care professional before taking medication if pulse rate is <60 or >100.
- ▫ Review signs and symptoms of digitalis toxicity with patient and family. Advise patient to notify health care professional immediately if these or symptoms of congestive heart failure occur. Inform patient that these symptoms may be mistaken for those of colds or flu.
- ▫ Instruct patient to keep digoxin tablets in their original container and not to mix in pill boxes with other medications, as they may look similar and may be mistaken for other medications.
- ▫ Advise patient that sharing of this medication can be dangerous.
- ▫ Caution patient to avoid concurrent use of OTC medications without consulting health care professional. Advise patient to avoid taking antacids or antidiarrheals within 2 hr of digoxin.
- ▫ Advise patient to notify health care professional of this medication regimen prior to treatment.
- ▫ Patients taking digoxin should carry identifi-

D

cation describing disease process and medication regimen at all times.

- Emphasize the importance of routine follow-up exams to determine effectiveness and to monitor for toxicity.

EVALUATION

Effectiveness of therapy can be demonstrated by: ▪ Decrease in severity of congestive heart failure ▪ Increase in cardiac output ▪ Decrease in ventricular response in atrial tachyarrhythmias ▪ Termination of paroxysmal atrial tachycardia.

DIGOXIN IMMUNE FAB

(di-**jox**-in im-**myoon** fab)
Digibind

CLASSIFICATION(S):
Antidote (for digoxin, digitoxin)

Pregnancy Category C

INDICATIONS

▪ Serious life-threatening overdosage with digoxin or digitoxin.

ACTION

▪ An antibody produced in sheep that binds antigenically to unbound digoxin or digitoxin in serum. **Therapeutic Effects:** ▪ Binding and subsequent removal of digoxin or digitoxin, preventing toxic effects in overdose.

PHARMACOKINETICS

Absorption: Administered IV only, resulting in complete bioavailability.
Distribution: Widely distributed throughout extracellular space.
Metabolism and Excretion: Excreted by the kidneys as the bound complex (digoxin immune Fab plus digoxin or digitoxin).
Half-life: 14–20 hr.

CONTRAINDICATIONS AND PRECAUTIONS

Contraindicated in: ▪ No known contraindications.
Use Cautiously in: ▪ Known hypersensitivity to sheep proteins or products ▪ Children, pregnancy, or lactation (safety not established).

ADVERSE REACTIONS AND SIDE EFFECTS*

CV: re-emergence of atrial fibrillation, re-emergence of congestive heart failure.
F and E: HYPOKALEMIA.

INTERACTIONS

Drug-Drug: ▪ Prevents response to digoxin or digitoxin.

ROUTE AND DOSAGE

38 mg of digoxin immune Fab will bind 0.5 mg of digitoxin or digoxin. Each vial contains 38 mg of digoxin immune Fab.

When Amount of Digitalis Glycoside Ingested (Administered) Is Known

- **IV (Adults and Children):** *For digitalis glycoside toxicity due to digoxin tablets, oral solution, or IM digoxin*—dose of digoxin ingested (mg) × 0.8 ÷ 1000 × 38. *For digitalis glycoside toxicity due to digitoxin tablets, digoxin capsules, IV digoxin*—dose of digoxin ingested (mg) ÷ 0.5 × 38.

When Serum Digoxin/Digitoxin Concentrations (SDCs) Are Known

- **IV (Adults and Children):** *For digoxin*—SDC (nanograms/ml) × body weight (kg) ÷ 100 × 38. *For digitoxin*—SDC (nanograms/ml) × body weight (kg) ÷ 1000 × 38.

When Amount Ingested Is Not Known or SDCs Are Unavailable

- **IV (Adults and Children):** 760 mg.

Skin Test

- **Intradermal (Adults):** 9.5 mcg.

AVAILABILITY

The following *approximate* doses of digoxin immune Fab would be administered when based on postdistribution serum *digoxin* concentration in children and adults:

*CAPITALS indicate life-threatening; underlines indicate most frequent.

BODY WEIGHT (in kg)	POSTDISTRIBUTION SERUM DIGOXIN CONCENTRATION (in ng/ml) 1	2	4	8	12	16	20
	DOSE OF DIGOXIN IMMUNE FAB (*in mg*)						
1	0.4	1	1.5	3	5	6	8
3	1	2	5	9	14	18	23
5	2	4	8	15	23	30	38
10	4	8	15	30	46	61	76
20	8	15	30	61	91	122	152
40	19	38	76	114	190	266	304
60	19	38	114	190	266	380	456
70	38	76	114	228	342	418	532
80	38	76	114	266	380	494	608
100	38	76	152	304	456	608	760

From *AHFS Drug Information® 97*. American Society of Health System Pharmacists, Bethesda, MD, 1997, with permission.

TIME/ACTION PROFILE (reversal of arrhythmias and hyperkalemia; reversal of inotropic effect may take several hr)

	ONSET	PEAK	DURATION
IV	30 min (variable)	UK	2–6 hr

NURSING IMPLICATIONS

ASSESSMENT

- Monitor ECG, pulse, blood pressure, and body temperature prior to and throughout treatment. Patients with atrial fibrillation may develop a rapid ventricular response as a result of decreased digoxin or digitoxin levels.
- Assess patient for increase in signs of congestive heart failure (peripheral edema, dyspnea, rales/crackles, weight gain).
- ***Lab Test Considerations:*** Monitor serum digoxin or digitoxin levels prior to administration.
- Monitor serum potassium levels frequently during treatment. Prior to treatment, hyperkalemia usually coexists with toxicity. Levels may decrease rapidly; hypokalemia should be treated promptly.
- Free serum digoxin or digitoxin levels fall rapidly following administration. Total serum concentrations rise suddenly after administration but are bound to the Fab molecule and are inactive. Total serum concentrations will decrease to undetectable levels within several days. Serum digoxin or digitoxin levels are not valid for 5–7 days following administration.

POTENTIAL NURSING DIAGNOSES

- Knowledge deficit, related to medication regimen (Patient/Family Teaching).

IMPLEMENTATION

- **General Info:** Cardiopulmonary resuscitation equipment and medications should be available during administration.
- Delay redigitalization for several days until the elimination of digoxin immune Fab from the body is complete.
- **Test Dose:** Patients with a high risk for allergy to digoxin immune Fab or sheep proteins should have skin testing for allergy prior to administration. Prepare skin test solution by diluting 0.1 ml of the reconstituted solution (10 mg/ml) in 9.9 ml of 0.9% NaCl to produce a 10-ml solution (100 mcg/ml). Testing may be administered by intradermal injection or scratch test. For intradermal use, inject 0.1 ml intradermally. For scratch test, place 1 drop of solution on the skin and make a ¼-in. scratch through the drop with a sterile needle. Following either method, inspect for urticarial wheal surrounded by erythema after 20 min. If a positive skin test occurs, use of digoxin immune Fab should be avoided unless absolutely necessary.
- **Intermittent Infusion:** Reconstitute each 38 mg for IV administration in 4 ml of sterile water for injection and mix gently. Solution will contain a concentration of 10 mg/ml. May be further diluted with 0.9% NaCl for IV infusion. Reconstituted solution should be used immediately but is stable for 4 hr if refrigerated.
- In infants and small children, monitor for fluid overload. For small doses, a reconstituted 38-mg vial can be diluted with 34 ml of 0.9% NaCl for a concentration of 1 mg/ml. Administer with a tuberculin syringe.
- ***Rate:*** Administer reconstituted solution by IV infusion through a 0.22-micron membrane filter over 15–30 min. If cardiac arrest is imminent, rapid direct IV injection may be used. Do not use rapid direct injection in other patients because of increased risk of adverse reactions.
- **Incompatibility:** Information unavailable. Do not mix with other drugs or solutions.

PATIENT/FAMILY TEACHING

□ Explain the procedure and purpose of the treatment to the patient.

EVALUATION

Effectiveness of therapy can be demonstrated by: ▪ Resolution of signs and symptoms of digoxin or digitoxin toxicity □ Decreased digoxin or digitoxin level without major side effects.

DILTIAZEM

(dil-**tye**-a-zem)

{Apo-Diltiaz}, Cardizem, Dilacor XR, Diltia XT, {Novo-Diltazem}, Nu-Diltiaz, {Syn-Diltiazem}, Tiamate, Tiazac

CLASSIFICATION(S):

Antianginal, Antiarrhythmic, Antihypertensive agent, Calcium channel blocker

Pregnancy Category C

INDICATIONS

▪ Management of: □ Hypertension □ Angina pectoris and vasospastic (Prinzmetal's) angina □ Management of supraventricular tachyarrhythmias and rapid ventricular rates in atrial flutter or fibrillation. **Unlabeled Uses:** ▪ Management of Raynaud's syndrome.

ACTION

▪ Inhibits the transport of calcium into myocardial and vascular smooth muscle cells, resulting in inhibition of excitation-contraction coupling and subsequent contraction. **Therapeutic Effects:** ▪ Systemic vasodilation resulting in decreased blood pressure ▪ Coronary vasodilation resulting in decreased frequency and severity of attacks of angina ▪ Suppression of arrhythmias.

PHARMACOKINETICS

Absorption: Well absorbed following oral administration but is rapidly metabolized.
Distribution: UK.
Metabolism and Excretion: Mostly metabolized by the liver.
Half-life: 3.5–9 hr.

CONTRAINDICATIONS AND PRECAUTIONS

Contraindicated in: ▪ Hypersensitivity ▪ Sick sinus syndrome ▪ 2nd- or 3rd-degree AV block (unless an artificial pacemaker is in place) ▪ Blood pressure <90 mm Hg ▪ Recent myocardial infarction (MI) or pulmonary congestion.
Use Cautiously in: ▪ Severe hepatic impairment (dosage reduction recommended for most agents) ▪ Geriatric patients (dosage reduction/slower IV infusion rate recommended; increased risk of hypotension) ▪ Severe renal impairment ▪ History of serious ventricular arrhythmias or congestive heart failure ▪ Pregnancy, lactation, or children (safety not established).

ADVERSE REACTIONS AND SIDE EFFECTS*

CNS: abnormal dreams, anxiety, confusion, dizziness, drowsiness, headache, nervousness, psychiatric disturbances, weakness.
EENT: blurred vision, disturbed equilibrium, epistaxis, tinnitus.
Resp: cough, dyspnea.
CV: ARRHYTHMIAS, CONGESTIVE HEART FAILURE, <u>peripheral edema</u>, bradycardia, chest pain, hypotension, palpitations, syncope, tachycardia.
GI: abnormal liver function studies, anorexia, constipation, diarrhea, dry mouth, dysgeusia, dyspepsia, nausea, vomiting.
GU: dysuria, nocturia, polyuria, sexual dysfunction, urinary frequency.
Derm: dermatitis, erythema multiforme, flushing, increased sweating, photosensitivity, pruritus/urticaria, rash.
Endo: gynecomastia, hyperglycemia.
Hemat: anemia, leukopenia, thrombocytopenia.
Metab: weight gain.
MS: joint stiffness, muscle cramps.
Neuro: paresthesia, tremor.
Misc: STEVENS-JOHNSON SYNDROME, gingival hyperplasia.

INTERACTIONS

Drug-Drug: ▪ Additive hypotension may occur when used concurrently with **fentanyl, other antihypertensives, nitrates,** acute ingestion of **alcohol,** or **quinidine** ▪ Antihypertensive ef-

{} = Available in Canada only.
*CAPITALS indicate life-threatening; <u>underlines</u> indicate most frequent.

fects may be decreased by concurrent use of **NSAIDs** ▪ Serum **digoxin** levels may be increased ▪ Concurrent use with **beta-adrenergic blockers, digoxin, disopyramide**, or **phenytoin** may result in bradycardia, conduction defects, or congestive heart failure ▪ **Phenobarbital** and **phenytoin** may increase metabolism and decrease effectiveness ▪ May decrease the metabolism of and increase the risk of toxicity from **cyclosporine, prazosin, quinidine**, or **carbamazepine.**

ROUTE AND DOSAGE

- **PO (Adults):** 30–120 mg 3–4 times daily or 60–120 mg twice daily as SR capsules or 180–240 mg once daily as CD or XR capsules (up to 360 mg/day).
- **IV (Adults):** 0.25 mg/kg; may repeat in 15 min with a dose of 0.35 mg/kg. May follow with continuous infusion at 10 mg/hr (range 5–15 mg/hr) for up to 24 hr.

AVAILABILITY

▪ ***Tablets:*** 30 mg[Rx], 60 mg[Rx], 90 mg[Rx], 120 mg[Rx] ▪ ***Extended (sustained)-release capsules:*** 60 mg[Rx], 90 mg[Rx], 120 mg[Rx], 180 mg[Rx], 240 mg[Rx], 300 mg[Rx] ▪ ***Injection:*** 5 mg/ml in 10-ml vials[Rx], 25 mg ready-to-use syringes (Lyo-Ject)[Rx] ▪ ***In combination with:*** enalapril (Teczem)[Rx]. See Appendix A.

TIME/ACTION PROFILE

	ONSET	PEAK	DURATION
PO	30 min	2–3 hr	6–8 hr
PO–SR	UK	UK	12 hr
PO–CD, XR	UK	14 days*	up to 24 hr
IV	2–5 min	2–4 hr	UK

*Maximum antihypertensive effect with chronic therapy.

NURSING IMPLICATIONS

ASSESSMENT

- **General Info:** Monitor blood pressure and pulse prior to therapy, during dosage titration, and periodically throughout therapy. Monitor ECG periodically during prolonged therapy. May cause prolonged PR interval.
  - Monitor intake and output ratios and daily weight. Assess for signs of congestive heart failure (peripheral edema, rales/crackles, dyspnea, weight gain, jugular venous distention).
  - Patients receiving digitalis glycosides concurrently with calcium channel blockers should have routine serum digitalis glycoside levels and be monitored for signs and symptoms of digitalis glycoside toxicity.
- **Angina:** Assess location, duration, intensity, and precipitating factors of patient's anginal pain.
- **Arrhythmias:** Monitor ECG continuously during administration. Report bradycardia or prolonged hypotension promptly. Emergency equipment and medication should be available. Monitor blood pressure and pulse before and frequently during administration.
- ***Lab Test Considerations:*** Total serum calcium concentrations are not affected by calcium channel blockers.
  - Monitor serum potassium periodically. Hypokalemia increases the risk of arrhythmias and should be corrected.
  - Monitor renal and hepatic functions periodically during long-term therapy. May cause increase in hepatic enzymes after several days of therapy, which return to normal on discontinuation of therapy.

POTENTIAL NURSING DIAGNOSES

- Cardiac output, decreased (Indications).
- Pain (Indications).
- Knowledge deficit, related to medication regimen (Patient/Family Teaching).

IMPLEMENTATION

- **PO:** May be administered without regard to meals. May be administered with meals if GI irritation becomes a problem.
  - Do not open, crush, break, or chew sustained-release capsules or tablets. Empty tablets that appear in stool are not significant. Crush and mix diltiazem with food or fluids for patients having difficulty swallowing.
- **Direct IV:** May be administered undiluted.
- ***Rate:*** Administer each dose as a bolus over 2 min.
- **Continuous Infusion:** Dilute 125 mg in 100 ml, 250 mg in 250 ml, or 250 mg in 500 ml of 0.9% NaCl, D5W, or D5/0.45% NaCl for concentrations of 1 mg/ml, 0.83 mg/ml, or

D

0.45 mg/ml, respectively. Solution is stable for 24 hr at room temperature or if refrigerated.

- ***Rate:*** Initial infusion should be administered at a rate of 10 mg/hr. May increase in increments of 5 mg/hr, up to 15 mg/hr if further reduction in heart rate is required. Some patients may respond to a rate of 5 mg/hr. Infusion may be continued up to 24 hr.
- **Y-Site Compatibility:** ▪ albumin ▪ amikacin ▪ amphotericin B deoxycholate ▪ aztreonam ▪ bretylium ▪ bumetanide ▪ cefazolin ▪ cefotaxime ▪ cefotetan ▪ cefoxitin ▪ ceftazidime ▪ ceftriaxone ▪ cefuroxime ▪ cimetidine ▪ ciprofloxacin ▪ clindamycin ▪ digoxin ▪ dobutamine ▪ dopamine ▪ doxycycline ▪ epinephrine ▪ erythromycin lactobionate ▪ esmolol ▪ fluconazole ▪ gentamicin ▪ hetastarch ▪ imipenem/cilastatin ▪ lidocaine ▪ lorazepam ▪ meperidine ▪ metoclopramide ▪ metronidazole ▪ morphine ▪ multivitamins ▪ nitroprusside ▪ nitroglycerin ▪ norepinephrine ▪ oxacillin ▪ penicillin G potassium ▪ pentamidine ▪ piperacillin ▪ potassium chloride ▪ potassium phosphate ▪ ranitidine ▪ theophylline ▪ ticarcillin ▪ ticarcillin/clavulanate ▪ tobramycin ▪ trimethoprim/sulfamethoxazole ▪ vancomycin.
- **Y-Site Incompatibility:** ▪ acetazolamide ▪ acyclovir ▪ aminophylline ▪ ampicillin ▪ ampicillin/sulbactam ▪ cefamandole ▪ cefoperazone ▪ diazepam ▪ furosemide ▪ hydrocortisone sodium succinate ▪ insulin ▪ methylprednisolone sodium succinate ▪ mezlocillin ▪ nafcillin ▪ phenytoin ▪ rifampin ▪ sodium bicarbonate.

PATIENT/FAMILY TEACHING

- **General Info:** Advise patient to take medication exactly as directed, even if feeling well. If a dose is missed, take as soon as possible unless almost time for next dose; do not double doses. May need to be discontinued gradually.
- □ Instruct patient on correct technique for monitoring pulse. Instruct patient to contact health care professional if heart rate is <50 bpm.
- □ Caution patient to change positions slowly to minimize orthostatic hypotension.
- □ May cause drowsiness or dizziness. Advise patient to avoid driving or other activities requiring alertness until response to the medication is known.
- □ Instruct patient on importance of maintaining good dental hygiene and seeing dentist frequently for teeth cleaning to prevent tenderness, bleeding, and gingival hyperplasia (gum enlargement).
- □ Instruct patient to avoid concurrent use of alcohol or OTC medications, especially cold preparations, without consulting health care professional.
- □ Advise patient to notify health care professional if irregular heartbeats, dyspnea, swelling of hands and feet, pronounced dizziness, nausea, constipation, or hypotension occurs or if headache is severe or persistent.
- □ Caution patient to wear protective clothing and use sunscreen to prevent photosensitivity reactions.
- **Angina:** Instruct patient on concurrent nitrate or beta-blocker therapy to continue taking both medications as directed and to use SL nitroglycerin as needed for anginal attacks.
- □ Advise patient to contact health care professional if chest pain does not improve, worsens after therapy, or occurs with diaphoresis; if shortness of breath occurs; or if severe, persistent headache occurs.
- □ Caution patient to discuss exercise restrictions with health care professional prior to exertion.
- **Hypertension:** Encourage patient to comply with other interventions for hypertension (weight reduction, low-sodium diet, smoking cessation, moderation of alcohol consumption, regular exercise, and stress management). Medication controls but does not cure hypertension.
- □ Instruct patient and family in proper technique for monitoring blood pressure. Advise patient to take blood pressure weekly and to report significant changes to health care professional.

EVALUATION

Effectiveness of therapy can be demonstrated by: ▪ Decrease in blood pressure ▪ Decrease in frequency and severity of anginal attacks □ Decrease in need for nitrate therapy □ Increase in activity tolerance and sense of well-being ▪ Suppression and prevention of atrial tachyarrhythmias.

DIMENHYDRINATE

(dye-men-**hye**-dri-nate)

{Apo-Dimenhydrinate}, Calm X, Children's Dramamine, Dimetabs, Dinate, Dommanate, Dramamine, Dramanate, Dramocen, Dramoject, Dymenate, {Gravol}, Hydrate, Marmine, {Nauseatol}, Nico-Vert, {Novo-Dimenate}, {PMS-Dimenhydrinate}, Tega-Vert, {Travamine}, {Traveltabs}, Triptone Caplets, Vertab

CLASSIFICATION(S):
Antiemetic, Antihistamine

Pregnancy Category B

INDICATIONS

▪ Treatment and prevention of nausea, vomiting, dizziness, and vertigo accompanying motion sickness.

ACTION

▪ Inhibits vestibular stimulation ▪ Has significant CNS depressant, anticholinergic, antihistaminic, and antiemetic properties. **Therapeutic Effects:** ▪ Decreased vestibular stimulation, which may prevent motion sickness.

PHARMACOKINETICS

Absorption: Well absorbed following oral or IM administration.
Distribution: UK. Probably crosses the placenta and enters breast milk.
Metabolism and Excretion: Metabolized by the liver.
Half-life: UK.

CONTRAINDICATIONS AND PRECAUTIONS

Contraindicated in: ▪ Hypersensitivity ▪ Alcohol intolerance (some liquid products).
Use Cautiously in: ▪ Narrow-angle glaucoma ▪ Seizure disorders ▪ Prostatic hypertrophy.

ADVERSE REACTIONS AND SIDE EFFECTS*

CNS: drowsiness, dizziness, headache, paradoxical excitation (children).
EENT: blurred vision, tinnitus.
CV: hypotension, palpitations.
GI: anorexia, constipation, diarrhea, dry mouth.
GU: dysuria, frequency.
Derm: photosensitivity.
Local: pain at IM site.

INTERACTIONS

Drug-Drug: ▪ Additive CNS depression with other **antihistamines, alcohol, opioids,** and **sedative/hypnotics** ▪ May mask signs or symptoms of ototoxicity in patients receiving **ototoxic drugs (aminoglycosides, ethacrynic acid)** ▪ Additive anticholinergic properties with **tricyclic antidepressants, quinidine,** or **disopyramide** ▪ **MAO inhibitors** intensify and prolong the anticholinergic effects of antihistamines.

ROUTE AND DOSAGE

- **PO (Adults):** 50–100 mg q 4 hr (not to exceed 400 mg/day).
- **PO (Children 6–12 yr):** 25–50 mg q 6–8 hr (not to exceed 300 mg/day).
- **Rect (Adults):** 50–100 mg q 6–8 hr.
- **Rect (Children 8–12 yr):** 25–50 mg q 8–12 hr.
- **Rect (Children 6–8 yr):** 12.5–25 mg q 8–12 hr.
- **IM, IV (Adults):** 50 mg q 4 hr as needed.
- **IM, IV (Children):** 1.25 mg/kg (37.5 mg/m^2) q 6 hr as needed (not to exceed 300 mg/day).

AVAILABILITY

▪ ***Tablets:*** 50 mg^{OTC} ▪ ***Chewable tablets:*** 50 mg^{OTC} ▪ ***Capsules:*** {50 mg^{OTC}} ▪ ***Extended-release capsules:*** {25 mg^{OTC}} ▪ ***Elixir:*** 12.5 mg/5 ml^{OTC}, {15 mg/5 ml^{OTC}} ▪ ***Liquid:*** 12.5 mg/4 ml^{OTC} ▪ ***Suppositories:*** {50 mg^{OTC}}, {100 mg^{OTC}} ▪ ***Injection:*** 50 mg/ml^{Rx}.

TIME/ACTION PROFILE (anti–motion sickness, antiemetic activity)

	ONSET	PEAK	DURATION
PO	15–60 min	1–2 hr	3–6 hr
Rect	30–45 min	UK	6–12 hr
IM	20–30 min	1–2 hr	3–6 hr
IV	rapid	UK	3–6 hr

{} = Available in Canada only.
***CAPITALS indicate life-threatening; underlines indicate most frequent.**

NURSING IMPLICATIONS

ASSESSMENT

- Assess nausea, vomiting, bowel sounds, and abdominal pain prior to and after the administration of this drug. Dimenhydrinate may mask the signs of an acute abdomen.
- Monitor intake and output, including emesis. Assess patient for signs of dehydration (excessive thirst, dry skin and mucous membranes, tachycardia, increased urine specific gravity, poor skin turgor).
- ***Lab Test Considerations:*** Will cause false-negative allergy skin tests; discontinue 72 hr prior to testing.

POTENTIAL NURSING DIAGNOSES

- Fluid volume deficit (Indications).
- Nutrition, altered, less than body requirements (Indications).
- Injury, risk for (Side Effects).

IMPLEMENTATION

- **General Info:** When used for prophylaxis of motion sickness, administer at least 30 min and preferably 1–2 hr before exposure to conditions that may precipitate motion sickness.
- **PO:** Use calibrated measuring device when administering liquid dose.
- **IM:** Administer into well-developed muscle; massage well.
- **Direct IV:** Dilute 50 mg in 10 ml of 0.9% NaCl for injection.
- ***Rate:*** Inject over 2 min.
- **Syringe Compatibility:** ▪ atropine ▪ droperidol ▪ fentanyl ▪ heparin ▪ hydromorphone ▪ meperidine ▪ metoclopromide ▪ morphine ▪ pentazocine ▪ perphenazine ▪ ranitidine ▪ scopolamine.
- **Syringe Incompatibility:** ▪ butorphanol ▪ glycopyrrolate ▪ midazolam ▪ pentobarbital ▪ thiopental.
- **Y-Site Compatibility:** ▪ acyclovir.
- **Y-Site Incompatibility:** ▪ aminophylline ▪ heparin ▪ hydrocortisone sodium succinate ▪ phenobarbital ▪ phenytoin ▪ prednisolone ▪ prochlorperazine edisylate ▪ promazine ▪ promethazine.
- **Solution Compatibility:** ▪ D5W, 0.45% NaCl, 0.9% NaCl, Ringer's solution, lactated Ringer's solution, dextrose/saline combinations, or dextrose/Ringer's combinations.

PATIENT/FAMILY TEACHING

- May cause drowsiness. Advise patient to avoid driving or other activities requiring alertness until response to the drug is known.
- Inform patient that this medication may cause dry mouth. Frequent oral rinses, good oral hygiene, and sugarless gum or candy may minimize this effect.
- Caution patient to avoid alcohol and other CNS depressants concurrently with this medication.
- Advise patient to use sunscreen and protective clothing to prevent photosensitivity reactions.

EVALUATION

Effectiveness of therapy can be demonstrated by: ▪ Prevention or decreased severity of nausea and vomiting, vertigo, or motion sickness.

DINOPROSTONE

(dye-noe-**prost**-one)
Cervidil Vaginal Insert, Prepidil Endocervical Gel, Prostin E_2 Vaginal Suppository

CLASSIFICATION(S):
Abortifacient (prostaglandin), Oxytocic, Cervical ripening agent (prostaglandin)

Pregnancy Category C

INDICATIONS

▪ **Endocervical Gel, Vaginal Insert:** □ Used to "ripen" the cervix in pregnancy at or near term, when induction of labor is indicated ▪ **Vaginal Suppository:** □ Induction of midtrimester abortion □ Management of missed abortion up to 28 wk □ Management of nonmetastatic gestational trophoblastic disease (benign hydatidiform mole).

ACTION

▪ Produces contractions similar to those occurring during labor at term by stimulating the myometrium (oxytocic effect) ▪ Initiates softening, effacement, and dilation of the cervix ("ripening") ▪ Also stimulates GI smooth muscle. **Ther-**

apeutic Effects: ■ Initiation of labor ■ Expulsion of fetus.

PHARMACOKINETICS

Absorption: Rapidly absorbed.
Distribution: Distribution not known. Action is mostly local.
Metabolism and Excretion: Metabolized by enzymes in lung, kidneys, spleen, and liver tissue.
Half-life: UK.

CONTRAINDICATIONS AND PRECAUTIONS

Contraindicated in: ■ Hypersensitivity to prostaglandins or additives in the gel or suppository ■ The gel/insert should be avoided in situations in which prolonged uterine contractions should be avoided including: ▫ Previous cesarean section or uterine surgery ▫ Cephalopelvic disproportion ▫ Traumatic delivery or difficult labor ▫ Multiparity (≥6 term pregnancies) ▫ Hyperactive or hypertonic uterus ▫ Fetal distress (if delivery is not imminent) ▫ Unexplained vaginal bleeding ▫ Placenta previa ▫ Vasa praevia ▫ Active herpes genitalis ▫ Obstetric emergency requiring surgical intervention ▫ Situations in which vaginal delivery is contraindicated ■ Presence of acute pelvic inflammatory disease or ruptured membranes ■ Concurrent oxytocic therapy (wait for 30 min after removing insert before using oxytocin).
Use Cautiously in: ■ Uterine scarring ■ Asthma ■ Hypotension ■ Cardiac disease ■ Adrenal disorders ■ Anemia ■ Jaundice ■ Diabetes mellitus ■ Epilepsy ■ Glaucoma ■ Pulmonary, renal, or hepatic disease ■ Multiparity (up to 5 previous term pregnancies).

ADVERSE REACTIONS AND SIDE EFFECTS*

▫ Endocervical Gel, Vaginal Insert

GU: uterine contractile abnormalities, warm feeling in vagina.
MS: back pain.
Misc: fever.

▫ Suppository

CNS: headache, drowsiness, syncope.
Resp: coughing, dyspnea, wheezing.
CV: hypotension, hypertension.
GI: diarrhea, nausea, vomiting.
GU: UTERINE RUPTURE, urinary tract infection, uterine hyperstimulation, vaginal/uterine pain.
Misc: allergic reactions including ANAPHYLAXIS, chills, fever.

INTERACTIONS

Drug-Drug: ■ Augments the effects of other **oxytocics.**

ROUTE AND DOSAGE

▫ Cervical Ripening

- **Vag (Adults, Cervical):** *Endocervical gel*—0.5 mg; if response is unfavorable, may repeat in 6 hr (not to exceed 1.5 mg/24 hr). *Vaginal insert*—one 10-mg insert.

▫ Abortifacient

- **Vag (Adults):** One 20-mg suppository, repeat q 3–5 hr (not to exceed 240 mg total).

AVAILABILITY

■ ***Endocervical gel (Prepidil):*** 0.5 mg dinoprostone in 3 g of gel vehicle in a prefilled syringe with catheters[Rx] ■ ***Vaginal insert (Cervidil):*** 10 mg[Rx] ■ ***Vaginal suppository (Prostin E Vaginal):*** 20 mg[Rx].

TIME/ACTION PROFILE

	ONSET	PEAK	DURATION
Cervical ripening (gel)	rapid	30–45 min	UK
Cervical ripening (insert)	rapid	UK	12 hr
Abortion time (suppository)	10 min	12–24 hr	2–3 hr

NURSING IMPLICATIONS

ASSESSMENT

- **Abortifacient:** Monitor frequency, duration, and force of contractions and uterine resting tone. Opioid analgesics may be administered for uterine pain.
- ▫ Monitor temperature, pulse, and blood pressure periodically throughout therapy. Dinoprostone-induced fever (elevation >1.1°C or 2°F) usually occurs within 15–45 min following insertion of suppository. This returns to

*CAPITALS indicate life-threatening; underlines indicate most frequent.

normal 2–6 hr after discontinuation or removal of suppository from vagina.
- ☐ Auscultate breath sounds. Wheezing and sensation of chest tightness may indicate hypersensitivity reaction.
- ☐ Assess for nausea, vomiting, and diarrhea in patients receiving suppository. Vomiting and diarrhea occur frequently. Patient should be premedicated with antiemetic and antidiarrheal.
- ☐ Monitor amount and type of vaginal discharge. Notify physician or other health care professional immediately if symptoms of hemorrhage (increased bleeding, hypotension, pallor, tachycardia) occur.
- ▪ **Cervical Ripening:** Monitor uterine activity, fetal status, and dilation and effacement of cervix continuously throughout therapy. Assess for hypertonus, sustained uterine contractility, and fetal distress. Insert should be removed at the onset of active labor.

POTENTIAL NURSING DIAGNOSES

- ▪ Knowledge deficit, related to medication regimen (Patient/Family Teaching).

IMPLEMENTATION

- ▪ **Abortifacient:** Warm the suppository to room temperature just prior to use.
- ☐ Wear gloves when handling unwrapped suppository to prevent absorption through skin.
- ☐ Patient should remain supine for 10 min following insertion of suppository; then she may be ambulatory.
- ▪ **Vaginal Insert:** Place vaginal insert transversely in the posterior vaginal fornix immediately after removing from foil package. Warming of insert and sterile conditions are not required. Use vaginal insert only with a retrieval system. Use minimal amount of water-soluble lubricant during insertion; avoid excess, as it may hamper release of dinoprostone from insert. Patient should remain supine for 2 hr after insertion, then may ambulate.
- ☐ Vaginal insert delivers dinoprostone 0.3 mg/hr over 12 hr. Remove insert at the onset of active labor, prior to amniotomy, or after 12 hr.
- ☐ Oxytocin should not be used during or less than 30 min following removal of insert.
- ▪ **Endocervical Gel:** Determine degree of effacement prior to insertion of the endocervical catheter. Do not administer above the level of the internal os. Use a 20-mm endocervical catheter if no effacement is present and a 10-mm catheter if the cervix is 50% effaced.
- ☐ Use caution to prevent contact of dinoprostone gel with skin. Wash hands thoroughly with soap and water after administration.
- ☐ Bring gel to room temperature just prior to administration. Do not force warming with external sources (water bath, microwave). Remove peel-off seal from end of syringe, then remove the protective end cap and insert end cap into plunger stopper assembly in barrel of syringe. Aseptically remove catheter from package. Firmly attach catheter hub to syringe tip; click is evidence of attachment. Fill catheter with sterile gel by pushing plunger to expel air from catheter prior to administration to patient. Gel is stable for 24 mo if refrigerated.
- ☐ Patient should be in dorsal position with cervix visualized using a speculum. Introduce gel with catheter into cervical canal using sterile technique. Administer gel by gentle expulsion from syringe and then remove catheter. Do not attempt to administer small amount of gel remaining in syringe. Use syringe for only 1 patient; discard syringe, catheter, and unused package contents after using.
- ☐ Patient should remain supine for 15–30 min following administration to minimize leakage from cervical canal.
- ☐ Oxytocin may be administered 6–12 hr following desired response from dinoprostone gel. If no cervical/uterine response to initial dose of dinoprostone is obtained, repeat dose may be administered in 6 hr.

PATIENT/FAMILY TEACHING

- ▪ **General Info:** Explain purpose of medication and vaginal exams.
- ▪ **Abortifacient:** Instruct patient to notify health care professional immediately if fever and chills, foul-smelling vaginal discharge, lower abdominal pain, or increased bleeding occurs.
- ☐ Provide emotional support throughout therapy.
- ▪ **Cervical Ripening:** Inform patient that she may experience a warm feeling in her vagina during administration.

□ Advise patient to notify health care professional if contractions become prolonged.

EVALUATION

Effectiveness of therapy can be demonstrated by: ▪ Complete abortion. Continuous administration for more than 2 days is not usually recommended ▪ Cervical ripening and induction of labor.

DIPHENHYDRAMINE

(dye-fen-**hye**-dra-meen)

{Allerdryl}, AllerMax, Allermed, Banophen, Benadryl, Benadryl Itch Relief Children's, Benadryl Itch Stopping Gel Children's Formula, Benadryl Itch Stopping Gel Maximum Strength, Benylin Cough, Bydramine Cough, Compoz, Diphen Cough, Diphenhist, Dormin, Genahist, {Insomnal}, Maximum Strength Benadryl Itch Relief, Nytol Maximum Strength, Siladril, Silphen, Sleep-Eze 3, Sominex, Tusstat, Twilite, Uni-Bent Cough, Unisom SleepGels Maximum Strength

CLASSIFICATION(S):

Antidyskinetic, Antihistamine, Antitussive, Sedative/hypnotic

Pregnancy Category B

INDICATIONS

▪ Relief of allergic symptoms caused by histamine release including: □ Anaphylaxis □ Seasonal and perennial allergic rhinitis □ Allergic dermatoses ▪ Parkinson's disease and dystonic reactions from medications ▪ Mild nighttime sedation ▪ Prevention of motion sickness ▪ Antitussive (syrup only) ▪ **Topical:** Temporary relief of minor skin irritation from: □ Insect bites □ Poison ivy, sumac, or oak.

ACTION

▪ Antagonizes the effects of histamine at H_1-receptor sites; does not bind to or inactivate histamine ▪ Significant CNS depressant and anticholinergic properties. **Therapeutic Effects:** ▪ Decreased symptoms of histamine excess (sneezing, rhinorrhea, nasal and ocular pruritus, ocular tearing and redness, urticaria) ▪ Relief of acute dystonic reactions ▪ Prevention of motion sickness ▪ Suppression of cough.

PHARMACOKINETICS

Absorption: Well absorbed following PO/IM administration. Minimally absorbed following topical use.
Distribution: Widely distributed. Crosses the placenta; enters breast milk.
Metabolism and Excretion: 95% metabolized by the liver.
Half-life: 2.4–7 hr.

CONTRAINDICATIONS AND PRECAUTIONS

Contraindicated in: ▪ Hypersensitivity ▪ Acute attacks of asthma ▪ Lactation ▪ Known alcohol intolerance (some liquid products).
Use Cautiously in: ▪ Geriatric patients (more susceptible to adverse drug reactions; dosage reduction recommended) ▪ Severe liver disease ▪ Narrow-angle glaucoma ▪ Seizure disorders ▪ Prostatic hypertrophy ▪ Pregnancy (safety not established).

ADVERSE REACTIONS AND SIDE EFFECTS*

CNS: <u>drowsiness</u>, dizziness, headache, paradoxical excitation (↑ in children).
EENT: blurred vision, tinnitus.
CV: hypotension, palpitations.
GI: <u>anorexia</u>, <u>dry mouth</u>, constipation, diarrhea.
GU: dysuria, frequency, urinary retention.
Derm: photosensitivity.
Local: pain at IM site.

INTERACTIONS

Drug-Drug: ▪ Additive CNS depression with other **antihistamines, alcohol, opioids,** and **sedative/hypnotics** ▪ Additive anticholinergic properties with **tricyclic antidepressants, quinidine,** or **disopyramide** ▪ **MAO inhibitors** intensify and prolong the anticholinergic effects of antihistamines.

{} = Available in Canada only.
***CAPITALS indicate life-threatening; <u>underlines</u> indicate most frequent.**

ROUTE AND DOSAGE

- **PO (Adults):** *Antihistaminic/antiemetic/antivertiginic*—25–50 mg q 4–6 hr. *Antitussive*—25 mg q 4 hr as needed. *Antidyskinetic*—25 mg 3 times daily (up to 50 mg 4 times daily). *Sedative/hypnotic*—50 mg 20–30 min before bedtime.
- **PO (Children >9.1 kg):** *Antihistaminic*—12.5–25 mg q 4–6 hr. *Antiemetic/antivertiginic*—1–1.5 mg/kg q 4–6 hr as needed (not to exceed 300 mg/day).
- **PO (Children <9.1 kg):** *Antihistaminic*—6.25–12.5 mg q 4–6 hr. *Antiemetic/antivertiginic*—1–1.5 mg/kg q 4–6 hr as needed (not to exceed 300 mg/day).
- **IM, IV (Adults):** 10–50 mg q 2–3 hr as needed (may need up to 100-mg dose, not to exceed 400 mg/day).
- **IM, IV (Children):** 1.25 mg/kg (37.5 mg/m^2) 4 times daily (not to exceed 300 mg/day).
- **Topical (Adults and Children ≥2 yr):** Apply 1–2% cream, gel, spray, or stick 3–4 times daily (2% strength should not be used in children <12 yr).

AVAILABILITY

▪ ***Capsules:*** 25 mg^{Rx,OTC}, 50 mg^{Rx,OTC} ▪ ***Tablets:*** 25 mg^{Rx,OTC}, 50 mg^{Rx,OTC} ▪ ***Chewable tablets:*** 25 mg^{Rx,OTC} ▪ ***Elixir:*** 12.5 mg/5 ml^{Rx,OTC} ▪ ***Syrup:*** 12.5 mg/5 ml^{Rx,OTC} ▪ ***Injection:*** 10 mg/ml^{Rx}, 50 mg/ml^{Rx} ▪ ***Cream:*** 1%^{OTC}, 2%^{OTC} ▪ ***Gel:*** 1%^{OTC}, 2%^{OTC} ▪ ***Stick:*** 2%^{OTC} ▪ ***Spray:*** 1%^{OTC} ▪ ***In combination with:*** analgesics, decongestants, and expectorants, in OTC pain, sleep, cough, and cold preparations. See Appendix A.

TIME/ACTION PROFILE (antihistaminic effects)

	ONSET	PEAK	DURATION
PO	15–60 min	1–4 hr	4–8 hr
IM	20–30 min	1–4 hr	4–8 hr
IV	rapid	UK	4–8 hr

NURSING IMPLICATIONS

ASSESSMENT

- **General Info:** Diphenhydramine has multiple uses. Determine why the medication was ordered and assess symptoms that apply to the individual patient.
- **Prevention and Treatment of Anaphylaxis:** Assess for urticaria and for patency of airway.
- **Allergic Rhinitis:** Assess degree of nasal stuffiness, rhinorrhea, and sneezing.
- **Parkinsonism and Extrapyramidal Reactions:** Assess movement disorder prior to and following administration.
- **Insomnia:** Assess sleep patterns.
- **Motion Sickness:** Assess nausea, vomiting, bowel sounds, and abdominal pain.
- **Cough Suppressant:** Assess frequency and nature of cough, lung sounds, and amount and type of sputum produced. Unless contraindicated, maintain fluid intake of 1500–2000 ml daily to decrease viscosity of bronchial secretions.
- **Pruritus:** Assess degree of itching, skin rash, and inflammation.
- ***Lab Test Considerations:*** Diphenhydramine may decrease skin response to allergy tests. Discontinue 4 days prior to skin testing.

POTENTIAL NURSING DIAGNOSES

- Sleep pattern disturbance (Indications).
- Fluid volume deficit, risk for (Indications).
- Injury, risk for (Side Effects).

IMPLEMENTATION

- **General Info:** When used for insomnia, administer 20 min before bedtime and schedule activities to minimize interruption of sleep.
- □ When used for prophylaxis of motion sickness, administer at least 30 min and preferably 1–2 hr before exposure to conditions that may precipitate motion sickness.
- **PO:** Administer with meals or milk to minimize GI irritation. Capsule may be emptied and contents taken with water or food.
- **IM:** Administer into well-developed muscle. Avoid SC injections.
- **Direct IV:** May give undiluted. May be further diluted in 0.9% NaCl, 0.45% NaCl, D5W, D10W, D5/0.9% NaCl, D5/0.45% NaCl, D5/0.25% NaCl, Ringer's solution, lactated Ringer's solution, and dextrose/Ringer's combinations.
- ***Rate:*** Inject 25 mg over at least 1 min.
- **Syringe Compatibility:** ▪ atropine ▪ butorphanol ▪ chlorpromazine ▪ cimetidine ▪ dimenhydrinate ▪ droperidol ▪ fentanyl ▪ fluphenazine ▪ glycopyrrolate ▪ hydromorphone ▪ hydroxyzine ▪ meperidine ▪ metoclopramide

▪ midazolam ▪ morphine ▪ nalbuphine ▪ pentazocine ▪ perphenazine ▪ prochlorperazine ▪ promazine ▪ promethazine ▪ ranitidine ▪ scopolamine ▪ sufentanil.

▪ **Syringe Incompatibility:** ▪ haloperidol ▪ pentobarbital ▪ phenobarbital ▪ phenytoin ▪ thiopental.

▪ **Y-Site Compatibility:** ▪ acyclovir ▪ aldesleukin ▪ amifostine ▪ aztreonam ▪ ciprofloxacin ▪ cisplatin ▪ cyclophosphamide ▪ cytarabine ▪ doxorubicin ▪ filgrastim ▪ fluconazole ▪ fludarabine ▪ gallium nitrate ▪ granisetron ▪ heparin ▪ hydrocortisone ▪ idarubicin ▪ melphalan ▪ meperidine ▪ methotrexate ▪ ondansetron ▪ paclitaxel ▪ piperacillin/tazobactam ▪ potassium chloride ▪ sargramostim ▪ sufentanil ▪ tacrolimus ▪ teniposide ▪ thiotepa ▪ vinorelbine ▪ vitamin B complex with C.

▪ **Y-Site Incompatibility:** ▪ foscarnet.

PATIENT/FAMILY TEACHING

- **General Info:** Instruct patient to take medication exactly as directed; do not exceed recommended amount.
- □ May cause drowsiness. Advise patient to avoid driving or other activities requiring alertness until response to drug is known.
- □ Inform patient that this drug may cause dry mouth. Frequent oral rinses, good oral hygiene, and sugarless gum or candy may minimize this effect. Notify dentist if dry mouth persists for more than 2 wk.
- □ Advise patient to use sunscreen and protective clothing to prevent photosensitivity reactions.
- □ Caution patient to avoid use of alcohol and other CNS depressants concurrently with this medication.
- □ Advise patients taking diphenhydramine in OTC preparations to notify health care professional if symptoms worsen or persist for more than 7 days.
- **Topical:** Instruct patient to cleanse affected skin prior to application, to avoid application to raw or blistered skin, and to discontinue use and contact health care professional if irritation occurs.
- □ Caution patient that medication should not be used on lesions of chickenpox or measles or on extensive areas of skin.

EVALUATION

Effectiveness of therapy can be demonstrated by: ▪ Prevention of or decreased urticaria in anaphylaxis or other allergic reactions ▪ Decreased dyskinesia in parkinsonism and extrapyramidal reactions ▪ Sedation when used as a sedative/hypnotic ▪ Prevention of or decrease in nausea and vomiting caused by motion sickness ▪ Decrease in frequency and intensity of cough without eliminating cough reflex.

DIPHENOXYLATE/ATROPINE

(dye-fen-**ox**-i-late/**a**-troe-peen)
Lofene, Logen, Lomocot, Lomotil, Lonox, Vi-Atro

DIFENOXIN/ATROPINE

(dye-fen-**ox**-in/**a**-troe-peen)
Motofen

CLASSIFICATION(S):
Antidiarrheals

Schedule V
Pregnancy Category C

INDICATIONS

▪ Adjunctive therapy in the treatment of diarrhea.

ACTION

▪ Inhibits excess GI motility ▪ Structurally related to opioid analgesics but has no analgesic properties ▪ Atropine added to discourage abuse. **Therapeutic Effects:** ▪ Decreased GI motility with subsequent decrease in diarrhea.

PHARMACOKINETICS

Absorption: Well absorbed from the GI tract.
Distribution: Enters breast milk.
Metabolism and Excretion: *Diphenoxylate*—mostly metabolized by the liver with some conversion to an active antidiarrheal compound (difenoxin). *Difenoxin*—metabolized by the liver. Minimal excretion in urine.
Half-life: *Diphenoxylate*—2.5 hr; *difenoxin*—4.5 hr.

CONTRAINDICATIONS AND PRECAUTIONS

Contraindicated in: ▪ Hypersensitivity ▪ Severe liver disease ▪ Infectious diarrhea (due to *E. Coli, Salmonella,* or *Shigella*) ▪ Diarrhea associated with pseudomembranous colitis ▪ Dehydrated patients ▪ Narrow-angle glaucoma

D

■ Children <2 yr ■ Known alcohol intolerance (some liquid diphenoxylate products only).

Use Cautiously in: ■ Patients physically dependent on opioids ■ Inflammatory bowel disease ■ Geriatric patients (more sensitive to effects) ■ Prostatic hypertrophy ■ Pregnancy, lactation, or children <12 yr (safety not established).

ADVERSE REACTIONS AND SIDE EFFECTS*

CNS: dizziness, confusion, drowsiness, headache, insomnia, nervousness.
EENT: blurred vision, dry eyes.
CV: tachycardia.
GI: constipation, dry mouth, epigastric distress, ileus, nausea, vomiting.
GU: urinary retention.
Derm: flushing.

INTERACTIONS

Drug-Drug: ■ Additive CNS depression with other **CNS depressants** including **alcohol, antihistamines, opioids,** and **sedative/hypnotics** ■ Additive anticholinergic properties with other **drugs having anticholinergic properties,** including **tricyclic antidepressants** and **disopyramide** ■ Use with **MAO inhibitors** may result in hypertensive crisis.

ROUTE AND DOSAGE

❑ Difenoxin/Atropine

Doses given are in terms of difenoxin tablets—each tablet contains 1 mg difenoxin with 0.025 mg of atropine.

- **PO (Adults):** 2 tablets initially, then 1 tablet after each loose stool or every 3–4 hr as needed (not to exceed 8 tablets/day).

❑ Diphenoxylate/Atropine

Doses given are in terms of diphenoxylate—each tablet contains 2.5 mg diphenoxylate with 0.025 mg of atropine; each 5 ml of liquid contains 2.5 mg diphenoxylate with 0.025 mg of atropine.

- **PO (Adults):** 5 mg 3–4 times daily initially, then 5 mg once daily as needed (not to exceed 20 mg/day).

AVAILABILITY

❑ Difenoxin/Atropine

■ ***Tablets:*** 1 mg difenoxin/0.025 mg atropine[Rx].

❑ Diphenoxylate/Atropine

■ ***Tablets:*** 2.5 mg diphenoxylate/0.025 mg atropine[Rx] ■ ***Liquid:*** 2.5 mg diphenoxylate/0.025 mg atropine per 5 ml[Rx].

TIME/ACTION PROFILE (antidiarrheal action)

	ONSET	PEAK	DURATION
Difenoxin–PO	45–60 min	2 hr	3–4 hr
Diphenoxylate–PO	45–60 min	2 hr	3–4 hr

NURSING IMPLICATIONS

ASSESSMENT

- ❑ Assess the frequency and consistency of stools and bowel sounds prior to and throughout therapy.
- ❑ Assess patient's fluid and electrolyte balance and skin turgor for dehydration.
- ■ ***Lab Test Considerations:*** Liver function tests should be evaluated periodically during prolonged therapy.
- ❑ Diphenoxylate/atropine may cause increased serum amylase concentrations.

POTENTIAL NURSING DIAGNOSES

- Diarrhea (Indications).
- Constipation (Side Effects).
- Knowledge deficit, related to medication regimen (Patient/Family Teaching).

IMPLEMENTATION

- **General Info:** Risk of dependence increases with high-dose, long-term use. Atropine has been added to discourage abuse.
- **PO:** Diphenoxylate/atropine tablets may be administered with food if GI irritation occurs. Tablets may be crushed and administered with patient's fluid of choice. Use calibrated measuring device for liquid preparations.

PATIENT/FAMILY TEACHING

- ❑ Instruct patient to take medication exactly as directed. Do not take more than the prescribed amount because of the habit-forming potential and risk of overdose in children. If on a scheduled dosing regimen, missed doses should be taken as soon as possible unless almost time for next dose. Do not double doses.

***CAPITALS indicate life-threatening; underlines indicate most frequent.**

- Medication may cause drowsiness. Advise patient to avoid driving or other activities requiring alertness until response to drug is known.
- Advise patient that frequent mouth rinses, good oral hygiene, and sugarless gum or candy may relieve dry mouth.
- Caution patient to avoid alcohol and other CNS depressants concurrently with this medication.
- Advise patient to inform health care professional of medication regimen prior to treatment or surgery.
- Instruct patient to notify health care professional if diarrhea persists or if fever, abdominal pain, or palpitations occur.

EVALUATION

Effectiveness of therapy can be demonstrated by: ▪ Decrease in diarrhea. Treatment of acute diarrhea should be continued for 24–36 hr before it is considered ineffective.

DIPYRIDAMOLE

(dye-peer-**id**-a-mole)

{Apo-Dipyridamole}, Dipridacot, {Novodipiradol}, Persantine, Persantine IV

CLASSIFICATION(S):

Antiplatelet agent, Diagnostic agent (coronary vasodilator)

Pregnancy Category B

INDICATIONS

▪ **PO:** Prevention of thromboembolism in patients with prosthetic heart valves (with warfarin) ▪ Maintains patency after surgical grafting procedures, including coronary artery bypass (with aspirin) ▪ **IV:** Diagnostic agent in lieu of exercise during thallium myocardial perfusion imaging.

ACTION

▪ **PO:** Decreases platelet aggregation by inhibiting the enzyme phosphodiesterase ▪ **IV:** Produces coronary vasodilation by inhibiting adenosine uptake. **Therapeutic Effects:** ▪ **PO:** Inhibition of platelet aggregation and subsequent thromboembolic events ▪ **IV:** In diagnostic thallium imaging, dipyridamole dilates normal coronary arteries, reducing flow to vessels that are narrowed and causing abnormal thallium distribution.

PHARMACOKINETICS

Absorption: Moderately absorbed (30–60%) after oral administration.
Distribution: Widely distributed. Crosses the placenta; enters breast milk.
Metabolism and Excretion: Metabolized by the liver; excreted in the bile.
Half-life: 10 hr.

CONTRAINDICATIONS AND PRECAUTIONS

Contraindicated in: ▪ Hypersensitivity.
Use Cautiously in: ▪ Hypotensive patients ▪ Patients with platelet defects ▪ Pregnancy (although safety not established, has been used without harm during pregnancy) ▪ Lactation or children <12 yr (safety not established).

ADVERSE REACTIONS AND SIDE EFFECTS*

CNS: dizziness, headache, syncope; *IV only*—transient cerebral ischemia, weakness.
Resp: *IV only*—bronchospasm.
CV: *IV only*—MYOCARDIAL INFARCTION, hypotension, arrhythmias, flushing.
GI: nausea, diarrhea, GI upset, vomiting.
Derm: rash.

INTERACTIONS

Drug-Drug: ▪ Additive effects with **aspirin** on platelet aggregation ▪ Risk of bleeding may be increased when used with **anticoagulants, thrombolytics, NSAIDs, cefamandole, cefoperazone, cefotetan, plicamycin, valproic acid,** or **sulfinpyrazone** ▪ Increased risk of hypotension with **alcohol** ▪ **Theophylline** may negate the effects of dipyridamole during diagnostic thallium imaging.

ROUTE AND DOSAGE

- **PO (Adults):** 75–100 mg 4 times daily.
- **IV (Adults):** 570 mcg/kg.

{} = **Available in Canada only.**
***CAPITALS indicate life-threatening; underlines indicate most frequent.**

AVAILABILITY

■ ***Tablets:*** 25 mg[Rx], 50 mg[Rx], 75 mg[Rx], {100 mg[Rx]} ■ ***Injection:*** 10 mg/2 ml[Rx].

TIME/ACTION PROFILE (PO = antiplatelet activity, IV = coronary vasodilation)

	ONSET	PEAK	DURATION
PO	UK	UK	UK
IV	UK	6.5 min*	30 min

*From start of infusion.

NURSING IMPLICATIONS

ASSESSMENT

- **PO:** Monitor blood pressure and pulse before instituting therapy and regularly during period of dosage adjustment.
- **IV:** Monitor vital signs during and for 10–15 min following infusion. Obtain ECG in at least 1 lead. If severe chest pain or bronchospasm occurs, administer IV aminophylline 50–250 mg at a rate of 50–100 mg over 30–60 sec. If hypotension is severe, place patient in a supine position with head tilting down. If chest pain is unrelieved with aminophylline 250 mg, administer nitroglycerin SL. If chest pain is still unrelieved, treat as myocardial infarction.
- ***Lab Test Considerations:*** Bleeding time should be monitored periodically throughout therapy.

POTENTIAL NURSING DIAGNOSES

- Cardiac output, decreased (Indications).
- Pain (Indications).
- Knowledge deficit, related to medication regimen (Patient/Family Teaching).

IMPLEMENTATION

- **PO:** Administer with a full glass of water at least 1 hr before or 2 hr after meals for faster absorption. If GI irritation occurs, may be administered with or immediately after meals. Tablets may be crushed and mixed with food if patient has difficulty swallowing. Pharmacist may make a suspension.
- **Intermittent Infusion:** Dilute in at least a 1:2 ratio of 0.45% NaCl, 0.9% NaCl, or D5W for a total volume of 20–50 ml. Undiluted dipyridamole may cause venous irritation.
- ***Rate:*** Infuse dose over 4 min.

PATIENT/FAMILY TEACHING

- **PO:** Instruct patient to take medication at evenly spaced intervals as directed. If a dose is missed, take as soon as remembered unless the next scheduled dose is within 4 hr. Do not double doses. Benefit of medication may not be apparent to patient; encourage patient to continue taking medication as directed.
- □ Caution patient to change positions slowly to minimize orthostatic hypotension.
- □ Advise patient to avoid the use of alcohol, as it may potentiate the hypotensive effects. Tobacco products should also be avoided because nicotine causes vasoconstriction.
- □ Advise patient to consult health care professional before taking OTC medications concurrently with this medication. Aspirin should be taken only if directed and only in dose prescribed. Advise patient to discuss alternatives for pain relief or fever.
- □ Instruct patient to notify health care professional if unusual bleeding or bruising occurs. Concurrent use of aspirin or warfarin may increase risk of bleeding but is commonly used with specific indications.
- □ Advise patient to notify health care professional of medication regimen and whether using concurrent aspirin or warfarin therapy.
- **IV:** Instruct patient to notify health care professional immediately if dyspnea or chest pain occurs.

EVALUATION

Effectiveness of therapy can be demonstrated by: ■ Prevention of postoperative thromboembolic complications associated with prosthetic heart valves ■ Maintenance of patency after surgical graft procedures ■ Coronary vasodilation in thallium myocardial perfusion imaging.

DISOPYRAMIDE

(dye-soe-**peer**-a-mide)

Norpace, Norpace CR, {Rythmodan}, {Rythmodan-LA}

CLASSIFICATION(S):

Antiarrhythmic (class I)

Pregnancy Category C

{} = Available in Canada only.

INDICATIONS

▪ Suppression/prevention of unifocal and multifocal PVCs, paired PVCs, and ventricular tachycardia. **Unlabeled Uses:** ▪ Treatment/prevention of supraventricular tachyarrhythmias.

ACTION

▪ Decreases myocardial excitability and conduction velocity ▪ Has anticholinergic properties ▪ Little effect on heart rate but has a direct negative inotropic effect. **Therapeutic Effects:** ▪ Suppression of ventricular arrhythmias.

PHARMACOKINETICS

Absorption: Well absorbed from the GI tract.
Distribution: Widely distributed; enters breast milk.
Metabolism and Excretion: Metabolized by the liver; 10% excreted unchanged in the feces, 50% excreted unchanged by the kidneys.
Half-life: 8–18 hr (increased in hepatic or renal impairment).

CONTRAINDICATIONS AND PRECAUTIONS

Contraindicated in: ▪ Hypersensitivity ▪ Cardiogenic shock ▪ 2nd-degree and 3rd-degree heart block ▪ Sick sinus syndrome (without a pacemaker).
Use Cautiously in: ▪ Congestive heart failure or left ventricular dysfunction (dosage reduction recommended) ▪ Hepatic or renal insufficiency (dosage reduction recommended if CCr ≤40 ml/min) ▪ Prostatic enlargement ▪ Myasthenia gravis ▪ Glaucoma ▪ Pregnancy or lactation (safety not established).

ADVERSE REACTIONS AND SIDE EFFECTS*

CNS: dizziness, fatigue, headache.
EENT: blurred vision, dry eyes, dry throat.
CV: CONGESTIVE HEART FAILURE, arrhythmias, AV block, dyspnea, edema, hypotension.
GI: constipation, dry mouth, abdominal pain, flatulence, nausea.
GU: urinary hesitancy, urinary retention.
Endo: hypoglycemia.
Misc: impaired temperature regulation.

INTERACTIONS

Drug-Drug: ▪ May potentiate anticoagulant effect of **warfarin** ▪ **Rifampin, phenobarbital,** and **phenytoin** may decrease blood levels and effectiveness ▪ **Cimetidine** may decrease metabolism and increase blood levels ▪ May have additive toxic cardiac effects when used with other **antiarrhythmics** (prolonged conduction and decreased cardiac output), especially **verapamil**—avoid using disopyramide for 48 hr before or 24 hr after ▪ Anticholinergic side effects may be additive with other **drugs having anticholinergic properties,** including **antihistamines** and **tricyclic antidepressants** ▪ Increased risk of arrhythmias with **pimozide.**

ROUTE AND DOSAGE

- **PO (Adults >50 kg):** 300 mg initially as immediate-release capsules followed by 150 mg q 6 hr (as immediate-release capsules) or 300 mg q 12 hr (as CR or LA dosage form; not to exceed 800 mg/day).
- **PO (Adults <50 kg or Patients with Poor Left Ventricular Function):** 200 mg initially as immediate-release capsules followed by 100 mg q 6–8 hr (as immediate-release capsules) or 200 mg q 12 hr (as CR or LA dosage form).
- **PO (Children 12–18 yr):** 6–15 mg/kg daily, in divided doses q 6 hr.
- **PO (Children 4–12 yr):** 10–15 mg/kg daily in divided doses q 6 hr.
- **PO (Children 1–4 yr):** 10–20 mg/kg daily in divided doses q 6 hr.
- **PO (Children <1 yr):** 10–30 mg/kg daily in divided doses q 6 hr.

AVAILABILITY

▪ ***Capsules:*** 100 mg[Rx], 150 mg[Rx] ▪ ***Extended-release capsules:*** 100 mg[Rx], 150 mg[Rx] ▪ ***Extended-release tablets:*** {150 mg[Rx]} ▪ ***Injection:*** {10 mg/ml[Rx]}.

TIME/ACTION PROFILE (antiarrhythmic effects)

	ONSET	PEAK	DURATION
PO	0.5–3.5 hr	2.5 hr	1.5–8.5 hr
PO-CR	0.5–3.5 hr	4.9 hr	12 hr

*CAPITALS indicate life-threatening; underlines indicate most frequent.

NURSING IMPLICATIONS

ASSESSMENT

- □ Monitor blood pressure, pulse, and ECG prior to and routinely throughout therapy. Check pulse prior to administering medication; withhold and notify physician or other health care professional if <60 or >120 bpm or if changes in rhythm occur.
- □ Monitor intake and output ratios and daily weight; assess for edema and urinary retention daily.
- □ Assess patient for signs of congestive heart failure (peripheral edema, rales/crackles, dyspnea, weight gain, jugular venous distention). Notify physician or other health care professional if these occur.
- ■ ***Lab Test Considerations:*** Renal and hepatic functions and serum potassium levels should be evaluated periodically throughout therapy.
- □ May cause elevated serum BUN, cholesterol, and triglyceride levels.
- □ May cause decreased blood glucose concentrations.

POTENTIAL NURSING DIAGNOSES

- ■ Cardiac output, decreased (Indications).
- ■ Oral mucous membrane, altered (Side Effects).
- ■ Knowledge deficit, related to medication regimen (Patient/Family Teaching).

IMPLEMENTATION

- ■ **General Info:** When changing from quinidine sulfate or procainamide to disopyramide, regular maintenance dose of disopyramide may be given 6–12 hr after last dose of quinidine sulfate or 3–6 hr after last dose of procainamide.
- □ Extended-release form (CR or LA formulations) is indicated for maintenance therapy only. When changing from regular form to extended-release forms, give the first dose of extended-release form 6 hr after the last regular dose.
- ■ **PO:** Administer medication on an empty stomach, 1 hr before or 2 hr after meals. Controlled-release capsules and long-acting tablets must be swallowed whole; do not break open, crush, or chew.
- □ Pharmacist may prepare a suspension with 100-mg capsules and cherry syrup.

PATIENT/FAMILY TEACHING

- □ Advise patient to take medication around the clock, exactly as directed. Do not discontinue medication without consulting health care professional. If a dose is missed, take as soon as remembered unless within 4 hr of next dose. Do not double doses.
- □ Medication may cause dizziness. Caution patients to avoid driving or other activities requiring alertness until response to medication is known.
- □ Instruct patient to change positions slowly to minimize orthostatic hypotension.
- □ Advise patient that frequent mouth rinses, good oral hygiene, and sugarless gum or candy may help relieve dry mouth.
- □ Caution patient to avoid extremes of temperature, as this medication may cause impairment of body temperature regulation. Patient should use sunscreen and protective clothing to prevent photosensitivity reactions.
- □ Advise patient to consult health care professional prior to taking OTC medications or alcohol concurrently with this medication.
- □ If constipation becomes a problem, advise patient that increasing bulk and fluids in the diet and exercising may minimize constipation.
- □ Instruct patient to notify health care professional if dry mouth, difficult urination, constipation, or blurred vision persists.

EVALUATION

Effectiveness of therapy can be demonstrated by: ■ Suppression of PVCs and ventricular tachycardia ■ Prevention of further arrhythmias.

DIURETICS (potassium-sparing)

amiloride
(a-**mill**-oh-ride)
Midamor

spironolactone
(speer-oh-no-**lak**-tone)
Aldactone, {Novospiroton}

{} = **Available in Canada only.**

triamterene
(trye-**am**-ter-een)
Dyrenium
CLASSIFICATION(S):
Diuretics (potassium-sparing)
Pregnancy Category C

INDICATIONS

▪ Counteracts potassium loss caused by other diuretics ▪ Commonly used with other agents (thiazides) to treat edema or hypertension ▪ Hyperaldosteronism (spironolactone only).

ACTION

▪ Causes loss of sodium bicarbonate and calcium while saving potassium and hydrogen ions. **Therapeutic Effects:** ▪ Weak diuretic and antihypertensive response when compared with other diuretics ▪ Conservation of potassium.

PHARMACOKINETICS

Absorption: *Amiloride*—15–25% absorbed from the GI tract; *spironolactone*—>90% absorbed after PO administration; *triamterene*—30–70% absorbed.
Distribution: *Amiloride* and *triamterene*—widely distributed; *spironolactone*—crosses the placenta; enters breast milk.
Metabolism and Excretion: *Amiloride*—50% eliminated unchanged in urine, 40% excreted unabsorbed in the feces; *spironolactone*—converted by the liver to its active diuretic compound (canrenone); *triamterene*—partially metabolized by the liver, some excretion of unchanged drug.
Half-life: *Amiloride*—6–9 hr; *spironolactone*—13–24 hr (canrenone); *triamterene*—100–150 min.

CONTRAINDICATIONS AND PRECAUTIONS

Contraindicated in: ▪ Hypersensitivity ▪ Hyperkalemia.
Use Cautiously in: ▪ Hepatic dysfunction ▪ Geriatric or debilitated patients or patients with diabetes mellitus (increased risk of hyperkalemia) ▪ Renal insufficiency (BUN >30 mg/dl or CCr <30 ml/min) ▪ History of gout or kidney stones (triamterene only) ▪ Pregnancy, lactation, or children (safety not established).

ADVERSE REACTIONS AND SIDE EFFECTS*

CNS: dizziness; *spironolactone only*—clumsiness, headache.
CV: arrhythmias.
GI: *amiloride*—constipation, GI irritation (↑ with spironolactone).
GU: impotence; *triamterene*—bluish urine, nephrolithiasis.
Derm: *triamterene* —photosensitivity.
Endo: *spironolactone*—gynecomastia.
F and E: <u>hyperkalemia</u>, hyponatremia.
Hemat: *spironolactone and triamterene*—dyscrasias.
MS: muscle cramps.
Misc: allergic reactions.

INTERACTIONS

Drug-Drug: ▪ Additive hypotension with acute ingestion of **alcohol**, other **antihypertensives**, or **nitrates** ▪ Use with **ACE inhibitors, indomethacin, potassium supplements,** or **cyclosporine** increases risk of hyperkalemia ▪ Decreases **lithium** excretion ▪ Effectiveness may be decreased by **NSAIDs** ▪ Spironolactone may increase the effects of **digoxin** ▪ Triamterene decreases the effects of **folic acid** (leucovorin should be used) ▪ Triamterene may increase risk of toxicity from **amantadine.**

ROUTE AND DOSAGE

❑ **Amiloride**
- **PO (Adults):** 5–10 mg/day (up to 20 mg).

❑ **Spironolactone**
- **PO (Adults):** 25–400 mg/day as a single dose or 2–4 divided doses.
- **PO (Children):** 1–3 mg/kg/day (30–90 mg/m^2/day as a single dose or 2–4 divided doses (not to exceed 3 times initial dose).

❑ **Triamterene**
- **PO (Adults):** 25–100 mg/day (not to exceed 300 mg/day).
- **PO (Children):** 2–4 mg/kg/day (120 mg/m^2/day) in divided doses given daily or every other day (not to exceed 6 mg/kg/day or 300 mg/day).

D

***CAPITALS indicate life-threatening; <u>underlines</u> indicate most frequent.**

AVAILABILITY

❑ Amiloride

▪ ***Tablets:*** 5 mg[Rx] ▪ ***In combination with:*** hydrochlorothiazide (Moduretic[Rx], {Moduret}[Rx]). See Appendix A.

❑ Spironolactone

▪ ***Tablets:*** 25 mg[Rx], 50 mg[Rx], 100 mg[Rx] ▪ ***In combination with:*** hydrochlorothiazide (Aldactazide, {Novo-Spirozine}, Spirazide)[Rx]. See Appendix A.

❑ Triamterene

▪ ***Capsules:*** 50 mg[Rx], 100 mg[Rx] ▪ ***Tablets:*** {50 mg[Rx]}, {100 mg[Rx]} ▪ ***In combination with:*** hydrochlorothiazide (Apo-Triazide, Dyazide, Maxzide, {Novo-Triamzide})[Rx]. See Appendix A.

TIME/ACTION PROFILE (diuretic effect)

	ONSET	PEAK	DURATION
Amiloride	2 hr*	6–10 hr*	24 hr*
Spironolactone	UK	2–3 days†	2–3 days†
Triamterene	2–4 hr*	1–several days†	7–9 hr*

*Single dose.
†Multiple doses.

NURSING IMPLICATIONS

ASSESSMENT

- Monitor intake and output ratios and daily weight throughout therapy.
- If medication is given as an adjunct to antihypertensive therapy, blood pressure should be evaluated before administering.
- Monitor response of signs and symptoms of hypokalemia (weakness, fatigue, U wave on ECG, arrhythmias, polyuria, polydipsia). Assess patient frequently for development of hyperkalemia (fatigue, muscle weakness, paresthesia, confusion, dyspnea, cardiac arrhythmias). Patients who have diabetes mellitus or kidney disease and elderly patients are at increased risk of developing these symptoms.
- Periodic ECGs are recommended in patients receiving prolonged therapy.
- ***Lab Test Considerations:*** Serum potassium levels should be evaluated prior to and routinely during therapy. Withhold drug and notify physician or other health care professional if patient becomes hyperkalemic.
- Monitor BUN, serum creatinine, and electrolytes prior to and periodically throughout therapy. May cause increased serum magnesium, uric acid, BUN, creatinine, potassium, plasma renin activity, and urinary calcium excretion levels. May also cause decreased sodium levels.
- Discontinue potassium-sparing diuretics 3 days prior to a glucose tolerance test because of risk of severe hyperkalemia.
- *Spironolactone* may cause false elevations of plasma cortisol concentrations. Spironolactone should be withdrawn 4–7 days before test.
- Monitor platelet count and total and differential leukocyte count prior to and periodically throughout therapy in patients taking *triamterene.*

POTENTIAL NURSING DIAGNOSES

- Fluid volume excess (Indications).
- Knowledge deficit, related to medication regimen (Patient/Family Teaching).

IMPLEMENTATION

- **PO:** Administer in AM to avoid interrupting sleep pattern.
- Administer with food or milk to minimize gastric irritation and to increase bioavailability.
- *Triamterene* capsules may be opened and contents mixed with food or fluids for patients with difficulty swallowing.

PATIENT/FAMILY TEACHING

- **General Info:** Emphasize the importance of continuing to take this medication, even if feeling well. Instruct patient to take medication at the same time each day. If a dose is missed, take as soon as remembered unless almost time for next dose. Do not double doses.
- Caution patient to avoid salt substitutes and foods that contain high levels of potassium or sodium unless prescribed by health care professional.
- May cause dizziness. Caution patient to avoid driving or other activities requiring alertness until response to medication is known.
- Advise patient to consult with health care professional before taking any OTC decongestants, cough or cold preparations, or appetite suppressants concurrently with this medication because of potential for increased blood pressure.
- Advise patients taking *triamterene* to use sun-

screen and protective clothing to prevent photosensitivity reactions.

- Instruct patient to notify health care professional of medication regimen prior to treatment or surgery.
- Inform patient that *triamterene* may cause bluish-colored urine.
- Advise patient to notify health care professional if muscle weakness or cramps; fatigue; or severe nausea, vomiting, or diarrhea occurs.
- Emphasize the need for follow-up exams to monitor progress.

▪ **Hypertension:** Reinforce need to continue additional therapies for hypertension (weight loss, restricted sodium intake, stress reduction, moderation of alcohol intake, regular exercise, and cessation of smoking). Medication helps control but does not cure hypertension.

- Teach patient and family the correct technique for checking blood pressure weekly.

EVALUATION

Effectiveness of therapy can be demonstrated by: ▪ Increase in diuresis and decrease in edema while maintaining serum potassium level in an acceptable range ▪ Decrease in blood pressure ▪ Prevention of hypokalemia in patients taking diuretics ▪ Treatment of hyperaldosteronism.

DIURETICS (thiazide)

chlorothiazide
(klor-oh-**thye**-a-zide)
Diuril

chlorthalidone
(klor-**thal**-i-doan)
{Apo-Chlorthalidone}, Hygroton, {Novo-Thalidone}, Thalitone, {Uridon}

hydrochlorothiazide
(hye-droe-klor-oh-**thye**-a-zide)
{Apo-Hydro}, {Duiclor H}, Esidrex, HCTZ, Hydro-Chlor, Hydro-D, HydroDIURIL, Microzide, {Neo-Codema}, Novo-Hydrazide, Oretic, {Urozide}

CLASSIFICATION(S):
Antihypertensive agents, Diuretics

Pregnancy Category B

INDICATIONS

▪ Management of mild to moderate hypertension ▪ Treatment of edema associated with: □ Congestive heart failure □ Renal dysfunction □ Cirrhosis □ Glucocorticoid therapy □ Estrogen therapy.

ACTION

▪ Increases excretion of sodium and water by inhibiting sodium reabsorption in the distal tubule ▪ Promotes excretion of chloride, potassium, magnesium, and bicarbonate ▪ May produce arteriolar dilation. **Therapeutic Effects:** ▪ Lowering of blood pressure in hypertensive patients and diuresis with mobilization of edema.

PHARMACOKINETICS

Absorption: All are rapidly absorbed following oral administration.

Distribution: Distributed into extracellular space. All cross the placenta and enter breast milk.

Metabolism and Excretion: All are excreted mainly unchanged by the kidneys.

Half-life: *Chlorothiazide*—1–2 hr; *chlorthalidone*—35–50 hr; *hydrochlorothiazide*—6–15 hr.

CONTRAINDICATIONS AND PRECAUTIONS

Contraindicated in: ▪ Hypersensitivity ▪ Cross-sensitivity with other thiazides or sulfonamides may exist ▪ Some products contain tartrazine and should be avoided in patients with known intolerance ▪ Anuria ▪ Lactation.

Use Cautiously in: ▪ Renal or severe hepatic impairment ▪ Pregnancy (jaundice or thrombocytopenia may be seen in the newborn).

ADVERSE REACTIONS AND SIDE EFFECTS*

CNS: dizziness, drowsiness, lethargy, weakness.
CV: hypotension.

{} = Available in Canada only.
*CAPITALS indicate life-threatening; underlines indicate most frequent.

GI: anorexia, cramping, hepatitis, nausea, vomiting.
Derm: photosensitivity, rashes.
Endo: hyperglycemia.
F and E: hypokalemia, dehydration, hypercalcemia, hypochloremic alkalosis, hypomagnesemia, hyponatremia, hypophosphatemia, hypovolemia.
Hemat: blood dyscrasias.
Metab: hyperuricemia, elevated lipids.
MS: muscle cramps.
Misc: pancreatitis.

INTERACTIONS

Drug-Drug: ▪ Additive hypotension with other **antihypertensive agents**, acute ingestion of **alcohol**, or **nitrates** ▪ Additive hypokalemia with **glucocorticoids, amphotericin B, mezlocillin, piperacillin**, or **ticarcillin** ▪ Decreases the excretion of **lithium** ▪ **Cholestyramine** or **colestipol** decreases absorption ▪ Hypokalemia increases risk of **digitalis glycoside** toxicity ▪ **NSAIDs** may decrease effectiveness ▪ **Allopurinol** may increase the risk of hypersensitivity reactions.

ROUTE AND DOSAGE

When used as a diuretic in adults, may be given every other day or 2–3 days/week.

❑ **Chlorothiazide**

- **PO (Adults):** 250 mg–1 g/day as a single dose or in divided doses.
- **PO (Children):** 10–20 mg/kg/day as a single dose or in 2 divided doses.
- **IV (Adults):** *Diuretic*—250 mg q 6–12 hr. *Antihypertensive*—500 mg–1 g/day as a single dose or 2 divided doses.

❑ **Chlorthalidone**

- **PO (Adults):** 25–100 mg once daily.

❑ **Hydrochlorothiazide**

- **PO (Adults):** 12.5–100 mg/day in 1–2 doses (up to 200 mg/day; not to exceed 50 mg/day for hypertension).
- **PO (Children >6 mo):** 1–2 mg/kg (30–60 mg/m²/day) in 1–2 divided doses.
- **PO (Children <6 mo):** Up to 3 mg/kg/day.

AVAILABILITY

❑ **Chlorothiazide**

▪ ***Tablets:*** 250 mg[Rx], 500 mg[Rx] ▪ ***Powder for injection:*** 500 mg[Rx] ▪ ***In combination with:*** methyldopa, reserpine[Rx]. See Appendix A.

❑ **Chlorthalidone**

▪ ***Tablets:*** 25 mg[Rx], 50 mg[Rx], 100 mg[Rx] ▪ ***In combination with:*** atenolol, clonidine, reserpine[Rx]. See Appendix A .

❑ **Hydrochlorothiazide**

▪ ***Tablets:*** 25 mg[Rx], 50 mg[Rx], 100 mg[Rx] ▪ ***Capsules*** : 12.5 mg[Rx] ▪ ***Oral solution:*** 10 mg/ml[Rx], 100 mg/ml[Rx] ▪ ***In combination with:*** spironolactone, triamterene, bisoprolol, hydralazine, moexipril, reserpine, timolol[Rx]. See Appendix A.

TIME/ACTION PROFILE (diuretic effect)

	ONSET	PEAK	DURATION
Chlorothiazide	2 hr	4 hr	6–12 hr
Chlorthalidone	2 hr	2 hr	48–72 hr
Hydrochlorothiazide*	2 hr	3–6 hr	6–12 hr

*Onset of antihypertensive effect is 3–4 days and does not become maximal for 7–14 days of dosing.

NURSING IMPLICATIONS

ASSESSMENT

- **General Info:** Monitor blood pressure, intake, output, and daily weight and assess feet, legs, and sacral area for edema daily.
- □ Assess patient, especially if taking digitalis glycosides, for anorexia, nausea, vomiting, muscle cramps, paresthesia, and confusion. Notify physician or other health care professional if these signs of electrolyte imbalance occur. Patients taking digitalis glycosides are at risk of digitalis toxicity due to the potassium-depleting effect of the diuretic.
- □ Assess patient for allergy to sulfonamides.
- **Hypertension:** Monitor blood pressure prior to and periodically throughout therapy.
- □ Monitor frequency of prescription refills to determine compliance.
- ***Lab Test Considerations:*** Monitor electrolytes (especially potassium), blood glucose, BUN, serum creatinine, and uric acid levels prior to and periodically throughout therapy.
- □ May cause increase in serum and urine glucose in diabetic patients.
- □ May cause an increase in serum bilirubin, calcium, creatinine, and uric acid, and a decrease in serum magnesium, potassium, sodium, and urinary calcium concentrations.

□ May cause decreased serum protein-bound iodine (PBI) concentrations.
□ May cause increased serum cholesterol, low-density lipoprotein, and triglyceride concentrations.

POTENTIAL NURSING DIAGNOSES

▪ Fluid volume excess (Indications).
▪ Fluid volume deficit (Side Effects).
▪ Knowledge deficit, related to medication regimen (Patient/Family Teaching).

IMPLEMENTATION

▪ **General Info:** Administer in the morning to prevent disruption of sleep cycle.
□ Intermittent dose schedule may be used for continued control of edema.
▪ **PO:** May give with food or milk to minimize GI irritation. Tablets may be crushed and mixed with fluid to facilitate swallowing.
▪ **Intermittent Infusion:** Reconstitute chlorthalidone with at least 18 ml of sterile water for injection for a concentration of 25 mg/ml. Shake to dissolve. Stable for 24 hr at room temperature. May be diluted further with D5W or 0.9% NaCl.

PATIENT/FAMILY TEACHING

▪ **General Info:** Instruct patient to take this medication at the same time each day. If a dose is missed, take as soon as remembered but not just before next dose is due. Do not double doses.
□ Instruct patient on use of calibrated dropper for measuring hydrochlorothiazide concentrated oral solution.
□ Instruct patient to monitor weight biweekly and notify health care professional of significant changes.
□ Caution patient to change positions slowly to minimize orthostatic hypotension. This may be potentiated by alcohol.
□ Advise patient to use sunscreen and protective clothing to prevent photosensitivity reactions.
□ Instruct patient to discuss dietary potassium requirements with health care professional (see Appendix K).
□ Instruct patient to notify health care professional of medication regimen prior to treatment or surgery.
□ Advise patient to report muscle weakness, cramps, nausea, vomiting, diarrhea, or dizziness to health care professional.
□ Emphasize the importance of routine follow-up exams.
▪ **Hypertension:** Advise patients to continue taking the medication even if feeling better. Medication controls but does not cure hypertension.
□ Encourage patient to comply with additional interventions for hypertension (weight reduction, low-sodium diet, regular exercise, smoking cessation, moderation of alcohol consumption, and stress management).
□ Instruct patient and family in correct technique for monitoring weekly blood pressure.
□ Advise patient to consult health care professional before taking OTC medication, especially cough or cold preparations, concurrently with this therapy.

EVALUATION

Effectiveness of therapy can be demonstrated by: ▪ Decrease in blood pressure ▪ Increase in urine output □ Decrease in edema.

DOBUTAMINE
(doe-**byoo**-ta-meen)
Dobutrex

CLASSIFICATION(S):
Inotropic agent

Pregnancy Category C

INDICATIONS

▪ Short-term management of heart failure due to depressed contractility from organic heart disease or surgical procedures.

ACTION

▪ Stimulates $beta_1$ (myocardial) -adrenergic receptors with relatively minor effect on heart rate or peripheral blood vessels. **Therapeutic Effects:** ▪ Increased cardiac output without significantly increased heart rate.

PHARMACOKINETICS

Absorption: Administered by IV infusion only, resulting in complete bioavailability.
Distribution: UK.

Metabolism and Excretion: Metabolized by the liver and other tissues.
Half-life: 2 min.

CONTRAINDICATIONS AND PRECAUTIONS

Contraindicated in: ▪ Hypersensitivity to dobutamine or bisulfites ▪ Idiopathic hypertrophic subaortic stenosis.
Use Cautiously in: ▪ Myocardial infarction ▪ Atrial fibrillation (pretreatment with digitalis glycosides recommended) ▪ Pregnancy, lactation, and children (safety not established).

ADVERSE REACTIONS AND SIDE EFFECTS*

CNS: headache.
Resp: dyspnea.
CV: hypertension, premature ventricular contractions, tachycardia, angina pectoris, arrhythmias.
GI: nausea, vomiting.
Misc: nonanginal chest pain.

INTERACTIONS

Drug-Drug: ▪ Use with **nitroprusside** may have a synergistic effect on increasing cardiac output ▪ **Beta-adrenergic blocking agents** may negate the effect of dobutamine ▪ Increased risk of arrhythmias or hypertension with some **anesthetics (cyclopropane, halothane), MAO inhibitors, oxytocics,** or **tricyclic antidepressants.**

ROUTE AND DOSAGE

See infusion rate chart in Appendix D.
- **IV (Adults):** 2.5–15 mcg/kg/min.
- **IV (Children):** 5–20 mcg/kg/min (unlabeled).

AVAILABILITY

- ***Injection:*** 12.5 mg/ml in 20-ml vial[Rx].

TIME/ACTION PROFILE (inotropic effects)

	ONSET	PEAK	DURATION
IV	1–2 min	10 min	brief (min)

NURSING IMPLICATIONS

ASSESSMENT

- □ Monitor blood pressure, heart rate, ECG, pulmonary capillary wedge pressure (PCWP), cardiac output, central venous pressure (CVP), and urinary output continuously during the administration. Report significant changes in vital signs or arrhythmias. Consult physician for parameters for pulse, blood pressure, or ECG changes for adjusting dosage or discontinuing medication.
- □ Palpate peripheral pulses and assess appearance of extremities routinely throughout dobutamine administration. Notify physician if quality of pulse deteriorates or if extremities become cold or mottled.
- ▪ ***Lab Test Considerations:*** Monitor potassium concentrations during therapy; may cause hypokalemia.
- □ Monitor electrolytes, BUN, creatinine, and prothrombin time weekly during prolonged therapy.
- ▪ ***Toxicity and Overdose:*** If overdose occurs, reduction or discontinuation of therapy is the only treatment necessary because of the short duration of dobutamine.

POTENTIAL NURSING DIAGNOSES

- ▪ Cardiac output, decreased (Indications).
- ▪ Tissue perfusion, altered (Indications).

IMPLEMENTATION

- ▪ **General Info:** Correct hypovolemia with volume expanders prior to initiating dobutamine therapy.
- □ Administer into a large vein, and assess administration site frequently. Extravasation may cause pain and inflammation.
- ▪ **IV:** Reconstitute 250-mg vial with 10 ml of sterile water or D5W for injection. If not completely dissolved, add another 10 ml of diluent. Dilute in at least 50 ml of D5W, 0.9% NaCl, sodium lactate, 0.45% NaCl, D5/0.45% NaCl, D5/0.9% NaCl, D5/LR, or lactated Ringer's solution. Standard concentrations range from 250 mcg/ml to 1000 mcg/ml. Concentrations should not exceed 5 mg of dobutamine per ml. Slight pink color of solution does not alter

*CAPITALS indicate life-threatening; underlines indicate most frequent.

potency. Solution is stable for 24 hr at room temperature.

- **Continuous Infusion:** Administer via infusion pump. Rate of administration is titrated according to patient response (heart rate, presence of ectopic activity, blood pressure, urine output, CVP, PCWP, cardiac output); see Appendix D.
- **Y-Site Compatibility:** ▪ amifostine ▪ amiodarone ▪ amrinone ▪ atracurium ▪ aztreonam ▪ bretylium ▪ calcium chloride ▪ calcium gluconate ▪ ciprofloxacin ▪ diazepam ▪ diltiazem ▪ dopamine ▪ enalaprilat ▪ famotidine ▪ fluconazole ▪ haloperidol ▪ insulin ▪ labetalol ▪ lidocaine ▪ magnesium sulfate ▪ meperidine ▪ nitroglycerin ▪ nitroprusside ▪ pancuronium ▪ potassium chloride ▪ protamine sulfate ▪ ranitidine ▪ streptokinase ▪ tacrolimus ▪ theophylline ▪ thiotepa ▪ tobramycin ▪ tolazoline ▪ vecuronium ▪ verapamil ▪ zidovudine.
- **Y-Site Incompatibility:** ▪ acyclovir ▪ alteplase ▪ aminophylline ▪ cefamandole ▪ cefazolin ▪ cephalothin ▪ cefepime ▪ ethacrynic acid ▪ foscarnet ▪ heparin ▪ hydrocortisone sodium succinate ▪ indomethacin ▪ penicillin ▪ phytonadione ▪ piperacillin/tazobactam.

PATIENT/FAMILY TEACHING

- □ Explain to patient the rationale for instituting this medication and the need for frequent monitoring.
- □ Advise patient to inform nurse immediately if chest pain; dyspnea; numbness, tingling, or burning of extremities occurs.
- □ Instruct patient to notify nurse immediately of pain or discomfort at the site of administration.
- ▪ **Home Care Issues:** Instruct caregiver on proper care of IV equipment.
- □ Instruct caregiver to report signs of worsening congestive heart failure (shortness of breath, orthopnea, decreased exercise tolerance), abdominal pain, and nausea or vomiting to health care professional promptly.

EVALUATION

Effectiveness of therapy can be demonstrated by: ▪ Increase in cardiac output □ Improved hemodynamic parameters □ Increased urine output.

DOCETAXEL
(doe-se-**tax**-el)
Taxotere

CLASSIFICATION(S):
Antineoplastic (taxoid)

Pregnancy Category D

INDICATIONS

▪ Management of locally advanced or metastatic breast cancer unresponsive to previous regimens that have included anthracyclines (doxorubicin or similar agents).

ACTION

▪ Interferes with normal cellular microtubule function required for interphase and mitosis. **Therapeutic Effects:** ▪ Death of rapidly replicating cells, particularly malignant ones.

PHARMACOKINETICS

Absorption: IV administration results in complete bioavailability.
Distribution: UK.
Metabolism and Excretion: Extensively metabolized by the liver; metabolites undergo fecal elimination.
Half-life: 11.1 hr.

CONTRAINDICATIONS AND PRECAUTIONS

Contraindicated in: ▪ Hypersensitivity ▪ Hypersensitivity to polysorbate 80 ▪ Known alcohol intolerance ▪ Neutrophil count $<1500/mm^3$ ▪ Liver impairment (serum bilirubin > upper limit of normal, ALT and/or AST >1.5 times upper limit of normal, with alkaline phosphatase >2.5 times upper limit of normal) ▪ Pregnancy or lactation.
Use Cautiously in: ▪ Patients with childbearing potential.

ADVERSE REACTIONS AND SIDE EFFECTS*

CNS: fatigue, weakness.
Resp: bronchospasm.
CV: ASCITES, CARDIAC TAMPONADE, PERICARDIAL EFFUSION, PULMONARY EDEMA, peripheral edema.

***CAPITALS indicate life-threatening; underlines indicate most frequent.**

GI: diarrhea, nausea, stomatitis, vomiting.
Derm: alopecia, rashes, dermatitis, desquamation, edema, erythema, nail disorders.
Hemat: anemia, thrombocytopenia, leukopenia.
Local: injection site reactions.
MS: myalgia, arthralgia.
Neuro: neurosensory deficits, peripheral neuropathy.
Misc: hypersensitivity reactions, including anaphylaxis

INTERACTIONS

Drug-Drug: ▪ Additive bone marrow depression may occur with other **antineoplastic agents** or **radiation therapy. Cyclosporine, ketoconazole, erythromycin,** or **troleandomycin** may significantly alter the effects of docetaxel.

ROUTE AND DOSAGE

- **IV (Adults):** 60–100 mg/m^2 q 3 wk.

AVAILABILITY

- ***Injection concentrate:*** 20 mg/0.5 ml polysorbate 80 with diluent (13% ethanol)^{Rx}, 80 mg/2 ml polysorbate 80 with diluent (13% ethanol)^{Rx}.

TIME/ACTION PROFILE (effect on blood counts)

	ONSET	PEAK	DURATION
IV	rapid	5–9 days	7 days

NURSING IMPLICATIONS

ASSESSMENT

- Monitor vital signs prior to and following administration.
- Assess infusion site for patency. Docetaxel is not a vessicant. If extravasation occurs, discontinue docetaxel immediately and aspirate the IV needle. Apply cold compresses to the site for 24 hr.
- Monitor for hypersensitivity reactions continuously during infusion. These are most common after first and second doses of docetaxel. Reactions may consist of bronchospasm, hypotension, and/or erythema. Mild to moderate reactions may be treated symptomatically and infusion slowed or stopped until reaction subsides. Severe reactions require discontinuation of therapy and symptomatic treatment. Do not readminister docetaxel to patients with previous severe reactions. Severe edema may also occur. Weigh patients before each treatment. Fluid accumulation may result in edema, ascites, and pleural or pericardial effusions. Pretreatment with glucocorticoids (such as dexamethasone 8 mg PO twice daily for 5 days, starting 1 day before docetaxel) is recommended to minimize edema and hypersensitivity reactions. PO furosemide may be used to treat edema.
- Monitor for bone marrow depression. Assess for bleeding (bleeding gums, bruising, petechiae, guaiac stools, urine, and emesis) and avoid IM injections and rectal temperatures if platelet count is low. Apply pressure to venipuncture sites for 10 min. Assess for signs of infection during neutropenia. Anemia may occur. Monitor for increased fatigue, dyspnea, and orthostatic hypotension.
- Assess patient for rash. May occur on feet or hands but may also occur on arms, face, or thorax, usually with pruritus. Rash usually occurs within 1 wk after infusion and resolves before next infusion.
- Assess for development of neurosensory deficit (paresthesia, dysesthesia, pain, burning). May also cause weakness. Pyridoxine may be used to minimize symptoms. Severe symptoms may require dose reduction or discontinuation.
- Assess patient for arthralgia and myalgia, which are usually relieved by nonopioid analgesics but may be severe enough to require treatment with opioid analgesics.
- ***Lab Test Considerations:*** Monitor CBC and differential prior to each treatment. Frequently causes neutropenia (<2000 neutrophils/mm^3); may require dose adjustment. If the neutrophil count is less than 1500/mm^3, dose should be held. Neutropenia is reversible and not cumulative. The nadir is 8 days, with a duration of 7 days. May also cause thrombocytopenia and anemia.
- Monitor liver function studies (AST, ALT, alkaline phosphatase, bilirubin) prior to each cycle. Doses are usually held if levels are elevated.

POTENTIAL NURSING DIAGNOSES

- Infection, risk for (Adverse Reactions).
- Injury, risk for (Adverse Reactions).
- Knowledge deficit, related to medication regimen (Patient/Family Teaching).

IMPLEMENTATION

- **General Info:** Solution should be prepared in a biologic cabinet. Wear gloves, gown, and mask while handling medication. Discard IV equipment in specially designated containers (see Appendix I).
- **Continuous Infusion:** Before dilution, allow vials to stand at room temperature for 5 min. Withdraw entire contents of diluent vial and transfer to vial of docetaxel. Rotate vial gently for 15 sec to mix. Do not shake. Solution should be clear but may contain foam at top. Allow to stand for a few minutes to allow foam to dissipate. All foam need not dissipate prior to continuing preparation. To prepare the solution for infusion, withdraw the required amount of 10 mg/ml solution into syringe and inject into 250 ml of 0.9% NaCl or D5W for a concentration of 0.3–0.9 mg/ml. Rotate infusion container to mix infusion thoroughly. Do not administer solutions that are cloudy or contain a precipitate. Solution does not require an in-line filter. Dilute solutions are stable for 8 hr if refrigerated or at room temperature.
- ***Rate:*** Administer over 1 hr.
- **Additive Incompatibility:** ▪ Information unavailable. Do not admix with other drugs or solutions.

PATIENT/FAMILY TEACHING

- Advise patient to notify health care professional if fever >101°F; chills; sore throat; signs of infection; bleeding gums; bruising; petechiae; or blood in urine, stool, or emesis occurs. Caution patient to avoid crowds and persons with known infections. Instruct patient to use soft toothbrush and electric razor.
- Patient should be cautioned not to drink alcoholic beverages or take products containing aspirin or NSAIDs.
- Fatigue is a frequent side effect of docetaxel. Advise patient that frequent rest periods and pacing of activities may minimize fatigue.
- Instruct patient to notify health care professional if abdominal pain, yellow skin, weakness, paresthesia, gait disturbances, swelling of the feet, or joint or muscle aches occur.
- Instruct patient to inspect oral mucosa for redness and ulceration. If mouth sores occur, advise patient to use sponge brush and rinse mouth with water after eating and drinking.
- Discuss with patient the possibility of hair loss. Complete hair loss usually begins after 1 or 2 treatments and is reversible after discontinuation of therapy. Explore coping strategies.
- Instruct patient not to receive any vaccinations without advice of health care professional.
- Emphasize the need for periodic lab tests to monitor for side effects.

EVALUATION

Effectiveness of therapy can be demonstrated by: ▪ Decrease in size or spread of malignancy in women with advanced breast cancer.

D

DOCUSATE
(**dok**-yoo-sate)

docusate calcium
DC Softgels, Pro-Cal-Sof, Sulfolax, Surfak

docusate potassium
Diocto-K, Kasof

docusate sodium
Afko-Lube, Colace, Correctol Stool Softener Soft Gels, Dialose, Diocto, Dioeze, Dio-Sosul, Diosuccin, DOK, DOSS, DSS, Duosol, Fleet Soflax Gelcaps, Laxinate, Modane Soft, Molatoc, Pro-Sof, {Regulex}, Silace, Soflax, Stulex, Therevac SB

CLASSIFICATION(S):
Laxative (stool softener)

Pregnancy Category C

INDICATIONS

▪ **PO:** Prevention of constipation (in patients who should avoid straining, such as after myocardial infarction or rectal surgery) ▪ **Rect:** Used by enema to soften fecal impaction.

ACTION

▪ Promotes incorporation of water into stool, resulting in softer fecal mass ▪ May also promote electrolyte and water secretion into the colon.

{} = Available in Canada only.

Therapeutic Effects: ▪ Softening and passage of stool.

PHARMACOKINETICS

Absorption: Small amounts may be absorbed from the small intestine after oral administration. Absorption from the rectum is not known.
Distribution: UK.
Metabolism and Excretion: Amounts absorbed after oral administration are eliminated in bile.
Half-life: UK.

CONTRAINDICATIONS AND PRECAUTIONS

Contraindicated in: ▪ Hypersensitivity ▪ Abdominal pain, nausea, or vomiting, especially when associated with fever or other signs of an acute abdomen.
Use Cautiously in: ▪ Excessive or prolonged use may lead to dependence ▪ Should not be used if prompt results are desired ▪ Has been used during pregnancy and lactation.

ADVERSE REACTIONS AND SIDE EFFECTS

EENT: throat irritation.
GI: mild cramps.
Derm: rashes.

INTERACTIONS

Drug-Drug: ▪ None significant.

ROUTE AND DOSAGE

❑ **Docusate Calcium**

- **PO (Adults):** 240 mg once daily.
- **PO (Children ≥6 yr and Adults with Minimal Requirements):** 50–150 mg once daily.

❑ **Docusate Potassium**

- **PO (Adults):** 100–300 mg once daily.
- **PO (Children ≥6 yr):** 100 mg once daily at bedtime.

❑ **Docusate Sodium**

- **PO (Adults and Children >12 yr):** 50–500 mg once daily.
- **PO (Children 6–12 yr):** 40–120 mg once daily.
- **PO (Children 3–6 yr):** 20–60 mg once daily.
- **PO (Children <3 yr):** 10–40 mg.
- **Rect (Adults):** 50–100 mg or 1 unit containing 283 mg docusate sodium, soft soap, and glycerin.

AVAILABILITY

❑ **Docusate Calcium**

▪ ***Capsules:*** 50 mg^{OTC}, 240 mg^{OTC}.

❑ **Docusate Potassium**

▪ ***Capsules:*** 100 mg^{OTC}.

❑ **Docusate Sodium**

▪ ***Tablets:*** 100 mg^{OTC} ▪ ***Capsules:*** 50 mg^{OTC}, 100 mg^{OTC}, 120 mg^{OTC}, 240 mg^{OTC}, 250 mg^{OTC} ▪ ***Syrup:*** 20 mg/5 ml^{OTC} ▪ ***Liquid:*** 150 mg/15 ml^{OTC} ▪ ***Solution:*** 50 mg/5 ml^{OTC} ▪ ***Enema:*** 283 mg/3.9-g capsule^{OTC} ▪ ***In combination with:*** stimulant laxatives^{OTC}. See Appendix A.

TIME/ACTION PROFILE (softening of stool)

	ONSET	PEAK	DURATION
PO	24–48 hr (up to 3–5 days)	UK	UK
Rectal	2–15 min	UK	UK

NURSING IMPLICATIONS

ASSESSMENT

- ❑ Assess patient for abdominal distention, presence of bowel sounds, and usual pattern of bowel function.
- ❑ Assess color, consistency, and amount of stool produced.

POTENTIAL NURSING DIAGNOSES

- Constipation (Indications).
- Knowledge deficit, related to medication regimen (Patient/Family Teaching).

IMPLEMENTATION

- **General Info:** This medication does not stimulate intestinal peristalsis.
- **PO:** Administer with a full glass of water or juice. May be administered on an empty stomach for more rapid results.
- ❑ Oral solution may be diluted in milk or fruit juice to decrease bitter taste.
- ❑ Do not administer within 2 hr of other laxatives, especially mineral oil. May cause increased absorption.

PATIENT/FAMILY TEACHING

- Advise patients that laxatives should be used only for short-term therapy. Long-term therapy may cause electrolyte imbalance and dependence.
- Encourage patients to use other forms of bowel regulation, such as increasing bulk in the diet, increasing fluid intake (6–8 full glasses/day), and increasing mobility. Normal bowel habits are variable and may vary from 3 times/day to 3 times/wk.
- Instruct patients with cardiac disease to avoid straining during bowel movements (Valsalva maneuver).
- Advise patient not to use laxatives when abdominal pain, nausea, vomiting, or fever is present.
- Advise patient not to take docusate within 2 hr of other laxatives.

EVALUATION

Effectiveness of therapy can be demonstrated by: ▪ A soft, formed bowel movement, usually within 24–48 hr. Therapy may take 3–5 days for results. Rectal dosage forms produce results within 2–15 min.

DOLASETRON

(dole-**ase**-tron)
Anzemet

CLASSIFICATION(S):
Antiemetic (5-HT_3 antagonist)

Pregnancy Category B

INDICATIONS

▪ Prevention of nausea and vomiting associated with emetogenic chemotherapy ▪ Prevention and treatment of postoperative nausea/vomiting.

ACTION

▪ Blocks the effects of serotonin at receptor sites (selective antagonist) located in vagal nerve terminals and in the chemoreceptor trigger zone in the CNS. **Therapeutic Effects:** ▪ Decreased incidence and severity of nausea/vomiting associated with emetogenic chemotherapy or surgery.

PHARMACOKINETICS

Absorption: Well absorbed but rapidly metabolized to hydrodolasetron, the active metabolite.
Distribution: UK.
Metabolism and Excretion: 61% of hydrodolasetron is excreted unchanged by the kidneys.
Half-life: *Hydrodolasetron*—8.1 hr (shorter in children).

CONTRAINDICATIONS AND PRECAUTIONS

Contraindicated in: ▪ Hypersensitivity.
Use Cautiously in: ▪ Patients with risk factors for prolongation of cardiac conduction intervals (hypokalemia, hypomagnesemia, concurrent diuretic or antiarrhythmic therapy, congenital QT syndrome, cumulative high-dose anthracycline therapy) ▪ Pregnancy or lactation (safety not established).

ADVERSE REACTIONS AND SIDE EFFECTS*

CNS: <u>headache</u> (↑ in cancer patients), dizziness, fatigue.
CV: bradycardia, ECG changes, hypertension, hypotension, tachycardia.
GI: diarrhea, dyspepsia.
GU: oliguria.
Derm: pruritus.
Misc: chills, fever, pain.

INTERACTIONS

Drug-Drug: ▪ Concurrent **diuretic** or **antiarrhythmic** therapy or cumulative **high-dose anthracycline therapy** may increase the risk of conduction abnormalities.

ROUTE AND DOSAGE

Prevention of Chemotherapy-Induced Nausea/Vomiting

- **PO (Adults):** 100 mg given within 1 hr before chemotherapy.
- **PO (Children 2–16 yr):** 1.8 mg/kg given within 1 hr before chemotherapy (not to exceed 100 mg).
- **IV (Adults and Children ≥2 yr):** 1.8 mg/kg given 30 min before chemotherapy (usual dose in adults is 100 mg; not to exceed 100 mg in children).

***CAPITALS indicate life-threatening; <u>underlines</u> indicate most frequent.**

D

❑ **Prevention/Treatment of Postoperative Nausea/Vomiting**

- **PO (Adults):** 100 mg given within 2 hr before surgery.
- **PO (Children 2–16 yr):** 1.2 mg/kg (up to 100 mg/dose) given within 2 hr before surgery.
- **IV (Adults):** 12.5 mg given 15 min before cessation of anesthesia (prevention) or as soon as nausea or vomiting begins (treatment).
- **IV (Children 2–16 yr):** 0.35 mg/kg (up to 12.5 mg) given 15 min before cessation of anesthesia (prevention) or as soon as nausea or vomiting begins (treatment).

AVAILABILITY

▪ ***Tablets:*** 50 mg[Rx], 100 mg[Rx] ▪ ***Injection:*** 12.5 mg/0.625 ml ampules[Rx], 20 mg/ml in 5-ml vials[Rx].

TIME/ACTION PROFILE (antiemetic effect)

	ONSET	PEAK	DURATION
PO	UK	1–2 hr	up to 24 hr
IV	UK	15–30 min	up to 24 hr

NURSING IMPLICATIONS

ASSESSMENT

❑ Assess patient for nausea, vomiting, abdominal distention, and bowel sounds prior to and following administration.

POTENTIAL NURSING DIAGNOSES

- Nutrition, altered, less than body requirements (Indications).
- Knowledge deficit, related to medication regimen (Patient/Family Teaching).

IMPLEMENTATION

- **PO:** Administer within 1 hr before chemotherapy or 2 hr prior to surgery.

❑ Injectable dolasetron may be mixed in apple or apple-grape juice for oral dosing for pediatric patients. May be stored at room temperature for 2 hr before use.

- **IV:** Administer 30 min before chemotherapy, 15 min before cessation of anesthesia, or postoperatively if nausea and vomiting occur shortly after surgery.
- **Direct IV:** May be administered undiluted.
- ***Rate:*** Administer over at least 30 sec.
- **Intermittent Infusion:** May be diluted in 50 ml of 0.9% NaCl, D5W, D5/0.45% NaCl, D5/LR, LR, or 10% mannitol solution. Solution is clear and colorless. Stable for 24 hr at room temperature or 48 hr if refrigerated following dilution.
- ***Rate:*** Administer each dose as an IV infusion over up to 15 min.
- **Y-Site Incompatibility:** ▪ Manufacturer recommends not admixing with other medications. Flush infusion line before and after administration.

PATIENT/FAMILY TEACHING

❑ Advise patient to notify health care professional if nausea or vomiting occurs.

EVALUATION

Effectiveness of therapy can be demonstrated by: ▪ Prevention of nausea and vomiting associated with emetogenic cancer chemotherapy ▪ Prevention and treatment of postoperative nausea and vomiting.

DONEPEZIL

(doe-**nep**-i-zill)

Aricept

CLASSIFICATION(S):

Cholinesterase inhibitor

Pregnancy Category C

INDICATIONS

▪ Treatment of mild to moderate dementia associated with Alzheimer's disease.

ACTION

▪ Improves cholinergic function by inhibiting acetylcholinesterase. **Therapeutic Effects:** ▪ May temporarily lessen some of the dementia associated with Alzheimer's disease ▪ Does not alter the course of the disease.

PHARMACOKINETICS

Absorption: Well absorbed following oral administration.

Distribution: UK.

Metabolism and Excretion: Partially metabolized by the liver and partially excreted by kid-

neys (17% unchanged). Two metabolites are pharmacologically active.
Half-life: 70 hr.

CONTRAINDICATIONS AND PRECAUTIONS

Contraindicated in: ▪ Hypersensitivity to donepezil or piperidine derivatives.
Use Cautiously in: ▪ Patients with underlying cardiac disease, especially sick sinus syndrome or supraventricular conduction defects ▪ Patients with a history of ulcer disease or those currently taking NSAIDs ▪ Patients with a history of seizures ▪ History of asthma or obstructive pulmonary disease ▪ Pregnancy, lactation, or children (safety not estabished).

ADVERSE REACTIONS AND SIDE EFFECTS*

CNS: headache, abnormal dreams, depression, dizziness, drowsiness, fatigue, insomnia, syncope.
CV: diarrhea, nausea, anorexia, vomiting.
GU: frequent urination.
Derm: ecchymoses.
Metab: weight loss.
MS: arthritis, muscle cramps.

INTERACTIONS

Drug-Drug: ▪ Exaggerates muscle relaxation from **succinylcholine** ▪ Interferes with the action of **anticholinergic agents** ▪ Increases the cholinergic effects of **bethanechol** ▪ May increase the risk of GI bleeding from **NSAIDs** ▪ **Quinidine** and **ketoconazole** decrease the metabolism of donepezil.

ROUTE AND DOSAGE

▪ **PO (Adults):** 5 mg once daily; after 4–6 wk may increase to 10 mg once daily.

AVAILABILITY

▪ ***Tablets:*** 5 mg[Rx], 10mg[Rx].

TIME/ACTION PROFILE (improvement in symptoms)

	ONSET	PEAK	DURATION
PO	UK	several wk	6 wk†

†Return to baseline following discontinuation.

NURSING IMPLICATIONS

ASSESSMENT

- Assess cognitive function (memory, attention, reasoning, language, ability to perform simple tasks) periodically throughout therapy.
- Monitor heart rate periodically during therapy. May cause bradycardia.

POTENTIAL NURSING DIAGNOSES

- Thought processes, altered (Indications).
- Injury, risk for (Indications).
- Knowledge deficit, related to medication regimen (Patient/Family Teaching).

IMPLEMENTATION

- **PO:** Administer in the evening just prior to going to bed. May be taken without regard to food.

PATIENT/FAMILY TEACHING

- Emphasize the importance of taking donepezil daily, as directed. Missed doses should be skipped and regular schedule returned to the following day. Do not take more than prescribed; higher doses do not increase effects but may increase side effects.
- Caution patient and caregiver that donepezil may cause dizziness.
- Advise patient and caregiver to notify health care professional if nausea, vomiting, diarrhea, or changes in the color of the stool occur or if new symptoms occur or previously noted symptoms increase in severity.
- Advise patient and caregiver to notify health care professional of medication regimen prior to treatment or surgery.
- Emphasize the importance of follow-up exams to monitor progress.

EVALUATION

Clinical response to therapy can be evaluated by: ▪ Improvement in cognitive function (memory, attention, reasoning, language, ability to perform simple tasks) in patients with Alzheimer's disease.

D

***CAPITALS indicate life-threatening; underlines indicate most frequent.**

DOPAMINE

(**dope**-a-meen)
Intropin, {Revimine}

CLASSIFICATION(S):
Inotropic agent, Vasopressor

Pregnancy Category C

INDICATIONS

■ Adjunct to standard measures to improve: □ Blood pressure □ Cardiac output □ Urine output in treatment of shock unresponsive to fluid replacement.

ACTION

■ Small doses (0.5–2 mcg/kg/min) stimulate dopaminergic receptors, producing renal vasodilation ■ Larger doses (2–10 mcg/kg/min) stimulate dopaminergic and $beta_1$-adrenergic receptors, producing cardiac stimulation and renal vasodilation ■ Doses greater than 10 mcg/kg/min stimulate alpha-adrenergic receptors and may cause renal vasoconstriction. **Therapeutic Effects:** ■ Increased cardiac output, increased blood pressure, and improved renal blood flow.

PHARMACOKINETICS

Absorption: Administered IV only, resulting in complete bioavailability.
Distribution: Widely distributed but does not cross the blood-brain barrier.
Metabolism and Excretion: Metabolized in liver, kidneys, and plasma.
Half-life: 2 min.

CONTRAINDICATIONS AND PRECAUTIONS

Contraindicated in: ■ Tachyarrhythmias ■ Pheochromocytoma ■ Hypersensitivity to bisulfites (some products).
Use Cautiously in: ■ Occlusive vascular diseases ■ Pregnancy, lactation, and children (safety not established).

ADVERSE REACTIONS AND SIDE EFFECTS*

CNS: headache.
EENT: mydriasis (high dose).
Resp: dyspnea.
CV: arrhythmias, hypotension, angina, ECG change, palpitations, vasoconstriction.
GI: nausea, vomiting.
Derm: piloerection.
Local: irritation at IV site.

INTERACTIONS

Drug-Drug: ■ Use with **MAO inhibitors, ergot alkaloids (ergotamine), guanethidine, guanadrel,** or some **antidepressants** results in severe hypertension ■ Use with **IV phenytoin** may cause hypotension and bradycardia ■ Use with **general anesthetics** may result in arrhythmias ■ **Beta-adrenergic blockers** may antagonize cardiac effects.

ROUTE AND DOSAGE

See infusion rate table in Appendix D.

- **IV (Adults):** *Dopaminergic (renal vasodilation) effects*—0.5–3 mcg/kg/min. *$Beta_1$-adrenergic (cardiac stimulation) effects*—2–10 mcg/kg/min. *Alpha-adrenergic (↑ peripheral vascular resistance) effects*—10 mcg/kg/min; infusion rate may be increased as needed.
- **IV (Children):** 5–20 mcg/kg/min, depending on desired response.

AVAILABILITY

■ ***Injection for dilution:*** 40 mg/ml^Rx, 80 mg/ml^Rx, 160 mg/ml^Rx ■ ***Premixed injection:*** 0.8 mg/ml, 1.6 mg/ml, and 3.2 mg/ml in 250- and 500-ml D5W^Rx.

TIME/ACTION PROFILE (hemodynamic effects)

	ONSET	PEAK	DURATION
IV	5 min	rapid	<10 min

NURSING IMPLICATIONS

ASSESSMENT

□ Monitor blood pressure, heart rate, pulse pressure, ECG, pulmonary capillary wedge pressure (PCWP), cardiac output, central venous pressure (CVP), and urinary output continuously during administration. Report significant changes in vital signs or arrhythmias.

{} = Available in Canada only.
*CAPITALS indicate life-threatening; underlines indicate most frequent.

Consult physician for parameters for pulse, blood pressure, or ECG changes for adjusting dosage or discontinuing medication.
- □ Monitor urine output frequently throughout administration. Report decreases in urine output promptly.
- □ Palpate peripheral pulses and assess appearance of extremities routinely throughout dopamine administration. Notify physician if quality of pulse deteriorates or if extremities become cold or mottled.
- □ If hypotension occurs, administration rate should be increased. If hypotension continues, more potent vasoconstrictors (norepinephrine) may be administered.
- ▪ ***Toxicity and Overdose:*** If excessive hypertension occurs, rate of infusion should be decreased or temporarily discontinued until blood pressure is decreased. Although additional measures are usually not necessary because of short duration of dopamine, phentolamine may be administered if hypertension continues.

POTENTIAL NURSING DIAGNOSES

- ▪ Cardiac output, decreased (Indications).
- ▪ Tissue perfusion, altered (Indications).

IMPLEMENTATION

- ▪ **General Info:** Correct hypovolemia with volume expanders prior to initiating dopamine therapy.
- □ Administer into a large vein, and assess administration site frequently. Extravasation may cause severe irritation, necrosis, and sloughing of tissue. If extravasation occurs, affected area should be infiltrated liberally with 10–15 ml of 0.9% NaCl containing 5–10 mg of phentolamine. Reduce proportionally for pediatric patients. Infiltration within 12 hr of extravasation produces immediate hyperemic changes.
- ▪ **Continuous Infusion:** Dilute 200–400 mg in 250–500 ml of 0.9% NaCl, D5W, D5/LR, D5/0.45% NaCl, D5/0.9% NaCl, or lactated Ringer's solution for IV infusion. Concentrations commonly used are 800 mcg/ml or 0.8 mg/ml (200 mg/250 ml) when fluid expansion is not problematic and 1.6 mg/ml (400 mg/250 ml) or 3.2 mg/ml (800 mg/250 ml) when patient is on fluid restriction or a slower rate is desired. Dilute immediately prior to administration. Yellow or brown discoloration indicates decomposition. Discard solution that is cloudy, discolored, or contains a precipitate. Solution is stable for 24 hr.
- ▪ ***Rate:*** Administer at a rate of 0.5–5 mcg/kg/min, and increase by 1–4 mcg/kg/min at 10- to 30-min intervals until desired dosage is obtained. Infusion must be administered via infusion pump to ensure precise amount delivered. Rate of administration is titrated according to patient response (blood pressure, heart rate, urine flow, peripheral perfusion, presence of ectopic activity, cardiac output); see infusion rate chart (Appendix D). Decrease rate gradually when discontinuing.
- ▪ **Y-Site Compatibility:** ▪ aldesleukin ▪ amifostine ▪ amiodarone ▪ amrinone ▪ atracurium ▪ aztreonam ▪ ciprofloxacin ▪ diltiazem ▪ dobutamine ▪ enalaprilat ▪ esmolol ▪ famotidine ▪ fluconazole ▪ foscarnet ▪ haloperidol ▪ heparin ▪ hydrocortisone sodium succinate ▪ labetalol ▪ lidocaine ▪ meperidine ▪ midazolam ▪ morphine ▪ nitroglycerin ▪ nitroprusside ▪ pancuronium ▪ piperacillin/tazobactam ▪ potassium chloride ▪ ranitidine ▪ sargramostim ▪ streptokinase ▪ tacrolimus ▪ theophylline ▪ thiotepa ▪ tolazoline ▪ vecuronium ▪ verapamil ▪ vitamin B complex with C ▪ zidovudine.
- ▪ **Y-Site Incompatibility:** ▪ acyclovir ▪ alteplase ▪ cefepime ▪ indomethacin ▪ insulin.

PATIENT/FAMILY TEACHING

- □ Explain to patient the rationale for instituting this medication and the need for frequent monitoring.
- □ Advise patient to inform nurse immediately if chest pain; dyspnea; numbness, tingling, or burning of extremities occurs.
- □ Instruct patient to inform nurse immediately of pain or discomfort at the site of administration.

EVALUATION

Effectiveness of therapy can be demonstrated by: ▪ Increase in blood pressure □ Increase in peripheral circulation □ Increase in urine output.

DOXAZOSIN
(dox-**ay**-zoe-sin)
Cardura

CLASSIFICATION(S):
Antihypertensive agent (peripherally acting antiadrenergic)

Pregnancy Category C

INDICATIONS

▪ Treatment of hypertension, alone or in combination with other agents ▪ Management of the symptoms of benign prostatic hyperplasia (BPH).

ACTION

▪ Dilates both arteries and veins by blocking postsynaptic $alpha_1$-adrenergic receptors. **Therapeutic Effects:** ▪ Lowering of blood pressure.

PHARMACOKINETICS

Absorption: Well absorbed following oral administration.
Distribution: Probably enters breast milk; remainder of distribution UK.
Metabolism and Excretion: Extensively metabolized by the liver.
Half-life: 22 hr.

CONTRAINDICATIONS AND PRECAUTIONS

Contraindicated in: ▪ Hypersensitivity.
Use Cautiously in: ▪ Hepatic dysfunction ▪ Geriatric patients or patients with impaired renal function (increased risk of hypotension) ▪ Pregnancy, lactation, or children (safety not established).

ADVERSE REACTIONS AND SIDE EFFECTS*

CNS: dizziness, headache, depression, drowsiness, fatigue, nervousness, weakness.
EENT: abnormal vision, blurred vision, conjunctivitis, epistaxis.
Resp: dyspnea.
CV: first-dose orthostatic hypotension, arrhythmias, chest pain, edema, palpitations.
GI: abdominal discomfort, constipation, diarrhea, dry mouth, flatulence, nausea, vomiting.
GU: decreased libido, sexual dysfunction.
Derm: flushing, rash.
MS: arthralgia, arthritis, gout, myalgia.

INTERACTIONS

Drug-Drug: ▪ Additive hypotension with acute ingestion of **alcohol,** other **antihypertensive agents,** or **nitrates** ▪ **NSAIDs** may decrease antihypertensive effects ▪ May decrease antihypertensive effect of **clonidine.**

ROUTE AND DOSAGE

▪ **PO (Adults):** *Hypertension*—1 mg once daily, may be gradually increased at 2-wk intervals to 2–16 mg/day; incidence of postural hypotension greatly increased at doses >4 mg/day. *BPH*—1 mg once daily, may be gradually increased to 8 mg/day.

AVAILABILITY

▪ ***Tablets:*** 1 mg[Rx], 2 mg[Rx], 4 mg[Rx], 8 mg[Rx].

TIME/ACTION PROFILE (antihypertensive effect)

	ONSET	PEAK	DURATION
PO	1–2 hr	2–6 hr	24 hr

NURSING IMPLICATIONS

ASSESSMENT

▪ **General Info:** Monitor blood pressure and pulse 2–6 hr after first dose, with each increase in dose, and periodically throughout course of therapy. Report significant changes.
□ Assess patient for first-dose orthostatic hypotension and syncope. Incidence may be dose related. Observe patient closely during this period and take precautions to prevent injury.
□ Monitor intake and output ratios and daily weight, and assess for edema daily, especially at beginning of therapy. Report weight gain or edema.
▪ **Benign Prostatic Hyperplasia:** Assess patient for symptoms of prostatic hyperplasia (urinary hesitancy, feeling of incomplete bladder emptying, interruption of urinary stream, impairment of size and force of urinary stream, terminal urinary dribbling, straining

*CAPITALS indicate life-threatening; underlines indicate most frequent.

to start flow, dysuria, urgency) prior to and periodically throughout therapy.

POTENTIAL NURSING DIAGNOSES

- Injury, risk for (Side Effects).
- Urinary elimination, altered patterns of (Indications).
- Knowledge deficit, related to medication regimen (Patient/Family Teaching).

IMPLEMENTATION

- **General Info:** Administer daily dose at bedtime.
- **Hypertension:** May be administered concurrently with a diuretic or other antihypertensive.

PATIENT/FAMILY TEACHING

- **General Info:** Emphasize the importance of continuing to take this medication, even if feeling well. Instruct patient to take medication at the same time each day. If a dose is missed, take as soon as remembered unless almost time for next dose. Do not double doses.
  - Doxazosin may cause drowsiness or dizziness. Advise patient to avoid driving or other activities requiring alertness until response to medication is known.
  - Caution patient to change positions slowly to decrease orthostatic hypotension.
  - Advise patient to consult health care professional before taking any cough, cold, or allergy remedies.
  - Emphasize the importance of follow-up visits to determine effectiveness of therapy.
- **Hypertension:** Instruct patient and family on proper technique for blood pressure monitoring. Advise them to check blood pressure at least weekly and report significant changes.
  - Encourage patient to comply with additional interventions for hypertension (weight reduction, low-sodium diet, smoking cessation, moderation of alcohol consumption, regular exercise, and stress management).

EVALUATION

Effectiveness of therapy can be demonstrated by: ▪ Decrease in blood pressure without appearance of side effects ▪ Decrease in urinary symptoms of BPH.

DOXEPIN

(**dox**-e-pin)

Sinequan, {Triadapin}, Zonalon

CLASSIFICATION(S):

Antianxiety agent, Antidepressant (tricyclic), Antipruritic (topical)

Pregnancy Category C (topical), UK (oral)

D

INDICATIONS

▪ **PO:** Management of various forms of endogenous depression (with psychotherapy) ▪ Treatment of anxiety ▪ **Top:** Short-term control of pruritus associated with: □ Eczematous dermatitis □ Lichen simplex chronicus. **Unlabeled Uses:** ▪ **PO:** Management of chronic pain syndromes □ Management of pruritus.

ACTION

PO: ▪ Prevents the reuptake of norepinephrine and serotonin by presynaptic neurons; resultant accumulation of neurotransmitters potentiates their activity ▪ Also possesses significant anticholinergic properties **Top:** ▪ Topical antipruritic action due to antihistaminic properties. **Therapeutic Effects: PO:** ▪ Relief of depression ▪ Decreased anxiety **Top:** ▪ Decreased pruritus.

PHARMACOKINETICS

Absorption: Well absorbed from the GI tract, although much is metabolized on first pass through the liver. Some systemic absorption follows topical application.

Distribution: Widely distributed. Enters breast milk; probably crosses the placenta.

Metabolism and Excretion: Metabolized by the liver. Some conversion to active antidepressant compound. May re-enter gastric juice via secretion from enterohepatic circulation, where more absorption may occur.

Half-life: 8–25 hr.

CONTRAINDICATIONS AND PRECAUTIONS

Contraindicated in: ▪ Hypersensitivity ▪ Some products contain bisulfites and should be

{} = Available in Canada only.

avoided in patients with known intolerance ▪ Untreated narrow-angle glaucoma ▪ Period immediately after myocardial infarction ▪ Pregnancy or lactation.

Use Cautiously in: ▪ Elderly patients (initial dosage reduction recommended) ▪ Pre-existing cardiovascular disease (increased risk of adverse reactions) ▪ Prostatic enlargement (more susceptible to urinary retention) ▪ Seizures.

ADVERSE REACTIONS AND SIDE EFFECTS*

CNS: fatigue, sedation, agitation, confusion, hallucinations.
EENT: blurred vision, increased intraocular pressure.
CV: hypotension, arrhythmias, ECG abnormalities.
GI: constipation, dry mouth, hepatitis, increased appetite, nausea, paralytic ileus.
GU: urinary retention.
Derm: photosensitivity, rashes.
Hemat: blood dyscrasias.
Misc: hypersensitivity reactions.

INTERACTIONS

Apply to both topical and oral use.
Drug-Drug: ▪ May cause hypotension, tachycardia, and potentially fatal reactions when used with **MAO inhibitors** (avoid concurrent use—discontinue 2 wk prior to doxepin) ▪ May prevent the therapeutic response to most **antihypertensives** ▪ May cause severe hypertension when used with **clonidine** (avoid concurrent use) ▪ Additive CNS depression with other **CNS depressants** including **alcohol, antihistamines, opioids,** and **sedative/hypnotics** ▪ **Adrenergic** and **anticholinergic** side effects may be additive with other agents having these properties ▪ **Cimetidine, fluoxetine, phenothiazines,** or **oral contraceptives** increase levels and may cause toxicity ▪ May produce transient delirium with **disulfiram** ▪ **Smoking** may increase metabolism and decrease effectiveness.

ROUTE AND DOSAGE

- **PO (Adults):** *Antidepressant/antianxiety*—25 mg 3 times daily, may be increased as needed (up to 150 mg/day in outpatients or 300 mg/day in inpatients; some patients may require only 25–50 mg/day). Once stabilized, entire daily dose may be given at bedtime. *Antipruritic*—10 mg at bedtime initially, may be increased up to 25 mg.
- **PO (Geriatric Patients):** *Antidepressant*—25–50 mg/day initially, may be increased as needed.
- **Topical (Adults):** Apply 4 times daily (wait 3–4 hr between applications) for up to 8 days.

AVAILABILITY

▪ ***Capsules:*** 10 mg[Rx], 25 mg[Rx], 50 mg[Rx], 75 mg[Rx], 100 mg[Rx], 150 mg[Rx] ▪ ***Oral concentrate:*** 10 mg/ml[Rx] ▪ ***Topical cream:*** 5%[Rx].

TIME/ACTION PROFILE (antidepressant activity)

	ONSET	PEAK	DURATION
PO	2–3 wk	up to 6 wk	days–wks

NURSING IMPLICATIONS

ASSESSMENT

- **General Info:** Monitor blood pressure and pulse rate prior to and during initial therapy. Patients taking high doses or with a history of cardiovascular disease should have ECG monitored prior to and periodically throughout therapy.
- **Depression:** Assess mental status frequently. Confusion, agitation, and hallucinations may occur during initiation of therapy and may require dosage reduction. Monitor mood changes. Assess for suicidal tendencies, especially during early therapy. Restrict amount of drug available to patient.
- **Anxiety:** Assess degree and manifestations of anxiety prior to and throughout therapy.
- **Pain:** Assess the type, location, and severity of pain prior to and periodically throughout therapy.
- **Topical:** Assess pruritic area prior to and periodically throughout therapy.
- ***Lab Test Considerations:*** Monitor leukocyte and differential blood counts, hepatic function, and serum glucose periodically. May cause elevated serum bilirubin and alkaline phosphatase levels. May cause bone marrow depression. Serum glucose may be increased or decreased.

*CAPITALS indicate life-threatening; underlines indicate most frequent.

POTENTIAL NURSING DIAGNOSES

- Coping, ineffective individual (Indications).
- Injury, risk for (Side Effects).
- Knowledge deficit, related to medication regimen (Patient/Family Teaching).

IMPLEMENTATION

- **General Info:** May be given as a single dose at bedtime to minimize sedation during the day. Dose increases should be made at bedtime because of sedation. Dose titration is a slow process; may take weeks to months.
- **PO:** Administer medication with or immediately following a meal to minimize gastric irritation. Capsules may be opened and mixed with foods or fluids if patient has difficulty swallowing.
- □ Oral concentrate must be diluted in at least 120 ml of water, milk, or fruit juice. Do not mix with carbonated beverages or grape juice. Use calibrated measuring device to ensure accurate amount.
- **Topical:** Apply thin film of doxepin cream only to affected areas, and rub in gently. Apply only to affected skin; not for ophthalmic, oral, or intravaginal use.

PATIENT/FAMILY TEACHING

- **General Info:** Inform patient that systemic side effects may occur with oral or topical use.
- □ May cause drowsiness and blurred vision. Caution patient to avoid driving and other activities requiring alertness until response to the medication is known.
- □ Orthostatic hypotension, sedation, and confusion are common during early therapy, especially in the elderly. Protect patient from falls and advise patient to change positions slowly.
- □ Advise patient to avoid alcohol or other CNS depressant drugs during and for at least 3–7 days after therapy has been discontinued.
- □ Instruct patient to notify health care professional if urinary retention occurs or if dry mouth or constipation persists. Sugarless candy or gum may diminish dry mouth, and an increase in fluid intake or bulk may prevent constipation. If symptoms persist, dosage reduction or discontinuation may be necessary. Consult health care professional if dry mouth persists for more than 2 weeks.
- □ Advise patient to notify health care professional of medication regimen prior to treatment or surgery.
- **PO:** Instruct patient to take medication exactly as directed. If a dose is missed, take as soon as possible unless almost time for next dose; if regimen is a single dose at bedtime, do not take in the morning because of side effects. Advise patient that drug effects may not be noticed for at least 2 wk. Abrupt discontinuation may cause nausea, vomiting, diarrhea, headache, trouble sleeping with vivid dreams, and irritability.
- □ Caution patient to use sunscreen and protective clothing to prevent photosensitivity reactions.
- □ Inform patient of need to monitor dietary intake. Increase in appetite is possible and may lead to undesired weight gain.
- □ Therapy for depression is usually prolonged. Emphasize the importance of follow-up exams to monitor effectiveness and side effects.
- **Topical:** Instruct patient to apply medication exactly as directed; do not use more medication than directed, apply to a larger area than directed, use more often than directed, or use longer than 8 days.
- □ Inform patient that topical preparation may cause burning, stinging, swelling, increased itching, or worsening of eczema. Notify health care professional if these symptoms become bothersome.
- □ Caution patient not to use occlusive dressings; may increase systemic absorption.
- □ Advise patient to notify health care professional if excessive drowsiness occurs with topical application. Number of applications per day, amount of cream applied, or area of application may be reduced. May require discontinuation of therapy.

EVALUATION

Effectiveness of therapy can be demonstrated by: ▪ Increased sense of well-being □ Renewed interest in surroundings □ Increased appetite □ Improved energy level □ Improved sleep ▪ Decrease in anxiety ▪ Decrease in chronic pain. Patients may require 2–6 wk of oral therapy before full therapeutic effects of medication are evident ▪ Decrease in pruritus associated with eczema.

D

DOXORUBICIN

doxorubicin hydrochloride
(dox-oh-**roo**-bi-sin)
Adriamycin PFS, Adriamycin RDF, Rubex

doxorubicin hydrochloride liposome
(dox-oh-**roo**-bi-sin **lye**-poe-sohm)
Doxil

CLASSIFICATION(S):
Antineoplastic (anthracycline)

Pregnancy Category D

INDICATIONS

▪ **Doxorubicin hydrochloride:** Alone and in combination with other modalities in the treatment of various solid tumors including: ▫ Breast ▫ Ovarian ▫ Bladder ▫ Bronchogenic carcinoma ▫ Malignant lymphomas and leukemias. ▪ **Doxorubicin hydrochloride liposome:** Management of AIDS-related Kaposi's sarcoma when disease has progressed despite or if patients cannot tolerate conventional therapy with combination antintineoplastic agents.

ACTION

▪ Inhibits DNA and RNA synthesis by forming a complex with DNA; action is cell-cycle S-phase–specific ▪ Also has immunosuppressive properties ▪ Encapsulation in a liposome increases uptake by tumors, prolongs action, and may decrease some toxicity. **Therapeutic Effects:** ▪ Death of rapidly replicating cells, particularly malignant ones.

PHARMACOKINETICS

Absorption: Administered IV only, resulting in complete bioavailability.
Distribution: Widely distributed; does not cross the blood-brain barrier. *Liposome*—higher concentrations are delivered to Kaposi's sarcoma lesions than to normal skin.
Metabolism and Excretion: Mostly metabolized by the liver. Converted by liver to an active compound. Excreted predominantly in the bile, 50% as unchanged drug. Less than 5% eliminated unchanged in the urine.
Half-life: 16.7 hr; *liposome*—55 hr.

CONTRAINDICATIONS AND PRECAUTIONS

Contraindicated in: ▪ Hypersensitivity ▪ Pregnancy or lactation.
Use Cautiously in: ▪ Pre-existing cardiac disease or previous high cumulative doses of anthracyclines ▪ Depressed bone marrow reserve ▪ Liver impairment (dosage reduction required if serum bilirubin >1.2 mg/dl) ▪ Patients with childbearing potential.

ADVERSE REACTIONS AND SIDE EFFECTS*

Doxorubicin hydrochloride
CV: CARDIOMYOPATHY, ECG changes.
GI: diarrhea, esophagitis, nausea, stomatitis, vomiting.
GU: red urine.
Derm: alopecia, photosensitivity.
Endo: gonadal suppression.
Hemat: anemia, leukopenia, thrombocytopenia.
Local: phlebitis at IV site, tissue necrosis.
Metab: hyperuricemia.
Misc: hypersensitivity reactions.
Doxorubicin hydrochloride liposome
CNS: weakness.
CV: CARDIOTOXICITY.
GI: nausea, diarrhea, increased alklaine phosphatase, moniliasis, stomatitis, vomiting.
Derm: alopecia, palmar-plantar erythrodysesthesia.
Hemat: anemia, leukopenia, thrombocytopenia.
Local: injection site reactions.
Misc: acute infusion-associated reactions, fever.

INTERACTIONS

Drug-Drug: ▪ Additive bone marrow depression with other **antineoplastics** or **radiation therapy** ▪ May aggravate skin reactions at previous **radiation therapy** sites ▪ May increase risk of hemorrhagic cystitis from **cyclophosphamide** or hepatitis from **mercaptopurine** ▪ Cardiac toxicity may be enhanced by **radiation therapy** or **cyclophosphamide** ▪ May decrease antibody response to **live virus vaccines** and increase the risk of adverse reactions.

***CAPITALS indicate life-threatening; underlines indicate most frequent.**

ROUTE AND DOSAGE

- **Doxorubicin Hydrochloride (Adriamycin, Rubex)**
  - **IV (Adults):** 60–75 mg/m^2 daily, repeat q 21 days; or 25–30 mg/m^2 daily for 2–3 days, repeat q 3–4 wk or 20 mg/m^2/wk. Total cumulative dose should not exceed 550 mg/m^2 without monitoring of cardiac function or 400 mg/m^2 in patients with previous chest radiation or other cardiotoxic chemotherapy.
  - **IV (Children):** 30 mg/m^2/day for 3 days, may be repeated q 4 wk.
- **Doxorubicin Hydrochloride Liposome (Doxil)**
  - **IV (Adults):** 20 mg/m^2 every 3 wk.

AVAILABILITY

- **Doxorubicin Hydrochloride (Adriamycin, Rubex)**

▪ ***Powder for injection:*** 10-mg, 20-mg, 50-mg, 100-mg, 150-mg vials[Rx] ▪ ***Injection:*** 2 mg/ml[Rx].

- **Doxorubicin Hydrochloride Liposome (Doxil)**

▪ ***Liposomal dispersion for injection:*** 20 mg/10 ml in 10-ml vials [Rx].

TIME/ACTION PROFILE (effect on blood counts)

	ONSET	PEAK	DURATION
IV	10 days	14 days	21–24 days

NURSING IMPLICATIONS

ASSESSMENT

- **General Info:** Monitor blood pressure, pulse, respiratory rate, and temperature frequently during administration. Report significant changes.
- Monitor for bone marrow depression. Assess for bleeding (bleeding gums, bruising, petechiae, guaiac stools, urine, and emesis) and avoid IM injections and rectal temperatures if platelet count is low. Apply pressure to venipuncture sites for 10 min. Assess for signs of infection during neutropenia. Anemia may occur. Monitor for increased fatigue, dyspnea, and orthostatic hypotension.
- Monitor intake and output ratios, and report occurrence of significant discrepancies. Encourage fluid intake of 2000–3000 ml/day. Allopurinol and alkalinization of the urine may be used to decrease serum uric acid levels and to help prevent urate stone formation.
- Severe and protracted nausea and vomiting may occur as early as 1 hr after therapy and may last 24 hr. Parenteral antiemetic agents should be administered 30–45 min prior to therapy and routinely around the clock for the next 24 hr as indicated. Monitor amount of emesis and notify physician or other health care professional if emesis exceeds guidelines to prevent dehydration.
- Monitor for development of signs of cardiac toxicity, which may be either acute and transient (ST segment depression, flattened T wave, sinus tachycardia, and extrasystoles) or late onset (usually occurs 1–6 mo after initiation of therapy) and characterized by intractable congestive heart failure (peripheral edema, dyspnea, rales/crackles, weight gain). Chest x ray, echocardiography, ECGs, and radionuclide angiography may be ordered prior to and periodically throughout therapy. Cardiotoxicity is more prevalent in children younger than 2 yr and geriatric patients. Dexrazoxane may be used to prevent cardiotoxicity in patients receiving cumulative doses of >300 mg/m^2. (see p. 254).
- Assess injection site frequently for redness, irritation, or inflammation. Doxorubicin is a vesicant but may infiltrate painlessly even if blood returns on aspiration of infusion needle. Severe tissue damage may occur if doxorubicin extravasates. If extravasation occurs, stop infusion immediately, restart, and complete dose in another vein. Local infiltration of antidote is not recommended. Apply ice packs and elevate and rest extremity for 24–48 hr to reduce swelling, then resume normal activity as tolerated. If swelling, redness, and/or pain persists beyond 48 hr, immediate consultation for possible debridement is indicated.
- Assess oral mucosa frequently for development of stomatitis. Increased dosing interval and/or decreased dosing is recommended if lesions are painful or interfere with nutrition.
- **Doxorubicin Hydrochloride Liposome:** Monitor for acute infusion-associated reactions consisting of flushing, shortness of breath, facial swelling, headache, chills, back pain, chest or throat tightness, which may be

D

accompanied by hypotension. Reactions usually resolve over 1 day and are usually limited to first dose. Slowing infusion rate may minimize this reaction. Reaction is thought to be due to liposome.

- Monitor for skin toxicity with prolonged use; palmar-plantar erythrodysesthesia usually occurs after 6 wk of treatment and consists of swelling, pain, and erythema of the hands and feet. This may progress to desquamation but usually regresses after 2 wk. In severe cases, modification of future doses of doxorubicin hydrochloride liposome may be necessary.
- ***Lab Test Considerations:*** Monitor CBC and differential prior to and periodically throughout therapy. The leukocyte count nadir occurs 10–14 days after administration, and recovery usually occurs by the 21st day. Thrombocytopenia and anemia may also occur. Increased dosing interval and/or decreased dose is recommended if ANC is $<$1000 cells/mm^3 and/or platelet count is $<$50,000 cells/mm^3.
- Monitor renal (BUN and creatinine) and hepatic (AST, ALT, LDH, and serum bilirubin) function prior to and periodically throughout therapy. Dose reduction is required for bilirubin $>$1.2 mg/dl or serum creatinine $>$3 mg/dl.
- May cause increased serum and urine uric acid concentrations.

POTENTIAL NURSING DIAGNOSES

- Infection, risk for (Adverse Reactions).
- Cardiac output, decreased (Adverse Reactions).
- Knowledge deficit, related to medication regimen (Patient/Family Teaching).

IMPLEMENTATION

- **General Info:** Do not confuse doxorubicin hydrochloride (Adriamycin, Rubex) with doxorubicin hydrochloride liposome (Doxil) or with daunorubicin (Cerubidine). To prevent confusion, orders should include generic and brand name.
- Solution should be prepared in a biologic cabinet. Wear gloves, gown, and mask while handling medication. Discard IV equipment in specially designated containers (see Appendix I).
- Aluminum needles may be used to administer doxorubicin but should not be used during storage, as prolonged contact results in discoloration of solution and formation of a dark precipitate. Solution is red.

Doxorubicin Hydrochloride

- **Direct IV:** Dilute each 10 mg with 5 ml of 0.9% NaCl (nonbacteriostatic) for injection. Shake to dissolve completely. Do not add to IV solution. Reconstituted medication is stable for 24 hr at room temperature and 48 hr if refrigerated. Protect from sunlight.
- ***Rate:*** Administer each dose over 3–5 minutes through Y-site of a free-flowing infusion of 0.9% NaCl or D5W. Facial flushing and erythema along involved vein frequently occur when administration is too rapid.
- **Syringe Compatibility:** ▪ bleomycin ▪ cisplatin ▪ cyclophosphamide ▪ droperidol ▪ leucovorin calcium ▪ methotrexate ▪ metoclopromide ▪ mitomycin ▪ vincristine.
- **Syringe Incompatibility:** ▪ furosemide ▪ heparin.
- **Y-Site Compatibility:** ▪ amifostine ▪ aztreonam ▪ bleomycin ▪ chlorpromazine ▪ cimetidine ▪ cisplatin ▪ cyclophosphamide ▪ dexamethasone ▪ diphenhydramine ▪ droperidol ▪ famotidine ▪ filgrastim ▪ fludarabine ▪ fluorouracil ▪ granisetron ▪ hydromorphone ▪ leucovorin calcium ▪ lorazepam ▪ melphalan ▪ methotrexate ▪ methylprednisolone ▪ metoclopromide ▪ mitomycin ▪ morphine ▪ ondansetron ▪ paclitaxel ▪ prochlorperazine edisylate ▪ ranitidine ▪ sargramostim ▪ sodium bicarbonate ▪ teniposide ▪ thioptepa ▪ vinblastine ▪ vincristine ▪ vinorelbine.
- **Y-Site Incompatibility:** ▪ cefepime ▪ gallium nitrate ▪ ganciclovir ▪ piperacillin/tazobactam.

Doxorubicin Hydrochloride Liposome

- **Intermittent Infusion:** Dilute the dose of doxorubicin hydrochloride liposome, up to 90 mg, in 250 ml of D5W. Do not dilute with other diluents or diluents containing a bacteriostatic agent. Solution is not clear, but a translucent red liposomal dispersion. Do not use in-line filters. Refrigerate diluted solutions and administer within 24 hr of dilution.
- ***Rate:*** Administer dose over 30 min. Do not administer as a bolus or undiluted solution. Rapid infusion may increase infusion-related reactions.
- **Additive Incompatibility:** ▪ Information un-

available. Do not admix with other solutions or medications.

PATIENT/FAMILY TEACHING

- ☐ Instruct patient to notify health care professional promptly if fever; sore throat; signs of infection; bleeding gums; bruising; petechiae; blood in stools, urine, or emesis; increased fatigue; dyspnea; or orthostatic hypotension occurs. Caution patient to avoid crowds and persons with known infections. Instruct patient to use soft toothbrush and electric razor and to avoid falls. Patient should be cautioned not to drink alcoholic beverages or take medication containing aspirin or NSAIDs, as these may precipitate gastric bleeding.
- ☐ Instruct patient to report pain at injection site immediately.
- ☐ Instruct patient to inspect oral mucosa for erythema and ulceration. If ulceration occurs, advise patient to use sponge brush, rinse mouth with water after eating and drinking, and confer with health care professional if mouth pain interferes with eating. Pain may require treatment with opioid analgesics. The risk of developing stomatitis is greatest 5–10 days after a dose; the usual duration is 3–7 days.
- ☐ Advise patient that this medication may have teratogenic effects. Contraception should be used during and for at least 4 mo after therapy is concluded. Inform patient before initiating therapy that this medication may cause irreversible gonadal suppression.
- ☐ Instruct patient to notify health care professional immediately if irregular heartbeat, shortness of breath, swelling of lower extremities, or skin irritation (swelling, pain, or redness of feet or hands) occurs.
- ☐ Discuss the possibility of hair loss with patient. Explore methods of coping. Regrowth usually occurs 2–3 mo after discontinuation of therapy.
- ☐ Instruct patient not to receive any vaccinations without advice of health care professional.
- ☐ Inform patient that medication may cause urine to appear red for 1–2 days.
- ☐ Instruct patient to notify health care professional if skin irritation occurs at site of previous radiation therapy.
- ☐ Emphasize the need for periodic lab tests to monitor for side effects.

EVALUATION

Effectiveness of therapy can be demonstrated by: ▪ Decrease in size or spread of malignancies in solid tumors ▪ Improvement of hematologic status in leukemias ▪ Arrested progression of Kaposi's sarcoma in patients with HIV infection.

DRONABINOL

(droe-**nab**-i-nol)
delta-9-tetrahydrocannabinol, THC, Marinol

CLASSIFICATION(S):
Antiemetic (cannabinoid)

Schedule II
Pregnancy Category C

D

INDICATIONS

▪ Prevention of serious nausea and vomiting from cancer chemotherapy when other more conventional agents have failed ▪ Management of wasting syndrome/anorexia, which may accompany HIV infection.

ACTION

▪ Active ingredient in marijuana ▪ Has a wide variety of CNS effects, including inhibition of the vomiting control mechanism in the medulla oblongata. **Therapeutic Effects:** ▪ Suppression of nausea and vomiting ▪ Increased appetite in patients with AIDS.

PHARMACOKINETICS

Absorption: Extensively metabolized following absorption, resulting in poor bioavailability (10–20%).
Distribution: Enters breast milk in high concentrations. Highly lipid-soluble. Persists in tissues for prolonged period of time.
Metabolism and Excretion: Extensively metabolized; 50% excreted via biliary elimination. At least 1 metabolite is psychoactive.
Half-life: 25–36 hr.

CONTRAINDICATIONS AND PRECAUTIONS

Contraindicated in: ▪ Hypersensitivity to dronabinol, marijuana, or sesame oil ▪ Nausea and vomiting due to any other causes ▪ Lactation.

Use Cautiously in: ▪ Patients who have abused drugs or have been drug-dependent in the past ▪ Chronic use may lead to withdrawal syndrome on discontinuation ▪ Geriatric patients ▪ Pregnancy (do not use unless clearly indicated) ▪ Safety in children <18 not established.

ADVERSE REACTIONS AND SIDE EFFECTS*

CNS: concentration difficulty, coordination impairment, dizziness, drowsiness, heightened awareness, perceptual difficulty, depression, disorientation, hallucinations, headache, impaired judgment, irritability, memory loss, nightmares, paranoia, speech difficulty, tinnitus, weakness.
EENT: dry mouth, visual distortion.
CV: syncope, tachycardia.
GI: diarrhea.
Derm: facial flushing, perspiration.
MS: muscular pain.
Neuro: ataxia, paresthesia.
Misc: physical dependence, psychological dependence (high doses or prolonged therapy).

INTERACTIONS

Drug-Drug: ▪ Additive CNS depression with **alcohol, antihistamines, opioids, tricyclic antidepressants,** and **sedative/hypnotics** ▪ Increased risk of tachycardia with **amphetamines, cocaine, sympathomimetics, anticholinergics, antihistamines,** and **tricyclic antidepressants.**

ROUTE AND DOSAGE

- **PO (Adults):** *Antiemetic*—5 mg/m² 1–3 hr prior to chemotherapy; may repeat every 2–4 hr after chemotherapy to a total of 4–6 doses/day. If initial dose is ineffective and no significant adverse reactions have occurred, dosage may be increased by 2.5 mg/m² to a maximum of 15 mg/m²/dose. *Appetite stimulant*—2.5 mg twice daily initially; may be increased as needed (up to 20 mg/day). May also be initiated with a 2.5-mg dose at bedtime.

AVAILABILITY

- ***Gelatin capsules:*** 2.5 mg^Rx^, 5 mg^Rx^, 10 mg^Rx^.

TIME/ACTION PROFILE (antiemetic effect)

	ONSET	PEAK	DURATION
PO	UK	2 hr	4–6 hr†

†Appetite stimulation lasts 24 hr or longer.

NURSING IMPLICATIONS

ASSESSMENT

- □ Assess nausea, vomiting, appetite, bowel sounds, and abdominal pain prior to and following the administration of this drug.
- □ Monitor hydration, nutritional status, and intake and output. Patients with severe nausea and vomiting may require IV fluids in addition to antiemetics.
- □ Monitor blood pressure and heart rate periodically throughout therapy.
- □ Patients on dronabinol therapy should be monitored closely for side effects because the effects of dronabinol vary with each patient.

POTENTIAL NURSING DIAGNOSES

- Fluid volume deficit, risk for (Indications).
- Nutrition, altered, less than body requirements (Indications).
- Injury, risk for (Side Effects).

IMPLEMENTATION

- **General Info:** Dronabinol capsules should be refrigerated (not frozen).
- □ Physical or psychological dependence may occur with high doses or prolonged therapy, causing a withdrawal syndrome (irritability, restlessness, insomnia, hot flashes, sweating, rhinorrhea, loose stools, hiccups, anorexia) when discontinued. This is unlikely to occur with therapeutic doses and short-term use of dronabinol.
- **Antiemetic:** This drug may be administered prophylactically 1–3 hr prior to chemotherapy and repeated every 2–4 hr after chemotherapy up to 4–6 doses daily.
- **Appetite Stimulant:** Give 2.5 mg bid before lunch and supper initially. Reduce dose to 2.5 mg/day in the evening or at bedtime for patients unable to tolerate 5 mg/day dose. May increase dose to 2.5 mg at lunch and 5 mg before supper or 5 mg at lunch and 5 mg after supper if further therapeutic effect is de-

*CAPITALS indicate life-threatening; underlines indicate most frequent.

sired and adverse effects are minimal. Most patients respond to 2.5-mg bid dose, but up to 10 mg bid have been tolerated in about 50% of patients. Adverse effects are usually dose related.

PATIENT/FAMILY TEACHING

- Instruct patient to take dronabinol exactly as directed. Take missed doses as soon as possible but not if almost time for next dose; do not double doses. Signs of overdose (mood changes, confusion, hallucinations, depression, nervousness, fast or pounding heartbeat) may occur with increased doses.
- Advise patient to call for assistance when ambulating, as this drug may cause dizziness, drowsiness, and impaired judgment and coordination. Avoid driving or other activities requiring alertness until response to the drug is known.
- Instruct patient to change positions slowly to minimize orthostatic hypotension.
- Caution patient to avoid taking alcohol or other CNS depressants during dronabinol therapy.
- Advise patient and family to use general measures to decrease nausea (begin with sips of liquids and small, nongreasy meals; provide oral hygiene; remove noxious stimuli from environment).

EVALUATION

Effectiveness of therapy can be demonstrated by: ▪ Prevention of and decrease in nausea and vomiting associated with chemotherapy ▪ Increased or maintained weight in patients with AIDS.

DROPERIDOL
(droe-**per**-i-dole)
Inapsine

CLASSIFICATION(S):
Antiemetic (butyrophenone), Tranquilizer (butyrophenone)

Pregnancy Category C

INDICATIONS

▪ Used to produce tranquilization and as an adjunct to general and regional anesthesia. **Unlabeled Uses:** ▪ Useful in decreasing postoperative or postprocedure nausea and vomiting.

ACTION

▪ Similar to haloperidol—alters the action of dopamine in the CNS. **Therapeutic Effects:** ▪ Tranquilization ▪ Suppression of nausea and vomiting in selected situations.

PHARMACOKINETICS

Absorption: Well absorbed following IM administration.
Distribution: Appears to cross the blood-brain barrier and placenta.
Metabolism and Excretion: Mainly metabolized by the liver. Only 10% excreted unchanged by the kidneys.
Half-life: 2.2 hr.

CONTRAINDICATIONS AND PRECAUTIONS

Contraindicated in: ▪ Hypersensitivity ▪ Known intolerance ▪ Narrow-angle glaucoma ▪ Bone marrow depression ▪ CNS depression ▪ Severe liver or cardiac disease.
Use Cautiously in: ▪ Elderly, debilitated, or severely ill patients (smaller doses should be used) ▪ Diabetics ▪ Respiratory insufficiency ▪ Prostatic hypertrophy ▪ CNS tumors ▪ Intestinal obstruction ▪ Cardiac disease ▪ Seizures (may lower seizure threshold) ▪ Severe liver disease ▪ Pregnancy, lactation, and children <2 yr (although safety not established, droperidol has been used during cesarean section without respiratory depression in the newborn).

ADVERSE REACTIONS AND SIDE EFFECTS*

CNS: SEIZURES, extrapyramidal reactions, abnormal EEG, anxiety, confusion, dizziness, excessive sedation, hallucinations, hyperactivity, mental depression, nightmares, restlessness, tardive dyskinesia.
EENT: blurred vision, dry eyes.
Resp: bronchospasm, laryngospasm.
CV: hypotension, tachycardia.
GI: constipation, dry mouth.
Misc: chills, facial sweating, shivering.

***CAPITALS indicate life-threatening; underlines indicate most frequent.**

INTERACTIONS

Drug-Drug: ▪ Additive hypotension with **antihypertensives** or **nitrates** ▪ Additive CNS depression with other **CNS depressants,** including **alcohol, antihistamines, antidepressants, opioids,** and other **sedatives.**

ROUTE AND DOSAGE

❑ Premedication/Use without Premedication in Diagnostic Procedures

- **IV, IM (Adults):** 2.5–10 mg 30–60 min prior to induction of anesthesia; additional doses of 1.25–2.5 mg IV may be needed.
- **IM, IV (Children 2–12 yr):** 1–1.5 mg/20–25 lb.

❑ Adjunct to General Anesthesia

- **IV (Adults):** 2.5 mg/20–25 lb; additional doses of 1.25–2.5 mg IV may be needed.
- **IM, IV (Children 2–12 yr):** 1–1.5 mg/20–25 lb.

❑ Adjunct in Regional Anesthesia

- **IM, IV (Adults):** 2.5–5 mg.

❑ Antiemetic

- **IV (Adults):** 0.5–1 mg q 4 hr as needed (unlabeled).

AVAILABILITY

- ***Injection:*** 2.5 mg/ml[Rx].

TIME/ACTION PROFILE (sedation)

	ONSET	PEAK	DURATION*
IM, IV	3–10 min	30 min	2–4 hr

*Listed as duration of tranquilization; alterations in consciousness may last up to 12 hr.

NURSING IMPLICATIONS

ASSESSMENT

- **General Info:** Monitor blood pressure and heart rate frequently throughout course of therapy. Report significant changes immediately. Hypotension may be treated with parenteral fluids if hypovolemia is a causal factor. Vasopressors (norepinephrine, phenylephrine) may be needed. Avoid use of epinephrine, as droperidol reverses its pressor effects and may cause paradoxical hypotension.
  - ❑ Assess patient for level of sedation following administration.
  - ❑ Observe patient for extrapyramidal symptoms (dystonia, oculogyric crisis, extended neck, flexed arms, tremor, restlessness, hyperactivity, anxiety) throughout therapy. Notify physician or other health care professional should these occur. An anticholinergic antiparkinsonian agent may be used to treat these symptoms.
- **Nausea and Vomiting:** Assess nausea, vomiting, hydration status, bowel sounds, and abdominal pain prior to and following administration.

POTENTIAL NURSING DIAGNOSES

- Injury, risk for (Side Effects).
- Knowledge deficit, related to medication regimen (Patient/Family Teaching).

IMPLEMENTATION

- **Direct IV:** Administer undiluted.
- ***Rate:*** Administer each dose slowly over at least 1 min.
- **Intermittent Infusion:** May be added to 250 ml of D5W, 0.9% NaCl, or lactated Ringer's solution.
- ***Rate:*** Administer by slow IV infusion. Titrate according to patient response.
- **Syringe Compatibility:** ▪ atropine ▪ bleomycin ▪ butorphanol ▪ chlorpromazine ▪ cimetidine ▪ cisplatin ▪ cyclophosphamide ▪ dimenhydrinate ▪ diphenhydramine ▪ doxorubicin ▪ fentanyl ▪ glycopyrrolate ▪ hydroxyzine ▪ meperidine ▪ metoclopramide ▪ midazolam ▪ mitomycin ▪ morphine ▪ nalbuphine ▪ pentazocine ▪ perphenazine ▪ prochlorperazine ▪ promazine ▪ promethazine ▪ scopolamine ▪ vinblastine ▪ vincristine.
- **Syringe Incompatibility:** ▪ fluorouracil ▪ furosemide ▪ heparin ▪ leucovorin calcium ▪ methotrexate ▪ pentobarbital.
- **Y-Site Compatibility:** ▪ aztreonam ▪ bleomycin ▪ buprenorphine ▪ cisplatin ▪ cyclophosphamide ▪ cytarabine ▪ doxorubicin ▪ filgrastim ▪ fluconazole ▪ fludarabine ▪ hydrocortisone sodium succinate ▪ idarubicin ▪ melphalan ▪ meperidine ▪ metoclopramide ▪ mitomycin ▪ ondansetron ▪ paclitaxel ▪ potassium chloride ▪ sargramostim ▪ teniposide ▪ vinblastine ▪ vincristine ▪ vinorelbine ▪ vitamin B complex with C.
- **Y-Site Incompatibility:** ▪ allopurinol sodium ▪ amifostine ▪ cefepime ▪ fluorouracil ▪ foscarnet ▪ furosemide ▪ leucovorin calcium

▪ methotrexate ▪ nafcillin ▪ piperacillin/tazobactam ▪ thiotepa.
▪ **Additive Incompatibility:** ▪ barbiturates.

PATIENT/FAMILY TEACHING

- Caution patient to change positions slowly to minimize orthostatic hypotension.
- Medication causes drowsiness. Advise patient to call for assistance during ambulation and transfer.

EVALUATION

Effectiveness of therapy can be demonstrated by: ▪ General quiescence and reduced motor activity ▪ Decreased nausea and vomiting.

EDROPHONIUM

(ed-roe-**fone**-ee-yum)
Enlon, Reversol, Tensilon

CLASSIFICATION(S):
Cholinergic (anticholinesterase)

Pregnancy Category C

INDICATIONS

▪ Diagnosis of myasthenia gravis ▪ Assessment of adequacy of anticholinesterase therapy in myasthenia gravis ▪ Differentiating myasthenic from cholinergic crisis ▪ Reversal of muscle paralysis from nondepolarizing neuromuscular blockers.

ACTION

▪ Inhibits the breakdown of acetylcholine so that it accumulates and has a prolonged effect. Effects include miosis; increased intestinal and skeletal muscle tone; bronchial and ureteral constriction; bradycardia; increased salivation, lacrimation, and sweating. **Therapeutic Effects:** ▪ Short-lived improvement in muscular function in patients with myasthenia gravis ▪ Reversal of nondepolarizing neuromuscular blockers.

PHARMACOKINETICS

Absorption: Absorption following IM and SC administration not known.
Distribution: UK.
Metabolism and Excretion: UK.
Half-life: 33–110 min.

CONTRAINDICATIONS AND PRECAUTIONS

Contraindicated in: ▪ Hypersensitivity ▪ Mechanical obstruction of the GI or GU tract ▪ Hypersensitivity to bisulfites ▪ Pregnancy (may cause uterine irritability after IV administration near term; newborns may display muscle weakness) ▪ Lactation.
Use Cautiously in: ▪ History of asthma ▪ Ulcer disease ▪ Cardiovascular disease ▪ Epilepsy ▪ Hyperthyroidism ▪ Because some patients may be extremely sensitive to the effects of anticholinesterases, atropine should be available in case of excessive dosage.

ADVERSE REACTIONS AND SIDE EFFECTS*

CNS: SEIZURES, dizziness, weakness.
EENT: lacrimation, miosis.
Resp: bronchospasm, excess secretions.
CV: bradycardia, hypotension.
GI: abdominal cramps, diarrhea, excess salivation, vomiting, nausea.
Derm: sweating, rashes.
MS: fasciculation.

INTERACTIONS

Drug-Drug: ▪ Action may be antagonized by **drugs possessing anticholinergic properties,** including **antihistamines, antidepressants, atropine, haloperidol, phenothiazines, quinidine,** and **disopyramide** ▪ Prolongs action of **depolarizing muscle-relaxing agents (succinylcholine, decamethonium)** ▪ May lead to excessive bradycardia in patients receiving **digitalis glycosides.**

ROUTE AND DOSAGE

Diagnosis of Myasthenia Gravis

- **IV (Adults):** 2 mg; if no response, administer an additional 8 mg after 45 sec; may repeat test in 30 min. If cholinergic response occurs, administer atropine 0.4 mg IV. Patients >50 yr should be pretreated with atropine to prevent bradycardia/hypotension.
- **IV (Children >34 kg):** 2 mg; if no response after 45 sec, may administer 1 mg q 30–45 sec to a total of 10 mg. If cholinergic response occurs, administer atropine IV.
- **IV (Children <34 kg):** 1 mg; if no response

***CAPITALS** indicate life-threatening; underlines indicate most frequent.**

after 45 sec, may administer 1 mg q 45 sec to a total of 5 mg. If cholinergic response occurs, administer atropine IV.

- **IV (Infants):** 0.5 mg.
- **IM (Adults):** 10 mg. If cholinergic response occurs, may repeat 2-mg dose in 30 min to rule out false-negative reaction. Patients >50 yr should be pretreated with atropine to prevent bradycardia/hypotension.
- **IM (Children >34 kg):** 5 mg.
- **IM (Children <34 kg):** 2 mg.

❑ **Assessment of Anticholinesterase Therapy**

- **IV (Adults):** 1–2 mg 1 hr after oral anticholinesterase dose.

❑ **Differentiation of Cholinergic from Myasthenic Crisis**

- **IV (Adults):** 1 mg; may give additional 1 mg 1 min later.

❑ **Reversal of Nondepolarizing Neuromuscular Blocking Agents**

- **IV (Adults):** 10 mg; may repeat as needed (not to exceed 40 mg). Doses of 0.5–1 mg/kg have been used.

AVAILABILITY

- ***Injection:*** 10 mg/ml[Rx] ▪ ***In combination with:*** atropine (Enlon-Plus)[Rx]. See Appendix A.

TIME/ACTION PROFILE (cholinergic activity)

	ONSET	PEAK	DURATION
IM	2–10 min	UK	5–30 min
IV	30–60 sec	UK	10 min

NURSING IMPLICATIONS

ASSESSMENT

- **General Info:** Assess neuromuscular status (ptosis, diplopia, vital capacity, ability to swallow, extremity strength) prior to and immediately after administration.
- ❑ To differentiate myasthenic from cholinergic crisis, assess for increased weakness, diaphoresis, increased saliva and bronchial secretions, dyspnea, nausea, vomiting, diarrhea, and bradycardia. If these symptoms occur, patient is in cholinergic crisis. If strength improves, patient is in myasthenic crisis.
- ***Toxicity and Overdose:*** Atropine may be used for treatment of cholinergic symptoms. Oxygen and resuscitation equipment should be available.

POTENTIAL NURSING DIAGNOSES

- Breathing pattern, ineffective (Indications).
- Knowledge deficit, related to medication regimen (Patient/Family Teaching).

IMPLEMENTATION

- **General Info:** For myasthenia gravis patients, diagnostic IV dose and dose to differentiate myasthenic from cholinergic crisis are administered by a physician.
- **Direct IV:** IV doses are administered undiluted with a tuberculin syringe.
- ***Rate:*** Administer doses over 30–45 sec.
- **Y-Site Compatibility:** ▪ heparin ▪ hydrocortisone ▪ potassium chloride ▪ vitamin B complex with C.

PATIENT/FAMILY TEACHING

- ❑ Inform patient that the effects of this medication last up to 30 min.

EVALUATION

Effectiveness of therapy can be demonstrated by: ▪ Relief of myasthenic symptoms ▪ Differentiation of myasthenic from cholinergic crisis ▪ Reversal of paralysis after anesthesia.

EPIDURAL LOCAL ANESTHETICS*

bupivacaine
(byoo-**pi**-vi-kane)
Marcaine, Sensorcaine

ropivacaine
(**roe**-pi-vi-kane)
Naropin

CLASSIFICATION(S):
Epidural anesthetics (analgesic adjuncts)

Pregnancy Category C

*Adapted with permission from Pasero, C, Portenoy, RK, and McCaffery, M: Opioid analgesics. In: McCaffery, M, and Pasero, C: *Pain: Clinical Manual,* St. Louis, Mosby, 1998.

INDICATIONS

▪ May be combined with epidural opioids in the management of severe acute or chronic pain. Low doses of epidural anesthetics act synergistically with opioids, allowing for use of lower doses of opioids and fewer systemic opioid side effects (constipation, nausea, respiratory depression, hypotension) ▫ Compared with other local anesthetics, these agents are better able to block nerve fibers that carry pain, with minimal effect on sensory and motor fibers.

ACTION

▪ Local anesthetics inhibit initiation and conduction of sensory nerve impulses by altering the influx of sodium and efflux of potassium in neurons, slowing or stopping pain transmission. Epidural administration allows action to take place at the level of the spinal nerve roots immediately adjacent to the site of administration. The catheter is placed as close as possible to the dermatomes (skin surface areas innervated by a single spinal nerve or group of spinal nerves) that, when blocked, will produce the most effective spread of analgesia for the site of injury. **Therapeutic Effects:** ▪ Decreased pain; low doses have minimal effect on sensory or motor function; higher doses may produce complete motor blockade. Catheter placement allows localization of effect.

PHARMACOKINETICS

Absorption: Systemic absorption of bupivacaine and ropivacaine follows epidural administration, but amount absorbed depends on dose.
Distribution: Both agents are lipid-soluble, which selectively keeps them in the epidural space and limits systemic absorption. If systemic absorption occurs, both agents are widely distributed and cross the placenta.
Metabolism and Excretion: Small amounts of bupivacaine and ropivacaine that may reach systemic circulation are mostly metabolized by the liver. Because only a small amount is cleared by the kidneys, renal function has minimal impact.
Half-life: *Bupivacaine*—5 hr (after epidural use); *ropivacaine*—3 hr (after epidural use).

CONTRAINDICATIONS AND PRECAUTIONS

Contraindicated in: ▪ Hypersensitivity; cross-sensitivity with other amide local anesthetics may occur (etidocaine, lidocaine, mepivacaine, prilocaine) ▪ Bupivacaine contains bisulfites and should be avoided in patients with known intolerance.
Use Cautiously in: ▪ Concurrent use of other local anesthetics ▪ Liver disease ▪ Concurrent use of anticoagulants (including low-dose heparin and low-molecular-weight heparins) increases the risk of spinal/epidural hematomas.

ADVERSE REACTIONS AND SIDE EFFECTS*

Ropivacaine has less CNS and cardiac toxicity than bupivacaine.
CNS: SEIZURES, irritability, slow speech, twitching.
EENT: tinnitus.
CV: CARDIOVASCULAR COLLAPSE, arrhythmias, bradycardia, hypotension.
GI: metallic taste.
GU: urinary retention.
F and E: acidosis.
Neuro: circumoral tingling/numbness.
Misc: allergic reactions.

INTERACTIONS

Drug-Drug: ▪ Additive toxicity may occur with concurrent use of other **amide local anesthetics.**

ROUTE AND DOSAGE

❑ Bupivacaine

- **Epidural (Adults):** *Epidural analgesia* 0.0625–0.125% solution (0.625–1.25 mg/ml). *Partial to moderate motor block*—25–50 mg as a 0.25% solution q 3 hr; *moderate to complete motor block*—50–100 mg as a 0.5% solution q 3 hr; *complete motor block*—75–150 mg as a 0.75% solution q 3 hr.

❑ Ropivacaine

- **Epidural (Adults):** *Postoperative pain*—0.2% solution (2 mg/ml). *Lumbar epidural continuous infusion*—12–20 mg/hr (6–10 ml/hr). *Thoracic epidural continuous infusion*—8–16 mg/hr (4–8 ml/hr).

*CAPITALS indicate life-threatening; underlines indicate most frequent.

AVAILABILITY

❑ **Bupivacaine**

▪ ***Solution for injection (with and without preservatives):*** 0.25%Rx, 0.5%Rx, 0.75%Rx ▪ ***In combination with:*** epinephrineRx.

❑ **Ropivacaine (Preservative-Free)**

▪ ***Solution for injection:*** 0.2 %Rx, 0.5%Rx, 0.75%Rx, 1%Rx.

TIME/ACTION PROFILE (analgesia)

	ONSET	PEAK	DURATION
bupivacaine, ropivacaine	5–20 min	UK	up to 6 hr*

*Duration of anesthetic block.

NURSING IMPLICATIONS

ASSESSMENT

- **Systemic Toxicity:** Assess for systemic toxicity (circumoral tingling and numbness, ringing in ears, metallic taste, slow speech, irritability, twitching, seizures, cardiac dysrhythmias) each shift. Report to anesthesiologist. Treatment includes removal of local anesthetic from analgesic solution.
- **Orthostatic Hypotension:** Assess heart rate and blood pressure, including orthostatic blood pressure prior to ambulation, regularly until dose is stabilized and it is clear that hypotension is not a problem. Mild hypotension is common because of the effect of local anesthetic block of nerve fibers on the sympathetic nervous system, causing vasodilation. Significant hypotension and bradycardia may occur, especially when rising from a prone position or following large dose increases or boluses. Treatment of unresolved hypotension may include hydration, decreasing the epidural infusion rate, and/or removal of local anesthetic from analgesic solution.
- **Unwanted Motor and Sensory Deficit:** The goal of adding low-dose local anesthetics to epidural opioids for pain management is to provide analgesia, not to produce anesthesia. Patients should be able to ambulate if their condition allows, and epidural analgesic should not hamper this important recovery activity. However, many factors, including location of the epidural catheter, local anesthetic dose, and variability in patient response, can result in patients experiencing unwanted motor and sensory deficits.
  - ❑ Assess for sensory deficit every shift. Ask patient to point to numb and tingling skin areas (numbness and tingling at the incision site is common and usually normal).
  - ❑ Assess patient for motor deficit. Ask patient to bend the knees and lift the buttocks off the mattress. Most are able to do this without difficulty. Determine patient's ability to bear weight. Provide assistance when ambulating as needed. Notify anesthesiologist of unwanted motor and sensory deficits.
  - ❑ Unwanted motor and sensory deficit often can be corrected with simple treatment. For example, a change in position may relieve temporary sensory loss in an extremity. Minor extremity muscle weakness is often treated by decreasing the epidural infusion rate and keeping the patient in bed until the weakness resolves. Sometimes removing the local anesthetic from the analgesic solution is necessary, such as when signs of local anesthetic toxicity are detected or when simple treatment of motor and sensory deficits has been unsuccessful.

POTENTIAL NURSING DIAGNOSES

- Pain, acute (Indications).
- Physical mobility, impaired (Adverse Reactions).
- Knowledge deficit, related to medication regimen (Patient/Family Teaching).

IMPLEMENTATION

- See Route and Dosage section.

PATIENT/FAMILY TEACHING

- ❑ Instruct patient to notify nurse if signs or symptoms of systemic toxicity occur.
- ❑ Advise patient to request assistance during ambulation until orthostatic hypotension and motor deficits are ruled out.

EVALUATION

Effectiveness of therapy can be demonstrated by: ▪ Decrease in postoperative pain without unwanted sensory or motor deficits.

EPINEPHRINE†

(e-pi-**nef**-rin)

Adrenalin, Ana-Gard, AsthmaHaler Mist, AsthmaNefrin (racepinephrine), Bronitin Mist, Bronkaid Mist, EpiPen, microNefrin, Nephron, Primatene, S-2, Sus-Phrine, Vaponefrin (racepinephrine)

CLASSIFICATION(S):

Antiglaucoma agent, Bronchodilator (adrenergic agonist), Vasopressor

Pregnancy Category C

†See Appendix O for ophthalmic use.

INDICATIONS

▪ **SC, IV, Inhalation:** Management of reversible airway disease due to asthma or COPD ▪ **SC, IV:** Management of severe allergic reactions ▪ **IV, Intracardiac:** Management of cardiac arrest ▪ **Local/Spinal:** Adjunct in the localization/prolongation of anesthesia.

ACTION

▪ Results in the accumulation of cyclic adenosine monophosphate (cAMP) at beta-adrenergic receptors ▪ Affects both $beta_1$ (cardiac) -adrenergic receptors and $beta_2$ (pulmonary) -adrenergic receptor sites ▪ Produces bronchodilation ▪ Also has alpha-adrenergic agonist properties, which result in vasoconstriction ▪ Inhibits the release of mediators of immediate hypersensitivity reactions from mast cells. **Therapeutic Effects:** ▪ Bronchodilation ▪ Maintenance of heart rate and blood pressure ▪ Localization/prolongation of local/spinal anesthetic.

PHARMACOKINETICS

Absorption: Well absorbed following SC administration; some absorption may occur following repeated inhalation of large doses.

Distribution: Does not cross the blood-brain barrier; crosses the placenta and enters breast milk.

Metabolism and Excretion: Action is rapidly terminated by metabolism and uptake by nerve endings.

Half-life: UK.

CONTRAINDICATIONS AND PRECAUTIONS

Contraindicated in: ▪ Hypersensitivity to adrenergic amines ▪ Some products may contain bisulfites or fluorocarbons (in some inhalers) and should be avoided in patients with known hypersensitivity or intolerance.

Use Cautiously in: ▪ Cardiac disease ▪ Hypertension ▪ Hyperthyroidism ▪ Diabetes ▪ Glaucoma (except for ophthalmic use) ▪ Elderly patients (more susceptible to adverse reactions; may require dosage reduction) ▪ Pregnancy (near term), lactation, and children <2 yr (safety not established) ▪ Excessive use may lead to tolerance and paradoxical bronchospasm (inhaler).

ADVERSE REACTIONS AND SIDE EFFECTS*

CNS: <u>nervousness</u>, <u>restlessness</u>, <u>tremor</u>, headache, insomnia.

Resp: paradoxical bronchospasm (excessive use of inhalers).

CV: <u>angina</u>, <u>arrhythmias</u>, <u>hypertension</u>, <u>tachycardia</u>.

GI: nausea, vomiting.

Endo: hyperglycemia.

INTERACTIONS

Drug-Drug: ▪ Concurrent use with other **adrenergic (sympathomimetic) agents** will have additive adrenergic side effects ▪ Use with **MAO inhibitors** may lead to hypertensive crisis ▪ **Beta-adrenergic blockers** may negate therapeutic effect.

ROUTE AND DOSAGE

- **SC, IM (Adults):** *Anaphylactic reactions/asthma*—0.1–0.5 mg (single dose not to exceed 1 mg); may repeat q 10–15 min for anaphylactic shock or q 20 min–4 hr for asthma. *Epinephrine suspension*—0.5 mg SC initially; may repeat 0.5–1.5 mg q 6 hr.
- **SC (Children):** *Anaphylactic reactions/asthma*—0.01 mg/kg or 0.3 mg/m² (not to exceed 0.5 mg/dose) q 15 min for 2 doses, then q 4 hr. *Epinephrine suspension*—0.025 mg/kg (0.625 mg/m²) SC; may be repeated q 6 hr (not to exceed 0.75 mg in children ≤30 kg).

*CAPITALS indicate life-threatening; <u>underlines</u> indicate most frequent.

E

- **IV (Adults):** *Severe anaphylaxis*—0.1–0.25 mg q 5–15 min; may be followed by 1–4 mcg/min continuous infusion. *Cardiopulmonary resuscitation*—0.5–1 mg q 3–5 min; may be followed by 1 mcg/min infusion (may be increased up to 4 mcg/min). *Bradycardia*—1 mcg/min initially; may be adjusted as needed (range 2–10 mcg/min).
- **IV (Children):** *Severe anaphylaxis*—0.1 mg (less in younger children); may be followed by 0.1 mcg/kg/min continuous infusion (may be increased up to 1.5 mcg/kg/min). *Cardiopulmonary resuscitation*—0.01 mg/kg, may be repeated q 3–5 min; may be followed by 0.1 mcg/kg/min infusion (may be gradually increased to 1 mcg/kg/min).
- **IV (Neonates):** *Cardiopulmonary resuscitation*—0.01–0.03 mg/kg; may be repeated q 3–5 min.
- **Inhalation (Adults and Children ≥4 yr):** *Metered-dose inhaler*—1 inhalation (160–250 mcg), may be repeated after 1–2 min; additional doses may be repeated q 3 hr. *Inhalation solution*—1 inhalation of 1% solution; may be repeated after 1–2 min; additional doses may be given q 3 hr. *Racepinephrine*—Via hand nebulizer, 2–3 inhalations of 2.25% solution; may repeat in 5 min with 2–3 more inhalations, up to 4–6 times daily.
- **Intracardiac (Adults):** 0.3–0.5 mg.
- **Endotracheal (Adults):** 1 mg.
- **Topical (Adults and Children ≥6 yr):** *Nasal decongestant*—Apply 1% solution as drops, spray, or with a swab.
- **Intraspinal (Adults and Children):** 0.2–0.4 ml of 1:1000 solution.
- **With Local Anesthetics (Adults and Children):** Use 1:200,000 solution with local anesthetic.

AVAILABILITY

▪ ***Inhalation aerosol:*** 0.125% (≥300 inhalations/15 ml)^OTC^, 0.5% (≥300 inhalations/15 ml)^OTC^, 300 mcg/spray (≥300 inhalations/15 ml)^OTC^ ▪ ***Inhalation solution:*** 1%^OTC^ ▪ ***Injection:*** 10 mcg/ml^Rx^, 100 mcg /ml^Rx^, 500 mcg/ml^Rx^, 1 mg/ml^Rx^ ▪ ***Suspension for injection:*** 5 mg/ml^Rx^ ▪ ***Auto-injector:*** 0.15 mg^Rx^, 0.3 mg^Rx^ ▪ ***Ophthalmic solution:*** 0.5%^Rx^, 1%^Rx^, 2%^Rx^ ▪ ***Topical solution:*** 0.1%^Rx^.

TIME/ACTION PROFILE (bronchodilation)

	ONSET	PEAK	DURATION
Inhaln	3–5 min	UK	1–3 hr
SC	6–12 min	20 min	<1–4 hr
IM	6–12 min	UK	<1–4 hr
IV	rapid	20 min	20–30 min

NURSING IMPLICATIONS

ASSESSMENT

- **Bronchodilator:** Assess lung sounds, respiratory pattern, pulse, and blood pressure before administration and during peak of medication. Note amount, color, and character of sputum produced, and notify physician or other health care professional of abnormal findings.
- □ Monitor pulmonary function tests before initiating therapy and periodically throughout course to determine effectiveness of medication.
- □ Observe for paradoxical bronchospasm (wheezing). If condition occurs, withhold medication and notify physician or other health care professional immediately.
- □ Observe patient for drug tolerance and rebound bronchospasm. Patients requiring more than 3 inhalation treatments in 24 hr should be under close supervision. If minimal or no relief is seen after 3–5 inhalation treatments within 6–12 hr, further treatment with aerosol alone is not recommended.
- □ Assess for hypersensitivity reaction (rash; urticaria; swelling of the face, lips, or eyelids). If condition occurs, withhold medication and notify physician or other health care professional immediately.
- **Vasopressor:** Monitor blood pressure, pulse, ECG, and respiratory rate frequently during IV administration. Continuous ECG monitoring, hemodynamic parameters, and urine output should be monitored continuously during IV administration.
- □ Monitor for chest pain, arrhythmias, heart rate >110 bpm, and hypertension. Consult physician for parameters of pulse, blood pressure, and ECG changes for adjusting dosage or discontinuing medication.
- **Shock:** Assess volume status. Hypovolemia should be corrected prior to administering isoproterenol IV.

- **Nasal Decongestant:** Assess patient for nasal and sinus congestion prior to and periodically during therapy.
- ***Lab Test Considerations:*** May cause transient decrease in serum potassium concentrations with nebulization or at higher than recommended doses.
- □ May cause an increase in blood glucose and serum lactic acid concentrations.
- ***Toxicity and Overdose:*** Symptoms of overdose include persistent agitation, chest pain or discomfort, decreased blood pressure, dizziness, hyperglycemia, hypokalemia, seizures, tachyarrhythmias, persistent trembling, and vomiting.
- □ Treatment includes discontinuing adrenergic bronchodilator and other beta-adrenergic agonists and symptomatic, supportive therapy. Cardioselective beta-adrenergic blocking agents are used cautiously, as they may induce bronchospasm.

POTENTIAL NURSING DIAGNOSES

- Airway clearance, ineffective (Indications).
- Tissue perfusion, altered (Indications).
- Knowledge deficit, related to medication regimen (Patient/Family Teaching).

IMPLEMENTATION

- **General Info:** Medication should be administered promptly at the onset of bronchospasm.
- □ Tolerance may develop with prolonged or excessive use. Effectiveness may be restored by discontinuing for a few days and then readministering.
- □ Check dose, concentration, and route of administration carefully prior to administration. Fatalities have occurred from medication errors. Use a tuberculin syringe with a 26-gauge, ½-in. needle for SC injection to ensure that correct amount of medication is administered. Suspension is for SC use *only*.
- □ Do not use solutions that are pinkish or brownish or that contain a precipitate.
- □ For anaphylactic shock, volume replacement should be administered concurrently with epinephrine. Antihistamines and glucocorticoids may be used in conjunction with epinephrine.
- **SC, IM:** Medication can cause irritation of tissue. Rotate injection sites to prevent tissue necrosis. Massage injection sites well after administration to enhance absorption and to decrease local vasoconstriction. Avoid IM administration in gluteal muscle. Shake suspension well before administering; inject promptly to prevent settling.
- **IV:** Dilute 1 mg (1 ml) of 1 : 1000 solution in at least 10 ml of 0.9% NaCl for injection to prepare a 1 : 10,000 solution. Discard any solution not used within 24 hr of preparation.
- **Direct IV:** Administer each 1 mg over at least 1 min; more rapid administration may be used during cardiac resuscitation.
- **Intermittent Infusion:** In severe anaphylactic shock, 0.1–0.25-mg dose may be repeated every 5–15 min.
- ***Rate:*** Administer over 5–10 min.
- **Continuous Infusion:** For maintenance, solution may be further diluted in 500 ml of D5W, D10W, 0.9% NaCl, D5/LR, D5/Ringer's solution, dextrose/saline combinations, or Ringer's or lactated Ringer's solution. Administer through Y-site via infusion pump to ensure accurate dosage.
- ***Rate:*** Administer at a rate of 1–4 mcg/min.
- **Syringe Compatibility:** ▪ doxapram ▪ heparin ▪ milrinone.
- **Y-Site Compatibility:** ▪ amrinone ▪ atracurium ▪ calcium chloride ▪ calcium gluconate ▪ diltiazem ▪ famotidine ▪ heparin ▪ hydrocortisone sodium succinate ▪ pancuronium ▪ phytonadione ▪ potassium chloride ▪ vecuronium ▪ vitamin B complex with C.
- **Y-Site Incompatibility:** ▪ ampicillin.
- **Additive Compatibility:** ▪ cimetidine ▪ ranitidine.
- **Additive Incompatibility:** ▪ aminophylline ▪ sodium bicarbonate.
- **Inhalation:** When using epinephrine inhalation solution, 10 drops of 1% base solution should be placed in the reservoir of the nebulizer.
- □ The 2.25% inhalation solution of racepinephrine must be diluted for use in the combination nebulizer/respirator.
- □ Allow 1–2 min to elapse between inhalations of epinephrine inhalation solution, epinephrine inhalation aerosol, or epinephrine bitartrate inhalation aerosol to make certain the second inhalation is necessary.
- □ When epinephrine is used concurrently with glucocorticoid or ipratropium inhalations, administer bronchodilator first and other med-

ications 5 min apart to prevent toxicity from inhaled fluorocarbon propellants.

- **Endotracheal:** Epinephrine can be injected directly into the bronchial tree via the endotracheal tube if the patient has been intubated. Perform 5 rapid insufflations; forcefully administer 10 ml containing 1 mg epinephrine (1 mg/ml) directly into tube; follow with 5 quick insufflations.

PATIENT/FAMILY TEACHING

- **General Info:** Instruct patient to take medication exactly as directed. If on a scheduled dosing regimen, take a missed dose as soon as possible; space remaining doses at regular intervals. Do not double doses. Caution patient not to exceed recommended dose; may cause adverse effects, paradoxical bronchospasm, or loss of effectiveness of medication.
- □ Instruct patient to contact health care professional immediately if shortness of breath is not relieved by medication or is accompanied by diaphoresis, dizziness, palpitations, or chest pain.
- □ Advise patient to consult health care professional before taking any OTC medications or alcoholic beverages concurrently with this therapy. Caution patient also to avoid smoking and other respiratory irritants.
- **Inhalation:** Review correct administration technique (aerosolization, IPPB, metered-dose inhaler) with patient. See Appendix H for administration with metered-dose inhaler. Wait 1–5 min before administering next dose. Mouthpiece should be washed after each use.
- □ Do not spray inhaler near eyes.
- □ Instruct patient to save inhaler; refill canisters may be available.
- □ Advise patients to use bronchodilator first if using other inhalation medications, and allow 5 min to elapse before administering other inhalant medications, unless otherwise directed.
- □ Advise patient to rinse mouth with water after each inhalation dose to minimize dry mouth.
- □ Advise patient to maintain adequate fluid intake (2000–3000 ml/day) to help liquefy tenacious secretions.
- □ Advise patient to consult health care professional if respiratory symptoms are not relieved or worsen after treatment or if chest pain, headache, severe dizziness, palpitations, nervousness, or weakness occurs.
- □ Instruct patient to notify health care professional if contents of one canister are used up in less than 2 wk.
- **Auto-injector:** Instruct patients using auto-injector for anaphylactic reactions to remove gray safety cap, placing black tip on thigh at right angle to leg. Press hard into thigh until auto-injector functions, hold in place several seconds, remove, and discard properly. Massage injected area for 10 sec.

EVALUATION

Effectiveness of therapy can be demonstrated by: ▪ Prevention or relief of bronchospasm □ Increase in ease of breathing □ Prevention of bronchospasm or reduction of frequency of acute asthma attacks in patients with chronic asthma □ Prevention of exercise-induced asthma ▪ Reversal of signs and symptoms of anaphylaxis ▪ Increase in cardiac rate and output, when used in cardiac resuscitation ▪ Increase in blood pressure, when used as a vasopressor ▪ Localization of local anesthetic ▪ Decrease in sinus and nasal congestion.

EPOETIN

(ee-**poe**-e-tin)

Epogen, EPO, erythropoietin, Procrit

CLASSIFICATION(S):

Antianemic, Hormone (erythropoietin, recombinant)

Pregnancy Category C

INDICATIONS

▪ Treatment of anemia associated with chronic renal failure ▪ Management of anemia secondary to zidovudine (AZT) therapy in HIV-infected patients ▪ Management of anemia from chemotherapy in patients with nonmyeloid malignancies ▪ Reduction of need for transfusions following surgery.

ACTION

▪ Stimulates erythropoiesis (production of red blood cells). **Therapeutic Effects:** ▪ Maintains and may elevate red blood cell counts, decreasing the need for transfusions.

PHARMACOKINETICS

Absorption: Well absorbed following SC administration.
Distribution: UK.
Metabolism and Excretion: UK.
Half-life: 4–13 hr.

CONTRAINDICATIONS AND PRECAUTIONS

Contraindicated in: ▪ Hypersensitivity to albumin or mammalian cell–derived products ▪ Uncontrolled hypertension ▪ Patients with erythropoietin levels >200 mU/ml.
Use Cautiously in: ▪ History of seizures ▪ Pregnancy, lactation, or children (safety not established).

ADVERSE REACTIONS AND SIDE EFFECTS*

CNS: SEIZURES, headache.
CV: hypertension, thrombotic events (hemodialysis patients).
Derm: transient rashes.
Endo: restored fertility, resumption of menses.

INTERACTIONS

Drug-Drug: ▪ May increase the requirement for **heparin** anticoagulation during hemodialysis.

ROUTE AND DOSAGE

❑ **Anemia of Chronic Renal Failure**

▪ **SC, IV (Adults):** 50–100 units/kg 3 times weekly initially, then adjust dosage based on hematocrit.

❑ **Anemia Secondary to Zidovudine (AZT) Therapy**

▪ **IV, SC (Adults):** 100 units/kg 3 times weekly for 8 wk; if inadequate response, may increase by 50–100 units/kg every 4–8 wk, up to 300 units/kg 3 times weekly.

❑ **Anemia from Chemotherapy**

▪ **SC (Adults):** 150 units/kg 3 times weekly; may increase after 8 wk up to 300 units/kg 3 times weekly.

❑ **Surgery**

▪ **SC (Adults):** 300 units/kg/day for 10 days before surgery, day of surgery, and 4 days after *or* 600 units/kg 21, 14, and 7 days before surgery and on day of surgery.

AVAILABILITY

▪ ***Injection:*** 2000 units/ml[Rx], 3000 units/ml[Rx], 4000 units/ml[Rx], 10,000 units/ml[Rx], 20,000 units/ml[Rx].

TIME/ACTION PROFILE (increase in RBCs)

	ONSET†	PEAK	DURATION
IV, SC	10 days	2–6 wk	2 wk‡

†Increase in reticulocytes.
‡Following discontinuation.

NURSING IMPLICATIONS

ASSESSMENT

□ Monitor blood pressure prior to and throughout therapy. Inform physician if severe hypertension is present or if blood pressure begins to increase. Additional antihypertensive therapy may be required during initiation of therapy.

□ Monitor response for symptoms of anemia (fatigue, dyspnea, pallor).

□ Monitor dialysis shunts (thrill and bruit) and status of artificial kidney during hemodialysis. Heparin dose may need to be increased to prevent clotting. Patients with underlying vascular disease should be monitored for impaired circulation.

▪ ***Lab Test Considerations:*** May cause increase in WBCs and platelets. May decrease bleeding times.

□ Serum ferritin, transferrin, and iron levels should also be monitored to assess need for concurrent iron therapy. Transferrin saturation should be at least 20% and ferritin should be at least 100 ng/ml.

▪ **Anemia of Chronic Renal Failure:** Hematocrit should be monitored prior to and twice weekly during initial therapy, for 2–6 wk after a change in dose, and regularly after target range (30–36%) has been reached and maintenance dose is determined. Other hematopoietic parameters (CBC with differential and platelet count) also should be monitored prior to and periodically throughout therapy. If hematocrit increases more than 4 points in a 2-wk period, the likelihood of hypertensive re-

E

action and seizures increases. Dose should be decreased and hematocrit monitored twice weekly for 2–6 wk. Dosage adjustment may be needed. If hematocrit is increasing and approaching 36%, dose is reduced to maintain suggested target hematocrit range. If increase in hematocrit continues and exceeds 36%, dose should be withheld until hematocrit begins to decrease; epoetin is then reinitiated at a lower dose. If hematocrit increase of 5–6 points is not achieved after an 8-wk period and iron stores are adequate, dose may be incrementally increased at 4–6 wk intervals until desired response is attained.

- □ Monitor renal function studies and electrolytes closely, as resulting increased sense of well-being may lead to decreased compliance with other therapies for renal failure. Increases in BUN, creatinine, uric acid, phosphorus, and potassium may occur.
- ▪ **Anemia Secondary to Zidovudine Therapy:** Before initiating therapy, determine serum erythropoietin level prior to transfusion. Patients receiving zidovudine with endogenous serum erythropoietin levels >500 mU/ml may not respond to therapy. Monitor hematocrit weekly during dosage adjustment. If response does not reduce transfusion requirements or increase hematocrit effectively after 8 wk of therapy, dose may be increased by 50–100 units/kg 3 times weekly. Evaluate response and adjust dose by 50–100 units/kg every 4–8 wk thereafter. If a satisfactory response is not obtained with a dose of 300 units/kg 3 times weekly, it is unlikely a higher dose will produce a response. Once desired response is attained, maintenance dose is titrated based on variations of zidovudine dose and intercurrent infections. If hematocrit exceeds 40%, discontinue dose until hematocrit drops to 36%, then decrease dose by 25%.
- ▪ **Anemia from Chemotherapy:** Monitor hematocrit weekly until stable. Patients with lower baseline serum erythropoietin levels may respond more rapidly; not recommended if levels >200 mU/ml. If response is not adequate after 8 wk of therapy, dose may be increased up to 300 units/kg 3 times weekly. If no response is obtained to this dose, it is unlikely that higher doses will produce a response. If hematocrit exceeds 40%, hold dose until it falls to 36%, then decrease dose by 25%. If initial dose response is >4 percentage points in any 2-wk period, reduce dose.
- ▪ **Surgery:** Determine that hematocrit is >10 to ≤13g/dl prior to therapy.

POTENTIAL NURSING DIAGNOSES

- ▪ Activity intolerance (Indications).
- ▪ Knowledge deficit, related to diet and medication regimen (Patient/Family Teaching).
- ▪ Noncompliance (Patient/Family Teaching).

IMPLEMENTATION

- ▪ **General Info:** Transfusions are still required for severe symptomatic anemia. Supplemental iron should be initiated with epoetin and continued throughout therapy.
- □ Institute seizure precautions in patients who experience greater than a 4-point increase in hematocrit in a 2-wk period or exhibit any change in neurologic status. Risk of seizures is greatest during the first 90 days of therapy.
- □ Do not shake vial; inactivation of medication may occur. Discard vial immediately after withdrawing dose from single-use 1-ml vial. Refrigerate multidose 2-ml vial; stable for 21 days after initial entry.
- ▪ **SC:** This route is often used for patients not requiring dialysis.
- □ May be admixed in syringe immediately prior to administration with 0.9% NaCl with benzyl alcohol 0.9% in a 1:1 ratio to prevent injection site discomfort.
- ▪ **Direct IV:** Administer undiluted.
- ▪ ***Rate:*** May be administered as direct injection or bolus into IV tubing or via venous line at end of dialysis session.

PATIENT/FAMILY TEACHING

- ▪ **General Info:** Explain rationale for concurrent iron therapy (increased red blood cell production requires iron).
- □ Discuss possible return of menses and fertility in women of childbearing age. Patient should discuss contraceptive options with health care professional.
- □ Discuss ways of preventing self-injury in patients at risk for seizures. Driving and activities requiring continuous alertness should be avoided.
- ▪ **Anemia of Chronic Renal Failure:** Stress importance of compliance with dietary restrictions, medications, and dialysis. Foods high in

iron and low in potassium include liver, pork, veal, beef, mustard and turnip greens, peas, eggs, broccoli, kale, blackberries, strawberries, apple juice, watermelon, oatmeal, and enriched bread. Epoetin will result in increased sense of well-being, but it does not cure underlying disease.

- **Home Care Issues:** Home dialysis patients determined to be able to safely and effectively administer epoetin should be taught proper dosage, administration technique, and proper disposal of equipment. *Information for Home Dialysis Patients* should be provided to patient along with medication.

EVALUATION

Clinical response to therapy can be evaluated by: ▪ Increase in hematocrit to 30–36% with improvement in symptoms of anemia in patients with chronic renal failure ▪ Increase in hematocrit in anemia secondary to zidovudine therapy ▪ Increase in hematocrit in patients with anemia due to chemotherapy ▪ Reduction of need for transfusions following surgery.

ERGONOVINE

(er-goe-**noe**-veen)

ergometrine, Ergotrate

CLASSIFICATION(S):

Oxytocic

Pregnancy Category UK

INDICATIONS

▪ Prevention and treatment of postpartum or postabortion hemorrhage caused by uterine atony or involution. **Unlabeled Uses:** ▪ As a diagnostic agent to provoke coronary artery spasm.

ACTION

▪ Directly stimulates uterine and vascular smooth muscle. **Therapeutic Effects:** ▪ Uterine contraction.

PHARMACOKINETICS

Absorption: Well absorbed following oral or IM administration.
Distribution: UK.
Metabolism and Excretion: UK. Probably metabolized by the liver.
Half-life: UK.

CONTRAINDICATIONS AND PRECAUTIONS

Contraindicated in: ▪ Hypersensitivity ▪ Avoid chronic use ▪ Should not be used to induce labor.

Use Cautiously in: ▪ Hypertensive or eclamptic patients (increased susceptibility to hypertensive and arrhythmogenic side effects) ▪ Severe hepatic or renal disease ▪ Sepsis ▪ Third stage of labor.

ADVERSE REACTIONS AND SIDE EFFECTS*

CNS: dizziness, headache.
EENT: tinnitus.
Resp: dyspnea.
CV: arrhythmias, chest pain, hypertension, palpitations.
GI: <u>nausea</u>, <u>vomiting</u>.
Derm: sweating.
Misc: allergic reactions.

INTERACTIONS

Drug-Drug: ▪ Excessive vasoconstriction may result when used with other **vasopressors,** such as **dopamine** or **nicotine.**

ROUTE AND DOSAGE

❑ Oxytocic

- **PO (Adults):** 0.2–0.4 mg q 6–12 hr (usual course is 48 hr).
- **IM, IV (Adults):** 200 mcg (0.2 mg) q 2–4 hr for up to 5 doses.

❑ Provocative Agent for Coronary Artery Spasm

- **IV (Adults):** 50 mcg (0.05 mg) q 5 min until chest pain occurs or a total dose of 400 mcg (0.4 mg) has been given (unlabeled).

AVAILABILITY

▪ ***Tablets:*** 0.2 mg[Rx] ▪ ***Injection:*** 0.2 mg/ml[Rx], {0.25 mg/ml[Rx]}.

*CAPITALS indicate life-threatening; <u>underlines</u> indicate most frequent.

E

TIME/ACTION PROFILE (uterine contractions)

	ONSET	PEAK	DURATION
PO	5–15 min	UK	3 hr or longer
IM	2–5 min	UK	3 hr or longer
IV	immediate	UK	45 min

NURSING IMPLICATIONS

ASSESSMENT

- Monitor blood pressure, pulse, and respirations every 15–30 min until transfer to the postpartum unit, then every 1–2 hr. Report hypertension, chest pain, arrhythmias, headache, or change in neurologic status.
- Monitor amount and type of vaginal discharge. Report symptoms of hemorrhage (increased bleeding, hypotension, pallor, tachycardia) immediately.
- Palpate uterine fundus, note position and consistency. Notify physician or other health care professional if fundus fails to contract in response to ergonovine. Assess patient for severe cramping; dose may be decreased.
- Assess for signs of ergotism (cold, numb fingers and toes; nausea; vomiting; diarrhea; headache; muscle pain; weakness).
- If patient fails to respond to ergonovine, check serum calcium level. Correction of hypocalcemia may restore responsiveness.
- ***Lab Test Considerations:*** May cause decreased serum prolactin level, which inhibits synthesis of breast milk.
- ***Toxicity and Overdose:*** Toxicity, initially manifested as ergotism, may cause seizures and gangrene. Seizures are treated with anticonvulsants. Vasodilators and heparin may be ordered to improve circulation to extremities.

POTENTIAL NURSING DIAGNOSES

- Tissue perfusion, altered (Indications).
- Injury, risk for (Side Effects).
- Knowledge deficit, related to medication regimen (Patient/Family Teaching).

IMPLEMENTATION

- **General Info:** Do not administer solution that is discolored or contains a precipitate.
- **PO:** Administration is usually limited to 48 hr postpartum, by which time the danger of hemorrhage from uterine atony has passed.
- Tablets may be administered SL.
- **IM:** The preferred route is IM. Firm uterine contractions are produced within a few minutes. Dose may need to be repeated every 2–4 hr for full therapeutic effect.
- **Direct IV:** The IV route is reserved for severe uterine bleeding. Dilute with 5 ml of 0.9% NaCl.
- ***Rate:*** Administer slow IV push over at least 1 min through Y-site injection of an IV of D5W or 0.9% NaCl.

PATIENT/FAMILY TEACHING

- Review symptoms of toxicity with patient. Instruct her to report occurrence of these immediately.
- Inform patient that uterine cramping demonstrates effectiveness of therapy.
- Explain need for pad count to determine degree of bleeding. Instruct patient to report immediately an increase in degree of bleeding or passage of clots.
- Instruct patient to report breast-feeding difficulties.
- Caution patient not to smoke while receiving ergonovine, as nicotine is also a vasoconstrictor.

EVALUATION

Effectiveness of therapy can be demonstrated by: ▪ Uterine contraction and cramping in the prevention or cessation of uterine hemorrhage after delivery or abortion ▪ Vasoconstriction of the coronary arteries when used as a diagnostic agent.

ERGOTAMINE

(er-**got**-a-meen)
{Ergomar}, Ergostat, {Gynergen}

DIHYDROERGOTAMINE

(dye-hye-droe-er-**got**-a-meen)
D.H.E. 45, {Dihydroergotamine-Sandoz}, Migranal

CLASSIFICATION(S):
Vascular headache suppressants (alpha-adrenergic blocking agents)

Pregnancy Category X

INDICATIONS

▪ Treatment of vascular headaches including: ▫ Migraine ▫ Cluster headaches.

ACTION

▪ In therapeutic doses produces vasoconstriction of dilated blood vessels by stimulating alpha-adrenergic and serotonergic (5-HT) receptors ▪ Larger doses may produce alpha-adrenergic blockade and vasodilation. **Therapeutic Effects:** ▪ Constriction of dilated carotid artery bed with resolution of vascular headache.

PHARMACOKINETICS

Absorption: Unpredictably absorbed (60%) from the GI tract. Oral absorption may be enhanced by caffeine. Sublingual absorption is very poor. Dihydroergotamine is rapidly absorbed following IM and SC administration. Dihydroergotamine is 32% absorbed from nasal mucosa.
Distribution: Ergotamine crosses the blood-brain barrier and enters breast milk.
Metabolism and Excretion: Both ergotamine and dihydroergotamine are highly metabolized (90%) by the liver. Some metabolites are active.
Half-life: *Ergotamine* (2 phases)—2.7 hr first phase; 21 hr second phase. *Dihydroergotamine* (2 phases)—2.3 min–1.45 hr first phase; 10–32 hr second phase.

CONTRAINDICATIONS AND PRECAUTIONS

Contraindicated in: ▪ Serious infections ▪ Peripheral vascular disease ▪ Cardiovascular disease ▪ Uncontrolled hypertension ▪ Severe renal or liver disease ▪ Malnutrition ▪ Pregnancy ▪ Lactation ▪ Known alcohol intolerance (dihydroergotamine injection only).
Use Cautiously in: ▪ Illnesses associated with peripheral vascular pathology such as diabetes mellitus ▪ Children <6 yr (safety not established).

ADVERSE REACTIONS AND SIDE EFFECTS*

CNS: dizziness.
EENT: rhinitus (nasal).
CV: MYOCARDIAL INFARCTION, angina pectoris, arterial spasm, intermittent claudication, sinus bradycardia, sinus tachycardia.
GI: abdominal pain, nausea, vomiting, altered taste (nasal), diarrhea, polydipsia.
MS: extremity stiffness, muscle pain, stiff neck, stiff shoulders.
Neuro: leg weakness, numbness or tingling in fingers or toes.
Misc: fatigue.

INTERACTIONS

Drug-Drug: ▪ Concurrent use with **beta-adrenergic blockers, oral contraceptives, vasoconstrictors, macrolide anti-infectives,** or **heavy smoking (nicotine)** may increase the risk of peripheral vasoconstriction ▪ When used concurrently with prophylactic **methysergide** (another ergot alkaloid), dosage of ergotamine should be decreased by 50% ▪ Dihydroergotamine antagonizes the antianginal effects of **nitrates** ▪ Concurrent use with **vasoconstrictors** may have additive effects (avoid concurrent use) ▪ Concurrent use with **sumatriptan** may result in prolonged vasoconstriction (allow 24 hr between use).

ROUTE AND DOSAGE

▫ **Ergotamine**

- **PO, SL (Adults):** 1–2 mg initially, then 1–2 mg q 30 min until attack subsides or a total of 6 mg has been given. Should not be used more than twice weekly, with at least 5 days between courses; 1–2 mg PO at bedtime daily for 10–14 days have been used to terminate series of cluster headaches.

▫ **Dihydroergotamine**

- **IM, SC (Adults):** 1 mg; may repeat in 1 hr to a total of 3 mg (not to exceed 3 mg/day or 6 mg/wk).
- **IM, SC (Children ≥6 yr):** 0.5 mg; may be repeated in 1 hr.
- **IV (Adults):** 0.5 mg; may repeat in 1 hr (not to exceed 2 mg/day or 6 mg/wk). For chronic intractable headache, 0.5–1 mg q 8 hr may be given until relief (not to exceed 6 mg/wk).
- **IV (Children ≥6 yr):** 0.25 mg; may be repeated in 1 hr.
- **IV (Children and Adolescents 12–16 yr):** *Severe, acute migraine*—0.25–0.5 mg; 1–2 more doses may be given q 20 min.
- **IV (Children 9–12 yr):** *Severe, acute mi-*

*CAPITALS indicate life-threatening; underlines indicate most frequent.

graine—0.2 mg; 1–2 more doses may be given q 20 min.
- **IV (Children 6–9 yr):** *Severe, acute migraine*—0.1–0.15 mg; 1–2 more doses may be given q 20 min.
- **Intranasal (Adults):** 1 spray (0.5 mg) in each nostril, repeat after 15 min (2 mg total dose); not to exceed 3 mg/24 hr or 4 mg/wk.

AVAILABILITY

❑ **Ergotamine**

▪ ***Sublingual tablets:*** 2 mg^Rx^ ▪ ***Tablets:*** 1 mg^Rx^.

❑ **Dihydroergotamine**

▪ ***Injection:*** 1 mg/ml (contains alcohol)^Rx^
▪ ***Nasal spray:*** 4 mg/1 ml in 1-ml ampules with nasal spray applicator
▪ ***In combination with:*** *Ergotamine*—caffeine, barbiturates, and belladonna alkaloids in preparations for vascular headaches^Rx^. See Appendix A.

TIME/ACTION PROFILE (relief of headache)

	ONSET	PEAK	DURATION
PO	1–2 hr (variable)	1–5 hr	UK
Nasal	within 30 min	UK	UK
SL	UK	UK	UK
IM, SC	15–30 min	15 min–2 hr	8 hr
IV	<5 min	15 min –2 hr	8 hr

NURSING IMPLICATIONS

ASSESSMENT

- Assess frequency, location, duration, and characteristics (pain, nausea, vomiting, visual disturbances) of chronic headaches. During acute attack, assess type, location, and intensity of pain prior to and 60 min after administration.
- Monitor blood pressure and peripheral pulses periodically during therapy. Report significant hypertension.
- Assess for signs of ergotism (cold, numb fingers and toes; nausea; vomiting; headache; muscle pain; weakness).
- Assess for nausea and vomiting. Ergotamine stimulates the chemoreceptor trigger zone. For adults, metoclopramide 10 mg IV may be administered 3–5 min prior to administration of dihydroergotamine IV. In children, metoclopramide or a phenothiazine antiemetic may be given orally as prophylaxis 1 hr prior to administration of dihydroergotamine IV. Oral administration may decrease risk of extrapyramidal and other side effects encountered with IV administration.
- ***Toxicity and Overdose:*** Toxicity is manifested by severe ergotism (chest pain, abdominal pain, persistent paresthesia in the extremities) and gangrene. Vasodilators, dextran, or heparin may be ordered to improve circulation.

POTENTIAL NURSING DIAGNOSES

- Pain, acute (Indications).
- Injury, risk for (Side Effects).
- Knowledge deficit, related to medication regimen (Patient/Family Teaching).

IMPLEMENTATION

- **General Info:** Administer as soon as patient reports prodromal symptoms or headache.
- **SL:** Allow tablet to dissolve under tongue. Do not allow patient to eat, drink, or smoke while tablet is dissolving.
- **Direct IV:** Dihydroergotamine may be administered undiluted.
- ***Rate:*** Administer over 1 min.

PATIENT/FAMILY TEACHING

- **General Info:** Instruct patient to take ergotamine at the first sign of an impending headache and not to exceed the maximum dose prescribed.
- Encourage patient to rest in a quiet, dark room after taking ergotamine.
- Review symptoms of toxicity. Instruct patient to report these promptly.
- Caution patient not to smoke and to avoid exposure to cold, as these vasoconstrictors may further impair peripheral circulation.
- May cause dizziness. Caution patient to avoid driving and other activities requiring alertness until response to the drug is known.
- Advise patient to avoid alcohol, as it may precipitate vascular headaches.
- Instruct female patients to inform health care professional if they plan or suspect pregnancy. Ergotamine should not be taken during pregnancy.
- **IM, SC:** Inject at the first sign of a headache and repeat at 1-hr intervals up to 3 doses.

Once minimal effective dose is determined, adjust dose for subsequent attacks.

- **Intranasal:** Instruct patient in proper use of nasal spray. Prime nasal sprayer 4 times prior to dose. Administer 1 spray to each nostril followed in 15 min by an additional spray in each nostril for a total of 4 sprays. Do not tilt head or sniff following spray. Do not use more than amount instructed. Discard ampule within 8 hr of opening. Do not refrigerate. Assembly may be used for 4 treatments, then discard.
- □ Advise patient not to use Migranal to prevent a headache if there are no symptoms or if headache is different from typical migraine.
- □ Instruct patient to notify health care professional if numbness or tingling in fingers or toes; pain, tightness, or discomfort in chest; muscle pain or cramps in arms or legs; weakness in legs; temporary speeding or slowing of heart rate; or swelling or itching occurs.

EVALUATION

Effectiveness of therapy can be demonstrated by: ▪ Prevention or relief of pain from vascular headaches.

ERYTHROMYCIN*

(eh-rith-roe-**mye**-sin)

erythromycin base

{Apo-Erythro-EC}, E-base, E-Mycin, {Erybid}, Eryc, Ery-Tab, {Erythromid}, Ilotycin, {Novo-rythro}, PCE

erythromycin estolate

Ilosone, {Novo-rythro}

erythromycin ethylsuccinate

{Apo-Erythro-ES}, E.E.S., EryPed, Erythro

erythromycin gluceptate

erythromycin lactobionate

Erythrocin

erythromycin stearate

Apo-Erythro-S, Erythrocin, {Novo-rythro}

erythromycin, ophthalmic

Ilotycin

erythromycin, topical

Akne-Mycin, A/T/S, Del-Mycin, E/Gel, Emgel, Erycette, Erygel, EryMax, Erysol, ETS, {Sans-Acne}, Staticin, Theramycin Z, T-Stat

CLASSIFICATION(S):

Anti-infective (macrolide)

Pregnancy Category B

*See Appendix O for ophthalmic use.

INDICATIONS

▪ **IV, PO:** Treatment of the following infections due to susceptible organisms: □ Upper and lower respiratory tract infections □ Otitis media (with sulfonamides) □ Skin and skin structure infections □ Pertussis □ Diphtheria □ Erythrasma □ Intestinal amebiasis □ Pelvic inflammatory disease □ Nongonococcal urethritis □ Syphilis □ Legionnaires' disease □ Rheumatic fever ▪ Useful in situations in which penicillin is the most appropriate drug but cannot be used because of previous hypersensitivity reactions, including: □ Streptococcal infections □ Treatment of syphilis or gonorrhea ▪ **Topical:** Treatment of acne.

ACTION

▪ Suppresses protein synthesis at the level of the 50S bacterial ribosome. **Therapeutic Effects:** ▪ Bacteriostatic action against susceptible bacteria. **Spectrum:** ▪ Active against many gram-positive cocci, including: □ Streptococci □ Staphylococci ▪ Gram-positive bacilli, including: □ *Clostridium* □ *Corynebacterium* ▪ Several gram-negative pathogens, notably: □ *Neisseria* □ *Legionella pneumophila* ▪ *Mycoplasma* and *Chlamydia* are also usually susceptible.

PHARMACOKINETICS

Absorption: Well absorbed from the duodenum following oral administration. Absorption of enteric-coated products is delayed. Minimal absorption may follow topical or ophthalmic use. **Distribution:** Widely distributed. Minimal penetration into CSF. Crosses the placenta; enters breast milk.

E

Metabolism and Excretion: Partially metabolized by the liver, excreted mainly unchanged in the bile; small amounts excreted unchanged in the urine.
Half-life: 1.4–2 hr.

CONTRAINDICATIONS AND PRECAUTIONS

Contraindicated in: ▪ Hypersensitivity ▪ Hepatic dysfunction (estolate salt) ▪ Pregnancy (estolate salt) ▪ Known alcohol intolerance (most topicals) ▪ Products containing benzyl alcohol should be avoided in neonates ▪ Tartrazine sensitivity (some products contain tartrazine—FDC yellow dye #5).
Use Cautiously in: ▪ Liver disease ▪ Salts other than the estolate may be used in pregnancy to treat chlamydial infections or syphilis.

ADVERSE REACTIONS AND SIDE EFFECTS*

EENT: ototoxicity.
GI: nausea, vomiting, abdominal pain, cramping, diarrhea, hepatitis.
Derm: rashes.
Local: phlebitis at IV site.
Misc: allergic reactions, superinfection.

INTERACTIONS

Drug-Drug: ▪ Increases activity and may increase the risk of toxicity from **alfentanil, clozapine, bromocriptine, theophylline, carbamazepine, cyclosporine, disopyramide, ergot alkaloids, warfarin, methylprednisolone,** or **triazolam** ▪ Concurrent use with **astemizole, pimozide,** or **cisapride** increases the risk of arrhythmias ▪ May increase serum **digoxin** levels in a small percentage of patients ▪ **Topical:** Concurrent use with **irritants, abrasives,** or **desquamating agents** may result in increased irritation ▪ **Topical clindamycin** may antagonize beneficial effects.

ROUTE AND DOSAGE

250 mg of erythromycin base, estolate, or stearate = 400 mg of erythromycin ethylsuccinate.

❑ **Most Infections**

- **PO (Adults):** *Base, estolate, stearate*—250 mg q 6 hr, 333 mg q 8 hr, or 500 mg q 12 hr. *Ethylsuccinate*—400 mg q 6 hr or 800 mg q 12 hr.
- **PO (Children):** 7.5–12.5 mg/kg q 6 hr or 12.5–25 mg/kg q 12 hr (up to 100 mg/kg/day).
- **IV (Adults):** *Gluceptate and lactobionate only*—250–500 mg (up to 1 g) q 6 hr.
- **IV (Children):** *Gluceptate and lactobionate only*—3.75–5 mg/kg q 6 hr.

❑ **Acne**

- **Topical (Adults and Children >12 yr):** 2% ointment, gel, or solution bid.

AVAILABILITY

❑ **Erythromycin Base**

▪ ***Enteric-coated tablets:*** 250 mg[Rx], 333 mg[Rx] ▪ ***Tablets with polymer-coated particles:*** 333 mg[Rx], 500 mg[Rx] ▪ ***Film-coated tablets:*** 500 mg[Rx] ▪ ***Delayed-release capsules:*** 250 mg[Rx].

❑ **Erythromycin Estolate**

▪ ***Tablets:*** 500 mg[Rx] ▪ ***Capsules:*** 250 mg[Rx] ▪ ***Oral suspension:*** 125 mg/5 ml[Rx], 250 mg/5 ml[Rx].

❑ **Erythromycin Stearate**

▪ ***Film-coated tablets:*** 250 mg[Rx], 500 mg[Rx].

❑ **Erythromycin Ethylsuccinate**

▪ ***Chewable tablets:*** 200 mg[Rx] ▪ ***Tablets:*** 400 mg[Rx] ▪ ***Oral suspension:*** 200 mg/5 ml[Rx], 400 mg/5 ml[Rx] ▪ ***Drops:*** 100 mg/2.5 ml[Rx].

❑ **Erythromycin Gluceptate**

▪ ***Powder for injection:*** 500 mg[Rx], 1 g[Rx].

❑ **Erythromycin Lactobionate**

▪ ***Powder for injection:*** 500 mg[Rx], 1 g[Rx].

❑ **Topical Preparations**

▪ ***Topical ointment:*** 2%[Rx] ▪ ***Topical gel:*** 2%[Rx] ▪ ***Topical solution:*** 2%[Rx] ▪ ***In combination with:*** sulfisoxazole (Eryzole, Pediazole)[Rx] and benzoyl peroxide (Benzamycin)[Rx]. See Appendix A.

TIME/ACTION PROFILE (blood levels)

	ONSET	PEAK	DURATION
PO	1 hr	1–4 hr	N/A
IV	rapid	end of infusion	N/A

***CAPITALS indicate life-threatening; underlines indicate most frequent.**

NURSING IMPLICATIONS

ASSESSMENT

- Assess patient for infection (vital signs; appearance of wound, sputum, urine, and stool; WBC) at beginning of and throughout therapy.
- Obtain specimens for culture and sensitivity prior to initiating therapy. First dose may be given before receiving results.
- ***Lab Test Considerations:*** Liver function tests should be performed periodically on patients receiving high-dose, long-term therapy.
- May cause increased serum bilirubin, AST, ALT, and alkaline phosphatase concentrations.
- May cause false elevations of urinary catecholamines.

POTENTIAL NURSING DIAGNOSES

- Infection, risk for (Indications, Side Effects).
- Knowledge deficit, related to medication regimen (Patient/Family Teaching).
- Noncompliance, related to medication regimen (Patient/Family Teaching).

IMPLEMENTATION

- **PO:** Administer around the clock. *Erythromycin film-coated tablets (base and stearate)* are absorbed better on an empty stomach, at least 1 hr before or 2 hr after meals; may be taken with food if GI irritation occurs. *Enteric-coated erythromycin (base and estolate)* may be taken without regard to meals. *Erythromycin ethylsuccinate* is best absorbed when taken with meals. Take each dose with a full glass of water.
- Use calibrated measuring device for liquid preparations. Shake well before using.
- Chewable tablets should be crushed or chewed and not swallowed whole.
- Do not crush or chew delayed-release capsules or tablets; swallow whole. *Erythromycin base delayed-release capsules* may be opened and sprinkled on applesauce, jelly, or ice cream immediately prior to ingestion. Entire contents of the capsule should be taken.
- **IV:** Add 10 ml of sterile water for injection without preservatives to 250- or 500-mg vials and 20 ml to 1-g vial. Solution is stable for 7 days after reconstitution if refrigerated.
- **Intermittent Infusion:** Dilute further in 100–250 ml of 0.9% NaCl or D5W.
- ***Rate:*** Administer slowly over 20–60 min to avoid phlebitis. Assess for pain along vein; slow rate if pain occurs; apply ice and notify physician or other health care professional if unable to relieve pain.
- **Continuous Infusion:** May also be administered as an infusion in a dilution of 1 g/liter of 0.9% NaCl, D5W, or lactated Ringer's solution over 4 hr.

Erythromycin Gluceptate

- **Syringe Incompatibility:** ▪ heparin.
- **Additive Compatibility:** ▪ calcium gluconate ▪ heparin ▪ hydrocortisone sodium succinate ▪ potassium chloride ▪ sodium bicarbonate.
- **Additive Incompatibility:** ▪ pentobarbital ▪ secobarbital.

Erythromycin Lactobionate

- **Syringe Incompatibility:** ▪ heparin.
- **Y-Site Compatibility:** ▪ acyclovir ▪ amiodarone ▪ cyclophosphamide ▪ diltiazem ▪ enalaprilat ▪ esmolol ▪ famotidine ▪ foscarnet ▪ heparin ▪ hydromorphone ▪ idarubicin ▪ labetalol ▪ lorazepam ▪ magnesium sulfate ▪ meperidine ▪ midazolam ▪ morphine ▪ multivitamins ▪ perphenazine ▪ tacrolimus ▪ theophylline ▪ vitamin B complex with C ▪ zidovudine.
- **Y-Site Incompatibility:** ▪ fluconazole.
- **Additive Compatibility:** ▪ cimetidine ▪ hydrocortisone sodium succinate ▪ pentobarbital ▪ potassium chloride ▪ prednisolone ▪ ranitidine ▪ sodium bicarbonate.
- **Additive Incompatibility:** ▪ heparin ▪ metoclopramide ▪ vitamin B complex with C.
- **Topical:** Cleanse area prior to application. Wear gloves during application.

PATIENT/FAMILY TEACHING

- Instruct patient to take medication around the clock and to finish the drug completely as directed, even if feeling better. Missed doses should be taken as soon as remembered, with remaining doses evenly spaced throughout day. Advise patient that sharing of this medication may be dangerous.
- May cause nausea, vomiting, diarrhea, or stomach cramps; notify health care professional if these effects persist or if severe abdominal pain, yellow discoloration of the skin or eyes, darkened urine, pale stools, or unusual tiredness develops.
- Advise patient to report signs of superinfection

(black, furry overgrowth on the tongue; vaginal itching or discharge; loose or foul-smelling stools).

- Instruct patient to notify health care professional if symptoms do not improve.

EVALUATION

Clinical response to therapy can be evaluated by: ▪ Resolution of the signs and symptoms of infection. Length of time for complete resolution depends on the organism and site of infection ▪ Improvement of acne lesions.

ESMOLOL

(**es**-moe-lole)

Brevibloc

CLASSIFICATION(S):

Antiarrhythmic (group II), Beta-adrenergic blocking agent (selective)

Pregnancy Category C

INDICATIONS

▪ Management of sinus tachycardia and supraventricular arrhythmias.

ACTION

▪ Blocks stimulation of $beta_1$ (myocardial) -adrenergic receptors. Does not usually affect $beta_2$ (pulmonary, vascular, or uterine) receptor sites. **Therapeutic Effects:** ▪ Decreased heart rate ▪ Decreased AV conduction.

PHARMACOKINETICS

Absorption: IV administration results in complete bioavailability.

Distribution: Rapidly and widely distributed.

Metabolism and Excretion: Metabolized by enzymes in red blood cells and liver.

Half-life: 9 min.

CONTRAINDICATIONS AND PRECAUTIONS

Contraindicated in: ▪ Uncompensated congestive heart failure ▪ Pulmonary edema ▪ Cardiogenic shock ▪ Bradycardia or heart block ▪ Known alcohol intolerance.

Use Cautiously in: ▪ Geriatric patients (increased sensitivity to the effects of beta-adrenergic blockers) ▪ Thyrotoxicosis (may mask symptoms) ▪ Diabetes mellitus (may mask symptoms of hypoglycemia) ▪ Patients with a history of severe allergic reactions (intensity of reactions may be increased) ▪ Pregnancy, lactation, or children (safety not established; neonatal bradycardia, hypotension, hypoglycemia, and respiratory depression may occur rarely).

ADVERSE REACTIONS AND SIDE EFFECTS*

CNS: fatigue, agitation, confusion, dizziness, drowsiness, weakness.

CV: hypotension, peripheral ischemia.

GI: nausea, vomiting.

Derm: sweating.

Local: injection site reactions.

INTERACTIONS

Drug-Drug: ▪ **General anesthesia, IV phenytoin,** and **verapamil** may cause additive myocardial depression ▪ Additive bradycardia may occur with **digitalis glycosides** ▪ Additive hypotension may occur with other **antihypertensives,** acute ingestion of **alcohol,** or **nitrates** ▪ Concurrent use with **amphetamines, cocaine, ephedrine, epinephrine, norepinephrine, phenylephrine,** or **pseudoephedrine** may result in unopposed alpha-adrenergic stimulation (excessive hypertension, bradycardia) ▪ Concurrent **thyroid** administration may decrease effectiveness ▪ May alter the effectiveness of **insulin** or **oral hypoglycemic agents** (dosage adjustments may be necessary) ▪ May decrease the effectiveness of **theophylline** ▪ May decrease the beneficial $beta_1$ cardiovascular effects of **dopamine** or **dobutamine** ▪ Use cautiously within 14 days of **MAO inhibitor** therapy (may result in hypertension).

ROUTE AND DOSAGE

▪ **IV (Adults):** *Antiarrhythmic*—500-mcg/kg loading dose over 1 min initially, followed by 50-mcg/kg/min infusion for 4 min; if no response within 5 min, give 2nd loading dose of 500 mcg/kg over 1 min, then increase infusion to 100 mcg/kg/min for 4 min. If no response, repeat loading dose of 500 mcg/kg over 1 min and increase infusion rate by 50-mcg/kg/min increments (not to exceed 200 mcg/kg/min for 48 hr). As therapeutic end point is

***CAPITALS indicate life-threatening; underlines indicate most frequent.**

achieved, eliminate loading doses and decrease dosage increments to 25 mg/kg/min. *Intraoperative antihypertensive/antiarrhythmic*—250–500-mcg/kg loading dose over 1 min initially, followed by 50-mcg/kg/min infusion for 4 min; if no response within 5 min, give 2nd loading dose of 250–500 mcg/kg over 1 min, then increase infusion to 100 mcg/kg/min for 4 min. If no response, repeat loading dose of 250–500 mcg/kg over 1 min and increase infusion rate by 50-mcg/kg/min increments (not to exceed 200 mcg/kg/min for 48 hr).

- **IV (Children):** *Antiarrhythmic*—50 mcg/kg/min, may be increased q 10 min up to 300 mcg/kg/min.

AVAILABILITY

Note differences in concentrations; errors may be fatal.

▪ ***Solution for injection (prediluted for use as loading dose):*** 10 mg/ml in 10-ml vials[Rx] ▪ ***Solution for injection (must be diluted before use):*** 250 mg/ml in 10-ml vials[Rx].

TIME/ACTION PROFILE (antiarrhythmic effect)

	ONSET	PEAK	DURATION
IV	within mins	UK	1–20 min

NURSING IMPLICATIONS

ASSESSMENT

- ▫ Monitor blood pressure, ECG, and pulse frequently during dosage adjustment period and periodically throughout therapy. The risk of hypotension is greatest within the first 30 min of initiating esmolol infusion.
- ▫ Monitor intake and output ratios and daily weights. Assess routinely for signs and symptoms of congestive heart failure (dyspnea, rales/crackles, weight gain, peripheral edema, jugular venous distention).
- ▫ Assess infusion site frequently throughout therapy. Concentrations >10 mg/ml may cause redness, swelling, skin discoloration, and burning at the injection site. Do not use butterfly needles for administration. If venous irritation occurs, stop the infusion and resume at another site.
- ***Toxicity and Overdose:*** Monitor patients receiving esmolol for signs of overdose (bradycardia, severe dizziness or fainting, severe drowsiness, dyspnea, bluish fingernails or palms, seizures). Notify physician immediately if these signs occur.
- ▫ IV glucagon and symptomatic care are used in the treatment of esmolol overdose. Because of the short action of esmolol, discontinuation of therapy may relieve acute toxicity.

POTENTIAL NURSING DIAGNOSES

- Cardiac output, decreased (Side Effects).
- Knowledge deficit, related to medication regimen (Patient/Family Teaching).

IMPLEMENTATION

- **General Info:** Available in different concentrations. Do not confuse; errors may be fatal.
- ▫ To convert to other antiarrhythmic agents following esmolol administration, administer the 1st dose of the antiarrhythmic agent and decrease the esmolol dose by 50% after 30 min. If an adequate response is maintained for 1 hr following the 2nd dose of the antiarrhythmic agent, discontinue the esmolol.
- **Direct IV:** The 10 mg/ml strength may be administered undiluted.
- **Intermittent Infusion:** To dilute for infusion, remove 20 ml from a 500-ml bottle of D5W, D5/LR, D5/0.45% NaCl, D5/0.9% NaCl, 0.45% NaCl, 0.9% NaCl, or lactated Ringer's solution. Add 5 g of esmolol to the bottle for a concentration of 10 mg/ml. Solution is clear, colorless to light yellow; stable for 24 hr at room temperature.
- ***Rate:*** The loading dose of esmolol is administered over 1 min, followed by a maintenance dose via IV infusion over 4 min. If the response is not adequate, procedure is repeated every 5 min with an increase in the maintenance dose. Titration of dose is based on desired heart rate or undesired decrease in blood pressure. The maintenance dose should not be >200 mcg/kg/min and can be administered for up to 48 hr. Esmolol infusions should not be abruptly discontinued; eliminate loading doses and decrease dosage by 25 mcg/kg/min (see Appendix D).
- **Y-Site Compatibility:** ▪ amikacin ▪ aminophylline ▪ ampicillin ▪ atracurium ▪ butorphanol ▪ calcium chloride ▪ cefazolin ▪ cefoperazone ▪ ceftazidime ▪ ceftizoxime

E

▪ chloramphenicol ▪ cimetidine ▪ clindamycin ▪ diltiazem ▪ dopamine ▪ enalaprilat ▪ erythromycin lactobionate ▪ famotidine ▪ fentanyl ▪ gentamicin ▪ heparin ▪ hydrocortisone sodium succinate ▪ magnesium sulfate ▪ methyldopate ▪ metronidazole ▪ morphine ▪ nafcillin ▪ pancuronium ▪ penicillin G potassium ▪ phenytoin ▪ piperacillin ▪ polymyxin B ▪ potassium chloride ▪ potassium phosphate ▪ ranitidine ▪ sodium acetate ▪ streptomycin ▪ tacrolimus ▪ tobramycin ▪ trimethoprim/sulfamethoxazole ▪ vancomycin ▪ vecuronium.
▪ **Y-Site Incompatibility:** ▪ furosemide.

PATIENT/FAMILY TEACHING

- May cause drowsiness. Caution patients receiving esmolol to call for assistance during ambulation or transfer.
- Advise patients to change positions slowly to minimize orthostatic hypotension.
- Diabetics should closely monitor blood sugar, especially if weakness, malaise, irritability, or fatigue occurs. Medication does not block dizziness or sweating as signs of hypoglycemia.

EVALUATION

Effectiveness of therapy can be demonstrated by: ▪ Control of arrhythmias without appearance of detrimental side effects.

ESTRADIOL

(ess-tra-**dye**-ole)
Estrace

estradiol cypionate
depGynogen, Depo-Estradiol, Depogen, Dura-Estrin, E-Cypionate, Estragyn LA 5, Estro-Cyp, Estrofem, Estroject-LA, Estro-L.A.

estradiol valerate
Clinagen LA, Delestrogen, Dioval, Duragen, Estra-L, Estro-Span, {Femogex}, Gynogen L.A., Menaval, Valergen

estradiol transdermal system
Alora, Climara, Estraderm, FemPatch, Vivelle

estradiol vaginal ring
Estring

CLASSIFICATION(S):
Hormone (estrogen)

Pregnancy Category X

INDICATIONS

▪ **PO, IM, Transdermal:** Replacement of estrogen (HRT) in the treatment of moderate to severe vasomotor symptoms of menopause and of various estrogen deficiency states including: □ Female hypogonadism □ Ovariectomy □ Primary ovarian failure ▪ Treatment and prevention of postmenopausal osteoporosis ▪ **PO:** Inoperable metastatic postmenopausal breast or prostate carcinoma ▪ **Vag:** Management of atrophic vaginitis that may occur with menopause ▪ Concurrent use of progestin is recommended during cyclical therapy to decrease the risk of endometrial carcinoma in patients with an intact uterus.

ACTION

▪ Estrogens promote the growth and development of female sex organs and the maintenance of secondary sex characteristics in women ▪ Metabolic effects include reduced blood cholesterol, protein synthesis, and sodium and water retention. **Therapeutic Effects:** ▪ Restoration of hormonal balance in various deficiency states ▪ Treatment of hormone-sensitive tumors.

PHARMACOKINETICS

Absorption: Well absorbed following oral administration. Readily absorbed through skin and mucous membranes.
Distribution: Widely distributed. Crosses the placenta and enters breast milk.
Metabolism and Excretion: Mostly metabolized by the liver and other tissues. Enterohepatic recirculation occurs, and more absorption may occur from the GI tract.
Half-life: UK.

CONTRAINDICATIONS AND PRECAUTIONS

Contraindicated in: ▪ Thromboembolic disease ▪ Undiagnosed vaginal bleeding ▪ Pregnancy (may result in harm to the fetus) ▪ Lactation.

Use Cautiously in: ▪ Underlying cardiovascular disease ▪ Severe hepatic or renal disease ▪ May increase the risk of endometrial carcinoma.

ADVERSE REACTIONS AND SIDE EFFECTS*

CNS: headache, dizziness, lethargy.
EENT: intolerance to contact lenses, worsening of myopia or astigmatism.
CV: MYOCARDIAL INFARCTION, THROMBOEMBOLISM, edema, hypertension.
GI: nausea, weight changes, anorexia, increased appetite, jaundice, vomiting.
GU: *women*—amenorrhea, dysmenorrhea, breakthrough bleeding, cervical erosions, loss of libido, vaginal candidiasis; *men*—impotence, testicular atrophy.
Derm: acne, oily skin, pigmentation, urticaria.
Endo: gynecomastia (men), hyperglycemia.
F and E: hypercalcemia, sodium and water retention.
MS: leg cramps.
Misc: breast tenderness.

INTERACTIONS

Drug-Drug: ▪ May alter requirement for **warfarin, oral hypoglycemic agents,** or **insulin** ▪ **Barbiturates** or **rifampin** may decrease effectiveness.

ROUTE AND DOSAGE

❑ **Symptoms of Menopause, Atrophic Vaginitis, Female Hypogonadism, Ovarian Failure/Osteoporosis**

- **PO (Adults):** 0.5–2 mg daily or in a cycle.
- **IM (Adults):** 1–5 mg monthly (estradiol cypionate) or 10–20 mg (estradiol valerate) monthly.
- **Transdermal (Adults):** *Alora, Estraderm*—50- or 100-mcg/24 hr transdermal patch applied twice weekly. *Climara*—50–100 mcg/24 patch applied weekly. *FemPatch*—25 mcg/24 hr patch applied q 7 days. *Vivelle*—37.5–100 mcg transdermal patch applied twice weekly. Progestin may be administered for 10–14 days of each month.
- **Vag (Adults):** 2–4 g cream (0.2–0.4 mg estradiol) daily for 1–2 wk, then decrease to 1–2 g/day for 1–2 wk; then maintenance dose of 1 g 1–3 times weekly for 3 wk, then off for 1 wk; then repeat cycle once vaginal mucosa has been restored *or* 2 mg vaginal ring q 3 mo.

❑ **Postmenopausal Breast Carcinoma**

- **PO (Adults):** 10 mg 3 times daily.

❑ **Prostate Carcinoma**

- **PO (Adults):** 1–2 mg 3 times daily.
- **IM (Adults):** 30 mg q 1–2 wk (estradiol valerate).

AVAILABILITY

▪ ***Tablets:*** 1 mg[Rx], 2 mg[Rx] ▪ ***Injection (valerate in oil):*** 10 mg/ml[Rx], 20 mg/ml[Rx], 40 mg/ml[Rx] ▪ ***Injection (cypionate in oil):*** 5 mg/ml[Rx] ▪ ***Transdermal system:*** 25 mcg/24 hr release rate (10.3 mg estradiol content)[Rx], 37.5 mcg /24 hr release rate (3.28 mg estradiol content)[Rx], 50 mcg/24 hr release rate (1.5–4.33 mg estradiol content)[Rx], 75 mcg/24 hr release rate (2.3–6.57 mg estradiol content)[Rx], 100 mcg/24 hr release rate (3.0–8.66 mg estradiol content)[Rx] ▪ ***Vaginal cream:*** 100 mcg/g[Rx] ▪ ***Vaginal ring:*** 2 mg released over 90 days[Rx].

TIME/ACTION PROFILE (estrogenic effects)

	ONSET	PEAK	DURATION
PO	UK	UK	UK
IM	UK	UK	UK
TD	UK	UK	3–4 days (Estraderm), 7 days (Climara)
Vaginal ring	UK	UK	90 days

NURSING IMPLICATIONS

ASSESSMENT

- ❑ Assess blood pressure prior to and periodically throughout therapy.
- ❑ Monitor intake and output ratios and weekly weight. Report significant discrepancies or steady weight gain.
- ▪ **Menopause:** Assess frequency and severity of vasomotor symptoms.
- ▪ ***Lab Test Considerations:*** May cause increased high-density lipoproteins (HDL), phospholipids, and triglycerides and decreased serum low-density lipoprotein (LDL) and total cholesterol concentrations.
- ❑ May cause increased serum glucose, sodium, cortisol, prolactin, prothrombin, and factor

*CAPITALS indicate life-threatening; underlines indicate most frequent.

VII, VIII, IX, and X levels. May decrease serum folate, pyridoxine, antithrombin III, and urine pregnanediol concentrations.
- Monitor hepatic function prior to and periodically throughout therapy.
- May cause false interpretations of thyroid function tests, false increases in norepinephrine platelet-induced aggregability, and false decreases in metyrapone tests.
- May cause hypercalcemia in patients with metastatic bone lesions.

POTENTIAL NURSING DIAGNOSES

- Sexual dysfunction (Indications).
- Knowledge deficit, related to medication regimen (Patient/Family Teaching).

IMPLEMENTATION

- **PO:** Administer with or immediately after food to reduce nausea.
- **Vag:** Manufacturer provides applicator with cream. Dosage is marked on the applicator. Wash applicator with mild soap and warm water after each use.
- **Transdermal:** When switching from PO form, begin transdermal therapy 1 wk after the last dose or when symptoms reappear.
- **IM:** Injection has oil base. Roll syringe to ensure even dispersion. Administer deep IM. Avoid IV administration.

PATIENT/FAMILY TEACHING

- **General Info:** Instruct patient to take medication as directed. If a dose is missed, take as soon as remembered as long as it is not just before next dose. Do not double doses.
- Explain dosage schedule and maintenance routine. Discontinuing medication suddenly may cause withdrawal bleeding.
- If nausea becomes a problem, advise patient that eating solid food often provides relief.
- Advise patient to report signs and symptoms of fluid retention (swelling of ankles and feet, weight gain), thromboembolic disorders (pain, swelling, tenderness in extremities, headache, chest pain, blurred vision), mental depression, or hepatic dysfunction (yellowed skin or eyes, pruritus, dark urine, light-colored stools) to health care professional.
- Instruct patient to stop taking medication and notify health care professional if pregnancy is suspected.
- Advise patient to notify health care professional of medication regimen prior to treatment or surgery.
- Caution patient that cigarette smoking during estrogen therapy may cause increased risk of serious side effects, especially for women over age 35.
- Caution patient to use sunscreen and protective clothing to prevent increased pigmentation.
- Advise patient treated for osteoporosis that exercise has been found to arrest and reverse bone loss. The patient should discuss any exercise limitations with health care professional before beginning program.
- Emphasize the importance of routine follow-up physical exams, including blood pressure; breast, abdomen, and pelvic examinations; PAP smears every 6–12 mo; and mammogram every 12 mo or as directed. Health care professional will evaluate possibility of discontinuing medication every 3–6 mo. If on continuous (not cyclical) therapy or without concurrent progestins, endometrial biopsy may be recommended, if uterus is intact.
- **Vag:** Instruct patient in the correct use of applicator. Patient should remain recumbent for at least 30 min after administration. May use sanitary napkin to protect clothing, but do not use tampon. If a dose is missed, do not use the missed dose, but return to regular dosing schedule.
- **Vaginal Ring:** Instruct patient to press ring into an oval and insert into the upper third of the vaginal vault. Exact position is not critical. Once ring is inserted, patient should not feel anything. If discomfort is felt, ring is probably not in far enough; gently push farther into vagina. Leave in place continuously for 90 days. Ring does not interfere with sexual intercourse. If straining at defecation makes ring move to lower vagina, push up with finger. If expelled totally, rinse ring with lukewarm water and reinsert. To remove, hook a finger through the ring and pull it out.
- **Transdermal:** Instruct patient to wash and dry hands first. Apply disk to intact skin on hairless portion of abdomen (do not apply to breasts or waistline). Press disk for 10 sec to ensure contact with skin (especially around edges). Avoid areas where clothing may rub disk loose. Change site with each administra-

tion to prevent skin irritation. Do not reuse site for 1 wk. Disk may be reapplied if it falls off.

EVALUATION

Effectiveness of therapy can be demonstrated by: ▪ Resolution of menopausal vasomotor symptoms ▪ Decreased vaginal and vulvar itching, inflammation, or dryness associated with menopause ▪ Normalization of estrogen levels in patients with ovariectomy or hypogonadism ▪ Control of the spread of advanced metastatic breast or prostate cancer ▪ Prevention of osteoporosis.

ESTRAMUSTINE

(ess-tra-**muss**-teen)
Emcyt

CLASSIFICATION(S):
Antineoplastic (hormone/alkylating agent)

Pregnancy Category UK

INDICATIONS

▪ Palliative treatment of advanced metastatic prostate cancer.

ACTION

▪ Consists of combination of mechlorethamine, an alkylating agent, and estradiol, an estrogenic compound. Antineoplastic activity may be due to either component or the combination ▪ Also decreases serum testosterone levels. **Therapeutic Effects:** ▪ Decreased spread of prostate cancer.

PHARMACOKINETICS

Absorption: Well absorbed (75%) following oral administration. During absorption, converted to estromustine and then to estrogenic compounds and mechlorethamine.
Distribution: Presence of estrogen enhances delivery to tissues with estrogen receptors. Concentrates in prostatic tissue.
Metabolism and Excretion: Eliminated primarily by biliary and fecal excretion. Small amounts excreted by kidneys.
Half-life: 20 hr.

CONTRAINDICATIONS AND PRECAUTIONS

Contraindicated in: ▪ Thromboembolism, recent stroke, or myocardial infarction ▪ Cross-sensitivity or tolerance to estradiol or mechlorethamine may exist.
Use Cautiously in: ▪ History of thromboembolic disorders ▪ Hypercalcemia ▪ Peptic ulcer ▪ Active infection including recent chickenpox or herpes zoster ▪ Renal or hepatic impairment ▪ Gallbladder disease ▪ Cardiovascular disease ▪ Cerebrovascular disease ▪ Migraine headaches ▪ Metabolic bone disease ▪ Epilepsy ▪ Asthma ▪ Bone marrow depression ▪ Patients with child-bearing potential.

ADVERSE REACTIONS AND SIDE EFFECTS*

CNS: insomnia.
CV: THROMBOEMBOLISM, edema, hypertension.
GI: diarrhea, nausea, vomiting.
Derm: rashes.
Endo: decreased libido, gynecomastia, gonadal suppression (azoospermia), hyperglycemia.
F and E: sodium and water retention, hypercalcemia.
Hemat: anemia, leukopenia, thrombocytopenia.
Misc: allergic reactions, fever.

INTERACTIONS

Drug-Drug: ▪ **Cigarette smoking (nicotine)** increases the risk of adverse vascular effects ▪ **Calcium supplements** form an insoluble complex with estramustine that cannot be absorbed ▪ Increases effects and risk of toxicity with **glucocorticoids** (dosage reduction may be necessary) ▪ May decrease appropriate immune response to **live virus vaccines** and increase risk of adverse reactions.
Drug-Food: ▪ **Calcium** in dairy foods forms an insoluble complex with estramustine that cannot be absorbed.

ROUTE AND DOSAGE

▪ **PO (Adults):** 600 mg/m²/day in 3 divided doses *or* 14 mg/kg/day (range 10–16 mg/kg) in 3–4 divided doses.

AVAILABILITY

▪ ***Capsules:*** 140 mg[Rx].

*CAPITALS indicate life-threatening; underlines indicate most frequent.

TIME/ACTION PROFILE (effect on tumor spread)

	ONSET	PEAK	DURATION
PO	30–90 days	UK	6 wk*

*Persistence of hematologic effects.

NURSING IMPLICATIONS

ASSESSMENT

- □ Monitor blood pressure periodically throughout therapy.
- □ Monitor intake and output ratios and weekly weight. Report significant discrepancies or steady weight gain.
- □ Monitor blood glucose closely in diabetic patients. May decrease glucose tolerance.
- ▪ ***Lab Test Considerations:*** Monitor hematologic and hepatic functions, serum calcium, and phosphorus periodically throughout therapy. May cause leukopenia and thrombocytopenia. May also cause elevated LDH, AST, and bilirubin levels.
- □ May cause increased serum glucose, sodium, triglyceride, phospholipid, cortisol, prolactin, prothrombin, and factor VII, VIII, IX, and X levels. May decrease serum folate, pyridoxine, antithrombin III, and pregnanediol excretion concentrations.
- □ May cause false interpretations of thyroid function tests, false increases in sulfobromophthalein (SBP) and norepinephrine platelet-induced aggregation, and false decreases in metyrapone tests.
- □ May cause hypercalcemia in patients with metastatic bone lesions.

POTENTIAL NURSING DIAGNOSES

- ▪ Knowledge deficit, related to medication regimen (Patient/Family Teaching).

IMPLEMENTATION

- ▪ **PO:** Administer with water 1 hr before or 2 hr after meals. Milk, milk products, and calcium-rich foods or calcium-containing antacids impair the absorption of estramustine and must not be taken simultaneously.
- □ Frequently causes nausea and sometimes causes vomiting. Phenothiazines may be administered to treat nausea and vomiting. May require discontinuation of therapy.

PATIENT/FAMILY TEACHING

- □ Instruct patient to take estramustine exactly as directed. If a dose is missed, omit; do not take at all. Do not double doses. Notify health care professional if vomiting occurs shortly after a dose is taken. Do not discontinue without consulting health care professional.
- □ Instruct patient to store capsules in the refrigerator, but they may be kept at room temperature for 24–48 hr without losing potency.
- □ Advise patient of the need for contraception throughout therapy, as sperm cells may be altered.
- □ Advise patient to report signs and symptoms of fluid retention (swelling of ankles and feet, weight gain) and thromboembolic disorders (pain, swelling, tenderness in extremities, headache, chest pain, blurred vision) to health care professional.
- □ Caution patient to avoid vaccinations without advice of health care professional.

EVALUATION

Effectiveness of therapy can be demonstrated by: ▪ Decrease in spread of prostate cancer. May require 30–90 days to determine maximum effects of therapy.

ESTROGENS, CONJUGATED

(**ess**-troe-jenz)

{C.E.S.}, {Congest}, Premarin

CLASSIFICATION(S):

Hormone (estrogen)

Pregnancy Category X

INDICATIONS

▪ **PO:** As part of replacement therapy (HRT) in the treatment of moderate to severe vasomotor symptoms of menopause ▪ Various estrogen deficiency states, including: □ Female hypogonadism □ Ovariectomy □ Primary ovarian failure ▪ Adjunctive therapy of postmenopausal osteoporosis ▪ Adjunctive therapy of advanced inoperable metastatic breast and prostatic carcinoma ▪ **IM, IV:** Uterine bleeding due to hormonal imbalance ▪ **Vag:** Management of atrophic vaginitis ▪ Concurrent use of progestin is recommended during cyclical therapy to decrease the risk of endometrial carcinoma in patients with an intact uterus.

ACTION

▪ Estrogens promote the growth and development of female sex organs and the maintenance of secondary sex characteristics in women ▪ Metabolic effects include reduced blood cholesterol, protein synthesis, and sodium and water retention. **Therapeutic Effects:** ▪ Restoration of hormonal balance in various deficiency states and treatment of hormone-sensitive tumors.

PHARMACOKINETICS

Absorption: Well absorbed following oral administration. Readily absorbed through skin and mucous membranes.
Distribution: Widely distributed. Crosses the placenta and enters breast milk.
Metabolism and Excretion: Mostly metabolized by the liver and other tissues. Enterohepatic recirculation occurs, and more absorption may occur from the GI tract.
Half-life: UK.

CONTRAINDICATIONS AND PRECAUTIONS

Contraindicated in: ▪ Thromboembolic disease ▪ Undiagnosed vaginal bleeding ▪ Pregnancy (may result in harm to the fetus) ▪ Lactation.
Use Cautiously in: ▪ Underlying cardiovascular disease ▪ Severe hepatic or renal disease ▪ May increase the risk of endometrial carcinoma.

ADVERSE REACTIONS AND SIDE EFFECTS* (systemic use)

CNS: headache, dizziness, lethargy, mental depression.
EENT: intolerance to contact lenses, worsening of myopia or astigmatism.
CV: MYOCARDIAL INFARCTION, THROMBOEMBOLISM, edema, hypertension.
GI: nausea, weight changes, anorexia, increased appetite, jaundice, vomiting.
GU: *women*—amenorrhea, breakthrough bleeding, dysmenorrhea, cervical erosion, loss of libido, vaginal candidiasis; *men*—impotence, testicular atrophy.
Derm: acne, oily skin, pigmentation, urticaria.
Endo: gynecomastia (men), hyperglycemia.
F and E: hypercalcemia, sodium and water retention.
MS: leg cramps.
Misc: breast tenderness.

INTERACTIONS

Drug-Drug: ▪ May alter requirement for **warfarin, oral hypoglycemic agents,** or **insulin** ▪ **Barbiturates** or **rifampin** may decrease effectiveness ▪ **Cigarette smoking** increases the risk of adverse cardiovascular reactions.

ROUTE AND DOSAGE

❑ **Ovariectomy, Primary Ovarian Failure**
- **PO (Adults):** 1.25 mg daily or in a cycle.

❑ **Osteoporosis/Menopausal Symptoms**
- **PO (Adults):** 0.3–1.25 mg daily or in a cycle.

❑ **Hypogonadism**
- **PO (Adults):** 2.5–7.5 mg daily or in a cycle.

❑ **Inoperable Breast Carcinoma—Men and Postmenopausal Women**
- **PO (Adults):** 10 mg tid.

❑ **Inoperable Prostate Carcinoma**
- **PO (Adults):** 1.25–2.5 mg tid.

❑ **Uterine Bleeding**
- **IM, IV (Adults):** 25 mg, may repeat in 6–12 hr if necessary.

❑ **Atrophic Vaginitis**
- **Vag (Adults):** 1.25–2.5 mg (2–4 g cream) daily for 3 wk, off for 1 wk, then repeat.

AVAILABILITY

▪ ***Tablets:*** 0.3 mg[Rx], 0.625 mg[Rx], 0.9 mg[Rx], 1.25 mg[Rx], 2.5 mg[Rx] ▪ ***Powder for injection:*** 25 mg/vial[Rx] ▪ ***Vaginal cream:*** 0.625 mg/g[Rx] ▪ ***In combination with:*** medroxyprogesterone in compliance package (Prempro and Premphase)[Rx]. See Appendix A.

TIME/ACTION PROFILE (estrogenic effects†)

	ONSET	PEAK	DURATION
PO	rapid	UK	24 hr
IM	delayed	UK	6–12 hr
IV	rapid	UK	6–12 hr

†Tumor response may take several weeks.

*CAPITALS indicate life-threatening; underlines indicate most frequent.

NURSING IMPLICATIONS

ASSESSMENT

- **General Info:** Assess blood pressure prior to and periodically throughout therapy.
- Monitor intake and output ratios and weekly weight. Report significant discrepancies or steady weight gain.
- **Menopause:** Assess frequency and severity of vasomotor symptoms.
- ***Lab Test Considerations:*** May cause increased high-density lipoproteins (HDL), phospholipids, and triglycerides, and decreased serum low-density lipoprotein (LDL) and total cholesterol concentrations.
- May cause increased serum glucose, sodium, cortisol, prolactin, prothrombin, and factor VII, VIII, IX, and X levels. May decrease serum folate, pyridoxine, antithrombin III, and urine pregnanediol concentrations.
- Monitor hepatic function prior to and periodically throughout therapy.
- May cause false interpretations of thyroid function tests, false increases in norepinephrine platelet-induced aggregability, and false decreases in metyrapone tests.
- May cause hypercalcemia in patients with metastatic bone lesions.

POTENTIAL NURSING DIAGNOSES

- Sexual dysfunction (Indications).
- Knowledge deficit, related to medication regimen (Patient/Family Teaching).

IMPLEMENTATION

- **PO:** Administer with or immediately after food to reduce nausea.
- **Vag:** Manufacturer provides applicator with cream. Dose is marked on the applicator. Wash applicator with mild soap and warm water after each use.
- **IM:** To reconstitute, withdraw at least 5 ml of air from dry container and then slowly introduce the sterile diluent against the container side. Gently agitate container to dissolve; do not shake vigorously. Solution is stable for 60 days if refrigerated. Do not use if precipitate is present or if solution is darkened.
- IV is preferred parenteral route because of rapid response.
- **Direct IV:** Reconstitute as for IM. Inject into distal port tubing of free-flowing IV of 0.9% NaCl, D5W, or lactated Ringer's solution.
- ***Rate:*** Administer slowly (no faster than 5 mg/min) to prevent flushing.
- **Y-Site Compatibility:** ▪ heparin ▪ potassium chloride ▪ vitamin B complex with C.
- **Additive Incompatibility:** ▪ ascorbic acid or acidic solutions.

PATIENT/FAMILY TEACHING

- **General Info:** Instruct patient to take oral medication as directed. If a dose is missed, take as soon as remembered, but not just before next dose. Do not double doses.
- Explain dosage schedule and maintenance routine. Discontinuing medication suddenly may cause withdrawal bleeding. Bleeding is anticipated during the week conjugated estrogens are withheld.
- If nausea becomes a problem, advise patient that eating solid food often provides relief.
- Advise patient to report signs and symptoms of fluid retention (swelling of ankles and feet, weight gain), thromboembolic disorders (pain, swelling, tenderness in extremities; headache; chest pain; blurred vision), depression, hepatic dysfunction (yellowed skin or eyes, pruritus, dark urine, light-colored stools), or abnormal vaginal bleeding to health care professional.
- Instruct patient to stop taking medication and notify health care professional if pregnancy is suspected.
- Caution patient that cigarette smoking during estrogen therapy may increase risk of serious side effects, especially for women over age 35.
- Caution patient to use sunscreen and protective clothing to prevent increased pigmentation.
- Advise patient to notify health care professional of medication regimen prior to treatment or surgery.
- Advise patient treated for osteoporosis that exercise has been found to arrest and reverse bone loss. The patient should discuss any exercise limitations with health care professional before beginning program.
- Emphasize the importance of routine follow-up physical exams, including blood pressure; breast, abdomen, and pelvic examinations; PAP smears every 6–12 mo; and mammogram every 12 mo or as directed. Health care

professional will evaluate possibility of discontinuing medication every 3–6 mo. If on continuous (not cyclical) therapy or without concurrent progestins, endometrial biopsy may be recommended, if uterus is intact.

- **Vag:** Instruct patient in the correct use of applicator. Patient should remain recumbent for at least 30 min after administration. May use sanitary napkin to protect clothing, but do not use tampon. If a dose is missed, do not use the missed dose, but return to regular dosing schedule.

EVALUATION

Effectiveness of therapy can be demonstrated by: ▪ Resolution of menopausal vasomotor symptoms ▫ Decreased vaginal and vulvar itching, inflammation, or dryness associated with menopause ▪ Normalization of estrogen levels in patients with ovariectomy or hypogonadism ▪ Control of the spread of advanced metastatic breast or prostate cancer ▪ Prevention of osteoporosis.

ESTROPIPATE

(ess-troe-**pi**-pate)

Ogen, Ortho-Est, piperazine estrone sulfate

CLASSIFICATION(S):

Hormone (estrogen)

Pregnancy Category X

INDICATIONS

▪ **PO:** As part of replacement therapy (HRT) in the treatment of vasomotor symptoms of menopause ▪ Treatment of various estrogen deficiency states, including: ▫ Female hypogonadism ▫ Ovariectomy ▫ Primary ovarian failure ▪ Adjunctive therapy of postmenopausal osteoporosis ▪ **Vag:** Management of atrophic vaginitis ▪ Concurrent use of progestin is recommended during cyclical therapy to decrease the risk of endometrial carcinoma in patients with an intact uterus.

ACTION

▪ Estrogens promote the growth and development of female sex organs and the maintenance of secondary sex characteristics in women ▪ Metabolic effects include reduced blood cholesterol, protein synthesis, and sodium and water retention. **Therapeutic Effects:** ▪ Restoration of hormonal balance in various deficiency states.

PHARMACOKINETICS

Absorption: Well absorbed following oral administration. Readily absorbed through skin and mucous membranes.

Distribution: Widely distributed. Crosses the placenta and enters breast milk.

Metabolism and Excretion: Mostly metabolized by the liver and other tissues. Enterohepatic recirculation occurs, and more absorption may occur from the GI tract.

Half-life: UK.

CONTRAINDICATIONS AND PRECAUTIONS

Contraindicated in: ▪ Thromboembolic disease ▪ Undiagnosed vaginal bleeding ▪ Pregnancy (may result in harm to the fetus) ▪ Lactation.

Use Cautiously in: ▪ Underlying cardiovascular disease ▪ Severe hepatic or renal disease ▪ May increase the risk of endometrial carcinoma.

ADVERSE REACTIONS AND SIDE EFFECTS* (systemic use)

CNS: headache, dizziness, lethargy, mental depression.

EENT: intolerance to contact lenses, worsening of myopia or astigmatism.

CV: MYOCARDIAL INFARCTION, THROMBOEMBOLISM, edema, hypertension.

GI: nausea, weight changes, anorexia, increased appetite, jaundice, vomiting.

GU: *women*—amenorrhea, breakthrough bleeding, dysmenorrhea, cervical erosion, loss of libido, vaginal candidiasis; *men*—impotence, testicular atrophy.

Derm: acne, oily skin, pigmentation, urticaria.

Endo: gynecomastia (men), hyperglycemia.

F and E: hypercalcemia, sodium and water retention.

MS: leg cramps.

Misc: breast tenderness.

INTERACTIONS

Drug-Drug: ▪ May alter requirement for **warfarin, oral hypoglycemic agents,** or **insulin**

***CAPITALS** indicate life-threatening; underlines indicate most frequent.**

▪ **Barbiturates** or **rifampin** may decrease effectiveness ▪ **Cigarette smoking** increases the risk of adverse cardiovascular reactions.

ROUTE AND DOSAGE

❑ Vasomotor Symptoms of Menopause/Atrophic Vaginitis/Osteoporosis

- **PO (Adults):** 0.75–6 mg daily or in a cycle.
- **Vag (Adults):** 3–6 mg (2–4 g of 0.15% cream) daily for 3 wk, then off for 1 wk, then repeat cycle.

❑ Female Hypogonadism/Ovarian Failure

- **PO (Adults):** 1.5–9 mg daily or in a cycle.

AVAILABILITY

▪ ***Tablets:*** 0.75 mg[Rx], 1.5 mg[Rx], 3 mg[Rx], 6 mg estropipate[Rx] ▪ ***Vaginal cream:*** 1.5 mg/g[Rx].

TIME/ACTION PROFILE (estrogenic effects)

	ONSET	PEAK	DURATION
PO	UK	UK	24 hr

NURSING IMPLICATIONS

ASSESSMENT

▪ **General Info:** Assess blood pressure prior to and periodically throughout therapy.

□ Monitor intake and output ratios and weekly weight. Report significant discrepancies or steady weight gain.

▪ **Menopause:** Assess frequency and severity of vasomotor symptoms.

▪ ***Lab Test Considerations:*** May cause increased high-density lipoproteins (HDL), phospholipids, and triglycerides, and decreased serum low-density lipoprotein (LDL) and total cholesterol concentrations.

□ May cause increased serum glucose, sodium, cortisol, prolactin, prothrombin, and factor VII, VIII, IX, and X levels. May decrease serum folate, pyridoxine, antithrombin III, and urine pregnanediol concentrations.

□ Monitor hepatic function prior to and periodically throughout therapy.

□ May cause false interpretations of thyroid function tests, false increases in norepinephrine platelet-induced aggregability, and false decreases in metyrapone tests.

POTENTIAL NURSING DIAGNOSES

- Sexual dysfunction (Indications).
- Knowledge deficit, related to medication regimen (Patient/Family Teaching).

IMPLEMENTATION

▪ **PO:** Administer PO doses with or immediately after food to reduce nausea.

▪ **Vag:** Manufacturer provides applicator with cream. Dose is marked on the applicator. Wash applicator with mild soap and warm water after each use.

PATIENT/FAMILY TEACHING

▪ **General Info:** Instruct patient to take oral medication as directed. If a dose is missed, take as soon as remembered as long as it is not just before next dose. Do not double doses.

□ Explain medication schedule to women on 21-day cycle followed by 7 days of not taking medication. Encourage patient to take medication at the same time each day.

□ If nausea becomes a problem, advise patient that eating solid food often provides relief.

□ Advise patient to report signs and symptoms of fluid retention (swelling of ankles and feet, weight gain), thromboembolic disorders (pain, swelling, or tenderness in extremities; headache; chest pain; blurred vision), mental depression, hepatic dysfunction (yellowed skin or eyes, pruritus, dark urine, light-colored stools), or abnormal vaginal bleeding to health care professional.

□ Instruct patient to stop taking medication and notify health care professional if pregnancy is suspected.

□ Caution patient that cigarette smoking during estrogen therapy may increase risk of serious side effects, especially for women over age 35.

□ Caution patient to use sunscreen and protective clothing to prevent increased pigmentation.

□ Advise patient to notify health care professional of medication regimen prior to treatment or surgery.

□ Advise patient treated for osteoporosis that exercise has been found to arrest and reverse bone loss. The patient should discuss any exercise limitations with health care professional before beginning program.

□ Emphasize the importance of routine follow-up physical exams, including blood pressure; breast, abdomen, and pelvic examinations; PAP smears every 6–12 mo; and mammogram every 12 mo or as directed. Health care professional will evaluate possibility of discontinuing medication every 3–6 mo. If on continuous (not cyclical) therapy or without concurrent progestins, endometrial biopsy may be recommended, if uterus is intact.

- **Vag:** Instruct patient in the correct use of applicator. Patient should remain recumbent for at least 30 min after administration. May use sanitary napkin to protect clothing, but do not use tampon. If a dose is missed, do not use the missed dose, but return to regular dosing schedule.

EVALUATION

Effectiveness of therapy can be demonstrated by: ▪ Resolution of menopausal vasomotor symptoms ▫ Decreased vaginal and vulvar itching, inflammation, or dryness associated with menopause ▪ Normalization of estrogen levels in patients with ovariectomy or hypogonadism ▪ Prevention of osteoporosis.

ETHAMBUTOL

(e-**tham**-byoo-tole)
{Etibi}, Myambutol

CLASSIFICATION(S):
Antitubercular

Pregnancy Category B

INDICATIONS

▪ Active tuberculosis or other mycobacterial diseases (with at least one other drug).

ACTION

▪ Inhibits the growth of mycobacteria. **Therapeutic Effects:** ▪ Tuberculostatic effect against susceptible organisms.

PHARMACOKINETICS

Absorption: Rapidly and well absorbed (80%) from the GI tract.
Distribution: Widely distributed into many body tissues and fluids. Crosses the blood-brain barrier in small amounts. Crosses the placenta; enters breast milk.
Metabolism and Excretion: 50% metabolized by the liver, 50% eliminated unchanged by the kidneys.
Half-life: 3.3 hr (increased in renal or hepatic impairment).

CONTRAINDICATIONS AND PRECAUTIONS

Contraindicated in: ▪ Hypersensitivity ▪ Optic neuritis.
Use Cautiously in: ▪ Renal and severe hepatic impairment (dosage reduction required) ▪ Children <13 yr (safety not established) ▪ Pregnancy (although safety not established, ethambutol has been used with isoniazid to treat tuberculosis in pregnant women without adverse effects on the fetus) ▪ Lactation.

ADVERSE REACTIONS AND SIDE EFFECTS*

CNS: confusion, dizziness, hallucinations, headache, malaise.
EENT: <u>optic neuritis</u>.
GI: abdominal pain, anorexia, hepatitis, nausea, vomiting.
Metab: hyperuricemia.
MS: joint pain.
Neuro: peripheral neuritis.
Misc: anaphylactoid reactions, fever.

INTERACTIONS

Drug-Drug: ▪ Neurotoxicity may be additive with other **neurotoxic agents.**

ROUTE AND DOSAGE

- **PO (Adults and Children >13 yr):** 15–25 mg/kg/day *or* 50 mg/kg (up to 2.5 g) twice weekly *or* 25–30 mg/kg 3 times weekly.

AVAILABILITY

- ***Tablets:*** 100 mg[Rx], 400 mg[Rx].

TIME/ACTION PROFILE (blood levels)

	ONSET	PEAK	DURATION
PO	rapid	2–4 hr	24 hr

{} = Available in Canada only.
*CAPITALS indicate life-threatening; underlines indicate most frequent.

E

NURSING IMPLICATIONS

ASSESSMENT

- Mycobacterial studies and susceptibility tests should be performed prior to and periodically throughout therapy to detect possible resistance.
- Assess lung sounds and character and amount of sputum periodically throughout therapy.
- Assessments of visual function should be made frequently during course of therapy. Advise patient to report blurring of vision, constriction of visual fields, or changes in color perception immediately. Visual impairment, if not identified early, may lead to permanent sight impairment.
- ***Lab Test Considerations:*** Renal and hepatic functions, CBC, and uric acid levels should be monitored routinely throughout therapy. Frequently causes elevated uric acid concentrations, which may precipitate an attack of gout.

POTENTIAL NURSING DIAGNOSES

- Infection, risk for (Indications).
- Sensory-perceptual alterations (Side Effects).
- Knowledge deficit, related to medication regimen (Patient/Family Teaching).

IMPLEMENTATION

- **General Info:** Ethambutol is given as a single daily dose and should be taken at the same time each day. Some regimens require dosing 2–3 times/week. Usually administered concurrently with other antitubercular medications to prevent development of bacterial resistance.
- **PO:** Administer with food or milk to minimize GI irritation.

PATIENT/FAMILY TEACHING

- Instruct patient to take medication exactly as directed. If a dose is missed, take as soon as possible unless almost time for next dose; do not double up on missed doses. A full course of therapy may take months to years. Do not discontinue without consulting health care professional, even though symptoms may disappear.
- Advise patient to notify health care professional if pregnancy is suspected.
- Instruct patient to notify health care professional if no improvement is seen in 2–3 wk. Health care professional should also be notified if unexpected weight gain or decreased urine output occurs.
- Emphasize the importance of routine exams to evaluate progress and ophthalmic examinations if signs of optic neuritis occur.

EVALUATION

Effectiveness of therapy can be demonstrated by: ▪ Resolution of clinical symptoms of tuberculosis ▫ Decrease in acid-fast bacteria in sputum samples ▫ Improvement in chest x rays. Therapy for tuberculosis is usually continued for at least 1–2 yr.

ETIDRONATE

(eh-tih-**droe**-nate)

Didronel

CLASSIFICATION(S):

Bone resorption inhibitor (biphosphonate), Electrolyte modifier (hypocalcemic)

Pregnancy Category B (PO), C (IV)

INDICATIONS

▪ Treatment of Paget's disease of bone ▪ Treatment and prophylaxis of heterotopic calcification associated with total hip replacement or spinal cord injury ▪ Used with other agents (saline diuresis) in the management of hypercalcemia associated with malignancies.

ACTION

▪ Blocks the growth of calcium hydroxyapatite crystals by binding to calcium phosphate. **Therapeutic Effects:** ▪ Decreased bone resorption and turnover.

PHARMACOKINETICS

Absorption: Absorption is generally poor (1–6%) following oral administration.

Distribution: Half of the absorbed dose is bound to hydroxyapatite crystals in areas of increased osteogenesis.

Metabolism and Excretion: Unabsorbed drug is eliminated in the feces; 50% of the absorbed dose is excreted unchanged by the kidneys.

Half-life: 5–7 hr.

CONTRAINDICATIONS AND PRECAUTIONS

Contraindicated in: ▪ Hypersensitivity ▪ Severe renal impairment (serum creatinine >5 mg/dl) ▪ Hypercalcemia due to hyperparathyroidism.
Use Cautiously in: ▪ Long bone fractures ▪ Congestive heart failure ▪ Hypocalcemia ▪ Hypovitaminosis D ▪ Moderate renal impairment (dosage reduction recommended if serum creatinine 2.5–4.9 mg/dl) ▪ Pregnancy, lactation, or children (safety not established).

ADVERSE REACTIONS AND SIDE EFFECTS*

GI: diarrhea, nausea; *IV*—loss of taste, metallic taste.
GU: nephrotoxicity.
Derm: rash.
MS: bone pain, bone tenderness, microfractures.

INTERACTIONS

Drug-Drug: ▪ **Antacids** or **mineral supplements** or **buffers** (as in didanosine) containing **calcium, aluminum, iron,** or **magnesium** may decrease the absorption of etidronate ▪ Hypocalcemic effect may be additive with **calcitonin.**
Drug-Food: ▪ Foods containing large amounts of **calcium, aluminum, iron,** or **magnesium** may decrease the absorption of etidronate.

ROUTE AND DOSAGE

❑ **Paget's Disease**

▪ **PO (Adults):** 5–10 mg/kg/day single dose for up to 6 mo *or* 11–20 mg/kg/day for not more than 3 mo.

❑ **Heterotopic Ossification (Hip Replacement)**

▪ **PO (Adults):** 20 mg/kg/day for 1 mo prior to and 3 mo following surgery.

❑ **Heterotopic Ossification (Spinal Cord Injury)**

▪ **PO (Adults):** 20 mg/kg/day for 2 wk, then decreased to 10 mg/kg/day for 10 wk.

❑ **Hypercalcemia**

▪ **PO (Adults):** 20 mg/kg/day for 30–90 days.
▪ **IV (Adults):** 7.5 mg/kg/day for 3 days. May be followed by oral therapy.

AVAILABILITY

▪ ***Tablets:*** 200 mg[Rx], 400 mg[Rx] ▪ ***Injection:*** 50 mg/ml in 6-ml ampules[Rx].

TIME/ACTION PROFILE

	ONSET	PEAK	DURATION
PO (Paget's disease)	1 mo†	UK	1 yr
PO (heterotopic calcification)	UK	UK	several mo
IV‡ (hypercalcemia)	24 hr	3 days	11 days

†As measured by decreased urinary hydroxyproline.
‡As measured by decreased urinary calcium excretion.

NURSING IMPLICATIONS

ASSESSMENT

▪ **General Info:** Assess patient for bone pain, weakness, or loss of function prior to and throughout therapy. Bone pain may persist or increase in patients with Paget's disease; it usually subsides days to months after therapy is discontinued. Confer with physician or other health care professional regarding analgesic to control pain.
▪ **Heterotopic Ossification:** Monitor for inflammation and pain at the site and loss of function if ossification occurs near a joint.
▪ **Hypercalcemia:** Monitor symptoms of hypercalcemia (nausea, vomiting, anorexia, weakness, constipation, thirst, and cardiac arrhythmias).
❑ Observe patient carefully for evidence of hypocalcemia (paresthesia, muscle twitching, laryngospasm, colic, cardiac arrhythmias, and Chvostek's or Trousseau's sign). Protect symptomatic patients by elevating and padding side rails; keep bed in low position. Risk of hypocalcemia is greatest after 3 days of continuous IV therapy.
▪ ***Lab Test Considerations:*** Etidronate interferes with bone uptake of technetium 99 in diagnostic scans.
❑ *Paget's disease:* Decreased urinary excretions of hydroxyproline and serum alkaline phosphatase are often the first clinical signs of ef-

*CAPITALS indicate life-threatening; underlines indicate most frequent.

E

fectiveness. These values are monitored every 3 mo. Treatment is restarted when levels return to 75% of pretreatment values. Serum phosphate levels are also monitored prior to and 4 wk after beginning therapy. Dosage may be reduced if serum phosphate is elevated without corresponding decrease in urinary excretion of hydroxyproline or serum alkaline phosphatase.

- *Hypercalcemia:* Monitor serum calcium and albumin levels to determine effectiveness of therapy.
- Monitor BUN and creatine prior to and periodically throughout course of therapy. Stable or reversible increases in BUN and creatinine may occur in patients with hypercalcemia.

POTENTIAL NURSING DIAGNOSES

- Pain (Indications, Side Effects).
- Injury, risk for (Indications).
- Knowledge deficit, related to medication regimen (Patient/Family Teaching).

IMPLEMENTATION

- **Hypercalcemia:** Used as adjunctive treatment after IV hydration and loop diuretics have restored urine output.
- Oral doses may be started on the day after the last IV infusion.
- **PO:** Administer on empty stomach, as food decreases absorption.
- **Intermittent Infusion:** Dilute in at least 250 ml of 0.9% NaCl or D5W. Solution is stable for 48 hr. Oral etidronate may be started on the day after last infusion.
- ***Rate:*** Infuse over at least 2 hr.

PATIENT/FAMILY TEACHING

- Advise patient to take as directed. If dose is missed, take as soon as remembered unless almost time for next dose. Do not double up on doses. Dose should not be taken within 2 hr of eating (especially products high in calcium) or taking vitamins or antacids, as absorption will be impaired.
- Instruct patient to notify health care professional if diarrhea occurs. Health care professional may divide the dose throughout the day to control diarrhea.
- Encourage patients to comply with diet recommendations. Diet should contain adequate amounts of calcium and vitamin D (see Appendix K).
- Advise patient to notify health care professional if pain appears or worsens during therapy.
- Explain to patient receiving IV dose that metallic taste is not uncommon and usually disappears in a few hours.
- Advise patient to report signs of hypercalcemic relapse (bone pain, anorexia, nausea, vomiting, thirst, lethargy) to health care professional promptly.
- Emphasize need for keeping follow-up appointments to monitor progress, even after medication is discontinued, to detect relapse.

EVALUATION

Effectiveness of therapy can be demonstrated by: ▪ Lowered serum calcium levels ▪ Decreased bone pain and fractures in Paget's disease ▪ Prevention or treatment of heterotopic ossification. Normal serum calcium levels are usually attained in 2–8 days in hypercalcemia associated with bony metastasis. Therapy may be repeated once after 1 wk.

ETODOLAC

(ee-**toe**-doe-lak)

Lodine, Lodine XL

CLASSIFICATION(S):

Nonopioid analgesic/Nonsteroidal anti-inflammatory agent

Pregnancy Category C

INDICATIONS

▪ Osteoarthritis ▪ Rheumatoid arthritis ▪ Mild to moderate pain (not XL tablets).

ACTION

▪ Inhibits prostaglandin synthesis ▪ Also has uricosuric action. **Therapeutic Effects:** ▪ Suppression of inflammation ▪ Decreased severity of pain.

PHARMACOKINETICS

Absorption: Well absorbed following oral administration.

Distribution: Widely distributed.

Metabolism and Excretion: Mostly metabo-

lized by the liver; <1% excreted unchanged in urine.
Half-life: 6–7 hr (single dose); 7.3 hr (chronic dosing).

CONTRAINDICATIONS AND PRECAUTIONS

Contraindicated in: ▪ Hypersensitivity ▪ Active GI bleeding or ulcer disease ▪ Cross-sensitivity may exist with other NSAIDs, including aspirin.
Use Cautiously in: ▪ Severe cardiovascular, renal, or hepatic disease ▪ History of ulcer disease ▪ Pregnancy (not recommended for use during second half of pregnancy) ▪ Lactation or children (safety not established).

ADVERSE REACTIONS AND SIDE EFFECTS*

CNS: depression, dizziness, drowsiness, insomnia, malaise, nervousness, syncope, weakness.
EENT: blurred vision, photophobia, tinnitus.
Resp: asthma.
CV: CONGESTIVE HEART FAILURE, edema, hypertension, palpitations.
GI: GI BLEEDING, <u>dyspepsia</u>, abdominal pain, constipation, diarrhea, drug-induced hepatitis, dry mouth, flatulence, gastritis, nausea, stomatitis, thirst, vomiting.
GU: dysuria, renal failure, urinary frequency.
Derm: ecchymoses, flushing, hyperpigmentation, pruritus, rashes, sweating.
Hemat: anemia, prolonged bleeding time, thrombocytopenia.
Misc: allergic reactions including ANAPHYLAXIS, ANGIOEDEMA, STEVENS-JOHNSON SYNDROME, chills, fever.

INTERACTIONS

Drug-Drug: ▪ Concurrent use with **aspirin** may decrease effectiveness ▪ Additive adverse GI effects with **aspirin**, other **NSAIDs, potassium supplements, glucocorticoids,** or **alcohol** ▪ Chronic use with **acetaminophen** may increase the risk of adverse renal reactions ▪ May decrease the effectiveness of **diuretic** or **antihypertensive** therapy ▪ May increase serum **lithium** levels and increase the risk of toxicity ▪ Increases the risk of toxicity from **methotrexate** ▪ Increased risk of bleeding with **cefamandole, cefotetan, cefoperazone, valproic acid, plicamycin, thrombolytic agents,** or **anticoagulants** ▪ Increased risk of adverse hematologic reactions with **antineoplastic agents** or **radiation therapy** ▪ May increase the risk of nephrotoxicity from **cyclosporine.**

ROUTE AND DOSAGE

- **PO (Adults):** *Analgesia*—200–400 mg q 6–8 hr (not to exceed 1200 mg/day). *Osteoarthritis/rheumatoid arthritis*—300 mg 2–3 times daily, 400 mg twice daily, or 500 mg twice daily; may also be given as 400–1000 mg once daily as XL (extended-release) tablets (not to exceed 1200 mg/day).

AVAILABILITY

▪ ***Capsules:*** 200 mg[Rx], 300 mg[Rx] ▪ ***Tablets:*** 400 mg[Rx], 500 mg[Rx] ▪ ***Extended-release tablets (XL):*** 400 mg[Rx], 600 mg[Rx].

TIME/ACTION PROFILE (analgesic effect)

	ONSET	PEAK	DURATION
PO (analgesic)	0.5 hr	1–2 hr	4–12 hr
PO (anti-inflammatory)	days–wks	UK	6–12† hr

†Up to 24 hr as XL (extended-release) tablet.

NURSING IMPLICATIONS

ASSESSMENT

- **General Info:** Patients who have asthma, aspirin-induced allergy, and nasal polyps are at increased risk for developing hypersensitivity reactions. Monitor for rhinitis, asthma, and urticaria.
- **Osteoarthritis/Rheumatoid Arthritis:** Assess pain and range of movement prior to and 1–2 hr following administration.
- **Pain:** Assess location, duration, and intensity of the pain prior to and 60 min following administration.
- ***Lab Test Considerations:*** May cause decreased hemoglobin, hematocrit, leukocyte, and platelet counts.
- ☐ Monitor liver function tests within 8 wk of initiating etodolac therapy and periodically during therapy. May cause elevated serum alkaline phosphatase, LDH, AST, and ALT concentrations.
- ☐ Monitor BUN, serum creatinine, and electrolytes periodically during therapy. May cause

*CAPITALS indicate life-threatening; <u>underlines</u> indicate most frequent.

increased BUN, serum creatinine, and electrolyte concentrations and decreased urine electrolyte concentrations.
- □ May cause decreased serum and increased urine uric acid concentrations.

POTENTIAL NURSING DIAGNOSES

- ▪ Pain (Indications).
- ▪ Physical mobility, impaired (Indications).
- ▪ Knowledge deficit, related to medication regimen (Patient/Family Teaching).

IMPLEMENTATION

- ▪ **General Info:** Administration in higher than recommended doses does not provide increased effectiveness but may cause increased side effects.
- ▪ **PO:** For rapid initial effect, administer 30 min before or 2 hr after meals. May be administered with food, milk, or antacids containing aluminum or magnesium to decrease GI irritation.
- □ Do not crush, break, or chew extended-release tablets.

PATIENT/FAMILY TEACHING

- □ Advise patients to take etodolac with a full glass of water and to remain in an upright position for 15–30 min after administration.
- □ Instruct patient to take medication exactly as directed. If a dose is missed, take as soon as possible within 1–2 hr if taking twice/day, or unless almost time for next dose if taking more than twice/day. Do not double doses.
- □ Etodolac may occasionally cause drowsiness or dizziness. Advise patient to avoid driving or other activities requiring alertness until response to the medication is known.
- □ Caution patient to avoid the concurrent use of alcohol, aspirin, acetaminophen, NSAIDs, or other OTC medications without consultation with health care professional.
- □ Advise patient to inform health care professional of medication regimen prior to treatment or surgery.
- □ Advise patient to consult health care professional if rash, itching, visual disturbances, tinnitus, weight gain, edema, black stools, persistent headache, or influenza-like syndrome (chills, fever, muscle aches, pain) occurs.

EVALUATION

Effectiveness of therapy can be demonstrated by: ▪ Decreased severity of pain ▪ Improved joint mobility. Patients who do not respond to one NSAID may respond to another. May require 2 wk or more for maximum anti-inflammatory effects.

ETOPOSIDES

(e-**toe**-poe-sides)

etoposide

VePesid, VP-16

etoposide phosphate

Etopophos

CLASSIFICATION(S):

Antineoplastic (podophyllotoxin derivative)

Pregnancy Category D

INDICATIONS

▪ Alone and in combination with other treatment modalities (other antineoplastic agents, radiation therapy, surgery) in the management of: □ Refractory testicular neoplasms □ Small cell lung carcinoma. **Unlabeled Uses:** ▪ Lymphomas and some leukemias.

ACTION

▪ Damages DNA prior to mitosis (cycle-dependent and phase-specific). **Therapeutic Effects:** ▪ Death of rapidly replicating cells, particularly malignant ones.

PHARMACOKINETICS

Absorption: Variably absorbed following oral administration. Following IV administration, etoposide phosphate is rapidly converted in plasma to etoposide.

Distribution: Rapidly distributed, does not appear to enter the CSF significantly but probably crosses placenta; enters breast milk.

Metabolism and Excretion: Some metabolism by the liver; 45% excreted unchanged by the kidneys.

Half-life: 7 hr (range 3–12 hr).

CONTRAINDICATIONS AND PRECAUTIONS

Contraindicated in: ▪ Hypersensitivity ▪ Pregnancy ▪ Lactation ▪ Known intolerance to benzyl alcohol, ethyl alcohol, polyethylene glycol (IV etoposide only), or dextran (IV etoposide phosphate only).

Use Cautiously in: ▪ Patients with childbearing potential ▪ Active infections ▪ Decreased bone marrow reserve ▪ Renal/hepatic impairment (dosage modification may be necessary) ▪ Other chronic debilitating illnesses.

ADVERSE REACTIONS AND SIDE EFFECTS*

CNS: drowsiness, fatigue, headache, vertigo.
Resp: PULMONARY EDEMA, bronchospasm.
CV: CONGESTIVE HEART FAILURE, MYOCARDIAL INFARCTION, hypotension (IV).
GI: nausea, vomiting.
Derm: alopecia.
Endo: gonadal suppression.
Hemat: leukopenia, thrombocytopenia.
Local: phlebitis at IV site.
MS: muscle cramps.
Neuro: peripheral neuropathy.
Misc: allergic reactions, including ANAPHYLAXIS, fever.

INTERACTIONS

Drug-Drug: ▪ Additive bone marrow depression with other **antineoplastics** or **radiation therapy** ▪ May impair normal immune response to **live virus vaccines** and increase the risk of adverse reactions.

ROUTE AND DOSAGE

❑ Testicular Neoplasms

- **IV (Adults):** 50–100 mg/m² daily for 5 days; repeat every 3–4 wk up to 100 mg/m² on days 1, 3, and 5 every 3–4 wk.

❑ Small Cell Carcinoma of the Lung

- **PO (Adults):** 35 mg/m² (rounded to the nearest 50 mg)/day for 4 days, repeated every 3–4 wk up to 50 mg/m² (rounded to the nearest 50 mg)/day for 5 days every 3–4 wk.
- **IV (Adults):** 35 mg/m² daily for 4 days up to 50 mg/m² daily for 5 days every 3–4 wk.

AVAILABILITY

❑ Etoposide

▪ ***Capsules:*** 50 mg^Rx ▪ ***Injection:*** 20 mg/ml^Rx.

❑ Etoposide Phosphate

▪ ***Powder for injection:*** 100 mg/vial (with dextran)^Rx.

TIME/ACTION PROFILE (noted as effects on blood counts)

	ONSET	PEAK	DURATION
PO	7–14 days	9–16 days	20 days
IV	7–14 days	9–16 days	20 days

NURSING IMPLICATIONS

ASSESSMENT

- ❑ Monitor blood pressure prior to and every 15 min during infusion. If hypotension occurs, stop infusion and notify physician or other health care professional. After stabilizing blood pressure with IV fluids and supportive measures, infusion may be resumed at slower rate.
- ❑ Monitor for hypersensitivity reaction (fever, chills, pruritus, urticaria, bronchospasm, tachycardia, hypotension). If these occur, stop infusion and notify physician. Keep epinephrine, an antihistamine, glucocorticoids, volume expanders, and resuscitative equipment close by in the event of an anaphylactic reaction.
- ❑ Assess for signs of infection (fever, chills, cough, hoarseness, lower back or side pain, sore throat, difficult or painful urination). Notify physician if these symptoms occur.
- ❑ Assess for bleeding (bleeding gums, bruising, petechiae, guaiac test stools, urine, and emesis). Avoid IM injections and rectal temperatures. Apply pressure to venipuncture sites for 10 min.
- ❑ Monitor intake and output, appetite, and nutritional intake. Etoposide causes nausea and vomiting in 30% of patients. Prophylactic antiemetics may decrease frequency and duration of nausea and vomiting.
- ❑ Adjust diet as tolerated to help maintain fluid and electrolyte balance and nutritional status.
- ▪ ***Lab Test Considerations:*** Monitor CBC and differential prior to and periodically

*CAPITALS indicate life-threatening; underlines indicate most frequent.

throughout therapy. The nadir of leukopenia occurs in 7–14 days. Notify physician if leukocyte count is <1000/mm³. The nadir of thrombocytopenia occurs in 9–16 days. Notify physician if the platelet count is <75,000/mm³. Recovery of leukopenia and thrombocytopenia occurs in 20 days.

- Monitor liver function studies (AST, ALT, LDH, bilirubin) and renal function studies (BUN, creatinine) prior to and periodically throughout therapy to detect hepatotoxicity and nephrotoxicity.
- May cause increased uric acid. Monitor levels periodically during therapy.

POTENTIAL NURSING DIAGNOSES

- Injury, risk for (Side Effects).
- Infection, risk for (Side Effects).
- Knowledge deficit, related to medication regimen (Patient/Family Teaching).

IMPLEMENTATION

- **General Info:** Avoid contact with skin. Use Luer-Lok tubing to prevent accidental leakage. If contact with skin occurs, immediately wash skin with soap and water.
- Solution should be prepared in a biologic cabinet. Wear gloves, gown, and mask while handling medication. Discard equipment in designated containers (see Appendix I).
- **PO:** Capsules should be refrigerated.

Etoposide (VePesid)

- **Intermittent Infusion:** Dilute 5-ml vial with 250–500 ml of D5W or 0.9% NaCl for a concentration of 200–400 mcg/ml. The 200-mcg/ml solution is stable for 96 hr. The 400-mcg/ml solution is stable for 48 hr. Concentrations >400 mcg/ml are not recommended, as crystallization is likely. Discard solution if crystals are present.
- ***Rate:*** Infuse slowly over 30–60 min. Temporary hypotension may occur with infusion rates shorter than 30 min.
- **Y-Site Compatibility:** ▪ fludarabine ▪ melphalan ▪ ondansetron ▪ paclitaxel ▪ piperacillin/tazobactam ▪ sargramostim ▪ teniposide ▪ vinorelbine.
- **Y-Site Incompatibility:** ▪ filgrastim ▪ gallium nitrate ▪ idarubicin.
- **Additive Compatibility:** ▪ cisplatin ▪ floxuridine ▪ fluorouracil ▪ ifosfamide.

Etoposide Phosphate (Etopophos)

- **Intermittent Infusion:** Reconstitute each vial with 5 or 10 ml of sterile water, D5W, or 0.9% NaCl for a concentration of 20 or 10 mg/ml, respectively.
- May be administered undiluted or diluted to a concentration as low as 0.1 mg/ml with D5W or 0.9% NaCl.
- Reconstituted solutions are stable for 24 hr at room temperature or if refrigerated.
- ***Rate:*** Administer over at least 5 min.

PATIENT/FAMILY TEACHING

- Instruct patient to take etoposide exactly as directed, even if nausea or vomiting occurs. If vomiting occurs shortly after dose is taken, consult physician. If a dose is missed, do not take at all.
- Advise patient to notify health care professional if fever; chills; sore throat or other signs of infection; bleeding gums; bruising; petechiae; or blood in urine, stool, or emesis occurs. Caution patient to avoid crowds and persons with known infections. Instruct patient to use soft toothbrush and electric razor. Patient should be cautioned not to drink alcoholic beverages or take products containing aspirin or NSAIDS.
- Instruct patient to notify health care professional if rapid heartbeat, difficulty breathing, abdominal pain, yellow skin, weakness, paresthesia, or gait disturbances occur.
- Instruct patient to inspect oral mucosa for redness and ulceration. If mouth sores occur, advise patient to use sponge brush and rinse mouth with water after eating and drinking. Viscous lidocaine swishes may be used if pain interferes with eating. Stomatitis pain may require treatment with opioid analgesics.
- Discuss with patient the possibility of hair loss. Explore coping strategies.
- Advise patient to use contraception.
- Instruct patient not to receive any vaccinations without advice of physician.
- Emphasize the need for periodic lab tests to monitor for side effects.

EVALUATION

Effectiveness of therapy can be demonstrated by: ▪ Decrease in size or spread of malignancies in solid tumors ▪ Improvement of hematologic status in leukemias.

FACTOR IX (human)

AlphaNine SD, Benefix, Hemonyne, Konyne 80, Mononine, Profilnine SD, Proplex T

CLASSIFICATION(S):
Blood derivative (clotting factor)

Pregnancy Category C

INDICATIONS

▪ Treatment of active or impending bleeding due to factor IX deficiency (hemophilia B, Christmas disease) ▪ Treatment of bleeding in patients with factor VIII inhibitors ▪ Prevention and treatment of bleeding in patients with factor VII deficiency (Proplex T only).

ACTION

▪ Factor IX complex preparations (AlphaNine SD, Konyne 80, Hemonyne, Profilnine SD, Proplex T) contain blood coagulation factors II, VII, IX, and X. Purified protein preparations (Benefix, Mononine) contain factor IX activity only. Benefix is made via recombinant DNA technology. **Therapeutic Effects:** ▪ Replacement of deficient factor IX in hemophilia B ▪ Restoration of hemostasis.

PHARMACOKINETICS

Absorption: Administered IV only, resulting in complete bioavailability.
Distribution: UK.
Metabolism and Excretion: Rapidly cleared from plasma by utilization in clotting process.
Half-life: *Factor IX*—24–32 hr; *factor VII*—3–6 hr.

CONTRAINDICATIONS AND PRECAUTIONS

Contraindicated in: ▪ Factor VII deficiency (except Proplex T) ▪ Intravascular coagulation or fibrinolysis associated with liver disease ▪ Allergy to mouse protein (Mononine).
Use Cautiously in: ▪ Postoperative period (increased risk of thrombosis) ▪ Blood groups A, B, or AB.

ADVERSE REACTIONS AND SIDE EFFECTS

CNS: drowsiness, headache, lethargy.
CV: changes in blood pressure, changes in heart rate.
GI: nausea, vomiting.
Derm: flushing, urticaria.
Hemat: disseminated intravascular coagulation, thrombosis.
Neuro: tingling.
Misc: chills, fever, risk of transmission of viral hepatitis, risk of transmission of HIV virus, hypersensitivity reactions.

INTERACTIONS

Drug-Drug: ▪ Use with **aminocaproic acid** may increase the risk of thrombosis.

ROUTE AND DOSAGE

The following general formula may be used: *Human derived products*—Dose (units) = body weight (kg) × 1 unit/kg × desired factor IX increase (% of normal). *Recombinant DNA product*—Dose (units) = body weight (kg) × 1.2 units/kg × desired factor IX increase (% of normal). Pre- and postoperatively maintain levels of >25% for at least 7 days. Calculate doses to increase levels to 40–60% of normal. High levels may require daily or twice daily dosing, while q 2–3 day dosing will maintain lower levels. A single dose may stop a minor bleed.

❑ **Hemophilia B**

▪ **IV (Adults and Children):** 40–60 units/kg initially, followed by 10–20 units/kg/day (maintain factor IX levels of >10–15% normal for minor spontaneous hemorrhage and >20–25% normal for major surgery or trauma).

❑ **Factor VIII Deficiency (Hemophilia A) (Proplex T, Konyne 80 only).**

▪ **IV (Adults and Children):** 75 units/kg.

AVAILABILITY

▪ ***Injection:*** Vials containing 250 units, 500 units, 1000 units, 1200 units, 1500 units[Rx].

TIME/ACTION PROFILE (hemostasis)

	ONSET	PEAK	DURATION
IV	immediate	10–30 min	1–2 days

F

NURSING IMPLICATIONS

ASSESSMENT

- □ Monitor blood pressure, pulse, and respirations frequently.
- □ Obtain history of current trauma; estimate amount of blood loss.
- □ Monitor for renewed or increased bleeding every 15–30 min. Immobilize and apply ice to affected joints.
- □ Monitor intake and output ratios; note urine color. Report significant discrepancies or urine becoming red or orange. Patients with type A, B, and AB blood are especially at risk for hemolytic reaction.
- □ If hypersensitivity reaction (fever, chills, tingling, headache, urticaria, changes in blood pressure or pulse, nausea and vomiting, lethargy) occurs, slow infusion and notify physician. Pyrogenic reactions (fever, chills) may also occur and are more common with high doses.
- ▪ ***Lab Test Considerations:*** Monitor coagulation studies (activated partial thromboplastin time [aPTT], plasma fibrinogen, platelet count, prothrombin time [PT], factor IX plasma concentrations) before, during, and after therapy to assess effectiveness of therapy.

POTENTIAL NURSING DIAGNOSES

- ▪ Tissue perfusion, altered (Indications).
- ▪ Injury, risk for (Indications).
- ▪ Knowledge deficit, related to medication regimen (Patient/Family Teaching).

IMPLEMENTATION

- ▪ **General Info:** Dosage varies with degree of clotting factor deficit, desired level of clotting factors, and weight.
- □ Obtain type and crossmatch of blood in case a transfusion is necessary.
- □ Hepatitis B vaccine may be given prior to therapy to prevent hepatitis.
- □ Inform all personnel of patient's bleeding tendency, to prevent further trauma. Apply pressure to all venipuncture sites for at least 5 min; avoid all IM injections.
- ▪ **Direct IV:** Refrigerate concentrate until just prior to reconstitution. Warm diluent (sterile water for injection) to room temperature before reconstituting. Use plastic syringe for preparation and administration. Use the filter needle provided by the manufacturer as an air vent to the vial when reconstituting. After adding diluent, rotate vial gently until contents are completely dissolved. Reconstitution generally requires 5–10 min for factor IX complex and 1–5 min for coagulation factor IX. Do not administer solutions that are discolored or contain particulate matter. Do not refrigerate after reconstitution. Begin administration within 3 hr.
- □ Dry concentrates should be refrigerated; however, do not refrigerate after reconstitution.
- □ Discard partially used vials.
- ▪ ***Rate:*** Rate of administration should be individualized according to specific product and response of the patient. Rates of 100–200 units/min or 2–3 ml/min are suggested. Temporarily stop infusion and resume at slower rate if headache, flushing, or changes in pulse or blood pressure occur.
- ▪ **Additive Incompatibility:** ▪ Reconstitute only with diluent provided. Administer through a separate line. Do not mix with other solutions or medications.

PATIENT/FAMILY TEACHING

- □ Instruct patient to notify nurse immediately if bleeding recurs.
- □ Advise patient to carry identification describing disease process at all times.
- □ Caution patient to avoid products containing aspirin or NSAIDs, as they may further impair clotting.
- □ Review with patient methods of preventing bleeding (use soft toothbrush, avoid IM and SC injections, avoid potentially traumatic activities).
- □ Advise patient that the risk of hepatitis or AIDS transmission may be decreased by use of heat-treated preparations. Current screening programs and vaccination with hepatitis B vaccine should help decrease the risk.
- □ Reinforce need for patients with hemophilia to receive close medical supervision.

EVALUATION

Effectiveness of therapy can be demonstrated by: ▪ Prevention of spontaneous bleeding or cessation of bleeding in patients with factor IX deficiency (hemophilia B, Christmas disease), factor VIII inhibitors, factor VII deficiency, or anticoagulant overdose.

FAMCICLOVIR
(fam-**sye**-kloe-veer)
Famvir

CLASSIFICATION(S):
Antiviral

Pregnancy Category B

INDICATIONS

- Acute herpes zoster infections (shingles)
- Treatment/suppression of recurrent herpes genitalis in immunocompetent patients.

ACTION

- Inhibits viral DNA synthesis in herpes-infected cells only. **Therapeutic Effects:** - Decreased duration of herpes zoster infection with decreased duration of viral shedding.

PHARMACOKINETICS

Absorption: Following absorption, famciclovir is rapidly converted in the intestinal wall to penciclovir, the active compound.
Distribution: UK.
Metabolism and Excretion: Penciclovir is mostly excreted by the kidneys.
Half-life: *Penciclovir*—2.1–3 hr (increased in renal impairment).

CONTRAINDICATIONS AND PRECAUTIONS

Contraindicated in: - Hypersensitivity.
Use Cautiously in: - Patients with impaired renal function (increased dosage interval recommended if CCr <60 ml/min in the treatment of herpes zoster or <40 ml/min in the treatment of herpes genitalis) - Geriatric patients (because of age-related decrease in renal function) - Pregnancy, lactation, or children <18 yr (safety not established).

ADVERSE REACTIONS AND SIDE EFFECTS*

CNS: <u>headache</u>, dizziness, fatigue.
GI: diarrhea, nausea, vomiting.

INTERACTIONS

Drug-Drug: - **Probenecid** increases plasma concentration of penciclovir.

ROUTE AND DOSAGE

- **PO (Adults):** *Herpes zoster*—500 mg every 8 hr for 7 days. *Herpes genitalis*—125 mg twice daily for 5 days (treatment); 250 mg twice daily (suppression).

AVAILABILITY

- ***Tablets:*** 125 mg[Rx], 250 mg[Rx], 500 mg[Rx].

TIME/ACTION PROFILE (penciclovir blood levels)

	ONSET	PEAK	DURATION
PO	rapid	0.9 hr	8–12 hr

NURSING IMPLICATIONS

F

ASSESSMENT

- ☐ Assess lesions prior to and daily during therapy.
- ☐ Assess patient for postherpetic neuralgia periodically during and following therapy.

POTENTIAL NURSING DIAGNOSES

- Skin integrity, impaired (Indications).
- Infection transmission, risk for (Indications, Patient/Family Teaching).
- Knowledge deficit, related to disease process and medication regimen (Patient/Family Teaching).

IMPLEMENTATION

- **General Info:** Famciclovir therapy should be started as soon as herpes zoster is diagnosed, at least within 72 hr, preferably within 48 hr.
- **PO:** Famciclovir may be administered without regard to meals.

PATIENT/FAMILY TEACHING

- ☐ Instruct patient to take famciclovir exactly as directed for the full course of therapy. If a dose is missed, take as soon as remembered if not just before next dose.
- ☐ Inform patient that famciclovir does not prevent the spread of infection to others. Precautions should be taken around others who have not had chickenpox or varicella vaccine or

*CAPITALS indicate life-threatening; <u>underlines</u> indicate most frequent.

people who are immunosuppressed until all lesions have crusted.

- Advise patient that condoms should be used during sexual contact and that no sexual contact should be made while lesions are present.
- Instruct women with genital herpes to have yearly PAP smears because these women may be more likely to develop cervical cancer.

EVALUATION

Effectiveness of therapy can be demonstrated by: ▪ Decrease in time to full crusting, loss of vesicles, loss of ulcers, and loss of crusts in patients with acute herpes zoster (shingles) ▪ Crusting over and healing of lesions in genital herpes ▪ Prevention of recurrence of herpes genitalis.

FAT EMULSION

(fat ee-**mul**-shun)

Intralipid, Liposyn II, Liposyn III

CLASSIFICATION(S):

Caloric agent (nonprotein)

Pregnancy Category C

INDICATIONS

▪ Provision of nonprotein calories to patients whose total caloric needs cannot be met by carbohydrates (glucose) alone, usually as part of parenteral nutrition ▪ Treatment and prevention of essential fatty acid deficiency in patients receiving long-term parenteral nutrition (provides linoleic acid).

ACTION

▪ Acts as a nonprotein calorie source. **Therapeutic Effects:** ▪ Provision of essential fatty acids and nonprotein calories.

PHARMACOKINETICS

Absorption: IV administration results in complete bioavailability.
Distribution: Distributes into intravascular space.
Metabolism and Excretion: Cleared by conversion to triglycerides, then to free fatty acids and glycerol by lipoprotein lipase. Free fatty acids are transported to tissues, where they may be oxidized as an energy source or re-stored as triglycerides.
Half-life: UK.

CONTRAINDICATIONS AND PRECAUTIONS

Contraindicated in: ▪ Hyperlipidemias ▪ Lipoid nephrosis ▪ Pancreatitis accompanied by lipemia ▪ Hypersensitivity to egg products (emulsifier is egg yolk phospholipid), legumes, soybeans, or fat emulsions.
Use Cautiously in: ▪ Thromboembolic disorders ▪ Severe liver or pulmonary disease ▪ Anemia or bleeding disorders ▪ Patients who are at risk for fat embolism.
Exercise Extreme Caution in: ▪ Preterm infants (decreased ability to clear fat emulsion).

ADVERSE REACTIONS AND SIDE EFFECTS*

CV: chest pain.
GI: hepatomegaly†, splenomegaly†, vomiting.
Derm: jaundice†.
Local: phlebitis at IV site.
Misc: fever, infection, chills, hypersensitivity reactions, overloading syndrome†, shivering.

INTERACTIONS

Drug-Drug: ▪ Concurrent use with **propofol** may increase the risk of hypertriglyceridemia.

ROUTE AND DOSAGE

Total Parenteral Nutrition

- **IV (Adults):** Not to exceed 3 g fat/kg/day.
- **IV (Children):** Not to exceed 4 g fat/kg/day.
- **IV (Infants, Premature):** 0.5 g fat/kg/day initially; may be increased as tolerated up to 3 g fat/kg/day.

Essential Fatty Acid Deficiency

- **IV (Adults and Children):** Provide 8–10% of caloric intake as fat.

AVAILABILITY

▪ ***Emulsion for IV Use:*** 10%[Rx], 20%[Rx], 30%[Rx].

TIME/ACTION PROFILE

	ONSET	PEAK	DURATION
IV	UK	UK	UK

***CAPITALS indicate life-threatening; underlines indicate most frequent.**
†Seen only with long-term use.

NURSING IMPLICATIONS

ASSESSMENT

- Monitor weight every other day in adults and daily in infants and children receiving fat emulsion to assist in meeting caloric requirements.
- Assess patient for allergy to eggs prior to therapy. Acute hypersensitivity reaction with pruritic urticaria may occur in patients allergic to eggs.
- ***Lab Test Considerations:*** Monitor triglyceride and fatty acid levels routinely to determine patient's capacity to eliminate infused fat from the circulation.
- Monitor hemoglobin, blood coagulation, and platelet count weekly, especially during continuous therapy. Report abnormalities promptly. Therapy may be discontinued.
- Monitor serum bilirubin, cholesterol, and phospholipid concentrations and hepatic function weekly, especially in premature infants to prevent hyperlipemia.
- ***Toxicity and Overdose:*** If signs of overloading syndrome (focal seizures, fever, leukocytosis, splenomegaly, shock) or elevated triglyceride or free fatty acid levels occur, infusion should be stopped and the patient reevaluated prior to reinstituting therapy.

POTENTIAL NURSING DIAGNOSES

- Nutrition, altered, less than body requirements (Indications).
- Knowledge deficit, related to medication regimen (Patient/Family Teaching).

IMPLEMENTATION

- **General Info:** Fat emulsion should compose no more than 60% of patient's total caloric intake. The remaining 40% should consist of carbohydrates and amino acids.
- Fat emulsion may be administered via peripheral or central venous catheter. Monitor peripheral sites for phlebitis.
- Infuse fat emulsion via Y-site near the infusion site. Because of the lower specific gravity, the fat emulsion solution must be hung higher than the amino acid and dextrose solutions to prevent the fat emulsion from backing up into the amino acid and dextrose line.
- Manufacturer does not recommend use of filters during administration, but 1.2-micron filters have been used.
- Use tubing provided by the manufacturer. Change IV tubing after each dose of fat emulsion.
- **Intermittent Infusion:** Emulsions that appear oily or that have separated should not be used.
- Maximum hang times are 12 hr for *Intralipid,* 24 hr for fat emulsion alone, and 24 hr for admixtures with dextrose and amino acids. Discard all unused portions.
- ***Rate:*** For adults, the initial infusion rate should be 1 ml/min for the 10% solution and 0.5 ml/min for the 20% solution for the first 15–30 min. If no adverse reactions occur, the rate may be increased to infuse 500 ml over 4–6 hr for the 10% solution and 250 ml over 4–6 hr or 500 ml over 8 hr for the 20% solution.
- No more than 500 ml of the 10% solution, 250 ml of *Liposyn II,* or 500 ml of *Intralipid 20%* solution should be infused the 1st day. Dose may be increased on subsequent days.
- For children, the initial infusion rate should be 0.1 ml/min of the 10% solution and 0.05 ml/min for the 20% solution for the first 10–15 min. If no adverse reactions occur, the rate may be increased to 1 g/kg over 4 hr. Do not exceed a rate of 100 ml/hr for the 10% solution or 50 ml/hr for the 20% solution.
- Administer via infusion pump to ensure accurate rate.
- **Y-Site Compatibility:** ▪ ampicillin ▪ cefamandole ▪ cefazolin ▪ cefoxitin ▪ cephapirin ▪ clindamycin ▪ digoxin ▪ dopamine ▪ erythromycin lactobionate ▪ furosemide ▪ gentamicin ▪ isoproterenol ▪ kanamycin ▪ lidocaine ▪ norepinephrine ▪ oxacillin ▪ penicillin G potassium ▪ ticarcillin ▪ tobramycin.
- **Y-Site Incompatibility:** ▪ amikacin.
- **Additive Compatibility:** ▪ Fat emulsion may be admixed ("3-in-1," all-in-one, triple mix total nutrient admixture [TNA]) or administered simultaneously with amino acid and dextrose solutions ▪ Intralipid is compatible with FreAmine II 8.5% ▪ Travasol without electrolytes 8.5% and 10% ▪ Veinamine 8% ▪ cimetidine ▪ diphenhydramine ▪ famotidine ▪ hydrocortisone ▪ multivitamins ▪ nizatidine ▪ dextrose 10% and 70% ▪ While not generally recommended, heparin may be added in a

F

concentration of 1–2 units/ml prior to administration to increase clearance rate of lipemia, minimize risks associated with hypercoagulability, and prevent catheter thrombosis.

- **Additive Incompatibility:** ▪ Although compatibility studies have been done, manufacturer recommends that fat emulsion not be admixed with any other medication.

PATIENT/FAMILY TEACHING

□ Explain the purpose of fat emulsion to the patient prior to administration.

EVALUATION

Effectiveness of therapy can be demonstrated by: ▪ Weight gain □ Maintenance of normal serum triglyceride and fatty acid levels.

FELODIPINE

(fe-**loe**-di-peen)
Plendil, {Renedil}

CLASSIFICATION(S):
Antianginal, Antihypertensive agent, Calcium channel blocker

Pregnancy Category C

INDICATIONS

▪ Management of hypertension, angina pectoris, and vasospastic (Prinzmetal's) angina.

ACTION

▪ Inhibits the transport of calcium into myocardial and vascular smooth muscle cells, resulting in inhibition of excitation-contraction coupling and subsequent contraction. **Therapeutic Effects:** ▪ Systemic vasodilation resulting in decreased blood pressure ▪ Coronary vasodilation resulting in decreased frequency and severity of attacks of angina.

PHARMACOKINETICS

Absorption: Well absorbed following oral administration, but extensively metabolized, resulting in decreased bioavailability.
Distribution: UK.
Metabolism and Excretion: Mostly metabolized; minimal amounts excreted unchanged by kidneys.
Half-life: 11–16 hr.

CONTRAINDICATIONS AND PRECAUTIONS

Contraindicated in: ▪ Hypersensitivity (cross-sensitivity may occur) ▪ Sick sinus syndrome ▪ 2nd- or 3rd-degree AV block (unless an artificial pacemaker is in place). ▪ Blood pressure <90 mm Hg.
Use Cautiously in: ▪ Severe hepatic impairment (dosage reduction recommended) ▪ Geriatric patients (dosage reduction recommended; increased risk of hypotension) ▪ Severe renal impairment ▪ History of serious ventricular arrhythmias or congestive heart failure ▪ Pregnancy, lactation, or children (safety not established).

ADVERSE REACTIONS AND SIDE EFFECTS*

CNS: headache, abnormal dreams, anxiety, confusion, dizziness, drowsiness, nervousness , psychiatric disturbances, weakness.
EENT: blurred vision, disturbed equilibrium, epistaxis, tinnitus.
Resp: cough, dyspnea.
CV: ARRHYTHMIAS, CONGESTIVE HEART FAILURE, peripheral edema, bradycardia, chest pain, hypotension, palpitations, syncope, tachycardia.
GI: abnormal liver function studies, anorexia, constipation, diarrhea, dry mouth, dysgeusia, dyspepsia, nausea, vomiting.
GU: dysuria, nocturia, polyuria, sexual dysfunction, urinary frequency.
Derm: dermatitis, erythema multiforme, flushing, increased sweating, photosensitivity, pruritus/urticaria, rash.
Endo: gynecomastia, hyperglycemia.
Hemat: anemia, leukopenia, thrombocytopenia.
Metab: weight gain.
MS: joint stiffness, muscle cramps.
Neuro: paresthesia, tremor.
Misc: STEVENS-JOHNSON SYNDROME, gingival hyperplasia.

INTERACTIONS

Drug-Drug: ▪ Additive hypotension may occur when used concurrently with **fentanyl, other antihypertensives, nitrates,** acute ingestion of

{} = Available in Canada only.
***CAPITALS indicate life-threatening; underlines indicate most frequent.**

alcohol, or **quinidine** ▪ Antihypertensive effects may be decreased by concurrent use of **NSAIDs** ▪ Concurrent use with **beta-adrenergic blockers, digoxin, disopyramide,** or **phenytoin** may result in bradycardia, conduction defects, or congestive heart failure ▪ **Cimetidine** and **propranolol** may decrease metabolism and increase the risk of toxicity.
Drug-Food: ▪ **Grapefruit juice** increases blood levels.

ROUTE AND DOSAGE

- **PO (Adults):** 5 mg/day (2.5 mg/day in geriatric patients); may increase q 2 wk (range 5–10 mg/day; not to exceed 20 mg/day).

AVAILABILITY

- ***Extended-release tablets:*** 5 mg[Rx], 10 mg[Rx].

TIME/ACTION PROFILE (antihypertensive effect)

	ONSET	PEAK	DURATION
PO	1 hr	2–4 hr	up to 24 hr

NURSING IMPLICATIONS

ASSESSMENT

- **General Info:** Monitor blood pressure and pulse prior to therapy, during dosage titration, and periodically throughout therapy. Monitor ECG periodically during prolonged therapy.
- □ Monitor intake and output ratios and daily weight. Assess for signs of congestive heart failure (peripheral edema, rales/crackles, dyspnea, weight gain, jugular venous distention).
- **Angina:** Assess location, duration, intensity, and precipitating factors of patient's anginal pain.
- ***Lab Test Considerations:*** Total serum calcium concentrations are not affected by calcium channel blockers.
- □ Monitor serum potassium periodically. Hypokalemia increases the risk of arrhythmias and should be corrected.
- □ Monitor renal and hepatic functions periodically during long-term therapy. May cause increase in hepatic enzymes after several days of therapy, which return to normal upon discontinuation of therapy.

POTENTIAL NURSING DIAGNOSES

- Tissue perfusion, altered (Indications).
- Pain (Indications).
- Knowledge deficit, related to medication regimen (Patient/Family Teaching).

IMPLEMENTATION

- **PO:** May be administered without regard to meals. May be administered with meals if GI irritation becomes a problem.
- □ Do not open, crush, break, or chew sustained-release tablets. Empty tablets that appear in stool are not significant.

PATIENT/FAMILY TEACHING

- **General Info:** Advise patient to take medication exactly as directed, even if feeling well. If a dose is missed, take as soon as possible unless almost time for next dose; do not double doses. May need to be discontinued gradually.
- □ Instruct patient on correct technique for monitoring pulse. Instruct patient to contact health care professional if heart rate is <50 bpm.
- □ Caution patient to change positions slowly to minimize orthostatic hypotension.
- □ May cause drowsiness or dizziness. Advise patient to avoid driving or other activities requiring alertness until response to the medication is known.
- □ Instruct patient on importance of maintaining good dental hygiene and seeing dentist frequently for teeth cleaning to prevent tenderness, bleeding, and gingival hyperplasia (gum enlargement).
- □ Instruct patient to avoid concurrent use of alcohol or OTC medications, especially cold preparations, without consulting health care professional.
- □ Advise patient to notify health care professional if irregular heartbeats, dyspnea, swelling of hands and feet, pronounced dizziness, nausea, constipation, or hypotension occurs or if headache is severe or persistent.
- □ Caution patient to wear protective clothing and to use sunscreen to prevent photosensitivity reactions.
- □ Advise patient to inform health care professional of medication regimen before treatment or surgery.
- **Angina:** Instruct patient on concurrent nitrate or beta-blocker therapy to continue taking

both medications as directed and to use SL nitroglycerin as needed for anginal attacks.
- □ Advise patient to contact health care professional if chest pain does not improve or worsens after therapy, occurs with diaphoresis or shortness of breath, or if severe, persistent headache occurs.
- □ Caution patient to discuss exercise restrictions with health care professional prior to exertion.
- ▪ **Hypertension:** Encourage patient to comply with other interventions for hypertension (weight reduction, low-sodium diet, smoking cessation, moderation of alcohol consumption, regular exercise, and stress management). Medication controls but does not cure hypertension.
- □ Instruct patient and family in proper technique for monitoring blood pressure. Advise patient to take blood pressure weekly and to report significant changes.

EVALUATION

Effectiveness of therapy can be demonstrated by: ▪ Decrease in blood pressure ▪ Decrease in frequency and severity of anginal attacks □ Decrease in need for nitrate therapy □ Increase in activity tolerance and sense of well-being.

FENOPROFEN

(fen-oh-**proe**-fen)
Nalfon

CLASSIFICATION(S):
Nonopioid analgesic/Nonsteroidal anti-inflammatory agent

Pregnancy Category B (first trimester)

INDICATIONS

▪ Rheumatoid arthritis ▪ Osteoarthritis ▪ Mild to moderate pain, including dysmenorrhea.

ACTION

▪ Inhibits prostaglandin synthesis. **Therapeutic Effects:** ▪ Suppression of pain and inflammation.

PHARMACOKINETICS

Absorption: Well absorbed from the GI tract.
Distribution: Does not cross the placenta; enters breast milk in low concentrations.
Metabolism and Excretion: Mostly metabolized by the liver. 2–5% excreted unchanged by the kidneys.
Half-life: 3 hr.

CONTRAINDICATIONS AND PRECAUTIONS

Contraindicated in: ▪ Hypersensitivity ▪ Cross-sensitivity may exist with other NSAIDs, including aspirin ▪ Active GI bleeding or ulcer disease.
Use Cautiously in: ▪ Severe cardiovascular, renal, or hepatic disease ▪ Patients with a history of ulcer disease ▪ Pregnancy (not recommended for use during second half of pregnancy) ▪ Lactation or children (safety not established).

ADVERSE REACTIONS AND SIDE EFFECTS*

CNS: drowsiness, headache, dizziness, psychic disturbances.
EENT: blurred vision, tinnitus.
CV: arrhythmias, edema.
GI: GI BLEEDING, HEPATITIS, constipation, dyspepsia, nausea, vomiting, discomfort.
GU: cystitis, hematuria, renal failure.
Derm: rashes.
Hemat: blood dyscrasias, prolonged bleeding time.
Misc: allergic reactions including ANAPHYLAXIS.

INTERACTIONS

Drug-Drug: ▪ Concurrent use with **aspirin** or **antacids** may decrease effectiveness ▪ Additive adverse GI effects with **aspirin,** other **NSAIDs, potassium supplements, glucocorticoids,** or **alcohol** ▪ Chronic use with **acetaminophen** may increase the risk of adverse renal reactions ▪ May increase the risk of hypoglycemia with **insulin** or **oral hypoglycemic agents** ▪ May decrease the effectiveness of **diuretics** or **antihypertensive** therapy ▪ May increase serum **lithium** levels and increase the risk of toxicity ▪ Increases the risk of toxicity from **methotrexate** ▪ Increased risk of bleeding with **cefamandole, cefotetan, cefoperazone, valproic**

***CAPITALS indicate life-threatening; underlines indicate most frequent.**

acid, plicamycin, heparin, thrombolytic agents, or **oral anticoagulants** ▪ Increased risk of adverse hematologic reactions with **antineoplastic agents** or **radiation therapy** ▪ **Phenobarbital** may increase metabolism and decrease effectiveness of fenoprofen ▪ May increase the risk of nephrotoxicity with **cyclosporine.**

ROUTE AND DOSAGE

❑ **Anti-inflammatory**

▪ **PO (Adults):** 300–600 mg 3–4 times daily (not to exceed 3.2 g/day).

❑ **Analgesic**

▪ **PO (Adults):** 200 mg q 4–6 hr.

AVAILABILITY

▪ ***Capsules:*** 200 mg[Rx], 300 mg[Rx] ▪ ***Tablets:*** 600 mg[Rx].

TIME/ACTION PROFILE

	ONSET	PEAK	DURATION
PO (analgesic activity)	15–30 min	1–2 hr	4–6 hr
PO (anti-inflammatory activity)	several days	2–3 wk	UK

NURSING IMPLICATIONS

ASSESSMENT

▪ **General Info:** Patients who have asthma, aspirin-induced allergy, and nasal polyps are at increased risk for developing hypersensitivity reactions. Monitor for rhinitis, asthma, and urticaria.

▪ **Arthritis:** Assess pain and range of movement prior to and 1–2 hr following administration.

▪ **Pain:** Assess pain (type, location, and intensity) prior to and 1–2 hr following administration.

▪ ***Lab Test Considerations:*** May cause prolonged bleeding time.

□ May cause decreased hemoglobin, hematocrit, leukocyte, and platelet counts.

□ Monitor liver function tests periodically during therapy. May cause elevated serum alkaline phosphatase, LDH, AST, and ALT concentrations.

□ Monitor BUN, serum creatinine, and electrolytes periodically during therapy. May cause increased BUN, serum creatinine, and electrolyte concentrations and decreased urine electrolyte concentrations.

□ May cause decreased serum and increased urine uric acid concentrations.

POTENTIAL NURSING DIAGNOSES

▪ Pain (Indications).

▪ Physical mobility, impaired (Indications).

▪ Knowledge deficit, related to medication regimen (Patient/Family Teaching).

IMPLEMENTATION

▪ **General Info:** Administration in higher than recommended doses does not provide increased effectiveness but may cause increased side effects.

□ Coadministration with opioid analgesics may have additive analgesic effects and may permit lower opioid doses.

▪ **PO:** For rapid initial effect, administer 30 min before or 2 hr after meals. Administer after meals or with food or an antacid containing aluminum or magnesium to minimize gastric irritation.

▪ **Dysmenorrhea:** Administer as soon as possible after the onset of menses. Prophylactic use has not been proved effective.

PATIENT/FAMILY TEACHING

□ Advise patient to take this medication with a full glass of water and to remain in an upright position for 15–30 min after administration.

□ Instruct patient to take medication exactly as directed. If a dose is missed, take as soon as remembered, but not if almost time for next dose. Do not double doses.

□ May cause drowsiness or dizziness. Advise patient to avoid driving or other activities requiring alertness until response to the medication is known.

□ Caution patient to avoid concurrent use of alcohol, aspirin, acetaminophen, other NSAIDs, or other OTC medications without consulting health care professional.

□ Instruct patient to notify health care professional of medication regimen prior to treatment or surgery.

□ Advise patient to consult health care professional if rash, itching, visual disturbances, tinnitus, weight gain, edema, black stools, persistent headache, or influenza-like syndrome (chills, fever, muscle aches, pain) occurs.

EVALUATION

Effectiveness of therapy can be demonstrated by: ▪ Decrease in severity of pain ▪ Improved joint mobility. Partial arthritic relief is usually seen within a few days, but maximum effects may require 2–3 wk of continuous therapy. Patients who do not respond to one NSAID may respond to another.

FENTANYL DERIVATIVES (parenteral)

alfentanil
(al-**fen**-ta-nil)
Alfenta

fentanyl
(**fen**-ta-nil)
Sublimaze

remifentanil
(re-mi-**fen**-ta-nill)
Ultiva

sufentanil
(soo-**fen**-ta-nil)
Sufenta

CLASSIFICATION(S):
Opioid analgesics (agonists)

Schedule II
Pregnancy Category C

INDICATIONS

▪ Analgesic supplement to general anesthesia; usually with other agents (ultra–short acting barbiturates, neuromuscular blockers, and inhalation anesthetics) to produce balanced anesthesia ▪ Induction/maintenance of anesthesia (with oxygen or oxygen/nitrous oxide and a neuromuscular blocker) ▪ **Fentanyl:** Neuroleptanalgesia/neuroleptanesthesia (with or without nitrous oxide) ▪ Supplement to regional/local anesthesia ▪ Pre- and postoperative analgesia (use limited by short duration of action) ▪ **Alfentanil, remifentanil:** Analgesic component for monitored anesthesia care (MAC).

ACTION

▪ Bind to opiate receptors in the CNS, altering the response to and perception of pain ▪ Produce CNS depression. **Therapeutic Effects:** ▪ Supplement in anesthesia ▪ Decreased pain.

PHARMACOKINETICS

Absorption: *Alfentanil, remifentanil, sufentanil*—IV administration results in complete bioavailability; *fentanyl*—well absorbed following IM administration.
Distribution: *Alfentanil, sufentanil*—do not readily penetrate adipose tissue; cross the placenta, enter breast milk. *Fentanyl*—UK; *remifentanil*—widely distributed.
Metabolism and Excretion: *Alfentanil*—>95% metabolized by the liver; *fentanyl*—mostly metabolized by the liver, 10–25% excreted unchanged by the kidneys; *remifentanil*—metabolized by blood and tissue esterases, metabolites are excreted by the kidneys; *sufentanil*—mostly metabolized by the liver, some metabolism in small intestine.
Half-life: *Alfentanil*—60–130 min; *fentanyl*—5–15 hr (increased after cardiopulmonary bypass and in elderly patients); *remifentanil*—3–10 min; *sufentanil*—2.7 hr (increased during cardiopulmonary bypass).

CONTRAINDICATIONS AND PRECAUTIONS

Contraindicated in: ▪ Hypersensitivity; cross-sensitivity among agents may occur ▪ Known intolerance ▪ Remifentanil is not to be given epidurally or intrathecally (because of glycine in the formulation).
Use Cautiously in: ▪ Geriatric, debilitated, or critically ill patients (decrease starting dose of remifentanil by 50% in patients >65 yr) ▪ *Remifentanil*—morbidly obese patients (determine dose by Ideal Body Weight (IBW) if >30% over IBW) ▪ Diabetics ▪ Severe pulmonary or hepatic disease ▪ CNS tumors ▪ Increased intracranial pressure ▪ Head trauma ▪ Adrenal insufficiency ▪ Undiagnosed abdominal pain ▪ Hypothyroidism ▪ Alcoholism ▪ Cardiac disease (arrhythmias) ▪ Pregnancy, lactation, and children <2 yr (safety not established in younger age groups for some agents; sufentanil has been used in women undergoing cesarean section—drowsiness may occur in infant).

ADVERSE REACTIONS AND SIDE EFFECTS*

CNS: confusion (↓ with alfentanil), paradoxical excitation/delirium, postoperative depression, postoperative drowsiness (↓ with alfentanil).
EENT: blurred/double vision.
Resp: APNEA, LARYNGOSPASM, allergic bronchospasm, respiratory depression.
CV: arrhythmias (↓ with sufentanil), bradycardia, circulatory depression, hypotension.
GI: biliary spasm, nausea/vomiting (↓ with sufentanil).
Derm: facial itching.
MS: skeletal and thoracic muscle rigidity.

INTERACTIONS

Drug-Drug: ▪ Avoid use in patients who have received **MAO inhibitors** within the previous 14 days (may produce unpredictable, potentially fatal reactions) ▪ Additive CNS and respiratory depression with other **CNS depressants**, including **alcohol, antihistamines, antidepressants**, other **sedative/hypnotics,** and other **opioids** ▪ Increased risk of hypotension with **benzodiazepines** ▪ **Cimetidine, erythromycin**, or other **agents that decrease hepatic metabolism** may prolong duration of recovery from alfentanil ▪ **Nalbuphine, buprenorphine, dezocine**, or **pentazocine** may decrease analgesia.

ROUTE AND DOSAGE

❑ **Alfentanil**

❑ ***Incremental Injection (Duration of Anesthesia ≤30 min)***

▪ **IV (Adults):** *Induction*—8–20 mcg/kg. *Maintenance*—3–5 mcg/kg increments or 0.5–1.0 mcg/kg/min (total dose 8–40 mcg/kg).

❑ ***Incremental Injection Period (Duration of Anesthesia 30–60 min)***

▪ **IV (Adults):** *Induction*—20–50 mcg/kg. *Maintenance*—5–15 mcg/kg increments (up to total dose of 75 mg/kg).

❑ ***Continuous Infusion (Duration of Anesthesia >45 min)***

▪ **IV (Adults):** *Induction*—50–75 mcg/kg. *Maintenance*—0.5–3.0 mcg/kg/min (average infusion rate 1–1.5 mcg/kg/min). Infusion rate should be decreased by 30–50% after 1st hour of maintenance. If lightening occurs, infusion rate may be increased up to 4 mcg/kg/min or boluses of 7 mcg/kg may be administered.

❑ ***Anesthetic Induction (Duration of Anesthesia >45 min)***

▪ **IV (Adults):** 130–245 mcg/kg followed by 0.5–1.5 mcg/kg/min or general anesthesia.

❑ ***Monitored Anesthesia Care (MAC)***

▪ **IV (Adults):** *Induction*—3–8 mcg/kg. *Maintenance*—3–5 mcg/kg q 20 min *or* 0.25–1 mcg/kg/min (total dose 3–40 mcg/kg).

❑ **Fentanyl**

❑ ***Preoperative Use***

▪ **IM (Adults):** 50–100 mcg (0.05–0.1 mg) or 0.7–1.4 mcg/kg 30–60 min before surgery.

❑ ***Adjunct to General Anesthesia***

▪ **IV (Adults):** *Low dose–minor surgery*—2 mcg (0.002 mg)/kg. *Moderate dose–major surgery*—2–20 mcg (0.002–0.02 mg)/kg. *High dose–major surgery*—20–50 mcg (0.02–0.05 mg)/kg.

❑ ***Adjunct to Regional Anesthesia***

▪ **IM, IV (Adults):** 50–100 mcg (0.05–0.1 mg) or 0.7–1.4 mcg/kg.

❑ ***Postoperative Use (Recovery Room)***

▪ **IM (Adults):** 50–100 mcg or 0.7–1.4 mcg/kg; may repeat in 1–2 hr.

❑ ***General Anesthesia***

▪ **IV (Adults):** 50–100 mcg (0.05–0.1 mg)/kg (up to 150 mcg/kg).
▪ **IV (Children 2–12 yr):** 2–3 mcg/kg.

❑ **Remifentanil**

❑ ***Induction of Anesthesia***

▪ **IV (Adults and Children ≥2 yr):** 0.5–1 mcg/kg/min continuous infusion (an initial dose of 1 mcg/kg may be given over 30–60 sec).

***CAPITALS indicate life-threatening; underlines indicate most frequent.**

F

❑ ***Maintenance of Anesthesia***

- **IV (Adults and Children ≥2 yr):** *With nitrous oxide 66%*—0.4 mcg/kg/min (range 0.1–2 mcg/kg/min); *with isoflurane (0.4–1.5 MAC) or propofol (100–200 mcg/kg/min)*—0.25 mcg/kg/min (range 0.05–2 mcg/kg/min). Supplemental bolus doses of 1 mcg/kg may be given.

❑ ***Continuation as an Analgesic in Immediately Postoperative Period***

- **IV (Adults and Children ≥2 yr):** 0.1 mcg/kg/min (range 0.025–0.2 mcg/kg/min).

❑ ***Monitored Anesthesia Care (Remifentanil Alone)***

- **IV (Adults and Children ≥2 yr):** *Single IV dose*—1 mcg/kg given 90 sec before local anesthetic *or continuous infusion*—0.1 mcg/kg/min beginning 5 min before local anesthetic, then 0.05 mcg/kg/min after local anesthetic (range 0.025–0.2 mcg/kg/min).

❑ ***Monitored Anesthesia Care (Remifentanil + Midazolam)***

- **IV (Adults and Children ≥2 yr):** *Single IV dose*—0.5 mcg/kg given 90 sec before local anesthetic *or continuous infusion*—0.05 mcg/kg/min beginning 5 min before local anesthetic, then 0.025 mcg/kg/min after local anesthetic (range 0.025–0.2 mcg/kg/min).

❑ **Sufentanil**

❑ ***Low-Dose Anesthesia Adjunct***

- **IV (Adults):** 0.5–1 mcg/kg initially, supplemental doses of 10–25 mcg may be given as needed (not to exceed 1 mcg/kg/hr when administered with nitrous oxide and oxygen).

❑ ***Moderate-Dose Anesthesia Adjunct***

- **IV (Adults):** 2–8 mcg/kg initially, supplemental doses of 10–50 mcg may be given as needed (not to exceed 1 mcg/kg/hr when administered with nitrous oxide and oxygen).

❑ ***Primary Anesthesia (with 100% Oxygen)***

- **IV (Adults):** 8–30 mcg/kg initially, supplemental doses of 25–50 mcg may be given as needed.
- **IV (Children):** *Cardiovascular surgery*—10–25 mcg/kg initially, followed by maintenance doses of up to 25–50 mcg.

AVAILABILITY

❑ **Alfentanil**

- ***Injection:*** 500 mg/ml[Rx].

❑ **Fentanyl**

- ***Injection:*** 0.05 mg/ml[Rx] ▪ ***In combination with:*** droperidol (Innovar)[Rx]. See Appendix A.

❑ **Remifentanil**

- ***Powder for injection:*** 1-mg, 2-mg, and 5-mg vials[Rx].

❑ **Sufentanil**

- ***Injection:*** 50 mcg/ml in 1-ml, 2-ml, and 5-ml ampules[Rx].

TIME/ACTION PROFILE (analgesia*)

	ONSET	PEAK	DURATION
Alfentanil IV	immediate	1–1.5 min	5–10 min†
Fentanyl IM	7–15 min	20–30 min	1–2 hr
Fentanyl IV	1–2 min	3–5 min	0.5–1 hr
Remifentanil IV	rapid	3–5 min	5–10 min
Sufentanil IV	within 1 min	UK	5 min

*Respiratory depression may last longer than analgesia.
†Longer in children.

NURSING IMPLICATIONS

ASSESSMENT

- **General Info:** Monitor respiratory rate and blood pressure frequently throughout therapy. Report significant changes immediately. The respiratory depressant effects of fentanyl derivatives may last longer than the analgesic effects. Initial doses of other opioids should be reduced by ¼–⅓ of the usually recommended dose. Monitor closely.
- **IM:** ❑ Assess type, location, and intensity of pain prior to and 30 min following IM administration or 3–5 min following IV administration when fentanyl derivatives are used to treat pain.
- ***Lab Test Considerations:*** May cause elevated serum amylase and lipase concentrations.
- ***Toxicity and Overdose:*** Symptoms of toxicity include respiratory depression, hypotension, arrhythmias, bradycardia, and asystole. Atropine may be used to treat bradycardia. If respiratory depression persists following surgery, prolonged mechanical ventilation may be required. If an opioid antagonist is required to reverse respiratory depression or coma, naloxone (Narcan) is the antidote. Dilute the

0.4-mg ampule of naloxone in 10 ml of 0.9% NaCl and administer 0.5 ml (0.02 mg) by direct IV push every 2 min. For children and patients weighing <40 kg, dilute 0.1 mg of naloxone in 10 ml of 0.9% NaCl for a concentration of 10 mcg/ml and administer 0.5 mcg/kg every 1–2 min. Titrate dose to avoid withdrawal, seizures, and severe pain. Administration of naloxone in these circumstances, especially in cardiac patients, has resulted in hypertension and tachycardia, occasionally causing left ventricular failure and pulmonary edema.

POTENTIAL NURSING DIAGNOSES

- Pain (Indications).
- Breathing pattern, ineffective (Adverse Reactions).
- Injury, risk for (Side Effects).

IMPLEMENTATION

- **General Info:** Benzodiazepines may be administered prior to or following administration of fentanyl derivatives to reduce the induction dose requirements, decrease the time to loss of consciousness, and produce amnesia. This combination may also increase the risk of hypotension.
- ☐ Opioid antagonist, oxygen, and resuscitative equipment should be readily available during the administration of fentanyl. Fentanyl derivatives should be administered IV only in monitored anesthesia care settings (operating room, emergency department, ICU) with immediate access to life support equipment and should be administered only by personnel trained in resuscitation and emergency airway management.
- **Direct IV:** Administer undiluted.
- ***Rate:*** Injections should be administered slowly over 1–3 min. Slow IV administration may reduce the incidence and severity of muscle rigidity, bradycardia, or hypotension. Neuromuscular blocking agents may be administered concurrently to decrease muscle rigidity.

☐ Alfentanil

- **Intermittent Infusion:** May also be diluted with D5W, 0.9% NaCl, D5/0.9% NaCl, D5/LR, or lactated Ringer's solution in a concentration of 25–80 mcg/ml.
- **Syringe Compatibility:** ▪ atracurium.
- **Y-Site Compatibility:** ▪ etomidate.
- **Y-Site Incompatibility:** ▪ thiopental.

☐ Fentanyl

- **Intermittent Infusion:** May be diluted in D5W or 0.9% NaCl.
- **Syringe Compatibility:** ▪ atracurium ▪ atropine ▪ butorphanol ▪ chlorpromazine ▪ cimetidine ▪ dimenhydrinate ▪ diphenhydramine ▪ droperidol ▪ heparin ▪ hydromorphone ▪ meperidine ▪ metoclopramide ▪ midazolam ▪ morphine ▪ pentazocine ▪ perphenazine ▪ prochlorperazine edisylate ▪ promazine ▪ promethazine ▪ ranitidine ▪ scopolamine.
- **Syringe Incompatibility:** ▪ pentobarbital.
- **Y-Site Compatibility:** ▪ atracurium ▪ enalaprilat ▪ esmolol ▪ etomidate ▪ heparin ▪ hydrocortisone sodium succinate ▪ labetalol ▪ lorazepam ▪ midazolam ▪ nafcillin ▪ pancuronium ▪ potassium chloride ▪ thiopental ▪ vecuronium ▪ vitamin B complex with C.
- **Additive Compatibility:** ▪ bupivacaine.
- **Additive Incompatibility:** ▪ methohexital ▪ pentobarbital ▪ thiopental.

☐ Remifentanil

- **Intermittent Infusion:** May be diluted in sterile water, D5W, D5/0.9% NaCl, 0.9% NaCl, or 0.45% NaCl in concentrations of 20–250 mcg/ml.
- **Y-Site Compatibility:** ▪ propofol.

☐ Sufentanil

- **Intermittent Infusion:** May be diluted with D5W.
- **Syringe Compatibility:** ▪ atracurium ▪ atropine ▪ dexamethasone ▪ diphenhydramine ▪ haloperidol ▪ hydroxyzine ▪ ketorolac ▪ methotrimeprazine ▪ metoclopramide ▪ midazolam ▪ prochlorperazine ▪ scopolamine.
- **Syringe Incompatibility:** ▪ diazepam ▪ lorazepam ▪ phenobarbital ▪ phenytoin.
- **Y-Site Compatibility:** ▪ atropine ▪ dexamethasone ▪ diazepam ▪ diphenhydramine ▪ etomidate ▪ haloperidol ▪ hydroxyzine ▪ ketorolac ▪ methotrimeprazine ▪ metoclopramide ▪ midazolam ▪ phenobarbital ▪ prochlorperazine ▪ scopolamine.
- **Y-Site Incompatibility:** ▪ lorazepam ▪ phenytoin ▪ thiopental.

PATIENT/FAMILY TEACHING

- ☐ Discuss the use of anesthetic agents and the sensations to expect with the patient prior to surgery.

- □ Explain pain assessment scale to patient.
- □ Caution patient to change positions slowly to minimize orthostatic hypotension.
- □ Medication causes dizziness and drowsiness. Advise patient to call for assistance during ambulation and transfer and to avoid driving or other activities requiring alertness for 24 hr after administration during outpatient surgery.
- □ Instruct patient to avoid alcohol or other CNS depressants for 24 hr after administration for outpatient surgery.

EVALUATION

Effectiveness of therapy can be demonstrated by: ▪ General quiescence □ Reduced motor activity ▪ Pronounced analgesia.

FENTANYL (transdermal)

(**fen**-ta-nil)

Duragesic

CLASSIFICATION(S):

Opioid analgesic (agonist)

Schedule II

Pregnancy Category C

INDICATIONS

▪ Management of chronic pain in patients requiring opioid analgesic therapy ▪ Transdermal fentanyl is not recommended for the control of postoperative, mild, or intermittent pain.

ACTION

▪ Binds to opiate receptors in the CNS, altering the response to and perception of pain. **Therapeutic Effects:** ▪ Decrease in severity of chronic pain.

PHARMACOKINETICS

Absorption: Well absorbed (92% of dose) through skin surface under transdermal patch, creating a depot in the upper skin layers. Release from transdermal system into systemic circulation increases gradually to a constant rate providing continuous delivery for 72 hr.

Distribution: Crosses the placenta; enters breast milk.

Metabolism and Excretion: Mostly metabolized by the liver; 10–25% excreted unchanged by the kidneys.

Half-life: 17 hr following removal of a single application patch, increases to 21 hr following removal of multiple patches (because of continued release from deposition of drug in skin layers).

CONTRAINDICATIONS AND PRECAUTIONS

Contraindicated in: ▪ Hypersensitivity to fentanyl or adhesives ▪ Known intolerance ▪ Acute pain (onset not rapid enough) ▪ Alcohol intolerance (small amounts of alcohol released into skin).

Use Cautiously in: ▪ Patients >60 yr, cachectic or debilitated patients (dosage reduction suggested because of altered drug disposition) ▪ Diabetics ▪ Patients with severe pulmonary or hepatic disease ▪ CNS tumors ▪ Increased intracranial pressure ▪ Head trauma ▪ Adrenal insufficiency ▪ Undiagnosed abdominal pain ▪ Hypothyroidism ▪ Alcoholism ▪ Cardiac disease (particularly bradyarrhythmias) ▪ Pregnancy, lactation, and children <2 yr (safety not established) ▪ Fever (increases release of fentanyl from delivery system) ▪ Titration period (additional analgesics may be required).

ADVERSE REACTIONS AND SIDE EFFECTS*

CNS: <u>confusion</u>, <u>sedation</u>, <u>weakness</u>, dizziness, restlessness.

Resp: APNEA, bronchoconstriction, laryngospasm, respiratory depression.

CV: bradycardia.

GI: <u>anorexia</u>, <u>constipation</u>, <u>dry mouth</u>, <u>nausea</u>, <u>vomiting</u>.

Derm: <u>sweating</u>, erythema.

Local: application site reactions.

MS: skeletal and thoracic muscle rigidity.

Misc: physical dependence, psychological dependence.

INTERACTIONS

Drug-Drug: ▪ Avoid use in patients who have received **MAO inhibitors** within the previous 14 days (may produce unpredictable, potentially fatal reations) ▪ Additive CNS and respiratory depression with other **CNS depressants,** in-

***CAPITALS indicate life-threatening; <u>underlines</u> indicate most frequent.**

cluding **alcohol, antihistamines, antidepressants, sedative/hypnotics,** and other **opioids.**

ROUTE AND DOSAGE

- **Transdermal (Adults):** 25 mcg/hr is the initial dose in patients who have not been receiving opioids prior to institution of transdermal fentanyl. To calculate the dosage of transdermal fentanyl required in patients who are already receiving opioid analgesics, assess the 24-hr requirement of currently used opioid. Using the equianalgesic table in Appendix B, convert this to an equivalent amount of morphine/24 hr. Conversion to fentanyl transdermal may be accomplished by using the fentanyl conversion table (Appendix B). During dosage titration, additional short-acting opioids should be available for any breakthrough pain that may occur. Morphine 10 mg IM or 60 mg PO q 4 hr (60 mg/24 hr IM or 360 mg/24 hr PO) is considered to be approximately equivalent to transdermal fentanyl 100 mcg/hr. Transdermal patch lasts 72 hr in most patients. Some patients require a new patch every 48 hr.
- **Transdermal (Adults >60 yr, Debilitated, or Cachectic Patients):** Initial dose should be 25 mcg/hr unless previous opioid use was >135 mg morphine PO/day (or other opioid equivalent).

AVAILABILITY

- ***Transdermal systems:*** 25 mcg/hr[Rx], 50 mcg/hr[Rx], 75 mcg/hr[Rx], 100 mcg/hr[Rx].

TIME/ACTION PROFILE (decreased pain)

	ONSET	PEAK	DURATION
Transdermal	6 hr*	12–24 hr	72 hr†

*Achievement of blood levels associated with analgesia. Maximal response and dose titration may take up to 6 days.
†While patch is worn.

NURSING IMPLICATIONS

ASSESSMENT

- ☐ Assess type, location, and intensity of pain prior to and 24 hr after application and periodically throughout therapy. Pain should be monitored frequently during initiation of therapy and dosage changes to assess need for supplementary analgesics for breakthrough pain.
- ☐ Assess blood pressure, pulse, and respirations before and periodically during administration. If respiratory rate is <10/min, assess level of sedation. Physical stimulation may be sufficient to prevent significant hypoventilation. Dose may need to be decreased by 25–50%. Initial drowsiness will diminish with continued use.
- ☐ Prolonged use may lead to physical and psychological dependence and tolerance. This should not prevent patient from receiving adequate analgesia. Most patients who receive opioid analgesics for pain do not develop psychological dependence.
- ☐ Progressively higher doses may be required to relieve pain with long-term therapy. It may take up to 6 days after increasing doses to reach equilibrium, so patients should wear higher dose through 2 applications before increasing dose again.
- ☐ Assess bowel function routinely. Prevention of constipation should be instituted with increased intake of fluids and bulk, and laxatives to minimize constipating effects. Stimulant laxatives should be administered routinely if opioid use exceeds 2–3 days, unless contraindicated.
- ***Lab Test Considerations:*** May increase plasma amylase and lipase levels.
- ***Toxicity and Overdose:*** If an opioid antagonist is required to reverse respiratory depression or coma, naloxone (Narcan) is the antidote. Dilute the 0.4-mg ampule of naloxone in 10 ml of 0.9% NaCl and administer 0.5 ml (0.02 mg) by direct IV push every 2 min. For patients weighing <40 kg, dilute 0.1 mg of naloxone in 10 ml of 0.9% NaCl for a concentration of 10 mcg/ml and administer 0.5 mcg/kg every 1–2 min. Titrate dose to avoid withdrawal, seizures, and severe pain. Monitor patient closely; dose may need to be repeated or may need to be administered as an infusion because of long duration of action despite removal of patch.

POTENTIAL NURSING DIAGNOSES

- Pain (Indications).
- Injury, risk for (Side Effects).
- Knowledge deficit, related to medication regimen (Patient/Family Teaching).

F

IMPLEMENTATION

- **General Info:** Supplemental doses of short-acting opioid analgesics should be used to manage pain until relief is obtained with the transdermal system. Patients may continue to require supplemental opioids for break-through pain. If >100 mcg/hr are required, use multiple systems.
- □ Dosage is titrated based on the patient's report of pain until adequate analgesia (50% reduction in patient's pain rating on numerical or visual analogue scale or patient reports satisfactory relief) is attained. Dose is determined by calculating the previous 24-hr analgesic requirement and converting to the equianalgesic morphine dose using Appendix B. The conversion ratio from morphine to transdermal fentanyl is conservative; 50% of patients may require a dose increase after initial application. Increase after 3 days based on required daily doses of supplemental analgesics. Increases should be based on ratio of 90 mg/24 hr of oral morphine to 25 mcg/hr increase in transdermal fentanyl dose. Patients requiring >300 mcg/hr may need other methods of opioid analgesic administration.
- □ Coadministration with nonopioid analgesics may have additive analgesic effects and permit lower opioid doses.
- □ To convert to another opioid analgesic, remove transdermal fentanyl system and begin treatment with half the equianalgesic dose of the new analgesic in 12–18 hr.
- □ Medication should be discontinued gradually after long-term use to prevent withdrawal symptoms.
- **Transdermal:** Apply system to upper torso on a flat, nonirritated, and nonirradiated site. If skin preparation is necessary, use clear water and clip, do not shave, hair. Allow skin to dry completely before application. Apply immediately after removing from package and press firmly in place with palm of hand for 10–20 sec, especially around the edges, to make sure contact is complete. For continued use, remove used system and fold so that adhesive edges are together. Flush system down toilet immediately upon removal. Apply new system to a different site. Discard unused systems by removing from pouch and flushing down toilet.

PATIENT/FAMILY TEACHING

- □ Instruct patient in how and when to ask for pain medication.
- □ Instruct patient in correct method for application and disposal of transdermal system.
- □ Medication may cause drowsiness or dizziness. Caution patient to call for assistance when ambulating or smoking and to avoid driving or other activities requiring alertness until response to medication is known.
- □ Advise patient to change positions slowly to minimize dizziness.
- □ Caution patient to avoid concurrent use of alcohol or other CNS depressants with this medication.
- □ Advise patient that fever, electric blankets, heating pads, saunas, hot tubs, and heated water beds increase the release of fentanyl from the patch.
- □ Advise patient that good oral hygiene, frequent mouth rinses, and sugarless gum or candy may decrease dry mouth.

EVALUATION

Effectiveness of therapy can be demonstrated by: ▪ Decrease in severity of pain without a significant alteration in level of consciousness, respiratory status, or blood pressure.

FEXOFENADINE

(fex-oh-**fen**-a-deen)
Allegra

CLASSIFICATION(S):
Antihistamine

Pregnancy Category C

INDICATIONS

▪ Relief of symptoms of seasonal allergic rhinitis.

ACTION

▪ Antagonizes the effects of histamine at peripheral histamine-1 (H_1) receptors, including pruritus and urticaria ▪ Also has a drying effect on the nasal musosa. **Therapeutic Effects:** ▪ Decreased sneezing, rhinorrhea, itchy eyes, nose/throat associated with seasonal allergies.

PHARMACOKINETICS

Absorption: Rapidly absorbed following oral administration.
Distribution: UK.
Metabolism and Excretion: 80% excreted in urine, 11% in feces.
Half-life: 14.4 hr (increased in renal impairment).

CONTRAINDICATIONS AND PRECAUTIONS

Contraindicated in: ▪ Hypersensitivity.
Use Cautiously in: ▪ Impaired renal function (increased dosing interval recommended) ▪ Pregnancy, lactation, or children <12 yr (safety not established).

ADVERSE REACTIONS AND SIDE EFFECTS

CNS: drowsiness, fatigue.
GI: dyspepsia.
Endo: dysmenorrhea.

INTERACTIONS

Drug-Drug: ▪ None significant.

ROUTE AND DOSAGE

▪ **PO (Adults and Children ≥12 yr):** 60 mg twice daily.

AVAILABILITY

▪ ***Capsules:*** 60 mg[Rx].

TIME/ACTION PROFILE (antihistaminic effect)

	ONSET	PEAK	DURATION
PO	within 1 hr	2–3 hr	12 hr

NURSING IMPLICATIONS

ASSESSMENT

- Assess allergy symptoms (rhinitis, conjunctivitis, hives) prior to and periodically throughout therapy.
- Assess lung sounds and character of bronchial secretions. Maintain fluid intake of 1500–2000 ml/day to decrease viscosity of secretions.

▪ ***Lab Test Considerations:*** Will cause false-negative reactions on allergy skin tests; discontinue 3 days prior to testing.

POTENTIAL NURSING DIAGNOSES

▪ Airway clearance, ineffective (Indications).
▪ Injury, risk for (Adverse Reactions).
▪ Knowledge deficit, related to medication regimen (Patient/Family Teaching).

IMPLEMENTATION

▪ **PO:** Administer with food or milk to decrease GI irritation.

PATIENT/FAMILY TEACHING

- Instruct patient to take medication as directed. If a dose is missed, take as soon as remembered unless almost time for next dose.
- Inform patient that drug may cause drowsiness, although it is less likely to occur than with other antihistamines. Avoid driving or other activities requiring alertness until response to drug is known.
- Instruct patient to contact health care professional if symptoms persist.

EVALUATION

Effectiveness of therapy can be demonstrated by: ▪ Decrease in allergic symptoms.

F

FILGRASTIM

(fill-**grass**-stim)
Neupogen, G-CSF, granulocyte-colony stimulating factor

CLASSIFICATION(S):
Colony-stimulating factor

Pregnancy Category C

INDICATIONS

▪ Prevention of febrile neutropenia and associated infection in patients who have received bone marrow–depressing antineoplastic agents for the treatment of nonmyeloid malignancies or acute myelocytic leukemia ▪ Adjunct therapy in bone marrow transplantation ▪ Management of patients with severe chronic neutropenia. **Unlabeled Uses:** ▪ Neutropenia associated with HIV infection.

ACTION

▪ A glycoprotein that binds to and stimulates immature neutrophils to divide and differentiate.

Also activates mature neutrophils. **Therapeutic Effects:** ▪ Decreased incidence of infection in patients who are neutropenic from chemotherapy or other causes.

PHARMACOKINETICS

Absorption: Well absorbed following subcutaneous administration.
Distribution: UK.
Metabolism and Excretion: UK.
Half-life: 3.5 hr.

CONTRAINDICATIONS AND PRECAUTIONS

Contraindicated in: ▪ Hypersensitivity to filgrastim or *Escherichia coli*–derived proteins.
Use Cautiously in: ▪ Pregnancy, lactation, or children (safety not established) ▪ Malignancy with myeloid characteristics ▪ Pre-existing cardiac disease.

ADVERSE REACTIONS AND SIDE EFFECTS*

Hemat: excessive leukocytosis.
Local: pain, redness at SC site.
MS: <u>medullary bone pain</u>.

INTERACTIONS

Drug-Drug: ▪ Simultaneous use with **antineoplastic agents** may have adverse effects on rapidly proliferating neutrophils—avoid use for 24 hr before and 24 hr following chemotherapy.

ROUTE AND DOSAGE

❑ Following Myelosuppressive Chemotherapy

- **IV, SC (Adults):** 5 mcg/kg/day as a single injection daily for up to 2 wk. Dosage may be increased by 5 mcg/kg during each cycle of chemotherapy depending on blood counts.

❑ Following Bone Marrow Transplantation

- **IV, SC (Adults):** 10 mcg/kg/day as a 4- or 24-hr IV infusion or as a continuous SC infusion; initiate at least 24 hr after chemotherapy and at least 24 hr following bone marrow transplantation. Subsequent dosage is adjusted according to blood counts.

❑ Severe Chronic Neutropenia

- **SC (Adults):** *Congenital neutropenia*—6 mcg/kg twice daily. *Idiopathic/cyclical neutropenia*—5 mcg/kg daily (decrease if ANC remains >10,000/mm³).

AVAILABILITY

- ***Injection:*** 300 mcg/ml in 1- and 1.6-ml vials[Rx].

TIME/ACTION PROFILE

	ONSET	PEAK	DURATION
IV, SC	UK	UK	4 days†

†Return of neutrophil count to baseline.

NURSING IMPLICATIONS

ASSESSMENT

- ❑ Monitor heart rate, blood pressure, and respiratory status prior to and periodically during therapy.
- ❑ Assess bone pain throughout therapy. Pain is usually mild to moderate and controllable with nonopioid analgesics but may require treatment with opioid analgesics, especially in patients receiving high-dose IV therapy.
- ▪ ***Lab Test Considerations:*** *Following chemotherapy,* obtain a CBC with differential, including examination for the presence of blast cells, and platelet count prior to chemotherapy and twice weekly during therapy to avoid leukocytosis. Monitor ANC. A transient rise is seen 1–2 days after initiation of therapy, but therapy should not be discontinued until ANC >10,000/mm³.
- ❑ *Following bone marrow transplant,* the daily dose is titrated by the neutrophil response. When the ANC is >1000/mm³ for 3 consecutive days, the dose should be reduced by 5 mcg/kg³/day. If the ANC remains >1000/mm³ for 3 or more consecutive days, filgrastim is discontinued. If the ANC decreases to <1000/mm³, filgrastim should be resumed at 5 mcg/kg/day.
- ❑ *For chronic severe neutropenia,* monitor CBC with differential and platelet count twice weekly during initial 4 wk of therapy and during 2 wk after any dose adjustment.
- ❑ May cause decreased platelet count and tran-

*CAPITALS indicate life-threatening; <u>underlines</u> indicate most frequent.

sient increases in uric acid, LDH, and alkaline phosphatase concentrations.

POTENTIAL NURSING DIAGNOSES

- Infection, risk for (Indications).
- Pain (Side Effects).
- Knowledge deficit, related to medication regimen (Patient/Family Teaching).

IMPLEMENTATION

- Administer no earlier than 24 hr following cytotoxic chemotherapy, at least 24 hr after bone marrow infusion, and not during the 24 hr before administration of chemotherapy.
- Refrigerate; do not freeze. Do not shake. May warm to room temperature for up to 6 hr prior to injection. Discard if left at room temperature for >6 hr. Vial is for 1-time use only.
- **SC:** If dose requires >1 ml of solution, may be divided into 2 injection sites.
- May also be administered as a continuous SC infusion over 24 hr following bone marrow transplantation.
- **Continuous Infusion:** Dilute in D5W to produce a concentration of >15 mcg of filgrastim/ml. If the final concentration is 2–15 mcg/ml, human albumin in a concentration of 2 mg/ml must be added to D5W before filgrastim to prevent adsorption of the components of the drug delivery system. Refrigerate; do not freeze. Do not shake. May warm to room temperature for up to 6 hr prior to injection. Vial is for 1-time use only.
- ***Rate:*** *Following chemotherapy,* dose is administered via infusion over 15–30 min.
- Dose *following chemotherapy* may also be administered as a continuous infusion.
- *Following bone marrow transplant,* dose should be administered as an infusion over 4 or 24 hr.
- **Y-Site Compatibility:** ▪ acyclovir ▪ amikacin ▪ aminophylline ▪ ampicillin ▪ ampicillin/sulbactam ▪ aztreonam ▪ bleomycin ▪ bumetanide ▪ buprenorphine ▪ butorphanol ▪ calcium gluconate ▪ carboplatin ▪ carmustine ▪ cefazolin ▪ cefotetan ▪ ceftazidime ▪ chlorpromazine ▪ cimetidine ▪ cisplatin ▪ cyclophosphamide ▪ cytarabine ▪ dacarbazine ▪ daunorubicin ▪ dexamethasone ▪ diphenhydramine ▪ doxorubicin ▪ doxycycline ▪ droperidol ▪ enalaprilat ▪ famotidine ▪ floxuridine ▪ fluconazole ▪ fludarabine ▪ gallium nitrate ▪ ganciclovir ▪ gentamicin ▪ haloperidol ▪ hydrocortisone ▪ hydromorphone ▪ idarubicin ▪ ifosfamide ▪ imipenem/cilastatin ▪ leucovorin calcium ▪ lorazepam ▪ mechlorethamine ▪ melphalan ▪ meperidine ▪ mesna ▪ methotrexate ▪ metoclopramide ▪ miconazole ▪ minocycline ▪ mitoxantrone ▪ morphine ▪ nalbuphine ▪ netilmicin ▪ ondansetron ▪ plicamycin ▪ potassium chloride ▪ promethazine ▪ ranitidine ▪ sodium bicarbonate ▪ streptozocin ▪ ticarcillin ▪ ticarcillin/clavulanate ▪ tobramycin ▪ trimethoprim/sulfamethoxazole ▪ vancomycin ▪ vinblastine ▪ vincristine ▪ vinorelbine ▪ zidovudine.
- **Y-Site Incompatibility:** ▪ amphotericin B ▪ cefepime ▪ cefonicid ▪ cefoperazone ▪ cefotaxime ▪ cefoxitin ▪ ceftizoxime ▪ ceftriaxone ▪ cefuroxime ▪ clindamycin ▪ dactinomycin ▪ etoposide ▪ fluorouracil ▪ furosemide ▪ heparin ▪ mannitol ▪ methylprednisolone sodium succinate ▪ metronidazole ▪ mezlocillin ▪ mitomycin ▪ piperacillin ▪ prochlorperazine ▪ thiotepa.

PATIENT/FAMILY TEACHING

- **Home Care Issues:** Instruct patient on correct technique and proper disposal for home administration. Caution patient not to reuse needle, vial, or syringe. Provide patient with a puncture-proof container for needle and syringe disposal.

EVALUATION

Effectiveness of therapy can be demonstrated by: ▪ Decreased incidence of infection in patients who receive bone marrow–depressing antineoplastic agents ▪ Reduction of duration and sequelae of neutropenia following bone marrow transplantation ▪ Reduction of the incidence and duration of sequelae of neutropenia in patients with severe chronic neutropenia.

F

FINASTERIDE

(fin-**ass**-te-ride)

Proscar

CLASSIFICATION(S):

Androgen inhibitor, Hair regrowth stimulant

INDICATIONS

■ Management of benign prostatic hyperplasia (BPH) ■ Treatment of androgenetic alopecia (male pattern baldness) in men only.

ACTION

■ Inhibits the enzyme 5alpha-reductase, which is responsible for converting testosterone to its potent metabolite 5alpha-dihydrotestosterone in prostate, liver, and skin; 5alpha-dihydrotestosterone is partially responsible for prostatic hyperplasia and hair loss. **Therapeutic Effects:** ■ Reduced prostate size with associated decrease in urinary symptoms ■ Decreases hair loss; promotes hair regrowth.

PHARMACOKINETICS

Absorption: Well absorbed following oral administration (63%).
Distribution: Enters prostatic tissue and crosses the blood-brain barrier. Remainder of distribution not known.
Metabolism and Excretion: Mostly metabolized; 39% excreted in urine as metabolites; 57% excreted in feces.
Half-life: 6 hr (range 6–15 hr; slightly increased in patients >70 yr).

CONTRAINDICATIONS AND PRECAUTIONS

Contraindicated in: ■ Hypersensitivity ■ Women.
Use Cautiously in: ■ Patients with hepatic impairment or obstructive uropathy.

ADVERSE REACTIONS AND SIDE EFFECTS

GU: decreased libido, decreased volume of ejaculate, impotence.

INTERACTIONS

Drug-Drug: ■ **Anticholinergics, adrenergic bronchodilators,** and **theophylline** may decrease the beneficial effects of finasteride.

ROUTE AND DOSAGE

■ **PO (Adult Males):** *BPH*—5 mg once daily; *androgenetic alopecia*—1 mg/day.

AVAILABILITY

■ ***Tablets:*** 5 mg[Rx].

TIME/ACTION PROFILE (reduction in dihydrotestosterone levels*)

	ONSET	PEAK	DURATION
PO	rapid	8 hr	2 wk

*Clinical effects as noted by urinary tract symptoms and hair regrowth may not be evident for several months and remain for 4 mo following discontinuation.

NURSING IMPLICATIONS

ASSESSMENT

- Assess patient for symptoms of prostatic hypertrophy (urinary hesitancy, feeling of incomplete bladder emptying, interruption of urinary stream, impairment of size and force of urinary stream, terminal urinary dribbling, straining to start flow, dysuria, urgency) prior to and periodically throughout therapy.
- Digital rectal examinations should be performed prior to and periodically throughout therapy.
- ***Lab Test Considerations:*** Serum prostate-specific antigen (PSA) concentrations, which are used to screen for prostate cancer, may be evaluated prior to and periodically throughout therapy. Finasteride may cause a decrease in serum PSA levels.

POTENTIAL NURSING DIAGNOSES

■ Urinary elimination, altered (Indications).
■ Knowledge deficit, related to medication regimen (Patient/Family Teaching).

IMPLEMENTATION

■ **PO:** Administer once daily with or without meals.

PATIENT/FAMILY TEACHING

- Instruct patient to take finasteride as directed, even if symptoms improve or are unchanged. At least 6–12 mo of therapy may be necessary to determine whether or not an individual will respond to finasteride.
- Inform patient that the volume of ejaculate may be decreased during therapy but that this will not interfere with normal sexual function.
- Caution patient that finasteride poses a potential risk to a male fetus. Women who are pregnant or may become pregnant should avoid exposure to semen of a partner taking finas-

teride and should not handle crushed finasteride because of the potential for absorption.

□ Emphasize the importance of periodic follow-up exams to determine whether a clinical response has occurred.

EVALUATION

Clinical response to therapy can be evaluated by: ▪ Decrease in urinary symptoms of benign prostatic hyperplasia ▪ Hair regrowth in androgenetic alopecia. Evidence of hair growth usually requires 3 mo or longer. Continued use is recommended to sustain benefit. Withdrawal leads to reversal of effect within 12 mo.

FLECAINIDE

(**flek**-a-nide)

Tambocor

CLASSIFICATION(S):

Antiarrhythmic (group IC)

Pregnancy Category C

INDICATIONS

▪ Treatment of life-threatening ventricular arrhythmias, including ventricular tachycardia ▪ Treatment of supraventricular tachyarrhythmias including: □ Paroxysmal supraventricular tachycardia (PSVT) □ Paroxysmal atrial fibrillation/flutter (PAF).

ACTION

▪ Slows conduction in cardiac tissue by altering transport of ions across cell membranes. **Therapeutic Effects:** ▪ Suppression of arrhythmias.

PHARMACOKINETICS

Absorption: Well absorbed from the GI tract following oral administration.

Distribution: Widely distributed.

Metabolism and Excretion: Mostly metabolized by the liver; 30% excreted unchanged by the kidneys.

Half-life: 11–14 hr.

CONTRAINDICATIONS AND PRECAUTIONS

Contraindicated in: ▪ Hypersensitivity ▪ Cardiogenic shock.

Use Cautiously in: ▪ Congestive heart failure (dosage reduction may be required) ▪ Pre-existing sinus node dysfunction or 2nd- or 3rd-degree heart block (without a pacemaker) ▪ Renal impairment (dosage reduction required if CCr <35 ml/min) ▪ Pregnancy, lactation, or children (safety not established).

ADVERSE REACTIONS AND SIDE EFFECTS*

CNS: dizziness, anxiety, fatigue, headache, mental depression.

EENT: blurred vision, visual disturbances.

CV: ARRHYTHMIAS, CHEST PAIN, CONGESTIVE HEART FAILURE.

GI: anorexia, constipation, drug-induced hepatitis, nausea, stomach pain, vomiting.

Derm: rashes.

Neuro: tremor.

INTERACTIONS

Drug-Drug: ▪ Increased risk of arrhythmias with other **antiarrhythmics,** including **calcium channel blockers** ▪ **Disopyramide, beta-adrenergic blockers,** or **verapamil** may have additive myocardial depressant effects; combination use should be undertaken cautiously ▪ **Amiodarone** doubles serum flecainide levels (decrease flecainide dose by 50%) ▪ Increases serum **digoxin** levels by a small amount (15–25%) ▪ Concurrent **beta-adrenergic blocker** therapy may result in increased levels of beta-adrenergic blocker and flecainide ▪ **Alkalinizing agents** promote reabsorption, increase blood levels, and may cause toxicity ▪ **Acidifying agents** increase renal elimination and may decrease effectiveness of flecainide (if urine pH <5).

Drug-Food: ▪ **Foods that increase urine pH** to >7 result in increased blood levels (strict **vegetarian diet)** ▪ **Foods or beverages that decrease urine pH** to <5 increase renal elimination and may decrease effectiveness of flecainide **(acidic juices).**

***CAPITALS indicate life-threatening; underlines indicate most frequent.**

ROUTE AND DOSAGE

- **PO (Adults):** *Ventricular tachycardia*—100 mg q 12 hr initially, increased by 50 mg bid until response is obtained or maximum total daily dose of 400 mg is reached. Some patients may require q 8 hr dosing. *PSVT/PAF*—50 mg q 12 hr initially, increased by 50 mg bid until response is obtained or maximum total daily dose of 300 mg is reached. Some patients may require q 8 hr dosing.

AVAILABILITY

- ***Tablets:*** 50 mg[Rx], 100 mg[Rx], 150 mg[Rx].

TIME/ACTION PROFILE (antiarrhythmic effects)

	ONSET	PEAK	DURATION
PO	days	days–wks	12 hr

NURSING IMPLICATIONS

ASSESSMENT

- □ Monitor ECG or Holter monitor prior to and periodically throughout therapy. May cause QRS widening, PR prolongation, and QT prolongation.
- □ Monitor blood pressure and pulse periodically throughout course of therapy.
- □ Monitor intake and output ratios and daily weight. Assess patient for signs of congestive heart failure (peripheral edema, rales/crackles, dyspnea, weight gain, jugular venous distention).
- ***Lab Test Considerations:*** Renal, pulmonary, and hepatic functions and CBC should be evaluated periodically on patients receiving long-term therapy. Flecainide should be discontinued if bone marrow depression occurs.
- □ May cause elevations in serum alkaline phosphatase during prolonged therapy.
- ***Toxicity and Overdose:*** Therapeutic blood levels range from 0.2 to 1.0 mcg/ml. Plasma trough levels should be monitored frequently during dosage adjustment in patients with severe renal or hepatic disease or in patients with congestive heart failure and moderate renal impairment.

POTENTIAL NURSING DIAGNOSES

- Cardiac output, decreased (Indications).
- Knowledge deficit, related to medication regimen (Patient/Family Teaching).

IMPLEMENTATION

- **General Info:** Previous antiarrhythmic therapy (except lidocaine) should be withdrawn 2–4 half-lives before starting flecainide.
- □ Therapy should be initiated in a hospital setting to monitor for increase in arrhythmias.
- □ Dosage adjustments should be at least 4 days apart because of the long half-life of flecainide.
- **PO:** May be administered with meals if GI irritation becomes a problem.

PATIENT/FAMILY TEACHING

- □ Instruct patient to take medication around the clock exactly as directed at evenly spaced intervals, even if feeling better. Missed doses should be taken as soon as remembered if within 6 hr; omit if remembered later. Gradual dosage reduction may be necessary.
- □ May cause dizziness or visual disturbances. Caution patient to avoid driving and other activities requiring alertness until response to medication is known.
- □ Advise patient to notify health care professional of medication regimen prior to treatment or surgery.
- □ Instruct patient to notify health care professional if chest pain, shortness of breath, or diaphoresis occurs.
- □ Advise patient to carry identification describing disease process and medication regimen at all times.
- □ Emphasize the importance of follow-up exams to monitor progress.

EVALUATION

Effectiveness of therapy can be demonstrated by: ▪ Decrease in frequency of life-threatening ventricular arrhythmias ▪ Decrease in supraventricular tachyarrhythmias.

FLUCONAZOLE

(floo-**kon**-a-zole)

Diflucan

CLASSIFICATION(S):

Antifungal

Pregnancy Category C

INDICATIONS

▪ **PO, IV:** Treatment of fungal infections due to susceptible organisms, including: ▫ Oropharyngeal or esophageal candidiasis ▫ Serious systemic candidal infections ▫ Urinary tract infections ▫ Peritonitis ▫ Cryptococcal meningitis ▪ Prevention of candidiasis in patients who have undergone bone marrow transplantation ▪ **PO:** Single-dose oral treatment of vaginal candidiasis.

ACTION

▪ Inhibits synthesis of fungal sterols, a necessary component of the cell wall. **Therapeutic Effects:** ▪ Fungistatic action against susceptible organisms ▪ May be fungicidal in higher concentrations. **Spectrum:** ▪ *Cryptococcus neoformans* ▪ *Candida* spp.

PHARMACOKINETICS

Absorption: Well absorbed following oral administration.
Distribution: Widely distributed, good penetration into cerebrospinal fluid, eye, and peritoneum.
Metabolism and Excretion: >80% excreted unchanged by the kidneys; <10% metabolized by the liver.
Half-life: 30 hr (increased in renal impairment).

CONTRAINDICATIONS AND PRECAUTIONS

Contraindicated in: ▪ Hypersensitivity to fluconazole or other azole antifungals.
Use Cautiously in: ▪ Renal impairment (dosage reduction required if CCr <50 ml/min) ▪ Underlying liver disease ▪ Pregnancy, lactation, or children (safety not established).

ADVERSE REACTIONS AND SIDE EFFECTS*

Incidence of adverse reactions is increased in HIV patients.
CNS: headache.
GI: HEPATOTOXICITY, abdominal discomfort, diarrhea, nausea, vomiting.
Derm: exfoliative skin disorders including STEVENS-JOHNSON SYNDROME.

INTERACTIONS

Drug-Drug: ▪ Increases the activity of **warfarin** ▪ **Rifampin** and **isoniazid** decrease blood levels ▪ Increases the hypoglycemic effects of **tolbutamide, glyburide,** or **glipizide** ▪ Increases blood levels of **cyclosporine** and **phenytoin.**

ROUTE AND DOSAGE

▫ Oropharyngeal Candidiasis

▪ **PO, IV (Adults):** 200 mg initially, then 100 mg daily for at least 2 wk.

▫ Esophageal Candidiasis

▪ **PO, IV (Adults):** 200 mg initially, then 100 mg once daily for at least 3 wk or 2 wk following symptomatic improvement (up to 400 mg/day).

▫ Other Candidiasis

▪ **PO, IV (Adults):** 50–400 mg/day.

▫ Cryptococcal Meningitis

▪ **PO, IV (Adults):** *Treatment*—400 mg once daily until favorable clinical response, then 200–400 mg once daily for at least 10–12 wk following clearing of cerebrospinal fluid; change to oral therapy as soon as possible. *Suppressive therapy*—200 mg once daily.

▫ Prevention of Candidiasis Following Bone Marrow Transplant

▪ **PO, IV (Adults):** 400 mg once daily; begin several days before procedure if severe neutropenia is expected, and continue for 7 days after ANC >1000 /mm³.

▫ Vaginal Candidiasis

▪ **PO (Adults):** 150 mg single dose.

AVAILABILITY

▪ ***Tablets:*** 50 mg[Rx], 100 mg[Rx], 150 mg[Rx], 200 mg[Rx] ▪ ***Oral suspension:*** 10 mg/ml[Rx] ▪ ***Injection:*** 2 mg/ml in 100- or 200-ml bottles/containers[Rx].

TIME/ACTION PROFILE (blood levels)

	ONSET	PEAK	DURATION
PO	UK	1–2 hr	24 hr
IV	rapid	end of infusion	24 hr

*CAPITALS indicate life-threatening; underlines indicate most frequent.

NURSING IMPLICATIONS

ASSESSMENT

- Assess infected area and monitor cerebrospinal fluid cultures prior to and periodically throughout therapy.
- Specimens for culture should be taken prior to instituting therapy. Therapy may be started before results are obtained.
- ***Lab Test Considerations:*** BUN and serum creatinine should be monitored prior to and periodically during therapy; patients with renal dysfunction will require dosage adjustment.
- Liver function tests should be monitored prior to and periodically throughout therapy. May cause increased AST, ALT, serum alkaline phosphate, and bilirubin concentrations.

POTENTIAL NURSING DIAGNOSES

- Infection, risk for (Indications).
- Knowledge deficit, related to medication regimen (Patient/Family Teaching).

IMPLEMENTATION

- **PO:** Shake oral suspension well prior to administration.
- **Intermittent Infusion:** Open overwrap immediately before infusion. Inner bag may have slight opacity that will diminish gradually. Do not administer solution that is cloudy or has a precipitate. Check for leaks by squeezing inner bag. If leaks are found, discard container as unsterile.
- Do not set tubing as part of a series of connections as this may cause air embolism.
- ***Rate:*** Infuse at a maximum rate of 200 mg/hr.
- **Y-Site Compatibility:** ▪ acyclovir ▪ aldesleukin ▪ amifostine ▪ amikacin ▪ aminophylline ▪ ampicillin/sulbactam ▪ aztreonam ▪ benztropine ▪ cefazolin ▪ cefepime ▪ cefotetan ▪ cefoxitin ▪ chlorpromazine ▪ cimetidine ▪ dexamethasone sodium phosphate ▪ diltiazem ▪ diphenhydramine ▪ dobutamine ▪ dopamine ▪ droperidol ▪ famotidine ▪ filgrastim ▪ fludarabine ▪ foscarnet ▪ gallium nitrate ▪ ganciclovir ▪ gentamicin ▪ heparin ▪ hydrocortisone ▪ immune globulin ▪ leucovorin ▪ lorazepam ▪ melphalan ▪ meperidine ▪ metoclopramide ▪ metronidazole ▪ midazolam ▪ morphine ▪ nafcillin ▪ ondansetron ▪ oxacillin ▪ paclitaxel ▪ pancuronium ▪ penicillin G potassium ▪ phenytoin ▪ piperacillin/tazobactam ▪ prochlorperazine ▪ promethazine ▪ ranitidine ▪ sargramostim ▪ tacrolimus ▪ teniposide ▪ theophylline ▪ thiotepa ▪ ticarcillin/clavulanate ▪ tobramycin ▪ vancomycin ▪ vecuronium ▪ vinorelbine ▪ zidovudine.
- **Y-Site Incompatibility:** ▪ amphotericin B ▪ ampicillin ▪ calcium gluconate ▪ cefotaxime ▪ ceftazidime ▪ ceftriaxone ▪ cefuroxime ▪ chloramphenicol ▪ clindamycin ▪ diazepam ▪ digoxin ▪ erythromycin lactobionate ▪ furosemide ▪ haloperidol ▪ hydroxyzine ▪ imipenem/cilastatin ▪ pentamidine ▪ piperacillin ▪ ticarcillin ▪ trimethoprim/sulfamethoxazole.
- **Additive Incompatibility:** ▪ Manufacturer does not recommend admixing.

PATIENT/FAMILY TEACHING

- Instruct patient to take medication exactly as directed, even if feeling better. Doses should be taken at the same time each day. If a dose is missed, take as soon as remembered, but not if almost time for next dose. Do not double doses.
- Instruct patient to notify health care professional if abdominal pain, fever, or diarrhea becomes pronounced or if signs and symptoms of liver dysfunction (unusual fatigue, anorexia, nausea, vomiting, jaundice, dark urine, or pale stools) occur or if no improvement is seen within a few days of therapy.

EVALUATION

Effectiveness of therapy can be demonstrated by: ▪ Resolution of clinical and laboratory indications of fungal infections. Full course of therapy may require weeks or months of treatment following resolution of symptoms ▪ Prevention of candidiasis in patients who have undergone bone marrow transplantation ▪ Decrease in skin irritation and vaginal discomfort in patients with vaginal candidiasis. Diagnosis should be reconfirmed with smears or cultures prior to a second course of therapy to rule out other pathogens associated with vulvovaginitis. Recurrent vaginal infections may be a sign of systemic illness.

FLUCYTOSINE
(floo-**sye**-toe-seen)
Ancobon, {Ancotil}, 5-FC

CLASSIFICATION(S):
Antifungal

Pregnancy Category C

INDICATIONS

■ Treatment of serious fungal infections including: □ Endocarditis □ Meningitis □ Septicemia □ Urinary tract infections □ Pulmonary infections.

ACTION

■ Following penetration into fungi, converted to fluorouracil, which interferes with fungal DNA and RNA synthesis ■ Synergistic action with amphotericin B against some fungi. **Therapeutic Effects:** ■ Fungicidal action against susceptible organisms. **Spectrum:** ■ Active against only a small number of fungi, mainly: □ *Candida* □ *Cryptococcus*.

PHARMACOKINETICS

Absorption: Well absorbed from the GI tract following oral administration.
Distribution: Widely distributed. Crosses the blood-brain barrier and placenta.
Metabolism and Excretion: 80–90% excreted unchanged by the kidneys.
Half-life: 2.5–8 hr (increased in renal impairment).

CONTRAINDICATIONS AND PRECAUTIONS

Contraindicated in: ■ Hypersensitivity ■ Pregnancy or lactation.
Use Cautiously in: ■ Renal impairment (blood level monitoring and increased dosage interval recommended if CCr <40 ml/min) ■ Bone marrow depression (especially following radiation therapy or antineoplastic drugs).

ADVERSE REACTIONS AND SIDE EFFECTS*

CNS: confusion, dizziness, drowsiness.
GI: diarrhea, nausea, vomiting, bloating.
Derm: photosensitivity.
Hemat: leukopenia, pancytopenia, anemia, thrombocytopenia.

INTERACTIONS

Drug-Drug: ■ Additive bone marrow depression with other **bone marrow depressant drugs,** including **antineoplastic agents** and **radiation therapy** ■ **Amphotericin B** may increase toxicity of flucytosine but may also increase antifungal activity ■ **Cytarabine** may decrease antifungal activity.

ROUTE AND DOSAGE

- **PO (Adults):** 12.5–37.5 mg/kg q 6 hr.
- **PO (Children):** 12.5–37.5 mg/kg q 6 hr or 375–562.5 mg/m² q 6 hr.

AVAILABILITY

■ ***Capsules:*** 250 mg[Rx], 500 mg[Rx].

TIME/ACTION PROFILE (antifungal blood levels)

	ONSET	PEAK	DURATION
PO	rapid	1–2 hr	6 hr

NURSING IMPLICATIONS

ASSESSMENT

□ Assess patient for signs and symptoms of systemic fungal infection prior to and periodically throughout therapy.
□ Obtain specimens for culture prior to initiating therapy. First dose may be given before receiving results.
■ ***Lab Test Considerations:*** Monitor AST, ALT, serum bilirubin, and alkaline phosphatase prior to and frequently during therapy.
□ Monitor BUN and serum creatinine prior to and periodically during therapy. Dosage should be reduced in renal impairment. Patients with renal impairment should have serum flucytosine concentrations monitored to prevent accumulation. Side effects are more common with serum concentrations >100 mcg/ml.
□ Monitor hematologic function periodically during therapy. May cause anemia, leukopenia, or thrombocytopenia.

{} = Available in Canada only.
***CAPITALS indicate life-threatening; underlines indicate most frequent.**

POTENTIAL NURSING DIAGNOSES

- Infection, risk for (Indications).
- Fluid volume deficit, potential (Adverse Reactions).
- Knowledge deficit, related to medication regimen (Patient/Family Teaching).

IMPLEMENTATION

- **General Info:** The number 5 in 5-FC is part of the drug name and not the dose.
- **PO:** To reduce nausea and vomiting, administer capsules a few at a time over 15 min.

PATIENT/FAMILY TEACHING

- □ Advise patient to take medication exactly as directed, even if feeling better. Missed doses should be taken as soon as remembered, if not almost time for next dose; do not double doses.
- □ May cause dizziness or drowsiness. Caution patient to avoid driving and other activities requiring alertness until response to medication is known.
- □ Caution patient to use sunscreen and wear protective clothing to prevent photosensitivity reactions.
- □ Instruct patient to notify health care professional promptly if rash, fever, sore throat, diarrhea, unusual bleeding or bruising, unusual tiredness, or weakness occurs.
- □ Emphasize the importance of follow-up exams to determine effectiveness of treatment.

EVALUATION

Effectiveness of therapy can be demonstrated by: ▪ Resolution of the signs and symptoms of fungal infection. Duration of therapy is generally 4–6 wk but may continue for several months.

FLUDROCORTISONE

(floo-droe-**kor**-ti-sone)
Florinef

CLASSIFICATION(S):
Mineralocorticoid

Pregnancy Category C

INDICATIONS

▪ Management of sodium loss and hypotension associated with adrenocortical insufficiency (given with hydrocortisone or cortisone) ▪ Management of sodium loss due to congenital adrenogenital syndrome (congenital adrenal hyperplasia). **Unlabeled Uses:** ▪ Management of idiopathic orthostatic hypotension (with ↑ sodium intake) ▪ Management of type IV renal tubular acidosis.

ACTION

▪ Causes sodium reabsorption, hydrogen and potassium excretion, and water retention by its effects on the distal renal tubule. **Therapeutic Effects:** ▪ Maintenance of sodium balance and blood pressure in patients with adrenocortical insufficiency.

PHARMACOKINETICS

Absorption: Well absorbed following oral administration.
Distribution: Appears to be widely distributed; probably enters breast milk.
Metabolism and Excretion: Mostly metabolized by the liver.
Half-life: 3.5 hr.

CONTRAINDICATIONS AND PRECAUTIONS

Contraindicated in: ▪ Hypersensitivity.
Use Cautiously in: ▪ Congestive heart failure ▪ Addison's disease (patients may have exaggerated response) ▪ Pregnancy, lactation, or children (safety not established).

ADVERSE REACTIONS AND SIDE EFFECTS*

CNS: dizziness, headache.
CV: CONGESTIVE HEART FAILURE, arrhythmias, edema, hypertension.
GI: anorexia, nausea.
Endo: adrenal suppression, weight gain.
F and E: hypokalemia, hypokalemic alkalosis.
MS: arthralgia, muscular weakness, tendon contractures.
Neuro: ascending paralysis.
Misc: hypersensitivity reactions.

***CAPITALS indicate life-threatening; underlines indicate most frequent.**

INTERACTIONS

Drug-Drug: ▪ Use with **diuretics, mezlocillin, piperacillin,** or **amphotericin B** may result in exaggerated hypokalemia ▪ Hypokalemia may increase the risk of **digitalis glycoside** toxicity ▪ May produce prolonged neuromuscular blockade following the use of **nondepolarizing neuromuscular blocking agents** ▪ **Phenobarbital** or **rifampin** may increase the metabolism and may decrease the effectiveness of fludrocortisone.

Drug-Food: ▪ Ingestion of large amounts of **salt** or **sodium-containing foods** may cause excessive sodium retention and potassium loss.

ROUTE AND DOSAGE

- **PO (Adults):** *Adrenocortical insufficiency*—100 mcg/day (range 100 mcg 3 times weekly—200 mcg daily). Doses as small as 50 mcg daily may be required by some patients. Use with 10–37.5 mg cortisone daily or 10–30 mg hydrocortisone daily. *Adrenogenital syndrome*—100–200 mcg/day. *Idiopathic hypotension*—50–200 mcg/day (unlabeled).
- **PO (Children):** 50–100 mcg/day.

AVAILABILITY

- ***Tablets:*** 100 mcg (0.1 mg)Rx.

TIME/ACTION PROFILE (mineralocorticoid activity)

	ONSET	PEAK	DURATION
PO	UK	UK	1–2 days

NURSING IMPLICATIONS

ASSESSMENT

- ▫ Monitor blood pressure periodically throughout therapy. Report significant changes. Hypotension may indicate insufficient dosage.
- ▫ Monitor for fluid retention (weigh daily, assess for edema, and auscultate lungs for rales/crackles).
- ▪ ***Lab Test Considerations:*** Monitor serum electrolytes periodically throughout therapy. Fludrocortisone causes decreased serum potassium levels.

POTENTIAL NURSING DIAGNOSES

- Fluid volume deficit (Indications).
- Fluid volume excess (Side Effects).
- Knowledge deficit, related to medication regimen (Patient/Family Teaching).

IMPLEMENTATION

- **PO:** Tablets are scored and may be broken if dosage adjustment is necessary.

PATIENT/FAMILY TEACHING

- ▫ Instruct patient to take medication exactly as directed. If a dose is missed, take as soon as remembered but not just before next dose is due. Explain that lifelong therapy may be necessary and that abrupt discontinuation may lead to addisonian crisis. Patient should keep an adequate supply available at all times.
- ▫ Advise patient to follow dietary modification prescribed by health care professional. Instruct patient to follow a diet high in potassium (see Appendix K). Amount of sodium allowed in diet varies with pathophysiology.
- ▫ Instruct patient to inform health care professional if weight gain or edema, muscle weakness, cramps, nausea, anorexia, or dizziness occurs.
- ▫ Advise patient to carry identification describing disease process and medication regimen at all times.

EVALUATION

Effectiveness of therapy can be demonstrated by: ▪ Normalization of fluid and electrolyte balance without the development of hypokalemia or hypertension.

FLUMAZENIL

(flu-**maz**-e-nil)
{Anexate}, Romazicon

CLASSIFICATION(S):
Antidote (benzodiazepine antagonist)

Pregnancy Category C

INDICATIONS

▪ Completely or partially reverses the effects of benzodiazepines used as general anesthetics, or during diagnostic or therapeutic procedures ▪ Management of intentional or accidental overdose of benzodiazepines.

ACTION

▪ Flumazenil is a benzodiazepine derivative that antagonizes the CNS depressant effects of benzodiazepine compounds. It has no effect on CNS depression of other causes, including opioids, alcohol, barbiturates, or general anesthetics. **Therapeutic Effects:** ▪ Reversal of benzodiazepine effects.

PHARMACOKINETICS

Absorption: IV administration results in complete bioavailability.
Distribution: UK.
Metabolism and Excretion: Metabolism of flumazenil occurs primarily in the liver.
Half-life: 41–79 min.

CONTRAINDICATIONS AND PRECAUTIONS

Contraindicated in: ▪ Hypersensitivity to flumazenil or benzodiazepines ▪ Patients receiving benzodiazepines for life-threatening medical problems including status epilepticus or increased intracranial pressure should not be given flumazenil ▪ Serious cyclic antidepressant overdosage.
Use Cautiously in: ▪ Mixed CNS depressant overdosage (effects of other agents may emerge when benzodiazepine effect is removed) ▪ History of seizures (seizures are more likely to occur in patients who are experiencing sedative/hypnotic withdrawal, patients who have recently received repeated doses of benzodiazepines, or those who have a prior history of seizure activity) ▪ Head injury (may increase intracranial pressure and risk of seizures) ▪ Pregnancy, lactation, or children (safety not established).

ADVERSE REACTIONS AND SIDE EFFECTS*

CNS: SEIZURES, dizziness, agitation, confusion, drowsiness, emotional lability, fatigue, headache, sleep disorders.
EENT: abnormal hearing, abnormal vision, blurred vision.
CV: arrhythmias, chest pain, hypertension.
GI: nausea, vomiting, hiccups.
Derm: flushing, sweating.
Local: pain/injection-site reactions, phlebitis.
Neuro: paresthesia.
Misc: rigors, shivering.

INTERACTIONS

Drug-Drug: ▪ None significant.

ROUTE AND DOSAGE

❑ **Reversal of Conscious Sedation or General Anesthesia**

- **IV (Adults):** 0.2 mg. Additional doses may be given at 1-min intervals until desired results are obtained, up to a total dose of 1 mg. If resedation occurs, regimen may be repeated at 20-min intervals, not to exceed 3 mg/hr.
- **IV (Children): Unlabeled:** 10 mcg (0.01 mg)/kg up to cumulative dose of 1 mg.

❑ **Suspected Benzodiazepine Overdose**

- **IV (Adults):** 0.2 mg. Additional 0.3 mg may be given 30 sec later. Further doses of 0.5 mg may be given at 1-min intervals, if necessary, to a total dose of 3 mg. Usual dose required is 1–3 mg. If resedation occurs, additional doses of 0.5 mg/min for 2 min may be given at 20-min intervals (given no more than 1 mg at a time, not to exceed 3 mg per hour).
- **IV (Children): Unlabeled:** 100 mcg (0.1 mg)/kg up to a cumulative dose of 1 mg.

AVAILABILITY

▪ ***Injection:*** 0.1 mg/ml[Rx].

TIME/ACTION PROFILE (reversal of benzodiazepine effects)

	ONSET	PEAK	DURATION
IV	1–2 min	6–10 min	1–2 hr†

†Depends on dose/concentration of benzodiazepine and dose of flumazenil.

NURSING IMPLICATIONS

ASSESSMENT

- **General Info:** Assess level of consciousness and respiratory status prior to and throughout therapy. Observe patient for at least 2 hr following administration for the appearance of resedation. Hypoventilation may occur.
- **Overdose:** Attempt to determine time of in-

*CAPITALS indicate life-threatening; underlines indicate most frequent.

gestion and amount and type of benzodiazepine taken. Knowledge of agent ingested allows an estimate of duration of CNS depression.

POTENTIAL NURSING DIAGNOSES

- Injury, risk for (Indications).
- Poisoning, risk for (Indications).

IMPLEMENTATION

- **General Info:** Ensure that patient has a patent airway before administration of flumazenil.
- □ Observe IV site frequently for redness or irritation. Administer through a free-flowing IV infusion into a large vein to minimize pain at the injection site.
- □ Optimal emergence should be undertaken slowly to decrease undesirable effects including confusion, agitation, emotional lability, and perceptual distortion.
- □ Institute seizure precautions. Seizures are more likely to occur in patients who are experiencing sedative/hypnotic withdrawal, patients who have recently received repeated doses of benzodiazepines, or those who have a prior history of seizure activity. Seizures may be treated with benzodiazepines, barbiturates, or phenytoin. Larger than normal doses of benzodiazepines may be required.
- **Suspected Benzodiazepine Overdose:** If no effects are seen following administration of flumazenil, consider other causes of decreased level of consciousness (alcohol, barbiturates, opioid analgesics).
- **Direct IV:** May be administered undiluted or diluted in syringe with D5W, 0.9% NaCl, or lactated Ringer's solution. Diluted solution should be discarded after 24 hr.
- ***Rate:*** Administer each dose over 15–30 sec into free-flowing IV in a large vein.

PATIENT/FAMILY TEACHING

- □ Flumazenil does not consistently reverse the amnestic effects of benzodiazepines. Provide patient and family with written instructions for postprocedure care. Inform family that patient may appear alert at the time of discharge but the sedative effects of the benzodiazepine may recur. Instruct patient to avoid driving or other activities requiring alertness for at least 24 hr after discharge.
- □ Instruct patient not to take any alcohol or nonprescription drugs for at least 18–24 hr after discharge.
- □ Resumption of usual activities should occur only when no residual effects of the benzodiazepine remain.

EVALUATION

Clinical response to therapy can be evaluated by: ▪ Improved level of consciousness □ Decrease in respiratory depression caused by benzodiazepines.

FLUORIDE SUPPLEMENTS

(**floor**-ide)

sodium fluoride (oral)

{Fluor-A-Day}, Fluoride Loz, Fluoritab, Flura, Flura-Drops, Flura-Loz, Karidium, Luride, Pediaflor, Pedi-Dent, Pharmaflur, Phos-Flur, {Solu-Flur}

fluoride (topical)

ACT, Fluorigard, Fluorinse, Gel Kam, Gel-Tin, Karigel, Listermint with Fluoride, Minute-Gel, MouthKote F/R, Point Two, Stop, Thera-Flur

CLASSIFICATION(S):
Dental caries prophylactic agents, Mineral supplements

Pregnancy Category UK

F

INDICATIONS

▪ Prevention of dental caries in children where insufficient fluoride is in drinking water.

ACTION

▪ Fluoride becomes incorporated into bone and teeth, where it serves to stabilize crystalline matrix. It promotes remineralization and may retard the growth of dental plaque. The presence of fluoride on the enamel surface of teeth promotes resistance to acid and prevents caries by interrupting the cariogenic microbial process. **Therapeutic Effects:** ▪ Decreased incidence of dental caries in children.

PHARMACOKINETICS

Absorption: Topical fluoride is taken up by enamel and plaque. Acidulated solutions are taken up by enamel to a greater extent than neutral solutions. Well absorbed following oral administration.
Distribution: Stored in bone and developing teeth. Readily crosses the placenta; small amounts enter breast milk.
Metabolism and Excretion: 50% excreted unchanged by the kidneys. Small amounts excreted in feces and sweat.
Half-life: UK.

CONTRAINDICATIONS AND PRECAUTIONS

Contraindicated in: ▪ Hypersensitivity ▪ Dietary sodium restriction ▪ Where fluoride in drinking water exceeds 0.7 parts per million (ppm) ▪ Some products contain tartrazine and other additives; avoid use in patients with known intolerance ▪ Severe renal impairment.
Use Cautiously in: ▪ Situations in which fluoride content of water is not known.

ADVERSE REACTIONS AND SIDE EFFECTS

CNS: headache, weakness.
GI: gastric distress.
Derm: atopic dermatitis, eczema, urticaria.
Misc: mottling of teeth (toxicity).

INTERACTIONS

Drug-Drug: ▪ If taken concurrently with **calcium supplements,** calcium fluoride will form and fluoride will not be absorbed. **Aluminum hydroxide** decreases absorption of fluoride.
Drug-Food: ▪ If taken concurrently with **dairy foods**, calcium fluoride will form and fluoride will not be absorbed.

ROUTE AND DOSAGE

❑ **Oral Fluoride—Fluoride Content of Drinking Water <0.3 ppm**

- **PO (Adults and Children >16 yr):** No supplementation.
- **PO (Children 6–16 yr):** 1 mg/day.
- **PO (Children 3–6 yr):** 0.5 mg/day.
- **PO (Children 6 mo–3 yr):** 0.25 mg/day.
- **PO (Children <6 mo):** No supplementation.

❑ **Oral Fluoride—Fluoride Content of Drinking Water 0.3–0.6 ppm**

- **PO (Adults and Children >16 yr):** No supplementation.
- **PO (Children 6–16 yr):** 0.5 mg/day.
- **PO (Children 3–6 yr):** 0.25 mg/day.
- **PO (Children <3 yr):** No supplementation.

❑ **Topical Fluoride**

- **Topical (Adults and Children >12 yr):** 10 ml/day. (Point-Two is used once weekly.)
- **Topical (Children 6–12 yr):** 5–10 ml/day. (Point-Two is used once weekly.)

AVAILABILITY

Listed as fluoride content.
▪ ***Tablets:*** 1 mg[Rx] ▪ ***Chewable tablets:*** 0.25 mg[Rx], 0.5 mg[Rx], 1 mg[Rx] ▪ ***Drops:*** 0.125 mg/drop[Rx], 0.25 mg/drop[Rx], 0.5 mg/drop[Rx] ▪ ***Lozenges:*** 1 mg[Rx] ▪ ***Solution:*** 0.2 mg/ml[Rx] ▪ ***Rinse:*** 0.01%[OTC], 0.02%[OTC], 0.04%[OTC], 0.09%[Rx] ▪ ***Gel:*** 0.1%[Rx,OTC], 0.5%[Rx], 1.2%[Rx], 1.23%[Rx] ▪ ***Gel drops:*** 0.5%[Rx].

TIME/ACTION PROFILE (blood levels)

	ONSET	PEAK	DURATION
PO	UK	30–60 min	UK

NURSING IMPLICATIONS

ASSESSMENT

- ❑ Examine teeth for staining or mottling periodically. Notify dentist if this occurs.

POTENTIAL NURSING DIAGNOSES

- ▪ Knowledge deficit, related to medication regimen.

IMPLEMENTATION

- ▪ Drops may be administered undiluted orally or mixed with food or fluids.
- ▪ Do not administer sodium fluoride within 2 hr of milk or other dairy products; will cause decreased absorption of sodium fluoride.

PATIENT/FAMILY TEACHING

- ❑ Instruct patient to take fluoride supplement as directed, according to directions included with each preparation.
- ❑ Rinses and gel are most effective if used immediately after brushing or flossing and just before sleep. Instruct patient to expectorate

any excess; *do not swallow.* Patient should not eat, drink, or rinse mouth for 30 min after application.

- Advise parents to keep fluoride out of reach of children.
- Encourage patient to have routine dental examinations to monitor dental hygiene.

EVALUATION

Effectiveness of therapy can be demonstrated by: ▪ Prevention of dental caries.

FLUOROQUINOLONES

(floor-oh-**kwin**-oh-lones)

alatrovafloxacin
(a-la-troe-va-**flox**-a-sin)
Trovan (oral)

ciprofloxacin*
(sip-roe-**flox**-a-sin)
Cipro

enoxacin
(ee-**nox**-a-sin)
Penetrex

grepafloxacin
(grepp-a-**flox**-a-sin)
Raxar

levofloxacin
(le-voe-**flox**-a-sin)
Levaquin

lomefloxacin
(loe-me-**flox**-a-sin)
Maxaquin

norfloxacin*
(nor-**flox**-a-sin)
Noroxin

ofloxacin*
(oh-**flox**-a-sin)
Floxin

sparfloxacin
(spar-**flox**-a-sin)
Zagam

trovafloxacin
(troe-va-**flox**-a-sin)
Trovan (IV)

CLASSIFICATION(S):
Anti-infectives

Pregnancy Category C

*See Appendix O for ophthalmic use.

INDICATIONS

▪ **PO, IV:** Treatment of the following infections: ▫ Urinary tract and gynecologic infections (not sparfloxacin) ▫ Gonorrhea (not levofloxacin or sparfloxacin) ▫ Prostatitis (ofloxacin) ▫ Respiratory tract infections (not enoxacin or norfloxacin) ▫ Skin and skin structure infections (alatrovafloxacin, trovafloxacin, ciprofloxacin, ofloxacin) ▫ Bone and joint infections (ciprofloxacin) ▫ Infectious diarrhea (ciprofloxacin) ▫ Intra-abdominal infections (ciprofloxacin with metronidazole, alatrovafloxacin, trovafloxacin) ▪ Perioperative prophylaxis before transurethral procedures (lomefloxacin) or colerectal procedures (alatrovafloxacin, trovafloxacin) ▪ Febrile neutropenia (ciprofloxacin).

ACTION

▪ Inhibit bacterial DNA synthesis by inhibiting DNA gyrase. **Therapeutic Effects:** ▪ Death of susceptible bacteria. **Spectrum:** ▪ Broad activity includes many gram-positive pathogens: ▫ Staphylococci including methicillin-resistant *Staphylococcus aureus* and *Staphylococcus epidermidis* (ciprofloxacin, grepafloxacin, alatrovafloxacin, trovafloxacin) ▫ *Streptococcus pneumoniae* (alatrovafloxacin, trovafloxacin) ▪ Gram-negative spectrum notable for activity against: ▫ *Escherichia coli* ▫ *Klebsiella* spp. ▫ *Enterobacter* ▫ *Salmonella* ▫ *Shigella* ▫ *Proteus vulgaris* ▫ *Providencia stuartii* ▫ *Providencia rettgeri* ▫ *Morganella morganii* ▫ *Pseudomonas aeruginosa* ▫ *Serratia* ▫ *Haemophilus* spp. ▫ *Acinetobacter* ▫ *Neisseria gonorrhoeae* and *Neisseria meningitidis* ▫ *Branhamela catarrhalis* ▫ *Yersinia* ▫ *Vibrio* ▫ *Brucella* ▫ *Campylobacter* ▫ *Aeromonas* spp. ▪ Active against the following anaerobic pathogens: ▫ *Bacteroides fragilis* and *Bacteroides intermedius* (alatrovafloxacin, sparfloxacin, trovafloxacin) ▫ *Clostridium perfringens* and *Clostridium welchii* ▫ *Gardnerella vaginalis* ▫ *Peptococcus niger* ▫ *Peptostreptococcus* spp. ▪ Additional spectrum includes: ▫ *Chlamydia pneumoniae* and *Chlamydia trachomatis* ▫ *Legionella pneu-*

F

moniae ▫ *Mycobacterium tuberculosis* ▫ *Mycoplasma pneumoniae* ▫ *Urea urealyticum*.

PHARMACOKINETICS

Absorption: Well absorbed following oral administration (*Ciprofloxacin, grepafloxacin*—70%; *enoxacin*—90%; *levofloxacin*—99%; *lomefloxacin*—95–98%; *norfloxacin*—30–40%; *ofloxacin*—89%; *sparfloxacin*—92%; *trovafloxacin*—88%; following IV administration alatrovafloxacin is rapidly converted to trovafloxacin).

Distribution: Widely distributed. High tissue and urinary levels are achieved. All agents appear to cross the placenta. *Ciprofloxacin, ofloxacin,* and *sparfloxacin* enter breast milk.

Metabolism and Excretion: *Ciprofloxacin*—15% metabolized by the liver, 40–50% excreted unchanged by the kidneys; *enoxacin*—>40% excreted unchanged by the kidneys, 20% metabolized by the liver; *grepafloxacin*—mostly metabolized by the liver, <10% excreted unchanged in urine; *levofloxacin*—87% excreted unchanged in urine, small amounts metabolized; *lomefloxacin*—65% excreted unchanged by the kidneys, 10% excreted unchanged in feces; *norfloxacin*—10% metabolized by the liver, 30% excreted unchanged by the kidneys, 30% excreted unchanged in feces; *ofloxacin*—70–80% excreted unchanged by the kidneys; *sparfloxacin*—partially metabolized by the liver, 10% excreted unchanged in urine; *trovafloxacin*—partially metabolized by the liver, 50% excreted unchanged in urine.

Half-life: *Ciprofloxacin*—4 hr, *enoxacin*—3–6 hr, *grepafloxacin*—16 hr, *levofloxacin*—6–8 hr, *lomefloxacin*—8 hr, *norfloxacin*—6.5 hr, *ofloxacin*—5–7 hr (all are increased in renal impairment), *sparfloxacin*—20 hr, *trovafloxacin*—11 hr.

CONTRAINDICATIONS AND PRECAUTIONS

Contraindicated in: ▪ Hypersensitivity. Cross-sensitivity among agents may occur (including cinoxacin and nalidixic acid) ▪ Children <18 yr ▪ Pregnancy ▪ *Sparfloxacin only:* ▫ Exposure to sun; bright, natural light; or UV rays ▫ Concurrent use of amiodarone, astemizole, bepridil, disopyramide, procainamide, quinidine, or sotalol ▫ Known QT_c prolongation or concurrent use of agents causing prolongation ▪ Hepatic failure (grepafloxacin only).

Use Cautiously in: ▪ Underlying CNS pathology ▪ Renal impairment (dosage reduction if CCr ≤80 ml/min for levofloxacin; ≤50 ml/min for ciprofloxacin, ofloxacin, sparfloxacin; ≤30 ml/min for enoxacin, norfloxacin; <40 ml/min for lomefloxacin) ▪ Cirrhosis (dose reduction for alatrovafloxacin/trovafloxacin recommended) ▪ Geriatric patients, dialysis patients (increased risk of tendon rupture and adverse CNS reactions) ▪ Lactation (safety not established).

ADVERSE REACTIONS AND SIDE EFFECTS*

CNS: SEIZURES, <u>dizziness</u>, <u>drowsiness</u>, <u>headache</u>, <u>insomnia</u>, acute psychoses, agitation, confusion, hallucinations, increased intracranial pressure, light-headedness, tremors.

CV: *sparfloxacin only*—ARRHYTHMIAS, QT_c prolongation, vasodilation.

GI: PSEUDOMEMBRANOUS COLITIS, <u>abdominal pain</u>, <u>diarrhea</u>, <u>nausea</u>, altered taste.

GU: interstitial cystitis, vaginitis.

Derm: photosensitivity (↑ with lomefloxacin), phototoxicity (sparfloxacin), rash.

Endo: hyperglycemia, hypoglycemia.

Local: phlebitis at IV site.

MS: tendinitis, tendon rupture.

Misc: hypersensitivity reactions including STEVENS-JOHNSON SYNDROME.

INTERACTIONS

Drug-Drug: ▪ Increased risk of serious adverse cardiovascular reactions with concurrent use of sparfloxacin and **amiodarone, astemizole, bepridil, disopyramide, procainamide, quinidine**, or **sotalol;** concurrent use is contraindicated ▪ Increases serum **theophylline** levels and may lead to toxicity ▪ Administration with **antacids, iron salts, bismuth subsalicylate, sucralfate**, and **zinc salts** decreases absorption of fluoroquinolones ▪ May increase the effects of **warfarin** ▪ Serum levels of fluoroquinolones may be decreased by **antineoplastic agents** ▪ **Cimetidine** may interfere with elimination of fluoroquinolones ▪ Beneficial effects of ciprofloxacin may be antagonized by **nitrofurantoin** ▪ **Probenecid** decreases renal elimination of fluoroquinolones ▪ **Digoxin** levels may be increased by concurrent enoxacin

*CAPITALS indicate life-threatening; <u>underlines</u> indicate most frequent.

▪ Fluoroquinolones may increase the risk of nephrotoxicity from **cyclosporine** ▪ Concurrent use of ciprofloxacin with **foscarnet** may increase the risk of seizures ▪ Concurrent **glucocorticoid** therapy may increase the risk of tendon rupture ▪ Concurrent use of grepafloxacin may increase the effects of **caffeine.**

Drug-Food: ▪ Absorption is impaired by concurrent tube feeding (because of metal cations).

ROUTE AND DOSAGE

❑ **Alatrovafloxacin**

- **IV (Adults):** *Serious infections*—300 mg q 24 hr. *Other infections*—200 mg q 24 hr. *Perioperative prophylaxis*—200 mg 30 min–4 hr prior to surgery.

❑ **Ciprofloxacin**

- **PO (Adults):** *Most infections*—500–750 mg q 12 hr. *Urinary tract infections*—250–500 mg q 12 hr. *Gonorrhea*—250 mg single dose.
- **IV (Adults):** *Most infections*—400 mg q 12 hr. *Urinary tract infections*—200 mg q 12 hr.

❑ **Enoxacin**

- **PO (Adults):** *Complicated urinary tract infections*—400 mg q 12 hr. *Uncomplicated urinary tract infections*—200 mg q 12 hr. *Gonorrhea*—400 mg single dose.

❑ **Grepafloxacin**

- **PO (Adults):** *Most infections*—400–600 mg once daily. *Gonorrhea*—400 mg single dose.

❑ **Levofloxacin**

- **PO, IV (Adults):** 250–500 mg q 24 hr.

❑ **Lomefloxacin**

- **PO (Adults):** *Bronchitis/urinary tract infections*—400 mg once daily. *Perioperative prophylaxis (transurethral surgery)*—400 mg 2–6 hr prior to surgery.

❑ **Norfloxacin**

- **PO (Adults):** *Urinary tract infections*—400 mg q 12 hr. *Gonorrhea*—800 mg single dose.

❑ **Ofloxacin**

- **PO, IV (Adults):** *Most infections*—400 mg q 12 hr. *Prostatitis/chlamydial infections*—300 mg q 12 hr. *Urinary tract infections*—200 mg q 12 hr. *Gonorrhea*—400 mg single dose.

❑ **Sparfloxacin**

- **PO (Adults):** 400 mg initially, then 200 mg q 24 hr for 10 days.

❑ **Trovafloxacin**

- **IV (Adults):** *Most infections*—100–200 mg q 24 hr. *Gonorrhea*—100 mg single dose. *Perioperative prophylaxis*—200 mg 30 min–4 hr prior to surgery.

AVAILABILITY

❑ **Alatrovafloxacin**

▪ ***Concentrated solution for injection:*** 200 mg/40 ml[Rx], 300 mg/60 ml[Rx].

❑ **Ciprofloxacin**

▪ ***Tablets:*** 250 mg[Rx], 500 mg[Rx], 750 mg[Rx] ▪ ***Injection:*** 200 mg/20 ml[Rx], 400 mg/40 ml[Rx].

❑ **Enoxacin**

▪ ***Tablets:*** 200 mg[Rx], 400 mg[Rx].

❑ **Grepafloxacin**

▪ ***Tablets:*** 200 mg[Rx].

❑ **Levofloxacin**

▪ ***Tablets:*** 250 mg[Rx], 500 mg[Rx] ▪ ***Concentrated solution for injection:*** 500 mg/20 ml[Rx] ▪ ***Premixed solution for injection:*** 250 mg[Rx], 500 mg[Rx].

❑ **Lomefloxacin**

▪ ***Tablets:*** 400 mg[Rx].

❑ **Norfloxacin**

▪ ***Tablets:*** 400 mg[Rx].

❑ **Ofloxacin**

▪ ***Tablets:*** 200 mg[Rx], 300 mg[Rx], 400 mg[Rx] ▪ ***Injection:*** 20 mg/ml[Rx], 40 mg/ml[Rx] ▪ ***Premixed injection:*** 200 mg/50 ml[Rx], 400 mg/100 ml[Rx].

❑ **Sparfloxacin**

▪ ***Tablets:*** 200 mg[Rx].

❑ **Trovafloxacin**

▪ ***Tablets:*** 100 mg[Rx], 200 mg[Rx].

F

TIME/ACTION PROFILE (blood levels)

	ONSET	PEAK	DURATION
Alatrovafloxacin IV	rapid	end of infusion	24 hr
Ciprofloxacin—PO	rapid	1–2 hr	12 hr
Ciprofloxacin—IV	rapid	end of infusion	12 hr
Enoxacin—PO	rapid	1–3 hr	12 hr
Grepafloxacin PO	rapid	2–3 hr	24 hr
Levofloxacin—PO	rapid	1–2 hr	24 hr
Levofloxacin—IV	rapid	end of infusion	24 hr
Lomefloxacin—PO	rapid	UK	24 hr
Norfloxacin—PO	rapid	2–3 hr	12 hr
Ofloxacin—PO	rapid	1–2 hr	12 hr
Ofloxacin—IV	rapid	end of infusion	12 hr
Sparfloxacin—PO	rapid	3–6 hr	24 hr
Trovafloxacin	rapid	1 hr	24 hr

NURSING IMPLICATIONS

ASSESSMENT

- Assess patient for infection (vital signs; appearance of wound, sputum, urine, and stool; WBC; urinalysis; frequency and urgency of urination; cloudy or foul-smelling urine) at beginning of and throughout therapy.
- Obtain specimens for culture and sensitivity prior to initiating therapy. First dose may be given before receiving results.
- ***Lab Test Considerations:*** May cause increased serum AST, ALT, LDH, bilirubin, and alkaline phosphatase.
- May also cause decreased WBC; increased or decreased serum glucose; and glucosuria, hematuria, proteinuria, and albuminuria.
- Ciprofloxacin and norfloxacin may also cause crystalluria and elevated BUN and serum creatinine concentrations.

POTENTIAL NURSING DIAGNOSES

- Infection, risk for (Patient/Family Teaching).
- Knowledge deficit, related to medication regimen (Patient/Family Teaching).

IMPLEMENTATION

- **PO:** Administer *norfloxacin, ofloxacin,* and *enoxacin* on an empty stomach 1 hr before or 2 hr after meals, with a full glass of water. *Alatrovafloxacin* and *grepafloxacin* may be administered without regard to meals. Antacids containing magnesium or aluminum, iron, or zinc preparations should not be taken within 4 hr before and 2 hr after administration.
- If gastric irritation occurs, ciprofloxacin and lomefloxacin may be administered with meals. Food slows and may slightly decrease absorption.
- Milk and yogurt decrease the absorption of ciprofloxacin. Do not administer concurrently.

Alatrovafloxacin

- **Intermittent Infusion:** Dilute with D5W, 0.45% NaCl, D5/0.45% NaCl, D5/0.9% NaCl, or D5/LR for a concentration of 1–2 mg/ml. Discard unused portion.
- ***Rate:*** Administer over 60 min.
- **Y-Site Incompatibility:** ▪ Temporarily discontinue other solutions when administering alatrovafloxacin. Flush line before and after administration.
- **Additive Incompatibility:** ▪ Do not admix with other medications.

Ciprofloxacin

- **Intermittent Infusion:** Dilute to a concentration of 1–2 mg/ml with 0.9% NaCl or D5W. Stable for 14 days at refrigerated or room temperature.
- ***Rate:*** Administer over 60 min into a large vein to minimize venous irritation.
- **Y-Site Incompatibility:** ▪ Temporarily discontinue other solutions when administering ciprofloxacin.

Levofloxacin

- **Intermittent Infusion:** Dilute to a concentration of 5 mg/ml with 0.9% NaCl, D5W, D5/0.9% NaCl, D5/0.45% NaCl, D5/LR, 5% sodium bicarbonate, D5, Plasmalyte 56, or sodium lactate. Also available in premixed bottles and flexible containers with D5W, which need no further dilution. Discard unused solution. Diluted solution is stable for 72 hr at room temperature and 14 days if refrigerated.
- ***Rate:*** Administer by infusion over at least 60 min. Avoid rapid bolus injection.
- **Additive Compatibility:** ▪ potassium chloride.

Ofloxacin

- **Intermittent Infusion:** Dilute to a concentration of 4 mg/ml with 0.9% NaCl, D5W, D5/0.9% NaCl, D5/LR, 5% sodium bicarbonate, D5, Plasmalyte 56, or sodium lactate. Also available in premixed bottles and flexible containers with D5W that need no further dilution. Discard unused solution.

- ***Rate:*** Administer by infusion only over at least 60 min.
- **Syringe Compatibility:** ▪ cefotaxime.
- **Y-Site Compatibility:** ▪ ampicillin.
- **Y-Site Incompatibility:** ▪ cefepime.
- **Additive Compatibility:** ▪ ceftazidime ▪ clindamycin ▪ gentamicin ▪ piperacillin ▪ tobramycin ▪ vancomycin.

PATIENT/FAMILY TEACHING

- □ Instruct patient to take medication as directed at evenly spaced times and to finish drug completely, even if feeling better. Missed doses should be taken as soon as possible, unless almost time for next dose. Do not double doses. Advise patient that sharing of this medication may be dangerous.
- □ Advise patients to notify health care professional immediately if they are taking theophylline.
- □ Encourage patient to maintain a fluid intake of at least 1500–2000 ml/day to prevent crystalluria.
- □ Advise patient that antacids or medications containing iron or zinc will decrease absorption and should not be taken within 2 hr before ***norfloxacin*** or ***ofloxacine,*** 4 hr before ***grepafloxacin*** or ***trovafloxacin,*** 6 hr before ***ciprofloxacin*** or ***lomefloxacin,*** or 8 hr before ***enoxacin*** and 2 hr (***grepafloxacin***—4 hr) after taking this medication.
- □ May cause dizziness and drowsiness. Caution patient to avoid driving or other activities requiring alertness until response to medication is known.
- □ Caution patient to use sunscreen and protective clothing to prevent phototoxicity reactions during and for 5 days following therapy.
- □ Advise patient that frequent mouth rinses, good oral hygiene, and sugarless gum or candy may minimize dry mouth.
- □ Instruct patients being treated for gonorrhea that partners also must be treated.
- □ Advise patient to report signs of superinfection (furry overgrowth on the tongue, vaginal itching or discharge, loose or foul-smelling stools).
- □ Instruct patient to notify health care professional immediately if rash or tendon pain or inflammation occurs or if symptoms do not improve within a few days of therapy.

EVALUATION

Clinical response to therapy can be evaluated by: ▪ Resolution of the signs and symptoms of infection. Time for complete resolution depends on organism and site of infection ▪ Resolution of the signs and symptoms of urinary tract infection □ Negative urine culture.

FLUOROURACIL

(flure-oh-**yoor**-a-sill)

Adrucil, Efudex, Fluoroplex, 5-FU

CLASSIFICATION(S):

Antineoplastic (antimetabolite)

Pregnancy Category D

INDICATIONS

▪ **IV:** Used alone and in combination with other modalities (surgery, radiation therapy, other antineoplastic agents) in the treatment of: □ Colon □ Breast □ Rectal □ Gastric □ Pancreatic carcinoma ▪ **Topical:** Management of multiple actinic (solar) keratoses and superficial basal cell carcinomas.

ACTION

▪ Inhibits DNA and RNA synthesis by preventing thymidine production (cell-cycle S-phase–specific). **Therapeutic Effects:** ▪ Death of rapidly replicating cells, particularly malignant ones.

PHARMACOKINETICS

Absorption: Minimal absorption (5–10%) following topical application.

Distribution: Widely distributed; concentrates and persists in tumors.

Metabolism and Excretion: Converted to an active metabolite; undergoes hepatic metabolism with small amounts excreted unchanged in urine.

Half-life: 20 hr.

F

CONTRAINDICATIONS AND PRECAUTIONS

Contraindicated in: ▪ Hypersensitivity ▪ Pregnancy or lactation.
Use Cautiously in: ▪ Patients with childbearing potential ▪ Infections ▪ Depressed bone marrow reserve ▪ Other chronic debilitating illnesses ▪ Obese patients, patients with edema or ascites (dose should be based on ideal body weight).

ADVERSE REACTIONS AND SIDE EFFECTS*

More likely to occur with systemic use than with topical use.
CNS: acute cerebellar dysfunction.
GI: diarrhea, nausea, stomatitis, vomiting.
Derm: alopecia, maculopapular rash, local inflammatory reactions (topical only), melanosis of nails, nail loss, palmar-plantar erythrodysesthesia, phototoxicity.
Endo: gonadal suppression.
Hemat: anemia, leukopenia, thrombocytopenia.
Local: thrombophlebitis.
Misc: fever.

INTERACTIONS

Drug-Drug: ▪ Additive bone marrow depression with other **bone marrow depressants** (other **antineoplastics** and **radiation therapy**) ▪ May decrease antibody response to **live virus vaccines** and increase risk of adverse reactions.

ROUTE AND DOSAGE

Doses may vary greatly, depending on tumor, patient condition, and protocol use.

❑ Advanced Colorectal Cancer

- **IV (Adults):** 370 mg/m² preceded by leucovorin or 425 mg/m² preceded by leucovorin daily for 5 days. May be repeated q 4–5 wk.

❑ Other Tumors

- **IV (Adults):** *Initial dose*—12 mg/kg/day for 4 days, then 1 day of rest, then 6 mg/kg every other day for 4–5 doses or 7–12 mg/kg/day for 4 days followed by 3-day rest, then 7–10 mg/kg q 3–4 days for 3 doses. *Maintenance*—7–12 mg/kg q 7–10 days or 300–500 mg/m²/day for 4–5 days, repeated monthly (no single daily dose should exceed 800 mg). **Poor-Risk Patients:** 3–6 mg/kg/day on days 1–3, 3 mg/kg/day on days 5, 7, 9 (not to exceed 400 mg/dose). Doses of 370–425 mg/m²/day for 5 days have been used in combination with leucovorin.

❑ Actinic (Solar) Keratoses/Superficial Basal Cell Carcinomas

- **Topical (Adults):** *Actinic/solar keratoses*—1% solution or cream 1–2 times daily to lesions on head, neck, or chest; 2–5% solution or cream may be needed for hands. *Superficial basal cell carcinomas*—5% solution or cream twice daily for 3–6 wk (up to 12 wk).

AVAILABILITY

▪ ***Injection:*** 50 mg/ml in 10-ml ampules or 10-, 20-, and 100-ml vials[Rx] ▪ ***Cream:*** 1%[Rx], 5%[Rx] ▪ ***Solution:*** 1%[Rx], 2%[Rx], 5%[Rx].

TIME/ACTION PROFILE (IV = effects on blood counts, Top = dermatologic effects)

	ONSET	PEAK	DURATION
IV	1–9 days	9–21 days (nadir)	30 days
Top	2–3 days	2–6 wk	1–2 mo

NURSING IMPLICATIONS

ASSESSMENT

- **General Info:** Monitor vital signs prior to and frequently during therapy.
- ☐ Assess mucous membranes, number and consistency of stools, and frequency of vomiting. Assess for signs of infection (fever, chills, sore throat, cough, hoarseness, pain in lower back or side, difficult or painful urination). Assess for bleeding (bleeding gums; bruising; petechiae; and guaiac test stools, urine, and emesis). Avoid IM injections and rectal temperatures. Apply pressure to venipuncture sites for 10 min. Notify physician if symptoms of toxicity (stomatitis or esophagopharyngitis, uncontrollable vomiting, diarrhea, GI bleeding, myocardial ischemia, leukocyte count <3500/mm³, platelet count <100,000/mm³, or hemorrhage from any site) occur; drug will need to be discontinued. May be reinitiated at a lower dose when side effects have subsided.
- ☐ Assess IV site frequently for inflammation or infiltration. Patient should notify nurse if pain

*CAPITALS indicate life-threatening; underlines indicate most frequent.

or irritation at injection site occurs. May cause thrombophlebitis. If extravasation occurs, infusion must be stopped and restarted in another vein to avoid damage to SC tissue. Report immediately. Standard treatment includes application of ice compresses.

- Assess skin for palmar-plantar erythrodysesthesia (tingling of hands and feet followed by pain, erythema, and swelling) throughout therapy.
- Monitor intake and output, appetite, and nutritional intake. GI effects usually occur on 4th day of therapy. Adjusting diet as tolerated may help maintain fluid and electrolyte balance and nutritional status.
- Monitor patient for cerebellar dysfunction (weakness, ataxia, dizziness). This may persist after discontinuation of therapy.

- **Topical:** Inspect involved skin prior to and throughout therapy.
- ***Lab Test Considerations:*** May cause a decrease in plasma albumin.
  - Hepatic (AST, ALT, LDH, and serum bilirubin), renal, and hematologic (hematocrit, hemoglobin, leukocyte, platelet count) functions should be monitored prior to and periodically throughout therapy. CBC should be monitored daily during IV therapy. Report WBC of $<3500/mm^3$ or platelets $<100,000/mm^3$ immediately; they are criteria for discontinuation. Nadir of leukopenia usually occurs in 9–14 days, with recovery by day 30. May also cause thrombocytopenia.
  - May cause an increase in urine excretion of 5-hydroxyindoleacetic acid (5-HIAA).

POTENTIAL NURSING DIAGNOSES

- Infection, risk for (Side Effects).
- Nutrition, altered, less than body requirements (Side Effects).
- Knowledge deficit, related to medication regimen (Patient/Family Teaching).

IMPLEMENTATION

- **General Info:** Solution should be prepared in a biologic cabinet. Wear gloves, gown, and mask while handling IV medication. Discard IV equipment in specially designated containers (see Appendix I).
  - The number 5 in 5-fluorouracil is part of the drug name and does not refer to the dosage.
- **Direct IV:** May be administered undiluted.
- ***Rate:*** Rapid IV push administration (over 1–2 min) is most effective, but there is a more rapid onset of toxicity.
- **Intermittent Infusion:** May be diluted with D5W or 0.9% NaCl.
  - Use plastic IV tubing and IV bags to maintain greater stability of medication. Solution is stable for 24 hr at room temperature; do not refrigerate. Solution is colorless to faint yellow. Discard highly discolored or cloudy solution. If crystals form, dissolve by warming solution to 140°F, shaking vigorously, and cooling to body temperature.
- ***Rate:*** Onset of toxicity is greatly delayed by administering an infusion over 2–8 hr.
- **Syringe Compatibility:** ▪ bleomycin ▪ cisplatin ▪ cyclophosphamide ▪ doxorubicin ▪ furosemide ▪ heparin ▪ leucovorin ▪ methotrexate ▪ metoclopramide ▪ mitomycin ▪ vinblastine ▪ vincristine.
- **Syringe Incompatibility:** ▪ droperidol.
- **Y-Site Compatibility:** ▪ amifostine ▪ aztreonam ▪ bleomycin ▪ cefepime ▪ cisplatin ▪ cyclophosphamide ▪ doxorubicin ▪ fludarabine ▪ furosemide ▪ granisetron ▪ heparin ▪ hydrocortisone ▪ leucovorin ▪ mannitol ▪ melphalan ▪ methotrexate ▪ metoclopramide ▪ mitomycin ▪ paclitaxel ▪ piperacillin/tazobactam ▪ potassium chloride ▪ sargramostim ▪ teniposide ▪ thiotepa ▪ vinblastine ▪ vincristine ▪ vitamin B complex with C.
- **Y-Site Incompatibility:** ▪ droperidol ▪ filgrastim ▪ gallium nitrate ▪ vinorelbine.
- **Additive Compatibility:** ▪ D5/LR ▪ bleomycin ▪ cyclophosphamide ▪ etoposide ▪ floxuridine ▪ ifosfamide ▪ leucovorin ▪ methotrexate ▪ mitoxantrone ▪ prednisolone ▪ vincristine.
- **Additive Incompatibility:** ▪ carboplatin ▪ cisplatin ▪ cytarabine ▪ diazepam ▪ doxorubicin ▪ leucovorin ▪ metoclopramide.
- **Topical:** Consult physician before administering topical preparations to determine what skin preparation regimen should be followed. Tight occlusive dressings are not advised because of irritation to surrounding healthy tissue. A loose gauze dressing for cosmetic purposes is usually preferred. Wear gloves when applying medication. Do not use metallic applicator.

F

PATIENT/FAMILY TEACHING

- **General Info:** Instruct patient to notify health care professional if fever; chills; sore throat; signs of infection; yellowing of skin or eyes; abdominal pain; joint or flank pain; swelling of feet or legs; bleeding gums; bruising; petechiae; or blood in urine, stool, or emesis occurs. Caution patient to avoid crowds and persons with known infections. Instruct patient to use soft toothbrush and electric razor. Patients should be cautioned not to drink alcoholic beverages or take products containing aspirin or NSAIDs.
  - Advise patient to rinse mouth with clear water after eating and drinking and to avoid flossing to minimize stomatitis. Viscous lidocaine may be used if mouth pain interferes with eating. Stomatitis pain may require treatment with opioid analgesics.
  - Discuss with patient the possibility of hair loss. Explore methods of coping.
  - Review with patient the need for contraception during therapy.
  - Caution patient to use sunscreen and protective clothing to prevent phototoxicity reactions.
  - Instruct patient not to receive any vaccinations without advice of health care professional.
  - Emphasize the importance of routine follow-up lab tests to monitor progress and to check for side effects.
- **Topical:** Instruct patient in correct application of solution or cream. Emphasize importance of avoiding the eyes; caution should also be used when applying medication near mouth and nose. If patient uses clean finger to self-administer, emphasize importance of washing hands thoroughly after application. Explain that erythema, scaling, and blistering with pruritus and burning sensation are expected. Therapy is discontinued when erosion, ulceration, and necrosis occur in 2–6 wk (10–12 wk for basal cell carcinomas). Skin heals 48 wk later.

EVALUATION

Effectiveness of therapy can be demonstrated by: ▪ Tumor regression ▪ Removal of solar keratoses or superficial basal cell skin cancers.

FLUOXETINE
(floo-**ox**-uh-teen)
Prozac

CLASSIFICATION(S):
Antidepressant (selective serotonin reuptake inhibitor [SSRI])

Pregnancy Category B

INDICATIONS

▪ Various forms of depression, often in conjunction with psychotherapy ▪ Obsessive-compulsive disorder (OCD) ▪ Bulimia nervosa. **Unlabeled Uses:** □ Anorexia nervosa □ Attention-deficit hyperactivity disorder □ Diabetic neuropathy □ Fibromyalgia □ Obesity □ Panic attacks □ Premenstrual syndrome □ Raynaud's phenomenon.

ACTION

▪ Selectively inhibits the reuptake of serotonin in the CNS. **Therapeutic Effects:** ▪ Antidepressant action.

PHARMACOKINETICS

Absorption: Well absorbed following oral administration.
Distribution: Crosses the blood-brain barrier.
Metabolism and Excretion: Converted by the liver to norfluoxetine, another antidepressant compound; fluoxetine and norfluoxetine are mostly metabolized by the liver; 12% excreted by kidneys as unchanged fluoxetine, 7% as unchanged norfluoxetine.
Half-life: 1–3 days (norfluoxetine 5–7 days).

CONTRAINDICATIONS AND PRECAUTIONS

Contraindicated in: ▪ Hypersensitivity ▪ Concurrent use of astemizole or cisapride.
Use Cautiously in: ▪ Severe hepatic or renal impairment (dosage adjustment may be necessary) ▪ History of seizures ▪ Debilitated patients (increased risk of seizures) ▪ Diabetes mellitus ▪ Geriatric patients and patients with impaired hepatic function, concurrent illness, or multiple drug therapy (lower doses/increased dosing interval may be necessary) ▪ Pregnancy or lactation (although safety not established, has been used without harm during pregnancy).

ADVERSE REACTIONS AND SIDE EFFECTS*

CNS: SEIZURES, anxiety, drowsiness, headache, insomnia, nervousness, abnormal dreams, dizziness, fatigue, hypomania, mania, weakness.
EENT: stuffy nose, visual disturbances.
Resp: cough.
CV: chest pain, palpitations.
GI: diarrhea, abdominal pain, abnormal taste, anorexia, constipation, dry mouth, dyspepsia, nausea, vomiting, weight loss.
GU: urinary frequency.
Derm: excessive sweating, pruritus, flushing, rashes.
Endo: dysmenorrhea.
MS: arthralgia, back pain, myalgia.
Neuro: tremor.
Misc: allergic reactions, fever, flu-like syndrome, hot flashes, sensitivity reaction, sexual dysfunction.

INTERACTIONS

Drug-Drug: ▪ **Discontinue use of MAO inhibitors** for 14 days prior to fluoxetine therapy; combined therapy may result in confusion, agitation, seizures, hypertension, hyperpyrexia (serotonin syndrome). Fluoxetine should be discontinued for at least 5 wk before MAO inhibitor therapy is initiated ▪ May increase the risk of serious adverse cardiovascular effects from **astemizole** or **cisapride** ▪ Additive CNS depression with **alcohol, antihistamines,** other **antidepressants, opioids,** or **sedative/hypnotics** ▪ Increased risk of side effects and adverse reactions with other **antidepressants, tryptophan,** or **phenothiazines** ▪ May increase effectiveness/risk of toxicity from **digitoxin, digoxin, phenytoin, lithium,** or **warfarin.**

ROUTE AND DOSAGE

- **PO (Adults):** *Depression, obsessive-compulsive disorder*—20 mg/day in the morning. After several weeks, may increase by 20 mg/day at weekly intervals. Doses greater than 20 mg/day should be given in 2 divided doses, in the morning and at noon (not to exceed 80 mg/day). *Bulimia nervosa*—60 mg/day (may need to titrate up to dosage over several days).
- **PO (Geriatric Patients):** 10 mg/day in the morning initially, may be increased (not to exceed 60 mg/day).

AVAILABILITY

▪ ***Capsules:*** 10 mg[Rx], 20 mg[Rx] ▪ ***Oral solution:*** 20 mg/5 ml[Rx].

TIME/ACTION PROFILE (antidepressant effect)

	ONSET	PEAK	DURATION
PO	1–4 wk	UK	2 wk

NURSING IMPLICATIONS

ASSESSMENT

- **General Info:** Monitor mood changes. Inform physician or other health care professional if patient demonstrates significant increase in anxiety, nervousness, or insomnia.
  - □ Assess for suicidal tendencies, especially during early therapy. Restrict amount of drug available to patient.
  - □ Monitor appetite and nutritional intake. Weigh weekly. Notify physician or other health care professional of continued weight loss. Adjust diet as tolerated to support nutritional status.
  - □ Assess patient for possible sensitivity reaction (urticaria, fever, arthralgia, edema, carpal tunnel syndrome, rash, hives, lymphadenopathy, respiratory distress) and notify physician or other health care professional if present; these symptoms usually resolve by stopping fluoxetine but may require administration of antihistamines or glucocorticoids.
- **Obsessive-Compulsive Disorder:** Assess patient for frequency of obsessive-compulsive behaviors. Note degree to which these thoughts and behaviors interfere with daily functioning.
- **Bulimia Nervosa:** Assess frequency of binge eating and vomiting throughout therapy.
- ***Lab Test Considerations:*** Monitor CBC and differential periodically during course of therapy. Notify physician or other health care professional if leukopenia, anemia, thrombocytopenia, or increased bleeding time occurs.

F

***CAPITALS indicate life-threatening; underlines indicate most frequent.**

- □ Proteinuria and mild increase in AST may occur during sensitivity reactions.
- □ May cause increase in serum alkaline phosphatase, ALT, BUN, creatine phosphokinase, hypouricemia, hypocalcemia, hypoglycemia or hyperglycemia, and hyponatremia.

POTENTIAL NURSING DIAGNOSES

- ■ Coping, ineffective individual (Indications).
- ■ Injury, risk for (Side Effects).
- ■ Knowledge deficit, related to medication regimen (Patient/Family Teaching).

IMPLEMENTATION

- ■ **PO:** Administer as a single dose in the morning. Some patients may require increased amounts, in divided doses, with a 2nd dose at noon.
- □ May be administered with food to minimize GI irritation.

PATIENT/FAMILY TEACHING

- □ Instruct patient to take fluoxetine exactly as directed. If a dose is missed, omit dose and return to regular dosing schedule. Do not double doses.
- □ May cause drowsiness, dizziness, impaired judgment, and blurred vision. Caution patient to avoid driving and other activities requiring alertness until response to the drug is known.
- □ Advise patient to avoid alcohol or other CNS depressant drugs during therapy and to consult health care professional before taking other medications with fluoxetine.
- □ Caution patient to change positions slowly to minimize dizziness.
- □ Inform patient that frequent mouth rinses, good oral hygiene, and sugarless gum or candy may minimize dry mouth. If dry mouth persists for more than 2 wk, consult health care professional regarding use of saliva substitute.
- □ Instruct female patients to inform health care professional if pregnancy is planned or suspected.
- □ Caution patient to wear protective clothing and use sunscreen to prevent photosensitivity reactions.
- □ Advise patient to notify health care professional if symptoms of sensitivity reaction occur or if headache, nausea, anorexia, anxiety, or insomnia persists.
- □ Emphasize the importance of follow-up exams to monitor progress. Encourage patient participation in psychotherapy.

EVALUATION

Effectiveness of therapy can be demonstrated by: ■ Increased sense of well-being □ Renewed interest in surroundings. May require 1–4 wk of therapy to obtain antidepressant effects ■ Decrease in obsessive-compulsive behaviors ■ Decrease in binge eating and vomiting in patients with bulimia nervosa.

FLUPHENAZINE
(floo-**fen**-a-zeen)

fluphenazine decanoate
{Modecate}, {Modecate Concentrate}, Prolixin Decanoate

fluphenazine enanthate
{Moditen Enanthate}, Prolixin Enanthate

fluphenazine hydrochloride
{Apo-Fluphenazine}, {Moditen HCl}, {Moditen HCl-HP}, Permitil, Prolixin

CLASSIFICATION(S):
Antipsychotic agents (phenothiazine)

Pregnancy Category C

INDICATIONS

■ Acute and chronic psychoses.

ACTION

■ Alter the effects of dopamine in the CNS ■ Possess anticholinergic and alpha-adrenergic blocking activity. **Therapeutic Effects:** ■ Diminished signs and symptoms of psychoses.

PHARMACOKINETICS

Absorption: Well absorbed following PO/IM administration. Decanoate and enanthate salts in sesame oil have delayed onset and prolonged action due to delayed release from oil vehicle and subsequent delayed release from fatty tissues.

{} = Available in Canada only.

Distribution: Widely distributed. Cross the blood-brain barrier. Cross the placenta; enter breast milk.
Protein Binding: ≥90%.
Metabolism and Excretion: Highly metabolized by the liver, undergo enterohepatic recirculation.
Half-life: *Fluphenazine hydrochloride*—4.7–15.3 hr; *fluphenazine enanthate*—3.7 days; *fluphenazine decanoate*—6.8–9.6 days.

CONTRAINDICATIONS AND PRECAUTIONS

Contraindicated in: ▪ Hypersensitivity ▪ Cross-sensitivity with other phenothiazines may exist ▪ Narrow-angle glaucoma ▪ Bone marrow depression ▪ Severe liver or cardiovascular disease ▪ Hypersensitivity to sesame oil (decanoate and enanthate salts) ▪ Some products contain alcohol or tartrazine and should be avoided in patients with known intolerance.
Use Cautiously in: ▪ Geriatric or debilitated patients (initial dosage reduction may be necessary) ▪ Diabetes mellitus ▪ Respiratory disease ▪ Prostatic hypertrophy ▪ CNS tumors ▪ Epilepsy ▪ Intestinal obstruction ▪ Pregnancy or lactation (safety not established).

ADVERSE REACTIONS AND SIDE EFFECTS*

CNS: extrapyramidal reactions, sedation, tardive dyskinesia.
EENT: blurred vision, dry eyes, lens opacities.
CV: hypotension, tachycardia.
GI: anorexia, constipation, drug-induced hepatitis, dry mouth, ileus.
GU: urinary retention.
Derm: photosensitivity, pigment changes, rashes.
Endo: galactorrhea.
Hemat: AGRANULOCYTOSIS, leukopenia.
Misc: allergic reactions, hyperthermia.

INTERACTIONS

Drug-Drug: ▪ Additive hypotension with **antihypertensive agents** ▪ Additive CNS depression with other **CNS depressants**, including **alcohol, antidepressants, antihistamines, MAO inhibitors, opioids, sedative/hypnotics**, or **general anesthetics** ▪ **Phenobarbital** may increase metabolism and decrease effectiveness ▪ Concurrent use with **lithium** may produce any of the following—decreased fluphenazine absorption, increased excretion of lithium, increased risk of extrapyramidal reactions, or masking of the early signs of lithium toxicity ▪ **Antacids** or **adsorbent antidiarrheals (kaolin)** may decrease oral absorption ▪ Increased risk of agranulocytosis with **antithyroid drugs** ▪ May decrease anti-Parkinson activity of **levodopa** and **bromocriptine** ▪ Decrease vasopressor response to **epinephrine** and **norepinephrine** ▪ Decrease antihypertensive effect of **guanethidine** ▪ Concurrent use with **beta blockers** may result in inhibition of metabolism of one or both drugs, producing an increased response ▪ Increased risk of anticholinergic effects with other **agents having anticholinergic properties**, including **antihistamines, tricyclic antidepressants, disopyramide**, or **quinidine.**

ROUTE AND DOSAGE

❑ **Fluphenazine Decanoate**

- **IM, SC (Adults):** 12.5–25 mg initially, may be repeated q 1–4 wk. Dosage may be slowly increased as needed (not to exceed 100 mg/dose).
- **IM, SC (Children ≥12 yr):** 6.25–18.75 mg initially, may be repeated q 1–3 wk. Dosage may be slowly increased as needed to 25 mg.
- **IM, SC (Children 5–12 yr):** 3.125–12.5 mg initially, may be repeated q 1–3 wk. Dosage may be slowly increased.

❑ **Fluphenazine Enanthate**

- **IM, SC (Adults):** 25 mg q 1–3 wk. May be slowly increased as needed (not to exceed 100 mg/dose).

❑ **Fluphenazine Hydrochloride**

- **PO (Adults):** *Initial dose*—2.5–10 mg/day in divided doses q 6–8 hr. *Maintenance dose*—1–5 mg/day.
- **PO, IM (Geriatric Patients or Debilitated Patients):** 1–2.5 mg/day initially.
- **IM (Adults):** 1.25–2.5 mg q 6–8 hr.

AVAILABILITY

▪ ***Fluphenazine decanoate injection:*** 25 mg/ml[Rx], {100 mg/ml[Rx]} ▪ ***Fluphenazine en-***

F

*CAPITALS indicate life-threatening; underlines indicate most frequent.

anthate injection: 25 mg/ml[Rx] ▪ {***Fluphenazine hydrochloride tablets:*** 1 mg[Rx], 2.5 mg[Rx], 5 mg[Rx], 10 mg[Rx]} ▪ ***Fluphenazine hydrochloride elixir:*** 2.5 mg/5 ml[Rx] ▪ ***Fluphenazine hydrochloride concentrate:*** 5 mg/ml[Rx] ▪ ***Fluphenazine hydrochloride injection:*** 2.5 mg/ml[Rx], {10 mg/ml[Rx]}.

TIME/ACTION PROFILE (antipsychotic activity)

	ONSET	PEAK	DURATION
PO hydrochloride	1 hr	UK	6–8 hr
IM hydrochloride	1 hr	1.5–2 hr	6–8 hr
IM enanthate	24–72 hr	UK	1–3 wk
IM decanoate	24–72 hr	UK	≥4 wk

NURSING IMPLICATIONS

ASSESSMENT

- Assess patient's mental status (orientation, mood, behavior) prior to and periodically throughout therapy.
- Monitor blood pressure (sitting, standing, lying), ECG, pulse, and respiratory rate prior to and frequently during the period of dosage adjustment. May cause Q-wave and T-wave changes in ECG.
- Observe patient carefully when administering oral medication to ensure medication is actually taken and not hoarded.
- Assess fluid intake and bowel function. Increased bulk and fluids in the diet help minimize constipation.
- Monitor patient for onset of akathisia (restlessness or desire to keep moving) and extrapyramidal side effects (*parkinsonian*—difficulty speaking or swallowing, loss of balance control, pill rolling, mask-like face, shuffling gait, rigidity, tremors; *dystonic*—muscle spasms, twisting motions, twitching, inability to move eyes, weakness of arms or legs) every 2 mo during therapy and 8–12 wk after therapy has been discontinued. Reduction in dosage or discontinuation of medication may be necessary. Trihexyphenidyl or diphenhydramine may be used to control these symptoms.
- Monitor for tardive dyskinesia (uncontrolled rhythmic movement of mouth, face, and extremities; lip smacking or puckering; puffing of cheeks; uncontrolled chewing; rapid or worm-like movements of tongue). Report immediately; may be irreversible.
- Monitor for development of neuroleptic malignant syndrome (fever, respiratory distress, tachycardia, convulsions, diaphoresis, hypertension or hypotension, pallor, tiredness, severe muscle stiffness, loss of bladder control). Report immediately.
- ***Lab Test Considerations:*** CBC, liver function tests, and ocular examinations should be evaluated periodically during therapy. May cause decreased hematocrit, hemoglobin, leukocytes, granulocytes, and platelets. May cause elevated bilirubin, AST, ALT, and alkaline phosphatase. Agranulocytosis may occur after 4–10 wk of therapy with recovery 1–2 wk following discontinuation. May recur if medication is restarted. Liver function abnormalities may require discontinuation of therapy.
- May cause false-positive or false-negative pregnancy tests and false-positive urine bilirubin test results.

POTENTIAL NURSING DIAGNOSES

- Thought processes, altered (Indications).
- Knowledge deficit, related to medication regimen (Patient/Family Teaching).
- Noncompliance (Patient/Family Teaching).

IMPLEMENTATION

- **General Info:** Slight yellow to amber color does not alter potency.
- To prevent contact dermatitis, avoid getting liquid preparations on hands and wash hands thoroughly if spillage occurs.
- Injectable forms must be drawn up with a dry syringe and dry 21-gauge needle to prevent clouding of the solution.
- **PO:** Dilute concentrate just prior to administration in 120–240 ml of water, milk, carbonated beverage, soup, or tomato or fruit juice. Do not mix with beverages containing caffeine (cola, coffee), tannics (tea), or pectinates (apple juice).
- **SC:** Fluphenazine decanoate and enanthate are dissolved in sesame oil for long duration of action. They may be administered SC or IM.
- **IM:** IM dose is usually ⅓–½ of oral dose. Because fluphenazine hydrochloride has a shorter duration of action, it is used initially to determine the patient's response to the drug and to treat the acutely agitated patient.
- Administer deep IM, using a dry syringe and

21-gauge needle, into dorsal gluteal site. Instruct patient to remain recumbent for 30 min to prevent hypotension.

PATIENT/FAMILY TEACHING

- Advise patient to take medication exactly as directed and not to skip doses or double up on missed doses. If a dose is missed, take within 1 hr or skip dose and return to regular schedule if taking more than 1 dose/day; take as soon as possible unless almost time for next dose if taking 1 dose/day. Abrupt withdrawal may lead to gastritis, nausea, vomiting, dizziness, headache, tachycardia, and insomnia.
- Inform patient of possibility of extrapyramidal symptoms and tardive dyskinesia. Caution patient to report these symptoms immediately to health care professional.
- Advise patient to change positions slowly to minimize orthostatic hypotension.
- Medication may cause drowsiness. Caution patient to avoid driving or other activities requiring alertness until response to medication is known.
- Caution patient to avoid taking alcohol or other CNS depressants concurrently with this medication.
- Advise patient to use sunscreen and protective clothing when exposed to the sun. Exposed surfaces may develop a blue-gray pigmentation, which may fade following discontinuation of the medication. Extremes of temperature should also be avoided, as this drug impairs body temperature regulation.
- Advise patient that good oral hygiene, frequent rinsing of mouth with water, and sugarless gum or candy may help relieve dry mouth. Health care professional should be notified if dry mouth persists beyond 2 wk.
- Inform patient that this medication may turn urine pink to reddish-brown.
- Instruct patient to notify health care professional promptly if sore throat, fever, unusual bleeding or bruising, rash, weakness, tremors, visual disturbances, dark-colored urine, or clay-colored stools occur.
- Advise patient to notify health care professional of medication regimen prior to treatment or surgery.
- Emphasize the importance of routine follow-up exams, including ocular exams, with long-term therapy and continued participation in psychotherapy.

EVALUATION

Effectiveness of therapy can be demonstrated by: ▪ Decrease in excitable, paranoic, or withdrawn behavior.

FLURAZEPAM

(flur-**az**-e-pam)

{Apo-Flurazepam}, Dalmane, {Novo-flupam}, {Somnol}

CLASSIFICATION(S):

Sedative/hypnotic (benzodiazepine)

Schedule IV

Pregnancy Category X

INDICATIONS

▪ Short-term management of insomnia (<4 wk).

ACTION

▪ Depresses the CNS, probably by potentiating gamma-aminobutyric acid (GABA), an inhibitory neurotransmitter. **Therapeutic Effects:** ▪ Relief of insomnia.

PHARMACOKINETICS

Absorption: Well absorbed following oral administration.

Distribution: Widely distributed; crosses blood-brain barrier. Probably crosses the placenta and enters breast milk. Accumulation of drug occurs with chronic dosing.

Metabolism and Excretion: Metabolized by the liver; some metabolites have hypnotic activity.

Half-life: 2.3 hr (half-life of active metabolite may be 30–200 hr).

CONTRAINDICATIONS AND PRECAUTIONS

Contraindicated in: ▪ Hypersensitivity ▪ Cross-sensitivity with other benzodiazepines may exist ▪ Pre-existing CNS depression ▪ Severe uncontrolled pain ▪ Narrow-angle glaucoma ▪ Pregnancy or lactation.

Use Cautiously in: ▪ Hepatic dysfunction (dosage reduction may be necessary) ▪ History of suicide attempt or drug dependence ▪ Geriatric or debilitated patients (initial dosage reduction may be necessary) ▪ Children <15 yr (safety not established).

ADVERSE REACTIONS AND SIDE EFFECTS

CNS: confusion, daytime drowsiness, decreased concentration, dizziness, headache, lethargy, mental depression, paradoxical excitation.
EENT: blurred vision.
GI: constipation, diarrhea, nausea, vomiting.
Derm: rashes.
Neuro: ataxia.
Misc: physical dependence, psychological dependence, tolerance.

INTERACTIONS

Drug-Drug: ▪ Concurrent use with **alcohol, antidepressants, antihistamines,** and **opioids** may result in additive CNS depression ▪ **Cimetidine, oral contraceptives, disulfiram, fluoxetine, isoniazid, ketoconazole, metoprolol, propoxyphene, propranolol,** or **valproic acid** may decrease the metabolism of flurazepam, enhancing its actions ▪ May decrease efficacy of **levodopa** ▪ **Rifampin** or **barbiturates** may increase the metabolism and decrease effectiveness of flurazepam ▪ Sedative effects may be decreased by **theophylline.**

ROUTE AND DOSAGE

- **PO (Adults):** 15–30 mg at bedtime.
- **PO (Geriatric Patients or Debilitated Patients):** 15 mg initially, may be increased.

AVAILABILITY

▪ ***Capsules:*** 15 mg[Rx], 30 mg[Rx] ▪ {***Tablets:*** 15 mg[Rx], 30 mg[Rx]}.

TIME/ACTION PROFILE (hypnotic activity)

	ONSET	PEAK	DURATION
PO	15–45 min	0.5–1 hr	7–8 hr

NURSING IMPLICATIONS

ASSESSMENT

- □ Assess sleep patterns prior to and periodically throughout therapy.
- □ Prolonged therapy may lead to psychological or physical dependence. Restrict amount of drug available to patient, especially if patient is depressed, suicidal, or has a history of addiction.

POTENTIAL NURSING DIAGNOSES

- Sleep pattern disturbance (Indications).
- Injury, risk for (Side Effects).
- Knowledge deficit, related to medication regimen (Patient/Family Teaching).

IMPLEMENTATION

- **General Info:** Supervise ambulation and transfer of patients following administration. Remove cigarettes. Side rails should be raised and call bell within reach at all times.
- **PO:** Capsules may be opened and mixed with food or fluids for patients having difficulty swallowing.

PATIENT/FAMILY TEACHING

- □ Advise patient to take medication exactly as directed. Discuss the importance of preparing environment for sleep (dark room, quiet, avoidance of nicotine and caffeine).
- □ Medication may cause daytime drowsiness. Caution patient to avoid driving and other activities requiring alertness until response to medication is known.
- □ Caution patient to avoid taking alcohol or other CNS depressants concurrently with this medication.
- □ Instruct patient to contact health care professional immediately if pregnancy is planned or suspected.

EVALUATION

Effectiveness of therapy can be demonstrated by: ▪ Improvement in sleep patterns. Maximum hypnotic properties are apparent 2–3 nights after initiating therapy and may last 1–2 nights after therapy is discontinued.

FLURBIPROFEN†

(flure-**bye**-proe-fen)
Ansaid, {Apo-Flurbiprofen}, {Froben}, {Novo-Flurprofen}, {Nu-Flurbiprofen}

{} = Available in Canada only.

CLASSIFICATION(S):
Nonsteroidal anti-inflammatory agent

Pregnancy Category B (first trimester)

†See Appendix O for ophthalmic use.

INDICATIONS

▪ **PO:** Inflammatory disorders including: ▫ Rheumatoid arthritis ▫ Osteoarthritis. **Unlabeled Uses:** ▪ **PO:** ▫ Nonopioid analgesic ▫ Antidysmenorrheal.

ACTION

▪ Inhibits prostaglandin synthesis, resulting in reduced inflammation and pain when administered orally. **Therapeutic Effects:** ▪ **PO:** Suppression of pain and inflammation.

PHARMACOKINETICS

Absorption: Well absorbed following oral administration.
Distribution: UK.
Metabolism and Excretion: Mostly metabolized by the liver; 20–25% excreted unchanged by the kidneys.
Half-life: 3–6 hr.

CONTRAINDICATIONS AND PRECAUTIONS

Contraindicated in: ▪ Hypersensitivity ▪ Cross-sensitivity may exist with other nonsteroidal anti-inflammatory agents, including aspirin ▪ Active GI bleeding or ulcer disease.
Use Cautiously in: ▪ Severe cardiovascular, renal, or hepatic disease ▪ History of ulcer disease ▪ Diabetes mellitus ▪ Bleeding disorders ▪ Pregnancy (not recommended for use during second half of pregnancy) ▪ Lactation or children (safety not established).

ADVERSE REACTIONS AND SIDE EFFECTS*

CNS: dizziness, drowsiness, headache, insomnia, mental depression, psychic disturbances.
EENT: blurred vision, corneal opacities, tinnitus.
CV: changes in blood pressure, edema, palpitations.
GI: GI BLEEDING, abdominal pain, heartburn, nausea, bloated feeling, constipation, diarrhea, drug-induced hepatitis, stomatitis.
GU: incontinence.
Derm: increased sweating, rashes.
Hemat: *PO*—blood dyscrasias, prolonged bleeding time.
MS: myalgia.
Misc: allergic reactions including ANAPHYLAXIS, and STEVENS-JOHNSON SYNDROME, chills, fever.

INTERACTIONS

Drug-Drug: ▪ Concurrent use with **aspirin** may decrease effectiveness ▪ Additive adverse GI effects with **aspirin**, other **NSAIDs, potassium supplements, glucocorticoids**, or **alcohol** ▪ Chronic use with **acetaminophen** may increase the risk of adverse renal reactions ▪ May decrease the effectiveness of **diuretics** or **antihypertensives** ▪ May increase the hypoglycemic response to **insulin** or **oral hypoglycemic** agents ▪ Increases the risk of toxicity from **methotrexate** ▪ **Probenecid** increases risk of toxicity from flurbiprofen ▪ Increased risk of bleeding with **cefamandole, cefotetan, cefoperazone, plicamycin, heparin, thrombolytic agents, valproic acid**, or **warfarin** ▪ Increased risk of adverse hematologic reactions with **antineoplastic agents** or **radiation therapy** ▪ Increased risk of nephrotoxicity with other **nephrotoxic agents.**

ROUTE AND DOSAGE

▪ **PO (Adults):** *Anti-inflammatory*—200–300 mg daily in 2–4 divided doses (not to exceed 300 mg/day or 100 mg/dose). *Nonopioid analgesic/antidysmenorrheal*—50 mg q 4–6 hr as needed (unlabeled).

AVAILABILITY

▪ ***Tablets:*** 50 mg[Rx], 100 mg[Rx] ▪ ***Extended-release capsules:*** {200 mg[Rx]}.

TIME/ACTION PROFILE

	ONSET	PEAK	DURATION
PO (anti-inflammatory)	few days–1 wk	1–2 wk	UK

F

*CAPITALS indicate life-threatening; underlines indicate most frequent.

NURSING IMPLICATIONS

ASSESSMENT

- **General Info:** Patients who have asthma, aspirin-induced allergy, and nasal polyps are at increased risk for developing hypersensitivity reactions. Monitor for rhinitis, asthma, and urticaria.
- **Arthritis:** Assess pain and range of movement prior to and periodically during therapy.
- ***Lab Test Considerations:*** May cause prolonged bleeding time; effects may persist for <1 day.
- May cause decreased hemoglobin, hematocrit, leukocyte, and platelet counts.
- Monitor liver function tests periodically during therapy. May cause elevated serum alkaline phosphatase, LDH, AST, and ALT concentrations.
- Monitor BUN, serum creatinine, and electrolytes periodically during therapy. May cause increased BUN, serum creatinine, and electrolyte concentrations and decreased urine electrolyte concentrations.

POTENTIAL NURSING DIAGNOSES

- Pain (Indications).
- Physical mobility, impaired (Indications).
- Knowledge deficit, related to medication regimen (Patient/Family Teaching).

IMPLEMENTATION

- **General Info:** Administration in higher than recommended doses does not provide increased effectiveness but may cause increased side effects.
- **PO:** For rapid initial effect, administer 30 min before or 2 hr after meals. Administer after meals or with food or an antacid containing aluminum or magnesium to minimize gastric irritation.

PATIENT/FAMILY TEACHING

- **Arthritis:** Advise patient to take this medication with a full glass of water and to remain in an upright position for 15–30 min after administration.
- Instruct patient to take medication exactly as prescribed. If a dose is missed, take as soon as remembered, but not if almost time for next dose. Do not double doses.
- May cause drowsiness or dizziness. Advise patient to avoid driving or other activities requiring alertness until response to medication is known.
- Caution patient to avoid the concurrent use of alcohol, aspirin, other NSAIDs, acetaminophen, or other OTC medications without consulting health care professional.
- Advise patient to inform health care professional of medication regimen prior to treatment or surgery.
- Advise patient to consult health care professional if rash, itching, visual disturbances, tinnitus, weight gain, edema, black stools, persistent headache, or influenza-like syndrome (chills, fever, muscle aches, pain) occurs.

EVALUATION

Effectiveness of therapy can be demonstrated by: ▪ Decreased pain ▫ Improved joint mobility. Patients who do not respond to one NSAID may respond to another.

FLUTAMIDE

(**floo**-ta-mide)
Eulexin

CLASSIFICATION(S):
Antineoplastic (hormone)

Pregnancy Category D

INDICATIONS

▪ Treatment of metastatic prostate carcinoma in conjunction with luteinizing hormone–releasing hormone analogues (LHRH) (leuprolide).

ACTION

▪ Antagonizes the effects of androgen (testosterone) at the cellular level. **Therapeutic Effects:** ▪ Decreased growth of prostate carcinoma, an androgen-sensitive tumor.

PHARMACOKINETICS

Absorption: Well absorbed following oral administration.
Distribution: UK.
Metabolism and Excretion: Mostly metabolized by the liver. Some conversion to another antiandrogenic compound (2-hydroxyflutamide).
Half-life: UK.

CONTRAINDICATIONS AND PRECAUTIONS

Contraindicated in: ▪ Hypersensitivity.
Use Cautiously in: ▪ Severe cardiovascular disease.

ADVERSE REACTIONS AND SIDE EFFECTS*

Side effects primarily due to LHRH antagonist.
CNS: anxiety, confusion, drowsiness, mental depression, nervousness.
CV: edema, hypertension.
GI: diarrhea, nausea, vomiting, hepatotoxicity.
GU: impotence, loss of libido.
Derm: photosensitivity, rash.
Endo: gynecomastia.
Misc: hot flashes.

INTERACTIONS

Drug-Drug: ▪ Acts synergistically with **luteinizing hormone–releasing hormone analogues (leuprolide).**

ROUTE AND DOSAGE

- **PO (Adults):** 250 mg q 8 hr; given concurrently with leuprolide.

AVAILABILITY

▪ ***Capsules:*** 125 mg[Rx], {250 mg[Rx]}.

TIME/ACTION PROFILE

	ONSET	PEAK	DURATION
PO	UK	UK	UK

NURSING IMPLICATIONS

ASSESSMENT

- Monitor for diarrhea, nausea, and vomiting. Adjust diet as tolerated. Notify physician if these symptoms become severe.
- ***Lab Test Considerations:*** May cause elevated AST, ALT, bilirubin, and serum creatinine values.
- May cause increased plasma estradiol and testosterone concentrations.

POTENTIAL NURSING DIAGNOSES

- Sexual dysfunction (Side Effects).
- Knowledge deficit, related to medication regimen (Patient/Family Teaching).

IMPLEMENTATION

- **General Info:** Used in combination with LHRH agonist, such as leuprolide.

PATIENT/FAMILY TEACHING

- Explain that flutamide must be taken in conjunction with leuprolide. Instruct patient to take flutamide exactly as directed. If a dose is missed, take as soon as possible unless almost time for next dose. Do not double doses.
- Warn patient that side effects such as hot flashes, loss of sex drive, impotence, and breast enlargement may be caused by the LHRH agonist. The primary side effect of flutamide alone is diarrhea, but the combination of drugs is necessary to achieve the therapeutic effect.
- Advise patient to notify health care professional immediately if dark urine, itching, loss of appetite, nausea, vomiting, pain in right side, or yellow eyes or skin occurs. Hepatotoxicity usually resolves when flutamide is discontinued, but it may be progressive and fatal; requires immediate medical attention.

EVALUATION

Effectiveness of therapy can be demonstrated by: ▪ Decrease in the spread of prostate cancer.

F

FLUVOXAMINE

(floo-**voks**-a-meen)
Luvox

CLASSIFICATION(S):
Antidepressant (selective serotonin reuptake inhibitor [SSRI]), Antiobsessive

Pregnancy Category C

INDICATIONS

▪ Obsessive-compulsive disorder. **Unlabeled Uses:** ▪ Depression.

*CAPITALS indicate life-threatening; underlines indicate most frequent.

ACTION

- Inhibits the reuptake of serotonin in the CNS.

Therapeutic Effects: - Decrease in obsessive-compulsive behaviors.

PHARMACOKINETICS

Absorption: 53% absorbed following oral administration.
Distribution: Excreted in breast milk; enters the CNS. Remainder of distribution not known.
Metabolism and Excretion: Eliminated mostly by the kidneys.
Half-life: 13.6–15.6 hr.

CONTRAINDICATIONS AND PRECAUTIONS

Contraindicated in: - Hypersensitivity to fluvoxamine or other selective serotonin reuptake inhibitors - Concurrent MAO inhibitor, cisapride, or astemizole therapy.
Use Cautiously in: - Geriatric patients or patients with impaired hepatic function (lower initial dose and slower dosage titration recommended) - Pregnancy, lactation, or children <18 yr (safety not established).

ADVERSE REACTIONS AND SIDE EFFECTS*

CNS: dizziness, drowsiness, headache, insomnia, nervousness, weakness, agitation, anxiety, apathy, emotional lability, manic reactions, mental depression, psychotic reactions, syncope.
EENT: sinusitis.
Resp: cough, dyspnea.
CV: edema, hypertension, palpitations, postural hypotension, tachycardia, vasodilation.
GI: constipation, diarrhea, dry mouth, dyspepsia, nausea, anorexia, dysphagia, elevated liver enzymes, flatulence, vomiting.
GU: decreased libido/sexual dysfunction.
Derm: excessive sweating.
Metab: weight gain, weight loss.
MS: hypertonia, myoclonus/twitching.
Neuro: hypokinesia/hyperkinesia, tremor.
Misc: allergic reactions, chills, flu-like symptoms, tooth disorder/caries, yawning.

INTERACTIONS

Drug-Drug: - Serious, potentially fatal reactions (serotonin syndrome) may occur with **MAO inhibitors** - May increase the risk of potentially fatal cardiac reactions to **astemizole** or **cisapride** - **Cigarette smoking** may decrease the effectiveness of fluvoxamine - Concurrent use with **tricyclic antidepressants** may increase plasma levels of fluvoxamine - Decreases metabolism and may increase effects of some **beta blockers (propranolol)**, some **benzodiazepines** (avoid concurrent **diazepam**), **carbamazepine, methadone, lithium, theophylline** (decrease dose to ⅓ of usual dose), **tolbutamide, warfarin,** and **L-tryptophan** - Increases blood levels and risk of toxicity from **clozapine** (dosage adjustments may be necessary).

ROUTE AND DOSAGE

- **PO (Adults):** *Initial dose*—50 mg daily at bedtime; increase by 50 mg q 4–7 days until desired effect is achieved. If daily dose >100 mg, give in two equally divided doses or give a larger dose at bedtime (not to exceed 300 mg/day). *Maintenance dose*—Make periodic adjustments to maintain lowest possible dose to control symptoms.
- **PO (Children 8–17 yr):** 25 mg at bedtime, may increase by 25 mg/day q 4–7 days (not to exceed 200 mg/day; daily doses >50 mg should be given in divided doses with a larger dose at bedtime).

AVAILABILITY

- ***Tablets:*** 25 mg[Rx], 50 mg[Rx], 100 mg[Rx].

TIME/ACTION PROFILE (improvement on obsessive-compulsive behaviors)

	ONSET	PEAK	DURATION
PO	within 2–3 wk	several mo	UK

NURSING IMPLICATIONS

ASSESSMENT

- ☐ Monitor mood changes. Assess patient for frequency of obsessive-compulsive behaviors. Note degree to which these thoughts and behaviors interfere with daily functioning. Inform physician or other health care professional if patient demonstrates significant increase in anxiety, nervousness, or insomnia.
- ☐ Assess for suicidal tendencies, especially dur-

*CAPITALS indicate life-threatening; underlines indicate most frequent.

ing early therapy. Restrict amount of drug available to patient.

- Monitor appetite and nutritional intake. Weigh weekly. Report significant changes in weight. Adjust diet as tolerated to support nutritional status.
- *Toxicity and Overdose:* Common symptoms of toxicity include drowsiness, vomiting, diarrhea, and dizziness. Coma, tachycardia, bradycardia, hypotension, ECG abnormalities, liver function abnormalities, and convulsions may also occur. Treatment is symptomatic and supportive.

POTENTIAL NURSING DIAGNOSES

- Coping, ineffective individual (Indications).
- Injury, risk for (Side Effects).
- Knowledge deficit, related to medication regimen (Patient/Family Teaching).

IMPLEMENTATION

- **PO:** Initial therapy is administered as a single bedtime dose. May be increased every 4–7 days as tolerated.
- Fluvoxamine may be given without regard to meals.

PATIENT/FAMILY TEACHING

- Instruct patient to take fluvoxamine exactly as directed. Do not skip or double up on missed doses. Improvement in symptoms may be noticed in 2–3 wk, but medication should be continued as directed.
- May cause drowsiness and dizziness. Caution patient to avoid driving and other activities requiring alertness until response to medication is known.
- Advise patient to avoid alcohol or other CNS depressants during therapy and to consult health care professional before taking other medications with fluvoxamine.
- Instruct female patients to notify health care professional if breast-feeding or if pregnancy is planned or suspected.
- Advise patient to notify health care professional if rash or hives occur or if headache, nausea, anorexia, anxiety, or insomnia persists.
- Emphasize the importance of follow-up exams to monitor progress.

EVALUATION

Effectiveness of therapy can be demonstrated by: ▪ Decrease in symptoms of obsessive-compulsive disorder.

FOLIC ACID

(foe-lik a-sid)

{Apo-Folic}, folate, Folvite, {Novofolacid}, vitamin B_9

CLASSIFICATION(S):

Antianemic, Vitamin (water-soluble)

Pregnancy Category A

INDICATIONS

▪ Prevention and treatment of megaloblastic and macrocytic anemias ▪ Given during pregnancy to promote normal fetal development.

ACTION

▪ Required for protein synthesis and red blood cell function. Stimulates the production of red blood cells, white blood cells, and platelets. Necessary for normal fetal development. **Therapeutic Effects:** ▪ Restoration and maintenance of normal hematopoiesis.

PHARMACOKINETICS

Absorption: Well absorbed from the GI tract and IM and SC sites.
Distribution: Half of all stores are in the liver. Enters breast milk. Crosses the placenta.
Metabolism and Excretion: Converted by the liver to its active metabolite, dihydrofolate reductase. Excess amounts are excreted unchanged by the kidneys.
Half-life: UK.

CONTRAINDICATIONS AND PRECAUTIONS

Contraindicated in: ▪ Uncorrected pernicious anemia (neurologic damage will progress despite correction of hematologic abnormalities) ▪ Preparations containing benzyl alcohol should not be used in newborns.
Use Cautiously in: ▪ Undiagnosed anemias.

F

ADVERSE REACTIONS AND SIDE EFFECTS

Derm: rashes.
Misc: fever.

INTERACTIONS

Drug-Drug: ▪ **Sulfonamides, methotrexate,** and **triamterene** prevent the activation of folic acid ▪ Absorption of folic acid is decreased by **sulfasalazine** ▪ Folic acid requirements are increased by **estrogens, phenytoin, carbamazepine,** or **glucocorticoids.**

ROUTE AND DOSAGE

□ **Therapeutic Dose**

- **PO, IM, IV, SC (Adults and Children):** Up to 1 mg/day.

□ **Maintenance Dose**

- **PO, IM, IV, SC (Adults and Children >4 yr):** 0.4 mg/day.
- **PO, IM, IV, SC (Adults, Pregnant and Lactating):** 0.8 mg/day.
- **PO, IM, IV, SC (Children <4 yr):** Up to 0.3 mg/day.
- **PO, IM, IV, SC (Infants):** 0.1 mg/day.

AVAILABILITY

▪ ***Tablets:*** 0.1 mg[Rx], 0.4 mg[Rx], 0.8 mg[Rx], 1 mg[Rx], {5 mg[Rx]} ▪ ***Injection:*** 5 mg/ml[Rx], 10 mg/ml[Rx] ▪ ***In combination with:*** other vitamins and minerals as multiple vitamins[Rx,OTC].

TIME/ACTION PROFILE (increase in reticulocyte count)

	ONSET	PEAK	DURATION
PO, IM, SC, IV	3–5 days	5–10 days	UK

NURSING IMPLICATIONS

ASSESSMENT

□ Assess patient for signs of megaloblastic anemia (fatigue, weakness, dyspnea) prior to and periodically throughout therapy.

▪ ***Lab Test Considerations:*** Monitor plasma folic acid levels, hemoglobin, hematocrit, and reticulocyte count prior to and periodically during therapy.

□ May cause decrease in serum concentrations of vitamin B_{12} when given in high continuous doses.

POTENTIAL NURSING DIAGNOSES

- Nutrition, altered, less than body requirements (Indications).
- Activity intolerance (Indications).
- Knowledge deficit, related to medication regimen (Patient/Family Teaching).

IMPLEMENTATION

▪ **General Info:** Because of infrequency of solitary vitamin deficiencies, combinations are commonly administered (see Appendix A).

□ May be given SC, deep IM, or IV when PO route is not feasible.

▪ **IV:** Solution ranges from yellow to orange-yellow in color.

▪ **Direct IV:** Administer at a rate of 5 mg over at least 1 min.

▪ **Continuous Infusion:** May be added to hyperalimentation solution.

▪ **Y-Site Compatibility:** ▪ famotidine.

▪ **Additive Compatibility:** ▪ D20W.

▪ **Additive Incompatibility:** ▪ D50W ▪ calcium gluconate.

PATIENT/FAMILY TEACHING

□ Encourage patient to comply with diet recommendations of health care professional. Explain that the best source of vitamins is a well-balanced diet with foods from the four basic food groups. A diet low in vitamin B_{12} and folate will be used to diagnose folic acid deficiency without concealing pernicious anemia.

□ Foods high in folic acid include vegetables, fruits, and organ meats; heat destroys folic acid in foods.

□ Patients self-medicating with vitamin supplements should be cautioned not to exceed RDA (see Appendix L). The effectiveness of megadoses for treatment of various medical conditions is unproven and may cause side effects.

□ Explain that folic acid may make urine more intensely yellow.

□ Instruct patient to notify health care professional if rash occurs, which may indicate hypersensitivity.

□ Emphasize the importance of follow-up exams to evaluate progress.

EVALUATION

Effectiveness of therapy can be demonstrated by: ▪ Reticulocytosis 2–5 days after beginning therapy ▫ Resolution of symptoms of megaloblastic anemia.

FOSCARNET
(foss-**kar**-net)
Foscavir

CLASSIFICATION(S):
Antiviral

Pregnancy Category C

INDICATIONS

▪ Treatment of cytomegalovirus (CMV) retinitis in HIV-infected patients (alone or with ganciclovir) ▪ Treatment of acyclovir-resistant mucocutaneous herpes simplex virus (HSV) infections in immunocompromised patients.

ACTION

▪ Prevents viral replication by inhibiting viral DNA-polymerase and reverse transcriptase. **Therapeutic Effects:** ▪ Virustatic action against susceptible viruses including CMV.

PHARMACOKINETICS

Absorption: Completely absorbed following IV administration.
Distribution: Variable penetration into CSF. May concentrate in and be slowly released from bone.
Metabolism and Excretion: 80–90% excreted unchanged in urine.
Half-life: 3 hr (in patients with normal renal function); longer half-life of 90 hr may reflect release of drug from bone.

CONTRAINDICATIONS AND PRECAUTIONS

Contraindicated in: ▪ Hypersensitivity.
Use Cautiously in: ▪ Renal impairment (dosage reduction required if CCr ≤1.4–1.6 ml/min/kg) ▪ History of seizures ▪ Pregnancy, lactation, or children (safety not established).

ADVERSE REACTIONS AND SIDE EFFECTS*

CNS: SEIZURES, headache, anxiety, confusion, dizziness, fatigue, malaise, mental depression, weakness.
EENT: conjunctivitis, eye pain, vision abnormalities.
Resp: coughing, dyspnea.
CV: chest pain, ECG abnormalities, edema, palpitations.
GI: diarrhea, nausea, vomiting, abdominal pain, abnormal taste sensation, anorexia, constipation, dyspepsia.
GU: renal failure, albuminuria, dysuria, nocturia, polyuria, urinary retention.
Derm: increased sweating, pruritus, rash, skin ulceration.
F and E: hypocalcemia, hypokalemia, hypomagnesemia, hyperphosphatemia, hypophosphatemia.
Hemat: anemia, granulocytopenia, leukopenia.
Local: pain/inflammation at injection site.
MS: arthralgia, myalgia, back pain, involuntary muscle contraction.
Neuro: ataxia, hypoesthesia, neuropathy, paresthesia, tremor.
Misc: fever, chills, flu-like syndrome, lymphoma, sarcoma.

INTERACTIONS

Drug-Drug: ▪ Concurrent use with parenteral **pentamidine** may result in severe, life-threatening hypocalcemia ▪ Risk of nephrotoxicity may be increased by concurrent use of other **nephrotoxic agents** (amphotericin B, aminoglycosides).

ROUTE AND DOSAGE

▪ **IV (Adults):** ***CMV retinitis***—60 mg/kg q 8 hr or 90 mg/kg q 12 hr for 2–3 wk, then 90–120 mg/kg/day as a single dose. Dosage reduction required for any degree of renal impairment; *HSV*—40 mg/kg q 8–12 hr for 2–3 wk or until healing occurs.

AVAILABILITY

▪ ***Injection:*** 6000 mg/250 ml[Rx], 12,000 mg/500 ml[Rx].

TIME/ACTION PROFILE

	ONSET	PEAK	DURATION
IV	rapid	end of infusion	8–24 hr

***CAPITALS indicate life-threatening; underlines indicate most frequent.**

F

NURSING IMPLICATIONS

ASSESSMENT

- **CMV Retinitis:** Diagnosis of CMV retinitis should be determined by ophthalmoscopy prior to treatment with foscarnet. Ophthalmologic examinations should also be performed at the conclusion of induction and every 4 wk during maintenance therapy.
  - Culture for CMV (urine, blood, throat) may be taken prior to administration. However, a negative CMV culture does not rule out CMV retinitis.
- **HSV Infections:** Assess lesions prior to and daily during therapy.
- ***Lab Test Considerations:*** Monitor serum creatinine prior to and 2–3 times weekly during induction therapy and at least once every 1–2 wk during maintenance therapy. Monitor 24-hr CCr prior to and periodically throughout therapy. If CCr drops below 0.4 ml/min/kg, foscarnet should be discontinued.
  - Monitor serum calcium, magnesium, potassium, and phosphorus prior to and 2–3 times weekly during induction therapy and at least weekly during maintenance therapy. May cause decreased concentrations.
  - May cause anemia, granulocytopenia, leukopenia, and thrombocytopenia.
  - May cause elevated AST and ALT levels and abnormal A-G ratios.

POTENTIAL NURSING DIAGNOSES

- Infection, risk for (Indications).
- Knowledge deficit, related to medication regimen (Patient/Family Teaching).

IMPLEMENTATION

- **General Info:** Patient should be adequately hydrated with 750–1000 ml of 0.9% NaCl or D5W prior to first infusion to establish diuresis and 750–1000 ml with 120 mg/kg of foscarnet or 500 ml with 40–60 mg/kg of foscarnet to prevent renal toxicity.
- **Intermittent Infusion:** May be administered via central line in standard 24 mg/ml solution undiluted. If administered via peripheral line, *must* be diluted to 12 mg/ml concentration with D5W or 0.9% NaCl to prevent vein irritation. Do not administer solution that is discolored or contains particulate matter. Use diluted solution within 24 hr.
  - Dose is based on patient weight; excess solution may be discarded from bottle prior to administration to prevent overdosage.
  - Patients who experience progression of CMV retinitis during maintenance therapy may be re-treated with induction therapy followed by maintenance therapy.
- ***Rate:*** Administer at a rate not to exceed 1 mg/kg/min. Doses of 40 or 60 mg/kg are infused over at least 1 hr; 90 mg/kg over 1.5–2 hr; and 90–120 mg/kg maintenance dose is infused over 2 hr.
  - Infuse solution via infusion pump to ensure accurate infusion rate.
- **Y-Site Incompatibility:** ▪ Manufacturer recommends that foscarnet not be administered concurrently with other drugs or solutions in the same IV catheter except D5W or 0.9% NaCl; precipitate will develop.

PATIENT/FAMILY TEACHING

- Inform patient that foscarnet is not a cure for CMV retinitis. Progression of retinitis may continue in immunocompromised patients during and following therapy. Advise patients to have regular ophthalmologic exams.
- Advise patient to notify health care professional immediately if perioral tingling or numbness in the extremities or paresthesia occurs during or after infusion. If these signs of electrolyte imbalance occur during administration, infusion should be stopped and lab samples for serum electrolyte concentrations obtained immediately.
- Emphasize the importance of frequent follow-up exams to monitor renal function and electrolytes.

EVALUATION

Effectiveness of therapy can be demonstrated by: ▪ Management of the symptoms of CMV retinitis in patients with AIDS ▪ Crusting over and healing of skin lesions in HSV infections.

FOSFOMYCIN TROMETHAMINE
(foss-foe-**mye**-sin troe-**meth**-a-meen)
Monurol

CLASSIFICATION(S):
Anti-infective (miscellaneous)

Pregnancy Category B

INDICATIONS
- Uncomplicated urinary tract infections in women (acute cystitis).

ACTION
- Inactivates an enzyme crucial for bacterial cell wall synthesis - Decreases adherence of bacteria to uroepithelial cells. **Therapeutic Effects:** - Bactericidal action against susceptible bacteria. **Spectrum:** - Active against: *Enterococcus faecalis* and *Escherichia coli*.

PHARMACOKINETICS
Absorption: Rapidly absorbed and converted to fosfomycin, its active component, resulting in 37% bioavailability.
Distribution: Distributes to kidneys and bladder wall; crosses the placenta.
Metabolism and Excretion: Excreted unchanged in urine (38%) and feces (18%).
Half-life: 5.7 hr.

CONTRAINDICATIONS AND PRECAUTIONS
Contraindicated in: - Hypersensitivity.
Use Cautiously in: - Pregnancy, lactation, or children <12 yr (safety not established; breastfeeding not recommended).

ADVERSE REACTIONS AND SIDE EFFECTS*
CNS: <u>headache</u> , dizziness, weakness.
EENT: rhinitis.
GI: <u>diarrhea</u>, dyspepsia, nausea.
GU: dysmenorrhea, vaginitis.
Derm: rash.
MS: back pain.

INTERACTIONS
Drug-Drug: - Urinary excretion and blood levels are decreased by **metoclopramide.**

ROUTE AND DOSAGE
- **PO (Adults and Children ≥12 yr):** 3 g single dose.

AVAILABILITY
- ***Sachet:*** 3 g[Rx].

TIME/ACTION PROFILE (bactericidal urine levels†)

	ONSET	PEAK	DURATION
PO	rapid	2–4 hr	UK

†Symptoms may take 24–48 hr to subside.

NURSING IMPLICATIONS

ASSESSMENT
- Assess patient for signs and symptoms of cystitis (frequency, urgency, painful urination).
- Obtain urine specimen for culture and sensitivity prior to administration.
- ***Lab Test Considerations:*** May cause increased eosinophil count, increased or decreased WBC, increased bilirubin, increased AST and ALT, increased alkaline phosphatase, decreased hemoglobin and hematocrit, and decreased platelet count.

POTENTIAL NURSING DIAGNOSES
- Infection, risk for (Indications).
- Pain (Indications).
- Knowledge deficit, related to medication regimen (Patient/Family Teaching).

IMPLEMENTATION
- **PO:** Do not take medication in dry form. Pour entire contents of single sachet into 3–4 oz (½ cup) water and stir to dissolve. Do not use hot water. Drink immediately after mixing. May be administered with or without food.

PATIENT/FAMILY TEACHING
- Instruct patient on correct preparation of sachet.
- Advise patient to notify health care professional if symptoms have not improved or persist more than 2–3 days after treatment.

F

***CAPITALS indicate life-threatening; <u>underlines</u> indicate most frequent.**

EVALUATION

Clinical response to therapy can be evaluated by: ▪ Improvement in symptoms of acute cystitis within 2–3 days.

FUROSEMIDE

(fur-**oh**-se-mide)

{Apo-Furosemide}, {Furoside}, Lasix, {Lasix Special}, {Myrosemide}, {Novosemide}, {Uritol}

CLASSIFICATION(S):

Antihypertensive agent, Diuretic (loop)

Pregnancy Category C

INDICATIONS

▪ Management of edema due to: ▫ Congestive heart failure ▫ Hepatic or renal disease ▪ Treatment of hypertension. **Unlabeled Uses:** ▪ Management of hypercalcemia of malignancy.

ACTION

▪ Inhibits the reabsorption of sodium and chloride from the loop of Henle and distal renal tubule ▪ Increases renal excretion of water, sodium, chloride, magnesium, hydrogen, and calcium ▪ May have renal and peripheral vasodilatory effects ▪ Effectiveness persists in impaired renal function. **Therapeutic Effects:** ▪ Diuresis and subsequent mobilization of excess fluid (edema, pleural effusions) ▪ Lowering of blood pressure.

PHARMACOKINETICS

Absorption: 60–75% absorbed from the GI tract following oral administration; also absorbed from IM sites.

Distribution: Crosses the placenta; enters breast milk.

Metabolism and Excretion: Some is metabolized by the liver (30–40%), some nonhepatic metabolism, and some renal excretion as unchanged drug.

Half-life: 30–60 min (increased in renal impairment and neonates, markedly increased in hepatic impairment).

CONTRAINDICATIONS AND PRECAUTIONS

Contraindicated in: ▪ Hypersensitivity ▪ Cross-sensitivity with thiazides and sulfonamides may exist ▪ Pre-existing uncorrected electrolyte imbalance, hepatic coma, or anuria ▪ Some liquid products may contain alcohol; avoid in patients with known alcohol intolerance.

Use Cautiously in: ▪ Severe liver disease accompanied by cirrhosis or ascites (may precipitate hepatic coma; concurrent use with potassium-sparing diuretics may be necessary) ▪ Electrolyte depletion ▪ Geriatric patients (difficulty assessing hearing status; increased risk of hypotension) ▪ Diabetes mellitus ▪ Increasing azotemia ▪ Pregnancy, lactation, or children (safety not established; has been used in children).

ADVERSE REACTIONS AND SIDE EFFECTS*

CNS: dizziness, encephalopathy, headache, insomnia, nervousness.

EENT: hearing loss, tinnitus.

CV: hypotension.

GI: constipation, diarrhea, dry mouth, dyspepsia, nausea, vomiting.

GU: excessive urination.

Derm: photosensitivity, rashes.

Endo: hyperglycemia.

F and E: dehydration, hypochloremia, hypokalemia, hypomagnesemia, hyponatremia, hypovolemia, metabolic alkalosis.

Hemat: blood dyscrasias.

Metab: hyperglycemia, hyperuricemia.

MS: arthralgia, muscle cramps, myalgia.

Misc: increased BUN.

INTERACTIONS

Drug-Drug: ▪ Additive hypotension with **antihypertensives** or **nitrates** ▪ Additive hypokalemia with other **diuretics, mezlocillin, piperacillin, amphotericin B,** and **glucocorticoids** ▪ Hypokalemia may increase **digitalis glycoside** toxicity ▪ Decreases **lithium** excretion, may cause toxicity ▪ Increased risk of ototoxicity with **aminoglycosides** ▪ May increase the effectiveness of **warfarin, thrombolytics,** or **anticoagulants.**

{} = Available in Canada only.

***CAPITALS indicate life-threatening; underlines indicate most frequent.**

ROUTE AND DOSAGE

- **PO, IM, IV (Adults):** *Diuretic*—20–80 mg/day initially (up to 600 mg may be necessary); may increase by 20–40 mg q 6–8 hr (up to 600 mg/day have been used in CHF and renal failure). When maintenance dose is determined, dose may be given every other day or 2–3 times weekly. *Antihypertensive*—40–80 mg (up to 200 mg if accompanied by pulmonary edema/acute renal failure). *Antihypercalcemic*—80–100 mg q 1–4 hr (IM, IV) or 120 mg/day as a single dose or 2 divided doses PO.
- **PO (Children):** 2 mg/kg as a single dose, may be increased by 1–2 mg/kg q 6–8 hr; 1–2 mg/kg/day initially (up to 5–6 mg/kg/day). Longer dosage intervals are recommended in neonates.
- **IM, IV (Children):** *Diuretic*—1 mg/kg, may increase by 1 mg/kg q 2 hr (not to exceed 6 mg/kg). *Antihypercalcemic*—25–50 mg, may be repeated q 4 hr.

AVAILABILITY

▪ ***Tablets:*** 20 mg[Rx], 40 mg[Rx], 80 mg[Rx], {500 mg[Rx]} ▪ ***Oral solution:*** 8 mg/ml[Rx], 10 mg/ml[Rx] ▪ ***Injection:*** 10 mg/ml[Rx].

TIME/ACTION PROFILE (diuretic effect)

	ONSET	PEAK	DURATION
PO	30–60 min	1–2 hr	6–8 hr
IM	10–30 min	UK	4–8 hr
IV	5 min	30 min	2 hr

NURSING IMPLICATIONS

ASSESSMENT

- Assess fluid status throughout therapy. Monitor daily weight, intake and output ratios, amount and location of edema, lung sounds, skin turgor, and mucous membranes. Report thirst, dry mouth, lethargy, weakness, hypotension, or oliguria.
- Monitor blood pressure and pulse before and during administration. Monitor frequency of prescription refills to determine compliance in patients treated for hypertension.
- Assess patients receiving digitalis glycosides for anorexia, nausea, vomiting, muscle cramps, paresthesia, and confusion. Patients taking digitalis glycosides are at increased risk of digitalis toxicity because of the potassium-depleting effect of the diuretic. Potassium supplements or potassium-sparing diuretics may be used concurrently to prevent hypokalemia.
- Assess patient for tinnitus and hearing loss. Audiometry is recommended for patients receiving prolonged high-dose IV therapy. Hearing loss is most common following rapid or high-dose IV administration in patients with decreased renal function or those taking other ototoxic drugs.
- Assess for allergy to sulfonamides.
- ***Lab Test Considerations:*** Monitor electrolytes, renal and hepatic function, serum glucose and uric acid levels prior to and periodically throughout therapy. May cause decreased serum potassium, calcium, and magnesium concentrations. May also cause increased BUN, serum glucose, creatinine, and uric acid levels.

F

POTENTIAL NURSING DIAGNOSES

- Fluid volume excess (Indications).
- Fluid volume deficit (Side Effects).
- Knowledge deficit, related to medication regimen (Patient/Family Teaching).

IMPLEMENTATION

- **General Info:** Administer medication in the morning to prevent disruption of sleep cycle.
- IV is preferred over IM for parenteral administration.
- When using furosemide for hypercalcemia, replace extracellular volume and sodium chloride to maintain fluid volume and increase calcium excretion effectively.
- **PO:** Administer orally with food or milk to minimize gastric irritation. Tablets may be crushed if patient has difficulty swallowing.
- Do not administer discolored solution or tablets.
- **Direct IV:** Administer undiluted.
- ***Rate:*** Administer slowly over 1–2 min.
- **Intermittent Infusion:** Dilute large doses in D5W, D10W, D20W, D5/0.9% NaCl, D5/LR, 0.9% NaCl, 3% NaCl, ⅙ M sodium lactate, or lactated Ringer's solution. Use reconstituted solution within 24 hr.
- ***Rate:*** Administer through Y-tubing at a rate not to exceed 4 mg/min in adults to prevent ototoxicity. Use an infusion pump to ensure accurate dosage.
- **Syringe Compatibility:** ▪ bleomycin ▪ cis-

platin ▪ cyclophosphamide ▪ fluorouracil ▪ heparin ▪ leucovorin calcium ▪ methotrexate ▪ miomycin.

- **Syringe Incompatibility:** ▪ doxapram ▪ doxorubicin ▪ droperidol ▪ metoclopramide ▪ milrinone ▪ vinblastine ▪ vincristine.
- **Y-Site Compatibility:** ▪ amifostine ▪ amikacin ▪ aztreonam ▪ bleomycin ▪ cefepime ▪ cisplatin ▪ cyclophosphamide ▪ cytarabine ▪ famotidine ▪ fludarabine ▪ fluorouracil ▪ foscarnet ▪ gallium nitrate ▪ granisetron ▪ heparin ▪ hydrocortisone sodium succinate ▪ indomethacin ▪ kanamycin ▪ leucovorin calcium ▪ lorazepam ▪ melphalan ▪ methotrexate ▪ mitomycin ▪ paclitaxel ▪ piperacillin/tazobactam ▪ potassium chloride ▪ sargramostim ▪ tacrolimus ▪ teniposide ▪ thiotepa ▪ tobramycin ▪ tolazoline ▪ vitamin B complex with C.
- **Y-Site Incompatibility:** ▪ ciprofloxacin ▪ diltiazem ▪ droperidol ▪ esmolol ▪ filgrastim ▪ fluconazole ▪ gentamicin ▪ hydralazine ▪ idarubicin ▪ metoclopramide ▪ midazolam ▪ milrinone ▪ morphine ▪ netilmicin ▪ ondansetron ▪ quinidine gluconate ▪ vinblastine ▪ vincristine ▪ vinorelbine.

PATIENT/FAMILY TEACHING

- **General Info:** Instruct patient to take furosemide exactly as directed. Missed doses should be taken as soon as possible; do not double doses.
- □ Caution patient to change positions slowly to minimize orthostatic hypotension. Caution patient that the use of alcohol, exercise during hot weather, or standing for long periods during therapy may enhance orthostatic hypotension.
- □ Instruct patient to consult health care professional regarding a diet high in potassium (see Appendix K).
- □ Advise patient to consult health care professional before taking OTC medication concurrently with this therapy.
- □ Instruct patient to notify health care professional of medication regimen prior to treatment or surgery.
- □ Caution patient to use sunscreen and protective clothing to prevent photosensitivity reactions.
- □ Advise patient to contact health care professional immediately if muscle weakness, cramps, nausea, dizziness, numbness, or tingling of extremities occurs.
- □ Advise patient taking furosemide not to change brands when refilling prescription; bioavailability among brands is variable.
- □ Emphasize the importance of routine follow-up exams.
- **Hypertension:** Advise patients on antihypertensive regimen to continue taking medication even if feeling better. Furosemide controls but does not cure hypertension.
- □ Reinforce the need to continue additional therapies for hypertension (weight loss, exercise, restricted sodium intake, stress reduction, regular exercise, moderation of alcohol consumption, cessation of smoking).

EVALUATION

Effectiveness of therapy can be demonstrated by: ▪ Decrease in edema □ Increase in urinary output ▪ Decrease in blood pressure ▪ Decrease in serum calcium when used to manage hypercalcemia.

GABAPENTIN
(ga-ba-**pen**-tin)
Neurontin

CLASSIFICATION(S):
Anticonvulsant (miscellaneous)

Pregnancy Category C

INDICATIONS

▪ Adjunctive treatment of adults with partial seizures with and without secondary generalization. **Unlabeled Uses:** ▪ Treatment of chronic pain.

ACTION

▪ Mechanism of action is not known. May affect transport of amino acids across neuronal membranes. **Therapeutic Effects:** ▪ Decreased incidence of seizures.

PHARMACOKINETICS

Absorption: Well absorbed following oral administration by an active transport system. At larger doses, system becomes saturated and absorption decreases (bioavailability ranges from 60% for a 300-mg dose to 35% for a 1600-mg dose).

Distribution: Crosses the blood-brain barrier.

Metabolism and Excretion: Eliminated almost entirely by the kidneys as unchanged drug.
Half-life: 5–7 hr in patients with normal renal function; up to 132 hr in anuric patients.

CONTRAINDICATIONS AND PRECAUTIONS

Contraindicated in: ▪ Hypersensitivity.
Use Cautiously in: ▪ Patients with renal insufficiency (decrease dose and/or increase dosing interval if CCr ≤60 ml/min) ▪ Geriatric patients (because of age-related decrease in renal function) ▪ Pregnancy, lactation, or children <12 yr (safety not established).

ADVERSE REACTIONS AND SIDE EFFECTS*

CNS: drowsiness, anxiety, dizziness, hostility, malaise, vertigo, weakness.
EENT: abnormal vision, nystagmus.
CV: hypertension.
GI: anorexia, flatulence, gingivitis.
MS: arthralgia.
Neuro: ataxia, altered reflexes, hyperkinesia, paresthesia.
Misc: facial edema.

INTERACTIONS

Drug-Drug: ▪ **Antacids** may decrease the absorption of gabapentin.

ROUTE AND DOSAGE

▪ **PO (Adults and Children >12 yr):** 300 mg once daily on 1st day, 300 mg twice a day on 2nd day, 300 mg 3 times daily on 3rd day. Rapid titration may be continued until desired effect is obtained (range is 900–1800 mg/day in 3 divided doses; doses should not be more than 12 hr apart).

AVAILABILITY

▪ ***Capsules:*** 100 mg^{Rx}, 300 mg^{Rx}, 400 mg^{Rx}.

TIME/ACTION PROFILE (blood levels)

	ONSET	PEAK	DURATION
PO	rapid	2–4 hr	8 hr

NURSING IMPLICATIONS

ASSESSMENT

▪ **Seizures:** Assess location, duration, and characteristics of seizure activity.
▪ **Chronic Pain:** Assess location, characteristics, and intensity of pain periodically during therapy.
▪ ***Lab Test Considerations:*** May cause false-positive readings when testing for urinary protein with *Ames N-Multistix SG* dipstick test; use sulfosalicylic acid precipitation procedure.
□ May cause leukopenia.

POTENTIAL NURSING DIAGNOSES

▪ Injury, risk for (Side Effects).
▪ Knowledge deficit, related to medication regimen (Patient/Family Teaching).

IMPLEMENTATION

▪ **PO:** May be administered without regard to meals.
□ Capsules may be opened and dissolved in juice or sprinkled on soft foods such as applesauce immediately before use. Do not store in solution; will degrade over time.
□ Gabapentin should be discontinued gradually over at least 1 wk. Abrupt discontinuation may cause increase in seizure frequency.

PATIENT/FAMILY TEACHING

□ Instruct patient to take medication exactly as directed. Patients on tid dosing should not exceed 12 hr between doses. If a dose is missed, take as soon as possible; if less than 2 hr until next dose, take dose immediately and take next dose 1–2 hr later, then resume regular dosing schedule. Do not double doses. Do not discontinue abruptly; may cause increase in frequency of seizures.
□ Advise patient not to take gabapentin within 2 hr of an antacid.
□ Gabapentin may cause dizziness and drowsiness. Caution patient to avoid driving or activities requiring alertness until response to medication is known. Do not resume driving until physician gives clearance based on control of seizure disorder.
□ Advise patient to notify health care profes-

G

*CAPITALS indicate life-threatening; underlines indicate most frequent.

sional if pregnancy is planned or suspected or if she intends to breast-feed or is breast-feeding an infant.

- Instruct patient to notify health care professional of medication regimen prior to treatment or surgery.
- Advise patient to carry identification describing disease process and medication regimen at all times.

EVALUATION

Effectiveness of therapy can be demonstrated by: ▪ Decrease in the frequency of or cessation of seizures ▪ Decrease in intensity of chronic pain.

GALLIUM NITRATE

(**gal**-ee-yum **nye**-trate)
Ganite

CLASSIFICATION(S):
Electrolyte modifier (hypocalcemic agent)

Pregnancy Category C

INDICATIONS

▪ Management of cancer-related hypercalcemia.

ACTION

▪ Inhibits calcium resorption from bone. Therapeutic Effects: ▪ Lowering of serum calcium levels.

PHARMACOKINETICS

Absorption: IV administration results in complete bioavailability.
Distribution: UK.
Metabolism and Excretion: Mostly excreted unchanged by the kidneys.
Half-life: 24 hr (increases to 72–115 hr with prolonged infusions).

CONTRAINDICATIONS AND PRECAUTIONS

Contraindicated in: ▪ Severe renal impairment (serum creatinine >2.5 mg%).
Use Cautiously in: ▪ Renal impairment ▪ Pregnancy, lactation, or children (safety not established).

ADVERSE REACTIONS AND SIDE EFFECTS*

EENT: hearing loss, optic neuritis, visual impairment.
GU: renal toxicity.
F and E: hypophosphatemia, hypocalcemia.

INTERACTIONS

Drug-Drug: ▪ Increased risk of nephrotoxicity with other **nephrotoxic agents,** including **amphotericin B** and **aminoglycosides** (discontinue gallium).

ROUTE AND DOSAGE

▪ **IV (Adults):** 100–200 mg/m^2 daily for 5 days; 2–4 wk rest recommended between courses of therapy.

AVAILABILITY

▪ ***Injection:*** 25 mg/ml in 20-ml vials^{Rx}.

TIME/ACTION PROFILE (effect on serum calcium)

	ONSET	PEAK	DURATION
IV	within 24 hr	5 days	7.5 days

NURSING IMPLICATIONS

ASSESSMENT

- Monitor symptoms of hypercalcemia (nausea, vomiting, anorexia, lethargy, fatigue, weakness, constipation, thirst, dehydration, impaired mental status, and cardiac arrhythmias).
- Observe patient carefully for evidence of hypocalcemia (paresthesia, muscle twitching, laryngospasm, colic, cardiac arrhythmias, and Chvostek's or Trousseau's sign). Protect symptomatic patients by elevating and padding side rails; keep bed in low position. If hypocalcemia occurs, stop gallium nitrate therapy. Temporary calcium therapy may be needed.
- If patient requires other nephrotoxic drugs, discontinue gallium nitrate and continue hydration for several days following administration of potentially nephrotoxic drug. Monitor serum creatinine and urine output during and after this period.

▪ ***Lab Test Considerations:*** Monitor BUN and serum creatinine prior to and every 2–3

*CAPITALS indicate life-threatening; underlines indicate most frequent.

days throughout therapy. Gallium nitrate therapy should be discontinued if serum creatinine is >2.5 mg/dl.

- Monitor serum calcium daily and serum phosphate levels twice weekly to determine effectiveness of therapy. Oral phosphate therapy may be needed for hypophosphatemia. May also cause decreased serum bicarbonate concentrations.
- Monitor serum albumin levels prior to and following each course of therapy.

POTENTIAL NURSING DIAGNOSES

- Injury, risk for (Indications).
- Urinary elimination, altered patterns of (Adverse Reactions).

IMPLEMENTATION

- **General Info:** Gallium nitrate should be instituted after adequate hydration with IV saline has been established. Saline promotes the renal excretion of calcium. Diuretics may also be used following correction of hypovolemia. Adequate hydration and urine output should be maintained at 2000 mg/day throughout therapy.
- **Direct IV:** May be administered undiluted via a metered ambulatory infusion pump.
- **Continuous Infusion:** Dilute daily dose in 1000 ml of 0.9% NaCl or D5W. Solution is clear and colorless. Solution is stable for 48 hr at room temperature and 7 days if refrigerated.
- ***Rate:*** Infuse over 24 hr.
- **Y-Site Compatibility:** ▪ acyclovir ▪ aminophylline ▪ amifostine ▪ ampicillin/sulbactam ▪ aztreonam ▪ cefazolin ▪ ceftazidime ▪ ceftriaxone ▪ cimetidine ▪ ciprofloxacin ▪ cyclophosphamide ▪ dexamethasone ▪ diphenhydramine ▪ filgrastim ▪ fluconazole ▪ furosemide ▪ heparin ▪ hydrocortisone sodium succinate ▪ ifosfamide ▪ magnesium sulfate ▪ mannitol ▪ melphalan ▪ meperidine ▪ mesna ▪ methotrexate ▪ metoclopramide ▪ ondansetron ▪ piperacillin ▪ piperacillin/tazobactam ▪ potassium chloride ▪ ranitidine ▪ sodium bicarbonate ▪ teniposide ▪ thiotepa ▪ ticarcillin/clavulanate ▪ trimethoprim/sulfamethoxazole ▪ vancomycin ▪ vinorelbine.
- **Y-Site Incompatibility:** ▪ cefepime ▪ cisplatin ▪ cytarabine ▪ doxorubicin ▪ etoposide ▪ fluorouracil ▪ haloperidol ▪ hydromorphone ▪ imipenem/cilastatin ▪ lorazepam ▪ morphine ▪ prochlorperazine edisylate.

PATIENT/FAMILY TEACHING

- Encourage patient to comply with physician's diet recommendations. Foods high in calcium that should be avoided include dairy products, canned salmon and sardines, broccoli, bok choy, tofu, molasses, and cream soups (see Appendix K).
- Emphasize need for keeping follow-up appointments to monitor progress, even after medication is discontinued, to detect relapse.

EVALUATION

Effectiveness of therapy can be demonstrated by: ▪ Lowered serum calcium levels in patients with cancer-related hypercalcemia.

GANCICLOVIR

(gan-**sye**-kloe-vir)
Cytovene, Vitrasert

CLASSIFICATION(S):
Antiviral

Pregnancy Category C

INDICATIONS

▪ **IV:** Treatment of cytomegalovirus (CMV) retinitis in immunocompromised patients, including HIV-infected patients (may be used with foscarnet) ▪ Prevention of CMV infection in transplant patients at risk ▪ **PO:** Maintenance treatment of stable CMV retinitis in immunocompromised patients following initial IV treatment and prevention of CMV retinitis in patients with advanced HIV infection.

ACTION

▪ CMV virus converts ganciclovir to its active form (ganciclovir phosphate) inside host cell, where it inhibits viral DNA polymerase. **Therapeutic Effects:** ▪ Antiviral effect directed preferentially against CMV-infected cells.

PHARMACOKINETICS

Absorption: 5–9% absorbed following oral administration. IV administration results in complete bioavailability. Action of intravitreal implant is local.

Distribution: Widely distributed; enters CSF.

Metabolism and Excretion: 90% excreted unchanged by the kidneys.
Half-life: 2.9 hr (increased in renal impairment).

CONTRAINDICATIONS AND PRECAUTIONS

Contraindicated in: ▪ Hypersensitivity to ganciclovir or acyclovir.
Use Cautiously in: ▪ Renal impairment (dosage reduction required if CCr <80 ml/min) ▪ Geriatric patients (dosage reduction recommended) ▪ Bone marrow depression or immunosuppression ▪ Pregnancy, lactation, or children (safety not established).

ADVERSE REACTIONS AND SIDE EFFECTS*

CNS: SEIZURES, abnormal dreams, coma, confusion, dizziness, drowsiness, headache, malaise, nervousness.
EENT: retinal detachment; *intravitreal only*—decreased visual acuity, vitreous hemorrhage, hyphema, intraocular pressure spikes, lens opacities, macular abnormalities, optic nerve changes, uveitis.
Resp: dyspnea.
CV: arrhythmias, edema, hypertension, hypotension.
GI: GI BLEEDING, abdominal pain, increased liver enzymes, nausea, vomiting.
GU: gonadal suppression, hematuria, renal toxicity.
Derm: alopecia, photosensitivity, pruritus, rash, urticaria.
Endo: hypoglycemia.
Hemat: neutropenia, thrombocytopenia, anemia, eosinophilia.
Local: pain/phlebitis at IV site.
Neuro: ataxia, tremor.
Misc: fever.

INTERACTIONS

Drug-Drug: ▪ Increased risk of bone marrow depression with **antineoplastic agents, radiation therapy**, or **zidovudine** ▪ Toxicity may be increased by **probenecid** ▪ Increased risk of seizures with **imipenem/cilastatin** ▪ Concurrent use of other **nephrotoxic drugs, cyclosporine**, or **amphotericin B** increases the risk of nephrotoxicity.

ROUTE AND DOSAGE

- **IV (Adults):** *Induction*—5 mg/kg q 12 hr for 14–21 days. *Maintenance regimen*—5 mg/kg/day or 6 mg/kg for 5 days of each week. If progression occurs, increase to q 12 hr regimen. *Prevention*—5 mg/kg q 12 hr for 7–14 days, then 5 mg/kg/day or 6 mg/kg for 5 days of each week.
- **PO (Adults):** *Maintenance regimen*—1000 mg 3 times daily (with food) or 500 mg q 3 hr while awake; *prevention of CMV retinitis in advanced HIV infection*—1000 mg 3 times daily.
- **Ophth (Adults, Intravitreal):** 4.5 mg implant.

AVAILABILITY

▪ ***Capsules:*** 250 mg[Rx], 500 mg[Rx] ▪ ***Powder for injection:*** 500 mg/vial[Rx] ▪ ***Intravitreal insert:*** at least 4.5 mg[Rx].

TIME/ACTION PROFILE (antiviral levels)

	ONSET	PEAK	DURATION
PO	rapid	1.8–3 hr	3–8 hr
IV	rapid	end of infusion	12–24 hr
Intravitreal	rapid	UK	5–8 mo

NURSING IMPLICATIONS

ASSESSMENT

- Diagnosis of CMV retinitis should be determined by ophthalmoscopy prior to treatment with ganciclovir.
- Culture for CMV (urine, blood, throat) may be taken prior to administration. However, a negative CMV culture does not rule out CMV retinitis. If symptoms do not respond after several weeks, resistance to ganciclovir may have occurred. Ophthalmologic exams should be performed weekly during induction and every 2 wk during maintenance or more frequently if the macula or optic nerve is threatened. Progression of CMV retinitis may occur during or following ganciclovir treatment.
- Assess for signs of infection (fever, chills, cough, hoarseness, lower back or side pain, sore throat, difficult or painful urination). No-

*CAPITALS indicate life-threatening; underlines indicate most frequent.

tify physician or other health care professional if these symptoms occur.

- Assess for bleeding (bleeding gums, bruising, petechiae, or guaiac stools, urine, and emesis). Avoid IM injections and rectal temperatures. Apply pressure to venipuncture sites for 10 min.
- ***Lab Test Considerations:*** Monitor neutrophil and platelet count at least every 2 days during bid therapy and weekly thereafter. Granulocytopenia usually occurs during the first 2 wk of treatment but may occur anytime during therapy. Do not administer if neutrophil count $<500/mm^3$ or platelet count $<25,000/mm^3$. Recovery begins within 3–7 days of discontinuation of therapy.
- Monitor BUN and serum creatinine at least once every 2 wk throughout therapy.
- Monitor liver function tests (AST, ALT, serum bilirubin, alkaline phosphatase) periodically during therapy. May cause elevated levels.
- May cause a decrease in blood glucose.

POTENTIAL NURSING DIAGNOSES

- Infection, risk for (Indications, Patient/Family Teaching).
- Knowledge deficit, related to medication regimen (Patient/Family Teaching).

IMPLEMENTATION

- **General Info:** Solution should be prepared in a biologic cabinet. Wear gloves, gown, and mask while handling medication. Discard IV equipment in specially designated containers (see Appendix I).
- Do not administer SC or IM, as severe tissue irritation may result.
- **PO:** Administer capsules with food.
- **IV:** Observe infusion site for phlebitis. Rotate infusion site to prevent phlebitis.
- Maintain adequate hydration throughout therapy.
- **Intermittent Infusion:** Reconstitute 500 mg with 10 ml of sterile water for injection for a concentration of 50 mg/ml. Do not reconstitute with bacteriostatic water with parabens; precipitation will occur. Shake well to dissolve completely. Discard vial if particulate matter or discoloration occurs. Reconstituted solution is stable for 12 hr at room temperature; do not refrigerate.
- Dilute in 100 ml of D5W, 0.9% NaCl, Ringer's or lactated Ringer's solution for a concentration not to exceed 10 mg/ml. Once diluted for infusion, solution should be used within 24 hr. Refrigerate but do not freeze.
- ***Rate:*** Administer slowly, via infusion pump, over 1 hr using an in-line filter. Rapid administration may increase toxicity.
- **Y-Site Compatibility:** ▪ cisplatin ▪ cyclophosphamide ▪ enalaprilat ▪ filgrastim ▪ fluconazole ▪ melphalan ▪ methotrexate ▪ paclitaxel ▪ tacrolimus ▪ teniposide ▪ thiotepa.
- **Y-Site Incompatibility:** ▪ aldesleukin ▪ amifostine ▪ aztreonam ▪ cytarabine ▪ doxorubicin ▪ fludarabine ▪ foscarnet ▪ ondansetron ▪ piperacillin/tazobactam ▪ sargramostim ▪ vinorelbine.

PATIENT/FAMILY TEACHING

- Instruct patient to take ganciclovir with food, exactly as directed.
- Inform patient that ganciclovir is not a cure for CMV retinitis. Progression of retinitis may continue in immunocompromised patients during and following therapy. Advise patients to have regular ophthalmic exams at least every 6 wk. Duration of therapy for CMV prevention is based on the duration and degree of immunosuppression.
- Advise patient to notify health care professional if fever; chills; sore throat; other signs of infection; bleeding gums; bruising; petechiae; or blood in urine, stool, or emesis occurs. Caution patient to avoid crowds and persons with known infections. Instruct patient to use soft toothbrush and electric razor. Patient should be cautioned not to drink alcoholic beverages or take products containing aspirin or NSAIDs.
- Advise patient that ganciclovir may have teratogenic effects. A nonhormonal method of contraception should be used during and for at least 90 days following therapy.
- Caution patient to use sunscreen and protective clothing to prevent photosensitivity reactions.
- Emphasize the importance of frequent follow-up exams to monitor blood counts.

EVALUATION

Effectiveness of therapy can be demonstrated by: ▪ Management of the symptoms of CMV retinitis in immunocompromised patients

G

▪ Prevention of CMV retinitis in transplant patients at risk.

GASTROINTESTINAL ANTI-INFLAMMATORIES

mesalamine
(me-**sal**-a-meen)
Asacol, Pentasa, Rowasa, {Salofalk}

olsalazine
(ole-**sal**-a-zeen)
{Dipentum}

sulfasalazine
(sul-fa-**sal**-a-zeen)
Azulfidine, {PMS-Sulfasalazine}, {Salazopyrin}, {S.A.S.}

CLASSIFICATION(S):
Anti-inflammatories (gastrointestinal/local)

Pregnancy Category B

INDICATIONS

▪ **Mesalamine, sulfasalazine:** Inflammatory bowel diseases including: ▫ Ulcerative colitis ▫ Proctitis ▫ Proctosigmoiditis ▪ **Olsalazine:** Ulcerative colitis in patients who cannot tolerate sulfasalazine ▪ **Sulfasalazine:** Rheumatoid arthritis in patients who do not respond to or are intolerant of analgesics and/or NSAIDs.

ACTION

▪ Locally acting anti-inflammatory action in the colon, where activity is probably due to inhibition of prostaglandin synthesis. **Therapeutic Effects:** ▪ Reduction in the symptoms of inflammatory bowel disease.

PHARMACOKINETICS

Absorption: *Mesalamine*—28% absorbed following oral administration; 10–30% absorbed from the colon, depending on retention time, following rectal administration. *Olsalazine*—acts locally in colon, where 98–99% is converted to mesalamine (5-aminosalicylic acid). *Sulfasalazine*—10–15% absorbed following oral administration.

Distribution: *Mesalamine*—UK. *Olsalazine*—action is primarily local and remains in the colon. *Sulfasalazine*—widely distributed; crosses the placenta and enters breast milk.

Metabolism and Excretion: *Mesalamine*—some metabolism occurs, site unknown; mostly eliminated unchanged in the feces. *Olsalazine*—2% absorbed into systemic circulation is rapidly metabolized; mostly eliminated as mesalamine in the feces. *Sulfasalazine*—split by intestinal bacteria into sulfapyridine and 5-aminosalicylic acid. Some of absorbed sulfasalazine is excreted by bile back into intestines; 15% excreted unchanged by the kidneys. Sulfapyridine also excreted mostly by the kidneys.

Half-life: *Mesalamine*—12 hr PO (range 2–15 hr); 0.5–1.5 hr rectal. *Olsalazine*—0.9 hr. *Sulfasalazine*—6 hr.

CONTRAINDICATIONS AND PRECAUTIONS

Contraindicated in: ▪ Hypersensitivity reactions to sulfonamides, salicylates, mesalamine, olsalazine, or sulfasalazine ▪ Cross-sensitivity with furosemide, sulfonylurea hypoglycemic agents, or carbonic anhydrase inhibitors may exist ▪ G6PD deficiency ▪ Hypersensitivity to bisulfites (mesalamine enema only) ▪ Urinary tract or intestinal obstruction ▪ Children <2 yr (sulfasalazine only; other agents are not labeled for pediatric use) ▪ Porphyria.

Use Cautiously in: ▪ Severe hepatic or renal impairment ▪ Pregnancy (sulfasalazine has been used safely) ▪ Renal impairment (increased risk of renal tubular damage with olsalazine) ▪ Lactation (safety not established).

ADVERSE REACTIONS AND SIDE EFFECTS*

CNS: *mesalamine*—headache, dizziness, malaise, weakness; *olsalazine*—depression, drowsiness, vertigo; *sulfasalazine*—ataxia, confusion, dizziness, drowsiness, headache, mental depression, psychosis, restlessness.

EENT: *mesalamine*—pharyngitis.

Resp: *sulfasalazine*—pneumonitis.

CV: *mesalamine*—pericarditis.

GI: *sulfasalazine*—anorexia, diarrhea, nausea, vomiting, drug-induced hepatitis; *mesalamine*—diarrhea, eructation (PO), flatulence,

{} = Available in Canada only.
***CAPITALS indicate life-threatening; underlines indicate most frequent.**

nausea, vomiting; *olsalazine*—diarrhea, abdominal pain, anorexia, exacerbation of colitis, drug-induced hepatitis, nausea, vomiting.
GU: *mesalamine*—interstitial nephritis, renal failure; *sulfasalazine*—crystalluria, oligospermia, orange-yellow discoloration of urine.
Derm: *mesalamine*—hair loss, rash; *olsalazine*—itching, rash; *sulfasalazine*—rashes, exfoliative dermatitis, photosensitivity, yellow discoloration.
Hemat: *olsalazine*—blood dyscrasias (less frequent than with sulfasalazine); *sulfasalazine*—AGRANULOCYTOSIS, APLASTIC ANEMIA, blood dyscrasias, eosinophilia, megaloblastic anemia, thrombocytopenia.
Local: *mesalamine*—anal irritation (mesalamine enema, suppository).
MS: *mesalamine*—back pain.
Neuro: *sulfasalazine*—peripheral neuropathy.
Misc: *mesalamine*—ANAPHYLAXIS, acute intolerance syndrome, fever; *sulfasalazine*—hypersensitivity reactions including SERUM SICKNESS and STEVENS-JOHNSON SYNDROME, fever.

INTERACTIONS

Drug-Drug: ▪ *Sulfasalazine*—May enhance the action and increase the risk of toxicity from **oral hypoglycemic agents, phenytoin, methotrexate, zidovudine,** or **warfarin** ▪ Increased risk of drug-induced hepatitis with other **hepatotoxic agents** ▪ Increased risk of crystalluria with **methenamine** ▪ *Mesalamine, olsalazine*—None significant.
Drug-Food: ▪ *Sulfasalazine*—May decrease **iron** and **folic acid** absorption.

ROUTE AND DOSAGE

❑ Mesalamine

- **PO (Adults):** 800 mg 3 times daily for 6 wk as delayed-release tablets or 1 g 4 times daily as extended-release capsules.
- **Rect (Adults):** 4-g enema (60 ml) at bedtime, retained for 8 hr for 3–6 wk or 500-mg suppository 2–3 times daily.

❑ Olsalazine

- **PO (Adults):** 500 mg twice daily.

❑ Sulfasalazine

- **PO (Adults):** *Inflammatory bowel disease*—1 g q 6–8 hr (may start with 500 mg q 6–12 hr), followed by maintenance dose of 500 mg q 6 hr. *Rheumatoid arthritis*—500 mg–1 g/day (as delayed-release tablets) for 1 wk, then increase by 500 mg/day q wk up to 2 g/day in 2 divided doses; if no benefit seen after 12 wk, increase to 3 g/day in 2 divided doses.
- **PO (Children >2 yr):** *Initial*—6.7–10 mg/kg q 4 hr or 10–15 mg/kg q 6 hr or 13.3–20 mg/kg q 8 hr. *Maintenance*—7.5 mg/kg q 6 hr (not to exceed 2 g/day).

AVAILABILITY

❑ Mesalamine

▪ ***Delayed-release tablets:*** {250 mg[Rx]}, 400 mg[Rx], {500 mg[Rx]} ▪ ***Extended-release capsules:*** 250 mg[Rx] ▪ ***Extended-release tablets:*** {250 mg[Rx]}, {500 mg[Rx]} ▪ ***Suppositories:*** 500 mg[Rx] ▪ ***Rectal suspension:*** 4 g/60 ml[Rx].

❑ Olsalazine

▪ ***Capsules:*** 250 mg[Rx].

❑ Sulfasalazine

▪ ***Tablets:*** 500 mg[Rx] ▪ ***Enteric-coated tablets:*** 500 mg[Rx] ▪ ***Oral suspension:*** {250 mg/5 ml[Rx]} ▪ ***Rectal suspension:*** {3 g[Rx]}.

TIME/ACTION PROFILE (levels [olsalazine, sulfasalazine]; clinical improvement [mesalamine])

	ONSET	PEAK	Duration
Mesalamine PO	UK	UK	6–8 hr
Mesalamine rectal	3–21 days	UK	24 hr
Olsalazine PO	UK	1 hr*4–8 hr†	12 hr†
Sulfasalazine PO	1 hr	1.5–6 hr	6–12 hr

*For olsalazine.
†For mesalamine.

NURSING IMPLICATIONS

ASSESSMENT

- **General Info:** Assess patient for allergy to sulfonamides and salicylates. Patients allergic to sulfasalazine may take mesalamine or olsalazine without difficulty, but therapy should be discontinued if rash or fever occurs.
- ❑ Monitor intake and output ratios. Fluid intake should be sufficient to maintain a urine output of at least 1200–1500 ml daily to prevent crystalluria and stone formation.
- **Inflammatory Bowel Disease:** Assess abdominal pain and frequency, quantity, and consistency of stools at the beginning of and throughout therapy.

G

- **Rheumatoid Arthritis:** Assess range of motion and degree of swelling and pain in affected joints prior to and periodically during therapy.
- ***Lab Test Considerations:*** Monitor urinalysis, BUN, and serum creatinine prior to and periodically during therapy. Mesalamine may cause renal toxicity. Sulfasalazine may cause crystalluria and urinary cell calculi formation.
- □ Olsalazine and mesalamine may cause elevated AST and ALT levels. Mesalamine may also cause elevated serum alkaline phosphatase, GGTP, LDH, amylase, and lipase.
- □ Monitor CBC prior to and every 3–6 mo during prolonged therapy. Discontinue olsalazine and sulfasalazine if blood dyscrasias occur.

POTENTIAL NURSING DIAGNOSES

- Pain (Indications).
- Diarrhea (Indications).
- Knowledge deficit, related to medication regimen (Patient/Family Teaching).

IMPLEMENTATION

- **General Info:** Varying dosing regimens of *sulfasalazine* may be used to minimize GI side effects.
- **PO:** Administer *mesalamine* before meals and at bedtime with a full glass of water. Tablets should be swallowed whole; do not break the outer coating, which is designed to remain intact. Intact or partially intact tablets may occasionally be found in the stool. If this occurs repeatedly, advise patient to notify health care professional.
- □ Administer *olsalazine* with food in evenly divided doses every 12 hr.
- □ Administer *sulfasalazine* after meals or with food to minimize GI irritation, with a full glass of water. Do not crush or chew enteric-coated tablets. Shake oral suspension well prior to administration. Use a calibrated measuring device to measure liquid preparations.
- **Rect:** Patient should empty bowel prior to administration of rectal dose forms.
- □ Avoid excessive handling of *suppository*. Remove foil wrapper and insert pointed end first into rectum with gentle pressure. Suppository should be retained for 1–3 hr or more for maximum benefit.
- □ Administer 60-ml retention enema once daily at bedtime. Solution should be retained for approximately 8 hr. Prior to administration of *rectal suspension,* shake bottle well and remove the protective cap. Have patient lie on left side with the lower leg extended and the upper leg flexed for support or place the patient in knee-chest position. Gently insert the applicator tip into the rectum, pointing toward the umbilicus. Squeeze the bottle steadily to discharge most of the preparation.

PATIENT/FAMILY TEACHING

- □ Instruct patient on the correct method of administration. Advise patient to take medication as directed, even if feeling better. If a dose is missed, it should be taken as soon as remembered unless almost time for next dose.
- □ May cause dizziness. Caution patient to avoid driving or other activities that require alertness until response to medication is known.
- □ Advise patient to notify health care professional if skin rash, sore throat, fever, mouth sores, unusual bleeding or bruising, wheezing, fever, or hives occur.
- □ Instruct patient to notify health care professional if symptoms do not improve after 1–2 mo of therapy.
- □ Instruct patient to notify health care professional if symptoms worsen or do not improve. If symptoms of acute intolerance (cramping, acute abdominal pain, bloody diarrhea, fever, headache, rash) occur, discontinue therapy and notify health care professional immediately.
- □ Inform patient that proctoscopy and sigmoidoscopy may be required periodically during treatment to determine response.
- **Rect:** Instruct patient to use *rectal suspension* at bedtime and retain suspension all night for best results.
- **Mesalamine:** Advise patient not to change brands of mesalamine without consulting health care professional.
- **Sulfasalazine:** Caution patient to use sunscreen and protective clothing to prevent photosensitivity reactions.
- □ Inform patient that this medication may cause orange-yellow discoloration of urine and skin, which is not significant. May permanently stain contact lenses yellow.

EVALUATION

Clinical response to therapy can be evaluated by: ▪ Decrease in diarrhea and abdominal pain ▪ Return to normal bowel pattern in patients with inflammatory bowel disease. Effects may be seen within 3–21 days. The usual course of therapy is 3–6 wk ▪ Maintenance of remission in patients with inflammatory bowel disease ▪ Decrease in pain and inflammation, and increase in mobility in patients with rheumatoid arthritis.

GEMCITABINE

(gem-**site**-a-been)
Gemzar

CLASSIFICATION(S):
Antineoplastic (nucleoside analogue)

Pregnancy Category D

INDICATIONS

▪ Locally advanced or metastatic carcinoma of the pancreas.

ACTION

▪ Interferes with DNA synthesis (cell-cycle phase–specific). **Therapeutic Effects:** ▪ Death of rapidly replicating cells, particularly malignant ones.

PHARMACOKINETICS

Absorption: IV administration results in complete bioavailability.
Distribution: UK.
Metabolism and Excretion: Converted in cells to active diphosphate and triphosphate metabolites; these are excreted primarily by the kidneys.
Half-life: 32–94 min.

CONTRAINDICATIONS AND PRECAUTIONS

Contraindicated in: ▪ Hypersensitivity ▪ Pregnancy or lactation.
Use Cautiously in: ▪ Impaired hepatic or renal function (increased risk of toxicity) ▪ Patients with childbearing potential ▪ Other chronic debilitating illness.

ADVERSE REACTIONS AND SIDE EFFECTS*

Resp: dyspnea, bronchospasm.
CV: edema.
GI: diarrhea, nausea, stomatitis, transient elevation of hepatic transaminases, vomiting.
GU: hematuria, proteinuria, hemolytic uremic syndrome.
Derm: alopecia, rash.
Hemat: anemia, leukopenia, thrombocytopenia.
Local: injection site reactions.
Neuro: paresthesias.
Misc: flu-like symptoms, fever, anaphylactoid reactions.

INTERACTIONS

Drug-Drug: ▪ Additive bone marrow depression with other **antineoplastic agents** or **radiation therapy.**

ROUTE AND DOSAGE

▪ **IV (Adults):** 1000 mg/m² once weekly for 7 wk, followed by a week of rest. May be followed by cycles of once weekly administration for 3 wk followed by a week of rest.

AVAILABILITY

▪ ***Powder for injection:*** 200 mg in 10-ml vial[Rx], 1 g in 50-ml vial[Rx].

TIME/ACTION PROFILE (effect on blood counts)

	ONSET	PEAK	DURATION
IV	UK	UK	UK

NURSING IMPLICATIONS

ASSESSMENT

- ☐ Monitor vital signs prior to and frequently during therapy.
- ☐ Monitor injection site during administration. Although gemcitabine is not considered a vesicant, local reactions may occur.
- ☐ Monitor for bone marrow depression. Assess for bleeding (bleeding gums, bruising, petechiae, guaiac stools, urine, and emesis) and avoid IM injections and rectal temperatures if platelet count is low. Apply pressure to venipuncture sites for 10 min. Assess for signs of infection during neutropenia. Anemia may occur. Monitor for increased fatigue, dyspnea, and orthostatic hypotension.
- ☐ Monitor intake and output, appetite, and nutritional intake. Mild to moderate nausea and

***CAPITALS indicate life-threatening; underlines indicate most frequent.**

G

vomiting occur frequently. Antiemetics may be used prophylactically.

- ***Lab Test Considerations:*** Monitor CBC, including differential and platelet count prior to each dose. Dose guidelines are based on the CBC. If the absolute granulocyte count is >1000 and platelet count is >100,000, full dose may be administered. If the absolute granulocyte count is 500–999 or platelet count is 50,000–99,000, 75% of dose may be given. If the absolute granulocyte count is <500 or platelet count is <50,000, further doses should be held.
- Monitor hepatic and renal function prior to and periodically during therapy. May cause transient elevations in serum AST, ALT, alkaline phosphatase, and bilirubin concentrations.
- May also cause elevated BUN and serum creatinine concentrations, proteinuria, and hematuria.

POTENTIAL NURSING DIAGNOSES

- Infection, risk for (Adverse Reactions).
- Knowledge deficit, related to medication regimen (Patient/Family Teaching).

IMPLEMENTATION

- **General Info:** Solution should be prepared in a biologic cabinet. Wear gloves, gown, and mask while handling IV medication. Discard IV equipment in specially designated containers (see Appendix I).
- **Intermittent Infusion:** To reconstitute, add 5 ml of 0.9% NaCl without preservatives to 200-mg vial or 25 ml of 0.9% NaCl to the 1-g vial of gemcitabine for a concentration of 40 mg/ml. Incomplete dissolution may result in concentrations greater than 40 mg/ml. May be further diluted with 0.9% NaCl for concentrations as low as 0.1 mg/ml. Solution is colorless to light straw color. Do not administer solutions that are discolored or contain particulate matter. Solution is stable for 24 hr at room temperature. Discard unused portions. Do not refrigerate; crystallization may occur.
- ***Rate:*** Administer dose over 30 min. Infusions longer than 60 min have a greater incidence of toxicity.
- **Additive Incompatibility:** ▪ Information unavailable. Do not admix with other solutions or medications.

PATIENT/FAMILY TEACHING

- Instruct patient to notify health care professional if fever; chills; sore throat; signs of infection; bleeding gums; bruising; petechiae; blood in urine, stool, or emesis occurs. Caution patient to avoid crowds and persons with known infections. Instruct patient to use soft toothbrush and electric razor. Patient should be cautioned not to drink alcoholic beverages or take products containing aspirin or NSAIDs.
- Instruct patient to inspect oral mucosa for erythema and ulceration. If ulceration occurs, advise patient to use sponge brush and rinse mouth with water after eating and drinking. Stomatitis pain may require management with opioid analgesics.
- Instruct patient to notify health care professional if flu-like symptoms (fever, anorexia, headache, cough, chills, myalgia), swelling of the feet or legs, or shortness of breath occurs.
- Discuss with patient possibility of hair loss. Explore methods of coping.
- Advise patient that this medication may have teratogenic effects. Contraception should be used during therapy.
- Instruct patient not to receive any vaccinations without advice of health care professional.
- Emphasize the need for periodic lab tests to monitor for side effects.

EVALUATION

Effectiveness of therapy can be demonstrated by: ▪ Palliative, symptomatic improvement in patients with pancreatic cancer.

GEMFIBROZIL

(gem-**fye**-broe-zil)
Lopid

CLASSIFICATION(S):
Lipid-lowering agent

Pregnancy Category C

INDICATIONS

▪ Management of type II-b hyperlipidemia (↓ high-density lipoproteins, ↑ low-density lipoproteins, ↑ triglycerides) in patients who do not yet have clinical coronary artery disease and have failed therapy with diet, exercise, weight loss, or other agents (niacin, bile acid sequestrants).

ACTION

■ Inhibits peripheral lipolysis ■ Decreases triglyceride production by the liver ■ Decreases production of the triglyceride carrier protein ■ Increases high-density lipoproteins (HDL).
Therapeutic Effects: ■ Decreased plasma triglycerides and increased HDL.

PHARMACOKINETICS

Absorption: Well absorbed following oral administration.
Distribution: UK.
Metabolism and Excretion: Some metabolism by the liver, 70% excreted by the kidneys (mostly unchanged), 6% excreted in feces.
Half-life: 1.3–1.5 hr.

CONTRAINDICATIONS AND PRECAUTIONS

Contraindicated in: ■ Hypersensitivity ■ Primary biliary cirrhosis.
Use Cautiously in: ■ Gallbladder disease ■ Liver disease ■ Severe renal impairment ■ Pregnancy, lactation, or children (safety not established).

ADVERSE REACTIONS AND SIDE EFFECTS*

CNS: dizziness, headache.
EENT: blurred vision.
GI: abdominal pain, diarrhea, epigastric pain, flatulence, gallstones, heartburn, nausea, vomiting.
Derm: alopecia, rashes, urticaria.
Hemat: anemia, leukopenia.
MS: myositis.

INTERACTIONS

Drug-Drug: ■ May increase the effect of **warfarin** ■ **Thiazide diuretics, methyldopa,** or **estrogens** may decrease the response to gemfibrozil ■ Concurrent use with **HMG-CoA reductase inhibitors** may increase the risk of rhabdomyolysis (avoid concurrent use).

ROUTE AND DOSAGE

■ **PO (Adults):** 600 mg twice daily 30 min before breakfast and dinner.

AVAILABILITY

■ ***Tablets:*** 600 mg[Rx] ■ ***Capsules:*** {300 mg[Rx]}.

TIME/ACTION PROFILE (triglyceride-VLDL–lowering effect)

	ONSET	PEAK	DURATION
PO	2–5 days	4 wk	several mo

NURSING IMPLICATIONS

ASSESSMENT

□ Obtain patient's diet history, especially regarding fat and alcohol consumption.
■ ***Lab Test Considerations:*** Serum triglyceride and cholesterol levels should be monitored prior to and periodically throughout therapy. LDL and VLDL levels should be assessed prior to and periodically throughout therapy. Medication should be discontinued if paradoxical increase in lipid levels occurs.
□ Liver function tests should be assessed prior to and periodically throughout therapy. May cause an increase in serum bilirubin, alkaline phosphatase, CK, LDH, AST, and ALT. If hepatic function tests rise significantly, therapy should be discontinued and not resumed.
□ CBC and electrolytes should be evaluated every 3–6 mo and then yearly throughout course of therapy. May cause mild decrease in hemoglobin, hematocrit, and leukocyte counts. May cause a decrease in serum potassium concentrations.
□ May cause slight increase in serum glucose.

POTENTIAL NURSING DIAGNOSES

■ Knowledge deficit, related to medication regimen (Patient/Family Teaching).
■ Noncompliance (Patient/Family Teaching).

IMPLEMENTATION

■ **PO:** Administer 30 min before breakfast or dinner.

PATIENT/FAMILY TEACHING

□ Instruct patient to take medication exactly as directed, not to skip doses or double up on missed doses. If a dose is missed, take as soon as remembered unless almost time for next dose.
□ Advise patient that this medication should be

G

***CAPITALS** indicate life-threatening; underlines indicate most frequent.**

used in conjunction with dietary restrictions (fat, cholesterol, carbohydrates, alcohol), exercise, and cessation of smoking.
- Instruct patient to notify health care professional promptly if any of the following symptoms occur: severe stomach pains with nausea and vomiting, fever, chills, sore throat, rash, diarrhea, muscle cramping, general abdominal discomfort, or persistent flatulence.

EVALUATION

Effectiveness of therapy can be demonstrated by: ▪ Decrease in serum triglyceride and cholesterol levels and improved HDL to total cholesterol ratios. If response is not seen within 3 mo, medication is usually discontinued.

GLUCAGON
(**gloo**-ka-gon)

CLASSIFICATION(S):
Hormone (pancreatic)

Pregnancy Category B

INDICATIONS

▪ Acute management of severe hypoglycemia when administration of glucose is not feasible ▪ Facilitation of radiographic examination of the GI tract. **Unlabeled Uses:** ▪ Antidote to: ▫ Beta-adrenergic blocking agents ▫ Calcium channel blockers.

ACTION

▪ Stimulates hepatic production of glucose from glycogen stores (glycogenolysis) ▪ Relaxes the musculature of the GI tract ▪ Has positive inotropic and chronotropic effects. **Therapeutic Effects:** ▪ Increase in blood sugar ▪ Relaxation of GI musculature, facilitating radiographic examination.

PHARMACOKINETICS

Absorption: Well absorbed following IM and SC administration.
Distribution: UK.
Metabolism and Excretion: Extensively metabolized by the liver and kidneys.
Half-life: 3–10 min.

CONTRAINDICATIONS AND PRECAUTIONS

Contraindicated in: ▪ Hypersensitivity to beef or pork protein ▪ Diluent contains glycerin and phenol—avoid use in patients with hypersensitivities to these ingredients.
Use Cautiously in: ▪ History of insulinoma or pheochromocytoma.

ADVERSE REACTIONS AND SIDE EFFECTS*

GI: <u>nausea</u>, <u>vomiting</u>.
Misc: hypersensitivity reactions.

INTERACTIONS

Drug-Drug: ▪ Large doses may enhance the effect of **warfarin** ▪ Negates the response to **insulin** or **oral hypoglycemic agents** ▪ Hyperglycemic effect is intensified and prolonged by **epinephrine.**

ROUTE AND DOSAGE

▫ Hypoglycemia, Terminating Insulin Shock

- **IV, IM, SC (Adults):** 0.5–1 mg; may repeat in 20 min.
- **IV, IM, SC (Children):** 25 mcg/kg (up to 1 mg); may repeat in 20 min.

▫ Radiographic Examination of the GI Tract

- **IV (Adults):** 0.25–1 mg.

▫ Antidote (unlabeled)

- **IV (Adults):** *To beta-adrenergic blockers*—50–150 mcg (0.05–0.15 mg)/kg, followed by 1–5 mg/hr infusion. *To calcium channel blockers*—2 mg; additional doses determined by response.

AVAILABILITY

▪ ***Powder for injection:*** 1-mg vials[Rx], 10-mg vials[Rx].

TIME/ACTION PROFILE

	ONSET	PEAK	DURATION
IV, SC (hyperglycemic action)	5–20 min	30 min	1–2 hr
IV (effect on GI musculature)	1 min	UK	9–25 min

***CAPITALS indicate life-threatening; <u>underlines</u> indicate most frequent.**

NURSING IMPLICATIONS

ASSESSMENT

- Assess patient for signs of hypoglycemia (sweating, hunger, weakness, headache, dizziness, tremor, irritability, tachycardia, anxiety) prior to and periodically during therapy.
- Assess neurologic status throughout therapy. Institute safety precautions to protect patient from injury caused by seizures, falling, or aspiration. For insulin shock therapy, 0.5–1 mg is administered after 1 hr of coma; patient usually awakens in 10–25 min. If no response occurs, repeat the dose. Feed patient orally as soon as possible after awakening.
- Assess nutritional status. Patients who lack liver glycogen stores (starvation, chronic hypoglycemia, adrenal insufficiency) will require glucose instead of glucagon.
- Assess for nausea and vomiting after administration of dose. Protect patients with depressed level of consciousness from aspiration by positioning on side; ensure that a suction unit is available. Notify physician if vomiting occurs; patient will require parenteral glucose to prevent recurrent hypoglycemia.
- ***Lab Test Considerations:*** Monitor serum glucose levels throughout episode, during treatment, and for 3–4 hr after patient regains consciousness. Use of bedside fingerstick blood glucose determination methods is recommended for rapid results. Follow-up lab results may be ordered to validate fingerstick values, but do not delay treatment while awaiting lab results, as this could result in neurologic injury or death.
- Large doses of glucagon may cause a decrease in serum potassium concentrations.

POTENTIAL NURSING DIAGNOSES

- Injury, risk for (Indications).
- Knowledge deficit, related to medication regimen (Patient/Family Teaching).
- Noncompliance (Patient/Family Teaching).

IMPLEMENTATION

- **General Info:** May be given SC, IM, or IV. Reconstitute with diluent supplied in kit by manufacturer. Inspect solution prior to use; use only clear, water-like solution. Solution is stable for 48 hr if refrigerated, 24 hr at room temperature. Unmixed medication should be stored at room temperature.
- Administer supplemental carbohydrates IV or orally to facilitate increase of serum glucose levels.
- **IV:** With doses >2 mg, use sterile water for injection instead of diluent supplied by manufacturer to minimize risk of thrombophlebitis, CNS toxicity, and myocardial depression from phenol preservative in diluent supplied by manufacturer. Use immediately after reconstituting. Final concentration should not exceed 1 mg/ml.
- **Direct IV:** Administer at a rate not exceeding 1 mg per min. May be administered through IV line containing D5W.
- May be given at the same time as a bolus of dextrose.
- **Additive Incompatibility:** ▪ 0.9% NaCl ▪ potassium chloride ▪ calcium chloride.

PATIENT/FAMILY TEACHING

- **General Info:** Teach patient and family signs and symptoms of hypoglycemia. Instruct patient to take oral glucose as soon as symptoms of hypoglycemia occur—glucagon is reserved for episodes when patient is unable to swallow because of decreased level of consciousness.
- **Home Care Issues:** Instruct family on correct technique to prepare, draw up, and administer injection. Health care professional must be contacted immediately after each dose for orders regarding further therapy or adjustment of insulin dose or diet.
- Advise family that patient should receive oral glucose when alertness returns.
- Instruct family to position patient on side until fully alert. Explain that glucagon may cause nausea and vomiting. Aspiration may occur if patient vomits while lying on back.
- Instruct patient to check expiration date monthly and to replace outdated medication immediately.
- Review hypoglycemic medication regimen, diet, and exercise programs.
- Patients with diabetes mellitus should carry a source of sugar (such as a packet of sugar or candy) and identification describing disease process and treatment regimen at all times.

EVALUATION

Effectiveness of therapy can be demonstrated by: ▪ Increase of serum glucose to nor-

G

mal levels with improved level of consciousness ▪ Smooth muscle relaxation of the stomach, duodenum, and small and large intestine in patients undergoing radiologic examination of the GI tract.

GLUCOCORTICOIDS (inhalation)

beclomethasone
(be-kloe-**meth**-a-sone)
{Beclodisk}, {Becloforte}, Beclovent, Vanceril, Vanceril Double Strength

budesonide
(byoo-**dess**-oh-nide)
Pulmicort

flunisolide
(floo-**niss**-oh-lide)
AeroBid, {Bronalide}

fluticasone
(floo-**ti**-ka-sone)
Flovent

triamcinolone
(trye-am-**sin**-oh-lone)
Azmacort

CLASSIFICATION(S):
Anti-inflammatories (pulmonary), Glucocorticoids (inhalation)

Pregnancy Category C

INDICATIONS

▪ Anti-inflammatory and immunosuppressant in the long-term control of asthma ▪ May decrease requirement for or avoid use of systemic glucocorticoids and delay pulmonary damage that occurs from chronic asthma.

ACTION

▪ Potent, locally acting anti-inflammatory and immune modifier. **Therapeutic Effects:** ▪ Decrease frequency and severity of asthma attacks ▪ Prevention of pulmonary damage associated with chronic asthma.

PHARMACOKINETICS

Absorption: *Beclomethasone, flunisolide*—rapidly absorbed from the lungs; *budesonide*—39% absorbed from the lungs; *fluticasone*—30% absorbed following inhalation; *triamcinolone*—more slowly absorbed following inhalation. Action of all agents is primarily local following inhalation; systemic absorption is minimal at recommended doses.
Distribution: 10–25% of inhaled glucocorticoids is deposited in the airways if a spacer device is not used. With the use of a spacer, a greater percentage may reach the respiratory tract. All agents cross the placenta and enter breast milk in small amounts.
Metabolism and Excretion: *Beclomethasone*—following inhalation, beclomethasone dipropionate is converted to beclomethasone monopropionate, an active metabolite that adds to its potency; *fluticasone*—UK; *triamcinolone*—rapidly and extensively metabolized by the liver following absorption from lungs.
Half-life: *Beclomethasone*—15 hr; *budesonide*—1.5 hr in children, 2 hr in adults; *fluticasone*—UK; *triamcinolone*—4 hr (due to prolonged absorption).

CONTRAINDICATIONS AND PRECAUTIONS

Contraindicated in: ▪ Some products contain fluorocarbon propellants, alcohol, propylene, or polyethylene glycol and should be avoided in patients with known hypersensitivity or intolerance. ▪ Acute attack of asthma/status asthmaticus.
Use Cautiously in: ▪ Active untreated infections ▪ Patients with diabetes or glaucoma ▪ Patients with underlying immunosuppression (due to disease or concurrent therapy) ▪ Systemic glucocorticoid therapy (should not be abruptly discontinued when inhalable therapy is started) ▪ Pregnancy, lactation, or children <6 yr (safety not established; prolonged or high-dose therapy may lead to complications).

ADVERSE REACTIONS AND SIDE EFFECTS*

CNS: *budesonide, fluticasone*—<u>headache</u>; *fluticasone*—agitation, depression, fatigue, insomnia, restlessness.

EENT: dysphonia, hoarseness, oropharyngeal fungal infections, cataracts; *fluticasone*—nasal stuffiness/sinusitis.
Resp: bronchospasm, cough, wheezing.
GI: dry mouth, esophageal candidiasis; *budesonide*—dyspepsia, gastroenteritis; *fluticasone*—nausea.
Endo: adrenal suppression (↑ dose, long-term therapy only).
MS: *budesonide*—back pain; *fluticasone*—muscle soreness.
Misc: *budesonide*—flu-like syndrome.

INTERACTIONS

Drug-Drug: ▪ **Ketoconazole** decreases metabolism and increases levels of budesonide.

ROUTE AND DOSAGE

❑ Beclomethasone

- **Inhalation (Adults and Children >12 yr):** *42–50 mcg/spray product*—2 metered sprays 3–4 times daily or 4 metered sprays twice daily. In severe asthma, up to 16 metered sprays/day in divided doses may be used but should be decreased according to response, or 1 metered spray 2–4 times a day, or 2 metered sprays twice daily (not to exceed 1 mg/day total by either route or combined); *84 mcg/spray product*—1 metered spray 3–4 times daily or 2 metered sprays twice daily. In severe asthma, up to 8 metered sprays/day in divided doses may be used but should be decreased (not to exceed 1 mg/day total by either route or combined).
- **Inhalation (Children 6–12 yr):** 1–2 metered sprays 3–4 times daily or 4 metered sprays twice daily (42–50 mcg/spray; not to exceed 10 metered sprays/day).

❑ Budesonide

- **Inhalation (Adults):** *Previously controlled on bronchodilators alone*—1–2 sprays twice daily (up to 2 sprays twice daily); *previously controlled on other inhaled glucocorticoids*—1–2 sprays twice daily (up to 4 sprays twice daily); *previously controlled on oral glucocorticoids*—2–4 sprays twice daily (up to 4 sprays twice daily).
- **Inhalation (Children ≥6 yr):** 1 spray twice daily (up to 2 sprays twice daily).

❑ Flunisolide

- **Inhalation (Adults and Children >4 yr):** 2 metered sprays twice daily (250 mcg/metered spray; not to exceed 8 metered sprays/day in adults or 4 metered sprays/day in children).

❑ Fluticasone (aerosol inhaler)

- **Inhalation (Adults and Adolescents):** *Patients whose previous asthma treatment did not include oral glucocorticoids*—88–440 mcg twice daily (some patients may require higher doses). *Patients whose previous asthma treatment did include oral glucocorticoids*—880 mcg twice daily (some patients may require higher doses); after 7 days, slow tapering of oral glucocorticoids may be considered.

❑ Fluticasone (dry powder inhaler)

- **Inhalation (Adults):** 50–250 mg twice daily.
- **Inhalation (Children ≥4 yr):** 50–100 mg twice daily.

❑ Triamcinolone

- **Inhalation (Adults and Children >12 yr):** 2 metered sprays 3–4 times daily; may be given in 2 divided doses (100 mcg/metered spray; not to exceed 16 metered sprays/day).
- **Inhalation (Children 6–12 yr):** 1–2 metered sprays 3–4 times daily; may be given in 2 divided doses (100 mcg/metered spray; not to exceed 12 metered sprays/day).

AVAILABILITY

❑ Beclomethasone

- ***Inhalation aerosol:*** 42 mcg/metered spray in 16.8-g canister (200 metered sprays)Rx, {50 mcg/metered spray in 16.8-g canister (200 metered sprays)Rx}, 84 mcg/metered spray in 5.4-g canister (40 metered sprays) or 12.2-g canister (120 metered sprays)Rx, {250 mcg/metered spray in 80- or 200-metered-spray canistersRx}
- ***Inhalation capsules:*** {100 mcgRx}, {200 mcgRx}.

❑ Budesonide

- ***Inhalation powder:*** 200 mcg/metered spray in 200-metered spray inhalerRx.

❑ Flunisolide

- ***Inhalation aerosol:*** 250 mcg/metered spray in 7-g canisters (100 metered sprays)Rx.

❑ Fluticasone

- ***Inhalation aerosol:*** 44 mcg/metered spray in 7.9-g (60 metered sprays) and 13-g (120

G

metered sprays) canisters[Rx], 110 mcg/metered spray in 13-g canisters (120 metered sprays)[Rx], 220 mcg/metered spray in 13-g canisters (120 metered sprays)[Rx].

- ***Dry powder inhaler (Diskhaler):*** 50 mcg[Rx], 100 mcg[Rx], 250 mcg[Rx] Rotadisk blister.

□ **Triamcinolone**

- ***Inhalation aerosol:*** 100 mcg/metered spray in 20-g canister (240 metered sprays)[Rx].

TIME/ACTION PROFILE (improvement in symptoms)

	ONSET	PEAK	DURATION
Inhalation	within 24 hr	1–4 wk*	UK

*Improvement in pulmonary function; ↓ airway responsiveness may take longer.

NURSING IMPLICATIONS

ASSESSMENT

- □ Monitor respiratory status and lung sounds. Pulmonary function tests may be assessed periodically during and for several months following a transfer from systemic to inhalation glucocorticoids.
- □ Assess patients changing from systemic glucocorticoids to inhalation glucocorticoids for signs of adrenal insufficiency (anorexia, nausea, weakness, fatigue, hypotension, hypoglycemia) during initial therapy and periods of stress. If these signs appear, notify physician or other health care professional immediately; condition may be life-threatening.
- □ Monitor for withdrawal symptoms (joint or muscular pain, lassitude, depression) during withdrawal from oral glucocorticoids.
- ***Lab Test Considerations:*** Periodic adrenal function tests may be ordered to assess degree of hypothalamic-pituitary-adrenal (HPA) axis suppression in chronic therapy. Children and patients using higher than recommended doses are at highest risk for HPA suppression.
- □ May cause increased serum and urine glucose concentrations if significant absorption occurs.

POTENTIAL NURSING DIAGNOSES

- Airway clearance, ineffective (Indications).
- Infection, risk for (Side Effects).
- Knowledge deficit, related to medication regimen (Patient/Family Teaching).

IMPLEMENTATION

- **General Info:** After the desired clinical effect has been obtained, attempts should be made to decrease dose to lowest amount required to control symptoms. Gradually decrease dose every 2–4 wk as long as desired effect is maintained. If symptoms return, dose may briefly return to starting dose.
- **Inhalation:** Allow at least 1 min between inhalations of aerosol medication.

PATIENT/FAMILY TEACHING

- **General Info:** Advise patient to take medication exactly as directed. If a dose is missed, take as soon as remembered unless almost time for next dose.
- □ Advise patients using inhalation glucocorticoids and bronchodilator to use bronchodilator first and to allow 5 min to elapse before administering the glucocorticoid, unless otherwise directed by health care professional.
- □ Advise patient that inhalation glucocorticoids should not be used to treat an acute asthma attack but should be continued even if other inhalation agents are used.
- □ Patients using inhalation glucocorticoids to control asthma may require systemic glucocorticoids for acute attacks. Advise patient to use peak flow monitoring to determine respiratory status.
- □ Caution patient to avoid smoking, known allergens, and other respiratory irritants.
- **Metered-Dose Inhaler:** Instruct patient in the proper use of the metered-dose inhaler. There are 3 methods of using a metered-dose inhaler. Shake inhaler well. (1) Take a drink of water to moisten the throat; place the inhaler mouthpiece 2 finger-widths away from mouth; tilt head back slightly; while activating inhaler, take a slow, deep breath for 3–5 sec, hold the breath for 10 sec, and breathe out slowly. (2) Exhale, close lips firmly around mouthpiece, administer during 2nd half of inhalation, and hold breath for as long as possible to ensure deep instillation of medication. (3) Use a spacer. Consult health care professional to determine method desired prior to instruction. Allow 1–2 min between inhalations. Rinse mouth with water or mouthwash after each use to minimize dry mouth and

hoarseness. Wash inhalation assembly at least daily in warm running water (see Appendix H).

- **Pulmicort Turbuhaler (budesonide):** Advise patient to follow instructions supplied. Prior to first-time use, prime unit by turning cover and lifting off; hold upright with mouthpiece up and twist brown grip fully to right, then to left; repeat. To administer dose, hold upright, twist brown grip fully to right, then to left, listening for click. Turn head away from inhaler and exhale (do not blow into inhaler). Do not shake. Place mouthpiece between lips and inhale forcefully. Repeat procedure if 2nd dose required. Replace cover; rinse mouth with water (do not swallow).
- **Flovent Rotadisk:** Advise patient to follow instructions for the administration of the contents of each blister via breath-activated Diskhaler device.

EVALUATION

Effectiveness of therapy can be demonstrated by: ▪ Management of the symptoms of chronic asthma ▪ Prevention of pulmonary damage that occurs from chronic asthma.

GLUCOCORTICOIDS (nasal)

beclomethasone
(be-kloe-**meth**-a-sone)
Beconase, Beconase AQ, Vancenase, Vancenase AQ

budesonide
(byoo-**dess**-oh-nide)
Rhinocort

dexamethasone
(dex-a-**meth**-a-sone)
Decadron

flunisolide
(floo-**niss**-oh-lide)
Nasalide, {Rhinalar}

fluticasone
(floo-**ti**-ka-sone)
Flonase

mometasone
(moe-**met**-a-sone)
Nasonex

triamcinolone
(trye-am-**sin**-oh-lone)
Nasacort

CLASSIFICATION(S):
Anti-inflammatories (nasal)

Pregnancy Category C

INDICATIONS

▪ Seasonal allergic rhinitis and other chronic nasal inflammatory conditions, including nasal polyps.

ACTION

▪ Potent, locally acting anti-inflammatory and immune modifier. **Therapeutic Effects:** ▪ Decrease in symptoms of allergic rhinitis.

PHARMACOKINETICS

Absorption: *Beclomethasone*—absorption is rapid; *budesonide*—small amounts absorbed; *flunisolide*—50% absorbed; *fluticasone*—<2% absorbed; *dexamethasone*—absorption is extensive and rapid. Action of all agents is primarily local following nasal use; systemic absorption is minimal at recommended doses; *mometasone*—negligible absorption.
Distribution: Small portions of glucocorticoids administered nasally are swallowed. All agents cross the placenta and enter breast milk in small amounts.
Metabolism and Excretion: Following absorption from nasal mucosa, glucocorticoids are rapidly and extensively metabolized by the liver.
Half-life: *Beclomethasone*—15 hr; *budesonide*—2 hr (plasma); *dexamethasone*—190 min; *flunisolide*—1–2 hr; *fluticasone*—3 hr; *mometasone*—5.8 hr; *triamcinolone*—4 hr (due to prolonged absorption).

CONTRAINDICATIONS AND PRECAUTIONS

Contraindicated in: ▪ Some products contain fluorocarbon propellants, alcohol, propylene, or

{} = **Available in Canada only.**

polyethylene glycol and should be avoided in patients with known hypersensitivity or intolerance.
Use Cautiously in: ▪ Active untreated infections ▪ Patients with diabetes or glaucoma ▪ Patients with underlying immunosuppression (due to disease or concurrent therapy) ▪ Systemic glucocorticoid therapy (should not be abruptly discontinued when intranasal therapy is started) ▪ Recent nasal trauma or surgery (wound healing may be impaired by nasal glucocorticoids) ▪ Pregnancy or lactation (safety not established; prolonged or high-dose therapy may lead to complications).

ADVERSE REACTIONS AND SIDE EFFECTS*

CNS: dizziness, headache (↑ with triamcinolone).
EENT: loss of sense of smell (dexamethasone and flunisolide only), nasal burning, nasal irritation, sneezing attacks, throat itching (budesonide only), nasal bleeding.
GI: abdominal pain, loss of sense of taste (dexamethasone and flunisolide only), esophageal candidiasis.
Endo: adrenal suppression (↑ dose, long-term therapy only).

INTERACTIONS

Drug-Drug: ▪ None significant at recommended doses.

ROUTE AND DOSAGE

❑ Beclomethasone

- **Intranasal (Adults and Children >12 yr):** *Nasal aerosol*—1 metered spray in each nostril 2–4 times daily (42–50 mcg/spray; not to exceed 1 mg/day total by either route or combined).
- **Intranasal (Children 6–12 yr):** *Nasal aerosol*—1 metered spray in each nostril 3–4 times daily (42–50 mcg/spray; not to exceed 500 mcg/day).
- **Intranasal (Adults and Children ≥6 yr):** *Nasal solution*—1–2 metered sprays twice daily (42–50 mcg/spray; not to exceed 12 metered sprays/day in adults or 8 metered sprays/day in children) or 1 spray (84 mcg/spray) once daily.

❑ Budesonide

- **Intranasal (Adults and Children ≥6 yr):** 2 metered sprays in each nostril twice daily or 4 metered sprays in each nostril in the morning; may be gradually decreased q 2–4 wk when desired effect has been achieved (32 mcg/metered spray).

❑ Dexamethasone

- **Intranasal (Adults and Children >12 yr):** 2 metered sprays in each nostril 2–3 times daily; dosage should be decreased as soon as possible and discontinued (100 mcg/metered spray; not to exceed 12 metered sprays/day).
- **Intranasal (Children 6–12 yr):** 1–2 metered sprays in each nostril twice daily; dosage should be decreased as soon as possible and discontinued (100 mcg/metered spray; not to exceed 8 metered sprays/day).

❑ Flunisolide

- **Intranasal (Adults and Children >14 yr):** 2 metered sprays in each nostril 2–3 times daily; dosage should be decreased to lowest effective amount and discontinued when possible (25 mcg/metered spray; not to exceed 16 metered sprays/day).
- **Intranasal (Children 6–14 yr):** 1 metered spray in each nostril twice daily; dosage should be decreased to lowest effective amount and discontinued when possible (25 mcg/metered spray; not to exceed 8 metered sprays/day).

❑ Fluticasone

- **Intranasal (Adults):** 2 metered sprays in each nostril once daily or 1 spray in each nostril twice daily after several days; decrease to 1 spray in each nostril once daily (50 mcg/metered spray; not to exceed 4 metered sprays/day).
- **Intranasal (Children >4 yr and Adolescents):** 1 spray in each nostril once daily (50 mcg/metered spray); not to exceed 200 mcg/day total dose.

❑ Mometasone

- **Intranasal (Adults and Children >12 yr):** 2 sprays in each nostril (50 mcg/spray) once daily.

*CAPITALS indicate life-threatening; underlines indicate most frequent.

❑ **Triamcinolone**

- **Intranasal (Adults):** 2 metered sprays in each nostril once daily (110 mcg/metered spray; not to exceed 8 metered sprays/day).
- **Intranasal (Children 6–11 yr):** 1 spray in each nostril once daily.

AVAILABILITY

❑ **Beclomethasone**

▪ ***Nasal aerosol:*** 42 mcg/metered spray in 16.8-g canister (200 metered sprays)[Rx], {50 mcg/metered spray in 16.8-g canister (200 metered sprays)[Rx]} ▪ ***Nasal solution:*** 42 mcg/metered spray in 25-g bottles (200 metered sprays)[Rx], 50 mcg/metered spray in 25-g bottles (200 metered sprays)[Rx], 84 mcg/metered spray in 25-g bottles (200 metered sprays)[Rx].

❑ **Budesonide**

▪ ***Nasal aerosol:*** 32 mcg/metered spray in 7-g canister (200 metered sprays)[Rx].

❑ **Dexamethasone**

▪ ***Nasal aerosol:*** {84 mcg/metered spray in 12.6-g canister (170 metered sprays)}.

❑ **Flunisolide**

▪ ***Nasal solution:*** 25 mcg/spray in 25-ml bottle (200 metered sprays)[Rx].

❑ **Fluticasone**

▪ ***Nasal spray:*** 50 mcg/metered spray in 9-g bottle (120 metered sprays)[Rx].

❑ **Mometasone**

▪ ***Nasal spray:*** 50 mcg/metered spray in 17-g bottle (120 sprays)[Rx].

❑ **Triamcinolone**

▪ ***Nasal spray:*** 55 mcg/metered spray in 15-g canister (100 metered sprays)[Rx].

TIME/ACTION PROFILE (improvement in symptoms)

	ONSET	PEAK	DURATION
Beclomethasone	5–7 days*	up to 3 wk	UK
Budesonide	24 hr	2–3* days	UK
Dexamethasone	few days	UK	UK
Flunisolide	few days	up to 3 wk	UK
Fluticasone	few days	UK	UK
Triamcinolone	few days	3–4 days	UK

*Up to 3 wk in some patients.

NURSING IMPLICATIONS

ASSESSMENT

- ❑ Monitor degree of nasal stuffiness, amount and color of nasal discharge, and frequency of sneezing.
- ❑ Patients on long-term therapy should have periodic otolaryngologic examinations to monitor nasal mucosa and passages for infection or ulceration.
- ▪ ***Lab Test Considerations:*** Periodic adrenal function tests may be ordered to assess degree of hypothalamic-pituitary-adrenal (HPA) axis suppression in chronic therapy. Children and patients using higher than recommended doses are at highest risk for HPA suppression.

POTENTIAL NURSING DIAGNOSES

- Airway clearance, ineffective (Indications).
- Infection, risk for (Side Effects).
- Knowledge deficit, related to medication regimen (Patient/Family Teaching).

IMPLEMENTATION

- **General Info:** After the desired clinical effect has been obtained, attempts should be made to decrease dose to lowest amount. Gradually decrease dose every 2–4 wk as long as desired effect is maintained. If symptoms return, dose may briefly return to starting dose.
- **Intranasal:** Patients also using a topical decongestant should be given decongestant 5–15 min before glucocorticoid nasal spray. If patient is unable to breathe freely through nasal passages, instruct patient to blow nose gently in advance of medication administration.

PATIENT/FAMILY TEACHING

- ❑ Advise patient to take medication exactly as directed. If a dose is missed, take as soon as remembered unless almost time for next dose.
- ❑ Caution patient not to exceed maximal daily dose of 4 sprays/nostril.
- ❑ Instruct patient in correct technique for administering nasal spray (see Appendix H). Shake well before use. Warn patient that temporary nasal stinging may occur.
- ❑ Advise patient to store canister with valve downward. Canister should not be stored in cold areas or in high humidity and should be used within 3 mo (beclomethasone, fluniso-

lide) or within 6 mo of opening aluminum pouch. Advise patient to save inhaler for beclomethasone or dexamethasone; refills may be available.

- Instruct patient to notify health care professional if symptoms do not improve within 1 mo or if nasal discharge becomes purulent.

EVALUATION

Effectiveness of therapy can be demonstrated by: ▪ Resolution of nasal stuffiness, discharge, and sneezing in seasonal or perennial rhinitis.

GLUCOCORTICOIDS (systemic)

SHORT-ACTING GLUCOCORTICOIDS

cortisone

(**kor**-ti-sone)
{Cortone}, Cortone Acetate

hydrocortisone

(hye-droe-**kor**-ti-sone)
A-hydroCort, Cortef, Cortenema, Cortifoam, Hydrocortone, Solu-Cortef

INTERMEDIATE-ACTING GLUCOCORTICOIDS

methylprednisolone

(meth-ill-pred-**niss**-oh-lone)
A-Methapred, depMedalone, Depoject, Depo-Medrol, Depopred, Depo-Predate, Duralone, Medralone, Medrol, Meprolone, Rep-Pred, Solu-Medrol

prednisolone

(pred-**niss**-oh-lone)
Articulose, Delta-Cortef, Hydeltrasol, Key-Pred, Pediapred, Predaject, Predate, Predicort, Prelone

prednisone

(**pred**-ni-sone)
Deltasone, Liquid Pred, Meticorten, Orasone, Prednicen-M, Sterapred, Winpred

triamcinolone

(trye-am-**sin**-oh-lone)
Amcort, Aristocort, Aristospan, Articulose LA, Cenocort, Cinalone, Cinonide, Kenacort, Kenaject, Kenalog, Triam-A, Triam-Forte, Triamolone, Triamonide, Tri-Kort, Trilog, Trilone, Tristoject

LONG-ACTING GLUCOCORTICOIDS

betamethasone

(bay-ta-**meth**-a-sone)
{Betnelan}, {Betnesol}, Celestone, {Selestoject}

dexamethasone

(dex-a-**meth**-a-sone)
AK-Dex, Dalalone, Decadrol, Decadron, Decaject, Dexacen, Dexasone, Dexone, Hexadrol, Mymethasone, Solurex

CLASSIFICATION(S):
Anti-inflammatories, Immunosuppressants

Pregnancy Category B, C

INDICATIONS

▪ **Cortisone, hydrocortisone:** Management of adrenocortical insufficiency; chronic use in other situations is limited because of mineralocorticoid activity. ▪ **Betamethasone, dexamethasone, prednisolone, prednisone, methylprednisolone, triamcinolone:** Used systemically and locally in a wide variety of chronic diseases including: □ Inflammatory □ Allergic □ Hematologic □ Neoplastic □ Autoimmune disorders ▪ Some agents are suitable for alternate-day dosing in the management of chronic illness (methylprednisolone, prednisolone, prednisone, triamcinolone) ▪ Replacement therapy in adrenal insufficiency (not dexamethasone) ▪ **Dexamethasone:** □ Management of cerebral edema □ Diagnostic agent in adrenal disorders. **Unlabeled Uses:** ▪ Short-term administration to high-risk mothers before delivery to prevent respiratory distress syndrome in the newborn (betamethasone, dexamethasone) ▪ Adjunctive therapy of hypercalcemia ▪ Management of acute spinal cord injury (meth-

{} = Available in Canada only.

ylprednisolone) ▪ Adjunctive management of nausea and vomiting from chemotherapy.

ACTION

▪ In pharmacologic doses, all agents suppress inflammation and the normal immune response ▪ All agents have numerous intense metabolic effects (see Adverse Reactions and Side Effects) ▪ Suppress adrenal function at chronic doses of *betamethasone*—0.6 mg/day; *cortisone, hydrocortisone*—20 mg/day; *dexamethasone*—0.75 mg/day; *methylprednisolone*—4 mg/day; *prednisone/prednisolone*—5 mg/day; *triamcinolone*—4 mg/day ▪ **Cortisone, hydrocortisone:** Replace endogenous cortisol in deficiency states ▪ **Cortisone, hydrocortisone:** Also have potent mineralocorticoid (sodium-retaining) activity ▪ **Prednisolone, prednisone:** Have minimal mineralocorticoid activity ▪ **Betamethasone, dexamethasone, methylprednisolone, triamcinolone:** Have negligible mineralocorticoid activity. **Therapeutic Effects:** ▪ Suppression of inflammation and modification of the normal immune response ▪ Replacement therapy in adrenal insufficiency.

PHARMACOKINETICS

Absorption: Well absorbed following oral administration. Sodium phosphate and sodium succinate salts are rapidly absorbed following IM administration. Acetate, acetonide, diacetate, hexacetonide, and tebutate salts are slowly but completely absorbed following IM administration. Absorption from local sites (intra-articular, intralesional) is slow but complete.

Distribution: All are widely distributed, cross the placenta, and probably enter breast milk.

Metabolism and Excretion: All are metabolized mostly by the liver. *Cortisone* is converted by the liver to hydrocortisone. *Prednisone* is converted by the liver to prednisolone, which is then metabolized by the liver.

Half-life: *Betamethasone*—3–5 hr (plasma), 36–54 hr (tissue); adrenal suppression lasts 3.25 days. *Cortisone*—0.5 hr (plasma), 8–12 hr (tissue); adrenal suppression lasts 1.25–1.5 days. *Dexamethasone*—3–4.5 hr (plasma), 36–54 hr (tissue); adrenal suppression lasts 2.75 days. *Hydrocortisone*—1.5–2 hr (plasma), 8–12 hr (tissue); adrenal suppression lasts 1.25–1.5 days. *Methylprednisolone*—>3.5 hr (plasma), 18–36 hr (tissue); adrenal suppression lasts 1.25–1.5 days. *Prednisolone*—2.1–3.5 hr (plasma), 18–36 hr (tissue); adrenal suppression lasts 1.25–1.5 days. *Prednisone*—3.4–3.8 hr (plasma), 18–36 hr (tissue); adrenal suppression lasts 1.25–1.5 days. *Triamcinolone*—2–>5 hr (plasma), 18–36 hr (tissue); adrenal suppression lasts 2.25 days.

CONTRAINDICATIONS AND PRECAUTIONS

Contraindicated in: ▪ Active untreated infections (may be used in patients being treated for tuberculous meningitis) ▪ Lactation (avoid chronic use) ▪ Known alcohol, bisulfite, or tartrazine hypersensitivity or intolerance (some products contain these and should be avoided in susceptible patients).

Use Cautiously in: ▪ Chronic treatment (will lead to adrenal suppression; use lowest possible dose for shortest period of time) ▪ Children (chronic use will result in decreased growth; use lowest possible dose for shortest period of time) ▪ Stress (surgery, infections); supplemental doses may be needed ▪ Potential infections may mask signs (fever, inflammation) ▪ Pregnancy (safety not established).

ADVERSE REACTIONS AND SIDE EFFECTS*

Adverse reactions/side effects are much more common with high-dose/long-term therapy.

CNS: depression, euphoria, headache, increased intracranial pressure (children only), personality changes, psychoses, restlessness.

EENT: cataracts, increased intraocular pressure.

CV: hypertension.

GI: PEPTIC ULCERATION, anorexia, nausea, vomiting.

Derm: acne, decreased wound healing, ecchymoses, fragility, hirsutism, petechiae.

Endo: adrenal suppression, hyperglycemia.

F and E: fluid retention (long-term high doses), hypokalemia, hypokalemic alkalosis.

Hemat: THROMBOEMBOLISM, thrombophlebitis.

Metab: weight gain, weight loss.

MS: muscle wasting, osteoporosis, aseptic necrosis of joints, muscle pain.

Misc: cushingoid appearance (moon face, buffalo hump), increased susceptibility to infection.

***CAPITALS indicate life-threatening; underlines indicate most frequent.**

G

INTERACTIONS

Drug-Drug: ▪ Additive hypokalemia with **thiazide** and **loop diuretics, amphotericin B, mezlocillin, piperacillin,** or **ticarcillin** ▪ Hypokalemia may increase the risk of **digitalis glycoside** toxicity ▪ May increase requirement for **insulin** or **oral hypoglycemic agents** ▪ **Phenytoin, phenobarbital,** and **rifampin** stimulate metabolism; may decrease effectiveness ▪ **Oral contraceptives** may block metabolism ▪ Increased risk of adverse GI effects with **NSAIDs** (including aspirin) ▪ At chronic doses that suppress adrenal function, may decrease the antibody response to and increase the risk of adverse reactions from **live virus vaccines** ▪ May increase the risk of tendon rupture from **fluoroquinolones.**

ROUTE AND DOSAGE

❑ Betamethasone

- **PO (Adults):** 0.6 mg–7.2 mg/day as single daily dose or in divided doses.
- **PO (Children):** *Adrenocortical insufficiency*—17.5 mcg/kg (500 mcg/m^2)/day in 3 divided doses. *Other uses*—62.5–250 mcg/kg (1.875–7.5 mg/m^2)/day in 3 divided doses.
- **IM, IV (Adults):** Up to 9 mg of betamethasone sodium phosphate or 0.5–9 mg IM as betamethasone sodium phosphate/acetate suspension. *Prevention of respiratory distress syndrome in newborn*—12 mg IM daily for 2–3 days before delivery (unlabeled).
- **IM (Children):** *Adrenocortical insufficiency*—17.5 mcg/kg (500 mcg/m^2)/day in 3 divided doses every 3rd day or 5.8–8.75 mcg/kg (166–250 mcg/m^2)/day as a single dose. *Other uses*—20.8–125 mcg/kg (0.625–3.75 mg/m^2) of the base q 12–24 hr.

❑ Cortisone

- **PO (Adults):** 25–300 mg/day as a single dose or in divided doses.
- **PO (Children):** *Adrenocortical insufficiency*—0.7 mg/kg (20–25 mg/m^2)/day in divided doses. *Other uses*—2.5–10 mg/kg (75–300 mg/m^2)/day as a single dose or in divided doses.
- **IM (Adults):** 20–300 mg/day.
- **IM (Children):** *Adrenocortical insufficiency*—0.7 mg/kg (37.5 mg/m^2) q 3 days or 0.23–0.35 mg/kg (12.5 mg/m^2)/day. *Other uses*—0.83–5 mg/kg (25–150 mg/m^2) q 12–24 hr.

❑ Dexamethasone (Adrenocortical Insufficiency/Anti-inflammatory/Most Other Uses)

- **PO (Adults):** 0.5–9 mg daily in single or divided doses.
- **PO (Children):** *Adrenocortical insufficiency*—23.3 mcg/kg (670 mcg/m^2/day) in 3 divided doses. *Other uses*—83.3–333.3 mcg/kg (2.5–10 mg/m^2)/day in 3–4 divided doses.
- **IV (Adults):** *Dexamethasone phosphate*—0.5–24 mg/day (up to 1mg/kg as a single dose has been used).
- **IM (Adults):** *Dexamethasone acetate*—8–16 mg q 1–3 wk.

❑ Dexamethasone (Cerebral Edema)

- **IM, IV (Adults):** *Dexamethasone phosphate*—10 mg initially IV, 4 mg q 6 hr, may be decreased to 2 mg q 8–12 hr, then change to PO.
- **PO (Adults):** 2 mg q 8–12 hr.

❑ Dexamethasone (Suppression Test)

- **PO (Adults):** 1 mg at 11 PM or 0.5 mg q 6 hr for 48 hr.

❑ Hydrocortisone

- **PO (Adults):** 20–240 mg/day in 1–4 divided doses.
- **PO (Children):** *Adrenocortical insufficiency*—0.56 mg/kg (15–20 mg/m^2)/day as a single dose or in divided doses. *Other uses*—2–8 mg/kg/day (60–240 mg/m^2/day) as a single dose or in divided doses.
- **Rect (Adults):** *Retention enema*—100 mg nightly for 21 days or until remission occurs; *aerosol foam*—90 mg 1–2 times/day for 2–3 wk; then adjusted.
- **IM, IV (Adults):** *Hydrocortisone sodium succinate/sodium phosphate*—100–500 mg q 2–6 hr (range 100–8000 mg/day). Hydrocortisone sodium phosphate may also be given SC.
- **IM, IV (Children):** *Adrenocortical insufficiency: hydrocortisone sodium succinate/sodium phosphate*—0.186–0.28 mg/kg/day

(10–12 mg/m²)/day in 3 divided doses. *Other uses: hydrocortisone sodium succinate/sodium phosphate*—0.666–4 mg/kg (20–120 mg/m²) q 12–24 hr (phosphate or succinate). Hydrocortisone sodium phosphate may also be given SC.

❑ Methylprednisolone

- **PO (Adults):** *Multiple sclerosis*—160 mg/day for 7 days, then 64 mg every other day for 1 mo. *Other uses*—4–48 mg/day as a single dose or in divided doses.
- **PO (Children):** *Adrenocortical insufficiency*—117 mcg/kg (3.33 mg/m²)/day in 3 divided doses. *Other uses*—0.417 mg/kg–1.67 mg/kg (12.5–50 mg/m²)/day in 3–4 divided doses.
- **Rect (Adults):** 40 mg 3–7 times weekly for at least 2 wk.
- **Rect (Children):** 0.5–1 mg/kg (15–30 mg/m²) daily or every other day for at least 1 wk.
- **IM, IV (Adults):** *Most uses: methylprednisolone sodium succinate*—10–40 mg, repeated as needed. *High-dose "pulse" therapy: methylprednisolone sodium succinate*—30 mg/kg IV q 4–6 hr for up to 72 hr. *Multiple sclerosis: methylprednisolone sodium succinate*—160 mg/day for 7 days, then 64 mg every other day for 1 mo. *Adjunctive therapy of* Pneumocystis carinii *pneumonia in AIDS patients: methylprednisolone sodium succinate*—30 mg twice daily for 5 days, then 30 mg once daily for 5 days, 15 mg once daily for 10 days. *Acute spinal cord injury: methylprednisolone sodium succinate*—30 mg/kg over 15 min initially, followed 45 min later with 5.4 mg/kg/hr for 23 hr (unlabeled).
- **IM, IV (Children):** *Adrenocortical insufficiency: methylprednisolone sodium succinate*—117 mcg/kg (3.33 mg/m²)/day in 3 divided doses. *Acute spinal cord injury: methylprednisolone sodium succinate*—30 mg/kg over 15 min initially, then 45 min later initiate continuous infusion of 5.4 mg/kg/hr for 23 hr (unlabeled). *Other uses: methylprednisolone sodium succinate*—139–835 mcg/kg (4.16–25 mg/m²) q 12–24 hr.
- **IM (Adults):** *Methylprednisolone acetate*—40–120 mg daily, weekly, or every 2 wk.

❑ Prednisolone

- **PO (Adults):** *Most uses*—5–60 mg/day single dose or divided doses. *Multiple sclerosis*—200 mg/day for 7 days, then 80 mg every other day for 1 mo.
- **PO (Children):** *Adrenocortical insufficiency*—0.14 mg/kg (4 mg/m²)/day in 3 divided doses. *Other uses*—0.5–2 mg/kg (15–60 mg/m²)/day in 3–4 divided doses.
- **IM, IV (Adults):** *Prednisolone sodium phosphate*—4–60 mg/day.
- **IM (Children):** *Adrenocortical insufficiency: prednisolone sodium phosphate/acetate*—0.14 mg/kg (4 mg/m²)/day in 3 divided doses q 3 days or 0.046–0.07 mg/kg (1.33–2 mg/m²) once daily. *Other uses*—0.166–1 mg/kg (5–30 mg/m²) q 12–24 hr.
- **IM (Adults):** *Prednisolone acetate*—4–60 mg/day. *Prednisolone sodium acetate/phosphate*—25–100 mg (total); may repeat q 3 days–4 wk.

❑ Prednisone

- **PO (Adults):** *Most uses*—5–60 mg/day single dose or divided doses. *Multiple sclerosis*—200 mg/day for 1 wk, then 80 mg every other day for 1 mo. *Adjunctive therapy of* Pneumocystis carinii *pneumonia in AIDS patients*—40 mg twice daily for 5 days, then 40 mg once daily for 5 days, then 20 mg once daily for 10 days.
- **PO (Children ≥10 yr):** *Nephrosis*—20 mg 4 times daily initially.
- **PO (Children 4–10 yr):** *Nephrosis*—15 mg 4 times daily initially.
- **PO (Children 18 mo–4 yr):** *Nephrosis*—7.5–10 mg 4 times daily initially.

❑ Triamcinolone

- **PO (Adults):** *Adrenocortical insufficiency*—4–12 mg/day as a single dose or in divided doses. *Other uses*—4–48 mg/day (up to 60 mg/day) as a single dose or in divided doses.
- **PO (Children):** *Adrenocortical insufficiency*—117 mcg/kg/day (3.3 mg/m²/day) as a single dose or in divided doses. *Other uses*—416 mcg–1.7 mg/kg /day (12.5–50 mg/m²/day) as a single dose or in divided doses. Some conditions may require up to 2 mg/kg/day.
- **IM (Adults):** *Triamcinolone acetonide*—40–80 mg q 4 wk. *Triamcinolone diacetate*—40 mg weekly.
- **IM (Children):** *Triamcinolone acetonide*—40 mg q 4 wk or 30–200 mcg/kg (1–

G

6.25 mg/m^2) q 1–7 days. *Triamcinolone diacetate*—40 mg weekly.

AVAILABILITY

❑ Betamethasone

▪ ***Tablets:*** {0.5 mg^{Rx}}, 0.6 mg^{Rx} ▪ ***Syrup:*** 0.6 mg/5 ml^{Rx} ▪ ***Effervescent tablets:*** {0.5 mg^{Rx}} ▪ {***Extended-release tablets:*** 1 mg^{Rx}} ▪ ***Solution for injection (sodium phosphate):*** 3 mg/ml^{Rx} ▪ ***Suspension for injection (Phosphate/acetate):*** 6 mg (total)/ml^{Rx}.

❑ Cortisone

▪ ***Tablets:*** 5 mg^{Rx}, 10 mg^{Rx}, 25 mg^{Rx} ▪ ***Suspension for injection:*** 50 mg/ml^{Rx}.

❑ Dexamethasone

▪ ***Tablets:*** 0.25 mg^{Rx}, 0.5 mg^{Rx}, 0.75 mg^{Rx}, 1 mg^{Rx}, 1.5 mg^{Rx}, 2 mg^{Rx}, 4 mg^{Rx}, 6 mg^{Rx} ▪ ***Elixir:*** 0.5 mg/5 ml^{Rx} ▪ ***Oral solution:*** 0.5 mg/5 ml^{Rx}, 1 mg/ml^{Rx} ▪ ***Solution for injection (sodium phosphate):*** 4 mg/ml^{Rx}, 10 mg/ml^{Rx}, 20 mg/ml^{Rx}, 24 mg/ml^{Rx} ▪ ***Suspension for injection (acetate):*** 8 mg/ml^{Rx}, 16 mg/ml^{Rx}.

❑ Hydrocortisone

▪ ***Tablets:*** 5 mg^{Rx}, 10 mg^{Rx}, 20 mg^{Rx} ▪ ***Oral suspension:*** 10 mg/5 ml^{Rx} ▪ ***Suspension for injection (base):*** 25 mg/ml^{Rx}, 50 mg/ml^{Rx} ▪ ***Suspension for injection (acetate):*** 25 mg/ml^{Rx}, 50 mg/ml^{Rx} ▪ ***Solution for injection (sodium phosphate):*** 50 mg/ml^{Rx} ▪ ***Enema:*** 100 mg^{Rx} ▪ ***Rectal aerosol:*** 90 mg^{Rx} ▪ ***Powder for injection (sodium succinate):*** 100 mg^{Rx}, 250 mg^{Rx}, 500 mg^{Rx}, 1 g^{Rx}.

❑ Methylprednisolone

▪ ***Tablets:*** 2 mg^{Rx}, 4 mg^{Rx}, 8 mg^{Rx}, 16 mg^{Rx}, 24 mg^{Rx}, 32 mg^{Rx} ▪ ***Solution for injection:*** 40 mg^{Rx}, 125 mg^{Rx}, 500 mg^{Rx}, 1 g^{Rx}, 2 g^{Rx} ▪ ***Suspension for injection:*** 20 mg/ml^{Rx}, 40 mg/ml^{Rx}, 80 mg/ml^{Rx} ▪ ***Enema:*** 40 mg^{Rx}.

❑ Prednisolone

▪ ***Tablets:*** 5 mg^{Rx} ▪ ***Syrup:*** 15 mg/5 ml^{Rx} ▪ ***Oral solution:*** 5 mg/ml^{Rx} ▪ ***Solution for injection (sodium phosphate):*** 20 mg/ml^{Rx} ▪ ***Suspension for injection (acetate):*** 25 mg/ml^{Rx}, 50 mg/ml^{Rx} ▪ ***Suspension for injection (sodium phosphate/acetate):*** 100 mg (total)/ml^{Rx} ▪ ***Suspension for injection (tebutate):*** 20 mg/ml^{Rx}.

❑ Prednisone

▪ ***Tablets:*** 1 mg^{Rx}, 2.5 mg^{Rx}, 5 mg^{Rx}, 10 mg^{Rx}, 20 mg^{Rx}, 50 mg^{Rx} ▪ ***Oral solution:*** 5 mg/5 ml^{Rx}, 5 mg/1 ml^{Rx} ▪ ***Syrup:*** 5 mg/5 ml^{Rx}.

❑ Triamcinolone

▪ ***Tablets:*** 1 mg^{Rx}, 2 mg^{Rx}, 4 mg^{Rx}, 8 mg^{Rx}, 16 mg^{Rx} ▪ ***Oral syrup:*** 2 mg/5 ml^{Rx}, 4 mg/5 ml^{Rx} ▪ ***Suspension for injection (acetonide):*** 3 mg/ml^{Rx}, 10 mg/ml^{Rx}, 40 mg/ml^{Rx} ▪ ***Suspension for injection (diacetate):*** 25 mg/ml^{Rx}, 40 mg/ml^{Rx} ▪ ***Suspension for injection (hexacetonide):*** 5 mg/ml^{Rx}, 20 mg/ml^{Rx}.

TIME/ACTION PROFILE (anti-inflammatory activity)

	ONSET	PEAK	DURATION
Betamethasone PO	UK	1–2 hr	3.25 days
Betamethasone sodium phosphate IM, IV	rapid	UK	UK
Betamethasone acetate/sodium phosphate IM	1–3 hr	UK	1 wk
Cortisone PO	rapid	2 hr	1.25–1.5 days
Cortisone IM	slow	20–48 hr	1.25–1.5 days
Dexamethasone PO	UK	1–2 hr	2.75 days
Dexamethasone IM, IV (phosphate)	rapid	UK	2.75 days
Dexamethasone IM (acetate)	UK	8 hr	6 days
Hydrocortisone PO	UK	1–2 hr	1.25–1.5 days
Hydrocortisone sodium succinate IM	rapid	1 hr	variable
Hydrocortisone IV	rapid	UK	UK
Methylprednisolone PO	UK	1–2 hr	1.25–1.5 days
Methylprednisolone IM (acetate)	6–48 hr	4–8 days	1–4 wk
Methylprednisolone IM, IV (succinate)	rapid	UK	UK
Prednisolone PO	UK	1–2 hr	1.25–1.5 days
Prednisolone IM, IV (phosphate)	rapid	1 hr	UK
Prednisolone IM (acetate)	slow	UK	UK
Prednisone PO	hr	UK	1.25–1.5 days
Triamcinolone PO	UK	1–2 hr	2.25 days
Triamcinolone IM (acetonide)	24–48 hr	UK	1–6 wk
Triamcinolone IM (diacetonide)	slow	UK	4 days–4 wk

NURSING IMPLICATIONS

ASSESSMENT

- ◻ These drugs are indicated for many conditions. Assess involved systems prior to and periodically throughout therapy.
- ◻ Assess patient for signs of adrenal insufficiency (hypotension, weight loss, weakness, nausea, vomiting, anorexia, lethargy, confusion, restlessness) prior to and periodically throughout therapy.
- ◻ Monitor intake and output ratios and daily weights. Observe patient for peripheral edema, steady weight gain, rales/crackles, or dyspnea. Notify physician or other health care professional should these occur.
- ◻ Children should have periodic evaluations of growth.
- ◻ Monitor for signs of anaphylaxis (swelling of face, nasal membranes, eyelids; hives; dyspnea; chest tightness; wheezing) in patients receiving high-dose pulse therapy. ECG should also be monitored. May cause convulsions, anaphylaxis, and arrhythmias. Resuscitation equipment, medications, and trained personnel should be readily available.
- ▪ **Cerebral Edema:** Assess patient for changes in level of consciousness and headache throughout therapy.
- ▪ ***Lab Test Considerations:*** *Systemic*—Monitor serum electrolytes and glucose. May cause hyperglycemia, especially in persons with diabetes. May cause hypokalemia. Patients on prolonged courses of therapy should routinely have hematologic values, serum electrolytes, and serum and urine glucose evaluated. May decrease WBC counts. May cause hyperglycemia, especially in persons with diabetes. May decrease serum potassium and calcium and increase serum sodium concentrations.
- ◻ Guaiac test stools. Promptly report presence of guaiac-positive stools.
- ◻ May increase serum cholesterol and lipid values. May decrease uptake of thyroid ^{123}I or ^{131}I.
- ◻ Suppress reactions to allergy skin tests.
- ◻ Periodic adrenal function tests may be ordered to assess degree of hypothalamic-pituitary-adrenal axis suppression in systemic and chronic topical therapy.
- ▪ **Dexamethasone Suppression Test:** To diagnose Cushing's syndrome: Obtain baseline cortisol level; administer dexamethasone at 11 PM and obtain cortisol levels at 8 AM the next day. Normal response is a decreased cortisol level.
- ◻ Alternative method: Obtain baseline 24-hr urine for 17-hydroxycorticosteroid (OHCS) concentrations, then begin 48-hr administration of dexamethasone. Second 24-hr urine for 17-OHCS is obtained after 24 hr of dexamethasone.

POTENTIAL NURSING DIAGNOSES

- ▪ Infection, risk for (Side Effects).
- ▪ Body image disturbance (Side Effects).
- ▪ Knowledge deficit, related to medication regimen (Patient/Family Teaching).

IMPLEMENTATION

- ▪ **General Info:** If dose is ordered daily or every other day, administer in the morning to coincide with the body's normal secretion of cortisol.
- ▪ **PO:** Administer with meals to minimize GI irritation.
- ◻ Tablets may be crushed and administered with food or fluids for patients with difficulty swallowing.
- ◻ Use calibrated measuring device to ensure accurate dosage of liquid forms.
- ▪ **IM, SC:** Shake suspension well before drawing up. IM doses should not be administered when rapid effect is desirable. Do not dilute with other solution or admix. Do not administer suspensions IV.

◻ Betamethasone

- ▪ **Direct IV:** Only betamethasone sodium phosphate may be given IV. Administer undiluted.
- ▪ ***Rate:*** Administer over at least 1 min.
- ▪ **Intermittent Infusion:** May be administered as infusion in D5W, 0.9% NaCl, Ringer's solution, D5/Ringer's solution, or D5/LR.
- ▪ **Y-Site Compatibility:** ▪ heparin ▪ potassium chloride ▪ vitamin B complex with C.

◻ Dexamethasone

- ▪ **Direct IV:** May be given undiluted. Do not administer suspension IV.
- ▪ ***Rate:*** Administer over 1 min.
- ▪ **Intermittent Infusion:** May be added to D5W or 0.9% NaCl solution. Administer infu-

G

sions at prescribed rate. Diluted solution should be used within 24 hr.

❑ Dexamethasone Sodium Phosphate

- **Syringe Compatibility:** ▪ granisetron ▪ metoclopramide ▪ ranitidine ▪ sufentanil.
- **Syringe Incompatibility:** ▪ doxapram ▪ glycopyrrolate.
- **Y-Site Compatibility:** ▪ acyclovir ▪ amifostine ▪ aztreonam ▪ cefepime ▪ cisplatin ▪ cyclophosphamide ▪ cytarabine ▪ doxorubicin ▪ famotidine ▪ filgrastim ▪ fluconazole ▪ fludarabine ▪ foscarnet ▪ granisetron ▪ heparin ▪ lorazepam ▪ melphalan ▪ meperidine ▪ methotrexate ▪ morphine ▪ ondansetron ▪ paclitaxel ▪ piperacillin/tazobactam ▪ potassium ▪ sargramostim ▪ sufentanil ▪ tacrolimus ▪ teniposide ▪ thiotepa ▪ vinorelbine ▪ vitamin B complex with C ▪ zidovudine.
- **Y-Site Incompatibility:** ▪ ciprofloxacin ▪ idarubicin ▪ midazolam.
- **Additive Compatibility:** ▪ aminophylline ▪ bleomycin ▪ cimetidine ▪ furosemide ▪ lidocaine ▪ nafcillin ▪ netilmicin ▪ ondansetron ▪ ranitidine
- **Additive Incompatibility:** ▪ daunorubicin ▪ doxorubicin ▪ metaraminol ▪ vancomycin.

❑ Hydrocortisone

- **Direct IV:** Reconstitute with provided solution (i.e., Act-O-Vials) or 2 ml of bacteriostatic water or saline for injection.
- ***Rate:*** Administer each 100 mg over at least 30 sec. Doses 500 mg and larger should be infused over at least 10 min.
- **Intermittent/Continuous Infusion:** May be added to 50–1000 ml of D5W, 0.9% NaCl, or D5/0.9% NaCl. Administer infusions at prescribed rate. Diluted solutions should be used within 24 hr.

❑ Hydrocortisone Sodium Phosphate

- **Syringe Compatibility:** ▪ metoclopramide.
- **Y-Site Compatibility:** ▪ amifostine ▪ aztreonam ▪ cefepime ▪ filgrastim ▪ fluconazole ▪ fludarabine ▪ melphalan ▪ ondansetron ▪ paclitaxel ▪ piperacillin/tazobactam ▪ teniposide ▪ thiotepa ▪ vinorelbine.
- **Y-Site Incompatibility:** ▪ sargramostim.
- **Additive Compatibility:** ▪ amikacin ▪ amphotericin B ▪ bleomycin ▪ cephapirin ▪ sodium bicarbonate.

❑ Hydrocortisone Sodium Succinate

- **Syringe Compatibility:** ▪ metoclopramide ▪ thiopental.
- **Y-Site Compatibility:** ▪ acyclovir ▪ amifostine ▪ aminophylline ▪ ampicillin ▪ amrinone ▪ atracurium ▪ atropine ▪ aztreonam ▪ calcium gluconate ▪ cefepime ▪ cephalothin ▪ cephapirin ▪ chlordiazepoxide ▪ chlorpromazine ▪ cyanocobalamin ▪ dexamethasone ▪ digoxin ▪ diphenhydramine ▪ dopamine ▪ droperidol ▪ droperidol/fentanyl ▪ edrophonium ▪ enalaprilat ▪ epinephrine ▪ esmolol ▪ conjugated estrogens ▪ ethacrynate ▪ famotidine ▪ fentanyl ▪ filgrastim ▪ fludarabine ▪ fluorouracil ▪ foscarnet ▪ furosemide ▪ gallium nitrate ▪ hydralazine ▪ insulin ▪ isoproterenol ▪ kanamycin ▪ lidocaine ▪ magnesium sulfate ▪ melphalan ▪ menadiol ▪ meperidine ▪ methicillin ▪ methoxamine ▪ methylergonovine ▪ minocycline ▪ morphine ▪ neostigmine ▪ norepinephrine ▪ ondansetron ▪ oxacillin ▪ oxytocin ▪ paclitaxel ▪ pancuronium ▪ penicillin G potassium ▪ pentazocine ▪ phytonadione ▪ piperacillin/tazobactam ▪ procainamide ▪ prochlorperazine edisylate ▪ propranolol ▪ pyridostigmine ▪ scopolamine ▪ sodium bicarbonate ▪ succinylcholine ▪ tacrolimus ▪ thiotepa ▪ trimethobenzamide ▪ trimethaphan camsylate ▪ vecuronium.
- **Y-Site Incompatibility:** ▪ ciprofloxacin ▪ diazepam ▪ ergotamine tartrate ▪ idarubicin ▪ phenytoin ▪ sargramostim.
- **Additive Compatibility:** ▪ amikacin ▪ aminophylline ▪ amphotericin ▪ daunorubicin ▪ diphenhydramine ▪ magnesium sulfate ▪ mitoxantrone ▪ potassium chloride ▪ vitamin B complex with C.
- **Additive Incompatibility:** ▪ bleomycin ▪ doxorubicin.

❑ Methylprednisolone

- **Direct IV:** Reconstitute with provided solution (Act-O-Vials, Univials, ADD-Vantage vials) or 2 ml of bacteriostatic water (with benzyl alcohol) for injection.
- ***Rate:*** May be administered direct IV push over 1 to several minutes.
- **Intermittent/Continuous Infusion:** May be diluted further in D5W, 0.9% NaCl, or D5/0.9% NaCl and administered as intermittent or continuous infusion at the prescribed rate. Solution may form a haze upon dilution.

❑ **Methylprednisolone Sodium Succinate**

- **Syringe Compatibility:** ▪ granisetron ▪ metoclopramide.
- **Y-Site Compatibility:** ▪ acyclovir ▪ amifostine ▪ amrinone ▪ aztreonam ▪ cefepime ▪ cisplatin ▪ cyclophosphamide ▪ cytarabine ▪ doxorubicin ▪ enalaprilat ▪ famotidine ▪ fludarabine ▪ heparin ▪ melphalan ▪ meperidine ▪ methotrexate ▪ midazolam ▪ morphine ▪ piperacillin/tazobactam ▪ sodium bicarbonate ▪ tacrolimus ▪ teniposide ▪ thiotepa.
- **Y-Site Incompatibility:** ▪ ciprofloxacin ▪ filgrastim ▪ ondansetron ▪ paclitaxel ▪ sargramostim.
- **Additive Compatibility:** ▪ cimetidine ▪ granisetron ▪ heparin ▪ ranitidine ▪ theophylline.

❑ **Prednisolone**

- **Direct IV:** Do not use the acetate form of this drug for IV administration.
- ***Rate:*** Prednisolone sodium phosphate IV may be administered direct IV push at a rate of no more than 10 mg/min.
- **Intermittent Infusion:** May be added to 50–1000 ml of D5W or 0.9% NaCl. Stable for 24 hr.
- ***Rate:*** Administer infusions at prescribed rate.
- **Y-Site Compatibility:** ▪ heparin ▪ potassium chloride ▪ vitamin B complex with C.
- **Additive Compatibility:** ▪ ascorbic acid ▪ cephalothin ▪ cytarabine ▪ erythromycin lactobionate ▪ fluorouracil ▪ heparin ▪ methicillin ▪ penicillin G potassium ▪ penicillin G sodium ▪ vitamin B complex with C.
- **Additive Incompatibility:** ▪ calcium gluceptate ▪ methotrexate ▪ polymyxin B sulfate.

PATIENT/FAMILY TEACHING

- **General Info:** Instruct patient on correct technique of medication administration. Advise patient to take medication as directed. Take missed doses as soon as remembered unless almost time for next dose. Do not double doses. Stopping the medication suddenly may result in adrenal insufficiency (anorexia, nausea, weakness, fatigue, dyspnea, hypotension, hypoglycemia). If these signs appear, notify health care professional immediately. This can be life-threatening.
- ❑ Glucocorticoids cause immunosuppression and may mask symptoms of infection. Instruct patient to avoid people with known contagious illnesses and to report possible infections immediately.
- ❑ Caution patient to avoid vaccinations without first consulting health care professional.
- ❑ Review side effects with patient. Instruct patient to inform health care professional promptly if severe abdominal pain or tarry stools occur. Patient should also report unusual swelling, weight gain, tiredness, bone pain, bruising, nonhealing sores, visual disturbances, or behavior changes.
- ❑ Advise patient to notify health care professional of medication regimen prior to treatment or surgery.
- ❑ Discuss possible effects on body image. Explore coping mechanisms.
- ❑ Instruct patient to inform health care professional if symptoms of underlying disease return or worsen.
- ❑ Advise patient to carry identification describing disease process and medication regimen in the event of emergency in which patient cannot relate medical history.
- ❑ Explain need for continued medical follow-up to assess effectiveness and possible side effects of medication. Periodic lab tests and eye exams may be needed.
- **Long-term Therapy:** Encourage patient to eat a diet high in protein, calcium, and potassium, and low in sodium and carbohydrates (see Appendix K). Alcohol should be avoided during therapy.

EVALUATION

Effectiveness of therapy can be demonstrated by: ▪ Decrease in presenting symptoms with minimal systemic side effects ▪ Suppression of the inflammatory and immune responses in autoimmune disorders, allergic reactions, and neoplasms ▪ Decrease in intracranial pressure ▪ Management of symptoms in adrenal insufficiency.

GLUCOCORTICOIDS (topical/local)

alclometasone

(al-kloe-**met**-a-sone)
Aclovate

amcinonide
(am-**sin**-oh-nide)
Cyclocort

betamethasone
(bay-ta-**meth**-a-sone)
Alphatrex, Beben, {Betacort}, {Betaderm}, Betatrex, Beta-Val, {Betnovate}, {Celestoderm}, Dermabet, Diprolene, Diprosone, {Ectosone}, Maxivate, {Metaderm}, {Novobetamet}, Occlucort, {Prevex}, Teladar, {Topilene}, {Topisone}, Uticort, Valisone, Valnac

clobetasol
(kloe-**bay**-ta-sol)
{Dermovate}, Temovate

clocortolone
(kloe-**kore**-toe-lone)
Cloderm

desonide
(**dess**-oh-nide)
DesOwen, Tridesilon

desoximetasone
(dess-ox-i-**met**-a-sone)
Topicort

dexamethasone
(dex-a-**meth**-a-sone)
Aeroseb-Dex, Decadron, Decaspray

diflorasone
(dye-**flor**-a-sone)
Florone, Maxiflor, Psorcon

fluocinolone
(floo-oh-**sin**-oh-lone)
Bio-Syn, Derma-Smoothe/FS, Fluocet, {Fluoderm}, {Fluolar}, Fluonid, {Fluonide}, Flurosyn, FS Shampoo, Synalar, {Synamol}, Synemol

fluocinonide
(floo-oh-**sin**-oh-nide)
Fluocin, Licon, {Lidemol}, Lidex, {Lyderm}, {Topsyn}

flurandrenolide
(floor-an-**dren**-oh-lide)
Cordran, {Drenison}

fluticasone
(floo-**tik**-a-sone)
Cutivate

halcinonide
(hal-**sin**-oh-nide)
Halog

halobetasol
(hal-oh-**bay**-ta-sol)
Ultravate

hydrocortisone
(hye-droe-**kor**-ti-sone)
Acticort, Aeroseb-HC, Ala-Cort, Ala-Scalp, Alphaderm, Anusol HC, Bactine, {Barriere-HC}, CaldeCORT Anti-Itch, Carmol HC, Cetacort, {Cortacet}, Cortaid, {Cortate}, Cort-Dome, {Cortef Feminine Itch}, Corticaine, {Corticreme}, Cortifair, Cortizone, Dermacort, DermiCort, Dermtex HC, {Emo-Cort}, FoilleCort, Gynecort, Hemril-HC, Hi-Cor, Hycort, {Hyderm}, Hydro-Tex, Hytone, LactiCare-HC, Lanacort 9-1-1, Lemoderm, Locoid, {Novohydrocort}, Nutracort, Orabase-HCA, Pandel, Penecort, Pharma-Cort, Prevex HC, Proctocort, Rhulicort, Synacort, Texacort, {Unicort}, Westcort

methylprednisolone
(meth-ill-pred-**niss**-oh-lone)
Medrol

mometasone
(moe-**met**-a-sone)
{Elocom}, Elocon

prednicarbate
(pred-ni-**kar**-bate)
Dermatop

triamcinolone
(trye-am-**sin**-oh-lone)
Aristocort, Delta-Tritex, Flutex, Kenalog, Kenonel, {Triaderm}, {Trianide}

{} = Available in Canada only.

CLASSIFICATION(S):
Anti-inflammatories (topical/local), Immunosuppressants (topical/local)
Pregnancy Category C

INDICATIONS

▪ Management of various allergic/immunologic skin problems.

ACTION

▪ Suppress normal immune response and inflammation. If systemically absorbed for prolonged periods of time may produce adrenal suppression. **Therapeutic Effects:** ▪ Suppression of dermatologic inflammation and immune processes.

PHARMACOKINETICS

Absorption: Prolonged use on large surface areas or large amounts applied or use of occlusive dressings will produce systemic absorption and adrenal suppression.
Distribution: Remain primarily at site of action.
Metabolism and Excretion: Usually metabolized in skin; some have been modified to resist local metabolism and have a prolonged local effect.
Half-life: *Betamethasone*—3–5 hr (plasma), 36–54 hr (tissue); adrenal suppression lasts 3.25 days. *Dexamethasone*—3–4.5 hr (plasma), 36–54 hr (tissue); adrenal suppression lasts 2.75 days. *Hydrocortisone*—1.5–2 hr (plasma), 8–12 hr (tissue); adrenal suppression lasts 1.25–1.5 days. *Methylprednisolone*—>3.5 hr (plasma), 18–36 hr (tissue); adrenal suppression lasts 1.25–1.5 days. *Triamcinolone*—2–>5 hr (plasma), 18–36 hr (tissue); adrenal suppression lasts 2.25 days.

CONTRAINDICATIONS AND PRECAUTIONS

Contraindicated in: ▪ Hypersensitivity or known intolerance to glucocorticoid or components of vehicles (ointment or cream base, preservative, alcohol) ▪ Untreated bacterial or viral infections.
Use Cautiously in: ▪ Hepatic dysfunction ▪ Diabetes mellitus, cataracts, glaucoma, or tuberculosis (use of large amounts of high-potency agents may worsen condition) ▪ Patients with pre-existing skin atrophy ▪ Pregnancy, lactation, or children (chronic high-dose usage may result in adrenal suppression in mother, growth suppression in children; children may be more susceptible to adrenal and growth suppression) ▪ Clobetasol not recommended for use in children <12 yr ▪ Desoximetasone not recommended in children <10 yr.

ADVERSE REACTIONS AND SIDE EFFECTS

Derm: allergic contact dermatitis, atrophy, burning, dryness, edema, folliculitis, hypersensitivity reactions, hypertrichosis, hypopigmentation, irritation, maceration, miliaria, perioral dermatitis, secondary infection, striae.
Misc: adrenal suppression (↑ dose, long-term therapy).

INTERACTIONS

Drug-Drug: ▪ None significant.

ROUTE AND DOSAGE

▪ **Topical (Adults and Children):** Apply 1–6 times daily (depends on product, preparation, and condition being treated).

AVAILABILITY

❑ **Alclometasone**
▪ ***Cream:*** 0.05%Rx ▪ ***Ointment:*** 0.05%Rx.

❑ **Amcinonide**
▪ ***Cream:*** 0.1%Rx ▪ ***Lotion:*** 0.1%Rx ▪ ***Ointment:*** 0.1%Rx.

❑ **Betamethasone**
▪ ***Cream:*** 0.01%Rx, 0.025%Rx, 0.05%Rx, 0.1%Rx ▪ ***Gel:*** 0.25%Rx, 0.05%Rx ▪ ***Lotion:*** 0.1%Rx, 0.025%Rx, 0.05%Rx ▪ ***Ointment:*** 0.05%Rx, 0.1%Rx ▪ ***Aerosol:*** 0.1%Rx.

❑ **Clobetasol**
▪ ***Cream:*** 0.05%Rx ▪ ***Ointment:*** 0.05%Rx ▪ ***Scalp solution:*** 0.05%Rx.

❑ **Clocortolone**
▪ ***Cream:*** 0.1%Rx.

❑ **Desonide**
▪ ***Cream:*** 0.05%Rx ▪ ***Ointment:*** 0.05%Rx ▪ ***Lotion:*** 0.05%Rx.

❑ **Desoximetasone**

▪ ***Cream:*** 0.25%^{Rx}, 0.05%^{Rx} ▪ ***Gel:*** 0.05%^{Rx} ▪ ***Ointment:*** 0.25%^{Rx}.

❑ **Dexamethasone**

▪ ***Cream:*** 1%^{Rx} ▪ ***Aerosol:*** 0.01%^{Rx}, 0.04%^{Rx}.

❑ **Diflorasone**

▪ ***Cream:*** 0.05%^{Rx} ▪ ***Ointment:*** 0.05%^{Rx}.

❑ **Fluocinolone**

▪ ***Cream:*** 0.01%^{Rx}, 0.02%^{Rx}, 0.025%^{Rx} ▪ ***Ointment:*** 0.025%^{Rx} ▪ ***Solution:*** 0.01%^{Rx} ▪ ***Shampoo:*** 0.01%^{Rx} ▪ ***Oil:*** 0.01%^{Rx}.

❑ **Fluocinonide**

▪ ***Cream:*** 0.05%^{Rx} ▪ ***Gel:*** 0.05%^{Rx} ▪ ***Ointment:*** 0.05%^{Rx} ▪ ***Solution:*** 0.05%^{Rx}.

❑ **Flurandrenolide**

▪ ***Cream:*** 0.025%^{Rx}, 0.05%^{Rx} ▪ ***Ointment:*** 0.025%^{Rx}, 0.05%^{Rx} ▪ ***Lotion:*** 0.05%^{Rx} ▪ ***Tape:*** 4 mcg/m$^{2 Rx}$.

❑ **Fluticasone**

▪ ***Cream:*** 0.05%^{Rx} ▪ ***Ointment:*** 0.005%^{Rx}.

❑ **Halcinonide**

▪ ***Cream:*** 0.025%^{Rx}, 0.1%^{Rx} ▪ ***Ointment:*** 0.1%^{Rx} ▪ ***Solution:*** 0.1%^{Rx}.

❑ **Halobetasol**

▪ ***Cream:*** 0.05%^{Rx} ▪ ***Ointment:*** 0.05%^{Rx}.

❑ **Hydrocortisone**

▪ ***Cream:*** 0.5%^{Rx,OTC}, 1%^{Rx,OTC}, 2.5%^{Rx} ▪ ***Gel:*** 0.5%^{Rx,OTC}, 1%^{Rx,OTC} ▪ ***Ointment:*** 0.5%^{Rx,OTC}, 1%^{Rx,OTC} ▪ ***Lotion:*** 0.25%^{Rx}, 0.5%^{Rx,OTC}, 1%^{Rx,OTC}, 2%^{Rx}, 2.5%^{Rx} ▪ ***Solution:*** 1%^{Rx} ▪ ***Spray:*** 0.5%^{Rx,OTC}, 1%^{Rx,OTC}.

❑ **Methylprednisolone**

▪ ***Ointment:*** 0.25%^{Rx}, 1%^{Rx}.

❑ **Mometasone**

▪ ***Cream:*** 0.1%^{Rx} ▪ ***Ointment:*** 0.1%^{Rx} ▪ ***Lotion:*** 0.1%^{Rx}.

❑ **Prednicarbate**

▪ ***Cream:*** 0.1%^{Rx}.

❑ **Triamcinolone**

▪ ***Cream:*** 0.025%^{Rx}, 0.1%^{Rx}, 0.5%^{Rx} ▪ ***Ointment:*** 0.025%^{Rx}, 0.1%^{Rx}, 0.5%^{Rx} ▪ ***Lotion:*** 0.025%^{Rx}, 0.1%^{Rx} ▪ ***Spray:*** 2 sec/spray^{Rx} ▪ ***In combination with:*** acetic acid, antifungals, anti-infectives, antihistamines, urea, and benzoyl peroxide in various otic and topical preparations. See Appendix A.

TIME/ACTION PROFILE (response depends on condition being treated)

	ONSET	PEAK	DURATION
Topical	min–hrs	hrs–days	hrs–days

NURSING IMPLICATIONS

ASSESSMENT

❑ Assess affected skin prior to and daily during therapy. Note degree of inflammation and pruritus. Notify physician or other health care professional if symptoms of infection (increased pain, erythema, purulent exudate) develop.

▪ ***Lab Test Considerations:*** Periodic adrenal function tests may be ordered to assess degree of hypothalamic-pituitary-adrenal (HPA) axis suppression in chronic topical therapy. Children and patients with dose applied to a large area, using an occlusive dressing, or using high-potency products are at highest risk for HPA suppression.

❑ May cause increased serum and urine glucose concentrations if significant absorption occurs.

POTENTIAL NURSING DIAGNOSES

▪ Skin integrity, impaired (Indications).
▪ Infection, risk for (Side Effects).
▪ Knowledge deficit, related to medication regimen (Patient/Family Teaching).

IMPLEMENTATION

▪ **General Info:** Choice of vehicle depends on site and type of lesion. Ointments are more occlusive and preferred for dry, scaly lesions. Creams should be used on oozing or intertriginous areas, where the occlusive action of ointments might cause folliculitis or maceration. Creams may be preferred for esthetic reasons even though they may be more drying to skin than ointments. Gels, aerosols, lotions, and solutions are useful in hairy areas.

▪ **Topical:** Apply *ointments, creams,* or *gels* sparingly as a thin film to clean, slightly moist skin. Wear gloves. Apply occlusive dressing only if specified by physician or other health care professional.

- ▫ Apply *lotion, solution,* or *gel* to hair by parting hair and applying a small amount to affected area. Rub in gently. Protect area from washing, clothing, or rubbing until medication has dried. Hair may be washed as usual but not right after applying medication.
- ▫ Use *aerosols* by shaking well and spraying on affected area, holding container 3–6 in. away. Spray for about 2 sec to cover an area the size of a hand. Do not inhale. If spraying near face, cover eyes.
- ▪ **Rect:** Applicator is provided by manufacturer. Do not insert aerosol container into rectum. Instructions are provided for correct usage of applicator. Clean applicator after each use. Advise patient to save applicator; refills may be available.

PATIENT/FAMILY TEACHING

- ▫ Instruct patient on correct technique of medication administration. Emphasize importance of avoiding the eyes. If a dose is missed, it should be applied as soon as remembered unless almost time for the next dose.
- ▫ Caution patient to use only as directed. Avoid using cosmetics, bandages, dressings, or other skin products over the treated area unless directed by health care professional.
- ▫ Advise parents of pediatric patients not to apply tight-fitting diapers or plastic pants on a child treated in the diaper area; these garments work like an occlusive dressing and may cause more of the drug to be absorbed.
- ▫ Advise patient to consult health care professional before using medicine for condition other than indicated.
- ▫ Instruct patient to inform health care professional if symptoms of underlying disease return or worsen or if symptoms of infection develop.

EVALUATION

Effectiveness of therapy can be demonstrated by: ▪ Resolution of skin inflammation, pruritus, or other dermatologic conditions.

GLYCERIN

(**gli**-ser-in)

Fleet Babylax, Glyrol, Osmoglyn, Sani-Supp

CLASSIFICATION(S):

Antiglaucoma agent, Diuretic (osmotic), Laxative (osmotic)

Pregnancy Category C

INDICATIONS

▪ **Rect:** Treatment of constipation ▪ **PO:** Short-term reduction of intraocular pressure. **Unlabeled Uses:** ▪ **PO:** Reduction of elevated intracranial pressure.

ACTION

▪ Draws water into the lumen of the colon ▪ Osmotically draws water from extravascular spaces, including the eye, into intravascular compartment. **Therapeutic Effects:** ▪ Relief of constipation ▪ Reduction of intraocular and intracranial pressure.

PHARMACOKINETICS

Absorption: Not significantly absorbed from colonic mucosa. Well absorbed following oral administration.

Distribution: Remains in the intravascular space.

Metabolism and Excretion: 80% metabolized by the liver, 10–20% metabolized by the kidneys.

Half-life: 30–45 min.

CONTRAINDICATIONS AND PRECAUTIONS

Contraindicated in: ▪ Hypersensitivity.

Use Cautiously in: ▪ Cardiovascular disease ▪ Mental confusion ▪ Severe dehydration ▪ Diabetes mellitus ▪ Hypervolemia ▪ Renal disease ▪ Elderly patients (increased risk of dehydration).

ADVERSE REACTIONS AND SIDE EFFECTS*

CNS: confusion, headache.

GI: <u>diarrhea</u>, nausea, vomiting.

*CAPITALS indicate life-threatening; <u>underlines</u> indicate most frequent.

G

F and E: dehydration.
Misc: thirst.

INTERACTIONS

Drug-Drug: ▪ **Diuretics** increase the intraocular pressure–lowering effects of glycerin.

ROUTE AND DOSAGE

❑ Laxative

- **Rect (Adults and Children >6 yr):** 2–3 g as a suppository or 5–15 ml as an enema.
- **Rect (Children <6 yr):** 1–1.7 g as a suppository or 2–5 ml as an enema.

❑ Reduction of Intraocular Pressure

- **PO (Adults):** 1–1.5 g/kg (up to 2 g/kg) as a single dose, may be followed by 500 mg/kg q 6 hr.
- **PO (Children):** 1–1.5 g/kg (40 g/m²) as a single dose, may be followed by 500 mg/kg 4–8 hr later.

AVAILABILITY

▪ ***Suppositories:*** Adult[OTC], pediatric[OTC] ▪ ***Liquid for rectal pediatric use:*** 4-ml applicators[OTC] ▪ ***Oral solution:*** 50%[Rx] ▪ ***Ophthalmic solution:*** 7.5-ml containers[Rx].

TIME/ACTION PROFILE

	ONSET	PEAK	DURATION
Rect (laxative effect)	UK	15–30 min	UK
PO (reduction of intraocular pressure)	within 10 min	60–90 min	5 hr
Ophth (reduced corneal swelling)	UK	UK	3–4 hr

NURSING IMPLICATIONS

ASSESSMENT

- **Laxative:** Assess patient for abdominal distention, presence of bowel sounds, and normal pattern of bowel function.
- ❑ Assess color, consistency, and amount of stool produced.
- ***Lab Test Considerations:*** May cause slightly elevated serum and urine glucose concentrations.

POTENTIAL NURSING DIAGNOSES

- Constipation (Indications).
- Knowledge deficit, related to medication regimen (Patient/Family Teaching).

IMPLEMENTATION

- **PO:** Solution is clear, colorless, and syrupy, with a sweet taste.
- ❑ Administer 50% glycerin solution with 0.9% NaCl flavored with lemon, lime, or orange juice or commercially prepared 50% or 75% flavored solution to improve taste and to minimize nausea and vomiting. May also be mixed with unsweetened fruit juice. Pour over cracked ice and sip through a straw.
- ❑ Have patient lie down during and after administration to prevent headache from cerebral dehydration.
- **Rect:** Glycerin suppository or enema usually causes evacuation of the colon in 15–30 min.

PATIENT/FAMILY TEACHING

- **General Info:** Instruct patient to take glycerin as directed. Do not take more than the amount prescribed.
- **Laxative:** Advise patient that laxatives should be used only for short-term therapy. Long-term therapy may cause electrolyte imbalance and dependence.
- ❑ Caution patients not to use laxatives when abdominal pain, nausea, vomiting, or fever is present.

EVALUATION

Effectiveness of therapy can be demonstrated by: ▪ Soft, formed bowel movement.

GLYCOPYRROLATE

(glye-koe-**pye**-roe-late)
Robinul, Robinul-Forte

CLASSIFICATION(S):
Anticholinergic

Pregnancy Category B

INDICATIONS

▪ Inhibits salivation and excessive respiratory secretions when given preoperatively ▪ Reverses some of the secretory and vagal actions of cholinesterase inhibitors used to treat nondepolarizing neuromuscular blockade (cholinergic adjunct) ▪ Adjunctive management of peptic ulcer disease.

ACTION

▪ Inhibits the action of acetylcholine at postganglionic sites located in smooth muscle, secretory glands, and the CNS (antimuscarinic activity) ▪ Low doses decrease sweating, salivation, and respiratory secretions ▪ Intermediate doses result in increased heart rate ▪ GI and GU tract motility are decreased at larger doses. **Therapeutic Effects:** ▪ Decreased GI and respiratory secretions.

PHARMACOKINETICS

Absorption: Incompletely absorbed following oral administration. Well absorbed following IM administration.
Distribution: Distribution not fully known. Does not significantly cross the blood-brain barrier or eye. Crosses the placenta.
Metabolism and Excretion: Eliminated primarily unchanged in the feces, via biliary excretion.
Half-life: 1.7 hr (0.6–4.6 hr).

CONTRAINDICATIONS AND PRECAUTIONS

Contraindicated in: ▪ Hypersensitivity ▪ Narrow-angle glaucoma ▪ Acute hemorrhage ▪ Tachycardia secondary to cardiac insufficiency or thyrotoxicosis ▪ Children <12 yr (for management of peptic ulcer only) ▪ Products containing benzyl alcohol should not be used in neonates.
Use Cautiously in: ▪ Elderly and the very young (increased susceptibility to adverse reactions) ▪ Patients who may have intra-abdominal infections ▪ Prostatic hypertrophy ▪ Chronic renal, hepatic, pulmonary, or cardiac disease ▪ Pregnancy and lactation (safety not established).

ADVERSE REACTIONS AND SIDE EFFECTS*

CNS: confusion, drowsiness.
EENT: blurred vision, cycloplegia, dry eyes, mydriasis.
CV: <u>tachycardia</u>, orthostatic hypotension, palpitations.
GI: <u>dry mouth</u>, constipation.
GU: <u>urinary hesitancy</u>, retention.

INTERACTIONS

Drug-Drug: ▪ Additive anticholinergic effects with other **anticholinergic compounds**, including **antihistamines, tricyclic antidepressants, quinidine**, and **disopyramide** ▪ May alter the absorption of other **orally administered drugs** by slowing motility of the GI tract ▪ **Antacids** or **adsorbent antidiarrheals** decrease the absorption of anticholinergics ▪ May increase GI mucosal lesions in patients taking **oral potassium chloride tablets** ▪ Increased risk of adverse cardiovascular reactions with **cyclopropane** anesthesia ▪ Concurrent use may decrease absorption of **ketoconazole** (administer 2 hr after ketoconazole).

ROUTE AND DOSAGE

❑ Control of Secretions during Surgery

- **IM (Adults):** 4.4 mcg/kg 30–60 min preop (not to exceed 0.1 mg).
- **IM (Children):** 4.4–8.8 mcg/kg 30–60 min preop.

❑ Cholinergic Adjunct

- **IV (Adults and Children):** 200 mcg for each 1 mg of neostigmine or 5 mg of pyridostigmine given at the same time.

❑ Antiarrhythmic

- **IV (Adults):** 100 mcg, may be repeated q 2–3 min.
- **IV (Children):** 4.4 mcg/kg (up to 100 mcg); may be repeated q 2–3 min.

❑ Peptic Ulcer

- **PO (Adults):** 1–2 mg 2–3 times daily. An additional 2 mg may be given at bedtime; may be decreased to 1 mg twice daily (not to exceed 8 mg/day).
- **IM, IV (Adults):** 100–200 mcg q 4 hr up to 4 times daily.

AVAILABILITY

▪ ***Tablets:*** 1 mg[Rx], 2 mg[Rx] ▪ ***Injection:*** 200 mcg (0.2 mg)/ml[Rx].

G

*CAPITALS indicate life-threatening; <u>underlines</u> indicate most frequent.

TIME/ACTION PROFILE (anticholinergic effects)

	ONSET	PEAK	DURATION
PO	UK	UK	8–12 hr
IM	15–30 min	30–45 min	2–7 hr*
IV	1 min	UK	2–7 hr*

*Antisecretory effect lasts up to 7 hr; vagal blockade lasts 2–3 hr.

NURSING IMPLICATIONS

ASSESSMENT

- Assess heart rate, blood pressure, and respiratory rate prior to and periodically during parenteral therapy.
- Monitor intake and output ratios in elderly or surgical patients; glycopyrrolate may cause urinary retention. Instruct patient to void prior to parenteral administration.
- Assess patient routinely for abdominal distention and auscultate for bowel sounds. If constipation becomes a problem, increasing fluids and adding bulk to the diet may help alleviate the constipating effects of the drug.
- Periodic intraocular pressure determinations should be made on patients receiving long-term therapy.
- ***Lab Test Considerations:*** Antagonizes effects of pentagastrin and histamine during the gastric acid secretion test. Avoid administration for 24 hr preceding the test.
- May cause decreased uric acid levels in patients with gout or hyperuricemia.
- ***Toxicity and Overdose:*** If overdosage occurs, neostigmine is the antidote.

POTENTIAL NURSING DIAGNOSES

- Oral mucous membrane, altered (Side Effects).
- Constipation (Side Effects).
- Knowledge deficit, related to medication regimen (Patient/Family Teaching).

IMPLEMENTATION

- **General Info:** Do not administer cloudy or discolored solution.
- **PO:** Administer 30–60 min before meals to maximize absorption.
- Do not administer within 1 hr of antacids or antidiarrheal medications.
- **IM:** May be administered undiluted or mixed and administered with D5W, D10W, or 0.9% NaCl.
- **Direct IV:** May be given undiluted through Y-site injection.
- ***Rate:*** Administer at a rate of 0.2 mg over 1–2 min.
- **Syringe Compatibility:** ▪ benzquinamide ▪ chlorpromazine ▪ cimetidine ▪ codeine ▪ diphenhydramine ▪ droperidol ▪ droperidol/fentanyl ▪ hydromorphone ▪ hydroxyzine ▪ levorphanol ▪ lidocaine ▪ meperidine ▪ midazolam ▪ morphine ▪ nalbuphine ▪ neostigmine ▪ oxymorphone ▪ prochlorperazine ▪ promazine ▪ promethazine ▪ propiomazine ▪ pyridostigmine ▪ ranitidine ▪ triflupromazine ▪ trimethobenzamide.
- **Syringe Incompatibility:** ▪ chloramphenicol ▪ dexamethasone ▪ diazepam ▪ dimenhydrinate ▪ methohexital ▪ pentazocine ▪ pentobarbital ▪ secobarbital ▪ sodium bicarbonate ▪ thiopental.
- **Solution Compatibility:** ▪ D5/0.45% NaCl ▪ D5W ▪ 0.9% NaCl ▪ Ringer's solution. Administer immediately after admixing.
- **Additive Incompatibility:** ▪ methylprednisolone sodium succinate.

PATIENT/FAMILY TEACHING

- **General Info:** Instruct patient to take glycopyrrolate exactly as directed and not to take more than the prescribed amount. Missed doses should be taken as soon as remembered if not just before next dose.
- Medication may cause drowsiness and blurred vision. Caution patient to avoid driving or other activities requiring alertness until response to the medication is known.
- Inform patient that frequent oral rinses, sugarless gum or candy, and good oral hygiene may help relieve dry mouth. Consult health care professional regarding use of saliva substitute if dry mouth persists for more than 2 wk.
- Advise patient to change positions slowly to minimize the effects of drug-induced orthostatic hypotension.
- Caution patient to avoid extremes of temperature. This medication decreases the ability to sweat and may increase the risk of heat stroke.
- Advise patient to notify health care professional immediately if eye pain or increased sensitivity to light occurs. Emphasize the importance of routine eye exams throughout therapy.

- ❑ Advise patient to consult health care professional prior to taking any OTC medications concurrently with this therapy.

EVALUATION

Effectiveness of therapy can be demonstrated by: ▪ Mouth dryness preoperatively ▪ Reversal of cholinergic medications ▪ Decrease in GI motility and pain in patients with peptic ulcer disease.

GOLD COMPOUNDS

auranofin
(au-**rane**-oh-fin)
Ridaura

aurothioglucose
(aur-oh-thye-oh-**gloo**-kose)
Solganol

gold sodium thiomalate
(gold **so**-dee-um thye-oh-**mah**-late)
Aurolate, aurothiomalate

CLASSIFICATION(S):
Anti-inflammatories

Pregnancy Category C

INDICATIONS

▪ Treatment of progressive rheumatoid arthritis resistant to conventional therapy.

ACTION

▪ Inhibit inflammatory process ▪ Modify immune response (immunomodulating properties). **Therapeutic Effects:** ▪ Relief of pain and inflammation ▪ Slowing of the disease process in rheumatoid arthritis.

PHARMACOKINETICS

Absorption: *Auranofin*—20–25% absorbed from the GI tract; *sodium gold thiomalate*—rapidly absorbed following IM administration; *aurothioglucose*—more slowly absorbed.
Distribution: Widely distributed, appears to concentrate in arthritic joints more than in uninvolved joints. Enters breast milk.
Metabolism and Excretion: 60–90% slowly excreted by the kidneys (up to 15 mo); 10–40% excreted in the feces.
Half-life: *Gold*—26 days in blood, 40–128 days in tissue.

CONTRAINDICATIONS AND PRECAUTIONS

Contraindicated in: ▪ Hypersensitivity ▪ Severe hepatic or renal dysfunction ▪ Previous heavy metal toxicity ▪ History of colitis or exfoliative dermatitis ▪ Uncontrolled diabetes mellitus ▪ Tuberculosis ▪ Congestive heart failure ▪ Systemic lupus erythematosus ▪ Recent radiation therapy ▪ Debilitated patients ▪ Pregnancy or lactation.
Use Cautiously in: ▪ History of blood dyscrasias ▪ Hypertension ▪ Rashes.

ADVERSE REACTIONS AND SIDE EFFECTS*

CNS: dizziness, headache, neuropathy, syncope.
EENT: corneal gold deposition, corneal ulcerations.
Resp: pneumonitis.
CV: bradycardia.
GI: abdominal pain, cramping, diarrhea, metallic taste, stomatitis, anorexia, difficulty swallowing, drug-induced hepatitis, dyspepsia, flatulence, nausea, vomiting.
Derm: dermatitis, rash, photosensitivity reactions, pruritus.
Hemat: AGRANULOCYTOSIS, APLASTIC ANEMIA, thrombocytopenia, eosinophilia, leukopenia.
Misc: allergic reactions, including ANAPHYLAXIS, angioneurotic edema, nitritoid reactions.

INTERACTIONS

Drug-Drug: ▪ Bone marrow toxicity may be additive with other **myelosuppressive agents (antineoplastic agents, radiation therapy)** ▪ Concurrent use with **penicillamine** increases the risk of adverse hematologic or renal reactions.

ROUTE AND DOSAGE

❑ **Auranofin**

- **PO (Adults):** 6 mg/day in 1–2 doses; may increase to 9 mg/day in 3 divided doses if no improvement after 6 mo.

❑ **Aurothioglucose**

- **IM (Adults):** 10 mg 1st wk, then 25 mg 2nd

***CAPITALS indicate life-threatening; underlines indicate most frequent.**

G

and 3rd wk, then 25–50 mg/wk until improvement or toxicity occurs (up to 1 g total). Maintenance dose is 25–50 mg q 2 wk for up to 20 wk then q 3–4 wk.

- **IM (Children 6–12 yr):** 2.5 mg 1st week, then 6.25 mg 2nd and 3rd wk, then 12.5 mg weekly until a total of 200–250 mg has been given. Maintenance dose is 6.25–12.5 mg q 3–4 wk.

❑ **Gold Sodium Thiomalate**

- **IM (Adults):** 10 mg initially, then 25 mg 1 wk later, followed by 25–50 mg weekly until improvement or toxicity occurs, up to 1 g total, then 25–50 mg q 2 wk for up to 20 wk, then q 3–4 wk. *History of a previous mild reaction*—Reinstitute with an initial dose of 5 mg, increasing by 5–10 mg weekly or monthly until a dose of 25–50 mg is reached.
- **IM (Children):** 10 mg initially, followed 1 wk later by 1 mg/kg q 2 wk for up to 20 wk, then q 3–4 wk.

AVAILABILITY

❑ **Auranofin**

- ***Capsules:*** 3 mg[Rx].

❑ **Aurothioglucose**

- ***Suspension for injection:*** 50 mg/ml[Rx].

❑ **Gold Sodium Thiomalate**

- ***Injection:*** 10 mg/ml[Rx], 25 mg/ml[Rx], 50 mg/ml[Rx].

TIME/ACTION PROFILE (anti-inflammatory activity)

	ONSET	PEAK	DURATION
PO	3–6 mo	UK	UK
IM	6–8 wk	UK	UK

NURSING IMPLICATIONS

ASSESSMENT

- **General Info:** Assess patient's range of motion and degree of swelling and pain in affected joints before and periodically throughout therapy.
- **IM:** Monitor patient for nitritoid reaction (flushing, fainting, dizziness, sweating, nausea, vomiting, headache, weakness, malaise) that may occur immediately to 10 min following injection. Reaction is transient and does not usually require discontinuation of therapy.
- ***Lab Test Considerations:*** Monitor renal, hepatic, and hematologic function and urinalysis prior to and periodically during therapy. Obtain urinalysis prior to each injection. Proteinuria or hematuria may necessitate discontinuation of therapy. Monitor CBC and platelets prior to every other injection or every 2–4 wk. May cause thrombocytopenia, leukopenia, and anemia. May also cause elevated liver enzymes.
- ***Toxicity and Overdose:*** Rapid decrease in hemoglobin, WBC $<4000/mm^3$, eosinophils $>5\%$, granulocytes $<1500/mm^3$, or platelets $<100{,}000–150{,}000/mm^3$, albuminuria, hematuria, rash, dermatitis, pruritus, skin eruption, stomatitis, persistent diarrhea, jaundice, or petechiae may indicate gold toxicity. Withhold therapy until toxicity has been ruled out. If signs of overdose occur, glucocorticoids are usually used to reverse effects. A chelating agent, dimercaprol (BAL), may be given to enhance gold excretion when glucocorticoids are ineffective.

POTENTIAL NURSING DIAGNOSES

- Physical mobility, impaired (Indications).
- Diarrhea (Side Effects).
- Knowledge deficit, related to medication regimen (Patient/Family Teaching).

IMPLEMENTATION

- **PO:** Administer with meals to minimize gastric irritation.
- **IM:** Using an 18-gauge, 1½–2 in. needle, inject deep into gluteal muscle.
  - Instruct patient to remain recumbent for 15 min after injection. Patient should be closely monitored for development of nitritoid or allergic reaction.
  - Injections may be followed by joint pain for 1–2 days. Never administer IV.
  - *Aurothioglucose:* Shake well. Vial may be immersed in warm water to facilitate withdrawing suspension. Change needles after withdrawal.
  - *Gold sodium thiomalate*—Solution is pale yellow; do not use solutions that have darkened or that contain a precipitate.

PATIENT/FAMILY TEACHING

- ▫ Concurrent therapy with salicylates or other NSAIDs or glucocorticoids is usually necessary, especially during the first few months of gold therapy. Patients should continue physical therapy and ensure adequate rest. Explain that joint damage will not be reversed; the goal is to slow or stop disease process.
- ▫ Emphasize the importance of good oral hygiene to reduce stomatitis.
- ▫ Caution patient to use sunscreen and protective clothing to prevent photosensitivity reactions. Chrysiasis (blue-gray pigmentation) may occur, especially on photoexposed areas.
- ▫ Instruct patient to report symptoms of leukopenia (fever, sore throat, signs of infection), thrombocytopenia (bleeding gums; bruising; petechiae; blood in stools, urine, or emesis), or gold toxicity immediately. Diarrhea may be resolved by decreasing the dose.
- ▫ Discuss the need for contraception while receiving this medication. Advise patient to notify health care professional promptly if pregnancy is suspected.
- ▫ Emphasize the importance of regular visits to health care professional to monitor progress and evaluate blood and urine tests for side effects.
- ▪ **PO:** Instruct patient to take medication exactly as directed; do not skip or double doses. Take missed dose as soon as possible except if next dose is almost due.
- ▪ **IM:** Discuss need for continued therapy. Initially, injections are given weekly. Later injections are spaced 3–4 wk apart.
- ▫ Inform patient that arthralgia may occur for a day or two after the first few injections. Increase in rheumatic symptoms is usually transient and mild but may be severe and require discontinuation of therapy.

EVALUATION

Effectiveness of therapy can be demonstrated by: ▪ Decrease in swelling, pain, and stiffness of joints ▫ Increase in mobility. Continuous therapy for 3–6 mo may be required before therapeutic effects are seen.

GOSERELIN

(**goe**-se-rel-lin)
Zoladex

CLASSIFICATION(S):
Antineoplastic (hormone), Hormone (gonadotropin-releasing hormone analogue)

Pregnancy Category D (breast cancer), X (endometriosis)

INDICATIONS

▪ Treatment (palliative) of prostate cancer in patients who cannot tolerate orchiectomy or estrogen therapy ▪ Palliative treatment of advanced breast cancer in peri- and postmenopausal women ▪ Management of endometriosis ▪ Used to thin the endometrium prior to endometrial ablation for dysfunctional uterine bleeding.

ACTION

▪ Acts as a synthetic form of luteinizing hormone–releasing hormone (LHRH, GnRH). Inhibits the production of gonadotropins by the pituitary gland. Initially, levels of luteinizing hormone (LH), follicle-stimulating hormone (FSH), and testosterone increase. Continued administration leads to decreased production of testosterone and estradiol. **Therapeutic Effects:** ▪ Decreased spread of cancer of the prostate or breast ▪ Regression of endometriosis with decreased pain ▪ Thinning of the endometrium.

PHARMACOKINETICS

Absorption: Well absorbed from SC implant. Absorption is slower in first 8 days, then is faster and continuous for remainder of 28-day dosing cycle.
Distribution: UK.
Metabolism and Excretion: Some metabolism by the liver, some excretion by kidneys.
Half-life: 4.2 hr.

CONTRAINDICATIONS AND PRECAUTIONS

Contraindicated in: ▪ Hypersensitivity ▪ Pregnancy or lactation ▪ Undiagnosed vaginal bleeding.

G

Use Cautiously in: ▪ Lactation or children <18 yr (safety not established).

ADVERSE REACTIONS AND SIDE EFFECTS*

CNS: headache, anxiety, depression, dizziness, fatigue, insomnia, weakness.
Resp: dyspnea.
CV: CEREBROVASCULAR ACCIDENT, MYOCARDIAL INFARCTION, vasodilation, chest pain, hypertension, palpitations.
GI: anorexia, constipation, diarrhea, nausea, ulcer, vomiting.
GU: renal insufficiency, urinary obstruction.
Derm: sweating, rashes.
Endo: decreased libido, impotence, breast swelling, breast tenderness, infertility.
F and E: peripheral edema.
Hemat: anemia.
Metab: gout, hyperglycemia, increased lipids.
MS: increased bone pain, arthralgia, decreased bone density.
Misc: hot flashes, chills, fever, weight gain.

INTERACTIONS

Drug-Drug: ▪ None significant.

ROUTE AND DOSAGE

- **SC (Adults):** 3.6 mg every 4 wk or 10.8 mg q 12 wk. *Endometrial thinning*—1 or 2 depots given 4 wk apart; if 1 depot used, surgery is performed at 4 wk; if 2 depots used, surgery is performed 2–4 wk after 2nd depot.

AVAILABILITY

▪ ***Implant:*** 3.6 mg[Rx], 10.8 mg[Rx].

TIME/ACTION PROFILE (decrease in serum testosterone levels)

	ONSET	PEAK	DURATION
SC	UK	2–4 wk	length of therapy

NURSING IMPLICATIONS

ASSESSMENT

- **Cancer:** Monitor patients with vertebral metastases for increased back pain and decreased sensory/motor function.
- □ Monitor intake and output ratios and assess for bladder distention in patients with urinary tract obstruction during initiation of therapy.
- **Endometriosis:** Assess patient for signs and symptoms of endometriosis prior to and periodically throughout therapy. Amenorrhea usually occurs within 8 wk of initial administration and menses usually resume 8 wk after completion.
- ***Lab Test Considerations:*** Initially increases, then decreases luteinizing hormone (LH) and follicle-stimulating hormone (FSH). This leads to castration levels of testosterone in men 2–4 wk after initial increase in concentrations.
- □ Monitor serum acid phosphatase and prostate-specific antigen concentrations periodically during therapy. May cause transient increases in serum acid phosphatase concentrations, which usually return to baseline by the 4th wk of therapy and may decrease to below baseline or return to baseline if elevated prior to therapy.
- □ May cause hypercalcemia in patients with breast or prostate cancer with bony metastases.
- □ May cause an increase in serum HDL, LDL, and triglycerides.

POTENTIAL NURSING DIAGNOSES

- Sexual dysfunction (Side Effects).
- Knowledge deficit, related to medication regimen (Patient/Family Teaching).

IMPLEMENTATION

- **SC:** Implant is inserted in upper SC tissue of abdominal wall every 28 days.
- □ If the implant needs to be removed for any reason, it can be located by ultrasound.

PATIENT/FAMILY TEACHING

- □ Advise patient that bone pain may increase at initiation of therapy. This will resolve with time. Patient should discuss use of analgesics to control pain with health care professional.
- □ Advise female patients to notify health care professional if regular menstruation persists.
- □ Advise patient that medication may cause hot flashes. Notify health care professional if these become bothersome.
- □ Instruct patient to notify health care professional promptly if difficulty urinating occurs.

***CAPITALS indicate life-threatening; underlines indicate most frequent.**

□ Emphasize the importance of adhering to the schedule of monthly or every 3 mo administration.

EVALUATION

Effectiveness of therapy can be demonstrated by: ▪ Decrease in the spread of prostate cancer ▪ Reduction of symptoms of advanced breast cancer in peri- and postmenopausal women ▪ Decrease in the signs and symptoms of endometriosis. Symptoms are usually reduced within 4 wk of implantation ▪ Thinning of the endometrium prior to endometrial ablation for dysfunctional uterine bleeding.

GRANISETRON

(gra-**nees**-e-tron)
Kytril

CLASSIFICATION(S):
Antiemetic (5-HT_3 antagonist)

Pregnancy Category B

INDICATIONS

▪ Prevention of nausea and vomiting associated with emetogenic chemotherapy. **Unlabeled Uses:** ▪ Management of acute nausea and vomiting following surgery.

ACTION

▪ Blocks the effects of serotonin at receptor sites (selective antagonist) located in vagal nerve terminals and in the chemoreceptor trigger zone in the CNS. **Therapeutic Effects:** ▪ Decreased incidence and severity of nausea and vomiting following emetogenic chemotherapy.

PHARMACOKINETICS

Absorption: 50% absorbed following oral administration.
Distribution: UK.
Metabolism and Excretion: Mostly metabolized by the liver; 12% excreted unchanged in urine.
Half-life: *Patients with cancer*—8–9 hr (range 0.9–31.1 hr); *healthy volunteers*—4.9 hr (range 0.9–15.2 hr); *geriatric patients*—7.7 hr (range 2.6–17.7 hr).

CONTRAINDICATIONS AND PRECAUTIONS

Contraindicated in: ▪ Hypersensitivity.
Use Cautiously in: ▪ Pregnancy or lactation (safety not established) ▪ Children <2 yr (safe use of IV route not established) ▪ Children <18 yr (safe use of PO route not established).

ADVERSE REACTIONS AND SIDE EFFECTS*

CNS: <u>headache</u>, agitation, anxiety, CNS stimulation, drowsiness, weakness.
CV: hypertension.
GI: constipation, diarrhea, elevated liver enzymes, taste disorder.
Misc: anaphylactoid reactions, fever.

INTERACTIONS

Drug-Drug: ▪ Concurrent use of **agents causing extrapyramidal reactions** may increase the risk of such reactions from granisetron.

ROUTE AND DOSAGE

- **PO (Adults):** 1 mg twice daily; 1st dose given at least 60 min prior to chemotherapy and 2nd dose 12 hr later only on days when chemotherapy is administered; may also be given as 2 mg once daily.
- **IV (Adults and Children 2–16 yr):** 10 mcg/kg within 30 min prior to chemotherapy.

AVAILABILITY

▪ ***Tablets:*** 1 mg[Rx] ▪ ***Injection:*** 1 mg/ml[Rx].

TIME/ACTION PROFILE

	ONSET	PEAK	DURATION
PO	rapid	60 min	24 hr
IV	rapid	30 min	up to 24 hr

NURSING IMPLICATIONS

ASSESSMENT

□ Assess patient for nausea, vomiting, abdominal distention, and bowel sounds prior to and following administration.
□ Assess for extrapyramidal symptoms (involuntary movements, facial grimacing, rigidity, shuffling walk, trembling of hands) throughout therapy. This occurs rarely and is usually

*CAPITALS indicate life-threatening; <u>underlines</u> indicate most frequent.

associated with concurrent use of other drugs known to cause this effect.

- *Lab Test Considerations:* May cause elevated AST and ALT levels.

POTENTIAL NURSING DIAGNOSES

- Nutrition, altered, less than body requirements (Indications).
- Pain, acute (Side Effects).
- Knowledge deficit, related to medication regimen (Patient/Family Teaching).

IMPLEMENTATION

- **General Info:** Granisetron is administered only on the day(s) chemotherapy is given. Continued treatment when not on chemotherapy has not been found useful.
- **PO:** Administer 1st dose up to 1 hr before chemotherapy and 2nd dose 12 hr after the first.
- **Direct IV:** May be administered undiluted or diluted in 20–50 ml of 0.9% NaCl or D5W. Solution should be prepared at time of administration but is stable for 24 hr at room temperature.
- *Rate:* Administer undiluted granisetron over 30 sec or as a diluted solution over 5 min.
- **Y-Site Compatibility:** ▪ carboplatin ▪ ceftazidime ▪ cimetidine ▪ cisplatin ▪ cyclophosphamide ▪ cytarabine ▪ dacarbazine ▪ dexamethasone ▪ diphenhydramine ▪ doxorubicin ▪ etoposide ▪ fluorouracil ▪ furosemide ▪ gentamicin ▪ hydromorphone ▪ ifosphamide ▪ lorazepam ▪ magnesium sulfate ▪ mechlorethamine ▪ mesna ▪ methotrexate ▪ methylprednisolone ▪ mezlocillin ▪ morphine ▪ paclitaxel ▪ potassium chloride ▪ sodium bicarbonate ▪ streptozocin ▪ thiotepa ▪ ticarcillin/clavulanate ▪ vincristine.
- **Additive Incompatibility:** ▪ Granisetron should not be admixed with other medications.

PATIENT/FAMILY TEACHING

- □ Advise patient to notify health care professional immediately if involuntary movement of eyes, face, or limbs occurs.

EVALUATION

Effectiveness of therapy can be demonstrated by: ▪ Prevention of nausea and vomiting associated with emetogenic cancer chemotherapy.

GRISEOFULVIN

(gris-ee-oh-**ful**-vin)

Fulvicin P/G, Fulvicin-U/F, Grifulvin V, Grisactin, Grisactin Ultra, Gris-PEG, {Grosovin-FP}

CLASSIFICATION(S):

Antifungal

Pregnancy Category C

INDICATIONS

▪ Treatment of various tinea infections ▪ Should not be used for superficial infections that may respond to topical antifungals.

ACTION

▪ Inhibits mitosis of fungal cells. Deposits in precursor cells of hair, skin, and nails, making them resistant to fungal invasion. **Therapeutic Effects:** ▪ Growth of new cells that are resistant to invasion by fungi.

PHARMACOKINETICS

Absorption: Microsize (Grisactin, Grisovin-FP, Grifulvin V, Fulvicin-U/F) preparations are variably (25–70%) absorbed following oral administration. Ultramicrosize products (Fulvicin P/G, Grisactin Ultra, Gris-PEG) are almost completely absorbed.

Distribution: Mostly deposited in keratin layer of skin; also found in liver, fat, and skeletal muscle.

Metabolism and Excretion: Metabolized by the liver, some excreted in feces and perspiration.

Half-life: 9–24 hr.

CONTRAINDICATIONS AND PRECAUTIONS

Contraindicated in: ▪ Hypersensitivity ▪ Severe liver disease or porphyria.

Use Cautiously in: ▪ Pregnancy or lactation (safety not established) ▪ Possible cross-sensitivity with penicillin.

ADVERSE REACTIONS AND SIDE EFFECTS*

CNS: headache, dizziness.
EENT: hearing loss.
GI: diarrhea, epigastric distress, extreme thirst, flatulence, nausea, vomiting.
Derm: photosensitivity, rashes.
Hemat: leukopenia.
Misc: hypersensitivity reactions including SERUM SICKNESS, lupus-like syndrome.

INTERACTIONS

Drug-Drug: ▪ Tachycardia, flushing, and increased CNS depression may result if taken concurrently with **alcohol** ▪ **Phenobarbital** decreases blood levels and may decrease effectiveness ▪ May decrease the effectiveness of **warfarin** ▪ May decrease the effectiveness of **oral contraceptive agents.**
Drug-Food: ▪ Absorption is increased by **fatty foods.**

ROUTE AND DOSAGE

❑ **Microsize**

- **PO (Adults):** *Tinea pedis, onychomycosis*—500 mg q 12 hr. *Tinea capitis, corporis, or cruris*—250 mg q 12 hr or 500 mg once daily.
- **PO (Children ≥23 kg):** 125–250 mg q 12 hr or 250–500 mg once daily.
- **PO (Children 14–23 kg):** 62.5–125 mg q 12 hr or 250 mg once daily.

❑ **Ultramicrosize**

- **PO (Adults):** *Tinea pedis, onychomycosis*—250–375 mg/day q 12 hr. *Tinea capitis, corporis, or cruris*—125–187.5 mg q 12 hr or 250–375 mg once daily.
- **PO (Children ≥23 kg):** 62.5–165 mg q 12 hr or 125–330 mg once daily.
- **PO (Children 14–23 kg):** 31.25–82.5 mg q 12 hr or 62.5–165 mg once daily.

AVAILABILITY

▪ ***Microsize tablets:*** 250 mg[Rx], 500 mg[Rx] ▪ ***Microsize capsules:*** 125 mg[Rx], 250 mg[Rx] ▪ ***Oral suspension (microsize):*** 125 mg/5 ml[Rx] ▪ ***Ultramicrosize tablets:*** 125 mg[Rx], 165 mg[Rx], 250 mg[Rx], 330 mg[Rx].

TIME/ACTION PROFILE (antifungal activity)

	ONSET	PEAK	DURATION
PO	4 hr	24 hr	2 days

NURSING IMPLICATIONS

ASSESSMENT

- ❑ Assess skin at site of fungal infection routinely throughout course of therapy.
- ❑ Assess patient for allergy to penicillin; potential cross-sensitivity exists.
- ▪ ***Lab Test Considerations:*** CBC, serum creatinine, and hepatic functions should be monitored periodically throughout treatment.
- ❑ Monitor urinalysis periodically during therapy. May rarely cause proteinuria.

POTENTIAL NURSING DIAGNOSES

- Skin integrity, impaired (Indications).
- Infection, risk for (Indications, Side Effects).
- Knowledge deficit, related to medication regimen (Patient/Family Teaching).

IMPLEMENTATION

- ▪ **General Info:** Concurrent use of a topical agent is usually required.
- ❑ Ultramicrosize griseofulvin 250–330 mg provides serum concentrations equal to that of microsize griseofulvin 500 mg.
- ▪ **PO:** Administer with or after meals, preferably meals with high fat content, to minimize GI irritation and increase absorption.

PATIENT/FAMILY TEACHING

- ❑ Instruct patient to complete full course of therapy; several weeks of therapy may be necessary. If a dose is missed, take as soon as remembered, but do not take if almost time for next dose.
- ❑ Instruct patient on hygiene to control sources of infection or reinfection.
- ❑ May cause dizziness. Caution patient to avoid driving or other activities requiring alertness until response to medication is known.
- ❑ Advise patient to wear sunscreen and protective clothing to prevent photosensitivity reaction.
- ❑ Caution patient not to drink alcohol while taking this medication.

***CAPITALS indicate life-threatening; underlines indicate most frequent.**

- Advise female patients taking oral contraceptives to use an additional nonhormonal form of contraception during therapy and until next menstrual period and to notify health care professional if pregnancy is planned or suspected.
- Advise patient to notify health care professional if rash, sore throat, fever, diarrhea, or soreness of mouth or tongue occurs.
- Emphasize importance of follow-up examinations to monitor progress of therapy.

EVALUATION

Effectiveness of therapy can be demonstrated by: ▪ Resolution of signs and symptoms of fungal infection. To prevent relapse, treatment may take weeks to months and should continue until organism is completely eradicated as determined by clinical or laboratory testing. Tinea capitis usually requires treatment for 8–10 wk; tinea corporis, 2–4 wk; tinea pedis, 4–8 wk; onychomycosis, at least 4 mo for fingernails and at least 6 mo for toenails (recurrence rates for toenails are very high).

GROWTH HORMONES

somatropin, recombinant

(soe-ma-**troe**-pin)

Genotropin, Humatrope, Norditropin, Nutropin, Nutropin AQ, Saizen, Serostim

somatrem, recombinant

(**soe**-ma-trem)

Protropin

CLASSIFICATION(S):

Growth hormones

Pregnancy Category B (Serostim), C (all other trade names)

INDICATIONS

▪ Management of growth failure in children due to chronic renal insufficiency ▪ Growth failure in children due to deficiency of growth hormone (not Serostim) ▪ Management of short stature associated with Turner's syndrome ▪ Growth hormone deficiency in adults (Humatrope, Nutropin) ▪ AIDS wasting or cachexia (Serostim only).

ACTION

▪ Produce growth (skeletal and cellular) ▪ Metabolic actions include: ▫ Increased protein synthesis ▫ Increased carbohydrate metabolism ▫ Lipid mobilization ▫ Retention of sodium, phosphorus, and potassium ▪ Somatropin has the same amino acid sequence as naturally occurring growth hormone; somatrem has 1 additional amino acid. Both are produced by recombinant DNA techniques. **Therapeutic Effects:** ▪ Increased skeletal growth in children with growth hormone deficiency ▪ Replacement of somatropin in deficient adults ▪ Decreased wasting in patients with AIDS.

PHARMACOKINETICS

Absorption: Well absorbed following SC or IM administration.

Distribution: Localize to highly perfused organs (liver, kidneys).

Metabolism and Excretion: Broken down in renal cells to amino acids that are recirculated; some liver metabolism.

Half-life: *SC*—3.8 hr; *IM*—4.9 hr.

CONTRAINDICATIONS AND PRECAUTIONS

Contraindicated in: ▪ Closure of epiphyses ▪ Tumors ▪ Hypersensitivity to *m*-cresol or glycerin (somatropin) or benzyl alcohol (somatrem).

Use Cautiously in: ▪ Growth hormone deficiency due to intracranial lesion ▪ Coexisting adrenocorticotropic hormone (ACTH) deficiency ▪ Diabetes (may cause insulin resistance) ▪ Thyroid dysfunction ▪ Pregnancy or lactation (safety not established).

ADVERSE REACTIONS AND SIDE EFFECTS

CV: edema of the hands and feet.

Endo: hyperglycemia, hypothyroidism, insulin resistance.

Local: pain at injection site.

MS: *Serostim only*—carpal tunnel syndrome, musculoskeletal pain.

INTERACTIONS

Drug-Drug: ▪ Excessive **glucocorticoid** use may decrease response to somatropin.

ROUTE AND DOSAGE

❑ **Somatropin/Genotropin**

- **SC (Adults):** 0.16–0.24 mg/kg/wk in 6–7 doses.

❑ **Humatrope**

- **SC (Adults):** 0.018 unit/kg/day (up to 0.0375 unit/day).
- **IM, SC (Children):** 0.18 mg/kg (0.54 unit/kg)/wk given in divided doses on 3 alternating days or 6 times weekly (up to 0.3 mg/kg [0.9 unit/kg]/wk).

❑ **Nutropin/Nutropin AQ**

- **SC (Children):** *Growth hormone inadequacy*—0.3 mg/kg (0.9 unit/kg)/wk. *Chronic renal insufficiency*—0.35 mg/kg (1.05 units/kg)/wk given as daily injections. *Turner's syndrome*—≤0.375 mg/kg (1.125 units/kg)/wk in 3–7 divided doses.

❑ **Norditropin**

- **SC (Children):** 0.024–0.034 mg/kg 6–7 times weekly.

❑ **Saizen**

- **SC, IM (Children):** 0.06 mg (0.18 unit/kg) 3 times weekly.

❑ **Serostim**

- **SC (Adults):** *>55 kg*—6 mg once daily; *45–55 kg*—5 mg once daily; *35–45 kg*—4 mg once daily; *<35 kg*—0.1 mg/kg once daily.

❑ **Somatrem**

- **IM, SC (Children):** Up to 0.1 mg/kg (0.26 unit/kg) 3 times weekly.

AVAILABILITY

❑ **Somatrem**

- ***Powder for injection:*** 5 mg (13 IU)/vial Rx, 10 mg (26 IU)/vial Rx.

❑ **Somatropin**

□ **Genotropin**

- ***Powder for injection:*** 1.5 mg intra-mix cartridge Rx, 5.8 mg intra-mix cartridge Rx.

□ **Humatrope**

- ***Powder for injection:*** 5 mg/vial Rx.

□ **Norditropin**

- ***Powder for injection:*** 4 mg (12 units)/vial Rx, 5 mg (13 units)/vial Rx, 8 mg (24 units)/vial Rx, 10 mg (26 units)/vial Rx.

□ **Nutropin**

- ***Powder for injection:*** 5 mg (13 units)/vial Rx, 10 mg (26 units)/vial) Rx.

□ **Nutropin AQ**

- ***Solution for injection (AQ):*** 5 mg (15 units)/ml in 2-ml vial Rx.

□ **Saizen**

- ***Powder for injection:*** 5 mg (15 units)/vial Rx, 6 mg (18 units)/vial Rx.

□ **Serostim**

- ***Powder for injection:*** 6 mg (15 units)/vial Rx.

TIME/ACTION PROFILE (growth)

	ONSET	PEAK	DURATION
IM, SC	within 3 mo	UK	UK

NURSING IMPLICATIONS

ASSESSMENT

- **Growth Failure:** Monitor bone age annually and growth rate determinations, height, and weight every 3–6 mo during therapy.
- **AIDS Wasting/Cachexia:** Re-evaluate treatment in patients who continue to lose weight in first 2 wk of treatment.
- ***Lab Test Considerations:*** Monitor thyroid function prior to and throughout therapy. May decrease T_4, radioactive iodine uptake, and thyroxine-binding capacity. Hypothyroidism necessitates concurrent thyroid replacement for growth hormone to be effective. Serum inorganic phosphorus, alkaline phosphatase, and parathyroid hormone may increase with somatropin therapy.

□ Monitor blood or urine glucose periodically throughout therapy. Diabetic patients may require increased insulin dose.

□ Monitor for development of neutralizing antibodies if growth rate does not exceed 2.5 cm/6 mo.

POTENTIAL NURSING DIAGNOSES

- Body image disturbance (Indications).
- Knowledge deficit, related to medication regimen (Patient/Family Teaching).

IMPLEMENTATION

- **Somatrem:** Reconstitute 5-mg vial with 1–5 ml and 10-mg vial with 1–10 ml of bacteriostatic water for injection, aiming the liquid against glass vial wall. Do not shake; swirl gently to dissolve. Solution is clear; do not use

G

cloudy solutions. Discard vial after withdrawing dose.

- **Somatropin:** Reconstitute 5-mg vial with 1.5–5 ml of sterile water for injection provided by manufacturer (contains preservative *m*-cresol), aiming the liquid against glass vial wall. Do not shake; swirl gently to dissolve. Solution is clear; do not use solutions that are cloudy or contain a precipitate. Stable for 14 days when refrigerated.
- □ *Genotropin:* Dissolve powder with solution provided with 2-chamber cartridge as directed. Gently tip cartridge upside down a few times until contents are completely dissolved. The 1.5-mg cartridge is stable following dilution for 24 hr if refrigerated. The 5.8-mg and 13.8-mg cartridges contain preservatives and are stable for 14 days if refrigerated.
- □ *Humatrope:* Reconstitute each 5-mg vial with 1.5 to 5 ml of diluent provided. Stable for 14 days if refrigerated.
- □ *Norditropin:* Reconstitute each 4-mg or 8-mg vial with 2 ml of diluent. Use reconstituted vials within 14 days.
- □ *Nutropin/Nutropin AQ:* Reconstitute 5-mg vial with 1–5 ml and 10-mg vial with 1–10 ml of bacteriostatic water for injection. Reconstituted vials are stable for 14 days (Nutropin) or 28 days (Nutropin AQ) if refrigerated.
- □ *Saizen:* Reconstitute each 5-mg vial with 1–3 ml of bacteriostatic water for injection. Reconsituted vials are stable for 14 days if refrigerated.
- □ *Serostim:* Reconstitute each vial with 1 ml of sterile water for injection. Use within 24 hr of reconstitution.
- **IM, SC:** Rotate injection sites with each injection.

PATIENT/FAMILY TEACHING

- □ Instruct patient and parents on correct procedure for reconstituting medication, site selection, technique for IM or SC injection, and disposal of needles and syringes. Review dosage schedule. Somatropin injections should be at least 48 hr apart. Parents should report persistent pain or edema at injection site.
- □ Explain rationale for prohibition of use for increasing athletic performance. Administration to persons without growth hormone deficiency or after epiphyseal closure may result in acromegaly (coarsening of facial features; enlarged hands, feet, and internal organs; increased blood sugar; hypertension).
- □ Emphasize need for regular follow-up with endocrinologist to ensure appropriate growth rate, to evaluate lab work, and to determine bone age by x-ray exam.
- □ Assure parents and child that these dosage forms are synthetic and therefore not capable of transmitting Creutzfeldt-Jakob disease, as was the original somatropin, which was extracted from human cadavers.

EVALUATION

Clinical response to therapy can be evaluated by: ▪ Child's attainment of adult height in growth failure secondary to pituitary growth hormone deficiency. Therapy is limited to period before closure of epiphyseal plates (approximately up to 14–15 yr in girls, 15–16 yr in boys) ▪ Replacement of somatropin in deficient adults ▪ Decreased wasting in patients with AIDS.

GUAIFENESIN

(gwye-**fen**-e-sin)

Anti-Tuss, {Balminil Expectorant}, {Benylin-E}, Breonesin, {Calmylin Expectorant}, Diabetic Tussin EX, Fenesin, Gee-Gee, Genatuss, GG-Cen, Glycotuss, Glytuss, Guiatuss, Halotussin, Humibid L.A., Humibid Sprinkle, Hytuss, Hytuss-2X, Naldecon Senior EX, Nortussin, Organidin NR, Pneumomist, {Resyl}, Robitussin, Scot-Tussin Expectorant, Sinumist-SR Caplets, Touro EX, Uni-tussin

CLASSIFICATION(S):
Expectorant

Pregnancy Category C

INDICATIONS

▪ Symptomatic management of coughs associated with viral upper respiratory tract infections.

ACTION

▪ Reduces viscosity of tenacious secretions by increasing respiratory tract fluid. **Therapeutic Effects:** ▪ Mobilization and subsequent expectoration of mucus.

PHARMACOKINETICS

Absorption: Well absorbed after oral administration.
Distribution: UK.
Metabolism and Excretion: Renally excreted as metabolites.
Half-life: UK.

CONTRAINDICATIONS AND PRECAUTIONS

Contraindicated in: ▪ Hypersensitivity ▪ Some products contain alcohol and should be avoided in patients with known intolerance.
Use Cautiously in: ▪ Cough lasting >1 wk or accompanied by fever, rash, or headache ▪ Pregnancy (although safety has not been established, guaifenesin has been used without adverse effects) ▪ Patients receiving disulfiram (liquid products may contain alcohol) ▪ Diabetics (products may contain sugar).

ADVERSE REACTIONS AND SIDE EFFECTS

CNS: dizziness, headache.
GI: diarrhea, nausea, stomach pain, vomiting.
Derm: rashes, urticaria.

INTERACTIONS

Drug-Drug: ▪ None significant.

ROUTE AND DOSAGE

- **PO (Adults):** 200–400 mg q 4 hr or 600–1200 mg q 12 hr as extended-release product (not to exceed 2400 mg/day).
- **PO (Children 6–12 yr):** 100–200 mg q 4 hr or 600 mg q 12 hr as extended-release product (not to exceed 1200 mg/day).
- **PO (Children 2–6 yr):** 50–100 mg q 4 hr (not to exceed 600 mg/day).

AVAILABILITY

▪ ***Syrup:*** 100 mg/5 ml[OTC] ▪ ***Oral solution:*** 100 mg/5 ml[OTC], 200 mg/5 ml[OTC] ▪ ***Capsules:*** 200 mg[OTC] ▪ ***Extended-release capsules:*** 300 mg[OTC] ▪ ***Tablets:*** 100 mg[OTC], 200 mg[OTC] ▪ ***Extended-release tablets:*** 600 mg[OTC] ▪ ***In combination with:*** analgesics/antipyretics, antihistamines, decongestants, and cough suppressants[Rx,OTC].

TIME/ACTION PROFILE (expectorant action)

	ONSET	PEAK	DURATION
PO	30 min	UK	4–6 hr
PO-ER	UK	UK	12 hr

NURSING IMPLICATIONS

ASSESSMENT

□ Assess lung sounds, frequency and type of cough, and character of bronchial secretions periodically throughout therapy. Maintain fluid intake of 1500–2000 ml/day to decrease viscosity of secretions.

POTENTIAL NURSING DIAGNOSES

- Airway clearance, ineffective (Indications).
- Knowledge deficit, related to medication regimen (Patient/Family Teaching).

IMPLEMENTATION

- **PO:** Administer each dose of guaifenesin followed by a full glass of water to decrease viscosity of secretions.

□ Sustained-release tablets and capsules should be swallowed whole; do not open, crush, break, or chew.

PATIENT/FAMILY TEACHING

□ Instruct patient to cough effectively. Patient should sit upright and take several deep breaths before attempting to cough.

□ Inform patient that drug may occasionally cause dizziness. Avoid driving or other activities requiring alertness until response to drug is known.

□ Advise patient to limit talking, stop smoking, maintain moisture in environmental air, and take some sugarless gum or hard candy to help alleviate the discomfort caused by a chronic nonproductive cough.

□ Instruct patient to contact health care professional if cough persists longer than 1 wk or is accompanied by fever, rash, or persistent headache or sore throat.

EVALUATION

Effectiveness of therapy can be demonstrated by: ▪ Decreased frequency of a dry,

G

nonproductive cough. Thick, viscous secretions are thinned, which allows easier expectoration.

GUANABENZ
(**gwahn**-a-benz)
Wytensin

CLASSIFICATION(S):
Antihypertensive agent (centrally acting alpha$_2$-adrenergic agonist)

Pregnancy Category C

INDICATIONS
▪ Management of hypertension.

ACTION
▪ Stimulates CNS alpha$_2$-adrenergic receptors, producing a decrease in sympathetic outflow to heart, kidneys, and blood vessels. Result is decreased blood pressure and peripheral resistance, a slight decrease in heart rate, and no change in cardiac output. **Therapeutic Effects:** ▪ Lowering of blood pressure.

PHARMACOKINETICS
Absorption: 70–80% absorbed following oral administration but undergoes extensive first-pass hepatic metabolism.
Distribution: Appears to be widely distributed.
Metabolism and Excretion: >95% metabolized by the liver.
Half-life: 6 hr.

CONTRAINDICATIONS AND PRECAUTIONS
Contraindicated in: ▪ Hypersensitivity.
Use Cautiously in: ▪ Serious cardiac or cerebrovascular disease, renal or hepatic insufficiency ▪ Geriatric patients (more prone to adverse reactions) ▪ Pregnancy, lactation, or children <12 yr (safety not established).

ADVERSE REACTIONS AND SIDE EFFECTS*
CNS: dizziness, drowsiness, weakness, headache, irritability, nervousness.
EENT: blurred vision, dry eyes, miosis, nasal congestion.
Resp: dyspnea.
CV: arrhythmias, bradycardia, chest pain, edema, hypotension, palpitations.
GI: dry mouth, abdominal pain, abnormal taste, anorexia, constipation, diarrhea, nausea, vomiting.
GU: impotence, urinary frequency.
Derm: pruritus, rashes, sweating.
Endo: gynecomastia.
MS: backache, painful extremities.
Misc: withdrawal phenomenon.

INTERACTIONS
Drug-Drug: ▪ Additive sedation with **CNS depressants**, including **alcohol, antihistamines, opioids,** and **sedative/hypnotics** ▪ **Tricyclic antidepressants** and **NSAIDs** may decrease antihypertensive effects ▪ **MAO inhibitors** decrease effectiveness ▪ Additive hypotension with other **antihypertensives, nitrates,** and acute ingestion of **alcohol.**

ROUTE AND DOSAGE
▪ **PO (Adults):** 4 mg bid; may increase q 1–2 wk in 4–8 mg increments (range 8–16 mg/day; not to exceed 32 mg/day).

AVAILABILITY
▪ ***Tablets:*** 4 mg[Rx], 8 mg[Rx].

TIME/ACTION PROFILE (antihypertensive effect†)

	ONSET	PEAK	DURATION
PO	1 hr	2–7 hr	12 hr

†After single dose.

NURSING IMPLICATIONS

ASSESSMENT
- Monitor blood pressure (lying and standing) and pulse frequently during initial dosage adjustment and periodically throughout therapy. Report significant changes.
- Monitor frequency of prescription refills to determine compliance.
- Monitor intake and output ratios and daily weight; assess for edema daily.
- ***Lab Test Considerations:*** With chronic use, may slightly decrease serum cholesterol and triglyceride levels.

***CAPITALS indicate life-threatening; underlines indicate most frequent.**

POTENTIAL NURSING DIAGNOSES

- Injury, risk for (Side Effects).
- Knowledge deficit, related to medication regimen (Patient/Family Teaching).
- Noncompliance (Patient/Family Teaching).

IMPLEMENTATION

- **PO:** Administer last dose at bedtime to minimize daytime sedation.
- May be used in conjunction with a thiazide diuretic in patients who fail to respond to diet, exercise, and initial antihypertensive drug therapy.

PATIENT/FAMILY TEACHING

- Emphasize the importance of continuing to take this medication as directed, even if feeling well. Medication controls but does not cure hypertension. Instruct patient to take medication at the same time each day. If a dose is missed, take as soon as remembered; do not double doses. Instruct patient to inform health care professional if more than one consecutive dose is missed. Do not discontinue abruptly; may cause sympathetic overstimulation (nervousness, anxiety, rebound hypertension).
- Advise patient to make sure enough medication is available for weekends, holidays, and vacations. A written prescription may be kept in wallet in case of emergency.
- Encourage patient to comply with additional interventions for hypertension (weight reduction, low-sodium diet, smoking cessation, moderation of alcohol consumption, regular exercise, and stress management).
- Instruct patient and family on proper technique for blood pressure monitoring. Advise them to check blood pressure at least weekly and report significant changes.
- Patients should weigh themselves twice weekly and assess feet and ankles for fluid retention.
- May cause drowsiness or dizziness. Caution patient to avoid driving or other activities requiring alertness until response to the medication is known. Drowsiness usually decreases with continued therapy.
- Advise patient to consult health care professional before taking any OTC medications, especially cough, cold, or allergy remedies.
- Caution patient to avoid alcohol and other CNS depressants while taking guanabenz.
- Frequent mouth rinses, good oral hygiene, and sugarless gum or candy may minimize dry mouth. If dry mouth persists for more than 2 wk, consult dentist regarding use of saliva substitute.
- Instruct patient to notify health care professional of medication regimen prior to treatment or surgery.
- Advise patient to notify health care professional if frequent dizziness or weakness, irritability or nervousness, slow heart rate, pinpoint pupils, unusual tiredness, or persistent dry mouth occurs.
- Emphasize the importance of follow-up exams to evaluate effectiveness of medication.

EVALUATION

Effectiveness of therapy can be demonstrated by: ▪ Decrease in blood pressure without appearance of excessive side effects.

G

GUANADREL

(**gwahn**-a-drel)
Hylorel

CLASSIFICATION(S):
Antihypertensive agent (peripherally acting antiadrenergic)

Pregnancy Category B

INDICATIONS

▪ Moderate to severe hypertension (with at least one other agent, usually a diuretic).

ACTION

▪ Prevents the release of norepinephrine from adrenergic nerve endings and the adrenal medulla in response to sympathetic (adrenergic) stimulation ▪ Depletes norepinephrine from nerve endings. Result is decreased sympathetically mediated vasoconstriction. **Therapeutic Effects:** ▪ Lowering of blood pressure.

PHARMACOKINETICS

Absorption: Well absorbed following oral administration.

Distribution: Widely distributed. CNS penetration is minimal.

Metabolism and Excretion: 50% metabolized

by the liver, 50% excreted unchanged by the kidneys.
Half-life: 12 hr (wide range).

CONTRAINDICATIONS AND PRECAUTIONS

Contraindicated in: ▪ Hypersensitivity ▪ Congestive heart failure ▪ Pheochromocytoma ▪ Lactation.
Use Cautiously in: ▪ Asthma ▪ Cardiovascular or cerebrovascular insufficiency ▪ Peptic ulcer disease ▪ Geriatric patients ▪ Patients with renal failure (increased dosing interval recommended if CCr <60 ml/min) ▪ Pregnancy, lactation, or children <18 yr (safety not established).

ADVERSE REACTIONS AND SIDE EFFECTS*

CNS: confusion, dizziness, drowsiness, fainting, fatigue, headaches, anxiety, depression, sleep disturbances.
EENT: nasal stuffiness, visual disturbances.
Resp: cough, shortness of breath.
CV: chest pain, edema, orthostatic hypotension, palpitations.
GI: anorexia, constipation, diarrhea, dry mouth, gas pain, indigestion, abdominal pain, nausea.
GU: ejaculation disturbances, impotence, nocturia, urinary frequency.
MS: aching limbs, leg cramps.
Neuro: paresthesia.

INTERACTIONS

Drug-Drug: ▪ Concurrent use with **beta-adrenergic blockers** or **vasodilators** increases the risk of excessive orthostatic hypotension (concurrent use with vasodilators is not recommended) ▪ Antihypertensive effects may be decreased by concurrent use of **phenothiazines** or **sympathomimetics.** Effects of direct-acting **sympathomimetics** may be increased by guanadrel ▪ **Tricyclic antidepressants** may diminish the antihypertensive effects of guanadrel ▪ Abrupt withdrawal of **tricyclic antidepressants** may enhance the effect of guanadrel ▪ **NSAIDs** may decrease the antihypertensive effects of guanadrel.

ROUTE AND DOSAGE

- **PO (Adults):** 5 mg bid, increased weekly or monthly as needed (range 20–75 mg/day in 2–4 divided doses).

AVAILABILITY

- ***Tablets:*** 10 mg[Rx], 25 mg[Rx].

TIME/ACTION PROFILE (antihypertensive effect†)

	ONSET	PEAK	DURATION
PO	2 hr	4–6 hr	9 hr

†Following single dose.

NURSING IMPLICATIONS

ASSESSMENT

- □ Monitor blood pressure (lying and standing) and pulse prior to administration, frequently during initial dosage adjustment, and periodically throughout therapy. Report significant changes.
- □ Monitor frequency of prescription refills to determine compliance.
- □ Monitor intake and output ratios and daily weight; assess for edema daily, especially at beginning of therapy.
- □ Monitor frequency and consistency of stools. Notify physician or other health care professional if excessive diarrhea occurs; may require dosage reduction.

POTENTIAL NURSING DIAGNOSES

- Injury, risk for (Side Effects).
- Knowledge deficit, related to medication regimen (Patient/Family Teaching).
- Noncompliance (Patient/Family Teaching).

IMPLEMENTATION

- **General Info:** Dosage adjustments should not be made unless there is no decrease in blood pressure when taken supine and after standing for 10 min.
- □ May be administered concurrently with diuretics to minimize tolerance and fluid retention.

PATIENT/FAMILY TEACHING

- □ Emphasize the importance of continuing to take this medication as directed, even if feel-

*CAPITALS indicate life-threatening; underlines indicate most frequent.

ing well. Medication controls but does not cure hypertension. Instruct patient to take medication at the same time each day. If a dose is missed, take as soon as remembered; do not double doses.

- ▫ Encourage patient to comply with additional interventions for hypertension (weight reduction, low-sodium diet, smoking cessation, moderation of alcohol consumption, regular exercise, and stress management).
- ▫ Instruct patient and family on proper technique for blood pressure monitoring. Advise them to check blood pressure at least weekly and report significant changes.
- ▫ Patients should weigh themselves twice weekly and assess feet and ankles for fluid retention.
- ▫ Inform patient that severity of side effects is usually reduced after the initial 8 wk of therapy.
- ▫ May cause drowsiness or dizziness. Advise patient to avoid driving or other activities requiring alertness until response to the medication is known.
- ▫ Caution patient to avoid sudden changes in position, especially upon arising in the morning, to minimize orthostatic hypotension. Alcohol and other CNS depressants, standing for long periods, hot showers, and exercising in hot weather should be avoided because of enhanced orthostatic effects.
- ▫ Advise patient to consult health care professional before taking any OTC medications, especially cough, cold, or allergy remedies.
- ▫ Caution patient to avoid alcohol and other CNS depressants while taking guanadrel.
- ▫ Instruct patient to notify health care professional of medication regimen prior to treatment or surgery.
- ▫ Advise patient to notify health care professional if severe diarrhea, frequent dizziness or fainting, fever, or swelling of feet or lower legs occurs. Dosage reduction may be required for excessive orthostatic hypotension, severe diarrhea, or normal supine blood pressure.
- ▫ Emphasize the importance of follow-up exams to evaluate effectiveness of medication.

EVALUATION

Effectiveness of therapy can be demonstrated by: ▪ Decrease in blood pressure without appearance of excessive side effects.

GUANFACINE

(**gwahn**-fa-seen)
Tenex

CLASSIFICATION(S):
Antihypertensive agent (centrally acting alpha-adrenergic agonist)

Pregnancy Category B

INDICATIONS

▪ Hypertension (with thiazide-type diuretics).

ACTION

▪ Stimulates CNS alpha$_2$-adrenergic receptors, producing a decrease in sympathetic outflow to heart, kidneys, and blood vessels. Result is decreased blood pressure and peripheral resistance, a slight decrease in heart rate, and no change in cardiac output. **Therapeutic Effects:** ▪ Lowering of blood pressure.

PHARMACOKINETICS

Absorption: Well absorbed (80%) following oral administration.
Distribution: Appears to be widely distributed.
Metabolism and Excretion: 50% metabolized by the liver, 50% excreted unchanged by the kidneys.
Half-life: 17 hr.

CONTRAINDICATIONS AND PRECAUTIONS

Contraindicated in: ▪ Hypersensitivity.
Use Cautiously in: ▪ Severe coronary artery disease or recent myocardial infarction ▪ Cerebrovascular disease ▪ Severe renal or liver disease ▪ Pregnancy, lactation, or children <12 yr (safety not established).

ADVERSE REACTIONS AND SIDE EFFECTS*

CNS: drowsiness, weakness, depression, dizziness, fatigue, headache, insomnia.
EENT: tinnitus.
Resp: dyspnea.
CV: bradycardia, chest pain, palpitations, rebound hypertension.

***CAPITALS indicate life-threatening; underlines indicate most frequent.**

G

GI: constipation, dry mouth, abdominal pain, nausea.
GU: impotence.

INTERACTIONS

Drug-Drug: ▪ Additive hypotension with other **antihypertensive agents, nitrates,** and acute ingestion of **alcohol** ▪ Additive CNS depression may occur with other **CNS depressants,** including **alcohol, antihistamines, opioids, tricyclic antidepressants,** and **sedative/hypnotics** ▪ **NSAIDs** may decrease effectiveness.

ROUTE AND DOSAGE

- **PO (Adults):** 1 mg daily given at bedtime, may be increased if necessary at 3–4 wk intervals up to 3 mg/day; may also be given in 2 divided doses.

AVAILABILITY

- ***Tablets:*** 1 mg[Rx], 2 mg[Rx], 3 mg[Rx].

TIME/ACTION PROFILE (antihypertensive effect)

	ONSET	PEAK	DURATION
PO (single dose)	UK	8–12 hr	24 hr
PO (multiple doses)	within 1 wk	1–3 mo	UK

NURSING IMPLICATIONS

ASSESSMENT

- Monitor blood pressure (lying and standing) and pulse frequently during initial dosage adjustment and periodically throughout therapy. Report significant changes.
- Monitor frequency of prescription refills to determine compliance.
- ***Lab Test Considerations:*** May cause temporary, clinically insignificant increase in plasma growth hormone levels.
- May cause decrease in urinary catecholamines and vanillylmandelic acid levels.

POTENTIAL NURSING DIAGNOSES

- Injury, risk for (Side Effects).
- Knowledge deficit, related to medication regimen (Patient/Family Teaching).
- Noncompliance (Patient/Family Teaching).

IMPLEMENTATION

- **PO:** Administer daily dose at bedtime to minimize daytime sedation.

PATIENT/FAMILY TEACHING

- Emphasize the importance of continuing to take medication as directed, even if feeling well. Medication controls but does not cure hypertension. Instruct patient to take medication at the same time each day. If a dose is missed, take as soon as remembered; do not double doses. If 2 or more doses are missed, consult health care professional. Do not discontinue abruptly; may cause sympathetic overstimulation (nervousness, anxiety, rebound hypertension, chest pain, tachycardia, increased salivation, nausea, trembling, stomach cramps, sweating, difficulty sleeping). These effects may occur 2–7 days after discontinuation, although rebound hypertension is rare and more likely to occur with high doses.
- Advise patient to make sure enough medication is available for weekends, holidays, and vacations. A written prescription may be kept in wallet in case of emergency.
- Encourage patient to comply with additional interventions for hypertension (weight reduction, low-sodium diet, smoking cessation, moderation of alcohol consumption, regular exercise, and stress management).
- Instruct patient and family on proper technique for blood pressure monitoring. Advise them to check blood pressure at least weekly and to report significant changes.
- May cause drowsiness or dizziness. Advise patient to avoid driving or other activities requiring alertness until response to the medication is known.
- Advise patient to consult health care professional before taking any OTC medications, especially cough, cold, or allergy remedies.
- Caution patient to avoid alcohol and other CNS depressants while taking guanfacine.
- Advise patient to notify health care professional if dry mouth or constipation persists. Frequent mouth rinses, good oral hygiene, and sugarless gum or candy may minimize dry mouth. Increase in fluid and fiber intake and exercise may decrease constipation.
- Instruct patient to notify health care profes-

sional of medication regimen prior to treatment or surgery.

- Advise patient to notify health care professional if dizziness, prolonged drowsiness, fatigue, weakness, depression, headache, sexual dysfunction, mental depression, or sleep pattern disturbance occurs. Discontinuation may be required if drug-related mental depression occurs.
- Emphasize the importance of follow-up exams to evaluate effectiveness of medication.

EVALUATION

Effectiveness of therapy can be demonstrated by: ▪ Decrease in blood pressure without excessive side effects.

HALOPERIDOL

(ha-loe-**per**-i-dole)

{Apo-Haloperidol}, Haldol, Haldol Decanoate, {Haldol LA}, {Novo-Peridol}, {Peridol}, {PMS Haloperidol}

CLASSIFICATION(S):

Antipsychotic agent (butyrophenone)

Pregnancy Category C

INDICATIONS

▪ Acute and chronic psychoses ▪ Tourette's syndrome ▪ Severe behavioral problems in children. **Unlabeled Uses:** ▪ Nausea and vomiting from surgery or chemotherapy.

ACTION

▪ Alters the effects of dopamine in the CNS ▪ Also has anticholinergic and alpha-adrenergic blocking activity. **Therapeutic Effects:** ▪ Diminished signs and symptoms of psychoses ▪ Improved behavior in children with Tourette's syndrome or other behavioral problems.

PHARMACOKINETICS

Absorption: Well absorbed following PO/IM administration. Decanoate salt is slowly absorbed and has a long duration of action.
Distribution: Concentrates in the liver. Crosses the placenta; enters breast milk.
Metabolism and Excretion: Mostly metabolized by the liver.
Half-life: 21–24 hr.

CONTRAINDICATIONS AND PRECAUTIONS

Contraindicated in: ▪ Hypersensitivity ▪ Narrow-angle glaucoma ▪ Bone marrow depression ▪ CNS depression ▪ Severe liver or cardiovascular disease ▪ Some products contain tartrazine, sesame oil, or benzyl alcohol and should be avoided in patients with known intolerance or hypersensitivity.
Use Cautiously in: ▪ Geriatric or debilitated patients (dosage reduction required) ▪ Cardiac disease ▪ Diabetes ▪ Respiratory insufficiency ▪ Prostatic hypertrophy ▪ CNS tumors ▪ Intestinal obstruction ▪ Seizures ▪ Pregnancy and lactation (safety not established).

ADVERSE REACTIONS AND SIDE EFFECTS*

CNS: SEIZURES, extrapyramidal reactions, confusion, drowsiness, restlessness, tardive dyskinesia.
EENT: blurred vision, dry eyes.
Resp: respiratory depression.
CV: hypotension, tachycardia.
GI: constipation, dry mouth, anorexia, drug-induced hepatitis, ileus.
GU: urinary retention.
Derm: diaphoresis, photosensitivity, rashes.
Endo: galactorrhea.
Hemat: anemia, leukopenia.
Metab: hyperpyrexia.
Misc: NEUROLEPTIC MALIGNANT SYNDROME, hypersensitivity reactions.

INTERACTIONS

Drug-Drug: ▪ Additive hypotension with **antihypertensives, nitrates**, or acute ingestion of **alcohol** ▪ Additive anticholinergic effects with **drugs having anticholinergic properties**, including **antihistamines, antidepressants, atropine, phenothiazines, quinidine,** and **disopyramide** ▪ Additive CNS depression with other **CNS depressants**, including **alcohol, antihistamines, opioids,** and **sedative/hypnotics** ▪ Concurrent use with **epinephrine** may result in severe hypotension and tachycardia

{} = Available in Canada only.
***CAPITALS indicate life-threatening; underlines indicate most frequent.**

H

▪ May decrease therapeutic effects of **levodopa** ▪ Acute encephalopathic syndrome may occur when used with **lithium** ▪ Dementia may occur with **methyldopa.**

ROUTE AND DOSAGE

❑ Haloperidol

- **PO (Adults):** 0.5–5 mg 2–3 times daily. Patients with severe symptoms may require up to 100 mg/day.
- **PO (Geriatric Patients or Debilitated Patients):** 0.5–2 mg twice daily initially; may be gradually increased as needed.
- **PO (Children 3–12 yr or 15–40 kg):** 50 mcg/kg/day in 2–3 divided doses; may increase by 500 mcg (0.5 mg)/day q 5–7 days as needed (up to 75 mcg/kg/day for nonpsychotic disorders or Tourette's syndrome or 150 mcg/kg/day for psychoses).
- **IM (Adults):** 2–5 mg q 1–8 hr (not to exceed 100 mg/day).
- **IV (Adults):** 0.5–5 mg, may be repeated q 30 min (unlabeled).

❑ Haloperidol Decanoate

- **IM (Adults):** 10–15 times the previous daily PO dose but not to exceed 100 mg initially, given monthly (not to exceed 300 mg/mo).

AVAILABILITY

▪ ***Tablets:*** 0.5 mg^{Rx}, 1 mg^{Rx}, 2 mg^{Rx}, 5 mg^{Rx}, 10 mg^{Rx}, 20 mg^{Rx} ▪ ***Oral concentrate:*** 2 mg/ml^{Rx} ▪ ***Haloperidol injection:*** 5 mg/ml^{Rx} ▪ ***Haloperidol decanoate injection:*** 50 mg/ml^{Rx}, 100 mg/ml^{Rx}.

TIME/ACTION PROFILE (antipsychotic activity)

	ONSET	PEAK	DURATION
PO	2 hr	2–6 hr	8–12 hr
IM	20–30 min	30–45 min	4–8 hr*
IM (decanoate)	3–9 days	UK	1 mo

*Effect may persist for several days.

NURSING IMPLICATIONS

ASSESSMENT

- □ Assess patient's mental status (orientation, mood, behavior) prior to and periodically throughout therapy.
- □ Monitor blood pressure (sitting, standing, lying) and pulse prior to and frequently during the period of dosage adjustment. May cause QT interval changes on ECG.
- □ Observe patient carefully when administering medication, to ensure that medication is actually taken and not hoarded.
- □ Monitor intake and output ratios and daily weight. Assess patient for signs and symptoms of dehydration (decreased thirst, lethargy, hemoconcentration), especially in geriatric patients.
- □ Assess fluid intake and bowel function. Increased bulk and fluids in the diet help minimize constipating effects.
- □ Monitor patient for onset of akathisia (restlessness or desire to keep moving), which may appear within 6 hr of 1st dose and may be difficult to distinguish from psychotic agitation; benztropine may be used to differentiate. Observe closely for extrapyramidal side effects (*parkinsonian*—difficulty speaking or swallowing, loss of balance control, pill rolling, mask-like face, shuffling gait, rigidity, tremors; and *dystonic*—muscle spasms, twisting motions, twitching, inability to move eyes, weakness of arms or legs).
- □ Monitor for tardive dyskinesia (uncontrolled rhythmic movement of mouth, face, and extremities; lip smacking or puckering; puffing of cheeks; uncontrolled chewing; rapid or worm-like movements of tongue). Report immediately; may be irreversible.
- □ Monitor for development of neuroleptic malignant syndrome (fever, respiratory distress, tachycardia, convulsions, diaphoresis, hypertension or hypotension, pallor, tiredness, severe muscle stiffness, loss of bladder control). Report symptoms immediately. May also cause leukocytosis, elevated liver function tests, elevated CPK.
- ▪ ***Lab Test Considerations:*** CBC with differential and liver function tests should be evaluated periodically throughout therapy.

POTENTIAL NURSING DIAGNOSES

- Thought processes, altered (Indications).
- Knowledge deficit, related to medication regimen (Patient/Family Teaching).

IMPLEMENTATION

- **PO:** Administer with food or full glass of water or milk to minimize GI irritation.
- □ Use calibrated measuring device for accurate dosage. Do not dilute concentrate with coffee or tea; may cause precipitation. Should be

given undiluted, but if necessary may dilute in at least 60 ml of liquid.

- **IM:** Inject slowly, using 2-in., 21-gauge needle into well-developed muscle via Z-track technique. Do not exceed 3 ml per injection site. Slight yellow color does not indicate altered potency. Keep patient recumbent for at least 30 min following injection to minimize hypotensive effects.
- **Direct IV:** May be administered undiluted for rapid control of acute psychosis or delirium.
- ***Rate:*** Administer at a rate of 5 mg/min.
- **Intermittent Infusion:** May be diluted in 30–50 ml of D5W.
- ***Rate:*** Infuse over 30 min.
- **Syringe Compatibility:** ▪ hydromorphone ▪ sufentanil.
- **Syringe Incompatibility:** ▪ heparin ▪ ketorolac.
- **Y-Site Compatibility:** ▪ amifostine ▪ aztreonam ▪ cimetidine ▪ dobutamine ▪ dopamine ▪ famotidine ▪ filgrastim ▪ fludarabine ▪ lidocaine ▪ lorazepam ▪ melphalan ▪ midazolam ▪ nitroglycerin ▪ norepinephrine ▪ ondansetron ▪ paclitaxel ▪ phenylephrine ▪ sufentanil ▪ tacrolimus ▪ teniposide ▪ theophylline ▪ thiotepa ▪ vinorelbine.
- **Y-Site Incompatibility:** ▪ cefepime ▪ fluconazole ▪ foscarnet ▪ gallium nitrate ▪ heparin ▪ piperacillin/tazobactam ▪ sargramostim.

PATIENT/FAMILY TEACHING

- □ Advise patient to take medication exactly as directed. Missed doses should be taken as soon as remembered, with remaining doses evenly spaced throughout the day. May require several weeks to obtain desired effects. Do not increase dose or discontinue medication without consulting health care professional. Abrupt withdrawal may cause dizziness; nausea; vomiting; GI upset; trembling; or uncontrolled movements of mouth, tongue, or jaw.
- □ Inform patient of possibility of extrapyramidal symptoms and tardive dyskinesia. Caution patient to report symptoms immediately.
- □ Advise patient to change positions slowly to minimize orthostatic hypotension.
- □ May cause drowsiness. Caution patient to avoid driving or other activities requiring alertness until response to medication is known.
- □ Caution patient to avoid taking alcohol or other CNS depressants concurrently with this medication.
- □ Advise patient to use sunscreen and protective clothing when exposed to the sun to prevent photosensitivity reactions. Extremes of temperature should also be avoided, as this drug impairs body temperature regulation.
- □ Instruct patient to use frequent mouth rinses, good oral hygiene, and sugarless gum or candy to minimize dry mouth.
- □ Advise patient to notify health care professional of medication regimen prior to treatment or surgery.
- □ Instruct patient to notify health care professional promptly if weakness, tremors, visual disturbances, dark-colored urine or clay-colored stools, sore throat, or fever is noted.
- □ Emphasize the importance of routine follow-up exams.

EVALUATION

Effectiveness of therapy can be demonstrated by: ▪ Decrease in hallucinations, insomnia, agitation, hostility, and delusions ▪ Decreased tics and vocalization in Tourette's syndrome. If no therapeutic effects are seen in 2–4 wk, dosage may be increased.

HEPARIN

(**hep**-a-rin)

{Calcilean}, {Hepalean}, {Heparin Leo}, Hep-Lock, Hep-Lock U/P

CLASSIFICATION(S):

Anticoagulant (antithrombotic)

Pregnancy Category C

INDICATIONS

▪ Prophylaxis and treatment of various thromboembolic disorders including: □ Venous thromboembolism □ Pulmonary emboli □ Atrial fibrillation with embolization □ Acute and chronic consumptive coagulopathies □ Peripheral arterial thromboembolism ▪ Used in very low doses (10–100 units) to maintain patency of IV catheters (heparin flush).

ACTION

▪ Potentiates the inhibitory effect of antithrombin on factor Xa and thrombin ▪ In low doses, prevents the conversion of prothrombin to thrombin by its effects on factor Xa ▪ Higher doses neutralize thrombin, preventing the conversion of fibrinogen to fibrin. **Therapeutc Effects:** ▪ Prevention of thrombus formation ▪ Prevention of extension of existing thrombi (full dose).

PHARMACOKINETICS

Absorption: Well absorbed following SC administration.
Distribution: Does not cross the placenta or enter breast milk.
Metabolism and Excretion: Probably removed by the reticuloendothelial system (lymph nodes, spleen).
Half-life: 1–2 hr (increases with increasing dosage).

CONTRAINDICATIONS AND PRECAUTIONS

Contraindicated in: ▪ Hypersensitivity ▪ Uncontrolled bleeding ▪ Severe thrombocytopenia ▪ Open wounds (full dose) ▪ Products containing benzyl alcohol should not be used in premature infants.
Use Cautiously in: ▪ Severe liver or kidney disease ▪ Retinopathy (hypertensive or diabetic) ▪ Untreated hypertension ▪ Ulcer disease ▪ Spinal cord or brain injury ▪ History of congenital or acquired bleeding disorder ▪ Malignancy ▪ Females >60 yr (increased risk of bleeding) ▪ May be used during pregnancy, but use with caution during the last trimester and in the immediate postpartum period. **Exercise Extreme Caution in:** ▪ Severe uncontrolled hypertension ▪ Bacterial endocarditis, bleeding disorders ▪ GI bleeding/ulceration/pathology ▪ Hemorrhagic stroke ▪ Recent CNS or ophthalmologic surgery ▪ Active GI bleeding/ulceration ▪ History of thrombocytopenia related to heparin.

ADVERSE REACTIONS AND SIDE EFFECTS*

GI: drug-induced hepatitis.
Derm: alopecia (long-term use), rashes, urticaria.
Hemat: BLEEDING, anemia, thrombocytopenia.
Local: pain at injection site.
MS: osteoporosis (long-term use).
Misc: fever, hypersensitivity.

INTERACTIONS

Heparin is frequently used concurrently or sequentially with other agents affecting coagulation. The risk of potentially serious interactions is greatest with full anticoagulation.
Drug-Drug: ▪ Risk of bleeding may be increased by concurrent use of **drugs that affect platelet function**, including **aspirin, NSAIDs, dipyridamole,** some **penicillins, ticlopidine,** and **dextran** ▪ Risk of bleeding may be increased by concurrent use of **drugs that cause hypoprothrombinemia,** including **quinidine, cefamandole, cefmetazole, cefoperazone, cefotetan, plicamycin,** and **valproic acid** ▪ Concurrent use of **thrombolytic agents** increases the risk of bleeding ▪ Heparins affect the prothrombin time used in assessing the response to **warfarin** ▪ **Digitalis glycosides, tetracyclines, nicotine,** and **antihistamines** may decrease the anticoagulant effect of heparin ▪ **Streptokinase** may be followed by relative resistance to heparin.

ROUTE AND DOSAGE

❑ Therapeutic Anticoagulation

- **IV (Adults):** *Intermittent boluses*—10,000 units, followed by 5000–10,000 units q 4–6 hr. *Continuous infusion*—5000 units (35–70 units/kg), followed by 20,000–40,000 units infused over 24 hr (approx 1000 units/hr or 15–18 units/kg/hr).
- **IV (Children):** *Intermittent boluses*—50 units/kg, followed by 50–100 units/kg q 4 hr. *Continuous infusion*—50 units/kg, followed by 100 units/kg/4 hr or 20,000 units/m^2/24 hr.
- **SC (Adults):** 5000 units IV, followed by initial SC dose of 10,000–20,000 units, then 8000–10,000 units q 8 hr or 15,000–20,000 units q 12 hr.

❑ Prophylaxis of Thromboembolism

- **SC (Adults):** 5000 units q 8–12 hr (may be started 2 hr prior to surgery).

❑ Cardiovascular Surgery

- **IV (Adults):** At least 150 units/kg (300 units/

***CAPITALS indicate life-threatening; underlines indicate most frequent.**

kg if procedure <60 min; 400 units/kg if >60 min).

- **"Flush"**
- **IV (Adults and Children):** 10–100 units/ml solution to fill heparin lock set to needle hub; replace after each use.

AVAILABILITY

- **Heparin Sodium**

▪ ***Solution for injection:*** 10 units/ml[Rx], 100 units/ml[Rx], 1000 units/ml[Rx], 5000 units/ml[Rx], 7500 units/ml[Rx], 10,000 units/ml[Rx], 20,000 units/ml[Rx], 40,000 units/ml[Rx] ▪ ***Premixed solution:*** 1000 units/500 ml[Rx], 2000 units/1000 ml[Rx], 12,500 units/250 ml[Rx], 25,000 units in 250 and 500 ml[Rx].

TIME/ACTION PROFILE (anticoagulant effect)

	ONSET	PEAK	DURATION
Heparin SC	20–60 min	2 hr	8–12 hr
Heparin IV	immediate	5–10 min	2–6 hr

NURSING IMPLICATIONS

ASSESSMENT

- **General Info:** Assess patient for signs of bleeding and hemorrhage (bleeding gums; nosebleed; unusual bruising; black, tarry stools; hematuria; fall in hematocrit or blood pressure; guaiac-positive stools). Notify physician if these occur.
- Assess patient for evidence of additional or increased thrombosis. Symptoms will depend on area of involvement.
- Monitor patient for hypersensitivity reactions (chills, fever, urticaria). Report signs to physician.
- **SC:** Observe injection sites for hematomas, ecchymosis, or inflammation.
- ***Lab Test Considerations:*** Activated partial thromboplastin time (aPTT) and hematocrit should be monitored prior to and periodically throughout therapy. When *intermittent IV* therapy is used, draw aPTT levels 30 min before each dose during initial therapy and then periodically. During *continuous* administration, monitor aPTT levels every 4 hr during early therapy. For *SC* therapy, draw blood 4–6 hr after injection.
- Monitor platelet count every 2–3 days throughout therapy. May cause mild thrombocytopenia, which appears on 4th day and resolves despite continued heparin therapy. Thrombocytopenia, which necessitates discontinuing medication, may develop on 8th day of therapy. Patients who have received a previous course of heparin may be at higher risk for severe thrombocytopenia for several months after the initial course.
- May cause prolonged PT levels, false elevations of serum thyroxine, T_3 resin, sulfobromopthalein (BSP), and false-negative ^{125}I fibrinogen uptake tests.
- May cause decreased serum triglyceride and cholesterol levels and increased plasma free fatty acid concentrations.
- May also cause hyperkalemia and elevated AST and ALT levels.
- ***Toxicity and Overdose:*** Protamine sulfate is the antidote. However, because of the short half-life, overdose can often be treated by withdrawing the drug.

POTENTIAL NURSING DIAGNOSES

- Tissue perfusion, altered (Indications).
- Injury, risk for (Side Effects).
- Knowledge deficit, related to medication regimen (Patient/Family Teaching).

IMPLEMENTATION

- Inform all personnel caring for patient of anticoagulant therapy. Venipunctures and injection sites require application of pressure to prevent bleeding or hematoma formation. IM injections of other medications should be avoided, as hematomas may develop.
- In patients requiring long-term anticoagulation, oral anticoagulant therapy should be instituted 4–5 days prior to discontinuing heparin therapy.
- Solution is colorless to slightly yellow.
- **SC:** Administer deep into SC tissue. Alternate injection sites between the left and right anterolateral and left and right posterolateral abdominal wall. Inject entire length of needle at a 45° or 90° angle into a skin fold held between thumb and forefinger; hold skin fold throughout injection. Do not aspirate or massage. Rotate sites frequently. Do not administer IM because of danger of hematoma formation. Solution should be clear; do not inject solution containing particulate matter.
- **Direct IV:** Loading dose usually precedes continuous infusion.

- *Rate:* May be given undiluted over at least 1 min.
- **Intermittent/Continuous Infusion:** Dilute in prescribed amount of 0.9% NaCl, D5W, or Ringer's solution for injection and give as a continuous or intermittent infusion. Ensure adequate mixing of heparin in solution by inverting container at least 6 times initially and periodically mixing during infusing.
- *Rate:* Infusion may be administered over 4–24 hr. Use an infusion pump to ensure accuracy. See infusion rate table in Appendix D.
- **Flush:** To prevent clot formation in intermittent infusion (heparin lock) sets, inject dilute heparin solution of 10–100 units/0.5–1 ml after each medication injection or every 8–12 hr. To prevent incompatibility of heparin with medication, flush lock set with sterile water or 0.9% NaCl for injection before and after medication is administered.
- **Syringe Compatibility:** ▪ ampicillin ▪ atropine ▪ bleomycin ▪ cefamandole ▪ cefazolin ▪ cefoperazone ▪ cefotaxime ▪ cefoxitin ▪ chloramphenicol ▪ cimetidine ▪ cisplatin ▪ clindamycin ▪ cyclophosphamide ▪ diazoxide ▪ digoxin ▪ dimenhydrinate ▪ fentanyl ▪ fluorouracil ▪ furosemide ▪ leucovorin ▪ lidocaine ▪ methotrexate ▪ metoclopramide ▪ mezlocillin ▪ mitomycin ▪ nafcillin ▪ naloxone ▪ neostigmine ▪ pancuronium ▪ penicillin G ▪ piperacillin ▪ succinylcholine ▪ trimethoprim/sulfamethoxazole ▪ verapamil ▪ vincristine.
- **Syringe Incompatibility:** ▪ amikacin ▪ amiodarone ▪ chlorpromazine ▪ diazepam ▪ doxorubicin ▪ droperidol ▪ droperidol/fentanyl ▪ erythromycin lactobionate ▪ gentamicin ▪ haloperidol ▪ kanamycin ▪ meperidine ▪ methicillin ▪ methotrimeprazine ▪ netilmicin ▪ pentazocine ▪ promethazine ▪ streptomycin ▪ tobramycin ▪ triflupromazine ▪ vancomycin.
- **Y-Site Compatibility:** ▪ acyclovir ▪ aldesleukin ▪ amifostine ▪ aminophylline ▪ ampicillin ▪ ampicillin/sulbactam ▪ atracurium ▪ atropine ▪ aztreonam ▪ betamethasone ▪ bleomycin ▪ calcium gluconate ▪ cefazolin ▪ cefotetan ▪ ceftazidime ▪ ceftriaxone ▪ cephalothin ▪ cephapirin ▪ chlordiazepoxide ▪ chlorpromazine ▪ cimetidine ▪ cisplatin ▪ cyanocobalamin ▪ cyclophosphamide ▪ cytarabine ▪ dexamethasone ▪ digoxin ▪ diphenhydramine ▪ dopamine ▪ droperidol/fentanyl ▪ edrophonium ▪ enalaprilat ▪ epinephrine ▪ esmolol ▪ conjugated estrogens ▪ ethacrynate ▪ famotidine ▪ fentanyl ▪ fluconazole ▪ fludarabine ▪ fluorouracil ▪ foscarnet ▪ furosemide ▪ gallium nitrate ▪ hydralazine ▪ insulin ▪ isoproterenol ▪ kanamycin ▪ leucovorin ▪ lidocaine ▪ lorazepam ▪ magnesium sulfate ▪ melphalan ▪ meperidine ▪ methicillin ▪ methotrexate ▪ methoxamine ▪ methyldopate ▪ methylergonovine ▪ metoclopramide ▪ metronidazole ▪ midazolam ▪ minocycline ▪ mitomycin ▪ morphine ▪ neostigmine ▪ nitroglycerin ▪ nitroprusside ▪ norepinephrine ▪ ondansetron ▪ oxacillin ▪ oxytocin ▪ paclitaxel ▪ pancuronium ▪ penicillin G potassium ▪ pentazocine ▪ piperacillin ▪ piperacillin/tazobactam ▪ potassium chloride ▪ prednisolone ▪ procainamide ▪ prochlorperazine ▪ propranolol ▪ pyridostigmine ▪ ranitidine ▪ sargramostim ▪ scopolamine ▪ sodium bicarbonate ▪ streptokinase ▪ succinylcholine ▪ tacrolimus ▪ teniposide ▪ theophylline ▪ thiotepa ▪ ticarcillin ▪ ticarcillin/clavulanate ▪ trimethobenzamide ▪ trimethophan camsylate ▪ vecuronium ▪ vinblastine ▪ vincristine ▪ vinorelbine ▪ zidovudine.
- **Y-Site Incompatibility:** ▪ alteplase ▪ amiodarone ▪ ciprofloxacin ▪ diazepam ▪ dobutamine ▪ doxycycline ▪ ergotamine tartrate ▪ filgrastim ▪ gentamicin ▪ haloperidol ▪ idarubicin ▪ methotrimeprazine ▪ phenytoin ▪ tobramycin ▪ triflupromazine ▪ vancomycin.
- **Additive Compatibility:** ▪ It is recommended that heparin not be mixed in solution with other medications when given for anticoagulation, even those that are compatible, because changes in rate of heparin infusion may be required that would also affect admixtures. If heparin is added to an admixture, the following drugs are compatible: ▪ amphotericin ▪ calcium gluconate ▪ cefepime ▪ cephapirin ▪ chloramphenicol ▪ clindamycin ▪ colistimethate ▪ dopamine ▪ erythromycin gluceptate ▪ fluconazole ▪ flumazenil ▪ furosemide ▪ methyldopate ▪ methylprednisolone ▪ nafcillin ▪ octreotide ▪ potassium chloride ▪ prednisolone ▪ promazine ▪ ranitidine ▪ sodium bicarbonate ▪ verapamil ▪ vitamin B complex ▪ vitamin B complex with C. Also compatible with TPN solutions or fat emulsion.
- **Additive Incompatibility:** ▪ alteplase ▪ amikacin ▪ cytarabine ▪ erythromycin lactobionate ▪ gentamicin ▪ kanamycin ▪ meperidine

▪ methadone ▪ morphine ▪ polymyxin B ▪ streptomycin.

PATIENT/FAMILY TEACHING

▪ **General Info:** Advise patient to report any symptoms of unusual bleeding or bruising to health care professional immediately.
□ Instruct patient not to take medications containing aspirin or NSAIDs while on heparin therapy.
□ Caution patient to avoid IM injections and activities leading to injury and to use a soft toothbrush and electric razor during heparin therapy.
□ Advise patient to inform health care professional of medication regimen prior to treatment or surgery.
□ Patients on anticoagulant therapy should carry an identification card with this information at all times.

EVALUATION

Clinical response to therapy can be evaluated by: ▪ Prolonged PTT of 1.5–2 times the control, without signs of hemorrhage ▪ Prevention of deep vein thrombosis and pulmonary emboli ▪ Patency of IV catheters.

HEPARINS (low molecular weight)/HEPARINOIDS

ardeparin
(ar-**dep**-a-rin)
Normiflo

dalteparin
(dal-**tep**-a-rin)
Fragmin

danaparoid
(da-**nap**-a-royd)
Orgaran

enoxaparin
(e-nox-a-**pa**-rin)
Lovenox

CLASSIFICATION(S):
Anticoagulants (antithrombotics)

Pregnancy Category B

INDICATIONS

▪ Prevention of thromboembolic phenomena including deep vein thrombosis and pulmonary emboli following surgical procedures known to increase the risk of such complications (knee/hip replacement, abdominal surgery) ▪ **Enoxaparin Only:** □ Treatment of deep vein thrombosis □ Prevention of clotting during extracorporeal circulation. **Unlabeled Uses:** ▪ Management of unstable angina.

ACTION

▪ Potentiate the inhibitory effect of antithrombin on factor Xa and thrombin ▪ Danaparoid is a heparinoid. **Therapeutic Effects:** ▪ Prevention of thrombus formation.

PHARMACOKINETICS

Absorption: All agents are destroyed by enzymes in the GI tract, necessitating parenteral administration. Well absorbed following SC administration (87% for dalteparin, 92% for ardeparin and enoxaparin, 100% for danaparoid).
Distribution: UK.
Metabolism and Excretion: *Ardeparin*—not renally excreted; *dalteparin*—UK; *danaparoid*—mostly renally excreted; *enoxaparin*—weakly metabolized by the liver; renally eliminated.
Half-life: *Ardeparin*—2.5–3.3 hr; *danaparoid*—24 hr; *dalteparin*—2.1–2.3 hr (increased in renal insufficiency); *enoxaparin*—3–6 hr.

CONTRAINDICATIONS AND PRECAUTIONS

Contraindicated in: ▪ Hypersensitivity to specific agents or pork products ▪ Uncontrolled bleeding ▪ Some products contain sulfites and should be avoided in patients with known hypersensitivity.
Use Cautiously in: ▪ Severe liver or kidney disease ▪ Retinopathy (hypertensive or diabetic) ▪ Untreated hypertension ▪ Recent history of ulcer disease ▪ Spinal/epidural anesthesia ▪ History of congenital or acquired bleeding disorder ▪ Elderly patients (enoxaparin elimination prolonged) ▪ Malignancy ▪ Pregnancy, lactation, or children (safety not established). **Exercise Extreme Caution in:** ▪ Severe uncontrolled hypertension ▪ Bacterial endocarditis, bleeding disorders ▪ GI bleeding/ulceration/pathology

▪ Hemorrhagic stroke ▪ Recent CNS or ophthalmologic surgery ▪ Active GI bleeding/ulceration ▪ History of thrombocytopenia related to heparin.

ADVERSE REACTIONS AND SIDE EFFECTS*

CNS: dizziness, headache, insomnia.
CV: edema.
GI: constipation, nausea, reversible increase in liver enzymes, vomiting.
GU: urinary retention.
Derm: ecchymoses, pruritus, rash, urticaria.
Hemat: BLEEDING, anemia, thrombocytopenia.
Local: erythema at injection site, hematoma, irritation, pain.
Misc: fever.

INTERACTIONS

Drug-Drug: ▪ Risk of bleeding may be increased by concurrent use of **warfarin** or **drugs that affect platelet function,** including **aspirin, NSAIDs, dipyridamole,** some **penicillins, ticlopidine,** and **dextran.**

ROUTE AND DOSAGE

❑ Ardeparin

▪ **SC (Adults):** 50 anti–factor Xa units/kg q 12 hr for 14 days or until ambulatory, starting evening of day of procedure or following morning.

❑ Dalteparin

▪ **SC (Adults):** 2500 IU/daily starting 1–2 hr preop, then daily for 5–10 days or until ambulatory. *Patients at high risk of thromboembolism*—5000 IU/daily starting evening before procedure, then daily for 5–10 days or until ambulatory; *patients with malignancies*—2500 IU 1–2 hr preop, then 2500 IU 12 hr postop, then 5000 IU daily for 5–10 days or until ambulatory; *systemic anticoagulation*—200 IU/kg once daily or 100 IU/kg q 12 hr.

❑ Danaparoid

▪ **SC (Adults):** 750 anti–factor Xa IU q 12 hr starting 1–4 hr preop and at least 2 hr postop for 7–10 days or until ambulatory (up to 14 days).

❑ Enoxaparin

▪ **SC (Adults):** *Prophylaxis before knee/hip surgery*—30 mg twice daily starting within 24 hr postop and continued for 7–10 days or until ambulatory (up to 14 days); *prophylaxis before abdominal surgery*—40 mg twice daily starting within 24 hr postop and continued for 7–10 days or until ambulatory (up to 14 days); *systemic anticoagulation*—1 mg/kg q 12 hr.

AVAILABILITY

❑ Ardeparin

▪ ***Solution for injection:*** 5000 anti–factor Xa IU/0.5 ml[Rx], 10,000 anti–factor Xa IU/0.5 ml[Rx].

❑ Dalteparin

▪ ***Solution for injection:*** 2500 anti–factor Xa IU/0.2 ml[Rx], 5000 anti–factor Xa IU/0.2 ml[Rx].

❑ Enoxaparin

▪ ***Solution for injection:*** 30 mg/0.3 ml (in prefilled syringes)[Rx], 40 mg/0.4 ml (in prefilled syringes)[Rx].

TIME/ACTION PROFILE (anticoagulant effect)

	ONSET	PEAK	DURATION
Ardeparin SC	UK	3 hr	12 hr
Danaparoid	UK	2–5 hr	12 hr
Dalteparin SC	rapid	4 hr	up to 24 hr
Enoxaparin SC	UK	UK	12 hr

NURSING IMPLICATIONS

ASSESSMENT

▪ **General Info:** Assess patient for signs of bleeding and hemorrhage (bleeding gums; nosebleed; unusual bruising; black, tarry stools; hematuria; fall in hematocrit or blood pressure; guaiac-positive stools); bleeding from surgical site. Notify physician if these occur.

❑ Assess patient for evidence of additional or increased thrombosis. Symptoms will depend on area of involvement.

❑ Monitor patient for hypersensitivity reactions (chills, fever, urticaria). Report signs to physician.

❑ Monitor patients with epidural catheters fre-

*CAPITALS indicate life-threatening; underlines indicate most frequent.

quently for signs and symptoms of neurologic impairment.

- **SC:** Observe injection sites for hematomas, ecchymosis, or inflammation.
- ***Lab Test Considerations:*** Monitor CBC, platelet count, and stools for occult blood periodically throughout therapy. If thrombocytopenia occurs, monitor closely. If hematocrit decreases unexpectedly, assess patient for potential bleeding sites.
  - Special monitoring of clotting times (aPTT) is not necessary.
  - May cause increases in AST and ALT levels.
- ***Toxicity and Overdose:*** For *ardeparin* overdose, protamine sulfate 1 mg for each 100 anti–Xa IU of ardeparin should be administered by slow IV injection. For *enoxaparin* overdose, protamine sulfate 1 mg for each mg of enoxaparin should be administered by slow IV injection. For *dalteparin* overdose, protamine sulfate 1 mg for each 100 anti–Xa IU of dalteparin should be administered by slow IV injection. If the aPTT measured 2–4 hr after protamine administration remains prolonged, a 2nd infusion of protamine 0.5 mg/100 anti–Xa IU of dalteparin may be administered.

POTENTIAL NURSING DIAGNOSES

- Tissue perfusion, altered (Indications).
- Injury, risk for (Side Effects).
- Knowledge deficit, related to medication regimen (Patient/Family Teaching).

IMPLEMENTATION

- **General Info:** Cannot be used interchangeably (unit for unit) with unfractionated heparin or other low-molecular-weight heparins.
- **SC:** Administer deep into SC tissue. Alternate injection sites daily between the left and right anterolateral and left and right posterolateral abdominal wall. Inject entire length of needle at a 45° or 90° angle into a skin fold held between thumb and forefinger; hold skin fold throughout injection. Do not aspirate or massage. Rotate sites frequently. Do not administer IM because of danger of hematoma formation. Solution should be clear; do not inject solution containing particulate matter.
  - If excessive bruising occurs, ice cube massage of site prior to injection may lessen bruising.
- **Ardeparin:** Dose may require only part of medication in Tubex. Extrude air and excess medication prior to administration.

PATIENT/FAMILY TEACHING

- Advise patient to report any symptoms of unusual bleeding or bruising, itching, rash, fever, swelling, or difficulty breathing to health care professional immediately.

EVALUATION

Effectiveness of therapy can be demonstrated by: ▪ Prevention of deep vein thrombosis and pulmonary emboli ▪ Treatment of deep vein thrombosis ▪ Prevention of clotting during extracorporeal circulation.

HETASTARCH

Hespan

CLASSIFICATION(S):

Volume expander

Pregnancy Category UK

H

INDICATIONS

▪ Adjunct for fluid replacement and volume expansion in the early management of shock or impending shock due to: ▫ Burns ▫ Hemorrhage ▫ Surgery ▫ Sepsis ▫ Trauma ▪ Adjunct in leukapheresis (improves collection of granulocytes).

ACTION

▪ A synthetic molecule that acts as a colloidal osmotic agent similar to albumin. **Therapeutic Effects:** ▪ Plasma volume expansion.

PHARMACOKINETICS

Absorption: Administered IV only, resulting in complete bioavailability.

Distribution: Distributes into intravascular space.

Metabolism and Excretion: Molecules with a molecular weight of 50,000 or less are excreted unchanged by the kidneys. Larger molecules are slowly degraded before excretion.

Half-life: 90% has half-life of 17 days, remaining 10% has half-life of 48 days.

CONTRAINDICATIONS AND PRECAUTIONS

Contraindicated in: ▪ Hypersensitivity ▪ Severe bleeding disorders ▪ Congestive heart failure ▪ Pulmonary edema ▪ Oliguric or anuric renal failure ▪ Early pregnancy.
Use Cautiously in: ▪ Thrombocytopenia ▪ Elderly patients ▪ Severe renal impairment (if CCr <10 ml/min, initial dose may be the same; subsequent doses should be decreased to 25–50% of usual dose) ▪ Lactation or children (safety not established).

ADVERSE REACTIONS AND SIDE EFFECTS*

CNS: headache.
CV: congestive heart failure, pulmonary edema.
GI: vomiting.
Derm: pruritus, urticaria.
F and E: fluid overload, peripheral edema of the lower extremities.
Hemat: decreased hematocrit, decreased platelet function.
MS: myalgia.
Misc: hypersensitivity reactions including ANAPHYLACTOID REACTIONS, chills, fever, parotid and submaxillary gland enlargement.

INTERACTIONS

Drug-Drug: ▪ No known interactions.

ROUTE AND DOSAGE

- **IV (Adults):** 30–60 g (500–1000 ml of 6% solution), may be repeated; not to exceed 90 g (1500 ml/day). In acute hemorrhagic shock, up to 20 ml/kg/hr may be used.

AVAILABILITY

▪ ***Injection:*** 6 g/100 ml in 0.9% saline in 250- and 500-ml infusion bottles[Rx].

TIME/ACTION PROFILE (volume expansion)

	ONSET	PEAK	DURATION
IV	rapid	end of infusion	24 hr or longer

NURSING IMPLICATIONS

ASSESSMENT

- Monitor vital signs, CVP, cardiac output, pulmonary capillary wedge pressure, and urinary output prior to and frequently throughout therapy. Assess patient for signs of vascular overload (elevated CVP, rales/crackles, dyspnea, hypertension, jugular venous distention) during and following administration.
- If fever, wheezing, flu-like symptoms, urticaria, periorbital edema, or submaxillary and parotid gland enlargement occurs, stop infusion and notify physician immediately. Antihistamines, epinephrine, glucocorticoids, and airway management may be required to suppress this response.
- Assess surgical patients for increased bleeding following administration caused by interference with platelet function and clotting factors (large volumes only).
- ***Lab Test Considerations:*** Monitor CBC with differential, hemoglobin, hematocrit, platelet count, prothrombin time (PT), partial thromboplastin time (PTT), and clotting time throughout therapy. Large volumes of hetastarch may cause hemodilution; do not allow hematocrit to drop below 30% by volume. May cause increased erythrocyte sedimentation rate, prolonged bleeding time, and prolonged prothrombin, partial thromboplastin, and clotting times.
- May cause elevated indirect serum bilirubin and amylase concentrations.
- During *leukapheresis,* monitor CBC, total leukocyte and platelet counts, leukocyte differential count, hemoglobin, hematocrit, PT, and PTT.

POTENTIAL NURSING DIAGNOSES

- Tissue perfusion, altered (Indications).
- Fluid volume deficit (Indications).
- Fluid volume excess (Side Effects).

IMPLEMENTATION

- **General Info:** Available in a 6% solution diluted with 0.9% NaCl. Solution should be clear pale yellow to amber; do not administer solution that is cloudy or that contains a precip-

*CAPITALS indicate life-threatening; underlines indicate most frequent.

itate. Store at room temperature. Discard unused solution.

- □ There is no danger of serum hepatitis or AIDS from hetastarch. Crossmatching is not required.
- ▪ **Intermittent Infusion:** For leukapheresis, 250–700 ml are infused at a constant ratio of 1:8–1:13 to venous whole blood.
- ▪ **Continuous Infusion:** Administer hetastarch undiluted by IV infusion.
- ▪ ***Rate:*** Rate of administration is determined by blood volume, indication, and patient response.
- □ In acute hemorrhagic shock, hetastarch may be administered up to 1.2 g/kg (20 ml/kg) per hr. Slower rates are generally used with burns and septic shock.
- ▪ **Y-Site Compatibility:** ▪ cimetidine ▪ diazepam ▪ doxycycline ▪ enalaprilat.
- ▪ **Y-Site Incompatibility:** ▪ amikacin ▪ cefamandole ▪ cefoperazone ▪ cefotaxime ▪ cefoxitin ▪ gentamicin ▪ theophylline ▪ tobramycin.

PATIENT/FAMILY TEACHING

- □ Explain to patient the rationale for use of this solution.
- □ Instruct patient to notify health care professional if dyspnea, itching, or flu-like symptoms occur.

EVALUATION

Effectiveness of therapy can be demonstrated by: ▪ Increase in blood pressure, blood volume, and urinary output when used to treat shock and burns ▪ Improved harvesting and increased yield of granulocytes during leukapheresis.

HISTAMINE H_2 ANTAGONISTS

cimetidine
(sye-**me**-ti-deen)
{Apo-Cimetidine}, {Novocimetine}, {Peptol}, Tagamet, Tagamet HB

famotidine
(fa-**moe**-ti-deen)
Mylanta AR, Pepcid, {Pepcid AC}

nizatidine
(ni-**za**-ti-deen)
Axid, Axid AR

ranitidine
(ra-**ni**-ti-deen)
Apo-Ranitidine, Zantac, {Zantac-C}, Zantac 75

ranitidine bismuth citrate
(ra-**ni**-ti-deen **biss**-muth **sye**-trate)
Tritec

CLASSIFICATION(S):
Antiulcer agents, Gastric acid secretion inhibitors

Pregnancy B

INDICATIONS

▪ Short-term treatment of active duodenal ulcers and benign gastric ulcers ▪ Prophylaxis of duodenal ulcers (at lower doses) ▪ Management of gastroesophageal reflux disease (GERD) ▪ Treatment of heartburn, acid indigestion, and sour stomach (OTC use) ▪ **Cimetidine, famotidine, ranitidine:** Management of gastric hypersecretory states (Zollinger-Ellison syndrome) ▪ **Cimetidine, famotidine, ranitidine IV:** Prevention and treatment of stress-induced upper GI bleeding in critically ill patients ▪ **Ranitidine bismuth citrate:** With clarithromycin to eradicate *Helicobacter pylori* in the treatment of duodenal ulcers. ▪ **Unlabeled Uses:** ▪ Management of GI symptoms associated with the use of NSAIDs ▪ Prevention of stress ulceration or aspiration pneumonitis ▪ Prevention of acid inactivation of supplemental pancreatic enzymes in patients with pancreatic insufficiency ▪ Management of urticaria.

ACTION

▪ Inhibits the action of histamine at the H_2-receptor site located primarily in gastric parietal cells, resulting in inhibition of gastric acid secretion ▪ In addition, ranitidine bismuth citrate has some antibacterial action against *Helicobacter pylori.* **Therapeutic Effects:** ▪ Healing and prevention of ulcers ▪ Decreased symptoms of

H

gastroesophageal reflux ▪ Decreased secretion of gastric acid.

PHARMACOKINETICS

Absorption: *Cimetidine*—well absorbed following oral and IM administration. *Famotidine*—40–45% absorbed following oral administration. *Nizatidine*—70–95% absorbed following oral administration. *Ranitidine*—50% absorbed following PO and IM administration. *Ranitidine bismuth citrate*—splits into ranitidine and bismuth in the GI tract; bismuth is not absorbed.
Distribution: All agents enter breast milk and cerebrospinal fluid.
Metabolism and Excretion: *Cimetidine*—30% metabolized by the liver; remainder is eliminated unchanged by the kidneys. *Famotidine*—up to 70% excreted unchanged by the kidneys, 30–35% metabolized by the liver. *Nizatidine*—60% excreted unchanged by the kidneys; some hepatic metabolism; at least 1 metabolite has histamine blocking activity. *Ranitidine*—metabolized by the liver, mostly on first pass; 30% excreted unchanged by the kidneys following PO administration, 70–80% following parenteral administration.
Half-life: *Cimetidine*—2 hr; *famotidine*—2.5–3.5 hr; *nizatidine*—1.6 hr; *ranitidine*—1.7–3 hr (all are increased in renal impairment).

CONTRAINDICATIONS AND PRECAUTIONS

Contraindicated in: ▪ Hypersensitivity ▪ Some oral liquids contain alcohol and should be avoided in patients with known intolerance ▪ Porphyria (ranitidine bismuth citrate only).
Use Cautiously in: ▪ Elderly patients (more susceptible to adverse CNS reactions; dosage reduction recommended) ▪ Renal impairment (more susceptible to adverse CNS reactions; increased dosage interval recommended for *cimetidine* if renal impairment is severe, for *famotidine* if CCr <10 ml/min, for *nizatidine* if CCr <50 ml/min, for *ranitidine* if CCr <50 ml/min, ranitidine bismuth citrate should not be used if CCr < 25 ml/min) ▪ Pregnancy or lactation.

ADVERSE REACTIONS AND SIDE EFFECTS*

CNS: <u>confusion</u>, dizziness, drowsiness, hallucinations, headache.
CV: ARRHYTHMIAS.
GI: black tongue (ranitidine bismuth citrate only), constipation, dark stools (ranitidine bismuth citrate only), diarrhea, drug-induced hepatitis (nizatidine, cimetidine), nausea.
GU: decreased sperm count, impotence.
Endo: gynecomastia.
Hemat: AGRANULOCYTOSIS, APLASTIC ANEMIA, anemia, neutropenia, thrombocytopenia.
Local: pain at IM site.
Misc: hypersensivity reactions.

INTERACTIONS

Drug-Drug: ▪ Cimetidine inhibits drug-metabolizing enzymes in the liver; may lead to increased blood levels and toxicity with the following—some **benzodiazepines** (especially chlordiazepoxide, diazepam, and midazolam), some **beta blockers** (labetalol, metoprolol, propranolol), **caffeine, calcium channel blockers, carbamazepine, chloroquine, lidocaine, metronidazole, moricizine, pentoxifylline, phenytoin, propafenone, quinidine, quinine, metformin, sulfonylureas, theophylline, triamterene, tricyclic antidepressants**, and **warfarin** ▪ Famotidine, nizatidine, and ranitidine have a much smaller and less significant effect on the metabolism of other drugs ▪ The effects of **succinylcholine, flecainide, procainamide, carmustine,** and **fluorouracil** are increased by cimetidine ▪ All agents decrease the absorption of **ketoconazole** ▪ **Antacids** and **sucralfate** decrease absorption of all agents ▪ **Clarithromycin** increases ranitidine levels.

ROUTE AND DOSAGE

❑ Cimetidine

- **PO (Adults):** *Short-term treatment of active ulcers*—300 mg 4 times daily or 800 mg at bedtime or 400–600 mg twice daily (not to exceed 2.4 g/day). *Duodenal ulcer prophylaxis*—300 mg twice daily or 400 mg at

*CAPITALS indicate life-threatening; <u>underlines</u> indicate most frequent.

bedtime. *GERD*—800–1600 mg/day in divided doses. *Gastric hypersecretory conditions*—300–600 mg q 6 hr (up to 12 g/day have been used). *OTC use*—up to 200 mg may be taken twice daily (not more than 2 wk).

- **PO (Children):** *Short-term treatment of active ulcers*—20–40 mg/kg/day in 4 divided doses (10–15 mg/kg/day if renal function is impaired).
- **IM, IV (Adults):** *Short-term treatment of active ulcers*—300 mg q 6 hr (not to exceed 2.4 g/day). *Continuous IV infusion*—900 mg infused over 24 hr (37.5 mg/hr); may be preceded by a 150-mg bolus dose. *Gastric hypersecretory conditions*—300–600 mg q 6 hr (up to 12 g/day have been used). *Prevention of aspiration pneumonitis*—300 mg IM 1 hr before anesthesia, then 300 mg IV q 4 hr until patient is conscious (unlabeled). *Prevention of upper GI bleeding in critically ill patients*—50 mg/hr (25 mg/hr if CCr <30 ml/min).
- **IM, IV (Children):** *Short-term treatment of active ulcers*—5–10 mg/kg q 6–8 hr.

❑ **Famotidine**

- **PO (Adults):** *Short-term treatment of active ulcers*—40 mg/day at bedtime or 20 mg twice daily for up to 8 wk. *Duodenal ulcer prophylaxis*—20 mg once daily at bedtime. *GERD*—20 mg twice daily for up to 6 wk; up to 40 mg twice daily for up to 12 wk for esophagitis with erosions, ulcerations, and continuing symptoms. *Gastric hypersecretory conditions*—20 mg q 6 hr initially, up to 160 mg q 6 hr. *OTC use*—10 mg for relief of symptoms; for prevention—10 mg 60 min before eating (not to exceed 20 mg/24 hr for up to 2 wk).
- **IV (Adults):** 20 mg q 12 hr.

❑ **Nizatidine**

- **PO (Adults):** *Short-term treatment of active ulcers*—300 mg once daily at bedtime. *Duodenal ulcer prophylaxis*—150 mg once daily at bedtime. *GERD*—150 mg twice daily. *OTC use*—75 mg 30–60 min before foods/beverages expected to cause symptoms.

❑ **Ranitidine**

- **PO (Adults):** *Short-term treatment of active ulcers*—100–150 mg twice daily or 300 mg once daily at bedtime. *Duodenal ulcer prophylaxis*—150 mg once daily at bedtime. *GERD*—150 mg twice daily. *Erosive esophagitis*—150 mg 4 times daily initially, then 150 mg twice daily as maintenance. *Gastric hypersecretory conditions*—150 mg twice daily initially; up to 6 g/day have been used. *OTC use*—75 mg when symptoms occur (up to twice daily).
- **IV, IM (Adults):** 50 mg q 6–8 hr (not to exceed 400 mg/day). *Continuous IV infusion*—6.25 mg/hr. *Gastric hypersecretory conditions* —1 mg/kg/hr; may be increased by 0.5 mg/kg/hr (not to exceed 2.5 mg/kg/hr).

❑ **Ranitidine Bismuth Citrate**

- **PO (Adults):** 400 mg twice daily for 4 wk with clarithromycin 500 mg 3 times daily for first 2 wk.

AVAILABILITY

❑ **Cimetidine**

- ***Tablets:*** 100 mg^{OTC}, 200 mg^{OTC}, 300 mg^{Rx}, 400 mg^{Rx}, {600 mg^{Rx}}, 800 mg^{Rx} ▪ ***Oral liquid:*** 300 mg/5 ml^{Rx} ▪ ***Solution for injection:*** 300 mg/2 ml-vials^{Rx}, 300 mg/50 ml 0.9% NaCl^{Rx}.

❑ **Famotidine**

- ***Tablets:*** 10 mg^{OTC}, 20 mg^{Rx}, 40 mg^{Rx} ▪ ***Oral suspension:*** 40 mg/5 ml^{Rx} ▪ ***Solution for injection:*** 10 mg/ml^{Rx}, 20 mg/50 ml 0.9% NaCl^{Rx}.

❑ **Nizatidine**

- ***Tablets:*** 75 mg^{OTC} ▪ ***Capsules:*** 150 mg^{Rx}, 300 mg^{Rx}

❑ **Ranitidine**

- ***Tablets:*** 75 mg^{OTC}, 150 mg^{Rx}, 300 mg^{Rx} ▪ ***Effervescent tablets (EFFERdose):*** 150 mg^{Rx} ▪ ***Effervescent granules (EFFERdose):*** 150 mg/packet^{Rx} ▪ ***Capsules (GELdose):*** 150 mg^{Rx}, 300 mg^{Rx} ▪ ***Syrup:*** 15 mg/ml^{Rx} ▪ ***Solution for injection:*** 25 mg/ml in 2-, 10-, and 40-ml vials^{Rx}, 50 mg/100-ml containers^{Rx}.

❑ **Ranitidine Bismuth Citrate**

- ***Tablets:*** 400 mg^{Rx}.

TIME/ACTION PROFILE

	ONSET	PEAK	DURATION
Cimetidine PO	30 min	45–90 min	4–5 hr
Cimetidine IM, IV	10 min	30 min	4–5 hr
Famotidine PO	within 60 min	1–4 hr	6–12 hr
Famotidine IV	within 60 min	0.5–3 hr	8–15 hr
Nizatidine PO	UK	UK	8–12 hr
Ranitidine PO	UK	1–3 hr	8–12 hr
Ranitidine IM	UK	15 min	8–12 hr
Ranitidine IV	UK	15 min	8–12 hr

NURSING IMPLICATIONS

ASSESSMENT

- Assess patient for epigastric or abdominal pain and frank or occult blood in the stool, emesis, or gastric aspirate.
- Assess elderly and debilitated patients routinely for confusion. Report promptly.
- ***Lab Test Considerations:*** CBC with differential should be monitored periodically throughout therapy.
- Antagonize effects of pentagastrin and histamine during gastric acid secretion testing. Avoid administration for 24 hr preceding the test.
- May cause false-negative results in skin tests using allergenic extracts. Histamine H_2 antagonists should be discontinued 24 hr prior to the test.
- May cause an increase in serum transaminases and serum creatinine.
- Serum prolactin concentration may be increased following IV bolus of *cimetidine.* May also cause decreased parathyroid concentrations.
- *Nizatidine* may cause elevated alkaline phosphatase concentrations or false-positive tests for urobilinogen.
- *Ranitidine* may cause false-positive results for urine protein; test with sulfosalicylic acid.

POTENTIAL NURSING DIAGNOSES

- Pain (Indications).
- Knowledge deficit, related to medication regimen (Patient/Family Teaching).

IMPLEMENTATION

- **General Info:**
- If antacids or sucralfate used concurrently for relief of pain, avoid administration of antacids within 30 min–1 hr of the histamine H_2 antagonist and take sucralfate 2 hr after histamine H_2 antagonist; may decrease the absorption of histamine H_2 antagonists.
- **PO:** Administer with meals or immediately afterward and at bedtime to prolong effect.
- Doses administered once daily should be administered at bedtime to prolong effect.
- Cimetidine tablets have a characteristic odor.
- Shake oral suspension prior to administration. Discard unused suspension after 30 days.
- Remove foil from *ranitidine effervescent tablets or granules* and dissolve in 6–8 oz water before drinking.

Cimetidine

- **Direct IV:** Dilute each 300 mg in 20 ml of 0.9% NaCl for injection.
- ***Rate:*** Administer over at least 5 min. Rapid administration may cause hypotension and arrhythmias.
- **Intermittent Infusion:** Dilute each 300 mg in 50 ml of 0.9% NaCl, D5W, D10W, D5/LR, D5/0.9% NaCl, D5/0.45% NaCl, D5/0.25% NaCl, Ringer's or lactated Ringer's solution, or sodium bicarbonate. Diluted solution is stable for 48 hr at room temperature. Refrigeration may cause cloudiness but will not affect potency. Do not use solution that is discolored or contains precipitate.
- ***Rate:*** Administer over 15–20 min.
- **Continuous Infusion:** Dilute cimetidine 900 mg in 100–1000 ml of compatible solution (see Intermittent Infusion).
- ***Rate:*** Usually infused at a rate of 37.5 mg/hr or greater but should be individualized.
- **Syringe Compatibility:** ▪ atropine ▪ butorphanol ▪ cephalothin ▪ diazepam ▪ diphenhydramine ▪ doxapram ▪ droperidol ▪ fentanyl ▪ glycopyrrolate ▪ heparin ▪ hydromorphone ▪ hydroxyzine ▪ lorazepam ▪ meperidine ▪ midazolam ▪ morphine ▪ nafcillin ▪ nalbuphine ▪ penicillin G potassium ▪ pentazocine ▪ perphenazine ▪ prochlorperazine ▪ prochlorperazine edisylate ▪ promazine ▪ promethazine ▪ scopolamine ▪ sodium acetate ▪ sodium chloride ▪ sodium lactate ▪ sterile water.
- **Syringe Incompatibility:** ▪ cefamandole ▪ cefazolin ▪ chlorpromazine ▪ indomethacin.
- **Y-Site Compatibility:** ▪ acyclovir ▪ amifostine ▪ aminophylline ▪ amrinone ▪ atracurium ▪ aztreonam ▪ cisplatin ▪ cyclophosphamide ▪ cytarabine ▪ diltiazem ▪ doxorubicin ▪ ena-

laprilat ▪ esmolol ▪ filgrastim ▪ fluconazole ▪ fludarabine ▪ foscarnet ▪ gallium nitrate ▪ granisetron ▪ haloperidol ▪ heparin ▪ hetastarch ▪ idarubicin ▪ labetalol ▪ melphalan ▪ methotrexate ▪ midazolam ▪ ondansetron ▪ paclitaxel ▪ pancuronium ▪ piperacillin/tazobactam ▪ sargramostim ▪ tacrolimus ▪ teniposide ▪ thiotepa ▪ tolazoline ▪ vecuronium ▪ vinorelbine ▪ zidovudine.

- **Y-Site Incompatibility:** ▪ cefepime ▪ indomethacin.

❑ Famotidine

- **Direct IV:** Dilute 2 ml (10 mg/ml solution) in 5 or 10 ml of 0.9% NaCl for injection.
- ***Rate:*** Administer over at least 2 min. Rapid administration may cause hypotension.
- **Intermittent Infusion:** Dilute each 20 mg in 100 ml of 0.9% NaCl, D5W, D10W, or lactated Ringer's solution for a concentration of 0.2 mg/ml. Diluted solution is stable for 48 hr at room temperature. Do not use solution that is discolored or contains a precipitate.
- ***Rate:*** Administer over 15–30 min.
- **Y-Site Compatibility:** ▪ amifostine ▪ aminophylline ▪ ampicillin ▪ ampicillin/sulbactam ▪ amrinone ▪ atropine ▪ aztreonam ▪ bretylium ▪ calcium gluconate ▪ cefazolin ▪ cefoperazone ▪ cefotaxime ▪ cefotetan ▪ cefoxitin ▪ ceftazidime ▪ ceftizoxime ▪ cefuroxime ▪ cephalothin ▪ cephapirin ▪ cisplatin ▪ cyclophosphamide ▪ cytarabine ▪ dexamethasone ▪ dextran 40 ▪ digoxin ▪ dobutamine ▪ dopamine ▪ doxorubicin ▪ enalaprilat ▪ epinephrine ▪ erythromycin lactobionate ▪ esmolol ▪ filgrastim ▪ fluconazole ▪ fludarabine ▪ folic acid ▪ furosemide ▪ gentamicin ▪ haloperidol ▪ heparin ▪ hydrocortisone sodium succinate ▪ imipenem/cilastatin ▪ insulin ▪ isoproterenol ▪ labetalol ▪ lidocaine ▪ magnesium sulfate ▪ melphalan ▪ meperidine ▪ methylprednisolone ▪ metoclopramide ▪ mezlocillin ▪ midazolam ▪ morphine ▪ nafcillin ▪ nitroglycerin ▪ nitroprusside ▪ norepinephrine ▪ ondansetron ▪ oxacillin ▪ paclitaxel ▪ perphenazine ▪ phenylephrine ▪ phenytoin ▪ phytonadione ▪ piperacillin ▪ potassium chloride ▪ potassium phosphate ▪ procainamide ▪ sargramostim ▪ sodium bicarbonate ▪ teniposide ▪ theophylline ▪ thiamine ▪ thiotepa ▪ ticarcillin ▪ ticarcillin/clavulanate ▪ verapamil ▪ vinorelbine.
- **Y-Site Incompatibility:** ▪ cefepime ▪ piperacillin/tazobactam.

❑ Ranitidine

- **Direct IV:** Dilute each 50 mg in 20 ml of 0.9% NaCl or D5W for injection.
- ***Rate:*** Administer over at least 5 min. Rapid administration may cause hypotension and arrhythmias.
- **Intermittent Infusion:** Dilute each 50 mg in 100 ml of 0.9% NaCl or D5W. Diluted solution is stable for 48 hr at room temperature. Do not use solution that is discolored or that contains precipitate.
- ***Rate:*** Administer over 15–20 min.
- **Continuous Infusion:** Add ranitidine to D5W for a concentration of 150 mg/250 ml (no greater than 2.5 mg/ml for Zollinger-Ellison patients).
- ***Rate:*** Administer at a rate of 6.25 mg/hr. In patients with Zollinger-Ellison syndrome, start infusion at 1 mg/kg/hr. If gastric acid output is >10 mEq/hr or patient becomes symptomatic after 4 hr, adjust dose by 0.5 mg/kg/hr increments and remeasure gastric output.
- **Syringe Compatibility:** ▪ atropine ▪ cyclizine ▪ dexamethasone ▪ dimenhydrinate ▪ diphenhydramine ▪ fentanyl ▪ glycopyrrolate ▪ hydromorphone ▪ meperidine ▪ metoclopramide ▪ morphine ▪ nalbuphine ▪ oxymorphone ▪ pentazocine ▪ perphenazine ▪ prochlorperazine ▪ promethazine ▪ scopolamine ▪ thiethylperazine.
- **Syringe Incompatibility:** ▪ hydroxyzine ▪ methotrimeprazine ▪ midazolam ▪ pentobarbital ▪ phenobarbital.
- **Y-Site Compatibility:** ▪ acyclovir ▪ aldesleukin ▪ amifostine ▪ aminophylline ▪ atracurium ▪ aztreonam ▪ bretylium ▪ cefepime ▪ cefmetazole ▪ ceftazidime ▪ ciprofloxacin ▪ cisplatin ▪ cyclophosphamide ▪ cytarabine ▪ diltiazem ▪ dobutamine ▪ dopamine ▪ doxorubicin ▪ enalaprilat ▪ esmolol ▪ filgrastim ▪ fluconazole ▪ fludarabine ▪ foscarnet ▪ gallium nitrate ▪ heparin ▪ idarubicin ▪ labetalol ▪ lorazepam ▪ melphalan ▪ meperidine ▪ methotrexate ▪ midazolam ▪ morphine ▪ nitroglycerin ▪ ondansetron ▪ paclitaxel ▪ pancuronium ▪ piperacillin ▪ piperacillin/tazobactam ▪ procainamide ▪ sargramostim ▪ tacrolimus ▪ teniposide ▪ thiotepa ▪ vecuronium ▪ vinorelbine ▪ zidovudine.
- **Additive Compatibility:** ▪ amikacin ▪ chlor-

H

amphenicol ▪ doxycycline ▪ furosemide ▪ gentamicin ▪ heparin ▪ lidocaine ▪ penicillin G sodium ▪ potassium chloride ▪ ticarcillin ▪ tobramycin ▪ vancomycin.

- **Additive Incompatibility:** ▪ amphotericin B ▪ clindamycin.

PATIENT/FAMILY TEACHING

- **General Info:** Instruct patient to take medication as directed for the full course of therapy, even if feeling better. If a dose is missed, it should be taken as soon as remembered but not if almost time for next dose. Do not double doses.
  - Advise patients taking OTC preparations not to take the maximum dose continuously for more than 2 wk without consulting health care professional. Notify health care professional if difficulty swallowing occurs or abdominal pain persists.
  - Inform patient that smoking interferes with the action of histamine antagonists. Encourage patient to quit smoking or at least not to smoke after last dose of the day.
  - May cause drowsiness or dizziness. Caution patient to avoid driving or other activities requiring alertness until response to the drug is known.
  - Advise patient to avoid alcohol, products containing aspirin or NSAIDs, and foods that may cause an increase in GI irritation.
  - Inform patient that increased fluid and fiber intake and exercise may minimize constipation.
  - Advise patient to report onset of black, tarry stools; fever; sore throat; diarrhea; dizziness; rash; confusion; or hallucinations to health care professional promptly.
- **Ranitidine bismuth citrate:** Inform patient that medication may temporarily cause stools and tongue to appear gray-black.

EVALUATION

Effectiveness of therapy can be demonstrated by: ▪ Decrease in abdominal pain ▪ Prevention of gastric irritation and bleeding. Healing of duodenal ulcers can be seen by x rays or endoscopy. Therapy is continued for at least 6 wk in treatment of ulcers but not usually longer than 8 wk ▪ Decreased symptoms of esophageal reflux ▪ Eradication of *Helicobacter pylori* in the treatment of duodenal ulcers.

HMG-CoA REDUCTASE INHIBITORS

atorvastatin
(a-**tore**-va-stat-in)
Lipitor

cerivastatin
(ser-**ee**-va-stat-in)
Baycol

fluvastatin
(**floo**-va-sta-tin)
Lescol

lovastatin
(**loe**-va-sta-tin)
Mevacor

pravastatin
(**pra**-va-sta-tin)
Pravachol

simvastatin
(**sim**-va-sta-tin)
Zocor

CLASSIFICATION(S):
Lipid-lowering agents

Pregnancy Category X

INDICATIONS

▪ Adjunct to dietary therapy in the management of primary hypercholesterolemia and mixed dyslipidemias ▪ Reduction of lipids/cholesterol reduces the risk of myocardial infarction and stroke sequelae.

ACTION

▪ Inhibit an enzyme, 3-hydroxy-3-methylglutaryl-coenzyme A (HMG-CoA) reductase, which is responsible for catalyzing an early step in the synthesis of cholesterol. **Therapeutic Effects:** ▪ Lowering of total and LDL cholesterol. Slightly increase HDL and decrease VLDL cholesterol and triglycerides ▪ Slowing of the progression of coronary artery disease with resultant decrease in myocardial infarction and need for myocardial revascularization.

PHARMACOKINETICS

Absorption: *Atorvastatin*—rapidly absorbed but undergoes extensive gastrointestinal and hepatic metabolism resulting in 14% bioavailability (30% for lipid-lowering activity); *cerivastatin*—60% absorbed following oral administration; *fluvastatin*—98% absorbed following oral administration; *lovastatin, pravastatin*—poorly and variably absorbed following oral administration; *simvastatin*—85% but rapidly metabolized.

Distribution: *Atorvastatin*—probably enters breast milk. *Cerivastatin and fluvastatin*—enter breast milk. *Lovastatin*—crosses the blood-brain barrier and placenta. *Pravastatin*—enters hepatocytes, where action occurs; small amounts enter breast milk.

Metabolism and Excretion: All agents are extensively metabolized by the liver, most during first pass; excreted in bile and feces. Small amounts (*atorvastatin*—<2%; *cerivastatin*—2%; *fluvastatin*—5%; *pravastatin*—20%; *lovastatin*—10%; *simvastatin*—13%) excreted unchanged by the kidneys. *Atorvastatin*—has 2 lipid-lowering metabolites.

Half-life: *Atorvastatin*—14 hr (lipid-lowering activity due to atorvastatin and its metabolites—20–30 hr; *cerivastatin*—2–3 hr; *fluvastatin*—1.2 hr; *lovastatin*—3 hr; *pravastatin*—1.3–2.7 hr; *simvastatin*—UK.

CONTRAINDICATIONS AND PRECAUTIONS

Contraindicated in: ▪ Hypersensitivity ▪ Cross-sensitivity among agents may occur ▪ Active liver disease ▪ Pregnancy or lactation ▪ Concurrent use of mibefradil (lovastatin and simvastatin only).

Use Cautiously in: ▪ History of liver disease ▪ Alcoholism ▪ Renal impairment (dosage reduction of cerivastatin recommended if CCr <60 ml/min) ▪ Severe acute infection ▪ Hypotension ▪ Major surgery ▪ Trauma ▪ Severe metabolic, endocrine, or electrolyte problems ▪ Uncontrolled seizures ▪ Visual disturbances ▪ Myopathy ▪ Children <18 yr (safety not established) ▪ Women of childbearing age.

ADVERSE REACTIONS AND SIDE EFFECTS*

CNS: dizziness, headache, insomnia, weakness.
EENT: *lovastatin*—blurred vision.
GI: abdominal cramps, constipation, diarrhea, flatus, heartburn, altered taste, drug-induced hepatitis, dyspepsia, elevated liver enzymes, nausea, pancreatitis.
GU: impotence.
Derm: rashes, pruritus.
MS: RHABDOMYOLYSIS, arthralgia, myalgia, myositis.
Misc: hypersensitivity reactions.

INTERACTIONS

Drug-Drug: ▪ Cholesterol-lowering effect may be additive with **bile acid sequestrants (cholestyramine, colestipol)** ▪ Bioavailability may be decreased by **bile acid sequestrants** ▪ Risk of myopathy is increased by concurrent **cyclosporine, gemfibrozil, clofibrate, erythromycin,** large doses of **niacin, mibefradil,** and **azole antifungals** (combined use with clofibrate, mibefradil, or gemfibrozil not recommended) ▪ Atorvastatin and simvastatin may slightly increase serum **digoxin** levels ▪ **Mibefradil** increases the risk of myopathy (lovastatin and simvatatin are contraindicated; atorvastatin and cerivastatin should be discouraged) ▪ Atorvastatin may increase levels of **oral contraceptives** ▪ May increase effects of **warfarin** ▪ Levels may be significantly increased by **azole antifungals** (temporarily discontinue HMG-CoA reductase inhibitor) ▪ Levels of cerivastatin are increased by **erythromycin** ▪ **Alcohol** decreases fluvastatin levels ▪ **Isradipine** may decrease the effectiveness of lovastatin ▪ **Digoxin, propranolol,** and **nicotinic acid** may decrease the effectiveness of fluvastatin.

Drug-Food: ▪ Food enhances blood levels of lovastatin.

ROUTE AND DOSAGE

❑ Atorvastatin

- **PO (Adults):** 10 mg once daily initially; may be increased q 2–4 wk up to 80 mg/day.

❑ Cerivastatin

- **PO (Adults):** 0.3 mg once daily in the evening; 0.2 mg for patients with decreased renal function.

❑ Fluvastatin

- **PO (Adults):** 20 mg once daily at bedtime; may be increased to 40 mg once daily or 20 mg twice daily.

***CAPITALS indicate life-threatening; underlines indicate most frequent.**

H

❑ **Lovastatin**

- **PO (Adults):** 20 mg once daily with evening meal. Increase at 4-wk intervals to a maximum of 80 mg/day in single or divided doses.

❑ **Pravastatin**

- **PO (Adults):** 10–20 mg once daily at bedtime.

❑ **Simvastatin**

- **PO (Adults):** 5–10 mg once daily in the evening. *Elderly patients, patients with LDL <190 mg/dl, or patients receiving cyclosporine*—5 mg/day initially. Increase at 4-wk intervals (not to exceed 10 mg/day in patients receiving cyclosporine).

AVAILABILITY

❑ **Atorvastatin**

- ***Tablets:*** 10 mg[Rx], 20 mg[Rx], 40 mg[Rx].

❑ **Cerivastatin**

- ***Tablets:*** 0.2 mg[Rx], 0.3 mg[Rx].

❑ **Fluvastatin**

- ***Capsules:*** 20 mg[Rx], 40 mg[Rx].

❑ **Lovastatin**

- ***Tablets:*** 10 mg[Rx], 20 mg[Rx], 40 mg[Rx].

❑ **Pravastatin**

- ***Tablets:*** 10 mg[Rx], 20 mg[Rx], 40 mg[Rx].

❑ **Simvastatin**

- ***Tablets:*** 5 mg[Rx], 10 mg[Rx], 20 mg[Rx], 40 mg[Rx].

TIME/ACTION PROFILE (cholesterol-lowering effect)

	ONSET	PEAK	DURATION
Atorvastatin	UK	UK	20–30 hr
Cerivastatin	UK	4 wk	UK
Fluvastatin	1–2 wk	4–6 wk	UK
Lovastatin	2 wk	4–6 wk	6 wk*
Pravastatin	UK	UK	UK
Simvastatin	UK	UK	UK

*Following discontinuation.

NURSING IMPLICATIONS

ASSESSMENT

- ❑ Obtain a diet history, especially with regard to fat consumption.
- ❑ Ophthalmic exams are recommended prior to and yearly throughout therapy.
- ***Lab Test Considerations:*** Serum cholesterol and triglyceride levels should be evaluated before initiating, after 4–6 wk of therapy, and periodically thereafter.
- ❑ Liver function tests, including AST, should be monitored prior to, at 6–12 wk after initiation of therapy or after dose elevation, and then every 6 mo. If AST levels increase to 3 times normal, HMG-CoA reductase inhibitor therapy should be discontinued. May also cause elevated alkaline phosphatase and bilirubin levels.
- ❑ If patient develops muscle tenderness during therapy, CK levels should be monitored. If CK levels are markedly increased or myopathy occurs, therapy should be discontinued.
- ❑ May cause thyroid function test abnormalities.

POTENTIAL NURSING DIAGNOSES

- Knowledge deficit, related to diet and medication regimen (Patient/Family Teaching).
- Noncompliance (Patient/Family Teaching).

IMPLEMENTATION

- **PO:** Administer *lovastatin* with food. Administration on an empty stomach decreases absorption by approximately 30%. Initial once-daily dose is administered with the evening meal.
- ❑ Administer *cerivastatin, fluvastatin, pravastatin,* and *simvastatin* once daily in the evening. May be administered without regard to food.
- ❑ If *cerivastatin, fluvastatin,* or *pravastatin* is administered in conjunction with bile acid sequestrants (cholestyramine, colestipol), administer 1 hr before or at least 2 hr *(cerivastatin, fluvastatin)* or 4 hr *(pravastatin)* after bile acid sequestrant.

PATIENT/FAMILY TEACHING

- ❑ Instruct patient to take medication exactly as directed, not to skip doses or double up on missed doses. Medication helps control but does not cure elevated serum cholesterol levels.
- ❑ Advise patient that this medication should be used in conjunction with diet restrictions (fat, cholesterol, carbohydrates, alcohol), exercise, and cessation of smoking.
- ❑ Instruct patient to notify health care professional if unexplained muscle pain, tenderness, or weakness occurs, especially if accompanied by fever or malaise.

- □ Advise patient to wear sunscreen and protective clothing to prevent photosensitivity reactions (rare).
- □ Instruct female patients to notify health care professional promptly if pregnancy is planned or suspected.
- □ Advise patient to notify health care professional of medication regimen prior to treatment or surgery.
- □ Emphasize the importance of follow-up exams to determine effectiveness and to monitor for side effects.

EVALUATION

Effectiveness of therapy can be demonstrated by: ▪ Decrease in serum LDL, VLDL, and total cholesterol levels □ Increase in HDL cholesterol levels □ Decrease in triglyceride levels ▪ Slowing of the progression of coronary artery disease.

HYDRALAZINE

(hyr-**dral**-a-zeen)

Apresoline, {Novo-Hylazin}

CLASSIFICATION(S):

Antihypertensive agent (vasodilator)

Pregnancy Category C

INDICATIONS

▪ Moderate to severe hypertension (with a diuretic). **Unlabeled Uses:** ▪ Congestive heart failure (CHF) unresponsive to conventional therapy with cardiac glycosides and diuretics.

ACTION

▪ Direct-acting peripheral arteriolar vasodilator. **Therapeutic Effects:** ▪ Lowering of blood pressure in hypertensive patients and decreased afterload in patients with CHF.

PHARMACOKINETICS

Absorption: Rapidly absorbed following oral administration; well absorbed from IM sites.
Distribution: Widely distributed. Crosses the placenta; enters breast milk in minimal concentrations.
Metabolism and Excretion: Mostly metabolized by the GI mucosa and liver.
Half-life: 2–8 hr.

CONTRAINDICATIONS AND PRECAUTIONS

Contraindicated in: ▪ Hypersensitivity ▪ Some products contain tartrazine and should be avoided in patients with known intolerance.
Use Cautiously in: ▪ Cardiovascular or cerebrovascular disease ▪ Severe renal and hepatic disease ▪ Pregnancy, lactation, or children (has been used safely during pregnancy).

ADVERSE REACTIONS AND SIDE EFFECTS*

CNS: dizziness, drowsiness, headache.
CV: tachycardia, angina, arrhythmias, edema, orthostatic hypotension.
GI: diarrhea, nausea, vomiting.
Derm: rashes.
F and E: sodium retention.
MS: arthralgias, arthritis.
Neuro: peripheral neuropathy.
Misc: drug-induced lupus syndrome.

INTERACTIONS

Drug-Drug: ▪ Additive hypotension with acute ingestion of **alcohol**, other **antihypertensive agents**, or **nitrates** ▪ **MAO inhibitors** may exaggerate hypotension ▪ May reduce the pressor response to **epinephrine** ▪ **NSAIDs** may decrease antihypertensive response ▪ **Beta-adrenergic blockers** decrease tachycardia from hydralazine (therapy may be combined for this reason) ▪ **Beta-adrenergic blockers** (metoprolol, propranolol) increase hydralazine levels ▪ Increases blood levels of **beta-adrenergic blockers** (metoprolol, propranolol).

ROUTE AND DOSAGE

- **PO (Adults):** *Hypertension*—10 mg 4 times daily initially. After 2–4 days may increase to 25 mg 4 times daily for the rest of the 1st week; may then increase to 50 mg 4 times daily (up to 300 mg/day). Once maintenance dose is established, twice daily dosing may be used. *CHF*—25–37.5 mg 4 times daily; may be increased up to 300 mg/day in 3–4 divided doses.

{} = Available in Canada only.
***CAPITALS indicate life-threatening; underlines indicate most frequent.**

- **PO (Children):** 0.75 mg/kg/day in 4 divided doses; may increase gradually to 7.5 mg/kg/day (200 mg/day) in 4 divided doses.
- **IM, IV (Adults):** *Hypertension*—5–40 mg repeated as needed. *Eclampsia*—5 mg q 15–20 min; if no response after a total of 20 mg, consider an alternative agent.
- **IM, IV (Children):** 1.7–3.5 mg/kg/day in 4–6 divided doses.

AVAILABILITY

▪ ***Tablets:*** 10 mg[Rx], 25 mg[Rx], 50 mg[Rx], 100 mg[Rx] ▪ ***Injection:*** 20 mg/ml[Rx] ▪ ***In combination with:*** hydrochlorothiazide and reserpine[Rx]. See Appendix A.

TIME/ACTION PROFILE (antihypertensive effect)

	ONSET	PEAK	DURATION
PO	45 min	2 hr	3–8 hr
IM	10–30 min	1 hr	3–8 hr
IV	10–20 min	15–30 min	3–8 hr

NURSING IMPLICATIONS

ASSESSMENT

- □ Monitor blood pressure and pulse frequently during initial dosage adjustment and periodically throughout therapy. Report significant changes.
- □ Monitor frequency of prescription refills to determine compliance.
- ▪ ***Lab Test Considerations:*** CBC, electrolytes, LE cell prep, and antinuclear antibody (ANA) titer should be monitored prior to and periodically during prolonged therapy.
- □ May cause a positive direct Coombs' test.

POTENTIAL NURSING DIAGNOSES

- Tissue perfusion, altered (Indications).
- Knowledge deficit, related to medication regimen (Patient/Family Teaching).
- Noncompliance (Patient/Family Teaching).

IMPLEMENTATION

- ▪ **General Info:** IM or IV route should be used only when drug cannot be given orally.
- □ May be administered concurrently with diuretics or beta-adrenergic blocking agents to permit lower doses and minimize side effects.
- ▪ **PO:** Administer with meals consistently to enhance absorption.
- □ Pharmacist may prepare oral solution from hydralazine injection for patients with difficulty swallowing.
- ▪ **Direct IV:** Administer undiluted. Use solution as quickly as possible after drawing through needle into syringe. Hydralazine changes color after contact with a metal filter.
- ▪ ***Rate:*** Administer at a rate of 10 mg over at least 1 min. Monitor blood pressure and pulse frequently after injection.
- ▪ **Y-Site Compatibility:** ▪ heparin ▪ hydrocortisone sodium succinate ▪ potassium chloride ▪ verapamil ▪ vitamin B complex with C.
- ▪ **Y-Site Incompatibility:** ▪ aminophylline ▪ ampicillin ▪ furosemide.
- ▪ **Solution Compatibility:** ▪ dextrose/saline combinations, dextrose/Ringer's solution combinations ▪ D5/LR ▪ D5W ▪ D10W ▪ D10/LR ▪ 0.45% NaCl ▪ 0.09% NaCl ▪ Ringer's or lactated Ringer's solution.

PATIENT/FAMILY TEACHING

- □ Emphasize the importance of continuing to take this medication, even if feeling well. Instruct patient to take medication at the same time each day; last dose of the day should be taken at bedtime. If a dose is missed, take as soon as remembered; do not double doses. If more than 2 doses in a row are missed, consult health care professional. Must be discontinued gradually to avoid sudden increase in blood pressure. Hydralazine controls but does not cure hypertension.
- □ Encourage patient to comply with additional interventions for hypertension (weight reduction, low-sodium diet, smoking cessation, moderation of alcohol intake, regular exercise, and stress management). Instruct patient and family on proper technique for blood pressure monitoring. Advise them to check blood pressure at least weekly and report significant changes.
- □ Patients should weigh themselves twice weekly and assess feet and ankles for fluid retention.
- □ May occasionally cause drowsiness. Advise patient to avoid driving or other activities requiring alertness until response to medication is known.

- Caution patient to avoid sudden changes in position to minimize orthostatic hypotension.
- Advise patient to consult health care professional before taking any cough, cold, or allergy remedies.
- Instruct patient to notify health care professional of medication prior to treatment or surgery.
- Advise patient to notify health care professional immediately if general tiredness; fever; muscle or joint aching; chest pain; skin rash; sore throat; or numbness, tingling, pain, or weakness of hands and feet occurs. Vitamin B_6 (pyridoxine) may be used to treat peripheral neuritis.
- Emphasize the importance of follow-up exams to evaluate effectiveness of medication.

EVALUATION

Effectiveness of therapy can be demonstrated by: ▪ Decrease in blood pressure without appearance of side effects ▪ Decreased afterload in patients with CHF.

HYDROCODONE

(hye-droe-**koe**-done)
Hycodan, {Robidone}, Tussigon
(U.S. antitussive formulations contain homatropine)

HYDROCODONE/ACETAMINOPHEN*
Allay, Anexsia, Anolor DH, Bancap HC, Co-Gesic, Dolacet, Dolagesic, Duocet, Hycomed, Hyco-Pap, Hydrocet, Hydrogesic, Hy-Phen, Lorcet, Lortab, Margesic-H, Oncet, Panacet, Panlor, Polygesic, Stagesic, T-Gesic, Ugesic, Vanacet, Vandone, Vicodin, Zydone

HYDROCODONE/ASPIRIN†
Azdone, Damason-P, Lortab ASA, Panasal

HYDROCODONE/IBUPROFEN‡
Vicoprofen

CLASSIFICATION(S):
Antitussive (opioid), Opioid analgesic (agonist), Opioid analgesic/nonopioid analgesic combination

Schedule III (in combination)
Pregnancy Category C

*For information on acetaminophen component of this formulation, see acetaminophen monograph on page 4.
†For information on aspirin component of this formulation, see salicylates monograph on page 900.
‡For information on ibuprofen component of this formulation, see ibuprofen monograph on page 501.

INDICATIONS

▪ Used mainly in combination with nonopioid analgesics (acetaminophen/aspirin) in the management of moderate to severe pain ▪ Antitussive (usually in combination products with decongestants).

ACTION

▪ Bind to opiate receptors in the CNS. Alter the perception of and response to painful stimuli while producing generalized CNS depression
□ Suppress the cough reflex via a direct central action. **Therapeutic Effects:** ▪ Decrease in severity of moderate pain ▪ Suppression of the cough reflex.

PHARMACOKINETICS

Absorption: Well absorbed following oral administration.
Distribution: UK.
Metabolism and Excretion: Mostly metabolized by the liver.
Half-life: 3.8 hr.

CONTRAINDICATIONS AND PRECAUTIONS

Contraindicated in: ▪ Hypersensitivity to hydrocodone ▪ Hypersensitivity to acetaminophen/aspirin (for combination products) ▪ Aspirin-containing products should be avoided in patients with bleeding disorders or thrombocytopenia ▪ Acetaminophen should be avoided in patients with severe hepatic or renal disease

▪ Pregnancy or lactation (avoid chronic use) ▪ Products containing alcohol, aspartame, saccharin, sugar, or tartrazine (FDC yellow dye #5) should be avoided in patients who have hypersensitivity or intolerance to these compounds.
Use Cautiously in: ▪ Head trauma ▪ Increased intracranial pressure ▪ Severe renal, hepatic, or pulmonary disease ▪ Hypothyroidism ▪ Adrenal insufficiency ▪ Alcoholism ▪ Geriatric or debilitated patients (initial dosage reduction required; more prone to CNS depression, constipation) ▪ Patients with undiagnosed abdominal pain ▪ Prostatic hypertrophy.

ADVERSE REACTIONS AND SIDE EFFECTS*

CNS: confusion, sedation, dysphoria, euphoria, floating feeling, hallucinations, headache, unusual dreams.
EENT: blurred vision, diplopia, miosis.
Resp: respiratory depression.
CV: hypotension, bradycardia.
GI: constipation, nausea, vomiting.
GU: urinary retention.
Derm: sweating.
Misc: physical dependence, psychological dependence, tolerance.

INTERACTIONS

Drug-Drug: ▪ Use with extreme caution in patients receiving **MAO inhibitors** (may produce severe, unpredictable reactions—reduce initial dose of hydrocodone to 25% of usual dose) ▪ Additive CNS depression with **alcohol, antihistamines,** and **sedative/hypnotics** ▪ Administration of **partial antagonist opioids (buprenorphine, butorphanol, nalbuphine,** or **pentazocine)** may precipitate opioid withdrawal in physically dependent patients ▪ **Buprenorphine** or **pentazocine** may decrease analgesia.

ROUTE AND DOSAGE

❑ Hydrocodone

- **PO (Adults):** *Analgesic*—5–10 mg q 4–6 hr as needed. *Antitussive*—5 mg q 4–6 hr as needed.
- **PO (Children):** *Analgesic*—0.2 mg/kg q 3–4 hr.

❑ Hydrocodone/Acetaminophen

- **PO (Adults):** *Tablets containing 2.5 mg hydrocodone/500 mg acetaminophen*—1–2 tablets q 4–6 hr. *Tablets/capsules containing 5 mg hydrocodone/500 mg acetaminophen*—1 tablet/capsule q 4–6 hr; may be increased to 2 q 6 hr. *Tablets containing 7.5 mg hydrocodone/650 mg acetaminophen*—1 tablet q 4–6 hr; may be increased to 2 q 6 hr. *Tablets containing 7.5 mg hydrocodone/750 mg acetaminophen*—1 tablet q 4–6 hr. *Tablets containing 10 mg hydrocodone/650 mg acetaminophen*—1 tablet q 4–6 hr. *Oral solution containing 2.5 mg hydrocodone plus 167 mg acetaminophen/5 ml*—15 ml q 4–6 hr; not to exceed 4 g acetaminophen/day.

❑ Hydrocodone/Aspirin

- **PO (Adults):** *Tablets containing 5 mg hydrocodone/500 mg aspirin*—1–2 tablets q 4–6 hr; not to exceed 4 g/day).

❑ Hydrocodone/Ibuprofen

- **PO (Adults):** *75 mg hydrocodone/200 mg ibuprofen (Vicoprofen) tablets*—1 tablet q 4–6 hr (initial) dosage not to exceed 5 tablets/24 hr.

AVAILABILITY

❑ Hydrocodone

▪ ***Hydrocodone tablets:*** {5 mg (Hycodan)Rx} ▪ ***Hydrocodone syrup:*** {5 mg/ml (Hycodan, Robidone)Rx}.

❑ Hydrocodone/Acetaminophen

▪ ***Tablets:*** 2.5 mg hydrocodone/500 mg acetaminophen (Lortab 2.5/500)Rx, 5 mg hydrocodone/500 mg acetaminophen (Anexsia 5/500, Co-Gesic, Dolacet, Hy-Phen, Lorcet, Lortab 5/500, Panacet 5/500, Vicodin)Rx, 7.5 mg hydrocodone/500 mg acetaminophen (Lortab 7.5/500Rx), 7.5 mg hydrocodone/650 mg acetaminophen (Anexsia 7.5/650, Lorcet PlusRx), 7.5 mg hydrocodone/750 mg acetaminophen (Vicodin ES)Rx, 10 mg hydrocodone/650 mg acetaminophen (Lorcet 10/650)Rx ▪ ***Capsules:*** 5 mg hydrocodone/500 mg acetaminophen (Allay, Anałor DH 5, Bancap-HC, Dolacet, Dolagesic, Hycomed, Hyco-Pap, Hydrocet, Hydrogesic, Lorcet-HD, Margesic-H, Panlor, Polygesic, Stagesic,

*CAPITALS indicate life-threatening; underlines indicate most frequent.

T-Gesic, Ugesic, Vendone, Zydone)[Rx] ▪ ***Elixir:*** 2.5 mg hydrocodone plus 167 mg acetaminophen/5 ml (Lortab elixir)[Rx].

❑ **Hydrocodone/Aspirin**

▪ ***Tablets:*** 5 mg hydrocodone/500 mg aspirin (Azdone, Damason-P, Lortab ASA, Panasal 5/500)[Rx] ▪ ***In combination with:*** antihistamines, caffeine, guaifenesin, decongestants[Rx]. See Appendix A.

❑ **Hydrocodone/Ibuprofen**

▪ ***Tablets:*** 7.5 mg hydrocodone/200 mg ibuprofen[Rx].

TIME/ACTION PROFILE (analgesic effect)

	ONSET	PEAK	DURATION
PO	10–30 min	30–60 min	4–6 hr

NURSING IMPLICATIONS

ASSESSMENT

- **General Info:** Assess blood pressure, pulse, and respirations before and periodically during administration. If respiratory rate is <10/min, assess level of sedation. Physical stimulation may be sufficient to prevent significant hypoventilation. Dose may need to be decreased by 25–50%. Initial drowsiness will diminish with continued use.
- ❑ Assess bowel function routinely. Prevention of constipation should be instituted with increased intake of fluids and bulk, and laxatives to minimize constipating effects. Stimulant laxatives should be administered routinely if opioid use exceeds 2–3 days, unless contraindicated.
- **Pain:** Assess type, location, and intensity of pain prior to and 1 hr (peak) following administration. When titrating opioid doses, increases of 25–50% should be administered until there is either a 50% reduction in the patient's pain rating on a numerical or visual analogue scale or the patient reports satisfactory pain relief. A repeat dose can be safely administered at the time of the peak if previous dose is ineffective and side effects are minimal.
- ❑ An equianalgesic chart (see Appendix B) should be used when changing routes or when changing from one opioid to another.
- ❑ Prolonged use may lead to physical and psychological dependence and tolerance. This should not prevent patient from receiving adequate analgesia. Most patients who receive opioids for pain do not develop psychological dependence. If progressively higher doses are required, consider conversion to a stronger opioid.
- **Cough:** Assess cough and lung sounds during antitussive use.
- ***Lab Test Considerations:*** May cause increased plasma amylase and lipase concentrations.
- ***Toxicity and Overdose:*** If an opioid antagonist is required to reverse respiratory depression or coma, naloxone (Narcan) is the antidote. Dilute the 0.4-mg ampule of naloxone in 10 ml of 0.9% NaCl and administer 0.5 ml (0.02 mg) by direct IV push every 2 min. For children and patients weighing <40 kg, dilute 0.1 mg of naloxone in 10 ml of 0.9% NaCl for a concentration of 10 mcg/ml and administer 0.5 mcg/kg every 1–2 min. Titrate dose to avoid withdrawal, seizures, and severe pain.

POTENTIAL NURSING DIAGNOSES

- Pain (Indications).
- Sensory-perceptual alterations: visual, auditory (Side Effects).
- Injury, risk for (Side Effects).

IMPLEMENTATION

- Explain therapeutic value of medication prior to administration to enhance the analgesic effect.
- ❑ Regularly administered doses may be more effective than prn administration. Analgesic is more effective if given before pain becomes severe.
- ❑ Combination with nonopioid analgesics may have additive analgesic effects and permit lower doses. Maximum doses of nonopioid agents limit the titration of hydrocodone doses.
- ❑ Medication should be discontinued gradually after long-term use to prevent withdrawal symptoms.
- **PO:** May be administered with food or milk to minimize GI irritation.

PATIENT/FAMILY TEACHING

- ❑ Advise patient to take medication exactly as directed and not to take more than the recommended amount. Severe and permanent liver damage may result from prolonged use or high doses of acetaminophen. Renal damage may occur with prolonged use of acetaminophen or aspirin. Doses of nonopioid agents should not exceed the maximum recommended daily dose.

- ☐ Instruct patient on how and when to ask for pain medication.
- ☐ May cause drowsiness or dizziness. Advise patient to call for assistance when ambulating or smoking. Caution patient to avoid driving or other activities requiring alertness until response to the medication is known.
- ☐ Advise patient to change positions slowly to minimize orthostatic hypotension.
- ☐ Caution patient to avoid concurrent use of alcohol or other CNS depressants with this medication.
- ☐ Encourage patient to turn, cough, and breathe deeply every 2 hr to prevent atelectasis.
- ☐ Advise patient that good oral hygiene, frequent mouth rinses, and sugarless gum or candy may decrease dry mouth.

EVALUATION

Effectiveness of therapy can be demonstrated by: ▪ Decrease in severity of pain without a significant alteration in level of consciousness or respiratory status ▪ Suppression of nonproductive cough.

HYDROMORPHONE

(hye-droe-**mor**-fone)
dihydromorphinone, Dilaudid, Dilaudid-HP, Hydrostat IR, PMS Hydromorphone

CLASSIFICATION(S):
Antitussive, Opioid analgesic (agonist)

Schedule II
Pregnancy Category C

INDICATIONS

▪ Moderate to severe pain (alone and in combination with nonopioid analgesics) ▪ Antitussive (lower doses).

ACTION

▪ Binds to opiate receptors in the CNS ▪ Alters the perception of and response to painful stimuli while producing generalized CNS depression ▪ Suppresses the cough reflex via a direct central action. **Therapeutic Effects:** ▪ Decrease in moderate to severe pain ▪ Suppression of cough.

PHARMACOKINETICS

Absorption: Well absorbed following oral, rectal, SC, and IM administration.
Distribution: Widely distributed. Crosses the placenta; enters breast milk.
Metabolism and Excretion: Mostly metabolized by the liver.
Half-life: 2–4 hr.

CONTRAINDICATIONS AND PRECAUTIONS

Contraindicated in: ▪ Hypersensitivity ▪ Avoid chronic use during pregnancy or lactation.
Use Cautiously in: ▪ Head trauma ▪ Increased intracranial pressure ▪ Severe renal, hepatic, or pulmonary disease ▪ Hypothyroidism ▪ Adrenal insufficiency ▪ Alcoholism ▪ Geriatric or debilitated patients (dosage reduction recommended) ▪ Undiagnosed abdominal pain ▪ Prostatic hypertrophy.

ADVERSE REACTIONS AND SIDE EFFECTS*

CNS: <u>confusion</u>, <u>sedation</u>, dizziness, dysphoria, euphoria, floating feeling, hallucinations, headache, unusual dreams.
EENT: blurred vision, diplopia, miosis.
Resp: respiratory depression.
CV: <u>hypotension</u>, bradycardia.
GI: <u>constipation</u>, nausea, vomiting.
GU: urinary retention.
Derm: flushing, sweating.
Misc: physical dependence, psychological dependence, tolerance.

INTERACTIONS

Drug-Drug: ▪ Exercise extreme caution with **MAO inhibitors** (may produce severe, unpredictable reactions—reduce initial dose of hydromorphone to 25% of usual dose) ▪ Additive CNS depression with **alcohol, antidepressants, antihistamines,** and **sedative/hypnot-**

***CAPITALS indicate life-threatening; <u>underlines</u> indicate most frequent.**

ics ▪ Administration of **partial antagonists (buprenorphine, butorphanol, dezocine, nalbuphine,** or **pentazocine)** may precipitate opioid withdrawal in physically dependent patients ▪ **Nalbuphine** or **pentazocine** may decrease analgesia.

ROUTE AND DOSAGE

Doses depend on level of pain and tolerance.

❑ **Analgesic**

- **PO (Adults ≥50 kg):** 6 mg q 3–4 hr initially.
- **PO (Adults <50 kg):** 0.06 mg/kg q 3–4 hr initially.
- **IV, IM, SC (Adults ≥50 kg):** 1.5 mg q 3–4 hr as needed initially; may be increased.
- **IV, IM, SC (Adults <50 kg):** 0.015 mg/kg mg q 3–4 hr as needed initially; may be increased.
- **IV (Adults):** *Continuous infusion (unlabeled)*—0.2–30 mg/hr depending on previous opioid use. An initial bolus of twice the hourly rate in mg may be given with subsequent "breakthrough" boluses of 50–100% of the hourly rate in mg.
- **Rect (Adults):** 3 mg q 4–8 hr initially as needed.

❑ **Antitussive**

- **PO (Adults):** 1 mg q 3–4 hr.
- **PO (Children 6–12 yr):** 0.5 mg q 3–4 hr.

AVAILABILITY

▪ ***Tablets:*** 1 mg[Rx], 2 mg[Rx], 3 mg[Rx], 4 mg[Rx], 8 mg[Rx] ▪ ***Oral solution:*** 5 mg/5 ml[Rx] ▪ ***Injection:*** 1 mg/ml[Rx], 2 mg/ml[Rx], 3 mg/ml[Rx], 4 mg/ml[Rx], 10 mg/ml[Rx] ▪ ***Suppositories:*** 3 mg[Rx] ▪ ***In combination with:*** guaifenesin and alcohol (Dilaudid Cough Syrup)[Rx]. See Appendix A.

TIME/ACTION PROFILE (analgesic effect)

	ONSET	PEAK	DURATION
PO	30 min	90–120 min	4 hr
SC	15 min	30–90 min	4–5 hr
IM	15 min	30–60 min	4–5 hr
IV	10–15 min	15–30 min	2–3 hr
Rect	15–30 min	30–90 min	4–5 hr

NURSING IMPLICATIONS

ASSESSMENT

- **General Info:** Assess blood pressure, pulse, and respirations before and periodically during administration. If respiratory rate is <10/min, assess level of sedation. Dose may need to be decreased by 25–50%. Initial drowsiness will diminish with continued use.
  - ▫ Assess bowel function routinely. Prevention of constipation should be instituted with increased intake of fluids and bulk, and laxatives to minimize constipating effects. Stimulant laxatives should be administered routinely if opioid use exceeds 2–3 days, unless contraindicated.
- **Pain:** Assess type, location, and intensity of pain prior to and 1 hr following IM and 5 min (peak) following IV administration. When titrating opioid doses, increases of 25–50% should be administered until there is either a 50% reduction in the patient's pain rating on a numerical or visual analogue scale or the patient reports satisfactory pain relief. A repeat dose can be safely administered at the time of the peak if previous dose is ineffective and side effects are minimal.
  - ▫ Patients on a continuous infusion should have additional bolus doses provided every 15–30 min, as needed, for breakthrough pain. The bolus dose is usually set to the amount of drug infused each hour by continuous infusion.
  - ▫ An equianalgesic chart (see Appendix B) should be used when changing routes or when changing from one opioid to another.
  - ▫ Prolonged use may lead to physical and psychological dependence and tolerance. This should not prevent patient from receiving adequate analgesia. Most patients who receive hydromorphone for pain do not develop psychological dependence. Progressively higher doses may be required to relieve pain with long-term therapy.
- **Cough:** Assess cough and lung sounds during antitussive use.
- ***Lab Test Considerations:*** May increase plasma amylase and lipase concentrations.
- ***Toxicity and Overdose:*** If an opioid antagonist is required to reverse respiratory depression or coma, naloxone (Narcan) is the antidote. Dilute the 0.4-mg ampule of naloxone in 10 ml of 0.9% NaCl and administer 0.5 ml (0.02 mg) by direct IV push every 2 min. For children and patients weighing <40 kg, dilute 0.1 mg of naloxone in 10 ml of 0.9% NaCl for a concentration of 10 mcg/ml and

H

administer 0.5 mcg every 2 min. Titrate dose to avoid withdrawal, seizures, and severe pain.

POTENTIAL NURSING DIAGNOSES

- Pain (Indications).
- Sensory-perceptual alterations: visual, auditory (Side Effects).
- Injury, risk for (Side Effects).

IMPLEMENTATION

- **General Info:** Do not confuse with meperidine or morphine; fatalities have occurred.
- □ Explain therapeutic value of medication prior to administration to enhance the analgesic effect.
- □ Regularly administered doses may be more effective than prn administration. Analgesic is more effective if given before pain becomes severe.
- □ Coadministration with nonopioid analgesics may have additive analgesic effects and permit lower opioid doses.
- □ Medication should be discontinued gradually after long-term use to prevent withdrawal symptoms.
- **PO:** May be administered with food or milk to minimize GI irritation.
- **Direct IV:** Dilute with at least 5 ml of sterile water or 0.9% NaCl for injection. Inspect solution for particulate matter. Slight yellow color does not alter potency. Store at room temperature.
- ***Rate:*** Administer slowly, at a rate not to exceed 2 mg over 3–5 min. Rapid administration may lead to increased respiratory depression, hypotension, and circulatory collapse.
- **Syringe Compatibility:** ▪ atropine ▪ chlorpromazine ▪ cimetidine ▪ diphenhydramine ▪ fentanyl ▪ glycopyrrolate ▪ hydroxyzine ▪ lorazepam ▪ midazolam ▪ pentobarbital ▪ promethazine ▪ ranitidine ▪ scopolamine ▪ teniposide ▪ thiethylperazine ▪ trimethobenzamide.
- **Y-Site Compatibility:** ▪ acyclovir ▪ amifostine ▪ amikacin ▪ aztreonam ▪ cefamandole ▪ cefepime ▪ cefoperazone ▪ cefotaxime ▪ cefoxitin ▪ ceftazidime ▪ ceftizoxime ▪ cefuroxime ▪ cephalothin ▪ cephapirin ▪ chloramphenicol ▪ cisplatin ▪ clindamycin ▪ cyclophosphamide ▪ cytarabine ▪ doxorubicin ▪ doxycycline ▪ erythromycin lactobionate ▪ filgrastim ▪ fludarabine ▪ foscarnet ▪ gentamicin ▪ granisetron ▪ kanamycin ▪ magnesium sulfate ▪ melphalan ▪ methotrexate ▪ metronidazole ▪ mezlocillin ▪ nafcillin ▪ ondansetron ▪ oxacillin ▪ paclitaxel ▪ penicillin G potassium ▪ piperacillin ▪ piperacillin/tazobactam ▪ thiotepa ▪ ticarcillin ▪ tobramycin ▪ trimethoprim/sulfamethoxazole ▪ vancomycin ▪ vinorelbine.
- **Y-Site Incompatibility:** ▪ diazepam ▪ gallium nitrate ▪ minocycline ▪ phenobarbital ▪ phenytoin ▪ sargramostim.
- **Additive Compatibility:** ▪ ondansetron.
- **Additive Incompatibility:** ▪ sodium bicarbonate ▪ thiopental.
- **Solution Compatibility:** ▪ D5W ▪ D5/0.45% NaCl ▪ D5/0.9% NaCl ▪ D5/LR ▪ D5/Ringer's solution ▪ 0.45% NaCl ▪ 0.9% NaCl ▪ Ringer's and lactated Ringer's solution.

PATIENT/FAMILY TEACHING

- □ Instruct patient on how and when to ask for pain medication.
- □ May cause drowsiness or dizziness. Advise patient to call for assistance when ambulating or smoking. Caution patient to avoid driving or other activities requiring alertness until response to medication is known.
- □ Advise patient to change positions slowly to minimize orthostatic hypotension.
- □ Instruct patient to avoid concurrent use of alcohol or other CNS depressants.
- □ Encourage patient to turn, cough, and breathe deeply every 2 hr to prevent atelectasis.

EVALUATION

Effectiveness of therapy can be demonstrated by: ▪ Decrease in severity of pain without a significant alteration in level of consciousness or respiratory status ▪ Suppression of cough.

HYDROXYCHLOROQUINE

(hye-drox-ee-**klor**-oh-kwin)
Plaquenil

CLASSIFICATION(S):
Antiarthritic, Antimalarial

Pregnancy Category C

INDICATIONS

- Suppression/chemoprophylaxis of malaria
- Treatment of severe rheumatoid arthritis/systemic lupus erythematosus.

ACTION

- Inhibits protein synthesis in susceptible organisms by inhibiting DNA and RNA polymerase.

Therapeutic Effects: ■ Death of plasmodia responsible for causing malaria ■ Also has anti-inflammatory properties.

PHARMACOKINETICS

Absorption: Appears to be well absorbed following oral administration.
Distribution: Appears to be widely distributed; high tissue concentrations achieved (especially liver). Probably enters breast milk.
Metabolism and Excretion: Partially metabolized by the liver; partially excreted unchanged by the kidneys.
Half-life: 72–120 hr.

CONTRAINDICATIONS AND PRECAUTIONS

Contraindicated in: ■ Hypersensitivity to hydroxychloroquine or chloroquine ■ Previous visual damage from hydroxychloroquine or chloroquine.
Use Cautiously in: ■ Concurrent use of hepatotoxic drugs ■ History of liver disease or alcoholism ■ G6PD deficiency ■ Psoriasis ■ Bone marrow depression ■ Obesity (determine dose by ideal body weight) ■ Pregnancy or lactation (avoid use unless treating/preventing malaria or treating amebic abscess).

ADVERSE REACTIONS AND SIDE EFFECTS*

CNS: SEIZURES, aggressiveness, anxiety, apathy, confusion, fatigue, headache, irritability, personality changes, psychoses.
EENT: keratopathy, ototoxicity, retinopathy, tinnitus, visual disturbances.
CV: ECG changes, hypotension.
GI: abdominal cramps, anorexia, diarrhea, epigastric discomfort, nausea, vomiting.
Derm: dermatoses.
Hemat: AGRANULOCYTOSIS, APLASTIC ANEMIA, leukopenia, thrombocytopenia.
Neuro: neuromyopathy, peripheral neuritis.

INTERACTIONS

Drug-Drug: ■ May increase the risk of hepatotoxicity when administered with **hepatotoxic drugs** ■ May increase the risk of hematologic toxicity when administered with **penicillamine** ■ May increase risk of dermatitis when administered with other **agents having dermatologic toxicity** ■ May decrease serum titers of rabies antibody when given concurrently with **human diploid cell rabies vaccine** ■ **Urinary acidifiers** may increase renal excretion ■ May increase serum levels of **digoxin.**

ROUTE AND DOSAGE

Antimalarial doses expressed as mg of base; antirheumatic doses expressed as mg of hydroxychloroquine sulfate (200 mg hydroxychloroquine sulfate = 155 mg of hydroxychloroquine base).

❑ Malaria

- **PO (Adults):** *Suppression or chemoprophylaxis*—310 mg once weekly; start 1–2 wk prior to entering malarious area; continue for 4 wk after leaving area. *Treatment*—620 mg, then 310 mg at 6 hr, 24 hr, and 48 hr after initial dose.
- **PO (Children):** *Suppression or chemoprophylaxis*—5 mg/kg once weekly; start 1–2 wk prior to entering malarious area; continue for 4 wk after leaving area. *Treatment*—10 mg/kg initially, then 5 mg/kg at 6 hr, 24 hr, and 48 hr after initial dose.

❑ Rheumatoid Arthritis

- **PO (Adults):** 400–600 mg/day initially, maintenance 200–400 mg/day.
- **PO (Children):** 3–5 mg/kg/day (not to exceed 7 mg/kg/day or 400 mg).

❑ Systemic Lupus Erythematosus

- **PO (Adults):** 400 mg 1–2 times daily initially; maintenance 200–400 mg/day.

AVAILABILITY

- ***Tablets:*** 200 mg (155-mg base)[Rx].

H

*CAPITALS indicate life-threatening; underlines indicate most frequent.

TIME/ACTION PROFILE (blood levels)

	ONSET	PEAK	DURATION
PO	rapid*	1–2 hr	days–wk

*Onset of antirheumatic action may take 6 wk.

NURSING IMPLICATIONS

ASSESSMENT

- **General Info:** Assess deep tendon reflexes periodically to determine muscle weakness. Therapy may be discontinued should this occur.
  - Patients on prolonged high-dose therapy should have eye exams prior to and every 3–6 mo during therapy to detect retinal damage.
- **Malaria or Lupus Erythematosus:** Assess patient for improvement in signs and symptoms of condition daily throughout course of therapy.
- **Rheumatoid Arthritis:** Assess patient monthly for pain, swelling, and range of motion.
- ***Lab Test Considerations:*** Monitor CBC and platelet count periodically throughout therapy. May cause decreased RBC, WBC, and platelet counts. If severe decreases occur that are not related to the disease process, hydroxychloroquine should be discontinued.

POTENTIAL NURSING DIAGNOSES

- Infection, risk for (Indications).
- Pain, chronic (Indications).
- Knowledge deficit, related to medication regimen (Patient/Family Teaching).

IMPLEMENTATION

- **PO:** Administer with milk or meals to minimize GI distress.
  - Tablets may be crushed and placed inside empty capsules for patients with difficulty swallowing. Contents of capsules may also be mixed with a teaspoonful of jam, jelly, or Jell-O prior to administration.
- **Malaria Prophylaxis:** Hydroxychloroquine therapy should be started 2 wk prior to potential exposure and continued for 4–6 wk after leaving the area.

PATIENT/FAMILY TEACHING

- Instruct patient to take medication exactly as directed and continue full course of therapy even if feeling better. Missed doses should be taken as soon as remembered unless it is almost time for next dose. Do not double doses.
- Advise patients to avoid use of alcohol while taking hydroxychloroquine.
- Caution patient to keep hydroxychloroquine out of reach of children; fatalities have occurred with ingestion of 3 or 4 tablets.
- Explain need for periodic ophthalmic exams for patients on prolonged high-dose therapy. Advise patient that the risk of ocular damage may be decreased by the use of dark glasses in bright light. Protective clothing and sunscreen should also be used to reduce risk of dermatoses.
- Advise patient to notify health care professional promptly if sore throat, fever, unusual bleeding or bruising, blurred vision, visual changes, ringing in the ears, difficulty hearing, or muscle weakness occurs.

- **Malaria Prophylaxis:** Review methods of minimizing exposure to mosquitoes with patients receiving hydroxychloroquine prophylactically (use repellent, wear long-sleeved shirt and long trousers, use screen or netting).
  - Advise patient to notify health care professional if fever develops while traveling or within 2 mo of leaving an endemic area.
- **Rheumatoid Arthritis:** Instruct patient to contact health care professional if no improvement is noticed within a few days. Treatment for rheumatoid arthritis may require up to 6 mo for full benefit.

EVALUATION

Effectiveness of therapy can be demonstrated by: ▪ Prevention or resolution of malaria ▪ Improvement in signs and symptoms of rheumatoid arthritis ▪ Improvement in symptoms of lupus erythematosus.

HYDROXYUREA

(hye-drox-ee-yoo-**ree**-ah)
Hydrea

CLASSIFICATION(S):
Antineoplastic (antimetabolite)

Pregnancy Category D

INDICATIONS

▪ Treatment of head and neck carcinoma ▪ Treatment of ovarian carcinoma ▪ Treatment of resistant chronic myelogenous leukemia ▪ Treatment of melanoma. **Unlabeled Uses:** ▪ Reduction of painful crises in sickle cell anemia.

ACTION

▪ Interferes with DNA synthesis (cell-cycle S phase–specific). **Therapeutic Effects:** ▪ Death of rapidly replicating cells, particularly malignant ones.

PHARMACOKINETICS

Absorption: Well absorbed following oral administration.
Distribution: Crosses the blood-brain barrier.
Metabolism and Excretion: 50% excreted unchanged by the kidneys; 50% metabolized by the liver and eliminated as respiratory CO_2.
Half-life: 3–4 hr.

CONTRAINDICATIONS AND PRECAUTIONS

Contraindicated in: ▪ Hypersensitivity ▪ Pregnancy or lactation ▪ Some products contain tartrazine (FDC yellow dye #5) and should be avoided in patients with known hypersensitivity.
Use Cautiously in: ▪ Patients with childbearing potential ▪ Active infections ▪ Decreased bone marrow reserve ▪ Other chronic debilitating illness ▪ Obese patients or patients with edema (dose should be determined using ideal body weight).

ADVERSE REACTIONS AND SIDE EFFECTS*

CNS: drowsiness (large doses).
GI: anorexia, diarrhea, nausea, vomiting, constipation, hepatitis, stomatitis.
GU: dysuria, gonadal suppression, renal tubular dysfunction.
Derm: alopecia, erythema, pruritus, rashes.
Hemat: leukopenia, anemia, thrombocytopenia.
Metab: hyperuricemia.
Misc: chills, fever, malaise.

INTERACTIONS

Drug-Drug: ▪ Additive bone marrow depression with **agents that depress bone marrow,** including **radiation therapy** ▪ May decrease the antibody response to and increase the risk of adverse reactions to **live virus vaccines.**

ROUTE AND DOSAGE

❑ Head and Neck Cancer, Ovarian Cancer, Malignant Melanoma

- **PO (Adults):** 60–80 mg/kg (2–3 g/m^2) as a single daily dose q 3 days or 20–30 mg/kg/day as a single dose. Therapy should be initiated 7 days prior to radiation and continued.

❑ Resistant Chronic Myelogenous Leukemia

- **PO (Adults):** 20–30 mg/kg/day in 1–2 divided doses.

❑ Sickle Cell Anemia (Unlabeled)

- **PO (Adults and Children):** 15–35 mg/kg/day.

AVAILABILITY

▪ ***Capsules:*** 500 mg^Rx^.

TIME/ACTION PROFILE (effects on blood counts)

	ONSET	PEAK	DURATION
PO	7 days	10 days	21 days

NURSING IMPLICATIONS

ASSESSMENT

- ☐ Assess for signs of infection (fever, sore throat, cough, hoarseness, pain in lower back or side, difficult or painful urination). If these symptoms occur, notify physician immediately.
- ☐ Anemia may occur. Monitor for increased fatigue, dyspnea, and orthostatic hypotension.
- ☐ Assess for bleeding (bleeding gums, bruising, petechiae, guaiac stools, urine, and emesis). Avoid IM injections and rectal temperatures. Hold pressure on all venipuncture sites for at least 10 min.
- ☐ Monitor intake and output, appetite, and nutritional intake. Adjust diet as tolerated to maintain nutritional status.
- ▪ ***Lab Test Considerations:*** Monitor CBC and differential prior to and periodically dur-

H

*CAPITALS indicate life-threatening; underlines indicate most frequent.

ing course of therapy. The onset of leukopenia occurs within 10 days of beginning therapy. Recovery usually occurs within 30 days. Notify physician if WBC <2500 mm³ or if a precipitous drop occurs. Institute thrombocytopenia precautions if platelet count <100,000/mm³. May cause temporary increase in mean corpuscular volume (MCV).

- □ Monitor renal (BUN, creatinine, and uric acid) and liver function tests (AST, ALT, bilirubin, and LDH) prior to and periodically during course of therapy. May cause increased BUN, creatinine, and uric acid concentrations.

POTENTIAL NURSING DIAGNOSES

- Injury, risk for (Side Effects).
- Infection, risk for (Side Effects).
- Knowledge deficit, related to medication regimen (Patient/Family Teaching).

IMPLEMENTATION

- **PO:** Capsules may be opened and contents mixed into a glass of water and taken immediately if patient has difficulty swallowing. Some inert powder may float on the surface.

PATIENT/FAMILY TEACHING

- **General Info:** Instruct patient to take medication exactly as directed, even if nausea, vomiting, or diarrhea is a problem. Consult health care professional if vomiting occurs shortly after dose is taken. If a dose is missed, do not take at all; do not double doses.
- □ Instruct patient to notify health care professional if fever; chills; sore throat; signs of infection; loss of appetite; nausea; vomiting; diarrhea; bleeding gums; bruising; petechiae; or blood in urine, stool, or emesis occurs. Caution patient to avoid crowds and persons with known infections. Instruct patient to use soft toothbrush and electric razor. Patients should be cautioned not to drink alcoholic beverages or to take products containing aspirin or NSAIDs.
- □ Instruct patient to inspect oral mucosa for erythema and ulceration. If ulceration occurs, advise patient to use sponge brush and rinse mouth with water after eating and drinking. Consult health care professional if mouth pain interferes with eating. Stomatitis pain may require treatment with opioid analgesics.
- □ Discuss possibility of drowsiness with patients receiving large doses. Advise patient to avoid driving or other activities until response to drug is known.
- □ Review with patient the need for contraception during therapy. Women need to use contraception even if amenorrhea occurs.
- □ Instruct patient not to receive any vaccinations without advice of health care professional.
- □ Discuss need for lab tests and follow-up visits to monitor progress and detect side effects.
- **Leukemia:** Encourage fluid intake of 2000–3000 ml/day. Allopurinol and alkalinization of the urine may be used to help prevent urate stone formation.

EVALUATION

Effectiveness of therapy can be demonstrated by: ▪ Decrease in size and spread of tumors ▪ Improved hematologic values in leukemia. Therapy is held if leukocytes are less than 2500/mm³ or platelets less than 100,000/mm³ and resumed when these values begin to return to normal limits, usually within 3 days ▪ Reduction in painful crisis of sickle cell anemia.

HYDROXYZINE

(hye-**drox**-i-zeen)

Anxanil, {Apo-Hydroxyzine}, Atarax, E-Vista, Hydroxacen, Hyzine, {Multipax}, {Novohydroxyzin}, Quiess, Vistaject, Vistaril, Vistazine

CLASSIFICATION(S):

Antihistamine, Sedative/hypnotic

Pregnancy Category C

INDICATIONS

▪ Treatment of anxiety ▪ Preoperative sedation ▪ Antiemetic ▪ Antipruritic ▪ Often combined with opioid analgesics.

ACTION

▪ Acts as a CNS depressant at the subcortical level of the CNS ▪ Has anticholinergic, antihistaminic, and antiemetic properties. **Therapeutic Effects:** ▪ Sedation ▪ Relief of anxiety ▪ Decreased nausea and vomiting ▪ Decreased allergic symptoms associated with release of histamine, including pruritus.

PHARMACOKINETICS

Absorption: Well absorbed following PO/IM administration.
Distribution: UK.
Metabolism and Excretion: Completely metabolized by the liver; eliminated in the feces via biliary excretion.
Half-life: 3 hr.

CONTRAINDICATIONS AND PRECAUTIONS

Contraindicated in: ▪ Hypersensitivity ▪ Pregnancy.
Use Cautiously in: ▪ Severe hepatic dysfunction ▪ Geriatric patients (dosage reduction recommended) ▪ Labor (has been used safely) ▪ Lactation (safety not established).

ADVERSE REACTIONS AND SIDE EFFECTS*

CNS: drowsiness, agitation, ataxia, dizziness, headache, weakness.
Resp: wheezing.
GI: dry mouth, bitter taste, constipation, nausea.
GU: urinary retention.
Derm: flushing.
Local: pain at IM site, abscesses at IM sites.
Misc: chest tightness.

INTERACTIONS

Drug-Drug: ▪ Additive CNS depression with other **CNS depressants**, including **alcohol, antidepressants, antihistamines, opioids,** and **sedative/hypnotics** ▪ Additive anticholinergic effects with other **drugs possessing anticholinergic properties,** including **antihistamines, antidepressants, atropine, haloperidol, phenothiazines, quinidine,** and **disopyramide.**

ROUTE AND DOSAGE

- **PO (Adults):** *Antianxiety, sedative/hypnotic*—50–100 mg single dose. *Antiemetic/antipruritic*—25–100 mg 3–4 times daily.
- **PO (Children):** *Antianxiety, sedative/hypnotic*—0.6 mg/kg single dose. *Antiemetic, antipruritic*—0.5 mg/kg (15 mg/m^2) q 6 hr.
- **PO (Children 6–12 yr):** *Antiemetic, antipruritic*—12.5–25 mg q 6 hr as needed.
- **PO (Children <6 yr):** *Antiemetic, antipruritic*—12.5 mg q 6 hr as needed.
- **IM (Adults):** *Antianxiety*—50–100 mg q 4–6 hr. *Sedative/hypnotic*—50 mg single dose. *Antiemetic, adjunct to opioid analgesics*—25–100 mg.
- **IM (Children):** *Antiemetic, adjunct to opioid analgesics*—1 mg/kg (30 mg/m^2).

AVAILABILITY

▪ ***Tablets:*** 10 mg[Rx], 25 mg[Rx], 50 mg[Rx], 100 mg[Rx] ▪ ***Capsules:*** 10 mg[Rx], 25 mg[Rx], 50 mg[Rx], 100 mg[Rx] ▪ ***Syrup:*** 10 mg/5 ml[Rx] ▪ ***Oral suspension:*** 25 mg/5 ml[Rx] ▪ ***Injection:*** 25 mg/ml[Rx], 50 mg/ml[Rx].

TIME/ACTION PROFILE (sedative, antiemetic, antipruritic effects)

	ONSET	PEAK	DURATION
PO	15–30 min	2–4 hr	4–6 hr
IM	15–30 min	2–4 hr	4–6 hr

NURSING IMPLICATIONS

ASSESSMENT

- **General Info:** Assess patient for profound sedation and provide safety precautions as indicated (side rails up, bed in low position, call bell within reach, supervision of ambulation and transfer).
- **Anxiety:** Assess mental status, mood, and behavior.
- **Nausea and Vomiting:** Assess degree of nausea and frequency and amount of emesis.
- **Pruritus:** Assess degree of itching and character of involved skin.
- ***Lab Test Considerations:*** May cause false-negative skin tests using allergen extracts. Discontinue hydroxyzine at least 72 hr prior to test.

POTENTIAL NURSING DIAGNOSES

- Anxiety (Indications).
- Skin integrity, impaired (Indications).
- Injury, risk for (Side Effects).

H

*CAPITALS indicate life-threatening; underlines indicate most frequent.

IMPLEMENTATION

- **PO:** Tablets may be crushed and capsules opened and administered with food or fluids for patients having difficulty swallowing.
- □ Shake suspension well before administration.
- **IM:** Administer IM deep into well-developed muscle, preferably with Z-track technique. Injection is extremely painful. Do not use deltoid site. Significant tissue damage, necrosis, and sloughing may result from SC or intra-arterial injections. Hemolysis may result from IV injections. Rotate injection sites frequently.
- **Syringe Compatibility:** ▪ atropine ▪ benzquinamide ▪ buprenorphine ▪ butorphanol ▪ chlorpromazine ▪ cimetidine ▪ codeine ▪ diphenhydramine ▪ doxapram ▪ droperidol ▪ fentanyl ▪ glycopyrrolate ▪ hydromorphone ▪ lidocaine ▪ meperidine ▪ methotrimeprazine ▪ metoclopramide ▪ midazolam ▪ morphine ▪ nalbuphine ▪ oxymorphone ▪ pentazocine ▪ procaine ▪ prochlorperazine ▪ promazine ▪ promethazine ▪ scopolamine ▪ sufentanil.
- **Syringe Incompatibility:** ▪ chloramphenicol ▪ dimenhydrinate ▪ heparin ▪ ketorolac ▪ penicillin G potassium ▪ pentobarbital ▪ phenobarbital ▪ phenytoin ▪ ranitidine ▪ vitamin B complex with C.

PATIENT/FAMILY TEACHING

- □ Instruct patient to take medication exactly as directed. Missed doses should be taken as soon as remembered unless almost time for next dose; do not double doses.
- □ May cause drowsiness or dizziness. Caution patient to avoid driving or other activities requiring alertness until response to medication is known.
- □ Advise patient to avoid concurrent use of alcohol or other CNS depressants with this medication.
- □ Inform patient that frequent mouth rinses, good oral hygiene, and sugarless gum or candy may help decrease dry mouth. If dry mouth persists for more than 2 wk, consult dentist regarding saliva substitute.

EVALUATION

Effectiveness of therapy can be demonstrated by: ▪ Decrease in anxiety ▪ Relief of nausea and vomiting ▪ Relief of pruritus ▪ Sedation when used as a sedative/hypnotic.

HYPOGLYCEMIC AGENTS, ORAL

glimepiride
(glye-**me**-pi-ride)
Amaryl

glipizide
(**glip**-i-zide)
Glucotrol, Glucotrol XL

glyburide
(**glye**-byoo-ride)
{Apo-Glyburide}, DiaBeta, {Euglucon}, {Gen-Glybe}, Glynase PresTab, Micronase, {Novo-Glyburide}, {Nu-Glyburide}

CLASSIFICATION(S):
Antidiabetic agents (sulfonylureas)

Pregnancy Category C

INDICATIONS

▪ **PO:** Control blood sugar in adult-onset non–insulin-dependent diabetes mellitus (NIDDM) when diet therapy fails. Require some pancreatic function.

ACTION

▪ Lower blood sugar by stimulating the release of insulin from the pancreas and increasing the sensitivity to insulin at receptor sites ▪ May also decrease hepatic glucose production. **Therapeutic Effects:** ▪ Lowering of blood sugar in diabetic patients.

PHARMACOKINETICS

Absorption: All agents are well absorbed following oral administration.
Distribution: *Glyburide*—reaches high concentrations in bile and crosses the placenta.
Metabolism and Excretion: All agents are mostly metabolized by the liver. *Glimepiride*—converted to a metabolite with hypoglycemic activity.
Half-life: *Glimepiride*—5–9.2 hr; *glipizide*—2.1–2.6 hr; *glyburide*—10 hr.

CONTRAINDICATIONS AND PRECAUTIONS

Contraindicated in: ▪ Hypersensitivity ▪ Cross-sensitivity with sulfonamides (including thiazide diuretics) may occur ▪ Insulin-dependent (type 1, juvenile-onset, ketosis-prone, brittle) diabetics ▪ Diabetic coma or ketoacidosis ▪ Severe renal, hepatic, thyroid, or other endocrine disease ▪ Uncontrolled infection, serious burns, or trauma.
Use Cautiously in: ▪ Severe cardiovascular or hepatic disease ▪ Geriatric patients (increased sensitivity; dosage reduction may be required) ▪ Severe renal disease (increased risk of hypoglycemia) ▪ Infection, stress, or changes in diet may alter requirements for control of blood sugar ▪ Impaired thyroid, pituitary, or adrenal function ▪ Malnutrition, high fever, prolonged nausea, or vomiting ▪ Pregnancy or lactation (safety not established; insulin recommended during pregnancy).

ADVERSE REACTIONS AND SIDE EFFECTS*

CNS: dizziness, drowsiness, headache, weakness.
GI: constipation, cramps, diarrhea, drug-induced hepatitis, heartburn, increased appetite, nausea, vomiting.
Derm: photosensitivity, rashes.
Endo: hypoglycemia.
F and E: hyponatremia.
Hemat: APLASTIC ANEMIA, agranulocytosis, leukopenia, pancytopenia, thrombocytopenia.

INTERACTIONS

Drug-Drug: ▪ Ingestion of **alcohol** may result in disulfiram-like reaction ▪ Effectiveness may be decreased by concurrent use of **diuretics, glucocorticoids, phenothiazines, oral contraceptives, estrogens, thyroid preparations, phenytoin, nicotinic acid, sympathomimetics,** and **isoniazid** ▪ **Alcohol, androgens (testosterone), chloramphenicol, clofibrate, guanethidine, MAO inhibitors, NSAIDs** (except diclofenac), **salicylates, sulfonamides,** and **warfarin** may increase the risk of hypoglycemia ▪ Concurrent use with **warfarin** may alter the response to both agents (increased effects of both initially, then decreased activity); close monitoring recommended during any changes in dosage ▪ **Beta-adrenergic blockers** may alter the response to oral hypoglycemic agents (increase or decrease requirements; nonselective agents may cause prolonged hypoglycemia).

ROUTE AND DOSAGE

❑ **Glimepiride**

- **PO (Adults):** 1–2 mg once daily initially; may increase q 1–2 wk up to 8 mg/day (usual range 1–4 mg/day).

❑ **Glipizide**

- **PO (Adults):** 5 mg/day initially, increased as needed (range 2.5–40 mg/day); XL dosage form is given once daily. Doses >15 mg/day should be given as 2 divided doses.
- **PO (Geriatric Patients):** 2.5 mg/day initially.

❑ **Glyburide**

- **PO (Adults):** *DiaBeta/Micronase*—2.5–5 mg once daily initially (range 1.25–20 mg/day). *Glynase PresTab*—1.5–3 mg/day initially (range 0.75–12 mg/day; doses >6 mg/day should be given as divided doses). Increments should not exceed 1.5 mg/wk.
- **PO (Geriatric Patients):** *DiaBeta/Micronase*—1.25–2.5 mg/day initially; may be increased by 2.5 mg/day weekly. *Glynase PresTab*—0.75–3 mg/day; may be increased by 1.5 mg/day weekly.

AVAILABILITY

❑ **Glimepiride**

- ***Tablets:*** 1 mg[Rx], 2 mg[Rx], 4 mg[Rx].

❑ **Glipizide**

- ***Tablets:*** 5 mg[Rx], 10 mg[Rx] ▪ ***Extended-release tablets:*** 5 mg[Rx], 10 mg[Rx].

❑ **Glyburide**

- ***Tablets:*** 1.25 mg[Rx], 2.5 mg[Rx], 5 mg[Rx] ▪ ***Micronized tablets:*** 1.5 mg[Rx], 3 mg[Rx], 6 mg[Rx].

TIME/ACTION PROFILE (hypoglycemic activity)

	ONSET	PEAK	DURATION
Glimepiride	UK	2–3 hr	24 hr
Glipizide	15–30 min	1–2 hr	up to 24 hr
Glyburide	45–60 min	1.5–3 hr	24 hr

***CAPITALS** indicate life-threatening; **underlines** indicate most frequent.

H

NURSING IMPLICATIONS

ASSESSMENT

- Observe patient for signs and symptoms of hypoglycemic reactions (sweating, hunger, weakness, dizziness, tremor, tachycardia, anxiety).
- Assess patient for allergy to sulfonamides.
- ***Lab Test Considerations:*** Monitor serum glucose and glycosylated hemoglobin periodically throughout therapy to evaluate effectiveness of treatment.
- Monitor CBC periodically throughout therapy. Report decrease in blood counts promptly.
- May cause an increase in AST, LDH, BUN, and serum creatinine.
- ***Toxicity and Overdose:*** Overdose is manifested by symptoms of hypoglycemia. Mild hypoglycemia may be treated with administration of oral glucose. Severe hypoglycemia should be treated with IV D50W followed by continuous IV infusion of more dilute dextrose solution at a rate sufficient to keep serum glucose at approximately 100 mg/dl.

POTENTIAL NURSING DIAGNOSES

- Nutrition, altered, more than body requirements (Indications).
- Knowledge deficit, related to medication regimen (Patient/Family Teaching).
- Noncompliance (Patient/Family Teaching).

IMPLEMENTATION

- **General Info:** Patients stabilized on a diabetic regimen who are exposed to stress, fever, trauma, infection, or surgery may require administration of insulin.
- To convert from other oral hypoglycemic agents, gradual conversion is not required. For insulin dosage of less than 20 units/day, change to oral hypoglycemic agents can be made without gradual dosage adjustment. Patients taking 20 or more units/day should convert gradually by receiving oral agent and a 25–30% reduction in insulin dose every day or every 2nd day with gradual insulin dosage reduction as tolerated. Monitor serum or urine glucose and ketones at least 3 times/day during conversion.
- **PO:** May be administered once in the morning or divided into 2 doses. Administer most sulfonylureas with meals to ensure best diabetic control and to minimize gastric irritation. Do not administer after last meal of the day.
- *Glipizide* should be taken 30 min before a meal.
- *Nonmicronized glyburide* should not be taken with a meal high in fat. *Micronized glyburide* cannot be substituted for *nonmicronized glyburide.* Preparations are not equivalent.
- Tablets may be crushed and taken with fluids if patient has difficulty swallowing.

PATIENT/FAMILY TEACHING

- Instruct patient to take medication at same time each day. If a dose is missed, take as soon as remembered unless almost time for next dose. Do not take if unable to eat.
- Explain to patient that this medication controls hyperglycemia but does not cure diabetes. Therapy is long term.
- Review signs of hypoglycemia and hyperglycemia with patient. If hypoglycemia occurs, advise patient to take a glass of orange juice or 2–3 tsp of sugar, honey, or corn syrup dissolved in water and notify health care professional.
- Encourage patient to follow prescribed diet, medication, and exercise regimen to prevent hypoglycemic or hyperglycemic episodes.
- Instruct patient in proper testing of serum glucose and ketones. These tests should be closely monitored during periods of stress or illness and health care professional notified if significant changes occur.
- May occasionally cause dizziness or drowsiness. Caution patient to avoid driving or other activities requiring alertness until response to medication is known.
- Caution patient to avoid other medications, especially aspirin and alcohol, while on this therapy without consulting health care professional.
- Concurrent use of alcohol may cause a disulfiram-like reaction (abdominal cramps, nausea, flushing, headaches, and hypoglycemia).
- Insulin is the recommended method of controlling blood sugar during pregnancy. Counsel female patients to use a form of contraception other than oral contraceptives and to notify health care professional promptly if pregnancy is planned or suspected.
- Caution patient to use sunscreen and protec-

tive clothing to prevent photosensitivity reactions.
- ▫ Advise patient to inform health care professional of medication regimen prior to treatment or surgery.
- ▫ Advise patient to carry a form of sugar (sugar packets, candy) and identification describing disease process and medication regimen at all times.
- ▫ Advise patient to notify health care professional promptly if unusual weight gain, swelling of ankles, drowsiness, shortness of breath, muscle cramps, weakness, sore throat, rash, or unusual bleeding or bruising occurs.
- ▫ Emphasize the importance of routine follow-up exams.

EVALUATION

Effectiveness of therapy can be demonstrated by: ▪ Control of blood glucose levels without the appearance of hypoglycemic or hyperglycemic episodes.

IBUPROFEN

(eye-byoo-**proe**-fen)
{Actiprofen}, Advil, {Apo-Ibuprofen}, Bayer Select Pain Relief, Children's Advil, Children's Motrin, Cramp End, Dolgesic, Excedrin IB, Genpril, Haltran, Ibuprin, Ibuprohm, Ibren, IBU, Ibu-Tab, Junior Strength Advil, Menadol, Medipren, Midol IB, Motrin, Motrin Drops, Motrin IB, Motrin Junior Strength, {Novo-Profen}, Nu-Ibuprofen, Nuprin, Pamprin-IB, PediaCare Children's Fever, Q-Profen, Rufen, Saleto, Trendar

CLASSIFICATION(S):
Antipyretic, Nonopioid analgesic/ Nonsteroidal anti-inflammatory agent

Pregnancy Category B (first trimester)

INDICATIONS

▪ Mild to moderate pain or dysmenorrhea ▪ Inflammatory disorders including: ▫ Rheumatoid arthritis ▫ Osteoarthritis ▪ Lowering of fever.

ACTION

▪ Inhibits prostaglandin synthesis. **Therapeutic Effects:** ▪ Decreased pain and inflammation ▪ Reduction of fever.

PHARMACOKINETICS

Absorption: Well absorbed from the GI tract.
Distribution: UK. Probably crosses the placenta; does not enter breast milk in significant amounts.
Metabolism and Excretion: Mostly metabolized by the liver; small amounts (10%) excreted unchanged by the kidneys.
Half-life: 2–4 hr.

CONTRAINDICATIONS AND PRECAUTIONS

Contraindicated in: ▪ Hypersensitivity ▪ Cross-sensitivity may exist with other NSAIDs, including aspirin ▪ Active GI bleeding or ulcer disease ▪ Chewable tablets contain aspartame and should not be used in patients with phenylketonuria.
Use Cautiously in: ▪ Severe cardiovascular, renal, or hepatic disease ▪ Geriatric patients (increased risk of adverse reactions; lower initial dose recommended) ▪ Chronic alcohol use/abuse ▪ History of ulcer disease ▪ Pregnancy (use not recommended) ▪ Lactation (has been used safely).

ADVERSE REACTIONS AND SIDE EFFECTS*

CNS: <u>headache</u>, dizziness, drowsiness, psychic disturbances.
EENT: amblyopia, blurred vision, tinnitus.
CV: arrhythmias, edema.
GI: GI BLEEDING, HEPATITIS, <u>constipation</u>, <u>dyspepsia</u>, <u>nausea</u>, <u>vomiting</u>, abdominal discomfort.
GU: cystitis, hematuria, renal failure.
Derm: rashes.
Hemat: blood dyscrasias, prolonged bleeding time.
Misc: allergic reactions including ANAPHYLAXIS.

INTERACTIONS

Drug-Drug: ▪ Concurrent use with **aspirin** may decrease effectiveness ▪ Additive adverse GI side effects with **aspirin**, other **NSAIDs, glucocorticoids**, or **alcohol** ▪ Chronic use with **acet-**

{} = Available in Canada only.
***CAPITALS indicate life-threatening; <u>underlines</u> indicate most frequent.**

aminophen may increase the risk of adverse renal reactions ▪ May decrease the effectiveness of **diuretics** or **antihypertensive therapy** ▪ May increase the hypoglycemic effects of **insulin** or **oral hypoglycemic agents** ▪ May slightly increase serum **digoxin** levels ▪ May increase serum **lithium** levels and increase the risk of toxicity ▪ Increases the risk of toxicity from **methotrexate** ▪ **Probenecid** increases risk of toxicity from ibuprofen ▪ Increased risk of bleeding with **cefamandole, cefotetan, cefoperazone, valproic acid, plicamycin, thrombolytic agents**, or **warfarin** ▪ Increased risk of adverse hematologic reactions with **antineoplastic agents** or **radiation therapy** ▪ Increased risk of nephrotoxicity with **cyclosporine.**

ROUTE AND DOSAGE

❑ Analgesia

- **PO (Adults):** *Anti-inflammatory*—400–800 mg 3–4 times daily (not to exceed 3600 mg/day). *Analgesic/antidysmenorrheal/antipyretic*—200–400 mg q 4–6 hr (not to exceed 1200 mg/day).
- **PO (Children 6 mo–12 yr):** *Anti-inflammatory*—20–40 mg/kg/day in divided doses (not to exceed 50 mg/kg/day). *Antipyretic*—5 mg/kg for temperature $<$102.5°F (39.17°C) or 10 mg/kg for higher temperatures (not to exceed 40 mg/kg/day); may be repeated q 4–6 hr.

❑ Pediatric OTC Dosing

- **PO (Children 11 yr—72–95 lb):** 300 mg q 6–8 hr.
- **PO (Children 9–10 yr —60–71 lb):** 250 mg q 6–8 hr.
- **PO (Children 6–8 yr—48–59 lb):** 200 mg q 6–8 hr.
- **PO (Children 4–5 yr—36–47 lb):** 150 mg q 6–8 hr.
- **PO (Children 2–3 yr—24–35 lb):** 100 mg q 6–8 hr.

AVAILABILITY

▪ ***Tablets:*** 200 mg^OTC^, 300 mg^Rx^, 400 mg^Rx^, 600 mg^Rx^, 800 mg^Rx^ ▪ ***Chewable tablets:*** 100 mg^OTC^ ▪ ***Oral suspension:*** 100 mg/5 ml^OTC^ ▪ ***Pediatric drops:*** 50 mg/1.25 ml^OTC^ ▪ ***In combination with:*** decongestants^OTC^, hydrocodone (Vicoprofen)^Rx^. See Appendix A.

TIME/ACTION PROFILE

	ONSET	PEAK	DURATION
PO (analgesic)	30 min	1–2 hr	4–6 hr
PO (anti-inflammatory)	7 days	1–2 wk	UK

NURSING IMPLICATIONS

ASSESSMENT

- **General Info:** Patients who have asthma, aspirin-induced allergy, and nasal polyps are at increased risk for developing hypersensitivity reactions. Assess for rhinitis, asthma, and urticaria.
- **Pain:** Assess pain (note type, location, and intensity) prior to and 1–2 hr following administration.
- **Arthritis:** Assess pain and range of motion prior to and 1–2 hr following administration.
- **Fever:** Monitor temperature; note signs associated with fever (diaphoresis, tachycardia, malaise).
- ***Lab Test Considerations:*** BUN, serum creatinine, CBC, and liver function tests should be evaluated periodically in patients receiving prolonged courses of therapy.
  - ▫ Serum potassium, BUN, serum creatinine, alkaline phosphatase, LDH, AST, and ALT tests may show increased levels. Blood glucose, hemoglobin, and hematocrit concentrations, leukocyte and platelet counts, and CCr may be decreased.
  - ▫ May cause prolonged bleeding time, which may persist for $<$1 day following discontinuation of therapy.

POTENTIAL NURSING DIAGNOSES

- Pain (Indications).
- Physical mobility, impaired (Indications).
- Knowledge deficit, related to medication regimen (Patient/Family Teaching).

IMPLEMENTATION

- **General Info:** Administration in higher than recommended doses does not provide increased effectiveness but may cause increased side effects.
  - ▫ Coadministration with opioid analgesics may have additive analgesic effects and may permit lower opioid doses.
- **PO:** For rapid initial effect, administer 30 min before or 2 hr after meals. May be adminis-

tered with food, milk, or antacids to decrease GI irritation. Tablets may be crushed and mixed with fluids or food; 800-mg tablet can be dissolved in water.

- **Dysmenorrhea:** Administer as soon as possible after the onset of menses. Prophylactic treatment has not been shown to be effective.

PATIENT/FAMILY TEACHING

- Advise patients to take this medication with a full glass of water and to remain in an upright position for 15–30 min after administration.
- Instruct patient to take medication exactly as directed. If dose is missed, it should be taken as soon as remembered but not if almost time for next dose. Do not double doses.
- May cause drowsiness or dizziness. Advise patient to avoid driving or other activities requiring alertness until response to medication is known.
- Caution patient to avoid the concurrent use of alcohol, aspirin, acetaminophen, or other OTC medications without consulting health care professional.
- Advise patient to inform health care professional of medication regimen prior to treatment or surgery.
- Caution patient to wear sunscreen and protective clothing to prevent photosensitivity reactions.
- Instruct patients not to take the OTC ibuprofen preparations for more than 10 days for pain or more than 3 days for fever and to consult health care professional if symptoms persist or worsen.
- Caution patient that use of ibuprofen with 3 or more glasses of alcohol per day may increase the risk of GI bleeding.
- Advise patient to consult health care professional if rash, itching, visual disturbances, tinnitus, weight gain, edema, black stools, persistent headache, or influenza-like syndrome (chills, fever, muscle aches, pain) occurs.

EVALUATION

Effectiveness of therapy can be demonstrated by: ▪ Decrease in severity of pain ▪ Improved joint mobility. Partial arthritic relief is usually seen within 7 days, but maximum effectiveness may require 1–2 wk of continuous therapy. Patients who do not respond to one NSAID may respond to another ▪ Reduction in fever.

IBUTILIDE

(eye-**byoo**-ti-lide)
Corvert

CLASSIFICATION(S):
Antiarrhythmic (group III)

Pregnancy Category C

INDICATIONS

▪ Rapid conversion of recent-onset atrial flutter or fibrillation to normal sinus rhythm.

ACTION

▪ Activates slow inward current of sodium in cardiac tissue, resulting in delayed repolarization, prolonged action potential duration, and increased refractoriness ▪ Mildly slows sinus rate and AV conduction. **Therapeutic Effects:** ▪ Conversion to normal sinus rhythm.

PHARMACOKINETICS

Absorption: IV administration results in complete bioavailability.
Distribution: UK.
Metabolism and Excretion: Highly metabolized by the liver, 1 metabolite is active; metabolites excreted by kidneys.
Half-life: 6 hr (2–12 hr).

CONTRAINDICATIONS AND PRECAUTIONS

Contraindicated in: ▪ Hypersensitivity.
Use Cautiously in: ▪ Congestive heart failure or left ventricular dysfunction (increased risk of more serious arrhythmias during infusion) ▪ Pregnancy, lactation, or children <18 yr (safety not established).

ADVERSE REACTIONS AND SIDE EFFECTS*

CNS: headache.
CV: arrhythmias.
GI: nausea.

I

*CAPITALS indicate life-threatening; underlines indicate most frequent.

INTERACTIONS

Drug-Drug: ▪ **Amiodarone, disopyramide, procainamide, quinidine,** and **sotalol** should not be given concurrently or within 4 hr because of additive effects on refractoriness ▪ Proarrhythmic effects may increased by **phenothiazines, tricyclic** and **tetracyclic antidepressants,** some **antihistamines,** and **histamine H_2-receptor blocking agents;** concurrent use should be avoided.

ROUTE AND DOSAGE

- **IV (Adults ≥60 kg):** 1 mg infusion; may be repeated 10 min following end of first infusion.
- **IV (Adults <60 kg):** 0.01 mg/kg infusion; may be repeated 10 min following end of first infusion.

AVAILABILITY

▪ ***Solution for injection:*** 0.1 mg/ml in 10-ml vial[Rx].

TIME/ACTION PROFILE (antiarrhythmic effect)

	ONSET	PEAK	DURATION
IV	within 30–90 min	UK	up to 24 hr

NURSING IMPLICATIONS

ASSESSMENT

□ Monitor ECG continuously throughout and for 4 hr following infusion or until QT_c interval normalizes. Discontinue if arrhythmia terminates or if sustained ventricular tachycardia, prolonged QT, or QT_c develops. Ibutilide may have proarrhythmic effects. These arrhythmias may be serious and potentially life-threatening. Clinicians trained to treat ventricular arrhythmias, medications, and equipment (defibrillator/cardioverter) should be available during therapy and monitoring of patient.

POTENTIAL NURSING DIAGNOSES

- Cardiac output, decreased (Indications).
- Knowledge deficit, related to medication regimen (Patient/Family Teaching).

IMPLEMENTATION

- **General Info:** Oral antiarrhythmic therapy may be instituted 4 hr following ibutilide infusion.
- **Intermittent Infusion:** May be administered undiluted or diluted in 50 ml of 0.9% NaCl or D5W for a concentration of approximately 0.017 mg/ml. Solution, diluted or undiluted, is stable for 24 hr at room temperature or 48 hr if refrigerated.
- ***Rate:*** Administer over 10 min.
- **Additive Incompatibility:** ▪ Information unavailable; do not admix with other solutions or medications.

PATIENT/FAMILY TEACHING

□ Inform patient of the purpose of ibutilide.

EVALUATION

Clinical response to therapy can be evaluated by: ▪ Conversion of recent-onset atrial flutter or fibrillation to normal sinus rhythm.

IDARUBICIN

(eye-da-**roo**-bi-sin)
Idamycin

CLASSIFICATION(S):
Antineoplastic (anthracycline)

Pregnancy Category D

INDICATIONS

▪ Part of combination chemotherapy for acute myelogenous leukemia in adults.

ACTION

▪ Inhibits nucleic acid synthesis. **Therapeutic Effects:** ▪ Death of rapidly replicating cells, particularly malignant ones.

PHARMACOKINETICS

Absorption: IV administration results in complete bioavailability.
Distribution: Rapidly distributed with extensive tissue binding. High degree of cellular uptake.
Metabolism and Excretion: Extensive hepatic and extrahepatic metabolism. One metabolite is active (idarubicinol). Primarily eliminated via biliary excretion.
Half-life: 22 hr (range 4–46 hr).

CONTRAINDICATIONS AND PRECAUTIONS

Contraindicated in: ▪ Pregnancy or lactation.
Use Cautiously in: ▪ Children (safety not es-

tablished) ▪ Patients with childbearing potential ▪ Active infection ▪ Decreased bone marrow reserve ▪ Geriatric patients ▪ Other chronic debilitating illnesses ▪ Hepatic impairment (dosage reduction may be required; avoid if bilirubin ≥5 mg/dl) ▪ Renal impairment ▪ Pre-existing cardiac disease ▪ Previous daunorubicin or doxorubicin therapy.

ADVERSE REACTIONS AND SIDE EFFECTS*

CNS: headache, mental status changes.
Resp: pulmonary toxicity, pulmonary allergic reactions.
CV: ARRHYTHMIAS, CARDIOTOXICITY, CONGESTIVE HEART FAILURE.
GI: abdominal cramps, diarrhea, mucositis, nausea, vomiting.
Derm: alopecia, photosensitivity, rashes.
Endo: gonadal suppression.
Hemat: BLEEDING, anemia, leukopenia, thrombocytopenia.
Local: phlebitis at IV site.
Metab: hyperuricemia.
Neuro: peripheral neuropathy.
Misc: fever.

INTERACTIONS

Drug-Drug: ▪ Additive myelosuppression with other **antineoplastic agents** or **radiation therapy** ▪ May decrease antibody response to and increase risk of adverse reactions from **live virus vaccines.**

ROUTE AND DOSAGE

- **IV (Adults):** 12 mg/m^2 daily for 3 days in combination with cytarabine.

AVAILABILITY

- ***Powder for injection:*** 5-mg vials[Rx], 10-mg vials[Rx].

TIME/ACTION PROFILE (effects on blood counts)

	ONSET	PEAK	DURATION
IV	UK	10–14 days	21 days

NURSING IMPLICATIONS

ASSESSMENT

- □ Monitor blood pressure, pulse, respiratory rate, and temperature frequently during administration. Report significant changes.
- □ Monitor for bone marrow depression. Assess for bleeding (bleeding gums, bruising, petechiae, guaiac stools, urine, and emesis) and avoid IM injections and rectal temperatures if platelet count is low. Apply pressure to venipuncture sites for 10 min. Assess for signs of infection during neutropenia. Anemia may occur. Monitor for increased fatigue, dyspnea, and orthostatic hypotension.
- □ Monitor intake and output ratios. Report significant discrepancies. Encourage fluid intake of 2000–3000 ml/day. Allopurinol and alkalinization of the urine may be used to decrease serum uric acid levels and to help prevent urate stone formation.
- □ Severe and protracted nausea and vomiting may occur as early as 1 hr after therapy and may last 24 hr. Parenteral antiemetic agents should be administered 30–45 min prior to therapy and routinely around the clock for the next 24 hr as indicated. Monitor amount of emesis; report emesis exceeding guidelines to prevent dehydration.
- □ Monitor for development of signs of myocardial toxicity manifested by life-threatening arrhythmias, cardiomyopathy, and congestive heart failure (peripheral edema, dyspnea, rales/crackles, weight gain). Chest x ray, ECG, echocardiography, and radionuclide angiography determinations of ejection fraction should be monitored prior to and periodically throughout therapy.
- □ Assess injection site frequently for redness, irritation, or inflammation. May infiltrate painlessly. If extravasation occurs, infusion must be stopped and restarted elsewhere to avoid damage to SC tissue. Treatment of extravasation includes rest and elevation of the extremity and application of intermittent ice packs (apply for 30 min immediately and 30 min qid for 3 days). If pain, erythema, or vesication persists longer than 48 hr, immediate plastic surgery may be warranted.
- ▪ ***Lab Test Considerations:*** Monitor CBC,

I

*CAPITALS indicate life-threatening; underlines indicate most frequent.

differential, and platelet count prior to and frequently throughout therapy. Nadirs of leukopenia and thrombocytopenia are 10–14 days, with recovery occurring 21 days after a dose.

- Monitor renal and hepatic function prior to and periodically throughout therapy. Idarubicin may cause hyperuricemia. May also cause transient increases in AST, ALT, LDH, serum alkaline phosphatase, and bilirubin.

POTENTIAL NURSING DIAGNOSES

- Infection, risk for (Adverse Reactions).
- Nutrition, altered, less than body requirements (Adverse Reactions).
- Knowledge deficit, related to medication regimen (Patient/Family Teaching).

IMPLEMENTATION

- **General Info:** Solution should be prepared in a biologic cabinet. Wear gloves, gown, and mask while handling medication. Discard IV equipment in specially designated containers (see Appendix I).
- See cytarabine monograph (p. 237) for specific information on administration of cytarabine with idarubicin.
- **Direct IV:** Reconstitute 5-mg and 10-mg vials with 5 ml and 10 ml, respectively, of 0.9% NaCl (nonbacteriostatic) for injection for a concentration of 1 mg/ml. Vial contents are under pressure; use care when inserting needle.
- Reconstituted medication is stable for 72 hr at room temperature and 7 days if refrigerated.
- ***Rate:*** Administer each dose slowly over 10–15 min through Y-site of a free-flowing infusion of 0.9% NaCl or D5W. Tubing may be attached to a butterfly needle and injected into a large vein.
- **Syringe Incompatibility:** ▪ heparin.
- **Y-Site Compatibility:** ▪ amikacin ▪ aztreonam ▪ cimetidine ▪ cyclophosphamide ▪ cytarabine ▪ diphenhydramine ▪ droperidol ▪ erythromycin lactobionate ▪ filgrastim ▪ imipenem/cilastatin ▪ magnesium sulfate ▪ mannitol ▪ melphalan ▪ metoclopramide ▪ potassium chloride ▪ ranitidine ▪ sargramostim ▪ vinorelbine.
- **Y-Site Incompatibility:** ▪ acyclovir ▪ ampicillin/sulbactam ▪ cefazolin ▪ cefepime ▪ ceftazidime ▪ clindamycin ▪ dexamethasone ▪ etoposide ▪ furosemide ▪ gentamicin ▪ heparin ▪ hydrocortisone sodium succinate ▪ lorazepam ▪ meperidine ▪ methotrexate ▪ mezlocillin ▪ piperacillin/tazobactam ▪ sodium bicarbonate ▪ teniposide ▪ vancomycin ▪ vincristine.

PATIENT/FAMILY TEACHING

- Instruct patient to notify health care professional promptly if fever; sore throat; signs of infection; bleeding gums; bruising; petechiae; blood in stools, urine, or emesis; increased fatigue; dyspnea; or orthostatic hypotension occurs. Caution patient to avoid crowds and persons with known infections. Instruct patient to use soft toothbrush and electric razor and to avoid falls. Patients should be cautioned not to drink alcoholic beverages or take medication containing aspirin or NSAIDs, as these may precipitate gastric bleeding.
- Instruct patient to report pain at injection site immediately.
- Instruct patient to inspect oral mucosa for erythema and ulceration. If ulceration occurs, advise patient to use sponge brush, rinse mouth with water after eating and drinking, and confer with health care professional if mouth pain interferes with eating. Further courses of idarubicin should be withheld until recovery from mucositis, and subsequent doses should be decreased by 25%. Stomatitis pain may require treatment with opioid analgesics.
- Advise patient that this medication may have teratogenic effects. Contraception should be practiced during and for at least 4 mo after therapy is concluded.
- Instruct patient to notify health care professional immediately if irregular heartbeat, shortness of breath, or swelling of lower extremities occurs.
- Advise patient to wear sunscreen and protective clothing to prevent photosensitivity reactions.
- Discuss with patient the possibility of hair loss. Explore methods of coping.
- Instruct patient not to receive any vaccinations without advice of health care professional.
- Inform patient that urine may turn a reddish color.
- Emphasize the need for periodic lab tests to monitor for side effects.

EVALUATION

Effectiveness of therapy can be demonstrated by: ▪ Improvement of hematologic status in leukemias.

IFOSFAMIDE

(**eye**-foss-fam-ide)
Ifex

CLASSIFICATION(S):
Antineoplastic (alkylating agent)

Pregnancy Category D

INDICATIONS

▪ In combination with other agents in the treatment of germ cell testicular carcinoma ▪ Used in combination with mesna, which prevents ifosfamide-induced hemorrhagic cystitis.

ACTION

▪ Following conversion to active compounds, interferes with DNA replication and RNA transcription, ultimately disrupting protein synthesis (cell-cycle phase–nonspecific). **Therapeutic Effects:** ▪ Death of rapidly replicating cells, particularly malignant ones.

PHARMACOKINETICS

Absorption: Administered IV only; inactive prior to conversion to metabolites.
Distribution: Excreted in breast milk.
Metabolism and Excretion: Metabolized by the liver to active antineoplastic compounds.
Half-life: 15 hr.

CONTRAINDICATIONS AND PRECAUTIONS

Contraindicated in: ▪ Hypersensitivity ▪ Pregnancy or lactation.
Use Cautiously in: ▪ Patients with childbearing potential ▪ Active infections ▪ Decreased bone marrow reserve ▪ Geriatric patients ▪ Other chronic debilitating illness ▪ Impaired renal function ▪ Children.

ADVERSE REACTIONS AND SIDE EFFECTS*

CNS: CNS toxicity (somnolence, confusion, hallucinations, coma), cranial nerve dysfunction, disorientation, dizziness.
CV: CARDIOTOXICITY.
GI: nausea, vomiting, anorexia, constipation, diarrhea, hepatotoxicity.
GU: hemorrhagic cystitis, dysuria, gonadal suppression, renal toxicity.
Derm: alopecia.
Hemat: anemia, leukopenia, thrombocytopenia.
Local: phlebitis.
Misc: allergic reactions.

INTERACTIONS

Drug-Drug: ▪ Additive myelosuppression with other **antineoplastic agents** or **radiation therapy** ▪ Toxicity may be increased by **allopurinol** or **phenobarbital** ▪ May decrease antibody response to and increase risk of adverse reactions from **live virus vaccines.**

ROUTE AND DOSAGE

▪ **IV (Adults):** 1.2 g/m²/day for 5 days; coadminister with mesna. May repeat cycle q 3 wk. Other regimens are used.

AVAILABILITY

▪ ***Injection:*** 1- and 3-g vials[Rx].

TIME/ACTION PROFILE (effects on blood counts)

	ONSET	PEAK	DURATION
IV	UK	7–14 days	21 days

NURSING IMPLICATIONS

ASSESSMENT

- ▫ Monitor blood pressure, pulse, respiratory rate, and temperature frequently during administration. Report significant changes.
- ▫ Monitor urinary output frequently throughout therapy. Notify physician if hematuria occurs. To reduce the risk of hemorrhagic cystitis, fluid intake should be at least 3000 ml/day for adults and 1000–2000 ml/day for children. Mesna is given concurrently to prevent hemorrhagic cystitis. (See mesna, p. 621.)
- ▫ Monitor neurologic status. Ifosfamide should be discontinued if severe CNS symptoms (agitation, confusion, hallucinations, unusual tiredness) occur. Symptoms usually return to normal within 3 days of discontinuation of ifosfamide but may persist for longer; fatalities have been reported.

I

*CAPITALS indicate life-threatening; underlines indicate most frequent.

- □ Assess nausea, vomiting, and appetite. Weigh weekly. Premedication with an antiemetic may be used to minimize GI effects. Adjust diet as tolerated.
- □ Monitor for bone marrow depression. Assess for bleeding (bleeding gums, bruising, petechiae, guaiac stools, urine, and emesis) and avoid IM injections and rectal temperatures if platelet count is low. Apply pressure to venipuncture sites for 10 min. Assess for signs of infection during neutropenia. Anemia may occur. Monitor for increased fatigue, dyspnea, and orthostatic hypotension.
- ▪ ***Lab Test Considerations:*** Monitor CBC, differential, and platelet count prior to and periodically throughout therapy. Withhold dose and notify physician if WBC $<2000/mm^3$ or platelet count is $<50{,}000/mm^3$. Nadir of leukopenia and thrombocytopenia occurs within 7–14 days and usually recovers within 21 days of a course of therapy.
- □ Urinalysis should be evaluated before each dose. Withhold dose and notify physician if urinalysis shows >10 RBCs per high-power field.
- □ May cause elevation in liver enzymes and serum bilirubin.
- □ Monitor AST, ALT, serum alkaline phosphatase, bilirubin, and LDH prior to and periodically during therapy. Ifosfamide may cause elevation in liver enzymes and serum bilirubin.
- □ Monitor BUN, serum creatinine, phosphate, and potassium periodically during therapy.

POTENTIAL NURSING DIAGNOSES

- ▪ Infection, risk for (Side Effects).
- ▪ Body image disturbance (Side Effects).
- ▪ Knowledge deficit, related to medication regimen (Patient/Family Teaching).

IMPLEMENTATION

- ▪ **General Info:** Solution should be prepared in a biologic cabinet. Wear gloves, gown, and mask while handling IV medication. Discard IV equipment in specially designated containers (see Appendix I).
- ▪ **IV:** Prepare solution by diluting each 1-g vial with 20 ml of sterile water or bacteriostatic water for injection containing parabens. Use solution prepared without bacteriostatic water within 6 hr. Solution prepared with bacteriostatic water is stable for 1 wk at 30°C or 6 wk at 5°C.
- ▪ **Intermittent Infusion:** May be further diluted to a concentration of 0.6 to 20 mg/ml in D5W, 0.9% NaCl, lactated Ringer's solution, or sterile water for injection.
- ▪ ***Rate:*** Administer over at least 30 min.
- ▪ **Syringe Compatibility:** ▪ mesna.
- ▪ **Continuous Infusion:** Has also been administered as a continuous infusion over 72 hr.
- ▪ **Y-Site Compatibility:** ▪ allopurinol sodium ▪ aztreonam ▪ filgrastim ▪ fludarabine ▪ gallium nitrate ▪ melphalan ▪ ondansetron ▪ paclitaxel ▪ piperacillin/tazobactam ▪ sargramostim ▪ sodium bicarbonate ▪ teniposide ▪ vinorelbine.
- ▪ **Y-Site Incompatibility:** ▪ cefepime ▪ methotrexate.
- ▪ **Additive Compatibility:** ▪ carboplatin ▪ cisplatin ▪ etoposide ▪ fluorouracil ▪ mesna.

PATIENT/FAMILY TEACHING

- □ Emphasize need for adequate fluid intake throughout therapy. Patient should void frequently to decrease bladder irritation from metabolites excreted by the kidneys. Health care professional should be notified immediately if hematuria is noted.
- □ Instruct patient to notify health care professional promptly if fever; chills; cough; hoarseness; sore throat; signs of infection; lower back or side pain; painful or difficult urination; bleeding gums; bruising; petechiae; blood in urine, stool, or emesis; or confusion occurs.
- □ Caution patient to avoid crowds and persons with known infections. Instruct patient to use soft toothbrush and electric razor and to avoid falls. Patients should also be cautioned not to drink alcoholic beverages or to take products containing aspirin or NSAIDs, as these may precipitate GI hemorrhage.
- □ Review with patient the need for contraception during therapy.
- □ Discuss with patient the possibility of hair loss. Explore methods of coping.
- □ Instruct patient not to receive any vaccinations without advice of health care professional; ifosfamide may decrease antibody response to and increase risk of adverse reactions from live virus vaccines.

EVALUATION

Effectiveness of therapy can be demonstrated by: ▪ Decrease in size or spread of malignant germ cell testicular carcinoma.

IMIPENEM/CILASTATIN

(i-me-**pen**-em/sye-la-**stat**-in)
Primaxin

CLASSIFICATION(S):
Anti-infective (carbapenem)

Pregnancy Category C

INDICATIONS

▪ Treatment of the following: ▫ Lower respiratory tract infections ▫ Urinary tract infections ▫ Abdominal infections ▫ Gynecologic infections ▫ Skin and skin structure infections ▫ Bone and joint infections ▫ Bacteremia ▫ Endocarditis ▫ Polymicrobic infections.

ACTION

▪ Imipenem binds to bacterial cell wall, resulting in cell death ▪ Combination with cilastatin prevents renal inactivation of imipenem, resulting in high urinary concentrations ▪ Imipenem resists the actions of many enzymes that degrade most other penicillins and penicillin-like anti-infectives. **Therapeutic Effects:** ▪ Bactericidal action against susceptible bacteria. **Spectrum:** ▪ Spectrum is broad ▪ Active against most gram-positive aerobic cocci: ▫ *Streptococcus pneumoniae* ▫ Group A beta-hemolytic streptococci ▫ *Enterococcus* ▫ *Staphylococcus aureus* ▪ Active against many gram-negative bacillary organisms: ▫ *Escherichia coli* ▫ *Klebsiella* ▫ *Acinetobacter* ▫ *Proteus* ▫ *Serratia* ▫ *Pseudomonas aeruginosa* ▪ Also displays activity against: ▫ *Salmonella* ▫ *Shigella* ▫ *Neisseria gonorrhoeae* ▫ Numerous anaerobes.

PHARMACOKINETICS

Absorption: Well absorbed following IM administration (imipenem 95%, cilastatin 75%). IV administration results in complete bioavailability.
Distribution: Widely distributed. Crosses the placenta; enters breast milk.
Metabolism and Excretion: *Imipenem and cilastatin*—70% excreted unchanged by the kidneys.
Half-life: *Imipenem and cilastatin*—1 hr (prolonged in renal impairment).

CONTRAINDICATIONS AND PRECAUTIONS

Contraindicated in: ▪ Hypersensitivity ▪ Cross-sensitivity may occur with penicillins and cephalosporins.
Use Cautiously in: ▪ Previous history of multiple hypersensitivity reactions ▪ Seizure disorders ▪ Geriatric patients ▪ Renal impairment (dosage reduction required if CCr $\leq$70 ml/min/1.73 m^2) ▪ Pregnancy, lactation, or children (safety not established).

ADVERSE REACTIONS AND SIDE EFFECTS*

CNS: SEIZURES, dizziness, somnolence.
CV: hypotension.
GI: <u>diarrhea</u>, <u>nausea</u>, <u>vomiting</u>.
Derm: <u>rash</u>, pruritus, sweating, urticaria.
Hemat: eosinophilia.
Local: phlebitis at IV site.
Misc: allergic reaction including ANAPHYLAXIS, fever, superinfection.

INTERACTIONS

Drug-Drug: ▪ Do not admix with **aminoglycosides** (inactivation may occur) ▪ **Probenecid** decreases renal excretion and increases blood levels ▪ Increased risk of seizures with **ganciclovir** (avoid concurrent use).

ROUTE AND DOSAGE

- **IV (Adults):** *Mild infections*—250–500 mg q 6 hr. *Moderate infections*—500 mg q 6–8 hr or 1 g q 8 hr. *Serious infections*—500 mg q 6 hr to 1 g q 6–8 hr.
- **IM (Adults):** 500–750 mg q 12 hr.

AVAILABILITY

▪ ***Powder for IV injection:*** 250 mg imipenem/250 mg cilastatin[Rx], 500 mg imipenem/500 mg cilastatin[Rx] ▪ ***Powder for IM injection:*** 500 mg imipenem/500 mg cilastatin[Rx], 750 mg imipenem/750 mg cilastatin[Rx].

***CAPITALS indicate life-threatening; <u>underlines</u> indicate most frequent.**

TIME/ACTION PROFILE (blood levels)

	ONSET	PEAK	DURATION
IM	rapid	1–2 hr	12 hr
IV	rapid	end of infusion	6–8 hr

NURSING IMPLICATIONS

ASSESSMENT

- Assess patient for infection (vital signs; appearance of wound, sputum, urine, and stool; WBC) at beginning of and throughout therapy.
- Obtain a history before initiating therapy to determine previous use of and reactions to penicillins. Persons with a negative history of penicillin sensitivity may still have an allergic response.
- Obtain specimens for culture and sensitivity prior to initiating therapy. First dose may be given before receiving results.
- Observe patient for signs and symptoms of anaphylaxis (rash, pruritus, laryngeal edema, wheezing). Discontinue the drug and notify the physician immediately if these occur. Have epinephrine, an antihistamine, and resuscitative equipment close by in the event of an anaphylactic reaction.
- ***Lab Test Considerations:*** BUN, AST, ALT, LDH, serum alkaline phosphatase, bilirubin, and creatinine may be transiently increased.
- Hemoglobin and hematocrit concentrations may be decreased.
- May cause positive direct Coombs' test.

POTENTIAL NURSING DIAGNOSES

- Infection, risk for (Indications, Side Effects).
- Knowledge deficit, related to medication regimen (Patient/Family Teaching).

IMPLEMENTATION

- **IM:** Reconstitute 500-mg vial with 2 ml and 750-mg vial with 3 ml of lidocaine without epinephrine. Shake well to form a suspension. Withdraw and inject entire contents of vial IM.
- **Intermittent Infusion:** Reconstitute each 250- or 500-mg vial with 10 ml of compatible diluent and shake well. Transfer the resulting solution to not less than 100 ml of compatible diluent. Add an additional 10 ml to each previously reconstituted vial and shake well to ensure all medication is used. Transfer the remaining contents of the vial to the infusion container.
- Reconstitute 120-ml infusion bottles with 100 ml of a compatible diluent. Shake well until clear.
- *Compatible diluents* include 0.9% NaCl, D5W, D10W, D5/0.2% sodium bicarbonate, D5/0.9% NaCl, D5/0.45% NaCl, D5/0.225% NaCl, or mannitol 2.5%, 5%, or 10%. Solution may range from clear to yellow in color. Do not administer cloudy solutions. Solution is stable for 4 hr at room temperature and 24 hr if refrigerated.
- ***Rate:*** Administer each 250- or 500-mg dose over 20–30 min and each 1-g dose over 40–60 min. Administer over 20–30 min for pediatric patients. Do not administer direct IV.
- Rapid infusion may cause nausea, vomiting, unusual tiredness or weakness, dizziness, or sweating. If these symptoms develop, slow infusion. Discontinuation of medication may be necessary.
- **Y-Site Compatibility:** ▪ acyclovir ▪ aztreonam ▪ cefepime ▪ diltiazem ▪ famotidine ▪ filgrastim ▪ fludarabine ▪ foscarnet ▪ idarubicin ▪ insulin ▪ melphalan ▪ methotrexate ▪ ondansetron ▪ tacrolimus ▪ teniposide ▪ vinorelbine ▪ zidovudine.
- **Y-Site Incompatibility:** ▪ fluconazole ▪ gallium nitrate ▪ meperidine ▪ sargramostim ▪ sodium bicarbonate.
- **Additive Incompatibility:** ▪ May be inactivated if administered concurrently with aminoglycosides. If administered concurrently, administer in separate sites, if possible, at least 1 hr apart. If second site is unavailable, flush lines between medications.

PATIENT/FAMILY TEACHING

- Advise patient to report the signs of superinfection (black, furry overgrowth on the tongue; vaginal itching or discharge; loose or foul-smelling stools) and allergy. Consult health care professional prior to treating with antidiarrheals.

EVALUATION

Clinical response to therapy can be evaluated by: ▪ Resolution of the signs and symptoms of infection. Length of time for complete resolution depends on the organism and site of infection.

IMIPRAMINE

(im-**ip**-ra-meen)
{Apo-Imipramine}, {Impril}, Norfranil, {Novopramine}, Tipramine, Tofranil, Tofranil PM

CLASSIFICATION(S):
Antidepressant (tricyclic)

Pregnancy Category C

INDICATIONS

▪ Various forms of depression (with psychotherapy) ▪ Enuresis in children. **Unlabeled Uses:** ▪ Adjunct in the management of chronic pain, incontinence (in adults), vascular headache prophylaxis, and cluster headache.

ACTION

▪ Potentiates the effect of serotonin and norepinephrine ▪ Has significant anticholinergic properties. **Therapeutic Effects:** ▪ Antidepressant action that develops slowly over several weeks.

PHARMACOKINETICS

Absorption: Well absorbed from the GI tract.
Distribution: Widely distributed. Probably crosses the placenta and enters breast milk.
Metabolism and Excretion: Extensively metabolized by the liver, mostly on first pass; some conversion to active compounds. Undergoes enterohepatic recirculation and secretion into gastric juices.
Half-life: 8–16 hr.

CONTRAINDICATIONS AND PRECAUTIONS

Contraindicated in: ▪ Hypersensitivity ▪ Cross-sensitivity with other antidepressants may occur ▪ Narrow-angle glaucoma ▪ Hypersensitivity to tartrazine or sulfites (in some preparations) ▪ Pregnancy and lactation.
Use Cautiously in: ▪ Geriatric patients (more susceptible to adverse reactions) ▪ Pre-existing cardiovascular disease ▪ Geriatric men with prostatic hyperplasia (more susceptible to urinary retention) ▪ Seizures or history of seizure disorder.

ADVERSE REACTIONS AND SIDE EFFECTS*

CNS: drowsiness, fatigue, agitation, confusion, hallucinations, insomnia.
EENT: blurred vision, dry eyes.
CV: ARRHYTHMIAS, hypotension, ECG changes.
GI: constipation, dry mouth, nausea, paralytic ileus.
GU: urinary retention.
Derm: photosensitivity.
Endo: gynecomastia.
Hemat: blood dyscrasias.

INTERACTIONS

Drug-Drug: ▪ May cause hypotension and tachycardia when used with **MAO inhibitors** (avoid concurrent use—discontinue 2 wk prior to imipramine) ▪ May cause severe hypertension when used with **clonidine** (avoid concurrent use) ▪ May prevent therapeutic response to most **antihypertensives** ▪ Additive CNS depression with other **CNS depressants**, including **alcohol, antihistamines, opioids,** and **sedative/hypnotics** ▪ **Adrenergic** and **anticholinergic** side effects may be additive with other agents having these properties ▪ **Cimetidine, fluoxetine, phenothiazines,** or **oral contraceptives** may increase levels and may cause toxicity ▪ May produce organic brain syndrome with **disulfiram** ▪ **Smoking** may increase metabolism and decrease effectiveness.

ROUTE AND DOSAGE

- **PO (Adults):** 25–50 mg 3–4 times daily (not to exceed 300 mg/day); total daily dose may be given at bedtime.
- **PO (Geriatric Patients):** 25 mg at bedtime initially, up to 100 mg/day in divided doses.
- **PO (Children >12 yr):** *Antidepressant*—25–50 mg/day in divided doses (not to exceed 100 mg/day).
- **PO (Children 6–12 yr):** *Antidepressant*—10–30 mg/day in 2 divided doses.
- **PO (Children >6 yr):** *Enuresis*—25 mg once daily 1 hr before bedtime; increase if necessary by 25 mg at weekly intervals to 50 mg in children <12 yr, up to 75 mg in children >12 yr.

I

{} = Available in Canada only.
***CAPITALS indicate life-threatening; underlines indicate most frequent.**

- **IM (Adults):** Up to 100 mg/day in divided doses (not to exceed 300 mg/day).

AVAILABILITY

- ***Tablets:*** 10 mg[Rx], 25 mg[Rx], 50 mg[Rx], {75 mg[Rx]} - ***Capsules:*** 75 mg[Rx], 100 mg[Rx], 125 mg[Rx], 150 mg[Rx] - ***Injection:*** 12.5 mg/ml[Rx].

TIME/ACTION PROFILE (antidepressant effect)

	ONSET	PEAK	DURATION
PO, IM	hr	2–6 wk	wks

NURSING IMPLICATIONS

ASSESSMENT

- **General Info:** Monitor blood pressure and pulse rate prior to and during initial therapy.
  - Monitor baseline and periodic ECGs in elderly or patients with heart disease and before increasing dosage with children treated for enuresis. May cause prolonged PR and QT intervals and may flatten T waves.
- **Depression:** Assess mental status frequently. Confusion, agitation, and hallucinations may occur during initiation of therapy and may require dosage reduction. Monitor mood changes. Assess for suicidal tendencies, especially during early therapy. Restrict amount of drug available to patient.
- **Enuresis:** Assess freqency of bed-wetting throughout therapy.
- **Pain:** Assess location, duration, and severity of pain periodically throughout therapy.
- ***Lab Test Considerations:*** Assess leukocyte and differential blood counts and renal and hepatic functions prior to and periodically during prolonged or high-dose therapy.
  - Serum levels may be monitored in patients who fail to respond to usual therapeutic dose. Therapeutic plasma concentration range for depression is 150–300 ng/ml.
  - May cause alterations in blood glucose levels.
- ***Toxicity and Overdose:*** Symptoms of acute overdose include disturbed concentration, confusion, restlessness, agitation, convulsions, drowsiness, mydriasis, arrhythmias, fever, hallucinations, vomiting, and dyspnea.
  - Treatment of overdose includes gastric lavage, activated charcoal, and a stimulant cathartic. Maintain respiratory and cardiac function (monitor ECG for at least 5 days) and temperature. Medications may include digoxin for congestive heart failure, antiarrhythmics, and anticonvulsants.

POTENTIAL NURSING DIAGNOSES

- Coping, ineffective individual (Indications).
- Urinary elimination, altered (Indications).
- Knowledge deficit, related to medication regimen (Patient/Family Teaching).

IMPLEMENTATION

- **General Info:** Dose increases should be made at bedtime because of sedation. Dose titration is a slow process; may take weeks to months. May be given as a single dose at bedtime to minimize sedation during the day.
- **PO:** Administer medication with or immediately following a meal to minimize gastric irritation.
- **IM:** May be slightly yellow or red in color. Crystals may develop if solution is cool; place ampule under warm running water for 1 min to dissolve.

PATIENT/FAMILY TEACHING

- **General Info:** Instruct patient to take medication exactly as directed. If a dose is missed, take as soon as possible unless almost time for next dose; if regimen is a single dose at bedtime, do not take in the morning because of side effects. Advise patient that drug effects may not be noticed for at least 2 wk. Abrupt discontinuation may cause nausea, vomiting, diarrhea, headache, trouble sleeping with vivid dreams, and irritability.
  - May cause drowsiness and blurred vision. Caution patient to avoid driving and other activities requiring alertness until response to drug is known.
  - Instruct patient to notify health care professional if visual changes occur. Inform patient that periodic glaucoma testing may be needed during long-term therapy.
  - Caution patient to change positions slowly to minimize orthostatic hypotension.
  - Advise patient to avoid alcohol or other CNS depressant drugs during therapy and for at least 3–7 days after therapy has been discontinued.

- ▫ Instruct patient to notify health care professional if urinary retention occurs or if dry mouth or constipation persists. Sugarless candy or gum may diminish dry mouth and an increase in fluid intake or bulk may prevent constipation. If symptoms persist, dose reduction or discontinuation may be necessary. Consult health care professional if dry mouth persists for more than 2 wk.
- ▫ Caution patient to use sunscreen and protective clothing to prevent photosensitivity reactions.
- ▫ Inform patient of need to monitor dietary intake, as possible increase in appetite may lead to undesired weight gain. Inform patient that increased amounts of riboflavin in the diet may be required; consult health care professional.
- ▫ Advise patient to notify health care professional of medication regimen prior to treatment or surgery.
- ▫ Therapy for depression is usually prolonged. Emphasize the importance of follow-up exams to evaluate progress.
- ▪ **Children:** Inform parents that the side effects most likely to occur include nervousness, insomnia, unusual tiredness, and mild nausea and vomiting. Notify health care professional if these symptoms become pronounced.
- ▫ Advise parents to keep medication out of reach of children to prevent inadvertent overdose.

EVALUATION

Effectiveness of therapy can be demonstrated by: ▪ Increased sense of well-being ▫ Renewed interest in surroundings ▫ Increased appetite ▫ Improved energy level ▫ Improved sleep in patients treated for depression. Patient may require 2–6 wk of therapy before full therapeutic effects of medication are noticeable ▪ Control of bed-wetting in children >6 yr ▪ Decrease in chronic neurogenic pain.

IMMUNE GLOBULIN

(im-**myoon glo**-byoo-lin)
gamma globulin, IG, ISG, immune serum globulin

immune globulin IM
Gamastan, Gammar, IGIM

immune globulin IV
Gamimune N, Gammagard S/D, Gammar-P IV, IG IV, Iveegam, Polygam, Polygam S/D, Sandoglobulin, Venoglobulin-I, Venoglobulin-S

CLASSIFICATION(S):
Serum (immune globulin)

Pregnancy Category C

INDICATIONS

▪ **IM:** Provide passive immunity to a variety of infections including: ▫ Hepatitis A ▫ Measles (rubeola) when immune sera are unavailable or when there is insufficient time for active immunization to take place ▪ **IV:** Useful in patients with immunodeficiency syndromes who are unable to produce IgG-type antibodies ▪ Prevention of bacterial infections in patients with B-cell chronic lymphocytic leukemia (Gammagard only) ▪ Prevention of bacterial infections in children infected with HIV ▪ Treatment of idiopathic thrombocytopenic purpura.

ACTION

▪ A human serum fraction containing gamma globulin antibodies (IgG). **Therapeutic Effects:** ▪ Provision of passive immunity against many infections.

PHARMACOKINETICS

Absorption: IV administration results in complete bioavailability. Well absorbed following IM administration.
Distribution: Rapidly and evenly distributed.
Metabolism and Excretion: Removed by redistribution, tissue binding, and catabolism.
Half-life: 21–24 days.

CONTRAINDICATIONS AND PRECAUTIONS

Contraindicated in: ▪ Hypersensitivity to immune globulins or additives (maltose, thimerisol, glycine, polyethylene glycol, albumin) ▪ Selective IgA deficiency.
Use Cautiously in: ▪ IM form in patients with thrombocytopenia ▪ Gamimune N product in patients with acid-base disorders ▪ Agammaglob-

ulinemia or hypogammaglobulinemia (increased risk of hypotension and anaphylaxis following rapid IV administration) ▪ Have been used during pregnancy, although safety is not established.

ADVERSE REACTIONS AND SIDE EFFECTS*

CNS: faintness, headache, light-headedness, malaise.
Resp: dyspnea, wheezing.
CV: chest pain.
GI: nausea.
GU: diuresis (if maltose in preparation), nephrotic syndrome.
Derm: cyanosis, urticaria.
Local: *at IM site*—muscle stiffness, pain, tenderness; *at IV site*—local inflammation, phlebitis, urticaria.
MS: arthralgia, back pain, hip pain.
Misc: allergic reactions including ANAPHYLAXIS, angioedema, chills, fever, sweating.

INTERACTIONS

Drug-Drug: ▪ May interfere with the normal immune response to some **live vaccines**, including **measles, mumps**, and **rubella virus vaccine** (do not administer within 3 mo of immune globulin).

ROUTE AND DOSAGE

❑ Hepatitis A Prophylaxis

- **IM (Adults and Children):** 0.02 ml/kg (for pre-exposure prophylaxis, higher doses—0.06 ml/kg q 4–6 mo are used if exposure will last >3 mo).

❑ Measles Prophylaxis

- **IM (Adults and Children):** 0.25 ml/kg (0.5 ml/kg if immunosuppressed; not to exceed 15 ml).

❑ Immunodeficiency

- **IV (Adults and Children):** 100–800 mg/kg q 3–4 wk (other regimens are used).

❑ Idiopathic Thrombocytopenic Purpura

- **IV (Adults and Children):** 400 mg/kg/day for 5 days; may be repeated as needed (other regimens are used).

❑ Prevention of Bacterial Infections in HIV-Infected Patients

- **IV (Adults and Children):** 400 mg/kg q 3–4 wk.

❑ Kawasaki Disease

- **IV (Children):** 400 mg/kg/day for 4 days or 2 g/kg single dose (unlabeled).

AVAILABILITY

- ***Injection (IM):*** 2-ml, 10-ml vials[Rx]
- ***Injection (IV):*** 5% solution[Rx], 10% solution[Rx], 0.5-g, 1-g, 2.5-g, 3-g, 6-g, 10-g vials[Rx].

TIME/ACTION PROFILE (antibody levels)

	ONSET	PEAK	DURATION
IM	5 days	UK	UK
IV	immediate	UK	3–4 wk

NURSING IMPLICATIONS

ASSESSMENT

- ❑ For passive immunity, determine the date of exposure to infection. Immune globulin should be administered within 2 wk of exposure to hepatitis A and within 6 days after exposure to measles.
- ❑ Monitor vital signs continuously during infusion of immune globulin IV and assess patient for signs of anaphylaxis (hypotension, flushing, chest tightness, wheezing, fever, dizziness, nausea, vomiting, diaphoresis) for 1 hr following initiation of infusion. Epinephrine and antihistamines should be available for treatment of anaphylactic reactions.
- **Leukemia:** Monitor patient for signs of infection (vital signs, WBC) throughout therapy.
- ***Lab Test Considerations:*** Monitor platelet counts in patients being treated for idiopathic thrombocytopenic purpura.

POTENTIAL NURSING DIAGNOSES

- Infection, risk for (Indications).
- Knowledge deficit, related to medication regimen (Patient/Family Teaching).

IMPLEMENTATION

- **IM:** Administer immune globulin IM (IGIM) in adults and children into the deltoid muscle

*CAPITALS indicate life-threatening; underlines indicate most frequent.

or anterolateral thigh. Volumes >10 ml should be divided into several injections to minimize local pain. Avoid IM administration of doses exceeding 20 ml. Use of the gluteal site should be reserved only for volumes >3 ml or when large volumes are divided into multiple injections to prevent damage to the sciatic nerve. Do not administer SC, intradermally, or IV. Solution of IGIM should be transparent or opalescent and may be colorless or brownish.

- **Intermittent Infusion:** Reconstituted solutions should be swirled to mix. Do not shake; foaming may occur. Immune globulin IV (IGIV) should be administered by IV infusion using separate tubing. Do not mix with other drugs or solutions. If adverse reactions occur during infusion, decrease the rate of infusion or stop the infusion until the adverse reactions subside. Most side effects subside within 30 min. The infusion may then be resumed at a rate of tolerance for the individual. Do not use turbid solution. Bring to room temperature prior to administration. Administer promptly, within 2–3 hr of dilution. Discard unused portions.
- □ Do not administer IGIV SC or IM.
- □ *Gamimune N* should be diluted with D5W and infused at a rate of 0.01–0.02 ml/kg/min for 30 min. If no adverse reactions occur, the infusion rate may be gradually increased to a maximum of 0.08 ml/kg/hr. Solutions of *Gamimune N* should be refrigerated but not frozen. Discard solution that has been frozen.
- □ *Gammagard S/D* or *Polygam* should be reconstituted with sterile water for injection for a solution containing 50 mg/ml. Administer solution as soon as possible within 2 hr of reconstitution. Infuse via the administration set containing an integral airway and 15-micron filter provided by the manufacturer. Infuse at a rate of 0.5 ml/kg/hr initially. If no adverse reactions occur, the rate of infusion may be increased gradually to a maximum of 4 ml/kg/hr.
- □ *Gammar-P IV* should be administered initially at a rate of 0.01 ml/kg/min of the 50 mg/ml solution for 15–30 min, increasing to 0.02 mg/kg/min, then gradually increasing to 0.03–0.06 ml/kg/min. Store at room temperature. Avoid freezing. Discard unused solution.
- □ *Iveegam* should be administered at a rate of 1 ml/min of the 5% solution up to a maximum of 2 ml/min.
- □ *Sandoglobulin* should be reconstituted with the 0.9% NaCl provided by the manufacturer for a solution containing 30 or 60 mg of protein per ml. For patients with agammaglobulinemia or hypogammaglobulinemia, use a solution containing 30 mg/ml for the initial dose. Infuse at an initial rate of 0.5–1 ml/min. After 15–30 min, the rate may be increased to 1.5–2.5 ml/min, and subsequent infusions may be given at a rate of 2–2.5 ml/min. Solutions of *Sandoglobulin* should be stored at room temperature.
- □ The 50 mg/ml solution of *Venoglobulin-I* or *Venoglobulin-S* should be administered at a rate of 0.01–0.02 ml/kg/min for 30 min. If patient does not experience discomfort, the rate may be gradually increased to 0.04 ml/kg/min. If patient tolerates higher rate, subsequent doses may be administered at the higher rate. Store at room temperature.
- **Y-Site Incompatibility:** ▪ It is recommended that IVIG be administered through a separate line, by itself, without mixing with other IV fluids, except those listed previously.

PATIENT/FAMILY TEACHING

- □ Explain the use and purpose of immune globulin therapy to the patient.
- □ Advise patient to report symptoms of anaphylaxis immediately.
- □ Inform patients that pain, tenderness, and muscle stiffness at the injection site may occur following IM injections of immune globulin. These may persist for several hours following administration.

EVALUATION

Effectiveness of therapy can be demonstrated by: ▪ Prevention of certain infectious diseases by provision of passive immunity in patients exposed to the infections or patients with immunodeficiency diseases ▪ Increased platelet counts in patients with idiopathic thrombocytopenic purpura ▪ Prevention of bacterial infections in patients with hypogammaglobulinemia associated with B-cell chronic lymphocytic leukemia.

INDAPAMIDE
(in-**dap**-a-mide)
{Lozide}, Lozol

CLASSIFICATION(S):
Antihypertensive agent, Diuretic (thiazide-like)

Pregnancy Category B

INDICATIONS

▪ Mild to moderate hypertension ▪ Edema associated with congestive heart failure and other causes.

ACTION

▪ Increases excretion of sodium and water by inhibiting sodium reabsorption in the distal tubule ▪ Promotes excretion of chloride, potassium, magnesium, and bicarbonate ▪ May produce arteriolar dilation. **Therapeutic Effects:** ▪ Lowering of blood pressure in hypertensive patients and diuresis with subsequent mobilization of edema.

PHARMACOKINETICS

Absorption: Well absorbed from the GI tract following oral administration.
Distribution: Widely distributed.
Metabolism and Excretion: Mostly metabolized by the liver. Small amounts (7%) excreted unchanged by the kidneys.
Half-life: 14–18 hr.

CONTRAINDICATIONS AND PRECAUTIONS

Contraindicated in: ▪ Hypersensitivity ▪ Cross-sensitivity with sulfonamides may occur ▪ Anuria ▪ Lactation.
Use Cautiously in: ▪ Renal or severe hepatic impairment ▪ Geriatric patients (increased sensitivity) ▪ Pregnancy or children (safety not established).

ADVERSE REACTIONS AND SIDE EFFECTS*

CNS: dizziness, drowsiness, lethargy.
CV: arrhythmias, hypotension.
GI: anorexia, cramping, nausea, vomiting.
Derm: photosensitivity, rashes.
Endo: hyperglycemia.
F and E: hypokalemia, dehydration, hypochloremic alkalosis, hyponatremia, hypovolemia.
Metab: hyperuricemia.
MS: muscle cramps.

INTERACTIONS

Drug-Drug: ▪ Additive hypotension with other **antihypertensives, nitrates,** or acute ingestion of **alcohol** ▪ Additive hypokalemia with **glucocorticoids, amphotericin B, mezlocillin, piperacillin,** or **ticarcillin** ▪ Decreases the excretion of **lithium;** may cause toxicity ▪ Hypokalemia may increase risk of **digitalis glycoside toxicity.**

ROUTE AND DOSAGE

▪ **PO (Adults):** *Hypertension*—1.25–5 mg daily in the morning; may be increased at 4-wk intervals up to 5 mg/day. *Edema secondary to congestive heart failure*—2.5 mg daily in the morning; may be increased after 1 wk to 5 mg/day.

AVAILABILITY

▪ ***Tablets:*** 1.25 mg[Rx], 2.5 mg[Rx].

TIME/ACTION PROFILE (antihypertensive effect)

	ONSET	PEAK	DURATION
PO (single dose)	UK	24 hr	UK
PO (multiple dose)	1–2 wk	8–12 wk	up to 8 wk

NURSING IMPLICATIONS

ASSESSMENT

□ Monitor blood pressure, intake and output, and daily weight and assess feet, legs, and sacral area for edema daily.
□ Assess patient, especially if taking digitalis glycosides, for anorexia, nausea, vomiting, muscle cramps, paresthesia, and confusion; report signs of electrolyte imbalance. Patients taking digitalis glycosides have an increased risk of digitalis toxicity due to the potassium-depleting effect of the diuretic.
□ Assess patient for allergy to sulfonamides.
▪ ***Lab Test Considerations:*** Monitor elec-

{} = Available in Canada only.
*CAPITALS indicate life-threatening; underlines indicate most frequent.

trolytes (especially potassium), blood glucose, BUN, serum creatinine, and uric acid levels prior to and periodically throughout therapy. May cause decreased potassium, sodium, and chloride concentrations. May increase serum glucose; diabetic patients may require increased oral hypoglycemic or insulin dosage. Increases uric acid level an average of 1.0 mg/100 ml; may precipitate an episode of gout.

POTENTIAL NURSING DIAGNOSES

- Fluid volume excess (Indications).
- Fluid volume deficit (Side Effects).
- Knowledge deficit, related to medication regimen (Patient/Family Teaching).

IMPLEMENTATION

- **General Info:** Administer in the morning to prevent disruption of sleep cycle.
- **PO:** May be given with food or milk to minimize GI irritation.

PATIENT/FAMILY TEACHING

- **General Info:** Instruct patient to take this medication at the same time each day. If a dose is missed, take as soon as remembered but not just before next dose is due. Do not double doses. Advise patients using indapamide for hypertension to continue taking the medication even if feeling well. Indapamide controls but does not cure hypertension.
- ◻ Caution patient to change positions slowly to minimize orthostatic hypotension. This may be potentiated by alcohol.
- ◻ Advise patient to use sunscreen (avoid those containing PABA) and protective clothing when in the sun to prevent photosensitivity reactions.
- ◻ Instruct patient to follow a diet high in potassium (see Appendix K).
- ◻ Advise patient to report muscle weakness, cramps, nausea, or dizziness to health care professional.
- ◻ Advise patient to consult health care professional before taking OTC medication concurrently with this therapy.
- ◻ Emphasize the importance of routine follow-up exams.
- **Hypertension:** Instruct patient and family on proper technique of blood pressure monitoring. Advise them to check blood pressure at least weekly and to report significant changes.
- ◻ Encourage patient to comply with additional interventions for hypertension (weight reduction, low-sodium diet, regular exercise, smoking cessation, moderation of alcohol consumption, and stress management).

EVALUATION

Effectiveness of therapy can be demonstrated by: ▪ Control of hypertension ▪ Decrease in edema secondary to congestive heart failure.

INDINAVIR

(in-**din**-a-veer)

Crixivan

CLASSIFICATION(S):

Antiretroviral (protease inhibitor)

Pregnancy Category C

INDICATIONS

▪ Management of HIV infection, usually in combination with other antiretroviral agents. **Unlabeled Uses:** ▪ Prevention of HIV infection following known exposure (with other antiretrovirals).

ACTION

▪ Inhibits the action of HIV protease and prevents the cleavage of viral polyproteins. **Therapeutic Effects:** ▪ Slowing of the progression of HIV infection and its sequelae.

PHARMACOKINETICS

Absorption: Rapidly absorbed following oral administration.

Distribution: UK.

Metabolism and Excretion: Mostly metabolized by the liver; <20% excreted unchanged by the kidneys.

Half-life: 1.8 hr.

CONTRAINDICATIONS AND PRECAUTIONS

Contraindicated in: ▪ Hypersensitivity ▪ Dehydration ▪ Concurrent astemizole, cisapride, dihydroergotamine, ergotamine, midazolam, rifampin, or triazolam.

Use Cautiously in: ▪ Hepatic impairment (dosage reduction recommended in moderate-to-severe hepatic insufficiency due to cirrhosis) ▪ Hemophilia (increased risk of bleeding)

■ Diabetes mellitus ■ Pregnancy, lactation, or children (safety not established; breast-feeding not recommended in HIV-infected patients).

ADVERSE REACTIONS AND SIDE EFFECTS*

CNS: dizziness, drowsiness, fatigue, headache, insomnia, weakness.
GI: abdominal pain, acid regurgitation, altered taste, asymptomatic hyperbilirubinemia, diarrhea, nausea, vomiting.
GU: nephrolithiasis.
Endo: hyperglycemia.
F and E: KETOACIDOSIS.
MS: back pain, flank pain.

INTERACTIONS

Drug-Drug: ■ Concurrent use with **astemizole, cisapride, dihydroergotamine, ergotamine, midazolam, rifampin,** or **triazolam** is contraindicated because of increased risk of serious or life-threatening adverse reactions, including arrhythmias, excessive sedation, vasoconstriction ■ **Rifampin** and **fluconazole** reduce blood levels; concurrent use should be avoided ■ Increases blood levels of **rifabutin** (decrease dosage of rifabutin) and **oral contraceptives** ■ Blood levels are increased by **ketoconazole** or **delavirdine** (decrease dose of indinavir) ■ Alters absorption of **didanosine** ■ Levels are decreased by **nevirapine** (increase indinavir dose).
Drug-Food: ■ **High-fat** or **high-protein meals** and **grapefruit juice** significantly decrease absorption.

ROUTE AND DOSAGE

■ **PO (Adults):** 800 mg q 8 hr.

AVAILABILITY

■ ***Capsules:*** 200 mg[Rx], 400 mg[Rx].

TIME/ACTION PROFILE (blood levels)

	ONSET	PEAK	DURATION
PO	rapid	0.8 hr	8 hr

NURSING IMPLICATIONS

ASSESSMENT

□ Assess patient for change in severity of symptoms of AIDS and for symptoms of opportunistic infections throughout therapy.
■ ***Lab Test Considerations:*** Monitor viral load and CD4 cell count periodically during therapy.
□ May cause hyperglycemia.
□ May cause elevated serum AST, ALT, total bilirubin, and amylase concentrations.

POTENTIAL NURSING DIAGNOSES

■ Infection, risk for (Indications).
■ Knowledge deficit, related to disease process and medication regimen (Patient/Family Teaching).
■ Noncompliance (Patient/Family Teaching).

IMPLEMENTATION

■ **PO:** Administer with water 1 hr before or 2 hr after a meal. May be taken with other liquids (skim milk, juice, coffee, tea) or a light meal (dry toast with jelly, coffee with skim milk and sugar, cornflakes with skim milk and sugar). Avoid high-fat, high-protein meals within 2 hr of indinavir.
□ Patients on concurrent didanosine therapy should take didanosine and indinavir at least 1 hr apart.

PATIENT/FAMILY TEACHING

□ Emphasize the importance of taking indinavir exactly as directed, at evenly spaced times throughout day. Do not take more than prescribed amount and do not stop taking without consulting health care professional. If a dose is missed, take as soon as remembered; do not double doses.
□ Instruct patient that indinavir should not be shared with others.
□ Instruct patient to store indinavir in original container with desiccant in bottle; indinavir is sensitive to moisture.
□ Indinavir may cause kidney stones. Advise patient to drink at least 1.5 liters of water each day. Kidney stones may require 1–3 day interruption of therapy.
□ Inform patient that indinavir may cause hy-

*CAPITALS indicate life-threatening; underlines indicate most frequent.

perglycemia. Advise patient to notify health care professional if increased thirst or hunger; unexplained weight loss; increased urination; fatigue; or dry, itchy skin occurs.

- □ Advise patient to avoid taking other medications, prescription or OTC, without consulting health care professional.
- □ Advise patients concurrently taking didanosine that both medications must be taken on an empty stomach, 1 hr apart.
- □ Inform patient that indinavir does not cure AIDS and does not reduce the risk of transmission of HIV to others through sexual contact or blood contamination. Caution patient to avoid using a condom and avoid sharing needles or donating blood to prevent spreading HIV to others.
- □ May cause drowsiness and dizziness. Advise patient to avoid driving and other activities requiring alertness until response to medication is known.
- □ Emphasize the importance of regular follow-up exams and blood counts to determine progress and monitor for side effects.

EVALUATION

Effectiveness of therapy can be demonstrated by: ▪ Delayed progression of AIDS and decreased opportunistic infections in patients with HIV ▪ Improved CD4 cell count and decrease in viral load.

INDOMETHACIN

(in-doe-**meth**-a-sin)

{Apo-Indomethacin}, {Indameth}, {Indocid}, Indocin, Indocin I.V., {Indocin PDA}, Indocin SR, {Novo-Methacin}, {Nu-Indo}

CLASSIFICATION(S):

Nonsteroidal anti-inflammatory agent

Pregnancy Category B (first trimester)

INDICATIONS

▪ **PO, Rect:** Inflammatory disorders including: □ Rheumatoid arthritis □ Gouty arthritis □ Osteoarthritis □ Ankylosing spondylitis ▪ Generally reserved for patients who do not respond to less toxic agents ▪ **IV:** Alternative to surgery in the management of patent ductus arteriosus in premature neonates.

ACTION

▪ Inhibits prostaglandin synthesis. **Therapeutic Effects:** ▪ **PO:** Suppression of pain and inflammation ▪ **IV:** Closure of patent ductus arteriosus.

PHARMACOKINETICS

Absorption: Well absorbed following PO/rectal administration.

Distribution: Crosses the blood-brain barrier and the placenta. Enters breast milk.

Metabolism and Excretion: Mostly metabolized by the liver.

Half-life: 2.6–11 hr (prolonged in neonates—up to 60 hr, average range 12–21 hr).

CONTRAINDICATIONS AND PRECAUTIONS

Contraindicated in: ▪ Hypersensitivity ▪ Known alcohol intolerance (suspension) ▪ Cross-sensitivity may exist with other NSAIDs, including aspirin ▪ Active GI bleeding ▪ Ulcer disease ▪ Proctitis or recent history of rectal bleeding.

Use Cautiously in: ▪ Severe cardiovascular, renal, or hepatic disease ▪ History of ulcer disease ▪ Geriatric patients (increased risk of adverse reactions) ▪ Pregnancy or lactation (not recommended during 2nd half of pregnancy) ▪ Lactation.

ADVERSE REACTIONS AND SIDE EFFECTS*

CNS: dizziness, drowsiness, headache, psychic disturbances.

EENT: blurred vision, tinnitus.

CV: arrhythmias, edema.

GI: *PO*—DRUG-INDUCED HEPATITIS, GI BLEEDING, constipation, dyspepsia, nausea, vomiting, discomfort; *rect*—rectal irritation, tenesmus.

GU: cystitis, hematuria, renal failure.

Derm: rashes.

F and E: hyperkalemia.

Hemat: blood dyscrasias, prolonged bleeding time.

Local: phlebitis at IV site.

{} = Available in Canada only.

***CAPITALS indicate life-threatening; underlines indicate most frequent.**

I

Misc: allergic reactions including ANAPHYLAXIS.

INTERACTIONS

Drug-Drug: ▪ Concurrent use with **aspirin** may decrease effectiveness ▪ Additive adverse GI effects with **aspirin**, other **NSAIDs, glucocorticoids**, or **alcohol** ▪ Chronic use of **acetaminophen** increases the risk of adverse renal reactions ▪ May decrease effectiveness of **diuretics** or **antihypertensives** ▪ May increase hypoglycemia from **insulin** or **oral hypoglycemic agents** ▪ May increase risk of toxicity from **lithium** or **zidovudine** (concurrent use with zidovudine should be avoided) ▪ Increases the risk of toxicity from **methotrexate** ▪ **Probenecid** increases risk of toxicity from indomethacin ▪ Increased risk of bleeding with **cefamandole, cefotetan, cefoperazone, valproic acid, plicamycin, thrombolytic agents**, or **anticoagulants** ▪ Increased risk of adverse hematologic reactions with **antineoplastic agents** or **radiation therapy** ▪ Increased risk of nephrotoxicity with **cyclosporine.**

ROUTE AND DOSAGE

❑ Anti-inflammatory

- **PO (Adults):** *Antiarthritic*—25–50 mg 2–4 times daily or 75-mg extended-release capsule once or twice daily (not to exceed 200 mg or 150 mg of SR/day). A single bedtime dose of 100 mg may be used. *Antigout*—100 mg initially, followed by 50 mg 3 times daily for relief of pain, then decreased further.
- **Rect (Adults):** 50 mg up to 4 times daily (not to exceed 200 mg/day by all routes).
- **PO, Rect (Children):** 1.5–2.5 mg/kg/day in 3–4 divided doses (not to exceed 4 mg/kg/day or 150–200 mg/day).

❑ Closure of Patent Ductus Arteriosus

- **IV, PO (Neonates):** 0.2 mg/kg initially, then 2 subsequent doses at 12–24 hr intervals of 0.1 mg/kg if age <48 hr at time of initial dose; 0.2 mg/kg if 2–7 days at initial dose; 0.25 mg/kg if >7 days at initial dose.

AVAILABILITY

▪ ***Capsules:*** 25 mg[Rx], 50 mg[Rx] ▪ ***Sustained-release capsules:*** 75 mg[Rx] ▪ ***Suppositories:*** 50 mg[Rx], {100 mg[Rx]} ▪ ***Oral suspension:*** 25 mg/5 ml[Rx] ▪ ***Powder for injection:*** 1-mg vials[Rx].

TIME/ACTION PROFILE

	ONSET	PEAK	DURATION
PO (analgesic)	30 min	0.5–2 hr	4–6 hr
PO-ER (analgesic)	30 min	UK	4–6 hr
PO (anti-inflammatory)	up to 7 days	1–2 wk	UK
PO-ER (anti-inflammatory)	up to 7 days	1–2 wk	UK
IV (closure of PDA)	up to 48 hr	UK	UK

NURSING IMPLICATIONS

ASSESSMENT

- **General Info:** Patients who have asthma, aspirin-induced allergy, and nasal polyps are at increased risk for developing hypersensitivity reactions. Monitor for rhinitis, asthma, and urticaria.
- **Arthritis:** Assess limitation of movement and pain—note type, location, and intensity prior to and 1–2 hr following administration.
- **Patent Ductus Arteriosus:** Monitor respiratory status and heart sounds routinely throughout therapy.
  - ▫ Monitor intake and output. Fluid restriction is usually instituted throughout therapy.
- ***Lab Test Considerations:*** BUN, serum creatinine, CBC, serum potassium levels, and liver function tests should be evaluated periodically in patients receiving prolonged therapy.
  - ▫ Serum potassium, BUN, serum creatinine, AST, and ALT tests may show increased levels. Blood glucose concentrations may be altered. Hemoglobin and hematocrit concentrations, leukocyte and platelet counts, and CCr may be decreased.
  - ▫ Urine glucose and urine protein concentrations may be increased.
  - ▫ Leukocyte and platelet count may be decreased. Bleeding time may be prolonged for several days after discontinuation.

POTENTIAL NURSING DIAGNOSES

- Pain (Indications).
- Physical mobility, impaired (Indications).
- Knowledge deficit, related to medication regimen (Patient/Family Teaching).

IMPLEMENTATION

- **General Info:** If prolonged therapy is used, dose should be reduced to the lowest level that controls symptoms.
- **PO:** Administer after meals, with food, or with antacids to decrease GI irritation. Do not crush, break, or chew sustained-release capsules.
- ▫ Shake suspension prior to administration. Do not mix with antacid or any other liquid.
- **Direct IV:** Reconstitute with 1 or 2 ml of preservative-free 0.9% NaCl or preservative-free sterile water for a concentration of 0.1 mg/ml or 0.05 mg/ml, respectively. Reconstitute immediately prior to use and discard any unused solution. Do not dilute further or admix.
- ***Rate:*** Administer over 5–10 sec. Avoid extravasation, as solution is irritating to tissues.
- **Y-Site Compatibility:** ▪ furosemide ▪ insulin ▪ nitroprusside ▪ potassium chloride ▪ sodium bicarbonate.
- **Y-Site Incompatibility:** ▪ calcium gluconate ▪ cimetidine ▪ dobutamine ▪ dopamine ▪ gentamicin ▪ tobramycin ▪ tolazoline.
- **Rect:** Encourage patient to retain suppository for 1 hr following administration.

PATIENT/FAMILY TEACHING

- **General Info:** Advise patient to take this medication with a full glass of water and to remain in an upright position for 15–30 min after administration.
- ▫ Instruct patient to take medication exactly as directed. Missed doses should be taken as soon as remembered if not almost time for next dose. Do not double doses.
- ▫ May cause drowsiness or dizziness. Advise patient to avoid driving or other activities requiring alertness until response to medication is known.
- ▫ Caution patient to avoid the concurrent use of alcohol, aspirin, other NSAIDs, acetaminophen, or other OTC medications without consulting health care professional.
- ▫ Caution patient to wear sunscreen and protective clothing to prevent photosensitivity reactions.
- ▫ Advise patient to inform health care professional of medication regimen prior to treatment or surgery.
- ▫ Instruct patient to notify health care professional if rash, itching, chills, fever, muscle aches, visual disturbances, weight gain, edema, abdominal pain, black stools, or persistent headache occurs.
- **Patent Ductus Arteriosus:** Explain to parents the purpose of medication and the need for frequent monitoring.

EVALUATION

Effectiveness of therapy can be demonstrated by: ▪ Decrease in severity of moderate pain ▫ Improved joint mobility. Partial arthritic relief is usually seen within 2 wk, but maximum effectiveness may require up to 1 mo of continuous therapy. Patients who do not respond to one NSAID may respond to another ▪ Successful closure of patent ductus arteriosus.

INSULINS
(**in**-su-lin)

insulin lispro, rDNA origin
Humalog

regular insulin (insulin injection, crystalline zinc insulin)
Humulin R, {Insulin-Toronto}, Novolin R, Novolin R PenFill, Regular Iletin I, Regular Pork Iletin II, Regular Purified Pork Insulin, Velosulin Human

NPH insulin (isophane insulin suspension)
Humulin N, NPH Iletin I, NPH-N, {Novolin ge NPH}, Novolin N, Novolin N PenFill, Pork NPH Iletin II

NPH/regular insulin mixtures
Humulin 50/50, Humulin 70/30, Novolin 70/30, Novolin 70/30 PenFill

insulin zinc suspension (lente insulin)
Humulin L, Lente Iletin I, Lente Iletin II, Lente L, {Novolin ge Lente}, Novolin L

I

{} = **Available in Canada only.**

insulin zinc suspension, extended (ultralente insulin)
Humulin U Ultralente, {Novolin de Ultralente}, Novolin U, Ultralente U

concentrated regular insulin
Regular (Concentrated) Iletin II U-500

CLASSIFICATION(S):
Hormones (pancreatic)

Pregnancy Category B

INDICATIONS

▪ Treatment of insulin-dependent diabetes mellitus (IDDM, type I) ▪ Management of non–insulin-dependent diabetes mellitus (NIDDM, type II) unresponsive to treatment with diet and/or oral hypoglycemic agents ▪ **Insulin lispro:** Produced by recombinant DNA technology, has a more rapid onset and shorter duration than regular insulin, and is usually used in combination with a longer-acting insulin ▪ **Concentrated insulin U-500 :** Only for use in patients with insulin requirements >200 units/day.

ACTION

▪ Lower blood glucose by increasing transport into cells and promoting the conversion of glucose to glycogen ▪ Promote the conversion of amino acids to proteins in muscle and stimulate triglyceride formation ▪ Inhibit the release of free fatty acids ▪ Sources include pork, beef/pork combinations, semisynthetic, biosynthetic, and recombinant DNA. **Therapeutic Effects:** ▪ Control of blood sugar in diabetic patients.

PHARMACOKINETICS

Absorption: Rapidly absorbed from SC administration sites. Absorption rate is determined by type of insulin, injection site, volume of injectate, and other factors.
Distribution: Widely distributed.
Metabolism and Excretion: Metabolized by liver, spleen, kidney, and muscle.
Half-life: 5–6 min (prolonged in diabetics; biological half-life is longer).

CONTRAINDICATIONS AND PRECAUTIONS

Contraindicated in: ▪ Allergy or hypersensitivity to a particular type of insulin, preservatives, or other additives.
Use Cautiously in: ▪ Stress, pregnancy, and infection (temporarily increase insulin requirements).

ADVERSE REACTIONS AND SIDE EFFECTS*

Derm: urticaria.
Endo: HYPOGLYCEMIA, rebound hyperglycemia (Somogyi effect).
Local: lipodystrophy, itching, lipohypertrophy, redness, swelling.
Misc: allergic reactions including ANAPHYLAXIS.

INTERACTIONS

Drug-Drug: ▪ **Beta-adrenergic blocking agents** may block some of the signs and symptoms of hypoglycemia and delay recovery from hypoglycemia ▪ **Thiazide diuretics, glucocorticoids, diltiazem, dobutamine, thyroid preparations, estrogens, nicotine, protease inhibitor antiretrovirals,** and **rifampin** may increase insulin requirements ▪ **Anabolic steroids (testosterone), alcohol, clofibrate, guanethidine, MAO inhibitors,** most **NSAIDs, oral hypoglycemic agents, sulfinpyrazone, tetracyclines, phenylbutazone,** and **warfarin** may decrease insulin requirements.

ROUTE AND DOSAGE

Dose depends on blood sugar, response, and many other factors.

❑ **Ketoacidosis—Regular Insulin Only**

- **IV (Adults):** 0.1 unit/kg/hr as a continuous infusion.
- **IV (Children):** Individualized on the basis of patient's size.

❑ **Maintenance Therapy**

- **SC (Adults and Children):** 0.5–1 unit/kg/day. *Adolescents during rapid growth*—0.8–1.2 units/kg/day.

***CAPITALS indicate life-threatening; underlines indicate most frequent.**

AVAILABILITY

■ ***Insulin injection (regular insulin):*** 100 units/ml[OTC] ■ ***Regular (concentrated) insulin injection:*** 500 units/ml[Rx] ■ ***Isophane insulin suspension (NPH insulin):*** 100 units/ml[Rx] ■ ***NPH insulin/regular insulin suspension:*** 70 units NPH/30 units regular insulin/ml (100 units/ml total)[OTC], 50 units NPH/50 units regular insulin/ml (100 units/ml total)[OTC] ■ ***Insulin zinc suspension (lente):*** 100 units/ml[OTC] ■ ***Insulin zinc suspension, extended (ultralente):*** 100 units/ml[OTC] ■ ***Insulin lispro:*** 100 units/ml in 10-ml vials and 1.5-ml cartridges.

TIME/ACTION PROFILE (hypoglycemic effect)

	ONSET	PEAK	DURATION
Insulin lispro SC	rapid	30–60 min	3–4 hr
Regular IV	10–30 min	15–30 min	30–60 min
Regular SC	0.5–1 hr	2–4 hr	5–7 hr
NPH 70/ regular 30 SC	30 min	4–8 hr	up to 24 hr
NPH SC	1–4 hr	6–12 hr	18–28 hr
Lente SC	1–3 hr	8–12 hr	18–28 hr
Ultralente SC	4–6 hr	18–24 hr	36 hr

NURSING IMPLICATIONS

ASSESSMENT

- □ Assess patient for signs and symptoms of hypoglycemia (anxiety; chills; cold sweats; confusion; cool, pale skin; difficulty in concentration; drowsiness; excessive hunger; headache; irritability; nausea; nervousness; rapid pulse; shakiness; unusual tiredness or weakness) and hyperglycemia (drowsiness; flushed, dry skin; fruit-like breath odor; frequent urination; loss of appetite; tiredness; unusual thirst) periodically throughout therapy.
- □ Monitor body weight periodically. Changes in weight may necessitate changes in insulin dose.
- ■ ***Lab Test Considerations:*** May cause decreased serum inorganic phosphate, magnesium, and potassium levels.
- □ Monitor blood glucose and ketones every 6 hr throughout therapy, more frequently in ketoacidosis and times of stress. Glycosylated hemoglobin may also be monitored to determine effectiveness of therapy.
- ■ ***Toxicity and Overdose:*** Overdose is manifested by symptoms of hypoglycemia. Mild hypoglycemia may be treated by ingestion of oral glucose. Severe hypoglycemia is a life-threatening emergency; treatment consists of IV glucose, glucagon, or epinephrine.

POTENTIAL NURSING DIAGNOSES

- ■ Knowledge deficit, related to medication regimen (Patient/Family Teaching).
- ■ Noncompliance (Patient/Family Teaching).

IMPLEMENTATION

- ■ **General Info:** Available in different types and strengths and from different species. Check type, species source, dose, and expiration date with another licensed nurse. Do not interchange insulins without consulting physician or other health care professional.
- □ Use *only* insulin syringes to draw up dose. The unit markings on the insulin syringe must match the insulin's units/ml. Special syringes for doses <50 units are available. Use *only* U-100 insulin syringes to draw up *insulin lispro* dose. Prior to withdrawing dose, rotate vial between palms to ensure uniform solution; do not shake.
- □ When mixing insulins, draw regular insulin or insulin lispro into syringe first to avoid contamination of regular insulin vial.
- □ Insulin should be stored in a cool place but does not need to be refrigerated.
- □ Because of short duration of insulin lispro, supplementation with longer-acting insulin may be necessary to control blood glucose levels.
- ■ **SC:** Administer insulin lispro within 15 min before a meal.
- ■ **IV:** Regular insulin is the *only* insulin that can be administered IV. Do not use if cloudy, discolored, or unusually viscous.
- □ Regular insulin U-500 is not intended for IV route.
- ■ **Direct IV:** May be administered IV undiluted directly into vein or through Y-site.
- ■ ***Rate:*** Administer up to 50 units over 1 min.
- ■ **Continuous Infusion:** May be diluted in commonly used IV solutions as an infusion; however, insulin potency may be reduced by at least 20–80% by the plastic or glass container or tubing before reaching the venous system.
- ■ ***Rate:*** When administered as an infusion, rate should be ordered by physician, and infusion

should be placed on an IV pump for accurate administration.

- □ Rate of administration should be decreased when serum glucose level reaches 250 mg/100 ml.

- ■ **Y-Site Compatibility:** ■ ampicillin ■ ampicillin/sulbactam ■ aztreonam ■ cefazolin ■ cefotetan ■ dobutamine ■ famotidine ■ gentamicin ■ heparin ■ imipenem/cilastatin ■ indomethacin ■ magnesium sulfate ■ meperidine ■ morphine ■ oxytocin ■ pentobarbital ■ potassium chloride ■ ritodrine ■ sodium bicarbonate ■ tacrolimus ■ terbutaline ■ ticarcillin ■ ticarcillin/clavulanate ■ tobramycin ■ vancomycin ■ vitamin B complex with C.
- ■ **Additive Compatibility:** ■ May be added to total parenteral nutrition (TPN) solutions.

PATIENT/FAMILY TEACHING

- □ Instruct patient on proper technique for administration. Include type of insulin, equipment (syringe, cartridge pens, alcohol swabs), storage, and place to discard syringes. Discuss the importance of not changing brands of insulin or syringes, selection and rotation of injection sites, and compliance with therapeutic regimen.
- □ Demonstrate technique for mixing insulins by drawing up regular insulin or insulin lispro first and rolling intermediate-acting insulin vial between palms to mix, rather than shaking (may cause inaccurate dose).
- □ Explain to patient that this medication controls hyperglycemia but does not cure diabetes. Therapy is long term.
- □ Instruct patient in proper testing of serum glucose and ketones. These tests should be closely monitored during periods of stress or illness and health care professional notified of significant changes.
- □ Emphasize the importance of compliance with nutritional guidelines and regular exercise as directed by health care professional.
- □ Advise patient to consult health care professional prior to using alcohol or other medications concurrently with insulin.
- □ Advise patient to notify health care professional of medication regimen prior to treatment or surgery.
- □ Advise patient to notify health care professional if nausea, vomiting, or fever develops, if unable to eat regular diet, or if blood sugar levels are not controlled.
- □ Instruct patient on signs and symptoms of hypoglycemia and hyperglycemia and what to do if they occur.
- □ Advise patient to notify health care professional if pregnancy is planned or suspected.
- □ Patients with diabetes mellitus should carry a source of sugar (candy, sugar packets) and identification describing their disease and treatment regimen at all times.
- □ Emphasize the importance of regular follow-up, especially during first few weeks of therapy.

EVALUATION

Effectiveness of therapy can be demonstrated by: ■ Control of blood glucose levels without the appearance of hypoglycemic or hyperglycemic episodes.

INTERFERONS, ALFA
(in-ter-**feer**-onz)

interferon alfa-2a, recombinant
Roferon-A

interferon alfa-2b, recombinant
a-2-interferon, Intron A

interferon alfa-n3, human
Alferon N

CLASSIFICATION(S):
Antineoplastics (miscellaneous), Immune modifiers

Pregnancy Category C

INDICATIONS

■ **Interferon alfa-2a:** Treatment of: □ Hairy cell leukemia □ AIDS-associated Kaposi's sarcoma □ Chronic myelogenous leukemia ■ **Interferon alfa-2b:** Treatment of: □ Hairy cell leukemia □ Malignant melanoma □ AIDS-associated Kaposi's sarcoma □ Condylomata acuminata (intralesional) □ Chronic hepatitis non-A, non-B/C □ Chronic hepatitis B ■ **Interferon alfa-n3:** Treatment of condylomata acuminata (intralesional).

ACTION

▪ Interferons are proteins capable of modifying the immune response and have antiproliferative action against tumor cells ▪ Interferon alfa-2a and interferon alfa-2b are produced by recombinant DNA techniques; interferon alfa-n3 is from pooled human leukocytes ▪ Interferons also have antiviral activity. **Therapeutic Effects:** ▪ Antineoplastic, antiviral, and antiproliferative activity.

PHARMACOKINETICS

Absorption: Not absorbed orally. Well absorbed (>80%) following IM and SC administration. Minimal systemic absorption follows intralesional administration.

Distribution: UK.

Metabolism and Excretion: Filtered by the kidneys and subsequently degraded in the renal tubule.

Half-life: *Interferon alfa-2a*—3.7–8.5 hr; *interferon alfa-2b*—2–3 hr.

CONTRAINDICATIONS AND PRECAUTIONS

Contraindicated in: ▪ Hypersensitivity to alfa interferons or human serum albumin ▪ Hypersensitivity to mouse immunoglobulin (interferon alfa-2a) ▪ Hypersensitivity to mouse immunoglobulin, neomycin, or egg protein (interferon alfa-n3).

Use Cautiously in: ▪ Severe cardiovascular, pulmonary, renal, or hepatic disease ▪ Active infections ▪ Underlying CNS pathology or psychiatric history ▪ Decreased bone marrow reserve or underlying immunosuppression ▪ Current history of chickenpox, herpes zoster, or herpes labialis (may reactivate or disseminate disease) ▪ Previous or concurrent radiation therapy ▪ Geriatric patients or patients with other debilitating illnesses ▪ History of suicide attempt ▪ Patients with childbearing potential ▪ Lactation and children <18 yr (safety not established).

ADVERSE REACTIONS AND SIDE EFFECTS*

All are more prominent with SC, IV, or IM administration.

CNS: dizziness, confusion, depression with suicidal ideation (↑ interferon alfa-2a), insomnia, nervousness, trouble concentrating, trouble thinking.

EENT: blurred vision.

CV: arrhythmias, chest pain.

GI: anorexia, decreased appetite, diarrhea, dry mouth, nausea, stomatitis, taste disorder, vomiting, weight loss, drug-induced hepatitis (↑ in Kaposi's sarcoma).

GU: gonadal suppression.

Derm: pruritus, rash, alopecia, dry skin, sweating.

Endo: thyroid disorders (↑ in Kaposi's sarcoma).

Hemat: anemia, leukopenia, thrombocytopenia.

MS: leg cramps.

Neuro: peripheral neuropathy.

Misc: chills, fever, flu-like syndrome.

INTERACTIONS

Drug-Drug: ▪ Additive myelosuppression with other **antineoplastic agents** or **radiation therapy** ▪ Additive CNS depression may occur with **CNS depressants,** including **alcohol, antihistamines, sedative/hypnotics,** and **opioids** ▪ May decrease metabolism and increase blood levels and toxicity of **theophylline.**

ROUTE AND DOSAGE

❑ Interferon Alfa-2a

▪ **IM, SC (Adults):** *Hairy cell leukemia (induction)*—3 million units/day for 16–24 wk. If severe adverse reactions occur, reduce dosage by 50%. *Hairy cell leukemia (maintenance)*—3 million units 3 times weekly. *Kaposi's sarcoma (induction)*—36 million units/day for 10–12 wk or 3 million units/day for 3 days, then 9 million units/day for next 3 days, then 18 million units/day for next 3 days, then 36 million units/day for rest of 10–12 wk course. *Kaposi's sarcoma (maintenance)*—36 million units 3 times weekly. *Chronic myelogenous leukemia*—9 million units/day (may be started as 3 million units/day for 3 days, then 6 million units/day for 3 days, then 9 million units/day).

❑ Interferon Alfa-2b

▪ **IV (Adults):** *Malignant melanoma*—20 million units/m^2/day for 5 days of each week

*CAPITALS indicate life-threatening; underlines indicate most frequent.

for 4 wk initially, followed by SC maintenance dosing.

- **IM, SC (Adults):** *Hairy cell leukemia*—2 million units/m^2 3 times weekly. *Malignant melanoma*—10 million units/m^2/day 3 times weekly for 48 wk, following initial IV dosing. *Kaposi's sarcoma*—30 million units/m^2 3 times weekly. *Chronic hepatitis non-A/non-B/C*—3 million units 3 times weekly for 24 mo. *Chronic hepatitis B*—5 million units/day or 10 million units 3 times weekly for 16 wk.
- **IL (Adults):** *Condylomata acuminata*—1 million units/lesion 3 times weekly for 3 wk; treat only 5 lesions per course.

❑ Interferon Alfa-n3

- **IL (Adults):** 250,000 units/lesion twice weekly for up to 8 wk; for large lesions, divide dose and inject at several sites.

AVAILABILITY

❑ Interferon Alfa-2a

- ***Solution for injection:*** 3 million units/ml[Rx], 6 million units/ml[Rx], 10 million units/ml[Rx], 36 million units/ml[Rx] ▪ ***Powder for injection:*** 18-million-unit vials[Rx].

❑ Interferon Alfa-2b

- ***Powder for injection:*** 3-million-unit vial[Rx], 5-million-unit vial[Rx], 10-million-unit vial[Rx], 18-million-unit vial[Rx], 25-million-unit vial[Rx], 50-million-unit vial[Rx] ▪ ***Solution for injection:*** 10 million units/2-ml vial[Rx], 18 million units/3.8-ml vial[Rx], 25 million units/5-ml vial[Rx].

❑ Interferon Alfa-n3

- ***Solution for injection:*** 5 million units/ml[Rx].

TIME/ACTION PROFILE (clinical effects)

	ONSET	PEAK	DURATION
Interferon alfa-2a IM, SC-BC	UK	17–19 days	several wks
Interferon alfa-2a IM, SC-CR	1–3 mo	UK	UK
Interferon alfa-2b IM, SC-CR	1–3 mo	UK	UK
Interferon alfa-2b IM, SC-BC	UK	3–5 days	3–5 days
Interferon alfa-2b IM, SC-LFT	2 wk	UK	UK
Interferon alfa-2b, n3 IL	UK	4–8 wk	UK

BC = effects on platelet counts; CR = clinical response; IL= regression of lesions; LFT = effects on liver function in patients with hepatitis.

NURSING IMPLICATIONS

ASSESSMENT

- **General Info:** Monitor vital signs prior to and periodically throughout therapy. Hypotension may occur up to 2 days after therapy.
- ❑ Assess patient for development of flu-like syndrome (fever, chills, myalgia, headache). Symptoms often appear suddenly 3–6 hr after therapy. Symptoms tend to decrease, even with continued therapy. Acetaminophen may be used for control of these symptoms.
- ❑ Monitor cardiac status, especially in patients with underlying cardiac disease or advanced malignancy. Assess heart sounds and chest pain, auscultate lung sounds for rales/crackles, and assess for edema. ECG may be monitored prior to and periodically during therapy.
- ❑ Monitor for bone marrow depression. Assess for bleeding (bleeding gums, bruising, petechiae, guaiac stools, urine, and emesis) and avoid IM injections and rectal temperatures if platelet count is low. Apply pressure to venipuncture sites for 10 min. Assess for signs of infection during neutropenia. Anemia may occur. Monitor for increased fatigue, dyspnea, and orthostatic hypotension.
- ❑ May cause nausea and vomiting. Antiemetics may be used prophylactically. Monitor intake and output, daily weight, and appetite. Adjust diet as tolerated for anorexia. Encourage fluid intake of at least 2 liters/day.
- ❑ Monitor neurologic status throughout therapy. Report confusion, decreased coordination, dizziness, gait disturbances, paresthesia, difficulty with speech, or psychological disturbances.
- ❑ Assess mental status throughout therapy. May cause depression and suicidal ideation. May require discontinuation of medication and continued treatment.
- **Kaposi's Sarcoma:** Monitor number, size, and character of lesions prior to and throughout therapy.
- ***Lab Test Considerations:*** **Systemic:** Monitor CBC and differential prior to and periodically throughout therapy. May cause leukopenia, neutropenia, thrombocytopenia, and decreased hemoglobin and hematocrit. The nadirs of leukopenia and thrombocytopenia from *interferon alfa-2a* occur in 17–19

days. Recovery from leukopenia and thrombocytopenia occurs a few weeks after withdrawal of *interferon alfa-2a.* The nadirs of leukopenia and thrombocytopenia occur in 3–5 days, with recovery 3–5 days after withdrawal of *interferon alfa-2b.* If granulocyte count <750 mm³ or platelet count <50,000/mm³, reduce interferon alfa-2b dose by 50%. If granulocyte count <500/mm³ or platelet count <30,000/mm³, discontinue *interferon alfa-2b* until platelet or granulocyte counts return to normal or baseline levels, then reinstitute at up to 100% of dose.

- Monitor liver function tests (AST, ALT, LDH, bilirubin, alkaline phosphatase) and renal function tests (BUN, creatinine, uric acid, urinalysis) prior to and periodically throughout therapy.
- **Hepatitis:** Monitor thyroid-stimulating hormone levels in patients treated for hepatitis non-A, non-B/C, or if thyroid function impairment occurs.
- **Hairy Cell Leukemia:** Monitor number of peripheral blood hairy cells and bone marrow hairy cells prior to and during therapy.

POTENTIAL NURSING DIAGNOSES

- Injury, risk for (Side Effects).
- Infection, risk for (Side Effects).
- Knowledge deficit, related to medication regimen (Patient/Family Teaching).

IMPLEMENTATION

- **General Info:** Solution should be prepared in a biologic cabinet. Wear gloves, gown, and mask while handling medication. Discard equipment in specially designated containers (see Appendix I).

Interferon Alfa-2a

- **SC, IM:** SC route is preferred for patients with a platelet count <50,000/mm³.
- Reconstitute the 18-million-unit vial of *interferon alfa-2a* with 3 ml of diluent provided for a concentration of 6 million units/ml. Refrigerate after reconstitution and use within 30 days.
- The 36 million unit/ml vial of *interferon alfa-2a* is for use in patients with AIDS-related Kaposi's sarcoma and should not be used for hairy cell leukemia.

Interferon Alfa-2b

- **SC, IM:** SC route is preferred for patients with a platelet count <50,000/mm³.
- Reconstitute 3-, 5-, and 50-million-unit vials with 1 ml, 10-million-unit dose with 2 ml, 18-million-unit vial with 3.8 ml, and 25-million-unit vial with 5 ml of diluent provided by manufacturer (bacteriostatic water for injection). Agitate gently. Solution may be colorless to light yellow. Refrigerate after reconstitution. Stable for 1 mo.
- **IL:** Reconstitute 10-million-unit vial with 1 ml of bacteriostatic water for injection. Use a TB syringe with 25–30-gauge needle to administer. Each 0.1-ml dose is injected into the center of the base of the wart using the intradermal injection approach. As many as 5 lesions can be treated at one time.

PATIENT/FAMILY TEACHING

- **General Info:** Advise patient to take medication exactly as directed. If a dose is missed, omit dose and return to the regular schedule. The patient should notify the health care professional if more than 1 dose is missed.
- **Home Care Issues:** Instruct patient and family on preparation and correct technique for administration of injection and care and disposal of equipment. Explain to patient that brands should not be switched without consulting health care professional; may result in a change of dosage.
- Discuss possibility of flu-like reaction 3–6 hr after dose. Acetaminophen may be taken prior to injection and every 3–4 hr afterward as needed to control symptoms.
- Review side effects with patient. Interferon may be temporarily discontinued or dose decreased by 50% if serious side effects occur.
- Instruct patient to notify health care professional promptly if fever; chills; cough; hoarseness; sore throat; signs of infection; lower back or side pain; painful or difficult urination; bleeding gums; bruising; petechiae; blood in stools, urine, or emesis; increased fatigue; dyspnea; or orthostatic hypotension occurs. Caution patient to avoid crowds and persons with known infections. Instruct patient to use soft toothbrush and electric razor and to avoid falls. Caution patient not to drink alcoholic beverages or take medication con-

taining aspirin or NSAIDS; may precipitate gastric bleeding.

- Inform patient of the potential for depression and advise patient to notify health care professional if depression occurs.
- Discuss with patient the possibility of hair loss. Explore coping strategies.
- Explain to patient that fertility may be impaired and that contraception is needed throughout course of treatment to prevent potential harm to the fetus.
- Instruct patient not to receive any vaccinations without advice of health care professional.
- Emphasize need for periodic lab tests to monitor for side effects.

EVALUATION

Effectiveness of therapy can be demonstrated by: ▪ Normalized blood parameters (hemoglobin, neutrophils, platelets, monocytes, and bone marrow and peripheral hairy cells) in hairy cell leukemia. Response may not be seen for 1–3 mo with *interferon alfa-2a* or for 6 mo with *interferon alfa-2b* ▪ Decrease in the size and number of lesions in Kaposi's sarcoma. Therapy may be required for 6 mo before full response is seen. Therapy is discontinued when there is no further clinical improvement and parameters have stabilized for 3 mo ▪ Improved hematologic parameters in patients with chronic myelogenous leukemia ▪ Increase in time to relapse and overall survival in patients with malignant melanoma ▪ Disappearance of or decrease in size and number of genital warts. Condylomata acuminata usually respond in 4–8 wk. The course of therapy may need to be extended to 16 wk; a second course may be required if genital warts persist and laboratory values remain in acceptable limits ▪ Decrease in symptoms and improvement in liver function tests in patients with hepatitis non-A, non-B/C, and hepatitis B.

INTERFERONS, BETA
(in-ter-**feer**-on)

inteferon beta-1a
Avonex

interferon beta-1b
Betaseron

CLASSIFICATION(S):
Immune modifiers

Pregnancy Category C

INDICATIONS

▪ **Interferon beta-1a:** Management of relapsing forms of multiple sclerosis in ambulatory patients ▪ **Interferon beta-1b:** Management of relapsing-remitting multiple sclerosis in ambulatory patients.

ACTION

▪ Have antiviral and immunoregulatory properties produced by interacting with specific receptor sites on cell surfaces ▪ Produced by recombinant DNA technology. **Therapeutic Effects:** ▪ Reduce incidence of relapse (neurologic dysfunction) and slow physical disability in patients with multiple sclerosis.

PHARMACOKINETICS

Absorption: *Interferon beta-1b*—50% absorbed following SC administration.
Distribution: UK.
Metabolism and Excretion: UK.
Half-life: *Interferon beta-1a*—8.6 hr (SC), 10 hr (IM); *interferon beta-1b*—8 min–4.3 hr.

CONTRAINDICATIONS AND PRECAUTIONS

Contraindicated in: ▪ Hypersensitivity to natural or recombinant interferon beta or human albumin.
Use Cautiously in: ▪ Patients with a history of suicide attempt or depression ▪ History of seizures ▪ Cardiovascular disease ▪ Patients with childbearing potential ▪ Pregnancy, lactation, or children <18 yr (safety not established).

ADVERSE REACTIONS AND SIDE EFFECTS*

CNS: SEIZURES, headache, weakness, anxiety, confusion, depersonalization, drowsiness, emotional lability, fainting, mental depression, sleep disorders, suicidal ideation.
EENT: conjunctivitis, laryngitis, otitis.
Resp: dyspnea, upper respiratory tract infection.
CV: chest pain, edema, hypertension, palpita-

*CAPITALS indicate life-threatening; underlines indicate most frequent.

tions, peripheral vascular disorders, tachycardia, vasodilation.
GI: constipation, diarrhea, dyspepsia, nausea, vomiting, abdominal pain, anorexia, elevated liver function studies, GI disorders.
GU: cystitis, ovarian cyst, pelvic pain.
Derm: sweating, alopecia, photosensitivity, phototoxicity.
Endo: menstrual disorders, breast pain, hypoglycemia, menorrhagia, spontaneous abortion.
Hemat: neutropenia, anemia, eosinophilia.
Local: injection-site reactions (↑ with interferon beta-1b), injection site necrosis.
Metab: weight loss.
MS: myalgia, arthralgia, muscle spasm.
Misc: chills, fever, flu-like symptoms, pain, hypersensitivity reactions.

INTERACTIONS

Drug-Drug: ▪ None significant.

ROUTE AND DOSAGE

❑ **Interferon Beta-1a**

▪ **IM (Adults):** 30 mcg once weekly.

❑ **Interferon Beta-1b**

▪ **SC (Adults):** 0.25 mg (8 million IU) every other day.

AVAILABILITY

❑ **Interferon Beta-1a**

▪ ***Powder for injection:*** 33 mcg (6.6 million IU/vial)Rx.

❑ **Interferon Beta-1b**

▪ ***Powder for injection:*** 0.3 mg (9.6 million IU)/vialRx.

TIME/ACTION PROFILE

	ONSET	PEAK	DURATION
Interferon beta-1a IM*	within 12 hr	48 hr	4 days
Interferon beta-1b SC†	rapid	1–8 hr	UK

*Biological response modifiers.
†Serum interferon levels.

NURSING IMPLICATIONS

ASSESSMENT

❑ Assess frequency of exacerbations of symptoms of multiple sclerosis periodically throughout therapy.

❑ Monitor patient for signs of depression throughout therapy. If depression occurs, notify physician or other health care professional immediately.

▪ ***Lab Test Considerations:*** Monitor hemoglobin, WBC, platelets, and blood chemistries including liver function tests prior to and periodically throughout therapy. Therapy may be temporarily discontinued if the absolute neutrophil count is $<750/mm^3$, if AST or ALT exceeds 10 times the upper limit of normal, or if serum bilirubin exceeds 5 times the upper limit of normal. Once the absolute neutrophil count is $>750/mm^3$ or the hepatic enzymes have returned to normal, therapy can be restarted at 50% of the original dose.

POTENTIAL NURSING DIAGNOSES

▪ Knowledge deficit, related to medication regimen (Patient/Family Teaching).

IMPLEMENTATION

▪ **General Info:** Do not confuse products. Interferon beta-1a and interferon beta-1b are not interchangeable.

▪ **Interferon Beta-1a:** Reconstitute with 1.1 ml of diluent and swirl gently to dissolve. Keep reconstituted solution in refrigerator; inject within 6 hr of reconstitution.

▪ **Interferon Beta-1b:** To reconstitute, inject 1.2 ml of diluent supplied into interferon beta-1b vial for a concentration of 0.25 mg (8 million IU)/ml. Swirl gently to dissolve completely; do not shake. Do not use solutions that are discolored or contain particulate matter. Keep reconstituted solution refrigerated; inject within 3 hr of reconstitution.

❑ Following reconstitution, withdraw 1 ml into a syringe with a 27-gauge needle and inject SC into arm, abdomen, hip, or thigh. Discard unused portion; vials are for single dose only.

PATIENT/FAMILY TEACHING

▪ **Home Care Issues:** Instruct patient in correct technique for injection and care and disposal of equipment. Caution patient not to reuse needles or syringes and provide patient with a puncture-resistant container for disposal.

❑ Instruct patient to take medication as directed; do not change dosage or schedule without consulting health care professional.

I

- Inform patient that flu-like symptoms (fever, chills, myalgia, sweating, malaise) may occur during therapy. Acetaminophen may be used for relief of fever and myalgias.
- Caution patient to use sunscreen and wear protective clothes to prevent photosensitivity reactions.
- Advise patient to notify health care professional if pregnancy is planned or suspected. May cause spontaneous abortion.

EVALUATION

Effectiveness of therapy can be demonstrated by: ▪ Decrease in the frequency of relapse (neurologic dysfunction) in patients with relapsing-remitting multiple sclerosis.

IODINE, IODIDE

potassium iodide, saturated solution
Pima, SSKI, Thyro-Block

sodium iodide
Iodopen

strong iodine solution
Lugol's solution

CLASSIFICATION(S):
Antithyroid agents

Pregnancy Category D

INDICATIONS

▪ Adjunct with other antithyroid drugs in preparation for thyroidectomy ▪ Treatment of thyrotoxic crisis ▪ Radiation protectant following radiation emergencies or administration of radioactive iodine ▪ Iodine replacement ▪ As a supplement during long-term parenteral nutrition.

ACTION

▪ Rapidly inhibit the release and synthesis of thyroid hormones ▪ Decrease the vascularity of the thyroid gland ▪ Decrease thyroidal uptake of radioactive iodine following radiation emergencies or administration of radioactive isotopes of iodine ▪ Iodine is a necessary component of thyroid hormone. **Therapeutic Effects:** ▪ Control of hyperthyroidism ▪ Decreased bleeding during thyroid surgery ▪ Replacement/supplementation of iodine ▪ Decreased incidence of thyroid cancer following radiation emergencies.

PHARMACOKINETICS

Absorption: Converted in the GI tract and enter the circulation as iodine; also absorbed through skin and lungs; may also be obtained via recycling of iodothyronines.
Distribution: Concentrate in the thyroid gland and muscle; also found in skin, skeleton, breasts, and hair. Cross the placenta; enter breast milk.
Metabolism and Excretion: Taken up by the thyroid gland, then eliminated via kidneys, liver, skin, lungs, and intestines.
Half-life: UK.

CONTRAINDICATIONS AND PRECAUTIONS

Contraindicated in: ▪ Hypersensitivity.
Use Cautiously in: ▪ Tuberculosis ▪ Bronchitis ▪ Hyperkalemia ▪ Impaired renal function ▪ Pregnancy or lactation (although iodine is required during pregnancy, excess amounts may cause thyroid abnormalities/goiter in the newborn; excess use during lactation may cause skin rash or thyroid suppression in the infant).

ADVERSE REACTIONS AND SIDE EFFECTS*

GI: diarrhea, GI irritation.
Derm: acneiform eruptions.
Endo: hypothyroidism, hyperthyroidism, thyroid hyperplasia.
F and E: hyperkalemia (potassium iodide only).
Misc: hypersensitivity, iodism.

INTERACTIONS

Drug-Drug: ▪ Use with **lithium** may cause additive hypothyroidism ▪ Increases the antithyroid effect of **antithyroid agents (methimazole, propylthiouracil)** ▪ Additive hyperkalemia may result from combined use of potassium iodide with **potassium-sparing diuretics**, **ACE inhibitors**, or **potassium supplements.**

ROUTE AND DOSAGE

SSKI = 1 g potassium iodide/ml; Lugol's solution = iodine 50 mg/ml plus potassium iodide

***CAPITALS indicate life-threatening; underlines indicate most frequent.**

100 mg/ml; sodium iodide =118 mcg sodium iodide (100 mcg iodide)/ml.

❑ **Preparation for Thyroidectomy**

- **PO (Adults and Children):** *Strong iodine solution*—3–5 drops (0.1–0.3 ml) 3 times daily for 10 days prior to surgery. *Potassium iodide saturated solution*—1–5 drops (50–250 mg) 3 times daily for 10–14 days prior to surgery.

❑ **Hyperthyroidism**

- **PO (Adults and Children):** *Strong iodine solution*—1 ml in water 3 times daily. *Potassium iodide saturated solution*—5 drops (250 mg) 3 times daily.

❑ **Radiation Protectant**

- **PO (Adults and Children ≥1 yr):** 130 mg potassium iodide/day for 3–14 days.
- **PO (Children <1 yr):** 65 mg potassium iodide/day for 3–14 days.

❑ **Replacement**

- **PO (Adults):** *Strong iodine solution*—0.3–1 ml 3–4 times daily.

❑ **Nutritional Supplement**

- **IV (Adults):** 1–2 mcg elemental iodide/kg/day added to parenteral nutrition. *Pregnant or lactating women*—2–3 mcg elemental iodide/kg/day added to parenteral nutrition.
- **IV (Children):** 2–3 mcg elemental iodide/kg/day added to parenteral nutrition.

AVAILABILITY

SSKI = Lugol's solution = sodium iodide = 118 sodium iodide (100 mcg iodide)/ml.

❑ **Potassium Iodide**

▪ ***Saturated solution:*** 1 g potassium iodide/ml in 30- and 240-ml bottles[Rx] ▪ ***Syrup:*** 325 mg potassium iodide/5 ml[Rx] ▪ ***Tablets:*** 130 mg[Rx] (available only through federal agencies).

❑ **Sodium Iodide**

▪ ***Solution for injection:*** 100 mcg iodide (118 mg sodium iodide)/ml in 10-ml vials[Rx].

❑ **Strong Iodine Solution**

▪ ***Oral solution:*** Iodine 50 mg/ml plus potassium iodide 100 mg/ml (5% iodine plus 10% potassium iodide) in 120-ml, pint, and gallon bottles.

TIME/ACTION PROFILE (effects on thyroid function)

	ONSET	PEAK	DURATION
PO	24 hr	10–15 days	variable
IV	rapid	UK	UK

NURSING IMPLICATIONS

ASSESSMENT

- ❑ Assess for signs and symptoms of iodism (metallic taste, stomatitis, skin lesions, cold symptoms, severe GI upset). Report these symptoms promptly to physician.
- ❑ Monitor response symptoms of hyperthyroidism (tachycardia, palpitations, nervousness, insomnia, diaphoresis, heat intolerance, tremors, weight loss).
- ❑ Monitor for hypersensitivity reaction (rash, pruritus, laryngeal edema, wheezing). Discontinue drug and notify physician immediately if these problems occur.
- ▪ ***Lab Test Considerations:*** Monitor thyroid function before and periodically during course of therapy. May alter results of radionuclide thyroid imaging and may decrease thyroidal uptake of ^{131}I, ^{123}I, and sodium pertechnetate Tc 99m in thyroid uptake tests.
- ❑ Monitor serum potassium levels periodically during course of therapy.

POTENTIAL NURSING DIAGNOSES

- ▪ Knowledge deficit, related to medication regimen (Patient/Family Teaching).

IMPLEMENTATION

- ▪ **PO:** Mix solutions in a full glass of fruit juice, water, broth, or milk. Administer after meals to minimize GI irritation.
- ❑ Solution is normally clear and colorless. Darkening upon standing does not affect potency of drug. Solutions that are brownish yellow should be discarded.
- ❑ Crystals may form, especially if refrigerated, but redissolve upon warming and shaking.
- ▪ **IV:** Parenteral administration should be used only when oral administration is not possible.
- ▪ **Continuous Infusion:** Sodium iodide is added to total parenteral nutrition solutions.
- ▪ **Additive Compatibility:** ▪ amino acid solutions ▪ dextrose solutions ▪ electrolytes ▪ trace metals.

PATIENT/FAMILY TEACHING

- □ Instruct patient to take medication exactly as directed. If a dose is missed, take as soon as possible but not just before next dose; do not double doses.
- □ Instruct patient to report suspected pregnancy to health care professional before therapy is initiated.
- □ Advise patient to consult health care professional about avoiding foods high in iodine (seafood, iodized salt, cabbage, kale, turnips) or potassium (see Appendix K).
- □ Advise patient to consult health care professional before using OTC cold remedies. Some cold remedies use iodide as an expectorant.
- ■ **Hyperthyroidism:** Instruct patient to take medication exactly as ordered. Missing a dose may precipitate hyperthyroidism.
- ■ **Nutritional Supplement:** Discuss the need for iodine in the body and identify food sources of iodine with patient.

EVALUATION

Effectiveness of therapy can be demonstrated by: ■ Resolution of the symptoms of thyroid crisis ■ Decrease in size and vascularity of the gland before thyroid surgery. Use of iodides in the treatment of hyperthyroidism is usually limited to 2 wk ■ Protection of the thyroid gland from the effects of radioactive iodine ■ Prevention and treatment of iodine deficiency.

IPECAC SYRUP

(ip-e-kak)

CLASSIFICATION(S):
Emetic

Pregnancy Category C

INDICATIONS

■ Induces vomiting in the early management of overdose/poisoning from noncaustic substances (in conscious patients).

ACTION

■ Stimulates the chemoreceptor trigger zone in the CNS and irritates the gastric mucosa. Action is due to 2 major alkaloids: emetine and cephaeline. **Therapeutic Effects:** ■ Induction of emesis in overdose situations.

PHARMACOKINETICS

Absorption: Absorption is minimal.
Distribution: UK.
Metabolism and Excretion: Excretion of emetine is very slow; detectable in urine for 60 days.
Half-life: UK.

CONTRAINDICATIONS AND PRECAUTIONS

Contraindicated in: ■ Semicomatose, inebriated, unconscious, or seizing patients ■ Shock ■ Patients who may not have a gag reflex ■ Ingestion of caustic substances ■ Alcohol intolerance.

Use Cautiously in: ■ Pregnancy, lactation, or children <6 mo (safety not established).

ADVERSE REACTIONS AND SIDE EFFECTS*

CNS: sedation.
CV: MYOCARDITIS (if drug is absorbed or overdosage ingested), arrhythmias.
GI: diarrhea.

INTERACTIONS

Drug-Drug: ■ Should not be given concurrently with **antiemetics** or **activated charcoal** (may reduce emetic efficacy).

Drug-Food: ■ Concurrent administration with **milk** decreases effectiveness ■ Avoid concurrent use of **carbonated beverages** (causes abdominal distention).

ROUTE AND DOSAGE

Ipecac syrup contains 7% powdered ipecac.

- ■ **PO (Adults):** 15–30 ml; if vomiting does not occur within 20–30 min, a 2nd dose of 15 ml may be given.
- ■ **PO (Children 1–12 yr):** 15 ml; if vomiting does not occur within 20–30 min, a 2nd dose may be given.
- ■ **PO (Children <1 yr):** 5–10 ml.

AVAILABILITY

■ ***Syrup (1% alcohol):*** 15-ml, 30-ml containers[OTC], pints[Rx], and gallons[Rx] ■ ***Syrup (2% alcohol):*** 15-ml, 30-ml containers[Rx].

***CAPITALS indicate life-threatening; underlines indicate most frequent.**

TIME/ACTION PROFILE (onset of emesis)

	ONSET	PEAK	DURATION
PO	20–30 min	UK	20–25 min

NURSING IMPLICATIONS

ASSESSMENT

- □ A history is essential in determining treatment and antidotes for accidental poisoning. Do not induce vomiting if patient has ingested petroleum distillates, volatile oils, or caustic substances.
- □ Assess level of consciousness prior to administration. Do not administer ipecac if patient is unconscious, semiconscious, or convulsing.

POTENTIAL NURSING DIAGNOSES

- ■ Injury, risk for (Indications).
- ■ Knowledge deficit, related to medication regimen (Patient/Family Teaching).

IMPLEMENTATION

- ■ **General Info:** If vomiting does not occur within 20–30 min, dose may be repeated. If vomiting does not occur within 30–45 min after 2nd dose, gastric lavage must be performed to recover the medication. No more than 2 doses should be administered; cardiotoxicity may occur.
- □ Administer activated charcoal only after vomiting has been induced and completed.
- □ Do not confuse ipecac syrup with ipecac fluid extract; fluid extract is 14 times stronger. Fatalities have occurred.
- ■ **PO:** Have patient sit up with head forward prior to administration. Ipecac syrup may not work on an empty stomach. Administer syrup followed immediately by adequate amounts of water (1 glass [240 ml] for adults, ½–1 glass [120–240 ml] for children). Children who are young and frightened may be given water before ipecac.
- □ Do not administer concurrently with milk, as it decreases the effectiveness of ipecac, or carbonated beverages, as they cause stomach distention.

PATIENT/FAMILY TEACHING

- ■ **Home Care Issues:** Advise parents with children >1 yr to keep a small amount of ipecac syrup on hand for emergency use. If child ingests a dangerous substance, the parents should contact a poison control center, physician, or emergency department for advice before administering this medication.
- □ Caution parents to avoid inducing emesis if child swallowed caustic substances, volatile oils, or petroleum distillates or if child is unconscious, semiconscious, or convulsing. Instruct parent to position child to avoid aspiration.
- □ Advise parents that the drug has a 1-yr shelf life and therefore needs to be replaced yearly. Advise parents to check expiration date of product before purchasing.

EVALUATION

Effectiveness of therapy can be demonstrated by: ■ Emesis within 30 min of administration.

IPRATROPIUM (inhalation)

(i-pra-**troe**-pee-um)

Atrovent

CLASSIFICATION(S):

Bronchodilator (anticholinergic), Nasal drying agent

Pregnancy Category B

INDICATIONS

■ **Inhalation:** Bronchodilator in maintenance therapy of reversible airway obstruction due to COPD ■ **Intranasal:** Management of rhinorrhea associated with allergic and nonallergic perennial rhinitis (0.03% solution) or the common cold (0.06% solution). **Unlabeled Uses:** ■ **Inhalation:** Adjunctive management of bronchospasm caused by asthma.

ACTION

■ **Inhalation:** Inhibits cholinergic receptors in bronchial smooth muscle, resulting in decreased concentrations of cyclic guanosine monophosphate (cGMP). Decreased levels of cGMP produce local bronchodilation. ■ **Intranasal:** Local application inhibits secretions from glands lining the nasal mucosa. **Therapeutic Effects:** ■ **Inhalation:** Bronchodilation without systemic anticholinergic properties ■ **Intranasal:** Decreased rhinorrhea.

PHARMACOKINETICS

Absorption: Minimal systemic absorption (2% for inhalation solution; 20% for inhalation aerosol; <20% following nasal use).
Distribution: Does not appear to cross the blood-brain barrier.
Metabolism and Excretion: Small amounts absorbed are metabolized by the liver.
Half-life: 2 hr.

CONTRAINDICATIONS AND PRECAUTIONS

Contraindicated in: ▪ Hypersensitivity to ipratropium, atropine, belladonna alkaloids, bromide, or fluorocarbons ▪ Avoid use during acute bronchospasm.
Use Cautiously in: ▪ Patients with bladder neck obstruction, prostatic hypertrophy, glaucoma, or urinary retention ▪ Geriatric patients (may be more sensitive to effects) ▪ Pregnancy, lactation, or children <5 hr (safety not established).

ADVERSE REACTIONS AND SIDE EFFECTS

CNS: dizziness, headache, nervousness.
EENT: blurred vision, sore throat; *nasal only*—epistaxis, nasal dryness/irritation.
Resp: bronchospasm, cough.
CV: hypotension, palpitations.
GI: GI irritation, nausea.
Derm: rash.
Misc: allergic reactions.

INTERACTIONS

Drug-Drug: ▪ Potential additive fluorocarbon toxicity when used with other **inhalation bronchodilators having a fluorocarbon propellant** ▪ Additive anticholinergic properties with other **drugs having anticholinergic properties** (antihistamines, phenothiazines, disopyramide).

ROUTE AND DOSAGE

- **Inhalation (Adults):** *Metered-dose inhaler*—1–4 inhalations 3–4 times daily (not to exceed 24 inhalations/24 hr or more frequently than q 4 hr). During initial therapy, up to 8 inhalations may be repeated. *Via nebulization*—250–500 mcg 3–4 times daily given q 6–8 hr as needed (up to 500 mcg q 4 hr).
- **Inhalation (Children 5–12 yr):** *Via nebulization*—125–250 mcg 3–4 times daily given q 4–6 hr as needed.
- **Intranasal (Adults and Children ≥12 yr):** *Perennial rhinitis*—2 sprays of 0.03% solution in each nostril 2–3 times daily (21 mcg/spray); *perennial rhinitis*—2 sprays of 0.06% solution in each nostril 3–4 times daily (42 mcg/spray) for up to 4 days.

AVAILABILITY

▪ ***Aerosol inhaler:*** 18 mcg/spray in 14-g canister (200 inhalations)[Rx] ▪ {***Inhalation solution:*** 0.0125%[Rx], 0.02% in single-dose vials containing 500 mcg[Rx], 0.025%[Rx]} ▪ ***Nasal spray:*** 0.03% solution—21 mcg/spray in 30-ml bottle (345 sprays/bottle)[Rx], 0.06% solution—42 mcg/spray in 15-ml bottle (165 sprays)[Rx] ▪ ***In combination with:*** albuterol (Combivent)[Rx]. See Appendix A.

TIME/ACTION PROFILE (bronchodilation)

	ONSET	PEAK	DURATION
Inhalation	5–15 min	1–2 hr	3–4 hr (up to 8 hr)
Intranasal	15 min	UK	6–12 hr

NURSING IMPLICATIONS

ASSESSMENT

- **General Info:** Assess for allergy to atropine and belladonna alkaloids; patients with these allergies may also be sensitive to ipratropium.
- **Inhalation:** Assess respiratory status (rate, breath sounds, degree of dyspnea, pulse) before administration and at peak of medication. Consult physician or other health care professional about alternative medication if severe bronchospasm is present; onset of action is too slow for patients in acute distress. If paradoxical bronchospasm (wheezing) occurs, withhold medication and notify physician or other health care professional immediately.
- **Nasal Spray:** Assess patient for rhinorrhea.

POTENTIAL NURSING DIAGNOSES

- Airway clearance, ineffective (Indications).
- Activity intolerance (Indications).
- Knowledge deficit, related to medication regimen (Patient/Family Teaching).

IMPLEMENTATION

- **Inhalation:** See Appendix H for administration of inhalation medications.

□ When ipratropium is administered concurrently with other inhalation medications, administer adrenergic bronchodilators first, followed by ipratropium, then glucocorticoids. Wait 5 min between medications.
□ Solution for *nebulization* can be diluted with preservative-free 0.9% NaCl. Diluted solution should be used within 24 hr at room temperature or 48 hr if refrigerated. Solution can be mixed with preservative-free albuterol, cromolyn, or metaproterenol if used within 1 hr of mixing.

PATIENT/FAMILY TEACHING

- **General Info:** Instruct patient in proper use of inhaler, nebulizer, or nasal spray and to take medication as directed. If a dose is missed, take as soon as remembered unless almost time for the next dose; space remaining doses evenly during day. Do not double doses.
□ Advise patient that rinsing mouth after using inhaler, good oral hygiene, and sugarless gum or candy may minimize dry mouth. Health care professional should be notified if stomatitis occurs or if dry mouth persists for more than 2 wk.
- **Inhalation:** Caution patient not to exceed 12 doses within 24 hr. Patient should notify health care professional if symptoms do not improve within 30 min after administration of medication or if condition worsens.
□ Explain need for pulmonary function tests prior to and periodically throughout therapy to determine effectiveness of medication.
□ Caution patient to avoid spraying medication in eyes; may cause blurring of vision or irritation.
□ Advise patient to inform health care professional if cough, nervousness, headache, dizziness, nausea, or GI distress occurs.
- **Nasal Spray:** Instruct patient in proper use of nasal spray. Clear nasal passages gently before administration. Do not inhale during administration, so medication remains in nasal passages. Prime pump initially with 7 actuations. If used regularly, no further priming is needed. If not used in 24 hr, prime with 2 actuations. If not used for >7 days, prime with 7 actuations.
□ Advise patient to contact health care professional if symptoms do not improve within 1–2 wk or if condition worsens.

EVALUATION

Effectiveness of therapy can be demonstrated by: ▪ Decreased dyspnea □ Improved breath sounds ▪ Decrease in rhinorrhea from perennial rhinitis or the common cold.

IRINOTECAN

(eye-ri-noe-**tee**-kan)
Camptosar

CLASSIFICATION(S):
Antineoplastic (enzyme inhibitor)

Pregnancy Category D

INDICATIONS

▪ Recurrent metastatic colon or rectal cancer that has not responded to previous therapy that included 5-fluorouracil.

ACTION

▪ Interferes with DNA synthesis by inhibiting the enzyme topoisomerase. **Therapeutic Effects:** ▪ Death of rapidly replicating cells, particularly malignant ones.

PHARMACOKINETICS

Absorption: IV administration results in complete bioavailability.
Distribution: UK.
Metabolism and Excretion: Converted by the liver to SN-38, its active metabolite, which is also metabolized by the liver. Small amounts excreted by kidneys.
Half-life: 6 hr.

CONTRAINDICATIONS AND PRECAUTIONS

Contraindicated in: ▪ Hypersensitivity ▪ Pregnancy or lactation.
Use Cautiously in: ▪ Previous pelvic or abdominal irradiation or age ≥65 yr (increased risk of myelosuppression) ▪ Presence of infection, underlying bone marrow depression, or concurrent chronic illness ▪ Previous severe myelosuppression or diarrhea (reinstitute at lower dose following resolution) ▪ Patients with childbearing potential ▪ Children (safety not established).

I

ADVERSE REACTIONS AND SIDE EFFECTS*

CNS: dizziness, headache, insomnia, weakness.
EENT: rhinitis.
Resp: coughing, dyspnea.
CV: edema, vasodilation.
GI: DIARRHEA, ELEVATED LIVER ENZYMES, abdominal pain/cramping, anorexia, constipation, dyspepsia, flatulence, nausea, stomatitis, vomiting, abdominal enlargement.
Derm: alopecia, rash, sweating.
F and E: dehydration.
Hemat: anemia, leukopenia, thrombocytopenia.
Local: injection site reactions.
Metab: weight loss.
MS: back pain.
Misc: chills, fever.

INTERACTIONS

Drug-Drug: ▪ Additive bone marrow depression may occur with other **antineoplastic agents** or **radiation therapy** ▪ **Laxatives** should be avoided (diarrhea may be exacerbated) ▪ **Diuretics** may increase the risk of dehydration if diarrhea occurs (may discontinue during therapy) ▪ **Dexamethasone** used as an antiemetic may increase the risk of hyperglycemia and lymphocytopenia ▪ **Prochlorperazine** given on the same day as irinotecan may increase the risk of akathisia.

ROUTE AND DOSAGE

- **IV (Adults):** 125 mg/m² once weekly for 4 wk, followed by a 2-wk rest period. Cycle may be repeated using doses ranging from 50–150 mg/m² depending on patient tolerance and degree of toxicity encountered.

AVAILABILITY

- ***Solution for injection:*** 20 mg/ml in 5-ml vials.

TIME/ACTION PROFILE (hematologic effects)

	ONSET	PEAK	DURATION
IV	UK	21–29 days	27–34 days

NURSING IMPLICATIONS

ASSESSMENT

- □ Monitor vital signs frequently during administration.
- □ Monitor for bone marrow depression. Assess for bleeding (bleeding gums, bruising, petechiae, guaiac stools, urine, and emesis) and avoid IM injections and rectal temperatures if platelet count is low. Apply pressure to venipuncture sites for 10 min. Assess for signs of infection during neutropenia. Anemia may occur. Monitor for increased fatigue, dyspnea, and orthostatic hypotension.
- □ Monitor closely for the development of diarrhea. Two types may occur. The early type occurs within 24 hr of administration and may be preceded by cramps and sweating. Atropine 0.25–1 mg IV may be given to decrease symptoms. Potentially life-threatening diarrhea may occur more than 24 hr after a dose and may be accompanied by severe dehydration and electrolyte imbalance. Loperamide 4 mg initially, followed by 2 mg every 2 hr until diarrhea ceases for at least 12 hr (or 4 mg every 4 hr if given during sleeping hours) should be administered promptly to treat late-occurring diarrhea. Careful fluid and electrolyte replacement should be instituted to prevent complications.
- □ Nausea and vomiting are common. Pretreatment with dexamethasone 10 mg along with agents such as ondansetron or granisetron should be started on the same day as irinotecan at least 30 min before administration. Prochlorperazine may be used on subsequent days but may increase risk of akathisia if given on the same day as irinotecan.
- □ Assess IV site frequently for inflammation. Avoid extravasation. If extravasation occurs, infusion must be stopped and restarted in another vein to avoid damage to SC tissue. Flushing site with sterile water and application of ice over the extravasated site are recommended.
- ▪ ***Lab Test Considerations:*** Monitor CBC with differential and platelet count prior to each dose. Temporarily discontinue irinotecan if absolute neutrophil count is <500 cells/mm³ or if neutropenic fever occurs. Admin-

*CAPITALS indicate life-threatening; underlines indicate most frequent.

istration of a colony-stimulating factor may be considered if clinically significant decreases in white blood cell count (<2000/mm^3), neutrophil count (<1000/mm^3), hemoglobin (<9 g/dl), or platelet count (<100,000 cells/mm^3) occur.

- May cause elevated serum alkaline phosphatase and AST concentrations.

POTENTIAL NURSING DIAGNOSES

- Infection, risk for (Adverse Reactions).
- Knowledge deficit, related to medication regimen (Patient/Family Teaching).

IMPLEMENTATION

- **General Info:** Solution should be prepared in a biologic cabinet. Wear gloves, gown, and mask while handling IV medication. Discard IV equipment in specially designated containers (see Appendix I).
- **Intermittent Infusion:** Dilute before infusion with D5W or 0.9% NaCl for a concentration of 0.12–1.1 mg/ml. Usual diluent is 500 ml of D5W. Solution is pale yellow. Do not administer solutions that are cloudy or contain particulate matter. Solution is stable for 24 hr at room temperature or 48 hr if refrigerated. To prevent microbial contamination, solutions should be used within 24 hr of dilution if refrigerated or 6 hr at room temperature. Do not refrigerate solutions diluted with 0.9% NaCl.
- ***Rate:*** Administer dose over 90 min.
- **Additive Incompatibility:** ▪ Information unavailable. Do not admix with other solutions or medications.

PATIENT/FAMILY TEACHING

- Instruct patient to report occurrence of diarrhea to health care professional immediately, especially if it occurs more than 24 hr after dose. Diarrhea may be accompanied by severe dehydration and electrolyte imbalance. It may be life-threatening and should be treated promptly.
- Instruct patient to notify health care professional if fever; chills; sore throat; signs of infection; bleeding gums; bruising; petechiae; blood in urine, stool, or emesis occurs. Caution patient to avoid crowds and persons with known infections. Instruct patient to use soft toothbrush and electric razor. Patient should be cautioned not to drink alcoholic beverages or take products containing aspirin or NSAIDs.
- Instruct patient to notify nurse of pain at injection site immediately.
- Instruct patient to notify health care professional if vomiting, fainting, or dizziness occurs.
- Discuss with patient possibility of hair loss. Explore methods of coping.
- Advise patient that this medication may have teratogenic effects. Contraception should be used during therapy.
- Instruct patient not to receive any vaccinations without consulting health care professional.
- Emphasize the need for periodic lab tests to monitor for side effects.

EVALUATION

Effectiveness of therapy can be demonstrated by: ▪ Decrease in size and and spread of malignancy.

IRON SUPPLEMENTS

ferrous fumarate

(**fer**-us **fyoo**-ma-rate)

Femiron, Feostat, Fumasorb, Fumerin, Hemocyte, Neo-Fer, {Nephro-Fer}, {Novofumar}, {Palafer}, Span-FF

ferrous gluconate

(**fer**-us **gloo**-koe-nate)

{Apo-Ferrous Gluconate}, Fergon, Ferralet, {Fertinic}, {Novoferrogluc}, Simron

ferrous sulfate

(**fer**-us **sul**-fate)

{Apo-Ferrous Sulfate}, Feosol, Feratab, Fer-gen-sol, Fer-In-Sol, Fer-Iron, {Fero-Grad}, Fero-Gradumet, Fero-space, Ferralyn, Ferra-TD, Mol-Iron, {Novoferrosulfa}, {PMS Ferrous Sulfate}, Slow Fe

iron dextran

(**eye**-ern **dex**-tran)

DexFerrum, InFeD

I

iron polysaccharide
(**eye**-ern poll-i-**sak**-a-ride)
Hytinic, Niferex, Nu-Iron

CLASSIFICATION(S):
Antianemics

Pregnancy Category C (iron dextran)

INDICATIONS

▪ **PO:** Prevention/treatment of iron-deficiency anemia ▪ **IM, IV:** Treatment/prevention of iron deficiency anemia in patients who cannot tolerate oral iron.

ACTION

▪ An essential mineral found in hemoglobin, myoglobin, and many enzymes ▪ Parenteral iron enters the bloodstream and organs of the reticuloendothelial system (liver, spleen, bone marrow), where iron is separated from the dextran complex and becomes part of iron stores. **Therapeutic Effects:** ▪ Prevention/treatment of iron deficiency.

PHARMACOKINETICS

Absorption: 5–10% of dietary iron is absorbed. In deficiency states this increases up to 30%. Therapeutically administered PO iron may be 60% absorbed; absorption is an active and passive transport process. Well absorbed following IM administration.
Distribution: Remain in the body for many months. Cross the placenta; enter breast milk.
Metabolism and Excretion: Mostly recycled; small daily losses occurring via desquamation, sweat, urine, and bile.
Half-life: *Iron dextran*—6 hr.

CONTRAINDICATIONS AND PRECAUTIONS

Contraindicated in: ▪ Primary hemochromatosis ▪ Hemolytic anemias and other anemias not due to iron deficiency.
Use Cautiously in: ▪ **PO**—Peptic ulcer ▪ Ulcerative colitis or regional enteritis (condition may be aggravated) ▪ Some products contain alcohol or tartrazine and should be avoided in patients with known intolerance/hypersensitivity ▪ Indiscriminate chronic use (may lead to iron overload) ▪ Autoimmune disorders and arthritis (more susceptible to allergic reactions following IM, IV use). **Use Extreme Caution in:** ▪ Patients with severe liver impairment (IM, IV only).

ADVERSE REACTIONS AND SIDE EFFECTS*

CNS: *IM, IV*— SEIZURES, dizziness, headache, syncope.
CV: *IM, IV*—hypotension, tachycardia.
GI: nausea; *PO*—constipation, dark stools, diarrhea, epigastric pain, GI bleeding; *IM, IV*—taste disorder, vomiting.
Derm: *IM, IV*—flushing, urticaria.
Local: pain at IM site, phlebitis at IV site, staining at IM site.
MS: *IM, IV*—arthralgia.
Misc: *PO*—staining of teeth (liquid preparations); *IM, IV*—allergic reactions including ANAPHYLAXIS, fever, lymphadenopathy.

INTERACTIONS

Drug-Drug: ▪ **Tetracycline** and **antacids** inhibit the absorption of iron by forming insoluble compounds ▪ **Tetracycline** absorption is also decreased by concurrent iron administration ▪ Iron decreases the absorption of **fluoroquinolones** or **penicillamine** ▪ **Chloramphenicol** and **vitamin E** may impair the hematologic response to iron therapy ▪ **Vitamin C** may slightly increase the absorption of PO iron.
Drug-Food: ▪ Iron absorption is decreased by ⅓–½ by concurrent administration of food.

ROUTE AND DOSAGE

❑ **Ferrous Fumarate**

▪ **PO (Adults):** *Prophylactic*—200 mg/day. *Therapeutic*—200 mg 3–4 times daily. Controlled-release capsules may be given twice daily.
▪ **PO (Children):** *Prophylactic*—3 mg/kg/day. *Therapeutic*—3–6 mg/kg 3 times daily.

❑ **Ferrous Gluconate**

▪ **PO (Adults):** *Prophylactic*—325 mg/day. *Therapeutic*—325–650 mg qid. Sustained-release capsules may be given twice daily.
▪ **PO (Children >2 yr):** *Prophylactic*—8 mg/kg/day. *Therapeutic*—16 mg/kg tid.

***CAPITALS indicate life-threatening; underlines indicate most frequent.**

❑ **Ferrous Sulfate**

- **PO (Adults):** *Prophylactic*—300–325 mg/day. *Therapeutic*—300 mg 2–4 times daily. Timed-release tablets may be given twice daily.
- **PO (Children):** *Prophylactic*—5 mg/kg/day. *Therapeutic*—10 mg/kg tid.

❑ **PO Dosage Expressed in mg Elemental Iron**

- **PO (Adults):** 50–100 mg 3 times daily.
- **PO (Children):** 4–6 mg/kg/day in 3 divided doses.
- **PO (Infants):** 1–2 mg/kg/day.
- **PO (Pregnant Women):** 30–60 mg/day.

❑ **Iron Dextran**

Test dose of 0.5 ml (25 mg) is given prior to therapy.

Iron Deficiency

- **IM, IV (Adults and Children >15 kg):** Total dose (ml) = 0.0442 (desired Hgb − actual Hgb) × lean body weight(kg) + (0.26 × lean body weight). Divided up and given in small daily doses until total is reached; not to exceed 100 mg/day. *Total dose IV infusion*—Total dose may be diluted and infused over 4–5 hr following a test dose of 10 drops (unlabeled).
- **IM, IV (Children 5–15 kg):** Total dose (ml) = 0.0442 (desired Hgb − actual Hgb) × weight(kg) + (0.26 × weight) (not to exceed 25 mg/day in children <5 kg; 50 mg/day in children <10 kg; or 100 mg/day in others).

Blood Loss

- **IM, IV (Adults):** Dose (ml) = (Blood loss [ml] × hematocrit) ÷ 50.

❑ **Iron Polysaccharide**

- **PO (Adults):** 50–100 mg 3 times daily.
- **PO (Children):** 4–6 mg/kg/day in 3 divided doses.
- **PO (Infants):** 1–2 mg/kg/day.
- **PO (Pregnant Women):** 30–60 mg/day.

AVAILABILITY

❑ **Ferrous Fumarate (33% Elemental Iron)**

▪ ***Tablets:*** 63 mg^{OTC}, 195 mg^{OTC}, 200 mg^{OTC}, 324 mg^{OTC}, 325 mg^{OTC} ▪ ***Chewable tablets:*** 100 mg^{OTC} ▪ ***Controlled-release capsules:*** 325 mg^{OTC} ▪ ***Suspension:*** 100 mg/5 ml^{OTC}, {300 mg/5 ml^{OTC}} ▪ ***Drops:*** 45 mg/0.6 ml^{OTC}, {60 mg/1 ml^{OTC}}.

❑ **Ferrous Gluconate (11.6% Elemental Iron)**

▪ ***Tablets:*** 300 mg^{OTC}, 320 mg^{OTC}, 325 mg^{OTC} ▪ ***Sustained-release tablets:*** 320 mg^{OTC} ▪ ***Soft gelatin capsules:*** 86 mg^{OTC} ▪ ***Elixir:*** 300 mg/5 ml^{OTC} ▪ ***Syrup:*** {300 mg/5 ml^{OTC}}.

❑ **Ferrous Sulfate (20–30% Elemental Iron)**

▪ ***Tablets:*** 195 mg^{OTC}, 300 mg^{OTC}, 325 mg^{OTC} ▪ ***Capsules:*** 150 mg^{OTC}, 250 mg^{OTC} ▪ ***Timed-release tablets:*** 525 mg^{OTC} ▪ ***Syrup:*** 90 mg/5 ml^{OTC} ▪ ***Elixir:*** 220 mg/5 ml^{OTC} ▪ ***Drops:*** 75 mg/0.6 ml^{OTC}, 125 mg/1 ml ^{OTC}.

❑ **Iron Dextran**

▪ ***Injection:*** 50 mg/ml^{Rx}.

❑ **Iron Polysaccharide (mg Iron)**

▪ ***Capsules:*** 150 mg^{OTC} ▪ ***Elixir:*** 100 mg/5 ml^{OTC} ▪ ***Tablets:*** 50 mg^{OTC} ▪ ***In combination with:*** ascorbic acid, antacids, multiple vitamins, and other minerals^{OTC}. See Appendix A.

TIME/ACTION PROFILE (effects on erythropoiesis)

	ONSET	PEAK	DURATION
PO	4 days	7–10 days	2–4 mo
IM, IV	4 days	1–2 wk	wks–mos

NURSING IMPLICATIONS

ASSESSMENT

- ❑ Assess patient's nutritional status and dietary history to determine possible cause of anemia and need for patient teaching.
- ❑ Assess bowel function for constipation or diarrhea. Notify physician or other health care professional and use appropriate nursing measures should these occur.
- ▪ **Iron Dextran:** Monitor blood pressure and heart rate frequently following IV administration until stable. Rapid infusion rate may cause hypotension and flushing.
- ❑ Assess patient for signs and symptoms of anaphylaxis (rash, pruritus, laryngeal edema, wheezing). Notify physician immediately if these occur. Keep epinephrine and resuscitation equipment close by in the event of an anaphylactic reaction.
- ▪ ***Lab Test Considerations:*** Hemoglobin, hematocrit, and reticulocyte values should be

monitored prior to and every 3 wk during the first 2 mo of therapy and periodically thereafter. Serum ferritin and iron levels may also be monitored to assess effectiveness of therapy.

- Occult blood in stools may be obscured by black coloration of iron in stool. Guaiac test results may occasionally be false-positive. Benzidine test results are not affected by iron preparations.
- **Iron Dextran:** Monitor hemoglobin, hematocrit, reticulocyte values, transferrin, ferritin, total iron-binding capacity, and plasma iron concentrations periodically throughout therapy. Serum ferritin levels peak in 7–9 days and return to normal in 3 wk. Serum iron determinations may be inaccurate for 1–2 wk after therapy with large doses; therefore, hemoglobin and hematocrit are used to gauge initial response. Normal hemoglobin concentrations of 14.8 g/100 ml should be used for patients weighing >15 kg, while 12 g/100 ml should be used for patients weighing 15 kg or less.
- May impart a brownish hue to blood drawn within 4 hr of administration. May cause false increase in serum bilirubin and false decrease in serum calcium values.
- Prolonged PTT may be calculated when blood sample is anticoagulated with citrate dextrose solution; use sodium citrate instead.

- ***Toxicity and Overdose:*** Early symptoms of overdose include stomach pain, fever, nausea, vomiting (may contain blood), and diarrhea. Late symptoms include bluish lips, fingernails, and palms; drowsiness; weakness; tachycardia; seizures; metabolic acidosis; hepatic injury; and cardiovascular collapse. The patient may appear to recover prior to the onset of late symptoms. Therefore, hospitalization continues for 24 hr after patient becomes asymptomatic to monitor for delayed onset of shock or GI bleeding. Late complications of overdose include intestinal obstruction, pyloric stenosis, and gastric scarring.
- Treatment includes inducing emesis with syrup of ipecac. If patient is comatose or seizing, gastric lavage with sodium bicarbonate is performed. Deferoxamine is the antidote. Additional supportive treatments to maintain fluid and electrolyte balance and correction of metabolic acidosis are also indicated.

POTENTIAL NURSING DIAGNOSES

- Activity intolerance (Indications).
- Knowledge deficit, related to medication and dietary regimen (Patient/Family Teaching).

IMPLEMENTATION

- **General Info:** Oral iron preparations should be discontinued prior to parenteral administration.
- Some parenteral products are for IV use only.
- **PO:** Oral preparations are most effectively absorbed if administered 1 hr before or 2 hr after meals. If gastric irritation occurs, administer with meals. Tablets and capsules should be taken with a full glass of water or juice. Do not crush or chew enteric-coated tablets and do not open capsules.
- Liquid preparations may stain teeth. Dilute water or fruit juice, full glass (240 ml) for adults and ½ glass (120 ml) for children, and administer with a straw or place drops at back of throat. Feosol elixir should be diluted in water only. Fer-In-Sol liquid or syrup may be diluted in water or fruit juice.
- Avoid using antacids, coffee, tea, dairy products, eggs, or whole-grain breads within 1 hr before and 2 hr after administration of ferrous salts.
- **Iron Dextran:** The 2-ml ampule may be used for IM or IV administration; the 10-ml multidose vials may be used only for IM administration.
- Prior to initial IM or IV dose, a test dose of 25 mg should be given by the same route as the dose is to be given, to determine reaction. The IV test dose should be administered over 5 min. The IM dose should be administered in the same injection site and by same technique as the therapeutic dose. The remaining portion may be administered after 1 hr, if no adverse symptoms have occurred.
- **IM:** Inject deeply via Z-track technique into upper outer quadrant of buttock, never into arm or other exposed areas. Use a 2–3 in., 19-gauge or 20-gauge needle. Change needles between withdrawal from container and injection to minimize staining of subcutaneous tissues. Stains are usually permanent.
- **IV:** Following IV administration, patient should remain recumbent for at least 30 min to prevent orthostatic hypotension.

- **Direct IV:** Administer undiluted.
- ***Rate:*** Administer slowly at a rate of 50 mg (1 ml) over at least 1 min.
- **Continuous Infusion:** May be diluted in 200–1000 ml of 0.9% NaCl or D5W; 0.9% NaCl is the preferred diluent; dilution in D5W increases incidence of pain and phlebitis.
- ***Rate:*** Administer over 1–8 hr following a test dose of 10 drops/min for 10 min. Flush line with 10 ml of 0.9% NaCl at completion of infusion.
- **Y-Site Incompatibility:** ▪ Discontinue other IV solutions during infusion.
- **Additive Incompatibility:** ▪ Manufacturer recommends that iron dextran not be mixed with other solutions; however, iron dextran has been added to total parenteral nutrition solutions.

PATIENT/FAMILY TEACHING

- ☐ Encourage patient to comply with medication regimen. If a dose is missed, take as soon as remembered within 12 hr; otherwise, return to regular dosing schedule. Do not double doses.
- ☐ Advise patient that stools may become dark green or black and that this change is harmless.
- ☐ Instruct patient to follow a diet high in iron (see Appendix K).
- ☐ Discuss with parents the risk of children overdosing on iron. Medication should be stored in the original childproof container and kept out of reach of children. Do not refer to vitamins as candy. Medical help should be sought immediately if overdose is suspected, as death may occur. Parents should have syrup of ipecac at home and call pediatrician, emergency department, or poison control center for instructions before administering.
- **Iron Dextran:** Delayed reaction may occur 1–2 days after administration and last 3–4 days if IV route used, 3–7 days with IM route. Instruct patient to contact physician if fever, chills, malaise, muscle and joint aches, nausea, vomiting, dizziness, and backache occur.

EVALUATION

Clinical response to therapy can be evaluated by: ▪ Increase in hemoglobin, which may reach normal parameters after 1–2 mo of therapy. May require 3–6 mo for normalization of body iron stores ▪ Increase in hemoglobin, hematocrit, and plasma iron levels with iron dextran. The diagnosis of iron-deficiency anemia should be reconfirmed if hemoglobin has not increased by 1 g/100 ml in 2 wk.

ISONIAZID

(eye-soe-**nye**-a-zid)

INH, {Isotamine}, Laniazid, Nydrazid, {PMS Isoniazid}

CLASSIFICATION(S):
Antitubercular

Pregnancy Category C

INDICATIONS

▪ First-line therapy of active tuberculosis, in combination with other agents ▪ Prevention of tuberculosis in patients exposed to active disease (alone).

ACTION

▪ Inhibits mycobacterial cell wall synthesis and interferes with metabolism. **Therapeutic Effects:** ▪ Bacteriostatic or bactericidal action against susceptible mycobacteria.

PHARMACOKINETICS

Absorption: Well absorbed following PO/IM administration.
Distribution: Widely distributed; readily crosses the blood-brain barrier. Crosses the placenta; enters breast milk in concentrations equal to plasma.
Metabolism and Excretion: 50% metabolized by the liver at rates that vary widely among individuals; 50% excreted unchanged by the kidneys.
Half-life: 1–4 hr.

CONTRAINDICATIONS AND PRECAUTIONS

Contraindicated in: ▪ Hypersensitivity ▪ Acute liver disease ▪ Previous hepatitis from isoniazid.
Use Cautiously in: ▪ History of liver damage or chronic alcohol ingestion ▪ Black and Hispanic women, women in the postpartum period, or patients >50 yr (increased risk of drug-in-

I

duced hepatitis) ▪ Severe renal impairment (dosage reduction may be necessary) ▪ Malnourished patients, diabetics, or chronic alcoholics (increased risk of neuropathy) ▪ Pregnancy and lactation (although safety is not established, isoniazid has been used with ethambutol to treat tuberculosis in pregnant women without harm to the fetus).

ADVERSE REACTIONS AND SIDE EFFECTS*

CNS: psychosis, seizures.
EENT: visual disturbances.
GI: DRUG-INDUCED HEPATITIS, nausea, vomiting.
Derm: rashes.
Endo: gynecomastia.
Hemat: blood dyscrasias.
Neuro: peripheral neuropathy.
Misc: fever.

INTERACTIONS

Drug-Drug: ▪ Additive CNS toxicity with other **antituberculars** ▪ **BCG vaccine** may not be effective during isoniazid therapy ▪ Isoniazid inhibits the metabolism of **phenytoin** ▪ **Aluminum-containing antacids** may decrease absorption ▪ Psychotic reactions and coordination difficulties may result with **disulfiram** ▪ Concurrent administration of **pyridoxine** may prevent neuropathy ▪ Increased risk of hepatotoxicity with other **hepatotoxic agents** including **alcohol** and **rifampin** ▪ Isoniazid may decrease blood levels and effectiveness of **ketoconazole** ▪ Concurrent use with **carbamazepine** increases carbamazepine blood levels and risk of hepatotoxicity.
Drug-Food: ▪ Severe reactions may occur with ingestion of foods containing high concentrations of **tyramine** (see Appendix K).

ROUTE AND DOSAGE

- **PO, IM (Adults):** 300 mg/day or 15 mg/kg (up to 900 mg) 2–3 times weekly.
- **PO, IM (Children):** 10–20 mg/kg/day (up to 300 mg/day) or 20–40 mg/kg (up to 900 mg) 2–3 times weekly.

AVAILABILITY

▪ ***Tablets:*** 50 mg[Rx], 100 mg[Rx], 300 mg[Rx] ▪ ***Syrup:*** 50 mg/5 ml[Rx] ▪ ***Injection:*** 100 mg/ml[Rx] ▪ ***In combination with:*** rifampin (Rifamate)[Rx] or with rifampin and pyrazinamide (Rifater)[Rx]. See Appendix A.

TIME/ACTION PROFILE (blood levels)

	ONSET	PEAK	DURATION
PO	rapid	1–2 hr	up to 24 hr
IM	rapid	1–2 hr	up to 24 hr

NURSING IMPLICATIONS

ASSESSMENT

- □ Mycobacterial studies and susceptibility tests should be performed prior to and periodically throughout therapy to detect possible resistance.
- ▪ ***Lab Test Considerations:*** Hepatic function should be evaluated prior to and monthly throughout therapy. Increased AST, ALT, and serum bilirubin may indicate drug-induced hepatitis. Black and Hispanic women, postpartal women, and patients >50 yr are at highest risk. The risk is lower in children; therefore, liver function tests are usually ordered less frequently for children.
- ▪ ***Toxicity and Overdose:*** If isoniazid overdosage occurs, treatment with pyridoxine (vitamin B_6) is instituted.

POTENTIAL NURSING DIAGNOSES

- Infection, risk for (Indications).
- Knowledge deficit, related to medication regimen (Patient/Family Teaching).
- Noncompliance (Patient/Family Teaching).

IMPLEMENTATION

- ▪ **PO:** May be administered with food or antacids if GI irritation occurs, although antacids containing aluminum should not be taken within 1 hr of administration.
- ▪ **IM:** Medication may cause discomfort at injection site. Massage site after administration and rotate injection sites.
- □ Solution may form crystals at low temperatures; crystals will redissolve upon warming to room temperature.

PATIENT/FAMILY TEACHING

- □ Advise patient to take medication exactly as directed. If a dose is missed, take as soon as possible unless almost time for next dose; do

*CAPITALS indicate life-threatening; underlines indicate most frequent.

not double up on missed doses. Emphasize the importance of continuing therapy even after symptoms have subsided. Therapy may be continued for 6 mo–2 yr.

- □ Advise patient to notify health care professional promptly if signs and symptoms of hepatitis (yellow eyes and skin, nausea, vomiting, anorexia, dark urine, unusual tiredness, or weakness) or peripheral neuritis (numbness, tingling, paresthesia) occurs. Pyridoxine may be used concurrently to prevent neuropathy. Any changes in visual acuity, eye pain, or blurred vision should also be reported immediately.
- □ Caution patient to avoid the use of alcohol during this therapy, as this may increase the risk of hepatotoxicity. Ingestion of Swiss or Cheshire cheeses, fish (tuna, skipjack, and sardinella), and possibly tyramine-containing foods (see Appendix K) should also be avoided, as they may result in redness or itching of the skin; hot feeling; rapid or pounding heartbeat; sweating; chills; cold, clammy feeling; headache; or light-headedness.
- □ Emphasize the importance of regular follow-up physical and ophthalmologic exams to monitor progress and to check for side effects.

EVALUATION

Effectiveness of therapy can be demonstrated by: ▪ Resolution of signs and symptoms of tuberculosis □ Negative sputum cultures ▪ Prevention of activation of tuberculosis in persons known to have been exposed.

ISOSORBIDE DINITRATE

(eye-soe-**sor**-bide dye-**nye**-trate)
{Apo-ISDN}, {Cedocard-SR}, {Coronex}, Dilatrate-SR, ISDN, Iso-Bid, Isonate, Isorbid, Isordil, Isotrate, {Novosorbide}, Sorbitrate, Sorbitrate SA

ISOSORBIDE MONONITRATE

(eye-soe-**sor**-bide mo-noe-**nye**-trate)
Imdur, Ismo, Monoket

CLASSIFICATION(S):
Antianginals, Vasodilators (nitrates)

Pregnancy Category C

INDICATIONS

▪ Acute treatment of anginal attacks (SL, chewable dinitrate only) ▪ Long-term prophylactic management of angina pectoris (dinitrate and mononitrate) ▪ Treatment of chronic congestive heart failure (dinitrate).

ACTION

▪ Produce vasodilation (venous greater than arterial) ▪ Decrease left ventricular end-diastolic pressure and left ventricular end-diastolic volume (preload). Net effect is reduced myocardial oxygen consumption ▪ Increase coronary blood flow by dilating coronary arteries and improving collateral flow to ischemic regions. **Therapeutic Effects:** ▪ Relief of anginal attacks and increase in cardiac output.

PHARMACOKINETICS

Absorption: Well absorbed following oral and sublingual administration.
Distribution: UK.
Metabolism and Excretion: Mostly metabolized by the liver.
Half-life: *Isosorbide dinitrate*—50 min; *isosorbide mononitrate*—5 hr.

CONTRAINDICATIONS AND PRECAUTIONS

Contraindicated in: ▪ Hypersensitivity ▪ Severe anemia.
Use Cautiously in: ▪ Head trauma or cerebral hemorrhage ▪ Pregnancy (may compromise maternal/fetal circulation) ▪ Children or lactation (safety not established).

ADVERSE REACTIONS AND SIDE EFFECTS*

CNS: dizziness, headache, apprehension, weakness.
CV: hypotension, tachycardia, paradoxical bradycardia, syncope.
GI: abdominal pain, nausea, vomiting.
Misc: cross-tolerance, flushing, tolerance.

I

{} = Available in Canada only.
*CAPITALS indicate life-threatening; underlines indicate most frequent.

INTERACTIONS

Drug-Drug: ▪ Additive hypotension with **antihypertensives,** acute ingestion of **alcohol, beta-adrenergic blocking agents, calcium channel blockers,** and **phenothiazines.**

ROUTE AND DOSAGE

❑ Isosorbide Dinitrate

- **SL, Chewable, Buccal (Adults):** *Acute attack of angina pectoris*—2.5–5 mg may be repeated q 5–10 min for 3 doses in 15–30 min. *Prophylaxis of angina pectoris*—2.5–10 mg may be repeated q 2–3 hr. Initial dose of chewable tablet is 5 mg.
- **PO (Adults):** *Prophylaxis of angina pectoris*—5–20 mg initially. Usual maintenance dose is 10–40 mg q 6 hr or 40–80 mg q 8–12 hr as sustained-release form.

❑ Isosorbide Mononitrate

- **PO (Adults):** *Ismo, Monoket*—20 mg twice daily (may start with 5 mg twice daily), 7 hr apart. *Imdur*—30–60 mg once daily; may increase to 120 mg once daily (up to 240 mg/day).

AVAILABILITY

❑ Isosorbide Dinitrate

▪ ***Sublingual tablets:*** 2.5 mgRx, 5 mgRx, 10 mgRx ▪ ***Chewable tablets:*** 5 mgRx, 10 mgRx ▪ ***Tablets:*** 2.5 mgRx, 5 mgRx, 10 mgRx, 20 mgRx, 30 mgRx, 40 mgRx ▪ ***Extended-release tablets:*** {20 mgRx}, 40 mgRx ▪ ***Capsules:*** 40 mgRx ▪ ***Extended-release capsules:*** 40 mgRx.

❑ Isosorbide Mononitrate

▪ ***Tablets:*** 10 mgRx, 20 mgRx ▪ ***Extended-release tablets (Imdur):*** 60 mgRx.

TIME/ACTION PROFILE (cardiovascular effects)

	ONSET	PEAK	DURATION
ISDN-SL, Chew	2–5 min	UK	1–2 hr
ISDN-PO	15–40 min	UK	4 hr
ISDN-PO-ER	30 min	UK	up to 12 hr
ISMN-PO	30–60 min	UK	7 hr
ISMN-ER	UK	UK	12 hr

NURSING IMPLICATIONS

ASSESSMENT

- ☐ Assess location, duration, intensity, and precipitating factors of anginal pain.
- ☐ Monitor blood pressure and pulse routinely during period of dosage adjustment.
- ▪ ***Lab Test Considerations:*** May cause falsely decreased serum cholesterol determinations.
- ☐ Excessive doses may increase methemoglobin concentrations.
- ☐ May cause increased urine vanillylmandelic acid (VMA) concentrations.

POTENTIAL NURSING DIAGNOSES

- ▪ Tissue perfusion, altered (Indications).
- ▪ Activity intolerance (Indications).
- ▪ Knowledge deficit, related to medication regimen (Patient/Family Teaching).

IMPLEMENTATION

❑ Isosorbide Dinitrate

- ▪ **PO:** Administer 1 hr before or 2 hr after meals with a full glass of water for faster absorption.
- ☐ Chewable tablets should be chewed well before swallowing and held in mouth for 2 min. Do not swallow whole.
- ☐ Extended-release tablets and capsules should be swallowed whole. Do not crush, break, or chew.
- ▪ **SL:** SL tablets should be held under tongue until dissolved.
- ☐ Avoid eating, drinking, or smoking until tablet is dissolved. Replace tablet if inadvertently swallowed.

❑ Isosorbide Mononitrate

- ▪ **PO:** Medication should be taken on an empty stomach with a full glass of water.

PATIENT/FAMILY TEACHING

- ☐ Instruct patient to take medication exactly as directed, even if feeling better. If a dose is missed, take as soon as remembered; doses of isosorbide dinitrate should be taken at least 2 hr apart (6 hr with extended-release preparations); daily doses of isosorbide mononitrate should be taken 7 hr apart. Do not double doses. Do not discontinue abruptly.
- ☐ Caution patient to make position changes slowly to minimize orthostatic hypotension.
- ☐ May cause dizziness. Caution patient to avoid driving or other activities requiring alertness until response to medication is known.
- ☐ Advise patient to avoid concurrent use of alcohol with this medication. Patients should

also consult health care professional before taking OTC medications while taking isosorbide.

- □ Inform patient that headache is a common side effect that should decrease with continuing therapy. Aspirin or acetaminophen may be ordered to treat headache. Notify health care professional if headache is persistent or severe. Do not alter dose to avoid headache.
- □ Advise patient to notify health care professional if dry mouth or blurred vision occurs or if undigested extended-release isosorbide dinitrate tablets are found in stool.

EVALUATION

Effectiveness of therapy can be demonstrated by: ▪ Decrease in frequency and severity of anginal attacks □ Increase in activity tolerance.

ISRADIPINE

(is-**ra**-di-peen)

DynaCirc, DynaCirc CR

CLASSIFICATION(S):

Antianginal, Antihypertensive agent, Calcium channel blocker

Pregnancy Category C

INDICATIONS

▪ Management of hypertension, angina pectoris, and vasospastic (Prinzmetal's) angina.

ACTION

▪ Inhibits the transport of calcium into myocardial and vascular smooth muscle cells, resulting in inhibition of excitation-contraction coupling and subsequent contraction. **Therapeutic Effects:** ▪ Systemic vasodilation resulting in decreased blood pressure ▪ Coronary vasodilation resulting in decreased frequency and severity of attacks of angina.

PHARMACOKINETICS

Absorption: Well absorbed following oral administration but extensively metabolized, resulting in decreased bioavailability.

Distribution: UK.

Metabolism and Excretion: Completely metabolized by the liver.

Half-life: 8 hr.

CONTRAINDICATIONS AND PRECAUTIONS

Contraindicated in: ▪ Hypersensitivity ▪ Sick sinus syndrome ▪ 2nd- or 3rd-degree AV block (unless an artificial pacemaker is in place) ▪ Blood pressure <90 mm Hg.

Use Cautiously in: ▪ Severe hepatic impairment (dosage reduction recommended) ▪ Geriatric patients (dosage reduction recommended for most agents; increased risk of hypotension) ▪ Severe renal impairment ▪ History of serious ventricular arrhythmias or congestive heart failure ▪ Pregnancy, lactation, or children (safety not established).

ADVERSE REACTIONS AND SIDE EFFECTS*

CNS: abnormal dreams, anxiety, confusion, dizziness, drowsiness, headache, nervousness, psychiatric disturbances, weakness.

EENT: blurred vision, disturbed equilibrium, epistaxis, tinnitus.

Resp: cough, dyspnea.

CV: ARRHYTHMIAS, CONGESTIVE HEART FAILURE, <u>peripheral edema</u>, bradycardia, chest pain, hypotension, palpitations, syncope, tachycardia.

GI: abnormal liver function studies, anorexia, constipation, diarrhea, dry mouth, dysgeusia, dyspepsia, nausea, vomiting.

GU: dysuria, nocturia, polyuria, sexual dysfunction, urinary frequency.

Derm: dermatitis, erythema multiforme, flushing, increased sweating, photosensitivity, pruritus/urticaria, rash.

Endo: gynecomastia, hyperglycemia.

Hemat: anemia, leukopenia, thrombocytopenia.

Metab: weight gain.

MS: joint stiffness, muscle cramps.

Neuro: paresthesia, tremor.

Misc: STEVENS-JOHNSON SYNDROME, gingival hyperplasia.

INTERACTIONS

Drug-Drug: ▪ Additive hypotension may occur when used concurrently with **fentanyl,** other **antihypertensives, nitrates,** acute ingestion of

I

***CAPITALS indicate life-threatening; <u>underlines</u> indicate most frequent.**

alcohol, or **quinidine** ▪ Antihypertensive effects may be decreased by concurrent use of **NSAIDs** ▪ Concurrent use with **beta-adrenergic blockers, digoxin, disopyramide**, or **phenytoin** may result in bradycardia, conduction defects, or congestive heart failure.

ROUTE AND DOSAGE

- **PO (Adults):** 2.5 mg twice daily; may be increased q 2–4 wk by 5 mg/day (not to exceed 20 mg/day) *or* 5 mg once daily as CR tablets; may be increased q 2–4 wk by 5 mg/day (not to exceed 20 mg/day).

AVAILABILITY

▪ ***Capsules:*** 2.5 mg[Rx], 5 mg[Rx] ▪ ***Controlled-release tablets:*** 5 mg[Rx], 10 mg[Rx].

TIME/ACTION PROFILE (cardiovascular effects*)

	ONSET	PEAK	DURATION
PO	<2 hr	2–3 hr	12 hr
PO-CR	2 hr	8–10 hr	24 hr

*For single doses, maximal antihypertensive effect during chronic dosing may take 2–4 wk.

NURSING IMPLICATIONS

ASSESSMENT

- □ Monitor blood pressure and pulse prior to and periodically throughout therapy. Monitor ECG periodically in patients receiving prolonged therapy.
- □ Monitor intake and output ratios and daily weight. Assess patient for signs of congestive heart failure (peripheral edema, rales/crackles, dyspnea, weight gain, jugular venous distention).
- ▪ **Angina:** Assess location, duration, intensity, and precipitating factors of patient's anginal pain.
- ▪ ***Lab Test Considerations:*** Total serum calcium concentrations are not affected by calcium channel blockers.
- □ Monitor serum potassium periodically. Hypokalemia increases risk of arrhythmias; should be corrected.
- □ Monitor renal and hepatic functions periodically during long-term therapy. Several days of therapy may cause increase in hepatic enzymes, which return to normal upon discontinuation of therapy.

POTENTIAL NURSING DIAGNOSES

- ▪ Cardiac output, decreased (Indications).
- ▪ Knowledge deficit, related to medication regimen (Patient/Family Teaching).

IMPLEMENTATION

- ▪ **PO:** May be administered without regard to meals. May be administered with meals if GI irritation becomes a problem.
- □ Do not open, crush, break, or chew controlled-release tablets.

PATIENT/FAMILY TEACHING

- □ Advise patient to take medication exactly as directed, even if feeling well. If a dose is missed, take as soon as possible unless almost time for next dose; do not double doses. May need to be discontinued gradually.
- □ Caution patient to change positions slowly to minimize orthostatic hypotension.
- □ May cause dizziness. Advise patient to avoid driving or other activities requiring alertness until response to the medication is known.
- □ Instruct patient to avoid concurrent use of alcohol or OTC medications without consulting health care professional.
- □ Caution patient to wear protective clothing and use sunscreen to prevent photosensitivity reactions.
- □ Advise patient to notify health care professional if irregular heartbeats, dyspnea, swelling of hands and feet, pronounced dizziness, nausea, constipation, or hypotension occurs.
- ▪ **Angina:** Instruct patient on concurrent nitrate or beta-blocker therapy to continue taking both medications as directed and to use SL nitroglycerin as needed for anginal attacks.
- □ Inform patient that anginal attacks may occur 30 min after administration because of reflex tachycardia. This is usually temporary and is not an indication for discontinuation.
- □ Advise patient to contact health care professional if chest pain does not improve, worsens after therapy, or occurs with diaphoresis or if shortness of breath or persistent headache occurs.
- □ Caution patient to discuss exercise restrictions with health care professional prior to exertion.
- ▪ **Hypertension:** Encourage patient to comply with other interventions for hypertension (weight reduction, low-sodium diet, smoking

cessation, moderation of alcohol consumption, regular exercise, and stress management). Medication controls but does not cure hypertension.

- Instruct patient and family in proper technique for monitoring BP. Advise patient to take BP weekly and to report significant changes to health care professional.

EVALUATION

Effectiveness of therapy can be demonstrated by: ▪ Decrease in blood pressure ▪ Decrease in frequency and severity of anginal attacks ▫ Decrease in need for nitrate therapy ▫ Increase in activity tolerance and sense of well-being.

ITRACONAZOLE
(it-tra-**kon**-a-zole)
Sporanox

CLASSIFICATION(S):
Antifungal (azole)

Pregnancy Category C

INDICATIONS

▪ Treatment of: ▫ Histoplasmosis ▫ Blastomycosis ▫ Aspergillosis ▫ Onychomycosis (fingernail, toenail fungus) ▫ Oropharyngeal candidiasis (oral solution only) ▫ Dermatophyte infections (in patients unable to comply with topical therapy).

ACTION

▪ Inhibits enzymes necessary for integrity of the fungal cell wall. **Therapeutic Effects:** ▪ Fungistatic effects against susceptible organisms. **Spectrum:** ▪ Active against *Histoplasma capsulatum, Blastomyces dermatitidis, Cryptococcus neoformans, Aspergillus fumigatus, Trichophyton* spp., *Candida,* and tinea unguium.

PHARMACOKINETICS

Absorption: Absorption following oral administration is enhanced by food.
Distribution: Tissue concentrations are higher than plasma concentrations. Does not enter CSF; enters breast milk.
Metabolism and Excretion: Mostly metabolized by the liver and excreted in feces. Hydroxyitraconazole, the major metabolite, has antifungal activity.
Half-life: 21 hr.

CONTRAINDICATIONS AND PRECAUTIONS

Contraindicated in: ▪ Hypersensitivity. Cross-sensitivity with other azole antifungals (miconazole, ketoconazole) may occur ▪ Lactation ▪ Concurrent astemizole or cisapride.
Use Cautiously in: ▪ Patients with hepatic impairment (dosage reduction may be required) ▪ Patients with achlorhydria or hypochlorhydria (absorption will be decreased) ▪ Pregnancy or children (safety not established).

ADVERSE REACTIONS AND SIDE EFFECTS*

CNS: dizziness, drowsiness, fatigue, headache, malaise.
EENT: tinnitus.
CV: edema, hypertension.
GI: <u>nausea</u>, abdominal pain, anorexia, diarrhea, drug-induced hepatitis, flatulence, vomiting.
GU: albuminuria, decreased libido, impotence.
Derm: TOXIC EPIDERMAL NECROLYSIS, pruritus, rash.
Endo: adrenal insufficiency.
F and E: hypokalemia.
MS: rhabdomyolysis.
Misc: fever.

INTERACTIONS

Drug-Drug: ▪ May increase the risk of serious arrhythmias with **astemizole** or **cisapride** (avoid concurrent use) ▪ **Phenytoin, phenobarbital, isoniazid, rifampin,** and **carbamazepine** increase metabolism of itraconazole. Increased dosage may be necessary ▪ Itraconazole decreases metabolism and may increase effects of **phenytoin, cyclosporine, tacrolimus, oral hypoglycemic agents,** and **warfarin** ▪ Itraconazole may increase serum **digoxin** levels ▪ If hypokalemia occurs, the risk of **cardiac glycoside** toxicity is increased ▪ Absorption may be decreased by **antacids, H_2 blockers,** or other **agents that increase gastric pH** ▪ Prolonged sedation may occur with

***CAPITALS indicate life-threatening; <u>underlines</u> indicate most frequent.**

I

midazolam or **triazolam** (avoid concurrent use).
Drug-Food: ▪ Food increases absorption.

ROUTE AND DOSAGE

Capsules and oral solution are not interchangeable; oral solution is only for oropharyngeal candidiasis.

- **PO (Adults):** *Aspergillosis*—200 mg once or twice daily for a minimum of 3 mo. *Blastomycosis, histoplasmosis*—200 mg once daily; may be increased by 100 mg/day up to 200 mg twice daily. *Toenail fungus with or without fingernail fungus*—200 mg/day for 12 consecutive wk. *Fingernail fungus*—200 mg twice daily for 1 wk, then 3 wk without therapy, then 200 mg twice daily an additional wk–6 mo. *Oropharyngeal candidiasis*—200 mg (20 ml) daily for 1–2 wk. *Oropharyngeal candidiasis unresponsive to fluconazole*—100 mg (10 ml) twice daily for at least 2–4 wk. *Esophageal candidiasis*—100 mg (10 ml) once daily for at least 3 wk.

AVAILABILITY

▪ ***Capsules:*** 100 mg[Rx] ▪ ***Oral solution:*** 10 mg/ml[Rx].

TIME/ACTION PROFILE (blood levels)

	ONSET	PEAK	DURATION
PO	rapid	4 hr	12–24 hr

NURSING IMPLICATIONS

ASSESSMENT

- □ Assess patient for signs and symptoms of infection (vital signs, lung sounds, sputum, WBC, oral and pharyngeal mucosa, nail beds) prior to and periodically throughout therapy.
- □ Specimens for culture should be taken prior to instituting therapy. Therapy may be started before results are obtained.
- ▪ ***Lab Test Considerations:*** Hepatic function tests should be monitored prior to and periodically throughout therapy, especially in patients with pre-existing hepatic function abnormalities. Discontinue itraconazole if abnormal values persist or worsen.
- □ Monitor serum potassium. May cause hypokalemia.

POTENTIAL NURSING DIAGNOSES

- Infection, risk for (Indications).
- Knowledge deficit, related to medication regimen (Patient/Family Teaching).
- Noncompliance, related to medication regimen (Patient/Family Teaching).

IMPLEMENTATION

- **General Info:** Do not interchange capsules and oral solution. Only oral solution is effective for oral pharyngeal candidiasis.
- **Capsules:** Administer with a full meal to minimize nausea and vomiting and to increase absorption.
- □ Do not administer with antacids or other medications that may increase gastric pH; may decrease absorption of itraconazole.
- **Oral Solution:** Administer without food, if possible. Swish solution in mouth vigorously, 10 ml at a time, for several seconds, then swallow.

PATIENT/FAMILY TEACHING

- □ Instruct patient to take medication exactly as directed, even if feeling better. Doses should be taken at the same time each day.
- □ May occasionally cause drowsiness. Caution patient to avoid driving or other activities requiring alertness until response to medication is known.
- □ Instruct patient to notify health care professional if signs and symptoms of liver dysfunction (unusual fatigue, anorexia, nausea, vomiting, jaundice, dark urine, or pale stools) occur.
- □ Advise patient to consult health care professional prior to taking any Rx or OTC medications concurrently with itraconazole.

EVALUATION

Effectiveness of therapy can be demonstrated by: ▪ Resolution of clinical and laboratory indications of fungal infections. Minimal treatment for systemic fungal infections is 3 mo. Inadequate period of treatment may lead to recurrence of active infection.

KAOLIN/PECTIN
(**kay**-oh-lin **pek**-tin)
{Donnagel-MB}, Kao-Spen, Kapectolin, K-P

CLASSIFICATION(S):
Antidiarrheal (adsorbent/protectant)

Pregnancy Category C

INDICATIONS
▪ Adjunctive therapy in the treatment of mild to moderate diarrhea.

ACTION
▪ Acts as an adsorbent and protectant ▪ Decreases stool fluid content, although total water loss does not change. **Therapeutic Effects:** ▪ Relief of diarrhea.

PHARMACOKINETICS
Absorption: Action is local, not systemically absorbed.
Distribution: UK.
Metabolism and Excretion: Pectin decomposes in the GI tract.
Half-life: UK.

CONTRAINDICATIONS AND PRECAUTIONS
Contraindicated in: ▪ Severe abdominal pain of unknown cause, especially when associated with fever ▪ Children <3 yr ▪ Some products contain alcohol and should be avoided in patients with known intolerance.
Use Cautiously in: ▪ Geriatric patients (>60 yr) ▪ Diarrhea continuing >48 hr (health care professional should be consulted).

ADVERSE REACTIONS AND SIDE EFFECTS
GI: constipation.

INTERACTIONS
Drug-Drug: ▪ May decrease the absorption of other **orally administered medications** (should not be administered for 2–3 hr before or after other medications).

ROUTE AND DOSAGE
Kaolin/pectin suspension contains 5.2–6 g kaolin/30 ml and 130–260 mg pectin/30 ml.
- **PO (Adults):** 60–120 ml after each loose stool.
- **PO (Children ≥12 yr):** 45–60 ml after each loose stool.
- **PO (Children 6–12 yr):** 30–60 ml after each loose stool.
- **PO (Children 3–6 yr):** 15–30 ml after each loose stool.

AVAILABILITY
▪ ***Suspension:*** 5.2 g kaolin plus 260 mg pectin/30 ml[OTC], 5.85 g kaolin plus 130 mg pectin/30 ml[OTC] ▪ ***In combination with:*** paregoric, bismuth, carboxymethylcellulose, and others[OTC]. See Appendix A.

TIME/ACTION PROFILE (relief of diarrhea)

	ONSET	PEAK	DURATION
PO	30 min	UK	4–6 hr

NURSING IMPLICATIONS

ASSESSMENT
- □ Assess the frequency and consistency of stools and bowel sounds prior to and throughout therapy.
- □ Assess fluid and electrolyte balance and skin turgor for dehydration.

POTENTIAL NURSING DIAGNOSES
- Diarrhea (Indications).
- Constipation (Side Effects).
- Knowledge deficit, related to medication regimen (Patient/Family Teaching).

IMPLEMENTATION
- **General Info:** Administer after each loose bowel movement until diarrhea is controlled.
- **PO:** Shake suspension well prior to administration.

PATIENT/FAMILY TEACHING
- □ Instruct patient to notify health care professional if diarrhea persists longer than 48 hr, if stool contains blood or mucus, or if fever or abdominal pain develops.

K

{} = Available in Canada only.

□ Advise patient to take other medications 2–3 hr before or after kaolin/pectin.

EVALUATION

Effectiveness of therapy can be demonstrated by: ▪ Decrease in frequency of loose stools ▪ Return to soft, formed stools.

KETOCONAZOLE†
(kee-toe-**koe**-na-zole)
Nizoral

CLASSIFICATION(S):
Antifungal

Pregnancy Category C

†For topical use, see page 69.

INDICATIONS

▪ Treatment of the following fungal infections: □ Candidiasis (disseminated and mucocutaneous) □ Chromomycosis □ Coccidioidomycosis □ Histoplasmosis □ Paracoccidioidomycosis. **Unlabeled Uses:** ▪ Treatment of advanced prostate cancer ▪ Treatment of Cushing's syndrome.

ACTION

▪ Disrupts fungal cell wall ▪ Interferes with fungal metabolism ▪ Also inhibits the production of adrenal steroids. **Therapeutic Effects:** ▪ Fungistatic or fungicidal action against susceptible organisms, depending on organism and site of infection. **Spectrum:** ▪ Active against many pathogenic fungi, including: □ *Blastomyces* □ *Candida* □ *Coccidioides* □ *Cryptococcus* □ *Histoplasma* □ Many dermatophytes.

PHARMACOKINETICS

Absorption: Absorption from the GI tract is pH dependent; increasing pH decreases absorption.
Distribution: Widely distributed. CNS penetration is unpredictable and minimal. Crosses the placenta; enters breast milk.
Metabolism and Excretion: Partially metabolized by the liver. Excreted in feces via biliary excretion.
Half-life: 8 hr.

CONTRAINDICATIONS AND PRECAUTIONS

Contraindicated in: ▪ Hypersensitivity ▪ Pregnancy or lactation ▪ Concurrent astemizole or cisapride.
Use Cautiously in: ▪ History of liver disease ▪ Achlorhydria or hypochlorhydria ▪ Alcoholism.

ADVERSE REACTIONS AND SIDE EFFECTS*

CNS: dizziness, drowsiness.
EENT: photophobia.
GI: DRUG-INDUCED HEPATITIS, nausea, vomiting, abdominal pain, constipation, diarrhea, flatulence.
GU: azoospermia, decreased male libido, menstrual irregularities, oligospermia.
Derm: rashes.
Endo: gynecomastia.

INTERACTIONS

Drug-Drug: ▪ Increased risk of serious, potentially life-threatening arrhythmias with **astemizole** or **cisapride** ▪ Drugs that increase gastric pH, including **antacids, histamine H_2 antagonists, didanosine** (because of buffer), and **gastric acid–pump inhibitors** decrease absorption (wait 2 hr before administration of ketoconazole) ▪ Additive hepatotoxicity with other **hepatotoxic agents,** including **alcohol** ▪ Disulfiram-like reaction may occur with **alcohol** ▪ **Rifampin** or **isoniazid** may decrease levels and effectiveness ▪ May increase effectiveness/risk of toxicity from **warfarin, phenytoin, cyclosporine,** or **glucocorticoids** ▪ Increases blood levels of **indinavir** (dosage reduction of indinavir recommended).

ROUTE AND DOSAGE

- **PO (Adults):** 200–400 mg/day, single dose. *Prostate cancer*—400 mg 3 times daily (unlabeled).
- **PO (Children >2 yr):** 3.3–6.6 mg/kg/day, single dose.

AVAILABILITY

▪ ***Tablets:*** 200 mg[Rx] ▪ ***Oral suspension:*** {100 mg/5 ml[Rx]}.

*CAPITALS indicate life-threatening; underlines indicate most frequent.

TIME/ACTION PROFILE (blood levels)

	ONSET	PEAK	DURATION
PO	rapid	1–4 hr	24 hr

NURSING IMPLICATIONS

ASSESSMENT

- Assess patient for symptoms of infection prior to and periodically throughout therapy.
- Specimens for culture should be taken prior to instituting therapy. Therapy may be started before results are obtained.
- ***Lab Test Considerations:*** Hepatic function tests should be monitored prior to and monthly for 3–4 mo and then periodically throughout course of therapy. May cause increased AST, ALT, serum alkaline phosphatase, and bilirubin concentrations. Ketoconazole should be discontinued if even minor abnormalities occur.
- May cause decreased serum testosterone concentrations.

POTENTIAL NURSING DIAGNOSES

- Infection, risk for (Indications).
- Knowledge deficit, related to medication regimen (Patient/Family Teaching).
- Noncompliance, related to medication regimen (Patient/Family Teaching).

IMPLEMENTATION

- **PO:** Administer with meals or snacks to minimize nausea and vomiting.
- Shake suspension well prior to administration.
- Do not administer histamine H_2 antagonists or antacids within 2 hr of ketoconazole.
- For patients with achlorhydria, dissolve each tablet in 4 ml of aqueous solution of 0.2 N hydrochloric acid. Use a glass or plastic straw to avoid contact with teeth and follow with a glass of water, swished in mouth and swallowed.

PATIENT/FAMILY TEACHING

- **General Info:** Instruct patient to take medication exactly as directed, even if feeling better. Doses should be taken at the same time each day. If a dose is missed, take as soon as remembered; if almost time for next dose, space missed dose and next dose 10–12 hr apart.
- May cause dizziness or drowsiness. Caution patient to avoid driving or other activities requiring alertness until response to medication is known.
- Advise patient to avoid taking OTC antacids within 2 hr of ketoconazole.
- Caution patient to wear sunglasses and to avoid prolonged exposure to bright light to prevent photophobic reactions.
- Advise patient to avoid concurrent use of alcohol while taking ketoconazole; may cause a disulfiram-like reaction (flushing, rash, peripheral edema, nausea, headache) and increase the risk of hepatotoxicity.
- Instruct patient to notify health care professional if abdominal pain, fever, or diarrhea becomes pronounced or if signs and symptoms of liver dysfunction (unusual fatigue, anorexia, nausea, vomiting, jaundice, dark urine, or pale stools) occur.

EVALUATION

Effectiveness of therapy can be demonstrated by: ▪ Resolution of clinical and laboratory indications of fungal infections ▪ Minimal treatment for candidiasis is 1–2 wk and for other systemic mycoses is 6 mo ▫ Chronic mucocutaneous candidiasis usually requires maintenance therapy.

KETOPROFEN

(kee-toe-**proe**-fen)

Actron, {Apo-Keto}, {Apo-Keto-E}, Orudis, {Orudis-E}, Orudis KT, {Orudis-SR}, Oruvail, {Rhodis}

CLASSIFICATION(S):

Nonopioid analgesic/Nonsteroidal anti-inflammatory agent

Pregnancy Category B (first trimester)

INDICATIONS

▪ Inflammatory disorders, including: ▫ Rheumatoid arthritis ▫ Osteoarthritis ▪ Mild to moderate pain, including dysmenorrhea and fever.

ACTION

▪ Inhibits prostaglandin synthesis. **Therapeutic Effects:** ▪ Suppression of pain and inflammation ▪ Reduction of fever.

PHARMACOKINETICS

Absorption: Well absorbed from the GI tract.
Distribution: UK.
Metabolism and Excretion: Mostly (60%) metabolized by the liver; some renal excretion.
Half-life: 2–4 hr.

CONTRAINDICATIONS AND PRECAUTIONS

Contraindicated in: ▪ Hypersensitivity ▪ Cross-sensitivity may exist with other NSAIDs, including aspirin ▪ Active GI bleeding ▪ Ulcer disease ▪ Some products contain tartrazine and should be avoided in patients with known intolerance.
Use Cautiously in: ▪ Severe cardiovascular, renal, or hepatic disease ▪ History of ulcer disease ▪ Renal impairment (dosage reduction suggested) ▪ Extended-release product should not be used in geriatric patients, patients of small stature, or patients with renal impairment ▪ Chronic alcohol use/abuse ▪ Pregnancy, lactation, or children (safety not established; avoid use during 2nd half of pregnancy).

ADVERSE REACTIONS AND SIDE EFFECTS*

CNS: drowsiness, headache, dizziness.
EENT: blurred vision, tinnitus.
CV: edema.
GI: DRUG-INDUCED HEPATITIS, GI BLEEDING, constipation, diarrhea, dyspepsia, nausea, vomiting, anorexia, discomfort, flatulence.
GU: cystitis, hematuria, renal failure.
Derm: photosensitivity, rashes.
Endo: gynecomastia.
Hemat: blood dyscrasias, prolonged bleeding time.
MS: myalgia.
Misc: allergic reactions including ANAPHYLAXIS, fever.

INTERACTIONS

Drug-Drug: ▪ **Aspirin** alters distribution, metabolism, and excretion of ketoprofen (concurrent use not recommended) ▪ Additive adverse GI effects with other **NSAIDs, glucocorticoids,** or **alcohol** ▪ Chronic use with **acetaminophen** may increase the risk of adverse renal reactions ▪ May decrease the effectiveness of **diuretics** or **antihypertensive therapy** ▪ May increase the hypoglycemic effects of **insulin** or **oral hypoglycemic agents** ▪ May increase serum **lithium** levels and increase the risk of toxicity ▪ Increases the risk of toxicity from **methotrexate** ▪ **Probenecid** increases risk of toxicity from ketoprofen (concurrent use not recommended) ▪ Increased risk of bleeding with **cefamandole, cefotetan, cefoperazone, valproic acid, plicamycin, thrombolytic agents,** or **anticoagulants** ▪ Increased risk of adverse hematologic reactions with **antineoplastic agents** or **radiation therapy** ▪ Increased risk of nephrotoxicity with **cyclosporine.**

ROUTE AND DOSAGE

- **PO (Adults):** *Anti-inflammatory*—150–300 mg/day in 3–4 divided doses or 150–200 mg once daily as extended-release product. *Analgesic*—25–50 mg q 6–8 hr. *OTC analgesic/antipyretic*—12.5 mg q 4–6 hr; if relief is not obtained 1 hr after first dose, an additional dose may be given. An initial dose of 25 mg may be used (not to exceed 25 mg/4–6 hr or 75 mg/24 hr).

AVAILABILITY

▪ ***Tablets:*** 12.5 mg[OTC] ▪ ***Capsules:*** 25 mg[Rx], 50 mg[Rx], 75 mg[Rx] ▪ ***Extended-release capsules:*** 100 mg[Rx], 150 mg [Rx], 200 mg[Rx].

TIME/ACTION PROFILE

	ONSET	PEAK	DURATION
PO (analgesic)	within 60 min	1 hr	4–6 hr
PO (anti-inflammatory)	few days–1 wk	UK	UK

NURSING IMPLICATIONS

ASSESSMENT

- **General Info:** Patients who have asthma, aspirin-induced allergy, and nasal polyps are at increased risk for developing hypersensitivity

*CAPITALS indicate life-threatening; underlines indicate most frequent.

reactions. Assess for rhinitis, wheezing, and urticaria.

- **Arthritis:** Assess pain and range of motion prior to and 1 hr following administration.
- **Pain:** Assess pain (note type, location, and intensity) prior to and 1 hr following administration.
- **Fever:** Monitor temperature; note signs associated with fever (diaphoresis, tachycardia, malaise).
- ***Lab Test Considerations:*** BUN, serum creatinine, CBC, and liver function tests should be evaluated periodically in patients receiving prolonged courses of therapy.
- □ Serum potassium, BUN, serum creatinine, alkaline phosphatase, LDH, AST, and ALT tests may show increased levels. Blood glucose, hemoglobin, and hematocrit concentrations, leukocyte and platelet counts, and CCr may be decreased.
- □ May prolong bleeding time by 3–4 min.
- □ May alter results of urine albumin, bilirubin, 17-ketosteroid, and 17-hydroxycorticosteroid determinations.

POTENTIAL NURSING DIAGNOSES

- Pain (Indications).
- Physical mobility, impaired (Indications).
- Knowledge deficit, related to medication regimen (Patient/Family Teaching).

IMPLEMENTATION

- **General Info:** Administration in higher than recommended doses does not provide increased effectiveness but may cause increased side effects.
- □ Coadministration with opioid analgesics may have additive analgesic effects and may permit lower opioid doses.
- □ Analgesic is more effective if given before pain becomes severe.
- **PO:** For rapid initial effect, administer 30 min before or 2 hr after meals. Capsules may be administered with food, milk, or antacids containing aluminum hydroxide and magnesium hydroxide to decrease GI irritation.
- □ Extended-release capsules should be swallowed whole; do not open or chew.
- **Dysmenorrhea:** Administer as soon as possible after the onset of menses. Prophylactic treatment has not been proved effective.

PATIENT/FAMILY TEACHING

- □ Advise patient to take this medication with a full glass of water and to remain in an upright position for 15–30 min after administration.
- □ Instruct patient to take medication exactly as directed. If a dose is missed, it should be taken as soon as remembered but not if almost time for the next dose. Do not double doses.
- □ May cause drowsiness or dizziness. Advise patient to avoid driving or other activities requiring alertness until response to medication is known.
- □ Caution patient to avoid the concurrent use of alcohol, aspirin, acetaminophen, or other OTC medications without consulting health care professional.
- □ Advise patient to inform health care professional of medication regimen prior to treatment or surgery.
- □ Caution patient to wear sunscreen and protective clothing to prevent photosensitivity reactions.
- □ Instruct patients not to take OTC ketoprofen preparations for more than 10 days for pain or more than 3 days for fever and to consult health care professional if symptoms persist or worsen.
- □ Caution patient that use of ketoprofen with 3 or more glasses of alcohol may increase risk of GI bleeding.
- □ Advise patient to consult health care professional if rash, itching, visual disturbances, tinnitus, weight gain, edema, black stools, persistent headache, or influenza-like syndrome (chills, fever, muscle aches, pain) occurs.

EVALUATION

Effectiveness of therapy can be demonstrated by: ▪ Improved joint mobility ▪ Decrease in severity of pain. Improvement in arthritis may be seen in a few days to 1 wk; 1–2 wk may be required for maximum effectiveness. Patients who do not respond to one NSAID may respond to another ▪ Reduction of fever.

KETOROLAC
(kee-**toe**-role-ak)
Toradol

CLASSIFICATION(S):
Nonopioid analgesic/Nonsteroidal anti-inflammatory agent

Pregnancy Category C (first trimester)

INDICATIONS

▪ Short-term management of pain (not to exceed 5 days total for all routes combined).

ACTION

▪ Inhibits prostaglandin synthesis, producing peripherally mediated analgesia ▪ Also has antipyretic and anti-inflammatory properties. **Therapeutic Effects:** ▪ **PO, IM:** Decreased pain.

PHARMACOKINETICS

Absorption: Rapidly and completely absorbed following all routes of administration.
Distribution: Enters breast milk in low concentrations.
Metabolism and Excretion: <50% metabolized by the liver. Ketorolac and its metabolites are excreted primarily by the kidneys (92%); 6% excreted in feces.
Half-life: 4.5 hr (range 3.8–6.3 hr; increased in geriatric patients and patients with impaired renal function).

CONTRAINDICATIONS AND PRECAUTIONS

Contraindicated in: ▪ Hypersensitivity ▪ Cross-sensitivity with other NSAIDs may exist ▪ Lactation ▪ Pre- or perioperative use ▪ Known alcohol intolerance (injection only) ▪ Patients wearing soft contact lenses (ophth only).
Use Cautiously in: ▪ History of GI bleeding ▪ Renal impairment (dosage reduction may be required) ▪ Cardiovascular disease ▪ Pregnancy and children (use not recommended during 2nd half of pregnancy).

ADVERSE REACTIONS AND SIDE EFFECTS*

CNS: drowsiness, abnormal thinking, dizziness, euphoria, headache.
Resp: asthma, dyspnea.
CV: edema, pallor, vasodilation.
GI: GI BLEEDING, abnormal taste, diarrhea, dry mouth, dyspepsia, GI pain, nausea.
GU: oliguria, renal toxicity, urinary frequency.
Derm: pruritus, purpura, sweating, urticaria.
Hemat: prolonged bleeding time.
Local: injection site pain.
Neuro: paresthesia.

INTERACTIONS

Drug-Drug: ▪ Concurrent use with **aspirin** may decrease effectiveness ▪ Additive adverse GI effects with **aspirin**, other **NSAIDs, potassium supplements, glucocorticoids,** or **alcohol** ▪ Chronic use with **acetaminophen** may increase the risk of adverse renal reactions ▪ May decrease the effectiveness of **diuretics** or **antihypertensive therapy** ▪ May increase serum **lithium** levels and increase the risk of toxicity ▪ Increases the risk of toxicity from **methotrexate** ▪ Increased risk of bleeding with **cefamandole, cefotetan, cefoperazone, valproic acid, plicamycin, thrombolytic agents,** or **anticoagulants** ▪ Increased risk of adverse hematologic reactions with **antineoplastic agents** or **radiation therapy** ▪ May increase the risk of nephrotoxicity from **cyclosporine** ▪ **Probenecid** increases ketorolac blood levels and the risk of adverse reactions (concurrent use should be avoided).

ROUTE AND DOSAGE

Oral therapy is indicated only as a continuation of parenteral therapy; parenteral therapy should not exceed 20 doses/5 days.

- **PO (Adults <65 yr):** 20 mg initially, followed by 10 mg q 4–6 hr as needed (not to exceed 40 mg/day).
- **PO (Adults ≥65 yr, <50 kg, or with Renal Impairment):** 10 mg q 4–6 hr as needed (not to exceed 40 mg/day).
- **IM (Adults <65 yr):** *Single dose*—60 mg. *Multiple dosing*—30 mg q 6 hr (not to exceed 120 mg/day; not to exceed 5 days combined PO/IM/IV).
- **IM (Adults ≥65 yr, <50 kg, or with Renal Impairment):** *Single dose*—30 mg. *Multiple dosing*—15 mg q 6 hr (not to exceed 60 mg/day; not to exceed 5 days combined PO/IM/IV).

***CAPITALS indicate life-threatening; underlines indicate most frequent.**

- **IV (Adults <65 yr):** *Single dose*—30 mg. *Multiple dosing*—30 mg q 6 hr (not to exceed 120 mg/day; not to exceed 5 days combined PO/IM/IV).
- **IV (Adults ≥65 yr, <50 kg, or with Renal Impairment):** *Single dose*—15 mg. *Multiple dosing*—15 mg q 6 hr (not to exceed 60 mg/day; not to exceed 5 days combined PO/IM/IV).

AVAILABILITY

▪ ***Tablets:*** 10 mg[Rx] ▪ ***Injection:*** 15 mg/ml in 1-ml preloaded syringes[Rx], 30 mg/ml in 1- and 2-ml preloaded syringes[Rx].

TIME/ACTION PROFILE (analgesic effects)

	ONSET	PEAK	DURATION
PO	UK	2–3 hr	4–6 hr or longer
IM, IV	10 min	1–2 hr	6 hr or longer

NURSING IMPLICATIONS

ASSESSMENT

- **General Info:** Patients who have asthma, aspirin-induced allergy, and nasal polyps are at increased risk for developing hypersensitivity reactions. Assess for rhinitis, asthma, and urticaria.
- **Pain:** Assess pain (note type, location, and intensity) prior to and 1–2 hr following administration.
- ***Lab Test Considerations:*** Liver function tests, especially AST and ALT, should be evaluated periodically in patients receiving prolonged courses of therapy. May cause increased levels.
  - May cause prolonged bleeding time that may persist for 24–48 hr following discontinuation of therapy.
  - May cause increased BUN, serum creatinine, or potassium concentrations.

POTENTIAL NURSING DIAGNOSES

- Pain (Indications).
- Knowledge deficit, related to medication regimen (Patient/Family Teaching).

IMPLEMENTATION

- **General Info:** Administration in higher than recommended doses does not provide increased effectiveness but may cause increased side effects. Duration of ketorolac therapy, by all routes combined, should not exceed 5 days.
  - Coadministration with opioid analgesics may have additive analgesic effects and may permit lower opioid doses.
- **PO:** Ketorolac therapy should always be given initially by the IM or IV route. Oral therapy should be used *only* as a continuation of parenteral therapy.
- **Direct IV:** Administer undiluted.
- ***Rate:*** Administer over at least 15 sec.
- **Syringe Compatibility:** ▪ sufentanil.
- **Syringe Incompatibility:** ▪ haloperidol ▪ hydroxyzine ▪ meperidine ▪ morphine ▪ nalbuphine ▪ prochlorperazine ▪ promethazine ▪ thiethylperazine.
- **Y-Site Compatibility:** ▪ sufentanil.
- **Solution Compatibility:** ▪ D5/0.9% NaCl ▪ D5W ▪ Ringer's injection ▪ lactated Ringer's injection ▪ 0.9% NaCl.

PATIENT/FAMILY TEACHING

- **General Info:** Instruct patient on how and when to ask for pain medication.
  - Instruct patient to take medication exactly as directed. If dose is missed, it should be taken as soon as remembered but not if almost time for next dose. Do not double doses.
  - May cause drowsiness or dizziness. Advise patient to avoid driving or other activities requiring alertness until response to the medication is known.
  - Caution patient to avoid the concurrent use of alcohol, aspirin, NSAIDs, acetaminophen, or other OTC medications without consulting health care professional.
  - Advise patient to inform health care professional of medication regimen prior to treatment or surgery.
  - Advise patient to consult health care professional if rash, itching, visual disturbances, tinnitus, weight gain, edema, black stools, persistent headache, or influenza-like syndrome (chills, fever, muscle aches, pain) occurs.

EVALUATION

Effectiveness of therapy can be demonstrated by: ▪ Decrease in severity of pain. Patients who do not respond to one NSAID may respond to another.

K

LABETALOL
(la-**bet**-oh-lole)
Normodyne, Trandate

CLASSIFICATION(S):
Antianginal, Antihypertensive agent, Beta-adrenergic blocking agent (nonselective)

Pregnancy Category C

INDICATIONS

▪ Management of hypertension.

ACTION

▪ Blocks stimulation of $beta_1$ (myocardial) and $beta_2$ (pulmonary, vascular, and uterine) -adrenergic receptor sites ▪ Also has $alpha_1$-adrenergic blocking activity, which may result in more orthostatic hypotension. **Therapeutic Effects:** ▪ Decreased blood pressure.

PHARMACOKINETICS

Absorption: Well absorbed but rapidly undergoes extensive first-pass hepatic metabolism, resulting in 25% bioavailability.
Distribution: Some CNS penetration; crosses the placenta.
Metabolism and Excretion: Undergoes extensive hepatic metabolism.
Half-life: 3–8 hr.

CONTRAINDICATIONS AND PRECAUTIONS

Contraindicated in: ▪ Uncompensated congestive heart failure ▪ Pulmonary edema ▪ Cardiogenic shock ▪ Bradycardia or heart block.
Use Cautiously in: ▪ Renal impairment ▪ Hepatic impairment ▪ Geriatric patients (increased sensitivity to beta-adrenergic blockers; initial dosage reduction recommended) ▪ Pulmonary disease (including asthma) ▪ Diabetes mellitus (may mask signs of hypoglycemia) ▪ Thyrotoxicosis (may mask symptoms) ▪ Patients with a history of severe allergic reactions (intensity of reactions may be increased) ▪ Pregnancy, lactation, or children (safety not established; may cause fetal/neonatal bradycardia, hypotension, hypoglycemia, or respiratory depression).

ADVERSE REACTIONS AND SIDE EFFECTS*

CNS: fatigue, weakness, anxiety, depression, dizziness, drowsiness, insomnia, memory loss, mental status changes, nightmares.
EENT: blurred vision, dry eyes, nasal stuffiness.
Resp: bronchospasm, wheezing.
CV: ARRHYTHMIAS, BRADYCARDIA, CONGESTIVE HEART FAILURE, PULMONARY EDEMA, orthostatic hypotension, peripheral vasoconstriction.
GI: constipation, diarrhea, nausea.
GU: impotence, decreased libido.
Derm: itching, rashes.
Endo: hyperglycemia, hypoglycemia.
MS: arthralgia, back pain, muscle cramps.
Neuro: paresthesia.

INTERACTIONS

Drug-Drug: ▪ **General anesthesia, IV phenytoin**, and **verapamil** may cause additive myocardial depression ▪ Additive bradycardia may occur with **digitalis glycosides** ▪ Additive hypotension may occur with other **antihypertensives**, acute ingestion of **alcohol**, or **nitrates** ▪ Concurrent **thyroid** administration may decrease effectiveness ▪ May alter the effectiveness of **insulin** or **oral hypoglycemic agents** (dosage adjustments may be necessary) ▪ May decrease the effectiveness of **beta-adrenergic bronchodilators** and **theophylline** ▪ May decrease the beneficial $beta_1$ cardiovascular effects of **dopamine** or **dobutamine** ▪ Use cautiously within 14 days of **MAO inhibitor therapy** (may result in hypertension) ▪ Effects may be increased by **propranolol** or **cimetidine** ▪ Concurrent **NSAIDs** may decrease antihypertensive action.

ROUTE AND DOSAGE

- **PO (Adults):** 100 mg twice daily initially, may be increased by 100 mg twice daily q 2–3 days as needed (usual range 400–800 mg/day in 2–3 divided doses; doses up to 1.2–2.4 g/day have been used).
- **IV (Adults):** 20 mg (0.25 mg/kg) initially, additional doses of 40–80 mg may be given q 10 min as needed (not to exceed 300 mg

*CAPITALS indicate life-threatening; underlines indicate most frequent.

total dose) *or* 2 mg/min infusion (range 50–300 mg total dose required).

AVAILABILITY

- ***Tablets:*** 100 mg[Rx], 200 mg[Rx], 300 mg[Rx]
- ***Injection:*** 5 mg/ml[Rx].

TIME/ACTION PROFILE (cardiovascular effects)

	ONSET	PEAK	DURATION
PO	20 min–2 hr	1–4 hr	8–12 hr
IV	2–5 min	5–15 min	2–4 hr

Up to 24 hr.

NURSING IMPLICATIONS

ASSESSMENT

- Monitor blood pressure and pulse frequently during dose adjustment and periodically during therapy. Assess for orthostatic hypotension when assisting patient up from supine position.
- Check frequency of refills to determine compliance.
- Patients receiving *labetalol IV* must be supine during and for 3 hr after administration. Vital signs should be monitored every 5–15 min during and for several hours after administration.
- Monitor intake and output ratios and daily weight. Assess patient routinely for evidence of fluid overload (peripheral edema, dyspnea, rales/crackles, fatigue, weight gain, jugular venous distention).
- ***Lab Test Considerations:*** May cause increased BUN, serum lipoprotein, potassium, triglyceride, and uric acid levels.
- May cause increased ANA titers.
- May cause increase in blood glucose levels.
- May cause increased serum alkaline phosphatase, LDH, AST, and ALT levels. Discontinue if jaundice or laboratory signs of hepatic function impairment occur.
- ***Toxicity and Overdose:*** Monitor patients receiving beta-adrenergic blocking agents for signs of overdose (bradycardia, severe dizziness or fainting, severe drowsiness, dyspnea, bluish fingernails or palms, seizures). Notify physician or other health care professional immediately if these signs occur.
- Glucagon has been used to treat bradycardia and hypotension.

POTENTIAL NURSING DIAGNOSES

- Cardiac output, decreased (Side Effects).
- Knowledge deficit, related to medication regimen (Patient/Family Teaching).
- Noncompliance, related to medication regimen (Patient/Family Teaching).

IMPLEMENTATION

- **General Info:** Discontinuation of concurrent clonidine should take place gradually, with beta blocker discontinued first. Then, after several days, discontinue clonidine.
- **PO:** Take apical pulse prior to administering. If <50 bpm or if arrhythmia occurs, withhold medication and notify physician or other health care professional.
- Administer with meals or directly after eating to enhance absorption.
- **Direct IV:** Administer undiluted.
- ***Rate:*** Administer slowly over 2 min.
- **Continuous Infusion:** Add 200 mg to 160 ml of diluent (1 mg/1 ml solution) or 200 mg to 250 ml of diluent (2 mg/3 ml solution). Compatible diluents include D5W, 0.9% NaCl, D5/0.25% NaCl, D5/0.9% NaCl, D5/Ringer's solution, D5/LR, Ringer's and lactated Ringer's solution.
- ***Rate:*** Administer at a rate of 2 mg/min and titrate for desired response. Infuse via infusion pump to ensure accurate dosage.
- **Y-Site Compatibility:** ▪ amikacin ▪ aminophylline ▪ amiodarone ▪ ampicillin ▪ butorphanol ▪ calcium gluconate ▪ cefazolin ▪ ceftazidine ▪ ceftizoxime ▪ chloramphenicol ▪ cimetidine ▪ clindamycin ▪ enalaprilat ▪ erythromycin lactobionate ▪ esmolol ▪ famotidine ▪ fentanyl ▪ gentamicin ▪ lidocaine ▪ magnesium sulfate ▪ meperidine ▪ metronidazole ▪ midazolam ▪ morphine ▪ nitroglycerin ▪ nitroprusside ▪ oxycillin ▪ penicillin G potassium ▪ piperacillin ▪ potassium chloride ▪ potassium phosphate ▪ ranitidine ▪ sodium acetate ▪ tobramycin ▪ trimethoprim/sulfamethoxazole ▪ vancomycin.
- **Y-Site Incompatibility:** ▪ cefoperazone ▪ nafcillin.
- **Additive Incompatibility:** ▪ sodium bicarbonate.

PATIENT/FAMILY TEACHING

- **General Info:** Instruct patient to take medication exactly as directed, at the same time each day, even if feeling well; do not skip or double up on missed doses. If a dose is missed, it should be taken as soon as possible up to 8 hr before next dose. Abrupt withdrawal may precipitate life-threatening arrhythmias, hypertension, or myocardial ischemia.

- Advise patient to make sure enough medication is available for weekends, holidays, and vacations. A written prescription may be kept in wallet in case of emergency.
- Teach patient and family how to check pulse and blood pressure. Instruct them to check pulse daily and blood pressure biweekly. Advise patient to hold dose and contact health care professional if pulse is <50 bpm or blood pressure changes significantly.
- May cause drowsiness or dizziness. Caution patients to avoid driving or other activities that require alertness until response to the drug is known. Caution patients receiving labetalol IV to call for assistance during ambulation or transfer.
- Advise patients to make position changes slowly to minimize orthostatic hypotension, especially during initiation of therapy or when dose is increased. Patients taking oral labetalol should be especially cautious when drinking alcohol, standing for long periods, or exercising, and during hot weather, as orthostatic hypotension is enhanced.
- Caution patient that this medication may increase sensitivity to cold.
- Instruct patient to consult health care professional before taking any OTC medications, especially cold preparations, concurrently with this medication.
- Diabetics should closely monitor blood sugar, especially if weakness, malaise, irritability, or fatigue occurs. Medication may mask tachycardia and increased blood pressure as signs of hypoglycemia, but dizziness and sweating may still occur.
- Advise patient to notify health care professional if slow pulse, difficulty breathing, wheezing, cold hands and feet, dizziness, lightheadedness, confusion, depression, rash, fever, sore throat, unusual bleeding, or bruising occurs.
- Instruct patient to inform health care professional of medication regimen prior to treatment or surgery.
- Advise patient to carry identification describing disease process and medication regimen at all times.
- **Hypertension:** Reinforce the need to continue additional therapies for hypertension (weight loss, sodium restriction, stress reduction, regular exercise, moderation of alcohol consumption, and smoking cessation). Medication controls but does not cure hypertension.

EVALUATION

Effectiveness of therapy can be demonstrated by: ▪ Decrease in blood pressure.

LACTULOSE

(**lak**-tyoo-lose)

Cholac, Chronulac, Constilac, Constulose, Duphalac, Enulose, Generlax, {Lactulax}, Lactulose PSE, Portalac

CLASSIFICATION(S):
Laxative (hyperosmotic)

Pregnancy Category B

INDICATIONS

▪ Treatment of chronic constipation in adults and in the elderly ▪ Adjunct in the management of portal-systemic (hepatic) encephalopathy (PSE).

ACTION

▪ Increases water content and softens the stool ▪ Lowers the pH of the colon, which inhibits the diffusion of ammonia from the colon into the blood, thereby reducing blood ammonia levels. **Therapeutic Effects:** ▪ Relief of constipation ▪ Decreased blood ammonia levels with improved mental status in PSE.

PHARMACOKINETICS

Absorption: Less than 3% absorbed following oral administration.
Distribution: UK.
Metabolism and Excretion: Absorbed lactulose is excreted unchanged in the urine. Unabsorbed lactulose is metabolized by colonic bacteria to lactic, acetic, and formic acids.
Half-life: UK.

CONTRAINDICATIONS AND PRECAUTIONS

Contraindicated in: ▪ Patients on low-galactose diets.
Use Cautiously in: ▪ Diabetes mellitus ▪ Pregnancy, lactation, or children (safety not established) ▪ Excessive or prolonged use (may lead to dependence).

ADVERSE REACTIONS AND SIDE EFFECTS*

GI: belching, cramps, distention, flatulence, diarrhea.
Endo: hyperglycemia (diabetic patients).

INTERACTIONS

Drug-Drug: ▪ Should not be used with other **laxatives** in the treatment of hepatic encephalopathy (leads to inability to determine optimal dose of lactulose) ▪ **Anti-infectives** may diminish effectiveness in hepatic encephalopathy ▪ **Antacids** may decrease the effect of lactulose on colonic pH.

ROUTE AND DOSAGE

❑ Constipation

- **PO (Adults):** 15–30 ml/day up to 60 ml/day.
- **PO (Children):** 7.5 ml daily (unlabeled).

❑ Portal-Systemic Encephalopathy

- **PO (Adults):** 30–45 ml 3–4 times/day; may be given q 1–2 hr initially to induce laxation.
- **PO (Infants):** 2.5–10 ml daily in divided doses (unlabeled).
- **PO (Children and Adolescents)**: 40–90 ml daily in divided doses (unlabeled).
- **Rect (Adults):** 300 ml diluted and administered as a retention enema q 4–6 hr.

AVAILABILITY

- ***Syrup:*** 10 g lactulose/15 ml[Rx].

TIME/ACTION PROFILE (relief of constipation)

	ONSET	PEAK	DURATION
PO	24–48 hr	UK	UK

NURSING IMPLICATIONS

ASSESSMENT

- **General Info:** Assess patient for abdominal distention, presence of bowel sounds, and normal pattern of bowel function.
- □ Assess color, consistency, and amount of stool produced.
- **Portal-Systemic Encephalopathy:** Assess mental status (orientation, level of consciousness) prior to and periodically throughout course of therapy.
- ***Lab Test Considerations:*** Decreases blood ammonia concentrations by 25–50%.
- □ May cause increased blood glucose levels in diabetic patients.
- □ Monitor serum electrolytes periodically when used chronically. May cause diarrhea with resulting hypokalemia and hypernatremia.

POTENTIAL NURSING DIAGNOSES

- Constipation (Indications).
- Knowledge deficit, related to medication regimen (Patient/Family Teaching).

IMPLEMENTATION

- **General Info:** When used in hepatic encephalopathy, dosage should be adjusted until patient averages 2–3 soft bowel movements per day. During initial therapy, 30–45 ml may be given hourly to induce rapid laxation.
- □ Darkening of solution does not alter potency.
- **PO:** Mix with fruit juice, water, milk, or carbonated citrus beverage to improve flavor. Administer with a full glass (240 ml) of water or juice. May be administered on an empty stomach for more rapid results.
- **Rect:** To administer enema, use rectal balloon catheter. Mix 300 ml of lactulose with 700 ml of water or 0.9% NaCl. Enema should be retained for 30–60 min. If inadvertently evacuated, may repeat administration.

PATIENT/FAMILY TEACHING

- □ Encourage patients to use other forms of bowel regulation, such as increasing bulk in the diet, increasing fluid intake, increasing mobility. Normal bowel habits are individualized and may vary from 3 times/day to 3 times/wk.

L

*CAPITALS indicate life-threatening; underlines indicate most frequent.

- Caution patients that this medication may cause belching, flatulence, or abdominal cramping. Health care professional should be notified if this becomes bothersome or if diarrhea occurs.

EVALUATION

Effectiveness of therapy can be demonstrated by: ▪ Passage of a soft, formed bowel movement, usually within 24–48 hr ▪ Clearing of confusion, apathy, and irritation and improved mental status in portal-systemic encephalopathy. Improvement may occur within 2 hr following enema and 24–48 hr following oral administration.

LAMIVUDINE
(la-**mi**-vue-deen)
Epivir, 3TC

CLASSIFICATION(S):
Antiretroviral (nucleoside reverse transcriptase inhibitor)

Pregnancy Category C

INDICATIONS

▪ Management of HIV infection (AIDS) in combination with other antiretrovirals. **Unlabeled Uses:** ▪ Part of HIV postexposure prophylaxis with zidovudine and indinavir.

ACTION

▪ Following intracellular conversion to its active form (lamivudine-5-triphosphate), inhibits viral DNA synthesis by inhibiting the enzyme reverse transcriptase. **Therapeutic Effects:** ▪ Slows the progression of HIV infection and decreases the occurrence of its sequelae ▪ Increases CD4 cell counts and decreases viral load.

PHARMACOKINETICS

Absorption: Well absorbed following oral administration (86% in adults, 66% in infants and children).
Distribution: Distributes into the extravascular space. Some penetration into CSF; remainder of distribution UK.
Metabolism and Excretion: Mostly excreted unchanged in urine; <5% metabolized by the liver.
Half-life: *Adults*—3.7 hr; *children*—2 hr.

CONTRAINDICATIONS AND PRECAUTIONS

Contraindicated in: ▪ Hypersensitivity ▪ Lactation.
Use Cautiously in: ▪ Impaired renal function (increased dosing interval/decreased dose recommended if CCr <50 ml/min) ▪ Geriatric patients (dosage reduction may be necessary) ▪ Coinfection with hepatitis B (hepatitis may recur following discontinuation of lamivudine) ▪ Pregnancy (safety not established). **Exercise Extreme Caution in:** ▪ Pediatric patients with a history of pancreatitis (use only if no alternative).

ADVERSE REACTIONS AND SIDE EFFECTS*

Noted for combination of lamivudine plus zidovudine.
CNS: fatigue, headache, insomnia, malaise, depression, dizziness.
Resp: cough.
GI: PANCREATITIS (↑ in pediatric patients), anorexia, diarrhea, nausea, vomiting, abdominal discomfort, abnormal liver function studies, dyspepsia.
Derm: rashes.
Hemat: anemia, neutropenia.
MS: musculoskeletal pain, arthralgia, myalgia.
Neuro: neuropathy.

INTERACTIONS

Drug-Drug: ▪ **Trimethoprim/sulfamethoxazole** increases lamivudine blood levels (dosage alteration may be necessary in renal impairment) ▪ Increased risk of pancreatitis with concurrent use of other **drugs causing pancreatitis** ▪ Increased risk of neuropathy with concurrent use of other **drugs causing neuropathy.**

ROUTE AND DOSAGE

Concurrent therapy with other antiretovirals is required.

- **PO (Adults and Children >12 yr and ≥50 kg):** 150 mg twice daily.

***CAPITALS indicate life-threatening; underlines indicate most frequent.**

- **PO (Adults <50 kg):** 2 mg/kg twice daily.
- **PO (Children 3 mo–12 yr):** 4 mg/kg twice daily (up to 150 mg twice daily).

AVAILABILITY

▪ ***Tablets:*** 150 mg[Rx] ▪ ***Oral solution:*** 10 mg/ml in 240-ml bottles[Rx] ▪ ***In combination with:*** zidovudine (Combivir[Rx]; see Appendix A).

TIME/ACTION PROFILE (blood levels)

	ONSET	PEAK	DURATION
PO	UK	0.9 hr*	12 hr

*On an empty stomach; peak levels occur at 3.2 hr if lamivudine is taken with food. Food does not affect total amount of drug absorbed.

NURSING IMPLICATIONS

ASSESSMENT

- ▫ Assess patient for change in severity of symptoms of HIV infection and for symptoms of opportunistic infection throughout therapy.
- ▫ Monitor patient for signs and symptoms of peripheral neuropathy (tingling, burning, numbness, or pain in hands or feet); may be difficult to differentiate from peripheral neuropathy of severe HIV disease. May require discontinuation of therapy.
- ▫ Assess patient, especially pediatric patients, for signs of pancreatitis (nausea, vomiting, abdominal pain) periodically throughout therapy. May require discontinuation of therapy.
- ***Lab Test Considerations:*** Monitor viral load and CD4 levels prior to and periodically throughout therapy.
- ▫ Monitor serum amylase, lipase, and triglycerides periodically during therapy. Elevated serum levels may indicate pancreatitis and require discontinuation.
- ▫ Monitor liver function periodically throughout therapy. May cause elevated AST, ALT, and bilirubin concentrations.
- ▫ May rarely cause neutropenia and anemia.

POTENTIAL NURSING DIAGNOSES

- Infection, risk for (Indications).
- Knowledge deficit, related to medication regimen (Patient/Family Teaching).

IMPLEMENTATION

- **PO:** May be administered without regard to food.

PATIENT/FAMILY TEACHING

- ▫ Instruct patient to take lamivudine exactly as directed, every 12 hr. Emphasize the importance of compliance with full course of therapy, not taking more than the prescribed amount and not discontinuing without consulting health care professional. If a dose is missed, take as soon as possible unless almost time for next dose. Do not double doses. Caution patient not to share medication with others.
- ▫ Inform patient that lamivudine does not cure HIV disease or prevent associated or opportunistic infections. Lamivudine does not reduce the risk of transmission of HIV to others through sexual contact or blood contamination. Caution patient to use a condom during sexual contact and avoid sharing needles or donating blood to prevent spreading HIV to others. Advise patient that the long-term effects of lamivudine are unknown at this time.
- ▫ Instruct patient to notify health care professional promptly if signs of peripheral neuropathy or pancreatitis occur.
- ▫ Advise patient not to take other OTC or prescription medications without consulting health care professional.
- ▫ Emphasize the importance of regular follow-up exams and blood tests to determine progress and monitor for side effects.

EVALUATION

Effectiveness of therapy can be demonstrated by: ▪ Slowing of the progression of HIV infection and its sequelae ▪ Decrease in viral load and improvement in CD4 levels in patients with advanced HIV infection.

LAMOTRIGINE

(la-**moe**-tri-jeen)
Lamictal

CLASSIFICATION(S):
Anticonvulsant (miscellaneous)

Pregnancy Category C

INDICATIONS

▪ Adjunct treatment of partial seizures in adults with epilepsy. **Unlabeled Uses:** ▪ Other seizure disorders in adults ▪ Infants and children with Lennox-Gastaut syndrome.

ACTION

▪ Stabilizes neuronal membranes by inhibiting sodium transport. **Therapeutic Effects:** ▪ Decreased incidence of seizures.

PHARMACOKINETICS

Absorption: 98% absorbed following oral administration.
Distribution: Enters breast milk. Highly bound to melanin-containing tissues (eyes, pigmented skin).
Metabolism and Excretion: Mostly metabolized by the liver to inactive metabolites; 10% excreted unchanged by the kidneys.
Half-life: 25.4 hr (during chronic therapy of lamotrigine alone).

CONTRAINDICATIONS AND PRECAUTIONS

Contraindicated in: ▪ Hypersensitivity ▪ Lactation.
Use Cautiously in: ▪ Patients with reduced renal function (lower maintenance doses may be required) ▪ Patients with impaired cardiac function ▪ Patients with impaired hepatic function ▪ Pregnancy or children <16 yr (safety not established).

ADVERSE REACTIONS AND SIDE EFFECTS*

CNS: ataxia, dizziness, headache, behavior changes, depression, drowsiness, insomnia, tremor.
EENT: blurred vision, double vision, rhinitis.
GI: nausea, vomiting.
GU: vaginitis.
Derm: photosensitivity, rash.
MS: arthralgia.

INTERACTIONS

Drug-Drug: ▪ Concurrent use with **carbamazepine** may result in decreased levels of lamotrigine and increased levels of an active metabolite of carbamazepine ▪ Lamotrigine levels are decreased by concurrent use of **phenobarbital**, **phenytoin**, or **primidone** ▪ Concurrent use with **valproic acid** results in a twofold increase in lamotrigine levels and a decrease in valproic acid levels.

ROUTE AND DOSAGE

▪ **PO (Adults >16 yrs):** *Patients taking carbamazepine, phenobarbital, phenytoin, or primidone*—50 mg daily as a single dose for first 2 wk, then 50 mg twice daily for next 2 wk; then increase by 100 mg/day on a weekly basis to maintenance dose of 150–250 mg twice daily (not to exceed 500 mg/day). *Patients taking carbamazepine, phenobarbital, phenytoin, or primidone with valproic acid*—25 mg every other day for first 2 wk, then 25 mg once daily for next 2 wk; then increase by 25–50 mg/day every 1–2 wk to maintenance dose of 50–75 mg twice daily (not to exceed 200 mg/day).

AVAILABILITY

▪ ***Tablets:*** 25 mg^{Rx}, 100 mg^{Rx}, 150 mg^{Rx}, 200 mg^{Rx}.

TIME/ACTION PROFILE (blood levels)

	ONSET	PEAK	DURATION
PO	UK	1.4–4.8 hr	UK

NURSING IMPLICATIONS

ASSESSMENT

- Assess location, duration, and characteristics of seizure activity.
- Assess patient for skin rash frequently throughout therapy. Lamotrigine should be discontinued at first sign of rash; may be life-threatening. Rash usually occurs during the initial 2–8 wk of therapy and is more frequent in patients taking multiple antiepileptic agents, including valproate, and much more frequent in patients <16 yrs.

▪ ***Lab Test Considerations:*** Lamotrigine plasma concentrations may be monitored periodically throughout therapy, especially in patients concurrently taking other anticonvulsants. Therapeutic plasma concentration range has not been established.

*CAPITALS indicate life-threatening; underlines indicate most frequent.

POTENTIAL NURSING DIAGNOSES

- Skin integrity, impaired, risk for (Adverse Reactions).
- Injury, risk for (Side Effects).
- Knowledge deficit, related to medication regimen (Patient/Family Teaching).

IMPLEMENTATION

- **PO:** May be administered without regard to meals.
- Lamotrigine should be discontinued gradually over at least 2 wk, unless safety concerns require a more rapid withdrawal. Abrupt discontinuation may cause increase in seizure frequency.

PATIENT/FAMILY TEACHING

- Instruct patient to take medication exactly as directed. If a dose is missed, take as soon as possible unless almost time for next dose. Do not double doses. Do not discontinue abruptly; may cause increase in frequency of seizures.
- Advise patient to notify health care professional immediately if skin rash occurs or if frequency of seizures increases.
- May cause dizziness, drowsiness, and blurred vision. Caution patient to avoid driving or activities requiring alertness until response to medication is known. Do not resume driving until physician gives clearance based on control of seizure disorder.
- Caution patient to wear sunscreen and protective clothing to prevent photosensitivity reactions.
- Advise patient to notify health care professional if pregnancy is planned or suspected or if patient intends to breast-feed or is breastfeeding.
- Instruct patient to notify health care professional of medication regimen prior to treatment or surgery.
- Advise patient to carry identification describing disease process and medication regimen at all times.

EVALUATION

Effectiveness of therapy can be demonstrated by: ▪ Decrease in the frequency of or cessation of seizures.

LANSOPRAZOLE

(lan-**soe**-pra-zole)
Prevacid

CLASSIFICATION(S):
Antiulcer agent (gastric acid–pump inhibitor)

Pregnancy Category B

INDICATIONS

▪ Treatment of erosive esophagitis ▪ Management of duodenal ulcers (with or without anti-infectives for *Helicobacter pylori*) ▪ Treatment of pathologic hypersecretory conditions, including Zollinger-Ellison syndrome.

ACTION

▪ Binds to an enzyme in the presence of acidic gastric pH, preventing the final transport of hydrogen ions into the gastric lumen. **Therapeutic Effects:** ▪ Diminished accumulation of acid in the gastric lumen, with lessened acid reflux ▪ Healing of duodenal ulcers and esophagitis.

PHARMACOKINETICS

Absorption: 80% absorbed following oral administration.
Distribution: UK.
Metabolism and Excretion: Extensively metabolized by the liver to inactive compounds. Converted intracellularly to at least two other antisecretory compounds.
Half-life: Less than 2 hr (increased in geriatric patients and patients with impaired hepatic function).

L

CONTRAINDICATIONS AND PRECAUTIONS

Contraindicated in: ▪ Hypersensitivity.
Use Cautiously in: ▪ Geriatric patients (maintenance dose should not exceed 30 mg/day unless additional acid suppression is required) ▪ Severe hepatic impairment (dosage reduction may be necessary) ▪ Pregnancy, lactation, or children (safety not established).

ADVERSE REACTIONS AND SIDE EFFECTS*

CNS: dizziness, headache.
GI: diarrhea, abdominal pain, nausea.
Derm: rash.

INTERACTIONS

Drug-Drug: ▪ **Sucralfate** decreases absorption of lansoprazole (take 30 min prior to sucralfate). May decrease absorption of drugs requiring acid pH, including **ketoconazole, ampicillin esters, iron salts,** and **digoxin.**

ROUTE AND DOSAGE

- **PO (Adults):** *Erosive esophagitis*—30 mg daily for 8 wk (additional 8 wk may be necessary). *Duodenal ulcers*—15 mg daily. *Duodenal ulcers associated with* H. pylori—30 mg twice daily with clarithromycin and amoxicillin or 30 mg 3 times daily with amoxicillin for 14 days. *Pathologic hypersecretory conditions*—60 mg once daily; may be increased up to 90 mg twice daily. If daily dose >120 mg, give in divided doses.

AVAILABILITY

- ***Delayed-release capsules:*** 15 mg[Rx], 30 mg[Rx] ▪ ***In combination with:*** amoxicillin and clarithromycin as part of a compliance package (Prevpac)[Rx]; see Appendix A.

TIME/ACTION PROFILE (acid suppression)

	ONSET	PEAK	DURATION
PO	rapid	UK	more than 24 hr

NURSING IMPLICATIONS

ASSESSMENT

- □ Assess patient routinely for epigastric or abdominal pain and for frank or occult blood in stool, emesis, or gastric aspirate.
- ▪ ***Lab Test Considerations:*** May cause abnormal liver function tests, including increased AST, ALT, alkaline phosphatase, LDH, and bilirubin.
- □ May cause increased serum creatinine and increased or decreased electrolyte levels.
- □ May alter RBC, WBC, and platelet levels.
- □ May also cause increased gastrin levels, abnormal A/G ratio, hyperlipidemia, and increased or decreased cholesterol.

POTENTIAL NURSING DIAGNOSES

- ▪ Pain (Indications).
- ▪ Knowledge deficit, related to medication regimen (Patient/Family Teaching).

IMPLEMENTATION

- ▪ **PO:** Administer before meals. Capsules may be opened and sprinkled on 1 tbs of applesauce and swallowed immediately for patients with difficulty swallowing. Do not crush or chew capsule contents.
- □ For patients with an NG tube, capsules may be opened and intact granules may be mixed in 40 ml of apple juice and injected through NG tube into stomach. Flush NG tube with additional apple juice to clear tube.
- □ Antacids may be used concurrently.

PATIENT/FAMILY TEACHING

- □ Instruct patient to take medication as directed for the full course of therapy, even if feeling better.
- □ Advise patient to avoid alcohol, products containing aspirin or NSAIDs, and foods that may cause an increase in GI irritation.
- □ May occasionally cause dizziness. Caution patient to avoid driving and other activities that require alertness until response to medication is known.
- □ Advise patient to report onset of black, tarry stools; diarrhea; or abdominal pain to health care professional promptly.

EVALUATION

Effectiveness of therapy can be demonstrated by: ▪ Decrease in abdominal pain or prevention of gastric irritation and bleeding. Healing of duodenal ulcers can be seen on x-ray examination or endoscopy. Therapy is continued for at least 2–4 wk. Therapy for pathologic hypersecretory conditions may be long term ▪ Healing in patients with erosive esophagitis. Therapy is continued for up to 8 wk, and an additional 8-wk course may be used for patients who do not heal in 8 wk or whose ulcer recurs.

***CAPITALS indicate life-threatening; underlines indicate most frequent.**

LETROZOLE
(**let**-roe-zole)
Femara

CLASSIFICATION(S):
Antineoplastic (aromatase inhibitor)

Pregnancy Category C

INDICATIONS
▪ Advanced breast cancer in postmenopausal patients with disease progression despite antiestrogen therapy.

ACTION
▪ Inhibits the enzyme aromatase, which is partially responsible for conversion of precursors to estrogen. **Therapeutic Effects:** ▪ Lowers levels of circulating estrogen, which may halt progression of estrogen-sensitive breast cancer.

PHARMACOKINETICS
Absorption: Rapidly and completely absorbed.
Distribution: UK.
Metabolism and Excretion: Mostly metabolized by the liver.
Half-life: 2 days.

CONTRAINDICATIONS AND PRECAUTIONS
Contraindicated in: ▪ Hypersensitivity ▪ Pregnancy.
Use Cautiously in: ▪ Severe hepatic impairment ▪ Lactation or children (safety not established).

ADVERSE REACTIONS AND SIDE EFFECTS*
CNS: anxiety, depression, dizziness, drowsiness, fatigue, headache, vertigo, weakness.
Resp: coughing, dyspnea, pleural effusion.
CV: chest pain, edema, hypertension.
GI: nausea, abdominal pain, anorexia, constipation, diarrhea, dyspepsia, vomiting.
Derm: alopecia, hot flashes, increased sweating, pruritus, rash.
F and E: hypercalcemia.
Metab: hypercholesterolemia, weight gain.
MS: musculoskeletal pain, arthralgia, fractures.

INTERACTIONS
Drug-Drug: ▪ None significant.

ROUTE AND DOSAGE
▪ **PO (Adults):** 2.5 mg daily.

AVAILABILITY
▪ ***Tablets:*** 2.5 mg[Rx].

TIME/ACTION PROFILE (effect on lowering of serum estradiol levels)

	ONSET	PEAK	DURATION
PO	UK	2–3 days	UK

NURSING IMPLICATIONS

ASSESSMENT
□ Assess patient for pain and other side effects periodically throughout therapy.
▪ ***Lab Test Considerations:*** May cause elevated GTT cholesterol levels.

POTENTIAL NURSING DIAGNOSES
▪ Pain (Side Effects).
▪ Knowledge deficit, related to medication regimen (Patient/Family Teaching).

IMPLEMENTATION
▪ May be taken without regard to food.

PATIENT/FAMILY TEACHING
□ Instruct patient to take medication as directed.
□ Inform patient of potential for adverse reactions and advise her to notify health care professional if side effects are problematic.

EVALUATION
Effectiveness of therapy can be demonstrated by: ▪ Slowing of disease progression in women with advanced breast cancer.

L

***CAPITALS indicate life-threatening; underlines indicate most frequent.**

LEUCOVORIN CALCIUM

(loo-koe-**vor**-in)
citrovorum factor, folinic acid, Wellcovorin

CLASSIFICATION(S):
Antidote (for methotrexate and folic acid antagonists), Vitamin (folic acid analogue)

Pregnancy Category C

INDICATIONS

▪ Used to minimize the hematologic effects of high-dose methotrexate therapy (leucovorin rescue) ▪ In combination with 5-fluorouracil in the management of advanced colorectal carcinoma ▪ Management of overdoses/prevention of toxicity from folic acid antagonists (pyrimethamine, trimethoprim, trimetrexate) ▪ Treatment of folic acid deficiency (megaloblastic anemia) unresponsive to oral replacement.

ACTION

▪ The reduced form of folic acid that serves as a cofactor in the synthesis of DNA and RNA. **Therapeutic Effects:** ▪ Reversal of toxic effects of folic acid antagonists ▪ Reversal of folic acid deficiency.

PHARMACOKINETICS

Absorption: Well absorbed following PO administration. Bioavailability decreases with larger doses. Oral absorption is saturated at doses >25 mg.
Distribution: Widely distributed. Concentrates in the CNS and liver.
Metabolism and Excretion: Extensively converted to tetrahydrofolic derivatives, including 5-methyltetrahydrofolate, a major storage form.
Half-life: 3.5 hr.

CONTRAINDICATIONS AND PRECAUTIONS

Contraindicated in: ▪ Hypersensitivity ▪ Preparations containing benzyl alcohol should not be used in neonates.
Use Cautiously in: ▪ Undiagnosed anemia (may mask the progression of pernicious anemia) ▪ Pregnancy and lactation (safety not established but has been used safely to treat megaloblastic anemia in pregnancy) ▪ Coadministration with high-dose methotrexate requires crucial timing of dosing and knowledge of methotrexate levels ▪ Ascites ▪ Renal failure ▪ Dehydration ▪ Pleural effusions ▪ Urine pH <7.

ADVERSE REACTIONS AND SIDE EFFECTS

Hemat: thrombocytosis (intra-arterial methotrexate only).
Misc: allergic reactions (rash, urticaria, wheezing).

INTERACTIONS

Drug-Drug: ▪ May decrease the anticonvulsant effect of **barbiturates**, **phenytoin**, or **primidone** ▪ High doses of the liquid contain significant amounts of **alcohol** and may result in additive CNS depression when used with **CNS depressants.**

ROUTE AND DOSAGE

❑ **High-Dose Methotrexate—Leucovorin Rescue**

Must start within 24 hr of methotrexate.

- **PO, IM, IV (Adults and Children):** *Normal methotrexate elimination*—10 mg/m² q 6 hr (1st dose IV/IM, then change to PO) until methotrexate level is $<10^{-8}$M. *CCr has increased to 50% above prior value or methotrexate level is* $>5 \times 10^{-6}$ *at 24 hr or if at 48 hr methotrexate level is* $>9 \times 10^{-7}$*M*—increase leucovorin to 100 mg/m² q 3 gr until methotrexate level $<10^{-8}$M. *Delayed late methotrexate elimination*—continue leucovorin 15 mg q 6 hr IM or IV until methotrexate level is <10 micromolars.

❑ **Advanced Colorectal Cancer**

- **IV (Adults):** 200 mg/m² followed by 5-fluorouracil 370 mg/m² or leucovorin 20 mg/m² is followed by 5-fluorouracil 425 mg/m². Regimen is given daily for 5 days q 4–5 wk.

❑ **Prevention of Hematologic Toxicity from Trimetrexate**

- **PO, IV (Adults and Children):** 20 mg/m² q 6 hr continued for 72 hr after last trimetrexate dose (oral doses should be rounded up to the next 25 mg); both trimetrexate and leucovorin doses require adjustment for hematologic toxicity.

❑ **Prevention of Hematologic Toxicity from Pyrimethamine**

- **PO, IV (Adults and Children):** 5–15 mg/day.

❑ **Inadvertent Overdose of Folic Acid Antagonists**

- **IM, IV (Adults and Children):** *Methotrexate–large doses*—75 mg IV followed by 12 mg IM q 6 hr for 4 doses; *methotrexate–average doses*—6–12 mg IM q 6 hr for 4 doses; *other folic acid antagonists*—amount equal in mg to folic acid antagonist.

❑ **Megaloblastic Anemia**

- **PO, IM, IV (Adults and Children):** Up to 1 mg/day (up to 6 mg/day for dihydrofolate reductase deficiency).

AVAILABILITY

- ***Tablets:*** 5 mg[Rx], 10 mg[Rx], 15 mg[Rx], 25 mg[Rx] - ***Solution for injection:*** 3 mg/ml in 1-ml ampules[Rx], 5 mg/ml[Rx] - ***Powder for injection:*** 50-, 100-, and 350-mg vials[Rx].

TIME/ACTION PROFILE (serum folate levels)

	ONSET	PEAK	DURATION
PO	20–30 min	UK	3–6 hr
IM	10–20 min	UK	3–6 hr
IV	$<$5 min	UK	3–6 hr

NURSING IMPLICATIONS

ASSESSMENT

- **General Info:** Assess patient for nausea and vomiting secondary to methotrexate therapy or folic acid antagonists (pyrimethamine and trimethoprim) overdose. Parenteral route may be necessary to ensure that patient receives dose.
  - Monitor for development of allergic reactions (rash, urticaria, wheezing). Notify physician if these occur.
- **Megaloblastic Anemia:** Assess degree of weakness and fatigue.
- ***Lab Test Considerations:*** *Leucovorin rescue*—Monitor serum methotrexate levels to determine dosage and effectiveness of therapy. Leucovorin calcium levels should be equal to or greater than methotrexate level. Rescue continues until serum methotrexate level is $<5 \times 10^{-8}$M.
  - Monitor CCr and serum creatinine prior to and every 24 hr during therapy to detect methotrexate toxicity. An increase $>$50% over the pretreatment concentration at 24 hr is associated with severe renal toxicity.
  - Monitor urine pH every 6 hr throughout therapy; pH should be maintained $>$7 to decrease nephrotoxic effects of high-dose methotrexate. Sodium bicarbonate or acetazolamide may be ordered to alkalinize urine.
  - *Megaloblastic anemia*—Monitor plasma folic acid levels, hemoglobin, hematocrit, and reticulocyte count prior to and periodically during therapy.

POTENTIAL NURSING DIAGNOSES

- Injury, risk for (Indications).
- Nutrition, altered, less than body requirements (Indications).
- Knowledge deficit, related to medication regimen (Patient/Family Teaching).

IMPLEMENTATION

- **General Info:** Make sure leucovorin calcium is available before administering high-dose methotrexate. Administration must be initiated within 24 hr of methotrexate therapy.
  - Administer as soon as possible after toxic dose of folic acid antagonists (pyrimethamine and trimethoprim). Effectiveness of therapy begins to decrease 1 hr after overdose.
- **PO:** Parenteral therapy should be used in patients with GI toxicity, with nausea and vomiting, or with doses $>$25 mg.
- **IM:** IM route is preferred for treatment of megaloblastic anemia. Ampules of leucovorin calcium injection for IM use do not require reconstitution.
- **Direct IV:** To reconstitute 50-mg vial of leucovorin calcium for injection, add 5 ml of bacteriostatic water or sterile water for injection for a concentration of 10 mg/ml. Use 10-ml diluent for 100-mg vial. The 350-mg vial should be reconstituted with 17 ml of diluent for a concentration of 20 mg/ml. If dose is >10 mg/m^2, do not use product containing benzyl alcohol. Use immediately if reconstituted with sterile water for injection. Stable for 7 days when reconstituted with bacteriostatic water.
- ***Rate:*** Rate should not exceed 160 mg/min (16 ml of 10 mg/ml solution per min).
- **Intermittent Infusion:** May be diluted in

L

100–500 ml of D5W, D10W, 0.9% NaCl, Ringer's or lactated Ringer's solution. Stable for 24 hr.

- **Y-Site Compatibility:** ▪ amifostine ▪ aztreonam ▪ bleomycin ▪ cefepime ▪ cisplatin ▪ cyclophosphamide ▪ doxorubicin ▪ filgrastim ▪ fluconazole ▪ fluorouracil ▪ furosemide ▪ heparin ▪ methotrexate ▪ metoclopramide ▪ mitomycin ▪ piperacillin/tazobactam ▪ tacrolimus ▪ teniposide ▪ thiotepa ▪ vinblastine ▪ vincristine.
- **Y-Site Incompatibility:** ▪ droperidol ▪ foscarnet ▪ sodium bicarbonate.

PATIENT/FAMILY TEACHING

- **General Info:** Explain purpose of medication to patient. Emphasize need to take exactly as ordered. Advise patient to contact health care professional if a dose is missed.
- **Leucovorin Rescue:** Instruct patient to drink at least 3 liters of fluid each day during leucovorin rescue.
- **Folic Acid Deficiency:** Encourage patient to eat a diet high in folic acid (meat proteins; bran; dried beans; and green, leafy vegetables).

EVALUATION

Effectiveness of therapy can be demonstrated by: ▪ Reversal of bone marrow and GI toxicity in patients receiving methotrexate or in overdose of folic acid antagonists ▪ Increased sense of well-being and increased production of normoblasts in patients with megaloblastic anemia.

LEUPROLIDE

(loo-**proe**-lide)

Lupron, Lupron Depot, Lupron Depot-PED, Lupron Depot-3 Month

CLASSIFICATION(S):

Antineoplastic (hormone), Hormone (gonadotropin-releasing hormone agonist)

Pregnancy Category X

INDICATIONS

▪ **Injection or depot:** Palliative treatment of advanced prostate cancer in patients who are unable to tolerate orchiectomy or estrogen therapy (may be used in combination with flutamide or bicalutamide) ▪ **3.75 mg depot only:** Endometriosis ▪ **Injection or depot:** Management of central precocious puberty (CPP) ▪ **3.75 mg depot only:** Uterine fibroids (with iron therapy).

ACTION

▪ A synthetic analogue of luteinizing hormone–releasing hormone (LHRH) ▪ Initially causes a transient increase in testosterone; however, with continuous administration, testosterone levels are decreased ▪ Reduces gonadotropins, testosterone, and estradiol. **Therapeutic Effects:** ▪ Decreased testosterone levels and resultant decrease in spread of prostate cancer ▪ Reduction of pain/lesions in endometriosis ▪ Decreased growth of fibroids ▪ Delayed puberty.

PHARMACOKINETICS

Absorption: Rapidly and almost completely absorbed following SC administration. More slowly absorbed following IM administration of depot form.

Distribution: UK.

Metabolism and Excretion: UK.

Half-life: 3 hr.

CONTRAINDICATIONS AND PRECAUTIONS

Contraindicated in: ▪ Intolerance to synthetic analogues of LHRH (GnRH) ▪ Pregnancy or lactation (depot form).

Use Cautiously in: ▪ Hypersensitivity to benzyl alcohol (results in induration and erythema at SC site).

ADVERSE REACTIONS AND SIDE EFFECTS*

CNS: dizziness, headache, syncope; *depot*—drowsiness, personality disorder; *SC*—anxiety, blurred vision, lethargy, memory disorder, mood swings.

EENT: blurred vision; *SC*—hearing disorder.

Resp: hemoptysis; *depot*—epistaxis, throat nodules; *SC*—cough, pleural rub, pulmonary fibrosis, pulmonary infiltrate.

CV: MYOCARDIAL INFARCTION, PULMONARY EMBOLI, angina, arrhythmias; *depot*—vasodilation; *SC*—transient ischemic attack/stroke.

***CAPITALS indicate life-threatening; underlines indicate most frequent.**

GI: anorexia, diarrhea, dysphagia, nausea, vomiting; *depot*—gingivitis; *SC*—GI BLEEDING, hepatic dysfunction, peptic ulcer, rectal polyps, taste disorders.
GU: dysuria, incontinence, testicular pain; *depot*—cervix disorder; *SC*—bladder spasm, penile swelling, prostate pain, urinary obstruction.
Derm: *depot*—hair growth, rash; *SC*—dry skin, hair loss, pigmentation, skin cancer, skin lesions.
Endo: breast swelling, breast tenderness, diabetes.
F and E: hypercalcemia, lower extremity edema.
Local: burning, itching, swelling at injection site.
Metab: *depot*—hyperuricemia, increased bone density.
MS: fibromyalgia, transient increase in bone pain (prostate cancer only); *SC*—ankylosing spondylitis, joint pain, pelvic fibrosis, temporal bone pain.
Neuro: *SC*—peripheral neuropathy.
Misc: hot flashes, chills, decreased libido, fever; *depot*—body odor, epistaxis.

INTERACTIONS

Drug-Drug: ▪ Additive antineoplastic effects with **antiandrogens (megestrol, flutamide).**

ROUTE AND DOSAGE

❑ Prostate Cancer

- **SC (Adults):** 1 mg/day.
- **IM (Adults):** 7.5 mg once monthly or 22.5 mg every 3 mo as depot injection.

❑ Endometriosis/Fibroids

- **IM (Adults):** 3.75 mg once monthly.

❑ Central Precocious Puberty

For IM dosing, may be increased by 3.75 mg q 4 wk as needed; further adjustments may be necessary.

- **SC (Children):** 50 mcg/kg/day, may be increased by 10 mcg/kg/day as required.
- **IM (Children >37.5 kg):** 15 mg q 4 wk.
- **IM (Children 25–37.5 kg):** 11.25 mg q 4 wk.
- **IM (Children ≤25 kg):** 7.5 mg q 4 wk.

AVAILABILITY

▪ ***Solution for injection:*** 5 mg/ml in 2.8-ml vial[Rx] ▪ ***Lyophilized microspheres for depot injection:*** 3.75-mg single-use vial[Rx], 7.5-mg single-use vial[Rx] ▪ ***Lyophilized microspheres for pediatric depot injection:*** 7.5 mg[Rx], 11.25 mg[Rx], 15-mg single-use kits[Rx] ▪ ***Lyophilized microspheres for 3-mo depot injection:*** 22.5-mg single-use kits[Rx].

TIME/ACTION PROFILE

	ONSET	PEAK	DURATION
SC*	1–2 wk	2–4 wk	UK
IM†	UK	4 hr	4 wk
IM-depot†	UK	4 hr	12 wk

*Decline in serum testosterone levels.
†Serum leuprolide levels.

NURSING IMPLICATIONS

ASSESSMENT

- **Prostate Cancer:** Assess patient for an increase in bone pain, especially during the first few weeks of therapy. Monitor patients with vertebral metastases for increased back pain and decreased sensory/motor function.
- ❑ Monitor intake and output ratios; assess for bladder distention in patients with urinary tract obstruction during initiation of therapy.
- **Endometriosis:** Assess patient for endometrial pain prior to and periodically throughout therapy.
- **Central Precocious Puberty (CPP):** Prior to therapy, diagnosis of CPP should be confirmed by onset of secondary sex characteristics in girls <8 yr or boys <9 yr; a complete physical and endocrinologic examination, including height, weight, hand and wrist x ray; total sex steroid level (estradiol or testosterone); adrenal steroid level; beta human chorionic gonadotropin level; GnRH stimulation test; and computerized tomography of the head must be performed. These parameters are monitored after 1–2 mo and every 6–12 mo during therapy.
- ❑ Assess patient for signs of precocious puberty (menses, breast development, testicular growth) periodically throughout therapy. Dose is increased until no progression of the disease is noted either clinically or by lab test parameters, then usually maintained throughout therapy. Discontinuation of therapy should be considered before age 11 in girls and age 12 in boys.
- ***Lab Test Considerations:*** Initially increases, then decreases luteinizing hormone (LH) and follicle-stimulating hormone (FSH).

L

This leads to castration levels of testosterone in boys 2–4 wk after initial increase in concentrations.

- Monitor testosterone, prostatic acid phosphate, and prostate-specific antigen (PSA) levels to evaluate response to therapy. Transient increase in levels may occur during the 1st month of therapy for prostate cancer.
- May cause increased BUN, serum calcium, uric acid, hypoproteinemia, LDH, alkaline phosphase, AST, hyperglycemia, hyperlipidemia, hyperphosphatemia, WBC, PT, or PTT. May also cause decreased platelets and serum potassium.

POTENTIAL NURSING DIAGNOSES

- Sexual dysfunction (Side Effects).
- Knowledge deficit, related to medication regimen (Patient/Family Teaching).

IMPLEMENTATION

- **SC, IM:** Use syringe supplied by manufacturer. Rotate sites.
- Leuprolide depot is *only* for IM injection.
- *Monthly formulation:* To reconstitute a single vial, use a 22-gauge needle; withdraw 1 ml of diluent and inject into vial to mix. To mix 2 or more vials, withdraw 0.5 ml and inject into each vial for a total volume of 1 ml. Shake each vial well; suspension will appear milky. Withdraw entire contents of all vials into syringe and inject immediately. Patients may store medication at room temperature.
- *3-mo formulation:* For single IM injection, reconstitute lyphosized microspheres using a 23-gauge needle; withdraw 1.5 ml of diluent and inject into vial. Shake well until suspension is uniformly milky. Withdraw entire contents and inject immediately.
- Store at room temperature; stable for 24 hr following reconstitution.

PATIENT/FAMILY TEACHING

- **General Info:** Advise patient that medication may cause hot flashes. Notify health care professional if these become bothersome.
- **Prostate Cancer:** Instruct patient and family on SC injection technique. Review patient insert provided with leuprolide patient-administration kit.
- Instruct patient to take medication exactly as directed. If a dose is missed, take as soon as remembered unless not remembered until next day.
- Advise patient that bone pain may increase at initiation of therapy. This will resolve with time. Patient should discuss with health care professional use of analgesics to control pain.
- Instruct patient to notify health care professional promptly if difficulty urinating, weakness, or numbness occurs.
- **Endometriosis:** Advise patient to use a form of contraception other than oral contraceptives during therapy. Inform patient that amenorrhea is expected but does not guarantee contraception.
- **Central Precocious Puberty:** Instruct patient and family on the proper technique for SC injection. Emphasize the importance of administering the medication at the same time each day. Rotate injection sites periodically.
- Inform patient and parents that if injections are not given daily, pubertal process may be reactivated.
- Advise patient and parents that during the first 2 mo of therapy patient may experience a light menstrual flow or spotting. Health care professional should be notified if this continues beyond 2nd mo.
- Instruct patient and parents to notify health care professional immediately if irritation at the injection site or unusual signs or symptoms occur.

EVALUATION

Effectiveness of therapy can be demonstrated by: ▪ Decrease in the spread of prostate cancer ▪ Decrease in lesions and pain in endometriosis ▪ Resolution of the signs of central precocious puberty ▪ Improvement in preoperative hematologic parameters in patients with anemia from uterine fibroids.

LEVAMISOLE

(lee-**vam**-i-sole)

Ergamisol

CLASSIFICATION(S):

Antineoplastic (immunomodulator)

Pregnancy Category C

INDICATIONS

■ Adjunctive treatment following surgery of Dukes' C colorectal carcinoma (with fluorouracil). **Unlabeled Uses:** ■ Advanced malignant melanoma.

ACTION

■ Restores depressed immune function including formation of antibodies, T-cell response, phagocytosis, and chemotaxis ■ Also has cholinergic activity. **Therapeutic Effects:** ■ Enhanced immunologic response to presence of tumor when used in conjunction with fluorouracil.

PHARMACOKINETICS

Absorption: Rapidly absorbed following oral administration.
Distribution: UK.
Metabolism and Excretion: Extensively metabolized by the liver.
Half-life: 3–4 hr.

CONTRAINDICATIONS AND PRECAUTIONS

Contraindicated in: ■ Hypersensitivity ■ Pregnancy.
Use Cautiously in: ■ Bone marrow depression ■ Other chronic debilitating illnesses ■ Patients with childbearing potential ■ Lactation or children (safety not established).

ADVERSE REACTIONS AND SIDE EFFECTS*

As occurring in combination with fluorouracil.
CNS: fatigue, anxiety, depression, dizziness, drowsiness, forgetfulness, headache, insomnia, nervousness.
EENT: abnormal tearing, altered sense of smell, blurred vision, conjunctivitis.
GI: diarrhea, nausea, stomatitis, vomiting, abdominal pain, abnormal taste, anorexia, dyspepsia, flatulence.
Derm: alopecia, dermatitis, pruritus, skin discoloration.
Hemat: AGRANULOCYTOSIS, anemia, leukopenia, thrombocytopenia.
MS: arthralgia, myalgia.
Neuro: ataxia, paresthesia.
Misc: chills, fever.

INTERACTIONS

Drug-Drug: ■ Increased bone marrow depression with other **antineoplastic agents** or **radiation therapy** ■ Ingestion of **alcohol** may produce disulfiram-like reaction ■ May increase blood levels and risk of toxicity with **phenytoin** ■ May increase effects of **warfarin.**

ROUTE AND DOSAGE

■ **PO (Adults):** 50 mg q 8 hr for 3 days every 2 wk with fluorouracil 450 mg/m²/day for 5 days initially, then followed 28 days later by fluorouracil 450 mg/m² once weekly.

AVAILABILITY

■ ***Tablets:*** 50 mg[Rx].

TIME/ACTION PROFILE (blood levels)

	ONSET	PEAK	DURATION
PO	UK	1.5–2 hr	UK

NURSING IMPLICATIONS

ASSESSMENT

□ Assess mucous membranes, number and consistency of stools, and frequency of vomiting. Assess for signs of infection (fever, chills, sore throat, cough, hoarseness, lower back or side pain, difficult or painful urination). Assess for bleeding (bleeding gums, bruising, petechiae, guaiac stools, urine, and emesis). Avoid IM injections and rectal temperatures. Apply pressure to venipuncture sites for 10 min. Report symptoms of toxicity (stomatitis, uncontrollable vomiting, diarrhea, gastrointestinal bleeding, leukocyte count of less than 3500/mm³, platelet count <100,000/mm³, or hemorrhage from any site); drug will need to be discontinued.

■ ***Lab Test Considerations:*** Hematologic functions should be monitored prior to and throughout therapy. CBC with differential and platelets, electrolytes, and liver function tests should be performed on the 1st day of therapy with levamisole and fluorouracil. Then, a CBC with differential should be performed weekly prior to each treatment with fluorouracil. Electrolytes and liver function should be monitored every 3 mo for 1 yr. If WBC is 2500–

L

*CAPITALS indicate life-threatening; underlines indicate most frequent.

3500/mm³, withhold fluorouracil until WBC >3500/mm³; if WBC <2500/mm³, withhold fluorouracil until WBC >3500/mm³ and decrease dose by 20%; if WBC remains <2500/mm³ for >10 days despite withholding fluorouracil, discontinue levamisole. Withhold both levamisole and fluorouracil if platelet count <100,000/mm³. Neutropenia is usually reversible upon discontinuation of therapy.

POTENTIAL NURSING DIAGNOSES

- Infection, risk for (Side Effects).
- Nutrition, altered, less than body requirements (Side Effects).
- Knowledge deficit, related to medication regimen (Patient/Family Teaching).

IMPLEMENTATION

- **General Info:** Levamisole therapy should be initiated no earlier than 7 days and no later than 30 days following surgery. Fluorouracil therapy should be initiated no earlier than 21 days and no later than 35 days following surgery in patients who are out of the hospital, ambulatory, maintaining oral nutrition, have well-healed wounds, and are fully recovered from postoperative complications. If levamisole has been initiated 7–20 days postoperatively, begin fluorouracil therapy with the 2nd course of levamisole therapy; if levamisole is initiated 21–30 days postoperatively, initiate fluorouracil with 1st course of levamisole therapy.
- □ Refer to fluorouracil monograph (p. 395) for specific information on administration of fluorouracil.
- **PO:** Administer levamisole every 8 hr for 3 days. Repeat course every 14 days for 1 yr.

PATIENT/FAMILY TEACHING

- □ Instruct patient to take medication exactly as directed. Consult health care professional if vomiting occurs shortly after taking dose. If dose is missed, omit dose and notify physician.
- □ Instruct patient to notify health care professional immediately if flu-like symptoms or malaise occurs or if fever; chills; sore throat; signs of infection; bleeding gums; bruising; petechiae; or blood in urine, stool, or emesis occurs. Caution patient to avoid crowds and persons with known infections. Instruct patient to use soft toothbrush and electric razor. Patients should be cautioned not to take products containing aspirin or NSAIDs.
- □ Caution patient that concurrent use of alcohol may cause a disulfiram-like reaction (abdominal cramps, nausea, headache, flushing, hypoglycemia).
- □ Advise patient to rinse mouth with clear water after eating and drinking and to avoid flossing to minimize stomatitis. Consult health care professional if mouth pain interferes with eating. Stomatitis pain may require treatment with opioid analgesics.
- □ Discuss with patient the possibility of hair loss. Explore methods of coping.
- □ Instruct patient not to receive any vaccinations without advice of health care professional.
- □ Review with patient the need for contraception during therapy.
- □ Emphasize the importance of routine follow-up lab tests to monitor progress and check for side effects.

EVALUATION

Effectiveness of therapy can be demonstrated by: ▪ Enhanced immunologic response to presence of tumor when used in conjunction with fluorouracil.

LEVODOPA

(**lee**-voe-doe-pa)
Dopar, Larodopa, L-dopa

CARBIDOPA/LEVODOPA

(**kar**-bi-doe-pa/**lee**-voe-doe-pa)
Sinemet, Sinemet CR

CLASSIFICATION(S):
Anti-Parkinson agent (dopamine agonist), Anti-Parkinson adjunct (decarboxylase inhibitor)

Pregnancy Category UK, C (carbidopa/levodopa)

INDICATIONS

▪ Parkinson's disease ▪ Not useful for drug-induced extrapyramidal reactions.

ACTION

▪ Levodopa is converted to dopamine in the CNS, where it serves as a neurotransmitter ▪ Carbidopa prevents peripheral destruction of levodopa. **Therapeutic Effects:** ▪ Relief of tremor and rigidity in Parkinson's syndrome.

PHARMACOKINETICS

Absorption: Well absorbed following oral administration.
Distribution: Widely distributed. *Levodopa*—enters the CNS in small concentrations. *Carbidopa*—does not cross the blood-brain barrier but does cross the placenta. Both enter breast milk.
Metabolism and Excretion: *Levodopa*—mostly metabolized by the GI tract and liver. *Carbidopa*—30% excreted unchanged by the kidneys.
Half-life: *Levodopa*—1 hr; *carbidopa*—1–2 hr.

CONTRAINDICATIONS AND PRECAUTIONS

Contraindicated in: ▪ Hypersensitivity ▪ Narrow-angle glaucoma ▪ MAO inhibitor therapy ▪ Malignant melanoma ▪ Undiagnosed skin lesions ▪ Lactation.
Use Cautiously in: ▪ History of cardiac, psychiatric, or ulcer disease ▪ Pregnancy or children <18 yr (safety not established).

ADVERSE REACTIONS AND SIDE EFFECTS*

CNS: involuntary movements, anxiety, dizziness, hallucinations, memory loss, psychiatric problems.
EENT: blurred vision, mydriasis.
GI: nausea, vomiting, anorexia, dry mouth, hepatotoxicity.
Derm: melanoma.
Hemat: hemolytic anemia, leukopenia.
Misc: darkening of urine or sweat.

INTERACTIONS

Drug-Drug: ▪ Use with **MAO inhibitors** may result in hypertensive reactions ▪ **Phenothiazines, haloperidol, papaverine, phenytoin,** and **reserpine** may reverse the effect of levodopa ▪ Large doses of **pyridoxine** may antagonize the beneficial effects of levodopa ▪ Concurrent use with **methyldopa** may alter the effectiveness of levodopa and increases the risk of CNS side effects ▪ Additive hypotension may result with concurrent **antihypertensives** ▪ **Anticholinergics** may decrease absorption of levodopa ▪ Increased risk of adverse reactions with **selegilene** or **cocaine.**
Drug-Food: ▪ Ingestion of foods containing large amounts of **pyridoxine** may reverse the effect of levodopa.

ROUTE AND DOSAGE

❑ Levodopa

- **PO (Adults):** 250 mg 2–4 times daily; may increase by 100–750 mg q 3–7 days until desired effect is achieved (not to exceed 8 g/day).

❑ Carbidopa/Levodopa

Tablets contain 10/100, 25/100, 25/250 mg.

- **PO (Adults):** *Patients not currently receiving levodopa*—10 mg carbidopa/100 mg levodopa 3–4 times daily or 25 mg carbidopa/100 mg levodopa 3 times daily; may be increased every 1–2 days until desired effect is achieved. *Conversion from levodopa alone (<1.5 g/day)*—25 mg carbidopa/100 mg levodopa 3–4 times daily; may be increased every 1–2 days until desired effect is achieved. *Conversion from levodopa alone (>1.5 g/day)*—25 mg carbidopa/250 mg levodopa 3–4 times daily; may be increased every 1–2 days until desired effect is achieved.

❑ Carbidopa/Levodopa Extended-Release

Extended-release (ER) tablets contain 25/100 or 50/200 of carbidopa and levodopa, respectively.

- **PO (Adults):** *Patients not currently receiving levodopa*—50 mg carbidopa/200 mg levodopa twice daily (minimum of 6 hr apart) initially. *Conversion from levodopa alone*—initiate therapy at 25% of the daily dose of levodopa; for moderate disease start with 50 mg carbidopa/200 mg levodopa twice daily. *Conversion from standard carbidopa/levodopa*—initiate therapy with at least 10% more levodopa content/day (may need up to 30% more) given at 4–8 hr intervals while awake. Allow 3 days between dosage changes; some patients may require larger doses and shorter dosing intervals.

L

***CAPITALS indicate life-threatening; underlines indicate most frequent.**

AVAILABILITY

❑ **Levodopa**

▪ ***Tablets:*** 100 mg[Rx], 250 mg[Rx], 500 mg[Rx] ▪ ***Capsules:*** 100 mg[Rx], 250 mg[Rx], 500 mg[Rx].

❑ **Carbidopa/Levodopa**

▪ ***Tablets:*** 10 mg carbidopa/100 mg levodopa[Rx], 25 mg carbidopa/100 mg levodopa[Rx], 25 mg carbidopa/250 mg levodopa[Rx] ▪ ***Extended-release tablets:*** 25 mg carbidopa/100 mg levodopa[Rx], 50 mg carbidopa/200 mg levodopa[Rx].

TIME/ACTION PROFILE (anti-Parkinson effects)

	ONSET	PEAK	DURATION
Carbidopa	UK	UK	5–24 hr
Levodopa	10–15 min	UK	5–24 hr or more
Carbidopa/Levodopa sustained release	UK	2 hr	12 hr

NURSING IMPLICATIONS

ASSESSMENT

- □ Assess parkinsonian symptoms (akinesia, rigidity, tremors, pill rolling, shuffling gait, mask-like facies, twisting motions, and drooling) throughout therapy. "On-off phenomenon" may cause symptoms to appear or improve suddenly.
- □ Assess blood pressure and pulse frequently during period of dose adjustment.
- ▪ ***Lab Test Considerations:*** May cause false-positive Coombs' test, serum and urine uric acid, serum gonadotropin, urine norepinephrine, and urine protein concentrations.
- □ Dipstick for urine ketones may reveal false-positive results.
- □ Patients on long-term therapy should have hepatic and renal function and CBC monitored periodically. May cause elevated BUN, AST, ALT, bilirubin, alkaline phosphatase, LDH, and serum protein-bound iodine concentrations.
- ▪ ***Toxicity and Overdose:*** Assess for signs of toxicity (involuntary muscle twitching, facial grimacing, spasmodic eye winking, exaggerated protrusion of tongue, behavioral changes). Consult physician or other health care professional if symptoms occur.

POTENTIAL NURSING DIAGNOSES

- ▪ Physical mobility, impaired (Indications).
- ▪ Injury, risk for (Indications).
- ▪ Knowledge deficit, related to medication regimen (Patient/Family Teaching).

IMPLEMENTATION

- ▪ **General Info:** In the carbidopa/levodopa combination, the number following the drug name represents the milligrams of each respective drug.
- □ Wait 8 hr after last levodopa dose before switching patient to carbidopa/levodopa. Carbidopa reduces the need for levodopa by 75%. Administering carbidopa shortly after a full dose of levodopa may result in toxicity.
- □ In preoperative patients or patients who are NPO, confer with physician or other health care professional about continuing medication administration.
- ▪ **PO:** Administer food shortly after medication to minimize gastric irritation; taking food before or concurrently may retard levodopa's effects but may be necessary to minimize GI irritation. If patient has difficulty swallowing, confer with pharmacist.
- □ Controlled-release tablets may be administered as whole or half tablets, but they should not be crushed or chewed.

PATIENT/FAMILY TEACHING

- □ Instruct patient to take this drug exactly as directed. If a dose is missed, take as soon as remembered, unless next scheduled dose is within 2 hr; do not double doses.
- □ Explain that gastric irritation may be decreased by eating food shortly after taking medications but that high-protein meals may impair levodopa's effects. Dividing the daily protein intake among all the meals may help ensure adequate protein intake and drug effectiveness. Do not drastically alter diet during levodopa therapy without consulting health care professional.
- □ May cause drowsiness or dizziness. Advise patient to avoid driving and other activities that require alertness until response to drug is known.
- □ Caution patient to change positions slowly to minimize orthostatic hypotension. Health care professional should be notified if orthostatic hypotension occurs.

- Instruct patient that frequent rinsing of mouth, good oral hygiene, and sugarless gum or candy may decrease dry mouth.
- Caution patient to monitor skin lesions for any changes. Health care professional should be notified promptly as carbidopa/levodopa may activate malignant melanoma.
- Advise patient to confer with health care professional before taking OTC medications, especially cold remedies. Patients receiving only levodopa should avoid multivitamins. Large amounts of vitamin B_6 (pyridoxine) may interfere with the action of levodopa.
- Inform patient that harmless darkening of urine or sweat may occur.
- Advise patient to notify health care professional if palpitations, urinary retention, involuntary movements, behavioral changes, severe nausea and vomiting, or new skin lesions occur. Dosage reduction may be required.

EVALUATION

Effectiveness of therapy can be demonstrated by: ▪ Resolution of parkinsonian signs and symptoms. Therapeutic effects usually become evident after 2–3 wk of therapy but may require up to 6 mo. Patients who take this medication for several years may experience a decrease in the effectiveness of this drug. Effectiveness may sometimes be restored after a "drug holiday."

LEVORPHANOL

(lee-**vor**-fan-ole)

Levo-Dromoran, Levorphan

CLASSIFICATION(S):
Opioid analgesic (agonist)

Schedule II
Pregnancy Category B

INDICATIONS

▪ Moderate to severe pain.

ACTION

▪ Binds to opiate receptors in the CNS, altering perception of and response to pain ▪ Produces generalized CNS depression. **Therapeutic Effects:** ▪ Decreased pain.

PHARMACOKINETICS

Absorption: Well absorbed following oral and SC administration.
Distribution: UK.
Metabolism and Excretion: Mostly metabolized by the liver.
Half-life: 12–16 hr.

CONTRAINDICATIONS AND PRECAUTIONS

Contraindicated in: ▪ Hypersensitivity ▪ Avoid chronic use during pregnancy or lactation.
Use Cautiously in: ▪ Head trauma ▪ Increased intracranial pressure ▪ Severe renal, hepatic, or pulmonary disease ▪ Hypothyroidism ▪ Adrenal insufficiency ▪ Alcoholism ▪ Undiagnosed abdominal pain ▪ Prostatic hypertrophy ▪ Geriatric or debilitated patients (dosage reduction suggested).

ADVERSE REACTIONS AND SIDE EFFECTS*

CNS: confusion, sedation, dysphoria, euphoria, floating feeling, hallucinations, headache, unusual dreams.
EENT: blurred vision, diplopia, miosis.
Resp: respiratory depression.
CV: hypotension, bradycardia.
GI: constipation, dry mouth, nausea, vomiting.
GU: urinary retention.
Derm: flushing, sweating.
Misc: physical dependence, psychological dependence, tolerance.

INTERACTIONS

Drug-Drug: ▪ Use with extreme caution in patients receiving **MAO inhibitors** (may result in unpredictable, severe reactions—decrease initial dose of levorphanol to 25% of usual dose) ▪ Additive CNS depression with **alcohol, antihistamines, antidepressants,** and **sedative/hypnotics** ▪ Administration of **partial-antagonist opioid analgesics** may precipitate withdrawal in physically dependent patients ▪ **Nalbuphine** or **pentazocine** may decrease analgesia.

ROUTE AND DOSAGE

Larger doses may be required during chronic use.

L

***CAPITALS indicate life-threatening; underlines indicate most frequent.**

- **PO (Adults ≥50 kg):** *Initial dosing in opioid-naive patients*—4 mg q 6–8 hr.
- **PO (Adults and Children <50 kg):** *Initial dosing in opioid-naive patients*—0.04 mg/kg q 6–8 hr (unlabeled for use in children).
- **SC, IV (Adults ≥50 kg):** *Initial dosing in opioid-naive patients*—2 mg q 6–8 hr. *Preoperative use*—1–2 mg SC 90 min prior to procedure.
- **SC, IV (Adults and Children <50 kg):** *Initial dosing in opioid-naive patients*—0.02 mg/kg mg q 6–8 hr (unlabeled for use in children).

AVAILABILITY

- ***Tablets:*** 2 mg[Rx] - ***Solution for injection:*** 2 mg/ml[Rx].

TIME/ACTION PROFILE (analgesic effect)

	ONSET	PEAK	DURATION
PO	10–60 min	90–120 min	4–5 hr
SC	UK	60–90 min	4–5 hr
IV	UK	within 20 min	4–5 hr

NURSING IMPLICATIONS

ASSESSMENT

- Assess type, location, and intensity of pain prior to and 90–120 min following PO, 60–90 min following SC, and 20 min (peak) following IV administration. When titrating opioid doses, increases of 25–50% should be administered until there is either a 50% reduction in the patient's pain rating on a numerical or visual analogue scale or the patient reports satisfactory pain relief. A repeat dose can be safely administered at the time of the peak if previous dose is ineffective and side effects are minimal.
- An equianalgesic chart (see Appendix B) should be used when changing routes or when changing from one opioid to another.
- Assess blood pressure, pulse, and respirations before and periodically during administration. If respiratory rate is <10/min, assess level of sedation. Dose may need to be decreased by 25–50%. Initial drowsiness will diminish with continued use.
- Assess bowel function routinely. Prevention of constipation should be instituted with increased intake of fluids and bulk and with laxatives to minimize constipating effects. Stimulant laxatives should be administered routinely if opioid use exceeds 2–3 days, unless contraindicated.
- Prolonged use may lead to physical and psychological dependence and tolerance. This should not prevent patient from receiving adequate analgesia. Most patients who receive levorphanol for pain do not develop psychological dependence. Progressively higher doses may be required to relieve pain with long-term therapy.
- ***Lab Test Considerations:*** May increase plasma amylase and lipase concentrations.
- ***Toxicity and Overdose:*** If an opioid antagonist is required to reverse respiratory depression or coma, naloxone (Narcan) is the antidote. Dilute the 0.4-mg ampule of naloxone in 10 ml of 0.9% NaCl and administer 0.5 ml (0.02 mg) by direct IV push every 2 min. For children and patients weighing <40 kg, dilute 0.1 mg of naloxone in 10 ml of 0.9% NaCl for a concentration of 10 mcg/ml and administer 0.5 mcg/kg every 1–2 min. Titrate dose to avoid withdrawal, seizures, and severe pain.

POTENTIAL NURSING DIAGNOSES

- Pain (Indications).
- Sensory-perceptual alterations: visual, auditory (Side Effects).
- Injury, risk for (Side Effects).

IMPLEMENTATION

- **General Info:** Explain therapeutic value of medication prior to administration to enhance the analgesic effect.
- Regularly administered doses may be more effective than prn administration. Analgesic is more effective if given before pain becomes severe.
- Coadministration with nonopioid analgesics may have additive analgesic effects and permit lower opioid doses.
- Medication should be discontinued gradually after long-term use to prevent withdrawal symptoms.
- **PO:** May be administered with food or milk to minimize GI irritation.
- **SC, IV:** Patients receiving parenteral therapy should be lying down and remain recumbent to minimize side effects for at least 30–60 min.

- **Direct IV:** May be administered undiluted.
- ***Rate:*** Administer slowly, over 3–5 min. Rapid administration may lead to increased respiratory depression, hypotension, and circulatory collapse.
- **Syringe Compatibility:** ▪ glycopyrrolate.

PATIENT/FAMILY TEACHING

- Instruct patient on how and when to ask for pain medication.
- Instruct patient to take levorphanol exactly as directed. If dose is less effective after a few weeks, do not increase dose without consulting health care professional.
- Medication may cause drowsiness or dizziness. Advise patient to call for assistance when ambulating or smoking. Caution patient to avoid driving or other activities that require alertness until response to the medication is known.
- Advise patient to change positions slowly to minimize orthostatic hypotension.
- Caution patient to avoid concurrent use of alcohol or other CNS depressants.
- Advise ambulatory patients that nausea and vomiting may be decreased by lying down.
- Encourage patient to turn, cough, and breathe deeply every 2 hr to prevent atelectasis.

EVALUATION

Effectiveness of therapy can be demonstrated by: ▪ Decrease in severity of pain without a significant alteration in level of consciousness or respiratory status.

LIDOCAINE (parenteral)
(**lye**-doe-kane)
LidoPen, Xylocaine, {Xylocard}

LIDOCAINE (local anesthetic)
Dilocaine, Lidoject, Nervocaine, Octocaine, Xylocaine

LIDOCAINE (mucosal)
Anestacon, Xylocaine Viscous

LIDOCAINE (topical)
DermaFlex, Solarcaine Aloe Extra Burn Relief, Xylocaine, Zilactin-L

CLASSIFICATION(S):
Anesthetic (local/mucosal/topical), Antiarrhythmic (group IB)

Pregnancy Category B

INDICATIONS

▪ **IV:** Ventricular arrhythmias ▪ **IM:** Self-injected or when IV unavailable (during transport to hospital facilities) ▪ **Local:** Infiltration/mucosal/topical anesthetic.

ACTION

▪ **IV, IM:** Suppresses automaticity and spontaneous depolarization of the ventricles during diastole by altering the flux of sodium ions across cell membranes with little or no effect on heart rate ▪ **Local:** Produces local anesthesia by inhibiting transport of ions across neuronal membranes, thereby preventing initiation and conduction of normal nerve impulses. **Therapeutic Effects:** ▪ Control of ventricular arrhythmias ▪ Local anesthesia.

PHARMACOKINETICS

Absorption: Well absorbed following IM administration into the deltoid muscle; some absorption follows local use.
Distribution: Widely distributed. Concentrates in adipose tissue. Crosses the blood-brain barrier and placenta.
Metabolism and Excretion: Mostly metabolized by the liver.
Half-life: Biphasic—initial phase, 7–30 min; terminal phase, 90–120 min.

CONTRAINDICATIONS AND PRECAUTIONS

Applies mainly to systemic use.
Contraindicated in: ▪ Hypersensitivity; cross-sensitivity may occur ▪ Advanced AV block.
Use Cautiously in: ▪ Liver disease, congestive heart failure, patients weighing <50 kg, and elderly patients (reduce bolus and/or maintenance dose) ▪ Respiratory depression, shock, or heart block ▪ Pregnancy or lactation (safety not established).

L

{} = **Available in Canada only.**

ADVERSE REACTIONS AND SIDE EFFECTS*

Applies mainly to systemic use.

CNS: SEIZURES, confusion, drowsiness, dizziness, nervousness, tremor.

EENT: *mucosal use*—decreased or absent gag reflex.

CV: CARDIAC ARREST, arrhythmias, bradycardia, hypotension.

GI: nausea, vomiting.

Local: stinging, burning, contact dermatitis, erythema.

Misc: allergic reactions, including ANAPHYLAXIS.

INTERACTIONS

Applies mainly to systemic use.

Drug-Drug: ▪ Additive cardiac depression and toxicity with **phenytoin, quinidine, procainamide,** or **propranolol** ▪ **Cimetidine** and **beta-adrenergic blockers** may decrease metabolism and increase risk of toxicity.

ROUTE AND DOSAGE

❑ Antiarrhythmic

See infusion rate table in Appendix D.

- **IV (Adults):** 50–100 mg (1 mg/kg) bolus (may be repeated in 5 min), then 1–4 mg/min (20–50 mcg/kg/min) infusion (up to 4.5 mg/kg or 300 mg in 1 hr).
- **IV (Children):** 1 mg/kg bolus; may be repeated after 5 min (not to exceed 3 mg/kg), followed by 30 mcg/kg/min infusion (range 20–50 mcg/kg/min).
- **IM (Adults and Children ≥50 kg):** 300 mg (4.5 mg/kg); may be repeated in 60–90 min.

❑ Local

- **Infiltration (Adults and Children):** Infiltrate affected area as needed (increased amount and frequency of use increases likelihood of systemic absorption and adverse reactions).
- **Topical (Adults):** Apply as needed (not to exceed 35 g/day as cream).
- **Mucosal (Adults):** *For anesthetizing oral surfaces*—20 mg as 2 sprays/quadrant (not to exceed 30 mg/quadrant) may be used. 15 ml of the viscous solution may be used q 3 hr for oral or pharyngeal pain. *For anesthetizing the female urethra* —3–5 ml of the jelly or 20 mg as 2% solution may be used. *For anesthetizing the male urethra*—5–10 ml of the jelly or 5–15 ml of 2% solution may be used before catheterization or 30 ml of jelly prior to cystoscopy or similar procedures. Topical solutions may be used to anesthetize mucous membranes of the larynx, trachea, or esophagus.

AVAILABILITY

▪ ***Auto-injector for IM injection:*** 300 mg/3 ml[Rx] ▪ ***Direct IV injection:*** 10 mg/ml (1%)[Rx], 20 mg/ml (2%)[Rx] ▪ ***For IV admixture:*** 40 mg/ml (4%)[Rx], 100 mg/ml (10%)[Rx], 200 mg/ml (20%)[Rx] ▪ ***Premixed solution for IV infusion:*** 2 mg/ml (0.2%)[Rx], 4 mg/ml (0.4%)[Rx], 8 mg/ml (0.8%)[Rx] ▪ ***Injection for local infiltration/nerve block:*** 0.5%[Rx], 1%[Rx], 1.5 %[Rx], 2%[Rx], 4%[Rx], 5%[Rx] ▪ ***In combination with:*** epinephrine for local infiltration[Rx] ▪ ***Jelly:*** 2%[Rx] ▪ ***Liquid:*** 5%[Rx] ▪ ***Ointment:*** 5%[Rx] ▪ ***Solution:*** 4%[Rx] ▪ ***Spray:*** 10%[Rx] ▪ ***Viscous solution:*** 2%[Rx] ▪ ***In combination with:*** in combination with prilocaine (see monograph on p. 579).

TIME/ACTION PROFILE (IV, IM = antiarrhythmic effects; Local = anesthetic effects)

	ONSET	PEAK	DURATION
IV	immediate	immediate	10–20 min
IM	5–15 min	20–30 min	60–90 min
Local	rapid	UK	1–3 hr

NURSING IMPLICATIONS

ASSESSMENT

- **Antiarrhythmic:** Monitor ECG continuously and blood pressure and respiratory status frequently throughout administration.
- **Anesthetic:** Assess degree of numbness of affected part.
- ***Lab Test Considerations:*** Serum electrolyte levels should be monitored periodically throughout prolonged therapy.
- ❑ IM administration may cause increased CPK levels.
- ***Toxicity and Overdose:*** Serum lidocaine levels should be monitored periodically throughout prolonged or high-dose therapy.

***CAPITALS indicate life-threatening; underlines indicate most frequent.**

Therapeutic serum lidocaine levels range from 1.5 to 5 mcg/ml.

- Signs and symptoms of toxicity include confusion, excitation, blurred or double vision, nausea, vomiting, ringing in ears, tremors, twitching, convulsions, difficulty breathing, severe dizziness or fainting, and unusually slow heart rate.
- If symptoms of overdose occur, stop infusion and monitor patient closely.

POTENTIAL NURSING DIAGNOSES

- Cardiac output, decreased (Indications).
- Pain (Indications).
- Knowledge deficit, related to medication regimen (Patient/Family Teaching).

IMPLEMENTATION

- **Throat Spray:** Ensure that gag reflex is intact before allowing patient to drink or eat.
- **IM:** IM injections are recommended only when ECG monitoring is not available and benefits outweigh risks. Administer IM injections only into deltoid muscle while frequently aspirating to prevent IV injection.
- **IV:** Only 1% and 2% solutions are used for direct IV injection.
- **Direct IV:** Administer undiluted IV loading dose of 1 mg/kg at a rate of 25–50 mg over 1 min. May repeat dose after 5 min. Follow by IV infusion. Do not use lidocaine with preservatives or other medications, such as epinephrine, for IV injection.
- **Continuous Infusion:** To prepare for IV infusion, add 1 g lidocaine to 250, 500, or 1000 ml of D5W. Solution is stable for 24 hr. Other compatible solutions include D5/LR, D5/0.45% NaCl, D5/0.9% NaCl, 0.45% NaCl, 0.9% NaCl, and lactated Ringer's solution.
- ***Rate:*** Administer via infusion pump for accurate dose at a rate of 1–4 mg/min (see Appendix D for infusion rate table).
- **Y-Site Compatibility:** ▪ alteplase ▪ amiodarone ▪ amrinone ▪ cefazolin ▪ ciprofloxacin ▪ diltiazem ▪ dobutamine ▪ dopamine ▪ enalaprilat ▪ famotidine ▪ haloperidol ▪ labetalol ▪ meperidine ▪ morphine ▪ nitroglycerin ▪ nitroprusside ▪ potassium chloride ▪ streptokinase ▪ theophylline ▪ vitamin B complex with C.
- **Infiltration:** Lidocaine with epinephrine may be used to minimize systemic absorption and prolong local anesthesia.

PATIENT/FAMILY TEACHING

- **General Info:** May cause drowsiness and dizziness. Advise patient to call for assistance during ambulation and transfer.
- **IM:** Available in LidoPen Auto-Injector for use outside the hospital setting. Advise patient to telephone health care professional immediately if symptoms of a heart attack occur. Do not administer unless instructed by health care professional. To administer, remove safety cap and place back end on thickest part of thigh or deltoid muscle. Press hard until needle prick is felt. Hold in place for 10 sec, then massage area for 10 sec. Do not drive after administration unless absolutely necessary.

EVALUATION

Effectiveness of therapy can be demonstrated by: ▪ Decrease in ventricular arrhythmias ▪ Local anesthesia.

LIDOCAINE/PRILOCAINE

(**lye**-doe-kane/**pri**-loe-kane)
Emla

CLASSIFICATION(S):
Local anesthetic combination

Pregnancy Category B

INDICATIONS

▪ Produces local anesthesia prior to minor painful procedures including: ▫ Insertion of cannulae or needles ▫ Arterial/venous/lumbar puncture ▫ Dermal procedures ▫ Laser treatments.

ACTION

▪ Produces local anesthesia by inhibiting transport of ions across neuronal membranes, thereby preventing initiation and conduction of normal nerve impulses. Combination of two anesthetics is applied as a system consisting of a cream under an occlusive dressing. Active drug is released into the dermal and epidermal skin layers, resulting in accumulation of local anesthetic in the regions of dermal pain receptors and nerve endings. **Therapeutic Effects:** ▪ Anesthetic action localized to the area of the application.

PHARMACOKINETICS

Absorption: Small amounts are systemically absorbed during 4-hr placement of Emla system.
Distribution: Small amounts absorbed are widely distributed and cross the placenta and blood-brain barrier.
Metabolism and Excretion: *Lidocaine*—mostly metabolized by the liver. *Prilocaine*—metabolized by the liver and kidneys.
Half-life: *Lidocaine*—7–30 min first phase, 90–120 min terminal phase; *prilocaine*—10–50 min.

CONTRAINDICATIONS AND PRECAUTIONS

Contraindicated in: ▪ Hypersensitivity to lidocaine, prilocaine, or any other amide-type local anesthetic ▪ Hypersensitivity to any other product in the formulation ▪ Should not be applied to middle ear ▪ Congenital or idiopathic methemoglobinemia ▪ Infants <6 mo who are receiving methemoglobin-inducing agents ▪ Infants <1 mo.
Use Cautiously in: ▪ Repeated use or use on large areas of skin (more likely to result in systemic absorption) ▪ Geriatric, acutely ill, or debilitated patients ▪ Severe liver disease ▪ Any conditions associated with methemoglobinemia (including glucose-6-phosphate dehydrogenase deficiency) ▪ Children<20 kg (area/duration of treatment should be limited) ▪ Lactation.

ADVERSE REACTIONS AND SIDE EFFECTS*

Local: blanching, redness, alteration in temperature sensation, edema, itching, rash.
Misc: allergic reactions including ANAPHYLAXIS.

INTERACTIONS

Drug-Drug: ▪ Concurrent use with **group I antiarrhythmics (tocainide, mexiletine)** may result in adverse cardiovascular effects ▪ Concurrent use with other **local anesthetics** may result in additive toxicity ▪ Concurrent use with **sulfonamides** in children increases the risk of methemoglobinemia (avoid concurrent use in children <12 mo).

ROUTE AND DOSAGE

Area covered should not exceed 2000 cm^2 in children >20 kg, 600 cm^2 in children 10–20 kg, or 100 cm^2 in children <10 kg.

❑ Minor Dermal Procedures (Venipuncture, IV Cannulation)

- **Topical (Adults and Children):** 2.5 g applied to 20–25 cm^2 (2 in. by 2 in.) area of skin, covered with an occlusive dressing for at least 1 hr. Area covered should not be >100 cm^2 in children weighing <10 kg or >600 cm^2 in children weighing 10–20 kg.

❑ Major Dermal Procedures (Split-Thickness Skin Graft Harvesting)

- **Topical (Adults and Children):** 2 g/10 cm^2 area of skin, covered with an occlusive dressing for at least 2 hr.

❑ Laser Treatments

- **Topical (Adults and Children):** 1–2 g/10 cm^2 area of skin.

AVAILABILITY

- ***Cream:*** 2.5% lidocaine with 2.5% prilocaine in 5- and 30-g tubes[Rx].

TIME/ACTION PROFILE (local anesthesia)

	ONSET	PEAK	DURATION†
Top	1–3 hr	3 hr	1–2 hr

†Following removal of occlusive dressing.

NURSING IMPLICATIONS

ASSESSMENT

- ❑ Assess application site for open wounds. Apply only to intact skin.
- ❑ Assess application site for anesthesia following removal of system and prior to procedure.

POTENTIAL NURSING DIAGNOSES

- Pain, acute (Indications).
- Knowledge deficit, related to medication regimen (Patient/Family Teaching).

IMPLEMENTATION

- **Topical:** When used for minor dermal procedures (venipuncture, IV cannulation, arte-

*CAPITALS indicate life-threatening; underlines indicate most frequent.

rial puncture, lumbar puncture), apply the 2.5-g tube of cream (½ of the 5-g tube) to each 2 in. by 2 in. area of skin in a *thick* layer at the site of the impending procedure. Remove the center cutout piece from an occlusive dressing (supplied with the 5-g tube) and peel the paper liner from the paper-framed dressing. Cover the lidocaine/prilocaine cream so that there is a *thick* layer of cream underneath the occlusive dressing. Do not spread out or rub in the cream. Smooth the dressing edges carefully and ensure it is secure to avoid leakage. Remove the paper frame and mark the time of application on the occlusive dressing. Lidocaine/prilocaine cream must be applied *at least 1 hr* before the start of a minor dermal procedure (venipuncture, IV cannulation). Anesthesia may be more profound with 90 min–2 hr application. Remove the occlusive dressing and wipe off the lidocaine/prilocaine cream. Clean the entire area with antiseptic solution and prepare the patient for the procedure.

□ For major dermal procedures (skin graft harvesting), follow the same procedure using larger amounts of lidocaine/prilocaine cream and the appropriate size occlusive dressing. Lidocaine/prilocaine cream must be applied *at least 2 hr* before major dermal procedures.

PATIENT/FAMILY TEACHING

□ Explain the purpose of cream and occlusive dressing to patient and parents. Inform the patient that lidocaine/prilocaine cream may block all sensations in the treated skin. Caution patient to avoid trauma to the area from scratching, rubbing, or exposure to extreme heat or cold temperatures until all sensation has returned.

▪ **Home Care Issues:** Instruct patient or parent in proper application. Provide a diagram of location for application.

EVALUATION

Clinical response to therapy can be evaluated by: ▪ Anesthesia in the area of application.

LINDANE

(**lin**-dane)

Bio-Well, gamma benzene hexachloride, {GBH}, G-Well, {Hexit}, Kildane, Kwell, {Kwellada}, Kwildane, {PMS Lindane}, Scabene, Thionex

CLASSIFICATION(S):
Pediculocide, Scabicide

Pregnancy Category B

INDICATIONS

▪ Second-line treatment of parasitic arthropod infestation (scabies and head, body, and crab lice) for use only in patients who are intolerant of or do not respond to less toxic agents.

ACTION

▪ Causes seizures and death in parasitic arthropods. **Therapeutic Effects:** ▪ Cure of infestation by parasitic arthropods.

PHARMACOKINETICS

Absorption: Significant systemic absorption (9–13%) occurs slowly following topical application.

Distribution: Stored in fat.

Metabolism and Excretion: Metabolized by the liver.

Half-life: 18 hr (infants and children).

CONTRAINDICATIONS AND PRECAUTIONS

Contraindicated in: ▪ Hypersensitivity ▪ Areas of skin rash, abrasion, or inflammation (absorption is increased) ▪ Children ≤2 yr (increased risk of CNS toxicity) ▪ Lactation ▪ History of seizures.

Use Cautiously in: ▪ Children (increased risk of systemic absorption and CNS side effects) ▪ Children ≤10 yr ▪ Pregnancy (do not exceed recommended dose; do not use >2 courses of therapy).

L

{} = **Available in Canada only.**

ADVERSE REACTIONS AND SIDE EFFECTS*

All adverse reactions except dermatologic are signs of systemic absorption and toxicity.

CNS: CNS TOXICITY.

CV: tachycardia.

GI: nausea, vomiting.

Derm: contact dermatitis (repeated application), local irritation.

INTERACTIONS

Drug-Drug: ▪ Simultaneous topical use of **skin, scalp,** or **hair preparations** may increase systemic absorption.

ROUTE AND DOSAGE

❑ **Scabies**

- **Topical (Adults and Children):** 1% cream or lotion applied to all skin surfaces from neck to toes; may require a 2nd treatment 1 wk later.
- **Topical (Children 2–10 yr):** 1% lotion applied to all skin surfaces from neck to toes; may require a 2nd treatment 1 wk later.

❑ **Head Lice or Crab Lice**

- **Topical (Adults):** 15–30 ml (up to 60 ml) of shampoo; may require a 2nd treatment 1 wk later.
- **Topical (Children 2–10 yr):** 15–30 ml of shampoo; may require a 2nd treatment 1 wk later.

AVAILABILITY

▪ ***Cream:*** 1%Rx ▪ ***Lotion:*** 1%Rx ▪ ***Shampoo:*** 1%Rx.

TIME/ACTION PROFILE (antiparasitic action)

	ONSET	PEAK	DURATION
Top	rapid	rapid	190 min

NURSING IMPLICATIONS

ASSESSMENT

- ❑ Assess skin and hair for signs of infestation before and after treatment.
- ❑ Examine family members and close contacts for infestation. When used in treatment of pediculosis pubis or scabies, sexual partners should receive concurrent prophylactic therapy.

POTENTIAL NURSING DIAGNOSES

- Skin integrity, impaired (Indications).
- Knowledge deficit, related to medication regimen (Patient/Family Teaching).

IMPLEMENTATION

- **Topical:** When applying medication to another person, wear gloves to prevent systemic absorption.
- ❑ Do not apply to open wounds (scratches, cuts, sores on skin or scalp) to minimize systemic absorption. Avoid contact with the eyes. If eye contact occurs, flush thoroughly with water and notify physician or other health care professional.
- ❑ Institute appropriate isolation techniques.
- **Cream/Lotion:** Instruct patient to bathe with soap and water. Dry skin well and allow to cool prior to application. Apply cream or lotion in amount sufficient to cover entire body surface with a thin film from neck down (60 ml for an adult). Leave medication on for 8–12 hr, then remove by washing. If rash, burning, or itching develops, wash off medication and notify physician or other health care professional.
- **Shampoo:** Use a sufficient amount of shampoo to wet hair and scalp (30 ml for short hair, 45 ml for medium hair, 60 ml for long hair). Rub thoroughly into hair and scalp and leave in place for 4 min. Then use enough water to work up a good lather; follow with thorough rinsing and drying. If applied in shower or bath, do not let shampoo run down on other parts of body or into water in which patient is sitting. When hair is dry, use fine-toothed comb to remove remaining nits or nit shells. Shampoo may also be used on combs and brushes to prevent spread of infestation.

PATIENT/FAMILY TEACHING

- **General Info:** Instruct patient on application technique. Patient should repeat therapy only at the recommendation of health care professional. Discuss hygienic measures to prevent and to control infestation. Discuss potential for infectious contacts with patient. Explain

*CAPITALS indicate life-threatening; underlines indicate most frequent.

why household members should be examined and sexual partners treated simultaneously.

- Instruct patient to wash all recently worn clothing and used bed linens and towels in very hot water or to dry-clean to prevent reinfestation or spreading.
- Instruct patient not to apply other oils or creams during therapy, as these increase the absorption of lindane and may lead to toxicity.
- Explain to patient that itching may persist after treatment; repeat treatment is necessary only if live mites are found.
- Advise patient that eyelashes can be treated by applying petroleum jelly 3 times/day for 1 wk.
- **Shampoo:** Advise patient that shampoo should not be used as a regular shampoo in the absence of infestation. Emphasize need to avoid contact with eyes.
- **Children:** Advise parents to monitor young children closely for evidence of CNS toxicity (seizures, dizziness, clumsiness, fast heartbeat, muscle cramps, nervousness, restlessness, irritability, nausea, vomiting) during and immediately after treatment.

EVALUATION

Effectiveness of therapy can be demonstrated by: ▪ Resolution of signs of infestation with scabies or lice.

LITHIUM

(**lith**-ee-um)

{Carbolith}, Cibalith-S, {Duralith}, Eskalith, Eskalith-CR, Lithane, {Lithizine}, Lithonate, Lithotabs

CLASSIFICATION(S):

Antimanic

Pregnancy Category D

INDICATIONS

▪ Treatment of a variety of psychiatric disorders, particularly bipolar affective disorders (treatment of acute manic episodes and prophylaxis against recurrence).

ACTION

▪ Alters cation transport in nerve and muscle ▪ May also influence reuptake of neurotransmitters. **Therapeutic Effects:** ▪ Antimanic and antidepressant properties.

PHARMACOKINETICS

Absorption: Completely absorbed following oral administration.

Distribution: Widely distributed into many tissues and fluids; CSF levels are 50% of plasma levels. Crosses the placenta; enters breast milk.

Metabolism and Excretion: Excreted almost entirely unchanged by the kidneys.

Half-life: 20–27 hr.

CONTRAINDICATIONS AND PRECAUTIONS

Contraindicated in: ▪ Hypersensitivity ▪ Severe cardiovascular or renal disease ▪ Dehydrated or debilitated patients ▪ Pregnancy or lactation ▪ Should be used only where therapy, including blood levels, may be closely monitored ▪ Some products contain alcohol or tartrazine and should be avoided in patients with known hypersensitivity or intolerance.

Use Cautiously in: ▪ Geriatric or debilitated patients (initial dosage reduction recommended) ▪ Any degree of cardiac, renal, or thyroid disease ▪ Diabetes mellitus ▪ Children (safety not established).

ADVERSE REACTIONS AND SIDE EFFECTS*

CNS: SEIZURES, fatigue, headache, impaired memory, ataxia, confusion, dizziness, drowsiness, psychomotor retardation, restlessness, stupor.

EENT: aphasia, blurred vision, dysarthria, tinnitus.

CV: ARRHYTHMIAS, ECG changes, edema, hypotension.

GI: abdominal pain, anorexia, bloating, diarrhea, nausea, dry mouth, metallic taste.

GU: polyuria, glycosuria, nephrogenic diabetes insipidus, renal toxicity.

Derm: acneiform eruption, folliculitis, alopecia, diminished sensation, pruritus.

Endo: hypothyroidism, goiter, hyperglycemia, hyperthyroidism.

F and E: hyponatremia.

Hemat: leukocytosis.

Metab: weight gain.

L

{} = Available in Canada only.

***CAPITALS indicate life-threatening; underlines indicate most frequent.**

MS: muscle weakness, hyperirritability, rigidity.
Neuro: tremors.

INTERACTIONS

Drug-Drug: ▪ May prolong the action of **neuromuscular blocking agents** ▪ Neurologic toxicity may occur with **haloperidol** or **molindone** ▪ **Diuretics, methyldopa, probenecid, fluoxetine,** and **NSAIDs** may increase the risk of toxicity ▪ Blood levels may be increased by **angiotensin-converting enzyme (ACE) inhibitors** ▪ Lithium may decrease the effects of **chlorpromazine** ▪ **Chlorpromazine** may mask early signs of lithium toxicity ▪ Hypothyroid effects may be additive with **potassium iodide** or **antithyroid drugs** ▪ **Aminophylline, phenothiazines,** and **drugs containing large amounts of sodium** increase renal elimination and may decrease effectiveness.
Drug-Food: ▪ Large changes in **sodium** intake may alter the renal elimination of lithium. Increasing sodium intake will increase renal excretion.

ROUTE AND DOSAGE

Precise dosing is based on serum lithium levels. 300 mg lithium carbonate contains 8–12 mEq lithium.

- **PO (Adults):** *Tablets/capsules*—300–600 mg 3 times daily initially; usual maintenance dose is 300 mg 3–4 times daily. *Slow-release capsules*—200–300 mg 3 times daily initially; increased up to 1800 mg/day in divided doses. Usual maintenance dose is 300–400 mg 3 times daily. *Extended-release tablets*—450–900 mg twice daily or 300–600 mg 3 times daily initially; usual maintenance dose is 450 mg twice daily or 300 mg 3 times daily.
- **PO (Children <12 yr):** 15–20 mg (0.4–0.5 mEq)/kg/day in 2–3 divided doses; dosage may be adjusted weekly.

AVAILABILITY

▪ ***Capsules:*** 150 mg[Rx], 300 mg[Rx], 600 mg[Rx] ▪ ***Tablets:*** 300 mg[Rx] ▪ ***Extended-release tablets:*** 300 mg[Rx], 450 mg[Rx] ▪ {***Slow-release capsules:*** 150 mg[Rx], 300 mg[Rx]} ▪ ***Syrup:*** 300 mg (8 mEq lithium)/5 ml[Rx].

TIME/ACTION PROFILE (antimanic effects)

	ONSET	PEAK	DURATION
PO, PO–ER	5–7 days	10–21 days	days

NURSING IMPLICATIONS

ASSESSMENT

- □ Assess mood, ideation, and behaviors frequently. Initiate suicide precautions if indicated.
- □ Monitor intake and output ratios. Report significant changes in totals. Unless contraindicated, fluid intake of at least 2000–3000 ml/day should be maintained. Weight should also be monitored at least every 3 mo.
- ▪ ***Lab Test Considerations:*** Renal and thyroid function, WBC with differential, serum electrolytes, and glucose should be evaluated periodically throughout therapy.
- ▪ ***Toxicity and Overdose:*** Serum lithium levels should be monitored twice weekly during initiation of therapy and every 2–3 mo during chronic therapy. Blood samples should be drawn in the morning immediately prior to next dose. Therapeutic levels range from 0.5 to 1.5 mEq/liter.
- □ Assess patient for signs and symptoms of lithium toxicity (vomiting, diarrhea, slurred speech, decreased coordination, drowsiness, muscle weakness, or twitching). If these occur, report prior to administering next dose.

POTENTIAL NURSING DIAGNOSES

- Thought processes, altered (Indications).
- Violence, risk for, directed at self or others (Indications).
- Noncompliance (Patient/Family Teaching).

IMPLEMENTATION

- **PO:** Administer with food or milk to minimize GI irritation. Extended-release preparations should be swallowed whole; do not break, crush, or chew.

PATIENT/FAMILY TEACHING

- □ Instruct patient to take medication exactly as directed, even if feeling well. If a dose is missed, take as soon as remembered unless within 2 hr of next dose (6 hr if extended release).
- □ Medication may cause dizziness or drowsiness. Caution patient to avoid driving or other activities requiring alertness until response to medication is known.
- □ Low sodium levels may predispose patient to toxicity. Advise patient to drink 2000–3000

ml fluid each day and eat a diet with consistent and moderate sodium intake. Excessive amounts of coffee, tea, and cola should be avoided because of diuretic effect. Avoid activities that cause excess sodium loss (heavy exertion, exercise in hot weather, saunas). Notify health care professional of fever, vomiting, and diarrhea, which also cause sodium loss.

- Advise patient that weight gain may occur. Review principles of a low-calorie diet.
- Instruct patient to consult health care professional prior to taking OTC medications concurrently with this therapy.
- Advise patient to use contraception and to consult health care professional if pregnancy is suspected.
- Review side effects and symptoms of toxicity with patient. Instruct patient to stop medication and report signs of toxicity to health care professional promptly.
- Explain to patients with cardiovascular disease or over 40 yr of age the need for ECG evaluation prior to and periodically during therapy. Patient should inform health care professional if fainting, irregular pulse, or difficulty breathing occurs.
- Emphasize the importance of periodic lab tests to monitor for lithium toxicity.

EVALUATION

Effectiveness of therapy can be demonstrated by: ▪ Resolution of the symptoms of mania (hyperactivity, pressured speech, poor judgment, need for little sleep) ▪ Decreased incidence of mood swings in bipolar disorders ▪ Improved affect in unipolar disorders. Improvement in condition may require 1–3 wk.

LOMUSTINE

(loe-**mus**-teen)
CCNU, CeeNu

CLASSIFICATION(S):
Antineoplastic (nitrosourea)

Pregnancy Category D

INDICATIONS

▪ Used alone or with other treatment modalities in the management of primary and metastatic brain tumors and Hodgkin's disease. **Unlabeled Uses:** ▪ Bronchogenic carcinoma ▪ Non-Hodgkin's lymphoma ▪ Malignant melanoma ▪ Breast carcinoma ▪ Renal cell carcinoma ▪ GI tract carcinoma.

ACTION

▪ Inhibits DNA and RNA synthesis by alkylation (cell-cycle phase–nonspecific). **Therapeutic Effects:** ▪ Death of rapidly replicating cells, particularly malignant ones.

PHARMACOKINETICS

Absorption: Rapidly absorbed following oral administration.
Distribution: Widely distributed. Active metabolites enter the CSF well. Enters breast milk.
Metabolism and Excretion: Mostly metabolized by the liver. Some metabolites are active antineoplastic agents.
Half-life: 1–2 days (active metabolites).

CONTRAINDICATIONS AND PRECAUTIONS

Contraindicated in: ▪ Hypersensitivity ▪ Pregnancy or lactation.
Use Cautiously in: ▪ Patients with childbearing potential ▪ Active infections ▪ Decreased bone marrow reserve (dosage reduction required) ▪ Geriatric patients or patients with other chronic debilitating illnesses ▪ Impaired liver function.

ADVERSE REACTIONS AND SIDE EFFECTS*

CNS: ataxia, disorientation, dysarthria, lethargy.
Resp: fibrosis, pulmonary infiltrates.
GI: <u>nausea</u>, <u>vomiting</u>, anorexia, hepatotoxicity, stomatitis.
GU: azotemia, renal failure.
Endo: gonadal suppression.
Hemat: <u>leukopenia</u>, <u>thrombocytopenia</u>, anemia.
Metab: hyperuricemia.
Misc: secondary malignancy (long-term use).

INTERACTIONS

Drug-Drug: ▪ Additive bone marrow depression with other **antineoplastic agents** or **radiation**

*CAPITALS indicate life-threatening; <u>underlines</u> indicate most frequent.

therapy ▪ May decrease antibody response to **live virus vaccines** and increase risk of adverse reactions.

ROUTE AND DOSAGE

- **PO (Adults and Children):** 100–130 mg/m² as a single dose every 6 wk. Dosage adjustments are required for concurrent therapy or decreased blood counts.

AVAILABILITY

- ***Capsules:*** 10 mg[Rx], 40 mg[Rx], 100 mg[Rx].

TIME/ACTION PROFILE (effects on blood counts)

	ONSET	PEAK	DURATION
PO	UK	4–7 wk	1–2 wk

NURSING IMPLICATIONS

ASSESSMENT

- Monitor for bone marrow depression. Assess for bleeding (bleeding gums, bruising, petechiae, guaiac stools, urine, and emesis) and avoid IM injections and rectal temperatures if platelet count is low. Apply pressure to venipuncture sites for 10 min. Assess for signs of infection during neutropenia. Anemia may occur. Monitor for increased fatigue, dyspnea, and orthostatic hypotension.
- Assess for nausea and vomiting, which usually begins within 3 hr of administration and persists for 24 hr. Prophylactic antiemetics may be used. Monitor intake and output, daily weight, and appetite. Adjust diet as tolerated for anorexia.
- Assess pulmonary function tests prior to initiation of therapy and periodically throughout therapy. Pulmonary toxicity may occur with cumulative doses of 600–1100 mg or with 6 mo or more of therapy.
- ***Lab Test Considerations:*** Monitor CBC and differential prior to and periodically throughout therapy. The nadir of leukopenia occurs in 4–6 wk. The nadir of thrombocytopenia occurs in 4 wk. Notify physician if leukocyte count is <4000/mm³ or platelet count is <100,000/mm³. Recovery from leukopenia and thrombocytopenia occurs in 1–2 wk. Myelosuppression is cumulative; subsequent courses of therapy should be delayed until recovery occurs.
- Monitor liver function studies (AST, ALT, LDH, bilirubin) and renal function studies (BUN, creatinine) prior to and periodically throughout therapy to detect hepatotoxicity and nephrotoxicity.
- May cause increased uric acid. Monitor periodically during therapy.

POTENTIAL NURSING DIAGNOSES

- Infection, risk for (Side Effects).
- Nutrition, altered, less than body requirements (Side Effects).
- Knowledge deficit, related to medication regimen (Patient/Family Teaching).

IMPLEMENTATION

- **PO:** Administer on empty stomach at bedtime. Preadministration of an antiemetic and a hypnotic may help control nausea.

PATIENT/FAMILY TEACHING

- Instruct patient to take lomustine exactly as directed, even if nausea and vomiting occur. If vomiting occurs shortly after dose is taken, consult health care professional.
- Inform patient that several different types of capsules may be found in medication container. Patient should take all the capsules at one time to receive the correct dose.
- Advise patient to notify health care professional promptly if fever; chills; sore throat; signs of infection; bleeding gums; bruising; petechiae; or blood in urine, stool, or emesis occurs. Caution patient to avoid crowds and persons with known infections. Instruct patient to use soft toothbrush and electric razor. Patient should be cautioned not to drink alcoholic beverages or take products containing aspirin or NSAIDs.
- Instruct patient to notify health care professional if abdominal pain, yellow skin, weakness, cough, slurred speech, or decreased urine output occurs.
- Instruct patient to inspect oral mucosa for redness and ulceration. If ulceration occurs, advise patient to use sponge brush and rinse mouth with water after eating and drinking. Consult health care professional if pain interferes with eating. Stomatitis pain may require treatment with opioid analgesics.
- Discuss with patient the possibility of hair loss. Explore coping strategies.
- Advise patient that, although lomustine may

cause infertility, contraception is necessary because of potential teratogenic effects in the fetus.
- Instruct patient not to receive any vaccinations without advice of health care professional.
- Emphasize need for periodic lab tests to monitor for side effects.

EVALUATION

Effectiveness of therapy can be demonstrated by: ▪ Decrease in size and spread of malignant tissue.

LOPERAMIDE

(loe-**per**-a-mide)

Diarrid, Imodium, Imodium A-D, Kaopectate II Caplets, Maalox Antidiarrheal Caplets, Pepto Diarrhea Control

CLASSIFICATION(S):
Antidiarrheal

Pregnancy Category B

INDICATIONS

▪ Adjunctive therapy of acute diarrhea ▪ Chronic diarrhea associated with inflammatory bowel disease ▪ Decreases the volume of ileostomy drainage.

ACTION

▪ Inhibits peristalsis and prolongs transit time by a direct effect on nerves in the intestinal muscle wall ▪ Reduces fecal volume, increases fecal viscosity and bulk while diminishing loss of fluid and electrolytes. **Therapeutic Effects:** ▪ Relief of diarrhea.

PHARMACOKINETICS

Absorption: Not well absorbed following oral administration.
Distribution: UK. Does not cross the blood-brain barrier.
Metabolism and Excretion: Metabolized partially by the liver, undergoes enterohepatic recirculation; 30% eliminated in the feces. Minimal excretion in the urine.
Half-life: 10.8 hr.

CONTRAINDICATIONS AND PRECAUTIONS

Contraindicated in: ▪ Hypersensitivity ▪ Patients in whom constipation must be avoided ▪ Abdominal pain of unknown cause, especially if associated with fever ▪ Alcohol intolerance (liquid only).
Use Cautiously in: ▪ Hepatic dysfunction ▪ Geriatric patients ▪ Pregnancy, lactation, or children <2 yr (safety not established).

ADVERSE REACTIONS AND SIDE EFFECTS*

CNS: drowsiness, dizziness.
GI: constipation, dry mouth, nausea.

INTERACTIONS

Drug-Drug: ▪ Additive CNS depression with other **CNS depressants**, including **alcohol, antihistamines, opioids**, and **sedative/hypnotics** ▪ Additive anticholinergic properties with other **drugs having anticholinergic properties**, including **antidepressants** and **antihistamines.**

ROUTE AND DOSAGE

- **PO (Adults):** 4 mg initially, then 2 mg after each loose stool. Maintenance dose usually 4–8 mg/day in divided doses (not to exceed 8 mg/day for OTC use or 16 mg/day for Rx use).
- **PO (Children 9–11 yr or 30–47 kg):** 2 mg initially; then 1 mg with each loose stool (not to exceed 6 mg/24 hr; OTC use should not exceed 2 days).
- **PO (Children 6–8 yr or 24–30 kg):** 1 mg initially, then 1 mg with each loose stool (not to exceed 4 mg/24 hr; OTC use should not exceed 2 days).

AVAILABILITY

▪ ***Tablets:*** 2 mg[OTC] ▪ ***Capsules:*** 2 mg[Rx] ▪ ***Liquid:*** 1 mg/5 ml[OTC] ▪ ***In combination with:*** simethicone (Immodium Advanced[OTC], see Appendix A).

TIME/ACTION PROFILE (relief of diarrhea)

	ONSET	PEAK	DURATION
PO	1 hr	2.5–5 hr	10 hr

*CAPITALS indicate life-threatening; underlines indicate most frequent.

L

NURSING IMPLICATIONS

ASSESSMENT

- □ Assess frequency and consistency of stools and bowel sounds prior to and throughout therapy.
- □ Assess fluid and electrolyte balance and skin turgor for dehydration.

POTENTIAL NURSING DIAGNOSES

- ▪ Diarrhea (Indications).
- ▪ Injury, risk for (Side Effects).
- ▪ Knowledge deficit, related to medication regimen (Patient/Family Teaching).

IMPLEMENTATION

- ▪ **PO:** Administer with clear fluids to help prevent dehydration, which may accompany diarrhea.

PATIENT/FAMILY TEACHING

- □ Instruct patient to take medication exactly as directed. Do not take missed doses, and do not double doses. In acute diarrhea, medication may be ordered after each unformed stool. Advise patient not to exceed the maximum number of doses.
- □ May cause drowsiness. Advise patient to avoid driving or other activities requiring alertness until response to drug is known.
- □ Advise patient that frequent mouth rinses, good oral hygiene, and sugarless gum or candy may relieve dry mouth.
- □ Caution patient to avoid using alcohol and other CNS depressants concurrently with this medication.
- □ Instruct patient to notify health care professional if diarrhea persists or if fever, abdominal pain, or distention occurs.

EVALUATION

Effectiveness of therapy can be demonstrated by: ▪ Decrease in diarrhea □ In acute diarrhea, treatment should be discontinued if no improvement is seen in 48 hr □ In chronic diarrhea, if no improvement has occurred after at least 10 days of treatment with maximum dose, loperamide is unlikely to be effective.

LORATADINE

(lor-**a**-ta-deen)
Claritin, Claritin Reditabs

CLASSIFICATION(S):
Antihistamine

Pregnancy Category B

INDICATIONS

▪ Relief of nasal and non-nasal symptoms of seasonal allergies ▪ Management of chronic idiopathic urticaria.

ACTION

▪ Blocks peripheral effects of histamine released during allergic reactions. **Therapeutic Effects:** ▪ Decreased symptoms of allergic reactions (nasal stuffiness; red, swollen eyes).

PHARMACOKINETICS

Absorption: Rapidly absorbed following oral administration (80%).
Distribution: UK.
Metabolism and Excretion: Rapidly and extensively metabolized during first pass through the liver. Much is converted to descarboethoxyloratadine, an active metabolite.
Half-life: *Loratadine*—7.8–11 hr; *descarboethoxyloratadine*—20 hr.

CONTRAINDICATIONS AND PRECAUTIONS

Contraindicated in: ▪ Hypersensitivity ▪ Lactation.
Use Cautiously in: ▪ Patients with hepatic impairment (dosage reduction to 10 mg every other day is recommended) ▪ Patients with renal impairment (dosage reduction to 10 mg every other day is recommended if CCr <30 ml/min) ▪ Patients receiving drugs known to affect hepatic metabolism of drugs ▪ Geriatric patients (increased risk of adverse reactions) ▪ Pregnancy or children <2 yr (safety not established).

ADVERSE REACTIONS AND SIDE EFFECTS

CNS: confusion, drowsiness (rare), paradoxical excitation.
EENT: blurred vision.

GI: dry mouth, GI upset.
Derm: photosensitivity, rash.
Metab: weight gain.

INTERACTIONS

Drug-Drug: ▪ Concurrent use of **drugs known to affect hepatic metabolism** may alter effectiveness.
Drug-Food: ▪ Food increases absorption.

ROUTE AND DOSAGE

- **PO (Adults and Children ≥12 yr):** 10 mg once daily.
- **PO (Children 2–11 yr):** 5 mg once daily.

AVAILABILITY

▪ ***Rapidly disintegrating tablets:*** 10 mg[Rx], {10 mg[OTC]} ▪ ***Tablets:*** 10 mg[Rx], {10 mg[OTC]} ▪ ***Syrup:*** {5 mg/5 ml[OTC]} ▪ ***In combination with:*** pseudoephedrine (Claritin-D)[Rx]. See Appendix A.

TIME/ACTION PROFILE (antihistaminic effects)

	ONSET	PEAK	DURATION
PO	1–3 hr	8–12 hr	>24 hr

NURSING IMPLICATIONS

ASSESSMENT

- Assess allergy symptoms (rhinitis, conjunctivitis, hives) prior to and periodically throughout course of therapy.
- Assess lung sounds and character of bronchial secretions. Maintain fluid intake of 1500–2000 ml/day to decrease viscosity of secretions.
- ***Lab Test Considerations:*** May cause false-negative allergy skin testing.

POTENTIAL NURSING DIAGNOSES

- Airway clearance, ineffective (Indications).
- Injury, risk for (Adverse Reactions).
- Knowledge deficit, related to medication regimen (Patient/Family Teaching).

IMPLEMENTATION

- **PO:** Administer once daily on an empty stomach.
- *For rapidly disintegrating tablets (Reditabs):* Place on tongue. Tablet disintegrates rapidly. May be taken with or without water.

PATIENT/FAMILY TEACHING

- Instruct patient to take medication 1 hr before or 2 hr after eating.
- May cause dizziness or drowsiness. Caution patient to avoid driving or other activities requiring alertness until response to medication is known.
- Caution patient to use sunscreen and protective clothing to prevent photosensitivity reactions.
- Advise patient to avoid taking alcohol or other CNS depressants concurrently with this drug.
- Advise patient that good oral hygiene, frequent rinsing of mouth with water, and sugarless gum or candy may minimize dry mouth. Patient should notify dentist if dry mouth persists >2 wk.
- Instruct patient to contact health care professional immediately if dizziness, fainting, or fast or irregular heartbeat occurs or if symptoms persist.

EVALUATION

Effectiveness of therapy can be demonstrated by: ▪ Decrease in allergic symptoms.

LORAZEPAM

(lor-**az**-e-pam)
{Apo-Lorazepam}, Ativan, {Novo-Lorazem}, {Nu-Loraz}

CLASSIFICATION(S):
Antianxiety agent, Anticonvulsant, Sedative/hypnotic (benzodiazepine)

Schedule IV
Pregnancy Category D

L

INDICATIONS

▪ Adjunct in the management of anxiety or insomnia ▪ Preoperative sedation ▪ Decreases preoperative anxiety and provides amnesia. **Unlabeled Uses:** ▪ **IV:** Antiemetic prior to chemotherapy ▪ Management of status epilepticus.

ACTION

▪ Depresses the CNS, probably by potentiating gamma-aminobutyric acid (GABA), an inhibitory neurotransmitter. **Therapeutic Effects:** ▪ Sedation ▪ Decreased anxiety ▪ Decreased seizures.

PHARMACOKINETICS

Absorption: Well absorbed following oral administration. Rapidly and completely absorbed following IM administration. Sublingual absorption is more rapid than oral and is similar to IM.
Distribution: Widely distributed. Crosses the blood-brain barrier. Crosses the placenta; enters breast milk.
Metabolism and Excretion: Highly metabolized by the liver.
Half-life: 10–20 hr.

CONTRAINDICATIONS AND PRECAUTIONS

Contraindicated in: ▪ Hypersensitivity ▪ Cross-sensitivity with other benzodiazepines may exist ▪ Comatose patients or those with pre-existing CNS depression ▪ Uncontrolled severe pain ▪ Narrow-angle glaucoma ▪ Pregnancy and lactation.
Use Cautiously in: ▪ Severe hepatic/renal/pulmonary impairment ▪ Myasthenia gravis ▪ History of suicide attempt or drug abuse ▪ Geriatric or debilitated patients (dosage reduction recommended) ▪ Hypnotic use should be short-term.

ADVERSE REACTIONS AND SIDE EFFECTS*

CNS: dizziness, drowsiness, lethargy, hangover, headache, mental depression, paradoxical excitation.
EENT: blurred vision.
Resp: respiratory depression.
CV: *rapid IV use only*—APNEA, CARDIAC ARREST, bradycardia, hypotension.
GI: constipation, diarrhea, nausea, vomiting.
Derm: rashes.
Misc: physical dependence, psychological dependence, tolerance.

INTERACTIONS

Drug-Drug: ▪ Additive CNS depression with other **CNS depressants** including **alcohol, antihistamines, antidepressants, opioids,** and other **sedative/hypnotics** including other benzodiazepines ▪ May decrease the efficacy of **levodopa** ▪ **Smoking** may increase metabolism and decrease effectiveness ▪ **Probenecid** may decrease metabolism of lorazepam, enhancing its actions.

ROUTE AND DOSAGE

- **PO (Adults):** *Anxiety*—1–3 mg 2–3 times daily (up to 10 mg/day). *Insomnia*—2–4 mg at bedtime.
- **PO (Geriatric Patients or Debilitated Patients):** *Anxiety*—0.5–2 mg/day in divided doses initially. *Insomnia*—0.25–1 mg initially, increased as needed.
- **IM (Adults):** *Preoperative sedation*—50 mcg (0.05 mg)/kg 2 hr before surgery (not to exceed 4 mg).
- **IV (Adults):** *Preoperative sedation*—44 mcg (0.044 mg)/kg (not to exceed 2 mg) 15–20 min before surgery. *Operative amnesia*—up to 50 mcg/kg (not to exceed 4 mg). *Antiemetic*—2 mg 30 min prior to chemotherapy; may be repeated q 4 hr as needed (unlabeled). *Anticonvulsant*—50 mcg (0.05 mg)/kg, up to 4 mg; may be repeated after 10–15 min (not to exceed 8 mg/12 hr; unlabeled).

AVAILABILITY

▪ ***Tablets:*** 0.5 mg^{Rx}, 1 mg^{Rx}, 2 mg^{Rx} ▪ ***Concentrated solution:*** 2 mg/ml^{Rx} ▪ ***Injection:*** 2 mg/ml^{Rx}, 4 mg/ml^{Rx}.

TIME/ACTION PROFILE (sedation)

	ONSET	PEAK	DURATION
PO	15–45 min	1–6 hr	up to 48 hr
IM	15–30 min	1–1.5 hr†	up to 48 hr
IV	5–15 min	UK†	up to 48 hr

†Peak amnestic response within 2 hr for IM, 15–20 min for IV.

NURSING IMPLICATIONS

ASSESSMENT

- **Anxiety:** Assess degree and manifestations of anxiety prior to and periodically throughout therapy.
- □ Prolonged high-dose therapy may lead to psychological or physical dependence. Restrict amount of drug available to patient.

*CAPITALS indicate life-threatening; underlines indicate most frequent.

- **Status Epilepticus:** Assess location, duration, characteristics, and frequency of seizures.
- ***Lab Test Considerations:*** Patients on high-dose therapy should receive routine evaluation of renal, hepatic, and hematologic function.

POTENTIAL NURSING DIAGNOSES

- Anxiety (Indications).
- Injury, risk for (Indications, Side Effects).
- Knowledge deficit, related to medication regimen (Patient/Family Teaching).

IMPLEMENTATION

- **General Info:** Following parenteral administration, keep patient supine for at least 8 hr and observe closely.
- **PO:** Tablet may also be given sublingually (unlabeled) for more rapid onset.
- **IM:** Administer IM doses deep into muscle mass at least 2 hr before surgery for optimum effect.
- **Direct IV:** Dilute immediately before use with an equal amount of sterile water, D5W, or 0.9% NaCl for injection. Do not use if solution is colored or contains a precipitate.
- ***Rate:*** Administer direct IV, through Y-site at a rate of 2 mg over 1 min. Rapid IV administration may result in apnea, hypotension, bradycardia, or cardiac arrest.
- **Y-Site Compatibility:** ▪ acyclovir ▪ albumin ▪ amifostine ▪ amikacin ▪ atracurium ▪ bumetanide ▪ cefotaxime ▪ ciprofloxacin ▪ cisplatin ▪ clonidine ▪ cyclophosphamide ▪ cytarabine ▪ dexamethasone sodium phosphate ▪ diltiazem ▪ doxorubicin ▪ erythromycin lactobionate ▪ fentanyl ▪ filgrastim ▪ fluconazole ▪ fludarabine ▪ furosemide ▪ gentamicin ▪ granisetron ▪ haloperidol ▪ heparin ▪ hydrocortisone sodium succinate ▪ melphalan ▪ methotrexate ▪ metronidazole ▪ morphine ▪ paclitaxel ▪ pancuronium ▪ piperacillin ▪ piperacillin/tazobactam ▪ potassium chloride ▪ ranitidine ▪ tacrolimus ▪ teniposide ▪ thiotepa ▪ trimethoprim/sulfamethoxazole ▪ vancomycin ▪ vecuronium ▪ vinorelbine ▪ zidovudine.
- **Y-Site Incompatibility:** ▪ aldesleukin ▪ gallium nitrate ▪ idarubicin ▪ imipenem/cilastatin ▪ omeprazole ▪ ondansetron ▪ sargramostim ▪ sufentanil ▪ thiopental.

PATIENT/FAMILY TEACHING

- □ Instruct patient to take medication exactly as directed and not to skip or double up on missed doses. If medication is less effective after a few weeks, check with health care professional; do not increase dose. Abrupt withdrawal may cause tremors, nausea, vomiting, and abdominal and muscle cramps.
- □ May cause drowsiness or dizziness. Advise patient to avoid driving or other activities requiring alertness until response to medication is known.
- □ Caution patient to avoid taking alcohol or other CNS depressants concurrently with this medication.
- □ Instruct patient to contact health care professional immediately if pregnancy is planned or suspected.
- □ Emphasize the importance of follow-up exams to determine effectiveness of the medication.

EVALUATION

Effectiveness of therapy can be demonstrated by: ▪ Increase in sense of well-being □ Decrease in subjective feelings of anxiety without excessive sedation ▪ Reduction of preoperative anxiety ▪ Postoperative amnesia ▪ Improvement in sleep patterns. Need for continued therapy should be re-evaluated regularly. Minimum effective dose should be used ▪ Cessation of seizures in status epilepticus.

LOXAPINE

(**lox**-a-peen)
{Loxapac}, Loxitane, Loxitane C, Loxitane IM

CLASSIFICATION(S):
Antipsychotic agent

Pregnancy Category C

INDICATIONS

▪ Psychoses. **Unlabeled Uses:** ▪ Depression and anxiety associated with depression.

L

ACTION

▪ Appears to block dopamine at postsynaptic receptor sites in the CNS. **Therapeutic Effects:** ▪ Diminution of psychotic behavior.

PHARMACOKINETICS

Absorption: Well absorbed following oral or IM administration.
Distribution: UK.
Metabolism and Excretion: Extensively metabolized by the liver; some conversion to active antipsychotic compounds.
Half-life: *PO*—3–4 hr; *IM*—12 hr.

CONTRAINDICATIONS AND PRECAUTIONS

Contraindicated in: ▪ Hypersensitivity or intolerance to loxapine or amoxapine ▪ Coma ▪ CNS depression ▪ Pregnancy or lactation.
Use Cautiously in: ▪ Glaucoma ▪ Geriatric men or males with prostatic hyperplasia (more prone to urinary retention) ▪ Geriatric patients (more susceptible to adverse reactions) ▪ Intestinal obstruction ▪ History of seizures ▪ Alcoholism ▪ Cardiovascular disease ▪ Impaired liver function ▪ Children <16 yr (safety not established).

ADVERSE REACTIONS AND SIDE EFFECTS*

CNS: NEUROLEPTIC MALIGNANT SYNDROME, confusion, dizziness, drowsiness, extrapyramidal reactions, headache, insomnia, syncope, tardive dyskinesia, weakness.
EENT: blurred vision, lens opacities, nasal congestion.
CV: orthostatic hypotension, tachycardia.
GI: constipation, drug-induced hepatitis, dry mouth, ileus, nausea, vomiting.
GU: urinary retention.
Derm: dermatitis, edema, facial photosensitivity, pigment changes, rashes, seborrhea.
Endo: galactorrhea.
Hemat: AGRANULOCYTOSIS.
Neuro: ataxia.
Misc: allergic reactions.

INTERACTIONS

Drug-Drug: ▪ Decreases the antihypertensive effects of **guanethidine** or **guanadrel** ▪ Blocks the alpha-adrenergic effects of **epinephrine** (may result in hypotension and tachycardia) ▪ Additive CNS depression with other **CNS depressants**, including **alcohol, antihistamines, opioids,** and **sedative/hypnotics** ▪ **Antacids** or **adsorbent antidiarrheals** may decrease absorption ▪ Use with **antidepressants** or **MAO inhibitors** may result in prolonged CNS depression and increased anticholinergic effects.

ROUTE AND DOSAGE

- **PO (Adults):** 10 mg bid, may be increased gradually over the first 7–10 days as needed and tolerated. Usual maintenance dose is 15–25 mg 2–4 times daily. Severely ill patients may require up to 50 mg/day initially and maintenance doses up to 250 mg/day.
- **IM (Adults):** 12.5–50 mg q 4–6 hr as needed and tolerated (up to 250 mg/day).

AVAILABILITY

▪ ***Capsules:*** 5 mg[Rx], 10 mg[Rx], 25 mg[Rx], 50 mg[Rx] ▪ ***Tablets:*** {5 mg[Rx]}, {10 mg[Rx]}, {25 mg[Rx]}, {50 mg[Rx]} ▪ ***Oral concentrate:*** 25 mg/ml[Rx] ▪ ***Injection:*** 50 mg/ml[Rx].

TIME/ACTION PROFILE (antipsychotic effect)

	ONSET	PEAK	DURATION
PO, IM	30 min	1.5–3 hr	12 hr

NURSING IMPLICATIONS

ASSESSMENT

- ▫ Monitor patient's mental status (delusions, hallucinations, and behavior) prior to and periodically throughout therapy.
- ▫ Monitor blood pressure (sitting, standing, lying) and pulse rate prior to and frequently during the period of dosage adjustment.
- ▫ Observe patient carefully when administering medication to ensure medication is actually taken and not hoarded.
- ▫ Monitor patient for onset of akathisia (restlessness or desire to keep moving) and extrapyramidal side effects (*parkinsonian*—difficulty speaking or swallowing, loss of balance control, pill rolling, mask-like face, shuffling gait, rigidity, tremors; and *dystonic*—muscle spasms, twisting motions, twitching, inability to move eyes, weakness of arms or legs) every

***CAPITALS indicate life-threatening; underlines indicate most frequent.**

2 mo during therapy and 8–12 wk after therapy has been discontinued. Report these symptoms; reduction in dosage or discontinuation of medication may be necessary. Trihexyphenidyl or diphenhydramine may be used to control symptoms.

- Monitor for tardive dyskinesia (uncontrolled rhythmic movement of mouth, face, and extremities; lip smacking or puckering; puffing of cheeks; uncontrolled chewing; rapid or worm-like movements of tongue). Tardive dyskinesia is dose related initially but may increase with cumulative dose. Report immediately; may be irreversible.
- Monitor frequency and consistency of bowel movements. Increasing bulk and fluids in the diet may help minimize constipation.
- Loxapine lowers the seizure threshold. Institute seizure precautions for patients with history of seizures.
- Monitor for development of neuroleptic malignant syndrome (fever, respiratory distress, tachycardia, convulsions, diaphoresis, hypertension or hypotension, pallor, tiredness, severe muscle stiffness, loss of bladder control). Report symptoms immediately.
- ***Lab Test Considerations:*** Monitor CBC and differential prior to and periodically throughout therapy.
- Monitor liver function studies and urine bilirubin and bile concentrations if patient develops jaundice.
- ***Toxicity and Overdose:*** Antiemetic effects of loxapine may block the action of ipecac. Overdose is treated by gastric lavage, barbiturates to control seizures, and supportive care for fluctuations in body temperature. Hypotension may be corrected by use of IV fluids, norepinephrine, or phenylephrine. Avoid use of epinephrine, as it may worsen hypotension.

POTENTIAL NURSING DIAGNOSES

- Thought processes, altered (Indications).
- Injury, risk for (Side Effects).
- Knowledge deficit, related to medication regimen (Patient/Family Teaching).

IMPLEMENTATION

- **PO:** Administer capsules with food or milk to decrease gastric irritation.
- Dilute oral solution with orange or grapefruit juice immediately prior to administration. Measure dose with provided dropper.
- Do not administer antacids or antidiarrheals within 2 hr of loxapine.
- **IM:** Do not inject SC. Inject slowly into deep, well-developed muscle. Light amber color does not alter potency of solution. Do not administer solution that is markedly discolored or that contains a precipitate.
- Keep patient recumbent for at least 30 min following parenteral administration to minimize hypotensive effects.

PATIENT/FAMILY TEACHING

- Instruct patient on need to take medication exactly as directed. If a dose is missed, it should be taken as soon as remembered, up to 1 hr before next scheduled dose. Patients on long-term high-dose therapy may need to discontinue gradually to avoid withdrawal symptoms (dyskinesia, tremors, dizziness, nausea, and vomiting).
- Instruct patient receiving oral solution on correct method of measuring dose with provided dropper.
- Inform patient of possibility of extrapyramidal symptoms and tardive dyskinesia. Instruct patient to report these symptoms immediately to health care professional.
- Advise patient to change positions slowly to minimize orthostatic hypotension.
- May cause drowsiness. Caution patient to avoid driving or other activities requiring alertness until response to the medication is known.
- Caution patient to use sunscreen and protective clothing to prevent photosensitivity reactions.
- Caution patient to avoid concurrent use of alcohol, other CNS depressants, and OTC medications without consulting health care professional.
- Instruct patient to use frequent mouth rinses, good oral hygiene, and sugarless gum or candy to minimize dry mouth. Consult health care professional if dry mouth continues for >2 wk.
- Advise patient to notify health care professional of medication regimen prior to treatment or surgery.
- Instruct patient to notify health care professional promptly if sore throat, fever, unusual bleeding or bruising, rash, weakness, tremors,

visual disturbances, dark-colored urine, or clay-colored stools occur.
- Advise patient of need for continued medical follow-up for psychotherapy, eye exams, and laboratory tests.

EVALUATION

Effectiveness of therapy can be demonstrated by: ▪ Decreased psychotic ideation.

MAGNESIUM AND ALUMINUM SALTS

aluminum hydroxide

(a-**loo**-mi-num hye-**drox**-ide)
Alu-Cap, {Alugel}, Alu-Tab, {Basalgel}, Dialume

magaldrate

(**mag**-al-drate)
{Losopan}, Lowsium, Riopan, {Riopan Extra Strength}

magnesium hydroxide/aluminum hydroxide

(mag-**nee**-zhum hye-**drox**-ide/a-**loo**-mi-num hye-**drox**-ide)
Alamag, {Diovol}, {Diovol Ex}, {Gelusil}, {Gelusil Extra Strength}, Maalox, Maalox TC, Mintox, Mylanta Double Strength, {Neutralca-S}, Rulox, Rulox No. 1, Rulox No. 2

CLASSIFICATION(S):
Antacids, Electrolyte modifiers (hypophosphatemic [aluminum hydroxide only])

Pregnancy Category UK

INDICATIONS

▪ Treat peptic ulcer pain and promote healing of duodenal and gastric ulcers ▪ Useful in a variety of GI complaints, including: □ Hyperacidity □ Indigestion □ Gastroesophageal reflux disease (GERD) □ Heartburn ▪ Aluminum hydroxide is also used to treat hyperphosphatemia associated with renal insufficiency.

ACTION

▪ Neutralize gastric acid following dissolution in gastric contents ▪ Inactivate pepsin if pH is raised to ≥4 ▪ Aluminum hydroxide combines with phosphates in the GI tract to form a nonabsorbable compound. **Therapeutic Effects:** ▪ Neutralization of gastric acid with healing of ulcers and decrease in associated pain ▪ Aluminum hydroxide lowers serum phosphate levels.

PHARMACOKINETICS

Absorption: During routine use, antacids are nonabsorbable. With chronic use, 15–30% of magnesium and smaller amounts of aluminum may be absorbed.
Distribution: Small amounts absorbed are widely distributed, cross the placenta, and appear in breast milk. Aluminum concentrates in the CNS.
Metabolism and Excretion: Excreted by the kidneys.
Half-life: UK.

CONTRAINDICATIONS AND PRECAUTIONS

Contraindicated in: ▪ Severe abdominal pain of unknown cause, especially if accompanied by fever ▪ Anuria (magnesium only) ▪ Products containing tartrazine or sugar in patients with known intolerance.
Use Cautiously in: ▪ Antacids containing magnesium in patients with any degree of renal insufficiency.

ADVERSE REACTIONS AND SIDE EFFECTS*

GI: *aluminum salts*—<u>constipation</u>; *magnesium salts*—<u>diarrhea</u>.
F and E: *magnesium salts*—hypermagnesemia; *aluminum salts*—hypophosphatemia.

INTERACTIONS

Drug-Drug: ▪ Magnesium and aluminum salts change the absorptive characteristics of many **orally administered drugs** ▪ Destroy coating of **enteric-coated drugs,** causing premature release into the stomach and resulting in altered absorption or side effects ▪ Absorption of **tet-**

{} = Available in Canada only.
***CAPITALS indicate life-threatening; <u>underlines</u> indicate most frequent.**

racyclines, phenothiazines, ketoconazole, iron salts, fluoroquinolones, and **isoniazid** may be decreased ▪ If urine pH is increased by large doses, **salicylate** blood levels may be decreased and **quinidine, flecainide,** and **amphetamine** levels may be increased.

ROUTE AND DOSAGE

Dosages vary, depending on concentration of ingredients in product chosen. Generally 5–30 ml or 1–2 tablets are given 1–3 hr after meals and at bedtime. In the early healing phase of peptic ulcer, more frequent administration may be necessary.

❑ Peptic Ulcer Disease

- **PO (Adults):** *Uncomplicated duodenal/gastric ulcers*—administer 1 and 3 hr after meals and at bedtime. Additional doses may be used for recurring symptoms; continue for 4–6 wk for duodenal ulcers and until healing is complete for gastric ulcers.

❑ Esophageal Reflux

- **PO (Adults):** *Acute management*—antacid suspension q 30–60 min. *Maintenance*—administer 1 and 3 hr after meals and at bedtime; additional doses may be used for recurring symptoms.

❑ GI Bleeding/Stress Ulceration

- **PO (Adults):** Administer q 1 hr or as needed to maintain pH of nasogastric aspirate >3.5.

❑ Prevention of Anesthesia-Induced GI Aspiration

- **PO (Adults):** Antacid suspension given 30 min prior to general anesthesia.

❑ Hyperphosphatemia (Aluminum Hydroxide Only)

- **PO (Adults):** 30–40 ml of aluminum hydroxide suspension 3–4 times daily.

AVAILABILITY

❑ Aluminum Hydroxide

▪ ***Tablets:*** 300 mg^{OTC}, 600 mg^{OTC} ▪ ***Capsules:*** 400 mg^{OTC}, 500 mg^{OTC} ▪ ***Suspension:*** 320 mg/5 ml^{OTC}, 450 mg/5 ml^{OTC}, 600 mg/5 ml^{OTC}, 675 mg/5 ml^{OTC}.

❑ Magaldrate

▪ ***Liquid:*** 540 mg/5 ml^{OTC} ▪ ***Suspension:*** 540 mg/5 ml^{OTC}.

❑ Magnesium Hydroxide/Aluminum Hydroxide

▪ ***Tablets:*** 200 mg aluminum hydroxide/200 mg magnesium hydroxide^{OTC}, 400 mg aluminum hydroxide/400 mg magnesium hydroxide^{OTC} ▪ ***Suspension:*** 200 mg aluminum hydroxide/225 mg magnesium hydroxide/5 ml^{OTC}, 300 mg aluminum hydroxide/600 mg magnesium hydroxide/5 ml^{OTC} ▪ ***In combination with:*** simethicone^{OTC}. See Appendix A.

TIME/ACTION PROFILE (effect on gastric pH)

	ONSET	PEAK	DURATION
Aluminum PO	slightly delayed	30 min	30 min–1 hr (empty stomach); 3 hr (after meals)
Magnesium PO	immediate	30 min	30 min–1 hr (empty stomach); 3 hr (after meals)

NURSING IMPLICATIONS

ASSESSMENT

- **Antacid:** Assess for heartburn and indigestion as well as location, duration, character, and precipitating factors of gastric pain.
- ***Lab Test Considerations:*** Monitor serum phosphate, potassium, and calcium levels periodically during chronic use. May cause increased serum calcium and decreased serum phosphate concentrations.
- ❑ May cause increased serum gastrin and systemic and urinary pH.
- ❑ Antagonize effects of pentagastrin and histamine during gastric acid secretion testing. Avoid administration for 24 hr preceding the test.

POTENTIAL NURSING DIAGNOSES

- Pain (Indications).
- Knowledge deficit, related to medication regimen (Patient/Family Teaching).

IMPLEMENTATION

- **General Info:** Magnesium and aluminum are combined as antacids to balance the constipating effects of aluminum with the laxative effects of magnesium.
- **PO:** To prevent tablets from entering small intestine in undissolved form, they must be

chewed thoroughly before swallowing. Follow with ½ glass of water.
- □ Shake suspensions well before administration.
- □ For an antacid effect, administer 1–3 hr after meals and at bedtime.
- □ Chewable tablets must be chewed thoroughly before swallowing. Follow with ½ glass (120 ml) of water. Shake suspension well.

PATIENT/FAMILY TEACHING

- □ Caution patient to consult health care professional before taking antacids for more than 2 wk if problem is recurring, if relief is not obtained, or if symptoms of gastric bleeding (black, tarry stools; coffee-ground emesis) occur.
- □ Advise patient not to take this medication within 2 hr of taking other medications.
- □ Some antacids contain large amounts of sodium. Caution patient on sodium-restricted diet to check sodium content when on long-term high-dose therapy.

EVALUATION

Effectiveness of therapy can be demonstrated by: ▪ Relief of gastric pain and irritation ▪ Decrease in serum phosphate levels.

MAGNESIUM SALTS

magnesium chloride
(12% Mg; 9.8 mEq Mg/g)
(mag-**nee**-zhum **klor**-ide)
Chloromag, Slo-Mag

magnesium citrate
(16.2% Mg; 4.4 mEq Mg/g)
(mag-**nee**-zhum **si**-trate)
Citrate of Magnesia, Citroma, {Citromag}, Evac-Q-Mag

magnesium hydroxide
(41.7% Mg; 34.3 mEq Mg/g)
(mag-**nee**-zhum hye-**drox**-ide)
Phillips Magnesia Tablets, Phillips Milk of Magnesia, MOM

magnesium oxide
(60.3% Mg; 49.6 mEq Mg/g)
(mag-**nee**-zhum **ox**-ide)
Mag-Ox 400, Maox, Uro-Mag

magnesium sulfate
(9.9% Mg; 8.1 mEq Mg/g)
(mag-**nee**-zhum **sul**-fate)
epsom salt

CLASSIFICATION(S):
Anticonvulsants, Electrolytes (magnesium), Laxatives (saline)

Pregnancy Category A

INDICATIONS

▪ **Magnesium sulfate IM, IV:** As a(n): □ Treatment/prevention of hypomagnesemia □ Anticonvulsant in severe eclampsia or pre-eclampsia ▪ **Magnesium salts PO :** As a: □ Laxative □ Bowel evacuant in preparation for surgical/radiographic procedures □ Prevention and treatment of magnesium deficiency ▪ Milk of Magnesia has also been used as an antacid. **Unlabeled Uses:** ▪ Preterm labor ▪ Treatment of torsades de pointes.

ACTION

▪ Essential for the activity of many enzymes ▪ Play an important role in neurotransmission and muscular excitability ▪ Are osmotically active in GI tract, drawing water into the lumen and causing peristalsis. **Therapeutic Effects:** ▪ Replacement in deficiency states ▪ Resolution of eclampsia ▪ Evacuation of the colon.

PHARMACOKINETICS

Absorption: Up to 30% may be absorbed orally. Well absorbed from IM sites.
Distribution: Widely distributed. Cross the placenta and are present in breast milk.
Metabolism and Excretion: Excreted primarily by the kidneys.
Half-life: UK.

CONTRAINDICATIONS AND PRECAUTIONS

Contraindicated in: ▪ Hypermagnesemia ▪ Hypocalcemia ▪ Anuria ▪ Heart block ▪ Active labor or within 2 hr of delivery (unless used for preterm labor).
Use Cautiously in: ▪ Any degree of renal insufficiency.

{} = Available in Canada only.

ADVERSE REACTIONS AND SIDE EFFECTS*

CNS: drowsiness.
Resp: decreased respiratory rate.
CV: arrhythmias, bradycardia, hypotension.
GI: diarrhea.
Derm: flushing, sweating.
Metab: hypothermia.

INTERACTIONS

Drug-Drug: ▪ Potentiate **neuromuscular blocking agents** ▪ May decrease absorption of **fluoroquinolones, nitrofurantoin,** and **tetracyclines** (oral magnesium).

ROUTE AND DOSAGE

❑ Prevention of Deficiency (in mg of magnesium)

- **PO (Adults and Children >10 yr):** *Adolescent and adult males*—270–400 mg/day; *adolescent and adult females*—280–300 mg/day; *pregnant females*—320 mg/day; *breast-feeding females*—340–355 mg/day.
- **PO (Children 7–10 yr):** 170 mg/day.
- **PO (Children 4–6 yr):** 120 mg/day.
- **PO (Children birth–3 yr):** 40–80 mg/day.

❑ Treatment of Deficiency (expressed as mg of magnesium)

- **PO (Adults):** 200–400 mg /day in 3–4 divided doses.
- **PO (Children 6–11 yr):** 3–6 mg/kg/day in 3–4 divided doses.
- **IM (Adults):** *Severe deficiency*—250 mg/kg over 4 hr; *mild deficiency*—1 g q 6 hr for 4 doses.
- **IV (Adults):** *Severe deficiency*—5 g

❑ Eclampsia/Pre-eclampsia (magnesium sulfate)

- **IV, IM (Adults):** 4–5 g by IV infusion, concurrently with up to 5g IM in each buttock; then 4–5 g IM q 4 hr *or* 4 g by IV infusion followed by 1–2 g/hr continuous infusion (not to exceed 40 g/day or 20 g/48 hr in the presence of severe renal insufficiency).

❑ Part of Parenteral Nutrition

- **IV (Adults):** 4–24 mEq/day.
- **IV (Children):** 0.25–0.5 mEq/kg/day.

❑ Laxative

- **PO (Adults):** *Magnesium citrate*—240 ml; *magnesium hydroxide (Milk of Magnesia)*—30–60 ml single or divided dose or 10–20 ml as concentrate; *magnesium sulfate*—10–30 g single or divided dose.
- **PO (Children 6–12 yr):** *Magnesium citrate*—100 ml; *magnesium hydroxide (Milk of Magnesia)*—15–30 ml single or divided dose; *magnesium sulfate*—5–10 g.
- **PO (Children 2–5 yr):** *magnesium hydroxide (Milk of Magnesia)*—5–15 ml single or divided dose.

AVAILABILITY

❑ Magnesium Chloride

▪ ***Sustained-release tablets:*** 535 mg (64 mg magnesium)^{OTC} ▪ ***Enteric-coated tablets:*** 833 mg (100 mg magnesium)^{OTC} ▪ ***Injection:*** 200 mg/ml in 50-ml vials^{Rx}.

❑ Magnesium Citrate

▪ ***Oral solution:*** 240-, 296-, and 300-ml bottles (77 mEq magnesium/100 ml)^{OTC}.

❑ Magnesium Hydroxide

▪ ***Liquid:*** 400 mg/5 ml (164 mg magnesium/5 ml)^{OTC} ▪ ***Concentrated liquid:*** 800 mg/5 ml (328 mg magnesium/5 ml)^{OTC} ▪ ***Chewable tablets:*** 300 mg (130 mg magnesium)^{OTC}, 600 mg (260 mg magnesium)^{OTC}.

❑ Magnesium Oxide

▪ ***Tablets:*** 400 mg (241.3 mg magnesium)^{OTC} ▪ ***Capsules:*** 140 mg (84.5 mg magnesium)^{OTC}.

❑ Magnesium Sulfate

▪ ***Powder for oral use:*** dry powder in bulk packages^{OTC} ▪ ***Epsom salts:*** any powder in bulk packages^{OTC} ▪ ***Injection:*** 10%^{Rx}, 12.5%^{Rx}, 25%^{Rx}, 50%^{Rx}.

TIME/ACTION PROFILE (PO = laxative effect; IM, IV = anticonvulsant effect)

	ONSET	PEAK	DURATION
PO	3–6 hr	UK	UK
IM	60 min	UK	3–4 hr
IV	immediate	UK	30 min

M

*CAPITALS indicate life-threatening; underlines indicate most frequent.

NURSING IMPLICATIONS

ASSESSMENT

- **Hypomagnesemia/Anticonvulsant:** Monitor pulse, blood pressure, respirations, and ECG frequently throughout administration of parenteral magnesium sulfate. Respirations should be at least 16/min before each dose.
- Monitor neurologic status before and throughout therapy. Institute seizure precautions. Patellar reflex (knee jerk) should be tested before each parenteral dose of magnesium sulfate. If response is absent, no additional doses should be administered until positive response is obtained.
- Monitor newborn for hypotension, hyporeflexia, and respiratory depression if mother has received magnesium sulfate.
- Monitor intake and output ratios. Urine output should be maintained at a level of at least 100 ml/4 hr.
- **Laxative:** Assess patient for abdominal distention, presence of bowel sounds, and usual pattern of bowel function.
- Assess color, consistency, and amount of stool produced.
- **Antacid:** Assess for heartburn and indigestion as well as location, duration, character, and precipitating factors of gastric pain.
- ***Lab Test Considerations:*** Serum magnesium levels and renal function should be monitored periodically throughout administration of parenteral magnesium sulfate.

POTENTIAL NURSING DIAGNOSES

- Injury, risk for (Indications, Side Effects).
- Constipation (Indications).
- Knowledge deficit, related to medication regimen (Patient/Family Teaching).

IMPLEMENTATION

- **PO:** To prevent tablets entering small intestine in undissolved form, they must be chewed thoroughly before swallowing. Follow with ½ glass of water.
- *Magnesium citrate:* Refrigerate solutions to ensure they retain potency and palatability. May be served over ice. Magnesium citrate in an open container will lose carbonation upon standing; this will not affect potency but may reduce palatability.
- *Magnesium hydroxide:* Shake solution well before administration.
- *Magnesium sulfate:* Dissolve in a full glass of water. May use lemon-flavored carbonated beverage to mask bitter taste. May be given as a single dose or several divided doses.
- **Antacid:** Administer 1–3 hr after meals and at bedtime.
- Powder and liquid forms are considered more effective than tablets.
- **Laxative:** Administer on empty stomach for more rapid results. Follow all oral laxative doses with a full glass of liquid to prevent dehydration and for faster effect. Do not administer at bedtime or late in the day.
- **IM:** Administer deep IM into gluteal sites. Administer subsequent injections in alternate sides.
- Use 25–50% concentrations for adults, 20% concentrations for children <14 yr.
- **Direct IV:** Administer 10% solution undiluted.
- ***Rate:*** Administer at a rate of 1.5 ml of a 10% solution (or its equivalent) over 1 min.
- **Continuous Infusion:** When given as an anticonvulsant, dilute 4 g in 250 ml of D5W or 0.9% NaCl.
- When given for hypomagnesemia, may dilute 5 g in 1000 ml of D5W, 0.9% NaCl, or Ringer's or lactated Ringer's solution.
- ***Rate:*** When given as an anticonvulsant, administer at a rate not to exceed 3 ml/min.
- When given for hypomagnesemia, administer slowly over 3 hr.
- Use infusion pump to accurately regulate rate.
- **Y-Site Compatibility:** ▪ acyclovir ▪ aldesleukin ▪ amifostine ▪ amikacin ▪ ampicillin ▪ aztreonam ▪ cefamandole ▪ cefazolin ▪ cefoperazone ▪ cefotaxime ▪ cefoxitin ▪ cephalothin ▪ cephapirin ▪ chloramphenicol ▪ clindamycin ▪ dobutamine ▪ doxycycline ▪ enalaprilat ▪ erythromycin lactobionate ▪ esmolol ▪ famotidine ▪ fludarabine ▪ gallium nitrate ▪ gentamicin ▪ granisetron ▪ heparin ▪ hydrocortisone sodium succinate ▪ hydromorphone ▪ idarubicin ▪ insulin ▪ kanamycin ▪ labetalol ▪ meperidine ▪ metronidazole ▪ minocycline ▪ morphine ▪ nafcillin ▪ ondansetron ▪ oxacillin ▪ paclitaxel ▪ penicillin G potassium ▪ piperacillin ▪ piperacillin/tazobactam ▪ potassium chloride ▪ sargramostim ▪ thiotepa ▪ ticarcillin ▪ tobramycin ▪ trimethoprim/sul-

famethoxazole ▪ vancomycin ▪ vitamin B complex with C.

▪ **Y-Site Incompatibility:** ▪ cefepime.

PATIENT/FAMILY TEACHING

▪ **General Info:** Advise patient not to take this medication within 2 hr of taking other medications.

▪ **Antacids:** Caution patient to consult health care professional before taking antacids for more than 2 wk if problem is recurring, if relief is not obtained, or if symptoms of gastric bleeding (black, tarry stools; coffee-ground emesis) occur.

▪ **Laxatives:** Advise patient that laxatives should be used only for short-term therapy. Long-term therapy may cause electrolyte imbalance and dependence.

□ Encourage patient to use other forms of bowel regulation, such as increasing bulk in the diet, fluid intake, and mobility. Normal bowel habits are individualized; frequency of bowel movement may vary from 3 times/day to 3 times/wk.

□ Advise patient to notify health care professional if unrelieved constipation, rectal bleeding, or symptoms of electrolyte imbalance (muscle cramps or pain, weakness, dizziness) occur.

EVALUATION

Effectiveness of therapy can be demonstrated by: ▪ Normal serum magnesium concentrations ▪ Control of seizures associated with toxemias of pregnancy ▪ Relief of gastric pain and irritation ▪ Passage of a soft, formed bowel movement, usually within 3–6 hr.

MANNITOL

(**man**-i-tol)

Osmitrol, Resectisol

CLASSIFICATION(S):

Diuretic (osmotic)

Pregnancy Category C

INDICATIONS

▪ **IV:** Adjunct in the treatment of: □ Acute oliguric renal failure □ Edema □ Increased intracranial or intraocular pressure □ Toxic overdose ▪ **GU irrigant:** During transurethral procedures (2.5–5% solution only).

ACTION

▪ Increases the osmotic pressure of the glomerular filtrate, thereby inhibiting reabsorption of water and electrolytes ▪ Causes excretion of: □ Water □ Sodium □ Potassium □ Chloride □ Calcium □ Phosphorus □ Magnesium □ Urea □ Uric acid. **Therapeutic Effects:** ▪ Mobilization of excess fluid in oliguric renal failure or edema ▪ Reduction of intraocular or intracranial pressure ▪ Increased urinary excretion of toxic materials ▪ Decreased hemolysis when used as an irrigant following transurethral prostatic resection.

PHARMACOKINETICS

Absorption: IV administration produces complete bioavailability. Some absorption may follow use as a GU irrigant.

Distribution: Confined to the extracellular space; does not usually cross the blood-brain barrier or eye.

Metabolism and Excretion: Excreted by the kidneys; minimal liver metabolism.

Half-life: 100 min.

CONTRAINDICATIONS AND PRECAUTIONS

Contraindicated in: ▪ Hypersensitivity ▪ Anuria ▪ Dehydration ▪ Active intracranial bleeding.

Use Cautiously in: ▪ Pregnancy and lactation (safety not established).

ADVERSE REACTIONS AND SIDE EFFECTS*

CNS: confusion, headache.

EENT: blurred vision, rhinitis.

CV: <u>transient volume expansion</u>, chest pain, congestive heart failure, pulmonary edema, tachycardia.

GI: nausea, thirst, vomiting.

GU: renal failure, urinary retention.

F and E: dehydration, hyperkalemia, hypernatremia, hypokalemia, hyponatremia.

Local: phlebitis at IV site.

***CAPITALS indicate life-threatening; <u>underlines</u> indicate most frequent.**

M

INTERACTIONS

Drug-Drug: ▪ Hypokalemia increases the risk of **digitalis glycoside** toxicity.

ROUTE AND DOSAGE

- **IV (Adults):** *Edema, oliguric renal failure*—50–100 g as a 5–25% solution; may precede with a test dose of 0.2 g/kg over 3–5 min. *Reduction of intracranial/intraocular pressure*—0.25–2 g/kg as 15–25% solution over 30–60 min (500 mg/kg may be sufficient in small or debilitated patients). *Diuresis in drug intoxications*—50–200 g as a 5–25% solution titrated to maintain urine flow of 100–500 ml/hr.
- **IV (Children):** *Edema, oliguric renal failure*—0.25–2 g/kg (60 g/m²) as a 15–20% solution over 2–6 hr; may precede with a test dose of 0.2 g/kg over 3–5 min. *Reduction of intracranial/intraocular pressure*—1–2 g/kg (30–60 g/m²) as a 15–20% solution over 30–60 min (500 mg/kg may be sufficient in small or debilitated patients). *Diuresis in drug intoxications*—up to 2 g/kg (60 g/m²) as a 5–10% solution.

AVAILABILITY

▪ ***IV injection:*** 5%[Rx], 10%[Rx], 15% [Rx], 20%[Rx] ▪ ***GU irrigant:*** 5%[Rx] ▪ ***In combination with:*** sorbitol for GU irrigation[Rx].

TIME/ACTION PROFILE (diuretic effect)

	ONSET	PEAK	DURATION
IV	30–60 min	1 hr	6–8 hr

NURSING IMPLICATIONS

ASSESSMENT

- **General Info:** Monitor vital signs, urine output, CVP, and pulmonary artery pressures (PAP) prior to and hourly throughout administration. Assess patient for signs and symptoms of dehydration (decreased skin turgor, fever, dry skin and mucous membranes, thirst) or signs of fluid overload (increased CVP, dyspnea, rales/crackles, edema).
  - Assess patient for anorexia, muscle weakness, numbness, tingling, paresthesia, confusion, and excessive thirst. Report signs of electrolyte imbalance.
- **Increased Intracranial Pressure:** Monitor neurologic status and intracranial pressure readings in patients receiving this medication to decrease cerebral edema.
- **Increased Intraocular Pressure:** Monitor for persistent or increased eye pain or decreased visual acuity.
- ***Lab Test Considerations:*** Renal function and serum electrolytes should be monitored routinely throughout course of therapy.

POTENTIAL NURSING DIAGNOSES

- Fluid volume excess (Indications).
- Fluid volume deficit, risk for (Side Effects).

IMPLEMENTATION

- **General Info:** Observe infusion site frequently for infiltration. Extravasation may cause tissue irritation and necrosis.
  - Do not administer electrolyte-free mannitol solution with blood. If blood must be administered simultaneously with mannitol, add at least 20 mEq NaCl to each liter of mannitol.
  - Confer with physician regarding placement of an indwelling Foley catheter (except when used to decrease intraocular pressure).
- **IV:** Administer by IV infusion undiluted. If solution contains crystals, warm bottle in hot water and shake vigorously. Do not administer solution in which crystals remain undissolved. Cool to body temperature. Use an in-line filter for 15%, 20%, and 25% infusions.
- **Test Dose:** Administer over 3–5 min to produce a urine output of 30–50 ml/hr. If urine flow does not increase, administer 2nd test dose. If urine output is not at least 30–50 ml/hr for 2–3 hr after 2nd test dose, patient should be re-evaluated.
- **Oliguria:** Administration rate should be titrated to produce a urine output of 30–50 ml/hr. Administer child's dose over 2–6 hr.
- **Increased Intracranial Pressure:** Infuse dose over 30–60 min in adults and children.
- **Intraocular Pressure:** Administer dose over 30 min. When used preoperatively, administer 60–90 min prior to surgery.
- **Y-Site Compatibility:** ▪ amifostine ▪ aztreonam ▪ fludarabine ▪ fluorouracil ▪ gallium nitrate ▪ idarubicin ▪ melphalan ▪ ondansetron ▪ paclitaxel ▪ piperacillin/tazobactam ▪ sargramostim ▪ teniposide ▪ thiotepa ▪ vinorelbine.
- **Y-Site Incompatibility:** ▪ cefepime ▪ filgrastim.

- **Irrigation:** Add contents of two 50-ml vials of 25% mannitol to 900 ml of sterile water for injection for a 2.5% solution for irrigation. Use only clear solutions.

PATIENT/FAMILY TEACHING

□ Explain purpose of therapy to patient.

EVALUATION

Effectiveness of therapy can be demonstrated by: ▪ Urine output of at least 30–50 ml/hr or an increase in urine output in accordance with parameters set by physician ▪ Reduction in intracranial pressure ▪ Reduction of intraocular pressure ▪ Excretion of certain toxic substances ▪ Irrigation during transurethral prostate resection.

MAPROTILINE

(ma-**proe**-ti-leen)
Ludiomil

CLASSIFICATION(S):
Antidepressant (tetracyclic)

Pregnancy Category B

INDICATIONS

▪ Depression and anxiety associated with depression (in conjunction with psychotherapy). **Unlabeled Uses:** ▪ Neurogenic pain.

ACTION

▪ Potentiates the effects of serotonin and norepinephrine ▪ Has significant anticholinergic properties. **Therapeutic Effects:** ▪ Antidepressant action, which may develop only over several weeks.

PHARMACOKINETICS

Absorption: Slowly but completely absorbed from the GI tract.
Distribution: Widely distributed. Probably crosses the placenta. Enters breast milk in concentrations similar to those in plasma.
Metabolism and Excretion: Slowly and extensively metabolized by the liver. Some conversion to active compounds; 30% excreted in the feces.
Half-life: 51 hr.

CONTRAINDICATIONS AND PRECAUTIONS

Contraindicated in: ▪ Narrow-angle glaucoma ▪ Pregnancy and lactation ▪ Acute myocardial infarction ▪ Seizure disorders (may lower seizure threshold) ▪ Some products contain tartrazine and should be avoided in patients with known intolerance.
Use Cautiously in: ▪ Geriatric patients (increased risk of adverse reactions; dosage reduction suggested) ▪ Patients with pre-existing cardiovascular disease ▪ Elderly men with prostatic hypertrophy (more susceptible to urinary retention).

ADVERSE REACTIONS AND SIDE EFFECTS*

CNS: SEIZURES, drowsiness, fatigue, lethargy, agitation, confusion, hallucinations.
EENT: blurred vision, dry eyes, dry mouth.
CV: ARRHYTHMIAS, hypotension, ECG changes.
GI: constipation, paralytic ileus.
GU: urinary retention.
Derm: photosensitivity.
Endo: gynecomastia.
Hemat: blood dyscrasias.

INTERACTIONS

Drug-Drug: ▪ May cause hyperpyrexia, seizures, hypertension, and death when used with **MAO inhibitors** (avoid concurrent use—discontinue 2 wk prior to maprotiline) ▪ May prevent the therapeutic response to **antihypertensives** ▪ Additive CNS depression with other **CNS depressants**, including **alcohol, antihistamines, opioid analgesics, clonidine**, and **sedative/hypnotics** ▪ Adrenergic effects may be additive with other **adrenergic agents**, including **vasoconstrictors** and **decongestants** ▪ Additive anticholinergic effects with other **drugs possessing anticholinergic properties**, including **antihistamines, atropine, haloperidol, phenothiazines, quinidine**, and **disopyramide** ▪ **Cimetidine, SSRI antidepressants**, or **oral contraceptives** increase levels and may cause toxicity ▪ **Sympathomimetics** increase risk of adverse cardiovascular reactions ▪ Increased risk of seizures with **phenothiazines.**

M

***CAPITALS indicate life-threatening; underlines indicate most frequent.**

ROUTE AND DOSAGE

- **PO (Adults):** 25–75 mg/day in divided doses initially; after 2 wk may increase by 25 mg/day (up to 150–225 mg/day); may be given as a single daily dose at bedtime when maintenance dose is determined.
- **PO (Geriatric Patients):** 25 mg/day initially; maintenance dose 50–75 mg/day.

AVAILABILITY

- ***Tablets:*** 25 mg[Rx], 50 mg[Rx], 75 mg[Rx].

TIME/ACTION PROFILE (antidepressant effect)

	ONSET	PEAK	DURATION
PO	3–7 days	1–3 wk	UK

NURSING IMPLICATIONS

ASSESSMENT

- □ Assess mental status frequently. Confusion, agitation, and hallucinations may occur during initiation of therapy and may require dosage reduction. Monitor mood changes. Assess for suicidal tendencies, especially during early therapy. Restrict amount of drug available to patient.
- □ Monitor blood pressure and pulse rate periodically during initial therapy. Report significant changes.
- □ Monitor for seizure activity in patients with a history of convulsions or alcohol abuse. Institute seizure precautions.
- ***Lab Test Considerations:*** Assess CBC and hepatic function prior to and periodically during therapy.

POTENTIAL NURSING DIAGNOSES

- Coping, ineffective individual (Indications).
- Anxiety (Indications).
- Knowledge deficit, related to medication regimen (Patient/Family Teaching).

IMPLEMENTATION

- **General Info:** May be given as a single dose at bedtime to minimize excessive drowsiness or dizziness.

PATIENT/FAMILY TEACHING

- □ Instruct patient to take medication exactly as directed. If a dose is missed, take as soon as remembered; if almost time for next dose, skip missed dose and return to regular schedule. If single bedtime dose regimen is used, do not take missed dose in morning; consult health care professional. Do not discontinue abruptly; gradual dosage reduction may be required.
- □ May cause drowsiness and blurred vision. Caution patient to avoid driving and other activities requiring alertness until response to drug is known.
- □ Caution patient to change positions slowly to minimize orthostatic hypotension.
- □ Advise patient to avoid alcohol or other CNS depressant drugs during and for at least 3–7 days after therapy has been discontinued.
- □ Advise patient to notify health care professional if dry mouth, urinary retention, or constipation occurs. Frequent rinses, good oral hygiene, and sugarless candy or gum may diminish dry mouth. An increase in fluid intake, fiber, and exercise may prevent constipation. Constipation may lead to paralytic ileus.
- □ Caution patient to use sunscreen and protective clothing to prevent photosensitivity reactions.
- □ Inform patient of need to monitor dietary intake. Increase in appetite may lead to undesired weight gain.
- □ Advise patient to consult health care professional before taking any OTC cold remedies with this medication.
- □ Advise patient to notify health care professional of medication regimen prior to treatment or surgery.
- □ Therapy for depression may be prolonged. Emphasize the importance of follow-up exams to monitor effectiveness and side effects.

EVALUATION

Effectiveness of therapy can be demonstrated by: ▪ Resolution of the symptoms of depression: □ Increased sense of well-being □ Renewed interest in surroundings □ Increased appetite □ Improved energy level □ Improved sleep ▪ Decrease in anxiety associated with depression. Therapeutic effects are sometimes seen in 3–7 days, although 2–3 wk are usually necessary before improvement is observed.

MAST CELL STABILIZERS

cromolyn†

Intal, Nasalcrom, {Rynacrom}

nedocromil

(ne-doe-**kroe**-mil)

Tilade

CLASSIFICATION(S):

Antihistamines

Pregnancy Category B

†For ophthalmic use, see ophthalmologic table on page 1114. For oral use, see infrequently used drug table on page 1129.

INDICATIONS

▪ Adjunct in the prophylaxis (long-term control) of allergic disorders including rhinitis and asthma ▪ Prevention of exercise-induced bronchospasm.

ACTION

▪ Prevents the release of histamine and slow-reacting substance of anaphylaxis (SRS-A) from sensitized mast cells. **Therapeutic Effects:** ▪ Decreased frequency and intensity of allergic reactions.

PHARMACOKINETICS

Absorption: *Cromolyn*—Poorly absorbed; action is local. Small amounts may reach systemic circulation after inhalation. *Nedocromil*—90% of the inhaled dose is swallowed; 2.5–3% of swallowed drug is absorbed. Inhaled drug that reaches the lung is completely absorbed (total bioavailability is 6–9%).

Distribution: Because only small amounts are absorbed, distribution of these agents is not known. They do not cross biologic membranes well and their action is primarily local.

Metabolism and Excretion: Small amounts absorbed are excreted unchanged in bile and urine.

Half-life: *Cromolyn*—80 min; *nedocromil*—1.5–2.3 hr.

CONTRAINDICATIONS AND PRECAUTIONS

Contraindicated in: ▪ Hypersensitivity ▪ Acute attacks of asthma (inhalation products).

Use Cautiously in: ▪ *Cromolyn*—Children <2 yr (safety not established) ▪ *Nedocromil*—Children <12 yr (safety not established) ▪ Will not relieve and may worsen acute attacks of bronchospasm (inhalation) ▪ Pregnancy and lactation (safety not established).

ADVERSE REACTIONS AND SIDE EFFECTS*

CNS: headache.

EENT: *intranasal*—nasal irritation, sneezing.

Resp: *inhalation*—irritation of the throat and trachea, bronchospasm, cough.

GI: unpleasant taste.

Derm: erythema, rash, urticaria.

Misc: allergic reactions including ANAPHYLAXIS or worsening of conditions being treated.

INTERACTIONS

Drug-Drug: ▪ None significant.

ROUTE AND DOSAGE

❑ **Cromolyn**

- **Inhalation (Adults and Children >5 yr):** 20-mg inhaler capsules or nebulizer solution or 2 sprays (0.8 mg/spray) as aerosol 4 times daily. For prevention of bronchospasm, use 2 aerosol sprays 10–15 min before exposure to known precipitating situation.
- **Intranasal (Adults and Children >6 yr):** 1 spray (5.2 mg/spray) each nostril 3–4 times daily (up to 6 times daily).

❑ **Nedocromil**

- **Inhalation (Adults and Children ≥6 yr):** 2 sprays (1.75 mg/spray) 4 times daily; decrease to 2–3 times daily as allowed. For prevention of bronchospasm, use 4 sprays up to 30 min before exposure to known precipitating situation (unlabeled).

AVAILABILITY

❑ **Cromolyn**

- ***Capsules for inhalation:*** 20 mg[Rx]
- ***Solution for nebulization:*** 20 mg/2 ml[Rx]

M

{} = Available in Canada only.

*CAPITALS indicate life-threatening; underlines indicate most frequent.

▪ ***Aerosol spray for inhalation:*** 800 mcg/spray in 8.1-g (112 sprays) or 14.2-g (≥200 sprays) containers[Rx] ▪ ***Nasal solution:*** 40 mg/ml (5.2 mg/spray) in 13-ml (≥100 sprays) or 26-ml (≥200 sprays) containers[OTC] ▪ ***Nasal insufflation:*** {10 mg/cartridge[Rx]}.

❑ **Nedocromil**

▪ ***Aerosol for inhalation:*** 1.75 mg/spray in 16.2-g canister (at least 112 inhalations)[Rx].

TIME/ACTION PROFILE (effects on symptoms)

	ONSET	PEAK	DURATION
Cromolyn—inhalation	<1 wk	2–4 wk	UK
Cromolyn—nasal	<1 wk	2–4 wk	UK
Nedocromil—inhalation	within 2 wk	UK	UK

NURSING IMPLICATIONS

ASSESSMENT

- **Inhalation:** Pulmonary function testing should be evaluated prior to initiating therapy in asthmatics.
- □ Assess lung sounds and respiratory function prior to and periodically throughout therapy.
- **Intranasal:** Assess for symptoms of rhinitis (stuffiness, rhinorrhea).

POTENTIAL NURSING DIAGNOSES

- Airway clearance, ineffective (Indications).
- Knowledge deficit, related to medication regimen (Patient/Family Teaching).

IMPLEMENTATION

- **General Info:** Reduction in dosage of other asthma medications may be possible after 2–4 wk of therapy.
- **Inhalation:** Medication should be used prophylactically, not during acute asthma attacks or status asthmaticus.
- □ Pretreatment with bronchodilator may be required to increase delivery of inhalation product.
- □ Do not use solution that is cloudy or contains a precipitate. Compatible with acetylcysteine, albuterol, epinephrine, isoetharine, isoproterenol, preservative-free ipratropium, metaproterenol, and terbutaline solutions for up to 60 min.
- □ Incompatible with bitolterol.

PATIENT/FAMILY TEACHING

- **General Info:** Medication must be used routinely and not more frequently than prescribed. If a dose is missed, take as soon as remembered and space other doses at regular intervals. Do not double doses. Do not discontinue therapy without consulting health care professional, or exacerbation of symptoms may occur.
- □ Instruct patient not to discontinue concurrent glucocorticoid or bronchodilator therapy without consulting health care professional.
- □ If cromolyn is prescribed before contact with known allergen or exercise, explain that it should be administered 10–15 min, and no earlier than 60 min, in advance.
- **Inhalation:** Inform patient that *Intal* capsules for inhalation are to be used for Spinhaler or Halermatic devices only.
- □ Instruct patient in the proper use of the metered-dose inhaler. See Appendix H for instructions.
- □ Advise patient that gargling and rinsing the mouth after each dose helps to decrease dryness of mouth, throat irritation, and hoarseness.
- □ Caution patient to notify health care professional if asthmatic symptoms do not improve within 4 wk, worsen, or recur.
- **Intranasal:** Instruct patient to clear nasal passages prior to administration and to inhale through nose during administration.

EVALUATION

Therapeutic effects, observable within 2–4 wk after beginning therapy, are demonstrated by: ▪ Reduction in symptoms of asthma ▪ Prevention of exercise-induced bronchospasm ▪ Decrease in the symptoms of rhinitis.

MEBENDAZOLE
(me-**ben**-da-zole)
Vermox

CLASSIFICATION(S):
Antihelmintic

Pregnancy Category C

INDICATIONS

▪ Treatment of: □ Whipworm (trichuriasis) □ Pinworm (enterobiasis) ▫ Roundworm (ascariasis) ▫ Hookworm (uncinariasis) infections.

ACTION

▪ Inhibits the uptake of glucose and other nutrients by susceptible helminths. **Therapeutic Effects:** ▪ Death of parasites, eggs, and hydatid cysts (vermicidal and ovacidal).

PHARMACOKINETICS

Absorption: Minimally (2–10%) absorbed following oral administration.
Distribution: UK.
Metabolism and Excretion: >95% eliminated in feces. Absorbed drug is mostly metabolized by the liver; small amounts excreted unchanged by the kidneys.
Half-life: 2.5–9 hr (increased in liver impairment).

CONTRAINDICATIONS AND PRECAUTIONS

Contraindicated in: ▪ Hypersensitivity.
Use Cautiously in: ▪ Impaired liver function ▪ Crohn's ileitis ▪ Ulcerative colitis ▪ Pregnancy, lactation, or children <2 yr (safety not established).

ADVERSE REACTIONS AND SIDE EFFECTS

Most side effects and adverse reactions are seen with high-dose therapy only.
CNS: dizziness, headache.
EENT: tinnitus.
GI: abdominal pain, diarrhea, nausea, vomiting.
Hemat: reversible myelosuppression (leukopenia, thrombocytopenia).
Neuro: numbness.
Misc: fever.

INTERACTIONS

Drug-Drug: ▪ **Carbamazepine** and **phenytoin** may increase the metabolism and decrease effectiveness of therapy in patients receiving high-dose therapy.
Drug-Food: ▪ Absorption may be increased by **fatty foods.**

ROUTE AND DOSAGE

▫ Enterobiasis

▪ **PO (Adults and Children >2 yr):** 100 mg as a single dose; repeat in 2–3 wk.

▫ Trichuriasis, Ascariasis, Hookworm, or Mixed Infections

▪ **PO (Adults and Children >2 yr):** 100 mg twice daily for 3 days. If not cured in 2–3 wk, a 2nd course is given.

AVAILABILITY

▪ ***Chewable tablets:*** 100 mg[Rx].

TIME/ACTION PROFILE (blood levels)

	ONSET	PEAK	DURATION
PO	UK	2–5 hr	UK

NURSING IMPLICATIONS

ASSESSMENT

▪ **Pinworm:** Perianal examinations should be performed to detect the presence of adult worms in the perianal area, and cellophane tape swabs of the perianal area should be taken prior to and starting 1 wk following treatment to detect the presence of ova. Swabs should be taken each morning prior to defecation or bathing for at least 3 days. Patients are not considered cured unless perianal swabs have been negative for 7 days.
▪ **Roundworm:** Stool examinations should be monitored prior to and 1–3 wk following treatment.
▪ ***Lab Test Considerations:*** May cause transient increase in serum BUN, AST, ALT, and alkaline phosphatase levels.
▫ CBC should be monitored prior to therapy and 2–3 times a week from day 10–25 and weekly thereafter in patients receiving high-dose therapy. Mebendazole may cause reversible leukopenia and thrombocytopenia.
▫ May cause decreased serum hemoglobin concentrations.

POTENTIAL NURSING DIAGNOSES

▪ Infection, risk for (Indications).
▪ Home maintenance management, impaired (Indications).
▪ Knowledge deficit (Patient/Family Teaching).

IMPLEMENTATION

▪ **General Info:** No special diets, fasting, laxatives, or enemas are required prior to administration of mebendazole.

- **PO:** Mebendazole tablet may be chewed, swallowed whole, or crushed and mixed with food. Patients on high-dose therapy should take tablets with high-fat meals to increase absorption.
- **Pinworm:** All members of the household should be treated concurrently, with treatment repeated in 2–3 wk.
- **Hookworm and Whipworm:** Patient may be required to take an iron supplement daily during treatment and for 6 mo following treatment if anemia occurs.

PATIENT/FAMILY TEACHING

- **General Info:** Instruct patient to take medication exactly as directed and to continue medication for full course of therapy, even if feeling better. If a dose is missed, take as soon as remembered; if on 2 doses/day schedule, space missed dose and next dose 4–5 hr apart or double next dose. A 2nd course of therapy may be required.
- □ Advise patient of hygienic precautions to minimize reinfection (wash hands with soap prior to eating and after using the toilet, disinfect toilet daily, keep hands away from mouth, wash all fruits and vegetables, wear shoes).
- □ May cause dizziness. Caution patient to avoid driving or activities requiring alertness until response to medication is known.
- □ Advise patient to consult health care professional if no improvement is seen within a few days.
- □ Emphasize the importance of follow-up exams to determine effectiveness, especially with high-dose therapy.
- **Pinworm:** Instruct patient to wash (do not shake) all bedding, undergarments, towels, and nightclothes after treatment to prevent reinfection.

EVALUATION

Effectiveness of therapy can be demonstrated by: ▪ Resolution of the signs and symptoms of infection or when stool specimens and perianal swabs are negative. Length of time for complete resolution depends on the parasite.

MECHLORETHAMINE

(me-klor-**eth**-a-meen)

Mustargen, nitrogen mustard

CLASSIFICATION(S):

Antineoplastic (alkylating agent)

Pregnancy Category D

INDICATIONS

▪ Part of combination therapy of Hodgkin's disease and malignant lymphomas ▪ Used palliatively in: □ Bronchogenic carcinoma □ Leukemias ▪ Administered into cavities (pleural, peritoneal) to prevent reaccumulation of malignant effusions.

ACTION

▪ Interferes with DNA and RNA synthesis by cross-linking strands (cell-cycle phase–nonspecific). **Therapeutic Effects:** ▪ Death of rapidly replicating cells, particularly malignant ones.

PHARMACOKINETICS

Absorption: Administered IV and intracavitary only. Some absorption occurs following intracavitary instillation.
Distribution: UK.
Metabolism and Excretion: Rapidly degraded in body tissues and fluids.
Half-life: UK.

CONTRAINDICATIONS AND PRECAUTIONS

Contraindicated in: ▪ Hypersensitivity ▪ Pregnancy ▪ Lactation.
Use Cautiously in: ▪ Patients with childbearing potential ▪ Infections ▪ Decreased bone marrow reserve ▪ Geriatric patients or patients with chronic debilitating illnesses ▪ Prior radiotherapy or chemotherapy (dosage reduction required).

ADVERSE REACTIONS AND SIDE EFFECTS*

CNS: SEIZURES, drowsiness, headache, vertigo, weakness.
GI: nausea, vomiting, anorexia, diarrhea.

*CAPITALS indicate life-threatening; underlines indicate most frequent.

GU: gonadal suppression.
Derm: rashes, alopecia.
Hemat: LEUKOPENIA, THROMBOCYTOPENIA, anemia.
Local: tissue necrosis, phlebitis at IV site.
Metab: hyperuricemia.
Misc: reactivation of herpes zoster.

INTERACTIONS

Drug-Drug: ▪ Additive myelosuppression with other **antineoplastic agents** or **radiation therapy** ▪ May decrease antibody response to **live virus vaccines** and increase the risk of adverse reactions.

ROUTE AND DOSAGE

- **IV (Adults and Children):** 0.4 mg/kg as single dose or divided over 2–4 days (not to exceed 0.2–0.3 mg/kg in patients who have received previous chemotherapy or radiation therapy); *as part of MOPP regimen for Hodgkin's lymphoma in adults*—6 mg/m² on days 1 and 8 of 28-day cycle; doses in subsequent cycles are determined by blood counts.
- **Intracavitary (Adults):** *Intrapericardial*—0.2 mg/kg; *intracavitary*—0.4 mg/kg.

AVAILABILITY

- ***Injection:*** 10-mg vials[Rx].

TIME/ACTION PROFILE (effects on blood counts)

	ONSET	PEAK	DURATION
WBCs	24 hr	7–14 days	10–21 days
Platelets	UK	9–16 days	20 days

NURSING IMPLICATIONS

ASSESSMENT

- □ Monitor blood pressure, pulse, and respiratory rate frequently during administration. Report significant changes.
- □ Assess injection site frequently for redness, irritation, or inflammation. If extravasation occurs, infusion must be stopped and restarted elsewhere to avoid damage to SC tissue. Infiltrate affected area promptly with isotonic sodium thiosulfate 1% or lidocaine and apply ice compresses for 6–12 hr as directed by physician.
- □ Monitor intake and output, appetite, and nutritional intake. Nausea and vomiting may occur 1–3 hr after therapy. Vomiting may persist for 8 hr; nausea may last 24 hr. Parenteral antiemetic agents should be administered 30–45 min prior to therapy and routinely around the clock for the next 24 hr as indicated. Adjust diet as tolerated to help maintain fluid and electrolyte balance and nutritional status.
- □ Monitor for bone marrow depression. Assess for bleeding (bleeding gums, bruising, petechiae, guaiac stools, urine, and emesis) and avoid IM injections and rectal temperatures if platelet count is low. Apply pressure to venipuncture sites for 10 min. Assess for signs of infection during neutropenia. Anemia may occur. Monitor for increased fatigue, dyspnea, and orthostatic hypotension.
- □ Monitor for symptoms of gout (increased uric acid, joint pain, edema). Encourage patient to drink at least 2 liters of fluid each day. Allopurinol may be given to decrease uric acid levels. Alkalinization of urine may be ordered to increase excretion of uric acid.
- ▪ **Intracavitary:** Pain frequently occurs following intracavitary injection and may persist for 2–3 days. Assess pain frequently and treat with analgesics as required.
- ▪ ***Lab Test Considerations:*** Monitor CBC and differential prior to and periodically throughout therapy. The nadir of leukopenia occurs in 7–14 days. Notify physician if leukocyte count is <1000/mm³. The nadir of thrombocytopenia occurs in 9–16 days. Notify physician if platelet count is <75,000/mm³. Recovery from leukopenia and thrombocytopenia occurs in 20 days.
- □ Monitor liver function studies (AST, ALT, LDH, bilirubin) and renal function studies (BUN, creatinine) prior to and periodically throughout therapy to detect hepatotoxicity and nephrotoxicity.
- □ Monitor uric acid concentrations prior to and periodically during therapy. May cause increased serum and urine uric acid levels.

POTENTIAL NURSING DIAGNOSES

- ▪ Infection, risk for (Adverse Reactions).
- ▪ Nutrition, altered, less than body requirements (Adverse Reactions).
- ▪ Knowledge deficit, related to medication regimen (Patient/Family Teaching).

IMPLEMENTATION

- **General Info:** Solution should be prepared in a biologic cabinet. Wear gloves, gown, and mask while handling medication. All equipment in contact with this medication must be decontaminated prior to disposal. Soak gloves, IV tubing, syringes, etc., in solution of 5% sodium thiosulfate and 5% sodium bicarbonate for 45 min. Unused portions of the drug must be mixed with equal amounts of this solution.
  - Discard all contaminated equipment in specially designated containers. If medication comes in contact with skin, flush with large volume of water for 15 min, followed by a 2% sodium thiosulfate solution. If eye contact occurs, flush eye with 0.9% NaCl and notify physician immediately (see Appendix I).
- **Direct IV:** Discard vial if droplets of water appear to be present prior to reconstitution. Dilute each 10 mg with 10 ml of 0.9% NaCl or sterile water for injection. Do not remove the needle from the vial stopper prior to agitating solution. Allow solution to dissolve completely. Reconstituted solution decomposes in 15 min. Administer immediately. Do not use a discolored solution or one that contains precipitates.
- ***Rate:*** Withdraw desired amount of drug and administer over 3–5 min via Y-tubing into a free-flowing solution of 0.9% NaCl.
- **Y-Site Compatibility:** ▪ amifostine ▪ aztreonam ▪ filgrastim ▪ fludarabine ▪ granisetron ▪ melphalan ▪ ondansetron ▪ sargramostim ▪ teniposide ▪ vinorelbine.
- **Y-Site Incompatibility:** ▪ cefepime.
- **Intracavitary:** May be further diluted in 50–100 ml of 0.9% NaCl. Consult physician regarding analgesia and schedule for repositioning patient to ensure mechlorethamine comes in contact with entire cavity surface. Remaining fluid may be removed after 24–36 hr.

PATIENT/FAMILY TEACHING

- Instruct patient to notify health care professional promptly if fever; chills; cough; hoarseness; sore throat; signs of infection; lower back or side pain; painful or difficult urination; bleeding gums; bruising; petechiae; blood in stools, urine, or emesis; increased fatigue; dyspnea; or orthostatic hypotension occurs. Caution patient to avoid crowds and persons with known infections. Instruct patient to use soft toothbrush and electric razor and to avoid falls. Caution patient not to drink alcoholic beverages or take medication containing aspirin or NSAIDS; may precipitate gastric bleeding.
- This drug may cause irreversible gonadal suppression; however, patient should still use birth control during and for at least 4 mo after therapy, as drug may have teratogenic effects.
- Discuss with patient the possibility of hair loss. Explore methods of coping.
- Instruct patient not to receive any vaccinations without advice of health care professional.
- Instruct patient to notify health care professional if skin rash occurs. Rash may indicate idiosyncratic reaction or reactivation of herpes zoster.
- Emphasize the need for periodic lab tests to monitor for side effects.

EVALUATION

Effectiveness of therapy can be demonstrated by: ▪ Decrease in size or spread of malignancies in solid tumors ▪ Improvement of hematologic status in leukemias.

MECLIZINE

(**mek**-li-zeen)

Antivert, {Bonamine}, Dramamine II, D-Vert, Meni-D, Ru-vert M

CLASSIFICATION(S):
Antiemetic, Antihistamine

Pregnancy Category B

INDICATIONS

▪ Management/prevention of: □ Motion sickness □ Vertigo.

ACTION

▪ Has central anticholinergic, CNS depressant, and antihistaminic properties ▪ Decreases excitability of the middle ear labyrinth and depresses conduction in middle ear vestibular-cerebellar pathways. **Therapeutic Effects:** ▪ Decreased motion sickness ▪ Decreased vertigo due to vestibular pathology.

PHARMACOKINETICS

Absorption: Absorbed following oral administration.
Distribution: UK.
Metabolism and Excretion: UK.
Half-life: 6 hr.

CONTRAINDICATIONS AND PRECAUTIONS

Contraindicated in: ▪ Hypersensitivity ▪ Pregnancy.
Use Cautiously in: ▪ Prostatic hypertrophy ▪ Narrow-angle glaucoma ▪ Geriatric or very young patients (increased sensitivity; increased risk of adverse reactions) ▪ Children or lactation (safety not established).

ADVERSE REACTIONS AND SIDE EFFECTS*

CNS: drowsiness, fatigue.
EENT: blurred vision.
GI: dry mouth.

INTERACTIONS

Drug-Drug: ▪ Additive CNS depression with other **CNS depressants**, including **alcohol**, other **antihistamines, opioids,** and **sedative/hypnotics** ▪ Additive anticholinergic effects with other **drugs possessing anticholinergic properties**, including **antihistamines, antidepressants, atropine, haloperidol, phenothiazines, quinidine**, and **disopyramide.**

ROUTE AND DOSAGE

- **PO (Adults):** *Motion sickness*—25–50 mg 1 hr before exposure; may repeat in 24 hr. *Vertigo*—25–100 mg/day in divided doses.

AVAILABILITY

▪ ***Tablets:*** 12.5 mg[Rx], 25 mg[Rx,OTC], 50 mg[Rx] ▪ ***Chewable tablets:*** 25 mg[Rx,OTC] ▪ ***Capsules:*** 15 mg[OTC], 25 mg[Rx], 30 mg[OTC].

TIME/ACTION PROFILE (antihistaminic effects)

	ONSET	PEAK	DURATION
PO	1 hr	UK	8–24 hr

NURSING IMPLICATIONS

ASSESSMENT

- **General Info:** Assess patient for level of sedation following administration.
- **Motion Sickness:** Assess patient for nausea and vomiting prior to and 60 min following administration.
- **Vertigo:** Assess degree of vertigo periodically in patients receiving meclizine for labyrinthitis.
- ***Lab Test Considerations:*** May cause false-negative results in skin tests using allergen extracts. Discontinue meclizine 72 hr prior to testing.

POTENTIAL NURSING DIAGNOSES

- Injury, risk for (Side Effects).
- Knowledge deficit, related to medication regimen (Patient/Family Teaching).

IMPLEMENTATION

- **PO:** Administer oral doses with food, water, or milk to minimize GI irritation. Chewable tablet may be chewed or swallowed whole.

PATIENT/FAMILY TEACHING

- **General Info:** Instruct patient to take meclizine exactly as directed. If a dose is missed, take as soon as possible unless almost time for next dose. Do not double doses.
- □ May cause drowsiness. Caution patient to avoid driving or other activities requiring alertness until response to the medication is known.
- □ Advise patient that frequent mouth rinses, good oral hygiene, and sugarless gum or candy may decrease dryness of mouth.
- □ Caution patient to avoid concurrent use of alcohol and other CNS depressants with this medication.
- **Motion Sickness:** When used as prophylaxis for motion sickness, advise patient to take medication at least 1 hr prior to exposure to conditions that may cause motion sickness.

EVALUATION

Effectiveness of therapy can be demonstrated by: ▪ Prevention and relief of symptoms in motion sickness ▪ Prevention and treatment of vertigo due to vestibular pathology.

M

***CAPITALS indicate life-threatening; underlines indicate most frequent.**

MECLOFENAMATE
(me-kloe-**fen**-am-ate)
Meclofen, Meclomen

CLASSIFICATION(S):
Nonopioid analgesic/Nonsteroidal anti-inflammatory agent

Pregnancy Category B (first trimester)

INDICATIONS

■ Management of inflammatory disorders, including: □ Rheumatoid arthritis □ Osteoarthritis ■ Management of mild to moderate pain, including dysmenorrhea ■ Management of excessive menstrual flow.

ACTION

■ Inhibits prostaglandin synthesis. **Therapeutic Effects:** ■ Suppression of pain and inflammation.

PHARMACOKINETICS

Absorption: Well absorbed from the GI tract.
Distribution: UK.
Metabolism and Excretion: Mostly metabolized by the liver.
Half-life: 40 min–2 hr.

CONTRAINDICATIONS AND PRECAUTIONS

Contraindicated in: ■ Hypersensitivity ■ Cross-sensitivity may occur with other NSAIDs, including aspirin ■ Active GI bleeding or ulcer disease.
Use Cautiously in: ■ Severe cardiovascular, renal, or hepatic disease ■ History of ulcer disease ■ Pregnancy, lactation, or children <14 yr (safety not established; avoid use during 2nd half of pregnancy).

ADVERSE REACTIONS AND SIDE EFFECTS*

CNS: dizziness, headache, drowsiness.
EENT: tinnitus, visual disturbances.
CV: edema.
GI: GI BLEEDING, DRUG-INDUCED HEPATITIS, diarrhea, dyspepsia, nausea, vomiting, anorexia, constipation, discomfort, flatulence, stomatitis.
GU: renal failure.
Derm: hives, itching.
Hemat: blood dyscrasias.
Misc: allergic reactions including ANAPHYLAXIS and STEVENS-JOHNSON SYNDROME, drug-induced systemic lupus erythematosus–like syndrome.

INTERACTIONS

Drug-Drug: ■ Concurrent use with **aspirin** may decrease meclofenamate blood levels and may decrease effectiveness ■ May increase risk of bleeding with **anticoagulants, thrombolytics, cefamandole, cefoperazone, cefotetan, valproic acid,** or **plicamycin** ■ Additive adverse GI side effects with **aspirin, alcohol, glucocorticoids, potassium supplements,** and other **NSAIDs** ■ **Probenecid** increases blood levels and may increase toxicity ■ Chronic use with **acetaminophen** or **gold compounds** may increase the risk of adverse renal reactions ■ May decrease the effectiveness of **antihypertensive agents** or **diuretics** ■ May increase hypoglycemia from **oral hypoglycemic agents** or **insulin** ■ Increased risk of hematologic adverse reactions with **antineoplastic agents** or **radiation therapy** ■ May increase blood levels and toxicity of **lithium** or **methotrexate** ■ Increased risk of nephrotoxicity with **cyclosporine.**

ROUTE AND DOSAGE

■ **PO (Adults):** *Anti-inflammatory*—200–400 mg/day in 3–4 divided doses. *Analgesic*—50–100 mg q 4–6 hr. *Dysmenorrhea/excessive menstrual flow*—100 mg 3 times daily for up to 6 days.

AVAILABILITY

■ ***Capsules:*** 50 mg[Rx], 100 mg[Rx].

TIME/ACTION PROFILE

	ONSET	PEAK	DURATION
PO (analgesic)	within 1 hr	UK	4–6 hr
PO (anti-inflammatory)	days	2–3 wk	days

NURSING IMPLICATIONS

ASSESSMENT

■ **General Info:** Patients who have asthma, aspirin-induced allergy, and nasal polyps are at

*CAPITALS indicate life-threatening; underlines indicate most frequent.

increased risk for developing hypersensitivity reactions. Monitor for rhinitis, asthma, and urticaria.

- **Arthritis:** Assess pain and range of movement prior to and periodically during therapy.
- **Pain:** Assess location, duration, and intensity of pain prior to and 1 hr following administration.
- ***Lab Test Considerations:*** BUN, serum creatinine, CBC, and liver function tests should be evaluated periodically in patients receiving prolonged therapy.
- □ Serum potassium, BUN, serum creatinine, alkaline phosphatase, LDH, AST, and ALT tests may show increased levels. Hemoglobin and hematocrit concentrations, leukocyte and platelet counts, and CCr may be decreased.
- □ Effects on bleeding time are minimal.

POTENTIAL NURSING DIAGNOSES

- Pain (Indications).
- Physical mobility, impaired (Indications).
- Knowledge deficit, related to medication regimen (Patient/Family Teaching).

IMPLEMENTATION

- **General Info:** Administration in higher than recommended doses does not provide increased effectiveness but may cause increased side effects.
- □ Coadministration with opioid analgesics may have additive analgesic effects and may permit lower opioid doses.
- **PO:** For rapid initial effect, administer 30 min before or 2 hr after meals. May be administered with food, milk, or antacids to decrease GI irritation.
- **Dysmenorrhea:** Administer as soon as possible after the onset of menses. Prophylactic treatment has not been shown to be effective.

PATIENT/FAMILY TEACHING

- □ Advise patients to take this medication with a full glass of water and to remain in an upright position for 15–30 min after administration.
- □ Instruct patient to take medication exactly as directed. If a dose is missed, take as soon as remembered but not if almost time for next dose. Do not double doses.
- □ May occasionally cause drowsiness or dizziness. Advise patient to avoid driving or other activities requiring alertness until response to the medication is known.
- □ Caution patient to avoid the concurrent use of alcohol, aspirin, acetaminophen, or other OTC medications without consulting health care professional.
- □ Advise patient to inform health care professional of medication regimen prior to treatment or surgery.
- □ Caution patient to wear sunscreen and protective clothing to prevent photosensitivity reactions.
- □ Advise patient to consult health care professional if rash, itching, visual disturbances, tinnitus, weight gain, edema, black stools, persistent headache, or influenza-like syndrome (chills, fever, muscle aches, pain) occurs.

EVALUATION

Effectiveness of therapy can be demonstrated by: ▪ Decrease in severity of pain ▪ Improved joint mobility. Partial arthritic relief is usually seen within a few days, but maximum effectiveness may require 2–3 wk of continuous therapy. Patients who do not respond to one NSAID may respond to another ▪ Decrease in menstrual flow.

MEDROXYPROGESTERONE*

(me-**drox**-ee-proe-jess-te-rone)

Amen, Curretab, Cycrin, Depo-Provera, Provera

CLASSIFICATION(S):

Antineoplastic (hormone), Hormone (progestin)

Pregnancy Category D

*For contraceptive use, see page 226.

INDICATIONS

▪ Treatment of secondary amenorrhea and abnormal uterine bleeding caused by hormonal imbalance ▪ Treatment of advanced unresponsive endometrial or renal carcinoma. **Unlabeled Uses:** ▪ Obesity-hypoventilation (pickwickian) syndrome ▪ Sleep apnea ▪ Hypersomnolence.

ACTION

▪ A synthetic form of progesterone—actions include secretory changes in the endometrium, increases in basal body temperature, histologic changes in vaginal epithelium, relaxation of uterine smooth muscle, mammary alveolar tissue growth, pituitary inhibition, and withdrawal bleeding in the presence of estrogen. **Therapeutic Effects:** ▪ Restoration of hormonal balance with control of uterine bleeding ▪ Management of endometrial or renal cancer ▪ Prevention of pregnancy.

PHARMACOKINETICS

Absorption: 0.6–10% absorbed following oral administration.
Distribution: Enters breast milk.
Metabolism and Excretion: Metabolized by the liver.
Half-life: *1st phase*—52 min; *2nd phase*—230 min; *biological*—14.5 hr.

CONTRAINDICATIONS AND PRECAUTIONS

Contraindicated in: ▪ Hypersensitivity ▪ Hypersensitivity to parabens (IM suspension only) ▪ Pregnancy ▪ Missed abortion ▪ Thromboembolic disease ▪ Cerebrovascular disease ▪ Severe liver disease ▪ Breast or genital cancer ▪ Porphyria.
Use Cautiously in: ▪ History of liver disease ▪ Renal disease ▪ Cardiovascular disease ▪ Seizure disorders ▪ Mental depression ▪ Lactation (when used as a contraceptive, wait until 6 wk after delivery if breast-feeding).

ADVERSE REACTIONS AND SIDE EFFECTS*

CNS: depression.
EENT: retinal thrombosis.
CV: PULMONARY EMBOLISM, thromboembolism, thrombophlebitis.
GI: drug-induced hepatitis, gingival bleeding.
GU: cervical erosions.
Derm: chloasma, melasma, rashes.
Endo: amenorrhea, breakthrough bleeding, breast tenderness, changes in menstrual flow, galactorrhea, hyperglycemia, spotting.
F and E: edema.
Misc: allergic reactions including ANAPHYLAXIS and ANGIOEDEMA, weight gain, weight loss.

INTERACTIONS

Drug-Drug: ▪ May decrease the effectiveness of **bromocriptine** when used concurrently for galactorrhea/amenorrhea ▪ Contraceptive effectiveness may be decreased by **carbamazepine, phenobarbital, phenytoin, rifampin,** or **rifabutin** ▪ **Aminoglutethimide** may decrease oral absorption.

ROUTE AND DOSAGE

❑ Secondary Amenorrhea

- **PO (Adults):** 5–10 mg/day for 5–10 days; start at any time in cycle.

❑ Dysfunctional Uterine Bleeding/Induction of Menses

- **PO (Adults):** 5–10 mg/day for 5–10 days, starting on day 16 or day 21 of menstrual cycle.

❑ Renal or Endometrial Carcinoma

- **IM (Adults):** 400–1000 mg, may be repeated weekly; if improvement occurs, attempt to decrease dosage to 400 mg monthly.

AVAILABILITY

▪ ***Tablets:*** 2.5 mg^{Rx}, 5 mg^{Rx}, 10 mg^{Rx}, {100 mg^{Rx}} ▪ ***Suspension for depot injection:*** {50 mg/ml^{Rx}}, {100 mg/ml^{Rx}}, 150 mg/ml^{Rx}, 400 mg/ml^{Rx} ▪ ***In combination with:*** conjugated estrogens (Prempro, Premphase) in convenience packages^{Rx}. See Appendix A..

TIME/ACTION PROFILE (IM = antineoplastic effects)

	ONSET	PEAK	DURATION
PO	UK	UK	UK
IM	wks–mos	mo	UK†

†Contraceptive effect lasts 3 mo.

NURSING IMPLICATIONS

ASSESSMENT

- **General Info:** Monitor blood pressure periodically throughout therapy.
- ❑ Assess patient's usual menstrual history. Administration of drug may begin on any day of cycle in patients with amenorrhea and on day 16 or 21 of cycle in patients with dysfunctional bleeding.
- ❑ Monitor intake and output ratios and weekly

*CAPITALS indicate life-threatening; underlines indicate most frequent.

weight. Report significant discrepancies or steady weight gain.

- ***Lab Test Considerations:*** Monitor hepatic function prior to and periodically throughout therapy.
- □ May cause increased alkaline phosphatase levels. May decrease pregnanediol excretion concentrations.
- □ May cause increased serum concentrations of low-density lipoproteins (LDL) and decreased concentrations of high-density lipoproteins (HDL).
- □ May alter thyroid hormone assays.

POTENTIAL NURSING DIAGNOSES

- Sexual dysfunction (Indications).
- Tissue perfusion, altered (Side Effects).
- Knowledge deficit, related to medication regimen (Patient/Family Teaching).

IMPLEMENTATION

- **General Info:** Only the 150 mg/ml vial should be used for contraception.
- **IM:** Shake vial vigorously before preparing IM dose. Administer deep IM.
- □ In patients with cancer, IM dose may initially be required weekly. Once stabilized, IM dose may be required only monthly.

PATIENT/FAMILY TEACHING

- **General Info:** Explain the dosage schedule. Instruct patient to take medication at the same time each day. If a dose is missed, patient should make up dose as soon as remembered, but do not double doses.
- □ Advise patients receiving medroxyprogesterone for menstrual dysfunction to anticipate withdrawal bleeding 3–7 days after discontinuing medication.
- □ Review patient package insert (PPI) with patient. Emphasize the importance of notifying health care professional if the following side effects occur: visual changes, sudden weakness, incoordination, difficulty with speech, headache, leg or calf pain, shortness of breath, chest pain, changes in vaginal bleeding pattern, yellow skin, swelling of extremities, depression, or rash. Patients receiving medroxyprogesterone for cancer may not receive PPI.
- □ Advise patient to keep a 1-mo supply of medroxyprogesterone available at all times.
- □ Instruct patient in correct method of monthly breast self-examination. Increased breast tenderness may occur.
- □ Advise patient that gingival bleeding may occur. Instruct patient to use good oral hygiene and to receive regular dental care and examinations.
- □ Instruct patient to notify health care professional if menstrual period is missed or if pregnancy is suspected. Patient should not attempt conception for 3 mo after discontinuing medication in order to decrease risk to fetus.
- □ Medroxyprogesterone may cause melasma (brown patches of discoloration) on face when patient is exposed to sunlight. Advise patient to avoid sun exposure and to wear sunscreen or protective clothing when outdoors.
- □ Emphasize the importance of routine follow-up physical exams, including blood pressure; breast, abdomen, and pelvic exams; and PAP smears every 6–12 mo.

EVALUATION

Effectiveness of therapy can be demonstrated by: ▪ Regular menstrual periods ▪ Control of the spread of endometrial or renal cancer.

MEGESTROL

(me-**jess**-trole)
Megace

CLASSIFICATION(S):
Antineoplastic (hormone), Hormone (progestin)

Pregnancy Category D (tablets), X (suspension)

INDICATIONS

▪ Palliative treatment of endometrial and breast carcinoma, either alone or with surgery or radiation ▪ Treatment of anorexia, weight loss, and cachexia associated with AIDS.

ACTION

▪ Antineoplastic effect may result from inhibition of pituitary function. **Therapeutic Effects:** ▪ Regression of tumor ▪ Increased appetite and weight gain in patients with AIDS.

PHARMACOKINETICS

Absorption: Well absorbed from the GI tract.
Distribution: UK.
Metabolism and Excretion: Completely metabolized by the liver.
Half-life: 38 hr (range 13–104 hr).

CONTRAINDICATIONS AND PRECAUTIONS

Contraindicated in: ▪ Hypersensitivity ▪ Pregnancy, missed abortion, or lactation ▪ Undiagnosed vaginal bleeding ▪ Severe liver disease.
Use Cautiously in: ▪ Diabetes ▪ Mental depression ▪ Renal disease ▪ History of thrombophlebitis ▪ Cardiovascular disease ▪ Seizure disorders.

ADVERSE REACTIONS AND SIDE EFFECTS*

CV: THROMBOEMBOLISM, edema.
GI: GI irritation.
Derm: alopecia.
Hemat: thrombophlebitis.
MS: carpal tunnel syndrome.

INTERACTIONS

Drug-Drug: ▪ None significant.

ROUTE AND DOSAGE

- **PO (Adults):** *Breast carcinoma*—160 mg/day single dose or divided doses; *endometrial/ovarian carcinoma*—40–320 mg/day in divided doses; *anorexia associated with AIDS*—800 mg day; may decrease to 400 mg/day after 1 mo (range 400–800 mg/day).

AVAILABILITY

▪ ***Tablets:*** 20 mg[Rx], 40 mg[Rx] ▪ ***Oral suspension:*** 200 mg/5 ml[Rx].

TIME/ACTION PROFILE (antineoplastic activity)

	ONSET	PEAK	DURATION
PO	wk–mos	2 mo	UK

NURSING IMPLICATIONS

ASSESSMENT

- **General Info:** Assess patient for swelling, pain, or tenderness in legs. Report these signs of deep vein thrombophlebitis.
- **Anorexia:** Monitor weight, appetite, and nutritional intake in patients with AIDS.

POTENTIAL NURSING DIAGNOSES

- Knowledge deficit, related to medication regimen (Patient/Family Teaching).

IMPLEMENTATION

- **General Info:** Because of high dose, suspension is most convenient form for patients with AIDS.
- **PO:** May be administered with meals if GI irritation becomes a problem.

PATIENT/FAMILY TEACHING

- Instruct patient to take medication exactly as directed; do not skip or double up on missed doses. Missed doses may be taken as long as it is not right before next dose.
- Advise patient to report to health care professional any unusual vaginal bleeding.
- Advise patient that this medication may have teratogenic effects. Contraception should be used during therapy and for at least 4 mo after therapy is completed.
- Discuss with patient the possibility of hair loss. Explore methods of coping.

EVALUATION

Effectiveness of therapy can be demonstrated by: ▪ Slowing or arresting the spread of endometrial or breast malignancy. Therapeutic effects usually occur within 2 mo of initiating therapy ▪ Increased appetite and weight gain in patients with AIDS.

MELPHALAN

(**mel**-fa-lan)
Alkeran, L-PAM, phenylalanine mustard

CLASSIFICATION(S):
Antineoplastic (alkylating agent)

Pregnancy Category D

INDICATIONS

▪ Used alone or with other treatment modalities in the management of: □ Multiple myeloma □ Ovarian cancer. **Unlabeled Uses:** ▪ Breast

*CAPITALS indicate life-threatening; underlines indicate most frequent.

cancer ▪ Prostate cancer ▪ Testicular carcinoma ▪ Chronic myelogenous leukemia ▪ Osteogenic sarcoma.

ACTION

▪ Inhibits DNA and RNA synthesis by alkylation (cell-cycle phase–nonspecific). **Therapeutic Effects:** ▪ Death of rapidly replicating cells, particularly malignant ones ▪ Also has immunosuppressive properties.

PHARMACOKINETICS

Absorption: Incompletely and variably absorbed following oral administration.
Distribution: Rapidly distributed throughout total body water.
Protein Binding: ≤30%.
Metabolism and Excretion: Rapidly metabolized in the bloodstream. Small amounts (10%) excreted unchanged by the kidneys.
Half-life: 1.5 hr.

CONTRAINDICATIONS AND PRECAUTIONS

Contraindicated in: ▪ Hypersensitivity to melphalan or chlorambucil ▪ Pregnancy or lactation.
Use Cautiously in: ▪ Patients with childbearing potential ▪ Active infections ▪ Decreased bone marrow reserve ▪ Geriatric patients or patients with other chronic debilitating illnesses ▪ Impaired renal function (dose reduction recommended if BUN ≥30 mg/dl) ▪ Children (safety not established).

ADVERSE REACTIONS AND SIDE EFFECTS*

Resp: bronchopulmonary dysplasia, pulmonary fibrosis.
GI: diarrhea, nausea, stomatitis, vomiting.
GU: gonadal suppression.
Derm: alopecia, pruritus, rashes.
Endo: menstrual irregularities.
Hemat: leukopenia, thrombocytopenia, anemia.
Metab: hyperuricemia.
Misc: allergic reactions, including ANAPHYLAXIS.

INTERACTIONS

Drug-Drug: ▪ Additive bone marrow depression with other **antineoplastic agents** or **radiation therapy** ▪ May decrease antibody response to **live virus vaccines** and increase the risk of adverse reactions ▪ May increase the risk of pulmonary toxicity with **carmustine** ▪ Concurrent IV use with **cyclosporine** may increase the risk of renal failure ▪ Risk of enterocolitis may be increased with concurrent **nalidixic acid.**

ROUTE AND DOSAGE

❑ Multiple Myeloma

- **PO (Adults):** 150 mcg (0.15 mg)/kg/day for 7 days, followed by 3-wk rest, then 50 mcg (0.05 mg)/kg/day maintenance dose *or* 100–150 mcg/kg/day or 250 mg (0.25 mg)/kg/day for 4 days for 2–3 wk followed by 2–4-wk rest, then 2–4 mg/day maintenance dose *or* 7 mg/m² *or* 250 mcg (0.25 mg)/kg daily for 5 days q 5–6 wk.

❑ Ovarian Carcinoma

- **IV (Adults):** 16 mg/m² q 2 wk for 4 doses, then q 4 wk.
- **PO (Adults):** 200 mcg (0.2 mg)/kg/day for 5 days given every 4–5 wk.

AVAILABILITY

▪ ***Tablets:*** 2 mg[Rx] ▪ ***Powder for injection:*** 50 mg[Rx].

TIME/ACTION PROFILE (effects on blood counts)

	ONSET	PEAK	DURATION
PO	5 days	2–3 wk	5–6 wk

NURSING IMPLICATIONS

ASSESSMENT

- ❑ Assess for signs of infection (fever, chills, sore throat, cough, hoarseness, lower back or side pain, difficult or painful urination). Notify physician if these symptoms occur.
- ❑ Assess for bleeding (bleeding gums, bruising, petechiae, guaiac stools, urine, and emesis). Avoid IM injections and rectal temperatures. Apply pressure to venipuncture sites for 10 min.
- ❑ May cause nausea and vomiting. Monitor intake and output, appetite, and nutritional intake. Prophylactic antiemetics may be used. Adjust diet as tolerated.
- ❑ Monitor for symptoms of gout (increased uric acid, joint pain, edema). Encourage patient to

M

*CAPITALS indicate life-threatening; underlines indicate most frequent.

drink at least 2 liters of fluid per day. Allopurinol may be given to decrease uric acid levels.

- Anemia may occur. Monitor for increased fatigue and dyspnea.
- Assess patient for allergy to chlorambucil. Patients may have cross-sensitivity.
- ***Lab Test Considerations:*** Monitor CBC and differential weekly throughout therapy. The nadir of leukopenia occurs in 2–3 wk. Notify physician if leukocyte count is <3000/mm³. The nadir of thrombocytopenia occurs in 2–3 wk. Notify physician if platelet count is <100,000/mm³. Recovery of leukopenia and thrombocytopenia occurs in 5–6 wk.
- Monitor liver function studies (AST, ALT, LDH, bilirubin) and renal function studies (BUN, creatinine) prior to and periodically throughout therapy to detect hepatotoxicity and nephrotoxicity.
- May cause increased uric acid. Monitor periodically during therapy.
- May cause elevated 5-hydroxyindoleacetic acid (5-HIAA) concentrations as a result of tumor breakdown.

POTENTIAL NURSING DIAGNOSES

- Injury, risk for (Side Effects).
- Infection, risk for (Side Effects).
- Knowledge deficit, related to medication regimen (Patient/Family Teaching).

IMPLEMENTATION

- **General Info:** Solution should be prepared in a biologic cabinet. Wear gloves, gown, and mask while handling medication. Discard IV equipment in specially designated container (see Appendix I).
- If solution contacts skin or mucosa, immediately wash skin or mucosa with soap and water.
- **PO:** May be ordered in divided doses or as a single daily dose.
- **Intermittent Infusion:** Reconstitute with 10 ml of diluent supplied for a concentration of 5 mg/ml and shake vigorously until solution is clear. Dilute dose immediately with 0.9% NaCl for a concentration of ≤0.45 mg/ml. Administer within 60 min of reconstitution.
- ***Rate:*** Administer over at least 15 min.
- **Y-Site Compatibility:** ▪ acyclovir ▪ amikacin ▪ aminophylline ▪ ampicillin ▪ aztreonam ▪ bleomycin ▪ bumetanide ▪ buprenorphine ▪ butorphanol ▪ calcium gluconate ▪ carboplatin ▪ carmustine ▪ cefazolin ▪ cefoperazone ▪ cefotaxime ▪ cefotetan ▪ ceftazidime ▪ ceftizoxime ▪ ceftriaxone ▪ cefuroxime ▪ cimetidine ▪ cisplatin ▪ clindamycin ▪ cyclophosphamide ▪ cytarabine ▪ dacarbazine ▪ dactinomycin ▪ daunorubicin ▪ dexamethasone ▪ diphenhydramine ▪ doxorubicin ▪ doxycycline ▪ droperidol ▪ enalaprilat ▪ etoposide ▪ famotidine ▪ floxuridine ▪ fluconazole ▪ fludarabine ▪ fluorouracil ▪ furosemide ▪ gallium nitrate ▪ ganciclovir ▪ gentamicin ▪ haloperidol ▪ heparin ▪ hydrocortisone ▪ hydromorphone ▪ idarubicin ▪ ifosfamide ▪ imipenem/cilastatin ▪ lorazepam ▪ mannitol ▪ mechlorethamine ▪ meperidine ▪ mesna ▪ methotrexate ▪ metoclopramide ▪ metronidazole ▪ miconazole ▪ minocycline ▪ mitomycin ▪ mitoxantrone ▪ morphine ▪ nalbuphine ▪ netilmicin ▪ ondansetron ▪ pentostatin ▪ piperacillin ▪ plicamycin ▪ potassium chloride ▪ prochlorperazine edisylate ▪ promethazine ▪ ranitidine ▪ sodium bicarbonate ▪ streptozocin ▪ teniposide ▪ thiotepa ▪ ticarcillin ▪ ticarcillin/clavulanate ▪ tobramycin ▪ trimethoprim/sulfamethoxazole ▪ vancomycin ▪ vinblastine ▪ vincristine ▪ vinorelbine ▪ zidovudine.
- **Y-Site Incompatibility:** ▪ amphotericin B ▪ chlorpromazine.

PATIENT/FAMILY TEACHING

- Instruct patient to take melphalan exactly as directed, even if nausea and vomiting occur. If vomiting occurs shortly after dose is taken, consult health care professional. If a dose is missed, do not take at all.
- Advise patient to notify physician if fever; chills; dyspnea; persistent cough; sore throat; signs of infection; bleeding gums; bruising; petechiae; or blood in urine, stool, or emesis occurs. Caution patient to avoid crowds and persons with known infections. Instruct patient to use soft toothbrush and electric razor. Caution patient not to drink alcoholic beverages or take products containing aspirin or NSAIDs.
- Instruct patient to notify health care professional if rash, itching, joint pain, or swelling occurs.
- Instruct patient to inspect oral mucosa for

redness and ulceration. If ulceration occurs, advise patient to use sponge brush and to rinse mouth with water after eating and drinking. Consult physician if pain interferes with eating. Stomatitis pain may require treatment with opioid analgesics.

- Advise patient that, although fertility may be decreased, contraception should be used during melphalan therapy because of potential teratogenic effects on the fetus.
- Instruct patient not to receive any vaccinations without advice of health care professional.
- Emphasize need for periodic lab tests to monitor for side effects.

EVALUATION

Effectiveness of therapy can be demonstrated by: ▪ Decrease in size and spread of malignant tissue.

MEPERIDINE

(me-**per**-i-deen)
Demerol, pethidine

CLASSIFICATION(S):
Opioid analgesic (agonist)

Schedule II
Pregnancy Category B (routine use)

INDICATIONS

▪ Moderate or severe pain (alone or with non-opioid agents) ▪ Anesthesia adjunct ▪ Analgesic during labor ▪ Preoperative sedation. **Unlabeled Uses:** ▪ Rigors.

ACTION

▪ Binds to opiate receptors in the CNS. Alters the perception of and response to painful stimuli, while producing generalized CNS depression. **Therapeutic Effects:** ▪ Decrease in severity of pain.

PHARMACOKINETICS

Absorption: 50% from the GI tract; well absorbed from IM sites. Oral and parenteral doses are not equal.
Distribution: Widely distributed. Crosses the placenta; enters breast milk.
Metabolism and Excretion: Mostly metabolized by the liver; some converted to normeperidine, which may accumulate and cause seizures. 5% excreted unchanged by the kidneys.
Half-life: 3–5 hr (prolonged in impaired renal or hepatic function).

CONTRAINDICATIONS AND PRECAUTIONS

Contraindicated in: ▪ Hypersensitivity ▪ Hypersensitivity to bisulfites (some injectable products) ▪ Pregnancy or lactation (chronic use) ▪ Recent (14–21 days) MAO inhibitor therapy.
Use Cautiously in: ▪ Head trauma ▪ Increased intracranial pressure ▪ Severe renal, hepatic, or pulmonary disease ▪ Hypothyroidism ▪ Adrenal insufficiency ▪ Alcoholism ▪ Geriatric or debilitated patients (dosage reduction suggested) ▪ Undiagnosed abdominal pain or prostatic hyperplasia ▪ Labor (respiratory depression may occur in the newborn) ▪ Patients with renal impairment, extensive burns ▪ High dose or prolonged therapy (>600 mg/day or >2 days; increased risk of CNS stimulation due to accumulation of normeperidine) ▪ Children (increased risk of seizures due to accumulation of normeperidine).

ADVERSE REACTIONS AND SIDE EFFECTS*

CNS: SEIZURES, <u>confusion</u>, <u>sedation</u>, dysphoria, euphoria, floating feeling, hallucinations, headache, unusual dreams.
EENT: blurred vision, diplopia, miosis.
Resp: respiratory depression.
CV: <u>hypotension</u>, bradycardia.
GI: <u>constipation</u>, <u>nausea</u>, <u>vomiting</u>.
GU: urinary retention.
Derm: flushing, sweating.
Misc: physical dependence, psychological dependence, tolerance.

INTERACTIONS

Drug-Drug: ▪ Use with extreme caution in patients receiving **MAO inhibitors** or **procarbazine** (may cause fatal reaction—contraindicated within 14–21 days of MAO inhibitor therapy) ▪ Additive CNS depression with **alcohol, antihistamines,** and **sedative/hypnotics** ▪ Administration of **partial-antagonist opioid analgesics** may precipitate opioid withdrawal in

***CAPITALS indicate life-threatening; <u>underlines</u> indicate most frequent.**

M

physically dependent patients ▪ **Nalbuphine** or **pentazocine** may decrease analgesia.

ROUTE AND DOSAGE

- **PO, IM, SC (Adults):** *Analgesia*—50–150 mg q 3–4 hr. *Analgesia during labor*—50–100 mg IM or SC when contractions become regular; may repeat q 1–3 hr. *Preoperative sedation*—50–100 mg IM or SC 30–90 min before anesthesia.
- **PO, IM, SC (Children):** *Analgesia*—1–1.8 mg/kg q 3–4 hr (should not exceed 100 mg/dose). *Preoperative sedation*—1–2.2 mg/kg 30–90 min before anesthesia (not to exceed adult dose).
- **IV (Adults):** 15–35 mg/hr as a continuous infusion.

AVAILABILITY

▪ ***Tablets:*** 50 mg[Rx], 100 mg[Rx] ▪ ***Syrup:*** 50 mg/5 ml[Rx] ▪ ***Injection:*** {10 mg/ml[Rx]}, 25 mg/ml[Rx], 50 mg/ml[Rx], 75 mg/ml[Rx], 100 mg/ml[Rx] ▪ ***In combination with:*** promethazine (Mepergan) and atropine[Rx]. See Appendix A.

TIME/ACTION PROFILE (analgesia)

	ONSET	PEAK	DURATION
PO	15 min	60 min	2–4 hr
IM	10–15 min	30–50 min	2–4 hr
SC	10–15 min	40–60 min	2–4 hr
IV	immediate	5–7 min	2–4 hr

NURSING IMPLICATIONS

ASSESSMENT

- Assess type, location, and intensity of pain prior to and 1 hr following PO, SC, and IM doses and 5 min (peak) following IV administration. When titrating opioid doses, increases of 25–50% should be administered until there is either a 50% reduction in the patient's pain rating on a numerical or visual analogue scale or the patient reports satisfactory pain relief. A repeat dose can be safely administered at the time of the peak if previous dose is ineffective and side effects are minimal.
- An equianalgesic chart (see Appendix B) should be used when changing routes or when changing from one opioid to another.
- Assess blood pressure, pulse, and respirations before and periodically during administration. If respiratory rate is <10/min, assess level of sedation. Dose may need to be decreased by 25–50%. Initial drowsiness will diminish with continued use.
- Assess bowel function routinely. Prevention of constipation should be instituted with increased intake of fluids and bulk and with laxatives to minimize constipating effects. Stimulant laxatives should be administered routinely if opioid use exceeds 2–3 days, unless contraindicated.
- Prolonged use may lead to physical and psychological dependence and tolerance. This should not prevent patient from receiving adequate analgesia. Most patients who receive meperidine for pain do not develop psychological dependence. Progressively higher doses may be required to relieve pain with long-term therapy.
- Monitor patients on chronic or high-dose therapy for CNS stimulation (restlessness, irritability, seizures) due to accumulation of normeperidine metabolite. Risk of toxicity increases with doses >600 mg/24 hr, chronic administration (>2 days), and renal impairment.
- ***Lab Test Considerations:*** May increase plasma amylase and lipase concentrations.
- ***Toxicity and Overdose:*** If an opioid antagonist is required to reverse respiratory depression or coma, naloxone (Narcan) is the antidote. Dilute the 0.4-mg ampule of naloxone in 10 ml of 0.9% NaCl and administer 0.5 ml (0.02 mg) by direct IV push every 2 min. For children and patients weighing <40 kg, dilute 0.1 mg of naloxone in 10 ml of 0.9% NaCl for a concentration of 10 mcg/ml and administer 0.5 mcg/kg every 1–2 min. Titrate dose to avoid withdrawal, seizures, and severe pain. In patients receiving meperidine chronically, naloxone may precipitate seizures by eliminating the effects of meperidine, allowing the convulsant activity of normeperidine to predominate. Monitor patient closely.

POTENTIAL NURSING DIAGNOSES

- Pain (Indications).
- Sensory-perceptual alterations: visual, auditory (Side Effects).
- Injury, risk for (Side Effects).

IMPLEMENTATION

- **General Info:** Do not confuse with morphine or hydromorphine; fatalities have occurred.
- □ Explain therapeutic value of medication prior to administration to enhance the analgesic effect.
- □ Regularly administered doses may be more effective than prn administration. Analgesic is more effective if given before pain becomes severe.
- □ Coadministration with nonopioid analgesics may have additive analgesic effects and permit lower doses.
- □ Oral dose is <50% as effective as parenteral. When changing to oral administration, dose may need to be increased (see Appendix B).
- □ Medication should be discontinued gradually after long-term use to prevent withdrawal symptoms.
- □ May be administered via patient-controlled analgesia (PCA) pump.
- **PO:** Doses may be administered with food or milk to minimize GI irritation. Syrup should be diluted in half-full glass of water.
- **IM:** Administration of repeated SC doses may cause local irritation.
- **Direct IV:** Dilute to a concentration of 10 mg/ml with sterile water or 0.9% NaCl for injection.
- ***Rate:*** Administer slowly. Rapid administration may lead to increased respiratory depression, hypotension, and circulatory collapse.
- **Continuous Infusion:** Dilute to a concentration of 1 mg/ml with D5W, D10W, dextrose/saline combinations, dextrose/Ringer's or lactated Ringer's injection combinations, 0.45% NaCl, 0.9% NaCl, or Ringer's or lactated Ringer's solution. Administer via infusion pump. Titrate according to patient needs.
- **Syringe Compatibility:** ▪ atropine ▪ benzquinamide ▪ chlorpromazine ▪ dimenhydrinate ▪ diphenhydramine ▪ droperidol ▪ glycopyrrolate ▪ hydroxyzine ▪ metoclopramide ▪ midazolam ▪ perphenazine ▪ prochlorperazine ▪ promazine ▪ promethazine ▪ scopolamine.
- **Syringe Incompatibility:** ▪ heparin ▪ pentobarbital.
- **Y-Site Compatibility:** ▪ amifostine ▪ amikacin ▪ ampicillin ▪ ampicillin/sulbactam ▪ atenolol ▪ aztreonam ▪ bumetanide ▪ cefamandole ▪ cefazolin ▪ cefotaxime ▪ cefotetan ▪ cefoxitin ▪ ceftazidime ▪ ceftizoxime ▪ ceftriaxone ▪ cefuroxime ▪ cephalothin ▪ cephapirin ▪ chloramphenicol ▪ clindamycin ▪ dexamethasone ▪ diltiazem ▪ diphenhydramine ▪ dobutamine ▪ dopamine ▪ doxycycline ▪ droperidol ▪ erythromycin lactobionate ▪ famotidine ▪ filgrastim ▪ fluconazole ▪ fludarabine ▪ gallium nitrate ▪ gentamicin ▪ heparin ▪ hydrocortisone sodium succinate ▪ insulin ▪ kanamycin ▪ labetalol ▪ lidocaine ▪ magnesium sulfate ▪ melphalan ▪ methyldopate ▪ methylprednisolone ▪ metoclopramide ▪ metoprolol ▪ metronidazole ▪ ondansetron ▪ oxacillin ▪ oxytocin ▪ paclitaxel ▪ penicillin G potassium ▪ piperacillin ▪ piperacillin/tazobactam ▪ potassium chloride ▪ propranolol ▪ ranitidine ▪ sargramostim ▪ teniposide ▪ thiotepa ▪ ticarcillin ▪ ticarcillin/clavulanate ▪ tobramycin ▪ trimethoprim/sulfamethoxazole ▪ vancomycin ▪ verapamil ▪ vinorelbine.
- **Y-Site Incompatibility:** ▪ cefepime ▪ cefoperazone ▪ idarubicin ▪ imipenem/cilastatin ▪ mezlocillin ▪ minocycline.

PATIENT/FAMILY TEACHING

- □ Instruct patient on how and when to ask for pain medication.
- □ Instruct patient to take meperidine exactly as directed. If dose is less effective after a few weeks, do not increase dose without consulting health care professional.
- □ May cause drowsiness or dizziness. Advise patient to call for assistance when ambulating or smoking. Caution patient to avoid driving or other activities requiring alertness until response to medication is known.
- □ Advise patient to change positions slowly to minimize orthostatic hypotension.
- □ Instruct patient to avoid concurrent use of alcohol or other CNS depressants.
- □ Advise ambulatory patients that nausea and vomiting may be decreased by lying down.
- □ Encourage patient to turn, cough, and breathe deeply every 2 hr to prevent atelectasis.

M

EVALUATION

Effectiveness of therapy can be demonstrated by: ▪ Decrease in severity of pain without a significant alteration in level of consciousness or respiratory status.

MEROPENEM
(mer-oh-**pen**-nem)
Merrem

CLASSIFICATION(S):
Anti-infective (carbapenem)

Pregnancy Category B

INDICATIONS
▪ Treatment of: ▫ Intra-abdominal infections ▫ Bacterial meningitis in pediatric patients ≥3 mo. **Unlabeled Uses:** ▪ ▫ Febrile neutropenia ▫ Hospital-acquired pneumonia and sepsis.

ACTION
▪ Binds to bacterial cell wall, resulting in cell death. **Therapeutic Effects:** ▪ Bactericidal action against susceptible bacteria. **Spectrum:** ▪ Active against the following gram-positive organisms: ▫ *Streptococcus pneumoniae* ▫ Viridans group streptococci ▪ Also active against the following gram-negative pathogens: ▫ *Escherichia coli* ▫ *Haemophilus influenzae* ▫ *Klebsiella pneumoniae* ▫ *Neisseria meningitidis* ▫ *Pseudomonas aeruginosa* ▪ Active against the following anaerobes: ▫ *Bacteroides fragilis* ▫ *Bacteroides thetaiotaomicron* ▫ *Peptostreptococcus* spp.

PHARMACOKINETICS
Absorption: IV administration results in complete bioavailability.
Distribution: Widely distributed into body tissues and fluids; enters CSF in bactericidal levels when meninges are inflamed.
Metabolism and Excretion: 65–83% excreted unchanged by the kidneys.
Half-life: 1 hr (increased in renal impairment).

CONTRAINDICATIONS AND PRECAUTIONS
Contraindicated in: ▪ Hypersensitivity to meropenem or imipenem ▪ Serious hypersensitivity to other beta-lactams (penicillins or cephalosporins; cross-sensitivity may occur).
Use Cautiously in: ▪ Renal impairment (increased risk of thrombocytopenia and seizures; dosage reduction recommended if CCr <50 ml/min) ▪ History of seizures, brain lesions, or meningitis ▪ Pregnancy, lactation, or children <3 mo (safety not established).

ADVERSE REACTIONS AND SIDE EFFECTS*
CNS: SEIZURES, dizziness, headache.
Resp: APNEA.
GI: PSEUDOMEMBRANOUS COLITIS, constipation, diarrhea, glossitis (↑ in children), nausea, thrush (↑ in children), vomiting.
Derm: moniliasis (children only), pruritus, rash.
Local: inflammation at injection site, phlebitis.

INTERACTIONS
Drug-Drug: ▪ **Probenecid** decreases renal excretion and increases blood levels (coadministration not recommended).

ROUTE AND DOSAGE
- **IV (Adults):** 1 g q 8 hr.
- **IV (Children ≥3 mo–12 yr):** *Intra-abdominal infections*—20 mg/kg q 8 hr; *meningitis*—40 mg/kg q 8 hr.

AVAILABILITY
▪ ***Powder for injection:*** 500 mg in 20- and 100-ml vials and 15-ml ADD-Vantage vials[Rx], 1 g in 30- and 100-ml vials and 15-ml ADD-Vantage vials[Rx].

TIME/ACTION PROFILE (blood levels)

	ONSET	PEAK	DURATION
IV	rapid	end of infusion	8 hr

NURSING IMPLICATIONS

ASSESSMENT
- ▫ Assess patient for infection (vital signs; appearance of wound, sputum, urine, and stool; WBC) at beginning of and throughout therapy.
- ▫ Obtain a history before initiating therapy to determine previous use of and reactions to penicillins. Persons with a negative history of penicillin sensitivity may still have an allergic response.
- ▫ Obtain specimens for culture and sensitivity prior to initiating therapy. First dose may be given before receiving results.

*CAPITALS indicate life-threatening; underlines indicate most frequent.

- □ Observe patient for signs and symptoms of anaphylaxis (rash, pruritus, laryngeal edema, wheezing). Discontinue the drug and notify physician immediately if these symptoms occur. Have epinephrine, an antihistamine, and resuscitative equipment close by in the event of an anaphylactic reaction.
- □ Assess injection site for phlebitis, pain, and swelling periodically during administration.
- ■ ***Lab Test Considerations:*** Monitor hematologic, hepatic, and renal functions periodically during therapy.
- □ BUN, AST, ALT, LDH, serum alkaline phosphatase, bilirubin, and creatinine may be transiently increased.
- □ Hemoglobin, hematocrit, and WBC concentrations may be decreased.
- □ May cause positive direct or indirect Coombs' test.

POTENTIAL NURSING DIAGNOSES

- ■ Infection, risk for (Indications, Side Effects).
- ■ Knowledge deficit, related to medication regimen (Patient/Family Teaching).

IMPLEMENTATION

- ■ **IV:** Reconstitute with 0.9% NaCl, D5W, D10W, D5/0.9% NaCl, D5/0.25% NaCl, sterile water for injection, 5% sodium bicarbonate, D5/LR, or lactated Ringer's injection.
- ■ **Direct IV:** Dilute in 5–20 ml of compatible solution.
- ■ ***Rate:*** May be administered as a bolus injection over 3–5 min.
- ■ **Intermittent Infusion:** Dilute in 5–20 ml of compatible solution.
- ■ ***Rate:*** Administer over 15–30 min.
- ■ **Additive Incompatibility:** ■ Information unavailable. Do not admix with other antibiotics.

PATIENT/FAMILY TEACHING

- □ Advise patient to report the signs of superinfection (black, furry overgrowth on the tongue; vaginal itching or discharge; loose or foul-smelling stools) and allergy.
- □ May cause dizziness. Caution patient to avoid driving or other activities requiring alertness until response to drug is known.

EVALUATION

Clinical response to therapy can be evaluated by: ■ Resolution of the signs and symptoms of infection. Length of time for complete resolution depends on the organism and site of infection.

MESNA

(**mes**-na)

Mesnex, {Uromitexan}

CLASSIFICATION(S):

Antidote (ifosfamide detoxifying agent)

Pregnancy Category B

INDICATIONS

■ Prevention of ifosfamide-induced hemorrhagic cystitis (see ifosfamide monograph, p. 507). **Unlabeled Uses:** ■ May also prevent hemorrhagic cystitis from cyclophosphamide.

ACTION

■ Binds to the toxic metabolites of ifosfamide in the kidneys. **Therapeutic Effects:** ■ Prevents hemorrhagic cystitis from ifosfamide.

PHARMACOKINETICS

Absorption: IV administration results in complete bioavailability; 76% absorbed following oral administration (unlabeled for oral use).
Distribution: UK.
Metabolism and Excretion: Rapidly converted to mesna disulfide, then converted back to mesna in the kidneys, where it is able to bind to the toxic metabolites of ifosfamide.
Half-life: *Mesna*—0.36 hr; *mesna disulfide*—1.17 hr.

CONTRAINDICATIONS AND PRECAUTIONS

Contraindicated in: ■ Hypersensitivity to mesna or other thiol (rubber) compounds.
Use Cautiously in: ■ Pregnancy or lactation (safety not established).

M

ADVERSE REACTIONS AND SIDE EFFECTS

GI: diarrhea, nausea, unpleasant taste, vomiting.

INTERACTIONS

Drug-Drug: ▪ None significant.

ROUTE AND DOSAGE

- **IV (Adults):** Give a dose of mesna equal to 20% of the ifosfamide dose at the same time as ifosfamide and 4 and 8 hr later.

AVAILABILITY

▪ ***Injection:*** 100 mg/ml in 2-, 4-, and 10-ml ampules[Rx].

TIME/ACTION PROFILE (detoxifying action)

	ONSET	PEAK	DURATION
IV	rapid	UK	4 hr

NURSING IMPLICATIONS

ASSESSMENT

- Monitor for development of hemorrhagic cystitis in patients receiving ifosfamide.
- ***Lab Test Considerations:*** Causes a false-positive result when testing urinary ketones.

POTENTIAL NURSING DIAGNOSES

- Knowledge deficit, related to medication regimen (Patient/Family Teaching).

IMPLEMENTATION

- **General Info:** Initial bolus is to be given at time of ifosfamide administration, 2nd dose is given 4 hr later, 3rd dose is given 8 hr after initial dose. This schedule must be repeated with each subsequent dose of ifosfamide.
- **PO:** Second and third doses have been administered orally (unlabeled use). Oral solution has been prepared with 20 or 50 mg of mesna/ml by diluting parenteral form with flavored syrup (stable for 7 days at room temperature). Has also been diluted in carbonated beverages or apple or orange juice for concentrations of 2, 10, or 50 mg/ml (stable for 24 hr if refrigerated).
- **Direct IV:** Dilute 2-, 4-, and 10-ml ampules, containing a concentration of 100 mg/ml in 8 ml, 16 ml, or 50 ml, respectively, of D5W, 0.9% NaCl, D5/0.9% NaCl, D5/0.2% NaCl, D5/0.33% NaCl, or lactated Ringer's solution, for a final concentration of 20 mg/ml. Refrigerate to store. Use within 6 hr. Discard unused solution.
- **Syringe Compatibility:** ▪ ifosfamide.
- **Y-Site Compatibility:** ▪ amifostine ▪ aztreonam ▪ cefepime ▪ filgrastim ▪ fludarabine ▪ gallium nitrate ▪ granisetron ▪ melphalan ▪ methotrexate ▪ ondansetron ▪ paclitaxel ▪ piperacillin/tazobactam ▪ sargramostim ▪ teniposide ▪ thiotepa ▪ vinorelbine.
- **Additive Compatibility:** ▪ cyclophosphamide ▪ ifosfamide.
- **Additive Incompatibility:** ▪ carboplatin ▪ cisplatin.

PATIENT/FAMILY TEACHING

- Inform patient that unpleasant taste may occur during administration.
- Advise patient to notify health care professional if nausea, vomiting, or diarrhea persists or is severe.

EVALUATION

Effectiveness of therapy can be demonstrated by: ▪ Prevention of hemorrhagic cystitis associated with ifosfamide therapy.

MESORIDAZINE

(mez-oh-**rid**-a-zeen)
Serentil

CLASSIFICATION(S):
Antipsychotic agent (phenothiazine)

Pregnancy Category C

INDICATIONS

- Acute and chronic psychoses.

ACTION

- Alters the effects of dopamine in the CNS
- Possesses anticholinergic and alpha-adrenergic blocking activity. **Therapeutic Effects:**
- Diminished signs and symptoms of psychoses.

PHARMACOKINETICS

Absorption: Appears to be well absorbed following oral administration.

Distribution: Widely distributed. Crosses the placenta. Crosses the blood-brain barrier and probably enters breast milk.

Metabolism and Excretion: Mostly metabolized by the liver.
Half-life: UK.

CONTRAINDICATIONS AND PRECAUTIONS

Contraindicated in: ▪ Hypersensitivity ▪ Cross-sensitivity with other phenothiazines may exist ▪ Narrow-angle glaucoma ▪ Bone marrow depression ▪ Severe liver or cardiovascular disease ▪ Known alcohol intolerance (oral concentrate only).
Use Cautiously in: ▪ Geriatric, emaciated, or debilitated patients (initial dosage reduction may be necessary) ▪ Diabetes mellitus ▪ Respiratory disease ▪ Prostatic hypertrophy ▪ CNS tumors ▪ Epilepsy ▪ Intestinal obstruction ▪ Pregnancy or lactation (safety not established).

ADVERSE REACTIONS AND SIDE EFFECTS*

CNS: NEUROLEPTIC MALIGNANT SYNDROME, drowsiness, extrapyramidal reactions, tardive dyskinesia.
EENT: blurred vision, dry eyes, lens opacities.
CV: hypotension, tachycardia.
GI: constipation, dry mouth, anorexia, ileus, drug-induced hepatitis.
GU: urinary retention.
Derm: photosensitivity, pigment changes, rashes.
Endo: galactorrhea.
Hemat: AGRANULOCYTOSIS, leukopenia.
Misc: allergic reactions, hyperthermia.

INTERACTIONS

Drug-Drug: ▪ Additive hypotension with acute ingestion of **alcohol, antihypertensive agents,** or **nitrates** ▪ Additive CNS depression with other **CNS depressants,** including **alcohol, antidepressants, antihistamines, MAO inhibitors, opioids, sedative/hypnotics,** or **general anesthetics** ▪ Concurrent use with **lithium** may produce any of the following—decreased mesoridazine absorption, increased excretion of lithium, increased risk of extrapyramidal reactions, or masking of the early signs of lithium toxicity ▪ **Antacids** or **adsorbent antidiarrheals (kaolin/attapulgite)** may decrease absorption ▪ Increased risk of agranulocytosis with **antithyroid drugs** ▪ May decrease antiparkinson activity of **levodopa** and **bromocriptine** ▪ Decreases vasopressor response to **epinephrine** and **norepinephrine** ▪ Decreases antihypertensive effect of **guanethidine** ▪ Concurrent use with **beta blockers** may result in inhibition of metabolism of one or both drugs, producing an increased response ▪ Increased risk of anticholinergic effects with other **agents having anticholinergic properties,** including **antihistamines, tricyclic antidepressants, quinidine,** or **disopyramide.**

ROUTE AND DOSAGE

- **PO (Adults and Children >12 yr):** 30–150 mg/day in 2–3 divided doses.
- **IM (Adults):** 25 mg; may be repeated in 30–60 min if needed and tolerated (range 25–200 mg/day).

AVAILABILITY

▪ ***Tablets:*** 10 mg^{Rx}, 25 mg^{Rx}, 50 mg^{Rx}, 100 mg^{Rx} ▪ ***Oral concentrate:*** 25 mg/ml^{Rx} ▪ ***Injection:*** 25 mg/ml^{Rx}.

TIME/ACTION PROFILE (blood levels)

	ONSET	PEAK	DURATION
PO	UK	4–7 days†	UK
IM	UK	4–7 days†	UK

†Steady-state levels during chronic dosing; full therapeutic effects may take 6 wk–6 mo.

NURSING IMPLICATIONS

ASSESSMENT

- ▫ Monitor patient's mental status (orientation to reality, anxiety, and behavior) prior to and periodically throughout therapy.
- ▫ Monitor blood pressure (sitting, standing, lying), ECG, pulse, and respiratory rate prior to and frequently during the period of dosage adjustment. May cause Q-wave and T-wave changes in ECG.
- ▫ Observe patient carefully when administering oral medication to ensure medication is actually taken and not hoarded.
- ▫ Assess patient for level of sedation following administration.
- ▫ Assess fluid intake and bowel function. Increased bulk and fluids in the diet may help minimize constipation.

*CAPITALS indicate life-threatening; underlines indicate most frequent.

- ☐ Monitor patient for onset of akathisia (restlessness or desire to keep moving) and extrapyramidal side effects (*parkinsonian*—difficulty speaking or swallowing, loss of balance control, pill rolling, mask-like face, shuffling gait, rigidity, tremors; and *dystonic*—muscle spasms, twisting motions, twitching, inability to move eyes, weakness of arms or legs) every 2 mo during therapy and 8–12 wk after therapy has been discontinued. Notify physician or other health care professional if these symptoms occur; reduction in dosage or discontinuation of medication may be necessary. Trihexyphenidyl or diphenhydramine may be used to control these symptoms.
- ☐ Monitor for tardive dyskinesia (uncontrolled rhythmic movement of mouth, face, and extremities; lip smacking or puckering; puffing of cheeks; uncontrolled chewing; rapid or worm-like movements of tongue). Report immediately; may be irreversible.
- ☐ Monitor for development of neuroleptic malignant syndrome (fever, respiratory distress, tachycardia, convulsions, diaphoresis, hypertension or hypotension, pallor, tiredness, severe muscle stiffness, loss of bladder control). Report immediately.
- ***Lab Test Considerations:*** CBC, liver function tests, and ocular examinations should be evaluated periodically throughout therapy. May cause decreased hematocrit, hemoglobin, leukocytes, granulocytes, and platelets. May cause elevated bilirubin, AST, ALT, and alkaline phosphatase. Agranulocytosis may occur after 4–10 wk of therapy, with recovery 1–2 wk following discontinuation. May recur if medication is restarted. Liver function abnormalities may require discontinuation of therapy.
- ☐ May cause false-positive or false-negative pregnancy tests and false-positive urine bilirubin test results.
- ☐ May cause increased serum prolactin levels.

POTENTIAL NURSING DIAGNOSES

- Thought processes, altered (Indications).
- Injury, risk for (Side Effects).
- Knowledge deficit, related to medication regimen (Patient/Family Teaching).

IMPLEMENTATION

- **General Info:** To prevent contact dermatitis, avoid getting liquid preparations on hands and wash hands thoroughly if spillage occurs.
- ☐ Phenothiazines should be discontinued 48 hr before and not resumed for 24 hr following myelography, because they lower the seizure threshold.
- **PO:** Administer capsules with food or milk to decrease gastric irritation.
- ☐ Dilute oral solution with 120 ml of acidified water, distilled water, or orange or grapefruit juice. Measure dose with provided dropper. Use just after diluting.
- **IM:** Should be administered deep into well-developed muscle. Do not use if precipitate is present; solution may be slightly yellow.

PATIENT/FAMILY TEACHING

- ☐ Instruct patient receiving parenteral mesoridazine to remain supine for 30 min after administration. Position changes should be made slowly to prevent orthostatic hypotension.
- ☐ Instruct patient on need to take medication exactly as directed. If a dose is missed, take within 1 hr or skip dose and return to regular schedule. Patients on long-term high-dose therapy may need to discontinue medication gradually to avoid withdrawal symptoms (dyskinesia, tremors, dizziness, nausea, and vomiting).
- ☐ Instruct patient receiving oral solution on correct method of measuring dose with provided dropper.
- ☐ Drowsiness may occur. Caution patient to avoid driving or other activities requiring alertness until response to medication is known.
- ☐ Instruct patient to use frequent mouth rinses, good oral hygiene, and sugarless gum or candy to minimize dry mouth. Consult health care professional if dry mouth continues for >2 wk.
- ☐ Advise patient to use sunscreen and protective clothing when exposed to the sun. Exposed surfaces may develop a temporary pigment change (ranging from yellow-brown to grayish purple). Extremes of temperature (exercise, hot weather, hot baths or showers) should also be avoided, because this drug impairs body temperature regulation.

- ☐ Caution patient to avoid concurrent use of alcohol, other CNS depressants, and OTC medications without consulting health care professional.
- ☐ Instruct patient to notify health care professional promptly if sore throat, fever, unusual bleeding or bruising, rash, weakness, tremors, visual disturbances, dark-colored urine, or clay-colored stools occur.
- ☐ Advise patient to notify health care professional of medication regimen prior to treatment or surgery.
- ☐ Inform patient of possibility of extrapyramidal symptoms and tardive dyskinesia. Caution patient to report these symptoms to health care professional immediately.
- ☐ Inform patient that increasing bulk and fluids in the diet and exercising regularly may minimize the constipating effects of this medication.
- ☐ Advise patient of need for continued medical follow-up for psychotherapy, eye exams, and laboratory tests.

EVALUATION

Effectiveness of therapy can be demonstrated by: ▪ Decreased psychotic ideation.

METAPROTERENOL

(met-a-proe-**ter**-e-nole)
Alupent

CLASSIFICATION(S):
Bronchodilator (adrenergic agonist)

Pregnancy Category C

INDICATIONS

▪ Management of reversible airway disease due to asthma or COPD.

ACTION

▪ Results in the accumulation of cyclic adenosine monophosphate (cAMP) at beta-adrenergic receptors ▪ Produces bronchodilation ▪ Inhibits the release of mediators of immediate hypersensitivity reactions from mast cells ▪ Relatively selective for $beta_2$ (pulmonary) -adrenergic receptor sites, with less effect on $beta_1$ (cardiac) -adrenergic receptors. **Therapeutic Effects:** ▪ Bronchodilation.

PHARMACOKINETICS

Absorption: Well absorbed following oral administration but rapidly undergoes extensive metabolism.
Distribution: UK.
Metabolism and Excretion: Extensively metabolized by the liver and other tissues.
Half-life: UK.

CONTRAINDICATIONS AND PRECAUTIONS

Contraindicated in: ▪ Hypersensitivity to adrenergic amines ▪ Selected products may contain bisulfites, alcohol (in some oral liquid preparations), or fluorocarbons (in some inhalers) and should be avoided in patients with known hypersensitivity or intolerance.
Use Cautiously in: ▪ Cardiac disease ▪ Hypertension ▪ Hyperthyroidism ▪ Diabetes ▪ Glaucoma ▪ Elderly patients (more susceptible to adverse reactions; may require dosage reduction) ▪ Excessive use may lead to tolerance and paradoxical bronchospasm (inhaler) ▪ Pregnancy (near term), lactation, and children <2 yr (safety not established).

ADVERSE REACTIONS AND SIDE EFFECTS*

CNS: <u>nervousness</u>, <u>restlessness</u>, <u>tremor</u>, headache, insomnia.
Resp: PARADOXICAL BRONCHOSPASM (excessive use of inhalers)
CV: angina, arrhythmias, hypertension, tachycardia.
GI: nausea, vomiting.
Endo: hyperglycemia.

INTERACTIONS

Drug-Drug: ▪ Concurrent use with other **adrenergic (sympathomimetic) agents** will have additive adrenergic side effects ▪ Use with **MAO inhibitors** may lead to hypertensive crisis ▪ **Beta-adrenergic blockers** may negate therapeutic effect.

M

***CAPITALS indicate life-threatening; underlines indicate most frequent.**

ROUTE AND DOSAGE

- **PO (Adults and Children >9 yr and >27 kg):** 20 mg 3–4 times daily.
- **PO (Children 6–9 yr and <27 kg):** 10 mg 3–4 times daily.
- **Inhalation (Adults >12 yr):** *Metered-dose inhaler*—2–3 inhalations q 3–4 hr (not to exceed 12 inhalations/day). *Hand-bulb nebulizer*—5–15 inhalations of undiluted 5% solution 3–4 times daily (not to exceed q 4 hr use). *IPPB*—0.2–0.3 ml of 5% solution or 2.5 ml of 0.4–0.6% solution for nebulization 3–4 times daily (not to exceed q 4 hr use).

AVAILABILITY

- ***Tablets:*** 10 mg[Rx], 20 mg[Rx] ▪ ***Syrup:*** 10 mg/5 ml[Rx] ▪ ***Inhalation aerosol:*** 650 mcg/spray (100 inhalations/5 ml)[Rx], {750 mcg/spray (100 inhalations/5 ml)[Rx]} ▪ ***Inhalation solution:*** 0.4%[Rx], 0.6%[Rx], 5%[Rx].

TIME/ACTION PROFILE (bronchodilation)

	ONSET	PEAK	DURATION
PO	within 15–30 min	within 1 hr	up to 4 hr
Inhaln-aerosol	within 1 min	1 hr	1–5 hr
Inhaln-IPPB	5–30 min	UK	2–6 hr

NURSING IMPLICATIONS

ASSESSMENT

- **Bronchodilator:** Assess lung sounds, respiratory pattern, pulse, and blood pressure before administration and during peak of medication. Note amount, color, and character of sputum produced. Report abnormal findings.
  - Monitor pulmonary function tests before initiating therapy and periodically throughout course to determine effectiveness of medication.
  - Observe for paradoxical bronchospasm (wheezing). If condition occurs, withhold medication and notify physician or other health care provider immediately.
  - Observe patient for drug tolerance and rebound bronchospasm. Patients requiring more than 3 inhalation treatments in 24 hr should be under close supervision. If minimal or no relief is seen after 3–5 inhalation treatments within 6–12 hr, further treatment with aerosol alone is not recommended.
- ***Lab Test Considerations:*** May cause decreased serum potassium concentrations, which are usually transient and dose related; rarely occurs at recommended doses and is more pronounced with frequent use of high doses.
- ***Toxicity and Overdose:*** Symptoms of overdose include persistent agitation, chest pain or discomfort, decreased blood pressure, dizziness, hyperglycemia, hypokalemia, seizures, tachyarrhythmias, persistent trembling, and vomiting.
  - Treatment includes discontinuing beta-adrenergic agonists and symptomatic, supportive therapy. Cardioselective beta-adrenergic blocking agents are used cautiously, as they may induce bronchospasm.

POTENTIAL NURSING DIAGNOSES

- Airway clearance, ineffective (Indications).
- Knowledge deficit, related to medication regimen (Patient/Family Teaching).

IMPLEMENTATION

- **PO:** Administer oral medication with meals to minimize gastric irritation.
- **Inhalation:** For IPPB administration, dilute each dose in 2.5 ml of 0.9% NaCl. Do not use if solution is brown or darker than slightly yellow, pinkish, or if it contains a precipitate.

PATIENT/FAMILY TEACHING

- **General Info:** Instruct patient to take medication exactly as directed. If on a scheduled dosing regimen, take a missed dose as soon as possible; space remaining doses at regular intervals. Do not double doses. Caution patient not to exceed recommended dose; may cause adverse effects, paradoxical bronchospasm, or loss of effectiveness of medication.
  - Instruct patient to contact health care professional immediately if shortness of breath is not relieved by medication or is accompanied by diaphoresis, dizziness, palpitations, or chest pain.
  - Advise patient to consult health care professional before taking any OTC medications or alcoholic beverages concurrently with this therapy. Caution patient also to avoid smoking and other respiratory irritants.
- **Inhalation:** Review correct administration technique (aerosolization, IPPB, metered-

dose inhaler) with patient. See Appendix H for administration with metered-dose inhaler. Wait 1–5 min before administering next dose. Mouthpiece should be washed after each use.

- □ Do not spray inhaler near eyes.
- □ Instruct patient to save inhaler; refill canisters may be available.
- □ Advise patient to use bronchodilator first if using other inhalation medications, and allow 5 min to elapse before administering other inhalant medications, unless otherwise directed.
- □ Advise patient to rinse mouth with water after each inhalation dose to minimize dry mouth.
- □ Advise patient to maintain adequate fluid intake (2000–3000 ml/day) to help liquefy tenacious secretions.
- □ Instruct patient to notify health care professional if contents of one canister are used up in less than 2 wk.

EVALUATION

Effectiveness of therapy can be demonstrated by: ▪ Prevention or relief of bronchospasm ▪ Increase in ease of breathing ▪ Prevention of exercise-induced asthma.

METFORMIN

(met-**for**-min)

CLASSIFICATION(S):
Oral hypoglycemic agent (biguanide)

Pregnancy Category B

INDICATIONS

▪ Adjunctive management of non–insulin-dependent diabetes mellitus (NIDDM). May be used with diet and/or sulfonylurea oral hypoglycemic agents.

ACTION

▪ Decreases hepatic production of glucose ▪ Decreases intestinal absorption of glucose ▪ Increases sensitivity to insulin. **Therapeutic Effects:** ▪ Maintenance of blood sugar.

PHARMACOKINETICS

Absorption: 50–60% absorbed following oral administration.

Distribution: Enters breast milk in concentrations similar to plasma.

Metabolism and Excretion: Eliminated almost entirely unchanged by the kidneys.

Half-life: 17.6 hr.

CONTRAINDICATIONS AND PRECAUTIONS

Contraindicated in: ▪ Hypersensitivity ▪ Metabolic acidosis of any cause ▪ Underlying renal dysfunction (serum creatinine >1.5 mg/dl in men or >1.4 mg/dl in women) ▪ Concurrent radiographic studies requiring IV administration of iodinated contrast media (temporarily withhold metformin) ▪ Hepatic impairment ▪ CHF requiring pharmacologic treatment.

Use Cautiously in: ▪ Any degree of renal impairment ▪ Geriatric or debilitated patients (lower doses may be required) ▪ Chronic alcohol use/abuse ▪ Dehydration, serious medical conditions (MI, stroke) ▪ Patients undergoing stress (infection, surgical procedures) ▪ Hypoxic patients ▪ Patients with pituitary deficiency or hyperthyroidism ▪ Pregnancy, lactation, or children (safety not established).

ADVERSE REACTIONS AND SIDE EFFECTS*

GI: abdominal bloating, diarrhea, nausea, vomiting, unpleasant metallic taste.

Endo: hypoglycemia.

F and E: LACTIC ACIDOSIS.

Misc: decreased vitamin B_{12} levels.

INTERACTIONS

Drug-Drug: ▪ **Iodinated contrast media** increase the risk of lactic acidosis ▪ **Amiloride, digoxin, morphine, procainamide, quinidine, ranitidine, triamterene, trimethoprim, calcium channel blockers,** and **vancomycin** may compete for elimination pathways with metformin. Altered responses may occur ▪ **Cimetidine** and **furosemide** may increase the effects of metformin ▪ **Nifedipine** increases absorption and may increase the effects of metformin.

ROUTE AND DOSAGE

▪ **PO (Adults):** 500 mg twice daily; may increase by 500 mg at weekly intervals up to

***CAPITALS indicate life-threatening; underlines indicate most frequent.**

M

2000 mg/day. If doses >2000 mg/day are required, give in 3 divided doses (not to exceed 2500 mg/day) or 850 mg once daily; may increase by 850 mg at 2-wk intervals (in divided doses) up to 2550 mg/day in divided doses (up to 850 mg 3 times daily).

AVAILABILITY

- ***Tablets:*** 500 mg^{Rx}, 850 mg^{Rx}.

TIME/ACTION PROFILE (control of blood sugar)

	ONSET	PEAK	DURATION
PO	several days	2–4 wk	UK

NURSING IMPLICATIONS

ASSESSMENT

- Observe patient for signs and symptoms of hypoglycemic reactions (abdominal pain, sweating, hunger, weakness, dizziness, headache, tremor, tachycardia, anxiety) when combined with oral sulfonylureas.
- Patients who have been well controlled on metformin who develop illness or laboratory abnormalities should be assessed for ketoacidosis or lactic acidosis. Assess serum electrolytes, ketones, glucose, and, if indicated, blood pH, lactate, pyruvate, and metformin levels. If either form of acidosis is present, discontinue metformin immediately and treat acidosis.
- ***Lab Test Considerations:*** Serum glucose and glycosylated hemoglobin should be monitored periodically throughout therapy to evaluate effectiveness of therapy. May cause false-positive results for urine ketones.
- Blood glucose concentrations should be monitored routinely by patient and every 3 mo by health care professional to determine effectiveness of therapy.
- Assess renal function prior to initiating and at least annually throughout therapy. Discontinue metformin if renal impairment occurs.
- Monitor serum folic acid and vitamin B_{12} every 1–2 yr in long-term therapy. Metformin may interfere with absorption.

POTENTIAL NURSING DIAGNOSES

- Nutrition, altered, more than body requirements (Indications).
- Knowledge deficit, related to diet and medication regimen (Patient/Family Teaching).
- Noncompliance (Patient/Family Teaching).

IMPLEMENTATION

- **General Info:** Patients stabilized on a diabetic regimen who are exposed to stress, fever, trauma, infection, or surgery may require administration of insulin. Withhold metformin and reinstitute after resolution of acute episode.
- Metformin therapy should be temporarily discontinued in patients requiring surgery involving restricted intake of food and fluids. Resume metformin when oral intake has resumed and renal function is normal.
- Withhold metformin during studies requiring IV administration of iodinated contrast media.
- **PO:** Administer metformin with meals to minimize GI effects.

PATIENT/FAMILY TEACHING

- Instruct patient to take metformin at the same time each day, exactly as directed. If a dose is missed, take as soon as possible unless almost time for next dose. Do not double doses.
- Explain to patient that metformin helps control hyperglycemia but does not cure diabetes. Therapy is usually long term.
- Encourage patient to follow prescribed diet, medication, and exercise regimen to prevent hyperglycemic or hypoglycemic episodes.
- Review signs of hypoglycemia and hyperglycemia with patient. If hypoglycemia occurs, advise patient to take a glass of orange juice or 2–3 tsp of sugar, honey, or corn syrup dissolved in water, and notify health care professional.
- Instruct patient in proper testing of blood glucose and urine ketones. These tests should be monitored closely during periods of stress or illness and health care professional notified if significant changes occur.
- Explain to patient the risk of lactic acidosis and the potential need for discontinuation of metformin therapy if a severe infection, dehydration, or severe or continuing diarrhea occurs or if medical tests or surgery is required. Symptoms of lactic acidosis (chills, diarrhea, dizziness, low blood pressure, muscle pain, sleepiness, slow heartbeat or pulse, dyspnea, or weakness) should be reported to health care professional immediately.

- Caution patient to avoid taking other prescription or OTC medications or alcohol during metformin therapy without consulting health care professional.
- Insulin is the recommended method of controlling blood sugar during pregnancy. Counsel female patients to use a form of contraception other than oral contraceptives and to notify health care professional promptly if pregnancy is planned or suspected.
- Inform patient that metformin may cause an unpleasant or metallic taste that usually resolves spontaneously.
- Advise patient to inform health care professional of medication regimen prior to treatment or surgery.
- Advise patient to carry a form of sugar (sugar packets, candy) and identification describing disease process and medication regimen at all times.
- Advise patient to report the occurrence of diarrhea, nausea, vomiting, and stomach pain or fullness to health care professional.
- Emphasize the importance of routine follow-up exams and regular testing of blood glucose, glycosylated hemoglobin, renal function, and hematologic parameters.

EVALUATION

Effectiveness of therapy can be demonstrated by: ▪ Control of blood glucose levels without the appearance of hypoglycemic or hyperglycemic episodes. Control may be achieved within a few days, but full effect of therapy may be delayed for up to 2 wk. If patient has not responded to metformin after 4 wk of maximum dose therapy, an oral sulfonylurea may be added. If satisfactory results are not obtained with 1–3 mo of concurrent therapy, oral agents may be discontinued and insulin therapy instituted.

METHADONE

(**meth**-a-done)
Dolophine, Methadose

CLASSIFICATION(S):
Opioid analgesic (agonist)

Schedule II
Pregnancy Category B

INDICATIONS

▪ Severe pain ▪ Suppresses withdrawal symptoms in opioid detoxification.

ACTION

▪ Binds to opiate receptors in the CNS ▪ Alters the perception of and response to painful stimuli, while producing generalized CNS depression. **Therapeutic Effects:** ▪ Decrease in severity of pain ▪ Suppression of withdrawal symptoms during detoxification and maintenance from heroin and other opioids.

PHARMACOKINETICS

Absorption: Well absorbed from all sites (50% absorbed following oral administration).
Distribution: Widely distributed. Crosses the placenta; enters breast milk.
Metabolism and Excretion: Mostly metabolized by the liver.
Half-life: 15–25 hr; increases with chronic use.

CONTRAINDICATIONS AND PRECAUTIONS

Contraindicated in: ▪ Hypersensitivity ▪ Known alcohol intolerance (some oral solutions) ▪ Pregnancy or lactation (chronic use) ▪ Concurrent MAO inhibitor therapy.
Use Cautiously in: ▪ Head trauma ▪ Increased intracranial pressure ▪ Severe renal, hepatic, or pulmonary disease ▪ Hypothyroidism ▪ Adrenal insufficiency ▪ Alcoholism ▪ Geriatric or debilitated patients (dosage reduction suggested) ▪ Undiagnosed abdominal pain ▪ Prostatic hypertrophy.

ADVERSE REACTIONS AND SIDE EFFECTS*

CNS: <u>confusion</u>, <u>sedation</u>, dizziness, dysphoria, euphoria, floating feeling, hallucinations, headache, unusual dreams.
EENT: blurred vision, diplopia, miosis.
Resp: respiratory depression.
CV: <u>hypotension</u>, bradycardia.
GI: <u>constipation</u>, nausea, vomiting.
GU: urinary retention.
Derm: flushing, sweating.
Misc: physical dependence, psychological dependence, tolerance.

M

***CAPITALS indicate life-threatening; <u>underlines</u> indicate most frequent.**

INTERACTIONS

Drug-Drug: ▪ Use with extreme caution in patients receiving **MAO inhibitors** (may result in severe, unpredictable reactions—reduce initial dose of methadone to 25% of usual dose) ▪ Additive CNS depression with **alcohol, antihistamines,** and **sedative/hypnotics** ▪ Administration of **partial-antagonist opioids** may precipitate opioid withdrawal in physically dependent patients ▪ **Nalbuphine** or **pentazocine** may decrease analgesia.

ROUTE AND DOSAGE

Larger doses may be required for analgesia during chronic therapy; interval may be decreased/dosage increased if pain recurs.

- **PO (Adults and Children ≥50 kg):** *Analgesic*—20 mg q 6–8 hr. *Opioid detoxification*—15–40 mg once daily or amount needed to prevent withdrawal. Dosage may be decreased q 1–2 days; maintenance dose is determined on an individual basis.
- **PO (Adults and Children <50 kg):** *Analgesic*—0.2 mg/kg q 6–8 hr.
- **IM, SC (Adults and Children ≥50 kg):** *Analgesic*—10 mg q 6–8 hr. *Opioid detoxification*—15–40 mg once daily or amount needed to prevent withdrawal. Dosage may be decreased q 1–2 days; maintenance dose is determined on an individual basis.
- **IM, SC (Adults and Children <50 kg):** 0.1 mg/kg mg q 6–8 hr.

AVAILABILITY

▪ ***Tablets:*** 5 mg[Rx], 10 mg[Rx] ▪ ***Dispersible tablets (diskettes):*** 40 mg (available only to licensed detoxification/maintenance programs)[Rx] ▪ ***Oral solution:*** 5 mg/5 ml[Rx], 10 mg/5 ml[Rx] ▪ ***Oral concentrate:*** 10 mg/ml[Rx].

TIME/ACTION PROFILE (analgesic effect)

	ONSET	PEAK	DURATION
PO	30–60 min	90–120 min	4–12 hr
IM, SC	10–20 min	60–120 min	4–6 hr

NURSING IMPLICATIONS

ASSESSMENT

- □ Assess type, location, and intensity of pain prior to and 1–2 hr (peak) following administration. When titrating opioid doses, increases of 25–50% should be administered until there is either a 50% reduction in the patient's pain rating on a numerical or visual analogue scale or the patient reports satisfactory pain relief. A repeat dose can be safely administered at the time of the peak if previous dose is ineffective and side effects are minimal. Cumulative effects of this medication may require periodic dosage adjustments.
- □ Doses of methadone for patients on methadone maintenance prevent only withdrawal symptoms; *no analgesia is provided.* Additional opioid doses are required for treatment of pain.
- □ An equianalgesic chart (see Appendix B) should be used when changing routes or when changing from one opioid to another.
- □ Assess blood pressure, pulse, and respirations before and periodically during administration. If respiratory rate is <10/min, assess level of sedation. Dose may need to be decreased by 25–50%. Initial drowsiness will diminish with continued use.
- □ Assess bowel function routinely. Prevention of constipation should be instituted with increased intake of fluids and bulk and with laxatives to minimize constipating effects. Stimulant laxatives should be administered routinely if opioid use exceeds 2–3 days, unless contraindicated.
- □ Prolonged use may lead to physical and psychological dependence and tolerance. This should not prevent patient from receiving adequate analgesia. Most patients who receive methadone for pain do not develop psychological dependence. Progressively higher doses may be required to relieve pain with long-term therapy.
- ▪ ***Lab Test Considerations:*** May increase plasma amylase and lipase levels.
- ▪ ***Toxicity and Overdose:*** If an opioid antagonist is required to reverse respiratory depression or coma, naloxone (Narcan) is the antidote. Dilute the 0.4-mg ampule of naloxone in 10 ml of 0.9% NaCl and administer 0.5 ml (0.02 mg) by direct IV push every 2 min. For children and patients weighing <40 kg, dilute 0.1 mg of naloxone in 10 ml of 0.9% NaCl for a concentration of 10 mcg/ml and administer 0.5 mcg/kg every 1–2 min. Titrate dose to avoid withdrawal, seizures, and severe pain.

POTENTIAL NURSING DIAGNOSES

- Pain (Indications).
- Sensory-perceptual alterations: visual, auditory (Side Effects).
- Injury, risk for (Side Effects).

IMPLEMENTATION

- **General Info:** Explain therapeutic value of medication prior to administration to enhance the analgesic effect.
  - Regularly administered doses may be more effective than prn administration. Analgesic is more effective if administered before pain becomes severe. For patients in chronic severe pain, the oral solution containing 5 or 10 mg/5 ml is recommended on a fixed dosage schedule.
  - Coadministration with nonopioid analgesics may have additive analgesic effects and may permit lower doses.
  - Medication should be discontinued gradually after long-term use to prevent withdrawal symptoms.
  - Diskettes (dispersible tablets) are to be dissolved and used for detoxification and maintenance treatment only.
- **PO:** Doses may be administered with food or milk to minimize GI irritation.
  - Dilute each dose of 10 mg/ml oral concentrate with at least 30 ml of water or other liquid prior to administration.
- **IM, SC:** IM is the preferred parenteral route for repeated doses. SC administration may cause tissue irritation.

PATIENT/FAMILY TEACHING

- Instruct patient on how and when to ask for pain medication.
- Instruct patient to take methadone exactly as directed. If dose is less effective after a few weeks, do not increase dose without consulting health care professional.
- May cause drowsiness or dizziness. Advise patient to call for assistance when ambulating or smoking and to avoid driving or other activities requiring alertness until response to medication is known.
- Advise patient to change positions slowly to minimize orthostatic hypotension.
- Caution patient to avoid concurrent use of alcohol or other CNS depressants with this medication.
- Encourage patient to turn, cough, and breathe deeply every 2 hr to prevent atelectasis.

EVALUATION

Effectiveness of therapy can be demonstrated by: ▪ Decrease in severity of pain without a significant alteration in level of consciousness or respiratory status ▪ Prevention of withdrawal symptoms in detoxification from heroin and other opioid analgesics.

METHIMAZOLE

(meth-**im**-a-zole)

Tapazole

CLASSIFICATION(S):

Antithyroid agent

Pregnancy Category D

INDICATIONS

▪ Palliative treatment of hyperthyroidism ▪ Used as an adjunct to control hyperthyroidism in preparation for thyroidectomy or radioactive iodine therapy.

ACTION

▪ Inhibits the synthesis of thyroid hormones. **Therapeutic Effects:** ▪ Decreased signs and symptoms of hyperthyroidism.

PHARMACOKINETICS

Absorption: Rapidly absorbed following oral administration.

Distribution: Crosses the placenta and enters breast milk in high concentrations.

Metabolism and Excretion: Mostly metabolized by the liver; $<10\%$ eliminated unchanged by the kidneys.

Half-life: 3–5 hr.

CONTRAINDICATIONS AND PRECAUTIONS

Contraindicated in: ▪ Hypersensitivity ▪ Lactation.

Use Cautiously in: ▪ Patients with decreased bone marrow reserve ▪ Patients >40 yr (increased risk of agranulocytosis) ▪ Pregnancy (may be used cautiously; however, thyroid problems may occur in the fetus).

ADVERSE REACTIONS AND SIDE EFFECTS*

CNS: drowsiness, headache, vertigo.
GI: diarrhea, drug-induced hepatitis, loss of taste, nausea, parotitis, vomiting.
Derm: rash, skin discoloration, urticaria.
Hemat: AGRANULOCYTOSIS, anemia, leukopenia, thrombocytopenia.
MS: arthralgia.
Misc: fever, lymphadenopathy.

INTERACTIONS

Drug-Drug: ▪ Additive bone marrow depression with **antineoplastic agents** or **radiation therapy** ▪ Antithyroid effect may be decreased by **potassium iodide** or **amiodarone** ▪ Increased risk of agranulocytosis with **phenothiazines** ▪ May alter response to **warfarin** and **digitalis glycosides.**

ROUTE AND DOSAGE

- **PO (Adults):** *Thyrotoxic crisis*—15–20 mg q 4 hr during the first 24 hr (with other interventions). *Hyperthyroidism*—15–60 mg/day as a single dose or divided doses for 6–8 wk.
- **PO (Children):** *Initial*—400 mcg (0.4 mg)/kg/day in single dose or 2 divided doses. *Maintenance*—200 mcg/kg/day in single dose or 2 divided doses.

AVAILABILITY

- ***Tablets:*** 5 mg[Rx], 10 mg[Rx].

TIME/ACTION PROFILE (effect on thyroid function)

	ONSET	PEAK	DURATION
PO	1 wk	4–10 wk	wks

NURSING IMPLICATIONS

ASSESSMENT

- □ Monitor response for symptoms of hyperthyroidism or thyrotoxicosis (tachycardia, palpitations, nervousness, insomnia, fever, diaphoresis, heat intolerance, tremors, weight loss, diarrhea).
- □ Assess patient for development of hypothyroidism (intolerance to cold, constipation, dry skin, headache, listlessness, tiredness, or weakness). Dosage adjustment may be required.
- □ Assess patient for skin rash or swelling of cervical lymph nodes. Treatment may be discontinued if this occurs.
- ▪ ***Lab Test Considerations:*** Thyroid function studies should be monitored prior to therapy, monthly during initial therapy, and every 2–3 mo throughout therapy.
- □ WBC and differential counts should be monitored periodically throughout therapy. Agranulocytosis may develop rapidly; it usually occurs during the first 2 mo and is more common in patients over 40 yr and those receiving >40 mg/day. This necessitates discontinuation of therapy.
- □ May cause increased AST, ALT, LDH, alkaline phosphatase, serum bilirubin, and prothrombin time.

POTENTIAL NURSING DIAGNOSES

- ▪ Knowledge deficit, related to medication regimen (Patient/Family Teaching).
- ▪ Noncompliance (Patient/Family Teaching).

IMPLEMENTATION

- ▪ **PO:** Administer at same time in relation to meals every day. Food may either increase or decrease absorption.

PATIENT/FAMILY TEACHING

- □ Instruct patient to take medication exactly as directed, around the clock. If a dose is missed, take as soon as remembered; take both doses together if almost time for next dose; check with health care professional if more than 1 dose is missed. Consult health care professional prior to discontinuing medication.
- □ Instruct patient to monitor weight 2–3 times weekly. Notify health care professional of significant changes.
- □ May cause drowsiness. Caution patient to avoid driving or other activities requiring alertness until response to medication is known.
- □ Advise patient to consult health care professional regarding dietary sources of iodine (iodized salt, shellfish).
- □ Advise patient to report sore throat, fever, chills, headache, malaise, weakness, yellowing of eyes or skin, unusual bleeding or bruising,

***CAPITALS indicate life-threatening; underlines indicate most frequent.**

rash, or symptoms of hyperthyroidism or hypothyroidism promptly.

- Instruct patient to consult health care professional before taking any OTC medications.
- Advise patient to carry identification describing medication regimen at all times.
- Advise patient to notify health care professional of medication regimen prior to treatment or surgery.
- Emphasize the importance of routine exams to monitor progress and to check for side effects.

EVALUATION

Effectiveness of therapy can be demonstrated by: ▪ Decrease in severity of symptoms of hyperthyroidism (lowered pulse rate and weight gain) ▪ Return of thyroid function studies to normal ▪ May be used as short-term adjunctive therapy to prepare patient for thyroidectomy or radiation therapy or may be used in treatment of hyperthyroidism. Treatment of 6 mo to several years may be necessary, usually averaging 1 yr.

METHOCARBAMOL

(meth-oh-**kar**-ba-mole)
Carbacot, Robaxin

CLASSIFICATION(S):
Skeletal muscle relaxant (centrally acting)

Pregnancy Category C

INDICATIONS

▪ Adjunctive treatment of muscle spasm associated with acute painful musculoskeletal conditions (with rest and physical therapy).

ACTION

▪ Skeletal muscle relaxation, probably due to CNS depression. **Therapeutic Effects:** ▪ Skeletal muscle relaxation.

PHARMACOKINETICS

Absorption: Rapidly absorbed from the GI tract.
Distribution: Widely distributed. Crosses the placenta; enters breast milk in small amounts.
Metabolism and Excretion: Metabolized by the liver.
Half-life: 1–2 hr.

CONTRAINDICATIONS AND PRECAUTIONS

Contraindicated in: ▪ Hypersensitivity ▪ Hypersensitivity to polyethylene glycol (parenteral only) ▪ Renal impairment (parenteral form).
Use Cautiously in: ▪ Pregnancy, lactation, and children (safety not established) ▪ Seizure disorders (parenteral form).

ADVERSE REACTIONS AND SIDE EFFECTS*

CNS: SEIZURES (IV, IM only), dizziness, drowsiness, light-headedness.
EENT: blurred vision, nasal congestion.
CV: *IV*—bradycardia, hypotension.
GI: anorexia, GI upset, nausea.
GU: brown, black, or green urine.
Derm: flushing (IV only), pruritus, rashes, urticaria.
Local: pain at IM site, phlebitis at IV site.
Misc: allergic reactions including ANAPHYLAXIS (IM, IV use only), fever.

INTERACTIONS

Drug-Drug: ▪ Additive CNS depression with other **CNS depressants**, including **alcohol, antihistamines, opioids,** and **sedative/hypnotics.**

ROUTE AND DOSAGE

- **PO (Adults):** 1.5 g qid initially (up to 8 g/day) for 2–3 days, then 4–4.5 g/day in 3–6 divided doses; may be followed by maintenance dosing of 750 mg q 4 hr or 1 g 4 times daily or 1.5 g 3 times daily.
- **IM, IV (Adults):** 1–3 g/day for not more than 3 days; course may be repeated after a 48-hr rest.

AVAILABILITY

▪ ***Tablets:*** {500 mg[OTC]}, {750 mg[OTC]} ▪ ***Injection:*** {100 mg/ml in 10-ml ampules[OTC]}, 100 mg/ml in 10-ml vials[Rx] ▪ ***In combination with:*** aspirin (Robaxisal)[Rx]. See Appendix A.

***CAPITALS indicate life-threatening; underlines indicate most frequent.**

M

TIME/ACTION PROFILE (skeletal muscle relaxation)

	ONSET	PEAK	DURATION
PO	30 min	2 hr	UK
IM	rapid	UK	UK
IV	immediate	end of infusion	UK

NURSING IMPLICATIONS

ASSESSMENT

- Assess patient for pain, muscle stiffness, and range of motion prior to and periodically throughout therapy.
- Monitor pulse and blood pressure every 15 min during parenteral administration.
- Assess patient for allergic reactions (skin rash, asthma, hives, wheezing, hypotension) following parenteral administration. Keep epinephrine and oxygen on hand in the event of a reaction.
- Monitor IV site. Injection is hypertonic and may cause thrombophlebitis. Avoid extravasation.
- ***Lab Test Considerations:*** Monitor renal function periodically during prolonged parenteral therapy (>3 days), as polyethylene glycol 300 vehicle is nephrotoxic.
- May cause falsely increased urinary 5-hydroxyindoleacetic acid (5-HIAA) and vanillylmandelic acid (VMA) determinations.

POTENTIAL NURSING DIAGNOSES

- Pain (Indications).
- Physical mobility, impaired (Indications).
- Injury, risk for (Side Effects).

IMPLEMENTATION

- **General Info:** Provide safety measures as indicated. Supervise ambulation and transfer of patients.
- **PO:** May be administered with food to minimize GI irritation. Tablets may be crushed and mixed with food or liquids to facilitate swallowing. For administration via NG tube, crush tablet and suspend in water or saline.
- **IM:** Do not administer SC. IM injections should contain no more than 5 ml (500 mg) at a time in the gluteal region.
- **Direct IV:** Administer undiluted.
- ***Rate:*** Administer at a rate of 3 ml (300 mg) over 1 min.
- **Intermittent Infusion:** Dilute each dose in no more than 250 ml of 0.9% NaCl or D5W for injection. Do not refrigerate after dilution.
- Have patient remain recumbent during and for at least 10–15 min following infusion to avoid orthostatic hypotension.

PATIENT/FAMILY TEACHING

- Advise patient to take medication exactly as directed. Missed doses should be taken within 1 hr; if not, return to regular dosing schedule. Do not double doses.
- Encourage patient to comply with additional therapies prescribed for muscle spasm (rest, physical therapy, heat).
- May cause dizziness, drowsiness, and blurred vision. Advise patient to avoid driving and other activities requiring alertness until response to drug is known.
- Instruct patient to change positions slowly to minimize orthostatic hypotension.
- Advise patient to avoid concurrent use of alcohol and other CNS depressants.
- Inform patient that urine may turn black, brown, or green, especially if left standing.
- Instruct patient to notify health care professional if skin rash, itching, fever, or nasal congestion occurs.
- Emphasize the importance of routine follow-up exams to monitor progress.

EVALUATION

Effectiveness of therapy can be demonstrated by: ▪ Decreased musculoskeletal pain and muscle spasticity ▫ Increased range of motion.

METHOTREXATE

(meth-o-**trex**-ate)

amethopterin, Folex, Folex PFS, Rheumatrex

CLASSIFICATION(S):

Antineoplastic (antimetabolite), Immunosuppressant

Pregnancy Category X

INDICATIONS

- Alone or in combination with other treatment modalities (other antineoplastic agents, surgery, or radiation therapy) in the treatment of:
  - Trophoblastic neoplasms (choriocarcinoma,

choriadenoma destruens, hydatidiform mole) ▫ Leukemias ▫ Breast carcinoma ▫ Head carcinoma ▫ Neck carcinoma ▫ Lung carcinoma ▪ Treatment of severe psoriasis and rheumatoid arthritis unresponsive to conventional therapy ▪ Treatment of mycosis fungoides.

ACTION

▪ Interferes with folic acid metabolism. Result is inhibition of DNA synthesis and cell reproduction (cell-cycle S phase–specific) ▪ Also has immunosuppressive activity. **Therapeutic Effects:** ▪ Death of rapidly replicating cells, particularly malignant ones, and immunosuppression.

PHARMACOKINETICS

Absorption: Small doses are well absorbed from the GI tract. Larger doses incompletely absorbed.

Distribution: Actively transported across cell membranes, widely distributed. Does not reach therapeutic concentrations in the CSF. Crosses the placenta; enters breast milk in low concentrations.

Metabolism and Excretion: Excreted mostly unchanged by the kidneys.

Half-life: 2–4 hr (increased in renal impairment).

CONTRAINDICATIONS AND PRECAUTIONS

Contraindicated in: ▪ Hypersensitivity ▪ Pregnancy or lactation.

Use Cautiously in: ▪ Renal impairment (CCr must be ≥60 ml/min prior to therapy) ▪ Patients with childbearing potential ▪ Active infections ▪ Decreased bone marrow reserve ▪ Geriatric patients or patients with other chronic debilitating illnesses.

ADVERSE REACTIONS AND SIDE EFFECTS*

CNS: arachnoiditis (IT use only), dizziness, drowsiness, headaches, malaise.

EENT: blurred vision.

Resp: PULMONARY FIBROSIS.

GI: anorexia, hepatotoxicity, nausea, stomatitis, vomiting.

GU: gonadal suppression.

Derm: alopecia, photosensitivity, pruritus, rashes, urticaria.

Hemat: anemia, leukopenia, thrombocytopenia.

Metab: hyperuricemia.

Misc: nephropathy, chills, fever.

INTERACTIONS

Drug-Drug: ▪ The following drugs may increase the toxicity of methotrexate: high-dose **salicylates, NSAIDs, sulfonylureas (oral hypoglycemic agents), phenytoin, tetracyclines, probenecid, trimethoprim/sulfamethoxazole, pyrimethamine**, and **chloramphenicol** ▪ Additive hepatotoxicity with other **hepatotoxic drugs** ▪ Additive nephrotoxicity with other **nephrotoxic drugs** ▪ Additive bone marrow depression with other **antineoplastic agents** or **radiation therapy** ▪ May decrease antibody response to **live virus vaccines** and increase the risk of adverse reactions ▪ Increased risk of neurologic reactions with **acyclovir** (IT methotrexate only) ▪ **Asparaginase** may decrease effects of methotrexate.

ROUTE AND DOSAGE

▫ Trophoblastic Neoplasms

- **PO, IM (Adults):** 15–30 mg/day for 5 days; repeat after 1 or more weeks for 3–5 courses.

▫ Breast Cancer

- **IV (Adults):** 40 mg/m² on days 1 and 8 (with other agents; many regimens are used).

▫ Leukemia

- **PO (Adults):** *Induction*—3.3 mg/m²/day, usually with prednisone.
- **PO, IM (Adults):** *Maintenance*—20–30 mg/m² twice weekly.
- **IV (Adults):** 2.5 mg/kg q 2 wk.
- **IT (Adults):** 12 mg/m² or 15 mg.
- **IT (Children ≥3 yr):** 12 mg.
- **IT (Children 2 yr):** 10 mg.
- **IT (Children 1 yr):** 8 mg.
- **IT (Children <1 yr):** 6 mg.

▫ Osteosarcoma

- **IV (Adults):** 12 g/m² as a 4-hr infusion followed by leucovorin rescue, usually as part of a combination chemotherapeutic regimen (or increase dose until peak serum methotrexate level is 1×10^{-3} M/liter but not to exceed 15 g/m²; 12 courses are given starting 4 wk

M

***CAPITALS indicate life-threatening; underlines indicate most frequent.**

after surgery and repeated at scheduled intervals.

❑ **Psoriasis**

Therapy may be preceded by a 5–10 mg test dose.

- **PO (Adults):** 2.5–5 mg q 12 hr for 3 doses or q 8 hr for 4 doses once weekly (not to exceed 30 mg/wk).
- **PO, IM, IV (Adults):** 10–25 mg/weekly (not to exceed 30 mg/wk).

❑ **Arthritis**

Therapy may be preceded by a 5–10 mg test dose.

- **PO (Adults):** 7.5 mg weekly (2.5 mg q 12 hr for 3 doses or single dose, not to exceed 20 mg/wk); when response is obtained, dosage should be decreased.

❑ **Mycosis Fungoides**

- **PO (Adults):** 2.5–10 mg/day for several weeks to months.
- **IM (Adults):** 50 mg once weekly or 25 mg twice weekly.

AVAILABILITY

▪ ***Tablets:*** 2.5 mg[Rx] ▪ ***Injection:*** 2.5 mg/ml[Rx], 25 mg/ml[Rx], 20 mg[Rx], 50 mg[Rx], 100 mg[Rx], 250 mg[Rx], 1 g[Rx] ▪ ***Preservative-free injection:*** 25 mg/ml[Rx].

TIME/ACTION PROFILE (effects on blood counts)

	ONSET	PEAK	DURATION
PO, IM, IV	4–7 days	7–14 days	21 days

NURSING IMPLICATIONS

ASSESSMENT

- **General Info:** Monitor blood pressure, pulse, and respiratory rate periodically during administration. Report significant changes.
- Monitor for abdominal pain, diarrhea, or stomatitis. Report occurrence; therapy may need to be discontinued.
- Monitor for bone marrow depression. Assess for bleeding (bleeding gums, bruising, petechiae, guaiac stools, urine, and emesis) and avoid IM injections and rectal temperatures if platelet count is low. Apply pressure to venipuncture sites for 10 min. Assess for signs of infection during neutropenia. Anemia may occur. Monitor for increased fatigue, dyspnea, and orthostatic hypotension.
- Monitor intake and output ratios and daily weights. Report significant changes in totals.
- Monitor for symptoms of pulmonary toxicity, which may manifest early as a dry, nonproductive cough.
- Monitor for symptoms of gout (increased uric acid, joint pain, edema). Encourage patient to drink at least 2 liters of fluid each day. Allopurinol and alkalinization of urine may be used to decrease uric acid levels.
- Assess patient's nutritional status. Administering an antiemetic prior to and periodically throughout therapy and adjusting diet as tolerated may help maintain fluid and electrolyte balance and nutritional status.
- **IT:** Assess for development of nuchal rigidity, headache, fever, confusion, drowsiness, dizziness, weakness, or seizures.
- **Rheumatoid Arthritis:** Assess patient for pain and range of motion prior to and periodically throughout therapy.
- **Psoriasis:** Assess skin lesions prior to and periodically throughout therapy.
- ***Lab Test Considerations:*** Monitor CBC and differential prior to and frequently throughout therapy. The nadir of leukopenia and thrombocytopenia occurs in 7–14 days. Leukocyte and thrombocyte counts usually recover 7 days after the nadirs. Notify physician of any sudden drop in values.
- Renal (BUN and creatinine) and hepatic function (AST, ALT, bilirubin, and LDH) should be monitored prior to and routinely throughout course of therapy. Urine pH should be monitored prior to high-dose methotrexate therapy and every 6 hr during leucovorin rescue. Urine pH should be kept above 7.0 to prevent renal damage.
- May cause elevated serum uric acid concentrations, especially during initial treatment of leukemia and lymphoma.
- ***Toxicity and Overdose:*** Serum methotrexate levels should be monitored every 12–24 hr during high-dose therapy until levels are $<5 \times 10^{-8}$ M. This monitoring is essential to plan correct leucovorin dose and determine duration of rescue therapy.
- With high-dose therapy, patient must receive leucovorin rescue within 24–48 hr to prevent fatal toxicity.

POTENTIAL NURSING DIAGNOSES

- Infection, risk for (Adverse Reactions).
- Nutrition, altered, less than body requirements (Adverse Reactions).
- Knowledge deficit, related to medication regimen (Patient/Family Teaching).

IMPLEMENTATION

- **General Info:** Solutions for injection should be prepared in a biologic cabinet. Wear gloves, gown, and mask while handling medication. Discard equipment in specially designated containers (see Appendix I).
- **Direct IV:** Reconstitute each vial with 25 ml of 0.9% NaCl for a concentration no greater than 25 mg/ml. Use sterile preservative-free diluents for high-dose regimens to prevent complications from large amounts of benzyl alcohol. Do not use preparations that are discolored or that contain a precipitate. Reconstitute immediately before use. Discard unused portion.
- ***Rate:*** Administer at a rate of 10 mg/min into Y-site of a free-flowing IV.
- **Intermittent/Continuous Infusion:** May also be diluted in D5W, D5/0.9% NaCl, or 0.9% NaCl and infused as intermittent or continuous infusion.
- ***Rate:*** Administration rates of 4–20 mg/hr have been used.
- **Y-Site Compatibility:** ▪ amifostine ▪ asparaginase ▪ bleomycin ▪ cefepime ▪ ceftriaxone ▪ cimetidine ▪ cisplatin ▪ cyclophosphamide ▪ cytarabine ▪ daunorubicin ▪ diphenhydramine ▪ doxorubicin ▪ etoposide ▪ famotidine ▪ filgrastim ▪ fludarabine ▪ fluorouracil ▪ furosemide ▪ gallium nitrate ▪ ganciclovir ▪ granisetron ▪ heparin ▪ hydromorphone ▪ imipenem/cilastatin ▪ leucovorin ▪ lorazepam ▪ melphalan ▪ mesna ▪ methylprednisolone sodium succinate ▪ metoclopramide ▪ mitomycin ▪ morphine ▪ ondansetron ▪ paclitaxel ▪ piperacillin/tazobactam ▪ prochlorperazine ▪ ranitidine ▪ sargramostim ▪ teniposide ▪ thiotepa ▪ vancomycin ▪ vinblastine ▪ vincristine ▪ vinorelbine.
- **Y-Site Incompatibility:** ▪ chlorpromazine ▪ idarubicin ▪ ifosfamide ▪ midazolam ▪ nalbuphine ▪ promethazine.
- **Additive Compatibility:** ▪ cyclophosphamide ▪ cytarabine ▪ fluorouracil ▪ sodium bicarbonate.
- **IT:** Reconstitute preservative-free methotrexate with preservative-free 0.9% NaCl, Elliot's B solution, or patient's CSF to a concentration of 1 mg/ml. May be administered via lumbar puncture or Ommaya reservoir. To prevent bacterial contamination, use immediately.

PATIENT/FAMILY TEACHING

- ☐ Instruct patient to take medication exactly as directed. If a dose is missed, it should be omitted. Health care professional should be consulted if vomiting occurs shortly after a dose is taken.
- ☐ Instruct patient to notify health care professional promptly if fever; chills; cough; hoarseness; sore throat; signs of infection; lower back or side pain; painful or difficult urination; bleeding gums; bruising; petechiae; blood in stools, urine, or emesis; increased fatigue; dyspnea; or orthostatic hypotension occurs. Caution patient to avoid crowds and persons with known infections. Instruct patient to use soft toothbrush and electric razor and to avoid falls. Caution patient not to drink alcoholic beverages or take medication containing aspirin or NSAIDS; may precipitate gastric bleeding.
- ☐ Instruct patient to inspect oral mucosa for erythema and ulceration. If ulceration occurs, advise patient to use sponge brush and to rinse mouth with water after eating and drinking. Topical therapy may be used if mouth pain interferes with eating. Stomatitis pain may require treatment with opioid analgesics.
- ☐ Instruct patient to avoid the use of OTC drugs without first consulting health care professional.
- ☐ Advise patient that this medication may have teratogenic effects. Contraception should be used during therapy and for at least 3 mo for men and 1 ovulatory cycle for women after completion of therapy.
- ☐ Discuss the possibility of hair loss with patient. Explore methods of coping.
- ☐ Instruct patient not to receive any vaccinations without advice of health care professional.
- ☐ Caution patient to use sunscreen and protective clothing to prevent photosensitivity reactions.
- ☐ Emphasize the need for periodic lab tests to monitor for side effects.

EVALUATION

Effectiveness of therapy can be demonstrated by: ▪ Improvement of hematopoietic values in leukemia ▫ Decrease in symptoms of meningeal involvement in leukemia ▪ Decrease in size and spread of non-Hodgkin's lymphomas and other solid cancers ▪ Resolution of skin lesions in severe psoriasis ▪ Decreased joint pain and swelling ▫ Improved mobility in patients with rheumatoid arthritis ▪ Regression of lesions in mycosis fungoides.

METHYLDOPA, oral
(meth-ill-**doe**-pa)
Aldomet, {Apo-Methyldopa}, {Dopamet}, {Novamedopa}, {Nu-Medopa}

METHYLDOPATE, intravenous
(meth-ill-**doe**-pate)
Aldomet

CLASSIFICATION(S):
Antihypertensive agent (centrally acting alpha-adrenergic agonist)

Pregnancy Category B

INDICATIONS

▪ Management of moderate to severe hypertension (with other agents) ▪ Due to delayed onset, parenteral form should not be used in emergencies.

ACTION

▪ Stimulates CNS alpha-adrenergic receptors, producing a decrease in sympathetic outflow to heart, kidneys, and blood vessels. Result is decreased blood pressure and peripheral resistance, a slight decrease in heart rate, and no change in cardiac output. **Therapeutic Effects:** ▪ Lowering of blood pressure.

PHARMACOKINETICS

Absorption: 50% absorbed from the GI tract. Parenteral form, methyldopate hydrochloride, is slowly converted to methyldopa.
Distribution: Crosses the blood-brain barrier. Crosses the placenta; small amounts enter breast milk.
Metabolism and Excretion: Partially metabolized by the liver, partially excreted unchanged by the kidneys.
Half-life: 1.7 hr.

CONTRAINDICATIONS AND PRECAUTIONS

Contraindicated in: ▪ Hypersensitivity ▪ Active liver disease ▪ Some products contain alcohol or bisulfites and should be avoided in patients with known intolerance.
Use Cautiously in: ▪ Previous history of liver disease ▪ Geriatric patients (increased risk of adverse reactions) ▪ Pregnancy (has been used safely) ▪ Lactation.

ADVERSE REACTIONS AND SIDE EFFECTS*

CNS: <u>sedation</u>, decreased mental acuity, depression.
EENT: nasal stuffiness.
CV: MYOCARDITIS, bradycardia, edema, orthostatic hypotension.
GI: DRUG-INDUCED HEPATITIS, diarrhea, dry mouth.
GU: <u>impotence</u>.
Hemat: eosinophilia, hemolytic anemia.
Misc: fever.

INTERACTIONS

Drug-Drug: ▪ Additive hypotension with other **antihypertensive agents,** acute ingestion of **alcohol, anesthesia,** and **nitrates** ▪ **Amphetamines, barbiturates, tricyclic antidepressants, NSAIDs,** and **phenothiazines** may decrease antihypertensive effect of methyldopa ▪ Increased effects and risk of psychoses with **haloperidol** ▪ Excess sympathetic stimulation may occur with concurrent use of **MAO inhibitors** or **sympathomimetics** ▪ May increase the effects of **tolbutamide** ▪ May increase **lithium** toxicity ▪ Additive hypotension and CNS toxicity with **levodopa** ▪ Additive CNS depression may occur with **alcohol, antihistamines, sedative/hypnotics,** some **antidepressants,** and **opioids.**

ROUTE AND DOSAGE

▪ **PO (Adults):** 250–500 mg 2–3 times daily (not to exceed 500 mg/day if used with other

{} = Available in Canada only.
*CAPITALS indicate life-threatening; <u>underlines</u> indicate most frequent.

agents); may be increased q 2 days as needed; usual maintenance dose is 500 mg–2 g/day (not to exceed 3 g/day).

- **PO (Children):** 10 mg/kg/day (300 mg/m²/day); may be increased q 2 days up to 65 mg/kg/day in divided doses (not to exceed 3 g/day).
- **IV (Adults):** 250–500 mg q 6 hr; up to 1 g q 6 hr.
- **IV (Children):** 5–10 mg/kg q 6 hr; up to 65 mg/kg/day in divided doses (not to exceed 3 g/day).

AVAILABILITY

■ ***Tablets:*** 125 mg[Rx], 250 mg[Rx], 500 mg[Rx] ■ ***Oral suspension:*** 250 mg/5 ml[Rx] ■ ***Injection:*** 250 mg/5 ml in 5- and 10-ml vials[Rx] ■ ***In combination with:*** hydrochlorothiazide (Aldoril) or chlorothiazide (Aldoclor[Rx]). See Appendix A.

TIME/ACTION PROFILE (antihypertensive effect)

	ONSET	PEAK	DURATION
PO	12–24 hr	4–6 hr	24–48 hr
IV	4–6 hr	UK	10–16 hr

NURSING IMPLICATIONS

ASSESSMENT

- □ Monitor blood pressure and pulse frequently during initial dosage adjustment and periodically throughout therapy. Report significant changes.
- □ Monitor frequency of prescription refills to determine compliance.
- □ Monitor intake and output ratios and weight and assess for edema daily, especially at beginning of therapy. Report weight gain or edema; sodium and water retention may be treated with diuretics.
- □ Assess patient for depression or other alterations in mental status. Notify physician or other health care professional promptly if these symptoms develop.
- □ Monitor temperature during therapy. Drug fever may occur shortly after initiation of therapy and may be accompanied by eosinophilia and hepatic function changes. Monitor hepatic function test if unexplained fever occurs.
- ■ ***Lab Test Considerations:*** Renal and hepatic function and CBC should be monitored prior to and periodically throughout therapy.
- □ Monitor direct Coombs' test prior to and after 6 and 12 mo of therapy. May cause a positive direct Coombs' test, rarely associated with hemolytic anemia.
- □ May cause increased BUN, serum creatinine, potassium, sodium, prolactin, uric acid, AST, ALT, alkaline phosphatase, and bilirubin concentrations.
- □ May cause prolonged prothrombin times.
- □ May interfere with serum creatinine and AST measurements.

POTENTIAL NURSING DIAGNOSES

- Injury, risk for (Side Effects).
- Knowledge deficit, related to medication regimen (Patient/Family Teaching).
- Noncompliance (Patient/Family Teaching).

IMPLEMENTATION

- ■ **General Info:** Fluid retention and expanded volume may cause tolerance to develop within 2–3 mo after initiation of therapy. Diuretics may be added to regimen at this time to maintain control.
- □ Dosage increases should be made with the evening dose to minimize drowsiness.
- □ When changing from IV to oral forms, dosage should remain consistent.
- ■ **PO:** Shake suspension prior to administration.
- ■ **Intermittent Infusion:** Dilute in 100 ml of D5W, 0.9% NaCl, D5/0.9% NaCl, 5% sodium bicarbonate, or Ringer's solution.
- ■ ***Rate:*** Infuse slowly over 30–60 min.
- ■ **Y-Site Compatibility:** ■ esmolol ■ heparin ■ meperidine ■ morphine ■ theophylline.

PATIENT/FAMILY TEACHING

- □ Emphasize the importance of continuing to take this medication, even if feeling well. Instruct patient to take medication at the same time each day; last dose of the day should be taken at bedtime. If a dose is missed, take as soon as remembered but not if almost time for next dose. Do not double doses.
- □ Encourage patient to comply with additional interventions for hypertension (weight reduction, low-sodium diet, smoking cessation, moderation of alcohol consumption, regular exercise, and stress management). Methyldopa controls but does not cure hypertension.
- □ Instruct patient and family on proper technique for monitoring blood pressure. Advise

them to check blood pressure at least weekly and to report significant changes.

- Inform patient that urine may darken or turn red-black when left standing.
- May cause drowsiness. Advise patient to avoid driving or other activities requiring alertness until response to medication is known. Drowsiness usually subsides after 7–10 days of continuous use.
- Caution patient to avoid sudden changes in position to decrease orthostatic hypotension.
- Advise patient that frequent mouth rinses, good oral hygiene, and sugarless gum or candy may minimize dry mouth. Notify health care professional if dry mouth continues for >2 wk.
- Caution patient to avoid concurrent use of alcohol or other CNS depressants.
- Advise patient to consult health care professional before taking any cough, cold, or allergy remedies.
- Advise patient to notify health care professional of medication regimen prior to treatment or surgery.
- Instruct patient to notify health care professional if fever, muscle aches, or flu-like syndrome occurs.

EVALUATION

Effectiveness of therapy can be demonstrated by: ▪ Decrease in blood pressure without appearance of side effects.

METHYLERGONOVINE

(meth-ill-er-goe-**noe**-veen)

Methergine

CLASSIFICATION(S):

Oxytocic

Pregnancy Category C

INDICATIONS

▪ Prevention and treatment of postpartum or postabortion hemorrhage caused by uterine atony or subinvolution.

ACTION

▪ Directly stimulates uterine and vascular smooth muscle. **Therapeutic Effects:** ▪ Uterine contraction.

PHARMACOKINETICS

Absorption: Well absorbed following oral or IM administration.

Distribution: UK. Enters breast milk in small quantities.

Metabolism and Excretion: Probably metabolized by the liver.

Half-life: 30–120 min.

CONTRAINDICATIONS AND PRECAUTIONS

Contraindicated in: ▪ Hypersensitivity ▪ Should not be used to induce labor.

Use Cautiously in: ▪ Hypertensive or eclamptic patients (more susceptible to hypertensive and arrhythmogenic side effects) ▪ Severe hepatic or renal disease ▪ Sepsis. **Exercise Extreme Caution in:** ▪ Third stage of labor.

ADVERSE REACTIONS AND SIDE EFFECTS*

CNS: dizziness, headache.

EENT: tinnitus.

Resp: dyspnea.

CV: HYPOTENSION, arrhythmias, chest pain, hypertension, palpitations.

GI: <u>nausea</u>, <u>vomiting</u>.

GU: <u>cramps</u>.

Derm: diaphoresis.

Misc: allergic reactions.

INTERACTIONS

Drug-Drug: ▪ Excessive vasoconstriction may result when used with heavy cigarette smoking **(nicotine)** or other **vasopressors** such as **dopamine.**

ROUTE AND DOSAGE

- **PO (Adults):** 200–400 mcg (0.4–0.6 mg) q 6–12 hr for 2–7 days.
- **IM, IV (Adults):** 200 mcg (0.2 mg) q 2–4 hr for up to 5 doses.

AVAILABILITY

▪ ***Tablets:*** 200 mcg (0.2 mg)[Rx] ▪ ***Injection:*** 200 mcg (0.2 mg)/ml in 1-ml ampules[Rx].

***CAPITALS** indicate life-threatening; **underlines** indicate most frequent.**

TIME/ACTION PROFILE (effects on uterine contractions)

	ONSET	PEAK	DURATION
PO	5–15 min	UK	3 hr
IM	2–5 min	UK	3 hr
IV	immediate	UK	45 min–3 hr

NURSING IMPLICATIONS

ASSESSMENT

- □ Monitor blood pressure, heart rate, and uterine response frequently during medication administration. Notify physician or other health care professional promptly if uterine relaxation becomes prolonged or if character of vaginal bleeding changes.
- □ Assess for signs of ergotism (cold, numb fingers and toes, chest pain, nausea, vomiting, headache, muscle pain, weakness).
- ▪ ***Lab Test Considerations:*** If no response to methylergonovine, calcium levels may need to be assessed. Effectiveness of medication is decreased with hypocalcemia.
- □ May cause decreased serum prolactin levels.

POTENTIAL NURSING DIAGNOSES

- ▪ Pain (Side Effects).
- ▪ Knowledge deficit, related to medication regimen (Patient/Family Teaching).

IMPLEMENTATION

- ▪ **IV:** IV administration is used for emergencies only. Oral and IM routes are preferred.
- ▪ **Direct IV:** May be given undiluted or diluted in 5 ml of 0.9% NaCl and administered through Y-site. Do not add to IV solutions. Do not mix in syringe with any other drug. Refrigerate; stable for storage at room temperature for 60 days; deteriorates with age. Use only solution that is clear and colorless and that contains no precipitate.
- ▪ ***Rate:*** Administer at a rate of 0.2 mg over at least 1 min.
- ▪ **Y-Site Compatibility:** ▪ heparin ▪ hydrocortisone sodium succinate ▪ potassium chloride ▪ vitamin B complex with C.

PATIENT/FAMILY TEACHING

- □ Instruct patient to take medication as directed; do not skip or double up on missed doses. If a dose is missed, omit it and return to regular dosage schedule.
- □ Advise patient that medication may cause menstrual-like cramps.
- □ Caution patient to avoid smoking, as nicotine constricts blood vessels.
- □ Instruct patient to notify health care professional if infection develops, as this may cause increased sensitivity to the medication.

EVALUATION

Effectiveness of therapy can be demonstrated by: ▪ Contractions that maintain uterine tone and prevent postpartum hemorrhage.

METHYLPHENIDATE

(meth-ill-**fen**-i-date)

PMS-Methylphenidate, Ritalin, Ritalin-SR

CLASSIFICATION(S):

CNS stimulant

Schedule II

Pregnancy Category C

INDICATIONS

▪ Adjunct in the treatment of attention-deficit hyperactivity disorder (ADHD) ▪ Symptomatic treatment of narcolepsy. **Unlabeled Uses:** ▪ Management of some forms of depression when more conventional antidepressants cannot be used.

ACTION

▪ Produces CNS and respiratory stimulation with weak sympathomimetic activity. **Therapeutic Effects:** ▪ Increased attention span in ADHD ▪ Increased motor activity, mental alertness, and diminished fatigue in narcoleptic patients.

PHARMACOKINETICS

Absorption: Well absorbed following oral administration; absorption of extended-release tablet (SR) is delayed.

Distribution: UK.

Metabolism and Excretion: Mostly metabolized (80%) by the liver.

Half-life: 1–3 hr.

CONTRAINDICATIONS AND PRECAUTIONS

Contraindicated in: ▪ Hypersensitivity ▪ Hyperexcitable states ▪ Hyperthyroidism ▪ Patients with

M

psychotic personalities or suicidal or homicidal tendencies ▪ Glaucoma ▪ Motor tics.

Use Cautiously in: ▪ History of cardiovascular disease ▪ Hypertension ▪ Diabetes mellitus ▪ Geriatric or debilitated patients ▪ Continual use (may result in psychological or physical dependence) ▪ Seizure disorders (may lower seizure threshold) ▪ Pregnancy or lactation (safety not established).

ADVERSE REACTIONS AND SIDE EFFECTS*

CNS: hyperactivity, insomnia, restlessness, tremor, dizziness, headache, irritability.
EENT: blurred vision.
CV: hypertension, palpitations, tachycardia, hypotension.
GI: anorexia, constipation, cramps, diarrhea, dry mouth, metallic taste, nausea, vomiting.
Derm: rashes.
Neuro: akathisia, dyskinesia.
Misc: fever, hypersensitivity reactions, physical dependence, psychological dependence, suppression of weight gain (children), tolerance.

INTERACTIONS

Drug-Drug: ▪ Additive sympathomimetic effects with other **sympathomimetics**, including **vasoconstrictors** and **decongestants** ▪ Use with **MAO inhibitors** or **vasopressors** may result in hypertensive crisis ▪ May antagonize the hypotensive effect of **guanethidine** ▪ Metabolism of **warfarin, anticonvulsants,** and **tricyclic antidepressants** may be inhibited and effects increased ▪ Avoid concurrent use with **pimozide** (may mask cause of tics).
Drug-Food: ▪ Excessive use of **caffeine**-containing foods or beverages (coffee, cola, tea) may cause additive CNS stimulation.

ROUTE AND DOSAGE

- **PO (Adults):** 5–20 mg 2–3 times daily. When maintenance dose is determined, may change to sustained-release formulation 20 mg 1–3 times daily at 8-hr intervals.
- **PO (Children >6 yr):** 5 mg before breakfast and lunch; increase by 5–10 mg at weekly intervals (not to exceed 60 mg/day). When maintenance dose is determined, may change to sustained-release formulation 20 mg 1–3 times daily at 8-hr intervals.

AVAILABILITY

- ***Tablets:*** 5 mg[Rx], 10 mg[Rx], 20 mg[Rx] ▪ ***Sustained-release tablets:*** 20 mg[Rx].

TIME/ACTION PROFILE (CNS stimulation)

	ONSET	PEAK	DURATION
PO	UK	1–3 hr	4–6 hr
PO-ER	UK	UK	up to 8 hr

NURSING IMPLICATIONS

ASSESSMENT

- **General Info:** Monitor blood pressure, pulse, and respiration before administering and periodically throughout therapy.
  - Monitor growth, both height and weight, in children on long-term therapy.
  - May produce a false sense of euphoria and well-being. Provide frequent rest periods and observe patient for rebound depression after the effects of the medication have worn off.
  - Methylphenidate has high dependence and abuse potential. Tolerance to medication occurs rapidly; do not increase dose.
- **Attention-Deficit Hyperactivity Disorder:** Assess attention span, impulse control, and interactions with others in children. Therapy may be interrupted at intervals to determine whether symptoms are sufficient to continue therapy.
- **Narcolepsy:** Observe and document frequency of episodes.
- ***Lab Test Considerations:*** Monitor CBC, differential, and platelet count periodically in patients receiving prolonged therapy.

POTENTIAL NURSING DIAGNOSES

- Thought processes, altered (Side Effects).
- Knowledge deficit, related to medication regimen (Patient/Family Teaching).

IMPLEMENTATION

- **PO:** Administer with or after a meal. Sustained-release tablets should be swallowed whole; do not crush, break, or chew.

PATIENT/FAMILY TEACHING

- **General Info:** Instruct patient to take medication exactly as directed. If a dose is missed, take the remaining doses for that day at reg-

***CAPITALS indicate life-threatening; underlines indicate most frequent.**

ularly spaced intervals; do not double doses. Take the last dose before 6 PM to minimize the risk of insomnia. Instruct patient not to alter dosage without consulting health care professional. Abrupt cessation of high doses may cause extreme fatigue and mental depression.

- ☐ Advise patient to check weight 2–3 times weekly and report weight loss to health care professional.
- ☐ May cause dizziness or blurred vision. Caution patient to avoid driving or activities requiring alertness until response to medication is known.
- ☐ Advise patient to avoid using caffeine-containing beverages concurrently with this therapy.
- ☐ Advise patient to notify health care professional if nervousness, insomnia, palpitations, vomiting, skin rash, or fever occurs.
- ☐ Inform patient that health care professional may order periodic holidays from the drug to assess progress and to decrease dependence.
- ☐ Emphasize the importance of routine follow-up exams to monitor progress.
- ▪ **Attention-Deficit Hyperactivity Disorder:** Advise parents to notify school nurse of medication regimen.

EVALUATION

Effectiveness of therapy can be demonstrated by: ▪ Decreased frequency of narcoleptic symptoms ▪ Improved attention span and social interactions in ADHD.

METOCLOPRAMIDE

(met-oh-kloe-**pra**-mide)

{Apo-Metoclop}, Clopra, {Emex}, {Maxeran}, Octamide, Octamide-PFS, Reclomide, Reglan

CLASSIFICATION(S):

Antiemetic, GI stimulant

Pregnancy Category B

INDICATIONS

▪ Prevention of chemotherapy-induced emesis ▪ Treatment of postsurgical and diabetic gastric stasis ▪ Facilitation of small bowel intubation in radiographic procedures ▪ Management of esophageal reflux ▪ Treatment and prevention of postoperative nausea and vomiting when nasogastric suctioning is undesirable. **Unlabeled Uses:** ▪ Treatment of hiccups ▪ Adjunct management of migraine headaches.

ACTION

▪ Blocks dopamine receptors in chemoreceptor trigger zone of the CNS ▪ Stimulates motility of the upper GI tract and accelerates gastric emptying. **Therapeutic Effects:** ▪ Decreased nausea and vomiting ▪ Decreased symptoms of gastric stasis ▪ Easier passage of nasogastric tube into small bowel.

PHARMACOKINETICS

Absorption: Well absorbed from the GI tract, from rectal mucosa, and from IM sites.
Distribution: Widely distributed into body tissues and fluids. Crosses blood-brain barrier and placenta. Enters breast milk in concentrations greater than plasma.
Metabolism and Excretion: Partially metabolized by the liver; 25% eliminated unchanged in the urine.
Half-life: 2.5–5 hr.

CONTRAINDICATIONS AND PRECAUTIONS

Contraindicated in: ▪ Hypersensitivity ▪ Possible GI obstruction or hemorrhage ▪ History of seizure disorders ▪ Pheochromocytoma ▪ Parkinson's disease.
Use Cautiously in: ▪ Children and geriatric patients (↑ incidence of extrapyramidal reactions) ▪ History of depression ▪ Diabetes (may alter response to insulin) ▪ Pregnancy and lactation (safety not established).

ADVERSE REACTIONS AND SIDE EFFECTS*

CNS: drowsiness, extrapyramidal reactions, restlessness, anxiety, depression, irritability, tardive dyskinesia.
CV: arrhythmias.
GI: constipation, diarrhea, dry mouth, nausea.
Endo: gynecomastia.

M

{} = Available in Canada only.
***CAPITALS indicate life-threatening; underlines indicate most frequent.**

INTERACTIONS

Drug-Drug: ▪ Additive CNS depression with other **CNS depressants**, including **alcohol**, **antidepressants**, **antihistamines**, **opioids**, and **sedative/hypnotics** ▪ May affect the GI absorption of other **orally administered drugs** as a result of effect on GI motility ▪ May exaggerate hypotension during **general anesthesia** ▪ Increased risk of extrapyramidal reactions with agents such as **haloperidol** or **phenothiazines** ▪ **Opioid analgesics** and **anticholinergics** may antagonize the GI effects of metoclopramide ▪ May increase absorption and risk of toxicity from **cyclosporine** ▪ Use cautiously with **MAO inhibitors** (causes release of catecholamines) ▪ May increase neuromuscular blockade from **succinylcholine** ▪ May decrease the effectiveness of **levodopa.**

ROUTE AND DOSAGE

❑ Prevention of Chemotherapy-Induced Vomiting

- **IV (Adults):** 1–2 mg/kg 30 min prior to chemotherapy. Additional doses of 1–2 mg/kg may be given q 2 hr for 2 doses, then q 3 hr for 3 additional doses. May also be given as 3 mg/kg before chemotherapy, followed by 0.5 mg/kg/hr for 8 hr (unlabeled).

❑ Facilitation of Small Bowel Intubation

- **IV (Adults):** 10 mg.
- **IV (Children 6–14 yr):** 2.5–5 mg (dose should not exceed 0.5 mg/kg).
- **IV (Children <6 yr):** 0.1 mg/kg.

❑ Diabetic Gastroparesis

- **PO (Adults):** 10 mg 30 min before meals and at bedtime.

❑ Gastroesophageal Reflux

- **PO (Adults):** 10–15 mg 30 min before meals and at bedtime (not to exceed 0.5 mg/kg/day). A single dose of 20 mg may be given preventively. Some patients may respond to doses as small as 5 mg.

❑ Postoperative Nausea/Vomiting

- **IM (Adults):** 10–20 mg.

❑ Treatment of Hiccups

- **PO, IM (Adults):** 10–20 mg 4 times daily PO; may be preceded by a single 10-mg dose IM (unlabeled).

AVAILABILITY

▪ ***Tablets:*** 5 mg[Rx], 10 mg[Rx] ▪ ***Concentrated solution:*** 10 mg/ml[Rx] ▪ ***Syrup:*** 5 mg/5 ml[Rx] ▪ ***Injection:*** 5 mg/ml[Rx].

TIME/ACTION PROFILE (effects on peristalsis)

	ONSET	PEAK	DURATION
PO	30–60 min	UK	1–2 hr
IM	10–15 min	UK	1–2 hr
IV	1–3 min	immediate	1–2 hr

NURSING IMPLICATIONS

ASSESSMENT

- ☐ Assess patient for nausea, vomiting, abdominal distention, and bowel sounds prior to and following administration.
- ☐ Assess patient for extrapyramidal side effects (*parkinsonian*—difficulty speaking or swallowing, loss of balance control, pill rolling, mask-like face, shuffling gait, rigidity, tremors; and *dystonic*—muscle spasms, twisting motions, twitching, inability to move eyes, weakness of arms or legs) periodically throughout course of therapy. May occur weeks to months after initiation of therapy and are reversible upon discontinuation. Dystonic reactions may occur within minutes of IV infusion and stop within 24 hr of discontinuation of metoclopramide. May be treated with 50 mg of IM diphenhydramine or diphenhydramine 1 mg/kg IV may be administered prophylactically 15 min prior to metoclopramide IV infusion.
- ☐ Monitor for tardive dyskinesia (uncontrolled rhythmic movement of mouth, face, and extremities; lip smacking or puckering; puffing of cheeks; uncontrolled chewing; rapid or worm-like movements of tongue). Usually occurs after a year or more of continued therapy. Report immediately; may be irreversible.
- ☐ Assess patient for signs of depression periodically throughout therapy.
- ▪ ***Lab Test Considerations:*** May alter hepatic function test results.
- ☐ May cause increased serum prolactin and aldosterone concentrations.

POTENTIAL NURSING DIAGNOSES

- Nutrition, altered, less than body requirements (Indications).
- Injury, risk for (Side Effects).

- Knowledge deficit, related to medication regimen (Patient/Family Teaching).

IMPLEMENTATION

- **PO:** Administer doses 30 min before meals and at bedtime.
- **IM:** For prevention of postoperative nausea and vomiting, inject IM near the end of surgery.
- **Rect:** Suppositories may be made by pharmacist. Administer 1 suppository 30–60 min before each meal and at bedtime.
- **Direct IV:** Administer IV dose 30 min prior to administration of chemotherapeutic agent.
- ***Rate:*** Doses may be given slowly over 1–2 min. Rapid administration causes a transient but intense feeling of anxiety and restlessness followed by drowsiness.
- **Intermittent Infusion:** May be diluted for IV infusion in 50 ml of D5W, 0.9% NaCl, D5/0.45% NaCl, Ringer's solution, or lactated Ringer's solution. Diluted solution is stable for 48 hr if protected from light or 24 hr under normal light.
- ***Rate:*** Infuse slowly over at least 15 min.
- **Syringe Compatibility:** ▪ bleomycin ▪ butorphanol ▪ cyclophosphamide ▪ cytarabine ▪ dexamethasone ▪ doxorubicin ▪ fluorouracil ▪ heparin ▪ hydrocortisone ▪ leucovorin ▪ meperidine ▪ methotrimeprazine ▪ methylprednisolone sodium succinate ▪ mitomycin ▪ morphine ▪ ranitidine ▪ vinblastine ▪ vincristine.
- **Y-Site Compatibility:** ▪ acyclovir ▪ aldesleukin ▪ amifostine ▪ aztreonam ▪ bleomycin ▪ ciprofloxacin ▪ cisplatin ▪ cyclophosphamide ▪ cytarabine ▪ diltiazem ▪ doxorubicin ▪ droperidol ▪ famotidine ▪ filgrastim ▪ fluconazole ▪ fludarabine ▪ fluorouracil ▪ foscarnet ▪ gallium nitrate ▪ heparin ▪ idarubicin ▪ leucovorin ▪ melphalan ▪ meperidine ▪ methotrexate ▪ mitomycin ▪ morphine ▪ ondansetron ▪ paclitaxel ▪ piperacillin/tazobactam ▪ sargramostim ▪ sufentanil ▪ tacrolimus ▪ teniposide ▪ thiotepa ▪ vinblastine ▪ vincristine ▪ vinorelbine ▪ zidovudine.
- **Y-Site Incompatibility:** ▪ cefepime ▪ furosemide.

PATIENT/FAMILY TEACHING

- ☐ Instruct patient to take metoclopramide exactly as directed. If a dose is missed, take as soon as remembered if not almost time for next dose.
- ☐ May cause drowsiness. Caution patient to avoid driving or other activities requiring alertness until response to medication is known.
- ☐ Advise patient to avoid concurrent use of alcohol and other CNS depressants while taking this medication.
- ☐ Advise patient to notify health care professional immediately if involuntary movement of eyes, face, or limbs occurs.

EVALUATION

Effectiveness of therapy can be demonstrated by: ▪ Prevention or relief of nausea and vomiting ▪ Decreased symptoms of gastric stasis ▪ Facilitation of small bowel intubation ▪ Decreased symptoms of esophageal reflux.

METOLAZONE

(me-**tole**-a-zone)
Mykrox, Zaroxolyn

CLASSIFICATION(S):
Antihypertensive agent, Diuretic (thiazide-like)

Pregnancy Category B

INDICATIONS

▪ Mild to moderate hypertension ▪ Edema associated with congestive heart failure or the nephrotic syndrome (Zaroxolyn only).

ACTION

▪ Increases excretion of sodium and water by inhibiting sodium reabsorption in the distal tubule ▪ Promotes excretion of chloride, potassium, magnesium, and bicarbonate ▪ May produce arteriolar dilation. **Therapeutic Effects:** ▪ Lowering of blood pressure in hypertensive patients ▪ Diuresis with subsequent mobilization of edema. Effect may continue in renal impairment.

PHARMACOKINETICS

Absorption: Absorption is more rapid and more complete with prompt tablet (Mykrox). Absorption is more variable with extended tablet (Zaroxolyn).

Distribution: UK.

Metabolism and Excretion: Excreted mainly unchanged by the kidneys.

Half-life: *Extended tablet*—8 hr; *prompt tablet*—14 hr.

CONTRAINDICATIONS AND PRECAUTIONS

Contraindicated in: ▪ Hypersensitivity ▪ Cross-sensitivity with other sulfonamides may exist ▪ Anuria ▪ Lactation.

Use Cautiously in: ▪ Severe hepatic impairment ▪ Geriatric patients (increased sensitivity). ▪ Pregnancy or children (safety not established).

ADVERSE REACTIONS AND SIDE EFFECTS*

CNS: drowsiness, lethargy.
CV: chest pain, hypotension, palpitations.
GI: anorexia, bloating, cramping, drug-induced hepatitis, nausea, vomiting.
Derm: photosensitivity, rashes.
Endo: hyperglycemia.
F and E: hypokalemia, dehydration, hypercalcemia, hypochloremic alkalosis, hypomagnesemia, hyponatremia, hypophosphatemia, hypovolemia.
Hemat: blood dyscrasias.
Metab: hyperuricemia.
MS: muscle cramps.
Misc: chills, pancreatitis.

INTERACTIONS

Drug-Drug: ▪ Additive hypotension with **nitrates, acute ingestion of alcohol,** or other **antihypertensives** ▪ Additive hypokalemia with **glucocorticoids, amphotericin B, mezlocillin, piperacillin,** or **ticarcillin** ▪ By causing hypokalemia, may increase the risk of **digitalis glycoside** toxicity ▪ Decreases the excretion of **lithium;** may cause toxicity ▪ May decrease the effectiveness of **methenamine.**

Drug-Food: ▪ **Food** may increase extent of absorption.

ROUTE AND DOSAGE

❑ **Mykrox**

▪ **PO (Adults):** *Hypertension*—0.5–1 mg/day.

❑ **Zaroxolyn**

▪ **PO (Adults):** *Hypertension*—2.5–5 mg/day; *edema*—5–20 mg/day.

AVAILABILITY

▪ ***Mykrox tablets:*** 0.5 mg[Rx] ▪ ***Zaroxolyn tablets:*** 2.5 mg[Rx], 5 mg[Rx], 10 mg[Rx].

TIME/ACTION PROFILE (diuretic effect†)

	ONSET	PEAK	DURATION
PO	1 hr	2 hr	12–24 hr

†Full antihypertensive effect may take days–weeks.

NURSING IMPLICATIONS

ASSESSMENT

▪ **General Info:** Monitor blood pressure, intake and output, and daily weight, and assess feet, legs, and sacral area for edema daily.
□ Assess patient, especially if taking digitalis glycosides, for anorexia, nausea, vomiting, muscle cramps, paresthesia, and confusion. Notify physician or other health care professional if these signs of electrolyte imbalance occur. Patients taking digitalis glycosides are at risk of digitalis toxicity due to the potassium-depleting effect of the diuretic.
□ Assess patient for allergy to sulfonamides.

▪ **Hypertension:** Monitor blood pressure prior to and periodically throughout therapy.
□ Monitor frequency of prescription refills to determine compliance.

▪ ***Lab Test Considerations:*** Monitor electrolytes (especially potassium), blood glucose, BUN, and serum creatinine and uric acid levels prior to and periodically throughout therapy.
□ May cause increase in serum and urine glucose in diabetic patients.
□ May cause an increase in serum bilirubin, calcium, creatinine, and uric acid, and a decrease in serum magnesium, potassium, and sodium and urinary calcium concentrations.
□ May cause decreased serum protein-bound iodine (PBI) concentrations.
□ May cause increased serum cholesterol, low-density lipoprotein, and triglyceride concentrations.

POTENTIAL NURSING DIAGNOSES

▪ Fluid volume excess (Indications).
▪ Fluid volume deficit (Side Effects).
▪ Knowledge deficit, related to medication regimen (Patient/Family Teaching).

IMPLEMENTATION

▪ **General Info:** Administer in the morning to prevent disruption of sleep cycle.

*CAPITALS indicate life-threatening; underlines indicate most frequent.

- □ Intermittent dose schedule may be used for continued control of edema.
- □ Extended (Zaroxolyn) and prompt (Mykrox) metolazone tablets are not equal. Do not substitute.
- ■ **PO:** May give with food or milk to minimize GI irritation.

PATIENT/FAMILY TEACHING

- ■ **General Info:** Instruct patient to take this medication at the same time each day. If a dose is missed, take as soon as remembered but not just before next dose is due. Do not double doses.
- □ Instruct patient to monitor weight biweekly and notify health care professional of significant changes.
- □ Caution patient to change positions slowly to minimize orthostatic hypotension. This may be potentiated by alcohol.
- □ Advise patient to use sunscreen and protective clothing in the sun to prevent photosensitivity reactions.
- □ Instruct patient to discuss dietary potassium requirements with health care professional (see Appendix K).
- □ Instruct patient to notify health care professional of medication regimen prior to treatment or surgery.
- □ Advise patient to report muscle weakness, cramps, nausea, vomiting, diarrhea, or dizziness to health care professional.
- □ Emphasize the importance of routine follow-up exams.
- ■ **Hypertension:** Advise patient to continue taking the medication even if feeling better. Medication controls but does not cure hypertension.
- □ Encourage patient to comply with additional interventions for hypertension (weight reduction, low-sodium diet, regular exercise, smoking cessation, moderation of alcohol consumption, and stress management).
- □ Instruct patient and family in correct technique for monitoring weekly blood pressure.
- □ Advise patient to consult health care professional before taking OTC medication, especially cough or cold preparations, concurrently with this therapy.

EVALUATION

Effectiveness of therapy can be demonstrated by: ■ Decrease in blood pressure ■ Increase in urine output ■ Decrease in edema.

METOPROLOL

(me-**toe**-proe-lole)
{Betaloc}, {Betaloc Durules}, {Lopresor}, {Lopresor SR}, Lopressor, {Novometoprol}, Toprol-XL

CLASSIFICATION(S):
Antianginal, Antiarrhythmic, Antihypertensive agent, Beta-adrenergic blocking agent (selective)

Pregnancy Category C

INDICATIONS

■ Hypertension ■ Angina pectoris ■ Prevention of MI and decreased mortality in patients with recent MI. **Unlabeled Uses:** ■ Ventricular arrhythmias/tachycardia ■ Migraine prophylaxis ■ Tremors ■ Aggressive behavior ■ Drug-induced akathisia ■ Anxiety.

ACTION

■ Blocks stimulation of $beta_1$ (myocardial) -adrenergic receptors. Does not usually affect $beta_2$ (pulmonary, vascular, uterine) receptor sites. **Therapeutic Effects:** ■ Decreased blood pressure and heart rate ■ Decreased frequency of attacks of angina pectoris.

PHARMACOKINETICS

Absorption: Well absorbed following oral administration.
Distribution: Crosses the blood-brain barrier, crosses the placenta; small amounts enter breast milk.
Metabolism and Excretion: Mostly metabolized by the liver.
Half-life: 3–7 hr.

CONTRAINDICATIONS AND PRECAUTIONS

Contraindicated in: ■ Uncompensated congestive heart failure (CHF) ■ Pulmonary edema

M

▪ Cardiogenic shock ▪ Bradycardia or heart block.

Use Cautiously in: ▪ Renal impairment ▪ Hepatic impairment ▪ Geriatric patients (increased sensitivity to beta-adrenergic blockers; initial dosage reduction recommended) ▪ Pulmonary disease (including asthma; beta$_1$ selectivity may be lost at higher doses) ▪ Diabetes mellitus (may mask signs of hypoglycemia) ▪ Thyrotoxicosis (may mask symptoms) ▪ Patients with a history of severe allergic reactions (intensity of reactions may be increased) ▪ Pregnancy, lactation, or children (safety not established; all agents cross the placenta and may cause fetal/neonatal bradycardia, hypotension, hypoglycemia, or respiratory depression).

ADVERSE REACTIONS AND SIDE EFFECTS*

CNS: fatigue, weakness, anxiety, depression, dizziness, drowsiness, insomnia, memory loss, mental status changes, nervousness, nightmares.
EENT: blurred vision, stuffy nose.
Resp: bronchospasm, wheezing.
CV: BRADYCARDIA, CHF, PULMONARY EDEMA, hypotension, peripheral vasoconstriction.
GI: constipation, diarrhea, nausea, vomiting.
GU: impotence, decreased libido, urinary frequency.
Derm: rashes.
Endo: hyperglycemia, hypoglycemia.
MS: arthralgia, back pain, joint pain.

INTERACTIONS

Drug-Drug: ▪ **General anesthesia, IV phenytoin,** and **verapamil** may cause additive myocardial depression ▪ Additive bradycardia may occur with **cardiac glycosides** ▪ Additive hypotension may occur with other **antihypertensives,** acute ingestion of **alcohol,** or **nitrates** ▪ Concurrent use with **amphetamines, cocaine, ephedrine, epinephrine, norepinephrine, phenylephrine,** or **pseudoephedrine** may result in unopposed alpha-adrenergic stimulation (excessive hypertension, bradycardia) ▪ Concurrent **thyroid** administration may decrease effectiveness ▪ May alter the effectiveness of **insulin** or **oral hypoglycemic agents** (dosage adjustments may be necessary) ▪ May decrease the effectiveness of **theophylline** ▪ May decrease the beneficial beta$_1$-cardiovascular effects of **dopamine** or **dobutamine** ▪ Use cautiously within 14 days of **MAO inhibitor therapy** (may result in hypertension).

ROUTE AND DOSAGE

- **PO (Adults):** *Antihypertensive/antianginal*—100 mg/day as a single dose or 2 divided doses; may be increased q 7 days as needed up to 450 mg/day (for angina, give in divided doses). Extended-release products are given once daily. *Myocardial infarction*—25–50 mg (starting 15 min after last IV dose) q 6 hr for 48 hr, then 100 mg twice daily for a minimum of 3 mo. *Migraine prevention*—50–100 mg 2–4 times daily (unlabeled).
- **IV (Adults):** *Myocardial infarction*—5 mg q 2 min for 3 doses, followed by oral dosing.

AVAILABILITY

▪ ***Tablets:*** 50 mg^{Rx}, 100 mg^{Rx} ▪ ***Extended-release tablets (succinate):*** {50 mg^{Rx}}, {100 mg^{Rx}}, {200 mg^{Rx}} ▪ ***Extended-release tablets (tartrate):*** {100 mg^{Rx}} ▪ ***Injection:*** 1 mg/ml^{Rx} ▪ ***In combination with:*** hydrochlorothiazide (Lopressor HCT)^{Rx}. See Appendix A.

TIME/ACTION PROFILE (cardiovascular effects)

	ONSET	PEAK	DURATION
PO†	15 min	UK	6–12 hr
PO–ER	UK	6–12 hr	24 hr
IV	immmediate	20 min	5–8 hr

†Maximal effects on BP (chronic therapy) may not occur for 1 wk. Hypotensive effects may persist for up to 4 wk after discontinuation.

NURSING IMPLICATIONS

ASSESSMENT

- ▫ Monitor blood pressure, ECG, and pulse frequently during dose adjustment and periodically throughout therapy.
- ▫ Vital signs and ECG should be monitored every 5–15 min during and for several hours after parenteral administration. If heart rate <40

*CAPITALS indicate life-threatening; underlines indicate most frequent.

bpm, especially if cardiac output is also decreased, administer atropine 0.25–0.5 mg IV.
- □ Monitor intake and output ratios and daily weights. Assess routinely for signs and symptoms of CHF (dyspnea, rales/crackles, weight gain, peripheral edema, jugular venous distention).
- ▪ **Angina:** Assess frequency and characteristics of anginal attacks periodically throughout therapy.
- ▪ ***Lab Test Considerations:*** May cause increased BUN, serum lipoprotein, potassium, triglyceride, and uric acid levels.
- □ May cause increased ANA titers.
- □ May cause increase in blood glucose levels.
- □ May cause increased serum alkaline phosphatase, LDH, AST, and ALT levels.

POTENTIAL NURSING DIAGNOSES

- ▪ Cardiac output, decreased (Side Effects).
- ▪ Knowledge deficit, related to medication regimen (Patient/Family Teaching).
- ▪ Noncompliance, related to medication regimen (Patient/Family Teaching).

IMPLEMENTATION

- ▪ **PO:** Take apical pulse prior to administering. If <50 bpm or if arrhythmia occurs, withhold medication and notify physician or other health care professional.
- □ Administer metoprolol with meals or directly after eating.
- □ Extended-release tablets should be swallowed whole; do not crush, break, or chew.
- ▪ **Direct IV:** May be administered by injecting 5 mg rapidly at 2-min intervals for 3 doses. Oral therapy should begin 15 min after last IV dose.
- ▪ **Y-Site Compatibility:** ▪ alteplase ▪ meperidine ▪ morphine.

PATIENT/FAMILY TEACHING

- ▪ **General Info:** Instruct patient to take medication exactly as directed, at the same time each day, even if feeling well; do not skip or double up on missed doses. If a dose is missed, it should be taken as soon as possible up to 8 hr before next dose. Abrupt withdrawal may precipitate life-threatening arrhythmias, hypertension, or myocardial ischemia.
- □ Teach patient and family how to check pulse and blood pressure. Instruct them to check pulse daily and blood pressure biweekly and to report significant changes to health care professional.
- □ May cause drowsiness. Caution patient to avoid driving or other activities that require alertness until response to the drug is known.
- □ Advise patient to change positions slowly to minimize orthostatic hypotension.
- □ Caution patient that this medication may increase sensitivity to cold.
- □ Instruct patient to consult health care professional before taking any OTC medications, especially cold preparations, concurrently with this medication. Patients on antihypertensive therapy should also avoid excessive amounts of coffee, tea, and cola.
- □ Diabetics should closely monitor blood sugar, especially if weakness, malaise, irritability, or fatigue occurs. Medication does not block sweating as a sign of hypoglycemia.
- □ Advise patient to notify health care professional if slow pulse, difficulty breathing, wheezing, cold hands and feet, dizziness, lightheadedness, confusion, depression, rash, fever, sore throat, unusual bleeding, or bruising occurs.
- □ Instruct patient to inform health care professional of medication regimen prior to treatment or surgery.
- □ Advise patient to carry identification describing disease process and medication regimen at all times.
- ▪ **Hypertension:** Reinforce the need to continue additional therapies for hypertension (weight loss, sodium restriction, stress reduction, regular exercise, moderation of alcohol consumption, and smoking cessation). Medication controls but does not cure hypertension.

EVALUATION

Effectiveness of therapy can be demonstrated by: ▪ Decrease in blood pressure ▪ Reduction in frequency of anginal attacks □ Increase in activity tolerance ▪ Prevention of myocardial infarction.

METRONIDAZOLE

(me-troe-**ni**-da-zole)
{Apo-Metronidazole}, Flagyl, Flagyl ER, Metric 21, MetroCream, MetroGel, MetroGel-Vaginal, Metro IV, Metryl, {Nidagel}, {Novonidazol}, Protostat, {Trikacide}

CLASSIFICATION(S):
Anti-infective (miscellaneous)

Pregnancy Category B

INDICATIONS

▪ **PO, IV:** Treatment of the following anaerobic infections: ▫ Intra-abdominal infections ▫ Gynecologic infections ▫ Skin and skin structure infections ▫ Lower respiratory tract infections ▫ Bone and joint infections ▫ CNS infections ▫ Septicemia ▫ Endocarditis ▪ **IV:** Perioperative prophylactic agent in colorectal surgery ▪ **PO:** ▫ Amebicide in the management of amebic dysentery, amebic liver abscess, and trichomoniasis ▫ Treatment of peptic ulcer disease due to *Helicobacter pylori* ▪ **Topical:** Treatment of acne rosacea ▪ **Vag:** Management of bacterial vaginosis. **Unlabeled Uses:** ▪ Treatment of giardiasis ▪ Treatment of anti-infective associated pseudomembranous colitis.

ACTION

▪ Disrupts DNA and protein synthesis in susceptible organisms. **Therapeutic Effects:** ▪ Bactericidal, trichomonacidal, or amebicidal action. **Spectrum:** ▪ Most notable for activity against anaerobic bacteria, including: ▫ *Bacteroides* ▫ *Clostridium* ▪ In addition, is active against: ▫ *Trichomonas vaginalis* ▫ *Entamoeba histolytica* ▫ *Giardia lamblia* ▫ *Helicobacter pylori* ▫ *Clostridium difficile*.

PHARMACOKINETICS

Absorption: 80% absorbed following oral administration. Minimal absorption following topical or vaginal application.
Distribution: Widely distributed into most tissues and fluids, including CSF. Crosses the placenta; enters breast milk in concentrations equal to plasma levels.
Metabolism and Excretion: Partially metabolized by the liver (30–60%), partially excreted unchanged in the urine, 6–15% eliminated in the feces.
Half-life: 6–8 hr.

CONTRAINDICATIONS AND PRECAUTIONS

Contraindicated in: ▪ Hypersensitivity ▪ Hypersensitivity to parabens (topical only) ▪ First trimester of pregnancy.
Use Cautiously in: ▪ History of blood dyscrasias ▪ History of seizures or neurologic problems ▪ Severe hepatic impairment (dosage reduction suggested) ▪ Children (safe use of IV form not established; safety of oral form for infections other than amebiasis in children not established) ▪ Pregnancy (although safety not established, has been used to treat trichomoniasis in 2nd- and 3rd-trimester pregnancy—but not as single-dose regimen) ▪ Lactation (if needed, use single dose and interrupt nursing for 24 hr thereafter).

ADVERSE REACTIONS AND SIDE EFFECTS*

CNS: SEIZURES, <u>dizziness</u>, <u>headache</u>.
EENT: tearing (topical only).
GI: <u>abdominal pain</u>, <u>anorexia</u>, <u>nausea</u>, diarrhea, dry mouth, furry tongue, glossitis, unpleasant taste, vomiting.
Derm: rashes, urticaria; *topical only*—burning, mild dryness, skin irritation, transient redness.
Hemat: leukopenia.
Local: phlebitis at IV site.
Neuro: peripheral neuropathy.
Misc: superinfection.

INTERACTIONS

Drug-Drug: ▪ **Cimetidine** may decrease the metabolism of metronidazole ▪ **Phenobarbital** increases metabolism and may decrease effectiveness ▪ Metronidazole increases the effects of **warfarin** ▪ Disulfiram-like reaction may occur with **alcohol** ingestion ▪ May cause acute psychosis and confusion with **disulfiram** ▪ In-

{} = Available in Canada only.
***CAPITALS indicate life-threatening; <u>underlines</u> indicate most frequent.**

creased risk of leukopenia with **fluorouracil** or **azathioprine.**

ROUTE AND DOSAGE

- **PO (Adults):** *Anaerobic infections*—7.5 mg/kg q 6 hr (not to exceed 4 g/day). *Trichomoniasis*—250 mg q 8 hr for 7 days or single 2-g dose or 1 g bid for 1 day. *Amebiasis*—500–750 mg q 8 hr for 5–10 days. *Helicobacter pylori*—250 mg 4 times daily or 500 mg twice daily for 1–2 wk (with other agents). *Bacterial vaginoses*—750 mg once daily as ER tables for 7 days.
- **PO (Children):** *Trichomoniasis*—5 mg/kg q 8 hr for 7–10 days. *Amebiasis*—11.6–16.7 mg/kg q 8 hr for 5–10 days (not to exceed 750 mg/dose)
- **IV (Adults):** *Anaerobic infections*—Initial dose 15 mg/kg, then 7.5 mg/kg q 6–8 hr or 500 mg q 6–8 hr (not to exceed 4 g/day). *Perioperative prophylaxis*—Initial dose 15 mg/kg 1 hr prior to surgery, then 7.5 mg/kg 6 and 12 hr later. *Amebiasis*—500–750 mg q 8 hr for 5–10 days.
- **Topical (Adults):** *Acne rosacea*—apply thin film to affected area bid.
- **Vag (Adults):** *Bacterial vaginosis*—one applicatorful (0.75% gel) 2 times daily for 5 days.

AVAILABILITY

■ ***Tablets:*** 250 mg^{Rx}, 500 mg^{Rx} ■ ***Extended-release (ER) tablets:*** 750 mg^{Rx} ■ ***Capsules:*** 375 mg^{Rx}, {500 mg^{Rx}} ■ ***Powder for injection:*** 500-mg vials^{Rx} ■ ***Premixed injection:*** 500 mg/100 ml^{Rx} RTU (ready to use) ■ ***Topical gel:*** 0.75% in 28.4-g tubes^{Rx} ■ ***Topical cream:*** 0.75% in 28.4-g tubes^{Rx} ■ ***Vaginal gel:*** 0.75% (37.5 mg/5 g applicatorful) in 70-g tubes^{Rx} ■ ***In combination with:*** bismuth subsalicylate tablets and tetracycline capsules (Helidac^{Rx}) as part of a compliance package (see Appendix A).

TIME/ACTION PROFILE (PO, IV = blood levels; topical = improvement in rosacea)

	ONSET	PEAK	DURATION
PO	rapid	1–3 hr	8 hr
PO-ER	rapid	UK	up to 24 hr
IV	rapid	end of infusion	6 hr
Topical	3 wk	9 wk	12 hr
Vaginal	UK	6–12 hr	12 hr

NURSING IMPLICATIONS

ASSESSMENT

- **General Info:** Assess patient for infection (vital signs; appearance of wound, sputum, urine, and stool; WBC) at beginning of and throughout therapy.
- □ Obtain specimens for culture and sensitivity prior to initiating therapy. First dose may be given before receiving results.
- □ Monitor neurologic status during and after IV infusions. Inform physician if numbness, paresthesia, weakness, ataxia, or convulsions occur.
- □ Monitor intake and output and daily weight, especially for patients on sodium restriction. Each 500 mg of Flagyl IV for dilution contains 5 mEq of sodium; each 500 mg of Flagyl RTU contains 14 mEq of sodium.
- **Giardiasis:** Monitor three stool samples taken several days apart, beginning 3–4 wk following treatment.
- ***Lab Test Considerations:*** May alter results of serum AST, ALT, and LDH tests.

POTENTIAL NURSING DIAGNOSES

- Infection, risk for (Indications).
- Diarrhea (Indications).
- Knowledge deficit, related to medication regimen (Patient/Family Teaching).

IMPLEMENTATION

- **PO:** Administer with food or milk to minimize GI irritation. Tablets may be crushed for patients with difficulty swallowing.
- **Intermittent Infusion:** Flagyl IV RTU is prediluted and ready to use (5 mg/ml). Prefilled plastic minibags should not be used in series connections; air embolism may result. Crystals may form during refrigeration but will dissolve when warmed to room temperature.
- □ Preparation of Flagyl IV requires a specific process. Do not use aluminum needles or hubs; color will turn orange/rust. Add 4.4 ml of sterile or bacteriostatic sterile water, or 0.9% or bacteriostatic 0.9% NaCl for injection (100 mg/ml). Solution should be clear, pale yellow-green. Do not use cloudy or precipitated solution. Dilute further to at least 8 mg/ml with 0.9% NaCl, D5W, or lactated Ringer's solution. Neutralize solution with 5 mEq so-

dium bicarbonate for each 500 mg. Mix thoroughly. Carbon dioxide gas will be generated and may require venting. Do not refrigerate. Stable for 24 hr at room temperature.

- *Rate:* Administer IV doses as a slow infusion, each single dose over 1 hr.
- **Y-Site Incompatibility:** ▪ Manufacturer recommends discontinuing primary IV during metronidazole infusion.
- **Additive Incompatibility:** ▪ Do not admix with other medications.
- **Topical:** Cleanse affected area prior to application. Apply and rub in a thin film twice daily, morning and evening. Avoid contact with eyes.

PATIENT/FAMILY TEACHING

- □ Instruct patient to take medication exactly as directed with evenly spaced times between doses, even if feeling better. Do not skip doses or double up on missed doses. If a dose is missed, take as soon as remembered if not almost time for next dose.
- □ Advise patients treated for trichomoniasis that sexual partners may be asymptomatic sources of reinfection and should be treated concurrently. Patient should also refrain from intercourse or use a condom to prevent reinfection.
- □ Caution patient to avoid intake of alcoholic beverages or preparations containing alcohol during and for at least 1 day following treatment with metronidazole, including vaginal gel. May cause a disulfiram-like reaction (flushing, nausea, vomiting, headache, abdominal cramps).
- □ May cause dizziness or light-headedness. Caution patient to avoid driving or other activities requiring alertness until response to medication is known.
- □ Inform patient that medication may cause an unpleasant metallic taste.
- □ Advise patient not to take OTC medications concurrently without consulting health care professional.
- □ Advise patient that frequent mouth rinses, good oral hygiene, and sugarless gum or candy may minimize dry mouth. Notify health care professional if dry mouth persists for more than 2 wk.
- □ Advise patient to inform health care professional if pregnancy is suspected prior to taking this medication.
- □ Inform patient that medication may cause urine to turn dark.
- □ Advise patient to consult health care professional if no improvement in a few days or if signs and symptoms of superinfection (black, furry overgrowth on tongue; vaginal itching or discharge; loose or foul-smelling stools) develop.
- **Vag:** Instruct patient in correct technique for intravaginal instillation. Advise patient to avoid intercourse during treatment with vaginal gel.
- **Topical:** Instruct patient on correct technique for application of topical gel. Cosmetics may be used following application of gel.

EVALUATION

Effectiveness of therapy can be demonstrated by: ▪ Resolution of the signs and symptoms of infection. Length of time for complete resolution depends on organism and site of infection □ Significant results should be seen within 3 wk of application of topical gel. Application may be continued for 9 wk.

MEXILETINE

(mex-**il**-e-teen)
Mexitil

CLASSIFICATION(S):
Antiarrhythmic (class type IB)

Pregnancy Category C

INDICATIONS

▪ Prophylaxis/treatment of serious ventricular arrhythmias, including VT and PVCs. **Unlabeled Uses:** ▪ Management of chronic neuropathic pain.

ACTION

▪ Decreases the duration of the action potential and effective refractory period in cardiac conduction tissue by altering transport of sodium across myocardial cell membranes ▪ Has little or no effect on heart rate. **Therapeutic Effects:** ▪ Control of ventricular arrhythmias.

PHARMACOKINETICS

Absorption: Well absorbed from the GI tract.
Distribution: Enters breast milk in concentrations similar to plasma.
Metabolism and Excretion: Mostly metabo-

lized by the liver; 10% excreted unchanged by the kidneys.
Half-life: 10–12 hr.

CONTRAINDICATIONS AND PRECAUTIONS

Contraindicated in: ▪ Hypersensitivity ▪ Cardiogenic shock ▪ 2nd- or 3rd-degree heart block (if a pacemaker has not been inserted) ▪ Lactation.
Use Cautiously in: ▪ Sinus node or intraventricular conduction abnormalities ▪ Hypotension ▪ Congestive heart failure ▪ Severe hepatic impairment (dosage reduction suggested) ▪ Pregnancy or children (safety not established).

ADVERSE REACTIONS AND SIDE EFFECTS*

CNS: dizziness, nervousness, confusion, fatigue, headache, sleep disorder.
EENT: blurred vision, tinnitus.
Resp: dyspnea.
CV: ARRHYTHMIAS, chest pain, edema, palpitations.
GI: HEPATIC NECROSIS, heartburn, nausea, vomiting.
Derm: rashes.
Hemat: blood dyscrasias.
Neuro: tremor, coordination difficulties, paresthesia.

INTERACTIONS

Drug-Drug: ▪ **Opioids, atropine,** and **antacids** may slow absorption ▪ **Metoclopramide** may speed absorption ▪ **Phenytoin, rifampin, cigarette smoking,** or **phenobarbital** may increase metabolism and decrease effectiveness ▪ **Cimetidine** may slow metabolism and increase toxicity ▪ Additive cardiac effects may occur with other **antiarrhythmics** ▪ **Drugs that drastically alter urine pH** may alter blood levels (alkalinization increases reabsorption and blood levels; acidification increases excretion and decreases blood levels).
Drug-Food: ▪ **Foods that drastically alter urine pH** may alter blood levels. Alkalinization increases reabsorption and increases blood levels. Acidification increases excretion and may decrease effectiveness (see Appendix K).

ROUTE AND DOSAGE

- **PO (Adults):** 400-mg loading dose initially, then 200 mg 8 hr later, then 200–400 mg q 8 hr; dosage alterations of 50–100 mg may be made q 2–3 days. If controlled on ≤300 mg q 8 hr, can give same daily dose at 12-hr intervals (not to exceed 1200 mg/day). Some patients may require q 6 hr dosing.

AVAILABILITY

- ***Capsules:*** {100 mg Rx}, 150 mg Rx, 200 mg Rx, 250 mg Rx.

TIME/ACTION PROFILE (antiarrhythmic effects†)

	ONSET	PEAK	DURATION
PO	30 min–2 hr	2–3 hr	8–12 hr

†Provided a loading dose has been given.

NURSING IMPLICATIONS

ASSESSMENT

- **General Info:** Monitor pulse, blood pressure, and ECG periodically throughout therapy. Continuous Holter monitoring and chest x-ray examinations may be necessary to determine efficacy and aid in dosage adjustment.
- **Pain:** Assess type, location, and severity of pain prior to and periodically throughout therapy.
- ***Lab Test Considerations:*** May occasionally cause a positive ANA test result.
  - May cause a transient increase in AST concentrations.
  - May cause thrombocytopenia within a few days after initiation of therapy. Blood counts usually return to normal within 1 mo after discontinuation of therapy.
- ***Toxicity and Overdose:*** Serum mexiletine concentrations may be determined during dosage adjustment. Incidence of side effects is greater with concentrations >2 mcg/ml.

POTENTIAL NURSING DIAGNOSES

- Cardiac output, decreased (Indications).
- Knowledge deficit, related to medication regimen (Patient/Family Teaching).

M

*CAPITALS indicate life-threatening; underlines indicate most frequent.

IMPLEMENTATION

- **General Info:** When changing from other antiarrhythmic therapy, give the 1st dose of mexiletine 6–12 hr after the last dose of quinidine, 3–6 hr after last dose of procainamide, or 8–12 hr after last dose of tocainide. When changing from parenteral lidocaine, decrease lidocaine dose or discontinue lidocaine 1–2 hr after administration of mexiletine or administer lower initial doses of mexiletine.
  - Transfer of patients with life-threatening arrhythmias from other antiarrhythmic agents to mexiletine should be managed in the hospital.
- **PO:** Administer with food or antacids to minimize GI irritation.

PATIENT/FAMILY TEACHING

- Advise patient to take medication exactly as directed, at evenly spaced intervals, even if feeling well. Missed doses should be taken within 4 hr or omitted. Do not skip or double up on missed doses.
- Teach patients to monitor pulse. Advise patient to contact health care professional if pulse rate is <50 bpm or becomes irregular.
- May cause dizziness and light-headedness. Caution patient to avoid driving and other activities requiring alertness until response to medication is known.
- Instruct patient to avoid changes in diet that may drastically acidify or alkalinize the urine (see Appendix K for foods included).
- Advise patient to notify health care professional of disease process and medication regimen prior to treatment or surgery.
- Advise patient to notify health care professional if general tiredness, yellowing of the skin or eyes, fever, sore throat, or persistent side effects occur.
- Patient should carry identification describing disease process and medication regimen at all times.

EVALUATION

Effectiveness of therapy can be demonstrated by: ▪ Decrease in frequency or resolution of serious ventricular arrhythmias ▪ Decrease in severity of chronic neurogenic pain.

MEZLOCILLIN

(mez-loe-**sill**-in)

Mezlin

CLASSIFICATION(S):

Anti-infective (extended-spectrum penicillin)

Pregnancy Category B

INDICATIONS

▪ Treatment of serious infections due to susceptible organisms, including: □ Skin and skin structure infections □ Bone and joint infections □ Septicemia □ Respiratory tract infections □ Intra-abdominal, gynecologic, and urinary tract infections ▪ Combination with an aminoglycoside may be synergistic against *Pseudomonas* ▪ Has been combined with other antibiotics in the treatment of infections in immunosuppressed patients.

ACTION

▪ Binds to bacterial cell wall membrane, causing cell death. **Therapeutic Effects:** ▪ Bactericidal against susceptible bacteria. **Spectrum:** ▪ Spectrum similar to penicillin but greatly extended to include several important gram-negative aerobic pathogens, notably: □ *Pseudomonas aeruginosa* □ *Escherichia coli* □ *Proteus mirabilis* □ *Providencia rettgeri* ▪ Also active against some anaerobic bacteria, including *Bacteroides*. Not active against penicillinase-producing staphylococci or beta-lactamase–producing Enterobacteriaceae.

PHARMACOKINETICS

Absorption: Well absorbed from IM sites.

Distribution: Widely distributed. Enters CSF well only when meninges are inflamed. Crosses the placenta; enters breast milk in low concentrations.

Metabolism and Excretion: 55–60% excreted unchanged by the kidneys. Small amounts metabolized by the liver; 15–30% excreted in the bile.

Half-life: 0.7–1.3 hr (increased in renal impairment).

CONTRAINDICATIONS AND PRECAUTIONS

Contraindicated in: ▪ Hypersensitivity to penicillins.

Use Cautiously in: ▪ Hypersensitivity to cephalosporins ▪ Severe renal impairment (increase dosing interval if CCr <30 ml/min) ▪ Pregnancy and lactation (safety not established) ▪ Severe liver disease.

ADVERSE REACTIONS AND SIDE EFFECTS*

CNS: SEIZURES (high doses), confusion, lethargy.
CV: ARRHYTHMIAS, CONGESTIVE HEART FAILURE.
GI: PSEUDOMEMBRANOUS COLITIS, diarrhea, nausea.
GU: hematuria (children only).
Derm: rashes, urticaria.
F and E: hypokalemia, hypernatremia.
Hemat: bleeding, blood dyscrasias, increased bleeding time.
Local: pain at IM site, phlebitis at IV site.
Metab: metabolic alkalosis.
Misc: hypersensitivity reactions including ANAPHYLAXIS and SERUM SICKNESS, superinfection.

INTERACTIONS

Drug-Drug: ▪ **Probenecid** decreases renal excretion and increases blood levels ▪ May alter excretion of **lithium** ▪ **Diuretics** may increase the risk of hypokalemia ▪ Hypokalemia increases the risk of **digitalis glycoside** toxicity.

ROUTE AND DOSAGE

Contains 1.85 mEq sodium/g.

- **IV, IM (Adults):** *Most infections*—3–4 g q 4–6 hr or 500 mg q 8 hr IV (up to 24 g/day). *Complicated urinary tract infections*—3 g q 6 hr. *Uncomplicated urinary tract infections*—1.5–2 g q 6 hr.
- **IM, IV (Children 1 mo–12 yr):** 50 mg/kg q 4 hr.
- **IM, IV (Neonates ≥2 kg):** 50 mg/kg q 8 hr for the first 7 days of life, then increase to 50 mg/kg q 6 hr.
- **IM, IV (Neonates <2 kg):** 50–75 mg/kg q 12 hr for the first 7 days of life, then increase to 50 mg/kg q 8 hr.

AVAILABILITY

▪ ***Powder for injection:*** 1 g/vial[Rx], 2 g/vial[Rx], 3 g/vial[Rx], 4 g/vial[Rx], 20 g/vial[Rx].

TIME/ACTION PROFILE (blood levels)

	ONSET	PEAK	DURATION
IM	rapid	45–90 min	4–6† hr
IV	rapid	end of infusion	4–6 hr†

†Longer in impaired renal function and neonates.

NURSING IMPLICATIONS

ASSESSMENT

- Assess patient for infection (vital signs; appearance of wound, sputum, urine, and stool; WBC) at beginning of and throughout therapy.
- Obtain a history before initiating therapy to determine previous use of and reactions to penicillins or cephalosporins. Persons with a negative history of penicillin sensitivity may still have an allergic response.
- Obtain specimens for culture and sensitivity prior to initiating therapy. First dose may be given before receiving results.
- Observe patient for signs and symptoms of anaphylaxis (rash, pruritus, laryngeal edema, wheezing). Discontinue the drug and notify the physician or other health care provider immediately if these occur. Keep epinephrine, an antihistamine, and resuscitation equipment close by in the event of an anaphylactic reaction.
- ▪ ***Lab Test Considerations:*** Renal and hepatic function, CBC, and serum potassium should be evaluated prior to and routinely throughout therapy.
- May cause false-positive urine protein test results.
- May cause elevated serum creatinine, AST, ALT, bilirubin, and alkaline phosphatase. May also cause elevated serum sodium and decreased serum potassium levels.
- May cause positive direct Coombs' test result.

M

POTENTIAL NURSING DIAGNOSES

- Infection, risk for (Indications, Side Effects).
- Knowledge deficit, related to medication regimen (Patient/Family Teaching).

***CAPITALS indicate life-threatening; underlines indicate most frequent.**

IMPLEMENTATION

- **General Info:** Reconstituted solution is stable for 48 hr at room temperature and 72 hr if refrigerated. Solution is colorless to pale yellow; darkened solution does not affect potency.
- **IM:** To constitute for IM use, add 3–4 ml of sterile water for injection or 0.5 or 1% lidocaine hydrochloride injection (without epinephrine) to each 1-g vial and shake vigorously. Inject deep into a well-developed muscle mass over 12–15 sec to minimize discomfort and massage well. IM injections should not exceed 2 g at each site.
- **IV:** The initial reconstitution is made with at least 10 ml of sterile water for injection, 0.9% NaCl, or D5W.
- □ Change IV sites every 48 hr to prevent phlebitis.
- **Direct IV:** Inject slowly, 1 g over 3–5 min to minimize vein irritation.
- **Intermittent Infusion:** Dilute in 50–100 ml of 0.9% NaCl, D5W, D10W, D5/0.25% NaCl, D5/0.45% NaCl, Ringer's, or lactated Ringer's solution.
- ***Rate:*** Administer over 30 min.
- **Y-Site Incompatibility:** ▪ Manufacturer recommends temporarily discontinuing primary infusion during mezlocillin infusion. If penicillins and aminoglycosides must be given concurrently, administer in separate sites at least 1 hr apart.
- **Additive Incompatibility:** ▪ Incompatible with aminoglycosides; do not admix.

PATIENT/FAMILY TEACHING

- □ Advise patient to report the signs of superinfection (black, furry overgrowth on the tongue; vaginal itching or discharge; loose or foul-smelling stools) and allergy.
- □ Advise patient to notify health care professional if fever and diarrhea develop, especially if stool contains blood, pus, or mucus. Instruct patient not to treat diarrhea without consulting health care professional.

EVALUATION

Clinical response to therapy can be evaluated by: ▪ Resolution of the signs and symptoms of infection. Length of time for complete resolution depends on the organism and site of infection.

MIBEFRADIL
(mye-**beff**-ra-dill)
Posicor

CLASSIFICATION(S):
Antianginal, Antihypertensive agent, Calcium channel blocker

Pregnancy Category C

INDICATIONS

▪ Management of: □ Hypertension □ Chronic stable angina pectoris.

ACTION

▪ Inhibits the transport of calcium into myocardial and vascular smooth muscle cells, resulting in inhibition of excitation-contraction coupling and subsequent contraction. **Therapeutic Effects:** ▪ Systemic vasodilation resulting in decreased blood pressure ▪ Coronary vasodilation resulting in decreased frequency and severity of attacks of angina.

PHARMACOKINETICS

Absorption: 64–90% absorbed following oral administration.
Distribution: Probably enters breast milk.
Metabolism and Excretion: Mostly metabolized by the liver; <3% excreted unchanged in urine.
Half-life: 17–25 hr.

CONTRAINDICATIONS AND PRECAUTIONS

Contraindicated in: ▪ Hypersensitivity (cross-sensitivity may occur) ▪ Sick sinus syndrome ▪ 2nd- or 3rd-degree AV block (unless an artificial pacemaker is in place) ▪ Blood pressure <90 mm Hg ▪ Lactation ▪ Lovastatin or simvastatin.
Use Cautiously in: ▪ Severe hepatic impairment (dosage reduction recommended for most agents) ▪ Geriatric patients (dosage reduction recommended; increased risk of hypotension) ▪ Severe renal impairment ▪ History of serious ventricular arrhythmias or congestive heart failure (CHF) ▪ Pregnancy or children (safety not established).

ADVERSE REACTIONS AND SIDE EFFECTS*

CNS: anxiety, headache, insomnia, light-headedness, mental depression, syncope, weakness.
EENT: otitis, rhinitis, tinnitus.
CV: CHF, arrhythmias, bradycardia, hypotension, leg edema.
GI: abdominal pain, constipation, diarrhea, dyspepsia, flatulence.
GU: impotence.
Derm: exfoliative dermatitis, increased sweating, rash.
MS: arthritis, back pain, muscle cramps.
Neuro: paresthesia.
Misc: allergic reactions including angioedema.

INTERACTIONS

Drug-Drug: ▪ Concurrent use of mibefradil with **astemizole** or **cisapride** may cause serious arrhythmias ▪ Additive hypotension may occur when used concurrently with **fentanyl,** other **antihypertensives, nitrates,** acute ingestion of **alcohol,** or **quinidine** ▪ Antihypertensive effects may be decreased by concurrent use of **NSAIDs** ▪ May decrease the metabolism of and increase the risk of toxicity from **cyclosporine** ▪ Mibefradil increases levels of **tricyclic antidepressants;** dosage reduction may be necessary ▪ Increased risk of myopathy with **simvastatin** or **lovastatin** (concurrent use contraindicated); concurrent use with **atorvastatin** or **cerivastatin** should be discouraged ▪ May increase blood levels and risk of toxicity from **cyclosporine** or **tacrolimus.**

ROUTE AND DOSAGE

- **PO (Adults):** 50 mg once daily; may be increased after 1–2 wk to 100 mg once daily.

AVAILABILITY

- ***Tablets:*** 50 mg Rx, 100 mg Rx.

TIME/ACTION PROFILE (cardiovascular effects)

	ONSET	PEAK	DURATION
PO	UK	7–14 days†	24 hr

†Maximum antihypertensive effect with chronic therapy.

NURSING IMPLICATIONS

ASSESSMENT

- **General Info:** Monitor BP and pulse prior to therapy, during dosage titration, and periodically throughout therapy. Monitor ECG periodically during prolonged therapy.
- □ Monitor intake and output ratios and daily weight. Assess for signs of CHF (peripheral edema, rales/crackles, dyspnea, weight gain, jugular venous distention).
- **Angina:** Assess location, duration, intensity, and precipitating factors of patient's anginal pain.
- ***Lab Test Considerations:*** Total serum calcium concentrations are not affected by calcium channel blockers.
- □ Monitor serum potassium periodically. Hypokalemia increases risk of arrhythmias; should be corrected.
- □ Monitor renal and hepatic functions periodically during long-term therapy. Several days of therapy may cause increase in hepatic enzymes, which return to normal upon discontinuation of therapy.

POTENTIAL NURSING DIAGNOSES

- Cardiac output, decreased (Indications).
- Pain (Indications).
- Knowledge deficit, related to medication regimen (Patient/Family Teaching).

IMPLEMENTATION

- **PO:** May be administered without regard to meals. Tablets should be swallowed whole and not crushed or chewed.

PATIENT/FAMILY TEACHING

- **General Info:** Advise patient to take medication exactly as directed, even if feeling well. If a dose is missed, take as soon as possible unless almost time for next dose; do not double doses. May need to be discontinued gradually.
- □ Instruct patient on technique for monitoring pulse. Instruct patient to contact health care professional if heart rate is <50 bpm.
- □ Caution patient to change positions slowly to minimize orthostatic hypotension.

M

*CAPITALS indicate life-threatening; underlines indicate most frequent.

- □ May cause drowsiness or dizziness. Advise patient to avoid driving or other activities requiring alertness until response to the medication is known.
- □ Instruct patient on importance of maintaining good dental hygiene and seeing dentist frequently for teeth cleaning to prevent tenderness, bleeding, and gingival hyperplasia (gum enlargement).
- □ Instruct patient to avoid concurrent use of alcohol or OTC medications, especially cold preparations, without consulting health care professional.
- □ Advise patient to notify health care professional if irregular heartbeats, dyspnea, swelling of hands and feet, pronounced dizziness, nausea, constipation, or hypotension occurs or if headache is severe or persistent.
- ▪ **Angina:** Instruct patient on concurrent nitrate or beta-blocker therapy to continue taking both medications as directed and use SL nitroglycerin as needed for anginal attacks.
- □ Advise patient to contact health care professional if chest pain does not improve, worsens after therapy, or occurs with diaphoresis or if shortness of breath or persistent headache occurs.
- □ Caution patient to discuss exercise restrictions with health care professional prior to exertion.
- ▪ **Hypertension:** Encourage patient to comply with other interventions for hypertension (weight reduction, low-sodium diet, smoking cessation, moderation of alcohol consumption, regular exercise, and stress management). Medication controls but does not cure hypertension.
- □ Instruct patient and family in proper technique for monitoring BP. Advise patient to take BP weekly and to report significant changes to health care professional.

EVALUATION

Effectiveness of therapy can be demonstrated by: ▪ Decrease in blood pressure ▪ Decrease in frequency and severity of anginal attacks □ Decrease in need for nitrate therapy □ Increase in activity tolerance and sense of well-being.

MICONAZOLE (systemic)*

(mi-**kon**-a-zole)

Monistat I.V.

CLASSIFICATION(S):

Antifungal (azole)

Pregnancy Category C

*For other miconazole dosage forms, see antifungals (topical) monograph on page 69 and antifungals (vaginal) monograph on page 72.

INDICATIONS

▪ **IV:** Treatment of severe fungal infections, including: □ Pulmonary infections □ Disseminated infections ▪ **IV:** Fungal meningitis ▪ **Bladder Irrigation:** *Candida* bladder infections.

ACTION

▪ Alters permeability of fungal cell membrane and function of fungal enzymes. **Therapeutic Effects:** ▪ Fungistatic or fungicidal action. **Spectrum:** ▪ Active against all pathogenic fungi and gram-positive bacteria ▪ Spectrum notable for activity against: □ *Aspergillus* □ *Coccidioides* □ *Cryptococcus* □ *Candida albicans* □ *Histoplasma* □ Dermatophytes.

PHARMACOKINETICS

Absorption: 50% absorbed following oral administration.

Distribution: Following IV administration is widely distributed. CSF penetration is poor, necessitating intrathecal administration in the treatment of meningitis.

Metabolism and Excretion: Mostly metabolized by the liver.

Half-life: 24 hr.

CONTRAINDICATIONS AND PRECAUTIONS

Contraindicated in: ▪ Hypersensitivity ▪ Hypersensitivity to castor oil or parabens (IV only) ▪ Concurrent use of cisapride.

Use Cautiously in: ▪ Pregnancy, lactation, or children <1 yr (safety not established).

ADVERSE REACTIONS AND SIDE EFFECTS*

CNS: anxiety, dizziness, drowsiness, headache.
EENT: blurred vision, dry eyes.
CV: arrhythmias.
GI: bitter taste, diarrhea, nausea, vomiting.
F and E: hyponatremia.
Hemat: anemia.
Local: *IV*—phlebitis, pruritus.
Misc: allergic reactions including ANAPHYLAXIS, fever, hyperlipidemia, increased libido.

INTERACTIONS

Drug-Drug: ▪ Increases blood levels and risk of potentially life-threatening arrythmias with **cisapride** ▪ Parenteral miconazole enhances the anticoagulant effect of **warfarin** ▪ Concurrent use with **rifampin** or **isoniazid** decreases blood levels and effectiveness of miconazole ▪ Increases blood levels and risk of toxicity with **cyclosporine** and **phenytoin.**

ROUTE AND DOSAGE

- **IV (Adults):** 200–3600 mg/day in divided doses q 8 hr.
- **IV (Children 1–12 yr):** 20–40 mg/kg/day in divided doses q 8 hr (not to exceed 15 mg/kg/dose).
- **IT (Adults):** 20 mg q 3–7 days.
- **Bladder Instillation (Adults):** 200 mg q 6–12 hr or by continuous irrigation.

AVAILABILITY

- ***Injection:*** 10 mg/ml in 20-ml vials[Rx].

TIME/ACTION PROFILE (blood levels)

	ONSET	PEAK	DURATION
IV	rapid	end of infusion	8 hr

NURSING IMPLICATIONS

ASSESSMENT

- □ Assess patient for infection prior to and throughout therapy.
- □ Obtain specimens for culture prior to treatment. First dose may be given before receiving results.
- □ Monitor IV site closely for phlebitis.
- ▪ ***Lab Test Considerations:*** Hemoglobin, hematocrit, serum electrolytes, and lipids should be monitored periodically throughout IV therapy.
- □ May cause abnormalities in tests of serum lipid concentrations.

POTENTIAL NURSING DIAGNOSES

- ▪ Infection, risk for (Indications).
- ▪ Skin integrity, impaired (Indications).
- ▪ Knowledge deficit, related to medication regimen (Patient/Family Teaching).

IMPLEMENTATION

- ▪ **Intermittent Infusion:** Dilute each dose in at least 200 ml of 0.9% NaCl or D5W. Solution is stable at room temperature for 48 hr. Darkened color of solution shows deterioration; discard.
- □ Initial dose of 200 mg should be administered under physician's supervision to determine hypersensitivity.
- ▪ ***Rate:*** Administer over at least 30–60 min. To minimize adverse reactions, a rate of 100 mg/hr is recommended. Rapid administration may cause transient tachycardia or arrhythmias.
- □ Nausea and vomiting may be minimized by reducing dose, slowing infusion rate, avoiding administration at mealtime, or administering antiemetics or antihistamines prior to IV miconazole infusion.
- ▪ **Y-Site Compatibility:** ▪ filgrastim ▪ foscarnet ▪ melphalan ▪ ondansetron ▪ sargramostim ▪ teniposide ▪ thiotepa ▪ vinorelbine.
- ▪ **Y-Site Incompatibility:** ▪ amifostine ▪ aztreonam ▪ cefepime ▪ fludarabine ▪ piperacillin/tazobactam.
- ▪ **Additive Incompatibility:** ▪ Manufacturer does not recommend admixing miconazole with other medications.
- ▪ **IT:** Administer undiluted. Intrathecal administration every 3–7 days may be used concurrently with IV administration for fungal meningitis.
- ▪ **Bladder Irrigation:** Bladder irrigation may be used concurrently with IV administration for bladder mycoses.

PATIENT/FAMILY TEACHING

- □ Explain purpose of medication to patient.

M

***CAPITALS indicate life-threatening; underlines indicate most frequent.**

EVALUATION

Effectiveness of therapy can be demonstrated by: ▪ Resolution of the signs and symptoms of infection. Length of time for complete resolution depends on organism and site of infection.

MIDAZOLAM

(mid-**ay**-zoe-lam)
Versed

CLASSIFICATION(S):
Sedative/hypnotic (benzodiazepine)

Schedule IV
Pregnancy Category D

INDICATIONS

▪ **IM, IV:** Preoperative sedation/anxiolysis/amnesia ▪ **IV:** Provides sedation/anxiolysis/amnesia during therapeutic, diagnostic, or radiographic procedures (conscious sedation) ▫ Aids in the induction of anesthesia and as part of balanced anesthesia ▫ As a continuous infusion, provides sedation of mechanically ventilated patients during anesthesia or in a critical care setting.

ACTION

▪ Acts at many levels of the CNS to produce generalized CNS depression ▪ Effects may be mediated by gamma-aminobutyric acid (GABA), an inhibitory neurotransmitter. **Therapeutic Effects:** ▪ Short-term sedation ▪ Postoperative amnesia.

PHARMACOKINETICS

Absorption: Well absorbed following IM administration.
Distribution: Crosses the blood-brain barrier and placenta.
Metabolism and Excretion: Almost exclusively metabolized by the liver.
Half-life: 1–12 hr (increased in renal impairment or congestive heart failure [CHF]).

CONTRAINDICATIONS AND PRECAUTIONS

Contraindicated in: ▪ Hypersensitivity ▪ Cross-sensitivity with other benzodiazepines may occur ▪ Shock ▪ Comatose patients or those with preexisting CNS depression ▪ Uncontrolled severe pain ▪ Products containing benzyl alcohol should not be used in neonates ▪ Pregnancy.
Use Cautiously in: ▪ Pulmonary disease ▪ CHF ▪ Renal impairment ▪ Severe hepatic impairment ▪ Geriatric or debilitated patients (more susceptible to depressant effects; dosage reduction required) ▪ Lactation (safety not established).

ADVERSE REACTIONS AND SIDE EFFECTS*

CNS: agitation, drowsiness, excess sedation, headache.
EENT: blurred vision.
Resp: APNEA, LARYNGOSPASM, RESPIRATORY DEPRESSION, bronchospasm, coughing.
CV: CARDIAC ARREST, arrhythmias.
GI: hiccups, nausea, vomiting.
Derm: rashes.
Local: <u>phlebitis</u> at IV site, pain at IM site.

INTERACTIONS

Drug-Drug: ▪ Additive CNS depression with **alcohol, antihistamines, opioids,** and other **sedative/hypnotics** (decrease midazolam dose by 30–50% if used concurrently) ▪ Increased risk of hypotension with **antihypertensives,** acute ingestion of **alcohol,** or **nitrates.**

ROUTE AND DOSAGE

Dosage must be individualized, taking caution to reduce dosage in geriatric patients and in those who are already sedated.

▫ Preoperative Sedation/Amnesia

- **IM (Adults Otherwise Healthy and <60 yr):** 70–80 mcg/kg 1 hr before surgery (usual dose 5 mg).
- **IM (Adults ≥60 yr, Debilitated or Chronically Ill):** 20–30 mcg/kg 1 hr before surgery (1–3 mg).
- **IM (Children):** 100–150 mcg (0.01–0.15 mg)/kg up to 500 mcg (0.5 mg)/kg; not to exceed 10 mg/dose.

▫ Conscious Sedation for Short Procedures

- **IV (Adults and Children Otherwise Healthy, >12 yr and <60 yr):** 1–1.5 mg initially; dosage may be increased further as

*CAPITALS indicate life-threatening; <u>underlines</u> indicate most frequent.

needed. Total doses >3.5 mg are rarely needed (reduce dose by 30% if other CNS depressants are used). Maintenance doses of 25% of the dose required for initial sedation may be given as necessary.

- **IV (Geriatric Patients ≥60 yr, Debilitated or Chronically Ill):** 1–2.5 mg initially; dosage may be increased further as needed. Total doses >5 mg are rarely needed (reduce dose by 50% if other CNS depressants are used). Maintenance doses of 25% of the dose required for initial sedation may be given as necessary.

❑ Conscious Sedation for Short Procedures or Prior to Anesthesia

- **IV (Children 6–12 yr):** 25–50 mcg/kg initially; up to 400 mcg/kg total dose may be required (not to exceed 10 mg total dose).
- **IV (Children 6 mo–5 yr):** 50–100 mcg/kg (not to exceed 600 mcg/kg [6 mg] total dose).

❑ Induction of Anesthesia (Adjunct)

May give additional dose of 25% of initial dose if needed.

- **IV (Adults Otherwise Healthy and <55 yr):** 300–350 mcg/kg initially (up to 600 mcg/kg total). If patient is premedicated, initial dose should be further reduced.
- **IV (Geriatric Patients >55 yr):** 150–300 mcg/kg as initial dose. If patient is premedicated, initial dose should be further reduced.
- **IV (Adults —Debilitated):** 150–250 mcg/kg initial dose. If patient is premedicated, initial dose should be further reduced.

❑ Sedation in Critical Care Settings

- **IV (Adults):** 10–50 mcg/kg (0.5–4 mg in most adults) initially if a loading dose is required; may repeat q 10–15 min until desired effect is obtained; may be followed by infusion at 20–100 mcg/kg/hr (1–7 mg/hr in most adults).
- **IV (Children):** *Intubated patients only*—50–200 mcg/kg initially as a loading dose; follow with infusion at 60–120 mcg/kg/min (1–2 mcg/kg/min).
- **IV (Neonates >32 wk):** *Intubated patients only*—60 mcg/kg/hr (1 mcg/kg/min).
- **IV (Neonates <32 wk):** *Intubated patients only*—30 mcg/kg/hr (0.5 mcg/kg/min).

AVAILABILITY

- ***Injection:*** 1 mg/ml[Rx], 5 mg/ml[Rx].

TIME/ACTION PROFILE (sedation)

	ONSET	PEAK	DURATION
IM	15 min	30–60 min	2–6 hr
IV	1.5–5 min	rapid	2–6 hr

NURSING IMPLICATIONS

ASSESSMENT

- ❑ Assess level of sedation and level of consciousness throughout and for 2–6 hr following administration.
- ❑ Monitor blood pressure, pulse, and respiration continuously throughout IV administration. Oxygen and resuscitative equipment should be immediately available.
- ***Toxicity and Overdose:*** If overdose occurs, monitor pulse, respiration, and blood pressure continuously. Maintain patent airway and assist ventilation as needed. If hypotension occurs, treatment includes IV fluids, repositioning, and vasopressors.
- ❑ The effects of midazolam can be reversed with flumazenil (Romazicon) (see p. 387).

POTENTIAL NURSING DIAGNOSES

- Breathing pattern, ineffective (Adverse Reactions).
- Injury, risk for (Side Effects).
- Knowledge deficit, related to medication regimen (Patient/Family Teaching).

IMPLEMENTATION

- **IM:** Administer IM doses deep into muscle mass.
- **Direct IV:** Administer undiluted or diluted with D5W, 0.9% NaCl, or lactated Ringer's injection through Y-site.
- ❑ When administered concurrently with opioid analgesics, dose should be reduced by 30–50%.
- ***Rate:*** Administer each dose slowly over at least 2 min. Monitor IV site closely to avoid extravasation. Titrate dose to patient response. Rapid injection, especially in neonates, has caused severe hypotension.
- **Continuous Infusion:** Dilute 5 mg/ml to a

concentration of 0.5 mg/ml with 0.9% NaCl or D5W.

- *Rate:* Usual infusion rate is 0.02–0.1 mg/kg/hr (1–7 mg/hr). Titrate to desired level of sedation. Assess sedation at regular intervals and adjust rate up or down by 25–50% as needed. Dose should also be decreased by 10–25% every few hours to find minimum effective infusion rate, which prevents accumulation of midazolam and provides more rapid recovery upon termination.
  - In pediatric patients, rate of 0.06–0.12 mg/kg/hr (1–2 mcg/kg/min) can be increased or decreased by 25% based on assessment of sedation.
  - In neonates, rate of 0.03 mg/kg/hr (0.5 mcg/kg/min) is used for neonates <32 weeks and rate of 0.06 mg/kg/hr (1 mcg/kg/min) is used for neonates >32 weeks of age.
- **Syringe Compatibility:** ▪ atropine ▪ benzquinamide ▪ buprenorphine ▪ butorphanol ▪ cimetidine ▪ fentanyl ▪ glycopyrrolate ▪ hydromorphone ▪ meperidine ▪ metoclopramide ▪ morphine ▪ nalbuphine ▪ scopolamine ▪ sufentanil ▪ thiethylperazine ▪ trimethobenzamide.
- **Syringe Incompatibility:** ▪ prochlorperazine ▪ ranitidine.
- **Y-Site Compatibility:** ▪ amikacin ▪ amiodarone ▪ atracurium ▪ bumetanide ▪ calcium gluconate ▪ cefazolin ▪ cefotaxime ▪ cimetidine ▪ ciprofloxacin ▪ clindamycin ▪ digoxin ▪ dopamine ▪ erythromycin lactobionate ▪ esmolol ▪ etomidate ▪ famotidine ▪ fentanyl ▪ fluconazole ▪ gentamicin ▪ haloperidol ▪ heparin ▪ insulin ▪ labetalol ▪ methylprednisolone ▪ metronidazole ▪ morphine ▪ nitroglycerin ▪ nitroprusside ▪ norepinephrine ▪ pancuronium ▪ piperacillin ▪ potassium chloride ▪ ranitidine ▪ sufentanil ▪ theophylline ▪ tobramycin ▪ vancomycin ▪ vecuronium.
- **Y-Site Incompatibility:** ▪ albumin ▪ ampicillin ▪ ceftazidime ▪ cefuroxime ▪ clinidine ▪ dexamethasone ▪ floxacillin ▪ foscarnet ▪ furosemide ▪ hydrocortisone ▪ imipenem/cilastatin ▪ methotrexate ▪ nafcillin ▪ omeprazole ▪ sodium bicarbonate ▪ trimethoprim/sulfamethoxazole.

PATIENT/FAMILY TEACHING

- Inform patient that this medication will decrease mental recall of the procedure.
- May cause drowsiness or dizziness. Advise patient to request assistance prior to ambulation and transfer and to avoid driving or other activities requiring alertness for 24 hr following administration.
- Instruct patient to inform health care professional prior to administration if pregnancy is suspected.
- Advise patient to avoid alcohol or other CNS depressants for 24 hr following administration of midazolam.

EVALUATION

Effectiveness of therapy can be demonstrated by: ▪ Sedation during and amnesia following surgical, diagnostic, and radiologic procedures ▪ Sedation and amnesia for mechanically ventilated patients in a critical care setting.

MIGLITOL

(**mi**-gli-tole)
Glyset

CLASSIFICATION(S):
Oral hypoglycemic agent (alpha-glucosidase inhibitor)

Pregnancy Category B

INDICATIONS

▪ Management of non–insulin-dependent diabetes mellitus (NIDDM) in conjunction with dietary therapy; may be used concurrently with sulfonylurea oral hypoglycemic agents.

ACTION

▪ Lowers blood sugar by inhibiting the enzyme alpha-glucosidase in the GI tract, resulting in delayed glucose absorption. **Therapeutic Effects:** ▪ Lowering of blood sugar in diabetic patients, especially postprandial hyperglycemia.

PHARMACOKINETICS

Absorption: Completely absorbed at lower doses (25 mg); 50–70% absorbed at higher doses (100 mg).
Distribution: Distributes primarily into extracellular fluid; small amounts enter breast milk.
Metabolism and Excretion: Not metabolized; action is primarily local in the GI tract; amounts that are absorbed are excreted mostly unchanged in urine.
Half-life: 2 hr.

CONTRAINDICATIONS AND PRECAUTIONS

Contraindicated in: ▪ Hypersensitivity ▪ Diabetic ketoacidosis ▪ Inflammatory bowel disease or other chronic intestinal conditions resulting in impaired absorption or predisposition to obstruction ▪ Lactation.

Use Cautiously in: ▪ Patients with: ▫ Fever ▫ Infection ▫ Trauma ▫ Stress (may cause hyperglycemia requiring alternate therapy) ▪ Renal impairment (use not recommended if creatinine >2 mg/dl) ▪ Pregnancy or children (safety not established).

ADVERSE REACTIONS AND SIDE EFFECTS*

GI: abdominal pain, diarrhea, flatulence.
Hemat: low serum iron.

INTERACTIONS

Drug-Drug: ▪ May decrease absorption of **ranitidine** and **propranolol** ▪ Effects may be decreased by **intestinal adsorbents** (such as **charcoal**) and **digestive enzyme products;** concurrent use should be avoided.
Drug-Food: ▪ Concurrent **carbohydrates** may increase diarrhea.

ROUTE AND DOSAGE

- **PO (Adults):** 25 mg 3 times daily; may begin with 25 mg once daily; may be increased up to 100 mg 3 times daily.

AVAILABILITY

- ***Tablets:*** 25 mg[Rx], 50 mg[Rx], 100 mg[Rx].

TIME/ACTION PROFILE (effect on glucose absorption)

	ONSET	PEAK	DURATION
PO	rapid	within 1 hr	UK

NURSING IMPLICATIONS

ASSESSMENT

- ▫ Observe patient for signs and symptoms of hypoglycemic reactions (sweating, hunger, weakness, dizziness, tremor, tachycardia, anxiety), especially when taking concurrently with other oral hypoglycemic agents.
- ***Lab Test Considerations:*** Serum glucose and glycosylated hemoglobin should be monitored periodically throughout therapy to evaluate effectiveness of therapy.
- ***Toxicity and Overdose:*** Symptoms of overdose are transient increase in flatulence, diarrhea, and abdominal discomfort. Miglitol alone does not cause hypoglycemia; however, other concurrently administered hypoglycemic agents may produce hypoglycemia requiring treatment. Mild hypoglycemia may be treated with administration of oral glucose.

POTENTIAL NURSING DIAGNOSES

- Nutrition, altered, more than body requirements (Indications).
- Knowledge deficit, related to medication regimen (Patient/Family Teaching).
- Noncompliance (Patient/Family Teaching).

IMPLEMENTATION

- **General Info:** Patients stabilized on a diabetic regimen who are exposed to stress, fever, trauma, infection, or surgery may require administration of insulin.
- ▫ Does not cause hypoglycemia when taken while fasting but may increase hypoglycemic effect of other hypoglycemic agents.
- **PO:** Administer miglitol 3 times daily with the first bite of each meal. Dose may be started lower and increased gradually to minimize GI effects.

PATIENT/FAMILY TEACHING

- ▫ Instruct patient to take miglitol at the same time each day, exactly as directed.
- ▫ Explain to patient that miglitol helps control hyperglycemia but does not cure diabetes. Therapy is usually long term.
- ▫ Encourage patient to follow prescribed diet, medication, and exercise regimen to prevent hyperglycemic or hypoglycemic episodes.
- ▫ Review signs of hypoglycemia and hyperglycemia with patient. If hypoglycemia occurs, advise patient to take a glass of orange juice, 2–3 tsp of sugar, honey, or corn syrup dissolved in water, and notify health care professional.
- ▫ Instruct patient in proper testing of blood glucose or urine ketones. These tests should be monitored closely during periods of stress or

M

***CAPITALS indicate life-threatening; underlines indicate most frequent.**

illness and health care professional notified of significant changes.

- Insulin is the recommended method of controlling blood sugar during pregnancy. Counsel female patients to use a form of contraception other than oral contraceptives and to notify health care professional promptly if pregnancy is planned or suspected.
- Advise patient to inform health care professional of medication regimen prior to treatment or surgery.
- Advise patient to carry a form of oral glucose (dextrose, D-glucose) and identification describing disease process and medication regimen at all times.
- Emphasize the importance of routine follow-up exams and regular testing of blood glucose and glycosylated hemoglobin.

EVALUATION

Effectiveness of therapy can be demonstrated by: ▪ Control of blood glucose levels without the appearance of hypoglycemic or hyperglycemic episodes.

MILRINONE

(**mill**-ri-none)

Primacor

CLASSIFICATION(S):

Inotropic agent

Pregnancy Category C

INDICATIONS

▪ Short-term treatment of congestive heart failure unresponsive to conventional therapy with digitalis glycosides, diuretics, and vasodilators.

ACTION

▪ Increases myocardial contractility ▪ Decreases preload and afterload by a direct dilating effect on vascular smooth muscle. **Therapeutic Effects:** ▪ Increased cardiac output (inotropic effect).

PHARMACOKINETICS

Absorption: IV administration results in complete bioavailability.

Distribution: UK.

Metabolism and Excretion: 80–90% excreted unchanged by the kidneys.

Half-life: 2.3 hr (increased in renal impairment).

CONTRAINDICATIONS AND PRECAUTIONS

Contraindicated in: ▪ Hypersensitivity ▪ Severe aortic or pulmonic valvular heart disease ▪ Hypertrophic subaortic stenosis (may increase outflow tract obstruction).

Use Cautiously in: ▪ History of arrhythmias, electrolyte abnormalities, abnormal digoxin levels, or insertion of vascular catheters (increased risk of ventricular arrhythmias) ▪ Renal impairment (reduced infusion rate recommended if CCr is <50 ml/min) ▪ Pregnancy, lactation, or children (safety not established).

ADVERSE REACTIONS AND SIDE EFFECTS*

CNS: headache, tremor.

CV: VENTRICULAR ARRHYTHMIAS, angina pectoris, chest pain, hypotension, supraventricular arrhythmias.

F and E: hypokalemia.

Hemat: thrombocytopenia.

INTERACTIONS

Drug-Drug: ▪ None significant.

ROUTE AND DOSAGE

- **IV (Adults):** *Loading dose*—50 mcg/kg followed by *infusion* at 0.50 mcg/kg/min (range 0.375–0.75 mcg/kg/min).

AVAILABILITY

▪ ***Injection:*** 1 mg/ml in 10- and 20-ml vials and 5-ml preloaded syringes[Rx].

TIME/ACTION PROFILE (hemodynamic effects)

	ONSET	PEAK	DURATION
IV	5–15 min	UK	3–6 hr

NURSING IMPLICATIONS

ASSESSMENT

- Monitor heart rate and blood pressure continuously during administration. Milrinone

*CAPITALS indicate life-threatening; underlines indicate most frequent.

should be slowed or discontinued if blood pressure drops excessively.

- □ Monitor intake and output and daily weight. Assess patient for resolution of signs and symptoms of congestive heart failure (peripheral edema, dyspnea, rales/crackles, weight gain) and improvement in hemodynamic parameters (increase in cardiac output and cardiac index, decrease in pulmonary capillary wedge pressure). The effects of previous aggressive diuretic therapy should be corrected to allow for optimal filling pressure.
- □ Monitor ECG continuously during infusion. Arrhythmias are common and may be life threatening. The risk of ventricular arrhythmias is increased in patients with a history of arrhythmias, electrolyte abnormalities, abnormal digoxin levels, or insertion of vascular catheters.
- ■ ***Lab Test Considerations:*** Monitor electrolytes and renal function frequently during administration. Hypokalemia should be corrected prior to administration to decrease the risk of arrhythmias.
- □ Monitor platelet count during therapy.
- ■ ***Toxicity and Overdose:*** Overdose manifests as hypotension. Dosage should be decreased or discontinued. Supportive measures may be necessary.

POTENTIAL NURSING DIAGNOSES

- ■ Cardiac output, decreased (Indications).
- ■ Knowledge deficit, related to medication regimen (Patient/Family Teaching).

IMPLEMENTATION

- ■ **Direct IV:** Loading dose may be administered undiluted.
- ■ ***Rate:*** Administer the loading dose over 10 min.
- ■ **Continuous Infusion:** The 20-mg vial may be diluted with 180 ml of diluent for a concentration of 100 mcg/ml, with 113 ml of diluent for a concentration of 150 mcg/ml, or with 80 ml of diluent for a concentration of 200 mcg/ml. Compatible diluents include 0.45% NaCl, 0.9% NaCl, and D5W. Do not use solutions that are discolored or contain particulate matter.
- ■ ***Rate:*** Infusion rate is titrated according to hemodynamic and clinical response. See infusion rate table in Appendix D.
- ■ **Syringe Compatibility:** ■ atropine ■ calcium chloride ■ digoxin ■ epinephrine ■ lidocaine ■ morphine ■ propranolol ■ sodium bicarbonate ■ verapamil.
- ■ **Syringe Incompatibility:** ■ furosemide.
- ■ **Y-Site Compatibility:** ■ digoxin ■ propranolol ■ quinidine gluconate.
- ■ **Y-Site Incompatibility:** ■ furosemide ■ procainamide.

PATIENT/FAMILY TEACHING

- □ Inform patient and family of reasons for administration. Milrinone is not a cure but is a temporary measure to control the symptoms of congestive heart failure.

EVALUATION

Clinical response to therapy can be evaluated by: ■ Decrease in the signs and symptoms of congestive heart failure □ Improvement in hemodynamic parameters.

MINERAL OIL

Agoral, Fleet Mineral Oil, {Kondremul}, Kondremul Plain, {Lansoyl}, Liqui-Doss, Milkinol, Neo-Cultol, Nujol, Petrogalar Plain, Zymenol

CLASSIFICATION(S):
Laxative (lubricant)

Pregnancy Category UK

INDICATIONS

■ Used to soften impacted feces in the management of constipation.

ACTION

■ Coats surface of stool and intestine with lubricant film to allow passage of stool through intestine ■ Improves water retention of stool. **Therapeutic Effects:** ■ Softening of fecal mass and subsequent passage.

PHARMACOKINETICS

Absorption: Minimally absorbed following oral administration.
Distribution: Distributes into mesenteric lymph nodes, intestinal mucosa, liver, and spleen.
Metabolism and Excretion: UK. Action is pri-

{} = Available in Canada only.

marily local; unabsorbed mineral oil is passed with fecal mass.
Half-life: UK.

CONTRAINDICATIONS AND PRECAUTIONS

Contraindicated in: ▪ Hypersensitivity ▪ Children <6 yr (oral) ▪ Children <2 yr (rect).
Use Cautiously in: ▪ Children, geriatric, or debilitated patients (increased risk of lipid pneumonia) ▪ Pregnancy (chronic use decreases absorption of fat-soluble vitamins; may cause hypoprothrombinemia in newborn).

ADVERSE REACTIONS AND SIDE EFFECTS

Resp: lipid pneumonia.
GI: anal irritation, rectal seepage of mineral oil.

INTERACTIONS

Drug-Drug: ▪ Decreases absorption of **fat-soluble vitamins (A, D, E, K)** ▪ Concurrent use with **stool softeners** may increase absorption of mineral oil.
Drug-Food: ▪ Decreases absorption of **fat-soluble vitamins (A, D, E, K).**

ROUTE AND DOSAGE

- **PO (Adults and Children >12 yr):** 5–45 ml.
- **PO (Children 6–12 yr):** 5–20 ml.
- **Rect (Adults and Children >12 yr):** 60–150 ml as a single dose.
- **Rect (Children 2–11 yr):** 30–60 ml as a single dose.

AVAILABILITY

▪ ***Liquid:*** in 30-ml, 180-ml, pint, and gallon containers[OTC] ▪ ***Jelly:*** 180-ml container[OTC] ▪ ***Emulsion:*** 480-ml containers[OTC] ▪ ***In combination with:*** magnesium hydroxide (Haley's M-O), cascara, and glycerin[OTC]. See Appendix A.

TIME/ACTION PROFILE (laxation)

	ONSET	PEAK	DURATION
PO	6–8 hr	UK	UK
Rect	2–15 min	UK	UK

NURSING IMPLICATIONS

ASSESSMENT

- □ Assess patient for abdominal distention, presence of bowel sounds, and usual pattern of bowel function.
- □ Assess color, consistency, and amount of stool produced.

POTENTIAL NURSING DIAGNOSES

- ▪ Constipation (Indications).
- ▪ Knowledge deficit, related to medication regimen (Patient/Family Teaching).

IMPLEMENTATION

- ▪ **General Info:** This medication does not stimulate intestinal peristalsis.
- □ Administer carefully to bedridden patients or children to prevent lipid pneumonia from aspiration of mineral oil. Do not administer to patients in a reclining position.
- ▪ **PO:** Usually administered at bedtime. Do not administer within 2 hr of meals; may interfere with absorption of nutrients and vitamins.
- □ Do not administer within 2 hr of stool softeners; may cause increased absorption of mineral oil.
- ▪ **Rect:** Do not lubricate suppositories containing mineral oil, as this may interfere with the action of the suppository. Moisten with water by placing under tap for 30 sec or in a cup of water for at least 10 sec prior to insertion.

PATIENT/FAMILY TEACHING

- □ Advise patients that laxatives should be used only for short-term therapy. Long-term therapy may interfere with absorption of nutrients and vitamins A, D, E, and K.
- □ Advise patients not to take this medication within 2 hr of food or other medications.
- □ Encourage patients to use other forms of bowel regulation, such as increasing bulk in the diet, increasing fluid intake, and increasing mobility. Normal bowel habits are variable and may vary from 3 times/day to 3 times/wk.
- □ Instruct patients with cardiac disease to avoid straining during bowel movements (Valsalva maneuver).
- □ Advise patients that large doses of mineral oil may cause leakage of mineral oil from the rectum; protection of clothing may be necessary. This may be prevented by reducing or

dividing the dose or by administering in emulsified form.

□ Advise patients not to use laxatives when abdominal pain, nausea, vomiting, or fever is present.

EVALUATION

Effectiveness of therapy can be demonstrated by: ▪ Soft, formed bowel movement, usually within 6–8 hr of an oral dose □ Results are usually obtained from rectal doses in 2–15 min.

MINOXIDIL (systemic)†

(mi-**nox**-i-dill)

Loniten

CLASSIFICATION(S):

Antihypertensive agent (vasodilator)

Pregnancy Category C

†For information on topical use, see the infrequent use table in Appendix Q.

INDICATIONS

▪ Management of severe symptomatic hypertension or hypertension associated with end-organ damage that has failed to respond to combinations of more conventional therapy.

ACTION

▪ Directly relaxes vascular smooth muscle, probably by inhibiting the enzyme phosphodiesterase. Results in vasodilation, which is more pronounced in arterioles than veins. **Therapeutic Effects:** ▪ Lowering of blood pressure.

PHARMACOKINETICS

Absorption: Well absorbed following oral administration.
Distribution: Widely distributed; enters breast milk.
Metabolism and Excretion: 90% metabolized by the liver.
Half-life: 4.2 hr.

CONTRAINDICATIONS AND PRECAUTIONS

Contraindicated in: ▪ Hypersensitivity ▪ Pheochromocytoma ▪ Patients currently receiving guanethidine.

Use Cautiously in: ▪ **PO**—Recent myocardial infarction ▪ Severe renal impairment (can be used in moderate renal impairment) ▪ Pregnancy or lactation (safety not established).

ADVERSE REACTIONS AND SIDE EFFECTS*

CNS: headache.
Resp: PULMONARY EDEMA.
CV: CONGESTIVE HEART FAILURE, ECG changes (alteration in T waves), tachycardia, angina, pericardial effusion.
GI: nausea.
Derm: hypertrichosis, pigment changes, rashes.
Endo: gynecomastia, menstrual irregularities.
F and E: sodium and water retention.
Misc: intermittent claudication.

INTERACTIONS

Drug-Drug: ▪ Additive hypotensive effects with other **antihypertensive agents,** acute ingestion of **alcohol,** or **nitrates** ▪ Severe hypotension may occur with **guanethidine** ▪ **NSAIDs** may decrease the antihypertensive effectiveness of minoxidil.

ROUTE AND DOSAGE

- **PO (Adults and Children >12 yr):** *Hypertension*—5 mg once daily or in 2 divided doses; may double at 3-day intervals; usual range 10–40 mg/day (for rapid control with careful monitoring, doses may be adjusted q 6 hr; up to 100 mg/day have been used).
- **PO (Children <12 yr):** *Hypertension*—0.2 mg/kg/day (5 mg maximum) as a single dose or 2 divided doses; may be gradually increased at 3-day intervals in increments of 50–100% until response is obtained; usual range 0.25–1 mg/kg/day (for rapid control, doses may be adjusted q 6 hr; not to exceed 50 mg/day).

AVAILABILITY

▪ ***Tablets:*** 2.5 mg[Rx], 10 mg[Rx].

TIME/ACTION PROFILE (antihypertensive effect)

	ONSET	PEAK	DURATION
PO	30 min	2–3 hr	2–5 days

*CAPITALS indicate life-threatening; underlines indicate most frequent.

M

NURSING IMPLICATIONS

ASSESSMENT

- **Hypertension:** Monitor blood pressure and pulse frequently during initial dosage adjustment and periodically throughout therapy. Report significant changes.
- □ Monitor frequency of prescription refills to determine compliance.
- □ Monitor intake and output ratios and daily weight and assess for edema daily, especially at beginning of therapy. Report weight gain or edema; sodium and water retention may be treated with diuretics.
- ***Lab Test Considerations:*** Renal and hepatic function, CBC, and electrolytes should be monitored prior to and periodically throughout therapy.
- □ May cause increased BUN, serum creatinine, alkaline phosphatase, plasma renin activity (PRA), and sodium levels. May also cause decreased RBC, hemoglobin, and hematocrit counts. Hematologic and renal values usually return to pretreatment levels with continued therapy.

POTENTIAL NURSING DIAGNOSES

- Tissue perfusion, altered (Indications).
- Knowledge deficit, related to medication regimen (Patient/Family Teaching).

IMPLEMENTATION

- **Hypertension:** Medication may need to be discontinued gradually to prevent rebound hypertension.
- □ Minoxidil is given concurrently with a diuretic unless patient is on hemodialysis.
- □ Dosage adjustments should not be made more frequently than every 3 days to allow for maximum effectiveness, unless rapid control is necessary.
- **PO:** May be administered without regard to meals or food.

PATIENT/FAMILY TEACHING

- □ Emphasize the importance of continuing to take this medication, even if feeling well. Instruct patient to take medication at the same time each day. If a dose is missed, take as soon as remembered if within a few hours; otherwise, omit dose and return to regular dosage schedule. Do not double doses. Advise patient not to discontinue minoxidil or other antihypertensive medications without consulting health care professional. Minoxidil helps control but does not cure hypertension.
- □ Encourage patient to comply with additional interventions for hypertension (weight reduction, low-sodium diet, smoking cessation, moderation of alcohol consumption, regular exercise, and stress management).
- □ Instruct patient and family on proper technique for pulse and blood pressure monitoring. Advise them to check blood pressure at least weekly and to report significant changes to health care professional, who should also be notified if resting pulse increases more than 20 bpm above baseline.
- □ Advise patient to check weight daily and to notify health care professional of rapid weight gain of >5 lb or if signs of fluid retention occur.
- □ Caution patient to change positions slowly to minimize orthostatic hypotension.
- □ Advise patient to consult health care professional before taking any cough, cold, or allergy remedies.
- □ Inform patient that depilatory creams may minimize increased hair growth. This is temporary and is reversible within 1–6 mo following discontinuation of minoxidil.
- □ Advise patient to notify health care professional if unusual swelling of face, extremities, or abdomen; difficulty breathing, especially when lying down; new or aggravated angina; severe indigestion; dizziness or fainting occurs.

EVALUATION

Effectiveness of therapy can be demonstrated by: ▪ Decrease in blood pressure without appearance of serious side effects.

MIRTAZAPINE
(meer-**taz**-a-peen)
Remeron

CLASSIFICATION(S):
Antidepressant (tetracyclic)

Pregnancy Category C

INDICATIONS

- Treatment of depression (with psychotherapy).

ACTION

▪ Potentiates the effects of norepinephrine and serotonin. **Therapeutic Effects:** ▪ Antidepressant action, which may develop only over several weeks.

PHARMACOKINETICS

Absorption: Well absorbed but rapidly metabolized, resulting in 50% bioavailability.
Distribution: UK.
Metabolism and Excretion: Extensively metabolized by the liver; metabolites excreted in urine (75%) and feces (15%).
Half-life: 20–40 hr.

CONTRAINDICATIONS AND PRECAUTIONS

Contraindicated in: ▪ Hypersensitivity.
Use Cautiously in: ▪ History of seizures ▪ History of suicide attempt ▪ History of mania/hypomania ▪ Geriatric patients or patients with hepatic or renal impairment (may need lower doses) ▪ Pregnancy, lactation, or children (safety not established).

ADVERSE REACTIONS AND SIDE EFFECTS*

CNS: drowsiness, abnormal dreams, abnormal thinking, agitation, anxiety, apathy, confusion, dizziness, malaise, weakness.
EENT: sinusitis.
Resp: dyspnea, increased cough.
CV: edema, hypotension, vasodilation.
GI: constipation, dry mouth, increased appetite, abdominal pain, anorexia, elevated liver enzymes, nausea, vomiting.
GU: urinary frequency.
Derm: pruritus, rash.
F and E: increased thirst.
Hemat: AGRANULOCYTOSIS.
Metab: weight gain, hypercholesterolemia, increased triglycerides.
MS: arthralgia, back pain, myalgia.
Neuro: hyperkinesia, hypesthesia, twitching.
Misc: flu-like syndrome.

INTERACTIONS

Drug-Drug: ▪ May cause hypertension, seizures, and death when used with **MAO inhibitors;** do not use within 14 days of MAO inhibitor therapy ▪ Additive CNS depression with other **CNS depressants,** including **alcohol** and **benzodiazepines** ▪ **Drugs affecting liver metabolism** may alter the effectiveness of mirtazapine.

ROUTE AND DOSAGE

▪ **PO (Adults):** 15 mg/day as a single bedtime dose initially; may be increased q 1–2 wk up to 45 mg/day.

AVAILABILITY

▪ ***Tablets:*** 15 mg[Rx], 30 mg[Rx].

TIME/ACTION PROFILE (antidepressant effect)

	ONSET	PEAK	DURATION
PO	1–2 wk	6 wk or more	UK

NURSING IMPLICATIONS

ASSESSMENT

□ Assess mental status frequently. Assess for suicidal tendencies, especially during early therapy. Restrict amount of drug available to patient.
□ Monitor blood pressure and pulse rate periodically during initial therapy. Report significant changes.
□ Monitor for seizure activity in patients with a history of convulsions or alcohol abuse. Institute seizure precautions.
▪ ***Lab Test Considerations:*** Assess CBC and hepatic function prior to and periodically during therapy.

POTENTIAL NURSING DIAGNOSES

▪ Coping, ineffective individual (Indications).
▪ Anxiety (Indications).
▪ Knowledge deficit, related to medication regimen (Patient/Family Teaching).

IMPLEMENTATION

▪ **General Info:** May be given as a single dose at bedtime to minimize excessive drowsiness or dizziness.
□ May be taken without regard to food.

M

***CAPITALS indicate life-threatening; underlines indicate most frequent.**

PATIENT/FAMILY TEACHING

- □ Instruct patient to take medication exactly as directed. If a dose is missed, take as soon as remembered; if almost time for next dose, skip missed dose and return to regular schedule. If single bedtime dose regimen is used, do not take missed dose in morning, but consult health care professional. Do not discontinue abruptly; gradual dosage reduction may be required.
- □ May cause drowsiness and dizziness. Caution patient to avoid driving and other activities requiring alertness until response to drug is known.
- □ Caution patient to change positions slowly to minimize orthostatic hypotension.
- □ Advise patient to avoid alcohol or other CNS depressant drugs during and for at least 3–7 days after therapy has been discontinued.
- □ Advise patient to notify health care professional if dry mouth, urinary retention, or constipation occurs. Frequent rinses, good oral hygiene, and sugarless candy or gum may diminish dry mouth. An increase in fluid intake, fiber, and exercise may prevent constipation.
- □ Inform patient of need to monitor dietary intake. Increase in appetite may lead to undesired weight gain.
- □ Advise patient to consult health care professional before taking any OTC cold remedies with this medication.
- □ Advise patient to notify health care professional of medication regimen prior to treatment or surgery.
- □ Therapy for depression may be prolonged. Emphasize the importance of follow-up exam to monitor effectiveness and side effects.

EVALUATION

Effectiveness of therapy can be demonstrated by: ▪ Resolution of the symptoms of depression: □ Increased sense of well-being □ Renewed interest in surroundings □ Increased appetite □ Improved energy level □ Improved sleep □ Therapeutic effects may be seen within 1 wk, although several wk are usually necessary before improvement is observed.

MISOPROSTOL

(mye-soe-**prost**-ole)
Cytotec

CLASSIFICATION(S):
Antiulcer agent (antisecretory), Antiulcer agent (cytoprotective)

Pregnancy Category X

INDICATIONS

▪ Prevention of gastric mucosal injury from NSAIDs, including aspirin, in high-risk patients (geriatric patients, debilitated patients, or those with a history of ulcers). **Unlabeled Uses:** ▪ Treatment of duodenal ulcers ▪ Induction of labor or ripening of cervix prior to labor induction.

ACTION

▪ Acts as a prostaglandin analogue, decreasing gastric acid secretion (antisecretory effect) and increasing the production of protective mucus (cytoprotective effect). **Therapeutic Effects:** ▪ Prevention of gastric ulceration from NSAIDs.

PHARMACOKINETICS

Absorption: Well absorbed following oral administration and rapidly converted to its active form (misoprostol acid).
Distribution: UK.
Metabolism and Excretion: Undergoes some metabolism and is then excreted by the kidneys.
Half-life: 20–40 min.

CONTRAINDICATIONS AND PRECAUTIONS

Contraindicated in: ▪ Hypersensitivity to prostaglandins ▪ Pregnancy or lactation.
Use Cautiously in: ▪ Patients with childbearing potential ▪ Children <18 yr (safety not established).

ADVERSE REACTIONS AND SIDE EFFECTS*

CNS: headache.
GI: abdominal pain, diarrhea, constipation, dyspepsia, flatulence, nausea, vomiting.
GU: miscarriage, menstrual disorders.

*CAPITALS indicate life-threatening; underlines indicate most frequent.

INTERACTIONS

Drug-Drug: ▪ Increased risk of diarrhea with **magnesium-containing antacids.**

ROUTE AND DOSAGE

- **PO (Adults):** 200 mcg 4 times daily with or after meals and at bedtime, or 400 mcg twice daily, with the last dose at bedtime. If intolerance occurs, dosage may be decreased to 100 mcg 4 times daily.

AVAILABILITY

▪ ***Tablets:*** 100 mcg (0.1 mg)Rx, 200 mcg (0.2 mg)Rx ▪ ***In combination with:*** 50 mg diclofenac/200 mcg misoprostol and 75 mg diclofenac/200 mcg misoprostol (ArthrotecRx); see Appendix A.

TIME/ACTION PROFILE (effect on gastric acid secretion)

	ONSET	PEAK	DURATION
PO	30 min	UK	3–6 hr

NURSING IMPLICATIONS

ASSESSMENT

- Assess patient routinely for epigastric or abdominal pain and frank or occult blood in the stool, emesis, or gastric aspirate.
- Assess women of childbearing age for pregnancy. Misoprostol is usually begun on 2nd or 3rd day of menstrual period following a negative pregnancy test.

POTENTIAL NURSING DIAGNOSES

- Pain (Indications).
- Knowledge deficit, related to medication regimen (Patient/Family Teaching).

IMPLEMENTATION

- **General Info:** Misoprostol therapy should be started at the onset of treatment with NSAIDs.
- **PO:** Administer medication with meals and at bedtime to reduce severity of diarrhea.
- Antacids may be administered before or after misoprostol for relief of pain. Avoid those containing magnesium, because of increased diarrhea with misoprostol.

PATIENT/FAMILY TEACHING

- Instruct patient to take medication as directed for the full course of therapy, even if feeling better. If a dose is missed, take as soon as possible unless almost time for next dose; do not double doses. Emphasize that sharing of this medication may be dangerous.
- Inform patient that misoprostol will cause spontaneous abortion. Women of childbearing age must be informed of this effect through verbal and written information and must use contraception throughout therapy. If pregnancy is suspected, the woman should stop taking misoprostol and immediately notify her health care professional.
- Inform patient that diarrhea may occur. Health care professional should be notified if diarrhea persists for more than 1 wk. Also advise patient to report onset of black, tarry stools or severe abdominal pain.
- Advise patient to avoid alcohol and foods that may cause an increase in GI irritation.

EVALUATION

Effectiveness of therapy can be demonstrated by: ▪ The prevention of gastric ulcers in patients receiving chronic NSAID therapy.

MITOMYCIN

(mye-toe-**mye**-sin)

Mutamycin

CLASSIFICATION(S):

Antineoplastic (antitumor antibiotic)

Pregnancy Category UK

INDICATIONS

▪ Used with other agents in the management of disseminated adenocarcinoma of the stomach or pancreas. **Unlabeled Uses:** ▪ Palliative treatment of: ▫ Carcinoma of the colon or breast ▫ Head and neck tumors ▫ Advanced biliary, lung, and cervical squamous cell carcinomas.

ACTION

▪ Primarily inhibits DNA synthesis by causing cross-linking; also inhibits RNA and protein synthesis (cell-cycle phase–nonspecific but is most active in S and G phases). **Therapeutic Effects:**

▪ Death of rapidly replicating cells, particularly malignant ones.

PHARMACOKINETICS

Absorption: IV administration results in complete bioavailability.
Distribution: Widely distributed, concentrates in tumor tissue. Does not enter CSF.
Metabolism and Excretion: Mostly metabolized by the liver. Small amounts (<10%) excreted unchanged by the kidneys and in bile.
Half-life: 50 min.

CONTRAINDICATIONS AND PRECAUTIONS

Contraindicated in: ▪ Hypersensitivity ▪ Pregnancy or lactation.
Use Cautiously in: ▪ Patients with childbearing potential ▪ Active infections ▪ Decreased bone marrow reserve ▪ Geriatric patients or patients with other chronic debilitating illnesses ▪ Impaired liver function ▪ History of pulmonary problems.

ADVERSE REACTIONS AND SIDE EFFECTS*

Resp: pulmonary toxicity.
CV: edema.
GI: nausea, vomiting, anorexia, stomatitis.
GU: gonadal suppression, renal failure.
Derm: alopecia, desquamation.
Hemat: leukopenia, thrombocytopenia, anemia.
Local: phlebitis at IV site.
Misc: HEMOLYTIC UREMIC SYNDROME, fever, prolonged malaise.

INTERACTIONS

Drug-Drug: ▪ Additive bone marrow depression with other **antineoplastic agents** or **radiation therapy** ▪ May decrease antibody response to **live virus vaccines** and increase the risk of adverse reactions ▪ Concurrent or sequential use with **vinca alkaloids** may result in respiratory toxicity.

ROUTE AND DOSAGE

▪ **IV (Adults):** 10–20 mg/m² every 6–8 wk.

AVAILABILITY

▪ ***Injection:*** 5-mg, 20-mg, and 40-mg vials[Rx].

TIME/ACTION PROFILE (effects on blood counts)

	ONSET	PEAK	DURATION
IV	3–8 wk	4–8 wk	up to 3 mo

NURSING IMPLICATIONS

ASSESSMENT

- Monitor vital signs periodically during administration.
- Monitor for bone marrow depression. Assess for bleeding (bleeding gums, bruising, petechiae, guaiac stools, urine, and emesis) and avoid IM injections and rectal temperatures if platelet count is low. Apply pressure to venipuncture sites for 10 min. Assess for signs of infection during neutropenia. Anemia may occur. Monitor for increased fatigue, dyspnea, and orthostatic hypotension.
- Monitor intake and output, appetite, and nutritional intake. Nausea and vomiting usually occur within 1–2 hr. Vomiting may stop within 3–4 hr; nausea may persist for 2–3 days. Antiemetics may be administered prophylactically. Adjust diet as tolerated to help maintain fluid and electrolyte balance and nutritional status.
- Assess respiratory status and chest x-ray examination prior to and periodically throughout course of therapy. Cough, bronchospasm, hemoptysis, or dyspnea usually occurs after several doses and may be indicative of pulmonary toxicity, which may be life-threatening.
- Monitor for potentially fatal hemolytic uremic syndrome in patients receiving long-term therapy. Symptoms include microangiopathic hemolytic anemia, thrombocytopenia, renal failure, and hypertension.
- ***Lab Test Considerations:*** Monitor CBC with differential, platelet count, and observation for fragmented red blood cells on peripheral blood smears prior to and periodically throughout therapy and for several months following therapy.
- The nadirs of leukopenia and thrombocytopenia occur in 4–8 wk. Notify physician if leukocyte count is <4000/mm³ or if platelet count is <150,000/mm³ or is progressively declining. Recovery from leukopenia and thrombocytopenia occurs within 10 wk after

*CAPITALS indicate life-threatening; underlines indicate most frequent.

cessation of therapy. Myelosuppression is cumulative and may be irreversible. Repeat courses of therapy are held until leukocyte count is $>4000/mm^3$ and platelet count is $>100,000/mm^3$.

- □ Monitor liver function studies (AST, ALT, LDH, bilirubin) and renal function studies (BUN, creatinine) prior to and periodically throughout therapy to detect hepatotoxicity and nephrotoxicity. Notify physician if creatinine is >1.7 mg/dl.

POTENTIAL NURSING DIAGNOSES

- Injury, risk for (Side Effects).
- Infection, risk for (Side Effects).
- Body image disturbance (Side Effects).

IMPLEMENTATION

- **General Info:** Solution should be prepared in a biologic cabinet. Wear gloves, gown, and mask while handling medication. Discard equipment in designated containers (see Appendix I).
- □ Ensure patency of IV. Extravasation may cause severe tissue necrosis. If patient complains of discomfort at IV site, discontinue immediately and restart infusion at another site. Promptly notify physician of extravasation.
- **Direct IV:** Reconstitute 5-mg vial with 10 ml and 10-mg vial with 40 ml of sterile water for injection. Shake the vial; may need to stand at room temperature for additional time to dissolve. Final solution is blue-gray. Reconstituted solution is stable for 7 days at room temperature, 14 days if refrigerated.
- ***Rate:*** May be administered IV push over 5–10 min through free-flowing IV of 0.9% NaCl or D5W.
- **Y-Site Compatibility:** ▪ amifostine ▪ bleomycin ▪ cisplatin ▪ cyclophosphamide ▪ doxorubicin ▪ droperidol ▪ fluorouracil ▪ furosemide ▪ heparin ▪ leucovorin ▪ melphalan ▪ methotrexate ▪ metoclopramide ▪ ondansetron ▪ teniposide ▪ thiotepa ▪ vinblastine ▪ vincristine.
- **Y-Site Incompatibility:** ▪ aztreonam ▪ cefepime ▪ filgrastim ▪ piperacillin/tazobactam ▪ sargramostim ▪ vinorelbine.

PATIENT/FAMILY TEACHING

- □ Instruct patient to notify health care professional promptly if fever; chills; cough; hoarseness; sore throat; signs of infection; lower back or side pain; painful or difficult urination; bleeding gums; bruising; petechiae; blood in stools, urine, or emesis; increased fatigue; dyspnea; or orthostatic hypotension occurs. Caution patient to avoid crowds and persons with known infections. Instruct patient to use soft toothbrush and electric razor and to avoid falls. Caution patient not to drink alcoholic beverages or take medication containing aspirin or NSAIDS; may precipitate gastric bleeding.
- □ Instruct patient to notify health care professional if decreased urine output, edema in lower extremities, shortness of breath, skin ulceration, or persistent nausea occurs.
- □ Instruct patient to inspect oral mucosa for redness and ulceration. If ulceration occurs, advise patient to use sponge brush and rinse mouth with water after eating and drinking. Topical agents may be used if pain interferes with eating. Stomatitis pain may require treatment with opioid analgesics.
- □ Discuss with patient the possibility of hair loss. Explore coping strategies.
- □ Advise patient that, although mitomycin may cause infertility, contraception during therapy is necessary because of teratogenic effects.
- □ Instruct patient not to receive any vaccinations without advice of health care professional.
- □ Emphasize need for periodic lab tests to monitor for side effects.

EVALUATION

Effectiveness of therapy can be demonstrated by: ▪ Decrease in size and spread of malignant tissue.

MITOXANTRONE

(mye-toe-**zan**-trone)

Novantrone

CLASSIFICATION(S):

Antineoplastic (antitumor antibiotic)

Pregnancy Category D

INDICATIONS

▪ Acute nonlymphocytic leukemia (ANLL) in adults (with other antineoplastic agents) ▪ Initial chemotherapy for patients with pain associated with advanced hormone-refractory prostate can-

M

cer. **Unlabeled Uses:** ▪ Breast cancer, liver cancer, and non-Hodgkin's lymphoma.

ACTION

▪ Inhibits DNA synthesis (cell-cycle phase–nonspecific). **Therapeutic Effects:** ▪ Death of rapidly replicating cells, particularly malignant ones ▪ Decreased pain in patients with advanced prostate cancer.

PHARMACOKINETICS

Absorption: IV administration results in complete bioavailability.
Distribution: Widely distributed; limited penetration of CSF.
Metabolism and Excretion: Mostly eliminated by hepatobiliary clearance; <10% excreted unchanged by the kidneys.
Half-life: 5.8 days.

CONTRAINDICATIONS AND PRECAUTIONS

Contraindicated in: ▪ Hypersensitivity ▪ Pregnancy or lactation.
Use Cautiously in: ▪ Previous cardiac disease ▪ Patients with childbearing potential ▪ Active infections ▪ Depressed bone marrow reserve ▪ Previous mediastinal radiation ▪ Geriatric patients or patients with other chronic debilitating illness ▪ Children (safety not established) ▪ Impaired hepatobiliary function or decreased blood counts (dosage reduction required).

ADVERSE REACTIONS AND SIDE EFFECTS*

CNS: SEIZURES, headache.
EENT: blue-green sclera, conjunctivitis.
Resp: cough, dyspnea.
CV: CARDIOTOXICITY, arrhythmias, ECG changes.
GI: abdominal pain, diarrhea, hepatic toxicity, nausea, stomatitis, vomiting.
GU: blue-green urine, gonadal suppression, renal failure.
Derm: alopecia, rashes.
Hemat: anemia, leukopenia, thrombocytopenia.
Metab: hyperuricemia.
Misc: fever, hypersensitivity reactions.

INTERACTIONS

Drug-Drug: ▪ Additive bone marrow depression with other **antineoplastics** or **radiation therapy** ▪ Risk of cardiomyopathy increased by previous **anthracycline antineoplastics** (daunorubicin, doxorubicin, idarubicin) or **mediastinal radiation** ▪ May decrease antibody response to **live virus vaccines** and increase the risk of adverse reactions.

ROUTE AND DOSAGE

❑ **Acute Nonlymphatic Leukemia**

▪ **IV (Adults):** *Induction*—12 mg/m²/day for 3 days (usually given with cytosine arabinoside 100 mg/m²/day for 7 days); if incomplete remission occurs, a 2nd induction may be given. *Consolidation*—12 mg/m²/day for 2 days (usually given with cytosine arabinoside 100 mg/m²/day for 5 days), given 6 wk after induction with another course 4 wk later.

❑ **Advanced Prostate Cancer**

▪ **IV (Adults):** 12–14 mg/m² single dose as a short infusion (with glucocorticoids).

AVAILABILITY

▪ ***Injection:*** 2 mg/ml in 10-, 12.5-, and 15-ml vials[Rx].

TIME/ACTION PROFILE (effects on blood counts)

	ONSET	PEAK	DURATION
IV	UK	10 days	21 days

NURSING IMPLICATIONS

ASSESSMENT

- Monitor for hypersensitivity reaction (rash, urticaria, bronchospasm, tachycardia, hypotension). If these occur, stop infusion and notify physician. Keep epinephrine, an antihistamine, and resuscitation equipment close by in the event of an anaphylactic reaction.
- Monitor for bone marrow depression. Assess for bleeding (bleeding gums, bruising, petechiae, guaiac stools, urine, and emesis) and avoid IM injections and rectal temperatures if platelet count is low. Apply pressure to venipuncture sites for 10 min. Assess for signs of infection during neutropenia. Anemia may occur. Monitor for increased fatigue, dyspnea, and orthostatic hypotension.
- Monitor intake and output, appetite, and nutritional intake. Assess patient for nausea and

*CAPITALS indicate life-threatening; underlines indicate most frequent.

vomiting. Antiemetics may be administered prophylactically. Adjust diet as tolerated to help maintain fluid and electrolyte balance and nutritional status.

- ☐ Monitor chest x ray, ECG, echocardiography, and radionuclide angiography to determine ejection fraction prior to and periodically during therapy. May cause cardiotoxicity, especially in patients who have received daunorubicin or doxorubicin. Assess for rales/crackles, dyspnea, edema, jugular vein distention, ECG changes, arrhythmias, and chest pain.
- ☐ Monitor for symptoms of gout (increased uric acid levels and joint pain and swelling). Encourage patient to drink at least 2 liters of fluid per day. Allopurinol may be given to decrease serum uric acid levels.
- ▪ ***Lab Test Considerations:*** Monitor CBC with differential and platelet count prior to and periodically throughout therapy. The nadir of leukopenia usually occurs within 10 days, and recovery usually occurs within 21 days.
- ☐ Monitor liver function studies (AST, ALT, LDH, bilirubin) and renal function studies (BUN, creatinine) prior to and periodically throughout therapy to detect hepatotoxicity and nephrotoxicity.
- ☐ May cause increased uric acid concentrations. Monitor periodically during therapy.

POTENTIAL NURSING DIAGNOSES

- ▪ Injury, risk for (Side Effects).
- ▪ Infection, risk for (Side Effects).
- ▪ Body image disturbance (Side Effects).

IMPLEMENTATION

- ▪ **General Info:** Solution should be prepared in a biologic cabinet. Wear gloves, gown, and mask while handling medication. Discard equipment in designated containers (see Appendix I).
- ☐ Avoid contact with skin. Use Luer-Lok tubing to prevent accidental leakage. If contact with skin occurs, immediately wash skin with soap and water.
- ☐ Clean all spills with an aqueous solution of calcium hypochlorite. Mix solution by adding 5.5 parts (per weight) of calcium hypochlorite to 13 parts water.
- ▪ **IV:** Monitor IV site. If extravasation occurs, discontinue IV and restart at another site. Mitoxantrone is not a vesicant.
- ▪ **Direct IV:** Dilute dark blue mitoxantrone solution in at least 50 ml of 0.9% NaCl or D5W. Discard unused solution appropriately.
- ▪ ***Rate:*** Administer slowly over at least 3 min into the tubing of a free-flowing IV of 0.9% NaCl or D5W.
- ▪ **Intermittent Infusion:** May be further diluted in D5W, 0.9% NaCl, or D5/0.9% NaCl and used immediately.
- ▪ **Y-Site Compatibility:** ▪ amifostine ▪ filgrastim ▪ fludarabine ▪ melphalan ▪ ondansetron ▪ sargramostim ▪ teniposide ▪ thiotepa ▪ vinorelbine.
- ▪ **Y-Site Incompatibility:** ▪ aztreonam ▪ cefepime ▪ paclitaxel ▪ piperacillin/tazobactam.
- ▪ **Additive Compatibility:** ▪ cyclophosphamide ▪ cytarabine ▪ fluorouracil ▪ hydrocortisone sodium succinate ▪ potassium chloride.
- ▪ **Additive Incompatibility:** ▪ heparin.

PATIENT/FAMILY TEACHING

- ☐ Instruct patient to notify health care professional promptly if fever; chills; cough; hoarseness; sore throat; signs of infection; lower back or side pain; painful or difficult urination; bleeding gums; bruising; petechiae; blood in stools, urine, or emesis; increased fatigue; dyspnea; or orthostatic hypotension occurs. Caution patient to avoid crowds and persons with known infections. Instruct patient to use soft toothbrush and electric razor and to avoid falls. Caution patient not to drink alcoholic beverages or take medication containing aspirin or NSAIDS; may precipitate gastric bleeding.
- ☐ Instruct patient to notify health care professional if abdominal pain, yellow skin, cough, diarrhea, or decreased urine output occurs.
- ☐ Inform patient that medication may cause the urine and sclera to turn blue-green.
- ☐ Instruct patient to inspect oral mucosa for redness and ulceration. If mouth sores occur, advise patient to use sponge brush and rinse mouth with water after eating and drinking. Topical agents may be used if pain interferes with eating. Stomatitis pain may require treatment with opioid analgesics.
- ☐ Discuss with patient the possibility of hair loss. Explore coping strategies.
- ☐ Advise patient that, although mitoxantrone may cause infertility, contraception during

therapy is necessary because of possible teratogenic effects.
- □ Instruct patient not to receive any vaccinations without advice of health care professional.
- □ Emphasize need for periodic lab tests to monitor for side effects.

EVALUATION

Effectiveness of therapy can be demonstrated by: ▪ Decrease in the production and spread of leukemic cells ▪ Decreased pain in patients with prostate cancer.

MONOAMINE OXIDASE (MAO) INHIBITORS

phenelzine
(**fen**-el-zeen)
Nardil

tranylcypromine
(tran-ill-**sip**-roe-meen)
Parnate

CLASSIFICATION(S):
Antidepressants

Pregnancy Category C

INDICATIONS

▪ Treatment of neurotic or atypical depression, usually in conjunction with psychotherapy, in patients who may not tolerate other more conventional modes of therapy (tricyclic antidepressants, selective serotonin reuptake inhibitors [SSRIs], or electroconvulsive therapy).

ACTION

▪ Inhibit the enzyme monoamine oxidase, resulting in an accumulation of various neurotransmitters (dopamine, epinephrine, norepinephrine, and serotonin) in the body. **Therapeutic Effects:** Improved mood in depressed patients.

PHARMACOKINETICS

Absorption: All are well absorbed from the GI tract.
Distribution: All cross the placenta and probably enter breast milk.
Metabolism and Excretion: All are mostly metabolized by the liver.
Half-life: UK.

CONTRAINDICATIONS AND PRECAUTIONS

Contraindicated in: ▪ Hypersensitivity ▪ Liver disease ▪ Severe renal disease ▪ Cerebrovascular disease ▪ Pheochromocytoma ▪ Congestive heart failure ▪ History of headache ▪ Concurrent meperidine, fluoxetine, fluvoxamine, paroxetine, sertraline, nefazodone, or trazodone administration.
Use Cautiously in: ▪ Patients who may be suicidal or have a history of drug dependency ▪ Symptomatic cardiovascular disease ▪ Geriatric patients (increased risk of adverse reactions) ▪ Hyperthyroidism ▪ Seizure disorders ▪ Pregnancy, lactation, or children (safety not established). **Exercise Extreme Caution in:** ▪ Surgery (should be discontinued several weeks prior to surgery if possible because of increased risk of unpredictable reactions).

ADVERSE REACTIONS AND SIDE EFFECTS*

CNS: SEIZURES, <u>dizziness</u>, <u>headache</u>, <u>insomnia</u>, <u>restlessness</u>, <u>weakness</u>, confusion, drowsiness.
EENT: <u>blurred vision</u>, glaucoma, nystagmus.
CV: HYPERTENSIVE CRISIS, <u>arrhythmias</u>, <u>orthostatic hypotension</u>, edema.
GI: <u>diarrhea</u>, abdominal pain, anorexia, constipation, dry mouth, nausea, vomiting.
GU: dysuria, urinary incontinence, urinary retention.
Derm: rashes.
Endo: hypoglycemia.
MS: arthralgia.

INTERACTIONS

Drug-Drug: ▪ Serious, potentially fatal adverse reactions may occur with concurrent use of other **antidepressants**. Avoid using within 2 wk of each other (wait 5 wk from end of **fluoxetine therapy**) ▪ Hypertensive crisis may occur with **amphetamines**, **methyldopa**, **levodopa**, **dopamine**, **epinephrine**, **norepinephrine**, **guanethidine**, **reserpine**, or **vasoconstrictors** ▪ Hypertension or hypotension, coma, convulsions, and death may occur with **opioids**

***CAPITALS indicate life-threatening; <u>underlines</u> indicate most frequent.**

(avoid use of **meperidine** within 14–21 days of MAO inhibitor therapy—decrease initial dose of other agents to 25% of usual dose) ▪ Additive hypotension with **antihypertensives** or **spinal anesthesia** ▪ Additive hypoglycemia with **insulin** or **oral hypoglycemic agents.**

Drug-Food: ▪ Hypertensive crisis may occur with ingestion of foods containing high concentrations of **tyramine** (see Appendix K).

ROUTE AND DOSAGE

❑ **Phenelzine**

- **PO (Adults):** 15 mg 3 times daily; increase to 60–90 mg/day in divided doses, then gradually reduce to smallest effective dose (15 mg/day or every other day).
- **PO (Geriatric Patients):** 15 mg/day initially, with slow dose titration.

❑ **Tranylcypromine**

- **PO (Adults):** 30 mg/day in 2 divided doses (morning and afternoon); after 2 wk can increase by 10 mg/day, at 1–3 wk intervals, up to 60 mg/day.
- **PO (Geriatric Patients):** 2.5–5 mg/day initially; increase every 3–4 days up to 45 mg/day.

AVAILABILITY

❑ **Phenelzine**

- ***Tablets:*** 15 mg[Rx].

❑ **Tranylcypromine**

- ***Tablets:*** 10 mg[Rx].

TIME/ACTION PROFILE (antidepressant effect)

	ONSET	PEAK	DURATION
Phenelzine	1–4 wk	2–6 wk	2 wk
Tranylcypromine	2 days–3 wk	2–3 wk	3–5 days

NURSING IMPLICATIONS

ASSESSMENT

- □ Assess mental status, mood changes, and anxiety level frequently. Assess for suicidal tendencies, especially during early therapy. Restrict amount of drug available to patient.
- □ Monitor blood pressure and pulse rate prior to and frequently throughout therapy. Report significant changes promptly.
- □ Monitor intake and output ratios and daily weight. Assess patient for peripheral edema and urinary retention.
- ▪ ***Lab Test Considerations:*** Assess hepatic function periodically during prolonged or high-dose therapy.
- □ Monitor serum or urine glucose closely in diabetic patients; hypoglycemia may occur.
- ▪ ***Toxicity and Overdose:*** Concurrent ingestion of tyramine-rich foods and many medications may result in a life-threatening hypertensive crisis. Signs and symptoms of hypertensive crisis include chest pain, tachycardia, severe headache, nausea and vomiting, photosensitivity, and enlarged pupils. Treatment includes IV phentolamine.
- □ Symptoms of overdose include anxiety, irritability, tachycardia, hypertension or hypotension, respiratory distress, dizziness, drowsiness, hallucinations, confusion, seizures, fever, and diaphoresis. Treatment includes induction of vomiting or gastric lavage and supportive therapy as symptoms arise.

POTENTIAL NURSING DIAGNOSES

- Coping, ineffective individual (Indications).
- Knowledge deficit, related to medication regimen (Patient/Family Teaching).
- Noncompliance (Patient/Family Teaching).

IMPLEMENTATION

- **General Info:** Do not administer these medications in the evening because the psychomotor stimulating effects may cause insomnia or other sleep disturbances.
- **PO:** Tablets may be crushed and mixed with food or fluids for patients with difficulty swallowing.

PATIENT/FAMILY TEACHING

- □ Instruct patient to take medication exactly as directed. If a dose is missed, take if remembered within 2 hr; otherwise, omit and return to regular dosage schedule. Medication should not be abruptly discontinued as withdrawal symptoms (nausea, vomiting, malaise, nightmares, agitation, psychosis, convulsions) may occur.
- □ Caution patient to avoid alcohol, CNS depressants, OTC drugs, and foods or beverages containing tyramine (see Appendix K) during and for at least 2 wk after therapy has been discontinued; they may precipitate a hypertensive

crisis. Contact health care professional immediately if symptoms of hypertensive crisis develop.
- May cause dizziness or drowsiness. Caution patient to avoid driving and other activities requiring alertness until response to medication is known.
- Caution patient to change positions slowly to minimize orthostatic hypotension. Geriatric patients are at increased risk for this side effect.
- Advise patient to notify health care professional if dry mouth, urinary retention, or constipation occurs. Frequent rinses, good oral hygiene, and sugarless candy or gum may diminish dry mouth. An increase in fluid intake, fiber, and exercise may prevent constipation.
- Instruct patient to notify health care professional of severe headache, palpitations, chest or throat tightness, sweating, dizziness, neck stiffness, nausea, or vomiting.
- Advise patient to notify health care professional of medication regimen prior to treatment or surgery. If possible, therapy should be discontinued at least 2 wk prior to surgery.
- Instruct patient to carry identification describing medication regimen at all times.
- Emphasize the importance of participation in psychotherapy if recommended by health care professional and follow-up exams to evaluate progress. Ophthalmic testing should also be done periodically during long-term therapy.

EVALUATION

Effectiveness of therapy can be demonstrated by: ▪ Improved mood in depressed patients □ Decreased anxiety □ Increased appetite □ Improved energy level □ Improved sleep. Patients may require 1–4 wk of therapy before therapeutic effects of medication are seen.

MORICIZINE

(more-**i**-sizz-een)

Ethmozine

CLASSIFICATION(S):

Antiarrhythmic (group I)

Pregnancy Category B

INDICATIONS

▪ Life-threatening ventricular arrhythmias, including sustained ventricular tachycardia.

ACTION

▪ Suppresses abnormal automaticity and prolongs PR and QRS intervals by blocking fast sodium channel in myocardial tissue ▪ Also has membrane stabilizing and local anesthetic properties. **Therapeutic Effects:** ▪ Suppression of life-threatening arrhythmias.

PHARMACOKINETICS

Absorption: Well absorbed but rapidly metabolized following oral administration.
Distribution: Enters breast milk.
Metabolism and Excretion: Extensively metabolized; <1% excreted unchanged in the urine. Metabolites may be active.
Half-life: 1.5–3.5 hr.

CONTRAINDICATIONS AND PRECAUTIONS

Contraindicated in: ▪ Hypersensitivity ▪ Cardiogenic shock ▪ 2nd- or 3rd-degree AV block or bundle branch block (unless a pacemaker has been placed).
Use Cautiously in: ▪ Electrolyte disturbances ▪ Severe renal or hepatic impairment (initial dosage reduction may be necessary) ▪ Congestive heart failure ▪ Pregnancy, lactation, or children (safety not established).
Use Extreme Caution in: ▪ Sick sinus syndrome.

ADVERSE REACTIONS AND SIDE EFFECTS*

CNS: <u>dizziness</u>, <u>fatigue</u>, <u>headache</u>, nervousness, sleep disorders, weakness.
EENT: blurred vision.
Resp: dyspnea.
CV: <u>ARRHYTHMIAS</u>, chest pain, congestive heart failure, palpitations.
GI: <u>nausea</u>, diarrhea, dry mouth, dyspepsia, vomiting.
Derm: sweating.
MS: musculoskeletal pain.
Neuro: paresthesia.
Misc: drug fever.

***CAPITALS indicate life-threatening; <u>underlines</u> indicate most frequent.**

INTERACTIONS

Drug-Drug: ▪ Decreases blood levels of **theophylline** ▪ **Cimetidine** increases blood levels of moricizine.

ROUTE AND DOSAGE

- **PO (Adults):** 600–900 mg/day given q 8 hr; within this range, dosage may be adjusted by 150 mg/day every 3 days as required and tolerated. Some patients may tolerate q 12 hr dosing (not to exceed 900 mg/day).

AVAILABILITY

- ***Tablets:*** 200 mg[Rx], 250 mg[Rx], 300 mg[Rx].

TIME/ACTION PROFILE (arrhythmia suppression)

	ONSET	PEAK	DURATION
PO	UK	0.5–2 hr	8–12 hr

NURSING IMPLICATIONS

ASSESSMENT

- □ Monitor ECG or Holter monitor prior to and periodically throughout therapy. May cause PR prolongation and QT prolongation.
- □ Monitor blood pressure and pulse periodically during therapy.
- □ Monitor intake and output ratios and daily weight. Assess patient for signs of congestive heart failure (peripheral edema, rales/crackles, dyspnea, weight gain, jugular venous distention).
- ***Lab Test Considerations:*** Renal, pulmonary, and hepatic function, and CBC should be evaluated periodically in patients receiving long-term therapy.

POTENTIAL NURSING DIAGNOSES

- Cardiac output, decreased (Indications).
- Knowledge deficit, related to medication regimen (Patient/Family Teaching).

IMPLEMENTATION

- **General Info:** Moricizine therapy should be initiated in a hospital with facilities for cardiac rhythm monitoring.
- □ Previous antiarrhythmic therapy should be withdrawn 1–2 half-lives before starting moricizine.
- □ Dosage adjustments should be at least 3 days apart because of the long half-life of moricizine.
- □ Pre-existing hypokalemia, hyperkalemia, or hypomagnesemia should be corrected prior to instituting therapy.
- **PO:** Tablets are usually administered every 8 hr. Total daily dose may be divided and administered every 12 hr for greater compliance, but risk of adverse reactions is greater with higher single dose.

PATIENT/FAMILY TEACHING

- □ Instruct patient to take medication around the clock exactly as directed, even if feeling better. Missed doses should be taken as soon as remembered if within 6 hr; omit if remembered later. Gradual dosage reduction may be necessary.
- □ May cause dizziness or visual disturbances. Caution patient to avoid driving and other activities requiring alertness until response to medication is known.
- □ Advise patient to notify health care professional of medication regimen prior to treatment or surgery.
- □ Instruct patient to notify health care professional if chest pain, shortness of breath, fever, or diaphoresis occurs.
- □ Advise patient to carry identification describing disease process and medication regimen at all times.
- □ Emphasize the importance of follow-up exams to monitor progress.

EVALUATION

Effectiveness of therapy can be demonstrated by: ▪ Decrease in frequency of ventricular arrhythmias.

MORPHINE

(**mor**-feen)

Astramorph, Astramorph PF, Duramorph, {Epimorph}, Infumorph, Kadian, {M-Eslon}, {Morphine H.P.}, {Morphitec}, {M.O.S.}, {M.O.S.-S.R.}, MS, MS Contin, {MS·IR}, MSIR, MSIR Capsules, MS/L Concentrate, MSO_4, MS/S, OMS Concentrate, Oramorph SR, RMS, Roxanol, Roxanol Rescudose, {Statex}

M

{} = Available in Canada only.

CLASSIFICATION(S):
Opioid analgesic (agonist)

Schedule II
Pregnancy Category C

INDICATIONS

■ Severe pain ■ Pulmonary edema ■ Pain associated with myocardial infarction.

ACTION

■ Binds to opiate receptors in the CNS. Alters the perception of and response to painful stimuli, while producing generalized CNS depression. **Therapeutic Effects:** ■ Decrease in severity of pain.

PHARMACOKINETICS

Absorption: Variably absorbed (about 30%) following oral administration. More reliably absorbed from rectal, SC, and IM sites.
Distribution: Widely distributed. Crosses the placenta; enters breast milk in small amounts.
Metabolism and Excretion: Mostly metabolized by the liver.
Half-life: 2–3 hr.

CONTRAINDICATIONS AND PRECAUTIONS

Contraindicated in: ■ Hypersensitivity ■ Some products contain bisulfites or alcohol and should be avoided in patients with known hypersensitivity.
Use Cautiously in: ■ Head trauma ■ Increased intracranial pressure ■ Severe renal, hepatic, or pulmonary disease ■ Hypothyroidism ■ Adrenal insufficiency ■ Alcoholism ■ Geriatric or debilitated patients (dosage reduction suggested) ■ Undiagnosed abdominal pain ■ Prostatic hypertrophy ■ Patients undergoing procedures that rapidly decrease pain (cordotomy, radiation); long-acting agents should be discontinued 24 hr prior and replaced with short-acting agent ■ Pregnancy or lactation (avoid chronic use; has been used during labor but may cause respiratory depression in the newborn).

ADVERSE REACTIONS AND SIDE EFFECTS*

CNS: confusion, sedation, dizziness, dysphoria, euphoria, floating feeling, hallucinations, headache, unusual dreams.
EENT: blurred vision, diplopia, miosis.
Resp: RESPIRATORY DEPRESSION.
CV: hypotension, bradycardia.
GI: constipation, nausea, vomiting.
GU: urinary retention.
Derm: flushing, itching, sweating.
Misc: physical dependence, psychological dependence, tolerance.

INTERACTIONS

Drug-Drug: ■ Use with **extreme caution** in patients receiving **MAO inhibitors** (may result in unpredictable, severe reactions—decrease initial dose of morphine to 25% of usual dose) ■ Additive CNS depression with **alcohol, sedative/hypnotics,** and **antihistamines** ■ Administration of **partial-antagonist opioid analgesics** may precipitate opioid withdrawal in physically dependent patients ■ **Buprenorphine, dezocine, nalbuphine,** or **pentazocine** may decrease analgesia.

ROUTE AND DOSAGE

Larger doses may be required during chronic therapy.

- **PO, Rect (Adults ≥50 kg):** *Usual starting dose for moderate-to-severe pain in opioid-naive patients*—30 mg q 3–4 hr initially *or* equivalent dose q 8–24 hr as controlled- or sustained-release morphine once 24-hr opioid requirement is determined (see equianalgesic chart, Appendix B).
- **PO, Rect (Adults and Children <50 kg):** *Usual starting dose for moderate-to-severe pain in opioid-naive patients*—0.3 mg/kg mg q 3–4 hr initially.
- **IM, IV, SC (Adults ≥50 kg):** *Usual starting dose for moderate-to-severe pain in opioid-naive patients*—10 mg q 3–4 hr.
- **IM, IV, SC (Adults and Children <50 kg):** *Usual starting dose for moderate-to-severe pain in opioid-naive patients*—0.1 mg/kg q 3–4 hr.

***CAPITALS indicate life-threatening; underlines indicate most frequent.**

- **IV, SC (Adults):** *Continuous infusion*—0.8–10 mg/hr; may be preceded by a bolus of 15 mg (infusion rates vary greatly; up to 400 mg/hr have been used).
- **IV, SC (Children):** *Continuous infusion*—0.025–2.6 mg/kg/hr (unlabeled).
- **IV (Neonates):** *Continuous infusion*—not to exceed 0.015–0.02 mg/kg/hr (unlabeled).
- **Epidural (Adults):** *Intermittent injection*—5 mg/day (initially); if relief is not obtained at 60 min, 1–2 mg increments may be made; not to exceed 10 mg/day. *Continuous infusion*—2–4 mg/24 hr; may increase by 1–2 mg/day (up to 30 mg/day).
- **IT (Adults):** 0.2–1 mg.

AVAILABILITY

▪ ***Soluble tablets:*** 10 mg^{Rx}, 15 mg^{Rx}, 30 mg^{Rx} ▪ ***Tablets:*** 15 mg^{Rx}, 30 mg^{Rx} ▪ ***Extended (controlled, sustained)-release tablets:*** 15 mg^{Rx}, 30 mg^{Rx}, 60 mg^{Rx}, 100 mg^{Rx}, 200 mg^{Rx} ▪ ***Extended (sustained)-release capsules:*** {10 mg^{Rx}}, 20 mg^{Rx}, {30 mg^{Rx}}, 50 mg^{Rx}, {60 mg^{Rx}}, 100 mg^{Rx} ▪ ***Oral solution:*** 10 mg/5 ml^{Rx}, 20 mg/5 ml^{Rx}, 100 mg/5 ml^{Rx}, 4 mg/ml^{Rx}, 20 mg/ml^{Rx} ▪ ***Rectal suppositories:*** 5 mg^{Rx}, 10 mg^{Rx}, 20 mg^{Rx}, 30 mg^{Rx} ▪ ***Solution for IM, SC, IV injection:*** 1 mg/ml^{Rx}, 2 mg/ml^{Rx}, 4 mg/ml^{Rx}, 5 mg/ml^{Rx}, 8 mg/ml^{Rx}, 10 mg/ml^{Rx}, 15 mg/ml^{Rx}, 25 mg/ml^{Rx}, 50 mg/ml^{Rx} ▪ ***Solution for epidural, intrathecal, IV injection (preservative-free):*** 0.5 mg/ml^{Rx}, 1 mg/ml^{Rx} ▪ ***Solution for epidural or intrathecal use (continuous microinfusion device; preservative-free):*** 10 mg/ml in 20-ml vial^{Rx}, 25 mg/ml in 20-ml vial^{Rx} ▪ ***Solution for IV injection (PCA device):*** 1 mg/ml^{Rx}, 2 mg/ml^{Rx}, 3 mg/ml^{Rx}, 5 mg/ml^{Rx} ▪ ***In combination with:*** atropine^{Rx}.

TIME/ACTION PROFILE (analgesia)

	ONSET	PEAK	DURATION
PO	UK	60–120 min	4–5 hr
PO-ER	UK	UK	8–24 hr
IM	10–30 min	30–60 min	4–5 hr
SC	20 min	50–90 min	4–5 hr
Rect	UK	20–60 min	4–5 hr
IV	rapid	20 min	4–5 hr
Epidural	6–30 min	UK	up to 24 hr
IT	rapid (min)	UK	up to 24 hr

NURSING IMPLICATIONS

ASSESSMENT

- □ Assess type, location, and intensity of pain prior to and 1 hr following PO, SC, IM, and 20 min (peak) following IV administration. When titrating opioid doses, increases of 25–50% should be administered until there is either a 50% reduction in the patient's pain rating on a numerical or visual analogue scale or the patient reports satisfactory pain relief. When titrating doses of short-acting morphine, a repeat dose can be safely administered at the time of the peak if previous dose is ineffective and side effects are minimal.
- □ Patients on a continuous infusion should have additional bolus doses provided every 15–30 min, as needed, for breakthrough pain. The bolus dose is usually set to the amount of drug infused each hour by continuous infusion.
- □ Patients taking sustained-release morphine may require additional short-acting opioid doses for breakthrough pain.
- □ An equianalgesic chart (see Appendix B) should be used when changing routes or when changing from one opioid to another.
- □ Assess blood pressure, pulse, and respirations before and periodically during administration. If respiratory rate is <10/min, assess level of sedation. Physical stimulation may be sufficient to prevent significant hypoventilation. Subsequent doses may need to be decreased by 25–50%. Initial drowsiness will diminish with continued use.
- □ Prolonged use may lead to physical and psychological dependence and tolerance. This should not prevent patient from receiving adequate analgesia. Most patients who receive morphine for pain do not develop psychological dependence. Progressively higher doses may be required to relieve pain with long-term therapy.
- □ Assess bowel function routinely. Prevention of constipation should be instituted with increased intake of fluids and bulk and with laxatives to minimize constipating effects. Stimulant laxatives should be administered routinely if opioid use exceeds 2–3 days, unless contraindicated.

▪ ***Lab Test Considerations:*** May increase plasma amylase and lipase levels.

M

- ***Toxicity and Overdose:*** If an opioid antagonist is required to reverse respiratory depression or coma, naloxone (Narcan) is the antidote. Dilute the 0.4-mg ampule of naloxone in 10 ml of 0.9% NaCl and administer 0.5 ml (0.02 mg) by direct IV push every 2 min. For children and adults weighing <40 kg, dilute 0.1 mg of naloxone in 10 ml of 0.9% NaCl for a concentration of 10 mcg/ml and administer 0.5 mcg/kg every 1–2 min. Titrate dose to avoid withdrawal, seizures, and severe pain.

POTENTIAL NURSING DIAGNOSES

- Pain (Indications).
- Sensory-perceptual alterations: visual, auditory (Side Effects).
- Injury, risk for (Side Effects).
- Knowledge deficit, related to medication regimen (Patient/Family Teaching).

IMPLEMENTATION

- **General Info:** Do not confuse with hydromorphone or meperidine; errors have resulted in fatalities.
  - Explain therapeutic value of medication prior to administration to enhance the analgesic effect.
  - Regularly administered doses may be more effective than prn administration. Analgesic is more effective if given before pain becomes severe.
  - Coadministration with nonopioid analgesics may have additive analgesic effects and may permit lower doses.
  - When transferring from other opioids or other forms of morphine to extended-release tablets, administer a total daily dose of oral morphine equivalent to previous daily dose (see Appendix B) and divided every 8 hr (Roxanol SR), every 12 hr (MS Contin, Oramorph SR), or every 12–24 hr (Kadian).
  - Morphine should be discontinued gradually to prevent withdrawal symptoms after long-term use.
- **Rect:** *MS Contin* and *Oramorph SR* have been administered rectally.
- **PO:** Doses may be administered with food or milk to minimize GI irritation.
  - Administer solution with properly calibrated measuring device. Solution may be diluted in a glass of fruit juice just prior to administration to improve taste.
  - Extended-release and controlled-release tablets should be swallowed whole; do not crush, break, or chew.
  - *MSIR* capsules may be swallowed whole or opened and the contents sprinkled on cool food (pudding, applesauce). As the coated beads inside capsule will not affect taste of food, the capsule may be opened and the contents added to liquid (e.g., juice) and administered immediately, or the capsule contents may be delivered via gastric or nasogastric tube by adding to or following with liquid. Coated beads inside capsule will not stick to tubes.
  - *Kadian* capsules may be opened and the pellets sprinkled onto applesauce immediately prior to administration. Pellets should not be chewed, crushed, or dissolved.
- **SC, IM:** Use IM route for repeated doses, as morphine is irritating to SC tissues.
- **IV:** Solution is colorless; do not administer discolored solution.
- **Direct IV:** Dilute with at least 5 ml of sterile water or 0.9% NaCl for injection.
- ***Rate:*** Administer 2.5–15 mg over 4–5 min. Rapid administration may lead to increased respiratory depression, hypotension, and circulatory collapse.
- **Continuous Infusion:** May be added to D5W, D10W, 0.9% NaCl, 0.45% NaCl, Ringer's or lactated Ringer's solution, dextrose/saline solution, or dextrose/Ringer's or lactated Ringer's solution in a concentration of 0.1–1 mg/ml or greater for continuous infusion.
- ***Rate:*** Administer via infusion pump to control the rate. Dose should be titrated to ensure adequate pain relief without excessive sedation, respiratory depression, or hypotension.
  - May be administered via patient-controlled analgesia (PCA) pump.
- **Syringe Compatibility:** ▪ atropine ▪ benzquinamide ▪ bupivicaine ▪ cimetidine ▪ dimenhydrinate ▪ diphenhydramine ▪ droperidol ▪ glycopyrrolate ▪ hydroxyzine ▪ metoclopramide ▪ midazolam ▪ milrinone ▪ perphenazine ▪ promazine ▪ ranitidine ▪ scopolamine.
- **Y-Site Compatibility:** ▪ amifostine ▪ amikacin ▪ aminophylline ▪ amiodarone ▪ ampicillin ▪ ampicillin/sulbactam ▪ atenolol ▪ atracurium ▪ aztreonam ▪ bumetanide ▪ calcium chloride ▪ cefamandole ▪ cefazolin ▪ cefoperazone

▪ cefotaxime ▪ cefotetan ▪ cefoxitin ▪ ceftazidime ▪ ceftizoxime ▪ ceftriaxone ▪ cefuroxime ▪ cephalothin ▪ cephapirin ▪ chloramphenicol ▪ cisplatin ▪ clindamycin ▪ cyclophosphamide ▪ cytarabine ▪ dexamethasone sodium phosphate ▪ digoxin ▪ diltiazem ▪ dopamine ▪ doxorubicin ▪ doxycycline ▪ enalaprilat ▪ erythromycin lactobionate ▪ esmololol ▪ famotidine ▪ filgrastim ▪ fluconazole ▪ fludarabine ▪ foscarnet ▪ gentamicin ▪ granisetron ▪ heparin ▪ hydrocortisone sodium succinate ▪ insulin ▪ kanamycin ▪ labetalol ▪ lidocaine ▪ lorazepam ▪ magnesium sulfate ▪ melphalan ▪ methotrexate ▪ methyldopate ▪ methylprednisolone ▪ metoclopramide ▪ metoprolol ▪ metronidazole ▪ mezlocillin ▪ midazolam ▪ nafcillin ▪ nitroprusside ▪ norepinephrine ▪ ondansetron ▪ oxacillin ▪ oxytocin ▪ paclitaxel ▪ pancuronium ▪ penicillin G potassium ▪ piperacillin ▪ piperacillin/tazobactam ▪ potassium chloride ▪ propranolol ▪ ranitidine ▪ sodium bicarbonate ▪ teniposide ▪ thiotepa ▪ ticarcillin ▪ ticarcillin/clavulanate ▪ tobramycin ▪ trimethoprim/sulfamethoxazole ▪ vancomycin ▪ vecuronium ▪ vinorelbine ▪ vitamin B complex with C ▪ zidovudine.

▪ **Y-Site Incompatibility:** ▪ cefepime ▪ furosemide ▪ gallium nitrate ▪ minocycline ▪ sargramostim ▪ thiopental.

PATIENT/FAMILY TEACHING

□ Instruct patient how and when to ask for pain medication.

□ May cause drowsiness or dizziness. Caution patient to call for assistance when ambulating or smoking and to avoid driving or other activities requiring alertness until response to medication is known.

□ Advise patient to change positions slowly to minimize orthostatic hypotension.

□ Caution patient to avoid concurrent use of alcohol or other CNS depressants with this medication.

□ Encourage patient to turn, cough, and breathe deeply every 2 hr to prevent atelectasis.

▪ **Home Care Issues:** Explain to patient and family how and when to administer morphine and how to care for infusion equipment properly.

□ Emphasize the importance of aggressive prevention of constipation with the use of morphine.

EVALUATION

Effectiveness of therapy can be demonstrated by: ▪ Decrease in severity of pain without a significant alteration in level of consciousness or respiratory status.

MULTIPLE VITAMINS, oral

Adavite, Certagen, Dayalets, Hexavitamin, LKV Drops, Multi-75, Multi-Day, Nutrox, One-A-Day, Optilets, Poly-Vi-Sol, Quintabs, Ru-lets, Sesame Street Vitamins, Sigtab, Syrvite, Tab-A-Vite, Therabid, Theragran, Thera Multi-Vitamin, Theravee, Theravim, Theravite, Therems, Unicaps, Vita-Bob, Vita-Kid, Zymacap

MULTIVITAMIN INFUSION, intravenous

B complex with C and B_{12}, Berocca Parenteral Nutrition, Multi Vitamin Concentrate, M.V.I.-12, M.V.I. Pediatric

CLASSIFICATION(S):
Vitamins (multiple, oral), Vitamins (multiple, parenteral)

Pregnancy Category UK

INDICATIONS

▪ **PO:** Treatment and prevention of vitamin deficiencies. Special formulations are available for patients with particular needs, including: □ Prenatal multiple vitamins (with larger doses of folic acid) □ Multiple vitamins with iron □ Multiple vitamins with fluoride □ Multiple vitamins with other minerals or trace elements ▪ **IV:** Treatment and prevention of vitamin deficiencies in patients who are unable to ingest oral feedings or vitamins.

ACTION

▪ Contain fat-soluble vitamins (A, D, and E) and most water-soluble vitamins (B-complex vitamins B_1, B_2, B_3, B_5, B_6, B_{12}, vitamin C, biotin, and folic acid). These vitamins are a diverse group of compounds necessary for normal

M

growth and development. Many act as coenzymes or catalysts in numerous metabolic processes ▪ Liquid products do not contain folic acid. **Therapeutic Effects:** ▪ **PO:** Prevention of deficiency or replacement in patients whose nutritional status is questionable ▪ **IV:** Replacement in patients who are unable to ingest oral feedings or vitamins.

PHARMACOKINETICS

Absorption: Well absorbed from the GI tract following oral administration; some processes are active, some are passive. Absorption of water-soluble vitamins generally increases in deficiency states. Absorption of some lipid-soluble vitamins may require bile acids.
Distribution: Widely distributed; cross the placenta and enter breast milk. Fat-soluble vitamins (A, D, and E) are stored in fatty tissues and the liver.
Metabolism and Excretion: Utilized in various biologic processes. Excess amounts of water-soluble vitamins (B vitamins, vitamin C, and folic acid) are excreted unchanged by the kidneys.
Half-life: UK.

CONTRAINDICATIONS AND PRECAUTIONS

Contraindicated in: ▪ Hypersensitivity to preservatives, colorants, or additives, including tartrazine, saccharin, and aspartame (oral forms) ▪ Some products contain alcohol and should be avoided in patients with known intolerance.
Use Cautiously in: ▪ Patients with anemia of undetermined cause.

ADVERSE REACTIONS AND SIDE EFFECTS

In recommended doses, adverse reactions are extremely rare.
Misc: allergic reactions to preservatives, additives, or colorants.

INTERACTIONS

Drug-Drug: ▪ Large amounts of vitamin B_6 may interfere with the beneficial effect of **levodopa.**

ROUTE AND DOSAGE

- **PO (Adults and Children):** 1 dosage unit (tablet/capsule/dropperful)/day or amount recommended by individual manufacturer.
- **IV (Adults and Children):** Amount sufficient to meet RDA (Recommended Daily Allowances—see Appendix L) for age group. Usually added to large-volume parenteral or total parenteral nutrition (hyperalimentation) solution.

AVAILABILITY

▪ ***Tablets***OTC ▪ ***Chewable tablets***OTC ▪ ***Chewable wafers***OTC ▪ ***Capsules***OTC ▪ ***Liquids***OTC ▪ ***Drops***OTC ▪ ***Injection***Rx ▪ ***In combination with:*** fluoride, minerals, and trace elements Rx,OTC.

TIME/ACTION PROFILE

	ONSET	PEAK	DURATION
PO	UK	UK	UK
IV	UK	UK	UK

NURSING IMPLICATIONS

ASSESSMENT

- ☐ Assess patient for signs of nutritional deficiency prior to and throughout therapy. Patients at risk include those who are elderly, debilitated, burned, or unable to take oral nutrition and those with malabsorption syndromes or chronic alcoholism.
- ▪ ***Toxicity and Overdose:*** Toxicity rarely occurs with multivitamin preparations because of the small amounts per unit of fat-soluble vitamins. For symptoms, see individual vitamin entries.
- ☐ If overdose occurs, treatment includes induction of emesis or gastric lavage, calcium gluconate IV if hypocalcemic, and maintenance of high urine output.

POTENTIAL NURSING DIAGNOSES

- Nutrition, altered, less than body requirements (Indications).
- Knowledge deficit, related to diet and medication regimen (Patient/Family Teaching).

IMPLEMENTATION

- ▪ **General Info:** Vitamins are usually given orally but may be given parenterally to patients in whom oral administration is not feasible.
- ☐ Combinations with >1 mg folic acid require a prescription.
- ▪ **PO:** Forms are not standardized.
- ☐ Chewable tablets should be crushed or chewed prior to swallowing.

- □ Liquid preparations may be dropped directly into mouth or mixed with juice or cereal.
- ■ **IV:** Administer multivitamin infusion by infusion only; do not use direct IV injection.
- □ Solution is bright yellow and will color IV solutions.
- ■ **Continuous Infusion:** Dilute each 5- or 10-ml ampule in 500–1000 ml of D5/LR, D5/0.9% NaCl, D5W, D10W, D20W, lactated Ringer's injection, 0.9% NaCl, 3% NaCl, or ⅙ M sodium lactate. Do not administer solution that has crystallized.
- ■ **Y-Site Compatibility:** ■ acyclovir ■ ampicillin ■ cefazolin ■ cephalothin ■ cephapirin ■ diltiazem ■ erythromycin lactobionate ■ fludarabine ■ gentamicin ■ tacrolimus.
- ■ **Additive Incompatibility:** ■ Incompatible in solution with many antibiotics.

PATIENT/FAMILY TEACHING

- □ Encourage patient to comply with recommendations of health care professional. Explain that the best source of vitamins is a well-balanced diet with foods from the 4 basic food groups.
- □ Advise parents not to refer to chewable multivitamins for children as candy.

EVALUATION

Effectiveness of therapy can be demonstrated by: ■ Prevention or decrease in the symptoms of vitamin deficiency.

MUPIROCIN

(myoo-**peer**-oh-sin)
Bactroban, Bactroban Nasal

CLASSIFICATION(S):
Anti-infective (topical)

Pregnancy Category B

INDICATIONS

■ **Topical:** Treatment of: □ Impetigo □ Secondarily infected traumatic skin lesions (up to 10 cm in length or 100 cm² area) caused by *Staphylococcus aureus* and *Staphylococcus pyogenes* ■ **Intranasal:** Eradicates nasal colonization with methicillin-resistant *Staphylococcus aureus*.

ACTION

■ Inhibits bacterial protein synthesis. **Therapeutic Effects:** ■ Inhibition of bacterial growth and reproduction. **Spectrum:** ■ Greatest activity against gram-positive organisms, including: □ *Staphylococcus aureus* □ Beta-hemolytic streptococci ■ Resolution of impetigo ■ Eradication of *Staphylococcus aureus* carrier state.

PHARMACOKINETICS

Absorption: Minimal systemic absorption.
Distribution: Remains in the stratum corneum following topical use for prolonged periods of time (72 hr).
Metabolism and Excretion: Metabolized in the skin, removed by desquamation.
Half-life: UK.

CONTRAINDICATIONS AND PRECAUTIONS

Contraindicated in: ■ Hypersensitivity to mupirocin or polyethylene glycol.
Use Cautiously in: ■ Pregnancy or lactation (safety not established).

ADVERSE REACTIONS AND SIDE EFFECTS

CNS: *nasal only*—headache.
EENT: *nasal only*—cough, itching, pharyngitis, rhinitis, upper respiratory tract congestion.
GI: nausea; *nasal only*—altered taste.
Derm: *topical only*—burning, itching, pain, stinging.

INTERACTIONS

Drug-Drug: ■ Nasal mupirocin should not be used concurrently with other **nasal products.**

ROUTE AND DOSAGE

- ■ **Topical (Adults and Children):** Apply 3 times daily.
- ■ **Intranasal (Adults):** Apply half of the contents of a single-use nasal ointment tube to each nostril twice daily for 5 days.

AVAILABILITY

■ ***Ointment:*** 2% in 15-g tubes^Rx, {2% in 15- and 30-g tubes^OTC} ■ ***Cream:*** 2% in 15- and 30-g tubes^Rx ■ ***Nasal ointment:*** 2% in 1-g single-use tubes^Rx.

M

TIME/ACTION PROFILE (anti-infective effect)

	ONSET	PEAK	DURATION
Nasal	UK	UK	12 hr
Top*	UK	3–5 days	72 hr

*Resolution of lesions.

NURSING IMPLICATIONS

ASSESSMENT

□ Assess lesions prior to and daily during therapy.

POTENTIAL NURSING DIAGNOSES

- Skin integrity, impaired (Indications).
- Infection, risk for (Indications, Patient/Family Teaching).
- Knowledge deficit, related to medication regimen (Patient/Family Teaching).

IMPLEMENTATION

- **Topical:** Wash affected area with soap and water and dry thoroughly. Apply a small amount of mupirocin to the affected area 3 times daily and rub in gently. Treated area may be covered with gauze, if desired.
- **Nasal:** Apply one-half of the ointment from the single-use tube to each nostril twice daily (morning and evening) for 5 days. After application, close nostrils by pressing together and releasing sides of the nose repeatedly for 1 min.

PATIENT/FAMILY TEACHING

- **General Info:** Instruct patient on the correct application of mupirocin. Advise patient to apply medication exactly as directed for the full course of therapy. If a dose is missed, apply as soon as possible unless almost time for next dose.
- **Topical:** Teach patient and family appropriate hygienic measures to prevent spread of impetigo.

□ Instruct parents to notify school nurse for screening and prevention of transmission.

□ Patient should consult health care professional if symptoms have not improved in 3–5 days.

EVALUATION

Effectiveness of therapy can be demonstrated by: ▪ Healing of skin lesions. If no clinical response is seen in 3–5 days, condition should be re-evaluated ▪ Eradication of methicillin-resistant *Staphylococcus aureus* carrier state in patients and health care workers during institutional outbreaks.

MUROMONAB-CD3

(myoor-oh-**mon**-ab CD3)

Orthoclone OKT3

CLASSIFICATION(S):

Immunosuppressant (monoclonal antibody)

Pregnancy Category C

INDICATIONS

▪ Acute renal allograft rejection reactions in transplant patients that have occurred despite conventional antirejection therapy ▪ Acute steroid-resistant hepatic or cardiac allograft rejection reactions.

ACTION

▪ A purified immunoglobulin antibody that acts as an immunosuppressant by interfering with normal T-cell function. **Therapeutic Effects:** ▪ Reversal of graft rejection in transplant patients.

PHARMACOKINETICS

Absorption: Administered IV only, resulting in complete bioavailability.
Distribution: UK.
Metabolism and Excretion: Eliminated by binding to T lymphocytes.
Half-life: 18 hr.

CONTRAINDICATIONS AND PRECAUTIONS

Contraindicated in: ▪ Hypersensitivity to muromonab-CD3, murine (mouse) proteins, or polysorbate ▪ Previous muromonab therapy ▪ Fluid overload ▪ Fever >37.8°C or 100°F ▪ Chickenpox or recent exposure to chickenpox ▪ Herpes zoster.
Use Cautiously in: ▪ Active infections ▪ Depressed bone marrow reserve ▪ Chronic debilitating illnesses ▪ Congestive heart failure ▪ Pregnancy, lactation, or children <2 yr (safety not established).

ADVERSE REACTIONS AND SIDE EFFECTS*

CNS: tremor, aseptic meningitis, dizziness.
Resp: PULMONARY EDEMA, dyspnea, shortness of breath, wheezing.
CV: chest pain.
GI: diarrhea, nausea, vomiting.
Misc: CYTOKINE RELEASE SYNDROME, INFECTIONS, chills, fever, hypersensitivity reactions, increased risk of lymphoma.

INTERACTIONS

Drug-Drug: ▪ Additive immunosuppression with other **immunosuppressive agents** ▪ Concurrent **prednisone** and **azathioprine** dosages should be reduced during muromonab therapy (increased risk of infection and lymphoproliferative disorders) ▪ **Cyclosporine** should be reduced or discontinued during muromonab-CD3 therapy (increased risk of infection and lymphoproliferative disorders) ▪ Increased risk of adverse CNS reactions with **indomethacin.**

ROUTE AND DOSAGE

- **IV (Adults):** 5 mg/day for 10–14 days (pretreatment with glucocorticoids, acetaminophen, and/or antihistamines recommended).
- **IV (Children):** 0.1 mg (100 mcg)/kg/day for 10–14 days.

AVAILABILITY

▪ ***Solution for injection:*** 1 mg/ml in 5-ml ampules[Rx].

TIME/ACTION PROFILE (noted as levels of circulating CD3-positive T cells)

	ONSET	PEAK	DURATION
IV	mins	2–7 days	1 wk

NURSING IMPLICATIONS

ASSESSMENT

- Assess for fluid overload (monitor weight and intake and output, assess for edema and rales/crackles). Notify physician if patient has experienced 3% or more weight gain in the previous week. Chest x-ray examination should be obtained within 24 hr prior to beginning therapy. Fluid-overloaded patients are at high risk of developing pulmonary edema. Monitor vital signs and breath sounds closely.
- Assess for cytokine release syndrome (CRS), usually manifested by high fever and chills, headache, tremor, nausea and vomiting, chest pain, muscle and joint pain, generalized weakness, shortness of breath, dizziness, abdominal pain, malaise, diarrhea, and trembling of hands, but may occasionally cause a severe, life-threatening, shock-like reaction. The severity of this reaction is greatest with initial dose. Reaction occurs within 30–48 hr and may persist for up to 6 hr. Acetaminophen and antihistamines may be used to treat early reactions. Patient temperature should be maintained below 37.8°C (100°F) at administration of each dose. Manifestations of CRS may be prevented or minimized by pretreatment with methylprednisolone sodium succinate 8 mg/kg IV given 1–4 hr prior to 1st dose of muromonab-CD3. Hydrocortisone 100 mg IV may also be given 30 min after the 1st and possibly 2nd dose to control respiratory side effects. Serious symptoms of CRS may require oxygen, IV fluids, glucocorticoids, vasopressors, antihistamines, and intubation.
- Monitor for signs of anaphylactic or hypersensitivity reactions at each dose. Resuscitation equipment should be readily available.
- Monitor for infection (fever, chills, rash, sore throat, purulent discharge, dysuria). Notify physician immediately if these symptoms occur; may necessitate discontinuation of therapy.
- Monitor for development of aseptic meningitis. Onset is usually within 3 days of beginning therapy. Assess for fever, headache, nuchal rigidity, and photophobia.

▪ ***Lab Test Considerations:*** Monitor CBC with differential and platelet count prior to and periodically throughout therapy.

- Monitor assays of T cells (CD3, CD4, CD8); target CD3 is <25 cells/mm^3 or plasma levels as determined by ELISA daily; target levels should be ≥800 ng/ml.
- Monitor BUN, serum creatinine, and hepatic enzymes (AST, ALT, alkaline phosphatase, bilirubin), especially during the first 1–3 days of therapy. May cause transient increases.

M

*CAPITALS indicate life-threatening; underlines indicate most frequent.

POTENTIAL NURSING DIAGNOSES

- Infection, risk for (Side Effects).
- Fluid volume excess (Side Effects).
- Knowledge deficit, related to medication regimen (Patient/Family Teaching).

IMPLEMENTATION

- **General Info:** Physician will reduce dosage of glucocorticoids and azathioprine and discontinue cyclosporine during 10–14-day course of muromonab-CD3. Cyclosporine may be resumed 3 days before end of therapy.
- □ Initial dose is administered during hospitalization; patient should be monitored closely for 48 hr. Subsequent doses may be administered on outpatient basis.
- □ Keep medication refrigerated at 2–8°C. Do not shake vial. Solution may contain a few fine translucent particles that do not affect potency. Discard unused portion.
- **Direct IV:** Draw solution into syringe via low-protein-binding 0.2- or 0.22-micrometer filter to ensure removal of translucent protein particles that may be present. Discard filter and attach 20-gauge needle for IV administration.
- ***Rate:*** Administer IV push over <1 min. Do not administer as an infusion.
- **Compatibility:** Do not admix; do not administer in IV line containing other medications. If line must be used for other medications, flush with 0.9% NaCl before and after muromonab–CD3.

PATIENT/FAMILY TEACHING

- □ Explain purpose of medication to patient. Inform patient of possible initial-dose side effects, which are markedly reduced in subsequent doses. Explain that patient will need to resume lifelong therapy with other immunosuppressive drugs after completion of muromonab course.
- □ Inform patient of potential for CRS. Describe reportable symptoms.
- □ Advise patient to notify health care professional at first sign of rash, urticaria, tachycardia, dyspnea, or difficulty swallowing.
- □ May cause dizziness. Caution patient to avoid driving or other activities requiring alertness until response is known.
- □ Instruct patient not to receive any vaccinations and to avoid contact with persons receiving oral polio vaccine without advice of health care professional.

PATIENT/FAMILY TEACHING

- □ Instruct patient to continue to avoid crowds and persons with known infections, as this drug also suppresses the immune system.

EVALUATION

Effectiveness of therapy can be demonstrated by: ▪ Reversal of the symptoms of acute organ rejection.

MYCOPHENOLATE

(mye-koe-**fee**-noe-late)

CellCept

CLASSIFICATION(S):

Immunosuppressant

Pregnancy Category C

INDICATIONS

▪ Prevention of rejection in patients who have undergone allogenic renal transplantation (used concurrently with cyclosporine and glucocorticoids).

ACTION

▪ Inhibits the enzyme inosine monophosphate dehydrogenase, which is involved in purine synthesis. This inhibition results in suppression of T- and B-lymphocyte proliferation. **Therapeutic Effects:** ▪ Prevention of kidney transplant rejection.

PHARMACOKINETICS

Absorption: Following oral administration, mycophenolate is rapidly hydrolyzed to mycophenolic acid (MPA), its active metabolite.

Distribution: UK.

Metabolism and Excretion: MPA is extensively metabolized; <1% excreted unchanged in urine. Some enterohepatic recirculation of MPA occurs.

Half-life: *MPA*—17.9 hr.

CONTRAINDICATIONS AND PRECAUTIONS

Contraindicated in: ▪ Hypersensitivity ▪ Pregnancy or lactation.

Use Cautiously in: ▪ Active serious pathology

of the GI tract (including history of ulcer disease or GI bleeding) ▪ Severe chronic renal impairment (dosage not to exceed 1 g twice daily if CCr <25 ml/min/1.73 m^2) ▪ Delayed graft function following transplantation (observe for increased toxicity) ▪ Patients with childbearing potential ▪ Children (safety not established).

ADVERSE REACTIONS AND SIDE EFFECTS*

GI: GI BLEEDING, diarrhea, vomiting.
Hemat: leukopenia.
Misc: sepsis, increased risk of malignancy.

INTERACTIONS

Drug-Drug: ▪ Combined use with **azathioprine** is not recommended (effects unknown) ▪ **Acyclovir** and **ganciclovir** compete with MPA for renal excretion and, in patients with renal failure, may increase each other's toxicity ▪ **Magnesium and aluminum hydroxide antacids** decrease the absorption of MPA (avoid simultaneous administration) ▪ **Cholestyramine** and **similar agents** decrease the absorption of MPA (avoid concurrent use) ▪ Toxicity may be increased by **salicylates.**
Drug-Food: ▪ When administered with food, peak blood levels of MPA were significantly decreased.

ROUTE AND DOSAGE

- **PO (Adults):** 1 g twice daily, to be started within 72 hr of transplantation.

AVAILABILITY

▪ ***Capsules:*** 250 mg^Rx^ ▪ ***Tablets:*** 250 mg^Rx^, 500 mg^Rx^.

TIME/ACTION PROFILE (blood levels of MPA)

	ONSET	PEAK	DURATION
PO	rapid	0.8–1.3 hr	N/A

NURSING IMPLICATIONS

ASSESSMENT

- □ Assess for symptoms of organ rejection throughout therapy.
- ▪ ***Lab Test Considerations:*** Monitor CBC with differential weekly during the 1st mo, twice monthly for the 2nd and 3rd mo of therapy, and then monthly throughout the 1st yr. Neutropenia occurs most frequently from 31–180 days post-transplant. If ANC is <1000/mm^3, dose should be reduced or discontinued.
- □ Monitor hepatic and renal status and electrolytes periodically during therapy. May cause increased serum alkaline phosphatase, AST, ALT, LDH, and creatinine. May also cause hypercalcemia, hypocalcemia, hyperuricemia, hyperlipidemia, hypoglycemia, and hypoproteinemia.

POTENTIAL NURSING DIAGNOSES

- ▪ Infection, risk for (Adverse Reactions).
- ▪ Knowledge deficit, related to medication regimen (Patient/Family Teaching).

IMPLEMENTATION

- ▪ **General Info:** The initial dose of mycophenolate should be given within 72 hr of transplant.
- □ Women of childbearing years should have a negative serum or urine pregnancy test within 1 wk prior to initiation of therapy.
- ▪ **PO:** Administer on an empty stomach, 1 hr before or 2 hr after meals. Capsules should be swallowed whole; do not open, crush, or chew.
- □ Do not administer mycophenolate concurrently with antacids containing magnesium or aluminum.

PATIENT/FAMILY TEACHING

- □ Instruct patient to take medication exactly as directed, at the same time each day. Do not skip or double up on missed doses. Do not discontinue without consulting health care professional.
- □ Reinforce the need for lifelong therapy to prevent transplant rejection. Review symptoms of rejection for the transplanted organ, and stress need to notify health care professional immediately if signs of rejection or infection occur.
- □ Inform female patients of the importance of simultaneously using two reliable forms of contraception, unless abstinence is the chosen method, prior to beginning, during, and for 6 wk following discontinuation of therapy.

M

- Advise patient to avoid contact with persons with contagious diseases.
- Inform patient of the increased risk of lymphoma and other malignancies.
- Advise patient to consult health care professional prior to taking other medications concurrently with mycophenolate.
- Emphasize the importance of routine follow-up laboratory tests.

EVALUATION

Effectiveness of therapy can be demonstrated by: ▪ Prevention of rejection of transplanted organs.

NABUMETONE

(na-**byoo**-me-tone)
Relafen

CLASSIFICATION(S):
Nonsteroidal anti-inflammatory agent

Pregnancy Category C (first trimester)

INDICATIONS

▪ Symptomatic management of rheumatoid arthritis and osteoarthritis.

ACTION

▪ Inhibits prostaglandin synthesis. **Therapeutic Effects:** ▪ Suppression of pain and inflammation.

PHARMACOKINETICS

Absorption: 80% absorbed following oral administration; 35% is rapidly converted to 6-methoxy-2-naphylacetic acid (6-MNA), which is the active metabolite.
Distribution: UK.
Metabolism and Excretion: 6-MNA is metabolized by the liver to inactive compounds.
Half-life: 24 hr (increased in severe renal impairment).

CONTRAINDICATIONS AND PRECAUTIONS

Contraindicated in: ▪ Hypersensitivity ▪ Cross-sensitivity may occur with other NSAIDs, including aspirin ▪ Active GI bleeding or ulcer disease.
Use Cautiously in: ▪ Severe cardiovascular, renal, or hepatic disease ▪ History of ulcer disease ▪ Pregnancy, lactation, or children (safety not established; avoid using during 2nd half of pregnancy).

ADVERSE REACTIONS AND SIDE EFFECTS*

CNS: agitation, anxiety, confusion, depression, dizziness, drowsiness, fatigue, headache, insomnia, malaise, weakness.
EENT: abnormal vision, tinnitus.
Resp: dyspnea, hypersensitivity pneumonitis.
CV: edema, fluid retention, vasculitis.
GI: GI BLEEDING, abdominal pain, diarrhea, abnormal liver function tests, anorexia, constipation, dry mouth, dyspepsia, flatulence, gastritis, gastroenteritis, increased appetite, nausea, stomatitis, vomiting.
GU: albuminuria, azotemia, interstitial nephritis.
Derm: increased sweating, photosensitivity, pruritus, rash.
Hemat: prolonged bleeding time.
Metab: weight gain.
Neuro: paresthesia, tremor.
Misc: allergic reactions including ANAPHYLAXIS, ANGIONEUROTIC EDEMA.

INTERACTIONS

Drug-Drug: ▪ Additive adverse GI effects with **aspirin**, other **NSAIDs**, **potassium supplements, glucocorticoids**, or **alcohol** ▪ Chronic use with **acetaminophen** may increase the risk of adverse renal reactions ▪ May decrease the effectiveness of **diuretics** or **antihypertensive therapy** ▪ May increase the hypoglycemic effects of **insulin** or **oral hypoglycemic agents** ▪ Increases the risk of toxicity from **methotrexate** ▪ Increased risk of bleeding with **cefamandole, cefotetan, cefoperazone, valproic acid, plicamycin, anticoagulants,** or **thrombolytic agents** ▪ Increased risk of adverse hematologic reactions with **antineoplastic agents** or **radiation therapy** ▪ Concurrent use with **cyclosporine** may increase the risk of renal toxicity.

ROUTE AND DOSAGE

▪ **PO (Adults):** 1000 mg/day as a single dose or divided dose twice daily; may be increased

*CAPITALS indicate life-threatening; underlines indicate most frequent.

up to 2000 mg/day; use lowest effective dose during chronic therapy.

AVAILABILITY

- ***Tablets:*** 500 mg[Rx], 750 mg[Rx].

TIME/ACTION PROFILE (analgesia/anti-inflammatory effects)

	ONSET	PEAK	DURATION
PO	1–2 days	few days–2 wk	UK

NURSING IMPLICATIONS

ASSESSMENT

- ▫ Patients who have asthma, aspirin-induced allergy, and nasal polyps are at increased risk for developing hypersensitivity reactions. Monitor for rhinitis, asthma, and urticaria.
- ▫ Assess pain and range of motion prior to and periodically throughout therapy.
- ***Lab Test Considerations:*** BUN, serum creatinine, CBC, and liver function tests should be evaluated periodically in patients receiving prolonged courses of therapy.
- ▫ Serum potassium, BUN, serum creatinine, alkaline phosphatase, LDH, AST, and ALT tests may show increased levels. Blood glucose, hemoglobin, and hematocrit concentrations, leukocyte and platelet counts, and CCr may be decreased.
- ▫ May cause prolonged bleeding time.

POTENTIAL NURSING DIAGNOSES

- Pain (Indications).
- Physical mobility, impaired (Indications).
- Knowledge deficit, related to medication regimen (Patient/Family Teaching).

IMPLEMENTATION

- **General Info:** Administration in higher than recommended doses does not provide increased effectiveness but may cause increased side effects.
- **PO:** Administer with meals or antacids to decrease GI irritation and increase absorption.

PATIENT/FAMILY TEACHING

- ▫ Advise patient to take this medication with a full glass of water and to remain in an upright position for 15–30 min after administration.
- ▫ Instruct patient to take medication exactly as directed. If a dose is missed, it should be taken as soon as remembered but not if almost time for the next dose. Do not double doses.
- ▫ May cause drowsiness, dizziness, or visual disturbances. Advise patient to avoid driving or other activities requiring alertness until response to the medication is known.
- ▫ Advise patient to use sunscreen and protective clothing to prevent photosensitivity reactions.
- ▫ Caution patient to avoid the concurrent use of alcohol, aspirin, acetaminophen, or other OTC medications without consulting health care professional.
- ▫ Advise patient to inform health care professional of medication regimen prior to treatment or surgery.
- ▫ Advise patient to consult health care professional if rash, itching, visual disturbances, tinnitus, weight gain, edema, black stools, persistent headache, or influenza-like syndrome (chills, fever, muscle aches, pain) occurs.

EVALUATION

Effectiveness of therapy can be demonstrated by: ▪ Decreased pain and improved joint mobility. Partial arthritic relief is usually seen within 1 wk, but maximum effectiveness may require 2 wk or more of continuous therapy. Patients who do not respond to one NSAID may respond to another.

NADOLOL

(**nay**-doe-lole)
Corgard, {Syn-Nadolol}

CLASSIFICATION(S):
Antianginal, Antihypertensive agent, Beta-adrenergic blocking agent (nonselective)

Pregnancy Category C

INDICATIONS

▪ Management of hypertension ▪ Management of angina pectoris. **Unlabeled Uses:** ▫ Arrhythmias ▫ Migraine prophylaxis ▫ Tremors (essential, lithium-induced, parkinsonian) ▫ Aggressive behavior ▫ Antipsychotic-associated akathisia

N

□ Situational anxiety □ Esophageal varices □ Reduction of intraocular pressure.

ACTION

▪ Blocks stimulation of $beta_1$ (myocardial) and $beta_2$ (pulmonary, vascular, and uterine) -adrenergic receptor sites. **Therapeutic Effects:** ▪ Decreased heart rate and blood pressure.

PHARMACOKINETICS

Absorption: 30% absorbed following oral administration.
Distribution: Minimal penetration of the CNS. Crosses the placenta and enters breast milk.
Metabolism and Excretion: 70% excreted unchanged by the kidneys.
Half-life: 10–24 hr (increased in renal impairment).

CONTRAINDICATIONS AND PRECAUTIONS

Contraindicated in: ▪ Uncompensated congestive heart failure ▪ Pulmonary edema ▪ Cardiogenic shock ▪ Bradycardia or heart block.
Use Cautiously in: ▪ Renal impairment ▪ Hepatic impairment ▪ Geriatric patients (increased sensitivity to beta-adrenergic blockers; initial dosage reduction recommended) ▪ Pulmonary disease (including asthma) ▪ Diabetes mellitus (may mask signs of hypoglycemia) ▪ Thyrotoxicosis (may mask symptoms) ▪ Patients with a history of severe allergic reactions (intensity of reactions may be increased) ▪ Pregnancy, lactation, or children (safety not established; crosses the placenta and may cause fetal/neonatal bradycardia, hypotension, hypoglycemia, or respiratory depression).

ADVERSE REACTIONS AND SIDE EFFECTS*

CNS: fatigue, weakness, anxiety, depression, dizziness, drowsiness, insomnia, memory loss, mental status changes, nightmares.
EENT: blurred vision, dry eyes, nasal stuffiness.
Resp: bronchospasm, wheezing.
CV: ARRHYTHMIAS, BRADYCARDIA, CONGESTIVE HEART FAILURE, PULMONARY EDEMA, orthostatic hypotension, peripheral vasoconstriction.
GI: constipation, diarrhea, nausea.
GU: impotence, decreased libido.
Derm: itching, rashes.
Endo: hyperglycemia, hypoglycemia.
MS: arthralgia, back pain, muscle cramps.
Neuro: paresthesia.

INTERACTIONS

Drug-Drug: ▪ **General anesthesia, IV phenytoin, diltiaziem,** and **verapamil** may cause additive myocardial depression ▪ Additive bradycardia may occur with **digitalis glycosides** ▪ Additive hypotension may occur with other **antihypertensives,** acute ingestion of **alcohol,** or **nitrates** ▪ Concurrent use with **amphetamines, cocaine, ephedrine, epinephrine, norepinephrine, phenylephrine,** or **pseudoephedrine** may result in unopposed alpha-adrenergic stimulation (excessive hypertension, bradycardia) ▪ Concurrent use with **clonidine** increases hypotension and bradycardia ▪ Concurrent **thyroid** administration may decrease effectiveness ▪ May alter the effectiveness of **insulin** or **oral hypoglycemic agents** (dosage adjustments may be necessary) ▪ May decrease the effectiveness of **theophylline** ▪ May decrease the beneficial $beta_1$ cardiovascular effects of **dopamine** or **dobutamine** ▪ Use cautiously within 14 days of **MAO inhibitor therapy** (may result in hypertension) ▪ Concurrent **NSAIDs** may decrease antihypertensive action.

ROUTE AND DOSAGE

▪ **PO (Adults):** *Antianginal*—40 mg once daily initially; may increase by 40–80 mg/day q 3–7 days as needed (up to 240 mg/day). *Antihypertensive*—40 mg once daily initially; may increase by 40–80 mg/day q 7 days as needed (up to 320 mg/day).

AVAILABILITY

▪ ***Tablets:*** 20 mg[Rx], 40 mg[Rx], 80 mg[Rx], 120 mg[Rx], 160 mg[Rx] ▪ ***In combination with:*** bendroflumethiazide (Corzide[Rx]). See Appendix A.

TIME/ACTION PROFILE (anithypertensive effects)

	ONSET	PEAK	DURATION
PO†	up to 5 days	6–9 days	24 hr

†With chronic dosing.

*CAPITALS indicate life-threatening; underlines indicate most frequent.

NURSING IMPLICATIONS

ASSESSMENT

- **General Info:** Monitor blood pressure and pulse frequently during dose adjustment and periodically during therapy. Assess for orthostatic hypotension when assisting patient up from supine position.
- Monitor intake and output ratios and daily weight. Assess patient routinely for evidence of fluid overload (peripheral edema, dyspnea, rales/crackles, fatigue, weight gain, jugular venous distention).
- **Hypertension:** Check frequency of refills to determine compliance.
- **Angina:** Assess frequency and characteristics of angina periodically during therapy.
- ***Lab Test Considerations:*** May cause increased BUN, serum lipoprotein, potassium, triglyceride, and uric acid levels.
- May cause increased ANA titers.
- May cause increase in blood glucose levels.
- ***Toxicity and Overdose:*** Monitor patients receiving beta-adrenergic blocking agents for signs of overdose (bradycardia, severe dizziness or fainting, severe drowsiness, dyspnea, bluish fingernails or palms, seizures). Notify physician or other health care professional immediately if these signs occur.

POTENTIAL NURSING DIAGNOSES

- Cardiac output, decreased (Side Effects).
- Knowledge deficit, related to medication regimen (Patient/Family Teaching).
- Noncompliance, related to medication regimen (Patient/Family Teaching).

IMPLEMENTATION

- **General Info:** Discontinuation of concurrent clonidine should be done gradually, with beta blocker discontinued first; then, after several days, discontinue clonidine.
- **PO:** Take apical pulse prior to administering. If <50 bpm or if arrhythmia occurs, withhold medication and notify physician or other health care professional.
- May be administered with food or on an empty stomach.
- Tablets may be crushed and mixed with food.

PATIENT/FAMILY TEACHING

- **General Info:** Instruct patient to take medication exactly as directed, at the same time each day, even if feeling well; do not skip or double up on missed doses. Take missed doses as soon as possible up to 8 hr before next dose. Abrupt withdrawal may precipitate life-threatening arrhythmias, hypertension, or myocardial ischemia.
- Advise patient to ensure enough medication is available for weekends, holidays, and vacations. A written prescription may be kept in wallet for emergency.
- Teach patient and family how to check pulse and BP. Instruct them to check pulse daily and BP biweekly. Advise patient to hold dose and contact health care professional if pulse is <50 bpm or if BP changes significantly.
- May cause drowsiness or dizziness. Caution patients to avoid driving or other activities that require alertness until response to the drug is known.
- Advise patients to make position changes slowly to minimize orthostatic hypotension, especially during initiation of therapy or when dose is increased.
- Caution patient that this medication may increase sensitivity to cold.
- Instruct patient to consult health care professional before taking any OTC medications, especially cold preparations, concurrently with this medication.
- Diabetics should closely monitor blood sugar, especially if weakness, malaise, irritability, or fatigue occurs. Medication may mask some signs of hypoglycemia, but dizziness and sweating may still occur.
- Advise patient to notify health care professional if slow pulse, difficulty breathing, wheezing, cold hands and feet, dizziness, confusion, depression, rash, fever, sore throat, unusual bleeding, or bruising occurs.
- Instruct patient to inform health care professional of medication regimen prior to treatment or surgery.
- Advise patient to carry identification describing disease process and medication regimen at all times.
- **Hypertension:** Reinforce the need to continue additional therapies for hypertension (weight loss, sodium restriction, stress reduction, regular exercise, moderation of alcohol consumption, and smoking cessation). Medication controls but does not cure hypertension.

- **Angina:** Caution patient to avoid overexertion with decrease in chest pain.

EVALUATION

Effectiveness of therapy can be demonstrated by: ▪ Decrease in blood pressure ▪ Reduction in frequency of angina ▫ Increase in activity tolerance. May require up to 5 days before therapeutic effects are seen.

NAFARELIN

(na-**fare**-e-lin)
Synarel

CLASSIFICATION(S):
Hormone (gonadotropin-releasing hormone)

Pregnancy Category X

INDICATIONS

▪ Management of endometriosis ▪ Management of central precocious puberty (gonadotropin-dependent) in children.

ACTION

▪ Acts as a synthetic analogue of gonadotropin-releasing hormone (GnRH). Initially increases pituitary production of luteinizing hormone (LH) and follicle-stimulating hormone (FSH), which cause ovarian steroid production. Chronic administration leads to decreased production of gonadotropins. Endometriotic lesions are sensitive to ovarian hormones. **Therapeutic Effects:** ▪ Reduction in lesions and associated pain in endometriosis ▪ Arrest and regression of puberty in children with central precocious puberty.

PHARMACOKINETICS

Absorption: Well absorbed following intranasal administration.
Distribution: UK.
Metabolism and Excretion: 20–40% excreted in feces; 3% excreted unchanged by the kidneys.
Half-life: 3 hr.

CONTRAINDICATIONS AND PRECAUTIONS

Contraindicated in: ▪ Hypersensitivity to gonadotropin-releasing hormone, its analogues, or sorbitol ▪ Pregnancy or lactation.
Use Cautiously in: ▪ Rhinitis.

ADVERSE REACTIONS AND SIDE EFFECTS*

CNS: emotional instability, headaches, depression, insomnia.
EENT: nasal irritation.
CV: edema.
GU: vaginal dryness.
Derm: acne, hirsutism, seborrhea.
Endo: cessation of menses, impaired fertility, reduced breast size.
MS: decreased bone density, myalgia.
Misc: decreased libido, hot flashes, hypersensitivity reactions, weight gain.

INTERACTIONS

Drug-Drug: ▪ Concurrent **topical nasal decongestants** may reduce absorption of nafarelin (administer decongestant at least 2 hr after nafarelin).

ROUTE AND DOSAGE

- **Intranasal (Adults):** *Endometriosis*—1 spray (200 mcg) in 1 nostril in the morning and 1 spray in the other nostril in the evening (400 mcg/day). May be increased to 1 spray in each nostril in the morning and evening (800 mcg/day).
- **Intranasal (Children):** *Central precocious puberty*—2 sprays in each nostril in the morning and in the evening (1600 mcg/day); may be increased up to 1800 mcg/day (3 sprays in alternating nostrils 3 times daily).

AVAILABILITY

- ***Nasal spray:*** 2 mg/ml 10-ml bottle (200 mcg/spray)[Rx].

TIME/ACTION PROFILE (decreased ovarian steroid production)

	ONSET	PEAK	DURATION
Intranasal	within 4 wk	3–4 wk	3–6 mo†

†Relief of symptoms of endometriosis following discontinuation.

*CAPITALS indicate life-threatening; underlines indicate most frequent.

NURSING IMPLICATIONS

ASSESSMENT

- **Endometriosis:** Assess patient for endometriotic pain periodically throughout therapy.
- **Central Precocious Puberty:** Prior to therapy, a complete physical and endocrinologic examination including height, weight, hand and wrist x ray, total sex steroid level (estradiol or testosterone), adrenal steroid level, beta human chorionic gonadotropin level, GnRH stimulation test, pelvic/adrenal/testicular ultrasound, and computerized tomography of the head must be performed. These parameters are monitored after 6–8 wk and every 3–6 mo during therapy.
- □ Assess patient for signs of precocious puberty (menses, breast development, testicular growth) periodically throughout therapy.
- □ Nafarelin is discontinued when the onset of normal puberty is desired. Monitor the onset of normal puberty and assess menstrual cycle, reproductive function, and final adult height.

POTENTIAL NURSING DIAGNOSES

- Pain (Indications).
- Sexual dysfunction (Indications, Side Effects).
- Knowledge deficit, related to medication regimen (Patient/Family Teaching).

IMPLEMENTATION

- **Endometriosis:** Treatment should be started between days 2 and 4 of the menstrual cycle and continued for up to 6 mo.

PATIENT/FAMILY TEACHING

- **General Info:** Instruct patient on the correct technique for nasal spray: The head should be tilted back slightly; wait 30 sec between sprays.
- □ Advise patient to consult health care professional if rhinitis occurs during therapy. If a topical decongestant is needed, do not use decongestant until 2 hr after nafarelin dosing. If possible, avoid sneezing during and immediately after nafarelin dose.
- **Endometriosis:** Inform patient that 1 spray should be administered into 1 nostril in the morning and 1 spray into the other nostril in the evening for the 400 mcg/day dose. If dose is increased to 800 mcg/day, administer 1 spray to each nostril (2 sprays) morning and evening; 1 bottle should provide a 30-day supply at the 400 mcg/day dose.
- □ Advise patient to use a form of contraception other than oral contraceptives during therapy. Inform patient that amenorrhea is expected. Instruct patient to notify health care professional if regular menstruation persists or if successive doses are missed.
- □ Advise patient that medication may cause hot flashes. Notify health care professional if these become bothersome.
- **Central Precocious Puberty:** Instruct patient on correct timing and number of sprays. The 1600 mcg/day dose is achieved by 2 sprays to each nostril in the morning (4 sprays) and 2 sprays to each nostril in the evening (4 sprays), for a total of 8 sprays. The 1800 mcg/day dose is achieved by 3 sprays into alternating nostrils 3 times per day, for a total of 9 sprays. Inform patient and parents that if doses are not taken as directed pubertal process may be reactivated. One bottle should provide a 7-day supply at the 1600 mcg/day dose.
- □ Advise patient and parents that during 1st mo of therapy some signs of puberty (vaginal bleeding, breast enlargement) may occur. These should resolve after the 1st mo of therapy. If these signs persist after the 2nd mo of therapy, notify health care professional.

EVALUATION

Clinical response to therapy can be evaluated by: ▪ Reduction in lesions and associated pain in endometriosis ▪ Resolution of the signs of precocious puberty.

NALBUPHINE

(**nal**-byoo-feen)

Nubain

CLASSIFICATION(S):

Opioid analgesic (agonist/antagonist)

Pregnancy Category C

INDICATIONS

▪ Moderate to severe pain ▪ Also provides: □ Analgesia during labor □ Sedation prior to surgery □ Supplement to balanced anesthesia.

ACTION

▪ Binds to opiate receptors in the CNS ▪ Alters the perception of and response to painful stimuli, while producing generalized CNS depression ▪ In addition, has partial antagonist properties, which may result in opioid withdrawal in physically dependent patients. **Therapeutic Effects:** ▪ Decreased pain.

PHARMACOKINETICS

Absorption: Well absorbed following IM and SC administration.
Distribution: Probably crosses the placenta and enters breast milk.
Metabolism and Excretion: Mostly metabolized by the liver and eliminated in the feces via biliary excretion. Minimal amounts excreted unchanged by the kidneys.
Half-life: 5 hr.

CONTRAINDICATIONS AND PRECAUTIONS

Contraindicated in: ▪ Hypersensitivity to nalbuphine or bisulfites ▪ Patients who are physically dependent on opioids and have not been detoxified (may precipitate withdrawal).
Use Cautiously in: ▪ Head trauma ▪ Increased intracranial pressure ▪ Severe renal, hepatic, or pulmonary disease ▪ Hypothyroidism ▪ Adrenal insufficiency ▪ Alcoholism ▪ Geriatric or debilitated patients (dosage reduction suggested) ▪ Undiagnosed abdominal pain ▪ Prostatic hypertrophy ▪ Pregnancy (has been used during labor but may cause respiratory depression in the newborn) ▪ Patients who have recently received opioid agonists ▪ Lactation or children (safety not established).

ADVERSE REACTIONS AND SIDE EFFECTS*

CNS: dizziness, headache, sedation, confusion, dysphoria, euphoria, floating feeling, hallucinations, unusual dreams.
EENT: blurred vision, diplopia, miosis (high doses).
Resp: respiratory depression.
CV: hypertension, orthostatic hypotension, palpitations.
GI: dry mouth, nausea, vomiting, constipation, ileus.
GU: urinary urgency.
Derm: clammy feeling, sweating.
Misc: physical dependence, psychological dependence, tolerance.

INTERACTIONS

Drug-Drug: ▪ Use with extreme caution in patients receiving **MAO inhibitors** (may result in unpredictable, severe reactions—reduce initial dose of nalbuphine to 25% of usual dose) ▪ Additive CNS depression with **alcohol, antihistamines,** and **sedative/hypnotics** ▪ May precipitate withdrawal in patients who are physically dependent on **opioid agonists** ▪ Avoid concurrent use with other **opioid analgesic agonists** (may diminish analgesic effect).

ROUTE AND DOSAGE

❑ **Analgesia**

- **IM, SC, IV (Adults):** Usual dose is 10 mg q 3–6 hr (single dose not to exceed 20 mg; total daily dose not to exceed 160 mg).

❑ **Supplement to Balanced Anesthesia**

- **IV (Adults):** *Initial*—0.3–3 mg/kg over 10–15 min. *Maintenance*—0.25–0.5 mg/kg as needed.

AVAILABILITY

▪ ***Injection:*** 10 mg/ml in 1- and 10-ml vials[Rx], 20 mg/ml in 1- and 10-ml vials and 1-ml preloaded syringes[Rx].

TIME/ACTION PROFILE (analgesia)

	ONSET	PEAK	DURATION
IM	<15 min	60 min	3–6 hr
SC	<15 min	UK	3–6 hr
IV	2–3 min	30 min	3–6 hr

NURSING IMPLICATIONS

ASSESSMENT

❑ Assess type, location, and intensity of pain prior to and 1 hr following IM or 30 min (peak) following IV administration. When titrating opioid doses, increases of 25–50% should be administered until there is either a 50% reduction in the patient's pain rating on a numerical or visual analogue scale or the patient reports satisfactory pain relief. A repeat dose can be safely administered at the time of

*CAPITALS indicate life-threatening; underlines indicate most frequent.

the peak if previous dose is ineffective and side effects are minimal. Patients requiring doses higher than 20 mg should be converted to an opioid agonist. Nalbuphine is not recommended for prolonged use or as first-line therapy for acute or cancer pain.

- An equianalgesic chart (see Appendix B) should be used when changing routes or when changing from one opioid to another.
- Assess blood pressure, pulse, and respirations before and periodically during administration. If respiratory rate is <10/min, assess level of sedation. Physical stimulation may be sufficient to prevent significant hypoventilation. Dose may need to be decreased by 25–50%. Nalbuphine produces respiratory depression, but this does not markedly increase with increased doses.
- Assess prior analgesic history. Antagonistic properties may induce withdrawal symptoms (vomiting, restlessness, abdominal cramps, and increased blood pressure and temperature) in patients physically dependent on opioids.
- Although this drug has a low potential for dependence, prolonged use may lead to physical and psychological dependence and tolerance. This should not prevent patient from receiving adequate analgesia. Most patients who receive nalbuphine for pain do not develop psychological dependence. If tolerance develops, changing to an opioid agonist may be required to relieve pain.
- ***Lab Test Considerations:*** May cause increased serum amylase and lipase concentrations.
- ***Toxicity and Overdose:*** If an opioid antagonist is required to reverse respiratory depression or coma, naloxone (Narcan) is the antidote. Dilute the 0.4-mg ampule of naloxone in 10 ml of 0.9% NaCl and administer 0.5 ml (0.02 mg) by direct IV push every 2 min. For children and patients weighing <40 kg, dilute 0.1 mg of naloxone in 10 ml of 0.9% NaCl for a concentration of 10 mcg/ml and administer 0.5 mcg/kg every 1–2 min. Titrate dose to avoid withdrawal, seizures, and severe pain.

POTENTIAL NURSING DIAGNOSES

- Pain (Indications).
- Injury, risk for (Side Effects).
- Sensory-perceptual alterations: visual, auditory (Side Effects).

IMPLEMENTATION

- **General Info:** Explain therapeutic value of medication prior to administration to enhance the analgesic effect.
- Regularly administered doses may be more effective than prn administration. Analgesic is more effective if administered before pain becomes severe.
- Coadministration with nonopioid analgesics may have additive effects and permit lower opioid doses.
- **IM:** Administer deep into well-developed muscle. Rotate sites of injections.
- **Direct IV:** May give IV undiluted.
- ***Rate:*** Administer slowly, each 10 mg over 3–5 min.
- **Syringe Compatibility:** ▪ atropine ▪ cimetidine ▪ diphenhydramine ▪ droperidol ▪ glycopyrrolate ▪ hydroxyzine ▪ lidocaine ▪ midazolam ▪ prochlorperazine ▪ ranitidine ▪ scopolamine ▪ trimethobenzamide.
- **Syringe Incompatibility:** ▪ diazepam ▪ ketorolac ▪ pentobarbital.
- **Y-Site Compatibility:** ▪ amifostine ▪ aztreonam ▪ filgrastim ▪ fludarabine ▪ melphalan ▪ paclitaxel ▪ teniposide ▪ thiotepa ▪ vinorelbine.
- **Y-Site Incompatibility:** ▪ cefepime ▪ methotrexate ▪ nafcillin ▪ piperacillin/tazobactam ▪ sargramostim ▪ sodium bicarbonate.

PATIENT/FAMILY TEACHING

- Instruct patient on how and when to ask for pain medication.
- May cause drowsiness or dizziness. Advise patient to call for assistance when ambulating and to avoid driving or other activities requiring alertness until response to the medication is known.
- Caution patient to change positions slowly to minimize orthostatic hypotension.
- Advise patient that frequent mouth rinses, good oral hygiene, and sugarless gum or candy may decrease dry mouth.
- Encourage patient to turn, cough, and breathe deeply every 2 hr to prevent atelectasis.
- Advise patient to avoid concurrent use of alcohol or other CNS depressants with this medication.

EVALUATION

Effectiveness of therapy can be demonstrated by: ▪ Decrease in severity of pain without a significant alteration in level of consciousness or respiratory status.

NALMEFENE
(**nal**-me-feen)
Revex

CLASSIFICATION(S):
Antidote (for opioids), Opioid antagonist

Pregnancy Category B

INDICATIONS

▪ Reversal (partial or complete) of opioid effects, including respiratory depression ▪ Management of known or suspected overdose of opioid agents.

ACTION

▪ Competitively blocks the effects of opioids, including CNS and respiratory depression, without producing any agonist (opioid-like) effects. **Therapeutic Effects:** ▪ Reversal of signs of opioid excess.

PHARMACOKINETICS

Absorption: IV administration results in complete bioavailability.
Distribution: Crosses the blood-brain barrier.
Metabolism and Excretion: Mostly metabolized by the liver; <5% excreted unchanged in urine, 17% in feces. Undergoes enterohepatic recycling.
Half-life: 10.8 hr.

CONTRAINDICATIONS AND PRECAUTIONS

Contraindicated in: ▪ Known hypersensitivity.
Use Cautiously in: ▪ Overdosage of long-acting opioids (methadone); repeat dosing may be required as emergence of signs of opioid excess recurs ▪ Patients with severe cardiovascular disease or those receiving cardioactive medications ▪ Overdosage of buprenorphine (may not completely reverse respiratory depression) ▪ Patients with renal failure (inject incremental doses more slowly) ▪ Pregnancy, lactation, or children (safe use not established). **Exercise Extreme Caution in:** ▪ Patients known to be physically dependent on opioid agents or who have undergone surgery with large doses of opioids (increased risk of withdrawal; increased risk of cardiovascular complications).

ADVERSE REACTIONS AND SIDE EFFECTS

Those listed are primarily due to the reversal of opioid effects.
CNS: dysphoria, headache.
CV: hypertension, hypotension, tachycardia, vasodilation.
GI: abdominal cramps, nausea.
MS: joint pain, myalgia.
Misc: chills, fever, postoperative pain.

INTERACTIONS

Drug-Drug: ▪ No significant interactions have been noted.

ROUTE AND DOSAGE

❑ **Reversal of Postoperative Opioid Depression**

▪ **IV (Adults):** 0.25 mcg/kg followed by incremental doses of 0.25 mcg/kg q 2–5 min (up to a total dose of 1 mcg/kg).

❑ **Known or Suspected Opioid Overdose**

▪ **IV (Adults):** *Patients not physically dependent on opioids*—0.5 mg/70 kg; may be followed 2–5 min later by 1 mg/70 kg (not to exceed 1.5 mg/70 kg total). *Patients suspected to be opioid dependent*—0.1 mg/70 kg is a challenge dose. If no signs of withdrawal occur in 2 min, regimen for non-opioid-dependent patients should be instituted.

AVAILABILITY

▪ ***Injection:*** 100 mcg/ml (blue label)^Rx^, 1 mg/ml (green label)^Rx^.

TIME/ACTION PROFILE (reversal of opioid effects)

	ONSET	PEAK	DURATION
IV	mins	UK	30–60 min*

*Following 1 mcg/kg dose; may last hours following larger doses.

NURSING IMPLICATIONS

ASSESSMENT

- Monitor respiratory rate, rhythm, and depth; pulse, ECG, and blood pressure; and level of sedation frequently until effects of opioid wear off. The effects of some opioids may last longer than the effects of nalmefene, and repeat doses may be necessary.
- Assess patient for intensity of pain when nalmefene is used to treat postoperative respiratory depression. Careful titration of nalmefene can reverse respiratory depression while maintaining analgesia.
- Assess patient for signs and symptoms of opioid withdrawal (vomiting, restlessness, anxiety, abdominal cramps, increased blood pressure and temperature). Symptoms may occur within a few min to 2 hr. Severity depends on dose of nalmefene, opioid involved, and degree of physical dependence. Patients tolerant of or physically dependent on opioids should be monitored closely following initial and subsequent doses.
- Lack of significant improvement indicates that symptoms are due to a disease process or to other nonopioid CNS depressants not affected by nalmefene.
- ***Lab Test Considerations:*** May cause elevated AST levels.

POTENTIAL NURSING DIAGNOSES

- Breathing pattern, ineffective (Indications).
- Coping, ineffective individual (Indications).
- Pain, acute (Interactions).

IMPLEMENTATION

- **General Info:** Resuscitation equipment, oxygen, vasopressors, and mechanical ventilation should be available to supplement nalmefene therapy as needed.
- Do not confuse blue-labeled ampule (100 mcg/ml) for reversal of postoperative respiratory depression with green-labeled ampule (1 mg/ml) for management of opioid overdose.
- Titrate doses slowly. Abrupt reversal of opioids in emergency or postoperative settings may cause pulmonary edema, cardiovascular instability, hypotension, hypertension, ventricular tachycardia, and ventricular fibrillation.
- Administration of higher doses or at shorter intervals than recommended may increase the incidence and severity of symptoms related to acute withdrawal (nausea, vomiting, hypertension, anxiety).
- If respiratory depression recurs, titrate repeat doses based on clinical effects to avoid over-reversal.
- Do not administer solutions that are discolored or contain particulate matter.
- If IV access is lost or not readily available, nalmefene has been administered IM or SC with effects of a 1-mg dose occurring within 5–15 min.

Reversal of Postoperative Respiratory Depression

- **Direct IV:** Dose is titrated to achieve reversal of excessive opioid effects without causing complete reversal and acute pain. Rapid complete reversal of opioid effects postoperatively has resulted in hypertension, tachycardia, and cardiovascular complications.
- Administer dose of 100 mcg/ml solution (blue-labeled ampule) undiluted in 0.25 mcg/kg increments every 2–5 min until desired degree of opioid reversal is obtained. Cumulative doses of >1.0 mcg/kg do not provide additional therapeutic effects.
- May dilute in 0.9% NaCl or sterile water for injection and administer in 0.1 mcg/kg increments in patients with increased cardiovascular risk.
- IV nalmefene has been used to reverse the effect of intrathecal opioids; recommended doses did not prevent analgesic response to subsequent doses.
- ***Rate:*** Administer as a bolus. Administer over 60 sec in patients with renal or hepatic disease.

Management of Known or Suspected Opioid Overdose

- **Direct IV:** If opioid dependency is suspected, administer a challenge dose and monitor for withdrawal symptoms. If no symptoms occur within 2 min, administer recommended dose.
- Administer dose using 1 mg/ml solution (green-labeled ampule). Administer only enough to restore normal respiratory rate to minimize cardiovascular stress and withdrawal symptoms.
- If no response is seen following administration of 1.5 mg/70 kg dose total, additional

doses are unlikely to have an effect, and other causes for CNS depression should be considered.

- *Rate:* Administer as a bolus. Administer over 60 sec in patients with renal or hepatic disease.
- **Syringe Incompatibility:** ▪ Information unavailable; do not mix with other medications.

PATIENT/FAMILY TEACHING

- ☐ Explain to family and patient, when awake, the rationale for use of nalmefene.

EVALUATION

Clinical response to therapy can be evaluated by: ▪ Reversal of respiratory depression, sedation, and hypotension caused by opioids.

NALOXONE

(nal-**ox**-one)

Narcan

CLASSIFICATION(S):

Antidote (for opioids), Opioid antagonist

Pregnancy Category B

INDICATIONS

▪ Reversal of CNS depression and respiratory depression because of suspected opioid overdosage. **Unlabeled Uses:** ▪ Management of refractory circulatory shock.

ACTION

▪ Competitively blocks the effects of opioids, including CNS and respiratory depression, without producing any agonist (opioid-like) effects. **Therapeutic Effects:** ▪ Reversal of signs of opioid excess.

PHARMACOKINETICS

Absorption: Well absorbed following IM or SC administration.

Distribution: Rapidly distributed to tissues. Crosses the placenta.

Metabolism and Excretion: Metabolized by the liver.

Half-life: 60–90 min (up to 3 hr in neonates).

CONTRAINDICATIONS AND PRECAUTIONS

Contraindicated in: ▪ Hypersensitivity.

Use Cautiously in: ▪ Cardiovascular disease ▪ Patients physically dependent on opioids (may precipitate severe withdrawal) ▪ Pregnancy (may cause withdrawal in mother and fetus if mother is opioid-dependent) ▪ Lactation (safety not established) ▪ Neonates of opioid-dependent mothers.

ADVERSE REACTIONS AND SIDE EFFECTS

CV: hypertension, hypotension, ventricular fibrillation, ventricular tachycardia.

GI: nausea, vomiting.

INTERACTIONS

Drug-Drug: ▪ Can precipitate withdrawal in patients physically dependent on **opioids** ▪ Larger doses may be required to reverse the effects of **buprenorphine, butorphanol, nalbuphine, pentazocine,** or **propoxyphene** ▪ Antagonizes postoperative **opioid analgesia.**

ROUTE AND DOSAGE

☐ Postoperative Opioid-Induced Respiratory Depression

- **IV (Adults):** 0.02–0.2 mg q 2–3 min until response obtained; repeat q 1–2 hr if needed.
- **IV (Children):** 5–10 mcg; may repeat q 2–3 min until response obtained. Additional doses may be given q 1–2 hr if needed.
- **IM, IV, SC (Neonates):** 10 mcg (0.01 mg)/kg; may repeat q 2–3 min until response obtained. Additional doses may be given q 1–2 hr if needed.

☐ Opioid-Induced Respiratory Depression during Chronic (>1 wk) Opioid Use

- **IV, IM, SC (Adults >40 kg):** 20–40 mcg (0.02–0.04 mg) given as small, frequent (q min) boluses or as an infusion titrated to improve respiratory function while not reversing analgesia.
- **IV, IM, SC (Adults and Children <40 kg):** 0.5–2 mcg/kg given as small, frequent (q min) boluses or as an infusion titrated to improve respiratory function while not reversing analgesia.

- **Overdose of Opioids**
- **IV, IM, SC (Adults):** *Patients not suspected of being opioid-dependent*—0.4 mg (10 mcg/kg); may repeat q 2–3 min (IV route is preferred). Some patients may require up to 2 mg. *Patients suspected to be opioid-dependent*—Initial dose should be decreased to 0.1–0.2 mg q 2–3 min. May also be given by IV infusion at rate adjusted to patient's response.
- **IV, IM, SC (Children):** 10 mcg (0.01 mg)/kg q 2–3 min; if no response occurs, dose may be increased to 100 mcg (0.1 mg)/kg.

AVAILABILITY

- ***Injection:*** 0.4 mg/ml[Rx] ▪ ***Neonatal injection:*** 0.02 mg/ml[Rx] ▪ ***In combination with:*** pentazocine (Talwin NX)[Rx]. See Appendix A.

TIME/ACTION PROFILE (reversal of opioid effects)

	ONSET	PEAK	DURATION
IV	1–2 min	UK	45 min
IM, SC	2–5 min	UK	>45 min

NURSING IMPLICATIONS

ASSESSMENT

- Monitor respiratory rate, rhythm, and depth; pulse, ECG, blood pressure; and level of consciousness frequently for 3–4 hr after the expected peak of blood concentrations. Following a moderate overdose of a short half-life opioid, physical stimulation may be enough to prevent significant hypoventilation. The effects of some opioids may last longer than the effects of naloxone, and repeat doses may be necessary.
- Patients who have been receiving opioids for >1 wk are extremely sensitive to the effects of naloxone. Dilute and administer carefully.
- Assess patient for level of pain following administration when used to treat postoperative respiratory depression. Naloxone decreases respiratory depression but also reverses analgesia.
- Assess patient for signs and symptoms of opioid withdrawal (vomiting, restlessness, abdominal cramps, increased blood pressure, and temperature). Symptoms may occur within a few minutes to 2 hr. Severity depends on dose of naloxone, opioid involved, and degree of physical dependence.
- Lack of significant improvement indicates that symptoms are due to a disease process or to other nonopioid CNS depressants not affected by naloxone.
- ***Toxicity and Overdose:*** Naloxone is a pure antagonist with no agonist properties and minimal toxicity.

POTENTIAL NURSING DIAGNOSES

- Breathing pattern, ineffective (Indications).
- Coping, ineffective individual (Indications).
- Pain (Interactions).

IMPLEMENTATION

- **General Info:** Larger doses of naloxone may be necessary when used to antagonize the effects of buprenorphine, butorphanol, nalbuphine, pentazocine, and propoxyphene.
- Resuscitation equipment, oxygen, vasopressors, and mechanical ventilation should be available to supplement naloxone therapy as needed.
- **Direct IV:** Administer undiluted for *suspected opioid overdose.*
- For patients with *opioid-induced respiratory depression,* dilute 0.4 mg of naloxone in 10 ml of sterile water or 0.9% NaCl for injection.
- For children or others weighing <40 kg, dilute 0.1 mg of naloxone in 10 ml of sterile water or 0.9% NaCl for injection for a concentration of 10 mcg/ml.
- ***Rate:*** Administer at a rate of 0.1–0.4 mg over 15 sec in patients with *suspected opioid overdose.*
- For patients who develop *opioid-induced respiratory depression,* administer dilute solution of 0.4 mg/10 ml at a rate of 0.5 ml (0.02 mg) by direct IV push every 2 min. Titrate dose to avoid withdrawal and severe pain. Excessive dose in postoperative patients may cause excitement, pain, hypotension, hypertension, pulmonary edema, ventricular tachycardia and fibrillation, and seizures.
- For children and others weighing <40 kg, administer 10 mcg/ml solution at a rate of 0.5 mcg/kg every 1–2 min. Titrate dose to avoid withdrawal, seizures, and severe pain.
- **Continuous Infusion:** Dilute in D5W or 0.9% NaCl for injection. Naloxone 2 mg in 500 ml equals a concentration of 4 mcg/ml. Mixture is stable for 24 hr; discard unused solution.

- *Rate:* Titrate dose according to patient response. Supplemental doses administered SC or IM, or a continuous infusion may provide longer-lasting effects.
- □ Doses should be titrated carefully in postoperative patients to avoid interference with control of postoperative pain.
- **Additive Incompatibility:** ▪ Incompatible with preparations containing bisulfite, sulfite, and solutions with an alkaline pH.

PATIENT/FAMILY TEACHING

- □ As medication becomes effective, explain purpose and effects of naloxone to patient.

EVALUATION

Clinical response to therapy can be evaluated by: ▪ Adequate ventilation □ Alertness without significant pain or withdrawal symptoms.

NAPROXEN

(na-**prox**-en)

{Apo-Naproxen}, EC-Naprosyn, Naprelan, Napron X, Naprosyn, {Naprosyn-E}, {Naprosyn-SR}, {Naxen}, {Novo-Naprox}, {Novo-Naprox Sodium}, {Nu-Naprox}

NAPROXEN SODIUM

(na-**prox**-en **soe**-dee-um)

Aleve, Anaprox, Anaprox DS, {Apo-Napro-Na}, Apo-Napro-Na DS, Naprelan, {Novo-Naprox Sodium}, {Novo-Naprox Sodium DS}, {Synflex}, {Synflex DS}

CLASSIFICATION(S):

Analgesics (nonopioid), Nonsteroidal anti-inflammatory agents

Pregnancy Category B (first trimester)

INDICATIONS

▪ Mild to moderate pain ▪ Dysmenorrhea ▪ Fever ▪ Inflammatory disorders, including: □ Rheumatoid arthritis □ Osteoarthritis.

ACTION

▪ Inhibit prostaglandin synthesis. **Therapeutic Effects:** ▪ Decreased pain ▪ Reduction of fever ▪ Suppression of inflammation.

PHARMACOKINETICS

Absorption: Completely absorbed from the GI tract. Sodium salt (Anaprox) is more rapidly absorbed.
Distribution: Cross the placenta; enter breast milk in low concentrations.
Metabolism and Excretion: Mostly metabolized by the liver.
Half-life: 10–20 hr.

CONTRAINDICATIONS AND PRECAUTIONS

Contraindicated in: ▪ Hypersensitivity ▪ Cross-sensitivity may occur with other NSAIDs, including aspirin ▪ Active GI bleeding ▪ Ulcer disease.
Use Cautiously in: ▪ Severe cardiovascular, renal, or hepatic disease ▪ History of ulcer disease ▪ Chronic alcohol use/abuse ▪ Pregnancy or lactation (safety not established; avoid using during 2nd half of pregnancy).

ADVERSE REACTIONS AND SIDE EFFECTS*

CNS: <u>dizziness</u>, <u>drowsiness</u>, <u>headache</u>.
EENT: tinnitus.
Resp: dyspnea.
CV: edema, palpitations, tachycardia.
GI: DRUG-INDUCED HEPATITIS, GI BLEEDING, <u>constipation</u>, <u>dyspepsia</u>, <u>nausea</u>, anorexia, diarrhea, discomfort, flatulence, vomiting.
GU: cystitis, hematuria, renal failure.
Derm: photosensitivity, rashes, sweating.
Hemat: blood dyscrasias, prolonged bleeding time.
Misc: allergic reactions including ANAPHYLAXIS.

INTERACTIONS

Drug-Drug: ▪ Concurrent use with **aspirin** decreases naproxen blood levels and may decrease effectiveness ▪ Increased risk of bleeding with **anticoagulants, thrombolytic agents, cefamandole, cefotetan, cefoperazone, valproic acid,** or **plicamycin** ▪ Additive adverse GI side effects with **aspirin, glucocorticoids,**

{} = Available in Canada only.
***CAPITALS indicate life-threatening; <u>underlines</u> indicate most frequent.**

and other **NSAIDs** ▪ **Probenecid** increases blood levels and may increase toxicity ▪ Increased risk of photosensitivity with other **photosensitizing agents** ▪ May increase the risk of toxicity from **methotrexate, antineoplastic agents,** or **radiation therapy** ▪ May increase serum levels and risk of toxicity from **lithium** ▪ Increased risk of adverse renal effects with **cyclosporine** or chronic use of **acetaminophen** ▪ May decrease response to **antihypertensives** or **diuretics** ▪ May increase risk of hypoglycemia with **insulin** or **oral hypoglycemic agents.**

ROUTE AND DOSAGE

275 mg naproxen sodium is equivalent to 250 mg naproxen.

❑ **Anti-inflammatory/Analgesic/Anti-dysmenorrheal**

- **PO (Adults):** *Naproxen*—250–500 mg naproxen bid (up to 1.5 g/day). *Delayed-release naproxen*—375–500 mg twice daily. *Naproxen sodium*—275–550 mg twice daily (up to 1.65 g/day).
- **PO (Children):** 5 mg/kg/day twice daily as naproxen suspension.

❑ **Antigout**

- **PO (Adults):** *Naproxen*—750 mg naproxen initially, then 250 mg q 8 hr. *Naproxen sodium*—825 mg initially, then 275 mg q 8 hr.

❑ **OTC Use**

- **PO (Adults):** 200 mg q 8–12 hr or 400 mg followed by 200 mg q 12 hr (not to exceed 600 mg/24 hr).
- **PO (Geriatric Patients >65 yr):** Not to exceed 200 mg q 12 hr.

AVAILABILITY

❑ **Naproxen**

▪ ***Tablets (Naprosyn, {Apo-Naproxen, Naxen, Novo-Naprox, Nu-Naprox}):*** {125 mg^{Rx}}, 250 mg^{Rx}, 375 mg^{Rx}, 500 mg^{Rx} ▪ ***Controlled-release tablets (Naprelan):*** 375 mg^{Rx}, 500 mg^{Rx} ▪ ***Delayed-release tablets (EC-Naprosyn, {Naprosyn-E}):*** {250 mg^{Rx}}, 375 mg^{Rx}, 500 mg^{Rx} ▪ ***Extended-release tablets {Naprosyn-SR}:*** {750 mg^{Rx}} ▪ ***Oral suspension (Naprosyn):*** 125 mg/5 ml^{Rx} ▪ ***Suppositories (Naprosyn, {Naxen}):*** {500 mg^{Rx}}.

❑ **Naproxen Sodium**

▪ ***Tablets (Aleve, Anaprox, Anaprox DS, {Apo-Napro-Na, Novo-Naprox Sodium, Novo-Naprox Sodium DS, Synaflex, Synaflex DS}):*** 220 mg^{OTC}, 275 mg^{Rx}, 550 mg^{Rx}.

TIME/ACTION PROFILE

	ONSET	PEAK	DURATION
PO (analgesic)	1 hr	UK	up to 7 hr
PO (anti-inflammatory)	14 days	2–4 wk	UK

NURSING IMPLICATIONS

ASSESSMENT

- **General Info:** Patients who have asthma, aspirin-induced allergy, and nasal polyps are at increased risk for developing hypersensitivity reactions. Assess for rhinitis, asthma, and urticaria.
- **Pain:** Assess pain (note type, location, and intensity) prior to and 1–2 hr following administration.
- **Arthritis:** Assess pain and range of motion prior to and 1–2 hr following administration.
- **Fever:** Monitor temperature; note signs associated with fever (diaphoresis, tachycardia, malaise).
- ***Lab Test Considerations:*** BUN, serum creatinine, CBC, and liver function tests should be evaluated periodically in patients receiving prolonged courses of therapy.
  - □ Serum potassium, BUN, serum creatinine, alkaline phosphatase, LDH, AST, and ALT tests may show increased levels. Blood glucose, hemoglobin, and hematocrit concentrations, leukocyte and platelet counts, and CCr may be decreased.
  - □ Bleeding time may be prolonged up to 4 days following discontinuation of therapy.
  - □ May alter test results for urine 5-HIAA and urine steroid determinations.

POTENTIAL NURSING DIAGNOSES

- Pain (Indications).
- Physical mobility, impaired (Indications).
- Knowledge deficit, related to medication regimen (Patient/Family Teaching).

IMPLEMENTATION

- **General Info:** Administration in higher than recommended doses does not provide increased effectiveness but may cause increased side effects.

- □ Coadministration with opioid analgesics may have additive analgesic effects and may permit lower opioid doses.
- □ Analgesic is more effective if given before pain becomes severe.
- ■ **PO:** For rapid initial effect, administer 30 min before or 2 hr after meals. May be administered with food, milk, or antacids to decrease GI irritation. Food slows but does not reduce the extent of absorption. Do not mix suspension with antacid or other liquid prior to administration.
- ■ **Dysmenorrhea:** Administer as soon as possible after the onset of menses. Prophylactic treatment has not been shown to be effective.

PATIENT/FAMILY TEACHING

- □ Advise patient to take this medication with a full glass of water and to remain in an upright position for 15–30 min after administration.
- □ Instruct patient to take medication exactly as directed. If a dose is missed, it should be taken as soon as remembered but not if almost time for the next dose. Do not double doses.
- □ May cause drowsiness or dizziness. Advise patient to avoid driving or other activities requiring alertness until response to the medication is known.
- □ Caution patient to avoid the concurrent use of alcohol, aspirin, acetaminophen, or other OTC medications without consulting health care professional. Use of naproxen with 3 or more glasses of alcohol per day may increase risk of GI bleeding.
- □ Advise patient to inform health care professional of medication regimen prior to treatment or surgery.
- □ Caution patient to wear sunscreen and protective clothing to prevent photosensitivity reactions.
- □ Instruct patients not to take OTC naproxen preparations for more than 3 days for fever and to consult health care professional if symptoms persist or worsen.
- □ Advise patient to consult health care professional if rash, itching, visual disturbances, tinnitus, weight gain, edema, black stools, persistent headache, or influenza-like syndrome (chills, fever, muscle aches, pain) occurs.

EVALUATION

Effectiveness of therapy can be demonstrated by: ■ Relief of pain ■ Improved joint mobility. Partial arthritic relief is usually seen within 2 wk, but maximum effectiveness may require 2–4 wk of continuous therapy. Patients who do not respond to one NSAID may respond to another ■ Reduction of fever.

NEFAZODONE

(neff-**a**-zoe-done)

Serzone

CLASSIFICATION(S):

Antidepressant (miscellaneous)

Pregnancy Category C

INDICATIONS

■ Major depression (in conjunction with psychotherapy).

ACTION

■ Inhibits the reuptake of serotonin and norepinephrine by neurons ■ Antagonizes $alpha_1$-adrenergic receptors. **Therapeutic Effects:** ■ Antidepressant action, which may develop only over several weeks.

PHARMACOKINETICS

Absorption: Well absorbed but undergoes extensive and variable first-pass hepatic metabolism (bioavailability about 20%).

Distribution: Widely distributed; enters the CNS.

Metabolism and Excretion: Extensively metabolized. One metabolite (hydroxynefazodone) has antidepressant activity.

Half-life: *Nefazodone*—2–4 hr; *hydroxynefazodone*—1.5–4 hr.

CONTRAINDICATIONS AND PRECAUTIONS

Contraindicated in: ■ Hypersensitivity ■ Concurrent astemizole, cisapride, or MAO inhibitor therapy.

Use Cautiously in: ■ Elderly patients (initiate therapy at lower doses) ■ History of suicide attempt or drug abuse ■ Underlying cardiovascular or cerebrovascular disease ■ History of mania

■ Pregnancy, lactation, or children <18 yr (safety not established).

ADVERSE REACTIONS AND SIDE EFFECTS*

CNS: dizziness, insomnia, somnolence, agitation, confusion, weakness.
EENT: abnormal vision, blurred vision, eye pain, tinnitus.
Resp: dyspnea.
CV: bradycardia, hypotension.
GI: constipation, dry mouth, nausea, gastroenteritis.
GU: impotence.
Derm: rashes.
Hemat: decreased hematocrit.

INTERACTIONS

Drug-Drug: ■ Concurrent use with **astemizole** or **cisapride** may result in serious, potentially fatal adverse cardiovascular reactions (avoid concurrent use) ■ Serious, potentially fatal reactions may occur during concurrent use with **MAO inhibitors** (do not use concurrently or within 2 wk of MAO inhibitors; discontinue nefazodone at least 7 days before starting MAO inhibitor therapy) ■ Additive CNS depression with other CNS depressants including **alcohol, antihistamines, opioid analgesics**, and **sedative/hypnotics** ■ May increase blood levels and effects of **alprazolam** or **triazolam** ■ May increase serum **digoxin** levels ■ Additive hypotension may occur with **antihypertensives, nitrates**, or acute ingestion of **alcohol** ■ May increase the risk of myopathy with **HMG-CoA reductase inhibitor.**

ROUTE AND DOSAGE

- **PO (Adults):** 100 mg twice daily initially; may be increased weekly up to 600 mg/day in 2 divided doses.
- **PO (Geriatric Patients):** 50 mg twice daily initially; may be increased weekly as tolerated.

AVAILABILITY

■ ***Tablets:*** 100 mg[Rx], 150 mg[Rx], 200 mg[Rx], 250 mg[Rx].

TIME/ACTION PROFILE (antidepressant actiion)

	ONSET	PEAK	DURATION
PO	days–wks	several wk	UK

NURSING IMPLICATIONS

ASSESSMENT

- □ Assess mental status and mood changes. Inform physician or other health care professional if patient demonstrates significant increase in anxiety, nervousness, or insomnia.
- □ Assess suicidal tendencies, especially in early therapy. Restrict amount of drug available to patient.
- □ Monitor blood pressure and pulse prior to and periodically throughout therapy.
- ■ ***Lab Test Considerations:*** May cause decrease in hematocrit and leukopenia.
- □ May cause elevated LDH, AST, and ALT.
- □ May also cause hypercholesterolemia and hypoglycemia.

POTENTIAL NURSING DIAGNOSES

- ■ Coping, ineffective individual (Indications).
- ■ Injury, risk for (Side Effects).
- ■ Knowledge deficit, related to medication regimen (Patient/Family Teaching).

IMPLEMENTATION

- ■ **PO:** Administer doses twice daily.

PATIENT/FAMILY TEACHING

- □ Instruct patient to take medication exactly as directed. Several weeks may be required to obtain a full antidepressant response. Once response is obtained, therapy should be continued for at least 6 mo. If a dose is missed, take as soon as possible unless almost time for next dose. Do not double doses.
- □ May cause drowsiness or dizziness. Caution patient to avoid driving or other activities requiring alertness until response to the drug is known.
- □ Advise patient to make position changes slowly to minimize orthostatic hypotension.
- □ Caution patient to avoid taking alcohol or other CNS depressant drugs during therapy and not to take other prescription or OTC medications without consulting health care professional.
- □ Inform patient that frequent mouth rinses, good oral hygiene, and sugarless gum or candy may minimize dry mouth. If dry mouth persists for more than 2 wk, consult health

N

*CAPITALS indicate life-threatening; underlines indicate most frequent.

care professional regarding use of saliva substitute.

- Instruct female patient to inform health care professional if pregnancy is planned or suspected or if breast-feeding.
- Instruct patient to notify health care professional of signs of allergy (rash, hives) or if agitation, blurred or other changes in vision, confusion, dizziness, unsteadiness, difficult or frequent urination, difficulty concentrating, or memory problems occur.
- Emphasize the importance of follow-up examinations to monitor progress. Encourage patient participation in psychotherapy.

EVALUATION

Effectiveness of therapy can be demonstrated by: ▪ Increased sense of well-being ▫ Renewed interest in surroundings. May require several weeks of therapy to obtain full response. Need for therapy should be periodically reassessed. Therapy is usually continued for 6 mo or more.

NEOSTIGMINE

(nee-oh-**stig**-meen)
Prostigmin

CLASSIFICATION(S):
Cholinergic (anticholinesterase agent)

Pregnancy Category C

INDICATIONS

▪ Improvement in muscle strength in symptomatic treatment of myasthenia gravis ▪ Prevention and treatment of postoperative bladder distention and urinary retention or ileus ▪ Reversal of nondepolarizing neuromuscular blockers.

ACTION

▪ Inhibits the breakdown of acetylcholine so that it accumulates and has a prolonged effect ▪ Effects include miosis, increased intestinal and skeletal muscle tone, bronchial and ureteral constriction, bradycardia, increased salivation, lacrimation, and sweating. **Therapeutic Effects:** ▪ Improved muscular function in patients with myasthenia gravis, improved bladder-emptying in patients with urinary retention, or reversal of nondepolarizing neuromuscular blockers.

PHARMACOKINETICS

Absorption: Poorly absorbed following oral administration, necessitating large oral doses as compared with parenteral doses.
Distribution: Probably doesn't cross the placenta or enter breast milk.
Metabolism and Excretion: Metabolized by plasma cholinesterases and the liver.
Half-life: *PO, IV*—40–60 min; *IM*—50–90 min.

CONTRAINDICATIONS AND PRECAUTIONS

Contraindicated in: ▪ Hypersensitivity ▪ Mechanical obstruction of the GI or GU tract.
Use Cautiously in: ▪ History of asthma ▪ Ulcer disease ▪ Cardiovascular disease ▪ Epilepsy ▪ Hyperthyroidism ▪ Pregnancy (may cause uterine irritability after IV administration near term; newborns may display muscle weakness) ▪ Lactation.

ADVERSE REACTIONS AND SIDE EFFECTS*

CNS: SEIZURES, dizziness, weakness.
EENT: lacrimation, miosis.
Resp: <u>bronchospasm</u>, <u>excess secretions</u>.
CV: <u>bradycardia</u>, hypotension.
GI: <u>abdominal cramps</u>, <u>diarrhea</u>, <u>excess salivation</u>, <u>nausea</u>, <u>vomiting</u>.
Derm: <u>sweating</u>, rashes.

INTERACTIONS

Drug-Drug: ▪ Action may be antagonized by **drugs possessing anticholinergic properties**, including **antihistamines, antidepressants, atropine, haloperidol, phenothiazines, quinidine**, and **disopyramide** ▪ Prolongs action of **depolarizing muscle-relaxing agents (succinylcholine, decamethonium)**.

ROUTE AND DOSAGE

▫ Myasthenia Gravis

▪ **PO (Adults):** 15 mg q 3–4 hr initially; increase at daily intervals until optimal response

*CAPITALS indicate life-threatening; <u>underlines</u> indicate most frequent.

NELFINAVIR
(nell-**finn**-a-veer)
Viracept
CLASSIFICATION(S):
Antiretroviral (protease inhibitor)
Pregnancy Category B

INDICATIONS
▪ Management of HIV infection in combination with other antiretrovirals.

ACTION
▪ Inhibits the action of HIV protease and prevents the cleavage of viral polyproteins. **Therapeutic Effects:** ▪ Increased CD4 cell count and decreased viral load ▪ Slowing of the progression of HIV infection and its sequelae.

PHARMACOKINETICS
Absorption: Well absorbed following oral administration.
Distribution: UK.
Protein Binding: >98%.
Metabolism and Excretion: Mostly metabolized and excreted in feces as metabolites (78%) or unchanged drug (22%); minimal amounts (1–2%) excreted unchanged in urine.
Half-life: 3.5–5 hr.

CONTRAINDICATIONS AND PRECAUTIONS
Contraindicated in: ▪ Hypersensitivity ▪ Concurrent use of astemizole, cisapride, midazolam, rifampin, or triazolam ▪ Lactation (breast-feeding should be avoided by HIV-infected patients).
Use Cautiously in: ▪ Hemophiliacs (increased risk of bleeding) ▪ Diabetes mellitus (may exacerbate condition) ▪ Patients with hepatic impairment.

ADVERSE REACTIONS AND SIDE EFFECTS*
CNS: SEIZURES, anxiety, depression, dizziness, drowsiness, emotional lability, headache, hyperkinesia, insomnia, malaise, migraine headache, sleep disorders, suicidal ideation, weakness.
EENT: acute iritis, pharyngitis, rhinitis, sinusitis.
Resp: dyspnea.
GI: diarrhea, anorexia, dyspepsia, elevated liver function studies, epigastric pain, flatulence, GI bleeding, hepatitis, nausea, oral ulcerations, pancreatitis, vomiting.
GU: nephrolithiasis, sexual dysfunction.
Derm: pruritus, rash, sweating, urticaria.
Endo: hyperglycemia.
F and E: dehydration.
Hemat: anemia, leukopenia, thrombocytopenia.
Metab: hyperlipidemia, hyperuricemia.
MS: arthralgia, arthritis, back pain, myalgia, myopathy.
Neuro: myasthenia, paresthesia.
Misc: allergic reactions, fever.

INTERACTIONS
Drug-Drug: ▪ Concurrent use of **astemizole, cisapride, dihydroergotamine** or **ergotamine, midazolam,** or **triazolam** should be avoided; may result in excess sedation, vasoconstriction, or serious cardiac arrhythmias ▪ Decreases metabolism and may increase effects of **rifabutin** (dosage of rifabutin should be reduced by **carbamazepine, phenobarbital, rifampin,** or **phenytoin** (concurrent use with rifampin should be avoided) ▪ Plasma levels and effectiveness may be increased by **ketoconazole, indinavir,** or **ritonavir** ▪ Increases plasma levels of **indinavir** and **saquinavir** ▪ May decrease plasma levels and effectiveness of **oral contraceptives.**
Drug-Food: ▪ **Food** enhances absorption.

ROUTE AND DOSAGE
- **PO (Adults and Children >13 yr):** 750 mg 3 times daily.
- **PO (Children 2–13 yr):** 20–30 mg/kg 3 times daily (not to exceed 750 mg 3 times daily).

AVAILABILITY
▪ ***Tablets:*** 250 mg[Rx] ▪ ***Oral powder:*** 50 mg nelfinavir/1 g powder (1 g powder/level scoopful).

TIME/ACTION PROFILE (plasma levels)

	ONSET	PEAK	DURATION
PO	rapid	2–4 hr	8 hr

*CAPITALS indicate life-threatening; underlines indicate most frequent.

N

NURSING IMPLICATIONS

ASSESSMENT

- □ Assess patient for change in severity of HIV symptoms and opportunistic infections throughout therapy.
- ■ ***Lab Test Considerations:*** Monitor viral load and CD4 cell counts regularly during therapy.
- □ May cause hyperglycemia.
- □ May cause elevated serum AST, ALT, total bilirubin, alkaline phosphatase, LDH, and CPK concentrations.
- □ May cause anemia, leukopenia, thrombocytopenia, hyperlipidemia, and hyperuricemia.

POTENTIAL NURSING DIAGNOSES

- ■ Infection, risk for (Indications).
- ■ Knowledge deficit, related to disease process and medication regimen (Patient/Family Teaching).
- ■ Noncompliance (Patient/Family Teaching).

IMPLEMENTATION

- ■ **PO:** Administer with a meal or light snack.
- □ Oral powder may be mixed with a small amount of water, milk, formula, soy formula, soy milk, or dietary supplements. Do not mix with acid food or juice (orange juice, apple juice, applesauce); results in a bitter taste. Do not reconstitute powder with water in its original container. Once mixed, the entire contents must be consumed to obtain the full dose. Mixture is stable for up to 6 hr.

PATIENT/FAMILY TEACHING

- □ Emphasize the importance of taking nelfinavir exactly as directed at evenly spaced times throughout the day. Do not take more than prescribed amount and do not stop taking without consulting health care professional. If a dose is missed, take as soon as remembered; do not double doses.
- □ Instruct patient that nelfinivir should not be shared with others.
- □ Advise patient to avoid taking other medications, prescription or OTC, without consulting health care professional.
- □ Inform patient that nelfinavir does not cure AIDS or prevent associated or opportunistic infections. Nelfinavir does not reduce the risk of transmission of HIV to others through sexual contact or blood contamination. Caution patient to avoid sexual contact or to use a condom and to avoid sharing needles or donating blood to prevent spreading the AIDS virus to others. Advise patient that the long-term effects of nelfinavir are unknown at this time.
- □ Inform patient that nelfinavir may cause hyperglycemia. Advise patient to notify health care professional if increased thirst or hunger; unexplained weight loss; increased urination; fatigue; or dry, itchy skin occurs.
- □ Advise patient that if diarrhea occurs, it can usually be controlled with OTC antidiarrheals, such as loperamide, which slow GI motility.
- □ Advise patient taking oral contraceptive to use a nonhormonal method of birth control during nelfinavir therapy.
- □ Emphasize the importance of regular follow-up and blood counts to determine progress and monitor for side effects.

EVALUATION

Effectiveness of therapy can be demonstrated by: ■ Delayed progression of AIDS and decreased opportunistic infections in patients with HIV ■ Improvement in CD4 cell count and decrease in viral load.

is achieved. Usual maintenance dose is 150 mg/day (up to 375 mg/day may be needed).
- **PO (Children):** 2 mg/kg/day (60 mg/m^2) in 6–8 divided doses.
- **SC, IM (Adults):** 0.5 mg.
- **SC, IM (Children):** 10–40 mcg/kg q 2–3 hr; may give with 10 mcg/kg atropine.

❑ **Bladder Atony, Abdominal Distention: Prevention**
- **IM, SC (Adults):** 250 mcg q 4–6 hr for 2–3 days.

❑ **Bladder Atony, Abdominal Distention: Treatment**
- **IM, SC (Adults):** 500 mcg as needed; may repeat q 3 hr for 5 doses after bladder has been emptied for bladder atony.

❑ **Antidote for Nondepolarizing Neuromuscular Blockers**
- **IV (Adults):** 0.5–2 mg slowly; pretreat with 0.6–1.2 mg atropine IV (may be repeated to a total dose of 5 mg).
- **IV (Children):** 40 mcg/kg with 20 mcg/kg atropine.

AVAILABILITY

▪ ***Tablets:*** 15 mg[Rx] ▪ ***Injection:*** 1:1000 in 10-ml vials[Rx], 1:2000 in 1-ml ampules and 10-ml vials[Rx], 1:4000 in 1-ml ampules[Rx] ▪ ***In combination with:*** atropine (Neostigmine Methylsulfate Min-I-Mix)[Rx].

TIME/ACTION PROFILE (cholinergic effects, increased muscle tone)

	ONSET	PEAK	DURATION
PO	45–75 min	UK	2–4 hr
IM	10–30 min	20–30 min	2–4 hr
IV	10–30 min	20–30 min	2–4 hr

NURSING IMPLICATIONS

ASSESSMENT

- **General Info:** Assess pulse, respiratory rate, and blood pressure prior to administration. Report significant changes in heart rate.
- **Myasthenia Gravis:** Assess neuromuscular status, including vital capacity, ptosis, diplopia, chewing, swallowing, hand grasp, and gait, prior to administering and at peak effect. Patients with myasthenia gravis may be advised to keep a daily record of their condition and the effects of this medication.
  - ❑ Assess patient for overdosage and underdosage or resistance. Both have similar symptoms (muscle weakness, dyspnea, dysphagia), but symptoms of overdosage usually occur within 1 hr of administration, whereas underdosage symptoms occur 3 or more hr after administration. Overdosage (cholinergic crisis) symptoms may also include increased respiratory secretions and saliva, bradycardia, nausea, vomiting, cramping, diarrhea, and diaphoresis. A Tensilon test (edrophonium chloride) may be used to distinguish between overdosage and underdosage.
- **Postoperative Ileus:** Monitor abdominal status (assess for distention, auscultate bowel sounds). A rectal tube may be inserted to facilitate expulsion of flatus.
- **Postoperative Urinary Retention:** Assess for bladder distention. Monitor intake and output. If patient is unable to void within 1 hr of neostigmine administration, consider catheterization.
- **Antidote to Nondepolarizing Neuromuscular Blocking Agents:** Monitor reversal of effects of neuromuscular blocking agents with a peripheral nerve stimulator. Recovery usually occurs consecutively in the following muscles: diaphragm, intercostal muscles, muscles of the glottis, abdominal muscles, limb muscles, muscles of mastication, and levator muscles of the eyelids. Closely observe the patient for residual muscle weakness and respiratory distress throughout the recovery period. Maintain airway patency and ventilation until recovery of normal respirations occurs.
- ***Toxicity and Overdose:*** If overdose occurs, atropine is the antidote.

POTENTIAL NURSING DIAGNOSES

- Physical mobility, impaired (Indications).
- Breathing pattern, ineffective (Indications).
- Knowledge deficit, related to medication regimen (Patient/Family Teaching).

IMPLEMENTATION

- **General Info:** Oral and parenteral doses are not interchangeable.

□ When used as an antidote to nondepolarizing neuromuscular blocking agents, atropine may be used prior to or currently with neostigmine to prevent or treat bradycardia.
■ **PO:** Administer with food or milk to minimize side effects. For patients who have difficulty chewing, neostigmine may be taken 30 min before meals.
■ **Direct IV:** Administer doses undiluted. May be given through Y-site of an IV of D5W, 0.9% NaCl, Ringer's solution, or lactated Ringer's solution.
■ ***Rate:*** Administer each 0.5 mg over 1 min.
■ **Syringe Compatibility:** ■ glycopyrrolate ■ heparin ■ pentobarbital ■ thiopental.
■ **Y-Site Compatibility:** ■ heparin ■ hydrocortisone sodium succinate ■ potassium chloride ■ vitamin B complex with C.

PATIENT/FAMILY TEACHING

□ Instruct patient to take medication exactly as directed. Do not skip or double up on missed doses. Patients with a history of dysphagia should have a nonelectric or battery-operated backup alarm clock to remind them of exact dose time. Patients with dysphagia may not be able to swallow the medication if the dose is not taken exactly on time. Taking the dose late may result in myasthenic crisis. Taking the dose early may result in cholinergic crisis. Patients with myasthenia gravis must continue this regimen as a lifelong therapy.
□ Instruct patient with myasthenia gravis to space activities to avoid fatigue.
□ Advise patient to carry identification describing disease and medication regimen at all times.

EVALUATION

Effectiveness of therapy can be demonstrated by: ■ Relief of ptosis and diplopia □ Improved chewing, swallowing, extremity strength, and breathing without the appearance of cholinergic symptoms in myasthenia gravis ■ Relief or prevention of postoperative gastrointestinal ileus ■ Relief of nonobstructive postoperative urinary retention ■ Reversal of nondepolarizing neuromuscular blocking agents in general anesthesia.

NEUROMUSCULAR BLOCKING AGENTS (nondepolarizing)

atracurium
(a-tra-**cure**-ee-um)
Tracrium

cisatracurium
(siss-a-tra-**kyoor**-ee-um)
Nimbex

doxacurium
(dox-a-**cure**-ee-yum)
Nuromax

gallamine
(**gal**-a-meen)
Flaxedil

metocurine
(me-toe-**cure**-een)
Metubine

mivacurium
(mi-va-**cure**-ee-um)
Mivacron

pancuronium
(pan-cure-**oh**-nee-yum)
Pavulon

pipecuronium
(pip-e-**kyoor**-oh-nee-um)
Arduan

rocuronium
(roe-kyoor-**own**-ee-um)
Zemuron

tubocurarine
(too-boh-**cure**-a-reen)
{Tubarine}

vecuronium
(ve-cure-**oh**-nee-yum)
Norcuron

CLASSIFICATION(S):
Neuromuscular blocking agents (nondepolarizing)

Pregnancy Category C

{} = Available in Canada only.

INDICATIONS

■ Induction of skeletal muscle paralysis and facilitation of intubation after induction of anesthesia in surgical procedures ■ Facilitation of compliance during mechanical ventilation ■ **Metocurine, tubocurarine:** Adjunct to electroconvulsive therapy ■ **Tubocurarine:** Diagnostic agent for myasthenia gravis.

ACTION

■ Prevent neuromuscular transmission by blocking the effect of acetylcholine at the myoneural junction. Have no analgesic or anxiolytic properties. **Therapeutic Effects:** ■ Skeletal muscle paralysis.

PHARMACOKINETICS

Absorption: Following IV administration, absorption is essentially complete. *Tubocurarine*—Although well absorbed following IM administration, effect is delayed as compared with IV administration.

Distribution: *Atracurium, gallamine*—Distribute into extracellular space; cross the placenta. *Metocurine*—Extensively distributed; crosses the placenta. *Mivacurium*—Tissue distribution is limited. *Pancuronium*—Rapidly distributes into extracellular fluid; small amounts cross the placenta. *Tubocurarine*—Extensively distributed and subsequently redistributed to various tissue compartments; saturation of compartments occurs, explaining prolonged duration of action following repeated doses. *Vecuronium*—Rapidly distributed in extracellular fluid; minimal penetration of the CNS.

Metabolism and Excretion: *Atracurium, mivacurium*—Metabolized in plasma. *Cisatracurium*—Undergoes pH-dependent breakdown, which is responsible for 80% of metabolism; remainder eliminated by liver and kidneys. *Doxacurium*—Excreted primarily unchanged in urine and bile. *Gallamine*—Excreted almost entirely unchanged by the kidneys. *Metocurine*—50% excreted unchanged in urine. *Pancuronium*—Excreted mostly unchanged by the kidneys; small amounts are eliminated in bile. *Pipecuronium*—>75% excreted by the kidneys, mostly as unmetabolized drug. *Rocuronium*—Mostly metabolized by the liver. *Tubocurarine*—30–75% excreted unchanged by the kidneys; 11% excreted in bile; small amounts are metabolized by the liver. *Vecuronium*—Some metabolism by the liver (20%), with conversion to at least one active metabolite; 35% excreted unchanged by the kidneys.

Half-life: *Atracurium*—20 min; *cisatracurium*—22–29 min; *doxacurium*—90–120 min (increased in kidney transplant patients); *gallamine*—2.5 hr; *metocurine*—3.6 hr; *mivacurium*—2 hr; *pancuronium*—2 hr; *pipecuronium*—1.7 hr (prolonged in renal impairment); *rocuronium*—1.4 hr (increased in hepatic impairment; *tubocurarine*—2 hr; *vecuronium*—31–80 min (decreased near term in pregnant patients, increased in patients with hepatic impairment).

CONTRAINDICATIONS AND PRECAUTIONS

Contraindicated in: ■ Hypersensitivity ■ Hypersensitivity to bromides (pancuronium, vecuronium only) ■ Hypersensitivity to iodides/iodine (gallamine, metocurine only) ■ Products containing benzyl alcohol should be avoided in neonates.

Use Cautiously in: ■ Patients with underlying cardiovascular disease (increased risk of arrhythmias; less with atracurium or vecuronium) ■ Dehydration or electrolyte abnormalities (should be corrected) ■ Situations in which histamine release would be problematic (worse with atracurium, mivacurium, and doxacurium; less with cisatracurium and vecuronium) ■ Fractures or muscle spasm ■ Geriatric patients or patients with impaired renal function (slower onset to complete paralysis with cisatracurium; decreased elimination of gallamine, metocurine, pancuronium, tubocurarine) ■ Hyperthermia (increased duration/intensity of paralysis) ■ Patients with significant hepatic impairment (decreased metabolism of vecuronium) ■ Shock (prolonged paralysis from gallamine, metocurine, tubocurarine) ■ Extensive burns (may be more resistant to effects of cisatracurium) ■ Low plasma pseudocholinesterase levels (may be seen in association with anemia, dehydration, cholinesterase inhibitors/insecticides, severe liver disease, pregnancy, or hereditary predisposition) ■ Pregnancy, lactation, or children (safety not established for some agents; most agents have been used safely in pregnant women undergoing cesarean section; selected agents have been used safely in children). **Exercise Extreme Caution in:** ▪ Patients with neuromuscular diseases such as myasthenia gravis (small test dose may be used to assess response).

ADVERSE REACTIONS AND SIDE EFFECTS*

Resp: bronchospasm.
CV: *tubocurarine*—arrhythmias; *atracurium, metocurine, tubocurarine*—hypotension (↑ with tubocurarine); *pancuronium, gallamine*—hypertension (↑ with gallamine); *atracurium, pancuronium, gallamine*—tachycardia (↑ with gallamine).
GI: *pancuronium*—excessive salivation.
Derm: rash; *atracurium*—skin flushing.
Misc: allergic reactions including ANAPHYLAXIS.

INTERACTIONS

Drug-Drug: ▪ Intensity and duration of paralysis may be prolonged by pretreatment with **succinylcholine, general anesthesia** (inhalation), **aminoglycosides, polymyxin B, colistin, clindamycin, lidocaine, quinidine, procainamide, beta-adrenergic blocking agents, potassium-losing diuretics**, or **magnesium** ▪ Effects of cisatracurium may be enhanced by concurrent **enflurane** or **isoflurane** (dosage requirements may be decreased by 30–40%; smaller boluses and lower infusion rates may be necessary) ▪ Higher infusion rates of cisatracurium may be required and duration of action may be shortened in patients receiving long-term **carbamazepine** or **phenytoin.**

ROUTE AND DOSAGE

❑ Atracurium

- **IV (Adults and Children >2 yr):** 0.3–0.5 mg/kg initially (0.25–0.35 mg/kg if administered after steady-state anesthesia with enflurane or isoflurane or 0.3–0.4 mg/kg following succinylcholine), then by continuous infusion at 2–15 mcg/kg/min.
- **IV (Children 1 mo–2 yr):** 0.3–0.4 mg/kg initially (while under halothane anesthesia).

❑ Cisatracurium

- **IV (Adults):** *Initial intubating dose*—0.15–0.2 mg/kg additional maintenance doses of 0.03 mg/kg may be used; *continuous infusion*—1–3 mcg/kg/min.
- **IV (Children 2–12 yr):** *Initial intubating dose*—0.1 mg/kg; *continuous infusion*—1–3 mcg/kg/min.

❑ Doxacurium

- **IV (Adults):** 50 mcg/kg (may need up to 80 mcg/kg for prolonged effect; 25 mcg/kg for succinylcholine-assisted intubation) initially, followed 60–100 min later by 5–10 mcg/kg, repeated as required.
- **IV (Children 2–12 yr):** 30–50 mcg/kg initially; maintenance doses may be required more frequently than in adults.

❑ Gallamine

- **IV (Adults and Children):** 1 mg/kg (not to exceed 100 mg/dose), then 0.5–1 mg/kg may be given 30–40 min later if needed during prolonged procedures; dose cautiously in patients <5 kg.

❑ Metocurine

- **IV (Adults):** 150–400 mcg/kg initially; may give additional doses of 0.5–1 mg q 30–90 min. *Adjunct to electroconvulsive therapy*—2–3 mg (range 1.75–5.5 mg).

❑ Mivacurium

- **IV (Adults):** 150–200 mcg/kg initially, then 100 mcg/kg as bolus doses every 15 min or as a continuous infusion at 9–10 mcg/kg/min. If infusion is begun at the same time as initial dose, start with rate of 4 mcg/kg/min. Infusion rates may range from 1–20 mcg/kg/min.
- **IV (Children 2–12 yr):** 200–250 mcg/kg initially; may be repeated as needed or continued as an infusion at 14 mcg/kg/min (range 5–31 mcg/kg/min).

❑ Pancuronium

- **IV (Adults and Children >1 mo):** 40–100 mcg/kg initially; incremental doses of 10 mcg/kg may be given q 20–60 min to maintain paralysis. *Provision of relaxation to allow mechanical ventilation*—15 mcg/kg.

***CAPITALS indicate life-threatening; underlines indicate most frequent.**

❑ **Pipecuronium**

- **IV (Adults):** 70–85 mcg/kg (if given following recovery from succinylcholine during intubation, decrease dose to 50 mcg/kg; 70–85 mcg/kg if longer paralysis desired). Additional doses of 10–15 mcg/kg may be required as maintenance (dosage reduction recommended if using concurrent inhalation anesthetics). Dose should be determined on the basis of ideal body weight in obese patients and may require adjustments in patients with renal impairment.
- **IV (Children 1–14 yr):** 57 mcg/kg initial dose.
- **IV (Infants 3 mo–1 yr):** 40 mcg/kg initial dose.

❑ **Rocuronium**

- **IV (Adults):** *Rapid sequence tracheal intubation*—600 mcg (0.6 mg)/kg; *maintenance dosing*—100–200 mcg (0.1–0.2 mg)/kg; *continuous infusion*—10–12 mcg (0.01–0.012 mg)/kg/min (range 4–16 mcg/kg/min).
- **IV (Children):** *Intubation dose*—600 mcg (0.6 mg)/kg; *maintenance dose*—75–125 mcg (0.075–0.125 mg)/kg; *continuous infusion*—12 mcg (0.012 mg)/kg/min.

❑ **Tubocurarine**

Preferred route is IV, but IM may be used in infants or other patients without venous access.

- **IM, IV (Adults):** 6–9 mg initially, followed by 3–4.5 mg after 3–5 min if needed. Additional doses of 3 mg (0.165 mg/kg) may be given as needed. *Provision of relaxation to allow mechanical ventilation*—1 mg IV (16.5 mcg/kg); subsequent doses may be given as necessary. *Adjunct to electroconvulsive therapy*—165 mcg/kg IV (initial doses should be 3 mg less than calculated dose). *Diagnosis of myasthenia gravis*—4–33 mcg/kg IV. Profound myasthenic symptoms may occur.
- **IV (Infants and Children):** 500 mcg/kg.
- **IV (Neonates–4 wk):** 250–500 mcg/kg initially, then additional increments of ⅕–⅙ of initial dose may be given.

❑ **Vecuronium**

- **IV (Adults and Children >10 yr):** *Intubation*—80–100 mcg/kg for intubation (60–85 mcg/kg if given after steady-state anesthesia achieved or 40–60 mcg/kg after succinylcholine-assisted intubation and anesthesia; wait for disappearance of succinylcholine effects; or 50–60 mcg/kg during balanced anesthesia). Up to 150–280 mcg/kg have been used in some patients. *Maintenance*—10–15 mcg/kg 25–40 min after initial dose, then q 12–15 min as needed or as a continuous infusion at 1 mcg/kg/min (range 0.8–1.2 mcg/kg/min).

AVAILABILITY

❑ **Atracurium**

- ***Injection:*** 10 mg/ml in 5-ml ampules and 10-ml vials[Rx].

❑ **Cisatracurium**

- ***Solution for injection:*** 2 mg/ml in 5-ml single-use vials[Rx] or 10-ml multiple-dose vials (with benzyl alcohol)[Rx].

❑ **Doxacurium**

- ***Injection:*** 1 mg/ml in 5-ml vials[Rx].

❑ **Gallamine**

- ***Injection:*** 20 mg/ml in 10-ml vials[Rx].

❑ **Metocurine**

- ***Injection:*** 2 mg/ml in 20-ml vials[Rx].

❑ **Mivacurium**

- ***Injection:*** 0.5 mg/ml premixed infusion in 50 ml D5W[Rx], 2 mg/ml in 5- and 10-ml vials[Rx].

❑ **Pancuronium**

- ***Injection:*** 1 mg/ml in 10-ml vials[Rx], 2 mg/ml in 2- and 5-ml ampules[Rx].

❑ **Pipecuronium**

- ***Powder for injection:*** 10 mg/vial[Rx].

❑ **Rocuronium**

- ***Injection:*** 10 mg/ml in 5-ml vials[Rx].

❑ **Tubocurarine**

- ***Injection:*** 3 mg (20 units)/min 10- and 20-ml vials and 5-ml syringes[Rx].

❑ **Vecuronium**

- ***Powder for injection:*** 10 mg in 5- and 10-ml vials[Rx].

TIME/ACTION PROFILE (neuromuscular blockade)

	ONSET	PEAK	DURATION
Atracurium IV	2–2.5 min	5 min	30–40 min
Cisatracurium IV	1.5–2.8 min	2.9–3.5 min	28–50 min
Doxacurium IV*	5 min	UK	100 min
Gallamine IV	1–2 min	3–5 min	15–30 min
Metocurine IV	within min	6 min	25–90 min†
Mivacurium IV (adults)	rapid	3.3 min	26 min
Mivacurium IV (children)	rapid	1.9 min	19 min
Pancuronium IV	30–45 sec	3–4.5 min	35–45 min
Pipecuronium IV	2.5–3 min	5 min	1–2 hr
Rocuronium IV	1 min	1.8 min	31 min‡
Tubocurarine IV	1 min	2–5 min	2–90 min
Tubocurarine IM	15–25 min	UK	UK
Vecuronium IV	1 min	3–5 min	15–25 min

*For a 0.05 mg/kg dose in an adult.
†Total recovery of function may take several hr.
‡Following 0.6 mg/kg dose in adult patients.

NURSING IMPLICATIONS

ASSESSMENT

- Assess respiratory status continuously throughout therapy with neuromuscular blocking agents. These medications should be used only to facilitate intubation or in patients already intubated.
- Neuromuscular response should be monitored with a peripheral nerve stimulator intraoperatively. Paralysis is initially selective and usually occurs sequentially in the following muscles: levator muscles of eyelids, muscles of mastication, limb muscles, abdominal muscles, muscles of the glottis, intercostal muscles, and the diaphragm. Recovery of muscle function usually occurs in reverse order.
- Monitor ECG, heart rate, and blood pressure throughout administration.
- Observe the patient for residual muscle weakness and respiratory distress during the recovery period.
- Monitor infusion site frequently. If signs of tissue irritation or extravasation occur, discontinue and restart in another vein.
- ***Toxicity and Overdose:*** If overdose occurs, use peripheral nerve stimulator to determine the degree of neuromuscular blockade. Maintain airway patency and ventilation until recovery of normal respirations occurs.
- Administration of anticholinesterase agents (neostigmine, pyridostigmine) may be used to antagonize the action of neuromuscular blocking agents once the patient has demonstrated some spontaneous recovery from neuromuscular block. Atropine is usually administered prior to or concurrently with anticholinesterase agents to counteract the muscarinic effects.
- Administration of fluids and vasopressors may be necessary to treat severe hypotension or shock.

POTENTIAL NURSING DIAGNOSES

- Breathing pattern, ineffective (Indications).
- Communication, impaired verbal (Side Effects).
- Fear (Side Effects).

IMPLEMENTATION

- **General Info:** Dose is titrated to patient response.
- Neuromuscular blocking agents have *no* effect on consciousness or pain threshold. Adequate anesthesia/analgesia should *always* be used when neuromuscular blocking agents are used as an adjunct to surgical procedures or when painful procedures are performed. Benzodiazepines and/or analgesics should be administered concurrently when prolonged neuromuscular blocker therapy is used for ventilator patients, because patient is awake and able to feel all sensations.
- If eyes remain open throughout prolonged administration, protect corneas with artificial tears.
- Store atracurium, cisatracurium, gallamine, metocurine, pancuronium, rocuronium, and vecuronium in refrigerator. To prevent absorption by plastic, pancuronium should not be stored in plastic syringes. May be administered in plastic syringes. Store doxacurium, mivacurium, and pipecuronium at room temperature.
- Most neuromuscular blocking agents are incompatible with barbiturates and sodium bicarbonate. Do not admix.

Atracurium

- **Direct IV:** May be administered undiluted.
- ***Rate:*** Administer initial IV dose as a bolus over 1 min.
- **Intermittent Infusion:** Maintenance dose is

usually required 20–45 min following initial dose.

- Dilute further in D5W, 0.9% NaCl, or D5/0.9% NaCl and administer every 15–25 min or by continuous infusion.
- **Continuous Infusion:** Maintenance dose is administered by infusion.
- ***Rate:*** Titrate according to patient response.
- **Syringe Compatibility:** ▪ alfentanil ▪ fentanyl ▪ midazolam ▪ sufentanil.
- **Y-Site Compatibility:** ▪ cefazolin ▪ cefuroxime ▪ cimetidine ▪ dobutamine ▪ dopamine ▪ epinephrine ▪ esmolol ▪ etomidate ▪ fentanyl ▪ gentamicin ▪ heparin ▪ hydrocortisone sodium succinate ▪ isoproterenol ▪ lorazepam ▪ midazolam ▪ morphine ▪ nitroglycerin ▪ nitroprusside ▪ ranitidine ▪ trimethoprim/sulfamethoxazole ▪ vancomycin.
- **Y-Site Incompatibility:** ▪ diazepam ▪ propofol ▪ thiopental.

❑ Cisatracurium

- **Direct IV:** May be administered undiluted.
- ***Rate:*** Administer over 5–10 sec.
- **Intermittent Infusion:** May be diluted in D5W, 0.9% NaCl, or D5/0.9% NaCl. Solution is stable for 24 hr at room temperature or if refrigerated.
- ***Rate:*** Administer at an initial rate of 3 mcg/kg/min, then decrease to 1–2 mcg/kg/min.
- **Y-Site Incompatibility:** ▪ ketorolac ▪ propofol.
- **Additive Compatibility:** ▪ droperidol ▪ fentanyl ▪ midazolam ▪ sufentanil.

❑ Doxacurium

- **Direct IV:** Administer initial IV dose as a bolus over 1 min. Maintenance dose is usually required 60 min following initial dose of 0.025 mg/kg or 100 min following initial dose of 0.05 mg/kg. May be diluted further in D5W or 0.9% NaCl. Use diluted doxacurium within 8 hr. Discard unused diluted doxacurium after 8 hr.
- ***Rate:*** Administer every 30–45 min.
- **Y-Site Compatibility:** ▪ D5/0.9% NaCl ▪ Lactated Ringer's (LR) ▪ D5/LR ▪ alfentanil ▪ fentanyl ▪ sufentanil.

❑ Gallamine

- **Direct IV:** Administer each single dose undiluted as a bolus over 30–60 sec.

❑ Metocurine

- **Direct IV:** Administer over 30–60 sec. Relaxation from initial dose lasts 25–90 min (average 60 min); administer supplemental doses of 0.5–1 mg as needed.
- **Syringe Incompatibility:** ▪ barbiturates ▪ meperidine ▪ morphine ▪ sodium bicarbonate.

❑ Mivacurium

- **Direct IV:** May be administered undiluted.
- ***Rate:*** Administer over 5–15 min.
- **Continuous Infusion:** May be diluted to 0.5 mg/ml in D5W, D5/0.9% NaCl, 0.9% NaCl, LR, or D5/LR. Solution is stable for 24 hr at room temperature. Discard unused portion after each use. Also available in premixed infusion of D5W.
- ***Rate:*** Titrate rate according to patient response and peripheral nerve stimulator.
- **Y-Site Compatibility:** ▪ alfentanil ▪ droperidol ▪ etomidate ▪ fentanyl ▪ midazolam ▪ sufentanil ▪ thiopental.
- **Y-Site Incompatibility:** ▪ barbiturates.

❑ Pancuronium

- **Direct IV:** Incremental doses may be administered every 20–60 min as needed. Dose is titrated to patient response.
- **Intermittent Infusion:** May be diluted in 0.9% NaCl, D5W, D5/0.9% NaCl, and LR injection. Solution is stable for 48 hr.
- ***Rate:*** Titrate rate according to patient response.
- **Syringe Compatibility:** ▪ heparin.
- **Y-Site Compatibility:** ▪ aminophylline ▪ cefazolin ▪ cefuroxime ▪ cimetidine ▪ dobutamine ▪ dopamine ▪ epinephrine ▪ esmolol ▪ etomidate ▪ fentanyl ▪ fluconazole ▪ gentamicin ▪ heparin ▪ hydrocortisone sodium succinate ▪ isoproterenol ▪ lorazepam ▪ midazolam ▪ morphine ▪ nitroglycerin ▪ nitroprusside ▪ ranitidine ▪ trimethoprim/sulfamethoxazole ▪ vancomycin.
- **Y-Site Incompatibility:** ▪ diazepam ▪ thiopental.

❑ Pipecuronium

- **Direct IV:** Reconstitute with 0.9% NaCl, D5W, D5/0.9% NaCl, LR, sterile water for injection, or bacteriostatic water for injection. Solution reconstituted with bacteriostatic water contains benzyl alcohol and should not be used for newborns; use within 5 days. Solution reconstituted with sterile water or other IV solutions should be refrigerated and used within 24 hr. Do not dilute into or administer from large-volume IV solutions.

❑ Rocuronium

- **Direct IV:** Administer undiluted.
- ***Rate:*** Titrate according to patient response.
- **Continuous Infusion:** May be diluted in solution with 0.9% NaCl, sterile water for injection, D5W, LR injection, and D5/0.9% NaCl for infusion. Solution is stable for 24 hr at room temperature.
- ***Rate:*** Infusion rates of 0.004–0.016 mg/kg/min have been used. Rate of infusion should be titrated according to patient's twitch response as monitored with a peripheral nerve stimulator.
- **Syringe/Y-Site Incompatibility:** ▪ alkaline solutions ▪ barbiturates.

❑ Tubocurarine

- **Direct IV:** Administer IV dose undiluted over 1–1.5 min. Rapid injection or large doses cause histamine release, resulting in hypotension and bronchospasm. Titrate dose to patient response.
- **Syringe Compatibility:** ▪ pentobarbital ▪ thiopental.
- **Solution Compatibility:** ▪ dextrose in Ringer's or LR combinations ▪ dextrose in saline combinations ▪ D5W ▪ D10W ▪ 0.45% NaCl ▪ 0.9% NaCl ▪ Ringer's and LR injection.
- **Additive Incompatibility:** ▪ Incompatible with most barbiturates, sodium bicarbonate, and trimethaphan.

❑ Vecuronium

- **IV:** Reconstitute vecuronium with bacteriostatic water (may be provided by manufacturer), D5W, 0.9% NaCl, D5/0.9% NaCl, or LR injection. Solution reconstituted with bacteriostatic water is stable if refrigerated for 5 days. If other diluents are used, solution is stable for 24 hr if refrigerated. Discard all unused solution.
- **Direct IV:** Reconstitute each dose in 5 ml. Titrate dose according to patient response.
- **Continuous Infusion:** Dilute vecuronium to a concentration of 10–20 mg/100 ml.
- ***Rate:*** Titrate rate of infusion according to patient response.
- **Syringe/Y-Site Incompatibility:** Incompatible in syringe or via Y-site injection with most barbiturates.
- **Y-Site Compatibility:** ▪ aminophylline ▪ cefazolin ▪ cefuroxime ▪ cimetidine ▪ dopamine ▪ epinephrine ▪ esmolol ▪ fentanyl ▪ gentamicin ▪ heparin ▪ hydrocortisone sodium succinate ▪ isoproterenol ▪ lorazepam ▪ midazolam ▪ morphine ▪ nitroglycerin ▪ nitroprusside ▪ ranitidine ▪ trimethoprim/sulfamethoxazole ▪ vancomycin.
- **Y-Site Incompatibility:** ▪ diazepam ▪ etomidate ▪ thiopental.

PATIENT/FAMILY TEACHING

- ❑ Explain all procedures to patient receiving neuromuscular blocker therapy without general anesthesia, because consciousness is not affected by neuromuscular blocking agents alone.
- ❑ Reassure patient that communication abilities will return as the medication wears off.

EVALUATION

Effectiveness of therapy can be demonstrated by: ▪ Adequate suppression of the twitch response when tested with peripheral nerve stimulation and subsequent muscle paralysis ▪ Diagnosis of myasthenia gravis.

NEVIRAPINE

(ne-**veer**-a-peen)
Viramune

CLASSIFICATION(S):
Antiretroviral (reverse transcriptase inhibitor)

Pregnancy Category C

INDICATIONS

▪ Management of HIV infection in combination with a nucleoside analogue.

ACTION

▪ Binds to the enzyme reverse transcriptase, which results in disruption of DNA synthesis. **Therapeutic Effects:** ▪ Slowed progression of HIV infection and decreased occurrence of sequelae.

PHARMACOKINETICS

Absorption: >90% absorbed following oral administration.
Distribution: Crosses the placenta and enters breast milk; enters CSF in levels that are 45% of those in plasma.
Metabolism and Excretion: Mostly metabolized by the liver; minor amounts excreted unchanged in urine.
Half-life: 25–30 hr (during multiple dosing).

CONTRAINDICATIONS AND PRECAUTIONS

Contraindicated in: ▪ Hypersensitivity.
Use Cautiously in: ▪ Hepatic or renal impairment ▪ Pregnancy, lactation, or children (safety not established; breast-feeding not recommended in HIV-infected patients).

ADVERSE REACTIONS AND SIDE EFFECTS*

Seen during combination therapy.
CNS: headache.
GI: abdominal pain, diarrhea, elevated liver enzymes, hepatitis, nausea, ulcerative stomatitis.
Derm: RASH.
MS: myalgia.
Neuro: paresthesia, peripheral neuropathy.
Misc: STEVENS-JOHNSON SYNDROME, fever.

INTERACTIONS

Drug-Drug: ▪ May decrease plasma levels and effectiveness of **protease inhibitor antiretrovirals** and **oral contraceptives** ▪ May alter blood levels and effectiveness of **rifampin** or **rifabutin** (use together only with careful monitoring).

ROUTE AND DOSAGE

- **PO (Adults):** 200 mg daily for the first 2 wk, then 200 mg twice daily (in combination with a nucleoside analogue antiretroviral).

AVAILABILITY

- ***Tablets:*** 200 mg[Rx].

TIME/ACTION PROFILE (blood levels)

	ONSET	PEAK	DURATION
PO	rapid	4 hr	12 hr

NURSING IMPLICATIONS

ASSESSMENT

- □ Assess patient for change in severity of HIV symptoms and for symptoms of opportunistic infections throughout therapy.
- □ Assess patient for rash, especially during 1st mo of therapy. If rash is severe or accompanied by systemic symptoms, therapy must be discontinued immediately.
- ▪ ***Lab Test Considerations:*** Monitor viral load and CD4 cell count regularly during therapy.
- □ May cause elevated serum AST, ALT, and GGT concentrations. If moderate to severe liver function test abnormalities occur, nevirapine doses should be held until levels return to normal. Discontinue if liver function abnormalities recur when therapy is resumed.

POTENTIAL NURSING DIAGNOSES

- ▪ Infection, risk for (Indications).
- ▪ Knowledge deficit, related to disease process and medication regimen (Patient/Family Teaching).
- ▪ Noncompliance (Patient/Family Teaching).

IMPLEMENTATION

- ▪ **PO:** May be administered with or without food.
- □ If therapy is interrupted for more than 7 days, restart therapy at 200 mg daily for 14 days, then increase dose to 200 mg twice daily.

PATIENT/FAMILY TEACHING

- □ Emphasize the importance of taking nevirapine exactly as directed, at evenly spaced times throughout day. Do not take more than prescribed amount and do not stop taking without consulting health care professional. If a dose is missed, take as soon as remembered; do not double doses.
- □ Instruct patient that nevirapine should not be shared with others.
- □ Advise patient to avoid taking other medications, prescription or OTC, without consulting health care professional.
- □ Inform patient that nevirapine does not cure AIDS or prevent associated or opportunistic infections. Nevirapine does not reduce the risk of transmission of HIV to others through sex-

N

*CAPITALS indicate life-threatening; underlines indicate most frequent.

ual contact or blood contamination. Caution patient to use a condom and avoid sharing needles or donating blood to prevent spreading the AIDS virus to others. Advise patient that the long-term effects of nevirapine are unknown at this time.

- □ Advise patients taking oral contraceptives to use a nonhormonal method of birth control during nevirapine therapy.
- □ Advise patient not to take other medications concurrently without consulting health care professional.
- □ Instruct patient to notify health care professional immediately if rash occurs.
- □ Emphasize the importance of regular follow-up exams and blood counts to determine progress and monitor for side effects.

EVALUATION

Effectiveness of therapy can be demonstrated by: ▪ Delayed progression of AIDS and decreased opportunistic infections in patients with HIV ▪ Decrease in viral load and increase in CD4 cell counts.

NIACIN

(**nye**-a-sin)
Edur-Acin, Nia-Bid, Niac, Niacels, Niacor, Nicobid, Nico-400, Nicolar, Nicotinex, nicotinic acid, {Novo-Niacin}, Slo-Niacin, vitamin B_3

NIACINAMIDE

(nye-a-**sin**-a-mide)
nicotinamide

CLASSIFICATION(S):
Lipid-lowering agents, Vitamins (water-soluble)

Pregnancy Category C

INDICATIONS

▪ Treatment and prevention of niacin deficiency (pellagra) ▪ Adjunctive therapy in certain hyperlipidemias (niacin only).

ACTION

▪ Required as coenzymes (for lipid metabolism, glycogenolysis, and tissue respiration) ▪ Large doses decrease lipoprotein and triglyceride synthesis by inhibiting the release of free fatty acids from adipose tissue and decreasing hepatic lipoprotein synthesis (niacin only) ▪ Causes peripheral vasodilation in large doses (niacin only). **Therapeutic Effects:** ▪ Decreased blood lipids (niacin only) ▪ Supplementation in deficiency states.

PHARMACOKINETICS

Absorption: Well absorbed following oral administration.
Distribution: Widely distributed following conversion to niacinamide. Enter breast milk.
Metabolism and Excretion: Amounts required for metabolic processes are converted to niacinamide. Large doses of niacin are excreted unchanged in the urine.
Half-life: 45 min.

CONTRAINDICATIONS AND PRECAUTIONS

Contraindicated in: ▪ Hypersensitivity to niacin ▪ Some products may contain tartrazine and should be avoided in patients with known hypersensitivity ▪ Alcohol intolerance (Nicotinex only).
Use Cautiously in: ▪ Liver disease ▪ Arterial bleeding ▪ History of peptic ulcer disease ▪ Gout ▪ Glaucoma ▪ Diabetes mellitus.

ADVERSE REACTIONS AND SIDE EFFECTS*

Adverse reactions and side effects refer to IV administration or doses used to treat hyperlipidemias.
CNS: nervousness, panic.
EENT: blurred vision, loss of central vision, proptosis, toxic amblyopia.
CV: orthostatic hypotension.
GI: HEPATOTOXICITY (ER oral form only), GI upset, bloating, diarrhea, dry mouth, flatulence, heartburn, hunger pains, nausea, peptic ulceration.
Derm: flushing of the face and neck, pruritus, burning, dry skin, hyperpigmentation, increased sebaceous gland activity, rashes, stinging or tingling of skin.
Metab: glycosuria, hyperglycemia, hyperuricemia.

{} = Available in Canada only.
***CAPITALS indicate life-threatening; underlines indicate most frequent.**

INTERACTIONS

Drug-Drug: ▪ Increased risk of myopathy with concurrent use of **HMG-CoA reductase inhibitors** ▪ Additive hypotension with **ganglionic blocking agents (guanethidine, guanadrel)** ▪ Large doses may decrease the uricosuric effects of **probenecid** or **sulfinpyrazone.**

ROUTE AND DOSAGE

- **PO (Adults and Children):** *Dietary supplement*—10–20 mg/day. *Dietary deficiency*—Up to 500 mg/day in divided doses. *Hyperlipidemias–Niacin only*—100–500 mg/day initially; increase slowly up to 1–2 g tid (up to 8 g/day).
- **PO (Children 7–10 yr):** *Prevention of deficiency*—13 mg/day.
- **PO (Children 4–6 yr):** *Prevention of deficiency*—12 mg/day.
- **PO (Children birth–3 yr):** *Prevention of deficiency*—5–9 mg/day.

AVAILABILITY

❑ **Niacin**

▪ ***Tablets:*** 25 mg[OTC], 50 mg[OTC], 100 mg[OTC], 125 mg[OTC], 250 mg[OTC], 400 mg[OTC], 500 mg[Rx,OTC] ▪ ***Extended-release tablets:*** 125 mg[Rx], 250 mg[Rx,OTC], 400 mg[OTC], 500 mg[Rx,OTC], 750 mg[Rx,OTC], 1000 mg[OTC] ▪ ***Extended-release capsules:*** 125 mg[Rx,OTC], 250 mg[Rx,OTC], 300 mg[Rx,OTC], 400 mg[Rx,OTC], 500 mg[Rx,OTC] ▪ ***Elixir:*** 50 mg/5 ml in pints and gallons[OTC].

❑ **Niacinamide**

▪ ***Tablets:*** 50 mg[OTC], 100 mg[OTC], 125 mg[OTC], 250 mg[OTC], 500 mg[Rx,OTC].

TIME/ACTION PROFILE (effects on blood lipids)

	ONSET	PEAK	DURATION
PO (cholesterol)	several days	UK	UK
PO (triglycerides)	several hr	UK	UK

NURSING IMPLICATIONS

ASSESSMENT

- **Vitamin Deficiency:** Assess patient for signs of niacin deficiency (*pellagra*—dermatitis, stomatitis, glossitis, anemia, nausea and vomiting, confusion, memory loss, and delirium) prior to and periodically throughout therapy.
- **Hyperlipidemia:** Obtain a diet history, especially in regard to fat consumption.
- ***Lab Test Considerations:*** Serum glucose and uric acid levels and hepatic function tests should be monitored periodically during prolonged high-dose therapy. Notify physician or other health care professional if AST, ALT, or LDH becomes elevated. May increase prothrombin times and decrease serum albumin.
  - ❑ High-dose therapy may cause elevated serum glucose and uric acid levels.
  - ❑ When niacin is used as a lipid-lowering agent, serum cholesterol and triglyceride levels should be monitored prior to and periodically throughout course of therapy.

POTENTIAL NURSING DIAGNOSES

- Nutrition, altered, less than body requirements (Indications).
- Knowledge deficit, related to medication regimen (Patient/Family Teaching).
- Noncompliance (Patient/Family Teaching).

IMPLEMENTATION

- **General Info:** Because of infrequency of single B-vitamin deficiencies, combinations are commonly administered.
- **PO:** Administer with meals or milk to minimize GI irritation.
  - ❑ Timed-release tablet and capsules should be swallowed whole, without crushing, breaking, or chewing. Use calibrated measuring device to ensure accurate dosage of solution.

PATIENT/FAMILY TEACHING

- **General Info:** Inform patient that cutaneous flushing and a sensation of warmth, especially in the face, neck, and ears; itching or tingling; and headache may occur within the first 2 hr after taking the drug. These effects are usually transient and subside with continued therapy. If flushing is distressing or persistent, aspirin 300 mg given 30 min before each dose or slow upward titration of dose may decrease flushing.
  - ❑ Emphasize the importance of follow-up examinations to evaluate progress.
  - ❑ Advise patient to change positions slowly to minimize orthostatic hypotension.
- **Vitamin Deficiency:** Encourage patient to comply with diet recommendations of health care professional. Explain that the best source of vitamins is a well-balanced diet with foods from the 4 basic food groups.

- □ Foods high in niacin include meats, eggs, milk, and dairy products; little is lost during ordinary cooking.
- □ Patients self-medicating with vitamin supplements should be cautioned not to exceed RDA (see Appendix L). The effectiveness of megadoses for treatment of various medical conditions is unproved and may cause side effects.
- ■ **Hyperlipidemia:** Advise patient that this medication should be used in conjunction with diet restrictions (fat, cholesterol, carbohydrates, alcohol), exercise, and cessation of smoking.

EVALUATION

Effectiveness of therapy can be demonstrated by: ■ Prevention and treatment of niacin deficiency ■ Decrease in serum cholesterol and triglyceride levels.

NICARDIPINE

(nye-**kar**-di-peen)

Cardene, Cardene IV, Cardene SR

CLASSIFICATION(S):
Antianginal, Antihypertensive agent, Calcium channel blocker

Pregnancy Category C

INDICATIONS

■ Management of: □ Hypertension □ Angina pectoris □ Vasospastic (Prinzmetal's) angina. **Unlabeled Uses:** ■ Management of congestive heart failure.

ACTION

■ Inhibits the transport of calcium into myocardial and vascular smooth muscle cells, resulting in inhibition of excitation-contraction coupling and subsequent contraction. **Therapeutic Effects:** ■ Systemic vasodilation resulting in decreased blood pressure ■ Coronary vasodilation resulting in decreased frequency and severity of attacks of angina.

PHARMACOKINETICS

Absorption: Well absorbed following oral administration but extensively metabolized, resulting in decreased bioavailability.

Distribution: UK.

Metabolism and Excretion: Mostly metabolized by the liver; ≤10% excreted unchanged by kidneys.

Half-life: 2–4 hr.

CONTRAINDICATIONS AND PRECAUTIONS

Contraindicated in: ■ Hypersensitivity ■ Sick sinus syndrome ■ 2nd- or 3rd-degree AV block (unless an artificial pacemaker is in place) ■ Blood pressure <90 mm Hg ■ Advanced aortic stenosis.

Use Cautiously in: ■ Severe hepatic impairment (dosage reduction recommended) ■ Geriatric patients (dosage reduction/slower IV infusion rates recommended for most agents; increased risk of hypotension) ■ Severe renal impairment (dosage reduction may be necessary) ■ History of serious ventricular arrhythmias or congestive heart failure ■ Pregnancy, lactation, or children (safety not established).

ADVERSE REACTIONS AND SIDE EFFECTS*

CNS: abnormal dreams, anxiety, confusion, dizziness, drowsiness, headache, jitteriness, nervousness, psychiatric disturbances, weakness.

EENT: blurred vision, disturbed equilibrium, epistaxis, tinnitus.

Resp: cough, dyspnea, shortness of breath.

CV: ARRHYTHMIAS, CONGESTIVE HEART FAILURE, peripheral edema, bradycardia, chest pain, hypotension, palpitations, syncope, tachycardia.

GI: abnormal liver function studies, anorexia, constipation, diarrhea, dry mouth, dysgeusia, dyspepsia, nausea, vomiting.

GU: dysuria, nocturia, polyuria, sexual dysfunction, urinary frequency.

Derm: dermatitis, erythema multiforme, flushing, increased sweating, photosensitivity, pruritus/urticaria, rash.

Endo: gynecomastia, hyperglycemia.

Hemat: anemia, leukopenia, thrombocytopenia.

Metab: weight gain.

MS: joint stiffness, muscle cramps.

Neuro: paresthesia, tremor.

Misc: STEVENS-JOHNSON SYNDROME, gingival hyperplasia.

***CAPITALS indicate life-threatening; underlines indicate most frequent.**

INTERACTIONS

Drug-Drug: ▪ Additive hypotension may occur when used concurrently with **fentanyl**, other **antihypertensives, nitrates**, acute ingestion of **alcohol**, or **quinidine** ▪ Antihypertensive effects may be decreased by concurrent use of **NSAIDs** ▪ Concurrent use with **beta-adrenergic blockers, digoxin, disopyramide**, or **phenytoin** may result in bradycardia, conduction defects, or congestive heart failure ▪ **Cimetidine** and **propranolol** may decrease metabolism and increase the risk of toxicity ▪ May decrease the metabolism of and increase the risk of toxicity from **cyclosporine, prazosin, quinidine**, or **carbamazepine.**

ROUTE AND DOSAGE

- **PO (Adults):** 20 mg 3 times daily, may increase q 3 days (range 20–40 mg 3 times daily); or 30 mg twice daily as sustained-release form (up to 60 mg twice daily).
- **IV (Adults):** *To replace PO use when PO route not feasible*—0.5–2.2 mg/hr continuous infusion. *For acute hypertensive episodes*—5 mg/hr titrated as needed (up to 15 mg/hr).

AVAILABILITY

▪ ***Capsules:*** 20 mg[Rx], 30 mg[Rx] ▪ ***Sustained-release capsules:*** 30 mg[Rx], 45 mg[Rx], 60 mg[Rx] ▪ ***Injection:*** 2.5 mg/ml in 10-ml amps[Rx].

TIME/ACTION PROFILE (cardiovascular effects)

	ONSET	PEAK	DURATION
PO	20 min	0.5–2 hr	8 hr
PO-ER	UK	UK	12 hr
IV	within min	45 min	50 hr*

*Following discontinuation.

NURSING IMPLICATIONS

ASSESSMENT

- **General Info:** Monitor blood pressure and pulse prior to therapy, during dosage titration, and periodically throughout therapy. Monitor ECG periodically during prolonged therapy.
- □ Monitor intake and output ratios and daily weight. Assess for signs of congestive heart failure (peripheral edema, rales/crackles, dyspnea, weight gain, jugular venous distention).
- **Angina:** Assess location, duration, intensity, and precipitating factors of patient's anginal pain.
- ***Lab Test Considerations:*** Total serum calcium concentrations are not affected by calcium channel blockers.
- □ Monitor serum potassium periodically. Hypokalemia increases risk of arrhythmias; should be corrected.
- □ Monitor renal and hepatic functions periodically during long-term therapy. Several days of therapy may cause increase in hepatic enzymes, which return to normal upon discontinuation of therapy.

POTENTIAL NURSING DIAGNOSES

- Cardiac output, decreased (Indications).
- Pain (Indications).
- Knowledge deficit, related to medication regimen (Patient/Family Teaching).

IMPLEMENTATION

- **General Info:** To transfer from IV nicardipine infusion to oral therapy with other antihypertensive, start oral therapy simultaneously with discontinuation of nicardipine infusion. If transferring to oral nicardipine therapy, administer 1st dose of a 3-times-a-day regimen 1 hr prior to discontinuation of infusion.
- □ Dosage adjustments of nicardipine should be made no more frequently than every 3 days.
- **PO:** May be administered without regard to meals. May be administered with meals if GI irritation becomes a problem.
- □ Do not open, crush, break, or chew sustained-release capsules.
- **Continuous Infusion:** Dilute each 25-mg ampule with 240 ml of D5W, D5/0.45% NaCl, D5/0.9% NaCl, D5/potassium chloride 40 mEq, 0.45% NaCl, or 0.9% NaCl for a concentration of 0.1 mg/ml. Stable for 24 hr at room temperature.
- ***Rate:*** Administer via slow infusion. Titrate rate according to blood pressure response. Continuous infusions of 0.5 mg/hr, 1.2 mg/hr, and 2.2 mg/hr produce average plasma concentrations equal to a 20-mg, 30-mg, and 40-mg oral dose, respectively, given every 8 hr at steady state.

PATIENT/FAMILY TEACHING

- **General Info:** Advise patient to take medication exactly as directed, even if feeling well.

If a dose is missed, take as soon as possible unless almost time for next dose; do not double doses. May need to be discontinued gradually.

- □ Instruct patient on technique for monitoring pulse. Instruct patient to contact health care professional if heart rate is <50 bpm.
- □ Caution patient to change positions slowly to minimize orthostatic hypotension.
- □ May cause drowsiness or dizziness. Advise patient to avoid driving or other activities requiring alertness until response to the medication is known.
- □ Instruct patient to avoid concurrent use of alcohol or OTC medications, especially cold preparations, without consulting health care professional.
- □ Advise patient to notify health care professional if irregular heartbeats, dyspnea, swelling of hands and feet, pronounced dizziness, nausea, constipation, or hypotension occurs or if headache is severe or persistent.
- □ Caution patient to wear protective clothing and to use sunscreen to prevent photosensitivity reactions.
- ■ **Angina:** Instruct patient on concurrent nitrate or beta-blocker therapy to continue taking both medications as directed and to use SL nitroglycerin as needed for anginal attacks.
- □ Advise patient to contact health care professional if chest pain does not improve, worsens after therapy, or occurs with diaphoresis; if shortness of breath; or if persistent headache occurs.
- □ Caution patient to discuss exercise restrictions with health care professional prior to exertion.
- ■ **Hypertension:** Encourage patient to comply with other interventions for hypertension (weight reduction, low-sodium diet, smoking cessation, moderation of alcohol consumption, regular exercise, and stress management). Medication controls but does not cure hypertension.
- □ Instruct patient and family in proper technique for monitoring blood pressure. Advise patient to take blood pressure weekly and to report significant changes to health care professional.

EVALUATION

Effectiveness of therapy can be demonstrated by: ■ Decrease in blood pressure ■ Decrease in frequency and severity of anginal attacks □ Decrease in need for nitrate therapy □ Increase in activity tolerance and sense of well-being.

NICOTINE

(**nik**-o-teen)

nicotine chewing gum
Nicorette

nicotine nasal spray
Nicotrol NS

nicotine transdermal
Habitrol, Nicoderm CQ, Nicotrol, Prostep

CLASSIFICATION(S):
Smoking deterrent

Pregnancy Category D

INDICATIONS

■ Adjunct therapy (with behavior modification) in the management of nicotine withdrawal in patients desiring to give up cigarette smoking.

ACTION

■ Provides a source of nicotine during controlled withdrawal from cigarette smoking. **Therapeutic Effects:** ■ Lessened sequelae of nicotine withdrawal (irritability, insomnia, somnolence, headache, and increased appetite).

PHARMACOKINETICS

Absorption: *Chewing gum*—Slowly absorbed from buccal mucosa during chewing. *Nasal spray*—93% absorbed from nasal mucosa. *Transdermal*—68% of nicotine released from the system is absorbed through the skin (Nicoderm).

Distribution: Enters breast milk.

Metabolism and Excretion: Mostly metabolized by the liver. Small amounts are metabolized by kidneys and lungs; 10–20% excreted unchanged by kidneys.

Half-life: 1–2 hr.

CONTRAINDICATIONS AND PRECAUTIONS

Contraindicated in: ▪ Severe cardiovascular disease ▪ Temporomandibular joint disease (gum only) ▪ Children ▪ Continued smoking.

Use Cautiously in: ▪ Cardiovascular disease including hypertension ▪ Diabetes mellitus ▪ Pheochromocytoma ▪ Peripheral vascular diseases ▪ Skin disorders (transdermal only) ▪ Dental disorders (gum only) ▪ History of chronic nasal disorders (nasal spray only) ▪ Esophagitis, pharyngitis, or stomatitis (gum only) ▪ Hyperthyroidism ▪ Lactation (potential for adverse effects in the newborn) ▪ Hepatic disease ▪ Patients <50 kg or who smoke <10 cigarettes/day (use lower initial dose) ▪ Pregnancy (cessation of all nicotine is preferred; safety not established).

ADVERSE REACTIONS AND SIDE EFFECTS*

CNS: headache, insomnia, abnormal dreams, dizziness, drowsiness, impaired concentration, nervousness, weakness.

EENT: sinusitus; *gum*—pharyngitis; *nasal spray*—nasopharyngeal irritation, rhinitis, sneezing, watering eyes, eye irritation.

Resp: increased cough (↑ with nasal spray).

CV: tachycardia, atrial fibrillation, chest pain, hypertension.

GI: abdominal pain, abnormal taste, constipation, diarrhea, dry mouth, dyspepsia, nausea, vomiting; *gum*—belching, increased appetite, increased salivation, oral injury, sore mouth, hiccups.

Derm: *transdermal*—burning at patch site, erythema, pruritus, cutaneous hypersensitivity, rash, sweating.

Endo: dysmenorrhea.

MS: arthralgia, back pain, myalgia; *gum*—jaw muscle ache.

Neuro: paresthesia.

Misc: allergy, pain.

INTERACTIONS

Drug-Drug: ▪ **Insulin** requirements may decrease during nicotine withdrawal ▪ Effects of **acetaminophen, furosemide, caffeine, imipramine, oxazepam, pentazocine, propranolol**, or other **beta blockers, adrenergic antagonists (prazosin, labetalol)**, and **theophylline** may be increased during nicotine withdrawal because of decreased metabolism; dosage reduction at cessation may be necessary ▪ Doses of **adrenergic agonists (isoproterenol, phenylephrine)** may need to be increased because of lower levels of circulation catecholamines at cessation.

ROUTE AND DOSAGE

- **Transdermal (Adults):** *Habitrol*—21 mg/day for 4–8 wk, 14 mg/day for 2–4 wk, then 7 mg/day for 2–4 wk (8–16 wk total); system is worn 24 hr. *Nicoderm CQ*—21 mg/day for 6 wk, 14 mg/day for 2 wk, then 7 mg/day for 2 wk (10 wk total); system is worn 24 hr. *Nicotrol*—15 mg (1 patch)/day for 6 wk; system is removed at bedtime (worn 16 hr/day). *Prostep*—22 mg/day for 4–8 wk, 11 mg/day for 2–4 wk (6–12 wk total).
- **Transdermal (Adults, Adolescents, or Children <100 Pounds Who Smoke <10 Cigarettes/Day or Who Have Underlying Cardiovascular Disease):** *Habitrol*—14 mg/day for 4–8 wk, then 7 mg/day for 2–4 wk (6–8 wk total); system is worn 24 hr. *Nicoderm CQ*—14 mg/day for 6 wk, then 7 mg/day for 2 wk (8 wk total); *Prostep*—11 mg/day for 4–8 wk. *Prostep*—11 mg/day for 2–4 wk.
- **Gum (Adults):** 2–4 mg as needed, amount needed determined by smoking urge or rate of chewing, or on a fixed schedule every 1–2 hr. Usual initial requirement 20 mg (not to exceed 60 mg/day).
- **Intranasal (Adults):** One spray in each nostril 1–2 times/hr (up to 5 times/hr) or 40 times/day (not to exceed 3 mo).

AVAILABILITY

▪ ***Chewing gum (Nicorette):*** 2 mg[OTC] ▪ ***Nasal spray (Nicotrol NS):*** 10 mg/ml (0.5 mg/spray) in 10-ml bottles (100 doses)[Rx], 4 mg[Rx] ▪ ***Transdermal patch (Habitrol):*** 7 mg/day[Rx], 14 mg/day[Rx], 21 mg/day[OTC,Rx] ▪ ***Transdermal patch (Nicotrol):*** 15 mg/day[OTC] ▪ ***Transdermal patch (Nicoderm CQ):*** 7 mg/day[OTC], 14 mg/day[OTC], 21 mg/day[OTC] ▪ ***Transdermal patch (Prostep):*** 11 mg/day[Rx], 22 mg/day[Rx].

***CAPITALS indicate life-threatening; underlines indicate most frequent.**

N

TIME/ACTION PROFILE (nicotine blood levels)

	ONSET	PEAK	DURATION
Nicorette—chew	rapid	15–30 min	UK
Nicoderm CQ—TD	rapid	2–4 hr	UK
Nicotrol NS	rapid	4–15 min	UK
Habitrol—TD	rapid	6–12 hr	UK
Prostep—TD	rapid	9 hr	UK

NURSING IMPLICATIONS

ASSESSMENT

- **General Info:** Prior to therapy, assess smoking history (number of cigarettes smoked daily, smoking patterns, nicotine content of preferred brand, degree to which patient inhales smoke).
- □ Assess patient for symptoms of smoking withdrawal (irritability, drowsiness, fatigue, headache, nicotine craving) periodically throughout therapy.
- □ Evaluate progress in smoking cessation periodically during therapy.
- **Gum:** Assess patient for history of temporomandibular joint pain or dysfunction.
- ***Toxicity and Overdose:*** Monitor for nausea, vomiting, diarrhea, increased salivation, abdominal pain, headache, dizziness, auditory and visual disturbances, weakness, dyspnea, hypotension, and irregular pulse.

POTENTIAL NURSING DIAGNOSES

- Coping, ineffective individual (Indications).
- Knowledge deficit, related to medication regimen (Patient/Family Teaching).

IMPLEMENTATION

- **Gum:** Protect gum from light; exposure to light causes gum to turn brown.
- **Transdermal:** Determine whether patch is to be worn for 16 or 24 hr. *Nicotrol* system should be applied upon awakening and removed at bedtime.
- **Nasal Spray:** Regular use of the spray during the 1st wk of therapy may help patient adjust to irritant effects of the spray.

PATIENT/FAMILY TEACHING

- **General Info:** Explain to patient the necessity of immediate cessation of smoking upon initiation and throughout therapy.
- □ Encourage patient to participate in a smoking cessation program while using this product.
- □ Review the patient instruction sheet enclosed in the package.
- □ Instruct patient in proper method of disposal of unit. Emphasize need to keep out of the reach of children.
- □ Emphasize the importance of regular visits to health care professional to monitor progress of smoking cessation.
- **Gum:** Explain purpose of nicotine gum to patient. The patient should chew 1 piece of gum whenever a craving for nicotine occurs or according to a fixed schedule (every 1–2 hr while awake) as directed. The gum should be chewed slowly until a tingling sensation is felt (about 15 chews). Then, patient should stop chewing and store the gum between the cheek and gums until the tingling sensation disappears (about 1 min). The process of stopping, then resuming chewing should be repeated for approximately 30 min. Rapid, vigorous chewing may result in side effects similar to those of smoking too many cigarettes (headache, dizziness, nausea, increased salivation, heartburn, and hiccups).
- □ Inform patient that the gum has a slight tobacco/pepper-like taste. Many patients initially find it unpleasant and slightly irritating to the mouth. This usually resolves after several days of therapy.
- □ Advise patient to carry gum at all times during therapy.
- □ Advise patient to avoid eating or drinking acidic beverages (coffee, juices, wine, soft drinks) for 15 min before and during chewing of nicotine gum; these interfere with buccal absorption of nicotine.
- □ The gum usually can be chewed by denture wearers. Contact dentist if the gum adheres to bridgework.
- □ Use of the gum may be discontinued when 1–2 pieces/day are sufficient to control the craving for nicotine. Gradual reduction of dose over 2–3 mo can be accomplished by decreasing daily dose by 1 or more every 4–7 days, decreasing chewing time with each piece from 30 min to 10–15 min for 4–7 days, and then decreasing number of pieces per day; substituting one or more pieces of sugarless gum for pieces of nicotine gum; increasing number of doses substituted every 4–7 days; replacing 4-mg dose with 2-mg dose; or applying any of these suggestions. The duration

of treatment is limited to 6 mo because physical and psychological dependence can occur. Discontinuing the gum too soon may result in withdrawal symptoms (anxiety, irritability, GI distress, headache, drowsiness, or tobacco craving).

- □ Instruct patient not to swallow gum.
- □ Dispose of the gum by wrapping in wrapper to prevent ingestion by children and animals. Call the poison control center, emergency department, or health care professional immediately if a child ingests the gum.
- □ Emphasize the need to discontinue the gum and to inform health care professional if pregnancy occurs.

- ▪ **Transdermal:** Instruct patient in application and use of patch. Apply patch at the same time each day. Keep patch in sealed pouch until ready to apply. Apply to clean, dry skin of upper arm or torso free of oil, hair, scars, cuts, burns, or irritation. Press patch firmly in place with palm for 10 sec, making sure there is good contact, especially around the edges. Keep patch in place during showering, bathing, or swimming; replace patches that have fallen off. Wash hands with plain water after handling patches; soap will increase absorption of nicotine. Do not trim or cut patch. Alternate application sites. Dispose of used patches by folding adhesive sides together and replacing in protective pouch or aluminum foil; keep out of reach of children.
- □ Advise patient that redness, itching, and burning at application site usually subside within 1 hr. Instruct patient to notify health care professional and not apply new patch if signs of allergic reaction (urticaria, generalized rash, hives) or persistent local skin reactions (severe erythema, pruritus, edema) occur.
- □ May cause drowsiness or dizziness. Caution patient to avoid driving or other activities requiring alertness until response to medication is known.

- ▪ **Nasal Spray:** Instruct patient in proper use of spray. Tilt head back slightly. Do not sniff, swallow, or inhale through nose as spray is being administered. Dose should be used for 8 wk, then discontinued over 4–6 wk.
- □ Discontinue nasal spray by using ½ dose (1 spray at a time), using the spray less frequently, skipping a dose by not using every hour, or setting a planned stop date for use of the spray.
- □ Patients who fail to stop smoking should be given a therapy holiday before another attempt.
- □ Instruct patient to replace child-resistant cap after using and before disposal.

EVALUATION

Effectiveness of therapy can be demonstrated by: ▪ Smoking cessation ▪ Decrease in nicotine withdrawal symptoms in patients participating in a supervised smoking cessation program. Therapy with nicotine gum is limited to 6 mo; most patients begin a gradual withdrawal after 3 mo of therapy. Nicotine transdermal should be discontinued if patient is unable to stop smoking by 4th wk of therapy, as patient is unlikely to quit on that attempt. Therapy with nicotine transdermal should not be used for longer than 20 wk. Treatment with nasal spray for longer than 3 mo has not been shown to improve outcome.

NIFEDIPINE

(nye-**fed**-i-peen)

Adalat, {Apo-Nifed}, {Novo-Nifedin}, {Nu-Nifed}, Procardia

CLASSIFICATION(S):

Antianginal, Antihypertensive agent, Calcium channel blocker

Pregnancy Category C

INDICATIONS

▪ Management of: □ Hypertension □ Angina pectoris □ Vasospastic (Prinzmetal's) angina. **Unlabeled Uses:** ▪ Prevention of migraine headache ▪ Management of congestive heart failure or cardiomyopathy.

ACTION

▪ Inhibits the transport of calcium into myocardial and vascular smooth muscle cells, resulting in inhibition of excitation-contraction coupling and subsequent contraction. **Therapeutic Effects:** ▪ Systemic vasodilation, resulting in decreased blood pressure ▪ Coronary vasodilation,

N

resulting in decreased frequency and severity of attacks of angina.

PHARMACOKINETICS

Absorption: Well absorbed following oral administration, but large amounts are rapidly metabolized, resulting in decreased bioavailability (45–70%); bioavailability is increased (80%) with long-acting (CC, PA, XL) forms.
Distribution: UK.
Metabolism and Excretion: Mostly metabolized by the liver.
Half-life: 2–5 hr.

CONTRAINDICATIONS AND PRECAUTIONS

Contraindicated in: ▪ Hypersensitivity ▪ Sick sinus syndrome ▪ 2nd- or 3rd-degree AV block (unless an artificial pacemaker is in place) ▪ Blood pressure <90 mm Hg.
Use Cautiously in: ▪ Severe hepatic impairment (dosage reduction recommended) ▪ Geriatric patients (dosage reduction recommended; increased risk of hypotension) ▪ Severe renal impairment (dosage reduction may be necessary) ▪ History of serious ventricular arrhythmias or congestive heart failure ▪ Pregnancy, lactation, or children (safety not established).

ADVERSE REACTIONS AND SIDE EFFECTS*

CNS: headache, abnormal dreams, anxiety, confusion, dizziness, drowsiness, jitteriness, nervousness, psychiatric disturbances, weakness.
EENT: blurred vision, disturbed equilibrium, epistaxis, tinnitus.
Resp: cough, dyspnea, shortness of breath.
CV: ARRHYTHMIAS, CONGESTIVE HEART FAILURE, peripheral edema, bradycardia, chest pain, hypotension, palpitations, syncope, tachycardia.
GI: abnormal liver function studies, anorexia, constipation, diarrhea, dry mouth, dysgeusia, dyspepsia, nausea, vomiting.
GU: dysuria, nocturia, polyuria, sexual dysfunction, urinary frequency.
Derm: flushing, dermatitis, erythema multiforme, increased sweating, photosensitivity, pruritus/urticaria, rash.
Endo: gynecomastia, hyperglycemia.
Hemat: anemia, leukopenia, thrombocytopenia.
Metab: weight gain.
MS: joint stiffness, muscle cramps.
Neuro: paresthesia, tremor.
Misc: STEVENS-JOHNSON SYNDROME, gingival hyperplasia.

INTERACTIONS

Drug-Drug: ▪ Additive hypotension may occur when used concurrently with **fentanyl,** other **antihypertensives, nitrates,** acute ingestion of **alcohol,** or **quinidine** ▪ Antihypertensive effects may be decreased by concurrent use of **NSAIDs** ▪ May increase serum levels and risk of toxicity from **digoxin** ▪ Concurrent use with **beta-adrenergic blockers, digoxin, disopyramide,** or **phenytoin** may result in bradycardia, conduction defects, or congestive heart failure ▪ **Cimetidine** and **propranolol** may decrease metabolism and increase the risk of toxicity ▪ May decrease the metabolism of and increase the risk of toxicity from **cyclosporine, prazosin, quinidine,** or **carbamazepine.**
Drug-Food: ▪ **Grapefruit juice** increases blood levels.

ROUTE AND DOSAGE

- **PO (Adults):** 10–30 mg 3 times daily (not to exceed 180 mg/day) or 30–90 mg once daily as sustained-release (CC, PA, XL) form (not to exceed 90–120 mg/day).
- **SL (Adults):** 10 mg; may be repeated in 15 min (unlabeled).

AVAILABILITY

▪ ***Capsules:*** {5 mg^{Rx}}, 10 mg^{Rx}, 20 mg^{Rx} ▪ ***Tablets:*** {10 mg^{Rx}} ▪ ***Extended-release tablets:*** {10 mg^{Rx}}, {20 mg^{Rx}}, 30 mg^{Rx}, 60 mg^{Rx}, 90 mg^{Rx}.

TIME/ACTION PROFILE

	ONSET	PEAK	DURATION
PO	20 min	UK	6–8 hr
PO–CC, PA, XL	UK	1 hr	24 hr

NURSING IMPLICATIONS

ASSESSMENT

- **General Info:** Monitor blood pressure and pulse prior to therapy, during dosage titration,

*CAPITALS indicate life-threatening; underlines indicate most frequent.

and periodically throughout therapy. Monitor ECG periodically during prolonged therapy.

- Monitor intake and output ratios and daily weight. Assess for signs of congestive heart failure (peripheral edema, rales/crackles, dyspnea, weight gain, jugular venous distention).
- Patients receiving digitalis glycosides concurrently with nifedipine should have routine serum digitalis glycoside level and be monitored for signs and symptoms of digitalis glycoside toxicity.

- **Angina:** Assess location, duration, intensity, and precipitating factors of patient's anginal pain.
- ***Lab Test Considerations:*** Total serum calcium concentrations are not affected by calcium channel blockers.
- Monitor serum potassium periodically. Hypokalemia increases risk of arrhythmias; should be corrected.
- Monitor renal and hepatic functions periodically during long-term therapy. Several days of therapy may cause increase in hepatic enzymes, which return to normal upon discontinuation of therapy.
- Nifedipine may cause positive antinuclear antibody (ANA) and direct Coombs' test results.

POTENTIAL NURSING DIAGNOSES

- Cardiac output, decreased (Indications).
- Pain (Indications).
- Knowledge deficit, related to medication regimen (Patient/Family Teaching).

IMPLEMENTATION

- **PO:** May be administered without regard to meals. May be administered with meals if GI irritation becomes a problem.
- Do not open, crush, break, or chew extended-release tablets. Empty tablets that appear in stool are not significant.
- Avoid administration with grapefruit juice.
- **SL:** Nifedipine may be administered by puncturing the capsule with a sterile needle and squeezing to administer the liquid into the buccal pouch. The dose used is the same as the oral dose. Chewing or puncturing and swallowing capsule has shown similar effectiveness as SL route for hypertensive emergencies.

PATIENT/FAMILY TEACHING

- **General Info:** Advise patient to take medication exactly as directed, even if feeling well. If a dose is missed, take as soon as possible unless almost time for next dose; do not double doses. May need to be discontinued gradually.
- Instruct patient on technique for monitoring pulse. Instruct patient to contact health care professional if heart rate is <50 bpm.
- Caution patient to change positions slowly to minimize orthostatic hypotension.
- May cause drowsiness or dizziness. Advise patient to avoid driving or other activities requiring alertness until response to the medication is known.
- Instruct patient on importance of maintaining good dental hygiene and seeing dentist frequently for teeth cleaning to prevent tenderness, bleeding, and gingival hyperplasia (gum enlargement).
- Instruct patient to avoid concurrent use of alcohol or OTC medications, especially cold preparations, without consulting health care professional.
- Advise patient to notify health care professional if irregular heartbeats, dyspnea, swelling of hands and feet, pronounced dizziness, nausea, constipation, or hypotension occurs or if headache is severe or persistent.
- Caution patient to wear protective clothing and use sunscreen to prevent photosensitivity reactions.
- **Angina:** Instruct patient on concurrent nitrate or beta-blocker therapy to continue taking both medications as directed and use SL nitroglycerin as needed for anginal attacks.
- Inform patient that anginal attacks may occur 30 min after administration because of reflex tachycardia. This is usually temporary and is not an indication for discontinuation.
- Advise patient to contact health care professional if chest pain does not improve, worsens after therapy, or occurs with diaphoresis; if shortness of breath occurs; or if persistent headache occurs.
- Caution patient to discuss exercise restrictions with health care professional prior to exertion.
- **Hypertension:** Encourage patient to comply with other interventions for hypertension (weight reduction, low-sodium diet, smoking

cessation, moderation of alcohol consumption, regular exercise, and stress management). Medication controls but does not cure hypertension.

□ Instruct patient and family in proper technique for monitoring blood pressure. Advise patient to take blood pressure weekly and to report significant changes to health care professional.

EVALUATION

Effectiveness of therapy can be demonstrated by: ▪ Decrease in blood pressure ▪ Decrease in frequency and severity of anginal attacks □ Decrease in need for nitrate therapy □ Increase in activity tolerance and sense of well-being.

NILUTAMIDE

(nye-**loot**-a-mide)

{Anandron}, Nilandron

CLASSIFICATION(S):

Antineoplastic (antiandrogen)

Pregnancy Category C

INDICATIONS

▪ Management of metastatic prostate cancer (with surgical castration).

ACTION

▪ Blocks the effects of androgen (testosterone) at the cellular level. **Therapeutic Effects:** ▪ Decreased spread of prostate cancer.

PHARMACOKINETICS

Absorption: Rapidly and completely absorbed following oral administration.
Distribution: UK.
Metabolism and Excretion: Extensively metabolized by the liver; 2 metabolites have antiandrogenic activity; <2% excreted unchanged in urine.
Half-life: 41–49 hr.

CONTRAINDICATIONS AND PRECAUTIONS

Contraindicated in: ▪ Hypersensitivity ▪ Severe hepatic impairment ▪ Severe respiratory insufficiency.
Use Cautiously in: ▪ History of liver disease or alcoholism ▪ History of respiratory problems ▪ Pregnancy, lactation, or children (safety not established).

ADVERSE REACTIONS AND SIDE EFFECTS*

CNS: dizziness.
EENT: impaired adaptation to dark, abnormal vision.
Resp: interstitial pneumonitis.
CV: hypertension.
GI: HEPATOTOXICITY, constipation, hepatitis, increased liver enzymes, nausea.
Derm: hot flushes, hair loss, sweating.

INTERACTIONS

Drug-Drug: ▪ May increase the effects of **warfarin, phenytoin,** and **theophylline** ▪ May cause **alcohol** intolerance.

ROUTE AND DOSAGE

▪ **PO (Adults):** 300 mg once daily for 30 days; then 150 mg once daily.

AVAILABILITY

▪ ***Tablets:*** 50 mg[Rx], {100 mg[Rx]}.

TIME/ACTION PROFILE (antiandrogenic effects)

	ONSET	PEAK	DURATION
PO	rapid	UK	24 hr

NURSING IMPLICATIONS

ASSESSMENT

□ Patients should have a chest x ray prior to initiation of therapy. Assess patient for symptoms of interstitial pneumonitis (dyspnea or worsening of pre-existing dyspnea). If symptoms occur, nilutamide should be discontinued until cause can be determined. Pneumonitis usually occurs during the first 3 mo of therapy and is almost always reversible when treatment is discontinued.

- ***Lab Test Considerations:*** Monitor hepatic function prior to and every 3 mo throughout therapy. If AST or ALT is elevated more than 2–3 times normal, treatment should be discontinued.
- May cause hyperglycemia; increased serum alkaline phosphatase, BUN, and creatinine; and leukopenia.

POTENTIAL NURSING DIAGNOSES

- Injury, risk for (Side Effects).
- Knowledge deficit, related to medication regimen (Patient/Family Teaching).

IMPLEMENTATION

- **PO:** May be taken without regard to food.

PATIENT/FAMILY TEACHING

- Instruct patient to take nilutamide exactly as directed. If a dose is missed, take as soon as possible unless almost time for next dose. Do not double doses.
- Caution patient that adaptation to dark may be impaired and may cause difficulty driving at night or through tunnels. Wearing tinted glasses may minimize this effect.
- Advise patient to notify physician immediately if dark urine, fatigue, abdominal pain, yellow eyes or skin, or unexplained GI symptoms occur. Hepatotoxicity usually resolves when nilutamide is discontinued but may be progressive and fatal; requires immediate medical attention.

EVALUATION

Effectiveness of therapy can be demonstrated by: ▪ Decrease in the spread of prostate cancer.

NIMODIPINE

(nye-**moe**-di-peen)
Nimotop

CLASSIFICATION(S):
Calcium channel blocker

Pregnancy Category C

INDICATIONS

- Management of subarachnoid hemorrhage.

ACTION

▪ Inhibits the transport of calcium into vascular smooth muscle cells, resulting in inhibition of excitation-contraction coupling and subsequent contraction ▪ Potent peripheral vasodilator. **Therapeutic Effects:** ▪ Prevention of vascular spasm after subarachnoid hemorrhage, resulting in decreased neurologic impairment.

PHARMACOKINETICS

Absorption: Well absorbed following oral administration but extensively metabolized, resulting in decreased bioavailability.
Distribution: Crosses the blood-brain barrier; remainder of distribution UK.
Metabolism and Excretion: Mostly metabolized by the liver; ≤10% excreted unchanged by kidneys.
Half-life: 1–2 hr.

CONTRAINDICATIONS AND PRECAUTIONS

Contraindicated in: ▪ Hypersensitivity ▪ Sick sinus syndrome ▪ 2nd- or 3rd-degree AV block (unless an artificial pacemaker is in place) ▪ Blood pressure <90 mm Hg.
Use Cautiously in: ▪ Severe hepatic impairment (dosage reduction recommended for most agents) ▪ Geriatric patients (dosage reduction recommended; increased risk of hypotension) ▪ Severe renal impairment ▪ History of serious ventricular arrhythmias or congestive heart failure ▪ Pregnancy, lactation, or children (safety not established).

ADVERSE REACTIONS AND SIDE EFFECTS*

CNS: abnormal dreams, anxiety, confusion, dizziness, drowsiness, headache, nervousness, psychiatric disturbances, weakness.
EENT: blurred vision, disturbed equilibrium, epistaxis, tinnitus.
Resp: cough, dyspnea.
CV: ARRHYTHMIAS, CONGESTIVE HEART FAILURE, bradycardia, chest pain, hypotension, palpitations, peripheral edema, syncope, tachycardia.
GI: abnormal liver function studies, anorexia,

N

***CAPITALS indicate life-threatening; underlines indicate most frequent.**

constipation, nausea, diarrhea, dry mouth, dysgeusia, dyspepsia, vomiting.
GU: dysuria, nocturia, polyuria, sexual dysfunction, urinary frequency.
Derm: dermatitis, erythema multiforme, flushing, increased sweating, photosensitivity, pruritus/urticaria, rash.
Endo: gynecomastia, hyperglycemia.
Hemat: anemia, leukopenia, thrombocytopenia.
Metab: weight gain.
MS: joint stiffness, muscle cramps.
Neuro: paresthesia, tremor.
Misc: STEVENS-JOHNSON SYNDROME, gingival hyperplasia.

INTERACTIONS

Drug-Drug: ▪ Additive hypotension may occur when used concurrently with **fentanyl,** other **antihypertensives, nitrates,** acute ingestion of **alcohol,** or **quinidine** ▪ Concurrent use with **beta-adrenergic blockers, digoxin, disopyramide,** or **phenytoin** may result in bradycardia, conduction defects, or congestive heart failure.

ROUTE AND DOSAGE

- **PO (Adults):** 60 mg q 4 hr for 21 days; therapy should be started within 96 hr of subarachnoid hemorrhage.

AVAILABILITY

- ***Capsules:*** 30 mg[Rx].

TIME/ACTION PROFILE (vasodilation)

	ONSET	PEAK	DURATION
PO	UK	1 hr	4 hr

NURSING IMPLICATIONS

ASSESSMENT

- □ Assess patient's neurologic status (level of consciousness, movement) prior to and periodically following administration.
- □ Monitor blood pressure and pulse prior to therapy and periodically throughout therapy.
- □ Monitor intake and output ratios and daily weight. Assess for signs of congestive heart failure (peripheral edema, rales/crackles, dyspnea, weight gain, jugular venous distention).
- ▪ ***Lab Test Considerations:*** Total serum calcium concentrations are not affected by calcium channel blockers.
- □ Monitor serum potassium periodically. Hypokalemia increases risk of arrhythmias; should be corrected.
- □ Monitor renal and hepatic functions periodically. Several days of therapy may cause increase in hepatic enzymes, which return to normal upon discontinuation of therapy.
- □ May occasionally cause decreased platelet count.

POTENTIAL NURSING DIAGNOSES

- ▪ Tissue perfusion, altered (Indications).
- ▪ Knowledge deficit, related to medication regimen (Patient/Family Teaching).

IMPLEMENTATION

- ▪ **General Info:** Begin administration within 96 hr of subarachnoid hemorrhage and continue every 4 hr for 21 consecutive days.
- ▪ **PO:** If patient is unable to swallow capsule, make a hole in both ends of the capsule with a sterile 18-gauge needle and extract the contents into a syringe. Empty contents into water or nasogastric tube and flush with 30 ml normal saline.

PATIENT/FAMILY TEACHING

- ▪ **General Info:** Advise patient to take medication exactly as directed, even if feeling well. If a dose is missed, take as soon as possible unless almost time for next dose; do not double doses. May need to be discontinued gradually.
- □ Caution patient to change positions slowly to minimize orthostatic hypotension.
- □ May cause drowsiness or dizziness. Advise patient to avoid driving or other activities requiring alertness until response to the medication is known.
- □ Instruct patient to avoid concurrent use of alcohol or OTC medications, especially cold preparations, without consulting health care professional.
- □ Advise patient to notify health care professional if irregular heartbeats, dyspnea, swelling of hands and feet, pronounced dizziness, nausea, constipation, or hypotension occurs or if headache is severe or persistent.
- □ Caution patient to wear protective clothing and

use sunscreen to prevent photosensitivity reactions.

EVALUATION

Effectiveness of therapy can be demonstrated by: ▪ Improvement in neurologic deficits due to vasospasm following subarachnoid hemorrhage.

NISOLDIPINE

(nye-**sole**-di-peen)
Sular

CLASSIFICATION(S):
Antihypertensive agent, Calcium channel blocker

Pregnancy Category C

INDICATIONS

▪ Management of hypertension.

ACTION

▪ Inhibits the transport of calcium into vascular smooth muscle cells, resulting in inhibition of vasoconstriction and dilation of arterioles. **Therapeutic Effects:** ▪ Systemic vasodilation, resulting in decreased blood pressure.

PHARMACOKINETICS

Absorption: Well absorbed (87%) following oral administration but rapidly and extensively metabolized in the gut wall, resulting in 5% bioavailability.
Distribution: UK.
Metabolism and Excretion: Highly metabolized.
Half-life: 7–12 hr.

CONTRAINDICATIONS AND PRECAUTIONS

Contraindicated in: ▪ Hypersensitivity ▪ Cross-sensitivity with calcium channel blockers may occur.
Use Cautiously in: ▪ Congestive heart failure/left ventricular dysfunction ▪ Hepatic impairment (dosage reduction may be necessary) ▪ Geriatric patients (dosage reduction may be necessary) ▪ Coronary artery disease (may precipitate angina) ▪ Pregnancy, lactation, or children (safety not established).

ADVERSE REACTIONS AND SIDE EFFECTS*

CNS: headache, dizziness.
EENT: pharyngitis, sinusitis.
CV: peripheral edema, chest pain, hypotension, palpitations.
GI: nausea.
Derm: rash.

INTERACTIONS

Drug-Drug: ▪ Additive hypotension may occur with other **antihypertensive agents,** acute ingestion of **alcohol,** or **nitrates.**
Drug-Food: ▪ **Grapefruit juice** significantly increases blood levels and effects of nisoldipine; concurrent ingestion should be avoided ▪ Blood levels are increased by concurrent ingestion of a **high-fat meal** and should be avoided.

ROUTE AND DOSAGE

▪ **PO (Adults):** 20 mg/day as a single dose initially; may be increased by 10 mg/day q 7 days, up to 60 mg/day (usual range 20–40 mg/day).

AVAILABILITY

▪ ***Extended-release tablets:*** 10 mg^{Rx}, 20 mg^{Rx}, 30 mg^{Rx}, 40 mg^{Rx}.

TIME/ACTION PROFILE (antihypertensive effects)

	ONSET	PEAK	DURATION
PO	UK	6–12 hr	24 hr

NURSING IMPLICATIONS

ASSESSMENT

- Monitor blood pressure and pulse prior to therapy, during dosage titration, and periodically throughout therapy. Monitor ECG periodically during prolonged therapy.
- Monitor intake and output ratios and daily weight. Assess for signs of congestive heart failure (peripheral edema, rales/crackles, dyspnea, weight gain, jugular venous distention).

N

*CAPITALS indicate life-threatening; underlines indicate most frequent.

- ***Lab Test Considerations:*** Total serum calcium concentrations are not affected by calcium channel blockers.

POTENTIAL NURSING DIAGNOSES

- Cardiac output, decreased (Indications).
- Knowledge deficit, related to medication regimen (Patient/Family Teaching).

IMPLEMENTATION

- **PO:** Avoid administration within 1 hr of high-fat meals or grapefruit products.
- □ Do not crush, break, or chew tablets.

PATIENT/FAMILY TEACHING

- □ Advise patient to take medication exactly as directed, even if feeling well. If a dose is missed, take as soon as possible unless almost time for next dose; do not double doses. May need to be discontinued gradually.
- □ Encourage patient to comply with other interventions for hypertension (weight reduction, low-sodium diet, smoking cessation, moderation of alcohol consumption, regular exercise, and stress management). Medication controls but does not cure hypertension.
- □ Instruct patient and family in proper technique for monitoring blood pressure. Advise patient to take blood pressure weekly and to report significant changes to health care professional.
- □ Caution patient to change positions slowly to minimize orthostatic hypotension.
- □ May cause dizziness. Advise patient to avoid driving or other activities requiring alertness until response to the medication is known.
- □ Instruct patient to avoid concurrent use of alcohol or OTC medications, especially cold preparations, without consulting health care professional.
- □ Advise patient to notify health care professional if irregular heartbeats, dyspnea, swelling of hands and feet, pronounced dizziness, nausea, constipation, or hypotension occurs or if headache is severe or persistent.

EVALUATION

Effectiveness of therapy can be demonstrated by: ▪ Decrease in blood pressure.

NITROFURANTOIN

(nye-troe-fyoor-**an**-toyn)
{Apo-Nitrofurantoin}, Furadantin, Furalan, Macrobid, Macrodantin, Nitrofuracot

CLASSIFICATION(S):
Anti-infective (miscellaneous)

Pregnancy Category B

INDICATIONS

▪ Urinary tract infections due to susceptible organisms; not effective in systemic bacterial infections ▪ Chronic suppressive therapy of urinary tract infections.

ACTION

▪ Interferes with bacterial enzymes. **Therapeutic Effects:** ▪ Bactericidal or bacteriostatic action against susceptible organisms. **Spectrum:** ▪ Many gram-negative and some gram-positive organisms, specifically: □ *Citrobacter* □ *Corynebacterium* □ *Enterobacter* □ *Escherichia coli* □ *Klebsiella* □ *Neisseria* □ *Salmonella* □ *Shigella* □ *Staphylococcus aureus* □ *Staphylococcus epidermidis* □ *Enterococcus*.

PHARMACOKINETICS

Absorption: Readily absorbed following oral administration. Absorption is slower but more complete with macrocrystals (Macrodantin).
Distribution: Crosses placenta; enters breast milk.
Metabolism and Excretion: Partially metabolized by the liver; 30–50% excreted unchanged by the kidneys.
Half-life: 20 min (increased in renal impairment).

CONTRAINDICATIONS AND PRECAUTIONS

Contraindicated in: ▪ Hypersensitivity ▪ Hypersensitivity to parabens (suspension) ▪ Oliguria or anuria ▪ Infants <1 mo and pregnancy near term (increased risk of hemolytic anemia in newborn) ▪ Glucose-6-phosphate dehydrogenase (G6PD) deficiency.

{} = Available in Canada only.

Use Cautiously in: ▪ Diabetics or debilitated patients (neuropathy may be more common) ▪ Pregnancy and lactation (safety not established but has been used safely in pregnant women; breast-feeding may cause hemolysis in G6PD-deficient infants).

ADVERSE REACTIONS AND SIDE EFFECTS*

CNS: dizziness, drowsiness, headache.
EENT: nystagmus.
Resp: pneumonitis.
CV: chest pain.
GI: anorexia, nausea, vomiting, abdominal pain, diarrhea, drug-induced hepatitis.
GU: rust/brown discoloration of urine.
Derm: photosensitivity.
Hemat: blood dyscrasias, hemolytic anemia.
Neuro: peripheral neuropathy.

INTERACTIONS

Drug-Drug: ▪ **Probenecid** and **sulfinpyrazone** prevent high urinary concentrations; may decrease effectiveness ▪ **Antacids** may decrease absorption ▪ Increased risk of neurotoxicity with **neurotoxic drugs** ▪ Increased risk of hepatotoxicity with **hepatotoxic drugs** ▪ Increased risk of pneumonitis with **drugs having pulmonary toxicity.**

ROUTE AND DOSAGE

- **PO (Adults):** *Treatment of active infection*—50–100 mg q 6–8 hr or 100 mg q 12 hr as extended-release product. *Chronic suppression*—50–100 mg single evening dose.
- **PO (Children >1 mo):** *Treatment of active infection*—0.75–1.75 mg/kg q 6 hr. *Chronic suppression*—1 mg/kg/day as a single dose at bedtime (unlabeled).

AVAILABILITY

▪ ***Tablets:*** 50 mg[Rx], 100 mg[Rx] ▪ ***Oral suspension:*** 25 mg/5 ml[Rx] ▪ ***Capsules:*** 25 mg[Rx], 50 mg[Rx], 100 mg[Rx] ▪ ***Extended-release capsules:*** 100 mg[Rx].

TIME/ACTION PROFILE (urine levels)

	ONSET	PEAK	DURATION
PO	UK	30 min	6–12 hr

NURSING IMPLICATIONS

ASSESSMENT

- □ Assess patient for signs and symptoms of urinary tract infection (frequency, urgency, pain, and burning on urination; fever; cloudy or foul-smelling urine) prior to and periodically throughout therapy.
- □ Obtain specimens for culture and sensitivity prior to and during drug administration.
- □ Monitor intake and output ratios. Report significant discrepancies in totals.
- ▪ ***Lab Test Considerations:*** CBC should be routinely monitored with patients on prolonged therapy.
- □ May cause elevated serum glucose, bilirubin, alkaline phosphatase, BUN, and creatinine.

POTENTIAL NURSING DIAGNOSES

- ▪ Infection, risk for (Indications).
- ▪ Knowledge deficit, related to medication regimen (Patient/Family Teaching).

IMPLEMENTATION

- ▪ **PO:** Administer with food or milk to minimize GI irritation, to delay and increase absorption, to increase peak concentration, and to prolong duration of therapeutic concentration in the urine.
- □ Do not crush tablets or open capsules.
- □ Administer liquid preparations with calibrated measuring device. Shake well prior to administration. Oral suspension may be mixed with water, milk, fruit juices, or infant formula. Rinse mouth with water following administration of oral suspension to avoid staining teeth.

PATIENT/FAMILY TEACHING

- □ Instruct patient to take medication around the clock, exactly as directed. If a dose is missed, take as soon as remembered and space next dose 2–4 hr apart. Do not skip or double up on missed doses.
- □ May cause dizziness or drowsiness. Caution patient to avoid driving or other activities requiring alertness until response to medication is known.

***CAPITALS indicate life-threatening; underlines indicate most frequent.**

- Inform patient that medication may cause a rust-yellow to brown discoloration of urine, which is not significant.
- Advise patient to notify health care professional if fever, chills, cough, chest pain, dyspnea, skin rash, numbness or tingling of the fingers or toes, or intolerable GI upset occurs. Signs of superinfection (milky, foul-smelling urine; perineal irritation; dysuria) should also be reported.
- Instruct patient to consult health care professional if no improvement is seen within a few days after initiation of therapy.

EVALUATION

Effectiveness of therapy can be demonstrated by: ▪ Resolution of the signs and symptoms of infection. Therapy should be continued for a minimum of 7 days and for at least 3 days after the urine has become sterile ▪ Decrease in the frequency of infections in chronic suppressive therapy.

NITROGLYCERIN
(nye-tro-**gli**-ser-in)

extended-release capsules
Nitrocap T.D., Nitroglyn, Nitrolin, Nitrospan, Nitro-Time

extended-release tablets
Nitrong

extended-release buccal tablets
Nitrogard, {Nitrogard SR}

intravenous
Nitro-Bid IV, Tridil

lingual spray
Nitrolingual

ointment
Nitro-Bid, Nitrol

sublingual
Nitrostat

transdermal system
Deponit, Minitran, Nitrek, Nitrocine, Nitrodisc, Nitro-Dur, Transderm-Nitro

CLASSIFICATION(S):
Antianginal, Coronary vasodilator, Vasodilator (nitrate)

Pregnancy Category C

INDICATIONS

▪ **Lingual, SL:** Acute treatment of angina pectoris ▪ **Lingual, SL; extended-release tablet; buccal tablet; capsules; ointment; transdermal:** Long-term prophylactic management of angina pectoris ▪ **PO, transdermal, ointment:** Adjunct treatment of congestive heart failure ▪ **IV:** Adjunct treatment of acute myocardial infarction ▪ Production of controlled hypotension during surgical procedures.

ACTION

▪ Increases coronary blood flow by dilating coronary arteries and improving collateral flow to ischemic regions ▪ Produces vasodilation (venous greater than arterial) ▪ Decreases left ventricular end-diastolic pressure and left ventricular end-diastolic volume (preload) ▪ Reduces myocardial oxygen consumption. **Therapeutic Effects:** ▪ Relief or prevention of anginal attacks ▪ Increased cardiac output ▪ Reduction of blood pressure.

PHARMACOKINETICS

Absorption: Well absorbed following oral, buccal, and sublingual administration. Also absorbed through skin. Orally administered nitroglycerin is rapidly metabolized, leading to decreased bioavailability.
Distribution: UK.
Metabolism and Excretion: Undergoes rapid and almost complete metabolism by the liver; also metabolized by enzymes in bloodstream.
Half-life: 1–4 min.

CONTRAINDICATIONS AND PRECAUTIONS

Contraindicated in: ▪ Hypersensitivity ▪ Severe anemia ▪ Pericardial tamponade ▪ Constrictive pericarditis ▪ Alcohol intolerance (large IV doses only).
Use Cautiously in: ▪ Head trauma or cerebral hemorrhage ▪ Pregnancy (may compromise maternal/fetal circulation) ▪ Children or lactation

{} = Available in Canada only.

(safety not established) ▪ Glaucoma ▪ Hypertrophic cardiomyopathy ▪ Severe liver impairment ▪ Malabsorption or hypermotility (PO) ▪ Hypovolemia (IV) ▪ Normal or decreased pulmonary capillary wedge pressure (IV) ▪ Cardioversion (remove transdermal patch prior to procedure).

ADVERSE REACTIONS AND SIDE EFFECTS*

CNS: dizziness, headache, apprehension, restlessness, weakness.
EENT: blurred vision.
CV: hypotension, tachycardia, syncope.
GI: abdominal pain, nausea, vomiting.
Derm: contact dermatitis (transdermal or ointment).
Misc: alcohol intoxication (large IV doses only), cross-tolerance, flushing, tolerance.

INTERACTIONS

Drug-Drug: ▪ Additive hypotension with **antihypertensives**, acute ingestion of **alcohol, beta-adrenergic blocking agents, calcium channel blockers, haloperidol**, or **phenothiazines** ▪ **Agents having anticholinergic properties (tricyclic antidepressants, antihistamines, phenothiazines)** may decrease absorption of lingual, sublingual, or buccal nitroglycerin.

ROUTE AND DOSAGE

- **SL (Adults):** 0.3–0.6 mg; may repeat q 5 min for 15 min for acute attack.
- **Lingual Spray (Adults):** (0.4 mg/spray) 1–2 sprays; may be repeated q 5 min for 15 min.
- **Buccal (Adults):** 1 mg q 5 hr; dosage and frequency may be increased as needed.
- **PO (Adults):** *Extended-release capsules*—2.5–9 mg q 8–12 hr. *Extended-release tablets*—1.3–6.5 mg q 8–12 hr.
- **IV (Adults):** 5 mcg/min; increase by 5 mcg/min q 3–5 min to 20 mcg/min, then increase by 10–20 mcg/min q 3–5 min (dosing determined by hemodynamic parameters).
- **Transdermal, Ointment (Adults):** *Ointment*—(1 in. = 15 mg) 1–2 in. q 8 hr (up to 5 in. q 4 hr). *Transdermal patch*—0.1–0.6 mg/hr, up to 0.8 mg/hr. Patch should be worn 12–14 hr/day.

AVAILABILITY

▪ ***Extended-release tablets:*** 2.6 mg^{Rx}, 6.5 mg^{Rx}, 9 mg^{Rx} ▪ ***Extended-release capsules:*** 2.5 mg^{Rx}, 6.5 mg^{Rx}, 9 mg^{Rx} ▪ ***Sublingual tablets:*** 0.3 mg^{Rx}, 0.4 mg^{Rx}, 0.6 mg^{Rx} ▪ ***Translingual spray:*** 0.4 mg/spray in 14.5-g canister (200 doses)^{Rx} ▪ ***Extended-release buccal tablets:*** 1 mg^{Rx}, 2 mg^{Rx}, 3 mg^{Rx}, {5 mg^{Rx}} ▪ ***Transdermal systems:*** 0.1 mg/hr^{Rx}, 0.2 mg/hr^{Rx}, 0.3 mg/hr^{Rx}, 0.4 mg/hr^{Rx}, 0.6 mg/hr^{Rx}, 0.8 mg/hr^{Rx} ▪ ***Transdermal ointment:*** 2%^{Rx} ▪ ***Injection:*** 0.5 mg/ml^{Rx}, 5 mg/ml^{Rx} ▪ ***Injection solution:*** 25 mg/250 ml^{Rx}, 50 mg/250 ml^{Rx}, 50 mg/500 ml^{Rx}, 100 mg/250 ml^{Rx}, 200 mg/500 ml^{Rx}.

TIME/ACTION PROFILE (cardiovascular effects)

	ONSET	PEAK	DURATION
SL	1–3 min	UK	30–60 min
Buccal-ER	UK	UK	5 hr
PO	40–60 min	UK	8–12 hr
TD-Oint	20–60 min	UK	4–8 hr
TD-Patch	40–60 min	UK	8–24 hr
IV	immediate	UK	several min

NURSING IMPLICATIONS

ASSESSMENT

□ Assess location, duration, intensity, and precipitating factors of patient's anginal pain.
□ Monitor blood pressure and pulse prior to and following administration. Patients receiving IV nitroglycerin require continuous ECG and blood pressure monitoring. Additional hemodynamic parameters may be monitored.
▪ ***Lab Test Considerations:*** May cause increased urine catecholamine and urine vanillylmandelic acid concentrations.
□ Excessive doses may cause increased methemoglobin concentrations.
□ May cause falsely elevated serum cholesterol levels.

POTENTIAL NURSING DIAGNOSES

- Pain (Indications).
- Tissue perfusion, altered (Indications).
- Knowledge deficit, related to medication regimen (Patient/Family Teaching).

N

***CAPITALS indicate life-threatening; underlines indicate most frequent.**

IMPLEMENTATION

- **PO:** Administer dose 1 hr before or 2 hr after meals with a full glass of water for faster absorption. Sustained-release preparations should be swallowed whole; do not crush, break, or chew.
- **SL:** Tablet should be held under tongue until dissolved. Avoid eating, drinking, or smoking until tablet is dissolved.
- **Buccal:** Place tablet under upper lip or between cheek and gum. Onset of action may be increased by touching the tablet with the tongue or by drinking hot liquids.
- **IV:** Doses must be diluted and administered as an infusion. Standard infusion sets made of polyvinyl chloride (PVC) plastic may absorb up to 80% of the nitroglycerin in solution. Use glass bottles only and special tubing provided by manufacturer.
- **Continuous Infusion:** Dilute in D5W or 0.9% NaCl in a concentration of 25–40 mcg/ml, dependent upon patient's fluid tolerance (see Appendix D for infusion rate chart). Solution is stable for 48 hr at room temperature. Solution is not explosive either before or after dilution.
- ***Rate:*** Administer via infusion pump to ensure accurate rate. Titrate rate according to patient response.
- **Y-Site Compatibility:** ▪ amiodarone ▪ amrinone ▪ atracurium ▪ diltiazem ▪ dobutamine ▪ dopamine ▪ esmolol ▪ famotidine ▪ haloperidol ▪ heparin ▪ insulin ▪ labetalol ▪ lidocaine ▪ midazolam ▪ nitroprusside ▪ pancuronium ▪ ranitidine ▪ streptokinase ▪ tacrolimus ▪ theophylline ▪ vecuronium.
- **Additive Incompatibility:** ▪ Manufacturer recommends that nitroglycerin not be admixed with other medications.
- **Topical:** Sites of topical application should be rotated to prevent skin irritation. Remove patch or ointment from previous site before application.
  - Doses may be increased to the highest dose that does not cause symptomatic hypotension.
  - Apply ointment by using dose-measuring application papers supplied with ointment. Squeeze ointment onto measuring scale printed on paper. Use paper to spread ointment onto nonhairy area of skin (chest, abdomen, thighs; avoid distal extremities) in a thin, even layer, covering a 2–3-in. area. Do not allow ointment to come in contact with hands. Do not massage or rub in ointment, as this will increase absorption and interfere with sustained action. Apply occlusive dressing if ordered.
  - Transdermal patches may be applied to any hairless site (avoid distal extremities or areas with cuts or calluses). Apply firm pressure over patch to ensure contact with skin, especially around edges. Apply a new dosage unit if the first one becomes loose or falls off. Units are waterproof and not affected by showering or bathing. Do not cut or trim system to adjust dosage. Do not alternate between brands of transdermal products; dosage may not be equivalent. Remove patches before cardioversion or defibrillation to prevent patient burns. Patch may be worn for 12–14 hr and removed for 10–12 hr at night to prevent development of tolerance.

PATIENT/FAMILY TEACHING

- **General Info:** Instruct patient to take medication exactly as directed, even if feeling better. If a dose is missed, take as soon as remembered unless next dose is scheduled within 2 hr (6 hr with extended-release preparations). Do not double doses. Do not discontinue abruptly; gradual dosage reduction may be necessary to prevent rebound angina.
  - Caution patient to change positions slowly to minimize orthostatic hypotension. First dose should be taken while in a sitting or reclining position, especially in geriatric patients.
  - Advise patient to avoid concurrent use of alcohol with this medication. Patient should also consult health care professional before taking OTC medications while taking nitroglycerin.
  - Inform patient that headache is a common side effect that should decrease with continuing therapy. Aspirin or acetaminophen may be ordered to treat headache. Notify health care professional if headache is persistent or severe.
  - Advise patient to notify health care professional if dry mouth or blurred vision occurs.
- **Acute Anginal Attacks:** Advise patient to sit down and use medication at first sign of attack. Relief usually occurs within 5 min. Dose may be repeated if pain is not relieved in 5–10 min. Call health care professional or go to

nearest emergency room if anginal pain is not relieved by 3 tablets in 15 min.

- **SL:** Inform patient that tablets should be kept in original glass container or in specially made metal containers, with cotton removed to prevent absorption. Tablets lose potency in containers made of plastic or cardboard or when mixed with other capsules or tablets. Exposure to air, heat, and moisture also causes loss of potency. Instruct patient not to open bottle frequently, handle tablets, or keep bottle of tablets next to body (i.e., shirt pocket) or in automobile glove compartment. Advise patient that tablets should be replaced 6 mo after opening to maintain potency.
- **Lingual Spray:** Instruct patient to lift tongue and spray dose under tongue.

EVALUATION

Effectiveness of therapy can be demonstrated by: ▪ Decrease in frequency and severity of anginal attacks ▫ Increase in activity tolerance. During chronic therapy, tolerance may be minimized by intermittent administration in 12–14 hr on/10–12 hr off intervals ▪ Controlled hypotension during surgical procedures.

NITROPRUSSIDE

(nye-troe-**pruss**-ide)
Nitropress

CLASSIFICATION(S):
Antihypertensive agent (vasodilator)

Pregnancy Category C

INDICATIONS

▪ Hypertensive crises ▪ Controlled hypotension during anesthesia ▪ Cardiac pump failure or cardiogenic shock (alone or with dopamine).

ACTION

▪ Produces peripheral vasodilation by a direct action on venous and arteriolar smooth muscle. **Therapeutic Effects:** ▪ Rapid lowering of blood pressure ▪ Decreased cardiac preload and afterload.

PHARMACOKINETICS

Absorption: IV administration results in complete bioavailability.
Distribution: UK.
Metabolism and Excretion: Rapidly metabolized in RBCs and tissues to cyanide and subsequently by the liver to thiocyanate.
Half-life: 2 min.

CONTRAINDICATIONS AND PRECAUTIONS

Contraindicated in: ▪ Hypersensitivity ▪ Decreased cerebral perfusion.
Use Cautiously in: ▪ Renal disease (increased risk of thiocyanate accumulation) ▪ Hepatic disease (increased risk of cyanide accumulation) ▪ Geriatric patients (increased sensitivity) ▪ Hypothyroidism ▪ Hyponatremia ▪ Vitamin B_{12} deficiency ▪ Pregnancy or lactation (safety not established).

ADVERSE REACTIONS AND SIDE EFFECTS*

CNS: dizziness, headache, restlessness.
EENT: blurred vision, tinnitus.
CV: dyspnea, hypotension, palpitations.
GI: abdominal pain, nausea, vomiting.
F and E: acidosis.
Local: phlebitis at IV site.
Misc: CYANIDE TOXICITY, thiocyanate toxicity.

INTERACTIONS

Drug-Drug: ▪ Increased hypotensive effect with **ganglionic blocking agents, general anesthetics**, and other **antihypertensives** ▪ **Estrogens** and **sympathomimetics** may decrease the response to nitroprusside.

ROUTE AND DOSAGE

- **IV (Adults and Children):** 0.3 mcg/kg/min initially; may be increased as needed up to 10 mcg/kg/min (usual dose is 3 mcg/kg/min; not to exceed 10 min of therapy at 10 mcg/kg/min infusion rate).

AVAILABILITY

▪ ***Powder for injection:*** 50 mg/vial[Rx].

N

***CAPITALS indicate life-threatening; underlines indicate most frequent.**

TIME/ACTION PROFILE (hypotensive effect)

	ONSET	PEAK	DURATION
IV	immediate	rapid	1–10 min

NURSING IMPLICATIONS

ASSESSMENT

- Monitor blood pressure, heart rate, and ECG frequently throughout therapy; continuous monitoring is preferred. Consult physician for parameters. Monitor for rebound hypertension following discontinuation of nitroprusside.
- Pulmonary capillary wedge pressure (PCWP) may be monitored in patients with myocardial infarction or congestive heart failure.
- ***Lab Test Considerations:*** May cause decrease in bicarbonate concentrations, Pco_2, and pH.
- May cause increased lactate concentrations.
- May cause increased serum cyanide and thiocyanate concentrations.
- Monitor serum methemoglobin concentrations in patients receiving >10 mg/kg and exhibiting signs of impaired oxygen delivery despite adequate cardiac output and arterial Pco_2 (blood is chocolate brown without change on exposure to air). Treatment of methemoglobinemia is 1–2 mg/kg of methylene blue IV administered over several minutes.
- ***Toxicity and Overdose:*** If severe hypotension occurs, drug effects are quickly reversed, within 1–10 min, by decreasing rate or temporarily discontinuing infusion. May place patient in Trendelenburg position to maximize venous return.
- Plasma thiocyanate levels should be monitored daily in patients receiving prolonged infusions at a rate >3 mcg/kg/min or 1 mcg/kg/min in patients with anuria. Thiocyanate levels should not exceed 1 millimole/liter.
- Signs and symptoms of thiocyanate toxicity include tinnitus, toxic psychoses, hyperreflexia, confusion, weakness, seizures, and coma.
- Cyanide toxicity may manifest as lactic acidosis, hypoxemia, tachycardia, altered consciousness, seizures, and characteristic breath odor similar to almonds.
- Acute treatment of cyanide toxicity includes 4–6 mg/kg of *sodium nitrite* (as a 3% solution) over 2–4 min. This acts as a buffer for cyanide by converting 10% of hemoglobin to methemoglobin. If administration of sodium nitrite is delayed, inhalation of crushed ampule (vaporole, aspirole) of *amyl nitrite* for 15–30 sec of every minute should be started until sodium nitrite is running. Following completion of sodium nitrite infusion, administer *sodium thiosulfate* 150–200 mcg/kg (available as 25% and 50% solutions). This will convert cyanide to thiocyanate, which may then be eliminated. If required, entire regimen may be repeated in 2 hr at 50% of the initial doses.

POTENTIAL NURSING DIAGNOSES

- Tissue perfusion, altered (Indications).

IMPLEMENTATION

- **General Info:** If infusion of 10 mcg/kg/min for 10 min does not produce adequate reduction in blood pressure, manufacturer recommends nitroprusside be discontinued.
- May be administered in left ventricular congestive heart failure concurrently with an inotropic agent (dopamine, dobutamine) when effective doses of nitroprusside restore pump function and cause excessive hypotension.
- **Continuous Infusion:** Reconstitute each 50 mg with 2–3 ml of D5W for injection without preservatives. Dilute further in 250–1000 ml of D5W for concentrations of 200–500 mcg/ml. Do not use other diluents for reconstitution or infusion. Wrap infusion bottle in aluminum foil to protect from light; administration set tubing need not be covered. Amber plastic bags do not offer sufficient protection from light; wrap must be opaque. Freshly prepared solution has a slight brownish tint; discard if solution is dark brown, orange, blue, green, or dark red. Solution must be used within 24 hr of preparation.
- Avoid extravasation.
- ***Rate:*** Administer via infusion pump to ensure accurate dosage rate (see Appendix D for dosage rate chart).
- **Y-Site Compatibility:** ▪ amrinone ▪ atracurium ▪ diltiazem ▪ dobutamine ▪ dopamine ▪ enalaprilat ▪ esmolol ▪ famotidine ▪ heparin ▪ indomethacin ▪ insulin ▪ labetalol ▪ lidocaine ▪ midazolam ▪ morphine ▪ nitroglycerin ▪ pancuronium ▪ tacrolimus ▪ theophylline ▪ vecuronium.

▪ **Additive Incompatibility:** ▪ Do not admix with other medications.

PATIENT/FAMILY TEACHING

□ Advise patient to report the onset of tinnitus, dyspnea, dizziness, headache, or blurred vision immediately.

EVALUATION

Effectiveness of therapy can be demonstrated by: ▪ Decrease in blood pressure without the appearance of side effects ▪ Treatment of cardiac pump failure or cardiogenic shock.

NORTRIPTYLINE

(nor-**trip**-ti-leen)

Aventyl, Pamelor

CLASSIFICATION(S):

Antidepressant (tricyclic)

Pregnancy Category UK

INDICATIONS

▪ Treatment of various forms of depression (with psychotherapy). **Unlabeled Uses:** ▪ Management of chronic neurogenic pain.

ACTION

▪ Potentiates the effect of serotonin and norepinephrine ▪ Has significant anticholinergic properties. **Therapeutic Effects:** ▪ Antidepressant action that develops slowly over several weeks.

PHARMACOKINETICS

Absorption: Well absorbed following oral administration.

Distribution: Widely distributed. Enters breast milk in small amounts; probably crosses the placenta.

Metabolism and Excretion: Extensively metabolized by the liver, much of it on its first pass. Some is converted to active compounds. Undergoes enterohepatic recirculation and secretion into gastric juices.

Half-life: 18–28 hr.

CONTRAINDICATIONS AND PRECAUTIONS

Contraindicated in: ▪ Hypersensitivity ▪ Narrow-angle glaucoma ▪ Pregnancy and lactation ▪ Alcohol intolerance (solution only).

Use Cautiously in: ▪ Geriatric patients (more susceptible to adverse reactions; dosage reduction recommended) ▪ Pre-existing cardiovascular disease ▪ Geriatric males with prostatic hyperplasia (more susceptible to urinary retention) ▪ History of seizures ▪ Asthma.

ADVERSE REACTIONS AND SIDE EFFECTS*

CNS: drowsiness, fatigue, lethargy, agitation, confusion, extrapyramidal reactions, hallucinations, headache, insomnia.

EENT: blurred vision, dry eyes, dry mouth.

CV: ARRHYTHMIAS, hypotension, ECG changes.

GI: constipation, nausea, paralytic ileus, unpleasant taste.

GU: urinary retention.

Derm: photosensitivity.

Endo: gynecomastia.

Hemat: blood dyscrasias.

Metab: weight gain.

INTERACTIONS

Drug-Drug: ▪ May cause hypertension, hyperpyrexia, seizures, and death when used with **MAO inhibitors** (avoid concurrent use—discontinue 2 wk prior to nortriptyline) ▪ May prevent the therapeutic response to most **antihypertensives** ▪ Hypertensive crisis may occur with **clonidine** ▪ Additive CNS depression with other **CNS depressants**, including **alcohol, antihistamines, opioids,** and **sedative/hypnotics** ▪ Sympathomimetic effects may be additive with other **adrenergic agents,** including **vasoconstrictors** and **decongestants** ▪ Additive anticholinergic effects with other **drugs possessing anticholinergic properties,** including **antihistamines, antidepressants, atropine, haloperidol, phenothiazines, quinidine,** and **disopyramide** ▪ **Cimetidine, fluoxetine,** or **oral contraceptives** increase blood levels and risk of toxicity ▪ Increased risk of agranulocytosis with **antithyroid agents.**

N

***CAPITALS indicate life-threatening; underlines indicate most frequent.**

ROUTE AND DOSAGE

- **PO (Adults):** 25 mg 3–4 times daily, up to 150 mg/day.
- **PO (Geriatric Patients):** 30–50 mg/day in divided doses.
- **PO (Children >12 yr):** 25–50 mg/day or 1–3 mg/kg/day in divided doses initially.
- **PO (Children 6–12 yr):** 10–20 mg/day or 1–3 mg/kg/day in divided doses.

AVAILABILITY

- ***Capsules:*** 10 mg^{Rx}, 25 mg^{Rx}, 50 mg^{Rx}, 75 mg^{Rx}
- ***Oral solution:*** 10 mg/5 ml^{Rx}.

TIME/ACTION PROFILE (antidepressant effect)

	ONSET	PEAK	DURATION
PO	2–3 wk	6 wk	UK

NURSING IMPLICATIONS

ASSESSMENT

- **General Info:** Monitor mental status and affect. Assess for suicidal tendencies, especially during early therapy. Restrict amount of drug available to patient.
- □ Monitor blood pressure and pulse rate prior to and during initial therapy. Report significant decreases in blood pressure or a sudden increase in pulse rate.
- □ Monitor baseline and periodic ECGs in elderly patients or patients with heart disease. May cause prolonged PR and QT intervals and may flatten T waves.
- **Pain:** Assess type, location, and severity of pain prior to and periodically throughout therapy.
- ***Lab Test Considerations:*** Assess leukocyte and differential blood counts, liver function, and serum glucose periodically. May cause elevated serum bilirubin and alkaline phosphatase. May cause bone marrow depression. Serum glucose may be increased or decreased.
- □ Serum levels may be monitored in patients who fail to respond to usual therapeutic dose. Therapeutic plasma concentration range is 50–150 ng/ml.
- □ May cause alterations in blood glucose levels.
- ***Toxicity and Overdose:*** Symptoms of acute overdose include disturbed concentration, confusion, restlessness, agitation, convulsions, drowsiness, mydriasis, arrhythmias, fever, hallucinations, vomiting, and dyspnea.
- □ Treatment of overdose includes gastric lavage, activated charcoal, and a stimulant cathartic. Maintain respiratory and cardiac function (monitor ECG for at least 5 days) and temperature. Medications may include digoxin for congestive heart failure, antiarrhythmics, and anticonvulsants.

POTENTIAL NURSING DIAGNOSES

- Coping, ineffective individual (Indications).
- Injury, risk for (Side Effects).
- Knowledge deficit, related to medication regimen (Patient/Family Teaching).

IMPLEMENTATION

- **PO:** Administer medication with meals to minimize gastric irritation.
- □ May be given as a single dose at bedtime to minimize sedation during the day. Dose increases should be made at bedtime because of sedation.

PATIENT/FAMILY TEACHING

- □ Instruct patient to take medication exactly as directed. If a dose is missed, take as soon as possible unless almost time for next dose; if regimen is a single dose at bedtime, do not take in the morning because of side effects. Advise patient that drug effects may not be noticed for at least 2 wk. Abrupt discontinuation may cause nausea, vomiting, diarrhea, headache, trouble sleeping with vivid dreams, and irritability.
- □ May cause drowsiness and blurred vision. Caution patient to avoid driving and other activities requiring alertness until response to drug is known.
- □ Instruct patient to notify health care professional if visual changes occur. Inform patient that periodic glaucoma testing may be required during long-term therapy.
- □ Caution patient to make position changes slowly to minimize orthostatic hypotension. (This side effect is less pronounced with this medication than with other tricyclic antidepressants.)
- □ Advise patient to avoid alcohol or other CNS depressant drugs during therapy and for at least 3–7 days after therapy has been discontinued.

- ▫ Instruct patient to notify health care professional if urinary retention occurs or if dry mouth or constipation persists. Sugarless candy or gum may diminish dry mouth, and an increase in fluid intake or bulk may prevent constipation. If symptoms persist, dose reduction or discontinuation may be necessary. Consult health care professional if dry mouth persists for more than 2 wk.
- ▫ Caution patient to use sunscreen and protective clothing to prevent photosensitivity reactions.
- ▫ Inform patient of need to monitor dietary intake. Increase in appetite may lead to undesired weight gain.
- ▫ May have teratogenic effects. Instruct patient to notify health care professional immediately if pregnancy is planned or suspected.
- ▫ Advise patient to notify health care professional of medication regimen prior to treatment or surgery.
- ▫ Therapy for depression is usually prolonged. Emphasize the importance of follow-up exams and participation in prescribed psychotherapy.

EVALUATION

Effectiveness of therapy can be demonstrated by: ▪ Increased sense of well-being ▫ Renewed interest in surroundings ▫ Increased appetite ▫ Improved energy level ▫ Improved sleep ▪ Decrease in severity of chronic neurogenic pain. Patients may require 2–6 wk of therapy before full therapeutic effects of medication are seen.

NYSTATIN, oral*

(nye-**stat**-in)

Mycostatin, {Nadostine}, Nilstat, Nystex, {PMS-Nystatin}

CLASSIFICATION(S):
Antifungal

Pregnancy Category B

*For other nystatin dosage forms, see antifungals (topical) on page 69 and antifungals (vaginal) on page 72.

INDICATIONS

▪ **Lozenges, oral suspension:** Local treatment of oropharyngeal candidiasis ▪ Treatment of intestinal candidiasis.

ACTION

▪ Binds to fungal cell membrane, allowing leakage of cellular contents. **Therapeutic Effects:** ▪ Fungistatic or fungicidal action. **Spectrum:** ▪ Active against most pathogenic *Candida* species, including *Candida albicans*.

PHARMACOKINETICS

Absorption: Poorly absorbed; action is primarily local.
Distribution: UK.
Metabolism and Excretion: Excreted unchanged in the feces following oral administration.
Half-life: UK.

CONTRAINDICATIONS AND PRECAUTIONS

Contraindicated in: ▪ Hypersensitivity ▪ Some products may contain ethyl alcohol or benzyl alcohol—avoid use in patients who may be hypersensitive to or intolerant of these additives.
Use Cautiously in: ▪ Children <5 yr (lozenges, pastilles, troches) ▪ Denture wearers (dentures require soaking in nystatin suspension).

ADVERSE REACTIONS AND SIDE EFFECTS

GI: *PO*—diarrhea, nausea, stomach pain (large doses), vomiting.

INTERACTIONS

Drug-Drug: ▪ None significant.

ROUTE AND DOSAGE

- **PO (Adults and Children):** 400,000–600,000 units 4 times daily as oral suspension or 200,000–400,000 units 4–5 times daily as pastilles (lozenges).
- **PO (Infants):** 200,000 units 4 times daily.
- **PO (Infants, Premature and Low Birth Weight):** 100,000 units 4 times daily.

N

{} = Available in Canada only.

AVAILABILITY

▪ ***Oral suspension:*** 100,000 units/ml in 5-, 60-, and 480-ml containers[Rx] ▪ ***Oral pastilles (lozenges, troches):*** 200,000 units/troche[Rx] ▪ ***Powder for oral suspension:*** ⅛ tsp = 500,000 units in 50-, 150-, and 500-million, 1-, 2-, and 5-billion-unit containers[Rx] ▪ ***Oral tablets:*** 500,000 units[Rx].

TIME/ACTION PROFILE (antifungal effects)

	ONSET	PEAK	DURATION
PO	rapid	UK	2 hr*

*Maintenance of saliva levels required to inhibit growth of *Candida* species following oral dissolution of 2 lozenges.

NURSING IMPLICATIONS

ASSESSMENT

□ Inspect mucous membranes prior to and frequently throughout therapy. Increased irritation of mucous membranes may indicate need to discontinue medication.

POTENTIAL NURSING DIAGNOSES

▪ Skin integrity, impaired, actual (Indications).
▪ Infection, risk for (Indications).
▪ Knowledge deficit, related to medication regimen (Patient/Family Teaching).

IMPLEMENTATION

▪ **PO:** Suspension should be administered by placing ½ of dose in each side of mouth. Patient should hold suspension in mouth or swish throughout mouth for several minutes prior to swallowing, then gargle and swallow. Use calibrated measuring device for liquid doses. Shake well prior to administration.

□ To prepare oral solution from powder, add ⅛ tsp (approximately 500,000 units) to 120 ml of water and stir well. Prepare immediately before use; contains no preservatives.

□ Lozenges (pastilles) should be allowed to dissolve slowly and completely in mouth; do not chew or swallow whole. Nystatin vaginal tablets can be administered orally for treatment of oral candidiasis.

PATIENT/FAMILY TEACHING

□ Instruct patient to take medication as directed. If a dose is missed, take as soon as remembered but not if almost time for next dose. Do not double doses. Therapy should be continued for at least 2 days after symptoms subside.

□ Advise patient to report increased irritation of mucous membranes or lack of therapeutic response to health care professional.

EVALUATION

Effectiveness of therapy can be demonstrated by: ▪ Decrease in stomatitis □ To prevent relapse following oral therapy, therapy should be continued for 48 hr after symptoms have disappeared and cultures are negative □ Therapy for a period of 2 wk is usually sufficient, but more prolonged therapy may be necessary.

OCTREOTIDE

(ok-**tree**-oh-tide)
Sandostatin

CLASSIFICATION(S):
Antidiarrheal, Hormone (gastrointestinal)

Pregnancy Category B

INDICATIONS

▪ Treatment of severe diarrhea and flushing episodes in patients with GI endocrine tumors, including metastatic carcinoid tumors and vasoactive intestinal peptide tumors (VIPomas). **Unlabeled Uses:** ▪ Relief of symptoms and suppressed tumor growth in patients with pituitary tumors associated with acromegaly ▪ Management of diarrhea in AIDS patients or patients with fistulas.

ACTION

▪ Suppresses secretion of serotonin and gastroenterohepatic peptides ▪ Increases absorption of fluid and electrolytes from the GI tract and increases transit time ▪ Decreases levels of serotonin metabolites ▪ Also suppresses growth hormone, insulin, and glucagon. **Therapeutic Effects:** ▪ Control of severe flushing and diarrhea associated with GI endocrine tumors.

PHARMACOKINETICS

Absorption: Well absorbed following SC administration.
Distribution: UK.
Protein Binding: 65%.

Metabolism and Excretion: 32% excreted unchanged in urine.
Half-life: 1.5 hr.

CONTRAINDICATIONS AND PRECAUTIONS

Contraindicated in: ▪ Hypersensitivity.
Use Cautiously in: ▪ Gallbladder disease (increased risk of stone formation) ▪ Renal impairment (dosage reduction may be necessary) ▪ Hyperglycemia or hypoglycemia (changes in blood sugar may occur) ▪ Fat malabsorption (may be aggravated) ▪ Pregnancy or lactation (safety not established).

ADVERSE REACTIONS AND SIDE EFFECTS

CNS: dizziness, drowsiness, fatigue, headache, weakness.
EENT: visual disturbances.
CV: edema, orthostatic hypotension, palpitations.
GI: abdominal pain, cholelithiasis, diarrhea, fat malabsorption, nausea, vomiting.
Derm: flushing.
Endo: hyperglycemia, hypoglycemia.
Local: injection site pain.

INTERACTIONS

Drug-Drug: ▪ May alter requirements for **insulin** or **oral hypoglycemic agents** ▪ May reduce blood levels of **cyclosporine.**

ROUTE AND DOSAGE

- **SC (Adults):** *Carcinoid tumors*—50 mcg initially, then 100–600 mcg/day in 2–4 divided doses during first 2 wk of therapy (range 50–1500 mcg/day). *VIPomas*—50 mcg initially, then 200–300 mcg/day in 2–4 divided doses during first 2 wk of therapy (range 150–750 mcg/day). *Suppression of growth hormone (acromegaly)*—50–100 mcg 2–3 times daily (unlabeled). *Antidiarrheal (AIDS patients)*—100–1800 mcg/day (unlabeled).

AVAILABILITY

▪ ***Injection:*** 0.05 mg/ml in 1-ml ampules[Rx], 0.1 mg/ml in 1-ml ampules[Rx], 0.2 mg/ml in 5-ml vials[Rx], 0.5 mg/ml in 1-ml ampules[Rx], 1 mg/ml in 5-ml vials[Rx].

TIME/ACTION PROFILE (control of symptoms)

	ONSET	PEAK	DURATION
SC	UK	UK	up to 12 hr

NURSING IMPLICATIONS

ASSESSMENT

- ▫ Assess frequency and consistency of stools and bowel sounds throughout therapy.
- ▫ Monitor pulse and blood pressure prior to and periodically throughout therapy.
- ▫ Assess patient's fluid and electrolyte balance and skin turgor for dehydration.
- ▫ Monitor diabetic patients for signs of hypoglycemia. May require reduction in requirements for insulin and sulfonylureas and treatment with diazoxide.
- ▫ Assess patient for gallbladder disease; assess for pain and monitor ultrasound examinations of gallbladder and bile ducts prior to and periodically throughout prolonged therapy.
- ▪ ***Lab Test Considerations:*** Monitor 5-HIAA (urinary 5-hydroxyindoleacetic acid), plasma serotonin, and plasma substance P in patients with carcinoid; VIP (plasma vasoactive intestinal peptide) in patients with VIPoma; and free T_4 and serum glucose concentrations prior to and periodically throughout therapy in all patients taking octreotide.
- ▫ Monitor quantitative 72-hr fecal fat and serum carotene determinations periodically for possible drug-induced aggravations of fat malabsorption.
- ▫ May cause a slight increase in liver enzymes.
- ▫ May cause decreased serum thyroxine (T_4) concentrations.

POTENTIAL NURSING DIAGNOSES

- Diarrhea (Indications).
- Knowledge deficit, related to medication regimen (Patient/Family Teaching).

IMPLEMENTATION

- **General Info:** Do not use solution that is discolored or contains particulate matter. Ampules should be refrigerated but may be stored at room temperature for the days they will be used. Discard unused solution.
- **SC:** Rotate injection sites; avoid multiple injections in same site within short periods of

time. Preferred injection sites are the hip, thigh, or abdomen.
- □ Administer injections between meals and at bedtime to avoid GI side effects.
- □ Allow medication to reach room temperature prior to injection to minimize local reactions at injection site.
- ■ **Direct IV:** Bolus injections have been used under emergency conditions.
- ■ ***Rate:*** Administer over 3 min.
- ■ **Intermittent Infusion:** Dilute in 50–200 ml of 0.9% NaCl or D5W.
- ■ ***Rate:*** Administer over 15–30 min.

PATIENT/FAMILY TEACHING

- ■ **General Info:** May cause dizziness, drowsiness, or visual disturbances. Caution patient to avoid driving or other activities requiring alertness until response to medication is known.
- □ Advise patient to change positions slowly to minimize orthostatic hypotension.
- ■ **Home Care Issues:** Instruct patients administering octreotide at home on correct technique for injection, storage, and disposal of equipment.
- □ Instruct patient to administer octreotide exactly as directed. If a dose is missed, administer as soon as possible, then return to regular schedule. Do not double doses.

EVALUATION

Effectiveness of therapy can be demonstrated by: ■ Decrease in severity of diarrhea and improvement of electrolyte imbalances in patients with carcinoid or VIP-secreting tumors ■ Relief of symptoms and suppressed tumor growth in patients with pituitary tumors associated with acromegaly ■ Management of diarrhea in patients with AIDS.

OLANZAPINE

(oh-**lan**-za-peen)
Zyprexa

CLASSIFICATION(S):
Antipsychotic agent (thienbenzodiazepine)

Pregnancy Category C

INDICATIONS

■ Management of psychotic disorders.

ACTION

■ Antagonizes dopamine and serotonin type 2 in the CNS ■ Also has anticholinergic, antihistaminic, and anti–alpha$_1$-adrenergic effects. **Therapeutic Effects:** ■ Decreased manifestations of psychoses.

PHARMACOKINETICS

Absorption: Well absorbed but rapidly metabolized by first-pass effect, resulting in 60% bioavailability.
Distribution: Extensively distributed.
Metabolism and Excretion: Highly metabolized; 7% excreted unchanged in urine.
Half-life: 21–54 hr.

CONTRAINDICATIONS AND PRECAUTIONS

Contraindicated in: ■ Hypersensitivity ■ Lactation.
Use Cautiously in: ■ Patients with hepatic impairment ■ Geriatric patients (may require smaller doses) ■ Cardiovascular or cerebrovascular disease ■ History of seizures ■ History of attemped suicide ■ Prostatic hypertrophy ■ Narrow-angle glaucoma ■ History of paralytic ileus ■ Pregnancy or children <18 yr (safety not established).

ADVERSE REACTIONS AND SIDE EFFECTS*

CNS: NEUROLEPTIC MALIGNANT SYNDROME, SEIZURES, agitation, dizziness, headache, restlessness, sedation, weakness, dystonia, insomnia, mood changes, personality disorder, speech impairment, tardive dyskinesia.
EENT: amblyopia, rhinitis, increased salivation, pharyngitis.
Resp: cough, dyspnea.
CV: orthostatic hypotension, tachycardia, chest pain.
GI: constipation, dry mouth, abdominal pain, increased appetite, nausea.
GU: decreased libido, urinary incontinence.
Derm: photosensitivity.
Endo: diabetes mellitus, goiter.
F and E: increased thirst.

***CAPITALS indicate life-threatening; underlines indicate most frequent.**

Metab: weight gain, weight loss.
MS: hypertonia, joint pain.
Neuro: tremor.
Misc: fever, flu-like syndrome.

INTERACTIONS

Drug-Drug: ▪ Effects may be decreased by concurrent **carbamazepine, omeprazole,** or **rifampin** ▪ Additive hypotension may occur with **antihypertensive agents** ▪ Additive CNS depression may occur with concurrent use of **alcohol** or other **CNS depressants** ▪ May antagonize the effects of **levodopa** or other **dopamine agonists.**

ROUTE AND DOSAGE

- **PO (Adults—Most Patients):** 5–10 mg/day initially; may increase at weekly intervals by 5 mg/day (not to exceed 15 mg/day).
- **PO (Adults—Debilitated or Nonsmoking Female Patients ≥65 yr):** Initiate therapy at 5 mg/day.

AVAILABILITY

- ***Tablets:*** 2.5 mg[Rx], 5 mg[Rx], 7.5 mg[Rx], 10 mg[Rx].

TIME/ACTION PROFILE (antipsychotic effects)

	ONSET	PEAK	DURATION
PO	UK	1 wk	UK

NURSING IMPLICATIONS

ASSESSMENT

- **General Info:** Assess patient's mental status (orientation, mood, behavior) prior to and periodically throughout therapy.
- Monitor blood pressure (sitting, standing, lying), ECG, pulse, and respiratory rate prior to and frequently during the period of dosage adjustment.
- Observe patient carefully when administering medication to ensure medication is actually taken and not hoarded.
- Assess fluid intake and bowel function. Increased bulk and fluids in the diet may help minimize constipation.
- Monitor patient for onset of akathisia (restlessness or desire to keep moving) and extrapyramidal side effects (*parkinsonian*—difficulty speaking or swallowing, loss of balance control, pill rolling, mask-like face, shuffling gait, rigidity, tremors; and *dystonic*—muscle spasms, twisting motions, twitching, inability to move eyes, weakness of arms or legs) every 2 mo during therapy and 8–12 wk after therapy has been discontinued. Report these symptoms if they occur, as reduction in dosage or discontinuation of medication may be necessary. Trihexyphenidyl or diphenhydramine may be used to control symptoms.
- Monitor for tardive dyskinesia (uncontrolled rhythmic movement of mouth, face, and extremities; lip smacking or puckering; puffing of cheeks; uncontrolled chewing; rapid or worm-like movements of tongue). Report immediately; may be irreversible.
- Monitor for development of neuroleptic malignant syndrome (fever, respiratory distress, tachycardia, convulsions, diaphoresis, hypertension or hypotension, pallor, tiredness, severe muscle stiffness, loss of bladder control). Notify physician or other health care professional immediately if these symptoms occur.
- ***Lab Test Considerations:*** CBC, liver function tests, and ocular examinations should be evaluated periodically throughout therapy. May cause decreased platelets. May cause elevated bilirubin, AST, ALT, GGT, CPK, and alkaline phosphatase.

POTENTIAL NURSING DIAGNOSES

- Thought processes, altered (Indications).
- Knowledge deficit, related to medication regimen (Patient/Family Teaching).
- Noncompliance (Patient/Family Teaching).

IMPLEMENTATION

- **PO:** May be administered without regard to meals.

PATIENT/FAMILY TEACHING

- Advise patient to take medication exactly as directed and not to skip doses or double up on missed doses. May need to discontinue gradually.
- Inform patient of possibility of extrapyramidal symptoms and tardive dyskinesia. Instruct patient to report these symptoms immediately to health care professional.
- Advise patient to change positions slowly to minimize orthostatic hypotension.
- Medication may cause drowsiness. Caution patient to avoid driving or other activities re-

quiring alertness until response to the medication is known.

- Caution patient to avoid taking alcohol or other CNS depressants concurrently with this medication.
- Advise patient to use sunscreen and protective clothing when exposed to the sun. Extremes of temperature (exercise, hot weather, hot baths or showers) should also be avoided, because this drug impairs body temperature regulation.
- Instruct patient to use frequent mouth rinses, good oral hygiene, and sugarless gum or candy to minimize dry mouth. Consult health care professional if dry mouth continues for >2 wk.
- Advise patient to notify health care professional of medication regimen prior to treatment or surgery.
- Instruct patient to notify health care professional promptly if sore throat, fever, unusual bleeding or bruising, rash, weakness, tremors, visual disturbances, dark-colored urine, or clay-colored stools occur.
- Emphasize the importance of routine follow-up exams and continued participation in psychotherapy as indicated.

EVALUATION

Effectiveness of therapy can be demonstrated by: ▪ Decrease in excitable, paranoic, or withdrawn behavior.

OMEPRAZOLE

(o-**mep**-ra-zole)
Prilosec

CLASSIFICATION(S):
Antiulcer agent (gastric acid–pump inhibitor)

Pregnancy Category C

INDICATIONS

▪ Management of gastroesophageal reflux disease (GERD) ▪ Management of duodenal ulcers (with or without anti-infectives for *Helicobacter pylori*) ▪ Treatment of pathologic hypersecretory conditions, including Zollinger-Ellison syndrome.

ACTION

▪ Binds to an enzyme on gastric parietal cells in the presence of acidic gastric pH, preventing the final transport of hydrogen ions into the gastric lumen. **Therapeutic Effects:** ▪ Diminished accumulation of acid in the gastric lumen with lessened gastroesophageal reflux ▪ Healing of duodenal ulcers.

PHARMACOKINETICS

Absorption: Rapidly absorbed following oral administration.
Distribution: Good distribution into gastric parietal cells.
Metabolism and Excretion: Extensively metabolized by the liver.
Half-life: 0.5–1 hr (increased in liver disease).

CONTRAINDICATIONS AND PRECAUTIONS

Contraindicated in: ▪ Hypersensitivity.
Use Cautiously in: ▪ Liver disease (dosage reduction may be necessary) ▪ Pregnancy, lactation, or children (safety not established).

ADVERSE REACTIONS AND SIDE EFFECTS*

CNS: dizziness, drowsiness, fatigue, headache, weakness.
CV: chest pain.
GI: abdominal pain, acid regurgitation, constipation, diarrhea, flatulence, nausea, vomiting.
Derm: itching, rash.

INTERACTIONS

Drug-Drug: ▪ Decreases metabolism and may increase effects of **phenytoin, diazepam,** and **warfarin** ▪ May interfere with absorption of drugs requiring acidic gastric pH, including **ketoconazole**, esters of **ampicillin**, and **iron salts** ▪ Has been used safely with **antacids.**

ROUTE AND DOSAGE

▪ **PO (Adults):** *GERD*—20 mg once daily. *Duodenal ulcers associated with* H. pylori—40 mg daily in the morning with clarithromycin for 2 wk, then 20 mg once daily for 2 wk. *Gastric ulcer*—40 mg once daily for 4–6 wk. *Gastric hypersecretory conditions*—60 mg once daily initially; may be increased

*CAPITALS indicate life-threatening; underlines indicate most frequent.

up to 120 mg 3 times daily. Doses >80 mg/day should be given in divided doses.

AVAILABILITY

- ***Delayed capsules:*** 10 mg[Rx], 20 mg[Rx].

TIME/ACTION PROFILE (antisecretory effects)

	ONSET	PEAK	DURATION
PO	within 1 hr	within 2 hr	72–96 hr

NURSING IMPLICATIONS

ASSESSMENT

- Assess patient routinely for epigastric or abdominal pain and frank or occult blood in the stool, emesis, or gastric aspirate.
- ***Lab Test Considerations:*** CBC with differential should be monitored periodically throughout therapy.
- May cause elevated AST, ALT, alkaline phosphatase, and bilirubin.
- May cause serum gastrin concentrations to increase during first 1–2 wk of therapy. Levels return to normal after discontinuation of omeprazole.

POTENTIAL NURSING DIAGNOSES

- Pain (Indications).
- Knowledge deficit, related to medication regimen (Patient/Family Teaching).

IMPLEMENTATION

- **PO:** Administer doses before meals, preferably in the morning. Capsules should be swallowed whole; do not crush, open, or chew.
- May be administered concurrently with antacids.

PATIENT/FAMILY TEACHING

- Instruct patient to take medication as directed for the full course of therapy, even if feeling better. If a dose is missed, it should be taken as soon as remembered but not if almost time for next dose. Do not double doses.
- May cause occasional drowsiness or dizziness. Caution patient to avoid driving or other activities requiring alertness until response to medication is known.
- Advise patient to avoid alcohol, products containing aspirin or NSAIDs, and foods that may cause an increase in GI irritation.
- Advise patient to report onset of black, tarry stools; diarrhea; abdominal pain; or persistent headache to health care professional promptly.

EVALUATION

Effectiveness of therapy can be demonstrated by: ▪ Decrease in abdominal pain or prevention of gastric irritation and bleeding. Healing of duodenal ulcers can be seen on x-ray examination or endoscopy ▪ Decrease in symptoms of gastroesophageal reflux disease (GERD). Therapy is continued for 4–8 wk after initial episode.

ONDANSETRON

(on-**dan**-se-tron)

Zofran

CLASSIFICATION(S):

Antiemetic (5-HT_3 antagonist)

Pregnancy Category B

INDICATIONS

▪ **PO, IV:** Prevention of nausea and vomiting associated with chemotherapy. Oral form to be used only for moderately emetogenic chemotherapy and not for high-dose regimens ▪ **IM, IV:** Treatment and prevention of postoperative nausea and vomiting ▪ **PO:** Management of nausea and vomiting associated with radiation therapy to the abdomen.

ACTION

▪ Blocks the effects of serotonin at 5-HT_3–receptor sites (selective antagonist) located in vagal nerve terminals and the chemoreceptor trigger zone in the CNS. **Therapeutic Effects:** ▪ Decreased incidence and severity of nausea and vomiting following chemotherapy or surgery.

PHARMACOKINETICS

Absorption: IV administration results in complete bioavailability; 50% absorbed following oral administration.

Distribution: UK.

Metabolism and Excretion: Extensively metabolized by the liver; 5% excreted unchanged by the kidneys.

Half-life: 3.5–5.5 hr.

CONTRAINDICATIONS AND PRECAUTIONS

Contraindicated in: ▪ Hypersensitivity.
Use Cautiously in: ▪ Liver impairment (use single doses not to exceed 8 mg) ▪ Abdominal surgery (may mask ileus) ▪ Pregnancy, lactation, or children ≤3 yr (safety not established).

ADVERSE REACTIONS AND SIDE EFFECTS*

CNS: headache, dizziness, drowsiness, fatigue, weakness.
GI: diarrhea, abdominal pain, constipation, dry mouth.
Neuro: extrapyramidal reactions.

INTERACTIONS

Drug-Drug: ▪ May be affected by **drugs altering the activity of liver enzymes.**

ROUTE AND DOSAGE

- **PO (Adults and Children ≥12 yr):** *Prevention of chemotherapy-induced nausea/vomiting*—8 mg 30 min prior to chemotherapy and repeated 8 hr later; 8 mg q 12 hr may be given for 1–2 days following chemotherapy. *Prevention of radiation-induced nausea/vomiting*—8 mg 1–2 hr prior to radiation; may be repeated q 8 hr, depending on type, location, and extent of radiation. *Prevention of postoperative nausea/vomiting*—16 mg 1 hr before induction of anesthesia.
- **PO (Children 4–11 yr):** *Prevention of chemotherapy-induced nausea/vomiting*—4 mg 30 min prior to chemotherapy and repeated 4 and 8 hr later; 4 mg q 8 hr may be given for 1–2 days following chemotherapy.
- **IV (Adults):** *Prevention of chemotherapy-induced nausea/vomiting*—0.15 mg/kg 15–30 min prior to chemotherapy, repeated 4 and 8 hr later, or 32-mg single dose 30 min prior to chemotherapy.
- **IM, IV (Adults):** *Prevention of postoperative nausea/vomiting*—4 mg before induction of anesthesia or postoperatively.
- **IV (Children 4–18 yr):** *Prevention of chemotherapy-induced nausea/vomiting*—0.15 mg/kg 15–30 min prior to chemotherapy, repeated 4 and 8 hr later.
- **IV (Children 2–12 yr and ≤40 kg):** *Prevention of postoperative nausea/vomiting*—0.1 mg/kg.
- **IV (Children >40 kg):** *Prevention of postoperative nausea/vomiting*—4 mg.

AVAILABILITY

▪ ***Tablets:*** 4 mg[Rx], 8 mg[Rx] ▪ ***Oral solution:*** 4 mg/5 ml[Rx] ▪ ***Injection:*** 2 mg/ml in 2- and 20-ml vials[Rx] ▪ ***Premixed injection:*** 32 mg/50 ml single-dose containers[Rx].

TIME/ACTION PROFILE (antiemetic effect)

	ONSET	PEAK	DURATION
PO, IV	rapid	15–30 min	4 hr
IM	rapid	40 min	UK

NURSING IMPLICATIONS

ASSESSMENT

- □ Assess patient for nausea, vomiting, abdominal distention, and bowel sounds prior to and following administration.
- □ Assess patient for extrapyramidal effects (involuntary movements, facial grimacing, rigidity, shuffling walk, trembling of hands) periodically throughout therapy.
- ***Lab Test Considerations:*** May cause transient elevations in serum bilirubin, AST, and ALT levels.

POTENTIAL NURSING DIAGNOSES

- Nutrition, altered, less than body requirements (Indications).
- Diarrhea or constipation (Side Effects).
- Knowledge deficit, related to medication regimen (Patient/Family Teaching).

IMPLEMENTATION

- **PO:** First dose is administered prior to emetogenic event.
- Administer undiluted.
- **Direct IV:** Administer 4 mg undiluted immediately before induction of anesthesia or postoperatively if nausea and vomiting occur shortly after surgery.
- ***Rate:*** Administer over at least 30 sec and preferably over 2–5 min.
- **Intermittent Infusion:** Dilute doses for prevention of nausea and vomiting associated with

***CAPITALS indicate life-threatening; underlines indicate most frequent.**

chemotherapy in 50 ml of D5W, 0.9% NaCl, D5/0.9% NaCl, D5/0.45% NaCl. Solution is clear and colorless. Stable for 7 days at room temperature following dilution.

- *Rate:* Administer each dose as an IV infusion over 15 min.
- **Y-Site Compatibility:** ▪ aldesleukin ▪ amifostine ▪ amikacin ▪ aztreonam ▪ bleomycin ▪ carboplatin ▪ carmustine ▪ cefazolin ▪ cefotaxime ▪ cefoxitin ▪ ceftazidime ▪ ceftizoxime ▪ cefuroxime ▪ cimetidine ▪ cisplatin ▪ clindamycin ▪ cyclophosphamide ▪ cytarabine ▪ dacarbazine ▪ dactinomycin ▪ daunorubicin ▪ dexamethasone sodium phosphate ▪ doxorubicin ▪ doxycycline ▪ droperidol ▪ etoposide ▪ famotidine ▪ filgrastim ▪ floxuridine ▪ fluconazole ▪ fludarabine ▪ gallium nitrate ▪ gentamicin ▪ heparin ▪ hydrocortisone sodium succinate ▪ hydrocortisone sodium phosphate ▪ hydromorphone ▪ ifosfamide ▪ imipenem/cilastatin ▪ magnesium sulfate ▪ mannitol ▪ mechlorethamine ▪ melphalan ▪ meperidine ▪ mesna ▪ methotrexate ▪ metoclopramide ▪ miconazole ▪ mitomycin ▪ mitoxantrone ▪ morphine ▪ paclitaxel ▪ pentostatin ▪ piperacillin/tazobactam ▪ potassium chloride ▪ ranitidine ▪ sodium acetate ▪ streptozocin ▪ teniposide ▪ thiotepa ▪ ticarcillin ▪ ticarcillin/clavulanate ▪ vancomycin ▪ vinblastine ▪ vincristine ▪ vinorelbine ▪ zidovudine.
- **Y-Site Incompatibility:** ▪ acyclovir ▪ aminophylline ▪ amphotericin B ▪ ampicillin ▪ ampicillin/sulbactam ▪ cefepime ▪ cefoperazone ▪ furosemide ▪ ganciclovir ▪ lorazepam ▪ methylprednisolone sodium succinate ▪ mezlocillin ▪ piperacillin ▪ sargramostim ▪ sodium bicarbonate.

PATIENT/FAMILY TEACHING

- ☐ Advise patient to notify health care professional immediately if involuntary movement of eyes, face, or limbs occurs.

EVALUATION

Effectiveness of therapy can be demonstrated by: ▪ Prevention of nausea and vomiting associated with initial and repeat courses of emetogenic cancer chemotherapy ▪ Prevention of postoperative nausea and vomiting ▪ Prevention of nausea and vomiting due to radiation therapy.

OPRELVEKIN

(o-**prell**-ve-kin)
Neumega

CLASSIFICATION(S):
Thrombopoietic growth factor

Pregnancy Category C

INDICATIONS

▪ Prevention of severe thrombocytopenia and reduction of the need for platelet transfusions following myelosuppressive chemotherapy in patients with nonmyeloid malignancies at risk for thrombocytopenia.

ACTION

▪ Stimulates production of megakaryocytes and platelets. **Therapeutic Effects:** ▪ Increased platelet count.

PHARMACOKINETICS

Absorption: >80% absorbed following SC administration.
Distribution: UK.
Metabolism and Excretion: Appears to be mostly metabolized, with metabolites eliminated by kidneys.
Half-life: 6.9 hr.

CONTRAINDICATIONS AND PRECAUTIONS

Contraindicated in: ▪ Hypersensitivity ▪ Lactation.
Use Cautiously in: ▪ Any condition in which sodium and water retention would pose problems (CHF, renal disease) ▪ Pre-existing pericardial effusion or ascites (may be exacerbated) ▪ History of atrial arrhythmias (especially if receiving cardiac medications or previous doxorubicin therapy) ▪ Pre-existing papilledema or tumors of the CNS ▪ Pregnancy or children (safety not established).

ADVERSE REACTIONS AND SIDE EFFECTS*

These effects occurred in patients who had recently received myelosuppressive chemotherapy.

*CAPITALS indicate life-threatening; underlines indicate most frequent.

CNS: dizziness, headache, insomnia, nervousness, weakness.
EENT: injected conjunctivae, blurred vision, papilledema, pharyngitis, rhinitis.
Resp: cough, dyspnea, pleural effusions.
CV: atrial fibrillation, edema, palpitations, syncope, tachycardia, vasodilation.
GI: anorexia, constipation, diarrhea, dyspepsia, mucositis, nausea, oral moniliasis, vomiting, abdominal pain.
Derm: alopecia, ecchymoses, rash.
F and E: sodium and water retention.
Local: injection site reactions.
MS: bone pain, myalgia.
Misc: chills, fever, infection, pain.

INTERACTIONS

Drug-Drug: ▪ None significant.

ROUTE AND DOSAGE

- **SC (Adults):** 50 mcg/kg once daily for 10–21 days.

AVAILABILITY

- ***Powder for injection:*** 5-mg vial[Rx].

TIME/ACTION PROFILE (increase in platelet count)

	ONSET	PEAK	DURATION
SC	5–9 days	UK	7–14 days*

*Counts continue to rise for 7 days following discontinuation and then return to baseline by 14 days.

NURSING IMPLICATIONS

ASSESSMENT

- ▫ Assess patient for signs of fluid retention (dyspnea on exertion, peripheral edema) during therapy. Fluid retention is a common side effect that usually resolves within several days following discontinuation of oprelvekin.
- ▪ ***Lab Test Considerations:*** Monitor platelet count prior to and periodically during therapy, especially at expected nadir. Therapy is continued until postnadir platelet count is ≥50,000 cells/ml.
- ▫ CBC should be monitored prior to and at regular intervals during therapy. Decrease in hemoglobin concentration, hematocrit, and red blood cell count may occur because of increased plasma volume (dilutional anemia); usually begins within 3–5 days of therapy and is reversible within a week of discontinuation of therapy.
- ▫ Monitor electrolyte concentrations in patients receiving chronic diuretic therapy. Hypokalemia may be fatal.
- ▫ May cause an increase in plasma fibrinogen.

POTENTIAL NURSING DIAGNOSES

- ▪ Fluid volume excess (Side Effects).
- ▪ Knowledge deficit, related to medication regimen (Patient/Family Teaching).

IMPLEMENTATION

- ▪ **General Info:** Therapy should be started within 6–24 hr after completion of chemotherapy and continued for 10–21 days.
- ▫ Treatment should be discontinued at least 2 days prior to next planned chemotherapy cycle.
- ▪ **SC:** Reconstitute with 1 ml of sterile water for injection without preservatives for a concentration of 5 mg/ml. Direct diluent to sides of vial and swirl gently. Solution is clear and colorless. Do not administer solutions that are discolored or contain particulate matter. Do not shake or agitate vigorously. Do not freeze. Do not reuse vials. Administer within 3 hr of reconstitution as a single injection in abdomen, hip, thigh, or upper arm.

PATIENT/FAMILY TEACHING

- ▫ Instruct patient in proper technique for preparation and administration of medication. Provide a puncture-resistant container for disposal of needles.
- ▫ May cause transient blurred vision or dizziness. Caution patient to avoid driving or other activities requiring alertness until response to medication is known.
- ▫ Advise patient to notify health care professional if pregnancy is planned or suspected.
- ▫ Inform patient of side effects and advise patient to notify health care professional if chest pain, shortness of breath, fatigue, blurred vision, or irregular heartbeat persists.

EVALUATION

Effectiveness of therapy can be demonstrated by: ▪ Increase in postnadir platelet count to ≥50,000 cells/ml.

O

OXAPROZIN

(ox-a-**proe**-zin)

Daypro

CLASSIFICATION(S):

Nonsteroidal anti-inflammatory agent

Pregnancy Category C (first trimester)

INDICATIONS

- Management of rheumatoid arthritis and osteoarthritis.

ACTION

- Inhibits prostaglandin synthesis. **Therapeutic Effects:** - Suppression of pain and inflammation.

PHARMACOKINETICS

Absorption: Well absorbed following oral administration (80%); 35% is rapidly converted to an active metabolite.

Distribution: UK.

Metabolism and Excretion: The active metabolite is metabolized by the liver to inactive compounds.

Half-life: 42–50 hr.

CONTRAINDICATIONS AND PRECAUTIONS

Contraindicated in: - Hypersensitivity - Cross-sensitivity may exist with other NSAIDs, including aspirin - Active GI bleeding or ulcer disease.

Use Cautiously in: - Severe cardiovascular or hepatic disease - Renal impairment (lower initial dose may be necessary) - History of ulcer disease - Pregnancy, lactation, or children (safety not established; not recommended for use during the 2nd half of pregnancy).

ADVERSE REACTIONS AND SIDE EFFECTS*

CNS: agitation, anxiety, confusion, depression, dizziness, drowsiness, fatigue, headache, insomnia, malaise, weakness.

EENT: abnormal vision, tinnitus.

Resp: dyspnea, hypersensitivity pneumonitis.

CV: edema, vasculitis.

GI: GI BLEEDING, <u>abdominal pain</u>, <u>diarrhea</u>, <u>dyspepsia</u>, abnormal liver function tests, anorexia, cholestatic jaundice, constipation, dry mouth, duodenal ulcer, flatulence, gastritis, increased appetite, nausea, stomatitis, vomiting.

GU: albuminuria, azotemia, interstitial nephritis.

Derm: increased sweating, photosensitivity, pruritus, rash.

Hemat: prolonged bleeding time.

Metab: weight gain.

Neuro: paresthesia, tremor.

Misc: allergic reactions including ANAPHYLAXIS, ANGIONEUROTIC EDEMA.

INTERACTIONS

Drug-Drug: - Additive adverse GI effects and toxicity with **aspirin**, other **NSAIDs, potassium supplements, glucocorticoids**, or **alcohol** - Chronic use with **acetaminophen** may increase the risk of adverse renal reactions - May decrease the effectiveness of **diuretics** or **antihypertensive** therapy - May increase the hypoglycemic effects of **insulin** or **oral hypoglycemic agents** - Increases the risk of toxicity from **methotrexate** - Increased risk of bleeding with **cefamandole, cefotetan, cefoperazone, plicamycin, thrombolytic agents**, or **anticoagulants** - Increased risk of adverse hematologic reactions with **antineoplastic agents** or **radiation therapy.**

ROUTE AND DOSAGE

- **PO (Adults):** 1200 mg once daily; onset may be more rapid with an initial 1800-mg dose. Patients with low body weight, mild disease, or renal impairment may be started at 600 mg/day (not to exceed 1800 mg/day or 26 mg/kg/day). Daily doses >1200 mg should be given in 2–3 divided doses.

AVAILABILITY

- ***Tablets:*** 600 mg[Rx].

TIME/ACTION PROFILE (antirheumatic action)

	ONSET	PEAK	DURATION
PO	within 7 days	UK	UK

*CAPITALS indicate life-threatening; <u>underlines</u> indicate most frequent.

NURSING IMPLICATIONS

ASSESSMENT

- □ Patients who have asthma, aspirin-induced allergy, and nasal polyps are at increased risk for developing hypersensitivity reactions. Monitor for rhinitis, asthma, and urticaria.
- □ Assess pain and range of motion prior to and periodically throughout therapy.
- ■ ***Lab Test Considerations:*** May cause prolonged bleeding time, which may persist for up to 2 wk following discontinuation of therapy.
- □ BUN, serum creatinine, CBC, and liver function tests should be evaluated periodically in patients receiving prolonged courses of therapy. Serum potassium, BUN, serum creatinine, alkaline phosphatase, LDH, AST, and ALT tests may show increased levels. Blood glucose, hemoglobin, and hematocrit concentrations, leukocyte and platelet counts, and CCr may be decreased.

POTENTIAL NURSING DIAGNOSES

- ■ Pain (Indications).
- ■ Knowledge deficit, related to medication regimen (Patient/Family Teaching).

IMPLEMENTATION

- ■ **General Info:** Administration in higher than recommended doses does not provide increased effectiveness but may cause increased side effects.
- ■ **PO:** Administer with food or antacids to decrease GI irritation.

PATIENT/FAMILY TEACHING

- □ Advise patient to take this medication with a full glass of water and to remain in an upright position for 15–30 min after administration.
- □ Instruct patient to take medication exactly as directed. If a dose is missed, it should be taken as soon as remembered but not if almost time for the next dose. Do not double doses.
- □ This medication may cause drowsiness and dizziness. Advise patient to avoid driving or other activities requiring alertness until response to the medication is known.
- □ Caution patient to avoid the concurrent use of alcohol, aspirin, acetaminophen, or other OTC medications without consulting health care professional.
- □ Advise patient to notify health care professional of medication regimen prior to treatment or surgery. Oxaprozin should be discontinued 2 wk prior to surgery.
- □ Caution patient to use sunscreen and protective clothing to prevent photosensitivity reactions.
- □ Advise patient to consult health care professional if rash, itching, visual disturbances, tinnitus, weight gain, edema, black stools, persistent headache, or influenza-like syndrome (chills, fever, muscle aches, pain) occurs.

EVALUATION

Effectiveness of therapy can be demonstrated by: ■ Decreased pain and improved joint mobility. Maximum effectiveness may require 2 wk or more of continuous therapy. Patients who do not respond to one NSAID may respond to another.

OXAZEPAM

(ox-**az**-e-pam)
{Apo-Oxazepam}, {Novoxapam}, Serax

CLASSIFICATION(S):
Antianxiety agent, Sedative/hypnotic (benzodiazepine)

Schedule IV
Pregnancy Category D

INDICATIONS

■ Management of anxiety ■ Symptomatic treatment of alcohol withdrawal.

ACTION

■ Depresses the CNS, probably by potentiating gamma-aminobutyric acid (GABA), an inhibitory neurotransmitter. **Therapeutic Effects:** ■ Relief of anxiety ■ Diminished symptoms of alcohol withdrawal.

PHARMACOKINETICS

Absorption: Well absorbed following oral administration. Absorption is slower than with other benzodiazepines.

Distribution: Widely distributed. Crosses the blood-brain barrier. May cross the placenta and enter breast milk.
Metabolism and Excretion: Metabolized by the liver to inactive compounds.
Half-life: 5–15 hr.

CONTRAINDICATIONS AND PRECAUTIONS

Contraindicated in: ▪ Hypersensitivity ▪ Cross-sensitivity with other benzodiazepines may exist ▪ Comatose patients or those with pre-existing CNS depression ▪ Uncontrolled severe pain ▪ Narrow-angle glaucoma ▪ Pregnancy and lactation ▪ Some products contain tartrazine and should be avoided in patients with known intolerance.
Use Cautiously in: ▪ Hepatic dysfunction ▪ History of suicide attempt or drug abuse ▪ Geriatric/debilitated patients (initial dosage reduction recommended) ▪ Severe chronic obstructive pulmonary disease ▪ Myasthenia gravis.

ADVERSE REACTIONS AND SIDE EFFECTS*

CNS: dizziness, drowsiness, confusion, hangover, headache, impaired memory, mental depression, paradoxical excitation, slurred speech.
EENT: blurred vision.
Resp: respiratory depression.
CV: tachycardia.
GI: constipation, diarrhea, drug-induced hepatitis, nausea, vomiting.
GU: urinary problems.
Derm: rashes.
Hemat: leukopenia.
Misc: physical dependence, psychological dependence, tolerance.

INTERACTIONS

Drug-Drug: ▪ Additive CNS depression with other **CNS depressants**, including **alcohol, antihistamines, antidepressants, opioids,** and other **sedative/hypnotics** (including other benzodiazepines) ▪ May decrease the therapeutic effectiveness of **levodopa** ▪ **Oral contraceptives** or **phenytoin** may decrease effectiveness ▪ **Theophylline** may decrease sedative effects of oxazepam.

ROUTE AND DOSAGE

- **PO (Adults):** *Antianxiety agent*—10–30 mg 3–4 times daily. *Sedative/hypnotic/management of alcohol withdrawal*—15–30 mg 3–4 times daily.
- **PO (Geriatric Patients):** 5 mg 1–2 times daily initially or 10 mg 3 times daily; may be increased as needed.

AVAILABILITY

- ***Capsules:*** 10 mg^Rx^, 15 mg^Rx^, 30 mg^Rx^
- ***Tablets:*** 10 mg^Rx^, 15 mg^Rx^, 30 mg^Rx^.

TIME/ACTION PROFILE (sedation)

	ONSET	PEAK	DURATION
PO	45–90 min	UK	6–12 hr

NURSING IMPLICATIONS

ASSESSMENT

- □ Assess patient for anxiety and level of sedation (ataxia, dizziness, slurred speech) periodically throughout therapy.
- □ Prolonged high-dose therapy may lead to psychological or physical dependence. Restrict the amount of drug available to patient.
- ▪ ***Lab Test Considerations:*** Monitor CBC and liver function tests periodically during prolonged therapy.
- □ May cause decreased thyroidal uptake of sodium iodide ^{123}I and ^{131}I.

POTENTIAL NURSING DIAGNOSES

- Anxiety (Indications).
- Injury, risk for (Side Effects).
- Knowledge deficit, related to medication regimen (Patient/Family Teaching).

IMPLEMENTATION

- **General Info:** Medication should be tapered at the completion of therapy. Sudden cessation of medication may lead to withdrawal (insomnia, irritability, nervousness, tremors).
- **PO:** Administer with food if GI irritation becomes a problem.

PATIENT/FAMILY TEACHING

- □ Instruct patient to take oxazepam exactly as directed. Missed doses should be taken within

*CAPITALS indicate life-threatening; underlines indicate most frequent.

1 hr; if remembered later, omit and return to regular dosing schedule. Do not double or increase doses. If dose is less effective after a few weeks, notify health care professional.

- ◻ May cause drowsiness or dizziness. Caution patient to avoid driving or other activities requiring alertness until response to medication is known.
- ◻ Advise patient to avoid the use of alcohol and to consult health care professional prior to the use of OTC preparations that contain antihistamines or alcohol.
- ◻ Advise patient to inform health care professional if pregnancy is planned or suspected.
- ◻ Advise patient to notify health care professional of medication regimen prior to treatment or surgery.
- ◻ Emphasize the importance of follow-up exams to monitor effectiveness of medication.

EVALUATION

Effectiveness of therapy can be demonstrated by: ▪ Decreased sense of anxiety ◻ Increased ability to cope ▪ Prevention or relief of acute agitation, tremor, and hallucinations during alcohol withdrawal.

OXYBUTYNIN

(ox-i-**byoo**-ti-nin)

Ditropan

CLASSIFICATION(S):

Antispasmodic (urinary)

Pregnancy Category B

INDICATIONS

▪ Treatment of the following urinary symptoms that may be associated with neurogenic bladder: ◻ Frequent urination ◻ Urgency ◻ Nocturia ◻ Incontinence.

ACTION

▪ Inhibits the action of acetylcholine at postganglionic receptors ▪ Has direct spasmolytic action on smooth muscle, including smooth muscle lining the GU tract, without affecting vascular smooth muscle. **Therapeutic Effects:** ▪ Increased bladder capacity ▪ Delayed desire to void.

PHARMACOKINETICS

Absorption: Rapidly absorbed following oral administration.

Distribution: UK.

Metabolism and Excretion: Metabolized by the liver; renally excreted.

Half-life: UK.

CONTRAINDICATIONS AND PRECAUTIONS

Contraindicated in: ▪ Hypersensitivity ▪ Glaucoma ▪ Intestinal obstruction or atony ▪ Toxic megacolon ▪ Paralytic ileus ▪ Severe colitis ▪ Myasthenia gravis ▪ Acute hemorrhage with shock ▪ Obstructive uropathy.

Use Cautiously in: ▪ Lactation (may be inhibited) ▪ Cardiovascular disease ▪ Reflux esophagitis ▪ Geriatric patients (increased risk of adverse reactions) ▪ Pregnancy or children <5 yr (safety not established).

ADVERSE REACTIONS AND SIDE EFFECTS

CNS: dizziness, drowsiness, hallucinations, insomnia, weakness.

EENT: blurred vision, cycloplegia, increased intraocular pressure, mydriasis, photophobia.

CV: palpitations, tachycardia.

GI: bloated feeling, constipation, dry mouth, nausea, vomiting.

GU: impotence, urinary hesitancy, urinary retention.

Derm: decreased sweating, urticaria.

Endo: suppressed lactation.

Metab: hyperthermia.

Misc: allergic reactions, fever, hot flashes.

INTERACTIONS

Drug-Drug: ▪ Additive anticholinergic effects with other **agents having anticholinergic properties**, including **antidepressants, phenothiazine, disopyramide**, and **haloperidol** ▪ Additive CNS depression with other **CNS depressants**, including **alcohol, antihistamines, antidepressants, opioids**, and **sedative/hypnotics** ▪ Concurrent use with **haloperidol** may result in tardive dyskinesia, worsening of schizophrenia, and decreased haloperidol levels ▪ May increase serum **digoxin** levels.

ROUTE AND DOSAGE

- **PO (Adults):** 5 mg 2–3 times daily (not to exceed 5 mg 4 times daily).
- **PO (Children >5 yr):** 5 mg 2–3 times daily (not to exceed 15 mg/day).

AVAILABILITY

- ***Tablets:*** 5 mg[Rx] ▪ ***Syrup:*** 5 mg/5 ml[Rx].

TIME/ACTION PROFILE (urinary spasmolytic effect)

	ONSET	PEAK	DURATION
PO	30–60 min	3–6 hr	6–10 hr

NURSING IMPLICATIONS

ASSESSMENT

- □ Monitor voiding pattern and intake and output ratios, and assess abdomen for bladder distention prior to and periodically throughout therapy. Catheterization may be used to assess postvoid residual. Cystometry, to diagnose type of bladder dysfunction, is usually performed prior to prescription of oxybutynin.

POTENTIAL NURSING DIAGNOSES

- Urinary elimination, altered patterns of (Indications).
- Pain (Indications).
- Knowledge deficit, related to medication regimen (Patient/Family Teaching).

IMPLEMENTATION

- **PO:** May be administered on an empty stomach or with meals or milk to prevent gastric irritation.

PATIENT/FAMILY TEACHING

- □ Instruct patient to take medication exactly as directed. If a dose is missed, it should be taken as soon as remembered unless almost time for next dose.
- □ Medication may cause drowsiness or blurred vision. Advise patient to avoid driving and other activities requiring alertness until response to medication is known.
- □ Advise patient to avoid concurrent use of alcohol and other CNS depressants while taking this medication.
- □ Instruct patient that frequent rinsing of mouth, good oral hygiene, and sugarless gum or candy may decrease dry mouth. Health care professional should be notified if mouth dryness persists >2 wk.
- □ Inform patient that oxybutynin decreases the body's ability to perspire. The patient should avoid strenuous activity in a warm environment because overheating may occur.
- □ Advise patient to wear sunglasses when out in bright sunlight, as increased sensitivity to light may occur.
- □ Advise patient to notify health care professional if urinary retention occurs or if constipation persists. Discuss with patient methods of preventing constipation, such as increasing bulk in the diet, increasing fluid intake, and increasing mobility.
- □ Discuss need for continued medical follow-up. Periodic cystometry may be used to evaluate effectiveness of medication. Ophthalmic exams should be performed periodically to detect glaucoma, especially in patients over 40 yr of age.

EVALUATION

Effectiveness of therapy can be demonstrated by: ▪ Relief of bladder spasm and associated symptoms (frequency, urgency, nocturia, and incontinence) in patients with a neurogenic bladder.

OXYCODONE

(ox-i-**koe**-done)

Oxycontin, Roxicodone, {Supeudol}

OXYCODONE/ACETAMINOPHEN*

{Endocet}, {Oxycocet}, Percocet, {Percocet-Demi}, Roxicet, Roxilox, Tylox

OXYCODONE/ASPIRIN†

{Endodan}, {Oxycodan}, Percodan, Percodan-Demi, Roxiprin

CLASSIFICATION(S):
Opioid analgesic (agonist)

Schedule II
Pregnancy Category C

*See also acetaminophen monograph on page 4.
†See also salicylates monograph on page 900.

INDICATIONS

▪ Management of moderate to severe pain.

ACTION

▪ Bind to opiate receptors in the CNS ▪ Alter the perception of and response to painful stimuli, while producing generalized CNS depression. **Therapeutic Effects:** ▪ Decreased pain.

PHARMACOKINETICS

Absorption: Well absorbed from the GI tract.
Distribution: Widely distributed. Cross the placenta; enter breast milk.
Metabolism and Excretion: Mostly metabolized by the liver.
Half-life: 2–3 hr.

CONTRAINDICATIONS AND PRECAUTIONS

Contraindicated in: ▪ Hypersensitivity ▪ Pregnancy or lactation (avoid chronic use) ▪ Some products contain alcohol or bisulfites and should be avoided in patients with known intolerance or hypersensitivity.
Use Cautiously in: ▪ Head trauma ▪ Increased intracranial pressure ▪ Severe renal, hepatic, or pulmonary disease ▪ Hypothyroidism ▪ Adrenal insufficiency ▪ Alcoholism ▪ Geriatric or debilitated patients (initial dosage reduction recommended) ▪ Undiagnosed abdominal pain ▪ Prostatic hypertrophy.

ADVERSE REACTIONS AND SIDE EFFECTS*

CNS: <u>confusion</u>, <u>sedation</u>, dizziness, dysphoria, euphoria, floating feeling, hallucinations, headache, unusual dreams.
EENT: blurred vision, diplopia, miosis.
Resp: RESPIRATORY DEPRESSION.
CV: orthostatic hypotension.
GI: <u>constipation</u>, dry mouth, nausea, vomiting.
GU: urinary retention.
Derm: flushing, sweating.
Misc: physical dependence, psychological dependence, tolerance.

INTERACTIONS

Drug-Drug: ▪ Use with caution in patients receiving **MAO inhibitors** (may result in unpredictable reactions—decrease initial dose of oxycodone to 25% of usual dose) ▪ Additive CNS depression with **alcohol, antihistamines,** and **sedative/hypnotics** ▪ Administration of **partial-antagonist opioid analgesics** may precipitate withdrawal in physically dependent patients ▪ **Nalbuphine, buprenorphine, dezocine,** or **pentazocine** may decrease analgesia.

ROUTE AND DOSAGE

Larger doses may be required during chronic therapy. Consider cumulative effects of additional acetaminophen/aspirin; if toxic levels are exceeded, change to pure oxycodone product.

- **PO (Adults ≥50 kg):** 5–10 mg q 3–4 hr initially, as needed. Controlled-release tablets (Oxycontin) may be given q 12 hr.
- **PO (Adults <50 kg or Children):** 0.2 mg/kg q 3–4 hr initially, as needed.
- **Rect (Adults):** 10–40 mg 3–4 times daily initially, as needed.

AVAILABILITY

❑ Oxycodone

▪ ***Oxycodone tablets:*** 5 mg (Roxicodone, Supeudol)Rx ▪ ***Oxycodone immediate-release capsules:*** 5 mg (OxyIR)Rx ▪ ***Oxycodone controlled-release tablets:*** 10 mgRx, 20 mgRx, 40 mgRx, 80 mg (OxyContin)Rx ▪ ***Oral solution:*** 5 mg/5 ml in 500-ml bottle (Roxicodone)Rx ▪ ***Concentrated oral solution:*** 20 mg/ml in 30-ml bottle with dropper (Roxicodone Intensol)Rx ▪ {***Suppositories:*** 10 mgRx, 20 mg (Supeudol)Rx}.

❑ Oxycodone/Acetaminophen

▪ ***Tablets:*** {2.5 mg oxycodone with 325 mg acetaminophen (Percocet-Demi)Rx}, 5 mg oxycodone with 325 mg acetaminophen (Endocet, Oxycet, Percocet, Roxicet)Rx ▪ ***Capsules:*** 5 mg oxycodone with 500 mg acetaminophen (Roxilox, Tylox)Rx ▪ ***Caplets:*** 5 mg oxycodone with 500 mg acetaminophen (Roxicet 5/500)Rx ▪ ***Oral solution:*** 5 mg oxycodone with 325 mg acetaminophen/5 ml (Roxicet Solution) in 500-ml bottlesRx.

❑ Oxycodone/Aspirin

▪ ***Tablets:*** 2.44 mg oxycodone with 325 mg aspirin (Percodan-Demi)Rx, 4.88 mg oxycodone

***CAPITALS indicate life-threatening; <u>underlines</u> indicate most frequent.**

with 325 mg aspirin (Endodan, Oxycodan, Percodan, Roxiprin)Rx.

TIME/ACTION PROFILE (analgesic effects)

	ONSET	PEAK	DURATION
PO	10–15 min	60–90 min	3–6 hr
PO-CR	10–15 min	3 hr	12 hr

NURSING IMPLICATIONS

ASSESSMENT

- Assess type, location, and intensity of pain prior to and 1 hr (peak) after administration. When titrating opioid doses, increases of 25–50% should be administered until there is either a 50% reduction in the patient's pain rating on a numerical or visual analogue scale or the patient reports satisfactory pain relief. A repeat dose can be safely administered at the time of the peak if previous dose is ineffective and side effects are minimal.
- Patients taking controlled-release tablets should also be given supplemental short-acting opioid doses for breakthrough pain.
- An equianalgesic chart (see Appendix B) should be used when changing routes or when changing from one opioid to another.
- Assess blood pressure, pulse, and respirations before and periodically during administration. If respiratory rate is <10/min, assess level of sedation. Physical stimulation may be sufficient to prevent significant hypoventilation. Dose may need to be decreased by 25–50%. Initial drowsiness will diminish with continued use.
- Prolonged use may lead to physical and psychological dependence and tolerance. This should not prevent patient from receiving adequate analgesia. Most patients who receive oxycodone for pain do not develop psychological dependence. Progressively higher doses may be required to relieve pain with long-term therapy.
- Assess bowel function routinely. Prevention of constipation should be instituted with increased intake of fluids and bulk, and laxatives to minimize constipating effects. Stimulant laxatives should be administered routinely if opioid use exceeds 2–3 days, unless contraindicated.
- ***Lab Test Considerations:*** May increase plasma amylase and lipase levels.
- ***Toxicity and Overdose:*** If an opioid antagonist is required to reverse respiratory depression or coma, naloxone (Narcan) is the antidote. Dilute the 0.4-mg ampule of naloxone in 10 ml of 0.9% NaCl and administer 0.5 ml (0.02 mg) by direct IV push every 2 min. For children and patients weighing <40 kg, dilute 0.1 mg of naloxone in 10 ml of 0.9% NaCl for a concentration of 10 mcg/ml and administer 0.5 mcg/kg every 1–2 min. Titrate dose to avoid withdrawal, seizures, and severe pain.

POTENTIAL NURSING DIAGNOSES

- Pain (Indications).
- Sensory-perceptual alterations: visual, auditory (Side Effects).
- Injury, risk for (Side Effects).

IMPLEMENTATION

- **General Info:** Explain therapeutic value of medication prior to administration to enhance the analgesic effect.
- Regularly administered doses may be more effective than prn administration. Analgesic is more effective if given before pain becomes severe.
- Coadministration with nonopioid analgesics may have additive analgesic effects and may permit lower doses.
- Medication should be discontinued gradually after long-term use to prevent withdrawal symptoms.
- **PO:** May be administered with food or milk to minimize GI irritation.
- Administer solution with properly calibrated measuring device.
- Controlled-release tablets should be swallowed whole; do not crush, break, or chew.

PATIENT/FAMILY TEACHING

- Instruct patient on how and when to ask for pain medication.
- Medication may cause drowsiness or dizziness. Advise patient to call for assistance when ambulating or smoking. Caution patient to avoid driving and other activities requiring alertness until response to medication is known.
- Advise patients taking Oxycontin tablets that empty matrix tablets may appear in stool.
- Advise patient to make position changes slowly to minimize orthostatic hypotension.

- Advise patient to avoid concurrent use of alcohol or other CNS depressants with this medication.
- Encourage patient to turn, cough, and breathe deeply every 2 hr to prevent atelectasis.

EVALUATION

Effectiveness of therapy can be demonstrated by: ▪ Decrease in severity of pain without a significant alteration in level of consciousness or respiratory status.

OXYMORPHONE

(ox-i-**mor**-fone)
Numorphan

CLASSIFICATION(S):
Opioid analgesic (agonist)

Schedule II
Pregnancy Category B (short-term use), D (used chronically, in high doses, or near term)

INDICATIONS

▪ Management of moderate to severe pain ▪ Supplement in balanced anesthesia.

ACTION

▪ Binds to opiate receptors in the CNS ▪ Alters the perception of and response to painful stimuli, while producing generalized CNS depression. **Therapeutic Effects:** ▪ Decrease in pain.

PHARMACOKINETICS

Absorption: Well absorbed following IM, SC, or rectal administration.
Distribution: Widely distributed; crosses the placenta and enters breast milk.
Metabolism and Excretion: Mostly metabolized by the liver.
Half-life: 2.6–4 hr.

CONTRAINDICATIONS AND PRECAUTIONS

Contraindicated in: ▪ Hypersensitivity ▪ Pregnancy or lactation (avoid chronic use) ▪ Children <12 yr.
Use Cautiously in: ▪ Head trauma ▪ Increased intracranial pressure ▪ Severe renal, hepatic, or pulmonary disease ▪ Hypothyroidism ▪ Adrenal insufficiency ▪ Alcoholism ▪ Geriatric or debilitated patients (initial dosage reduction recommended) ▪ Undiagnosed abdominal pain ▪ Prostatic hypertrophy.

ADVERSE REACTIONS AND SIDE EFFECTS*

CNS: confusion, sedation, dizziness, dysphoria, euphoria, floating feeling, hallucinations, headache, unusual dreams.
EENT: blurred vision, diplopia, miosis.
Resp: RESPIRATORY DEPRESSION.
CV: orthostatic hypotension.
GI: constipation, dry mouth, nausea, vomiting.
GU: urinary retention.
Derm: flushing, sweating.
Misc: physical dependence, psychological dependence, tolerance.

INTERACTIONS

Drug-Drug: ▪ Use with caution in patients receiving **MAO inhibitors** (may result in unpredictable reactions—decrease initial dose of oxymorphone to 25% of usual dose) ▪ Additive CNS depression with **alcohol, antihistamines,** and **sedative/hypnotics** ▪ Administration of **partial-antagonist opioid analgesics** may precipitate withdrawal in physically dependent patients ▪ **Nalbuphine, buprenorphine, dezocine,** or **pentazocine** may decrease analgesia.

ROUTE AND DOSAGE

Larger doses may be required during chronic therapy.

- **SC, IM (Adults):** 1–1.5 mg q 3–6 hr as needed. *Analgesia during labor*—0.5–1 mg.
- **IV (Adults):** 0.5 mg q 3–6 hr as needed; increase as needed.
- **Rect (Adults):** 5 mg q 4–6 hr as needed.

AVAILABILITY

▪ ***Injection:*** 1 mg/ml in 1-ml ampules[Rx], 1.5 mg/ml in 1-ml ampules and 10-ml vials[Rx] ▪ ***Suppositories:*** 5 mg[Rx].

***CAPITALS indicate life-threatening; underlines indicate most frequent.**

TIME/ACTION PROFILE (analgesic effects)

	ONSET	PEAK	DURATION
IM	10–15 min	30–90 min	3–6 hr
IV	5–10 min	15–30 min	3–6 hr
SC	10–20 min	UK	3–4 hr
Rect	15–30 min	120 min	3–6 hr

NURSING IMPLICATIONS

ASSESSMENT

- Assess type, location, and intensity of pain prior to and 1 hr following IM and 15–30 min (peak) following IV administration. When titrating opioid doses, increases of 25–50% should be administered until there is either a 50% reduction in the patient's pain rating on a numerical or visual analogue scale or the patient reports satisfactory pain relief. A repeat dose can be safely administered at the time of the peak if previous dose is ineffective and side effects are minimal.
- An equianalgesic chart (see Appendix B) should be used when changing routes or when changing from one opioid to another.
- Assess blood pressure, pulse, and respirations before and periodically during administration. If respiratory rate is <10/min, assess level of sedation. Physical stimulation may be sufficient to prevent significant hypoventilation. Dose may need to be decreased by 25–50%. Initial drowsiness will diminish with continued use.
- Prolonged use may lead to physical and psychological dependence and tolerance. This should not prevent patient from receiving adequate analgesia. Most patients who receive oxymorphone for pain do not develop psychological dependence. Progressively higher doses may be required to relieve pain with long-term therapy.
- Assess bowel function routinely. Prevention of constipation should be instituted with increased intake of fluids and bulk, and laxatives. Stimulant laxatives should be administered routinely if opioid use exceeds 2–3 days, unless contraindicated.
- ***Lab Test Considerations:*** May increase plasma amylase and lipase levels.
- ***Toxicity and Overdose:*** If an opioid antagonist is required to reverse respiratory depression or coma, naloxone (Narcan) is the antidote. Dilute the 0.4-mg ampule of naloxone in 10 ml of 0.9% NaCl and administer 0.5 ml (0.02 mg) by direct IV push every 2 min. For children and patients weighing <40 kg, dilute 0.1 mg of naloxone in 10 ml of 0.9% NaCl for a concentration of 10 mcg/ml and administer 0.5 mcg/kg every 1–2 min. Titrate dose to avoid withdrawal, seizures, and severe pain.

POTENTIAL NURSING DIAGNOSES

- Pain (Indications).
- Sensory-perceptual alterations: visual, auditory (Side Effects).
- Injury, risk for (Side Effects).

IMPLEMENTATION

- **General Info:** Explain therapeutic value of medication prior to administration to enhance the analgesic effect.
- Regularly administered doses may be more effective than prn administration. Analgesic is more effective if given before pain becomes severe.
- Coadministration with nonopioid analgesics may have additive analgesic effects and may permit lower doses.
- Medication should be discontinued gradually after long-term use to prevent withdrawal symptoms.
- **Rect:** Suppositories should be stored in the refrigerator.
- **Direct IV:** Administer undiluted over 2–3 min.
- **Y-Site Compatibility:** ▪ glycopyrrolate ▪ ranitidine.

PATIENT/FAMILY TEACHING

- Instruct patient on how and when to ask for pain medication.
- Medication may cause drowsiness or dizziness. Advise patient to call for assistance when ambulating or smoking. Caution patient to avoid driving and other activities requiring alertness until response to medication is known.
- Advise patient to make position changes slowly to minimize orthostatic hypotension.
- Advise patient to avoid concurrent use of alcohol or other CNS depressants with this medication.
- Encourage patient to turn, cough, and breathe deeply every 2 hr to prevent atelectasis.

EVALUATION

Effectiveness of therapy can be demonstrated by: ▪ Decrease in severity of pain without a significant alteration in level of consciousness or respiratory status.

OXYTOCIN
(ox-i-**toe**-sin)
Pitocin, Syntocinon

CLASSIFICATION(S):
Hormone (oxytocic)

Pregnancy Category X (intranasal), UK (IV, IM)

INDICATIONS

▪ **IV:** Induction of labor at term ▪ Facilitation of uterine contractions at term ▪ Facilitation of threatened abortion ▪ Postpartum control of bleeding after expulsion of the placenta ▪ **Intranasal:** Used to promote milk letdown in lactating women. **Unlabeled Uses:** ▪ Evaluation of fetal competence (fetal stress test).

ACTION

▪ Stimulates uterine smooth muscle, producing uterine contractions similar to those in spontaneous labor ▪ Stimulates mammary gland smooth muscle, facilitating lactation ▪ Has vasopressor and antidiuretic effects. **Therapeutic Effects:** ▪ Induction of labor (IV) ▪ Milk letdown (intranasal).

PHARMACOKINETICS

Absorption: Well absorbed from the nasal mucosa.
Distribution: Widely distributed in extracellular fluid. Small amounts reach fetal circulation.
Metabolism and Excretion: Rapidly metabolized by liver and kidneys.
Half-life: 3–9 min.

CONTRAINDICATIONS AND PRECAUTIONS

Contraindicated in: ▪ Hypersensitivity ▪ Anticipated nonvaginal delivery ▪ Pregnancy (intranasal).
Use Cautiously in: ▪ First and second stages of labor.

ADVERSE REACTIONS AND SIDE EFFECTS*

Maternal adverse reactions are noted for IV use only.
CNS: *maternal*—COMA, SEIZURES; *fetal*—INTRACRANIAL HEMORRHAGE.
Resp: *fetal*—ASPHYXIA, hypoxia.
CV: *maternal*—hypotension; *fetal*—arrhythmias.
F and E: *maternal*—hypochloremia, hyponatremia, water intoxication.
Misc: *maternal*—increased uterine motility, painful contractions, abruptio placentae, decreased uterine blood flow, hypersensitivity.

INTERACTIONS

Drug-Drug: ▪ Severe hypertension may occur if oxytocin follows administration of **vasopressors** ▪ Concurrent use with **cyclopropane anesthesia** may result in excessive hypotension.

ROUTE AND DOSAGE

❑ Induction/Stimulation of Labor

- **IV (Adults):** 0.5–2 milliunits/min; increase by 1–2 milliunits/min q 15–60 min until pattern established (usually 5–6 milliunits/min; maximum 20 milliunits/min), then decrease dose.

❑ Postpartum Hemorrhage

- **IV (Adults):** 10 units infused at 20–40 milliunits/min.
- **IM (Adults):** 10 units after delivery of placenta.

❑ Incomplete/Inevitable Abortion

- **IV (Adults):** 10 units at a rate of 20–40 milliunits/min.

❑ Promotion of Milk Letdown

- **Intranasal (Adults):** 1 spray in 1 or both nostrils 2–3 min before breast-feeding or pumping breasts.

❑ Fetal Stress Test

- **IV (Adults):** 0.5 milliunits/min; may be doubled q 20 min until 3 moderate contractions occur in one 10-min period (usually 5–6 mil-

***CAPITALS indicate life-threatening; underlines indicate most frequent.**

liunits/min) to a maximum of 20 milliunits with maternal/fetal monitoring.

AVAILABILITY

▪ ***Solution for injection:*** 10 units/ml in 0.5- and 1-ml ampules[Rx], 1-ml prefilled syringes[Rx], 1-ml and 10-ml vials[Rx] ▪ ***Nasal spray:*** 40 units/ml in 2- and 5-ml containers[Rx].

TIME/ACTION PROFILE (IV = uterine contractions; intranasal = milk letdown)

	ONSET	PEAK	DURATION
IV	immediate	UK	1 hr
IM	3–5 min	UK	30–60 min
Intranasal	few min	UK	20 min

NURSING IMPLICATIONS

ASSESSMENT

- Fetal maturity, presentation, and pelvic adequacy should be assessed prior to administration of oxytocin for induction of labor.
- Assess character, frequency, and duration of uterine contractions; resting uterine tone; and fetal heart rate frequently throughout administration. If contractions occur <2 min apart and are >50–65 mm Hg on monitor, if they last 60–90 sec or longer, or if a significant change in fetal heart rate develops, stop infusion and turn patient on her left side to prevent fetal anoxia. Notify physician or other health care professional immediately.
- Monitor maternal blood pressure and pulse frequently and fetal heart rate continuously throughout administration.
- This drug occasionally causes water intoxication. Monitor patient for signs and symptoms (drowsiness, listlessness, confusion, headache, anuria) and notify physician or other health care professional if they occur.
- ***Lab Test Considerations:*** Monitor maternal electrolytes. Water retention may result in hypochloremia or hyponatremia.

POTENTIAL NURSING DIAGNOSES

- Knowledge deficit, related to medication regimen (Patient/Family Teaching).

IMPLEMENTATION

- **General Info:** Do not administer oxytocin simultaneously by more than one route.
- **Continuous Infusion:** Rotate infusion container to ensure thorough mixing. Store solution in refrigerator, but do not freeze.
- Infuse via infusion pump for accurate dosage. Oxytocin should be connected via Y-site injection to an IV of 0.9% NaCl for use during adverse reactions.
- Magnesium sulfate should be available if needed for relaxation of the myometrium.
- **Induction of Labor:** Dilute 1 ml (10 units) in 1 liter of compatible infusion fluid for a concentration of 10 milliunits/ml.
- ***Rate:*** Begin infusion at 0.5–2 milliunits/min (0.05–0.2 ml); increase in increments of 1–2 milliunits/min at 15–30 min intervals until contractions simulate normal labor.
- **Postpartum Bleeding:** For control of postpartum bleeding, dilute 1–4 ml (10–40 units) in 1 liter of compatible infusion fluid (10–40 milliunits/ml).
- ***Rate:*** Begin infusion at a rate of 20–40 milliunits/min to control uterine atony. Adjust rate as indicated.
- **Incomplete or Inevitable Abortion:** For incomplete or inevitable abortion, dilute 1 ml (10 units) in 500 ml of compatible infusion fluid for a concentration of 20 milliunits/ml.
- ***Rate:*** Infuse at a rate of 20–40 milliunits/min.
- **Y-Site Compatibility:** ▪ heparin ▪ hydrocortisone sodium succinate ▪ insulin ▪ meperidine ▪ morphine ▪ potassium chloride ▪ vitamin B complex with C.
- **Solution Compatibility:** ▪ dextrose/Ringer's or lactated Ringer's combinations ▪ dextrose/saline combinations ▪ Ringer's or lactated Ringer's injection ▪ D5W ▪ D10W ▪ 0.45% NaCl ▪ 0.9% NaCl.
- **Intranasal:** Hold squeeze bottle upright while patient is in sitting position. Patient should clear nasal passages prior to administration.

PATIENT/FAMILY TEACHING

- **General Info:** Advise patient to expect contractions similar to menstrual cramps after administration has started.
- **Nasal Spray:** Advise patient to administer nasal spray 2–3 min prior to planned breastfeeding. Patient should notify health care professional if milk drips from non-nursed breast or if uterine cramps occur.

EVALUATION

Effectiveness of therapy can be demonstrated by: ▪ Onset of effective contractions ▪ Increase in uterine tone ▪ Effective letdown reflex.

PACLITAXEL
(pa-kli-**tax**-el)
Taxol

CLASSIFICATION(S):
Antineoplastic (antimicrotubule agent)

Pregnancy Category D

INDICATIONS

▪ Metastatic ovarian cancer that has been unresponsive to first-line or other therapy ▪ Metastatic breast cancer that has been unresponsive to first-line or other therapy ▪ Second-line treatment of AIDS-related Kaposi's sarcoma.

ACTION

▪ Interferes with the normal cellular microtubule function that is required for interphase and mitosis. **Therapeutic Effects:** ▪ Death of rapidly replicating cells, particularly malignant ones.

PHARMACOKINETICS

Absorption: IV administration results in complete bioavailability.
Distribution: UK.
Metabolism and Excretion: Probably highly metabolized by the liver.
Half-life: 5.3–17.4 hr.

CONTRAINDICATIONS AND PRECAUTIONS

Contraindicated in: ▪ Hypersensitivity to paclitaxel or to castor oil (vehicle contains polyoxyethylated castor oil) ▪ Known alcohol intolerance ▪ Pregnancy or lactation ▪ WBC $\leq$1500/mm^3 in patients with ovarian or breast cancer ▪ WBC $\leq$1000/mm^3 in patients with AIDS-related Kaposi's sarcoma.
Use Cautiously in: ▪ Severe hepatic impairment ▪ Childbearing potential ▪ Active infection ▪ Decreased bone marrow reserve ▪ Chronic debilitating illnesses ▪ Children (safety not established).

ADVERSE REACTIONS AND SIDE EFFECTS*

CNS: abnormal ECG, bradycardia, hypotension.
GI: diarrhea, nausea, vomiting, abnormal liver function tests, stomatitis.
Derm: alopecia.
Hemat: anemia, leukopenia, thrombocytopenia.
MS: arthralgia, myalgia.
Neuro: peripheral neuropathy.
Misc: hypersensitivity reactions including ANAPHYLAXIS.

INTERACTIONS

Drug-Drug: ▪ **Ketoconazole** may inhibit metabolism and increase the risk of serious toxicity; concurrent use should be undertaken with caution ▪ Increased risk of myelosuppression with other **antineoplastic agents** or **radiation therapy** ▪ Myelosuppression increases when given after **cisplatin** ▪ May decrease antibody response to and increase risk of adverse reactions from **live virus vaccines.**

ROUTE AND DOSAGE

Other regimens have been used.

❑ **Ovarian Carcinoma**

- **IV (Adults):** 135 mg/m^2 over 24 hr every 3 wk. (Canadian labeling recommends a dosage of 170 mg/m^2.)

❑ **Breast Carcinoma**

- **IV (Adults):** 175 mg/m^2 over 3 hr every 3 wk.

❑ **AIDS-Related Kaposi's Sarcoma**

- **IV (Adults):** 135 mg/m^2 q 3 wk or 100 mg/m^2 q 2 wk (dosage reduction/adjustment may be necessary in patients with advanced HIV infection).

AVAILABILITY

▪ ***Concentrate for injection:*** 30 mg/5-ml vials[Rx].

TIME/ACTION PROFILE (effect on WBC counts)

	ONSET	PEAK	DURATION
IV	UK	11 days	3 wk

*CAPITALS indicate life-threatening; underlines indicate most frequent.

NURSING IMPLICATIONS

ASSESSMENT

- Monitor vital signs frequently, especially during 1st hr of 24-hr infusion.
- Monitor for hypersensitivity reactions continuously during the first 30 min and frequently thereafter. These occur frequently (19%), usually during the first 10 min of paclitaxel infusion, after the 1st or 2nd dose. Pretreatment is recommended for *all* patients and should include dexamethasone 20 mg PO 12 and 6 hours prior to paclitaxel, diphenhydramine 50 mg IV 30–60 min prior to paclitaxel, and cimetidine 300 mg or ranitidine 50 mg IV 30–60 min prior to paclitaxel. Most common manifestations are dyspnea, hypotension, and chest pain. If these occur, stop infusion and notify physician. Treatment may include bronchodilators, epinephrine, antihistamines, and glucocorticoids. Keep these agents and resuscitative equipment close by in the event of an anaphylactic reaction. Other manifestations of hypersensitivity reactions include flushing and rash.
- Monitor cardiovascular status especially during 1st hr of infusion. Hypotension and bradycardia are common but usually do not require treatment. Continuous ECG monitoring is recommended only for patients with serious underlying conduction abnormalities.
- Monitor for bone marrow depression. Assess for bleeding (bleeding gums, bruising, petechiae, guaiac stools, urine, and emesis) and avoid IM injections and rectal temperatures if platelet count is low. Apply pressure to venipuncture sites for 10 min. Assess for signs of infection during neutropenia. Anemia may occur. Monitor for increased fatigue, dyspnea, and orthostatic hypotension.
- Assess for development of peripheral neuropathy. If severe symptoms occur, subsequent dosage should be reduced by 20%.
- Monitor intake and output, appetite, and nutritional intake. Paclitaxel causes nausea and vomiting in 60% of patients. Prophylactic antiemetics may be used. Adjust diet as tolerated to help maintain fluid and electrolyte balance and nutritional status.
- Assess patient for arthralgia and myalgia, which usually begin 2–3 days after therapy and resolve within 5 days. Pain is usually relieved by nonopioid analgesics but may be severe enough to require treatment with opioid analgesics.
- ***Lab Test Considerations:*** Monitor CBC and differential prior to and periodically throughout therapy. The nadir of leukopenia occurs in 11 days, with recovery by days 15–21. Notify physician if the leukocyte count is $<1500/mm^3$ ($1000/mm^3$ in AIDS-related Kaposi's sarcoma) or if the platelet count is $<100,000/mm^3$. Subsequent doses are usually held until leukocyte count is $>1500/mm^3$ ($1000/mm^3$ in AIDS-related Kaposi's sarcoma) and platelet count is $>100,000/mm^3$.
- Monitor liver function studies (AST, ALT, LDH, bilirubin) prior to and periodically throughout therapy to detect hepatotoxicity.
- May cause elevated serum triglycerides.

P

POTENTIAL NURSING DIAGNOSES

- Infection, risk for (Adverse Reactions).
- Injury, risk for (Adverse Reactions).
- Knowledge deficit, related to medication regimen (Patient/Family Teaching).

IMPLEMENTATION

- **Continuous Infusion:** Paclitaxel must be diluted prior to injection. Dilute contents of 5-ml (30-mg) vials to a concentration of 0.3–1.2 mg/ml with the following diluents: 0.9% NaCl, D5W, D5/0.9% NaCl, or dextrose in Ringer's solution. Although haziness in the solution is normal, inspect for particulate matter or discoloration before use. Use an in-line filter of not >0.22-micron pore size. Solutions are stable for 27 hr at room temperature and lighting. Do not use PVC containers or administration sets.
- ***Rate:*** Dose for ***breast cancer or AIDS-related Kaposi's sarcoma*** is administered over 3 hr. Dose for ***ovarian cancer*** is administered as a 24-hr infusion.
- **Y-Site Compatibility:** ▪ acyclovir ▪ amikacin ▪ aminophylline ▪ ampicillin/sulbactam ▪ bleomycin ▪ butorphanol ▪ calcium chloride ▪ carboplatin ▪ cefepime ▪ cefotetan ▪ ceftazidime ▪ ceftriaxone ▪ cimetidine ▪ cisplatin ▪ cyclophosphamide ▪ cytarabine ▪ dacarbazine ▪ dexamethasone ▪ diphenhydramine ▪ doxorubicin ▪ droperidol ▪ etoposide ▪ famotidine ▪ floxuridine ▪ fluconazole ▪ fluorouracil ▪ furosemide ▪ ganciclovir ▪ gentamicin ▪ grani-

setron ▪ haloperidol ▪ heparin ▪ hydrocortisone ▪ hydromorphone ▪ ifosfamide ▪ lorazepam ▪ magnesium sulfate ▪ mannitol ▪ meperidine ▪ mesna ▪ methotrexate ▪ metoclopramide ▪ morphine ▪ nalbuphine ▪ ondansetron ▪ pentostatin ▪ potassium chloride ▪ prochlorperazine edisylate ▪ ranitidine ▪ sodium bicarbonate ▪ thiotepa ▪ vancomycin ▪ vinblastine ▪ vincristine ▪ zidovudine.
▪ **Y-Site Incompatibility:** ▪ amphotericin B ▪ chlorpromazine ▪ methylprednisolone sodium succinate ▪ mitoxantrone.

PATIENT/FAMILY TEACHING

- Instruct patient to notify health care professional promptly if fever; chills; cough; hoarseness; sore throat; signs of infection; lower back or side pain; painful or difficult urination; bleeding gums; bruising; petechiae; blood in stools, urine, or emesis; increased fatigue; dyspnea; or orthostatic hypotension occurs. Caution patient to avoid crowds and persons with known infections. Instruct patient to use soft toothbrush and electric razor and to avoid falls. Caution patient not to drink alcoholic beverages or to take medication containing aspirin or NSAIDS; may precipitate gastric bleeding.
- Instruct patient to notify health care professional if abdominal pain, yellow skin, weakness, paresthesia, gait disturbances, or joint or muscle aches occur.
- Instruct patient to inspect oral mucosa for redness and ulceration. If mouth sores occur, advise patient to use sponge brush and rinse mouth with water after eating and drinking. Stomatitis usually resolves in 5–7 days.
- Discuss with patient the possibility of hair loss. Complete hair loss usually occurs between days 14 and 21 and is reversible after discontinuation of therapy. Explore coping strategies.
- Advise patient to use a nonhormonal method of contraception.
- Instruct patient not to receive any vaccinations without advice of health care professional.
- Emphasize the need for periodic lab tests to monitor for side effects.

EVALUATION

Effectiveness of therapy can be demonstrated by: ▪ Decrease in size or spread of malignancy.

PAMIDRONATE
(pa-**mid**-roe-nate)
Aredia

CLASSIFICATION(S):
Bone resorption inhibitor, Electrolyte modifier (hypocalcemic), Hypocalcemic (biphosphonate)

Pregnancy Category C

INDICATIONS

▪ Management of moderate to severe hypercalcemia associated with malignancy ▪ Management of osteolytic bone lesions associated with multiple myeloma or breast cancer ▪ Management of moderate to severe Paget's disease.

ACTION

▪ Inhibits resorption of bone. **Therapeutic Effects:** ▪ Decreased serum calcium ▪ Decreased skeletal destruction in multiple myeloma or breast cancer ▪ Decreased skeletal complications in Paget's disease.

PHARMACOKINETICS

Absorption: IV administration results in complete bioavailability.
Distribution: Rapidly absorbed by bone. Reaches high concentrations in bone, liver, spleen, teeth, and tracheal cartilage. Approximately 50% of a dose is retained by bone and then slowly released.
Metabolism and Excretion: 50% is excreted unchanged in the urine.
Half-life: Elimination half-life from plasma is biphasic—1st phase 1.6 hr, 2nd phase 27.2 hr. Elimination half-life from bone is 300 days.

CONTRAINDICATIONS AND PRECAUTIONS

Contraindicated in: ▪ Hypersensitivity to pamidronate, other biphosphonates, or mannitol.
Use Cautiously in: ▪ Underlying cardiovascular disease, especially congestive heart failure (initiate saline hydration cautiously) ▪ Renal impairment (dosage reduction recommended) ▪ Pregnancy, lactation, or children (safety not established).

ADVERSE REACTIONS AND SIDE EFFECTS*

CNS: fatigue.
EENT: rhinitis.
Resp: rales.
CV: arrhythmias, hypertension, syncope, tachycardia.
GI: nausea, abdominal pain, anorexia, constipation, vomiting.
F and E: hypocalcemia, hypokalemia, hypomagnesemia, hypophosphatemia, fluid overload.
Hemat: leukopenia, anemia.
Local: phlebitis at injection site.
Metab: hypothyroidism.
MS: muscle stiffness, bone pain.
Misc: fever, generalized pain.

INTERACTIONS

Drug-Drug: ▪ Hypokalemia and hypomagnesemia may increase the risk of **digitalis glycoside** toxicity ▪ **Calcium** and **vitamin D** will antagonize the beneficial effects of pamidronate.

ROUTE AND DOSAGE

❑ **Hypercalcemia of Malignancy**
- **IV (Adults):** *Moderate hypercalcemia*—30–90 mg; may be repeated after 7 days.

❑ **Osteolytic Lesions from Multiple Myeloma**
- **IV (Adults):** 90 mg monthly.

❑ **Osteolytic Lesions from Metastatic Breast Cancer**
- **IV (Adults):** 90 mg q 3–4 wk.

❑ **Paget's Disease**
- **IV (Adults):** 90–180 mg/treatment; may be given as 30 mg daily for 3 days up to 30 mg/wk for 6 wk. Single doses of 60–90 mg may also be effective.

AVAILABILITY

▪ ***Injection:*** 30 mg/vial[Rx], 60 mg/vial[Rx], 90 mg/vial[Rx].

TIME/ACTION PROFILE (effect on serum calcium)

	ONSET	PEAK	DURATION
IV	24 hr	7 days	UK

NURSING IMPLICATIONS

ASSESSMENT

- ☐ Monitor intake/output ratios and blood pressure frequently during therapy. Assess for signs of fluid overload (edema, rales/crackles).
- ☐ Monitor symptoms of hypercalcemia (nausea, vomiting, anorexia, weakness, constipation, thirst, and cardiac arrhythmias).
- ☐ Observe for evidence of hypocalcemia (paresthesia, muscle twitching, laryngospasm, and Chvostek's or Trousseau's sign). Protect symptomatic patients by elevating and padding side rails; keep bed in low position.
- ☐ Monitor IV site for phlebitis (pain, redness, swelling). Symptomatic treatment should be used if this occurs.
- ☐ Assess patient for bone pain. Treatment with nonopioid or opioid analgesics may be necessary.
- ▪ ***Lab Test Considerations:*** Electrolytes (including calcium, phosphate, potassium, and magnesium), hemoglobin, and creatinine should be monitored closely. CBC and platelet count should be monitored during the first 2 wk of therapy.

POTENTIAL NURSING DIAGNOSES

- Pain (Indications, Side Effects).
- Injury, risk for (Indications).
- Knowledge deficit, related to medication regimen (Patient/Family Teaching).

IMPLEMENTATION

- ▪ **General Info:** Vigorous saline hydration, maintaining a urine output of 2000 ml/24 hr, should be undertaken concurrently with pamidronate therapy. Initiate saline hydration cautiously in patients with underlying cardiovascular disease, especially congestive heart failure.
- ☐ Patients with severe hypercalcemia should be started at the 90-mg dose.
- ▪ **IV:** Reconstitute by adding 10 ml of sterile water for injection to each vial for a concentration of 30 mg/10 ml, 60 mg/ml, or 90 mg/ml. Allow drug to dissolve before withdrawing. Solution is stable for 24 hr if refrigerated.
- ▪ **Hypercalcemia:** Dilute further in 1000 ml of

***CAPITALS indicate life-threatening; underlines indicate most frequent.**

0.45% NaCl, 0.9% NaCl, or D5W. Solution is stable for 24 hr at room temperature.

- *Rate:* Administer 60-mg infusion over at least 4 hr and 90-mg infusion over 24 hr.
- **Multiple Myeloma:** Dilute reconstituted solution in 500 ml of 0.45% NaCl, 0.9% NaCl, or D5W.
- *Rate:* Administer over 4 hr.
- **Paget's Disease:** Dilute reconstituted solution in 500 ml of 0.45% NaCl, 0.9% NaCl, or D5W.
- *Rate:* Administer over 4 hr.
- **Additive Incompatibility:** ■ Calcium-containing solutions, such as Ringer's solution.

PATIENT/FAMILY TEACHING

□ Advise patient to report signs of hypercalcemic relapse (bone pain, anorexia, nausea, vomiting, thirst, lethargy) to health care professional promptly.
□ Advise patient to notify nurse of pain at the infusion site.
□ Encourage patient to comply with dietary recommendations. Diet should contain adequate amounts of calcium and vitamin D (see Appendix K).
□ Advise patient to notify health care professional if bone pain is severe or persistent.
□ Emphasize the need for keeping follow-up exams to monitor progress, even after medication is discontinued, to detect relapse.

EVALUATION

Effectiveness of therapy can be demonstrated by: ■ Lowered serum calcium levels ■ Decreased pain from lytic lesions.

PANCRELIPASE

(pan-kree-**li**-pase)

Cotazym, {Cotazym-65 B}, Cotazym E.C.S. 8, Cotazym E.C.S. 20, Cotazym-S, Enzymase-16, Ilozyme, Ku-Zyme HP, Pancoate, Pancrease, Pancrease MT 4, Pancrease MT 10, Pancrease MT 16, Pancrease MT 20, Pancrebarb MS-8, Protilase, Ultrase MT 12, Ultrase MT 20, Viokase, Zymase

CLASSIFICATION(S):
Pancreatic enzyme

Pregnancy Category C

INDICATIONS

■ Pancreatic insufficiency associated with: □ Chronic pancreatitis □ Pancreatectomy □ Cystic fibrosis □ GI bypass surgery □ Ductal obstruction secondary to tumor.

ACTION

■ Contains lipolytic, amylolytic, and proteolytic activity. **Therapeutic Effects:** ■ Increased digestion of fats, carbohydrates, and proteins in the GI tract.

PHARMACOKINETICS

Absorption: UK.
Distribution: UK.
Metabolism and Excretion: UK.
Half-life: UK.

CONTRAINDICATIONS AND PRECAUTIONS

Contraindicated in: ■ Hypersensitivity to hog proteins.
Use Cautiously in: ■ Pregnancy or lactation (safety not established).

ADVERSE REACTIONS AND SIDE EFFECTS*

EENT: nasal stuffiness.
Resp: dyspnea, shortness of breath, wheezing.
GI: abdominal pain (high doses only), diarrhea, nausea, stomach cramps, oral irritation.
GU: hematuria.
Derm: hives, rash.
Metab: hyperuricemia.
Misc: allergic reactions.

INTERACTIONS

Drug-Drug: ■ **Antacids (calcium carbonate** or **magnesium hydroxide)** may decrease effectiveness of pancrelipase ■ May decrease the absorption of concurrently administered **iron preparations.**
Drug-Food: ■ **Alkaline foods** destroy coating on enteric-coated products.

{} = Available in Canada only.
***CAPITALS indicate life-threatening; underlines indicate most frequent.**

ROUTE AND DOSAGE

- **PO (Adults):** 1–3 capsule(s) before or with meals; dosage may be increased as needed (up to 8 capsules may be needed), or 1–2 delayed-release capsule(s), or 0.7 g powder.
- **PO (Children):** 1–3 capsule(s) before or with meals; dosage may be increased as needed, or 1–2 delayed-release capsule(s), or 0.7 g powder.

AVAILABILITY

▪ ***Capsules:*** 8000 units lipase/30,000 units protease and amylase[Rx] ▪ ***Delayed-release capsules:*** 4000 units lipase/12,000 units protease and amylase[Rx], 4000 units lipase/25,000 units protease/20,000 units amylase[Rx], 5000 units lipase/20,000 units protease and amylase[Rx], {8000 units lipase/30,000 units protease and amylase[Rx]}, 10,000 units lipase/30,000 units protease and amylase[Rx], 12,000 units lipase/24,000 units protease and amylase[Rx], 12,000 units lipase/39,000 units protease and amylase[Rx], 16,000 units lipase/48,000 units protease and amylase[Rx], {20,000 units lipase/55,000 units protease and amylase[Rx]}, 20,000 units lipase/65,000 units protease and amylase[Rx], 24,000 units lipase/78,000 units protease and amylase[Rx] ▪ ***Powder:*** 16,800 units lipase/70,000 units protease and amylase[Rx].

TIME/ACTION PROFILE (digestant effects)

	ONSET	PEAK	DURATION
PO	rapid	UK	UK

NURSING IMPLICATIONS

ASSESSMENT

- ▫ Assess patient's nutritional status (height, weight, skin fold thickness, arm muscle circumference, and lab values) prior to and periodically throughout therapy.
- ▫ Monitor stools for high fat content (steatorrhea). Stools will be foul-smelling and frothy.
- ▫ Assess patient for allergy to pork; sensitivity to pancrelipase may exist.
- ***Lab Test Considerations:*** May cause elevated serum and urine uric acid concentrations.

POTENTIAL NURSING DIAGNOSES

- Nutrition, altered, less than body requirements (Indications).
- Knowledge deficit, related to medication regimen (Patient/Family Teaching).

IMPLEMENTATION

- **PO:** Administer immediately before or with meals and snacks.
- ▫ Capsules may be opened and sprinkled on foods. Capsules filled with enteric-coated beads should not be chewed (sprinkle on soft foods that can be swallowed without chewing, such as applesauce or Jell-O).
- ▫ Pancrelipase is destroyed by acid. Concurrent sodium bicarbonate or aluminum-containing antacids may be used with nonenteric-coated preparations to neutralize gastric pH. Enteric-coated beads are designed to withstand the acid pH of the stomach. These medications should not be chewed or mixed with alkaline foods prior to ingestion or coating will be destroyed.

PATIENT/FAMILY TEACHING

- ▫ Encourage patients to comply with diet recommendations of health care professional (generally high-calorie, high-protein, low-fat). Dosage should be adjusted for fat content of diet. Usually 300 mg of pancrelipase is necessary to digest every 17 g of dietary fat. If a dose is missed, it should be omitted.
- ▫ Instruct patient not to chew tablets and to swallow them quickly with plenty of liquid to prevent mouth and throat irritation. Patient should be sitting upright to enhance swallowing. Eating immediately after taking medication helps further ensure that the medication is swallowed and does not remain in contact with mouth and esophagus for a prolonged period. Patient should avoid sniffing powdered contents of capsules, as sensitization of nose and throat may occur (nasal stuffiness or respiratory distress).
- ▫ Instruct patient to notify health care professional if joint pain, swelling of legs, gastric distress, or rash occurs.

EVALUATION

Effectiveness of therapy can be demonstrated by: ▪ Improved nutritional status in patients with pancreatic insufficiency ▫ Normalization of stools in patients with steatorrhea.

P

PAROXETINE
(par-**ox**-e-teen)
Paxil

CLASSIFICATION(S):
Antidepressant (selective serotonin reuptake inhibitor)

Pregnancy Category C

INDICATIONS

▪ Treatment of: ▫ Depression ▫ Panic disorder ▫ Obsessive-compulsive disorder (often in conjunction with psychotherapy).

ACTION

▪ Inhibits neuronal reuptake of serotonin in the CNS, thus potentiating the activity of serotonin; has little effect on norepinephrine or dopamine. **Therapeutic Effects:** ▪ Antidepressant action ▪ Decreased frequency of panic attacks or obsessive-compulsive behavior.

PHARMACOKINETICS

Absorption: Well absorbed following oral administration.
Distribution: Widely distributed throughout body fluids and tissues, including the CNS; enters breast milk.
Metabolism and Excretion: Highly metabolized by the liver; 2% excreted unchanged in urine.
Half-life: 21 hr.

CONTRAINDICATIONS AND PRECAUTIONS

Contraindicated in: ▪ Hypersensitivity ▪ Concurrent MAO inhibitor therapy (may result in serious, potentially fatal reactions).
Use Cautiously in: ▪ Severe renal or hepatic impairment, geriatric or debilitated patients (start with smaller doses; daily dose should not be >40 mg) ▪ History of mania ▪ History or risk of suicide attempt ▪ Pregnancy, lactation, or children (safety not established).

ADVERSE REACTIONS AND SIDE EFFECTS*

CNS: anxiety, dizziness, drowsiness, headache, insomnia, weakness, agitation, amnesia, confusion, emotional lability, hangover, impaired concentration, malaise, mental depression, syncope.
EENT: blurred vision, rhinitis.
Resp: cough, pharyngitis, respiratory disorders, yawning.
CV: chest pain, edema, hypertension, palpitations, postural hypotension, tachycardia, vasodilation.
GI: constipation, diarrhea, dry mouth, nausea, abdominal pain, decreased appetite, dyspepsia, flatulence, increased appetite, taste disturbances, vomiting.
GU: ejaculatory disturbance, decreased libido, genital disorders, urinary disorders, urinary frequency.
Derm: sweating, photosensitivity, pruritus, rash.
Metab: weight gain, weight loss.
MS: back pain, myalgia, myasthenia, myopathy.
Neuro: tremor, myoclonus, paresthesia.
Misc: chills, fever.

INTERACTIONS

Drug-Drug: ▪ Serious, potentially fatal reactions (hyperthermia, rigidity, myoclonus, autonomic instability, with fluctuating vital signs and extreme agitation, which may proceed to delirium and coma) may occur with concurrent **MAO inhibitor** therapy. MAO inhibitors should be stopped at least 14 days prior to paroxetine therapy. Paroxetine should be stopped at least 14 days prior to MAO inhibitor therapy ▪ May decrease the metabolism and increase the effects of certain **drugs that are metabolized by the liver,** including other **antidepressants, phenothiazines, group IC antiarrhythmics, procyclidine,** and **quinidine.** Concurrent use should be undertaken with caution ▪ **Cimetidine** increases blood levels ▪ **Phenobarbital** and **phenytoin** may decrease effectiveness ▪ Concurrent use with **alcohol** is not recommended ▪ May decrease the effectiveness of **digoxin** ▪ Concurrent use with **tryptophan** may result in headache, nausea, sweating, and dizziness ▪ May increase the risk of bleeding with **warfarin** without altering prothrombin time.

ROUTE AND DOSAGE

▫ **Depression**

- **PO (Adults):** 20 mg as a single dose in the morning; may be increased by 10 mg/day at weekly intervals (range 20–50 mg).

*CAPITALS indicate life-threatening; underlines indicate most frequent.

- **PO (Geriatric Patients/Debilitated Patients/Patients with Severe Hepatic or Renal Impairment):** 10 mg/day initially; may be slowly increased (not to exceed 40 mg/day).

□ **Obsessive-Compulsive Disorder**

- **PO (Adults):** 20 mg/day initially; increase by 10 mg/day q wk up to 40 mg (range 40–60 mg/day).

□ **Panic Disorder**

- **PO (Adults):** 10 mg/day initially; increase by 10 mg/day q wk up to 40 mg (range 10–60 mg/day).

AVAILABILITY

- ***Tablets:*** 20 mg[Rx], 30 mg[Rx].

TIME/ACTION PROFILE (antidepressant action)

	ONSET	PEAK	DURATION
PO	1–4 wk	UK	UK

NURSING IMPLICATIONS

ASSESSMENT

- **General Info:** Monitor appetite and nutritional intake. Weigh weekly. Notify physician or other health care professional of continued weight loss. Adjust diet as tolerated to support nutritional status.
- **Depression:** Monitor mood changes. Inform physician or other health care professional if patient demonstrates significant increase in anxiety, nervousness, or insomnia.

□ Assess for suicidal tendencies, especially during early therapy. Restrict amount of drug available to patient.

- **Obsessive-Compulsive Disorder:** Assess patient for frequency of obsessive-compulsive behaviors. Note degree to which these thoughts and behaviors interfere with daily functioning.
- **Panic Attacks:** Assess frequency and severity of panic attacks.
- ***Lab Test Considerations:*** Monitor CBC and differential periodically during therapy. Report leukopenia or anemia.

POTENTIAL NURSING DIAGNOSES

- Coping, ineffective individual (Indications).
- Injury, risk for (Side Effects).
- Knowledge deficit, related to medication regimen (Patient/Family Teaching).

IMPLEMENTATION

- **General Info:** Periodically reassess dose and continued need for therapy.
- **PO:** Administer as a single dose in the morning. May administer with food to minimize GI irritation.

PATIENT/FAMILY TEACHING

□ Instruct patient to take paroxetine exactly as directed. If a dose is missed, take as soon as possible and return to regular dosing schedule. Do not double doses.

□ May cause drowsiness or dizziness. Caution patient to avoid driving and other activities requiring alertness until response to the drug is known.

□ Advise patient to avoid alcohol or other CNS-depressant drugs during therapy and to consult with health care professional before taking other medications with paroxetine.

□ Inform patient that frequent mouth rinses, good oral hygiene, and sugarless gum or candy may minimize dry mouth. If dry mouth persists for more than 2 wk, consult health care professional regarding use of saliva substitute.

□ Advise patient to wear sunscreen and protective clothing to prevent photosensitivity reactions.

□ Instruct female patient to inform health care professional if pregnancy is planned or suspected or if she is breast-feeding.

□ Advise patient to notify health care professional if headache, weakness, nausea, anorexia, anxiety, or insomnia persists.

□ Emphasize the importance of follow-up exams to monitor progress. Encourage patient participation in psychotherapy.

EVALUATION

Effectiveness of therapy can be demonstrated by: ▪ Increased sense of well-being □ Renewed interest in surroundings. May require 1–4 wk of therapy to obtain antidepressant effects ▪ Decrease in obsessive-compulsive behaviors ▪ Decrease in frequency and severity of panic attacks.

PEGASPARGASE
(peg-ass-**par**-jase)
Oncaspar, PEG-L-asparaginase

CLASSIFICATION(S):
Antineoplastic (enzyme)

Pregnancy Category C

INDICATIONS

▪ Treatment (usually with other agents) of acute lymphoblastic leukemia (ALL) in patients who have had a previous hypersensitivity reaction to native asparaginase.

ACTION

▪ Consists of L-asparaginase bound to polyethylene glycol (PEG). This compound depletes asparagine, which leukemic cells cannot synthesize. Normal cells are able to produce their own asparagine and are less susceptible to the effects of asparaginase. Binding to PEG renders asparaginase less antigenic and therefore less likely to induce hypersensitivity reactions. **Therapeutic Effects:** ▪ Death of leukemic cells.

PHARMACOKINETICS

Absorption: IV administration results in complete bioavailability.
Distribution: UK.
Metabolism and Excretion: Metabolized by serum proteases and in the reticuloendothelial system.
Half-life: 5.7 days (less in patients with previous hypersensitivity to native L-asparaginase).

CONTRAINDICATIONS AND PRECAUTIONS

Contraindicated in: ▪ Pancreatitis or history of pancreatitis ▪ History of previous hemorrhagic reaction to asparaginase therapy ▪ Previous hypersensitivity reactions to pegaspargase.
Use Cautiously in: ▪ History of previous hypersensitivity reactions to other drugs ▪ Patients with childbearing potential ▪ Pregnancy or lactation (safety not established).

ADVERSE REACTIONS AND SIDE EFFECTS*

CNS: SEIZURES, headache, malaise.
GI: PANCREATITIS, abdominal pain, abnormal liver function tests, anorexia, diarrhea, lip edema, nausea, vomiting.
Derm: jaundice.
Endo: hyperglycemia.
F and E: peripheral edema.
Hemat: decreased fibrinogen, disseminated intravascular coagulation, hemolytic anemia, increased thromboplastin, leukopenia, pancytopenia, thrombocytopenia.
Local: injection site hypersensitivity, injection site pain, thrombosis.
MS: arthralgia, myalgia, pain in extremities.
Neuro: paresthesia.
Misc: chills, hypersensitivity reactions, night sweats.

INTERACTIONS

Drug-Drug: ▪ May alter response to **anticoagulants** or **antiplatelet agents** ▪ May alter the response to other **drugs that are metabolized by the liver.**

ROUTE AND DOSAGE

- **IM, IV (Adults and Children with Body Surface Area ≥0.6 m²):** 2500 IU/m² q 14 days (usually in combination with other agents).
- **IM, IV (Children with Body Surface Area <0.6 m²):** 82.5 IU/kg q 14 days (usually in combination with other agents).

AVAILABILITY

▪ ***Injection:*** 750 IU/ml[Rx].

TIME/ACTION PROFILE (hematologic effects)

	ONSET	PEAK	DURATION
IV	rapid	UK	14 days

NURSING IMPLICATIONS

ASSESSMENT

□ Assess patient for previous hypersensitivity reactions to native L-asparaginase. Monitor for hypersensitivity reaction (urticaria, diaphore-

*CAPITALS indicate life-threatening; underlines indicate most frequent.

sis, facial swelling, joint pain, hypotension, bronchospasm). Epinephrine and resuscitation equipment should be readily available. Reaction may occur up to 2 hr after administration.

- ▫ Monitor for development of bone marrow depression. Assess for fever, sore throat, and signs of infection. Monitor platelet count throughout therapy. Assess for bleeding (bleeding gums, bruising, petechiae, guaiac test stools, urine, and emesis). Avoid giving IM injections and taking rectal temperatures. Apply pressure to venipuncture sites for 10 min. Anemia may occur. Monitor for increased fatigue, dyspnea, and orthostatic hypotension.
- ▫ Monitor patient frequently for signs of pancreatitis (nausea, vomiting, abdominal pain).
- ▫ Assess nausea, vomiting, and appetite. Weigh patient weekly. Prophylactic antiemetics may be used prior to administration.
- ▪ ***Lab Test Considerations:*** Monitor CBC prior to and periodically throughout therapy. May alter coagulation studies. Fibrinogen may be decreased; prothrombin time (PT) and partial thromboplastin time (PTT) may be increased.
- ▫ Monitor serum amylase frequently to detect pancreatitis.
- ▫ Monitor blood glucose; may cause hyperglycemia.
- ▫ May cause elevated BUN and serum creatinine.
- ▫ Hepatotoxicity may be manifested by increased AST, ALT, or bilirubin. Liver function tests usually return to normal after therapy.
- ▫ May cause decreased serum calcium.
- ▫ May cause elevated serum and urine uric acid and hyponatremia.

POTENTIAL NURSING DIAGNOSES

- ▪ Infection, risk for (Adverse Reactions).
- ▪ Knowledge deficit, related to medication regimen (Patient/Family Teaching).

IMPLEMENTATION

- ▪ **General Info:** IM is the preferred route because of a lower incidence of adverse reactions.
- ▫ Solutions should be prepared in a biologic cabinet. Wear gloves, gown, and mask while handling medication. Discard equipment in specially designated containers (see Appendix I).
- ▪ **IM:** Limit single injection volume to 2 ml. If volume of injection is >2 ml, use multiple injection sites.
- ▪ **Intermittent Infusion:** Dilute each dose in 100 ml of 0.9% NaCl or D5W. Do not shake or agitate. Do not use if solution is cloudy or has formed a precipitate.
- ▫ Use only 1 dose per vial; do not re-enter the vial. Discard unused portions.
- ▫ Keep refrigerated but do not freeze. Freezing destroys activity but does not change the appearance of pegaspargase.
- ▪ ***Rate:*** Administer over 1–2 hr via Y-site through an infusion that is already running.
- ▪ **Additive Incompatibility:** ▪ Information unavailable. Do not admix with other medications or solutions.

PATIENT/FAMILY TEACHING

- ▫ Inform patient of the possibility of hypersensitivity reactions, including anaphylaxis.
- ▫ Advise patient that concurrent use of other medications may increase the risk of bleeding and the toxicity of pegaspargase. Consult health care professional before taking any other medications, including OTC drugs.
- ▫ Instruct patient to notify health care professional if abdominal pain, severe nausea and vomiting, jaundice, fever, chills, sore throat, bleeding or bruising, excess thirst or urination, or mouth sores occur. Caution patient to avoid crowds and persons with known infections. Instruct patient to use soft toothbrush, electric razor, and to be especially careful to avoid falls. Patients should also be cautioned not to drink alcoholic beverages or take medications containing aspirin or NSAIDs because these may precipitate gastric bleeding.
- ▫ Instruct patient not to receive any vaccinations without advice of health care professional. Advise parents that this may alter child's immunization schedule.
- ▫ Emphasize the need for periodic lab tests to monitor for side effects.

EVALUATION

Effectiveness of therapy can be demonstrated by: ▪ Improvement of hematologic status in patients with leukemia.

PEMOLINE
(pem-oh-leen)
Cylert

CLASSIFICATION(S):
CNS stimulant

Schedule IV
Pregnancy Category B

INDICATIONS

▪ Adjunct in the management of attention-deficit hyperactivity disorder (ADHD) in children >6 yr. **Unlabeled Uses:** ▪ Treatment of fatigue or mental depression ▪ Schizophrenia ▪ As a stimulant in geriatric patients.

ACTION

▪ Produces CNS stimulation, which may be mediated by dopamine ▪ Causes increased motor activity and mental alertness, decreased fatigue, mild euphoria, and decreased appetite. **Therapeutic Effects:** ▪ Increased attention span in children with ADHD.

PHARMACOKINETICS

Absorption: Absorbed from the GI tract.
Distribution: UK.
Metabolism and Excretion: Partially (50%) metabolized by the liver; 40% excreted unchanged by the kidneys.
Half-life: 9–14 hr.

CONTRAINDICATIONS AND PRECAUTIONS

Contraindicated in: ▪ Hypersensitivity ▪ Liver disease.
Use Cautiously in: ▪ Renal impairment ▪ Unstable emotional status or psychoses ▪ History of seizure disorders ▪ Tics ▪ Pregnancy or lactation (safety not established).

ADVERSE REACTIONS AND SIDE EFFECTS*

CNS: SEIZURES, insomnia, dizziness, dyskinetic movements, headache, irritability, mental depression, nervousness (↑ doses).
CV: tachycardia (↑ doses).
GI: anorexia, drug-induced hepatitis.
Derm: rash, sweating.
Metab: weight loss.
Misc: fever.

INTERACTIONS

Drug-Drug: ▪ May have additive CNS stimulation with other **CNS stimulants** or **adrenergics,** including **decongestants.**

ROUTE AND DOSAGE

▪ **PO (Children >6 yr):** 37.5 mg initially as single morning dose; may be increased by 18.75 mg at weekly intervals until optimum response is achieved (range 56.25–75 mg/day, not to exceed 112.5 mg/day).

AVAILABILITY

▪ ***Tablets:*** 18.75 mg[Rx], 37.5 mg[Rx], 75 mg[Rx] ▪ ***Chewable tablets:*** 37.5 mg[Rx].

TIME/ACTION PROFILE (ADHD = effects in attention-deficit hyperactivity disorder)

	ONSET	PEAK	DURATION
PO (ADHD)	days–wks	2–3 wk	days
PO (CNS stimulation)	UK	4 hr	8 hr

NURSING IMPLICATIONS

ASSESSMENT

□ Assess attention span, motor or vocal tics, impulse control, and interactions with others in children with ADHD. Therapy may be interrupted at intervals to determine whether symptoms are sufficient to continue therapy.
□ Monitor growth, both height and weight, in children on long-term therapy. Inform physician or other health care professional if growth inhibition occurs.
▪ ***Lab Test Considerations:*** Hepatic function should be monitored prior to and periodically throughout therapy. May cause elevated LDH, alkaline phosphatase, AST, and ALT levels.

POTENTIAL NURSING DIAGNOSES

▪ Sleep pattern disturbance (Side Effects).
▪ Knowledge deficit, related to medication regimen (Patient/Family Teaching).

*CAPITALS indicate life-threatening; underlines indicate most frequent.

IMPLEMENTATION

- **General Info:** When symptoms of ADHD are controlled in children, dosage reduction or interruption of therapy may be possible during summer months, on weekends, or when child is under less stress.
- **PO:** Administer daily dose in the morning. Chewable tablets must be chewed well before swallowing.

PATIENT/FAMILY TEACHING

- **General Info:** Instruct patient to take medication in morning to avoid sleep disturbances. If a dose is missed, take as soon as remembered; if remembered the next day, omit and continue on dosage schedule. Do not double doses. Pemoline has a high dependence and abuse potential. Tolerance occurs rapidly; do not increase dose. Consult health care professional before discontinuing. In long-term therapy, dosage should be reduced gradually to prevent withdrawal symptoms. Abrupt cessation of high doses may cause extreme fatigue and mental depression.
- □ May cause dizziness. Caution patient to avoid driving or other activities requiring alertness until response to medication is known.
- □ Advise patient to avoid intake of large amounts of caffeine.
- □ Advise patient to notify health care professional if yellow skin or sclera, pale stools or dark urine, palpitations, sweating, fever, or uncontrolled tremors develop or if nervousness, restlessness, insomnia, dizziness, or anorexia becomes severe.
- □ Inform patient that periodic holidays from the drug may be used to assess progress and to decrease dependence.
- □ Emphasize the importance of routine follow-up exams to monitor progress.
- **Attention-Deficit Hyperactivity Disorder:** Advise parents to notify school nurse of medication regimen.

EVALUATION

Effectiveness of therapy can be demonstrated by: ▪ Calming effect with decreased hyperactivity and prolonged attention span in children with ADHD. Significant beneficial effects may not be evident until the 3rd or 4th wk of therapy, because clinical improvement is gradual.

PENBUTOLOL

(pen-**byoo**-toe-lole)

Levatol

CLASSIFICATION(S):

Antihypertensive agent, Beta-adrenergic blocking agent (nonselective)

Pregnancy Category C

INDICATIONS

▪ Management of hypertension.

ACTION

▪ Blocks stimulation of $beta_1$ (myocardial) and $beta_2$ (pulmonary, vascular, and uterine) -adrenergic receptor sites ▪ Also has intrinsic sympathomimetic activity (ISA), which may produce less bradycardia. **Therapeutic Effects:** ▪ Decreased heart rate and blood pressure.

PHARMACOKINETICS

Absorption: Well absorbed following oral administration.
Distribution: Moderate CNS penetration; crosses the placenta.
Metabolism and Excretion: Mostly metabolized by the liver.
Half-life: 5 hr.

CONTRAINDICATIONS AND PRECAUTIONS

Contraindicated in: ▪ Uncompensated congestive heart failure ▪ Pulmonary edema ▪ Cardiogenic shock ▪ Bradycardia or heart block.
Use Cautiously in: ▪ Renal impairment ▪ Hepatic impairment (lower doses may be necessary) ▪ Geriatric patients (increased sensitivity to beta-adrenergic blockers; initial dosage reduction recommended) ▪ Pulmonary disease (including asthma) ▪ Diabetes mellitus (may mask signs of hypoglycemia) ▪ Thyrotoxicosis (may mask symptoms) ▪ Patients with a history of severe allergic reactions (intensity of reactions may be increased) ▪ Pregnancy, lactation, or children (safety not established; all agents cross the placenta and may cause fetal/neonatal bradycardia,

hypotension, hypoglycemia, or respiratory depression).

ADVERSE REACTIONS AND SIDE EFFECTS*

CNS: fatigue, weakness, anxiety, depression, dizziness, drowsiness, insomnia, memory loss, mental status changes, nervousness, nightmares.
EENT: blurred vision, dry eyes, nasal stuffiness.
Resp: bronchospasm, wheezing.
CV: ARRHYTHMIAS, BRADYCARDIA, CONGESTIVE HEART FAILURE, PULMONARY EDEMA, orthostatic hypotension, peripheral vasoconstriction.
GI: constipation, diarrhea, nausea.
GU: impotence, decreased libido.
Derm: itching, rashes.
Endo: hyperglycemia, hypoglycemia.
MS: arthralgia, back pain, muscle cramps.
Neuro: paresthesia.

INTERACTIONS

Drug-Drug: ▪ **General anesthesia, IV phenytoin,** and **verapamil** may cause additive myocardial depression ▪ Additive bradycardia may occur with **digitalis glycosides** ▪ Additive hypotension may occur with other **antihypertensives**, acute ingestion of **alcohol**, or **nitrates** ▪ Concurrent use with **amphetamines, cocaine, ephedrine, epinephrine, norepinephrine, phenylephrine**, or **pseudoephedrine** may result in unopposed alpha-adrenergic stimulation (excessive hypertension, bradycardia) ▪ Concurrent **thyroid** administration may decrease effectiveness ▪ May alter the effectiveness of **insulin** or **oral hypoglycemic agents** (dosage adjustments may be necessary) ▪ May decrease the effectiveness of **beta-adrenergic bronchodilators** and **theophylline** ▪ May decrease the beneficial $beta_1$-cardiovascular effects of **dopamine** or **dobutamine** ▪ Use cautiously within 14 days of **MAO inhibitor** therapy (may result in hypertension) ▪ Concurrent **NSAIDs** may decrease antihypertensive action.

ROUTE AND DOSAGE

- **PO (Adults):** 20 mg once daily.

AVAILABILITY

- ***Tablets:*** 20 mg[Rx].

TIME/ACTION PROFILE (cardiovascular effects)

	ONSET	PEAK	DURATION
PO	1 hr	1.5–3 hr†	24 hr

†Following single dose, full effect not seen until several weeks of therapy.

NURSING IMPLICATIONS

ASSESSMENT

- **General Info:** Monitor blood pressure and pulse frequently during dosage adjustment period and periodically throughout therapy. Assess for orthostatic hypotension when assisting patient up from supine position.
  - Monitor intake and output ratios and daily weight. Assess patient routinely for evidence of fluid overload (peripheral edema, dyspnea, rales/crackles, fatigue, weight gain, jugular venous distention).
- ***Lab Test Considerations:*** May cause increased BUN, serum lipoprotein, potassium, triglyceride, and uric acid levels.
  - May cause increased ANA titers.
  - May cause increase in blood glucose levels.

POTENTIAL NURSING DIAGNOSES

- Cardiac output, decreased (Side Effects).
- Knowledge deficit, related to medication regimen (Patient/Family Teaching).
- Noncompliance, related to medication regimen (Patient/Family Teaching).

IMPLEMENTATION

- **General Info:** Take apical pulse prior to administering. If <50 bpm or if arrhythmia occurs, withhold medication and notify physician or other health care professional.
- **PO:** May be administered with food or on an empty stomach.

PATIENT/FAMILY TEACHING

- **General Info:** Instruct patient to take medication exactly as directed, at the same time each day, even if feeling well; do not skip or double up on missed doses. If a dose is missed, it should be taken as soon as possible up to 8 hr before next dose. Abrupt withdrawal may precipitate life-threatening arrhythmias, hypertension, or myocardial ischemia.

***CAPITALS indicate life-threatening; underlines indicate most frequent.**

- Advise patient to make sure enough medication is available for weekends, holidays, and vacations. A written prescription may be kept in wallet in case of emergency.
- Teach patient and family how to check pulse and blood pressure. Instruct them to check pulse daily and blood pressure biweekly. Advise patient to hold dose and contact health care professional if pulse is $<$50 bpm or if blood pressure changes significantly.
- May cause drowsiness or dizziness. Caution patient to avoid driving or other activities that require alertness until response to the drug is known.
- Advise patient to change positions slowly to minimize orthostatic hypotension, especially during initiation of therapy or upon dose increase.
- Caution patient that this medication may increase sensitivity to cold.
- Instruct patient to consult health care professional before taking any OTC medications, especially cold preparations, concurrently with this medication.
- Diabetics should closely monitor blood sugar, especially if weakness, malaise, irritability, or fatigue occurs. Medication may mask tachycardia and increased blood pressure as signs of hypoglycemia, but dizziness and sweating may still occur.
- Advise patient to notify health care professional if slow pulse, difficulty breathing, wheezing, cold hands and feet, dizziness, confusion, depression, rash, fever, sore throat, unusual bleeding, or bruising occurs.
- Instruct patient to inform health care professional of medication regimen prior to treatment or surgery.
- Advise patient to carry identification describing disease process and medication regimen at all times.

- **Hypertension:** Reinforce the need to continue additional therapies for hypertension (weight loss, sodium restriction, stress reduction, regular exercise, moderation of alcohol consumption, and smoking cessation). Medication controls but does not cure hypertension.

EVALUATION

Effectiveness of therapy can be demonstrated by: ■ Decrease in blood pressure. Maximum antihypertensive effects are usually seen by the end of week 2. Full effects of lower doses may not be seen for 4–6 wk.

PENCICLOVIR

(pen-**sye**-kloe-veer)

Denavir

CLASSIFICATION(S):

Antiviral (topical)

Pregnancy Category B

INDICATIONS

■ Recurrent herpes labialis (cold sores).

ACTION

■ Inhibits viral DNA synthesis and replication. **Therapeutic Effects:** ■ Death of herpes virus ■ Decreased lesion duration and pain ■ Active against herpes viruses.

PHARMACOKINETICS

Absorption: Not absorbed following topical use.

Distribution: UK.

Metabolism and Excretion: Converted intracellularly to active triphosphate form; excreted in urine.

Half-life: 2–2.5 hr.

CONTRAINDICATIONS AND PRECAUTIONS

Contraindicated in: ■ Hypersensitivity to penciclovir or other components of the formulation.

Use Cautiously in: ■ Pregnancy, lactation, or children (safety not established).

ADVERSE REACTIONS AND SIDE EFFECTS

CNS: headache.

Local: application site reactions.

INTERACTIONS

Drug-Drug: ■ None significant.

ROUTE AND DOSAGE

- **PO (Adults):** Apply 1% cream q 2 hr for 4 days while awake.

AVAILABILITY

- *Cream:* 1% in 2-g tubes[Rx].

TIME/ACTION PROFILE

	ONSET	PEAK	DURATION
Top	UK	UK	UK

NURSING IMPLICATIONS

ASSESSMENT

- Assess lesions prior to and daily during therapy.

POTENTIAL NURSING DIAGNOSES

- Skin integrity, impaired (Indications).
- Infection transmission, risk for (Indications, Patient/Family Teaching).
- Knowledge deficit, related to medication regimen (Patient/Family Teaching).

IMPLEMENTATION

- **General Info:** Begin treatment as early as possible, during prodrome or when lesions appear
- **Topical:** Apply to lesions every 2 hr for 4 days while awake.
- Apply to lips and face only; avoid application to mucous membranes or near the eyes.

PATIENT/FAMILY TEACHING

- Advise patient to apply medication exactly as directed for the full course of therapy. If a dose is missed, apply as soon as possible but not just before next dose is due; do not double doses. Penciclovir should not be used more frequently or longer than prescribed.
- Advise patients that the additional use of OTC creams, lotions, and ointments may delay healing and may cause spreading of lesions.

EVALUATION

Effectiveness of therapy can be demonstrated by: ▪ More rapid healing of lesions and relief of pain in herpes labialis.

PENICILLAMINE

(pen-i-**sill**-a-meen)
Cuprimine, Depen

CLASSIFICATION(S):
Antirheumatic (disease-modifying), Antiurolithic, Chelating agent

Pregnancy Category D

INDICATIONS

▪ Progressive rheumatoid arthritis resistant to conventional therapy ▪ Management of copper deposition in Wilson's disease ▪ Management of recurrent cystine calculi. **Unlabeled Uses:** ▪ Adjunct in the treatment of heavy metal poisoning.

ACTION

▪ Antirheumatic effect, probably due to enhanced lymphocyte function ▪ Chelates heavy metals, including copper, mercury, lead, and iron, into complexes that are excreted by the kidneys ▪ Forms a soluble complex with cystine that is readily excreted by the kidneys. **Therapeutic Effects:** ▪ Decreased disease progression in rheumatoid arthritis ▪ Decreased copper deposition in Wilson's disease ▪ Decreased cystine renal calculi formation.

PHARMACOKINETICS

Absorption: Well absorbed following oral administration.
Distribution: Crosses the placenta.
Metabolism and Excretion: Some excreted in urine as heavy metal–penicillamine complex, some excreted in urine as cystine-penicillamine complex, some metabolized by the liver.
Half-life: 1–7.5 hr (4–6 days during long-term use).

CONTRAINDICATIONS AND PRECAUTIONS

Contraindicated in: ▪ Hypersensitivity ▪ Cross-sensitivity with penicillin may exist ▪ Patients currently receiving gold salts, antimalarials, antineoplastic agents, oxyphenbutazone, or phenylbutazone ▪ Concurrent use of iron supplements ▪ Pregnancy (penicillamine should be avoided in pregnant patients with rheumatoid arthritis or cystinuria) ▪ Lactation.

Use Cautiously in: ▪ Geriatric patients (increased risk of hematologic toxicity; dosage reduction recommended) ▪ Renal impairment (increased risk of adverse renal reactions in patients with rheumatoid arthritis) ▪ History of aplastic anemia due to penicillamine ▪ Patients requiring surgery (may impair wound healing) ▪ Pregnancy (for patients with Wilson's disease, limit daily dose to <1 g. If cesarean section is planned, decrease daily dose to 250 mg for last 6 wk of pregnancy and until incision is healed).

ADVERSE REACTIONS AND SIDE EFFECTS*

EENT: blurred vision, eye pain.
Resp: coughing, shortness of breath, wheezing.
GI: altered taste, anorexia, cholestatic jaundice, diarrhea, drug-induced pancreatitis, dyspepsia, epigastric pain, hepatic dysfunction, nausea, oral ulceration, vomiting.
GU: proteinuria.
Derm: pemphigus, ecchymoses, hives, itching, rashes, wrinkling.
Hemat: APLASTIC ANEMIA, anemia, eosinophilia, leukopenia, thrombocytopenia, thrombocytosis.
MS: arthralgia, migratory polyarthritis.
Neuro: myasthenia gravis syndrome.
Misc: GOODPASTURE'S SYNDROME (GLOMERULONEPHRITIS AND INTRA-ALVEOLAR HEMORRHAGE), allergic reactions, fever, lymphadenopathy, systemic lupus erythematosus–like syndrome.

INTERACTIONS

Drug-Drug: ▪ Increased risk of adverse hematologic effects with **antineoplastic agents, immunosuppressive agents,** or **gold salts** (avoid concurrent use) ▪ Concurrent administration of **iron supplements** decreases absorption of penicillamine ▪ May decrease serum **digoxin** levels.
Drug-Food: ▪ May increase requirements for **pyridoxine** (vitamin B_6).

ROUTE AND DOSAGE

- **PO (Adults):** *Antirheumatic*—125–250 mg/day as a single dose; may be slowly increased up to 1.5 g/day. *Chelating agent (Wilson's disease)*—250 mg qid. *Antiurolithic*—500 mg qid.
- **PO (Children >6 mo):** *Chelating agent (Wilson's disease)*—250 mg/day as a single dose; older children may receive the adult dose. *Antiurolithic*—7.5 mg/kg qid.

AVAILABILITY

▪ ***Capsules:*** 125 mg[Rx], 250 mg[Rx] ▪ ***Tablets:*** 250 mg[Rx].

TIME/ACTION PROFILE

	ONSET	PEAK	DURATION
PO (antirheumatic)	1–3 mo	UK	1–3 mo
PO (Wilson's disease)	1–3 mo	UK	UK

NURSING IMPLICATIONS

ASSESSMENT

- **General Info:** Monitor intake and output and daily weight, and assess patient for edema throughout therapy. Notify physician or other health care professional if edema or weight gain occurs.
- ▫ Monitor patient for allergic reactions (rash, fever). Discontinue treatment and reinstitute at lower dose (250 mg/day), increasing gradually. Prednisone 20 mg/day may be administered for the first few weeks of therapy to decrease severity of reactions. Antihistamines may be used to control pruritus.
- **Arthritis:** Assess pain and range of motion periodically throughout therapy.
- **Cystinuria:** X-ray examinations for renal calculi should be monitored annually for stone formation.
- ***Lab Test Considerations:*** Monitor CBC with differential, platelet counts, and urinalysis (especially for protein and cells) at least every 2 wk during the first 6 mo of therapy or following dose increases and monthly thereafter. May cause leukopenia, anemia, and thrombocytopenia. Discontinue therapy if WBC <3500/mm^3, neutrophils <2000/mm^3, monocytes <500/mm^3, platelet count <100,000/mm^3, or if hematuria occurs.
- ▫ Monitor liver function tests every 6 mo during the first 18 mo of therapy.
- ▫ May cause a positive antinuclear antibody (ANA) test.
- ▫ May cause hypoglycemia.
- ▫ *Arthritis:* Monitor 24-hr urinary protein levels

***CAPITALS indicate life-threatening; underlines indicate most frequent.**

every 1–2 wk in patients with moderate proteinuria.

- *Wilson's disease:* Monitor urinary copper levels prior to and soon after initiation of therapy and every 3 mo during continued therapy.
- *Cystinuria:* Monitor urinary cystine levels. Urinary cystine excretion should be maintained at <100 mg in patients with a history of pain or calculi or at 100–200 mg in patients without a history of calculi.

POTENTIAL NURSING DIAGNOSES

- Pain (Indications).
- Knowledge deficit, related to medication regimen (Patient/Family Teaching).

IMPLEMENTATION

- **PO:** Administer on an empty stomach, at least 1 hr before or 2 hr after meals. Other medications should be administered at least 1 hr apart from penicillamine to maximize absorption.
- Do not administer concurrently with iron-containing products.
- Penicillamine increases the daily requirements for pyridoxine. Supplemental doses of pyridoxine 25 mg/day (vitamin B_6) may be required in patients with impaired nutrition.
- **Arthritis:** Dosage adjustments may be required every 2–3 mo during therapy.
- If no improvement is seen after 3–4 mo of therapy with doses of 1–1.5 g daily, medication should be discontinued.
- **Wilson's Disease:** Sulfurated potash (10–40 mg) may be administered with meals to minimize copper absorption.

PATIENT/FAMILY TEACHING

- **General Info:** Instruct patient to take penicillamine exactly as directed. If on once-daily schedule, missed doses should be taken as soon as remembered unless remembered the next day; if on twice-daily schedule, take missed doses as soon as remembered unless almost time for next dose; if on more than twice-daily dosing schedule, take missed doses within 1 hr or omit. Do not double doses.
- Consult health care professional prior to discontinuation of therapy, as interruption of therapy may cause sensitivity reactions when therapy is resumed. Therapy should be resumed starting with smaller dose and increasing gradually.
- Inform patient that penicillamine may alter taste acuity, which may be restored by administration of copper 5–10 mg daily. Cupric sulfate 4% solution 5–10 drops may be mixed in fruit juice and taken bid. This is contraindicated in patients with Wilson's disease.
- Advise patient to notify health care professional of medication regimen prior to surgery or treatment. Dose of penicillamine should be reduced until wound healing is complete.
- Instruct patient to notify health care professional of skin rash, unusual bleeding or bruising, sore throat, exertional dyspnea, unexplained coughing or wheezing, fever, chills, or any unusual effects.
- Emphasize the importance of follow-up exams to check progress.
- **Wilson's Disease:** Advise patient to discuss dietary restrictions with health care professional. A low-copper diet may be required. Chocolate, nuts, shellfish, mushrooms, liver, molasses, broccoli, and cereals enriched with copper should be avoided. If drinking water contains >100 mcg/liter of copper, distilled or demineralized water should be used.
- **Crystinuria:** Advise patient to maintain a fluid intake of at least 2000–3000 ml/day, with increased fluids at night.
- Advise patient to discuss dietary restrictions with health care professional. Low-methionine diet may be required to minimize cystine production but is contraindicated in growing children or pregnancy because of low protein content.

EVALUATION

Effectiveness of therapy can be demonstrated by: ▪ Decreased pain and increased range of motion in patients with rheumatoid arthritis ▪ Prevention and treatment of symptoms of Wilson's disease ▪ Prevention and treatment of renal calculi in patients with excessive urinary cystine levels.

PENICILLINS
(pen-i-**sill**-in)

penicillin G potassium
Pfizerpen

penicillin G sodium

P

penicillin V
{Apo-Pen VK}, Beepen-VK, Betapen-VK, Ledercillin VK, {Nadopen-V}, {Novo-Pen-VK}, {Nu-Pen-VK}, {Pen·Vee}, Pen·Vee K, {PVF K}, V-Cillin K, Veetids

procaine penicillin G
{Ayercillin}, Crysticillin A.S., Pfizerpen-AS, Wycillin

benzathine penicillin G
Bicillin, Bicillin L-A, {Megacillin}, Permapen

CLASSIFICATION(S):
Anti-infectives (penicillins)

Pregnancy Category B

INDICATIONS

▪ Treatment of a wide variety of infections, including: ▫ Pneumococcal pneumonia ▫ Streptococcal pharyngitis ▫ Syphilis ▫ Gonorrhea ▪ Treatment of enterococcal infections (requires the addition of an aminoglycoside) ▪ Prevention of rheumatic fever.

ACTION

▪ Bind to bacterial cell wall, resulting in cell death. **Therapeutic Effects:** ▪ Bactericidal action against susceptible bacteria. **Spectrum:** ▪ Active against: ▫ Most gram-positive organisms, including many streptococci (*Streptococcus pneumoniae*, group A beta-hemolytic streptococci) and staphylococci (non–penicillinase-producing strains) ▫ Some gram-negative organisms, such as *Neisseria meningitidis* and *Neisseria gonorrhoeae* ▫ Some anaerobic bacteria and spirochetes.

PHARMACOKINETICS

Absorption: Variably absorbed from the GI tract. *Penicillin V*—resists acid degradation in the GI tract. *Procaine and benzathine penicillin*—IM absorption is delayed and prolonged and results in sustained therapeutic blood levels.
Distribution: Widely distributed, although CNS penetration is poor in the presence of uninflamed meninges. Cross the placenta and enter breast milk.
Protein Binding: 60%.
Metabolism and Excretion: Minimally metabolized by the liver, excreted mainly unchanged by the kidneys.
Half-life: 30–60 min.

CONTRAINDICATIONS AND PRECAUTIONS

Contraindicated in: ▪ Previous hypersensitivity to penicillins (cross-sensitivity may exist with cephalosporins) ▪ Hypersensitivity to procaine or benzathine (procaine and benzathine preparations only) ▪ Some products may contain tartrazine and should be avoided in patients with known hypersensitivity.
Use Cautiously in: ▪ Severe renal insufficiency (dosage reduction recommended) ▪ Pregnancy (although safety not established, has been used safely) ▪ Lactation.

ADVERSE REACTIONS AND SIDE EFFECTS*

CNS: SEIZURES.
GI: <u>diarrhea</u>, <u>epigastric distress</u>, <u>nausea</u>, <u>vomiting</u>, pseudomembranous colitis.
GU: interstitial nephritis.
Derm: <u>rashes</u>, urticaria.
Hemat: eosinophilia, hemolytic anemia, leukopenia.
Local: <u>pain</u> at IM site, <u>phlebitis</u> at IV site.
Misc: allergic reactions including ANAPHYLAXIS and SERUM SICKNESS, superinfection.

INTERACTIONS

Drug-Drug: ▪ Penicillin V may decrease the effectiveness of **oral contraceptive agents** ▪ **Probenecid** decreases renal excretion and increases blood levels of penicillin (therapy may be combined for this purpose) ▪ **Cholestyramine** and **colestipol** may decrease the absorption of oral penicillin G ▪ **Neomycin** may decrease the absorption of penicillin V ▪ Concurrent use with **methotrexate** decreases methotrexate elimination and increases the risk of serious toxicity.

ROUTE AND DOSAGE

1 mg = 1600 units; penicillin G sodium contains 2 mEq sodium/million units; penicillin G potas-

{} = Available in Canada only.
***CAPITALS indicate life-threatening; <u>underlines</u> indicate most frequent.**

sium contains 1.7 mEq and 0.3 mEq sodium/million units.

❑ Penicillin G

- **IM, IV (Adults):** 1–5 million units q 4–6 hr.
- **IM, IV (Children):** 8333–16,667 units/kg q 4 hr; 12,550–25,000 units/kg q 6 hr.
- **IM, IV (Infants):** *Most infections*—30,000 units/kg q 12 hr (up to 1 million units/day have been used for listeriosis).
- **IM, IV (Neonates ≥2 kg):** *Meningitis*—50,000 units/kg q 8 hr for the first 7 days of life, then 50,000 units/kg q 6 hr.
- **IM, IV (Neonates <2 kg):** *Meningitis*—25,000–50,000 units/kg q 12 hr for the first 7 days of life, then 50,000 units/kg q 8 hr.

❑ Penicillin V

- **PO (Adults and Children ≥12 yr):** *Most infections*—125–500 mg q 6–8 hr. *Rheumatic fever prevention*—125–250 mg q 12 hr.
- **PO (Children <12 yr):** 2.5–8.3 mg/kg q 4 hr *or* 3.75–12.5 mg/kg q 6 hr *or* 5–16.7 mg/kg q 8 hr.

❑ Benzathine Penicillin G

- **IM (Adults):** *Streptococcal infections/erysipeloid*—1.2 million units single dose. *Primary, secondary, and early latent syphilis*—2.4 million units single dose. *Tertiary and late latent syphilis (not neurosyphilis)*—2.4 million units once weekly for 3 wk. *Prevention of rheumatic fever*—1.2 million units q 3–4 wk.
- **IM (Children >27 kg):** *Streptococcal infections/erysipeloid*—900,000–1.2 million units (single dose). *Primary, secondary, and early latent syphilis*—up to 2.4 million units single dose. *Late latent or latent syphilis of undetermined duration*—50,000 units/kg weekly for 3 wk. *Prevention of rheumatic fever*—1.2 million units q 2–3 wk.
- **IM (Children <27 kg):** *Streptococcal infections/erysipeloid*—300,000–600,000 units single dose. *Primary, secondary, and early latent syphilis*—up to 2.4 million units single dose. *Late latent or latent syphilis of undetermined duration*—50,000 units/kg weekly for 3 wk. *Prevention of rheumatic fever*—1.2 million units q 2–3 wk.

❑ Procaine Penicillin G

- **IM (Adults):** *Moderate or severe infections*—600,000–1.2 million units/day, single dose or 2 divided doses. *Neurosyphilis*—2.4 million units/day with 500 mg probenecid PO 4 times daily for 10–14 days.
- **IM (Children):** *Congenital syphilis*—50,000 units/kg/day for 10–14 days.

AVAILABILITY

❑ Penicillin G Potassium

▪ ***Powder for injection:*** 1 million units/vial^Rx^, 5 million units/vial^Rx^, 10 million units/vial^Rx^, 20 million units/vial^Rx^ ▪ ***Premixed solution for injection:*** 1 million units/50 ml^Rx^, 2 million units/50 ml^Rx^, 3 million units/50 ml^Rx^.

❑ Penicillin G Sodium

▪ ***Powder for injection:*** 5 million units/vial^Rx^.

❑ Penicillin V Potassium

▪ ***Tablets:*** 400,000 units (250 mg)^Rx^, {500,000 units (300 mg)^Rx^}, 800,000 units (500 mg)^Rx^ ▪ ***Oral solution:*** 200,000 units (125 mg)/5 ml^Rx^, 400,000 units (250 mg)/5 ml^Rx^, 500,000 units (300 mg)/5 ml^Rx^.

❑ Procaine Penicillin G

▪ ***Suspension for IM injection:*** 300,000 units/ml in 10-ml vials^Rx^, 500,000 units/ml in 12-ml vials^Rx^, 600,000 units/ml in 1-, 2-, and 4-ml prefilled syringes^Rx^.

❑ Benthazine Penicillin G

▪ ***Suspension for IM injection:*** 300,000 units/ml in 10-ml vials^Rx^, 600,000 units/ml in 1-, 2-, and 4-ml prefilled syringes^Rx^.

TIME/ACTION PROFILE (blood levels)

	ONSET	PEAK	DURATION
Penicillin PO	rapid	0.5–1 hr	4–6 hr
Penicillin G IM	rapid	0.25–0.5 hr	4–6 hr
Benzathine penicillin IM	delayed	12–24 hr	3 wk
Procaine penicillin IM	delayed	1–4 hr	12 hr
Penicillin G IV	rapid	end of infusion	4–6 hr

NURSING IMPLICATIONS

ASSESSMENT

- ❑ Assess patient for infection (vital signs; appearance of wound, sputum, urine, and stool; WBC) at beginning of and throughout therapy.

- Obtain a history to determine previous use of and reactions to penicillins or cephalosporins. Persons with a negative history of penicillin sensitivity may still have an allergic response.
- Obtain specimens for culture and sensitivity before initiating therapy. First dose may be given before receiving results.
- Observe patient for signs and symptoms of anaphylaxis (rash, pruritus, laryngeal edema, wheezing). Discontinue drug and notify physician or other health care professional immediately if these symptoms occur. Keep epinephrine, an antihistamine, and resuscitation equipment close by in case of an anaphylactic reaction.
- ***Lab Test Considerations:*** May cause positive direct Coombs' test results.
- Hyperkalemia may develop following large doses of penicillin G potassium.
- Monitor serum sodium concentrations in patient with hypertension or congestive heart failure. Hypernatremia may develop following large doses of penicillin sodium.
- May cause elevated AST, ALT, LDH, and serum alkaline phosphatase concentrations.
- May cause leukopenia and neutropenia, especially with prolonged therapy or hepatic impairment.

POTENTIAL NURSING DIAGNOSES

- Infection, risk for (Indications, Side Effects).
- Knowledge deficit, related to medication regimen (Patient/Family Teaching).
- Noncompliance, related to medication regimen (Patient/Family Teaching).

IMPLEMENTATION

- **PO:** Administer around the clock. Penicillin V may be administered without regard for meals.
- Use calibrated measuring device for liquid preparations. Solution is stable for 14 days if refrigerated.
- **IM, IV:** Reconstitute according to manufacturer's directions with sterile water for injection, D5W, or 0.9% NaCl.
- **IM:** Shake medication well before injection. Inject penicillin deep into a well-developed muscle mass at a slow, consistent rate to prevent blockage of the needle. Massage well. Accidental injury near or into a nerve can result in severe pain and dysfunction.
- Penicillin G potassium or sodium may be diluted with lidocaine (without epinephrine) 1 or 2% to minimize pain from IM injection.
- Never give penicillin G benzathine or penicillin G procaine suspensions IV. May cause embolism or toxic reactions.
- **IV:** Change IV sites every 48 hr to prevent phlebitis.
- Administer slowly and observe patient closely for signs of hypersensitivity.
- **Intermittent Infusion:** Doses of 3 million units or less should be diluted in at least 50 ml of D5W or 0.9% NaCl; doses of more than 3 million units should be diluted with 100 ml.
- ***Rate:*** Infuse over 1–2 hr in adults or 15–30 min in children.
- **Continuous Infusion:** Doses of 10 million units or more may be diluted in 1 or 2 liters.
- ***Rate:*** Infuse over 24 hr.

Penicillin G Potassium

- **Y-Site Compatibility:** ▪ acyclovir ▪ amiodarone ▪ cyclophosphamide ▪ diltiazem ▪ enalaprilat ▪ esmolol ▪ fluconazole ▪ foscarnet ▪ heparin ▪ hydromorphone ▪ labetalol ▪ magnesium sulfate ▪ meperidine ▪ morphine ▪ perphenazine ▪ potassium chloride ▪ tacrolimus ▪ verapamil ▪ vitamin B complex with C.
- **Y-Site Incompatibility:** ▪ If aminoglycosides and penicillins must be administered concurrently, administer in separate sites at least 1 hr apart.
- **Additive Incompatibility:** ▪ Incompatible with aminoglycosides; do not admix.

Penicillin G Sodium

- **Y-Site Incompatibility:** ▪ If aminoglycosides and penicillins must be administered concurrently, administer in separate sites at least 1 hr apart.
- **Additive Incompatibility:** ▪ Incompatible with aminoglycosides; do not admix.

PATIENT/FAMILY TEACHING

- Instruct patient to take medication around the clock and to finish drug completely as directed, even if feeling better. Advise patient that sharing this medication may be dangerous.
- Advise patient to report signs of superinfection (black, furry overgrowth on tongue; vaginal itching or discharge; loose or foul-smelling stools) and allergy.

- □ Instruct patient to notify health care professional if fever and diarrhea develop, especially if stool contains blood, pus, or mucus. Advise patient not to treat diarrhea without consulting health care professional.
- □ Instruct patient to notify health care professional if symptoms do not improve.
- □ Advise patient taking oral contraceptives to use an additional nonhormonal method of contraception during therapy with penicillin V and until next menstrual period.
- □ Patient with an allergy to penicillin should be instructed to always carry an identification card with this information.

EVALUATION

Clinical response to therapy can be evaluated by: ▪ Resolution of signs and symptoms of infection. Length of time for complete resolution depends on the organism and site of infection ▪ Prevention of rheumatic fever.

PENICILLINS, PENICILLINASE RESISTANT

cloxacillin
(klox-a-**sill**-in)
{Apo-Cloxi}, Cloxapen, {Novo-Cloxin}, {Nu-Cloxi}, {Orbenin}, Tegopen

dicloxacillin
(dye-klox-a-**sill**-in)
Dycill, Dynapen, Pathocil

methicillin
(meth-i-**sill**-in)
Staphcillin

nafcillin
(naf-**sill**-in)
Nafcil, Nallpen, Unipen

oxacillin
(ox-a-**sill**-in)
Bactocill, Prostaphlin

CLASSIFICATION(S):
Anti-infectives (penicillinase-resistant penicillins)

Pregnancy Category B

INDICATIONS

▪ Treatment of the following infections due to penicillinase-producing staphylococci: □ Respiratory tract infections □ Sinusitis □ Skin and skin structure infections ▪ **Methicillin, nafcillin, oxacillin:** Are also used to treat: □ Bone and joint infections □ Urinary tract infections □ Endocarditis □ Septicemia □ Meningitis.

ACTION

▪ Bind to bacterial cell wall, leading to cell death. Resist the action of penicillinase, an enzyme capable of inactivating penicillin. **Therapeutic Effects:** ▪ Bactericidal action. **Spectrum:** ▪ Active against most gram-positive aerobic cocci but less so than penicillin ▪ Spectrum is notable for activity against: □ Penicillinase-producing strains of *Staphylococcus aureus* □ *Staphylococcus epidermidis* ▪ Not active against methicillin-resistant staphylococci.

PHARMACOKINETICS

Absorption: *Cloxacillin*—Moderately absorbed (37–60%) following oral administration. *Dicloxacillin*—Rapidly but incompletely (35–76%) absorbed from the GI tract. *Methicillin*—Well absorbed from IM sites. *Nafcillin*—Poorly and erratically absorbed from the GI tract; well absorbed from IM sites. *Oxacillin*—Rapidly but incompletely absorbed from the GI tract; well absorbed from IM sites.
Distribution: *Cloxacillin, dicloxacillin*—Widely distributed; penetration into CSF is minimal; cross the placenta and enter breast milk. *Methicillin, nafcillin, oxacillin*—Widely distributed; penetration into CSF is minimal but sufficient in the presence of inflamed meninges; cross the placenta and enter breast milk.
Metabolism and Excretion: *Cloxacillin*—Some metabolism by the liver (9–22%) and some renal excretion of unchanged drug (30–45%). *Dicloxacillin*—Some metabolism by the liver (6–10%) and some renal excretion of unchanged drug (60%); small amounts eliminated in the feces via the bile. *Methicillin*—Excreted mostly unchanged by the kidneys. *Nafcillin, oxacillin*—Partially metabolized by the liver (nafcillin 60%, oxacillin 49%), partially excreted unchanged by the kidneys.
Half-life: *Cloxacillin*—0.5–1.1 hr (increased

in severe hepatic and renal dysfunction); *dicloxacillin*—0.5–1 hr (increased in severe hepatic and renal dysfunction); *methicillin*—0.3–0.5 hr (increased in renal impairment); *nafcillin*—0.5–1.5 hr (increased in renal impairment); *oxacillin*—0.3–0.8 hr (increased in severe hepatic impairment).

CONTRAINDICATIONS AND PRECAUTIONS

Contraindicated in: ▪ Hypersensitivity to penicillins (cross-sensitivity with cephalosporins may exist).

Use Cautiously in: ▪ Severe renal or hepatic impairment (dosage reduction recommended for methicillin if CCr ≤10 ml/min) ▪ Pregnancy or lactation (safety not established).

ADVERSE REACTIONS AND SIDE EFFECTS*

CNS: SEIZURES (high doses).

GI: PSEUDOMEMBRANOUS COLITIS, diarrhea, nausea, drug-induced hepatitis (↑ with cloxacillin, dicloxacillin, nafcillin, oxacillin), vomiting.

GU: interstitial nephritis (↑ with methicillin, nafcillin, oxacillin).

Derm: rashes, urticaria.

Hemat: blood dyscrasias.

Local: pain at IM sites, phlebitis at IV sites.

Misc: allergic reactions including ANAPHYLAXIS and SERUM SICKNESS, superinfection.

INTERACTIONS

Drug-Drug: ▪ **Probenecid** decreases renal excretion and increases blood levels ▪ May alter the effect of **warfarin.**

Drug-Food: ▪ **Food** and **acidic juices** decrease absorption of cloxacillin, dicloxacillin, nafcillin, and oxacillin.

ROUTE AND DOSAGE

❑ Cloxacillin

- **PO (Adults and Children >20 kg):** 250–500 mg q 6 hr.
- **PO (Children >1 mo and <20 kg):** 6.25–12.5 mg/kg q 6 hr.

❑ Dicloxacillin

- **PO (Adults and Children ≥40 kg):** 125–250 mg q 6 hr (up to 6 g/day).
- **PO (Children <40 kg):** 3.125–6.25 mg/kg q 6 hr (up to 25 mg/kg q 6 hr in cystic fibrosis patients).

❑ Methicillin

1 g contains 2.6–3.1 mEq of sodium.

- **IM (Adults):** 1 g q 4–6 hr (up to 24 g/day).
- **IM, IV (Children):** 25 mg/kg q 6 hr (up to 50 mg/kg q 6 hr in cystic fibrosis patients).
- **IV (Adults):** 1 g q 6 hr (up to 24 g/day).
- **IM, IV (Neonates ≥2000 g):** *Meningitis*—50 mg/kg q 8 hr for the first 7 days of life, then 50 mg/kg q 6 hr.
- **IM, IV (Neonates <2000 g):** *Meningitis*—25–50 mg/kg q 12 hr for the first 7 days of life, then 50 mg/kg q 8 hr.

❑ Nafcillin

Parenteral nafcillin contains 2.9 mEq sodium/g.

- **PO (Adults):** 250–1000 mg q 4–6 hr.
- **PO (Children and Infants):** *Most infections*—6.25–12.5 mg/kg q 6 hr. *Pharyngitis*—250 mg q 8 hr.
- **PO (Neonates):** 10 mg/kg q 6–8 hr.
- **IM (Adults):** 500 mg q 4–6 hr.
- **IM (Children and Infants):** 25 mg/kg q 12 hr.
- **IM (Neonates):** 10 mg/kg q 12 hr.
- **IV (Adults):** 500–1500 mg q 4–6 hr.
- **IV (Children, Infants, and Neonates):** *Most infections*—10–20 mg/kg q 4 hr or 20–40 mg/kg q 8 hr (up to 200 mg/kg/day).
- **IM, IV (Neonates ≥2 kg):** *Meningitis*—50 mg/kg q 8 hr for the first 7 days of life, then 50 mg/kg q 6 hr.
- **IM, IV (Neonates <2 kg):** *Meningitis*—25–50 mg/kg q 12 hr for the first 7 days of life, then 50 mg/kg q 8 hr.

❑ Oxacillin

Injection contains 2.5–3.1 mEq sodium/g.

- **PO (Adults and Children ≥40 kg):** 500–1000 mg q 4–6 hr.
- **PO (Children <40 kg):** 12.5–25 mg/kg q 6 hr.
- **IM, IV (Adults and Children ≥40 kg):** 250–2000 mg q 4–6 hr (up to 20 g/day).
- **IM, IV (Children <40 kg):** 12.5–25 mg/kg q 6 hr or 16.7 mg/kg q 4 hr.
- **IM, IV (Neonates and Premature Infants):** *Most infections*—6.25 mg/kg q 6 hr.
- **IM, IV (Neonates ≥2 kg):** *Meningitis*—

***CAPITALS indicate life-threatening; underlines indicate most frequent.**

50 mg/kg q 8 hr for the first 7 days of life, then 50 mg/kg q 6 hr.

- **IM, IV (Neonates <2 kg):** *Meningitis*—25–50 mg/kg q 12 hr for the first 7 days of life, then 50 mg/kg q 8 hr.

AVAILABILITY

Cloxacillin

- ***Capsules:*** 250 mg[Rx], 500 mg[Rx] - ***Oral solution:*** 125 mg/5 ml[Rx] - ***Powder for injection:*** {250-mg}, {500-mg}, {and 2-g vials[Rx]}.

Dicloxacillin

- ***Capsules:*** 125 mg[Rx], 250 mg[Rx], 500 mg[Rx] - ***Oral suspension:*** 62.5 mg/5 ml[Rx].

Methicillin

- ***Powder for injection:*** 1-, 4-, 6-, 10-g vials[Rx].

Nafcillin

- ***Tablets:*** 500 mg[Rx] - ***Capsules:*** 250 mg[Rx] - ***Powder for injection:*** 1-, 2-, and 10-g vials[Rx].

Oxacillin

- ***Capsules:*** 250 mg[Rx], 500 mg[Rx] - ***Oral solution:*** 250 mg/5 ml[Rx] - ***Powder for injection:*** 250-mg, 500-mg, 2-g, 4-g, and 10-g vials[Rx].

TIME/ACTION PROFILE (blood levels)

	ONSET	PEAK	DURATION
Cloxacillin PO	30 min	30–120 min	6 hr
Dicloxacillin PO	30 min	30–120 min	6 hr
Methicillin IM	rapid	30–60 min	4–6 hr
Methicillin IV	rapid	end of infusion	4–6 hr
Nafcillin PO, IM	30 min	60–120 min	4–6 hr
Nafcillin IV	rapid	end of infusion	4–6 hr
Oxacillin PO	rapid	30–60 min	4–6 hr
Oxacillin IM	rapid	30 min	4–6 hr
Oxacillin IV	rapid	end of infusion	4–6 hr

NURSING IMPLICATIONS

ASSESSMENT

- Assess patient for infection (vital signs; appearance of wound, sputum, urine, and stool; WBC) at beginning of and throughout therapy.
- Obtain a history before initiating therapy to determine previous use of and reactions to penicillins or cephalosporins. Persons with a negative history of penicillin sensitivity may still have an allergic response.
- Obtain specimens for culture and sensitivity prior to initiating therapy. First dose may be given before receiving results.
- Observe patient for signs and symptoms of anaphylaxis (rash, pruritus, laryngeal edema, wheezing, abdominal pain). Discontinue the drug and notify the physician or other health care professional immediately if these occur. Keep epinephrine, an antihistamine, and resuscitation equipment close by in the event of an anaphylactic reaction.
- Assess vein for signs of irritation and phlebitis. Change IV site every 48 hr to prevent phlebitis.
- ***Lab Test Considerations:*** May cause leukopenia and neutropenia, especially with prolonged therapy or hepatic impairment.
- May cause positive direct Coombs' test result.
- May cause elevations in AST, ALT, LDH, and serum alkaline phosphatase concentrations.

POTENTIAL NURSING DIAGNOSES

- Infection, risk for (Indications, Side Effects).
- Knowledge deficit, related to medication regimen (Patient/Family Teaching).
- Noncompliance, related to medication regimen (Patient/Family Teaching).

IMPLEMENTATION

- **PO:** Administer around the clock on an empty stomach at least 1 hr before or 2 hr after meals. Take with a full glass of water; acidic juices may decrease absorption of penicillins.
- Use calibrated measuring device for liquid preparations. Shake well. Solution stable for 14 days if refrigerated.

Methicillin

- **General Info:** To reconstitute for IM or IV use, add 1.5 ml of sterile water or 0.9% NaCl for injection to each 1-g vial, 5.7 ml to each 4-g vial, and 8.6 ml to each 6-g vial, for a concentration of 500 mg/ml. Solution is straw-colored.
- **IM:** Administer slowly by deep intragluteal injection.
- **Direct IV:** Each ml (500 mg) of reconstituted solution should be further diluted in 25 ml of sterile water or 0.9% NaCl for injection.
- ***Rate:*** Administer at a rate of 10 ml over 1 min.
- **Intermittent Infusion:** Dilute in 0.9% NaCl, D5W, D10W, D5/0.9% NaCl, D5/LR, Ringer's or lactated Ringer's solution, for a concentration of 2–20 mg/ml. Constituted solution is

stable for 24 hr at room temperature and for 4 days if refrigerated.

- ***Rate:*** Infuse over 20–30 min.
- **Y-Site Compatibility:** ▪ heparin ▪ hydrocortisone sodium succinate ▪ potassium chloride ▪ verapamil ▪ vitamin B complex with C.
- **Y-Site Incompatibility:** ▪ If penicillins and aminoglycosides must be administered concurrently, administer at separate sites at least 1 hr apart.
- **Additive Incompatibility:** ▪ Manufacturer recommends that methicillin not be admixed with other drugs.

❑ Nafcillin

- **IM, IV:** To reconstitute, add 3.4 ml to each 1-g vial or 6.8 ml to each 2-g vial, for a concentration of 250 mg/ml. Stable for 2–7 days if refrigerated.
- **Direct IV:** Dilute reconstituted solution with 15–30 ml of sterile water, 0.45% NaCl, or 0.9% NaCl for injection.
- ***Rate:*** Administer over 5–10 min.
- **Intermittent Infusion:** Dilute to a concentration of 2–40 mg/ml with sterile water for injection, 0.9% NaCl, D5W, D10W, D5/0.25% NaCl, D5/0.45% NaCl, D5/0.9% NaCl, D5/LR, Ringer's or lactated Ringer's solution. Stable for 24 hr at room temperature, 96 hr if refrigerated.
- ***Rate:*** Infuse over at least 30–60 min to avoid vein irritation.
- **Y-Site Compatibility:** ▪ acyclovir ▪ atropine ▪ cyclophosphamide ▪ diazepam ▪ enalaprilat ▪ esmolol ▪ famotidine ▪ fentanyl ▪ fluconazole ▪ foscarnet ▪ hydromorphone ▪ magnesium sulfate ▪ morphine ▪ perphenazine ▪ zidovudine.
- **Y-Site Incompatibility:** ▪ droperidol ▪ droperidol/fentanyl ▪ insulin ▪ labetalol ▪ nalbuphine ▪ pentazocine ▪ verapamil. If penicillins and aminoglycosides must be administered concurrently, administer at separate sites.

❑ Oxacillin

- **IM, IV:** To reconstitute for IM or IV use, add 1.4 ml of sterile water for injection to each 250-mg vial, 2.7 ml to each 500-mg vial, 5.7 ml to each 1-g vial, 11.5 ml to each 2-g vial, and 23 ml to each 4-g vial, for a concentration of 250 mg/1.5 ml. Stable for 3 days at room temperature or 7 days if refrigerated.
- **Direct IV:** Further dilute each reconstituted 250-mg or 500-mg vial with 5 ml of sterile water or 0.9% NaCl for injection, 10 ml for each 1-g vial, 20 ml for each 2-g vial, and 40 ml for each 4-g vial.
- ***Rate:*** Administer slowly over 10 min.
- **Intermittent Infusion:** Dilute to a concentration of 0.5–40 mg/ml with 0.9% NaCl, D5W, D5/0.9% NaCl, or lactated Ringer's solution.
- ***Rate:*** May be infused for up to 6 hr.
- **Y-Site Compatibility:** ▪ acyclovir ▪ cyclophosphamide ▪ diltiazem ▪ famotidine ▪ fluconazole ▪ foscarnet ▪ heparin ▪ hydrocortisone sodium succinate ▪ hydromorphone ▪ labetalol ▪ magnesium sulfate ▪ meperidine ▪ methotrexate ▪ morphine ▪ perphenazine ▪ potassium chloride ▪ tacrolimus ▪ vitamin B complex with C ▪ zidovudine.
- **Y-Site Incompatibility:** ▪ sodium bicarbonate ▪ verapamil. If penicillins and aminoglycosides must be administered concurrently, administer at separate sites.

PATIENT/FAMILY TEACHING

- ❑ Instruct patient to take medication around the clock and to finish the drug completely as directed, even if feeling better. Missed doses should be taken as soon as remembered. Advise patient that sharing of this medication may be dangerous.
- ❑ Advise patient to report signs of superinfection (black, furry overgrowth on the tongue; vaginal itching or discharge; loose or foul-smelling stools) and allergy.
- ❑ Instruct patient to notify health care professional if fever and diarrhea develop, especially if stool contains blood, pus, or mucus. Advise patient not to treat diarrhea without consulting health care professional.
- ❑ Instruct patient to notify health care professional if symptoms do not improve.

EVALUATION

Clinical response to therapy can be evaluated by: ▪ Resolution of the signs and symptoms of infection. Length of time for complete resolution depends on the organism and site of infection.

P

PENTAMIDINE

(pen-**tam**-i-deen)

NebuPent, Pentam 300, {Pentacarinat}, {Pneumopent}

CLASSIFICATION(S):

Anti-infective (antiprotozoal)

Pregnancy Category C

INDICATIONS

▪ **IV:** Treatment of *Pneumocystis carinii* pneumonia (PCP) ▪ **Inhalation:** Prevention of PCP in AIDS or HIV-positive patients who have had PCP or who have a peripheral CD4 lymphocyte count of $\leq 200/mm^3$. **Unlabeled Uses:** ▪ **Inhalation:** Treatment of *Pneumocystis carinii* pneumonia.

ACTION

▪ Appears to disrupt DNA or RNA synthesis in protozoa ▪ Also has a direct toxic effect on pancreatic islet cells. **Therapeutic Effects:** ▪ Death of susceptible protozoa.

PHARMACOKINETICS

Absorption: Minimal systemic absorption occurs following inhalation.
Distribution: Widely and extensively distributed but does not cross the blood-brain barrier. Concentrates in liver, kidneys, lungs, and spleen, with prolonged storage in some tissues.
Metabolism and Excretion: 1–30% excreted unchanged by the kidneys. Remainder of metabolic fate unknown.
Half-life: 6.4–9.4 hr (increased in renal impairment).

CONTRAINDICATIONS AND PRECAUTIONS

Contraindicated in: ▪ History of previous anaphylactic reaction to pentamidine.
Use Cautiously in: ▪ Hypotension ▪ Hypertension ▪ Hypoglycemia ▪ Hyperglycemia ▪ Hypocalcemia ▪ Leukopenia ▪ Thrombocytopenia ▪ Anemia ▪ Renal impairment (dosage reduction required) ▪ Diabetes mellitus ▪ Liver impairment ▪ Cardiovascular disease ▪ Bone marrow depression, previous antineoplastic therapy, or radiation therapy ▪ Pregnancy or lactation (safety not established during pregnancy; breast-feeding not recommended).

ADVERSE REACTIONS AND SIDE EFFECTS*

For parenteral form, unless otherwise indicated.
CNS: anxiety, headache, confusion, dizziness, hallucinations.
EENT: *inhalation*—burning in throat.
Resp: *inhalation*—bronchospasm, cough.
CV: ARRHYTHMIAS, HYPOTENSION.
GI: PANCREATITIS, abdominal pain, anorexia, drug-induced hepatitis, nausea, unpleasant metallic taste, vomiting.
GU: nephrotoxicity.
Derm: pallor, rash.
Endo: HYPOGLYCEMIA, hyperglycemia.
F and E: hyperkalemia, hypocalcemia.
Hemat: anemia, leukopenia, thrombocytopenia.
Local: *IV*—phlebitis, pruritus, urticaria at IV site; *IM*—sterile abscesses at IM sites.
Misc: allergic reactions including ANAPHYLAXIS, STEVENS-JOHNSON SYNDROME, chills, fever.

INTERACTIONS

Listed for parenteral administration.
Drug-Drug: ▪ Concurrent use with erythromycin IV may increase the risk of potentially fatal arrhythmias ▪ Additive nephrotoxicity with other **nephrotoxic agents**, including **aminoglycosides, amphotericin B**, and **vancomycin** ▪ Additive bone marrow depression with **antineoplastic agents** or previous **radiation therapy** ▪ Increased risk of pancreatitis with **didanosine** ▪ Increased risk of nephrotoxicity, hypocalcemia, and hypomagnesemia with **foscarnet.**

ROUTE AND DOSAGE

- **IV (Adults and Children):** 4 mg/kg once daily for 14–21 days (longer treatment may be required in AIDS patients; some patients may respond to 3 mg/kg/day).
- **Inhalation (Adults):** *NebuPent, Pentacarinat*—300 mg q 4 wk, using a Respirgard II jet nebulizer (150 mg q 2 wk have also been used). *Pneumopent*—60 mg q 24–72 hr for 5 doses over a 2-wk period, then q 2 wk using a Fisoneb ultrasonic nebulizer.

{} = Available in Canada only.
*CAPITALS indicate life-threatening; underlines indicate most frequent.

- **Inhalation (Children >5 yr):** *NebuPent, Pentacarinat*—300 mg q 4 wk, using a Respirgard II jet nebulizer (for patients who cannot tolerate trimethoprim/sulfamethoxazole; unlabeled).

AVAILABILITY

- ***Injection:*** 300 mg/vial[Rx] - ***Solution for aerosol use (NebuPent, Pentacarinat):*** 300 mg/vial[Rx] - ***Solution for aerosol use (Pneumopent):*** {60 mg/vial[Rx]}.

TIME/ACTION PROFILE (blood levels)

	ONSET	PEAK	DURATION
IV	UK	end of infusion	24 hr
Inhaln	UK	UK	UK

NURSING IMPLICATIONS

ASSESSMENT

- **General Info:** Assess patient for infection (vital signs, sputum, WBC) and monitor respiratory status (rate, character, lung sounds, dyspnea, sputum) at beginning of and throughout therapy.
- □ Obtain specimens for culture and sensitivity prior to initiating therapy. First dose may be given before receiving results.
- **IM, IV:** Monitor blood pressure frequently during and following IM or IV administration of pentamidine. Patient should be lying down during administration. Sudden, severe hypotension may occur following a single dose. Resuscitation equipment should be immediately available.
- □ Assess patient for signs of hypoglycemia (anxiety; chills; diaphoresis; cold, pale skin; headache; increased hunger; nausea; nervousness; shakiness) and hyperglycemia (drowsiness; flushed, dry skin; fruit-like breath odor; increased thirst; increased urination; loss of appetite), which may occur up to several months after therapy is discontinued.
- □ Pulse and ECG should be monitored prior to and periodically during course of therapy. Fatalities due to cardiac arrhythmias, tachycardia, and cardiotoxicity have been reported.
- **Inhalation:** A tuberculin skin test, chest x ray, and sputum culture should be performed prior to administration to rule out tuberculosis.
- ***Lab Test Considerations:*** *IM, IV*—Blood glucose concentrations should be monitored prior to, daily during, and for several months following therapy. Severe hypoglycemia and permanent diabetes mellitus have occurred.
- □ Monitor BUN and serum creatinine prior to and daily during therapy to monitor for nephrotoxicity. Concentrations may be increased.
- □ Monitor CBC and platelet count prior to and every 3 days during therapy. Pentamidine may cause leukopenia, anemia, and thrombocytopenia.
- □ May cause elevated serum bilirubin, alkaline phosphatase, AST, and ALT concentrations. These liver function tests should be monitored prior to and every 3 days during therapy.
- □ Serum calcium and magnesium concentrations should be monitored prior to and every 3 days during therapy, as pentamidine may cause hypocalcemia and hypomagnesemia.
- □ May cause elevated serum potassium concentrations.

POTENTIAL NURSING DIAGNOSES

- Infection, risk for (Indications, Side Effects).
- Knowledge deficit, related to medication regimen (Patient/Family Teaching).

IMPLEMENTATION

- **General Info:** Pentamidine must be given on a regular schedule for the full course of therapy. If a dose is missed, administer as soon as remembered. If almost time for the next dose, skip the missed dose and return to the regular schedule. Do not double doses.
- **IM:** Dilute 300 mg of pentamidine with 3 ml of sterile water for injection for a concentration of 100 mg/ml. IM administration should be used only for patients with adequate muscle mass and given deep IM via Z-track technique. May cause sterile abscesses.
- **Intermittent Infusion:** To reconstitute, add 3–5 ml of sterile water for injection or D5W to each 300-mg vial for a concentration of 100, 75, or 60 mg/ml, respectively. Withdraw dose and dilute further in 50–250 ml of D5W. Solution is stable for 48 hr at room temperature. Discard unused portions.
- ***Rate:*** Administer slowly over 1–2 hr.
- **Y-Site Compatibility:** - diltiazem - zidovudine.
- **Y-Site Incompatibility:** - aldesleukin - cefazolin - cefoperazone - cefotaxime - cefoxitin

▪ ceftazidime ▪ ceftriaxone ▪ fluconazole ▪ foscarnet.

▪ **Inhalation:** If using inhalation bronchodilator, administer bronchodilator 5–10 min prior to pentamidine administration.
□ Administer in a well-ventilated area.
□ Administration with patient in supine or recumbent position appears to provide a more uniform distribution of pentamidine.
□ *NebuPent* or *Pentacarinat:* Dilute 300 or 600 mg (for prophylaxis or treatment, respectively) in 6 ml of sterile water for injection. Place reconstituted solution into Respirgard II nebulizer. Do not dilute with 0.9% NaCl or admix with other medications, as solution will form a precipitate. Do not use Respirgard II nebulizer for other medications.
□ Administer inhalation dose through nebulizer until chamber is empty, approximately 30–45 min.
□ *Pneumopent:* Remove rubber stopper and set upside down on a clean surface for use later. Add 3–5 ml of sterile water for inhalation or injection to vial and replace rubber stopper. Do not use tap water or 0.9% NaCl. Powder should dissolve immediately; if not, shake gently to mix. Solution should be clear and colorless; do not use if cloudy. Solution is stable for 24 hr at room temperature or 48 hr if refrigerated. Place entire reconstituted contents into Fisoneb ultrasonic nebulizer
□ Administer with the flow rate of the nebulizer at the midflow mark over approximately 15 min until the chamber is empty.

PATIENT/FAMILY TEACHING

▪ **General Info:** Inform patient of the importance of completing the full course of pentamidine therapy, even if feeling better.

▪ **IV:** Instruct patient to notify health care professional promptly if fever; sore throat; signs of infection; bleeding of gums; unusual bruising; petechiae; or blood in stool, urine, or emesis occurs. Caution patient to avoid crowds and persons with known infections. Instruct patient to use soft toothbrush and electric razor and to avoid falls. Patient should not be given IM injections or rectal thermometers. Patient should be cautioned not to drink alcoholic beverages or take medication containing aspirin or NSAIDs, as these may precipitate gastric bleeding.
□ Caution patient to make position changes slowly to minimize orthostatic hypotension.

▪ **Inhalation:** Advise patient that an unpleasant metallic taste may occur with pentamidine administration but is not significant.
□ Inform patients who continue to smoke that bronchospasm and coughing during therapy are more likely.

EVALUATION

Clinical response to therapy can be evaluated by: ▪ Prevention or resolution of the signs and symptoms of *Pneumocystis carinii* pneumonia in HIV-positive patients.

PENTAZOCINE

(pen-**taz**-oh-seen)
Talwin, Talwin NX

CLASSIFICATION(S):
Opioid analgesic (agonist/antagonist)

Schedule IV
Pregnancy Category C

INDICATIONS

▪ Moderate to severe pain ▪ Also used for: □ Analgesia during labor □ Sedation prior to surgery □ Supplemention in balanced anesthesia.

ACTION

▪ Binds to opiate receptors in the CNS ▪ Alters perception of and response to painful stimuli, while producing generalized CNS depression ▪ Has partial antagonist properties, which may result in opioid withdrawal in physically dependent patients. **Therapeutic Effects:** ▪ Decrease in moderate to severe pain.

PHARMACOKINETICS

Absorption: Well absorbed following oral, IM, and SC administration. Small amount (0.5 mg) of naloxone in tablets included to prevent parenteral abuse.
Distribution: Widely distributed. Crosses the placenta.
Metabolism and Excretion: Mostly metabolized by the liver. Small amounts excreted unchanged by the kidneys.
Half-life: 2–3 hr.

CONTRAINDICATIONS AND PRECAUTIONS

Contraindicated in: ▪ Hypersensitivity ▪ Patients who are physically dependent on opioids (may precipitate withdrawal).
Use Cautiously in: ▪ Head trauma ▪ History of drug abuse ▪ Increased intracranial pressure ▪ Severe renal, hepatic, or pulmonary disease ▪ Hypothyroidism ▪ Adrenal insufficiency ▪ Alcoholism ▪ Geriatric, debilitated patients, or patients with severe liver impairment (dosage reduction recommended) ▪ Undiagnosed abdominal pain ▪ Prostatic hypertrophy ▪ Patients who have recently received opioid agonists ▪ Pregnancy (has been used during labor but may cause respiratory depression in the newborn) ▪ Lactation or children (safety not established).

ADVERSE REACTIONS AND SIDE EFFECTS*

CNS: dizziness, euphoria, hallucinations, headache, sedation, confusion, dysphoria, floating feeling, unusual dreams.
EENT: blurred vision, diplopia, miosis (high doses).
Resp: respiratory depression.
CV: hypertension, hypotension, palpitations.
GI: nausea, constipation, dry mouth, ileus, vomiting.
GU: urinary retention.
Derm: clammy feeling, sweating.
Local: severe tissue damage at SC sites.
Misc: physical dependence, psychological dependence, tolerance.

INTERACTIONS

Drug-Drug: ▪ Use with caution in patients receiving **MAO inhibitors** (may result in unpredictable reactions—decrease initial dose of pentazocine to 25% of usual dose) ▪ Additive CNS depression with **alcohol, antihistamines,** and **sedative/hypnotics** ▪ May precipitate withdrawal in patients who are physically dependent on **opioid analgesic agonists** ▪ May diminish analgesic effects of other **opioid analgesics.**

ROUTE AND DOSAGE

▪ **PO (Adults):** 50–100 mg q 3–4 hr (not to exceed 600 mg/day).
▪ **SC, IV, IM (Adults):** 30 mg q 3–4 hr (not to exceed 30 mg/dose IV or 60 mg/dose IM or SC; not to exceed 360 mg/day SC, IV, or IM). ***Obstetrical use***—20 mg IV or 30 mg IM. When contractions become regular, q 2–3 hr for 2–3 doses.

AVAILABILITY

▪ ***Tablets:*** 50 mg (with 0.5 mg naloxone)[Rx], {50 mg[Rx]} ▪ ***Injection:*** 30 mg/ml[Rx] ▪ ***In combination with:*** acetaminophen (Talacen) or aspirin (Talwin compound)[Rx]. See Appendix A.

TIME/ACTION PROFILE (analgesia)

	ONSET	PEAK	DURATION
PO	15–30 min	60–90 min	3 hr
IM, SC	15–20 min	30–60 min	2–3 hr
IV	2–3 min	15–30 min	2–3 hr

NURSING IMPLICATIONS

ASSESSMENT

- Assess type, location, and intensity of pain prior to and 1 hr following PO, SC, or IM and 15–30 min (peak) following IV administration. When titrating opioid doses, increases of 25–50% should be administered until there is either a 50% reduction in the patient's pain rating on a numerical or visual analogue scale or the patient reports satisfactory pain relief. A repeat dose can be safely administered at the time of the peak if previous dose is ineffective and side effects are minimal. Patients requiring doses higher than 100 mg should be converted to an opioid agonist. Pentazocine is not recommended for prolonged use or as first-line therapy for acute or cancer pain.
- An equianalgesic chart (see Appendix B) should be used when changing routes or when changing from one opioid to another.
- Assess blood pressure, pulse, and respirations before and periodically during administration. If respiratory rate is $<$10/min, assess level of sedation. Physical stimulation may be sufficient to prevent significant hypoventilation. Dose may need to be decreased by 25–50%. Pentazocine produces respiratory depression, but it does not markedly increase with increased doses.
- Assess prior analgesic history. Antagonistic

*CAPITALS indicate life-threatening; underlines indicate most frequent.

properties may induce withdrawal symptoms (vomiting, restlessness, abdominal cramps, and increased blood pressure and temperature) in patients physically dependent on opioids.

- Although this drug has a low potential for dependence, prolonged use may lead to physical and psychological dependence and tolerance. This should not prevent patient from receiving adequate analgesia. Most patients receiving pentazocine for pain do not develop psychological dependence. If tolerance develops, changing to an opioid agonist may be required to relieve pain.

- ***Lab Test Considerations:*** May cause elevated serum amylase and lipase levels.
- ***Toxicity and Overdose:*** If an opioid antagonist is required to reverse respiratory depression or coma, naloxone (Narcan) is the antidote. Dilute the 0.4-mg ampule of naloxone in 10 ml of 0.9% NaCl and administer 0.5 ml (0.02 mg) by direct IV push every 2 min. For patients weighing <40 kg, dilute 0.1 mg of naloxone in 10 ml of 0.9% NaCl for a concentration of 10 mcg/ml and administer 0.5 mcg/kg every 1–2 min. Titrate dose to avoid withdrawal, seizures, and severe pain.

POTENTIAL NURSING DIAGNOSES

- Pain (Indications).
- Injury, risk for (Side Effects).
- Sensory-perceptual alterations: visual, auditory (Side Effects).

IMPLEMENTATION

- **General Info:** Explain therapeutic value of medication prior to administration to enhance the analgesic effect.
- Regularly administered doses may be more effective than prn administration. Analgesic is more effective if administered before pain becomes severe.
- Coadministration with nonopioid analgesics may have additive effects and may permit lower opioid doses.
- **PO:** Talwin NX contains 0.5 mg of naloxone, which has no pharmacologic activity when administered orally. If the product is abused by injection, naloxone antagonizes pentazocine. Parenteral use of oral pentazocine may lead to severe, potentially fatal reactions (pulmonary emboli, vascular occlusion, ulceration and abscess, and withdrawal symptoms in opioid-dependent individuals).
- **IM, SC:** Administer IM injections deep into well-developed muscle. Rotate sites of injections. SC route may cause tissue damage with repeated injections.
- **Direct IV:** Manufacturer recommends diluting each 5 mg with at least 1 ml of sterile water for injection.
- ***Rate:*** Administer slowly, each 5 mg over at least 1 min.
- **Syringe Compatibility:** ▪ atropine ▪ benzquinamide ▪ chlorpromazine ▪ cimetidine ▪ dimenhydrinate ▪ diphenhydramine ▪ droperidol ▪ hydroxyzine ▪ metoclopramide ▪ perphenazine ▪ prochlorperazine edisylate ▪ promazine ▪ promethazine ▪ propiomazine ▪ ranitidine ▪ scopolamine.
- **Syringe Incompatibility:** ▪ glycopyrrolate ▪ heparin ▪ pentobarbital.
- **Y-Site Compatibility:** ▪ heparin ▪ hydrocortisone sodium succinate ▪ potassium chloride ▪ vitamin B complex with C.
- **Y-Site Incompatibility:** ▪ nafcillin.

PATIENT/FAMILY TEACHING

- Instruct patient on how and when to ask for pain medication.
- Medication may cause drowsiness, dizziness, or hallucinations. Advise patient to call for assistance when ambulating and to avoid driving or other activities requiring alertness until response to medication is known.
- Caution patient to change positions slowly to minimize orthostatic hypotension.
- Advise patient to avoid concurrent use of alcohol and other CNS depressants.
- Encourage patient to turn, cough, and breathe deeply every 2 hr to prevent atelectasis.
- Advise patient that frequent mouth rinses, good oral hygiene, and sugarless gum or candy may decrease dry mouth.

EVALUATION

Effectiveness of therapy can be demonstrated by: ▪ Decrease in severity of pain without a significant alteration in level of consciousness or respiratory status.

PENTOBARBITAL

(pen-toe-**bar**-bi-tal)
Nembutal, {Novopentobarb}, {Nova Rectal}

CLASSIFICATION(S):
Anticonvulsant, Sedative/hypnotic (barbiturate)

Schedule II (oral and parenteral), III (rectal)
Pregnancy Category D

INDICATIONS

▪ Hypnotic agent (short-term) ▪ Preoperative sedation and other situations in which sedation is required ▪ Treatment of seizures. **Unlabeled Uses:** ▪ **IV:** Induction of coma in selected patients with cerebral ischemia and management of increased intracranial pressure (high doses).

ACTION

▪ Depresses the CNS, probably by potentiating gamma-aminobutyric acid (GABA), an inhibitory neurotransmitter ▪ Produces all levels of CNS depression, including the sensory cortex, motor activity, and altered cerebellar function ▪ Anticonvulsant effect due to decreased synaptic transmission and increased seizure threshold ▪ May decrease cerebral blood flow, cerebral edema, and intracranial pressure (IV only). **Therapeutic Effects:** ▪ Sedation and/or induction of sleep.

PHARMACOKINETICS

Absorption: Well absorbed following all routes.
Distribution: Widely distributed; highest concentrations in brain and liver. Crosses the placenta; small amounts enter breast milk.
Metabolism and Excretion: Metabolized by the liver. Minimal renal excretion.
Half-life: 35–50 hr.

CONTRAINDICATIONS AND PRECAUTIONS

Contraindicated in: ▪ Hypersensitivity ▪ Some products contain tartrazine, alcohol, or propylene glycol and should be avoided in patients with known hypersensitivity or intolerance ▪ Comatose patients or those with pre-existing CNS depression (unless used to induce coma) ▪ Uncontrolled severe pain ▪ Pregnancy or lactation.
Use Cautiously in: ▪ Hepatic dysfunction ▪ Severe renal impairment ▪ Patients who may be suicidal or who may have been addicted to drugs previously ▪ Geriatric or debilitated patients (initial dosage reduction recommended) ▪ Hypnotic use should be short-term (chronic use may lead to dependence).

ADVERSE REACTIONS AND SIDE EFFECTS*

CNS: drowsiness, hangover, lethargy, delirium, excitation, mental depression, vertigo.
Resp: respiratory depression; *IV*—LARYNGOSPASM, bronchospasm.
CV: *IV*—hypotension.
GI: constipation, diarrhea, nausea, vomiting.
Derm: rashes, urticaria.
Local: phlebitis at IV site.
MS: arthralgia, myalgia, neuralgia.
Misc: hypersensitivity reactions including ANGIOEDEMA and SERUM SICKNESS, physical dependence, psychological dependence.

INTERACTIONS

Drug-Drug: ▪ Additive CNS depression with other **CNS depressants**, including **alcohol, antihistamines, opioids**, and other **sedative/hypnotics** ▪ May induce hepatic enzymes, which metabolize other drugs, decreasing their effectiveness, including **oral contraceptives, oral anticoagulants, chloramphenicol, cyclosporine, dacarbazine, glucocorticoids, tricyclic antidepressants**, and **quinidine** ▪ May increase the risk of hepatic toxicity of **acetaminophen** ▪ **MAO inhibitors, valproic acid**, or **divalproex** may decrease the metabolism of pentobarbital, increasing sedation.

ROUTE AND DOSAGE

- **PO (Adults):** *Sedative*—20 mg 3–4 times daily. *Hypnotic/preoperative sedative*—100 mg.
- **PO (Children):** *Sedative*—2–6 mg/kg/day in divided doses. *Preoperative sedative*—2–6 mg/kg (up to 100 mg/dose).
- **IM (Adults):** *Hypnotic/preoperative sedative*—150–200 mg.

{} = Available in Canada only.
***CAPITALS indicate life-threatening; underlines indicate most frequent.**

- **IM (Children):** *Sedative*—2–6 mg/kg/day in divided doses. *Preoperative sedative*—2–6 mg/kg (up to 100 mg/dose).
- **IV (Adults):** *Hypnotic/anticonvulsant*—100 mg initially; additional small doses may be given q min up to 500 mg total. *Induction of coma*—5–7 mg/kg, then 3–4 mg/kg q 3–4 hr adjusted by serum label (unlabeled).
- **IV (Children):** *Hypnotic/anticonvulsant*—50 mg; additional, smaller doses may be given q min.
- **Rect (Adults):** *Sedative*—30 mg 2–4 times daily. *Hypnotic*—120–200 mg at bedtime.
- **Rect (Children):** *Sedative*—2 mg/kg (60 mg/m^2) 3 times daily.
- **Rect (Children 12–14 yr):** *Preoperative sedative/hypnotic*—60–120 mg.
- **Rect (Children 5–12 yr):** *Preoperative sedative/hypnotic*—60 mg.
- **Rect (Children 1–4 yr):** *Preoperative sedative/hypnotic*—30–60 mg.
- **Rect (Children 2 mo–1 yr):** *Preoperative sedative/hypnotic*—30 mg.

AVAILABILITY

▪ ***Capsules:*** 50 mg^{Rx}, 100 mg^{Rx} ▪ ***Elixir:*** 20 mg/5 ml^{Rx} ▪ ***Suppositories:*** {25 mg^{Rx}}, 30 mg^{Rx}, {50 mg^{Rx}}, 60 mg^{Rx}, 120 mg^{Rx}, 200 mg^{Rx} ▪ ***Injection:*** 50 mg/ml in 2-ml ampules, prefilled syringes, and 20- and 50-ml vials^{Rx}.

TIME/ACTION PROFILE (sedation)

	ONSET	PEAK	DURATION*
PO	15–60 min	3–4 hr	1–4 hr
Rectal	15–60 min	UK	1–4 hr
IM	10–25 min	UK	1–4 hr
IV	immediate	1 min	15 min

*Noted as hypnotic effect; sedative effects are longer lasting.

NURSING IMPLICATIONS

ASSESSMENT

- **General Info:** Monitor respiratory status, pulse, and blood pressure frequently in patients receiving pentobarbital IV. Equipment for resuscitation and artificial ventilation should be readily available. Respiratory depression is dose-dependent.
  - Prolonged therapy may lead to psychological or physical dependence. Restrict amount of drug available to patient, especially if depressed, suicidal, or previously addicted.
  - Assess postoperative patients for pain. Pentobarbital may increase responsiveness to painful stimuli.
- **Sleep:** Assess sleep patterns prior to and periodically throughout course of therapy. Hypnotic doses of pentobarbital suppress REM sleep. Patient may experience an increase in dreaming upon discontinuation of medication.
- **Cerebral Edema:** Monitor intracranial pressure and level of consciousness in patients in barbiturate coma.
- **Seizures:** Assess location, duration, and characteristics of seizure activity. Implement seizure precautions.

POTENTIAL NURSING DIAGNOSES

- Sleep pattern disturbance (Indications).
- Injury, risk for (Side Effects).
- Knowledge deficit, related to medication regimen (Patient/Family Teaching).

IMPLEMENTATION

- **General Info:** Supervise ambulation and transfer of patients following administration. Remove cigarettes. Side rails should be raised and call bell within reach at all times. Keep bed in low position.
- **PO:** Elixir may be administered undiluted or diluted in water, milk, or fruit juice. Use calibrated measuring device for accurate dosage. Do not use cloudy solutions.
- **IM:** Do not administer SC. IM injections should be given deep into the gluteal muscle to minimize tissue irritation. Do not inject more than 5 ml into any one site because of tissue irritation.
- **Direct IV:** Doses may be given undiluted or diluted with sterile water, 0.45% NaCl, 0.9% NaCl, D5W, D10W, Ringer's or lactated Ringer's solution, dextrose/saline combinations, or dextrose/Ringer's or lactated Ringer's combinations. Do not use solution that is discolored or that contains particulate matter.
  - Solution is highly alkaline; avoid extravasation, which may cause tissue damage and necrosis. If extravasation occurs, infiltration of 5% procaine solution into affected area and application of moist heat may be used.
- ***Rate:*** Administer each 50 mg over at least 1 min. Titrate slowly for desired response. Rapid administration may result in respiratory de-

pression, apnea, laryngospasm, bronchospasm, or hypertension.

- **Syringe Compatibility:** ▪ scopolamine.
- **Syringe Incompatibility:** ▪ glycopyrrolate.
- **Y-Site Compatibility:** ▪ acyclovir ▪ regular insulin.
- **Rect:** To ensure accurate dose, do not divide rectal suppository. Suppositories should be refrigerated.

PATIENT/FAMILY TEACHING

- Advise patient to take medication exactly as prescribed. Do not increase dose of the drug without consulting health care professional.
- Discuss the importance of preparing environment for sleep (dark room, quiet, avoidance of nicotine and caffeine).
- Advise patients on prolonged therapy not to discontinue medication without consulting health care professional. Abrupt withdrawal may precipitate withdrawal symptoms.
- May cause daytime drowsiness. Caution patient to avoid driving and other activities requiring alertness until response to medication is known.
- Caution patient to avoid taking alcohol or other CNS depressants concurrently with this medication.
- Instruct patient to contact health care professional immediately if pregnancy is suspected.

EVALUATION

Effectiveness of therapy can be demonstrated by: ▪ Improvement in sleep pattern without excessive daytime sedation. Therapy is usually limited to a 2-wk period ▪ Prevention of cerebral anoxia ▪ Decrease or cessation of seizures without excessive sedation.

PENTOXIFYLLINE

(pen-tox-**if**-i-lin)
Trental

CLASSIFICATION(S):
Blood viscosity–reducing agent

Pregnancy Category C

INDICATIONS

▪ Management of symptomatic peripheral vascular disease (intermittent claudication).

ACTION

▪ Increases the flexibility of red blood cells by increasing levels of cyclic adenosine monophosphate (cAMP) ▪ Decreases blood viscosity by inhibiting platelet aggregation and decreasing fibrinogen. **Therapeutic Effects:** ▪ Increased blood flow.

PHARMACOKINETICS

Absorption: Well absorbed following oral administration.
Distribution: Bound to erythrocyte membrane. Enters breast milk.
Metabolism and Excretion: Metabolized by red blood cells and the liver.
Half-life: 25–50 min.

CONTRAINDICATIONS AND PRECAUTIONS

Contraindicated in: ▪ Hypersensitivity ▪ Intolerance to other xanthine derivatives (caffeine and theophylline).
Use Cautiously in: ▪ Coronary artery or cerebrovascular disease ▪ Renal disease (lower doses may be used) ▪ Geriatric patients (increased risk of adverse reactions) ▪ Pregnancy, lactation, or children (safety not established).

ADVERSE REACTIONS AND SIDE EFFECTS

CNS: agitation, dizziness, drowsiness, headache, insomnia, nervousness.
EENT: blurred vision.
Resp: dyspnea.
CV: angina, arrhythmias, edema, flushing, hypotension.
GI: abdominal discomfort, belching, bloating, diarrhea, dyspepsia, flatus, nausea, vomiting.
Neuro: tremor.

INTERACTIONS

Drug-Drug: ▪ Additive hypotension may occur with **antihypertensives** and **nitrates** ▪ May increase the risk of bleeding with **warfarin, heparin, aspirin, NSAIDs, cefamandole, cefoperazone, cefotetan, plicamycin, valproic acid**, or **thrombolytic agents** ▪ May increase the risk of theophylline toxicity ▪ **Smoking** (nicotine) may decrease the beneficial effects of pentoxifylline.

ROUTE AND DOSAGE

- **PO (Adults):** 400 mg 3 times daily.

AVAILABILITY

- ***Controlled-release tablets:*** 400 mg[Rx].

TIME/ACTION PROFILE (improvement in blood flow)

	ONSET	PEAK	DURATION
PO	2–4 wk	8 wk	8 hr

NURSING IMPLICATIONS

ASSESSMENT

- Assess patient for intermittent claudication prior to and periodically throughout therapy.
- Monitor blood pressure periodically in patients on concurrent antihypertensive therapy.

POTENTIAL NURSING DIAGNOSES

- Pain (Indications).
- Activity intolerance (Indications).
- Knowledge deficit, related to medication regimen (Patient/Family Teaching).

IMPLEMENTATION

- **PO:** Administer with meals to minimize GI irritation. Tablets should be swallowed whole; do not crush, break, or chew.
- If GI and CNS side effects occur, decrease dose to twice daily. Discontinue if side effects persist.

PATIENT/FAMILY TEACHING

- Instruct patient to take medication exactly as directed. If a dose is missed, it should be taken as soon as remembered unless almost time for next dose. Consult health care professional before discontinuing medication, because several weeks of therapy may be required before effects are seen.
- May cause dizziness and blurred vision. Caution patient to avoid driving and other activities requiring alertness until response to medication is known.
- Advise patient to avoid smoking, as nicotine constricts blood vessels.
- Instruct patient to notify health care professional if nausea, vomiting, GI upset, drowsiness, dizziness, or headache persists.

EVALUATION

Effectiveness of therapy can be demonstrated by: ▪ Relief from cramping in calf muscles, buttocks, thighs, and feet during exercise ▫ Improvement in walking endurance. Therapeutic effects may be seen in 2–4 wk, but therapy should be continued for ≥8 wk.

PERGOLIDE

(**per**-goe-lide)
Permax

CLASSIFICATION(S):
Anti-Parkinson agent (dopamine agonist)

Pregnancy Category B

INDICATIONS

- Management of Parkinson's disease in conjunction with levodopa/carbidopa.

ACTION

- Acts as a dopamine agonist, directly stimulating postsynaptic dopaminergic receptors in the CNS. **Therapeutic Effects:** ▪ Continued relief of symptoms of Parkinson's disease at a lower dosage of levodopa/carbidopa.

PHARMACOKINETICS

Absorption: Well absorbed following oral administration.
Distribution: UK.
Metabolism and Excretion: Highly metabolized by the liver. Metabolites are excreted by the kidneys.
Half-life: UK.

CONTRAINDICATIONS AND PRECAUTIONS

Contraindicated in: ▪ Hypersensitivity to pergolide or ergot derivatives ▪ Lactation (may inhibit lactation).
Use Cautiously in: ▪ Arrhythmias ▪ History of psychiatric disorders ▪ Pregnancy or children (safety not established).

ADVERSE REACTIONS AND SIDE EFFECTS*

CNS: drowsiness, dyskinesia, hallucinations, confusion, insomnia.
EENT: rhinitis.
Resp: dyspnea.
CV: orthostatic hypotension, arrhythmias (atrial premature contractions, sinus tachycardia), hypertension, palpitations.
GI: constipation, nausea, abdominal pain, diarrhea, dry mouth, dyspepsia.

INTERACTIONS

Drug-Drug: ▪ **Phenothiazines, metoclopramide, reserpine,** or **haloperidol** may decrease effectiveness by antagonizing the effects of dopamine ▪ Additive hypotension may occur with **antihypertensives.**

ROUTE AND DOSAGE

- **PO (Adults):** 50 mcg/day for 2 days; increase by 100–150 mcg/day every 3rd day for 12 days, then may increase by 250 mcg/day every 3rd day until optimal response is obtained. Usual dose is 1 mg 3 times daily (not to exceed 5 mg/day). Usually given in 3 divided doses.

AVAILABILITY

▪ ***Tablets:*** 50 mcg (0.05 mg)^{Rx}, 250 mcg (0.25 mg)^{Rx}, 1 mg^{Rx}.

TIME/ACTION PROFILE (anti-Parkinson effects)

	ONSET	PEAK	DURATION
PO	UK	UK	UK

NURSING IMPLICATIONS

ASSESSMENT

- Assess patient for signs and symptoms of Parkinson's disease (tremor, muscle weakness and rigidity, ataxic gait) prior to and throughout therapy.
- Assess patient for confusion or hallucinations. Notify physician or other health care professional if these occur.
- Monitor ECG and blood pressure frequently during dosage adjustment and periodically throughout therapy.

POTENTIAL NURSING DIAGNOSES

- Physical mobility, impaired (Indications).
- Injury, risk for (Indications, Side Effects).
- Knowledge deficit, related to medication regimen (Patient/Family Teaching).

IMPLEMENTATION

- **PO:** An attempt to reduce the dose of levodopa/carbidopa may be made cautiously during pergolide therapy.
- Administer with meals to minimize nausea; usually resolves with continued therapy.

PATIENT/FAMILY TEACHING

- Instruct patient to take medication exactly as directed. Missed doses should be taken as soon as remembered if not almost time for next dose. Do not double doses. Consult health care professional before reducing dose or discontinuing medication.
- May cause drowsiness. Caution patient to avoid driving or other activities requiring alertness until response to medication is known.
- Advise patient to change positions slowly to minimize orthostatic hypotension. Initial dose may be administered at bedtime to minimize this effect.
- Inform patient that frequent mouth rinses, good oral hygiene, and sugarless gum or candy may minimize dry mouth. Advise patient to consult health care professional if dry mouth persists for longer than 2 wk.

EVALUATION

Effectiveness of therapy can be demonstrated by: ▪ Improved response to levodopa/carbidopa in patients with Parkinson's disease.

PERMETHRIN

(per-**meth**-rin)
Elimite, Nix

CLASSIFICATION(S):
Anti-infective (pediculocide)

Pregnancy Category B

INDICATIONS

▪ **1% lotion:** Eradication of *Pediculus humanus capitis* (head lice and their eggs) ▫ Pre-

*CAPITALS indicate life-threatening; underlines indicate most frequent.

vention of infestation of head lice during epidemics ▪ **5% cream:** Eradication of *Sarcoptes scabiei* (scabies).

ACTION

▪ Causes repolarization and paralysis in lice by disrupting sodium transport in normal nerve cells. **Therapeutic Effects:** ▪ Death of parasites.

PHARMACOKINETICS

Absorption: Small amounts (<2%) systemically absorbed. Remains on hair for 10 days.
Distribution: UK.
Metabolism and Excretion: Rapidly inactivated by enzymes.
Half-life: UK.

CONTRAINDICATIONS AND PRECAUTIONS

Contraindicated in: ▪ Hypersensitivity to permethrin, pyrethrins (insecticides or veterinary pesticides), chrysanthemums, or isopropyl alcohol.
Use Cautiously in: ▪ Pregnancy or lactation ▪ Children <2 yr (1% lotion) ▪ Children <2 mo (5% cream).

ADVERSE REACTIONS AND SIDE EFFECTS

Derm: burning, itching, rash, redness, stinging, swelling.
Neuro: numbness, tingling.

INTERACTIONS

Drug-Drug: ▪ No significant interactions.

ROUTE AND DOSAGE

☐ Head Lice (Treatment and Prevention)

- **Topical (Adults and Children >2 yr):** 1% lotion applied to the hair, left on for 10 min, then rinsed, for 1 application.

☐ Scabies

- **Topical (Adults and Children):** Massage 5% cream into all skin surfaces. Leave on for 8–14 hr, then wash off.
- **Topical (Infants >2 mo):** Massage 5% cream into hairline, scalp, neck, temple, and forehead. Leave on for 8–14 hr, then wash off.

AVAILABILITY

▪ ***Liquid cream rinse (lotion):*** 1% in 60-ml containers[OTC] ▪ ***Cream:*** 5% in 60-g tube[Rx].

TIME/ACTION PROFILE (pediculocidal action)

	ONSET	PEAK	DURATION
Top	10 min	UK	14 days

NURSING IMPLICATIONS

ASSESSMENT

- **Head Lice:** Assess scalp for presence of lice and their ova (nits) prior to and 1 wk after application of permethrin.
- **Scabies:** Assess skin for scabies prior to and following therapy.

POTENTIAL NURSING DIAGNOSES

- Home maintenance management, impaired (Indications).
- Self-care deficit (Indications).
- Knowledge deficit, related to medication regimen (Patient/Family Teaching).

IMPLEMENTATION

- **Topical:** For topical application only.

PATIENT/FAMILY TEACHING

- **General Info:** Instruct patient to notify health care professional if scalp itching, numbness, redness, or rash occurs.
- ☐ Instruct patient to avoid getting Elimite cream in eyes. If this occurs, eyes should be flushed thoroughly with water. Health care professional should be contacted if eye irritation persists.
- ☐ Advise patient that others residing in the home should also be checked for lice.
- ☐ Instruct patient on methods of preventing reinfestation. All clothes, including outdoor apparel and household linens, should be machine-washed using very hot water and dried for at least 20 min in a hot dryer. Dry-clean nonwashable clothes. Brushes and combs should be soaked in hot (130°F), soapy water for 5–10 min. Remind patient that brushes and combs should not be shared. Wigs and hairpieces should be shampooed. Rugs and upholstered furniture should be vacuumed. Toys should be washed in hot, soapy water.

Items that cannot be washed should be sealed in a plastic bag for 2 wk.

- □ If patient is a child, instruct parents to notify school nurse or day care center so that classmates and playmates can be checked.
- ■ **Head Lice:** Instruct patient to wash hair with regular shampoo, rinse, and towel dry. Each container holds enough medication for one treatment. Shake the container well. Thoroughly wet scalp and hair with the lotion. The patient should use as much of the solution as needed to coat entire head of hair, then discard remainder of solution. Allow lotion to remain on hair for 10 min, then thoroughly rinse hair and towel dry with a clean towel. Comb hair with a fine-toothed comb to remove dead lice and eggs (not necessary but may be desired for cosmetic effects).
- □ Explain to patient that permethrin will protect from reinfestation for 2 wk. These effects continue even when the patient resumes regular shampooing.
- ■ **Scabies:** Instruct patient to massage thoroughly into the skin from head to soles of feet. Treat infants on the hairline, neck, scalp, temple, and forehead. Remove the cream by washing after 8–14 hr. Usually 30 g (½ tube) is sufficient for adults. One application is curative.

EVALUATION

Effectiveness of therapy can be demonstrated by: ■ The absence of lice and eggs 1 wk after therapy. A 2nd application is indicated if lice are detected at this time □ Prevention of infestation of head lice during epidemics ■ Eradication of scabies following one application.

PERPHENAZINE

(per-**fen**-a-zeen)

{Apo-Perphenazine}, {PMS Perphenazine}, Trilafon

CLASSIFICATION(S):

Antiemetic, Antipsychotic agent (phenothiazine)

Pregnancy Category C

INDICATIONS

■ Acute and chronic psychoses ■ Nausea, vomiting, or intractable hiccups.

ACTION

■ Alters the effects of dopamine in the CNS ■ Possesses significant anticholinergic and alpha-adrenergic blocking activity ■ Blocks dopamine in the chemoreceptor trigger zone (CTZ). **Therapeutic Effects:** ■ Diminished signs and symptoms of psychoses ■ Decreased nausea, vomiting, or hiccups.

PHARMACOKINETICS

Absorption: Absorption from tablet is variable; may be better with oral liquid formulations; well absorbed following IM administration.

Distribution: Widely distributed, high concentrations in the CNS; crosses the placenta and enters breast milk.

Metabolism and Excretion: Highly metabolized by the liver and GI mucosa; some conversion to active compounds.

Half-life: 8.4–12.3 hr.

CONTRAINDICATIONS AND PRECAUTIONS

Contraindicated in: ■ Hypersensitivity ■ Hypersensitivity to bisulfites (injection only) ■ Known alcohol intolerance (concentrate only) ■ Cross-sensitivity with other phenothiazines may occur ■ Narrow-angle glaucoma ■ Bone marrow depression ■ Severe liver or cardiovascular disease ■ Intestinal obstruction.

Use Cautiously in: ■ Geriatric, emaciated, or debilitated patients (lower initial dose recommended) ■ Pregnancy, lactation, or children <12 yr (safety not established) ■ Diabetes mellitus ■ Respiratory disease ■ Prostatic hypertrophy ■ CNS tumors ■ History of seizure disorder.

ADVERSE REACTIONS AND SIDE EFFECTS*

CNS: NEUROLEPTIC MALIGNANT SYNDROME, extrapyramidal reactions, sedation, tardive dyskinesia.

EENT: blurred vision, dry eyes, lens opacities.

CV: hypotension, tachycardia.

GI: constipation, dry mouth, anorexia, drug-induced hepatitis, ileus.

{} = Available in Canada only.

***CAPITALS indicate life-threatening; underlines indicate most frequent.**

GU: discoloration of urine, urinary retention.
Derm: photosensitivity, pigment changes, rashes.
Endo: galactorrhea.
Hemat: AGRANULOCYTOSIS, leukopenia.
Metab: hyperthermia.
Misc: allergic reactions.

INTERACTIONS

Drug-Drug: ▪ Additive hypotension with **antihypertensive agents**, acute ingestion of **alcohol**, or **nitrates** ▪ Additive CNS depression with **MAO inhibitors** or other **CNS depressants**, including **alcohol, antihistamines, opioids, sedative/hypnotics**, and **general anesthetics** ▪ Additive anticholinergic effects with other **drugs possessing anticholinergic properties**, including **antihistamines, antidepressants, atropine, disopyramide, haloperidol**, and **other phenothiazines** ▪ Hypotension and tachycardia may occur with **epinephrine** ▪ Increased risk of agranulocytosis with **antithyroid agents** ▪ Increased risk of extrapyramidal reactions with **lithium** ▪ May mask **lithium** toxicity ▪ **Antacids** or **lithium** may decrease absorption of perphenazine ▪ May decrease antiparkinson effect of **levodopa** or **bromocriptine.**

ROUTE AND DOSAGE

- **PO (Adults):** *Psychoses*—2–16 mg 2–4 times daily (not to exceed 64 mg/day). *Nausea/vomiting*—8–16 mg/day in divided doses (not to exceed 24 mg/day).
- **IM (Adults):** *Psychoses*—5–10 mg initially; may repeat q 6 hr (not to exceed 15–30 mg/day). *Nausea/vomiting*—5 mg initially; may be increased to 10 mg if needed.
- **IV (Adults):** *Severe nausea/vomiting/hiccups*—1 mg at 1–2-min intervals to a total of 5 mg or as an infusion at a rate not to exceed 1 mg/min (not to exceed 5 mg total dose).

AVAILABILITY

▪ ***Tablets:*** 2 mg[Rx], 4 mg[Rx], 8 mg[Rx], 16 mg[Rx] ▪ ***Syrup:*** {2 mg/5 ml[Rx]} ▪ ***Oral concentrate:*** 16 mg/5 ml[Rx] ▪ ***Injection:*** 5 mg/ml in 1-ml ampules[Rx] ▪ ***In combination with:*** amitriptyline (Etrafon, Triavil)[Rx]. See Appendix A.

TIME/ACTION PROFILE (PO, IM = antipsychotic effect*; IV = antiemetic effect)

	ONSET	PEAK	DURATION
PO	2–6 hr	UK	6–12 hr
IM	2–6 hr	UK	6–12 hr
IV	rapid	UK	UK

*Optimal antipsychotic response may not occur for several weeks.

NURSING IMPLICATIONS

ASSESSMENT

- **General Info:** Assess patient's mental status (orientation, mood, behavior) prior to and periodically throughout therapy.
- Monitor blood pressure (sitting, standing, lying), ECG, pulse, and respiratory rate prior to and frequently during the period of dosage adjustment. May cause Q-wave and T-wave changes in ECG.
- Observe patient carefully when administering medication to ensure that medication is actually taken and not hoarded.
- Assess fluid intake and bowel function. Increased bulk and fluids in the diet may help minimize constipation.
- Monitor patient for onset of akathisia (restlessness or desire to keep moving) and extrapyramidal side effects (*parkinsonian*—difficulty speaking or swallowing, loss of balance control, pill rolling, mask-like face, shuffling gait, rigidity, tremors; and *dystonic*—muscle spasms, twisting motions, twitching, inability to move eyes, weakness of arms or legs) every 2 mo during therapy and 8–12 wk after therapy has been discontinued. Report these symptoms; reduction in dosage or discontinuation of medication may be necessary. Trihexyphenidyl or diphenhydramine may be used to control these symptoms.
- Monitor for tardive dyskinesia (uncontrolled rhythmic movement of mouth, face, and extremities; lip smacking or puckering; puffing of cheeks; uncontrolled chewing; rapid or worm-like movements of tongue). Notify physician or other health care professional immediately if these symptoms occur, as these side effects may be irreversible.
- Monitor for development of neuroleptic malignant syndrome (fever, respiratory distress, tachycardia, convulsions, diaphoresis, hypertension or hypotension, pallor, tiredness, se-

vere muscle stiffness, loss of bladder control). Notify physician or other health care professional immediately if these symptoms occur.

- **Antiemetic:** Assess nausea and vomiting prior to and following perphenazine administration.
- □ Monitor intake and output. Patients with severe nausea and vomiting may require IV fluids with electrolytes in addition to antiemetics.
- ***Lab Test Considerations:*** CBC, liver function tests, and ocular examinations should be evaluated periodically throughout therapy. May cause decreased hematocrit, hemoglobin, leukocytes, granulocytes, or platelets. May cause elevated bilirubin, AST, ALT, and alkaline phosphatase. Agranulocytosis occurs after 4–10 wk of therapy, with recovery 1–2 wk following discontinuation. May recur if medication is restarted. Liver function abnormalities may require discontinuation of therapy.
- □ May cause false-positive or false-negative pregnancy tests and false-positive urine bilirubin test results.

POTENTIAL NURSING DIAGNOSES

- Thought processes, altered (Indications).
- Knowledge deficit, related to medication regimen (Patient/Family Teaching).
- Noncompliance (Patient/Family Teaching).

IMPLEMENTATION

- **General Info:** To prevent contact dermatitis, avoid getting liquid preparations on hands, and wash hands thoroughly if spillage occurs.
- □ Keep patient recumbent for at least 30 min following parenteral administration to minimize hypotensive effects.
- □ Phenothiazines should be discontinued 48 hr before and not resumed for 24 hr following myelography, because they lower the seizure threshold.
- **PO:** Dilute concentrate just prior to administration in water, milk, carbonated beverage, soup, or tomato or fruit juice. Do not mix with beverages containing caffeine (cola, coffee), tannics (tea), or pectinates (apple juice). The concentration should be 5 ml of perphenazine oral concentrate to 60 ml of diluent.
- **IM:** Inject deep into well-developed muscle. Keep patient in recumbent position and monitor for at least 30 min following injection. Slight yellow color will not alter potency; do not use if solution is dark or contains a precipitate.
- **Direct IV:** Dilute to a concentration of 0.5 mg/ml with 0.9% NaCl.
- ***Rate:*** Administer each 1 mg over at least 1 min.
- **Syringe Compatibility:** ▪ atropine ▪ butorphanol ▪ cimetidine ▪ dimenhydrinate ▪ diphenhydramine ▪ droperidol ▪ fentanyl ▪ meperidine ▪ metoclopramide ▪ morphine ▪ pentazocine ▪ ranitidine ▪ scopolamine.
- **Syringe Incompatibility:** ▪ midazolam ▪ pentobarbital.
- **Y-Site Compatibility:** ▪ acyclovir ▪ amikacin ▪ ampicillin ▪ cefamandole ▪ cefazolin ▪ cefotaxime ▪ cefoxitin ▪ cefuroxime ▪ cephalothin ▪ cephapirin ▪ chloramphenicol ▪ clindamycin ▪ doxycycline ▪ erythromycin lactobionate ▪ famotidine ▪ gentamicin ▪ kanamycin ▪ metronidazole ▪ mezlocillin ▪ minocycline ▪ nafcillin ▪ oxacillin ▪ penicillin G potassium ▪ piperacillin ▪ tacrolimus ▪ ticarcillin ▪ ticarcillin/clavulanate ▪ tobramycin ▪ trimethoprim/sulfamethoxazole ▪ vancomycin.
- **Y-Site Incompatibility:** ▪ cefoperazone.

PATIENT/FAMILY TEACHING

- □ Advise patient to take medication exactly as directed and not to skip doses or double up on missed doses. If a dose is missed, it should be taken as soon as remembered unless almost time for the next dose. If more than 2 doses a day are ordered, the missed dose should be taken within 1 hr of the scheduled time or omitted. Abrupt withdrawal may lead to gastritis, nausea, vomiting, dizziness, headache, tachycardia, and insomnia.
- □ Inform patient of possibility of extrapyramidal symptoms and tardive dyskinesia. Instruct patient to report these symptoms immediately.
- □ Advise patient to make position changes slowly to minimize orthostatic hypotension.
- □ Medication may cause drowsiness. Caution patient to avoid driving or other activities requiring alertness until response to medication is known.
- □ Caution patient to avoid taking alcohol or other CNS depressants concurrently with this medication.
- □ Advise patient to use sunscreen and protective clothing when exposed to the sun. Exposed surfaces may develop a blue-gray pigmentation, which may fade following discontinuation of the medication. Extremes in temperature

should also be avoided, as this drug impairs body temperature regulation.

- ▫ Instruct patient to use frequent mouth rinses, good oral hygiene, and sugarless gum or candy to minimize dry mouth. Consult health care professional if dry mouth continues for >2 wk.
- ▫ Advise patient not to take perphenazine within 2 hr of antacids or antidiarrheal medication.
- ▫ Inform patient that this medication may turn urine a pink to reddish-brown color.
- ▫ Advise patient to notify health care professional of medication regimen prior to treatment or surgery.
- ▫ Instruct patient to notify health care professional promptly if sore throat, fever, unusual bleeding or bruising, rash, weakness, tremors, visual disturbances, dark-colored urine, or clay-colored stools occur.
- ▫ Emphasize the importance of routine follow-up exams and continued participation in psychotherapy as indicated.

EVALUATION

Effectiveness of therapy can be demonstrated by: ▪ Decrease in excitable, paranoic, or withdrawn behavior ▪ Relief of nausea and vomiting ▪ Relief of intractable hiccups.

PHENAZOPYRIDINE

(fen-az-oh-**peer**-i-deen)

Azo-Standard, Baridium, Eridium, Geridium, {Phenazo}, Phenazodine, Prodium, Pyridiate, Pyridium, Urodine, Urogesic, Viridium

CLASSIFICATION(S):

Nonopioid analgesic (urinary tract analgesic)

Pregnancy Category B

INDICATIONS

▪ Provides relief from the following urinary tract symptoms, which may occur in association with infection or following urologic procedures: ▫ Pain ▫ Itching ▫ Burning ▫ Urgency ▫ Frequency.

ACTION

▪ Acts locally on the urinary tract mucosa to produce analgesic or local anesthetic effects ▪ Has no antimicrobial activity. **Therapeutic Effects:** ▪ Diminished urinary tract discomfort.

PHARMACOKINETICS

Absorption: Appears to be well absorbed following oral administration.
Distribution: UK. Small amounts cross the placenta.
Metabolism and Excretion: Rapidly excreted unchanged in the urine.
Half-life: UK.

CONTRAINDICATIONS AND PRECAUTIONS

Contraindicated in: ▪ Hypersensitivity ▪ Glomerulonephritis ▪ Severe hepatitis, uremia, or renal failure ▪ Renal insufficiency ▪ G6PD deficiency.
Use Cautiously in: ▪ Hepatitis. ▪ Pregnancy or lactation (safety not established).

ADVERSE REACTIONS AND SIDE EFFECTS*

CNS: headache, vertigo.
GI: hepatotoxicity, nausea.
GU: bright-orange urine, renal failure.
Derm: rash.
Hemat: hemolytic anemia, methemoglobinemia.

INTERACTIONS

Drug-Drug: ▪ None significant.

ROUTE AND DOSAGE

- ▪ **PO (Adults):** 200 mg 3 times daily for 2 days.
- ▪ **PO (Children):** 4 mg/kg 3 times daily for 2 days.

AVAILABILITY

▪ ***Tablets:*** 95 mg[OTC], 100 mg[Rx], {100 mg[OTC]}, {200 mg[OTC]}, 200 mg[Rx].

TIME/ACTION PROFILE (urinary analgesia)

	ONSET	PEAK	DURATION
PO	UK	5–6 hr	6–8 hr

{} = Available in Canada only.
***CAPITALS indicate life-threatening; underlines indicate most frequent.**

P

NURSING IMPLICATIONS

ASSESSMENT

- □ Assess patient for urgency, frequency, and pain on urination prior to and throughout therapy.
- ▪ ***Lab Test Considerations:*** Renal function should be monitored periodically during course of therapy.
- □ Interferes with urine tests based on color reactions (glucose, ketones, bilirubin, steroids, protein).

POTENTIAL NURSING DIAGNOSES

- ▪ Pain (Indications).
- ▪ Urinary elimination, altered patterns of (Indications).
- ▪ Knowledge deficit, related to medication regimen (Patient/Family Teaching).

IMPLEMENTATION

- ▪ **General Info:** Medication should be discontinued after pain or discomfort is relieved (usually 2 days for treatment of urinary tract infection). Concurrent antibiotic therapy should continue for full prescribed duration.
- ▪ **PO:** Administer medication with or following meals to decrease GI irritation. Do not crush or chew tablet.

PATIENT/FAMILY TEACHING

- □ Instruct patient to take medication exactly as directed. If a dose is missed, take as soon as remembered unless almost time for next dose.
- □ Advise patient that while phenazopyridine administration is stopped once pain or discomfort is relieved, concurrent antibiotic therapy must be continued for full duration of therapy. Do not save unused portion of phenazopyridine without consulting health care professional.
- □ Inform patient that drug causes reddish-orange discoloration of urine that may stain clothing or bedding. Sanitary napkin may be worn to avoid clothing stains. May also cause staining of soft contact lenses.
- □ Instruct patient to notify health care professional if rash, skin discoloration, or unusual tiredness occurs.

EVALUATION

Effectiveness of therapy can be demonstrated by: ▪ Decrease in pain and burning on urination.

PHENOBARBITAL

(fee-noe-**bar**-bi-tal)

{Ancalixir}, Barbita, Luminal, Solfoton

CLASSIFICATION(S):

Anticonvulsant (barbiturate), Sedative/hypnotic

Schedule IV

Pregnancy Category D

INDICATIONS

▪ Anticonvulsant in tonic-clonic (grand mal), partial, and febrile seizures in children ▪ Preoperative sedative and in other situations in which sedation may be required ▪ Hypnotic (short-term). **Unlabeled Uses:** ▪ Prevention/treatment of hyperbilirubinemia.

ACTION

▪ Produces all levels of CNS depression ▪ Depresses the sensory cortex, decreases motor activity, and alters cerebellar function ▪ Inhibits transmission in the nervous system and raises the seizure threshold ▪ Capable of inducing (speeding up) enzymes in the liver that metabolize drugs, bilirubin, and other compounds. **Therapeutic Effects:** ▪ Anticonvulsant activity ▪ Sedation.

PHARMACOKINETICS

Absorption: Absorption is slow but relatively complete (70–90%).

Distribution: UK.

Metabolism and Excretion: 75% metabolized by the liver, 25% excreted unchanged by the kidneys.

Half-life: 2–6 days.

CONTRAINDICATIONS AND PRECAUTIONS

Contraindicated in: ▪ Hypersensitivity ▪ Comatose patients or those with pre-existing CNS depression ▪ Uncontrolled severe pain ▪ Lactation ▪ Known alcohol intolerance (elixir only).

Use Cautiously in: ▪ Hepatic dysfunction ▪ Severe renal impairment ▪ History of suicide attempt or drug abuse ▪ Geriatric patients (initial dosage reduction recommended) ▪ Hypnotic use should be short-term. Chronic use may lead to dependence ▪ Pregnancy (chronic use results in drug dependency in the infant; may result in coagulation defects and fetal malformation; acute use at term may result in respiratory depression in the newborn).

ADVERSE REACTIONS AND SIDE EFFECTS*

CNS: hangover, delirium, depression, drowsiness, excitation, lethargy, vertigo.

Resp: respiratory depression; *IV*—LARYNGOSPASM, bronchospasm.

CV: *IV*—hypotension.

GI: constipation, diarrhea, nausea, vomiting.

Derm: photosensitivity, rashes, urticaria.

Local: phlebitis at IV site.

MS: arthralgia, myalgia, neuralgia.

Misc: hypersensitivity reactions including ANGIOEDEMA and SERUM SICKNESS, physical dependence, psychological dependence.

INTERACTIONS

Drug-Drug: ▪ Additive CNS depression with other **CNS depressants**, including **alcohol, antihistamines, opioids**, and other **sedative/hypnotics** ▪ May induce hepatic enzymes that metabolize other drugs, decreasing their effectiveness, including **oral contraceptives, warfarin, chloramphenicol, cyclosporine, dacarbazine, glucocorticoids, tricyclic antidepressants,** and **quinidine** ▪ May increase the risk of hepatic toxicity of **acetaminophen** ▪ **MAO inhibitors, valproic acid,** or **divalproex** may decrease the metabolism of phenobarbital, increasing sedation ▪ May increase the risk of hematologic toxicity with **cyclophosphamide.**

ROUTE AND DOSAGE

- **PO (Adults):** *Anticonvulsant*—60–250 mg/day as a single dose or 2–3 divided doses. *Sedative*—30–120 mg/day in 2–3 divided doses. *Hypnotic*—100–320 mg at bedtime. *Hyperbilirubinemia*—30–60 mg 3 times daily.
- **PO (Children):** *Anticonvulsant*—1–6 mg/kg/day, single dose or divided doses. *Sedative*—2 mg/kg (60 mg/m²) 3 times daily. *Hyperbilirubinemia*—1–4 mg/kg 3 times daily.
- **PO, IM, IV (Children):** *Preoperative sedative*—1–3 mg/kg 60–90 min preop.
- **PO, IM (Neonates):** *Hyperbilirubinemia*—5–10 mg/kg/day.
- **IM, IV (Adults):** *Sedative*—30–120 mg/day in 2–3 divided doses. *Preoperative sedative*—130–200 mg 60–90 min preop. *Hypnotic*—100–325 mg at bedtime.
- **IV (Adults):** *Anticonvulsant*—100–320 mg as needed initially (total of 600 mg/24-hr period). *Status epilepticus*—10–20 mg/kg.
- **IV (Children):** *Anticonvulsant*—10–20 mg/kg initially, followed by 1–6 mg/kg/day. *Status epilepticus*—15–20 mg/kg.

AVAILABILITY

▪ ***Tablets:*** 8 mg[Rx], 15 mg[Rx], 30 mg[Rx], 60 mg[Rx], 100 mg[Rx] ▪ ***Capsules:*** 15 mg[Rx] ▪ ***Elixir:*** 20 mg/5 ml[Rx] ▪ ***Injection:*** 30 mg/ml in 1-ml prefilled syringes[Rx], 60 mg/ml in 1-ml prefilled syringes[Rx], 65 mg/ml in 1-ml vials[Rx], 130 mg/ml in 1-ml prefilled syringes, 1-ml vials, and 1-ml ampules[Rx] ▪ ***In combination with:*** phenytoin[Rx]. See Appendix A.

TIME/ACTION PROFILE (sedation†)

	ONSET	PEAK	DURATION
PO	30–60 min	UK	>6 hr
IM, SC	10–30 min	UK	4–6 hr
IV	5 min	30 min	4–6 hr

†Full anticonvulsant effects occur after 2–3 wk of chronic dosing unless a loading dose has been used.

NURSING IMPLICATIONS

ASSESSMENT

- **General Info:** Monitor respiratory status, pulse, and blood pressure frequently in patients receiving phenobarbital IV. Equipment for resuscitation and artificial ventilation should be readily available. Respiratory depression is dose-dependent.
- □ Prolonged therapy may lead to psychological or physical dependence. Restrict amount of

*CAPITALS indicate life-threatening; underlines indicate most frequent.

drug available to patient, especially if depressed, suicidal, or with a history of addiction.

- **Seizures:** Assess location, duration, and characteristics of seizure activity.
- **Sedation:** Assess level of consciousness and anxiety when used as a preoperative sedative.
- □ Assess postoperative patients for pain. Phenobarbital may increase sensitivity to painful stimuli.
- ***Lab Test Considerations:*** Patients on prolonged therapy should have hepatic and renal function and CBC evaluated periodically.
- □ Serum folate concentrations should be monitored periodically during therapy because of increased folate requirements of patients on long-term anticonvulsant therapy with phenobarbital.
- □ May cause decreased serum bilirubin concentrations in neonates, in patients with congenital nonhemolytic unconjugated hyperbilirubinemia, and in epileptics.
- ***Toxicity and Overdose:*** Serum phenobarbital levels may be monitored when used as an anticonvulsant. Therapeutic blood levels are 10–40 mcg/ml. Symptoms of toxicity include confusion, drowsiness, dyspnea, slurred speech, and staggering.

POTENTIAL NURSING DIAGNOSES

- Injury, risk for (Indications, Side Effects).
- Knowledge deficit, related to medication regimen (Patient/Family Teaching).

IMPLEMENTATION

- **General Info:** Supervise ambulation and transfer of patients following administration. Remove cigarettes. Side rails should be raised and call bell within reach at all times. Keep bed in low position. Institute seizure precautions.
- □ When changing from phenobarbital to another anticonvulsant, gradually decrease phenobarbital dose while concurrently increasing dose of replacement medication to maintain anticonvulsant effects.
- **PO:** Tablets may be crushed and mixed with food or fluids (do not administer dry) for patients with difficulty swallowing. Oral solution may be taken undiluted or mixed with water, milk, or fruit juice. Use calibrated measuring device for accurate measurement of liquid doses.
- **IM:** Injections should be given deep into the gluteal muscle to minimize tissue irritation. Do not inject >5 ml into any one site, because of tissue irritation.
- **IV:** Doses may require 15–30 min to reach peak concentrations in the brain. Administer minimal dose and wait for effectiveness before administering 2nd dose to prevent cumulative barbiturate-induced depression.
- **Direct IV:** Reconstitute sterile powder for IV dose with a minimum of 3 ml of sterile water for injection. Dilute further with 10 ml of sterile water. Do not use solution that is not absolutely clear within 5 min after reconstitution or that contains a precipitate. Discard powder or solution that has been exposed to air for longer than 30 min.
- □ Solution is highly alkaline; avoid extravasation, which may cause tissue damage and necrosis. If extravasation occurs, injection of 5% procaine solution into affected area and application of moist heat may be ordered.
- ***Rate:*** Administer each 60 mg over at least 1 min. Titrate slowly for desired response. Rapid administration may result in respiratory depression.
- **Y-Site Compatibility:** ▪ enalaprilat ▪ sufentanil.
- **Y-Site Incompatibility:** ▪ hydromorphone.

PATIENT/FAMILY TEACHING

- □ Advise patient to take medication exactly as directed. If a dose is missed, take as soon as remembered if not almost time for next dose; do not double doses.
- □ Advise patients on prolonged therapy not to discontinue medication without consulting health care professional. Abrupt withdrawal may precipitate seizures or status epilepticus.
- □ Medication may cause daytime drowsiness. Caution patient to avoid driving and other activities requiring alertness until response to medication is known. Do not resume driving until physician gives clearance based on control of seizure disorder.
- □ Caution patient to avoid taking alcohol or other CNS depressants concurrently with this medication.
- □ Advise female patients using oral contraceptives to use an additional nonhormonal contraceptive during therapy and until next menstrual period. Instruct patient to contact health

P

care professional immediately if pregnancy is suspected.

- Advise patient to notify health care professional if fever, sore throat, mouth sores, unusual bleeding or bruising, nosebleeds, or petechiae occur.

EVALUATION

Effectiveness of therapy can be demonstrated by: ▪ Decrease or cessation of seizure activity without excessive sedation. Several weeks may be required to achieve maximum anticonvulsant effects ▪ Preoperative sedation ▪ Improvement in sleep patterns ▪ Decrease in serum bilirubin levels.

PHENTOLAMINE
(fen-**tole**-a-meen)
Regitine, {Rogitine}

CLASSIFICATION(S):
Alpha-adrenergic blocking agent

Pregnancy Category C

INDICATIONS

▪ **IV:** Control of blood pressure during surgical removal of a pheochromocytoma ▪ **IV, Infiltration:** Prevention and treatment of dermal necrosis and sloughing following extravasation of norepinephrine, phenylephrine, or dopamine. **Unlabeled Uses:** ▪ **IM, IV:** Treatment of hypertension associated with pheochromocytoma or adrenergic (sympathetic) excess, such as administration of phenylephrine, tyramine-containing foods in patients on MAO inhibitor therapy, or clonidine withdrawal.

ACTION

▪ Produces incomplete and short-lived blockade of alpha-adrenergic receptors located primarily in smooth muscle and exocrine glands ▪ Induces hypotension by direct relaxation of vascular smooth muscle and by alpha blockade. **Therapeutic Effects:** ▪ Reduction of blood pressure in situations in which hypertension is due to adrenergic (sympathetic) excess ▪ When infiltrated locally, reverses vasoconstriction caused by norepinephrine or dopamine.

PHARMACOKINETICS

Absorption: Well absorbed following IM administration.
Distribution: UK.
Metabolism and Excretion: 10% excreted unchanged by kidneys.
Half-life: UK.

CONTRAINDICATIONS AND PRECAUTIONS

Contraindicated in: ▪ Hypersensitivity ▪ Coronary or cerebral arteriosclerosis ▪ Renal impairment.
Use Cautiously in: ▪ Peptic ulcer disease ▪ Geriatric patients (more susceptible to hypotensive effects; dosage reduction recommended) ▪ Pregnancy or lactation (safety not established).

ADVERSE REACTIONS AND SIDE EFFECTS*

With parenteral use.
CNS: CEREBROVASCULAR SPASM, dizziness, weakness.
EENT: nasal stuffiness.
CV: HYPOTENSION, MYOCARDIAL INFARCTION, angina, arrhythmias, tachycardia.
GI: abdominal pain, diarrhea, nausea, vomiting, aggravation of peptic ulcer.
Derm: flushing.

INTERACTIONS

Drug-Drug: ▪ Antagonizes the effects of **alpha-adrenergic stimulants** ▪ May decrease the pressor response to **ephedrine, phenylephrine,** or **metaraminol** ▪ Severe hypotension may occur with concurrent use of **epinephrine** or **methoxamine** ▪ Use with **guanethidine** or **guanadrel** may result in exaggerated hypotension and bradycardia ▪ Decreases peripheral vasoconstriction from high doses of **dopamine.**

ROUTE AND DOSAGE

- **Hypertension Associated with Pheochromocytoma—before/during Surgery**
  - **IV (Adults):** 5 mg given 1–2 hr preop, repeated as necessary. May be infused at a rate of 0.5–1 mg/min during surgery.
  - **IV, IM (Children):** 1 mg or 0.1 mg/kg (3

{} = Available in Canada only.
*CAPITALS indicate life-threatening; underlines indicate most frequent.

mg/m²) given 1–2 hr preop, repeated IV as necessary during surgery.

- **Prevention of Dermal Necrosis during Infusion of Norepinephrine, Phenylephrine, or Dopamine**
- **IV (Adults):** Add 10 mg phentolamine to every 1000 ml of fluid containing norepinephrine.
- **Treatment of Dermal Necrosis Following Extravasation of Norepinephrine, Phenylephrine, or Dopamine**
- **Infiltrate (Adults):** 5–10 mg.
- **Infiltrate (Children):** 0.1–0.2 mg/kg (up to 10 mg).

AVAILABILITY

- ***Powder for injection:*** 5 mg/vial[Rx].

TIME/ACTION PROFILE (alpha-adrenergic blockade)

	ONSET	PEAK	DURATION
IM	UK	20 min	30–45 min
IV	immediate	2 min	15–30 min

NURSING IMPLICATIONS

ASSESSMENT

- Monitor blood pressure, pulse, and ECG every 2 min until stable during IV administration. If hypotensive crisis occurs, epinephrine is contraindicated and may cause paradoxical further decrease in blood pressure; norepinephrine may be used.

POTENTIAL NURSING DIAGNOSES

- Tissue perfusion, altered (Indications).
- Injury, risk for (Indications).
- Knowledge deficit, related to medication regimen (Patient/Family Teaching).

IMPLEMENTATION

- **General Info:** Patient should remain supine throughout parenteral administration.
- **IV:** Reconstitute each 5 mg with 1 ml of sterile water for injection or 0.9% NaCl. Discard unused solution.
- Inject each 5 mg over 1 min.
- **Continuous Infusion:** Dilute 5–10 mg in 500 ml of D5W.
- ***Rate:*** Titrate infusion rate according to patient response.
- May also add 10 mg to every 1000 ml of fluid containing norepinephrine for prevention of dermal necrosis and sloughing. Does not affect pressor effect of norepinephrine.
- **Syringe Compatibility:** ■ papaverine.
- **Y-Site Compatibility:** ■ amiodarone.
- **Additive Compatibility:** ■ dobutamine ■ norepinephrine.
- **Infiltration:** Dilute 5–10 mg of phentolamine in 10 ml of 0.9% NaCl. For children, use 0.1–0.2 mg/kg up to a maximum of 10 mg. Infiltrate site of extravasation promptly. Must be given within 12 hr of extravasation to be effective.

PATIENT/FAMILY TEACHING

- Advise patient to change positions slowly to minimize orthostatic hypotension.
- Instruct patient to notify health care professional if chest pain occurs during IV infusion.

EVALUATION

Clinical response to therapy can be evaluated by: ■ Decrease in blood pressure ■ Prevention of dermal necrosis and sloughing in extravasation of norepinephrine, dopamine, and phenylephrine.

PHENYLPROPANOLAMINE

(fen-il-proe-pa-**nole**-a-meen)

Acutrim 16 hr, Acutrim Late Day, Acutrim II Maximum Strength, Control, Dexatrim Maximum Strength, Eped-II Yellow, PPA, Prolamine, Propagest, Rhinedecon

CLASSIFICATION(S):

Appetite suppressant, Decongestant

Pregnancy Category C

INDICATIONS

■ Short-term adjunct therapy in the management of exogenous obesity in conjunction with behavior modification, diet, and exercise ■ Short-term management of nasal congestion. **Unlabeled Uses:** ■ Management of urinary incontinence.

ACTION

■ Acts as an agonist of dopamine and norepinephrine ■ Suppresses appetite by depressing CNS appetite control center ■ Stimulates alpha-adrenergic receptors in nasal mucosa, producing vasoconstriction ▪ Stimulates alpha-adrenergic receptors in bladder and urethra; produces contraction of smooth muscle. **Therapeutic Effects:** ▪ Decreased appetite ▪ Nasal decongestion ▪ Decreased urinary incontinence.

PHARMACOKINETICS

Absorption: Well absorbed following oral administration.
Distribution: UK.
Metabolism and Excretion: 80–90% excreted unchanged by the kidneys. Small amounts metabolized by the liver.
Half-life: 3–4 hr.

CONTRAINDICATIONS AND PRECAUTIONS

Contraindicated in: ▪ Hypersensitivity ▪ Children <12 yr (appetite suppressant use only) ▪ Pregnancy or lactation.
Use Cautiously in: ▪ Glaucoma ▪ Prostatic hypertrophy ▪ Hyperthyroidism ▪ Cardiovascular disease, including hypertension ▪ Diabetes mellitus.

ADVERSE REACTIONS AND SIDE EFFECTS

CNS: dizziness, drowsiness, headache, nervousness, restlessness.
EENT: rebound congestion (decongestant use).
CV: arrhythmias, chest pain, hypertension.
GI: anorexia, nausea.
Misc: tachyphylaxis (decongestant use).

INTERACTIONS

Drug-Drug: ▪ Additive sympathomimetic effects with other **adrenergic (sympathomimetic) agents** ▪ Vasopressor effects are increased by concurrent administration of **MAO inhibitors** ▪ Increased risk of arrhythmias with some **general anesthetics** ▪ Increased risk of hypertension with **reserpine, tricyclic antidepressants,** or **ganglionic blocking agents.**

ROUTE AND DOSAGE

- **PO (Adults):** *Appetite suppressant*—25 mg tid or 75 mg of extended-release preparation once daily. *Decongestant*—25 mg q 4 hr (not to exceed 150 mg/day) or 75 mg of extended-release preparation q 12 hr. *Incontinence*—50–150 mg/day in divided doses.
- **PO (Children 6–12 yr):** *Decongestant*—12.5 mg q 4 hr (not to exceed 75 mg/day).
- **PO (Children 2–6 yr):** *Decongestant*—6.25 mg q 4 hr (not to exceed 37.5 mg/day).

AVAILABILITY

▪ ***Tablets:*** 25 mg^{OTC}, 50 mg^{OTC} ▪ ***Extended-release tablets:*** 75 mg^{OTC} ▪ ***Capsules:*** 25 mg^{OTC}, 37.5 mg^{OTC} ▪ ***Extended-release capsules:*** 75 mg^{OTC} ▪ ***In combination with:*** vitamins and/or grapefruit extract, antihistamines, cough suppressants^{OTC} (see Appendix A).

TIME/ACTION PROFILE (nasal decongestion)

	ONSET	PEAK	DURATION
PO	15–30 min	UK	3 hr
PO-ER	UK	UK	12–16 hr

NURSING IMPLICATIONS

ASSESSMENT

- **Obesity:** Monitor patient's weight and nutritional intake periodically throughout therapy.
- **Nasal Congestion:** Assess patient for nasal congestion periodically throughout therapy.

POTENTIAL NURSING DIAGNOSES

- Nutrition, altered, more than body requirements (Indications).
- Knowledge deficit, related to medication regimen (Patient/Family Teaching).

IMPLEMENTATION

- **General Info:** Administer last dose a few hours prior to sleep (12 hr with extended-release forms) to minimize insomnia.
- **PO:** Administer extended-release tablets once daily, in the morning after breakfast. Extended-release tablets should be swallowed whole; do not crush or chew.
- **Obesity:** Do not administer to children under 12 yr. Administer to children 12–18 yr according to recommendations of physician or other health care professional.

PATIENT/FAMILY TEACHING

- **General Info:** Instruct patient to take only as directed. Do not take more medication or for a longer time than directed; tolerance may develop.
- □ Advise patient not to drink large amounts of coffee, tea, or colas containing caffeine.

- **Obesity:** Instruct patient on modification of caloric intake and exercise program.
- **Nasal Decongestant:** Advise patient to consult health care professional if symptoms do not improve within 7 days or if a fever is present.

EVALUATION

Effectiveness of therapy can be demonstrated by: ▪ Decrease in appetite and subsequent decrease in weight when used for obesity. Should be used no longer than a few weeks for obesity ▪ Decrease in nasal congestion.

PHENYTOIN/FOSPHENYTOIN

phenytoin
(**fen**-i-toyn)
Dilantin, Diphenylan, diphenylhydantoin, DPH

fosphenytoin
(foss-**fen**-i-toyn)
Cerebyx

CLASSIFICATION(S):
Antiarrhythmic (group IB), Anticonvulsant (hydantoin)

Pregnancy Category C, D

INDICATIONS

▪ **Phenytoin:** Treatment/prevention of tonic-clonic (grand mal) seizures and complex partial seizures ▪ **Fosphenytoin:** ▫ Short-term (<5 day) management of seizures when oral phenytoin use is not feasible ▫ Treatment/prevention of seizures during neurosurgery. **Unlabeled Uses:** ▪ **Phenytoin:** As an antiarrhythmic, particularly for arrhythmias associated with cardiac glycoside toxicity ▪ Management of painful syndromes, including trigeminal neuralgia.

ACTION

▪ Limit seizure propagation by altering ion transport ▪ Antiarrhythmic properties as a result of improvement in AV conduction ▪ May also decrease synaptic transmission ▪ Fosphenytoin is rapidly converted to phenytoin, which is responsible for its pharmacologic effects. **Therapeutic Effects:** ▪ Diminished seizure activity ▪ Control of arrhythmias ▪ Decreased pain.

PHARMACOKINETICS

Absorption: *Phenytoin*—absorbed slowly from the GI tract. Bioavailability differs among products; only Dilantin preparation is considered to be an "extended" product. Other products are considered to be prompt release. *Fosphenytoin*—rapidly converted to phenytoin following IV administration and completely absorbed following IM administration.

Distribution: Distribute into CSF and other body tissues and fluids. Enter breast milk; cross the placenta, achieving similar maternal/fetal levels. Preferentially distribute into fatty tissue.

Metabolism and Excretion: Mostly metabolized by the liver; minimal amounts excreted in the urine.

Half-life: *Fosphenytoin*—15 min; *phenytoin*—22 hr (longer at higher blood levels).

CONTRAINDICATIONS AND PRECAUTIONS

Contraindicated in: ▪ Hypersensitivity ▪ Hypersensitivity to propylene glycol (phenytoin injection only) ▪ Alcohol intolerance (phenytoin injection and liquid only) ▪ Sinus bradycardia, sinoatrial block, 2nd- or 3rd-degree heart block or Stokes-Adams syndrome.

Use Cautiously in: ▪ Hepatic or renal disease (increased risk of adverse reactions; dosage reduction recommended for hepatic impairment) ▪ Geriatric patients or those with severe cardiac or respiratory disease (parenteral use—increased risk of serious adverse reactions, especially with IV phenytoin) ▪ Obese patients (initial dose of IV phenytoin should be based on ideal body weight + 1.33 times excess weight) ▪ Pregnancy (safety not established; may result in fetal hydantoin syndrome if used chronically or hemorrhage in the newborn if used at term) ▪ Lactation (safety not established).

ADVERSE REACTIONS AND SIDE EFFECTS*

Most listed are for chronic use of phenytoin.

CNS: ataxia, agitation, cerebral edema, coma, dizziness, drowsiness, dysarthria, dyskinesia, extrapyramidal syndrome, headache, nervousness, weakness.

*CAPITALS indicate life-threatening; underlines indicate most frequent.

EENT: diplopia, nystagmus, tinnitus.
CV: hypotension (↑ with IV phenytoin), tachycardia, vasodilation.
GI: gingival hyperplasia, nausea, altered taste, anorexia, constipation, drug-induced hepatitis, dry mouth, vomiting, weight loss.
GU: pink, red, reddish-brown discoloration of urine.
Derm: hypertrichosis, rashes, exfoliative dermatitis, pruritus.
F and E: hypocalcemia.
Hemat: AGRANULOCYTOSIS, APLASTIC ANEMIA, leukopenia, megaloblastic anemia, thrombocytopenia.
MS: back pain, osteomalacia, pelvic pain.
Misc: allergic reactions including STEVENS-JOHNSON SYNDROME, fever, lymphadenopathy.

INTERACTIONS

Drug-Drug: ▪ **Phenylbutazone, disulfiram,** acute ingestion of **alcohol, amiodarone, isoniazid, chloramphenicol, influenza vaccine, sulfonamides, disulfiram, fluoxetine, benzodiazepines, omeprazole, metronidazole, ketoconazole, fluconazole, miconazole, estrogens, succinamides, halothane, methylphenidate, phenothiazines, salicylates, tolbutamide, trazodone, felbamate,** and **cimetidine** may increase phenytoin blood levels ▪ **Barbiturates, carbamazepine, reserpine,** chronic ingestion of **alcohol,** and **warfarin** may decrease phenytoin blood levels ▪ Phenytoin may alter the effects of **digitoxin, warfarin, felbamate, glucocorticoids, doxycycline, rifampin, quinidine, methadone, cyclosporine,** and **estrogens** ▪ IV phenytoin and **dopamine** may cause additive hypotension ▪ Additive CNS depression with other **CNS depressants,** including **alcohol, antihistamines, antidepressants, opioids,** and **sedative/hypnotics** ▪ **Antacids** may decrease absorption of orally administered phenytoin ▪ May decrease the effectiveness of **streptozocin** or **theophylline** ▪ Additive cardiac depression may occur with **propranolol** or **lidocaine** ▪ **Calcium** and **sucralfate** decrease phenytoin absorption.
Drug-Food: ▪ Phenytoin may decrease absorption of **folic acid** ▪ Concurrent administration of **enteral tube feedings** may decrease phenytoin absorption.

ROUTE AND DOSAGE

❑ Fosphenytoin

All doses are expressed as phenytoin sodium equivalents (PE).

❑ ***Status Epilepticus***

- **IV (Adults and Children):** 15–20 mg PE/kg

❑ ***Nonemergent and Maintenance Dosing***

- **IV, IM (Adults and Children):** *Loading dose*—10–20 mg PE/kg. *Maintenance dose*—4–6 mg PE/kg/day.

❑ Phenytoin

IM administration should be a last resort. Dosage should be increased by 50% over previously established daily oral dosage.

❑ ***Anticonvulsant***

- **PO (Adults):** Loading dose 1 g or 20 mg/kg as extended capsules in 3–4 divided doses at 2-hr intervals or as 400 mg, then 300 mg q 2 hr for 2 doses; maintenance dose 300–400 mg/day. May be given once daily as extended (Dilantin Kapseals) or in 3 divided capsules; usual maximum dose 600 mg/day.
- **PO (Geriatric Patients):** 3 mg/kg/day in divided doses.
- **PO (Children):** Initially 5 mg/kg/day; maintenance dose 4–8 mg/kg/day (250 mg/m^2) in 2–3 divided doses (not to exceed 300 mg/day).
- **IV (Adults):** 15–20 mg/kg. Rate not to exceed 25–50 mg/min, followed by 100 mg q 6–8 hr.
- **IV (Children):** 15–20 mg/kg (250 mg/m^2) at 1–3 mg/kg/min.

❑ ***Antiarrhythmic***

- **IV (Adults):** 50–100 mg q 10–15 min until arrhythmia is abolished, 15 mg/kg have been given, or toxicity occurs.

❑ ***Antineuralgic***

- **PO (Adults):** 200–600 mg/day in divided doses.

AVAILABILITY

❑ Fosphenytoin

▪ ***Injection:*** 150 mg (100 mg phenytoin equivalent) in 2-ml vials^{Rx}, 750 mg (500 mg phenytoin equivalent) in 10-ml vials^{Rx}.

P

□ **Phenytoin**

▪ ***Chewable tablets:*** 50 mgRx ▪ ***Oral suspension:*** 30 mg/5 mlRx, 125 mg/5 mlRx ▪ ***Prompt-release capsules:*** 30 mgRx, 100 mgRx ▪ ***Extended capsules:*** 30 mgRx, 100 mgRx ▪ ***Injection:*** 50 mg/ml in 2- and 5-ml ampules, 2- and 5-ml vials, and 2-ml prefilled syringesRx ▪ ***In combination with:*** phenobarbitalRx. See Appendix A.

TIME/ACTION PROFILE (anticonvulsant effect)

	ONSET*	PEAK	DURATION
Fosphenytoin IM	UK	30 min	up to 24 hr
Fosphenytoin IV	15–45 min	15–60 min	up to 24 hr
Phenytoin PO	2–24 hr (1 wk)	1.5–3 hr	6–12 hr
Phenytoin PO-ER	2–24 hr (1 wk)	4–12 hr	12–36 hr
Phenytoin IV	1–2 hr (1 wk)	rapid	12–24 hr
Phenytoin IM	UK (erratic)	erratic	12–24 hr

*( ) = time required for onset of action without a loading dose.

NURSING IMPLICATIONS

ASSESSMENT

- **Seizures:** Assess location, duration, frequency, and characteristics of seizure activity. EEG may be monitored periodically throughout therapy.
- **Arrhythmias:** Monitor ECG continuously during treatment of arrhythmias.
- **Neuralgia:** Assess pain (location, duration, intensity, precipitating factors) prior to and periodically throughout therapy.
- **Phenytoin:** Assess oral hygiene. Vigorous cleaning beginning within 10 days of initiation of phenytoin therapy may help control gingival hyperplasia.
  - □ Assess patient for phenytoin hypersensitivity syndrome (fever, skin rash, lymphadenopathy). Rash usually occurs within the first 2 wk of therapy. Hypersensitivity syndrome usually occurs at 3–8 wk but may occur up to 12 wk after initiation of therapy. May lead to renal failure, rhabdomyolysis, or hepatic necrosis; may be fatal.
- **Fosphenytoin:** Monitor blood pressure, ECG, and respiratory function continuously during administration of fosphenytoin and throughout period when peak serum plasma occurs (10–20 min following infusion).
  - □ Observe patient for development of rash. Fosphenytoin should be discontinued at the first sign of skin reactions. Serious adverse reactions such as exfoliative, purpuric, or bullous rashes or the development of lupus erythematosus, Stevens-Johnson syndrome, or toxic epidermal necrolysis precludes further use of phenytoin or fosphenytoin. If less serious skin eruptions (measles-like or scarlatiniform) occur, fosphenytoin may be resumed after complete clearing of the rash. If rash reappears, further use of fosphenytoin or phenytoin should be avoided.
- ***Lab Test Considerations:*** *Phenytoin:* CBC and platelet count, serum calcium, albumin, urinalysis, and hepatic and thyroid function tests should be monitored prior to and monthly for the first several months, then periodically throughout therapy.
  - □ May cause increased serum alkaline phosphatase, GTT, and glucose levels.
  - □ Serum folate concentrations should be monitored periodically during prolonged therapy.
- ***Toxicity and Overdose:*** *Phenytoin:* Serum phenytoin levels should be routinely monitored. Therapeutic blood levels are 10–20 mcg/ml in patients with normal serum albumin and renal function. In patients with altered protein binding (neonates, patients with renal failure, hypoalbuminemia, acute trauma), free phenytoin serum concentrations should be monitored. Therapeutic serum free phenytoin levels are 0.8–2 mcg/ml.
  - □ Progressive signs and symptoms of phenytoin toxicity include nystagmus, ataxia, confusion, nausea, slurred speech, and dizziness.

POTENTIAL NURSING DIAGNOSES

- Injury, risk for (Indications).
- Oral mucous membrane, altered (Side Effects).
- Knowledge deficit, related to medication regimen (Patient/Family Teaching).

IMPLEMENTATION

- **General Info:** Implement seizure precautions.
  - □ When transferring from phenytoin to another anticonvulsant, dosage adjustments are made gradually over several weeks.
  - □ When substituting *fosphenytoin* for oral *phenytoin* therapy, the same total daily dose may

be given as a single dose. Unlike parenteral phenytoin, fosphenytoin may be given safely by the IM route.

- The anticonvulsant effect of fosphenytoin is not immediate. Additional measures (including parenteral benzodiazepines) are usually required in the immediate management of status epilepticus. Loading dosage of *fosphenytoin* should be followed with the institution of maintenance anticonvulsant therapy.
- **PO:** Administer with or immediately after meals to minimize GI irritation. Shake liquid preparations well before pouring. Use a calibrated measuring device for accurate dosage. Chewable tablets must be crushed or chewed well before swallowing. Capsules may be opened and mixed with food or fluids for patients with difficulty swallowing. To prevent direct contact of alkaline drug with mucosa, have patient swallow a liquid first, follow with mixture of medication, then follow with a full glass of water or milk or with food.
- If patient is receiving enteral tube feedings, 2 hr should elapse between feeding and phenytoin administration. If phenytoin is administered via nasogastric tube, flush tube with 2–4 oz water before and after administration.
- Do not interchange chewable phenytoin tablets with phenytoin sodium capsules, as they are not bioequivalent.
- Capsules labeled "extended" may be used for once-a-day dosage (Dilantin Kapseals only); those labeled "prompt" may result in toxic serum levels if used for once-a-day dosage.

Phenytoin

- **IV:** Slight yellow color will not alter solution potency. If refrigerated, may form precipitate, which dissolves after warming to room temperature. Discard solution that is not clear.
- To prevent precipitation and minimize local venous irritation, follow infusion with 0.9% NaCl. Avoid extravasation; phenytoin is caustic to tissues.
- **Direct IV:** Administer at a rate not to exceed 50 mg over 1 min (25 mg/min [may be as low as 5–10 mg/min] in patients who may develop hypotension, patients who are on sympathomimetic medication, patients with cardiovascular disease, or geriatric patients; 1–3 mg/kg/min in neonates). Rapid administration may result in severe hypotension, cardiovascular collapse, or CNS depression.
- **Intermittent Infusion:** Administer by mixing with no more than 50 ml of 0.9% NaCl in a concentration of 1–10 mg/ml. Administer immediately following admixture. Use tubing with a 0.45- to 0.22-micron in-line filter.
- ***Rate:*** Complete infusion within 1 hr at a rate not to exceed 50 mg/min. Monitor cardiac function and blood pressure throughout infusion.
- **Y-Site Compatibility:** ▪ esmolol ▪ famotidine ▪ fluconazole ▪ foscarnet ▪ tacrolimus.
- **Y-Site Incompatibility:** ▪ ciprofloxacin ▪ diltiazem ▪ enalaprilat ▪ hydromorphone ▪ potassium chloride ▪ sufentanil ▪ vitamin B complex with C.
- **Additive Incompatibility:** ▪ Do not admix with other solutions or medications, especially dextrose, as precipitation will occur.

Fosphenytoin

- **Direct IV:** Dilute fosphenytoin in D5W or 0.9% NaCl for a concentration of 1.5–25 mg PE/kg. May be refrigerated for up to 48 hours.
- ***Rate:*** Administer at a rate of <150 mg PE/min to minimize risk of hypotension.
- **Additive Incompatibility:** ▪ Information unavailable. Do not admix with other solutions or medications.

PATIENT/FAMILY TEACHING

- **General Info:** May cause drowsiness or dizziness. Caution patient to avoid driving or other activities requiring alertness until response to medication is known. Do not resume driving until physician gives clearance based on control of seizure disorder.
- Advise patient to carry identification describing disease process and medication regimen at all times.
- Advise patient to notify health care professional if skin rash, severe nausea or vomiting, drowsiness, slurred speech, unsteady gait, swollen glands, bleeding or tender gums, yellow skin or eyes, joint pain, fever, sore throat, unusual bleeding or bruising, or persistent headache occurs.
- Emphasize the importance of routine exams to monitor progress. Patient should have routine physical exams, especially monitoring skin and lymph nodes, and EEG testing.

- **Phenytoin:** Instruct patient to take medication exactly as directed, at the same time each day. If a dose is missed from a once-a-day schedule, take as soon as possible and return to regular dosing schedule. If taking several doses a day, take missed dose as soon as possible within 4 hr of next scheduled dose; do not double doses. Consult health care professional if doses are missed for 2 consecutive days. Abrupt withdrawal may lead to status epilepticus.
- Caution patient to avoid taking alcohol or OTC medications concurrently with phenytoin without consulting health care professional.
- Instruct patient on importance of maintaining good dental hygiene and seeing dentist frequently for teeth cleaning to prevent tenderness, bleeding, and gingival hyperplasia. Institution of oral hygiene program within 10 days of initiation of phenytoin therapy may minimize growth rate and severity of gingival enlargement. Patients under 23 yr of age and those taking doses >500 mg/day are at increased risk for gingival hyperplasia.
- Advise patient that brands of phenytoin may not be equivalent. Check with health care professional if brand or dosage form is changed.
- Inform patient that phenytoin may color urine pink, red, or reddish brown, but color change is not significant.
- Advise diabetic patients to monitor blood glucose carefully and to notify health care professional of significant changes.
- Instruct patient to notify health care professional of medication regimen prior to treatment or surgery.
- Advise patient not to take phenytoin within 2–3 hr of antacids or antidiarrheals.
- Advise female patients to use an additional nonhormonal method of contraception during therapy and until next menstrual period. Instruct patient to notify health care professional if pregnancy is planned or suspected.

EVALUATION

Effectiveness of therapy can be demonstrated by: ▪ Decrease or cessation of seizures without excessive sedation ▪ Suppression of arrhythmias ▪ Relief of pain due to neuralgia.

PHOSPHATE/BIPHOSPHATE

(**foss**-fate/bye-**foss**-fate)

Fleet Enema, Phospho-Soda

CLASSIFICATION(S):

Laxative (saline)

Pregnancy Category UK

INDICATIONS

▪ Preparation of the bowel prior to surgery or radiologic studies ▪ Intermittent treatment of chronic constipation.

ACTION

▪ Osmotically active in the lumen of the GI tract ▪ Produces laxative effect by causing water retention and stimulation of peristalsis ▪ Stimulates motility and inhibits fluid and electrolyte absorption from the small intestine. **Therapeutic Effects:** ▪ Relief of constipation ▪ Emptying of the bowel.

PHARMACOKINETICS

Absorption: 1–20% of rectally administered sodium and phosphate may be absorbed.
Distribution: UK.
Metabolism and Excretion: Excreted by the kidneys.
Half-life: UK.

CONTRAINDICATIONS AND PRECAUTIONS

Contraindicated in: ▪ Abdominal pain, nausea, or vomiting, especially when associated with fever or other signs of an acute abdomen ▪ Renal disease ▪ Severe cardiac disease ▪ Intestinal obstruction ▪ Pregnancy (at term).
Use Cautiously in: ▪ Excessive or chronic use (may lead to dependence) ▪ Pregnancy (may cause sodium retention and edema).

ADVERSE REACTIONS AND SIDE EFFECTS*

GI: <u>cramping</u>, <u>nausea</u>.
F and E: hyperphosphatemia, hypocalcemia, sodium retention.

***CAPITALS indicate life-threatening; <u>underlines</u> indicate most frequent.**

INTERACTIONS

Drug-Drug: ▪ None significant.

ROUTE AND DOSAGE

Each Fleet Enema contains 4.4 g sodium/118 ml. Each 20 ml of Fleet Phospho-Soda oral solution contains 96.4 mEq sodium.

- **PO (Adults):** 20–30 ml Phospho-Soda.
- **PO (Children):** 5–15 ml Phospho-Soda.
- **Rect (Adults and Children >12 yr):** 118 ml Fleet Enema.
- **Rect (Children >2 yr):** ½ of the adult dose.

AVAILABILITY

▪ ***Oral solution:*** 18 g sodium phosphate and 48 g sodium biphosphate/100 ml in 45-, 90-, and 237-ml containers[OTC] ▪ ***Enema:*** 7 g sodium phosphate and 19 g sodium biphosphate/118 ml in 67.5- and 133-ml containers[OTC].

TIME/ACTION PROFILE (laxative effect)

	ONSET	PEAK	DURATION
PO	0.5–3 hr	UK	UK
Rect	2–5 min	UK	UK

NURSING IMPLICATIONS

ASSESSMENT

- ▫ Assess patient for fever, abdominal distention, presence of bowel sounds, and usual pattern of bowel function.
- ▫ Assess color, consistency, and amount of stool produced.
- ▪ ***Lab Test Considerations:*** May cause increased serum sodium and phosphorus levels, decreased serum calcium levels, and acidosis.

POTENTIAL NURSING DIAGNOSES

- Constipation (Indications).
- Knowledge deficit, related to medication regimen (Patient/Family Teaching).

IMPLEMENTATION

- **General Info:** Do not administer at bedtime or late in the day.
- **PO:** Administer on an empty stomach for more rapid results. Mix dose in at least ½ glass cold water. May be followed by carbonated beverage or fruit juice to improve flavor.
- **Rect:** Position patient on left side with knee slightly flexed. Insert prelubricated tip about 2 in. into rectum, aiming toward the umbilicus. Gently squeeze bottle until empty. Discontinue if resistance is met, as perforation may occur if contents are forced into rectum.

PATIENT/FAMILY TEACHING

- ▫ Advise patient that laxatives should be used only for short-term therapy. Long-term therapy may cause electrolyte imbalance and dependence.
- ▫ Caution patient on sodium restriction that this product has a high sodium content.
- ▫ Advise patient not to take oral form of this medication within 2 hr of other medications.
- ▫ Encourage patient to use other forms of bowel regulation, such as increasing bulk in the diet, fluid intake, and mobility. Normal bowel habits may vary from 3 times/day to 3 times/wk.
- ▫ Advise patient to notify health care professional if unrelieved constipation, rectal bleeding, or symptoms of electrolyte imbalance (muscle cramps or pain, weakness, dizziness, and so forth) occur.

EVALUATION

Effectiveness of therapy can be demonstrated by: ▪ Soft, formed bowel movement ▪ Evacuation of the bowel.

PHYTONADIONE

(fye-toe-na-**dye**-one)
AquaMEPHYTON, Mephyton, vitamin K_1

CLASSIFICATION(S):
Vitamin (fat-soluble)

Pregnancy Category UK

INDICATIONS

▪ Prevention and treatment of hypoprothrombinemia, which may be associated with: ▫ Excessive doses of oral anticoagulants ▫ Salicylates ▫ Certain anti-infective agents ▫ Nutritional deficiencies ▫ Prolonged total parenteral nutrition ▪ Prevention of hemorrhagic disease of the newborn.

ACTION

▪ Required for hepatic synthesis of blood coagulation factors II (prothrombin), VII, IX, and X.

Therapeutic Effects: ▪ Prevention of bleeding due to hypoprothrombinemia.

PHARMACOKINETICS

Absorption: Well absorbed following oral, IM, or SC administration. Oral absorption requires presence of bile salts. Some vitamin K is produced by bacteria in the GI tract.
Distribution: Crosses the placenta; does not enter breast milk.
Metabolism and Excretion: Rapidly metabolized by the liver.
Half-life: UK.

CONTRAINDICATIONS AND PRECAUTIONS

Contraindicated in: ▪ Hypersensitivity ▪ Hypersensitivity or intolerance to benzyl alcohol (injection only).
Use Cautiously in: ▪ Impaired liver function.

ADVERSE REACTIONS AND SIDE EFFECTS

GI: gastric upset, unusual taste.
Derm: flushing, rash, urticaria.
Hemat: hemolytic anemia.
Local: erythema, pain at injection site, swelling.
Misc: allergic reactions, hyperbilirubinemia (large doses in very premature infants), kernicterus.

INTERACTIONS

Drug-Drug: ▪ Large doses will counteract the effect of **warfarin** ▪ Large doses of **salicylates** or broad-spectrum **anti-infectives** may increase vitamin K requirements ▪ **Cholestyramine, colestipol, mineral oil,** and **sucralfate** may decrease vitamin K absorption from the GI tract.

ROUTE AND DOSAGE

IV use of phytonadione should be reserved for emergencies.

❑ Treatment of Hypoprothrombinemia

- **PO, SC, IM, IV (Adults):** 2.5–10 mg; repeat PO in 12–48 hr if necessary or in 6–8 hr after parenteral dose (up to 25–50 mg; smaller doses have been used to partially reverse the effects of warfarin).
- **PO, SC, IM, IV (Children):** 5–10 mg.
- **PO, IM, SC, IV (Infants):** 1–2 mg.

❑ Prevention of Hypoprothrombinemia during Total Parenteral Nutrition

- **IM, IV (Adults):** 5–10 mg once weekly.
- **IM, IV (Children):** 2–5 mg once weekly.

❑ Prevention of Hemorrhagic Disease of Newborn

- **IM (Neonates):** 0.5–1 mg, within 1 hr of birth. May be repeated in 2–3 wk if mother received previous anticonvulsant/anticoagulant/anti-infective/antitubercular therapy. 1–5 mg may be given IM to mother 12–24 hr before delivery.

❑ Treatment of Hemorrhagic Disease of Newborn

- **IM, SC (Neonates):** 1 mg.

AVAILABILITY

▪ ***Tablets:*** 5 mg[Rx] ▪ ***Injection (aqueous colloid solution):*** 2 mg/ml in 0.5-ml ampules[Rx] ▪ ***Injection (aqueous dispersion):*** 10 mg/ml in 1-ml ampules and 2.5- and 5-ml vials[Rx].

TIME/ACTION PROFILE

	ONSET	PEAK*	DURATION†
PO	6–12 hr	UK	UK
IM, SC	1–2 hr	3–6 hr	12–14 hr
IV	1–2 hr	3–6 hr	12 hr

*Control of hemorrhage.
†Normal prothrombin time achieved.

NURSING IMPLICATIONS

ASSESSMENT

- ▫ Monitor for frank and occult bleeding (guaiac stools, Hematest urine and emesis). Monitor pulse and blood pressure frequently; notify physician immediately if symptoms of internal bleeding or hypovolemic shock develop. Inform all personnel of patient's bleeding tendency to prevent further trauma. Apply pressure to all venipuncture sites for at least 5 min; avoid unnecessary IM injections.
- ***Lab Test Considerations:*** Prothrombin time (PT) should be monitored prior to and throughout vitamin K therapy to determine response to and need for further therapy.

POTENTIAL NURSING DIAGNOSES

- Nutrition, altered, less than body requirements (Indications).
- Tissue perfusion, altered (Indications).

- Knowledge deficit, related to medication regimen (Patient/Family Teaching).

IMPLEMENTATION

- **General Info:** The parenteral route is preferred for phytonadione therapy but, because of severe hypersensitivity reactions, IV vitamin K is not recommended.
  - Administration of whole blood or plasma may also be required in severe bleeding because of the delayed onset of this medication.
  - Phytonadione is an antidote for warfarin overdose but does not counteract the anticoagulant activity of heparin.
- **Direct IV:** May be administered undiluted.
- ***Rate:*** If IV administration is unavoidable, administer very slowly, at a rate not to exceed 1 mg/min.
- **Intermittent Infusion:** May also be diluted in 0.9% NaCl, D5W, or D5/0.9% NaCl.
- ***Rate:*** If IV administration is unavoidable, administer very slowly, at a rate not to exceed 1 mg/min.
- **Y-Site Compatibility:** ▪ ampicillin ▪ epinephrine ▪ famotidine ▪ heparin ▪ hydrocortisone sodium succinate ▪ potassium chloride ▪ tolazoline ▪ vitamin B complex with C.
- **Y-Site Incompatibility:** ▪ dobutamine.

PATIENT/FAMILY TEACHING

- Instruct patient to take this medication as ordered. If a dose is missed, take as soon as remembered unless almost time for next dose. Notify health care professional of missed doses.
- Cooking does not destroy substantial amounts of vitamin K. Patient should not drastically alter diet while taking vitamin K. See Appendix K for foods high in vitamin K.
- Caution patient to avoid IM injections and activities leading to injury. Use a soft toothbrush, do not floss, and shave with an electric razor until coagulation defect is corrected.
- Advise patient to report any symptoms of unusual bleeding or bruising (bleeding gums; nosebleed; black, tarry stools; hematuria; excessive menstrual flow).
- Patients receiving vitamin K therapy should be cautioned not to take OTC medications without advice of health care professional.
- Advise patient to inform health care professional of medication regimen prior to treatment or surgery.
- Advise patient to carry identification describing disease process at all times.
- Emphasize the importance of frequent lab tests to monitor coagulation factors.

EVALUATION

Effectiveness of therapy can be demonstrated by: ▪ Prevention of spontaneous bleeding or cessation of bleeding in patients with hypoprothrombinemia secondary to impaired intestinal absorption or oral anticoagulant, salicylate, or antibiotic therapy ▪ Prevention of hemorrhagic disease in the newborn.

PILOCARPINE (oral)*

(pye-loe-**kar**-peen)

Salagen

CLASSIFICATION(S):

Cholinergic (direct-acting)

Pregnancy Category C

*For ophthalmic use of pilocarpine, see ophthalmics table in Appendix O.

INDICATIONS

▪ Management of xerostomia, which may occur as a consequence of radiation therapy for cancer of the head and neck.

ACTION

▪ Stimulates cholinergic receptors, resulting in primarily muscarinic action, including stimulation of exocrine glands ▪ Other effects include: □ Increased sweating, gastric secretions □ Increased bronchial secretions □ Increased tone and motility of the urinary tract, gallbladder, and biliary duct smooth muscle. **Therapeutic Effects:** ▪ Increased salivary gland secretion.

PHARMACOKINETICS

Absorption: Well absorbed following oral administration.

Distribution: UK.

Metabolism and Excretion: Inactivated at neuronal synapses and in plasma. Some unchanged pilocarpine and metabolites are excreted in urine.

Half-life: *After 5-mg dose for 2 days*—0.8 hr; *after 10-mg dose for 2 days*—1.3 hr.

CONTRAINDICATIONS AND PRECAUTIONS

Contraindicated in: ▪ Hypersensitivity ▪ Uncontrolled asthma ▪ Angle-closure glaucoma ▪ Iritis. **Use Cautiously in:** ▪ History of pulmonary disease (asthma, bronchitis, or chronic obstructive pulmonary disease) ▪ Biliary tract disease or cholelithiasis ▪ Cardiovascular disease ▪ Retinal disease ▪ Nephrolithiasis ▪ History of psychiatric or cognitive disorders ▪ Pregnancy, lactation, or children (safety not established).

ADVERSE REACTIONS AND SIDE EFFECTS*

CNS: dizziness, headache, weakness.
EENT: amblyopia, epistaxis, rhinitis.
CV: edema, hypertension, tachycardia.
GI: nausea, vomiting, dyspepsia, dysphagia.
GU: urinary frequency.
Derm: flushing, sweating.
Neuro: tremors.
Misc: chills, voice change.

INTERACTIONS

Drug-Drug: ▪ Concurrent use of **anticholinergics** will decrease the effectiveness of pilocarpine ▪ Concurrent use of **bethanechol** or **ophthalmic cholinergics** may result in additive cholinergic effects ▪ Concurrent use with **beta-adrenergic blocking agents** may increase the risk of adverse cardiovascular reactions (conduction disturbances).

ROUTE AND DOSAGE

- **PO (Adults):** 5 mg 3 times daily; may be increased to 10 mg 3 times daily.

AVAILABILITY

- ***Tablets:*** 5 mg[Rx].

TIME/ACTION PROFILE

	ONSET	PEAK	DURATION
PO	20 min	1 hr	3–5 hr

NURSING IMPLICATIONS

ASSESSMENT

- ☐ Assess oral mucosa for dryness and ulceration periodically throughout therapy.

POTENTIAL NURSING DIAGNOSES

- Oral mucous membrane, altered (Indications).
- Knowledge deficit, related to medication regimen (Patient/Family Teaching).

IMPLEMENTATION

- **PO:** Use lowest dose that is tolerated and effective for maintenance.

PATIENT/FAMILY TEACHING

- ☐ Instruct patient to take medication exactly as directed.
- ☐ Caution patient that pilocarpine may cause visual changes, especially at night; avoid driving or other activities requiring alertness until effects of medication are known.
- ☐ Advise patient to drink adequate daily fluids (1500–2000 ml/day), especially if sweating occurs. Less than adequate fluid intake may lead to dehydration.

EVALUATION

Effectiveness of therapy can be demonstrated by: ▪ Increased salivary gland secretion in patients with xerostomia.

PINDOLOL
(**pin**-doe-lole)
{Novo-Pindol}, {Syn-Pindolol}, Visken

CLASSIFICATION(S):
Antihypertensive agent, Beta-adrenergic blocking agent (nonselective)

Pregnancy Category B

INDICATIONS

- Management of hypertension. **Unlabeled Uses:** ▪ Management of angina pectoris.

ACTION

- Blocks stimulation of $beta_1$ (myocardial) and $beta_2$ (pulmonary, vascular, and uterine) -adrenergic receptor sites ▪ Has intrinsic sympathomimetic activity (ISA), which may produce less bradycardia. **Therapeutic Effects:** ▪ Decreased heart rate and blood pressure.

*CAPITALS indicate life-threatening; underlines indicate most frequent.
{} = Available in Canada only.

PHARMACOKINETICS

Absorption: Well absorbed following oral administration.
Distribution: Moderate CNS penetration. Crosses the placenta; enters breast milk.
Metabolism and Excretion: Partially metabolized by the liver; 50% excreted unchanged by the kidneys.
Half-life: 3–4 hr.

CONTRAINDICATIONS AND PRECAUTIONS

Contraindicated in: ▪ Uncompensated congestive heart failure ▪ Pulmonary edema ▪ Cardiogenic shock ▪ Bradycardia or heart block.
Use Cautiously in: ▪ Renal impairment ▪ Hepatic impairment ▪ Geriatric patients (increased sensitivity to beta-adrenergic blockers; initial dosage reduction recommended) ▪ Pulmonary disease (including asthma) ▪ Diabetes mellitus (may mask signs of hypoglycemia) ▪ Thyrotoxicosis (may mask symptoms) ▪ Patients with a history of severe allergic reactions (intensity of reactions may be increased) ▪ Pregnancy, lactation, or children (safety not established; may cause fetal/neonatal bradycardia, hypotension, hypoglycemia, or respiratory depression).

ADVERSE REACTIONS AND SIDE EFFECTS*

CNS: fatigue, weakness, anxiety, depression, dizziness, drowsiness, insomnia, memory loss, mental status changes, nervousness, nightmares.
EENT: blurred vision, dry eyes, nasal stuffiness.
Resp: bronchospasm, wheezing.
CV: ARRHYTHMIAS, BRADYCARDIA, CONGESTIVE HEART FAILURE, PULMONARY EDEMA, orthostatic hypotension, peripheral vasoconstriction.
GI: constipation, diarrhea, nausea.
GU: impotence, decreased libido.
Derm: itching, rashes.
Endo: hyperglycemia, hypoglycemia.
MS: arthralgia, back pain, muscle cramps.
Neuro: paresthesia.

INTERACTIONS

Drug-Drug: ▪ **General anesthesia, IV phenytoin,** and **verapamil** may cause additive myocardial depression ▪ Additive bradycardia may occur with **digitalis glycosides** ▪ Additive hypotension may occur with other **antihypertensives,** acute ingestion of **alcohol,** or **nitrates** ▪ Concurrent use with **amphetamines, cocaine, ephedrine, epinephrine, norepinephrine, phenylephrine,** or **pseudoephedrine** may result in unopposed alpha-adrenergic stimulation (excessive hypertension, bradycardia) ▪ Concurrent **thyroid** administration may decrease effectiveness ▪ May alter the effectiveness of **insulin** or **oral hypoglycemic agents** (dosage adjustments may be necessary) ▪ May decrease the effectiveness of **beta-adrenergic bronchodilators** and **theophylline** ▪ May decrease the beneficial beta$_1$ cardiovascular effects of **dopamine** or **dobutamine** ▪ Use cautiously within 14 days of **MAO inhibitor** therapy (may result in hypertension) ▪ Concurrent **NSAIDs** may decrease antihypertensive action.

ROUTE AND DOSAGE

- **PO (Adults):** 5 mg twice daily initially; may be increased by 10 mg/day q 2–3 wk as needed (up to 45–60 mg/day).

AVAILABILITY

▪ ***Tablets:*** 5 mg^{Rx}, 10 mg^{Rx}, {15 mg^{Rx}}.

TIME/ACTION PROFILE (cardiovascular effects)

	ONSET	PEAK	DURATION
Pindolol–PO	7 days	2 wk	8–24 hr

NURSING IMPLICATIONS

ASSESSMENT

- **General Info:** Monitor blood pressure and pulse frequently during dosage adjustment period and periodically throughout therapy. Assess for orthostatic hypotension when assisting patient up from supine position.
- □ Monitor intake and output ratios and daily weight. Assess patient routinely for evidence of fluid overload (peripheral edema, dyspnea, rales/crackles, fatigue, weight gain, jugular venous distention).
- **Angina:** Assess frequency and characteristics of anginal attacks periodically throughout therapy.
- ***Lab Test Considerations:*** May cause increased BUN, serum lipoprotein, potassium, triglyceride, and uric acid levels.

***CAPITALS indicate life-threatening; underlines indicate most frequent.**

□ May cause increased ANA titers.
□ May cause increase in blood glucose levels.

POTENTIAL NURSING DIAGNOSES

- Cardiac output, decreased (Side Effects).
- Knowledge deficit, related to medication regimen (Patient/Family Teaching).
- Noncompliance, related to medication regimen (Patient/Family Teaching).

IMPLEMENTATION

- **PO:** Take apical pulse prior to administering. If <50 bpm or if arrhythmia occurs, withhold medication and notify physician or other health care professional.

□ May be administered with food or on an empty stomach.

PATIENT/FAMILY TEACHING

- **General Info:** Instruct patient to take medication exactly as directed, at the same time each day, even if feeling well; do not skip or double up on missed doses. If a dose is missed, it should be taken as soon as possible up to 4 hr before next dose. Abrupt withdrawal may precipitate life-threatening arrhythmias, hypertension, or myocardial ischemia.

□ Advise patient to make sure enough medication is available for weekends, holidays, and vacations. A written prescription may be kept in wallet in case of emergency.
□ Teach patient and family how to check pulse and blood pressure. Instruct them to check pulse daily and blood pressure biweekly. Advise patient to hold dose and contact health care professional if pulse is <50 bpm or blood pressure changes significantly.
□ May cause drowsiness or dizziness. Caution patients to avoid driving or other activities that require alertness until response to the drug is known.
□ Advise patients to change positions slowly to minimize orthostatic hypotension, especially during initiation of therapy or when dose is increased.
□ Caution patient that this medication may increase sensitivity to cold.
□ Instruct patient to consult health care professional before taking any OTC medications, especially cold preparations, concurrently with this medication.
□ Diabetics should closely monitor blood sugar, especially if weakness, malaise, irritability, or fatigue occurs. Medication may mask tachycardia and increased blood pressure as signs of hypoglycemia, but dizziness and sweating may still occur.
□ Advise patient to notify health care professional if slow pulse, difficulty breathing, wheezing, cold hands and feet, dizziness, confusion, depression, rash, fever, sore throat, unusual bleeding or bruising occurs.
□ Instruct patient to inform health care professional of medication regimen prior to treatment or surgery.
□ Advise patient to carry identification describing disease process and medication regimen at all times.

- **Hypertension:** Reinforce the need to continue additional therapies for hypertension (weight loss, sodium restriction, stress reduction, regular exercise, moderation of alcohol consumption, and smoking cessation). Medication controls but does not cure hypertension.
- **Angina:** Caution patient to avoid overexertion with decrease in chest pain.

EVALUATION

Effectiveness of therapy can be demonstrated by: ▪ Decrease in blood pressure ▪ Reduction in frequency of anginal attacks □ Increase in activity tolerance.

PIPERACILLIN

(pi-**per**-a-sill-in)
Pipracil

PIPERACILLIN/TAZOBACTAM

(pi-**per**-a-sill-in/tay-zoe-**bak**-tam)
Zosyn

CLASSIFICATION(S):
Anti-infectives (extended-spectrum penicillin)

Pregnancy Category B

INDICATIONS

- ***Piperacillin:*** Treatment of serious infections due to susceptible organisms, including: □ Skin and skin structure infections □ Bone and joint infections ▫ Septicemia ▫ Respiratory tract infections ▫ Intra-abdominal infections ▫ Gynecologic and urinary tract infections ▪ Combination with an aminoglycoside may be synergistic against *Pseudomonas* ▪ Has been combined with other antibiotics in the treatment of infections in immunosuppressed patients ▪ Perioperative prophylactic anti-infective in abdominal, genitourinary, and head and neck surgery ▪ ***Piperacillin/Tazobactam:*** ▫ Appendicitis ▫ Skin and skin structure infections ▫ Gynecologic infections ▫ Pneumonia caused by piperacillin-resistant, beta-lactamase–producing bacteria.

ACTION

▪ ***Piperacillin:*** Binds to bacterial cell wall membrane, causing cell death. Spectrum is extended when compared with other penicillins ▪ ***Tazobactam:*** Inhibits beta-lactamase, an enzyme that can destroy penicillins. **Therapeutic Effects:** ▪ Death of susceptible bacteria. **Spectrum:** ▪ ***Piperacillin:*** Spectrum similar to penicillin but greatly extended, including several important gram-negative aerobic pathogens, notably ▫ *Pseudomonas aeruginosa* ▫ *Escherichia coli* ▫ *Proteus mirabilis* ▫ *Providencia rettgeri* ▫ *Neisseria gonorrhoeae* ▪ Also active against some anaerobic bacteria, including ▫ *Bacteroides* ▪ Not active against penicillinase-producing staphylococci or beta-lactamase–producing ▫ Enterobacteriaceae ▪ ***Piperacillin/Tazobactam:*** Active against piperacillin-resistant, beta-lactamase–producing ▫ *Bacteroides fragilis* ▫ *E. coli* ▫ *Staphylococcus aureus* ▫ *Haemophilus influenzae*.

PHARMACOKINETICS

Absorption: Piperacillin is well absorbed (80%) from IM sites.

Distribution: Widely distributed. Enter CSF well only when meninges are inflamed. Cross the placenta and enter breast milk in low concentrations.

Metabolism and Excretion: Piperacillin is mostly (90%) excreted unchanged by the kidneys; 10% excreted in bile. Tazobactam is 80% renally excreted.

Half-life: 0.7–1.2 hr.

CONTRAINDICATIONS AND PRECAUTIONS

Contraindicated in: ▪ Hypersensitivity to penicillins or tazobactam (cross-sensitivity with cephalosporins may occur).

Use Cautiously in: ▪ Renal impairment (dosage reduction or increased interval recommended if CCr <40 ml/min) ▪ Sodium restriction ▪ Pregnancy and lactation (safety not established).

ADVERSE REACTIONS AND SIDE EFFECTS*

CNS: SEIZURES (↑ doses), confusion, lethargy.

CV: arrhythmias, congestive heart failure.

GI: pseudomembranous colitis, diarrhea, drug-induced hepatitis, nausea.

GU: hematuria (children only), interstitial nephritis.

Derm: rashes, urticaria.

F and E: hypokalemia, hypernatremia.

Hemat: bleeding, blood dyscrasias, increased bleeding time.

Local: pain at IM site, phlebitis at IV site.

Metab: metabolic alkalosis.

Misc: hypersensitivity reactions, including ANAPHYLAXIS and SERUM SICKNESS, superinfection.

INTERACTIONS

Drug-Drug: ▪ **Probenecid** decreases renal excretion and increases blood levels ▪ May alter excretion of **lithium** ▪ **Diuretics, glucocorticoids**, or **amphotericin B** may increase the risk of hypokalemia ▪ Additive risk of hepatotoxicity with other **hepatotoxic agents** ▪ May decrease the half-life of **aminoglycosides** in patients with renal impairment.

ROUTE AND DOSAGE

Contains 1.85 mEq sodium/g of piperacillin.

▫ Piperacillin

- **IM, IV (Adults):** *Most infections*—3–4 g q 4–6 hr (up to 24 g/day). *Complicated urinary tract infections*—3–4 g q 6–8 hr. *Uncomplicated urinary tract infections*—1.5–2 g q 6 hr or 3–4 g q 12 hr.
- **IM, IV (Neonates ≥2 kg):** *Meningitis*—50 mg/kg q 8 hr for the first 7 days of life, then 50 mg/kg q 6 hr.

***CAPITALS indicate life-threatening; underlines indicate most frequent.**

- **IM, IV (Neonates <2 kg):** *Meningitis*—50 mg/kg q 12 hr for the first 7 days of life, then 50 mg/kg q 8 hr.

❑ **Piperacillin/Tazobactam**

- **IV (Adults):** 3–4 g piperacillin with 0.375–0.5 g tazobactam q 6–8 hr.

AVAILABILITY

❑ **Piperacillin**

- ***Powder for injection:*** 2-, 3-, and 4-g vials and infusion bottles[Rx], 40-g bulk vials[Rx].

❑ **Piperacillin/Tazobactam**

- ***Powder for injection:*** 2 g piperacillin/0.25-g tazobactam vials[Rx], 3 g piperacillin/0.375-g tazobactam vials[Rx], 4 g piperacillin/0.5-g tazobactam vials[Rx].

TIME/ACTION PROFILE (piperacillin blood levels)

	ONSET	PEAK	DURATION
IM	rapid	30–50 min	4–6 hr
IV	rapid	end of infusion	4–6 hr

NURSING IMPLICATIONS

ASSESSMENT

- Assess patient for infection (vital signs; appearance of wound, sputum, urine, and stool; WBC) at beginning of and throughout therapy.
- Obtain a history before initiating therapy to determine previous use of and reactions to penicillins or cephalosporins. Persons with a negative history of penicillin sensitivity may still have an allergic response.
- Obtain specimens for culture and sensitivity prior to initiating therapy. First dose may be given before receiving results.
- Observe patient for signs and symptoms of anaphylaxis (rash, pruritus, laryngeal edema, wheezing). Discontinue the drug and notify the physician or other health care professional immediately if these occur. Keep epinephrine, an antihistamine, and resuscitation equipment close by in the event of an anaphylactic reaction.
- ***Lab Test Considerations:*** Renal and hepatic function, CBC, serum potassium, and bleeding times should be evaluated prior to and routinely throughout therapy.
- May cause positive direct Coombs' test results.
- May cause elevated BUN, creatinine, AST, ALT, serum bilirubin, alkaline phosphatase, and LDH.
- May cause leukopenia and neutropenia, especially with prolonged therapy or hepatic impairment.
- May cause prolonged prothrombin and partial thromboplastin time.
- *Piperacillin* may cause elevated serum sodium and decreased serum potassium concentrations.
- *Piperacillin/tazobactam* may also cause decreased hemoglobin and hematocrit and thrombocytopenia, eosinophilia, leukopenia, and neutropenia. It also may cause proteinuria; hematuria; pyuria; hyperglycemia; decreases in total protein or albumin; and abnormalities in sodium, potassium, and calcium levels.

POTENTIAL NURSING DIAGNOSES

- Infection, risk for (Indications, Side Effects).
- Knowledge deficit, related to medication regimen (Patient/Family Teaching).

IMPLEMENTATION

- **IM:** To constitute for IM use, add 4 ml of sterile water, bacteriostatic water, 0.9% NaCl for injection, or 0.5 or 1% lidocaine hydrochloride injection (without epinephrine) to each 2-g vial, 6 ml to each 3-g vial, and 8 ml to each 4-g vial for a concentration of 1 g/2.5 ml.
- Inject deep into a well-developed muscle mass and massage well. IM injections should not exceed 2 g at each site.

❑ **Piperacillin**

- **IV:** The initial reconstitution for IV use is made with at least 5 ml of sterile water for injection, 0.9% NaCl, or bacteriostatic water. Shake well until dissolved. Reconstituted solution is stable for 24 hr at room temperature and 7 days if refrigerated.
- Change IV sites every 48 hr to prevent phlebitis.
- **Direct IV:** Inject slowly, over 3–5 min, to minimize vein irritation.
- **Intermittent Infusion:** Dilute in at least 50 ml of 0.9% NaCl, D5W, D5/0.9% NaCl, or lactated Ringer's solution.
- ***Rate:*** Administer over 20–30 min for adults and 30 min for children.
- **Y-Site Compatibility:** ▪ acyclovir ▪ amifos-

tine ▪ aztreonam ▪ ciprofloxacin ▪ cyclophosphamide ▪ diltiazem ▪ enalaprilat ▪ esmolol ▪ famotidine ▪ fludarabine ▪ foscarnet ▪ gallium nitrate ▪ heparin ▪ hydromorphone ▪ labetalol ▪ lorazepam ▪ magnesium sulfate ▪ melphalan ▪ meperidine ▪ midazolam ▪ morphine ▪ perphenazine ▪ ranitidine ▪ tacrolimus ▪ teniposide ▪ theophylline ▪ thiotepa ▪ verapamil ▪ zidovudine.

- **Y-Site Incompatibility:** ▪ filgrastim ▪ fluconazole ▪ ondansetron ▪ sargramostim ▪ vinorelbine. If aminoglycosides and penicillins must be administered concurrently, administer in separate sites at least 1 hr apart.

❑ **Piperacillin/Tazobactam**

- **Intermittent Infusion:** Reconstitute with 5 ml of 0.9% NaCl, sterile or bacteriostatic water for injection, or D5W. Do not use lactated Ringer's solution—incompatible. Shake well until dissolved. Dilute further in at least 50 ml of diluent. Discard any unused solution after 24 hr at room temperature or 48 hr if refrigerated.
- ***Rate:*** Administer over at least 30 min.
- **Y-Site Compatibility:** ▪ aminophylline ▪ aztreonam ▪ bleomycin ▪ bumetanide ▪ buprenorphine ▪ butorphanol ▪ calcium gluconate ▪ carboplatin ▪ carmustine ▪ cefepime ▪ cimetidine ▪ clindamycin ▪ cyclophosphamide ▪ cytarabine ▪ dexamethasone ▪ diphenhydramine ▪ dopamine ▪ enalaprilat ▪ etoposide ▪ floxuridine ▪ fluconazole ▪ fludarabine ▪ fluorouracil ▪ furosemide ▪ gallium nitrate ▪ heparin ▪ hydrocortisone ▪ hydromorphone ▪ ifosfamide ▪ leucovorin calcium ▪ lorazepam ▪ magnesium sulfate ▪ mannitol ▪ meperidine ▪ mesna ▪ methotrexate ▪ methylprednisolone sodium succinate ▪ metoclopramide ▪ metronidazole ▪ morphine ▪ ondansetron ▪ plicamycin ▪ potassium chloride ▪ ranitidine ▪ sargramostim ▪ sodium bicarbonate ▪ thiotepa ▪ trimethoprim/sulfamethoxazole ▪ vinblastine ▪ vincristine ▪ zidovudine.
- **Y-Site Incompatibility:** ▪ acyclovir ▪ amphotericin B ▪ chlorpromazine ▪ cisplatin ▪ dacarbazine ▪ daunorubicin ▪ dobutamine ▪ doxorubicin ▪ doxycycline ▪ droperidol ▪ famotidine ▪ ganciclovir ▪ haloperidol ▪ idarubicin ▪ miconazole ▪ minocycline ▪ mitomycin ▪ mitoxantrone ▪ nalbuphine ▪ prochlorperazine edisylate ▪ promethazine ▪ streptozocin ▪ vancomycin.

PATIENT/FAMILY TEACHING

❑ Advise patient to report the signs of superinfection (black, furry overgrowth on the tongue; vaginal itching or discharge; loose or foul-smelling stools) and allergy.

EVALUATION

Clinical response to therapy can be evaluated by: ▪ Resolution of the signs and symptoms of infection. Length of time for complete resolution depends on the organism and site of infection.

PIRBUTEROL

(peer-**byoo**-ter-ole)
Maxair

CLASSIFICATION(S):
Bronchodilator (adrenergic agonist)

Pregnancy Category C

INDICATIONS

▪ Used as a bronchodilator (quick-relief agent) in the management of reversible airway disease due to intermittent asthma or COPD.

ACTION

▪ Results in the accumulation of cyclic adenosine monophosphate (cAMP) at beta-adrenergic receptors ▪ Produces bronchodilation ▪ Inhibits the release of mediators of immediate hypersensitivity reactions from mast cells ▪ Relatively selective for $beta_2$ (pulmonary) -adrenergic receptor sites with less effect on $beta_1$ (cardiac) -adrenergic receptors. **Therapeutic Effects:** ▪ Bronchodilation.

PHARMACOKINETICS

Absorption: Minimal systemic absorption occurs following inhalation.
Distribution: UK.
Metabolism and Excretion: Metabolized by the liver.
Half-life: 2 hr.

CONTRAINDICATIONS AND PRECAUTIONS

Contraindicated in: ▪ Hypersensitivity to adrenergic amines ▪ Known hypersensitivity or intolerance to fluorocarbons.

Use Cautiously in: ▪ Cardiac disease ▪ Hypertension ▪ Hyperthyroidism ▪ Diabetes ▪ Glaucoma ▪ Elderly patients (more susceptible to adverse reactions; may require dosage reduction) ▪ Excessive use may lead to tolerance and paradoxical bronchospasm (inhaler) ▪ Pregnancy (near term), lactation, and children <2 yr (safety not established).

ADVERSE REACTIONS AND SIDE EFFECTS*

CNS: nervousness, restlessness, tremor, headache, insomnia.
Resp: PARADOXICAL BRONCHOSPASM.
CV: angina, arrhythmias, hypertension, tachycardia.
GI: nausea, vomiting.
Endo: hyperglycemia.

INTERACTIONS

Drug-Drug: ▪ Concurrent use with other **adrenergic (sympathomimetic) agents** will have additive adrenergic side effects ▪ Use with **MAO inhibitors** may lead to hypertensive crisis ▪ **Beta-adrenergic blockers** may negate therapeutic effect.

ROUTE AND DOSAGE

- **Inhalation (Adults):** 1–2 inhalations q 4–6 hr (not to exceed 12 inhalations/day).

AVAILABILITY

- ***Inhalation aerosol:*** 200 mcg/spray (≥300 inhalations/25.6-g canister)Rx.

TIME/ACTION PROFILE (bronchodilation)

	ONSET	PEAK	DURATION
Inhaln	within 5 min	1.5 hr	6–8 hr

NURSING IMPLICATIONS

ASSESSMENT

- **Bronchodilator:** Assess lung sounds, respiratory pattern, pulse, and blood pressure before administration and during peak of medication. Note amount, color, and character of sputum produced, and report abnormal findings.
- □ Monitor pulmonary function tests before initiating therapy and periodically throughout course to determine effectiveness of medication.
- □ Observe for paradoxical bronchospasm (wheezing). If condition occurs, withhold medication and notify physician or other health care professional immediately.
- □ Observe patient for drug tolerance and rebound bronchospasm. Patients requiring more than 3 inhalation treatments in 24 hr should be under close supervision. If minimal or no relief is seen after 3–5 inhalation treatments within 6–12 hr, further treatment with aerosol alone is not recommended.

POTENTIAL NURSING DIAGNOSES

- Airway clearance, ineffective (Indications).
- Knowledge deficit, related to medication regimen (Patient/Family Teaching).

IMPLEMENTATION

- **Inhalation:** When pirbuterol is used concurrently with glucocorticoid or ipratropium inhalations, administer bronchodilator first and other medications 5 min apart to prevent toxicity from inhaled fluorocarbon propellants.

PATIENT/FAMILY TEACHING

- **General Info:** Instruct patient to take medication exactly as directed. If on a scheduled dosing regimen, take a missed dose as soon as possible; space remaining doses at regular intervals. Do not double doses. Caution patient not to exceed recommended dose; may cause adverse effects, paradoxical bronchospasm, or loss of effectiveness of medication.
- □ Instruct patient to contact health care professional immediately if shortness of breath is not relieved by medication or is accompanied by diaphoresis, dizziness, palpitations, or chest pain.
- □ Advise patient to consult health care professional before taking any OTC medications or alcoholic beverages concurrently with this therapy. Caution patient also to avoid smoking and other respiratory irritants.
- **Inhalation:** Review correct administration technique with patient. See Appendix H for administration with metered-dose inhaler. Wait 1–5 min before administering next dose. Mouthpiece should be washed after each use.
- □ Do not spray inhaler near eyes.

***CAPITALS indicate life-threatening; underlines indicate most frequent.**

P

- Instruct patient to save inhaler; refill canisters may be available.
- Advise patient to use bronchodilator first if using other inhalation medications, and allow 5 min to elapse before administering other inhalant medications, unless otherwise directed.
- Advise patient to rinse mouth with water after each inhalation dose to minimize dry mouth.
- Advise patient to maintain adequate fluid intake (2000–3000 ml/day) to help liquefy tenacious secretions.
- Advise patient to consult health care professional if respiratory symptoms are not relieved or worsen after treatment or if chest pain, headache, severe dizziness, palpitations, nervousness, or weakness occurs.
- Instruct patient to notify health care professional if contents of one canister are used up in less than 2 wk.

EVALUATION

Effectiveness of therapy can be demonstrated by: ▪ Prevention or relief of bronchospasm ▪ Increase in ease of breathing.

PIROXICAM

(peer-**ox**-i-kam)
{Apo-Piroxicam}, Feldene, {Novo-Pirocam}, Nu-Pirox, PMS-Piroxicam

CLASSIFICATION(S):
Nonsteroidal anti-inflammatory agent (NSAID)

Pregnancy Category B

INDICATIONS

▪ Management of inflammatory disorders, including: □ Rheumatoid arthritis □ Osteoarthritis. **Unlabeled Uses:** ▪ Management of dysmenorrhea.

ACTION

▪ Inhibits prostaglandin synthesis. **Therapeutic Effects:** ▪ Suppression of pain and inflammation.

PHARMACOKINETICS

Absorption: Well absorbed from the GI tract.
Distribution: UK. Enters breast milk in small amounts.
Metabolism and Excretion: Mostly metabolized by the liver. Minimal amounts excreted unchanged by the kidneys.
Half-life: 50 hr.

CONTRAINDICATIONS AND PRECAUTIONS

Contraindicated in: ▪ Hypersensitivity ▪ Cross-sensitivity may exist with other NSAIDs, including aspirin ▪ Active GI bleeding or ulcer disease ▪ Lactation.
Use Cautiously in: ▪ Severe cardiovascular or hepatic disease ▪ History of ulcer disease ▪ Renal impairment (dosage reduction recommended) ▪ Pregnancy or children (safety not established; avoid use during 2nd half of pregnancy).

ADVERSE REACTIONS AND SIDE EFFECTS*

CNS: drowsiness, headache, dizziness.
EENT: blurred vision, tinnitus.
CV: edema.
GI: DRUG-INDUCED HEPATITIS, GI BLEEDING, discomfort, dyspepsia, nausea, vomiting, anorexia, constipation, diarrhea, flatulence.
GU: renal failure.
Derm: rashes.
Hemat: blood dyscrasias, prolonged bleeding time.
Misc: allergic reactions including ANAPHYLAXIS.

INTERACTIONS

Drug-Drug: ▪ Concurrent use with **aspirin** decreases piroxicam blood levels and may decrease effectiveness ▪ Increased risk of bleeding with **anticoagulants, cefamandole, cefoperazone, cefotetan, heparin, thrombolytic agents, valproic acid,** or **plicamycin** ▪ Additive adverse GI side effects with **aspirin, glucocorticoids,** and other **NSAIDs** ▪ **Probenecid** increases blood levels and may increase toxicity ▪ May decrease response to **antihypertensives** or **diuretics** ▪ May increase serum levels and risk of toxicity from **lithium** ▪ May increase risk of hypoglycemia from **insulin** or

{} = Available in Canada only.
*CAPITALS indicate life-threatening; underlines indicate most frequent.

oral hypoglycemic agents ▪ Increased risk of adverse renal effects with **gold compounds, cyclosporine,** or chronic use of **acetaminophen** ▪ May increase the risk of hematologic toxicity from **antineoplastic agents** or **radiation therapy.**

ROUTE AND DOSAGE

- **PO (Adults):** *Anti-inflammatory*—10–20 mg/day; may be given as single dose or 2 divided doses. *Antidysmenorrheal*—40 mg initially, then 20 mg/day.
- **PO (Geriatric Patients):** 10 mg/day initially.

AVAILABILITY

▪ ***Capsules:*** 10 mg[Rx], 20 mg[Rx] ▪ ***Suppositories:*** {10 mg[Rx]}, {20 mg[Rx]}.

TIME/ACTION PROFILE

	ONSET	PEAK	DURATION
PO (analgesic effect)	1 hr	UK	48–72 hr
PO (anti-inflammatory effect)	7–12 days	2–3 wk*	UK

*May take up to 12 wk.

NURSING IMPLICATIONS

ASSESSMENT

- **General Info:** Patients who have asthma, aspirin-induced allergy, and nasal polyps are at increased risk for developing hypersensitivity reactions. Monitor for rhinitis, asthma, and urticaria.
- **Arthritis:** Assess pain and range of motion prior to and 1–2 hr following administration.
- ***Lab Test Considerations:*** Bleeding time may be prolonged for up to 2 wk following discontinuation of therapy.
- □ May cause decreased hemoglobin, hematocrit, leukocyte, and platelet counts.
- □ Monitor liver function tests periodically during therapy. May cause elevated serum alkaline phosphatase, LDH, AST, and ALT concentrations.
- □ Monitor BUN, serum creatinine, and electrolytes periodically during therapy. May cause increased BUN, serum creatinine, and electrolyte concentrations and decreased urine electrolyte concentrations.

POTENTIAL NURSING DIAGNOSES

- Pain (Indications).
- Physical mobility, impaired (Indications).
- Knowledge deficit, related to medication regimen (Patient/Family Teaching).

IMPLEMENTATION

- **General Info:** Administration in higher than recommended doses does not provide increased effectiveness but may cause increased side effects.
- **PO:** Administer after meals or with food or an antacid containing aluminum or magnesium to minimize gastric irritation.
- Administer as soon as possible after the onset of menses. Prophylactic use has not been proved effective.

PATIENT/FAMILY TEACHING

- □ Advise patient to take this medication with a full glass of water and to remain in an upright position for 15–30 min after administration.
- □ Instruct patient to take medication exactly as directed. If a dose is missed, it should be taken as soon as remembered but not if almost time for the next dose. Do not double doses.
- □ May cause drowsiness or dizziness. Advise patient to avoid driving or other activities requiring alertness until response to the medication is known.
- □ Caution patient to avoid the concurrent use of alcohol, aspirin, acetaminophen, or other OTC medications without consulting health care professional.
- □ Advise patient to inform health care professional of medication regimen prior to treatment or surgery.
- □ Caution patient to use sunscreen and protective clothing to prevent photosensitivity reaction (rare).
- □ Advise patient to consult health care professional if rash, itching, visual disturbances, tinnitus, weight gain, edema, black stools, persistent headache, or influenza-like syndrome (chills, fever, muscle aches, pain) occurs.

EVALUATION

Effectiveness of therapy can be demonstrated by: ▪ Decreased pain and improved joint mobility. Partial arthritic relief is usually seen within 2 wk, but maximum effectiveness may require up to 12 wk of continuous therapy. Patients who do not respond to one NSAID may respond to another.

PLASMA PROTEIN FRACTION

(**plaz**-ma **proe**-teen **frak**-shun)
Plasmanate, Plasma-Plex, Plasmatein, Protenate

CLASSIFICATION(S):
Volume expander

Pregnancy Category C

INDICATIONS

▪ Expansion of plasma volume and maintenance of cardiac output in situations associated with deficiencies in circulatory volume, including: ▫ Shock ▫ Hemorrhage ▫ Burns ▪ Temporary replacement therapy in edema associated with low plasma proteins, such as the nephrotic syndrome and end-stage liver disease.

ACTION

▪ Provides colloidal osmotic pressure (in the form of albumin and globulins) within the intravascular space, causing the shift of water from extravascular tissues back into the intravascular space. **Therapeutic Effects:** ▪ Mobilization of fluid from extravascular tissue into intravascular space.

PHARMACOKINETICS

Absorption: Administered IV only, resulting in complete bioavailability.
Distribution: Stays mainly in the intravascular space.
Metabolism and Excretion: UK.
Half-life: UK.

CONTRAINDICATIONS AND PRECAUTIONS

Contraindicated in: ▪ Allergic reactions to albumin ▪ Severe anemia ▪ Congestive heart failure ▪ Normal or increased intravascular volume ▪ Cardiopulmonary bypass procedures.
Use Cautiously in: ▪ Severe hepatic or renal disease ▪ Rapid infusion (may cause hypotension or hypertension) ▪ Dehydration (additional fluids may be required) ▪ Large doses (may cause anemia, requiring transfusion).

ADVERSE REACTIONS AND SIDE EFFECTS

CNS: headache.
CV: hypotension, tachycardia, vascular overload.
GI: excess salivation, nausea, vomiting.
Derm: erythema, urticaria.
MS: back pain.
Misc: chills, fever, flushing.

INTERACTIONS

Drug-Drug: ▪ None significant.

ROUTE AND DOSAGE

Dose is highly individualized and depends on condition being treated. Contains 130–160 mEq sodium/liter. Not to exceed 250 g/24 hr.

- **IV (Adults):** *Hypovolemia*—250–500 ml (12.5–25 g protein). *Hypoproteinemia*—1000–1500 ml (50–75 g protein).
- **IV (Infants and Young Children):** *Hypovolemia*—10–30 ml/kg (0.5–1.5 g protein/kg).

AVAILABILITY

▪ ***Injection:*** 5% in 50-, 250-, and 500-ml containers[Rx].

TIME/ACTION PROFILE (intravascular volume expansion)

	ONSET	PEAK	DURATION
IV	15–30 min	UK	UK

NURSING IMPLICATIONS

ASSESSMENT

- ▫ Monitor vital signs, CVP, pulmonary capillary wedge pressure (PCWP), and intake and output prior to and frequently throughout therapy. Hypotension may result from too rapid infusion.
- ▫ Assess patient for signs of vascular overload (elevated CVP, elevated PCWP, rales/crackles, dyspnea, hypertension, jugular venous distention) during and following administration.
- ▫ Assess surgical patients for increased bleeding following administration caused by increased blood pressure and circulating blood volume. Plasma protein fraction does not contain clotting factors.

- ***Lab Test Considerations:*** Monitor hemoglobin, hematocrit, serum protein, and electrolytes throughout therapy.

POTENTIAL NURSING DIAGNOSES

- Cardiac output, decreased (Indications).
- Fluid volume deficit (Indications).
- Fluid volume excess (Side Effects).

IMPLEMENTATION

- **General Info:** Administer through a large-gauge (at least 20-gauge) needle. Use administration set provided by manufacturer.
- Solution may vary from nearly colorless to straw to brownish. Do not use cloudy solution. Store at room temperature. Do not administer more than 250 g (5000 ml 5%) in 48 hr.
- There is no danger of serum hepatitis from plasma protein fraction. Crossmatching is not required.
- Dehydration should be corrected by additional IV fluids.
- **Intermittent Infusion:** Administer plasma protein fraction undiluted by IV infusion. Infusion must be completed within 4 hr.
- ***Rate:*** Rate of administration is determined by blood volume, indication, and patient response but should not exceed 10 ml/min, to minimize the possibility of hypotension. As the plasma volume approaches normal, the rate of administration should not exceed 5–8 ml/min. The rate for infants and children should not exceed 5–10 ml/min. Monitor the patient for signs of hypervolemia.
- **Additive Compatibility:** ▪ carbohydrate and electrolyte solutions ▪ whole blood ▪ packed red blood cells ▪ chloramphenicol.
- **Additive Incompatibility:** ▪ solutions containing protein hydrolysates ▪ amino acids ▪ alcohol ▪ norepinephrine.

PATIENT/FAMILY TEACHING

- Explain the rationale for use of this solution to the patient.

EVALUATION

Effectiveness of therapy can be demonstrated by: ▪ Increase in blood pressure and blood volume ▪ Elevated serum plasma protein in patients with hypoproteinemia.

PLICAMYCIN

(plye-ka-**mye**-sin)
Mithramycin, Mithracin

CLASSIFICATION(S):
Antineoplastic (antitumor antibiotic), Electrolyte modifier (hypocalcemic agent)

Pregnancy Category X

P

INDICATIONS

▪ Treatment of advanced unresponsive testicular carcinoma ▪ Management of hypercalcemia and hypercalciuria associated with malignancy.

ACTION

▪ Forms a complex with DNA that subsequently inhibits RNA synthesis ▪ Antagonizes the action of vitamin D and inhibits the action of parathyroid hormone on osteoclasts. **Therapeutic Effects:** ▪ Death of rapidly replicating cells, particularly malignant ones ▪ Lowering of serum calcium.

PHARMACOKINETICS

Absorption: Administered IV only, resulting in complete bioavailability.
Distribution: Appears to concentrate in the liver, renal tubule, and bone surface. Crosses the blood-brain barrier.
Metabolism and Excretion: Excreted primarily by the kidneys.
Half-life: UK.

CONTRAINDICATIONS AND PRECAUTIONS

Contraindicated in: ▪ Hypersensitivity ▪ Bleeding disorders ▪ Depressed bone marrow reserve ▪ Hypocalcemia ▪ Severe renal or liver disease ▪ Pregnancy or lactation.
Use Cautiously in: ▪ Patients with childbearing potential ▪ Active infections ▪ Other chronic debilitating illnesses ▪ Renal or hepatic impairment (dosage reduction required) ▪ Children (safety not established).

ADVERSE REACTIONS AND SIDE EFFECTS*

CNS: dizziness, drowsiness, fatigue, headache, irritability, malaise, mental depression, nervousness, weakness.
EENT: epistaxis.
GI: anorexia, diarrhea, drug-induced hepatitis, nausea, stomatitis, vomiting.
GU: gonadal suppression, renal failure.
Derm: facial flushing, rashes.
F and E: hypocalcemia, hypokalemia, hypophosphatemia, rebound hypercalcemia.
Hemat: BLEEDING, thrombocytopenia, anemia, leukopenia.
Local: phlebitis at IV site.
Misc: fever.

INTERACTIONS

Drug-Drug: ▪ Additive myelosuppression with other **antineoplastic agents** or **radiation therapy** ▪ Increased risk of bleeding with **aspirin, warfarin, thrombolytic agents, heparin, some cephalosporins, NSAIDs, sulfinpyrazone, valproic acid**, or **dextran** ▪ Increased risk of hepatotoxicity with other **hepatotoxic agents** ▪ Increased risk of renal toxicity with other **nephrotoxic agents.**

ROUTE AND DOSAGE

❑ Testicular Tumors

- **IV (Adults):** 25–30 mcg/kg once daily for 8–10 days or 25–50 mcg/kg every other day for up to 8 doses. May be repeated monthly.

❑ Hypercalcemia/Hypercalciuria

- **IV (Adults):** 15–25 mcg/kg once daily for 3–4 days; may be repeated after 7 days or 1–3 times weekly.

AVAILABILITY

- ***Powder for injection:*** 2500 mcg/vial[Rx].

TIME/ACTION PROFILE

	ONSET	PEAK	DURATION
IV (hematologic effects)	UK	7–10 days	3–4 wk
IV (hypocalcemic effects)	24–48 hr	72 hr	7–10 days

NURSING IMPLICATIONS

ASSESSMENT

- **General Info:** Monitor closely for bleeding (bleeding gums, bruising, petechiae, guaiac test stools, urine, and emesis). May begin as epistaxis and progress to severe generalized or GI bleeding. May require blood transfusions, fresh frozen plasma, vitamin K, or aminocaproic acid to control bleeding. Avoid IM injections and rectal temperatures. Apply pressure to venipuncture sites for 10 min.
- ❑ Monitor intake and output, appetite, and nutritional intake. Dehydration or volume depletion should be corrected prior to initiating plicamycin therapy. May cause nausea and vomiting, which usually occurs 1–2 hr after therapy is initiated, persists 12–24 hr, and should be treated with prophylactic antiemetics. Adjust diet as tolerated to help maintain fluid and electrolyte balance and nutritional status.
- ❑ Assess for signs of infection (fever, chills, sore throat, cough, hoarseness, pain in lower back or side, difficult or painful urination). Notify physician if these symptoms occur.
- **Hypercalcemia:** Monitor symptoms of hypercalcemia (nausea, vomiting, anorexia, thirst, weakness, constipation, paralytic ileus, and bradycardia). Observe patient for evidence of hypocalcemia (paresthesia, muscle twitching, laryngospasm, colic, cardiac arrhythmias, and Chvostek's or Trousseau's sign).
- ***Lab Test Considerations:*** Monitor CBC with differential, platelet count, prothrombin time, and bleeding time prior to and periodically throughout therapy. May cause thrombocytopenia, leukemia, and anemia. Notify physician if platelet count is $<150,000/mm^3$, prothrombin time is elevated 4 or more sec above control, or leukocyte count is $<4000/mm^3$.
- ❑ Monitor serum electrolytes prior to and daily during course of therapy. May cause hypocalcemia, hypokalemia, and hypophosphatemia. Correct electrolyte imbalances before beginning therapy. Calcium and phosphate levels may rebound after therapy.
- ❑ Monitor liver function studies (AST, ALT, LDH, bilirubin) and renal function studies (BUN, creatinine, urinalysis) prior to and periodi-

***CAPITALS indicate life-threatening; underlines indicate most frequent.**

cally throughout therapy to detect hepatotoxicity and nephrotoxicity.

POTENTIAL NURSING DIAGNOSES

- Injury, risk for (Side Effects).
- Infection, risk for (Side Effects).
- Body image disturbance (Side Effects).

IMPLEMENTATION

- **General Info:** Solution should be prepared in a biologic cabinet. Wear gloves, gown, and mask while handling medication. Discard equipment in designated containers (see Appendix I).
- Ensure patency of the IV. If patient complains of discomfort at the IV site or if extravasation occurs, discontinue IV and restart at another site. Extravasation may cause irritation and cellulitis. Apply ice to site to prevent pain and swelling. If swelling occurs, application of moderate heat to site may help disperse medication and decrease discomfort.
- **IV:** To reconstitute, add 4.9 ml of sterile water for injection to the 2.5-mg vial of plicamycin to yield a final concentration of 500 mcg/ml. Shake vial to dissolve drug. Use immediately after reconstitution. Discard unused portions.
- **Direct IV:** May be administered undiluted IV push to decrease risk of extravasation.
- ***Rate:*** Administer over 20–30 min.
- **Intermittent Infusion:** Add to 1000 ml of D5W or 0.9% NaCl.
- ***Rate:*** Infuse over 4–6 hr. Rapid infusion rate will increase incidence and severity of GI side effects.
- **Y-Site Compatibility:** ▪ allopurinol sodium ▪ amifostine ▪ aztreonam ▪ filgrastim ▪ melphalan ▪ piperacillin/tazobactam ▪ teniposide ▪ thiotepa ▪ vinorelbine.

PATIENT/FAMILY TEACHING

- Advise patient to notify health care professional promptly if fever; chills; sore throat; signs of infection; bleeding gums; bruising; petechiae; or blood in urine, stool, or emesis occurs. Caution patient to avoid crowds and persons with known infections. Instruct patient to use soft toothbrush and electric razor. Patients should be cautioned not to drink alcoholic beverages or take products containing aspirin or NSAIDs.
- Instruct patient to notify health care professional if weakness, rash, persistent nausea or vomiting, or depression occurs.
- Instruct patient to inspect oral mucosa for redness and ulceration. If mouth sores occur, advise patient to use sponge brush and rinse mouth with water after eating and drinking. Topical medications may be used if pain interferes with eating. Stomatitis pain may require treatment with opioid analgesics.
- Advise patient that, although fertility may be decreased with plicamycin, contraception should be used during therapy because of potential teratogenic effects on the fetus.
- Instruct patient not to receive any vaccinations without advice of health care professional.
- Emphasize need for periodic lab tests to monitor for side effects.

EVALUATION

Effectiveness of therapy can be demonstrated by: ▪ Decrease in size and spread of malignant tissue ▪ Normalization of elevated calcium levels in hypercalcemia and hypercalciuria within 24–48 hr.

POLYCARBOPHIL

(pol-i-**kar**-boe-fil)

Equalactin, Fiberall, FiberCon, Fiber-Lax, Mitrolan

CLASSIFICATION(S):

Antidiarrheal, Laxative (bulk-forming agent)

Pregnancy Category UK

INDICATIONS

▪ Treatment of constipation or diarrhea that may be associated with diverticulosis or irritable bowel syndrome.

ACTION

▪ Acts as a bulk laxative by keeping water within the bowel lumen ▪ Acts as an antidiarrheal by taking on water within the bowel lumen to create a formed stool. **Therapeutic Effects:** ▪ Normalization of bowel water content while adding bulk, treating both diarrhea and constipation.

PHARMACOKINETICS

Absorption: Minimal systemic absorption.
Distribution: UK.

Metabolism and Excretion: Complex plus absorbed water are excreted in the feces.
Half-life: UK.

CONTRAINDICATIONS AND PRECAUTIONS

Contraindicated in: ▪ Hypersensitivity ▪ Abdominal pain ▪ Nausea or vomiting (especially when associated with fever or other signs of acute abdomen) ▪ Serious intra-abdominal adhesions ▪ Dysphagia.
Use Cautiously in: ▪ Pregnancy or lactation (has been used safely).

ADVERSE REACTIONS AND SIDE EFFECTS

GI: abdominal fullness.

INTERACTIONS

Drug-Drug: ▪ May decrease the absorption of concurrently administered **tetracycline.**

ROUTE AND DOSAGE

- **PO (Adults):** 1 g 1–4 times daily or as needed (not to exceed 6 g/24 hr); for severe diarrhea, may repeat q 30 min.
- **PO (Children 6–12 yr):** 500 mg 1–3 times daily or as needed (not to exceed 3 g/24 hr); for severe diarrhea, may repeat q 30 min.
- **PO (Children 2–6 yr):** 500 mg 1–2 times daily or as needed (not to exceed 1.5 g/24 hr); for severe diarrhea, may repeat q 30 min.

AVAILABILITY

▪ ***Tablets:*** 500 mg[OTC] ▪ ***Chewable tablets:*** 500 mg[OTC], 1000 mg[OTC].

TIME/ACTION PROFILE (effect on bowel function)

	ONSET	PEAK	DURATION
PO	12–24 hr*	UK	UK

*May take as long as 72 hr.

NURSING IMPLICATIONS

ASSESSMENT

- **General Info:** Assess for fever, nausea, vomiting, abdominal distention, and pain. Notify health care professional if present. Auscultate bowel sounds. Inquire about patient's usual diet, fluid intake, activity level, and bowel function.
- □ Monitor for color, consistency, and amount of stool produced.
- **Diarrhea:** Monitor for signs of dehydration (decreased skin turgor, dry mucous membranes, weight loss, decreased urine output, tachycardia, and hypotension).

POTENTIAL NURSING DIAGNOSES

- Constipation (Indications).
- Diarrhea (Indications).
- Knowledge deficit, related to medication regimen (Patient/Family Teaching).

IMPLEMENTATION

- **General Info:** Administer 1 hr before or 2 hr after tetracycline.
- **Diarrhea:** For treatment of severe diarrhea, dose may be repeated every 30 min. Do not exceed total daily prescribed dose.
- □ Chewable tablets consume up to 60 times their weight in water.
- **Constipation:** For treatment of constipation, administer with 8 oz water or juice.

PATIENT/FAMILY TEACHING

- □ Encourage patients with constipation to use other forms of bowel regulation, such as increasing bulk in diet, fluid intake, and mobility. Normal bowel habits are individualized and may vary from 3 times/day to 3 times/wk.
- □ Instruct patients with sudden onset of constipation to notify health care professional; medical evaluation may be necessary.
- □ Instruct patients with diarrhea to notify health care professional if fever or bloody stools occur or if diarrhea persists or worsens. Discuss need for fluids and diet modifications during episodes of diarrhea.

EVALUATION

Effectiveness of therapy can be demonstrated by: ▪ Soft, formed bowel movement. May require 3 days for therapeutic effect to occur.

POLYETHYLENE GLYCOL/ ELECTROLYTE

(po-lee-**eth**-e-leen **glye**-kole/e-**lek**-troe-lite)

Colovage, Colyte, GoLYTELY, {Klean-Prep}, NuLytely, OCL, Peglyte

CLASSIFICATION(S):
Laxative (osmotic)

Pregnancy Category C

INDICATIONS

▪ Bowel cleansing in preparation for GI examination. **Unlabeled Uses:** ▪ Treatment of acute iron overdose in children.

ACTION

▪ Polyethylene glycol (PEG) in solution acts as an osmotic agent, drawing water into the lumen of the GI tract. **Therapeutic Effects:** ▪ Evacuation of the GI tract without water or electrolyte imbalance.

PHARMACOKINETICS

Absorption: Ions in the solution are nonabsorbable.
Distribution: UK.
Metabolism and Excretion: Solution is excreted in fecal contents.
Half-life: UK.

CONTRAINDICATIONS AND PRECAUTIONS

Contraindicated in: ▪ GI obstruction ▪ Gastric retention ▪ Toxic colitis ▪ Megacolon.
Use Cautiously in: ▪ Patients with absent or diminished gag reflex ▪ Unconscious or semicomatose states, in which administration is via nasogastric tube ▪ Barium enema using double-contrast technique (may not allow proper barium coating of mucosa) ▪ Abdominal pain of uncertain cause, particularly if accompanied by fever ▪ Children (safety not established).

ADVERSE REACTIONS AND SIDE EFFECTS*

GI: abdominal fullness, diarrhea, bloating, cramps, nausea, vomiting.

INTERACTIONS

Drug-Drug: ▪ Interferes with the absorption of **orally administered medications** by decreasing transit time (do not administer within 1 hr of start of therapy).

ROUTE AND DOSAGE

- **PO (Adults):** 240 ml q 10 min (up to 4 liters) until fecal discharge appears clear and has no solid material; may be given through nasogastric tube at 20–30 ml/min.
- **PO (Children):** 25–40 ml/kg/hr until fecal discharge is clear and has no solid material; may also be given through a nasogastric tube (unlabeled).

AVAILABILITY

▪ ***Oral solution***[Rx,OTC] ▪ ***Powder for oral solution***[Rx,OTC].

TIME/ACTION PROFILE

	ONSET	PEAK	DURATION
PO	1 hr	UK	4 hr

NURSING IMPLICATIONS

ASSESSMENT

- □ Assess patient for abdominal distention, presence of bowel sounds, and usual pattern of bowel function.
- □ Assess color, consistency, and amount of stool produced.
- □ Monitor semiconscious or unconscious patients closely for regurgitation when administering via nasogastric tube.

POTENTIAL NURSING DIAGNOSES

- Diarrhea (Side Effects).
- Knowledge deficit, related to medication regimen (Patient/Family Teaching).

IMPLEMENTATION

- **General Info:** Do not add flavorings or additional ingredients to solution prior to administration.
- □ Patient should fast for 3–4 hr prior to administration and should never have solid food within 2 hr of administration.

{} = Available in Canada only.
*CAPITALS indicate life-threatening; underlines indicate most frequent.

- Patient should be allowed only clear liquids after administration.
- May be administered on the morning of the examination as long as time is allotted to drink solution (3 hr) and evacuate bowel (1 additional hr). For barium enema, administer solution early evening (6 PM) prior to exam to allow proper mucosal coating by barium.
- **PO:** Solution may be reconstituted with tap water. Shake vigorously until powder is dissolved.
- May be administered via nasogastric tube at a rate of 20–30 ml/min.

PATIENT/FAMILY TEACHING

- Instruct patient to drink 240 ml every 10 min until 4 liters have been consumed or fecal discharge is clear and free of solid matter. Rapidly drinking each 240 ml is preferred over drinking small amounts continuously.

EVALUATION

Effectiveness of therapy can be demonstrated by: ▪ Diarrhea, which cleanses the bowel within 4 hr. The first bowel movement usually occurs within 1 hr of administration.

POTASSIUM AND SODIUM PHOSPHATES

(**foss**-fates)

monobasic potassium and sodium phosphates

K-Phos M.F., K-Phos Neutral, K-Phos No. 2

potassium and sodium phosphates

Neutra-Phos, Uro-KP Neutral

CLASSIFICATION(S):

Antiurolithics, Electrolytes (phosphate supplements), Urinary acidifiers

Pregnancy Category C

INDICATIONS

▪ Treatment and prevention of phosphate depletion in patients who are unable to ingest adequate dietary potassium (potassium and sodium phosphate) ▪ Adjunct therapy of urinary tract infections with methenamine hippurate or mandelate (potassium and sodium phosphates or monobasic potassium phosphate) ▪ Prevention of calcium urinary stones (potassium and sodium phosphates or monobasic potassium phosphate) ▪ Phosphate salts of potassium may be used in hypokalemic patients with metabolic acidosis or coexisting phosphorus deficiency.

ACTION

▪ Phosphate is present in bone and is involved in energy transfer and carbohydrate metabolism ▪ Serves as a buffer for the excretion of hydrogen ions by the kidneys ▪ Dibasic potassium phosphate is converted in renal tubule to monobasic salt, resulting in urinary acidification, which is required for methenamine hippurate or mandelate to be active as urinary anti-infectives ▪ Acidification of urine increases solubility of calcium, decreasing calcium stone formation. **Therapeutic Effects:** ▪ Replacement of phosphorus in deficiency states ▪ Urinary acidification ▪ Increased efficacy of methenamine ▪ Decreased formation of calcium urinary tract stones.

PHARMACOKINETICS

Absorption: Well absorbed following oral administration. Vitamin D promotes GI absorption of phosphates.

Distribution: Phosphates enter extracellular fluids and are then actively transported to sites of action.

Metabolism and Excretion: Excreted mainly (>90%) by the kidneys.

Half-life: UK.

CONTRAINDICATIONS AND PRECAUTIONS

Contraindicated in: ▪ Hyperkalemia (potassium salts) ▪ Hyperphosphatemia ▪ Hypocalcemia ▪ Severe renal impairment ▪ Untreated Addison's disease (potassium salts) ▪ Severe tissue trauma (potassium salts) ▪ Hyperkalemic familial periodic paralysis (potassium salts).

Use Cautiously in: ▪ Hyperparathyroidism ▪ Cardiac disease ▪ Hypernatremia (sodium phosphate only) ▪ Hypertension (sodium phosphate only) ▪ Renal impairment.

P

ADVERSE REACTIONS AND SIDE EFFECTS*

Related to hyperphosphatemia, unless otherwise indicated.

CNS: confusion, listlessness, weakness.
CV: ARRHYTHMIAS, CARDIAC ARREST, ECG changes (absent P waves, widening of the QRS complex with biphasic curve), hypotension; *hyperkalemia*—ARRHYTHMIAS, ECG changes (prolonged PR interval, ST segment depression, tall-tented T waves); *hypernatremia*—edema.
GI: diarrhea, abdominal pain, nausea, vomiting.
F and E: hyperkalemia, hypernatremia, hyperphosphatemia, hypocalcemia, hypomagnesemia.
Local: irritation at IV site, phlebitis.
MS: *hypocalcemia*—tremors; *hyperkalemia*—muscle cramps.
Neuro: flaccid paralysis, heaviness of legs, paresthesias.

INTERACTIONS

Drug-Drug: ▪ Concurrent use of **potassium-sparing diuretics** or **ACE inhibitors** with potassium phosphates may result in hyperkalemia ▪ Concurrent use of **glucocorticoids** with sodium phosphate may result in hypernatremia ▪ Concurrent administration of **calcium-, magnesium-, or aluminum-containing compounds** decreases absorption of phosphates by formation of insoluble complexes ▪ **Vitamin D** enhances the absorption of phosphates.
Drug-Food: ▪ **Oxalates** (in spinach and rhubarb) and **phytates** (in bran and whole grains) may decrease the absorption of phosphates by binding them in the GI tract.

ROUTE AND DOSAGE

❑ **Monobasic Potassium and Sodium Phosphates**

- **PO (Adults and Children >4 yr):** 250 mg (8 mmol) 4 times daily; may be increased to 250 mg (8 mmol) q 2 hr (not to exceed 2 g phosphorus/24 hr).
- **PO (Children <4 yr):** 200 mg (6.4 mmol) 4 times daily.

❑ **Potassium and Sodium Phosphates**

- **PO (Adults and Children >4 yr):** 250 mg (8 mmol) phosphorus 4 times daily.
- **PO (Children <4 yr):** 200 mg (6.4 mmol) 4 times daily.

AVAILABILITY

❑ **Monobasic Potassium and Sodium Phosphates**

▪ ***Tablets for oral solution:*** 125.6 mg (4 mmol) phosphorus[Rx], 250 mg (8 mmol) phosphorus[Rx].

❑ **Potassium and Sodium Phosphates**

▪ ***Capsules for oral solution:*** 250 mg (8 mmol) phosphorus[Rx] ▪ ***Tablets for oral solution:*** 250 mg (8 mmol) phosphorus[Rx] ▪ ***Powder for oral solution:*** 250 mg (8 mmol)/75 ml when reconstituted[Rx].

TIME/ACTION PROFILE (effects on serum phosphate levels)

	ONSET	PEAK	DURATION
PO	UK	UK	UK

NURSING IMPLICATIONS

ASSESSMENT

- ❑ Assess patient for signs and symptoms of hypokalemia (weakness, fatigue, arrhythmias, presence of U waves on ECG, polyuria, polydipsia) and hypophosphatemia (anorexia, weakness, decreased reflexes, bone pain, confusion, blood dyscrasias) throughout therapy.
- ❑ Monitor intake and output ratios and daily weight. Report significant discrepancies.
- ▪ ***Lab Test Considerations:*** Monitor serum phosphate, potassium, sodium, and calcium levels prior to and periodically throughout therapy. Increased phosphate may cause hypocalcemia.
- ❑ Monitor renal function studies prior to and periodically throughout therapy.
- ❑ Monitor urinary pH in patients receiving potassium and sodium phosphate as a urinary acidifier.

POTENTIAL NURSING DIAGNOSES

- Nutrition, altered, less than body requirements (Indications).
- Knowledge deficit, related to medication regimen (Patient/Family Teaching).

***CAPITALS indicate life-threatening; underlines indicate most frequent.**

IMPLEMENTATION

- **PO:** Tablets should be dissolved in a full glass of water. Capsules should be opened and mixed thoroughly in ⅓ cup of water each. Allow mixture to stand for 2–5 min to ensure it is fully dissolved. Solutions prepared by pharmacy should not be further diluted.
- □ Medication should be administered after meals to minimize gastric irritation and laxative effect.
- □ Do not administer simultaneously with antacids containing aluminum, magnesium, or calcium.

PATIENT/FAMILY TEACHING

- □ Explain to the patient the purpose of the medication and the need to take as directed. If a dose is missed, it should be taken as soon as remembered unless within 1 or 2 hr of the next dose. Explain that the tablets and capsules should not be swallowed whole. Tablets should be dissolved in water; capsules should be opened and the contents mixed in water.
- □ Instruct patients in low-sodium diet (see Appendix K).
- □ Advise patient of the importance of maintaining a high fluid intake (drinking at least one 8-oz glass of water each hr) to prevent kidney stones.
- □ Instruct the patient to promptly report diarrhea, weakness, fatigue, muscle cramps, unexplained weight gain, swelling of lower extremities, shortness of breath, unusual thirst, or tremors.

EVALUATION

Effectiveness of therapy can be demonstrated by: ▪ Prevention and correction of serum phosphate and potassium deficiencies ▪ Maintenance of acid urine ▪ Decreased urine calcium, which prevents formation of renal calculi.

POTASSIUM PHOSPHATES

(poe-**tass**-ee-um **foss**-fates)

monobasic potassium phosphate

K-Phos Original

potassium phosphates

Neutra-Phos-K

potassium phosphate

CLASSIFICATION(S):

Antiurolithics, Electrolytes (phosphate supplements), Urinary acidifiers

Pregnancy Category C

INDICATIONS

▪ Treatment and prevention of phosphate depletion in patients who are unable to ingest adequate dietary potassium ▪ Adjunct therapy of urinary tract infections with methenamine hippurate or mandelate (potassium and sodium phosphates or monobasic potassium phosphate) ▪ Prevention of calcium urinary stones (potassium and sodium phosphates or monobasic potassium phosphate) ▪ Phosphate salts of potassium may be used in hypokalemic patients with metabolic acidosis or coexisting phosphorus deficiency.

ACTION

▪ Phosphate is present in bone and is involved in energy transfer and carbohydrate metabolism ▪ Serves as a buffer for the excretion of hydrogen ions by the kidney ▪ Dibasic potassium phosphate is converted in renal tubule to monobasic salt by hydrogen ions, resulting in urinary acidification ▪ Acidification of urine is required for methenamine hippurate or mandelate to be active as a urinary anti-infective ▪ Acidification of urine increases solubility of calcium, decreasing calcium stone formation. **Therapeutic Effects:** ▪ Replacement of phosphorus in deficiency states ▪ Urinary acidification ▪ Increased efficacy of methenamine ▪ Decreased formation of calcium urinary tract stones.

PHARMACOKINETICS

Absorption: Well absorbed following oral administration. Vitamin D promotes GI absorption of phosphates.
Distribution: Phosphates enter extracellular fluids and are then actively transported to sites of action.
Metabolism and Excretion: Excreted mainly (>90%) by the kidneys.
Half-life: UK.

P

CONTRAINDICATIONS AND PRECAUTIONS

Contraindicated in: ▪ Hyperkalemia ▪ Hyperphosphatemia ▪ Hypocalcemia ▪ Severe renal impairment ▪ Untreated Addison's disease ▪ Severe tissue trauma ▪ Hyperkalemic familial periodic paralysis.
Use Cautiously in: ▪ Hyperparathyroidism ▪ Cardiac disease ▪ Renal impairment.

ADVERSE REACTIONS AND SIDE EFFECTS*

Related to hyperphosphatemia, unless otherwise indicated.
CNS: confusion, listlessness, weakness.
CV: ARRHYTHMIAS, CARDIAC ARREST, ECG changes (absent P waves, widening of the QRS complex with biphasic curve), hypotension; *hyperkalemia*—arrhythmias, ECG changes (prolonged PR interval, ST segment depression, tall-tented T waves).
GI: diarrhea, abdominal pain, nausea, vomiting.
F and E: hyperkalemia, hyperphosphatemia, hypocalcemia, hypomagnesemia.
Local: irritation at IV site, phlebitis.
MS: *hyperkalemia*—muscle cramps; *hypercalcemia*—tremors.
Neuro: flaccid paralysis, heaviness of legs, paresthesias.

INTERACTIONS

Drug-Drug: ▪ Concurrent use of **potassium-sparing diuretics** or **ACE inhibitors** may result in hyperkalemia ▪ Concurrent administration of **calcium-** or **aluminum-containing compounds** decreases absorption of phosphates by formation of insoluble complexes ▪ **Vitamin D** enhances the absorption of phosphates.
Drug-Food: ▪ **Oxalates** (in spinach and rhubarb) and **phytates** (in bran and whole grains) may decrease the absorption of phosphates by binding them in the GI tract.

ROUTE AND DOSAGE

❑ **Monobasic Potassium Phosphate**

- **PO (Adults and Children >4 yr):** 1 g (7.4 mmol) in water 4 times daily.
- **PO (Children <4 yr):** 200 mg (6.4 mmol) in water 4 times daily.

❑ **Potassium Phosphates**

- **PO (Adults and Children >4 yr):** 1.45 g (8 mmol) 4 times daily.
- **PO (Children <4 yr):** 200 mg (6.4 mmol) phosphorus 4 times daily.
- **IV (Adults):** 10 mmol phosphorus/day as an infusion.
- **IV (Infants):** 1.5–2 mmol phosphorus/day as an infusion.

AVAILABILITY

❑ **Monobasic Potassium Phosphate**

▪ ***Tablets for oral solution:*** 500 mg (contains 114 mg or 3.7 mmol phosphorus)Rx.

❑ **Potassium Phosphates**

▪ ***Capsules for oral solution:*** 1.45 g (contains 1.45 g or 8 mmol phosphorus)Rx ▪ ***Concentrate for injection:*** 93 mg (3 mmol) phosphorus/ml in 5-, 10-, 15-, 30-, and 50-ml vialsRx ▪ ***In combination with:*** sodium phosphatesRx.

TIME/ACTION PROFILE (effects on serum phosphate levels)

	ONSET	PEAK	DURATION
PO	UK	UK	UK
IV	rapid (min–hr)	end of infusion	UK

NURSING IMPLICATIONS

ASSESSMENT

- ❑ Assess patient for signs and symptoms of hypokalemia (weakness, fatigue, arrhythmias, presence of U waves on ECG, polyuria, polydipsia) and hypophosphatemia (anorexia, weakness, decreased reflexes, bone pain, confusion, blood dyscrasias) throughout therapy.
- ❑ Monitor pulse, blood pressure, and ECG prior to and periodically throughout IV therapy.
- ❑ Monitor intake and output ratios and daily weight. Report significant discrepancies.
- ▪ ***Lab Test Considerations:*** Monitor serum phosphate, potassium, and calcium levels prior to and periodically throughout therapy. Increased phosphate may cause hypocalcemia.
- ❑ Monitor renal function studies prior to and periodically throughout course of therapy.

***CAPITALS indicate life-threatening; underlines indicate most frequent.**

□ Monitor urinary pH in patients receiving potassium phosphate as a urinary acidifier.

■ ***Toxicity and Overdose:*** Symptoms of toxicity are those of hyperkalemia (fatigue, muscle weakness, paresthesia, confusion, dyspnea, peaked T waves, depressed ST segments, prolonged QT segments, widened QRS complexes, loss of P waves, and cardiac arrhythmias) and hyperphosphatemia or hypocalcemia (paresthesia, muscle twitching, laryngospasm, colic, cardiac arrhythmias, or Chvostek's or Trousseau's sign).

□ Treatment includes discontinuation of infusion, calcium replacement, and lowering serum potassium (dextrose and insulin to facilitate passage of potassium into cells, sodium polystyrene as an exchange resin, and/or dialysis in patients with impaired renal function).

POTENTIAL NURSING DIAGNOSES

■ Nutrition, altered, less than body requirements (Indications).

■ Knowledge deficit, related to medication regimen (Patient/Family Teaching).

IMPLEMENTATION

■ **PO:** Tablets should be dissolved in a full glass of water. Capsules should be opened and mixed thoroughly in ⅓ cup water each. Allow mixture to stand for 2–5 min to ensure that it is fully dissolved.

□ Medication should be administered after meals to minimize gastric irritation and laxative effect.

□ Do not administer simultaneously with antacids containing aluminum, magnesium, or calcium.

■ **IV:** Administer only in dilute concentration. Common component of total parenteral nutrition. Do not administer IM.

■ **Continuous Infusion:** Dilute to a concentration no greater than 160 mEq/liter with 0.45% NaCl, 0.9% NaCl, D5W, D10W, D5/0.45% NaCl, D5/0.9% NaCl, or TPN solutions.

■ ***Rate:*** Infuse as a continuous infusion at a slow rate.

■ **Y-Site Compatibility:** ■ ciprofloxacin ■ diltiazem ■ enalaprilat ■ esmolol ■ famotidine ■ labetalol.

■ **Additive Compatibility:** ■ magnesium sulfate.

■ **Solution Incompatibility:** ■ Ringer's or lactated Ringer's injection ■ D10/0.9% NaCl ■ D5/LR.

PATIENT/FAMILY TEACHING

□ Explain to patient purpose of the medication and the need to take as directed. If a dose is missed, it should be taken as soon as remembered unless within 1–2 hr of the next dose. Explain that the tablets and capsules should not be swallowed whole. Tablets should be dissolved in water; capsules should be opened and the contents mixed in water.

□ Advise patient of the importance of maintaining a high fluid intake (drinking at least one 8-oz glass of water each hr) to prevent kidney stones.

□ Instruct the patient to report diarrhea, weakness, fatigue, muscle cramps, or tremors promptly.

EVALUATION

Effectiveness of therapy can be demonstrated by: ■ Prevention and correction of serum phosphate and potassium deficiencies ■ Maintenance of acid urine ■ Decrease in urine calcium, which prevents formation of renal calculi.

POTASSIUM SUPPLEMENTS
(poe-**tass**-ee-um)

potassium acetate

potassium bicarbonate
K+Care ET, K-Electrolyte, K-Ide, Klor-Con/EF, K-Lyte, K-Vescent

potassium bicarbonate/ potassium chloride
Klorvess, Klorvess Effervescent Granules, K-Lyte/Cl, {Neo-K}, {Potassium Sandoz}

potassium bicarbonate/ potassium citrate
Effer-K, K-Lyte DS

{} = Available in Canada only.

potassium chloride
{Apo-K}, Cena-K, Gen-K, K+ Care, K+ 10, {Kalium Durules}, Kaochlor, Kaochlor S-F, Kaon-Cl, Kay Ciel, KCl, K-Dur, K-Lease, {K-Long}, K-Lor, Klor-Con, Klorvess Liquid, Klotrix, K-Lyte/Cl Powder, K-Med, K-Norm, K-Sol, K-Tab, Micro-K, Micro-LS, Potasalan, Roychlor, Rum-K, Slow-K, Ten-K

potassium chloride/potassium bicarbonate/potassium citrate
Kaochlor Eff

potassium gluconate
Kaon, Kaylixir, K-G Elixir, {Potassium-Rougier}

potassium gluconate/potassium chloride
Kolyum

potassium gluconate/potassium citrate
Twin-K

trikates (potassium acetate/potassium bicarbonate/potassium citrate)
Tri-K

CLASSIFICATION(S):
Electrolytes (potassium supplements)

Pregnancy Category C

INDICATIONS

▪ **PO, IV:** Treatment or prevention of potassium depletion ▪ **IV:** Treatment of certain arrhythmias due to cardiac glycoside toxicity.

ACTION

▪ Maintain acid-base balance, isotonicity, and electrophysiologic balance of the cell ▪ Activator in many enzymatic reactions; essential to transmission of nerve impulses; contraction of cardiac, skeletal, and smooth muscle; gastric secretion; renal function; tissue synthesis; and carbohydrate metabolism. **Therapeutic Effects:** ▪ Replacement ▪ Prevention of deficiency.

PHARMACOKINETICS

Absorption: Well absorbed following oral administration.
Distribution: Enter extracellular fluid; then actively transported into cells.
Metabolism and Excretion: Excreted by the kidneys.
Half-life: UK.

CONTRAINDICATIONS AND PRECAUTIONS

Contraindicated in: ▪ Hyperkalemia ▪ Severe renal impairment ▪ Untreated Addison's disease ▪ Severe tissue trauma ▪ Hyperkalemic familial periodic paralysis ▪ Some products may contain tartrazine (FDC yellow dye #5) or alcohol; avoid using in patients with known hypersensitivity or intolerance.
Use Cautiously in: ▪ Cardiac disease ▪ Renal impairment ▪ Diabetes mellitus (liquids may contain sugar) ▪ GI hypomotility including dysphagia or esophageal compression from left atrial enlargement (tablets, capsules).

ADVERSE REACTIONS AND SIDE EFFECTS*

CNS: confusion, restlessness, weakness.
CV: ARRHYTHMIAS, ECG changes.
GI: abdominal pain, diarrhea, nausea, vomiting, GI ulceration (tablets only).
Local: irritation at IV site.
Neuro: paralysis, paresthesia.

INTERACTIONS

Drug-Drug: ▪ Use with **potassium-sparing diuretics** or **ACE inhibitors** may lead to hyperkalemia ▪ **Anticholinergics** may increase GI mucosal lesions in patients taking wax-matrix potassium chloride preparations.

ROUTE AND DOSAGE

Expressed as mEq of potassium. Potassium acetate contains 10.2 mEq/g; potassium bicarbonate contains 10 mEq potassium/g; potassium chloride contains 13.4 mEq potassium/g; potassium gluconate contains 4.3 mEq/g.

❑ **Prevention/Treatment**

▪ **PO (Adults):** 20 mEq 2–4 times daily (range 6.7–80 mEq/day).

{} = Available in Canada only.
***CAPITALS indicate life-threatening; underlines indicate most frequent.**

- **PO (Children):** 2–3 mEq/kg/day or 20–40 mEq/m²/day in divided doses.
- **IV (Adults):** *Serum potassium >2.5 mEq/liter*—Up to 200 mEq/day as an infusion (not to exceed 10 mEq/hr or a concentration of 40 mEq/liter via peripheral line (up to 100 mEq/liter have been used via central line [unlabeled]). *Serum potassium <2 mEq/liter with symptoms*—Up to 400 mEq/day as an infusion (rate should generally not exceed 20 mEq/hr).
- **IV (Children):** Up to 3 mEq/kg/day (40 mEq/m²/day) as an infusion.

AVAILABILITY

❑ Potassium Acetate

▪ ***Concentrate for injection:*** 2 mEq/ml in 20-, 50-, and 100-ml vials^Rx^, 40 mEq/ml in 50-ml vials^Rx^.

❑ Potassium Bicarbonate

▪ ***Tablets for effervescent oral solution:*** 25 mEq^Rx^.

❑ Potasssium Bicarbonate/Potassium Chloride

▪ ***Packets for effervescent oral solution:*** 20 mEq/2.8-g packet^Rx^ ▪ ***Tablets for effervescent oral solution:*** {12 mEq^Rx^}, 20 mEq^Rx^, 25 mEq^Rx^, 50 mEq^Rx^.

❑ Potassium Bicarbonate/Potassium Citrate

▪ ***Tablets for effervescent oral solution:*** 25 mEq^Rx^, 50 mEq^Rx^.

❑ Potassium Chloride

▪ ***Extended-release tablets:*** 6.7 mEq^Rx^, 8 mEq^Rx^, 10 mEq^Rx^, 20 mEq^Rx^ ▪ ***Extended-release capsules:*** 8 mEq^Rx^, 10 mEq^Rx^ ▪ ***Oral solution:*** 10 mEq/15 ml^Rx^, 20 mEq/15 ml^Rx^, 30 mEq/15 ml^Rx^, 40 mEq/15 ml^Rx^ ▪ ***Powder/packets for oral solution:*** 15 mEq/1.2-g packet^Rx^, 20 mEq/1.5-g packet^Rx^, 25 mEq/1.8-g packet^Rx^ ▪ ***Packets for oral suspension:*** 20 mEq/1.5-g packet^Rx^ ▪ ***Concentrate for injection:*** 0.1 mEq/ml in 10-mEq ampules and vials^Rx^, 0.2 mEq/ml in 10- and 20-mEq ampules and vials^Rx^, 0.3 mEq/ml in 30-mEq ampules and vials^Rx^, 0.4 mEq/ml in 20- and 40-mEq ampules and vials^Rx^, 1.5 mEq/ml^Rx^, 2 mEq/ml^Rx^, 3 mEq/ml^Rx^ ▪ ***Solution for IV infusion:*** 10 mEq/liter in various dextrose and saline solutions in 250-, 500-, and 100-ml containers^Rx^, 20 mEq/liter in dextrose/saline/Lactated Ringer's solutions in 250-, 500-, and 100-ml containers^Rx^, 30 mEq/liter in various dextrose and saline solutions in 250-, 500-, and 100-ml containers^Rx^, 40 mEq/liter in various dextrose and saline solutions in 250-, 500-, and 100-ml containers^Rx^.

❑ Potassium Chloride/Potassium Bicarbonate/Potassium Citrate

▪ ***Tablets for effervescent oral solution:*** 20 mEq^Rx^.

❑ Potasssium Gluconate

▪ ***Tablets:*** 2 mEq^Rx^, 5 mEq^Rx^ ▪ ***Elixir:*** 20 mEq/15 ml^Rx^.

❑ Potassium Gluconate/Potassium Chloride

▪ ***Oral solution:*** 20 mEq/15 ml^Rx^ ▪ ***Powder for oral solution:*** 20 mEq/5-g packet^Rx^.

❑ Potassium Gluconate/Potassium Citrate

▪ ***Oral solution:*** 20 mEq/15 ml^Rx^.

❑ Trikates (Potassium Acetate, Potassium Bicarbonate/Potassium Citrate)

▪ ***Oral solution:*** 15 mEq/5 ml^Rx^.

TIME/ACTION PROFILE (increase in serum potassium levels)

	ONSET	PEAK	DURATION
PO	UK	1–2 hr	UK
IV	rapid	end of infusion	UK

NURSING IMPLICATIONS

ASSESSMENT

- ❑ Assess patient for signs and symptoms of hypokalemia (weakness, fatigue, U wave on ECG, arrhythmias, polyuria, polydipsia) and hyperkalemia (see Toxicity and Overdose).
- ❑ Monitor pulse, blood pressure, and ECG periodically throughout IV therapy.
- ▪ ***Lab Test Considerations:*** Monitor serum potassium before and periodically throughout therapy. Monitor renal function, serum bicarbonate, and pH. Determine serum magnesium level if patient has refractory hypokalemia; hypomagnesemia should be corrected to facilitate effectiveness of potassium replacement. Monitor serum chloride because hypochlo-

remia may occur if replacing potassium without concurrent chloride.

- ***Toxicity and Overdose:*** Symptoms of toxicity are those of hyperkalemia (slow, irregular heartbeat; fatigue; muscle weakness; paresthesia; confusion; dyspnea; peaked T waves; depressed ST segments; prolonged QT segments; widened QRS complexes; loss of P waves; and cardiac arrhythmias).
- Treatment includes discontinuation of potassium, administration of sodium bicarbonate to correct acidosis, dextrose and insulin to facilitate passage of potassium into cells, calcium salts to reverse ECG effects (in patients who are not receiving cardiac glycosides), sodium polystyrene used as an exchange resin, and/or dialysis for patient with impaired renal function.

POTENTIAL NURSING DIAGNOSES

- Nutrition, altered, less than body requirements (Indications).
- Knowledge deficit, related to medication regimen (Patient/Family Teaching).

IMPLEMENTATION

- **PO:** Administer with or after meals to decrease GI irritation.
- Administer tablets with full glass of water. Do not chew or crush enteric-coated or extended-release tablets or capsules. Dissolve effervescent tablets in 3–8 oz cold water. Ensure effervescent tablet is fully dissolved. Powders and solutions should be diluted in 3–8 oz cold water or juice (do not use tomato juice if patient is on sodium restriction). Instruct patient to drink slowly over 5–10 min.
- **IV:** Avoid extravasation; severe pain and tissue necrosis may occur.

Potassium Acetate

- **Continuous Infusion:** Do not administer undiluted. Each single dose *must* be diluted and thoroughly mixed in 100–1000 ml of dextrose, saline, Ringer's or lactated Ringer's solution, dextrose/saline, dextrose/Ringer's, or lactated Ringer's solution combinations. Usually limited to 40 mEq/liter via peripheral line (100 mEq/liter via central line).
- ***Rate:*** Infuse slowly, at a rate up to 20 mEq/hr. Do not exceed 1 mEq/min in adults and 0.02 mEq/kg/min in children.
- **Y-Site Compatibility:** ▪ ciprofloxacin.

Potassium Chloride

- **Continuous Infusion:** Do not administer concentrations of 1.5 or 2 mEq/ml undiluted; fatalities have occurred. Concentrated products have black caps on vials or black stripes above constriction on ampules and are labeled with a warning regarding dilution requirement. Each single dose must be diluted and thoroughly mixed in 100–1000 ml of IV solution. Usually limited to 40 mEq/liter via peripheral line (100 mEq/liter via central line).
- Concentrations of 0.1 and 0.4 mEq/ml are intended for administration via calibrated infusion device and do not require dilution.
- ***Rate:*** Infuse slowly, at a rate up to 20 mEq/hr. Do not exceed 1 mEq/min in adults and 0.02 mEq/kg/min in children.
- **Solution Compatibility:** ▪ May be diluted in dextrose, saline, Ringer's solution, lactated Ringer's solution, dextrose/saline, dextrose/Ringer's solution, and dextrose/lactated Ringer's solution combinations. Commercially available premixed with many of the above IV solutions.
- **Y-Site Compatibility:** ▪ acyclovir ▪ aldesleukin ▪ amifostine ▪ aminophylline ▪ amiodarone ▪ ampicillin ▪ amrinone ▪ atropine ▪ aztreonam ▪ betamethasone ▪ calcium gluconate ▪ cephalothin sodium neutral ▪ cephapirin ▪ chlordiazepoxide ▪ chlorpromazine ▪ ciprofloxacin ▪ cyanocobalamin ▪ dexamethasone ▪ digoxin ▪ diltiazem ▪ diphenhydramine ▪ dobutamine ▪ dopamine ▪ droperidol ▪ droperidol/fentanyl ▪ edrophonium ▪ enalaprilat ▪ epinephrine ▪ esmolol ▪ conjugated estrogens ▪ ethacrynate sodium ▪ famotidine ▪ fentanyl ▪ filgrastim ▪ fludarabine ▪ fluorouracil ▪ furosemide ▪ gallium nitrate ▪ granisetron ▪ hydralazine ▪ idarubicin potassium ▪ indomethacin ▪ insulin ▪ isoproterenol ▪ kanamycin ▪ labetalol ▪ lidocaine ▪ lorazepam ▪ magnesium sulfate ▪ melphalan ▪ menadiol ▪ meperidine ▪ methicillin ▪ methoxamine ▪ methylergonovine ▪ midazolam ▪ minocycline ▪ morphine ▪ neostigmine ▪ norepinephrine ▪ ondansetron ▪ oxacillin ▪ oxytocin ▪ paclitaxel ▪ penicillin G potassium ▪ pentazocine ▪ phytonadione ▪ piperacillin/tazobactam ▪ prednisolone ▪ procainamide ▪ prochlorperazine edisylate ▪ propranolol ▪ pyridostigmine ▪ sargramostim ▪ scopolamine ▪ sodium bicarbonate ▪ succinylcholine ▪ tacrolimus

▪ teniposide ▪ theophylline ▪ thiotepa ▪ trimethaphan ▪ trimethobenzamide ▪ vinorelbine ▪ zidovudine.

- **Y-Site Incompatibility:** ▪ diazepam ▪ ergotamine tartrate ▪ phenytoin.
- **Additive Compatibility:** ▪ calcium gluconate ▪ cimetidine ▪ lidocaine ▪ ranitidine ▪ sodium bicarbonate ▪ vitamin B complex with C.

PATIENT/FAMILY TEACHING

- ☐ Explain to patient purpose of the medication and the need to take as directed, especially when concurrent cardiac glycosides or diuretics are taken. A missed dose should be taken as soon as remembered within 2 hr; if not, return to regular dosage schedule. Do not double dose.
- ☐ Emphasize correct method of administration. GI irritation or ulceration may result from chewing enteric-coated tablets or insufficient dilution of liquid or powder forms.
- ☐ Some extended-release tablets are contained in a wax matrix that may be expelled in the stool. This occurrence is not significant.
- ☐ Instruct patient to avoid salt substitutes or low-salt milk or food unless approved by health care professional. Patient should be advised to read all labels to prevent excess potassium intake.
- ☐ Advise patient regarding sources of dietary potassium (see Appendix K). Encourage compliance with recommended diet.
- ☐ Instruct patient to report dark, tarry, or bloody stools; weakness; unusual fatigue; or tingling of extremities. Notify health care professional if nausea, vomiting, diarrhea, or stomach discomfort persists. Dosage may require adjustment.
- ☐ Emphasize the importance of regular follow-up exams to monitor serum levels and progress.

EVALUATION

Effectiveness of therapy can be demonstrated by: ▪ Prevention and correction of serum potassium depletion ▪ Cessation of arrhythmias caused by cardiac glycoside toxicity.

PRAMIPEXOLE
(pra-mi-**pex**-ole)

CLASSIFICATION(S): *Anti-Parkinson agent (dopamine agonist)*

Pregnancy Category C

INDICATIONS

▪ Management of idiopathic Parkinson's disease.

ACTION

▪ Stimulates dopamine receptors in the striatum of the brain. **Therapeutic Effects:** ▪ Decreased tremor and rigidity in Parkinson's disease.

PHARMACOKINETICS

Absorption: >90% absorbed following oral administration.
Distribution: Widely distributed.
Metabolism and Excretion: 90% excreted unchanged in urine.
Half-life: 8 hr (increased in geriatric patients and patients with renal impairment).

CONTRAINDICATIONS AND PRECAUTIONS

Contraindicated in: ▪ Hypersensitivity.
Use Cautiously in: ▪ Geriatric patients (increased risk of hallucinations) ▪ Renal impairment (increased dosing interval recommended if CCr <60 ml/min) ▪ Pregnancy, lactation, or children (safety not established).

ADVERSE REACTIONS AND SIDE EFFECTS*

CNS: amnesia, dizziness, drowsiness, hallucinations, weakness, abnormal dreams, confusion, dyskinesia, extrapyramidal syndrome, headache, insomnia.
CV: postural hypotension.
GI: constipation, dry mouth, dyspepsia, nausea.
GU: urinary frequency.
MS: leg cramps.
Neuro: hypertonia.

***CAPITALS indicate life-threatening; underlines indicate most frequent.**

INTERACTIONS

Drug-Drug: ▪ Concurrent **levodopa** increases the risk of hallucinations and dyskinesia ▪ Effectiveness may be increased by **cimetidine** ▪ Effectiveness may be decreased by **dopamine antagonists**, including **phenothiazines, butyrophenones, thioxanthenes,** or **metoclopramide.**

ROUTE AND DOSAGE

- **PO (Adults):** 0.125 mg 3 times daily initially; may be increased q 5–7 days (range 1.5–4.5 mg/day in 3 divided doses).

AVAILABILITY

▪ ***Tablets:*** 0.125 mg[Rx], 0.25 mg[Rx], 1 mg[Rx], 1.5 mg[Rx].

TIME/ACTION PROFILE (blood levels)

	ONSET	PEAK	DURATION
PO	UK	2 hr	8 hr

NURSING IMPLICATIONS

ASSESSMENT

- □ Assess patient for signs and symptoms of Parkinson's disease (tremor, muscle weakness and rigidity, ataxia) prior to and throughout therapy.
- □ Assess patient for confusion or hallucinations. Notify physician or other health care professional if these occur.
- □ Monitor ECG and blood pressure frequently during dosage adjustment and periodically throughout therapy.

POTENTIAL NURSING DIAGNOSES

- Physical mobility, impaired (Indications).
- Injury, risk for (Indications, Side Effects).
- Knowledge deficit, related to medication regimen (Patient/Family Teaching).

IMPLEMENTATION

- **PO:** An attempt to reduce the dose of levodopa/carbidopa may be made cautiously during pramipexole therapy.
- □ Administer with meals to minimize nausea; usually resolves with continued therapy.

PATIENT/FAMILY TEACHING

- □ Instruct patient to take medication exactly as directed. Missed doses should be taken as soon as remembered if not almost time for next dose. Do not double doses. Consult health care professional before reducing dose or discontinuing medication.
- □ May cause drowsiness. Caution patient to avoid driving or other activities requiring alertness until response to medication is known.
- □ Advise patient to change positions slowly to minimize orthostatic hypotension. May occur more frequently during initial therapy.
- □ Advise patient to notify health care professional if pregnancy is planned or suspected or if currently or planning breast-feeding.

EVALUATION

Effectiveness of therapy can be demonstrated by: ▪ Decreased tremor and rigidity in Parkinson's disease.

PRAZOSIN

(**pra**-zoe-sin)
Minipress

CLASSIFICATION(S):
Antihypertensive agent (peripherally acting antiadrenergic)

Pregnancy Category C

INDICATIONS

▪ Mild to moderate hypertension. **Unlabeled Uses:** ▪ Management of urinary outflow obstruction in patients with benign prostatic hyperplasia.

ACTION

▪ Dilates both arteries and veins by blocking postsynaptic $alpha_1$-adrenergic receptors ▪ Decreases contractions in smooth muscle of prostatic capsule. **Therapeutic Effects:** ▪ Lowering of blood pressure ▪ Decreased cardiac preload and afterload ▪ Decreased symptoms of prostatic hyperplasia (urinary urgency, urinary hesitancy, nocturia).

PHARMACOKINETICS

Absorption: 60% absorbed following oral administration.

Distribution: Widely distributed.
Metabolism and Excretion: Extensively metabolized by the liver. Minimal (5–10%) renal excretion of unchanged drug.
Half-life: 2–3 hr.

CONTRAINDICATIONS AND PRECAUTIONS

Contraindicated in: ▪ Hypersensitivity.
Use Cautiously in: ▪ Renal insufficiency (increased sensitivity to effects; dosage reduction may be required) ▪ Pregnancy, lactation, or children (safety not established) ▪ Angina pectoris ▪ When adding diuretics (reduce dose of prazosin).

ADVERSE REACTIONS AND SIDE EFFECTS*

CNS: dizziness, headache, weakness, drowsiness, mental depression, syncope.
EENT: blurred vision.
CV: first-dose orthostatic hypotension, palpitations, angina, edema.
GI: abdominal cramps, diarrhea, dry mouth, nausea, vomiting.
GU: impotence, priapism.

INTERACTIONS

Drug-Drug: ▪ Additive hypotension with acute ingestion of **alcohol,** other **antihypertensive agents,** or **nitrates** ▪ Antihypertensive effects may be decreased by **NSAIDs.**

ROUTE AND DOSAGE

❑ Hypertension

- **PO (Adults):** 1 mg 2–3 times daily (give 1st dose at bedtime) for initial 3 days of therapy, then 1 mg 2–3 times daily for 3 days, then increase gradually to maintenance dose of 6–15 mg/day in 2–3 divided doses (not to exceed 20–40 mg/day).
- **PO (Children):** 50–400 mcg (0.05–0.4 mg)/kg/day in 2–3 divided doses (not to exceed 7 mg/dose or 15 mg/day).

❑ Benign Prostatic Hyperplasia

- **PO (Adults):** 1–5 mg twice daily.

AVAILABILITY

▪ ***Capsules:*** 1 mg^{Rx}, 2 mg^{Rx}, 5 mg^{Rx} ▪ ***Tablets:*** 1 mg^{Rx}, 2 mg^{Rx}, 5 mg^{Rx} ▪ ***In combination with:*** polythiazide (Minizide)^{Rx}. See Appendix A.

TIME/ACTION PROFILE (antihypertensive effects)

	ONSET	PEAK	DURATION
PO	2 hr	2–4 hr†	10 hr

†Following single dose; maximal antihypertensive effects occur after 3–4 wk of chronic dosing.

NURSING IMPLICATIONS

ASSESSMENT

- **General Info:** Monitor intake and output ratios and daily weight and assess for edema daily, especially at beginning of therapy. Report significant weight gain or edema.
- **Hypertension:** Monitor blood pressure and pulse frequently during initial dosage adjustment and periodically throughout therapy. Report significant changes.
- ❑ Monitor frequency of prescription refills to determine compliance.
- **Benign Prostatic Hypertrophy:** Assess patient for urinary symptoms (retention, dribbling, hesitancy, urgency) periodically during therapy.
- ***Lab Test Considerations:*** May cause elevated serum sodium levels.
- ❑ May cause increased vanillylmandelic acid (VMA) concentrations; false-positive results may occur in screening tests for pheochromocytoma.

POTENTIAL NURSING DIAGNOSES

- Injury, risk for (Side Effects).
- Knowledge deficit, related to medication regimen (Patient/Family Teaching).
- Noncompliance (Patient/Family Teaching).

IMPLEMENTATION

- **General Info:** Following initial dose, patient may develop 1st-dose orthostatic hypotensive reaction, which most frequently occurs 30–90 min after initial dose and may be manifested by dizziness, weakness, and syncope. Observe patient closely during this period, and take precautions to prevent injury. The first

*CAPITALS indicate life-threatening; underlines indicate most frequent.

dose may be given at bedtime to minimize this reaction.

- Commonly administered concurrently with a thiazide diuretic or a beta-adrenergic blocker for treatment of hypertension.

PATIENT/FAMILY TEACHING

- Emphasize the importance of continuing to take this medication, even if feeling well. Instruct patient to take medication at the same time each day. If a dose is missed, take as soon as remembered unless almost time for next dose. Do not double doses.
- Encourage patient to comply with additional interventions for hypertension (weight reduction, low-sodium diet, smoking cessation, moderation of alcohol consumption, regular exercise, stress management).
- Instruct patient and family on proper technique for blood pressure monitoring. Advise them to check blood pressure at least weekly and to report significant changes.
- May cause drowsiness or dizziness. Advise patient to avoid driving or other activities requiring alertness until response to medication is known.
- Caution patient to change positions slowly to decrease orthostatic hypotension.
- Advise patient to consult health care professional before taking any OTC medications, especially cough, cold, or allergy remedies.
- Emphasize the importance of follow-up visits to determine effectiveness of therapy.

EVALUATION

Effectiveness of therapy can be demonstrated by: ▪ Decrease in blood pressure without appearance of side effects ▪ Decrease in symptoms of prostatic hypertrophy.

PRIMIDONE

(**pri**-mi-done)

{Apo-Primidone}, Myidone, Mysoline, {PMS-Primidone}, {Sertan}

CLASSIFICATION(S):

Anticonvulsant

Pregnancy Category D

INDICATIONS

▪ Management of tonic-clonic, complex partial, and focal seizures. **Unlabeled Uses:** ▪ Management of essential (familial) tremor.

ACTION

▪ Decreases neuronal excitability ▪ Increases the threshold of electric stimulation of the motor cortex. **Therapeutic Effects:** ▪ Prevention of seizures.

PHARMACOKINETICS

Absorption: 60–80% absorbed from the GI tract.

Distribution: Widely distributed. Crosses the placenta and enters breast milk.

Metabolism and Excretion: Converted to phenobarbital and another active anticonvulsant compound (PEMA) by the liver.

Half-life: 3–24 hr.

CONTRAINDICATIONS AND PRECAUTIONS

Contraindicated in: ▪ Previous hypersensitivity ▪ Porphyria.

Use Cautiously in: ▪ Severe liver disease (dosage adjustment required) ▪ Pregnancy and lactation (safety not established; may cause hemorrhage in the newborn).

ADVERSE REACTIONS AND SIDE EFFECTS*

CNS: <u>ataxia</u>, <u>drowsiness</u>, <u>vertigo</u>, excitement (↑ children).

EENT: visual changes.

Resp: dyspnea.

CV: edema, orthostatic hypotension.

GI: <u>anorexia</u>, drug-induced hepatitis, nausea, vomiting.

Derm: alopecia, rashes.

Hemat: blood dyscrasias, megaloblastic anemia.

Misc: folic acid deficiency.

INTERACTIONS

Drug-Drug: ▪ Induces liver enzymes and may hasten metabolism and decrease the effectiveness of other drugs metabolized by the liver, including **oral contraceptives, chloramphenicol, acebutolol, propranolol, metoprolol,**

{} = Available in Canada only.
***CAPITALS indicate life-threatening; <u>underlines</u> indicate most frequent.**

timolol, doxycycline, glucocorticoids, tricyclic antidepressants, phenothiazines, phenylbutazone, and **quinidine** ▪ Additive CNS depression with other **CNS depressants,** including **alcohol, antihistamines, opioids,** and **sedative/hypnotics** ▪ Concurrent use with **phenobarbital** may lead to phenobarbital toxicity.

Drug-Food: ▪ Decreases the absorption of **folic acid.**

ROUTE AND DOSAGE

- **PO (Adults and Children >8 yr):** Initial dose of 100–125 mg hs for 3 days, then 100–125 mg bid for 3 days, then 100–125 mg tid for 3 days, then maintenance dose of 250 mg 3 times daily (not to exceed 2 g/day).
- **PO (Children <8 yr):** Initial dose of 50 mg hs for 3 days, then 50 mg bid for next 3 days, then 100 mg bid for 3 days, then maintenance dose of 125–250 mg tid (10–25 mg/kg/day).

AVAILABILITY

- ***Tablets:*** 50 mg[Rx], {125 mg[Rx]}, 250 mg[Rx]
- ***Oral suspension:*** 250 mg/5 ml[Rx]
- {***Chewable tablets:*** 125 mg[Rx]}.

TIME/ACTION PROFILE (anticonvulsant effect)

	ONSET	PEAK	DURATION
PO	4–7 days	7–10 days	8–12 hr

NURSING IMPLICATIONS

ASSESSMENT

- □ Assess location, duration, frequency, and characteristics of seizure activity. Institute seizure precautions.
- □ Assess patient for allergy to phenobarbital, as it is a metabolite of primidone.
- □ Assess patient for signs of folic acid deficiency (mental dysfunction, unusual tiredness or weakness, psychiatric disorders, neuropathy, megaloblastic anemia). May be treated with folic acid.
- ▪ ***Lab Test Considerations:*** CBC and sequential multiple analysis–12 (SMA-12) tests should be monitored every 6 mo throughout course of therapy. May cause leukopenia and thrombocytopenia. May cause decreased serum bilirubin concentrations.
- □ Monitor serum folate concentrations periodically during therapy.
- ▪ ***Toxicity and Overdose:*** Serum primidone and phenobarbital (a major metabolite of primidone) levels should be routinely monitored. Therapeutic blood levels for primidone—5–10 mcg/ml; for phenobarbital—15–40 mcg/ml.
- □ Signs of primidone toxicity include ataxia, lethargy, changes in vision, confusion, and dyspnea.

POTENTIAL NURSING DIAGNOSES

- ▪ Injury, risk for (Indications).
- ▪ Knowledge deficit, related to medication regimen (Patient/Family Teaching).

IMPLEMENTATION

- ▪ **General Info:** When switching from alternative anticonvulsant medication to primidone or when adding primidone to regimen, increase primidone dose gradually while decreasing or continuing other anticonvulsant dosages to maintain seizure control. The switch to primidone alone should take at least 2 wk. Dosage adjustment is usually made at bedtime.
- ▪ **PO:** May be administered with food to minimize GI irritation. Low initial doses (25 mg twice daily) have been used in patients experiencing nausea and vomiting. Tablets may be crushed and mixed with food or fluids for patients with difficulty swallowing. Shake liquid preparations well before pouring. Use calibrated measuring device to ensure accurate dosage.

PATIENT/FAMILY TEACHING

- □ Instruct patient to take medication at the same time each day exactly as directed. If a dose is missed, take as soon as remembered unless within 1 hr of next dose. Abrupt withdrawal may lead to status epilepticus.
- □ May cause drowsiness or dizziness. Caution patient to avoid driving or other activities requiring alertness until response to medication is known. These symptoms usually diminish in frequency and intensity with continued use of the medication. Do not resume driving until physician gives medical clearance based on control of seizure disorder.
- □ Caution patient to avoid taking alcohol or other CNS depressants concurrently with this medication.

- ☐ Caution patient to avoid sudden changes in position to decrease orthostatic hypotension.
- ☐ Instruct patient to notify health care professional of medication regimen prior to treatment or surgery.
- ☐ Advise patient to carry identification describing medication regimen at all times.
- ☐ Advise patient to notify health care professional if skin rash, unsteady gait, joint pain, fever, changes in vision, dyspnea, pregnancy, or paradoxical excitement (especially in children or the elderly) occurs.
- ☐ Emphasize the importance of routine exams to monitor progress.

EVALUATION

Effectiveness of therapy can be demonstrated by: ▪ Decrease or cessation of seizures without excessive sedation. May require 1 wk or more of therapy before therapeutic response is seen.

PROBENECID
(proe-**ben**-e-sid)
Benemid, {Benuryl}, Probalan

CLASSIFICATION(S):
Antigout agent (uricosuric)

Pregnancy Category B

INDICATIONS

▪ Prevention of recurrences of gouty arthritis ▪ Treatment of hyperuricemia secondary to thiazide therapy ▪ Used to increase and prolong serum levels of penicillin and related anti-infectives.

ACTION

▪ Inhibits renal tubular reabsorption of uric acid, thus promoting its renal excretion. **Therapeutic Effects:** ▪ Reduction of serum uric acid levels.

PHARMACOKINETICS

Absorption: Well absorbed following oral administration.
Distribution: Crosses the placenta.
Metabolism and Excretion: Mostly metabolized by the liver; 10% excreted unchanged in the urine.
Half-life: 4–17 hr.

CONTRAINDICATIONS AND PRECAUTIONS

Contraindicated in: ▪ Hypersensitivity ▪ Chronic high-dose salicylate therapy ▪ Children <2 yr. **Use Cautiously in:** ▪ Peptic ulcer ▪ Blood dyscrasias ▪ Uric acid kidney stones ▪ Renal impairment (dosage reduction recommended; may not be effective if CCr ≤30 ml/min) ▪ Pregnancy or lactation (has been used safely during pregnancy; safety during lactation not established).

ADVERSE REACTIONS AND SIDE EFFECTS*

CNS: headache, dizziness.
GI: nausea, vomiting, abdominal pain, diarrhea, drug-induced hepatitis, sore gums.
GU: uric acid stones, urinary frequency.
Derm: flushing, rashes.
Hemat: APLASTIC ANEMIA, anemia.

INTERACTIONS

Drug-Drug: ▪ Increases blood levels of **acyclovir, allopurinol, barbiturates, benzodiazepines, cephalosporins, clofibrate, dapsone, dyphylline, methotrexate, NSAIDs, pantothenic acid, penicillamine, penicillins, rifampin, sulfonamides, sulfonylureas,** or **zidovudine** ▪ Large doses of **salicylates** may decrease uricosuric activity.

ROUTE AND DOSAGE

- **PO (Adults and Children >50 kg):** *Hyperuricemia*—250 mg bid for 1 wk; increase to 500 mg twice daily, then may increase by 500 mg/day every 4 wk (not to exceed 3 g/day). *Augmentation of penicillin/cephalosporins*—500 mg 4 times daily. *Single-dose therapy of gonorrhea*—1 g with amoxicillin or penicillin.
- **PO (Children 2–14 yr and ≤50kg):** 25 mg/kg (700 mg/m^2) initially; then 10 mg/kg (300 mg/m^2) 4 times daily.

AVAILABILITY

▪ ***Tablets:*** 0.5 g^{Rx} ▪ ***In combination with:*** 0.5 mg colchicine (ColBenemid, Col-Probene-

{} = Available in Canada only.
*CAPITALS indicate life-threatening; underlines indicate most frequent.

cid, Proben-C) and ampicillin (Polycillin-PRB, Probampacin)Rx. See Appendix A.

TIME/ACTION PROFILE (effects on serum uric acid levels)

	ONSET	PEAK	DURATION
PO	30 min	2–4 hr	8 hr

NURSING IMPLICATIONS

ASSESSMENT

- **Gout:** Assess involved joints for pain, mobility, and edema throughout course of therapy.
- Monitor intake and output ratios. Fluids should be encouraged to prevent urate stone formation (2000–3000 ml/day). Alkalinization of the urine with sodium bicarbonate, potassium citrate, or acetazolamide may also be used for this purpose.
- ***Lab Test Considerations:*** CBC, serum uric acid levels, and renal function should be monitored routinely during long-term therapy.
- Serum and urine uric acid determinations may be measured periodically when probenecid is used to treat hyperuricemia.

POTENTIAL NURSING DIAGNOSES

- Pain (Indications).
- Physical mobility, impaired (Indications).
- Knowledge deficit, related to medication regimen (Patient/Family Teaching).

IMPLEMENTATION

- **General Info:** Probenecid therapy is not used to treat gouty arthritis but, rather, to prevent it. If acute attacks occur during therapy, probenecid is usually continued at full dose along with colchicine or NSAIDs.
- **PO:** Administer with food or antacid to minimize gastric irritation.
- Gradual dosage reduction should be attempted if uric acid levels remain stable following 6 mo of therapy.

PATIENT/FAMILY TEACHING

- Instruct patient to take medication exactly as directed, not to discontinue without consulting health care professional. Irregular dosage schedules may cause elevation of uric acid levels and precipitate an acute gout attack.
- Explain purpose of the medication to patients taking probenecid with penicillin.
- Advise patient to follow recommendations of health care professional regarding weight loss, diet, and alcohol consumption.
- Caution patient not to take aspirin or other salicylates, as they decrease the effects of probenecid.
- Instruct patient to report nausea, vomiting, loss of appetite, abdominal pain, unusual bleeding or bruising, sore throat, fatigue, malaise, or yellowing of the skin or eyes promptly.

EVALUATION

Effectiveness of therapy can be demonstrated by: ▪ Decrease in pain and swelling in affected joints and subsequent decrease in frequency of gout attacks. May require several months of continuous therapy for maximum effects ▪ Decrease in serum uric acid levels ▪ Prolonged serum levels of penicillins and other related antibiotics.

PROCAINAMIDE

(proe-**kane**-ah-mide)

Procanbid, Promine, Pronestyl, Pronestyl-SR

CLASSIFICATION(S):

Antiarrhythmic (group IA)

Pregnancy Category C

INDICATIONS

▪ Treatment of a wide variety of ventricular and atrial arrhythmias, including: ▫ Atrial premature contractions ▫ Premature ventricular contractions ▫ Ventricular tachycardia ▫ Paroxysmal atrial tachycardia ▪ Maintenance of normal sinus rhythm after conversion from atrial fibrillation or flutter.

ACTION

▪ Decreases myocardial excitability ▪ Slows conduction velocity ▪ May depress myocardial contractility. **Therapeutic Effects:** ▪ Suppression of arrhythmias.

PHARMACOKINETICS

Absorption: Well absorbed (75–90%) following oral and IM administration. Sustained-release oral preparation is more slowly absorbed.
Distribution: Rapidly and widely distributed.
Metabolism and Excretion: Converted by the

liver to *N*-acetylprocainamide (NAPA), an active antiarrhythmic compound. Remainder (40–70%) excreted unchanged by the kidneys.
Half-life: 2.5–4.7 hr (NAPA—7 hr), prolonged in renal impairment.

CONTRAINDICATIONS AND PRECAUTIONS

Contraindicated in: ▪ Hypersensitivity ▪ AV block ▪ Myasthenia gravis ▪ Hypersensitivity to tartrazine (FDC yellow dye #5; present in some oral products).
Use Cautiously in: ▪ Myocardial infarction or cardiac glycoside toxicity ▪ Congestive heart failure, renal or hepatic insufficiency, geriatric patients (dosage reduction or increased dosing intervals recommended) ▪ Pregnancy, lactation, or children (safety not established).

ADVERSE REACTIONS AND SIDE EFFECTS*

CNS: SEIZURES, confusion, dizziness.
CV: ASYSTOLE, HEART BLOCK, VENTRICULAR ARRHYTHMIAS, hypotension.
GI: diarrhea, anorexia, bitter taste, nausea, vomiting.
Derm: rashes.
Hemat: AGRANULOCYTOSIS, eosinophilia, leukopenia, thrombocytopenia.
Misc: chills, drug-induced systemic lupus syndrome, fever.

INTERACTIONS

Drug-Drug: ▪ May have additive or antagonistic effects with other **antiarrhythmics** ▪ Additive neurologic toxicity (confusion, seizures) with **lidocaine** ▪ **Antihypertensives** and **nitrates** may potentiate hypotensive effect ▪ Potentiates **neuromuscular blocking agents** ▪ May partially antagonize the therapeutic effects of **anticholinesterase agents** in myasthenia gravis ▪ Increased risk of arrhythmias with **pimozide** ▪ Additive anticholinergic effects with other **drugs possessing anticholinergic properties**, including **antihistamines, antidepressants, atropine, haloperidol,** and **phenothiazines** ▪ Effects of procainamide may be increased by **cimetidine, quinidine,** or **trimethoprim.**

ROUTE AND DOSAGE

See infusion rate chart in Appendix D.

- **PO (Adults):** *Atrial arrhythmias*—1.25 g initially, then 750 mg 2 hr later, then 0.5–1 g q 2–3 hr followed by maintenance dosing of 0.5–1 g q 4–6 hr or 1 g q 12 hr as sustained-release tablets. *Ventricular arrhythmias*—50 mg/kg/day in divided doses q 3 hr or q 12 hr for sustained-release tablets. Lower doses/longer dosing intervals are recommended for geriatric patients or those with renal, hepatic, or cardiac insufficiency.
- **PO (Children):** 12.5 mg/kg (375 mg/m²) 4 times daily.
- **IM (Adults):** 50 mg/kg/day in divided doses q 3–6 hr.
- **IV (Adults):** 100 mg q 5 min until arrhythmia is abolished or 1000 mg have been given; wait at least 10 min until further dosing *or* loading infusion of 500–600 mg over 25–30 min followed by maintenance infusion of 2–6 mg/min.

AVAILABILITY

▪ ***Tablets:*** 250 mg^Rx^, 375 mg^Rx^, 500 mg^Rx^ ▪ ***Sustained-release tablets:*** 500 mg^Rx^, 1000 mg^Rx^ ▪ ***Capsules:*** 250 mg^Rx^, 375 mg^Rx^, 500 mg^Rx^ ▪ ***Injection:*** 100 mg/ml in 10-ml vials^Rx^, 500 mg/ml in 2-ml vials and 2- and 4-ml prefilled syringes^Rx^.

TIME/ACTION PROFILE (antiarrhythmic effects)

	ONSET	PEAK	DURATION
PO	30 min	60–90 min	3–4 hr
PO-ER	UK	UK	6–12 hr
IV	immediate	25–60 min	3–4 hr
IM	10–30 min	15–60 min	3–4 hr

NURSING IMPLICATIONS

ASSESSMENT

- ☐ Monitor ECG, pulse, and blood pressure continuously throughout IV administration. Parameters should be monitored periodically during oral administration. IV administration is usually discontinued if any of the following occur: arrhythmia is resolved, QRS complex widens by 50%, PR interval is prolonged, blood pressure drops >15 mm Hg, or toxic side effects develop. Patient should remain su-

*CAPITALS indicate life-threatening; underlines indicate most frequent.

pine throughout IV administration to minimize hypotension.

- ***Lab Test Considerations:*** CBC should be monitored every 2 wk during the first 3 mo of therapy. May cause decreased leukocyte, neutrophil, and platelet counts. Therapy may be discontinued if leukopenia occurs. Blood counts usually return to normal within 1 mo of discontinuation of therapy.
- □ Monitor antinuclear antibody (ANA) periodically during prolonged therapy or if symptoms of lupus-like reaction occur. Therapy is discontinued if a steady increase in ANA titer occurs.
- □ May cause an increase in AST, ALT, alkaline phosphatase, LDH, bilirubin, and a positive Coombs' test result.
- ***Toxicity and Overdose:*** Serum procainamide and NAPA levels may be monitored periodically during dosage adjustment. Therapeutic blood level of procainamide is 4–8 mcg/ml.
- □ Toxicity may occur with procainamide blood levels of 8–16 mcg/ml or greater.
- □ Signs of toxicity include confusion, dizziness, drowsiness, decreased urination, nausea, vomiting, and tachyarrhythmias.

POTENTIAL NURSING DIAGNOSES

- Cardiac output, decreased (Indications).
- Knowledge deficit, related to medication regimen (Patient/Family Teaching).

IMPLEMENTATION

- **General Info:** When converting from IV to oral dose regimen, allow 3–4 hr to elapse between last IV dose and administration of first oral dose.
- **PO:** Administer with a full glass of water on an empty stomach either 1 hr before or 2 hr after meals for faster absorption. If GI irritation becomes a problem, may be administered with or immediately after meals. Tablets may be crushed and capsules opened and mixed with food or fluids for patients with difficulty swallowing. Do not break, crush, or chew sustained-release tablets (Procan SR, Pronestyl-SR). Wax matrix of sustained-release tablets may be found in stool but is not significant.
- **IM:** Used only when oral and IV routes are not feasible.
- **Direct IV:** Dilute each 100 mg with 10 ml of D5W or sterile water for injection.
- ***Rate:*** Administer at a rate not to exceed 25–50 mg/min. Rapid administration may cause ventricular fibrillation or asystole.
- **Intermittent Infusion:** Prepare IV infusion by adding 200 mg–1 g to 50–500 ml of D5W for a concentration of 2–4 mg/ml. Slight yellow color of solution will not alter potency; do not use when darker than light amber or if solution contains a precipitate.
- ***Rate:*** Administer initial infusion over 30 min. Maintenance infusion should infuse at 2–6 mg/min to maintain control of arrhythmia. Use infusion pump to ensure accurate dosage (see Appendix D for infusion rate chart).
- **Y-Site Compatibility:** ▪ amiodarone ▪ famotidine ▪ heparin ▪ hydrocortisone sodium succinate ▪ potassium chloride ▪ ranitidine ▪ vitamin B complex with C.
- **Y-Site Incompatibility:** ▪ milrinone.

PATIENT/FAMILY TEACHING

- □ Instruct patient to take medication around the clock, exactly as directed, even if feeling well. If a dose is missed, take as soon as remembered within 2 hr (4 hr for sustained-release tablets); omit if remembered later. Do not double doses. Consult health care professional prior to discontinuing medication, as gradual reduction in dosage may be needed to prevent worsening of condition.
- □ Instruct patient or family member on how to take pulse. Advise patient to report changes in pulse rate or rhythm to health care professional.
- □ May cause dizziness. Caution patient to avoid driving or other activities requiring alertness until response to medication is known.
- □ Advise patient to notify health care professional immediately if signs of drug-induced lupus syndrome (fever, chills, joint pain or swelling, pain with breathing, skin rash), leukopenia (sore throat, mouth, or gums), or thrombocytopenia (unusual bleeding or bruising) occur. Medication may be discontinued if these occur.
- □ Caution patient not to take OTC medications with procainamide without consulting health care professional.
- □ Advise patient to inform health care professional of medication regimen prior to treatment or surgery.
- □ Advise patient to carry identification describ-

ing disease process and medication regimen at all times.
- Emphasize the importance of routine follow-up exams to monitor progress.

EVALUATION

Effectiveness of therapy can be demonstrated by: ▪ Resolution of cardiac arrhythmias without detrimental side effects.

PROCARBAZINE

(proe-**kar**-ba-zeen)
Matulane, {Natulan}

CLASSIFICATION(S):
Antineoplastic (alkylating agent)

Pregnancy Category D

INDICATIONS

▪ In combination with other antineoplastic agents and modalities in the treatment of Hodgkin's disease. **Unlabeled Uses:** ▪ Other lymphomas ▪ Brain and lung tumors ▪ Multiple myeloma ▪ Malignant melanoma ▪ Polycythemia vera.

ACTION

▪ Appears to inhibit DNA, RNA, and protein synthesis (cell-cycle S phase–specific). **Therapeutic Effects:** ▪ Death of rapidly replicating cells, particularly malignant ones.

PHARMACOKINETICS

Absorption: Well absorbed following oral administration.
Distribution: Widely distributed; crosses the blood-brain barrier.
Metabolism and Excretion: Metabolized by the liver; <5% excreted unchanged by the kidneys; some respiratory elimination as methane and carbon dioxide.
Half-life: 1 hr.

CONTRAINDICATIONS AND PRECAUTIONS

Contraindicated in: ▪ Hypersensitivity ▪ Pregnancy or lactation ▪ Alcoholism ▪ Severe renal or liver impairment ▪ Pheochromocytoma ▪ Congestive heart failure.

Use Cautiously in: ▪ Patients with childbearing potential ▪ Infections ▪ Decreased bone marrow reserve ▪ Other chronic debilitating illnesses ▪ Headaches ▪ Psychiatric illness ▪ Liver impairment ▪ Cardiovascular disease.

ADVERSE REACTIONS AND SIDE EFFECTS*

CNS: SEIZURES, confusion, dizziness, drowsiness, hallucinations, headache, mania, mental depression, nightmares, psychosis, syncope, tremor.
EENT: nystagmus, photophobia, retinal hemorrhage.
Resp: cough, pleural effusions.
CV: edema, hypotension, tachycardia.
GI: nausea, vomiting, anorexia, diarrhea, dry mouth, dysphagia, hepatic dysfunction, stomatitis.
GU: gonadal suppression.
Derm: alopecia, photosensitivity, pruritus, rashes.
Endo: gynecomastia.
Hemat: anemia, leukopenia, thrombocytopenia.
Neuro: neuropathy, paresthesia.
Misc: ascites.

INTERACTIONS

Drug-Drug: ▪ Concurrent use with **indirect-acting sympathomimetic amines** may produce life-threatening hypertension ▪ Deep coma and death may result from concurrent use of **opioids**; avoid meperidine. Use small incremental doses of other agents and titrate to effect ▪ Additive bone marrow depression may occur with other **antineoplastic agents** or **radiation therapy** ▪ Seizures and hyperpyrexia may occur with concurrent use of **MAO inhibitors, tricyclic antidepressants, SSRI antidepressants** (should not be used within 5 wk of fluoxetine), or **carbamazepine** ▪ May decrease serum **digoxin** levels ▪ Concurrent use with **levodopa** may result in flushing and hypertension ▪ Additive CNS depression with other **CNS depressants**, including **alcohol, antidepressants, antihistamines, opioids, phenothiazines**, and **sedative/hypnotics** ▪ Disulfiram-like reaction may occur with **alcohol.**
Drug-Food: ▪ Ingestion of foods high in **tyramine** content (see Appendix K) may result in

hypertension ▪ Ingestion of foods high in **caffeine** content may result in arrhythmias.

ROUTE AND DOSAGE

- **PO (Adults):** 2–4 mg/kg/day as a single dose or in divided doses for 1 wk, then 4–6 mg/kg/day until response is obtained; then maintenance dose of 1–2 mg/kg/day. Dosage should be rounded off to the nearest 50 mg.
- **PO (Children):** 50 mg/m^2/day for 7 days, then 100 mg/m^2/day, maintenance dose of 50 mg/m^2/day.

AVAILABILITY

- ***Capsules:*** 50 mg[Rx].

TIME/ACTION PROFILE (effects on blood counts)

	ONSET	PEAK	DURATION
PO	14 days	2–8 wk	28 days or more (up to 6 wk)

NURSING IMPLICATIONS

ASSESSMENT

- □ Monitor blood pressure, pulse, and respiratory rate periodically during course of therapy. Report significant changes to health care professional.
- □ Assess patient's nutritional status (appetite, intake and output ratios, weight, frequency and amount of emesis). Anorexia and weight loss can be decreased by feeding light, frequent meals. Nausea and vomiting can be minimized by administering an antiemetic at least 1 hr prior to receiving medication. Phenothiazine antiemetics should be avoided.
- □ Monitor for bone marrow depression. Assess for bleeding (bleeding gums, bruising, petechiae, guaiac stools, urine, and emesis) and avoid IM injections and rectal temperatures if platelet count is low. Apply pressure to venipuncture sites for 10 min. Assess for signs of infection during neutropenia. Anemia may occur. Monitor for increased fatigue, dyspnea, and orthostatic hypotension.
- □ Concurrent ingestion of tyramine-rich foods and many medications may result in life-threatening hypertensive crisis. Signs and symptoms of hypertensive crisis include chest pain, severe headache, nausea and vomiting, photosensitivity, and enlarged pupils. Treatment includes IV phentolamine.
- □ Procarbazine should be discontinued until side effects clear and then resumed at a lower dose if leukopenia, thrombocytopenia, hypersensitivity reaction, stomatitis (first small ulceration or persistent soreness), diarrhea, hemorrhage, or bleeding tendencies occur.
- ▪ ***Lab Test Considerations:*** Monitor hemoglobin, hematocrit, WBC, differential, reticulocytes, and platelet count prior to and every 3–4 days throughout therapy. Notify physician if WBC $<4000/mm^3$ or platelet count $<100,000/mm^3$. Therapy should be discontinued and resumed at a lower dose when counts improve. The nadir of leukopenia and thrombocytopenia occurs in approximately 2–8 wk, and recovery usually occurs in about 6 wk. Anemia also may occur.
- □ Assess hepatic and renal function prior to therapy. Monitor urinalysis, AST, ALT, alkaline phosphatase, and BUN at least weekly during therapy.
- □ Closely monitor serum glucose in diabetic patients. Oral hypoglycemics or insulin dosage may need to be reduced, as hypoglycemic effects are enhanced.
- □ Bone marrow aspiration studies are recommended prior to initiation of therapy and at time of maximum hematologic response to ensure adequate bone marrow reserve.

POTENTIAL NURSING DIAGNOSES

- Infection, risk for (Adverse Reactions).
- Nutrition, altered, less than body requirements (Adverse Reactions).
- Knowledge deficit, related to medication regimen (Patient/Family Teaching).

IMPLEMENTATION

- **PO:** Administer with food or fluids if GI irritation occurs. Confer with pharmacist regarding opening of capsules if patient has difficulty swallowing.

PATIENT/FAMILY TEACHING

- □ Emphasize the need to take medication exactly as directed. If a dose is missed, it should be taken as soon as remembered within a few hours but not if several hours have passed or if almost time for next dose. Health care professional should be consulted if vomiting occurs shortly after a dose is taken.
- □ Instruct patient to notify health care profes-

sional promptly if signs of infection (fever, sore throat, chills, cough, thickened bronchial secretions, hoarseness, pain in lower back or side, difficult or painful urination); bleeding gums; bruising; petechiae; or blood in stool, urine, or emesis occurs. Caution patient to avoid crowds and persons with known infections. Instruct patient to use soft toothbrush and electric razor and to avoid falls. Patient should not receive IM injections or rectal temperatures. Patient should also be cautioned not to drink alcoholic beverages or take medication containing aspirin or NSAIDs; may precipitate gastric bleeding.

- ☐ Caution patient to avoid alcohol, caffeinated beverages, CNS depressants, OTC drugs, and foods or beverages containing tyramine (see Appendix K for foods included) during therapy and for at least 2 wk after therapy has been discontinued, as they may precipitate a hypertensive crisis.
- ☐ Advise patient that an additional interaction of alcohol with procarbazine is a disulfiram-like reaction (flushing, nausea, vomiting, headache, abdominal cramps).
- ☐ Instruct patient to inspect oral mucosa for erythema and ulceration. If ulceration occurs, advise patient to notify health care professional and to use sponge brush and rinse mouth with water after eating and drinking. Topical agents may be used if mouth pain interferes with eating. Stomatitis pain may require treatment with opioid analgesics.
- ☐ May cause drowsiness or dizziness. Caution patient to avoid driving or other activities that require alertness until response to medication is known.
- ☐ Advise patient that this medication may have teratogenic effects. Contraception should be practiced during therapy and for at least 4 mo after therapy is concluded.
- ☐ Discuss the possibility of hair loss with patient. Explore methods of coping.
- ☐ Caution patient to use sunscreen and protective clothing to prevent photosensitivity reactions.
- ☐ Instruct patient not to receive any vaccinations without advice of health care professional.
- ☐ Advise patient to notify health care professional of medication regimen prior to treatment or surgery. This therapy usually should be withdrawn at least 2 wk prior to surgery.
- ☐ Instruct patient to inform health care professional if muscle or joint pain, nausea, vomiting, sweating, tiredness, weakness, constipation, headache, difficulty swallowing, or loss of appetite becomes pronounced.
- ☐ Advise patient to carry identification describing medication regimen at all times.
- ☐ Emphasize the need for periodic lab tests to monitor for side effects.

EVALUATION

Effectiveness of therapy can be demonstrated by: ▪ Decrease in size and spread of malignant tissue in Hodgkin's disease.

PROCHLORPERAZINE

(proe-klor-**pair**-a-zeen)

Chlorpazine, Compa-Z, Compazine, Cotranzine, {PMS-Prochlorperazine}, {Prorazin}, {Stemetil}, Ultrazine

CLASSIFICATION(S):

Antiemetic (phenothiazine), Antipsychotic agent

Pregnancy Category C

INDICATIONS

▪ Management of nausea and vomiting ▪ Treatment of psychoses.

ACTION

▪ Alters the effects of dopamine in the CNS ▪ Possesses significant anticholinergic and alpha-adrenergic blocking activity ▪ Depresses the chemoreceptor trigger zone (CTZ) in the CNS. **Therapeutic Effects:** ▪ Diminished nausea and vomiting ▪ Diminished signs and symptoms of psychoses.

PHARMACOKINETICS

Absorption: Absorption from tablet is variable; may be better with oral liquid formulations. Well absorbed following IM administration.

Distribution: Widely distributed, high concentrations in the CNS. Crosses the placenta and probably enters breast milk.

Metabolism and Excretion: Highly metabolized by the liver and GI mucosa. Converted to some compounds with antipsychotic activity.
Half-life: UK.

CONTRAINDICATIONS AND PRECAUTIONS

Contraindicated in: ▪ Hypersensitivity ▪ Cross-sensitivity with other phenothiazines may exist ▪ Narrow-angle glaucoma ▪ Bone marrow depression ▪ Severe liver or cardiovascular disease ▪ Hypersensitivity to bisulfites or benzyl alcohol (some parenteral products) ▪ Children <2 yr or 9.1 kg.
Use Cautiously in: ▪ Geriatric or debilitated patients (dosage reduction recommended) ▪ Diabetes mellitus ▪ Respiratory disease ▪ Prostatic hypertrophy ▪ CNS tumors ▪ Epilepsy ▪ Intestinal obstruction ▪ Pregnancy or lactation (safety not established).

ADVERSE REACTIONS AND SIDE EFFECTS*

CNS: NEUROLEPTIC MALIGNANT SYNDROME, extrapyramidal reactions, sedation, tardive dyskinesia.
EENT: blurred vision, dry eyes, lens opacities.
CV: ECG changes, hypotension, tachycardia.
GI: constipation, dry mouth, anorexia, drug-induced hepatitis, ileus.
GU: pink or reddish-brown discoloration of urine, urinary retention.
Derm: photosensitivity, pigment changes, rashes.
Endo: galactorrhea.
Hemat: AGRANULOCYTOSIS, leukopenia.
Metab: hyperthermia.
Misc: allergic reactions.

INTERACTIONS

Drug-Drug: ▪ Additive hypotension with **antihypertensive agents**, **nitrates**, or acute ingestion of **alcohol** ▪ Additive CNS depression with other **CNS depressants**, including **alcohol**, **antidepressants**, **antihistamines**, **opioids**, **sedative/hypnotics**, or **general anesthetics** ▪ Additive anticholinergic effects with other **drugs possessing anticholinergic properties**, including **antihistamines**, **antidepressants**, **atropine**, **haloperidol**, and other **phenothiazines** ▪ **Lithium** increases the risk of extrapyramidal reactions ▪ May mask early signs of **lithium** toxicity ▪ Increased risk of agranulocytosis with **antithyroid agents** ▪ Decreases the beneficial effects of **levodopa** ▪ **Antacids** may decrease absorption.

ROUTE AND DOSAGE

Pediatric dose should not exceed 10 mg on the 1st day and then should not exceed 20 mg/day in children 2–5 yr or 25 mg/day in children 6–12 yr.

❑ Antiemetic

- **PO (Adults and Children ≥12 yr):** 5–10 mg 3–4 times daily; may also be given as 15–30 mg once daily or 10 mg twice daily as ER capsules (up to 40 mg/day).
- **PO (Children 18–39 kg):** 2.5 mg 3 times daily or 5 mg twice daily (not to exceed 15 mg/day).
- **PO (Children 14–17 kg):** 2.5 mg 2–3 times daily (not to exceed 10 mg/day).
- **PO (Children 9–13 kg):** 2.5 mg 1–2 times daily (not to exceed 7.5 mg/day).
- **IM (Adults and Children ≥12 yr):** 5–10 mg q 3–4 hr as needed. *Nausea/vomiting associated with surgery*—5–10 mg; may be repeated once.
- **IM (Children 2–12 yr):** 132 mcg (0.132 mg)/kg; usually only 1 dose is required.
- **IV (Adults and Children ≥12 yr):** 2.5–10 mg (not to exceed 40 mg/day). *Nausea/vomiting associated with surgery*—5–10 mg; may be repeated once.
- **Rect (Adults):** 25 mg twice daily.
- **Rect (Children 18–39 kg):** 2.5 mg 3 times daily or 5 mg twice daily (not to exceed 15 mg/day).
- **Rect (Children 14–17 kg):** 2.5 mg 2–3 times daily (not to exceed 10 mg/day).
- **Rect (Children 9–13 kg):** 2.5 mg 1–2 times daily (not to exceed 7.5 mg/day).

❑ Antipsychotic

- **PO (Adults and Children ≥12 yr):** 5–10 mg 3–4 times daily; may be increased q 2–3 days (up to 150 mg/day).
- **PO (Children 2–12 yr):** 2.5 mg 2–3 times daily.
- **IM (Adults):** 10–20 mg q 2–4 hr for up to 4 doses, then 10–20 mg q 4–6 hr (up to 200 mg/day).

*CAPITALS indicate life-threatening; underlines indicate most frequent.

- **IM (Children 2–12 yr):** 132 mcg (0.132 mg)/kg (not to exceed 10 mg/dose).
- **IV (Adults and Children ≥12 yr):** 2.5–10 mg (up to 40 mg/day).
- **Rect (Adults):** 10 mg 3–4 times daily; may be increased by 5–10 mg q 2–3 days as needed.

❑ **Antianxiety**

- **PO (Adults and Children ≥12 yr):** 5 mg 3–4 times daily (not to exceed 20 mg/day or longer than 12 wk); may also be given as 15 mg once daily or 10 mg twice daily as ER capsules.
- **IM (Adults and Children ≥12 yr):** 5–10 mg q 3–4 hr as needed (up to 40 mg/day).
- **IM (Children 2–12 yr):** 132 mcg (0.132 mg)/kg.
- **IV (Adults):** 2.5–10 mg (up to 40 mg/day).

AVAILABILITY

▪ ***Tablets:*** 5 mg[Rx], 10 mg[Rx], 25 mg[Rx] ▪ ***Syrup:*** 5 mg/5 ml (edisylate)[Rx], {5 mg/5 ml (mesylate)[Rx]} ▪ ***Extended-release capsules:*** 10 mg[Rx], 15 mg[Rx], 30 mg[Rx] ▪ ***Injection:*** 5 mg/ml (edisylate)[Rx], {5 mg/ml (mesylate)[Rx]} ▪ ***Suppositories:*** 2.5 mg[Rx], 5 mg[Rx], 25 mg[Rx].

TIME/ACTION PROFILE (antiemetic effect)

	ONSET	PEAK	DURATION
PO	30–40 min	UK	3–4 hr
PO-ER	30–40 min	UK	10–12 hr
Rect	60 min	UK	3–4 hr
IM	10–20 min	10–30 min	3–4 hr
IV	rapid (mins)	10–30 min	3–4 hr

NURSING IMPLICATIONS

ASSESSMENT

- **General Info:** Monitor blood pressure (sitting, standing, lying), ECG, pulse, and respiratory rate prior to and frequently during the period of dosage adjustment. May cause Q-wave and T-wave changes in ECG.
- ❑ Assess patient for level of sedation following administration.
- ❑ Monitor patient for onset of akathisia (restlessness or desire to keep moving) and extrapyramidal side effects (*parkinsonian*—difficulty speaking or swallowing, loss of balance control, pill rolling, mask-like face, shuffling gait, rigidity, tremors; and *dystonic*—muscle spasms, twisting motions, twitching, inability to move eyes, weakness of arms or legs) every 2 mo during therapy and 8–12 wk after therapy has been discontinued. Report these symptoms; reduction in dosage or discontinuation may be necessary. Trihexyphenidyl or diphenhydramine may be used to control these symptoms.
- ❑ Monitor for tardive dyskinesia (uncontrolled rhythmic movement of mouth, face, and extremities; lip smacking or puckering; puffing of cheeks; uncontrolled chewing; rapid or worm-like movements of tongue). Report immediately; may be irreversible.
- ❑ Monitor for development of neuroleptic malignant syndrome (fever, respiratory distress, tachycardia, convulsions, diaphoresis, hypertension or hypotension, pallor, tiredness, severe muscle stiffness, loss of bladder control). Notify physician or other health care professional immediately if these symptoms occur.
- **Antiemetic:** Assess patient for nausea and vomiting prior to and 30–60 min following administration.
- **Antipsychotic:** Monitor patient's mental status (orientation to reality and behavior) prior to and periodically throughout therapy.
- ❑ Observe patient carefully when administering oral medication to ensure that medication is actually taken and not hoarded.
- ❑ Assess fluid intake and bowel function. Increased bulk and fluids in the diet may help minimize constipation.
- ***Lab Test Considerations:*** CBC and liver function tests should be evaluated periodically throughout course of therapy. May cause blood dyscrasias, especially between wk 4 and 10 of therapy. Hepatotoxicity is more likely to occur between wk 2 and 4 of therapy. May recur if medication is restarted. Liver function abnormalities may require discontinuation of therapy.
- ❑ May cause false-positive or false-negative pregnancy test results and false-positive urine bilirubin test results.
- ❑ May cause increased serum prolactin levels and interfere with gonadorelin test results.

POTENTIAL NURSING DIAGNOSES

- Fluid volume deficit (Indications).
- Thought processes, altered (Indications).
- Knowledge deficit, related to medication regimen (Patient/Family Teaching).

IMPLEMENTATION

- **General Info:** To prevent contact dermatitis, avoid getting solution on hands.
- □ Phenothiazines should be discontinued 48 hr before and not resumed for 24 hr following myelography, as they lower seizure threshold.
- **PO:** Do not crush or chew extended-release capsules. Administer with food, milk, or a full glass of water to minimize gastric irritation.
- □ Dilute syrup in citrus or chocolate-flavored drinks.
- □ Do not open, crush, or chew extended-release capsules.
- **IM:** Do not inject SC. Inject slowly, deep into well-developed muscle. Keep patient recumbent for at least 30 min following injection to minimize hypotensive effects. Slight yellow color will not alter potency. Do not administer solution that is markedly discolored or that contains a precipitate.
- **Direct IV:** Dilute to a concentration of 1 mg/ml.
- ***Rate:*** Administer at a rate of 1 mg/min; not to exceed 5 mg/min.
- **Intermittent Infusion:** Dilute 20 mg in up to 1 liter dextrose, saline, Ringer's or lactated Ringer's solution, dextrose/saline, dextrose/Ringer's, or lactated Ringer's combinations.
- **Syringe Incompatibility:** ▪ Manufacturer does not recommend mixing prochlorperazine with other medications in syringe.
- **Y-Site Compatibility:** ▪ cisplatin ▪ cyclophosphamide ▪ cytarabine ▪ doxorubicin ▪ fluconazole ▪ fludarabine ▪ heparin ▪ hydrocortisone sodium succinate ▪ melphalan ▪ methotrexate ▪ ondansetron ▪ paclitaxel ▪ potassium chloride ▪ sargramostim ▪ sufentanil ▪ teniposide ▪ thiotepa ▪ vinorelbine ▪ vitamin B complex with C.
- **Y-Site Incompatibility:** ▪ aldesleukin ▪ amifostine ▪ aztreonam ▪ cefepime ▪ filgrastim ▪ fludarabine ▪ foscarnet ▪ gallium nitrate ▪ piperacillin/tazobactam.

PATIENT/FAMILY TEACHING

- □ Instruct patient to take medication exactly as directed, not to skip doses or double up on missed doses. If a dose is missed, it should be taken as soon as remembered unless almost time for next dose. If more than 2 doses are scheduled each day, missed dose should be taken within about 1 hr of the ordered time. Abrupt withdrawal may lead to gastritis, nausea, vomiting, dizziness, headache, tachycardia, and insomnia.
- □ Inform patient of possibility of extrapyramidal symptoms and tardive dyskinesia. Instruct patient to report these symptoms immediately to health care professional.
- □ Advise patient to change positions slowly to minimize orthostatic hypotension.
- □ May cause drowsiness. Caution patient to avoid driving or other activities requiring alertness until response to medication is known.
- □ Caution patient to avoid taking alcohol or other CNS depressants concurrently with this medication.
- □ Advise patient to use sunscreen and protective clothing when exposed to the sun to prevent photosensitivity reactions. Extremes in temperature should also be avoided, as this drug impairs body temperature regulation.
- □ Instruct patient to use frequent mouth rinses, good oral hygiene, and sugarless gum or candy to minimize dry mouth. Consult health care professional if dry mouth continues for >2 wk.
- □ Advise patient not to take prochlorperazine within 2 hr of antacids or antidiarrheal medication.
- □ Advise patient that increasing bulk and fluids in the diet and exercise may help minimize the constipating effects of this medication.
- □ Inform patient that this medication may turn urine pink to reddish-brown.
- □ Advise patient to notify health care professional of medication regimen prior to treatment or surgery.
- □ Instruct patient to notify health care professional promptly if sore throat, fever, unusual bleeding or bruising, skin rashes, weakness, tremors, visual disturbances, dark-colored urine, or clay-colored stools are noted.
- □ Emphasize the importance of routine follow-up exams to monitor response to medication and detect side effects. Periodic ocular exams are indicated. Encourage continued participation in psychotherapy as ordered by health care professional.

EVALUATION

Effectiveness of therapy can be demonstrated by: ▪ Relief of nausea and vomiting

■ Decrease in excitable, paranoic, or withdrawn behavior when used as an antipsychotic.

PROMAZINE
(**proe**-ma-zeen)
Primazine, Prozine, Sparine

CLASSIFICATION(S):
Antipsychotic agent (phenothiazine)

Pregnancy Category UK

INDICATIONS

■ Treatment of psychoses.

ACTION

■ Alters the effects of dopamine in the CNS ■ Possesses significant anticholinergic and alpha-adrenergic blocking activity. **Therapeutic Effects:** ■ Diminished signs and symptoms of psychoses.

PHARMACOKINETICS

Absorption: Absorption from tablets is variable; well absorbed following IM administration.
Distribution: Widely distributed, high concentrations in the CNS; crosses placenta; probably enters breast milk.
Metabolism and Excretion: Highly metabolized by the liver and GI mucosa.
Half-life: UK.

CONTRAINDICATIONS AND PRECAUTIONS

Contraindicated in: ■ Hypersensitivity ■ Cross-sensitivity with other phenothiazines may occur ■ Narrow-angle glaucoma ■ Bone marrow depression ■ Severe liver or cardiovascular disease ■ Hypersensitivity to bisulfites or formaldehyde (injection only).
Use Cautiously in: ■ Geriatric or debilitated patients (dosage reduction may be required) ■ Pregnancy or lactation (safety not established) ■ Diabetes mellitus ■ Respiratory disease ■ Prostatic hypertrophy ■ CNS tumors ■ Epilepsy ■ Intestinal obstruction.

ADVERSE REACTIONS AND SIDE EFFECTS*

CNS: NEUROLEPTIC MALIGNANT SYNDROME, extrapyramidal reactions, sedation, tardive dyskinesia.
EENT: blurred vision, dry eyes, lens opacities.
CV: hypotension, tachycardia.
GI: constipation, dry mouth, anorexia, drug-induced hepatitis, ileus.
GU: urinary retention.
Derm: photosensitivity, pigment changes, rashes.
Endo: galactorrhea.
Hemat: AGRANULOCYTOSIS, leukopenia.
Metab: hyperthermia.
Misc: allergic reactions.

INTERACTIONS

Drug-Drug: ■ Additive hypotension with **antihypertensive agents, nitrates,** or acute ingestion of **alcohol** ■ Additive CNS depression with other **CNS depressants,** including **alcohol, antihistamines, opioids, sedative/hypnotics,** or **general anesthetics** ■ Additive anticholinergic effects with other **drugs possessing anticholinergic properties,** including **antihistamines, antidepressants, atropine, haloperidol,** and other **phenothiazines** ■ **Lithium** decreases absorption and increases the risk of extrapyramidal reactions ■ May mask early signs of **lithium** toxicity ■ Decreases beneficial effects of **levodopa** ■ Increased risk of agranulocytosis with **antithyroid agents.**

ROUTE AND DOSAGE

- **PO (Adults):** 10–200 mg q 4–6 hr up to 1 g/day.
- **PO, IM (Children >12 yr):** 10–25 mg q 4–6 hr.
- **IM, IV (Adults):** 50–150 mg initially; if required, additional doses may be given after 30 min up to a total of 300 mg; when desired effect is achieved, change to PO (not to exceed 1 g/24 hr; initial dose in inebriated patients should not exceed 50 mg).

AVAILABILITY

■ ***Tablets:*** 25 mg[Rx], 50 mg[Rx], 100 mg[Rx] ■ ***Injection:*** 25 mg/ml in 10-ml vials[Rx], 50 mg/ml in 2- and 10-ml vials and 1-ml prefilled syringes[Rx].

***CAPITALS indicate life-threatening; underlines indicate most frequent.**

TIME/ACTION PROFILE (antipsychotic effects)

	ONSET	PEAK	DURATION
PO	30 min	UK	4–6 hr
IM	within 30 min	UK	UK

NURSING IMPLICATIONS

ASSESSMENT

- Monitor patient's mental status (orientation to reality and behavior) prior to and periodically during therapy.
- Monitor blood pressure (sitting, standing, lying), ECG, pulse, and respiratory rate prior to and frequently during the period of dosage adjustment. May cause Q-wave and T-wave changes in ECG.
- Observe patient carefully when administering oral medication to ensure medication is actually taken and not hoarded.
- Assess patient for level of sedation following administration.
- Monitor patient for onset of akathisia (restlessness or desire to keep moving) and extrapyramidal side effects (*parkinsonian*—difficulty speaking or swallowing, loss of balance control, pill rolling, mask-like face, shuffling gait, rigidity, tremors; and *dystonic*—muscle spasms, twisting motions, twitching, inability to move eyes, weakness of arms or legs) every 2 mo during therapy and 8–12 wk after therapy has been discontinued. Report symptoms; reduction in dosage or discontinuation of medication may be necessary. Trihexyphenidyl or diphenhydramine may be used to control these symptoms.
- Monitor for tardive dyskinesia (uncontrolled rhythmic movement of mouth, face, and extremities; lip smacking or puckering; puffing of cheeks; uncontrolled chewing; rapid or worm-like movements of tongue). Report immediately; may be irreversible.
- Monitor for development of neuroleptic malignant syndrome (fever, respiratory distress, tachycardia, convulsions, diaphoresis, hypertension or hypotension, pallor, tiredness, severe muscle stiffness, loss of bladder control). Notify physician or other health care professional immediately if these symptoms occur.
- Assess fluid intake and bowel function. Increased bulk and fluids in the diet help minimize the constipating effects of this medication.
- ***Lab Test Considerations:*** CBC and liver function tests should be evaluated periodically throughout course of therapy. May cause blood dyscrasias, especially between wk 4 and 10 of therapy. Hepatotoxicity is more likely to occur between wk 2 and 4 of therapy. May recur if medication is restarted. Liver function abnormalities may require discontinuation of therapy.
- May cause false-positive or false-negative pregnancy test results and false-positive urine bilirubin test results.
- May cause increased serum prolactin levels, thereby interfering with gonadorelin test results.

POTENTIAL NURSING DIAGNOSES

- Thought processes, altered (Indications).
- Knowledge deficit, related to medication regimen (Patient/Family Teaching).
- Noncompliance (Patient/Family Teaching).

IMPLEMENTATION

- **General Info:** To prevent contact dermatitis, avoid getting solution on hands.
- Phenothiazines should be discontinued 48 hr before and not resumed for 24 hr following myelography, as they lower the seizure threshold.
- **PO:** Administer with food, milk, or a full glass of water to minimize gastric irritation.
- **IM:** Do not inject SC. Inject slowly into deep, well-developed muscle. Keep patient recumbent for at least 30 min following injection to minimize hypotensive effects. Slight yellow color will not alter potency. Do not administer solution that is markedly discolored or that contains a precipitate.
- **Direct IV:** Administer in a concentration not to exceed 25 mg/ml.
- ***Rate:*** Administer slowly.
- **Syringe Compatibility:** ▪ atropine ▪ cimetidine ▪ diphenhydramine ▪ metoclopramide ▪ midazolam ▪ scopolamine.

PATIENT/FAMILY TEACHING

- Instruct patient to take medication exactly as directed, not to skip doses or double up on missed doses. If a dose is missed, it should be taken as soon as remembered unless almost time for next dose. If more than 2 doses are scheduled each day, the missed dose should be taken within about 1 hr of the ordered time. Abrupt withdrawal may lead to gastritis, nausea, vomiting, dizziness, headache, tachycardia, and insomnia.

- □ Inform patient of possibility of extrapyramidal symptoms, tardive dyskinesia, and neuroleptic malignant syndrome. Caution patient to report these symptoms immediately.
- □ Advise patient to change positions slowly to minimize orthostatic hypotension.
- □ May cause drowsiness. Caution patient to avoid driving or other activities requiring alertness until response to medication is known.
- □ Caution patient to avoid taking alcohol or other CNS depressants concurrently with this medication.
- □ Advise patient to use sunscreen and protective clothing when exposed to the sun to prevent photosensitivity reactions. Extremes in temperature should also be avoided, as this drug impairs body temperature regulation.
- □ Advise patient not to take promazine within 2 hr of antacids or antidiarrheal medication.
- □ Instruct patient to use frequent mouth rinses, good oral hygiene, and sugarless gum or candy to minimize dry mouth. Consult health care professional if dry mouth continues for >2 wk.
- □ Advise patient to notify health care professional of medication regimen prior to treatment or surgery.
- □ Instruct patient to notify health care professional promptly if sore throat, fever, unusual bleeding or bruising, skin rashes, weakness, tremors, visual disturbances, dark-colored urine, or clay-colored stools are noted.
- □ Emphasize the importance of routine follow-up examinations to monitor response to medication and detect side effects. Periodic ocular examinations are indicated. Encourage continued participation in psychotherapy.

EVALUATION

Effectiveness of therapy can be demonstrated by: ▪ Decrease in excitable, paranoic, or withdrawn behavior.

PROMETHAZINE

(proe-**meth**-a-zeen)

Anergan, Antinaus, {Histanil}, Pentazine, Phenazine, Phencen-50, Phenergan, Phenergan Fortis, Phenergan Plain, Phenerzine, Phenoject, Pro-50, Promacot, Pro-Med, Promet, Prorex, Prothazine, Shogan, V-Gan

CLASSIFICATION(S):

Antiemetic, Antihistamine (phenothiazine), Sedative/hypnotic

Pregnancy Category C

INDICATIONS

▪ Treatment of various allergic conditions and motion sickness ▪ Preoperative sedation ▪ Treatment and prevention of nausea and vomiting ▪ Adjunct to anesthesia and analgesia.

ACTION

▪ Blocks the effects of histamine ▪ Has inhibitory effect on the chemoreceptor trigger zone in the medulla, resulting in antiemetic properties ▪ Alters the effects of dopamine in the CNS ▪ Possesses significant anticholinergic activity ▪ Produces CNS depression by indirectly decreased stimulation of the CNS reticular system. **Therapeutic Effects:** ▪ Relief of symptoms of histamine excess usually seen in allergic conditions ▪ Diminished nausea or vomiting ▪ Sedation.

PHARMACOKINETICS

Absorption: Well absorbed following oral and IM administration; rectal administration may be less reliable.

Distribution: Widely distributed; crosses the blood-brain barrier and the placenta.

Metabolism and Excretion: Metabolized by the liver.

Half-life: UK.

CONTRAINDICATIONS AND PRECAUTIONS

Contraindicated in: ▪ Hypersensitivity ▪ Comatose patients ▪ Prostatic hypertrophy ▪ Bladder neck obstruction ▪ Some liquid products contain

{} = Available in Canada only.

alcohol and should be avoided in patients with known intolerance ▪ Narrow-angle glaucoma.
Use Cautiously in: ▪ Hypertension ▪ Sleep apnea ▪ Epilepsy ▪ Underlying bone marrow depression ▪ Pregnancy (has been used safely during labor; avoid chronic use during pregnancy) ▪ Lactation (safety not established; may cause drowsiness in infant).

ADVERSE REACTIONS AND SIDE EFFECTS*

CNS: NEUROLEPTIC MALIGNANT SYNDROME, <u>confusion</u>, <u>disorientation</u>, <u>sedation</u>, dizziness, extrapyramidal reactions, fatigue, insomnia, nervousness.
EENT: blurred vision, diplopia, tinnitus.
CV: bradycardia, hypertension, hypotension, tachycardia.
GI: constipation, drug-induced hepatitis, dry mouth.
Derm: photosensitivity, rashes.
Hemat: blood dyscrasias.

INTERACTIONS

Drug-Drug: ▪ Additive CNS depression with other **CNS depressants**, including **alcohol**, other **antihistamines**, **opioids**, and other **sedative/hypnotics** ▪ Additive anticholinergic effects with other **drugs possessing anticholinergic properties**, including other **antihistamines**, **antidepressants**, **atropine**, **haloperidol**, other **phenothiazines**, **quinidine**, and **disopyramide** ▪ Concurrent use with **MAO inhibitors** may result in increased sedation and anticholinergic side effects.

ROUTE AND DOSAGE

❑ Antihistamine

- **PO (Adults):** 25 mg at bedtime or 10–12.5 mg 4 times daily.
- **PO (Children ≥2 yr):** 5–12.5 mg 3 times daily or 25 mg at bedtime.
- **IM, IV, Rect (Adults):** 25 mg; may repeat in 2 hr.
- **Rect (Children ≥2 yr):** 0.125 mg/kg (3.75 mg/m^2) q 4–6 hr or 0.5 mg/kg (15 mg/m^2) at bedtime; may also be given as 6.25–12.5 mg 3 times daily or 25 mg at bedtime.

❑ Antivertigo (Motion Sickness)

- **PO (Adults):** 25 mg 30–60 min prior to departure; may be repeated in 8–12 hr.
- **PO (Children ≥2 yr):** 10–25 mg or 0.5 mg/kg 30–60 min prior to departure; may be given twice daily.

❑ Sedation

- **PO, Rect, IM, IV (Adults):** 25–50 mg.
- **PO, Rect, IM (Children >2 yr):** 10–25 mg or 0.5–1.1 mg/kg.

❑ Sedation during Labor

- **IM, IV (Adults):** 50 mg in early labor; when labor is established, additional doses of 25–75 mg may be given 1–2 times at 4-hr intervals (24-hr dose should not exceed 100 mg).

❑ Antiemetic

- **PO, Rect, IM, IV (Adults):** 10–25 mg q 4 hr as needed; initial PO dose should be 25 mg.
- **PO, Rect, IM (Children ≥2 yr):** 0.25–0.5 mg/kg (7.5–15 mg/m^2) q 4–6 hr or 10–25 mg q 4–6 hr.

AVAILABILITY

▪ ***Tablets:*** 10 mg ^{OTC}, 12.5 mg^{Rx}, {12.5 mg^{OTC}}, 25 mg^{Rx}, {25 mg^{OTC}}, 50 mg^{Rx}, {50 mg^{OTC}} ▪ ***Syrup:*** 6.25 mg/5 ml^{Rx}, {10 mg/5 ml^{OTC}}, 25 mg/5 ml^{Rx} ▪ ***Injection:*** 25 mg/ml in 1-ml ampules and 1- and 10-ml vials^{Rx}, 50 mg/ml in 1-ml ampules and 10-ml vials^{Rx} ▪ ***Suppositories:*** 12.5 mg^{Rx}, 25 mg^{Rx}, 50 mg^{Rx} ▪ ***In combination with:*** codeine, dextromethorphan, phenylephrine, and/or pseudoephedrine in a variety of cough and cold preparations^{Rx}. See Appendix A.

TIME/ACTION PROFILE (noted as antihistaminic effects; sedative effects last 2–8 hr)

	ONSET	PEAK	DURATION
PO, IM	20 min	UK	4–12 hr
Rectal	20 min	UK	4–12 hr
IV	3–5 min	UK	4–12 hr

NURSING IMPLICATIONS

ASSESSMENT

- **General Info:** Monitor blood pressure, pulse, and respiratory rate frequently in patients receiving IV doses.

*CAPITALS indicate life-threatening; <u>underlines</u> indicate most frequent.

- Assess patient for level of sedation following administration.
- Monitor patient for onset of extrapyramidal side effects (*akathisia*—restlessness; *dystonia*—muscle spasms and twisting motions; *pseudoparkinsonism*—mask facies, rigidity, tremors, drooling, shuffling gait, dysphagia). Notify physician or other health care professional if these symptoms occur.
- **Allergy:** Assess allergy symptoms (rhinitis, conjunctivitis, hives) prior to and periodically throughout course of therapy.
- **Antiemetic:** Assess patient for nausea and vomiting prior to and following administration.
- ***Lab Test Considerations:*** May cause false-positive or false-negative pregnancy tests.
- CBC should be evaluated periodically during chronic therapy, as blood dyscrasias may occur.
- May cause increased serum glucose.
- May cause false-negative results in skin tests using allergen extracts. Promethazine should be discontinued 72 hr prior to the test.

POTENTIAL NURSING DIAGNOSES

- Fluid volume deficit (Indications).
- Injury, risk for (Side Effects).
- Knowledge deficit, related to medication regimen (Patient/Family Teaching).

IMPLEMENTATION

- **General Info:** When administering promethazine concurrently with opioid analgesics, supervise ambulation closely to prevent injury due to increased sedation.
- **PO:** Administer with food, water, or milk to minimize GI irritation. Tablets may be crushed and mixed with food or fluids for patients with difficulty swallowing.
- **IM:** Administer deep into well-developed muscle. SC administration may cause tissue necrosis.
- **Direct IV:** Doses should not exceed a concentration of 25 mg/ml. Slight yellow color does not alter potency. Do not use if precipitate is present.
- ***Rate:*** Administer each 25 mg slowly, over at least 1 min. Rapid administration may produce a transient fall in blood pressure.
- **Solution Compatibility:** ▪ dextrose ▪ saline ▪ Ringer's or lactated Ringer's solution ▪ dextrose/saline ▪ dextrose/Ringer's ▪ lactated Ringer's combinations.
- **Syringe Compatibility:** ▪ atropine ▪ butorphanol ▪ cimetidine ▪ droperidol ▪ fentanyl ▪ glycopyrrolate ▪ hydromorphone ▪ meperidine ▪ metoclopramide ▪ midazolam ▪ pentazocine ▪ ranitidine ▪ scopolamine.
- **Syringe Incompatibility:** ▪ heparin ▪ ketorolac ▪ pentobarbital ▪ thiopental.
- **Y-Site Compatibility:** ▪ amifostine ▪ aztreonam ▪ ciprofloxacin ▪ cisplatin ▪ cyclophosphamide ▪ cytarabine ▪ doxorubicin ▪ filgrastim ▪ fluconazole ▪ fludarabine ▪ melphalan ▪ ondansetron ▪ sargramostim ▪ teniposide ▪ thiotepa ▪ vinorelbine.
- **Y-Site Incompatibility:** ▪ aldesleukin ▪ cefepime ▪ cefoperazone ▪ cefotetan ▪ foscarnet ▪ methotrexate ▪ piperacillin/tazobactam.

PATIENT/FAMILY TEACHING

- **General Info:** Review dosage schedule with patient. If medication is ordered regularly and a dose is missed, take as soon as remembered unless time for next dose.
- May cause drowsiness. Caution patient to avoid driving or other activities requiring alertness until response to medication is known.
- Advise patient that frequent mouth rinses, good oral hygiene, and sugarless gum or candy may decrease dry mouth. Health care professional should be notified if dry mouth persists >2 wk.
- Caution patient to use sunscreen and protective clothing to prevent photosensitivity reactions.
- Advise patient to change positions slowly to minimize orthostatic hypotension. Geriatric patients are at increased risk for this side effect.
- Caution patient to avoid concurrent use of alcohol and other CNS depressants with this medication.
- Instruct patient to notify health care professional if sore throat, fever, jaundice, or uncontrolled movements are noted.
- **Motion Sickness:** When used as prophylaxis for motion sickness, advise patient to take medication at least 30 min and preferably 1–2 hr prior to exposure to conditions that may cause motion sickness.

EVALUATION

Effectiveness of therapy can be demonstrated by: ▪ Relief from allergic symptoms ▪ Prevention of motion sickness ▪ Sedation ▪ Relief from nausea and vomiting.

PROPAFENONE

(proe-**paff**-e-nown)

Rhythmol

CLASSIFICATION(S):

Antiarrhythmic (group IC)

Pregnancy Category C

INDICATIONS

▪ Treatment of life-threatening ventricular arrhythmias, including ventricular tachycardia.

ACTION

▪ Slows conduction in cardiac tissue by altering transport of ions across cell membranes. **Therapeutic Effects:** ▪ Suppression of ventricular arrhythmias.

PHARMACOKINETICS

Absorption: Although well absorbed following oral administration, undergoes rapid hepatic metabolism (bioavailability 3–11%).

Distribution: Widely distributed; crosses the placenta.

Metabolism and Excretion: Extensively metabolized by the liver, some metabolites have antiarrhythmic activity. >90% of patients are considered extensive metabolizers. Others metabolize propafenone more slowly.

Half-life: 2–10 hr in extensive metabolizers, 10–32 hr in slow metabolizers.

CONTRAINDICATIONS AND PRECAUTIONS

Contraindicated in: ▪ Hypersensitivity ▪ Cardiogenic shock ▪ Conduction disorders including sick sinus syndrome and AV block (without a pacemaker) ▪ Bradycardia ▪ Severe hypotension ▪ Nonallergic bronchospasm ▪ Electrolyte disturbances ▪ Uncontrolled congestive heart failure.

Use Cautiously in: ▪ Severe hepatic or renal impairment (dosage reduction may be necessary) ▪ Geriatric patients (lower doses may be necessary) ▪ Pregnancy, lactation, or children (safety not established).

ADVERSE REACTIONS AND SIDE EFFECTS*

CNS: dizziness, shaking, weakness.

EENT: blurred vision.

CV: SUPRAVENTRICULAR ARRHYTHMIA, VENTRICULAR ARRHYTHMIAS, conduction disturbances, angina, bradycardia, hypotension.

GI: altered taste, constipation, nausea, vomiting, diarrhea, dry mouth.

Derm: rash.

MS: joint pain.

INTERACTIONS

Drug-Drug: ▪ Increases serum **digoxin** levels by 35–85% (dosage reduction may be required) ▪ Increases blood levels of **metoprolol** and **propranolol** (dosage reduction may be required) ▪ Concurrent use of **local anesthetics** may increase the risk of CNS adverse reactions ▪ Increases the effects of **warfarin** (decrease warfarin dose by 25–50%) ▪ May increase **cyclosporine** through blood levels and risk of nephrotoxicity ▪ **Rifampin** may decrease serum levels and effectiveness of propafenone.

ROUTE AND DOSAGE

▪ **PO (Adults):** 150 mg q 8 hr; may be gradually increased at 3–4-day intervals as required up to 300 mg q 8–12 hr.

AVAILABILITY

▪ ***Tablets:*** 150 mg^{Rx}, 225 mg^{Rx}, 300 mg^{Rx}.

TIME/ACTION PROFILE (antiarrhythmic effects)

	ONSET	PEAK	DURATION
PO	hrs–days	4–5 days†	hrs

†Chronic dosing.

NURSING IMPLICATIONS

ASSESSMENT

□ Monitor ECG or use Holter monitor prior to and periodically throughout therapy. May cause PR prolongation and QT prolongation.

□ Monitor blood pressure and pulse periodically throughout therapy.

*CAPITALS indicate life-threatening; underlines indicate most frequent.

- □ Monitor intake and output ratios and daily weight. Assess patients for signs of congestive heart failure (peripheral edema, rales/crackles, dyspnea, weight gain, jugular venous distention). May require reduction or discontinuation of therapy.
- ▪ ***Lab Test Considerations:*** May cause elevated antinuclear antibody (ANA) titer, which is usually asymptomatic and reversible.
- ▪ ***Toxicity and Overdose:*** Signs of toxicity include hypotension, excessive drowsiness, and decreased or abnormal heart rate. Notify physician or other health care professional if these signs occur.

POTENTIAL NURSING DIAGNOSES

- ▪ Cardiac output, decreased (Indications).
- ▪ Knowledge deficit, related to medication regimen (Patient/Family Teaching).

IMPLEMENTATION

- ▪ **PO:** Propafenone therapy should be initiated in a hospital with facilities for cardiac rhythm monitoring. Most serious proarrhythmic effects are seen in the first 2 wk of therapy.
- □ Previous antiarrhythmic therapy should be withdrawn 2–5 half-lives before starting propafenone.
- □ Dosage adjustments should be at least 3–4 days apart because of the long half-life of propafenone.
- □ Pre-existing hypokalemia or hyperkalemia should be corrected prior to instituting therapy.

PATIENT/FAMILY TEACHING

- □ Instruct patient to take medication around the clock exactly as directed, even if feeling better. Missed doses should be taken as soon as remembered if within 4 hr; omit if remembered later. Gradual dosage reduction may be necessary.
- □ May cause dizziness. Caution patient to avoid driving and other activities requiring alertness until response to medication is known.
- □ Advise patient to notify health care professional of medication regimen prior to treatment or surgery.
- □ Instruct patient to notify health care professional if fever, sore throat, chills, or unusual bleeding or bruising occurs or if chest pain, shortness of breath, diaphoresis, palpitations, or visual changes become bothersome.
- □ Advise patient to carry identification describing disease process and medication regimen at all times.
- □ Emphasize the importance of follow-up exams to monitor progress.

EVALUATION

Effectiveness of therapy can be demonstrated by: ▪ Decrease in frequency of ventricular arrhythmias.

PROPANTHELINE

(proe-**pan**-the-leen)

{Probanthel}, Pro-Banthine

CLASSIFICATION(S):

Anticholinergic (antimuscarinic)

Pregnancy Category C

INDICATIONS

▪ Adjunctive therapy in the treatment of peptic ulcer disease. **Unlabeled Uses:** ▪ Antisecretory or antispasmodic agent.

ACTION

▪ Competitively inhibits the muscarinic action of acetylcholine, resulting in decreased GI secretions. **Therapeutic Effects:** ▪ Reduction of signs and symptoms of peptic ulcer disease.

PHARMACOKINETICS

Absorption: Incompletely absorbed from the GI tract.

Distribution: Distribution not known. Does not cross the blood-brain barrier.

Metabolism and Excretion: Inactivated in the upper small intestine.

Half-life: UK.

CONTRAINDICATIONS AND PRECAUTIONS

Contraindicated in: ▪ Hypersensitivity ▪ Narrow-angle glaucoma ▪ Tachycardia secondary to cardiac insufficiency or thyrotoxicosis ▪ Myasthenia gravis.

Use Cautiously in: ▪ Geriatric patients or patients of small stature (dosage reduction required) ▪ Prostatic hypertrophy ▪ Chronic renal, cardiac, or pulmonary disease ▪ Patients who may have intra-abdominal infections ▪ Pregnancy, lactation, or children (safety not established).

ADVERSE REACTIONS AND SIDE EFFECTS*

CNS: confusion, dizziness, drowsiness, excitement.
EENT: blurred vision, mydriasis, photophobia.
CV: tachycardia, orthostatic hypotension, palpitations.
GI: constipation, dry mouth.
GU: urinary hesitancy, urinary retention.
Derm: rash.
Misc: decreased sweating.

INTERACTIONS

Drug-Drug: ▪ Additive anticholinergic effects with other **drugs possessing anticholinergic properties**, including **antihistamines, antidepressants, atropine, haloperidol, phenothiazines, quinidine**, and **disopyramide** ▪ May alter the absorption of other **orally administered drugs** by slowing motility of the GI tract ▪ **Antacids** and **adsorbent antidiarrheals** decrease the absorption of anticholinergics (avoid taking within 2–3 hr of propantheline) ▪ May increase GI mucosal lesions in patients taking **wax-matrix potassium chloride preparations.**

ROUTE AND DOSAGE

- **PO (Adults):** 15 mg 3 times daily, 30 mg at bedtime.
- **PO (Geriatric Patients, Patients with Mild Symptoms or Small Stature):** 7.5 mg 3–4 times daily.
- **PO (Children):** 0.375 mg/kg (10 mg/m^2) 4 times daily.

AVAILABILITY

- ***Tablets:*** 7.5 mg[Rx], 15 mg[Rx].

TIME/ACTION PROFILE (anticholinergic effects)

	ONSET	PEAK	DURATION
PO	30–60 min	2–6 hr	6 hr

NURSING IMPLICATIONS

ASSESSMENT

- ▫ Assess for abdominal pain prior to and periodically throughout therapy.
- ▪ ***Lab Test Considerations:*** Antagonizes effects of pentagastrin and histamine during gastric acid secretion test. Avoid administration for 24 hr preceding the test.

POTENTIAL NURSING DIAGNOSES

- ▪ Pain (Indications).
- ▪ Constipation (Side Effects).
- ▪ Knowledge deficit, related to medication regimen (Patient/Family Teaching).

IMPLEMENTATION

- ▪ **PO:** Administer 30 min before meals. Bedtime dose should be administered at least 2 hr after last meal of the day.
- ▫ Do not administer within 1 hr of antacids or antidiarrheal medications.

PATIENT/FAMILY TEACHING

- ▫ Instruct patient to take medication as directed. If a dose is missed, take as soon as remembered unless almost time for next dose. Do not double doses.
- ▫ May cause drowsiness or blurred vision. Caution patient to avoid driving or other activities requiring alertness until response to medication is known.
- ▫ Instruct patient that frequent oral rinses, sugarless gum or candy, and good oral hygiene may help relieve dry mouth. Consult health care professional regarding use of saliva substitute if dry mouth persists >2 wk.
- ▫ Advise patient that increasing fluid intake, adding bulk to the diet, and exercise may help alleviate the constipating effects of the drug.
- ▫ Advise elderly patients to change positions slowly to minimize the effects of drug-induced orthostatic hypotension.
- ▫ Caution patient to avoid extremes of temperature. This medication decreases the ability to sweat and may increase the risk of heat stroke.
- ▫ Advise patient to wear sunglasses and avoid bright lights to prevent photosensitivity.
- ▫ Instruct patient to notify health care professional if confusion, excitement, dizziness,

*CAPITALS indicate life-threatening; underlines indicate most frequent.

rash, difficulty with urination, or eye pain occurs. Health care professional may recommend periodic ophthalmic examinations to monitor intraocular pressure, especially in the elderly.

EVALUATION

Effectiveness of therapy can be demonstrated by: ▪ Decrease in GI pain in patients with peptic ulcer disease.

PROPOFOL

(**proe**-poe-fol)

Diprivan, disoprofol

CLASSIFICATION(S):

Anesthetic (general)

Pregnancy Category B

INDICATIONS

▪ Induction of general anesthesia ▪ Maintenance of balanced anesthesia when used with other agents ▪ Initiation and maintenance of monitored anesthesia care (MAC) ▪ Sedation of intubated, mechanically ventilated patients in intensive care units.

ACTION

▪ Short-acting hypnotic. Mechanism of action is unknown ▪ Produces amnesia ▪ Has no analgesic properties. **Therapeutic Effects:** ▪ Induction and maintenance of anesthesia.

PHARMACOKINETICS

Absorption: Administered IV only, resulting in complete absorption.
Distribution: Rapidly and widely distributed. Crosses the blood-brain barrier well; rapidly redistributed to other tissues. Crosses the placenta and enters breast milk.
Metabolism and Excretion: Rapidly metabolized by the liver.
Half-life: 3–12 hr (blood-brain equilibration half-life 2.9 min).

CONTRAINDICATIONS AND PRECAUTIONS

Contraindicated in: ▪ Hypersensitivity to propofol, soybean oil, egg lecithin, or glycerol ▪ Labor and delivery.

Use Cautiously in: ▪ Cardiovascular disease ▪ Lipid disorders (emulsion may have detrimental effect) ▪ Increased intracranial pressure ▪ Cerebrovascular disorders ▪ Geriatric, debilitated, or hypovolemic patients (dosage reduction recommended) ▪ Children or lactation (safety not established).

ADVERSE REACTIONS AND SIDE EFFECTS*

CNS: dizziness, headache.
Resp: APNEA, cough.
CV: bradycardia, hypotension, hypertension.
GI: abdominal cramping, hiccups, nausea, vomiting.
Derm: flushing.
Local: burning, pain, stinging, coldness, numbness, tingling at IV site.
MS: involuntary muscle movements, perioperative myoclonia.
Misc: fever.

INTERACTIONS

Drug-Drug: ▪ Additive CNS and respiratory depression with **alcohol, antihistamines, opioids,** and **sedative/hypnotics** (dosage reduction may be required) ▪ Increased risk of hypertriglyceridemia with **intravenous fat emulsion.**

ROUTE AND DOSAGE

❑ General Anesthesia

- **IV (Adults <55 yr):** *Induction*—40 mg (2–2.5 mg/kg) q 10 sec until induction achieved. *Maintenance*—100–200 mcg/kg/min. Rates of 150–200 mcg/kg/min are usually required during first 10–15 min after induction, then decreased by 30–50% during first 30 min of maintenance. Rates of 50–100 mcg/kg/min are associated with optimal recovery time. May also be given intermittently in increments of 25–50 mg.
- **IV (Geriatric Patients, Debilitated Patients, or Hypovolemic Patients):** *Induction*—20 mg (1–1.5 mg/kg) q 10 sec until induction achieved. *Maintenance*—50–100 mcg/kg/min.
- **IV (Adults Undergoing Neurosurgical Procedures):** *Induction*—20 mg q 10 sec

*CAPITALS indicate life-threatening; underlines indicate most frequent.

until induction achieved (1–2 mg/kg). *Maintenance*—100–200 mg/kg/min.

- **IV (Children ≥3 yr):** *Induction*—2.5–3.5 mg/kg. *Maintenance*—125–300 mcg/kg/min.

❑ **Monitored Anesthesia Care (MAC) Sedation**

- **IV (Adults <55 yr):** *Initiation*—100–150 mcg/kg/min infusion or 0.5 mg/kg as slow injection. *Maintenance*—25–75 mg/kg/min infusion or incremental boluses of 10–20 mg.
- **IV (Geriatric Patients, Debilitated Patients, or ASA III/IV Patients):** *Initiation*—Use slower infusion or injection rates. *Maintenance*—20% less than the usual adult infusion dose; rapid/repeated bolus dosing should be avoided.

❑ **ICU Sedation**

- **IV (Adults):** 5 mcg/kg/min for a minimum of 5 min. Additional increments of 5–10 mcg/kg/min over 5–10 min may be given until desired response is obtained. (Range 5–50 mcg/kg/min.) Dose should be reassessed every 24 hr.

AVAILABILITY

- ***Injection:*** 10 mg/ml in 20-ml ampules, 50- and 100-ml infusion vials[Rx].

TIME/ACTION PROFILE (loss of consciousness)

	ONSET	PEAK	DURATION*
IV	40 sec	UK	3–5 min

*Time to recovery is 8 min (up to 19 min if opioid analgesics have been used).

NURSING IMPLICATIONS

ASSESSMENT

- ❑ Assess respiratory status, pulse, and blood pressure continuously throughout propofol therapy. Frequently causes apnea lasting ≥60 sec. Maintain patent airway and adequate ventilation. Propofol should be used only by individuals experienced in endotracheal intubation, and equipment for this procedure should be readily available.
- ❑ Assess level of sedation and level of consciousness throughout and following administration.
- ***Toxicity and Overdose:*** If overdose occurs, monitor pulse, respiration, and blood pressure continuously. Maintain patent airway and assist ventilation as needed. If hypotension occurs, treatment includes IV fluids, repositioning, and vasopressors.

POTENTIAL NURSING DIAGNOSES

- Breathing pattern, ineffective (Adverse Reactions).
- Injury, risk for (Side Effects).
- Knowledge deficit, related to medication regimen (Patient/Family Teaching).

IMPLEMENTATION

- **General Info:** Dose is titrated to patient response.
- ❑ Propofol has no effect on the pain threshold. Adequate analgesia should *always* be used when propofol is used as an adjunct to surgical procedures.
- **Direct IV:** Shake well before use. If diluted prior to administration, use only D5W and dilute to a concentration not less than 2 mg/ml. Solution is opaque, making detection of contaminants difficult. Do not use if separation of the emulsion is evident. Contains no preservatives; maintain sterile technique and administer immediately after preparation. Discard unused portions and IV lines at the end of procedure or within 6 hr. For ICU sedation, discard after 12 hr if administered directly from vial or after 6 hr if transferred to a syringe or other container.
- ❑ Aseptic technique is essential. Vehicle is capable of rapid growth of bacterial contaminants. Infections and subsequent deaths have been reported.
- ❑ Frequently causes pain, burning, and stinging at injection site; use larger veins of the forearm, antecubital fossa, or a dedicated IV catheter. Lidocaine 10–20 mg IV may be administered prior to injection to minimize pain.
- ***Rate:*** Administer over 3–5 min. Titrate to desired level of sedation.
- **Intermittent/Continuous Infusion:** May be administered as an intermittent or continuous infusion (see Route and Dosage for rate). Administer via infusion pump to ensure accurate rate. Wake-up and assessment of CNS function should be done daily throughout maintenance to determine minimum dose required for sedation. Maintain a light level of sedation during these assessments; do not discontinue.

Abrupt discontinuation may cause rapid awakening with anxiety, agitation, and resistance to mechanical ventilation.

- **Solution Compatibility:** ▪ D5W ▪ LR ▪ D5/LR ▪ D5/0.45% NaCl ▪ D5/0.2% NaCl.
- **Y-Site Incompatibility:** ▪ atracurium ▪ blood ▪ plasma.
- **Additive Incompatibility:** ▪ Manufacturer does not recommend admixing propofol with other medications.

PATIENT/FAMILY TEACHING

- □ Inform patient that this medication will decrease mental recall of the procedure.
- □ May cause drowsiness or dizziness. Advise patient to request assistance prior to ambulation and transfer and to avoid driving or other activities requiring alertness for 24 hr following administration.
- □ Advise patient to avoid alcohol or other CNS depressants for 24 hr following administration.

EVALUATION

Effectiveness of therapy can be demonstrated by: ▪ Induction and maintenance of anesthesia □ Amnesia ▪ Sedation in mechanically ventilated patients in an intensive care setting.

PROPOXYPHENE

(pro-**pox**-i-feen)

Darvon, Darvon-N, Dolene, PP-Cap, {642}

PROPOXYPHENE/ACETAMINOPHEN†

Darvocet-N, E-Lor, Genagesic, Propacet, Propoxyphene with APAP, Wygesic

PROPOXYPHENE/ASPIRIN‡

{Darvon-N with ASA}

PROPOXYPHENE/ASPIRIN/CAFFEINE‡

Darvon Compound-65, {Darvon-N Compound}, PC-Cap, Propoxyphene Compound, {692}

CLASSIFICATION(S):
Opioid analgesics (agonist)

Schedule IV
Pregnancy Category C

†See also acetaminophen monograph on page 4.
‡See also salicylates monograph on page 900.

INDICATIONS

▪ Mild to moderate pain.

ACTION

▪ Binds to opiate receptors in the CNS ▪ Alters the perception of and response to painful stimuli, while producing generalized CNS depression. **Therapeutic Effects:** ▪ Decrease in mild to moderate pain.

PHARMACOKINETICS

Absorption: Well absorbed following oral administration. Napsylate salt is more slowly absorbed.
Distribution: Widely distributed. Probably crosses the placenta. Enters breast milk in small amounts.
Metabolism and Excretion: Mostly metabolized by the liver. Some conversion to norpropoxyphene, a toxic metabolite.
Half-life: 6–12 hr.

CONTRAINDICATIONS AND PRECAUTIONS

Contraindicated in: ▪ Hypersensitivity ▪ Pregnancy or lactation (avoid chronic use) ▪ Children.
Use Cautiously in: ▪ Head trauma ▪ Increased intracranial pressure ▪ Severe renal, hepatic, or pulmonary disease ▪ Hypothyroidism ▪ Adrenal insufficiency ▪ Alcoholism ▪ Geriatric or debilitated patients (dosage reduction recommended) ▪ Undiagnosed abdominal pain ▪ Prostatic hypertrophy ▪ Lactation (has been used safely).

ADVERSE REACTIONS AND SIDE EFFECTS*

CNS: dizziness, weakness, dysphoria, euphoria, headache, insomnia, paradoxical excitement, sedation.

{} = Available in Canada only.
*CAPITALS indicate life-threatening; underlines indicate most frequent.

EENT: blurred vision.
CV: hypotension.
GI: nausea, abdominal pain, constipation, vomiting.
Derm: rashes.
Misc: physical dependence, psychological dependence, tolerance.

INTERACTIONS

Drug-Drug: ▪ Use with extreme caution in patients receiving **MAO inhibitors** (may result in unpredictable, severe, and potentially fatal reactions—decrease initial dose to 25% of usual dose) ▪ Additive CNS depression with **alcohol, antidepressants,** and **sedative/hypnotics** ▪ **Smoking (nicotine)** increases metabolism and may decrease analgesic effectiveness ▪ Administration of **partial-antagonist opioid analgesics** may precipitate withdrawal in physically dependent patients ▪ **Nalbuphine, buprenorphine, dezocine,** or **pentazocine** may decrease analgesia.

ROUTE AND DOSAGE

Consider cumulative effects of additional acetaminophen/aspirin; if toxic levels are exceeded, change to pure proxyphene product.

- **PO (Adults):** 65 mg q 4 hr (hydrochloride—Darvon) or 100 mg q 4 hr (napsylate—Darvon-N) as needed (not to exceed 390 mg/day as hydrochloride or 600 mg/day as napsylate). 100 mg propoxyphene napsylate = 65 mg propoxyphene hydrochloride.

AVAILABILITY

❑ **Propoxyphene Hydrochloride**

▪ ***Capsules:*** 65 mg[Rx] ▪ {***Tablets:*** 65 mg[Rx]}.

❑ **Propoxyphene Napsylate**

▪ {***Capsules:*** 100 mg[Rx]} ▪ ***Tablets:*** 50 mg[Rx], 100 mg[Rx].

❑ **Propoxyphene Hydrochloride/Acetaminophen**

▪ ***Tablets:*** propoxyphene 65 mg/acetaminophen 650 mg[Rx].

❑ **Propoxyphene Napsylate/Acetaminophen**

▪ ***Tablets:*** propoxyphene 50 mg/acetaminophen 325 mg[Rx], propoxyphene 100 mg/acetaminophen 650 mg[Rx].

❑ **Propoxyphene Hydrochloride/Aspirin/Caffeine**

▪ ***Capsules:*** propoxyphene 65 mg, aspirin 389 mg, caffeine 32.4 mg[Rx] ▪ ***Tablets:*** {propoxyphene 65 mg, aspirin 375 mg, caffeine 30 mg[Rx]}.

❑ **Propoxyphene Napsylate/Aspirin**

▪ ***Tablets:*** {propoxyphene 100 mg/aspirin 325 mg[Rx]}.

❑ **Propoxyphene Napsylate/Aspirin/Caffeine**

▪ ***Tablets:*** {propoxyphene 100 mg/aspirin 375 mg/caffeine 30 mg[Rx]}.

TIME/ACTION PROFILE (analgesic effect)

	ONSET	PEAK	DURATION
PO	15–60 min	2–3 hr	4–6 hr

NURSING IMPLICATIONS

ASSESSMENT

- ❑ Assess type, location, and intensity of pain prior to and 2 hr (peak) following administration. When titrating opioid doses, increases of 25–50% should be administered until there is either a 50% reduction in the patient's pain rating on a numerical or visual analogue scale or the patient reports satisfactory pain relief. A repeat dose can be safely administered at the time of the peak if previous dose is ineffective and side effects are minimal.
- ❑ An equianalgesic chart (see Appendix B) should be used when changing routes or when changing from one opioid to another.
- ❑ Prolonged, high-dose therapy may lead to physical and psychological dependence and tolerance. This should not prevent patient from receiving adequate analgesia. Most patients who receive propoxyphene for pain do not develop psychological dependence. Progressively higher doses or change to a stronger opioid may be required to relieve pain with long-term therapy.
- ❑ Assess blood pressure, pulse, and respirations before and periodically during administration. If respiratory rate is <10/min, assess level of sedation. Physical stimulation may be sufficient to prevent significant hypoventilation. Dose may need to be decreased by 25–50%. Initial drowsiness will diminish with continued use.

□ Assess bowel function routinely. Prevention of constipation should be instituted with increased intake of fluids and bulk, and laxatives to minimize constipating effects. Stimulant laxatives should be administered routinely if opioid use exceeds 2–3 days, unless contraindicated.

- ***Lab Test Considerations:*** May cause elevated serum amylase and lipase levels.

□ May cause increased AST, ALT, serum alkaline phosphatase, LDH, and bilirubin concentrations.

- ***Toxicity and Overdose:*** If an opioid antagonist is required to reverse respiratory depression or coma, naloxone (Narcan) is the antidote. Dilute the 0.4-mg ampule of naloxone in 10 ml of 0.9% NaCl and administer 0.5 ml (0.02 mg) by direct IV push every 2 min. For patients weighing <40 kg, dilute 0.1 mg of naloxone in 10 ml of 0.9% NaCl for a concentration of 10 mcg/ml and administer 0.5 mcg/kg every 1–2 min. Titrate dose to avoid withdrawal, seizures, and severe pain.

POTENTIAL NURSING DIAGNOSES

- Pain (Indications).
- Sensory-perceptual alterations: visual, auditory (Side Effects).
- Injury, risk for (Side Effects).

IMPLEMENTATION

- **General Info:** Explain therapeutic value of medication prior to administration, to enhance the analgesic effect.

□ Regularly administered doses may be more effective than prn administration. Analgesic is more effective if given before pain becomes severe.

□ Coadministration with nonopioid analgesics may have additive analgesic effects and may permit lower opioid doses.

□ Medication should be discontinued gradually after long-term use to prevent withdrawal symptoms.

- **PO:** Doses may be administered with food or milk to minimize GI irritation.

PATIENT/FAMILY TEACHING

□ Advise patient to take medication exactly as directed and not to take more than the recommended amount. Severe and permanent liver damage may result from prolonged use or high doses of acetaminophen. Renal damage may occur with prolonged use of acetaminophen or aspirin. Doses of nonopioid agents should not exceed the maximum recommended daily dose.

□ Instruct patient on how and when to ask for pain medication.

□ Medication may cause drowsiness or dizziness. Caution patient to avoid driving and other activities requiring alertness until response to the drug is known.

□ Advise patient to change positions slowly to minimize orthostatic hypotension.

□ Caution patient to avoid concurrent use of alcohol or other CNS depressants with this medication.

□ Encourage patient to turn, cough, and breathe deeply every 2 hr to prevent atelectasis.

□ Advise patient that good oral hygiene, frequent mouth rinses, and sugarless gum or candy may decrease dry mouth.

EVALUATION

Effectiveness of therapy can be demonstrated by: ■ Decrease in severity of pain without a significant alteration in level of consciousness.

PROPRANOLOL

(proe-**pran**-oh-lole)
{Apo-Propranolol}, {Detensol}, Inderal, Inderal LA, {Novopranol}, {pms Propranolol}

CLASSIFICATION(S):
Antianginal, Antiarrhythmic, Antihypertensive agent, Beta-adrenergic blocking agent (nonselective)

Pregnancy Category C

INDICATIONS

■ Management of hypertension ■ Management of angina pectoris ■ Management of arrhythmias ■ Prevention and management of myocardial infarction ■ Also used to: □ Prevent vascular headaches □ Manage thyrotoxicosis □ Manage pheochromocytoma □ Treat essential tremors □ Manage hypertrophic cardiomyopathy. **Unla-**

{} = **Available in Canada only.**

beled Uses: ▪ Also used to manage: ▫ Alcohol withdrawal ▫ Aggressive behavior ▫ Antipsychotic-associated akathisia ▫ Situational anxiety ▫ Esophageal varices.

ACTION

▪ Blocks stimulation of $beta_1$ (myocardial) and $beta_2$ (pulmonary, vascular, and uterine) -adrenergic receptor sites. **Therapeutic Effects:** ▪ Decreased heart rate and blood pressure ▪ Suppression of arrhythmias ▪ Prevention of myocardial infarction.

PHARMACOKINETICS

Absorption: Well absorbed but undergoes extensive first-pass hepatic metabolism.
Distribution: Moderate CNS penetration. Crosses the placenta; enters breast milk.
Metabolism and Excretion: Almost completely metabolized by the liver.
Half-life: 3.4–6 hr.

CONTRAINDICATIONS AND PRECAUTIONS

Contraindicated in: ▪ Uncompensated congestive heart failure ▪ Pulmonary edema ▪ Cardiogenic shock ▪ Bradycardia or heart block.
Use Cautiously in: ▪ Renal impairment ▪ Hepatic impairment ▪ Geriatric patients (increased sensitivity to beta-adrenergic blockers; initial dosage reduction recommended) ▪ Pulmonary disease (including asthma) ▪ Diabetes mellitus (may mask signs of hypoglycemia) ▪ Thyrotoxicosis (may mask symptoms) ▪ Patients with a history of severe allergic reactions (intensity of reactions may be increased) ▪ Pregnancy, lactation, or children (safety not established; all agents cross the placenta and may cause fetal/neonatal bradycardia, hypotension, hypoglycemia, or respiratory depression).

ADVERSE REACTIONS AND SIDE EFFECTS*

CNS: <u>fatigue</u>, <u>weakness</u>, anxiety, dizziness, drowsiness, insomnia, memory loss, mental depression, mental status changes, nervousness, nightmares.
EENT: blurred vision, dry eyes, nasal stuffiness.
Resp: bronchospasm, wheezing.
CV: ARRHYTHMIAS, BRADYCARDIA, CONGESTIVE HEART FAILURE, PULMONARY EDEMA, orthostatic hypotension, peripheral vasoconstriction.
GI: constipation, diarrhea, nausea.
GU: <u>impotence</u>, decreased libido.
Derm: itching, rashes.
Endo: hyperglycemia, hypoglycemia (↑ in children).
MS: arthralgia, back pain, muscle cramps.
Neuro: paresthesia.

INTERACTIONS

Drug-Drug: ▪ **General anesthesia, IV phenytoin,** and **verapamil** may cause additive myocardial depression ▪ Additive bradycardia may occur with **digitalis glycosides** ▪ Additive hypotension may occur with other **antihypertensives,** acute ingestion of **alcohol,** or **nitrates** ▪ Concurrent use with **amphetamines, cocaine, ephedrine, epinephrine, norepinephrine, phenylephrine,** or **pseudoephedrine** may result in unopposed alpha-adrenergic stimulation (excessive hypertension, bradycardia) ▪ Concurrent **thyroid** administration may decrease effectiveness ▪ May alter the effectiveness of **insulin** or **oral hypoglycemic agents** (dosage adjustments may be necessary) ▪ May decrease the effectiveness of **beta-adrenergic bronchodilators** and **theophylline** ▪ May decrease the beneficial $beta_1$ cardiovascular effects of **dopamine** or **dobutamine** ▪ Use cautiously within 14 days of **MAO inhibitor** therapy (may result in hypertension) ▪ **Cimetidine** may increase toxicity from labetalol, timolol, or propranolol ▪ Concurrent **NSAIDs** may decrease antihypertensive action.

ROUTE AND DOSAGE

- **PO (Adults):** *Antianginal*—80–320 mg/day in 2–4 divided doses or once daily as extended-release capsules. *Antihypertensive*—40 mg twice daily initially; may be increased as needed (usual range 120–240 mg/day; doses up to 1 g/day have been used); or 80 mg once daily as extended-release capsules, increased as needed. *Antiarrhythmic*—10–30 mg 3–4 times daily. *Prevention of myocardial infarction*—180–240 mg/day in divided doses. *Hypertrophic cardiomyopathy*—20–40 mg 3–4 times daily. *Adjunct therapy of pheochromocytoma*—20 mg 3 times daily to 40 mg 3–4 times daily

*CAPITALS indicate life-threatening; <u>underlines</u> indicate most frequent.

concurrently with alpha-blocking therapy, started 3 days before surgery is planned. *Vascular headache prevention*—20 mg 4 times daily or 80 mg/day as extended-release capsules; may be increased as needed up to 240 mg/day. *Management of tremor*—40 mg twice daily; may be increased up to 120 mg/day (up to 320 mg have been used).

- **PO (Children):** *Antihypertensive/antiarrhythmic*—0.5–1 mg/kg/day in 2–4 divided doses; may be increased as needed (usual range for maintenance dose is 2–4 mg/kg/day in 2 divided doses).
- **IV (Adults):** *Antiarrhythmic*—1–3 mg; may be repeated after 2 min and again in 4 hr if needed.
- **IV (Children):** *Antiarrhythmic*—10–100 mcg (0.01–0.1 mg)/kg (up to 1 mg/dose); may be repeated q 6–8 hr if needed.

AVAILABILITY

▪ ***Oral solution:*** 4 mg/ml^Rx^, 8 mg/ml^Rx^, 80 mg/ml^Rx^ ▪ ***Tablets:*** 10 mg^Rx^, 20 mg^Rx^, 40 mg^Rx^, 60 mg^Rx^, 90 mg^Rx^, {120 mg^Rx^} ▪ ***Extended-release capsules:*** 60 mg^Rx^, 80 mg^Rx^, 120 mg^Rx^, 160 mg^Rx^ ▪ ***Injection:*** 1 mg/ml^Rx^ ▪ ***In combination with:*** hydrochlorothiazide (Inderide^Rx^, Inderide LA^Rx^). See Appendix A.

TIME/ACTION PROFILE (cardiovascular effects)

	ONSET	PEAK	DURATION
PO	30 min	60–90 min*	6–12 hr
PO–ER	UK	6 hr	24 hr
IV	immediate	1 min	4–6 hr

*Following single dose, full effect not seen until several weeks of therapy.

NURSING IMPLICATIONS

ASSESSMENT

- **General Info:** Monitor blood pressure and pulse frequently during dosage adjustment period and periodically throughout therapy. Assess for orthostatic hypotension when assisting patient up from supine position.
  - Patients receiving *propranolol IV* must have continuous ECG monitoring and may have pulmonary capillary wedge pressure (PCWP) or central venous pressure (CVP) monitoring during and for several hours after administration.
  - Monitor intake and output ratios and daily weight. Assess patient routinely for evidence of fluid overload (peripheral edema, dyspnea, rales/crackles, fatigue, weight gain, jugular venous distention).
- **Angina:** Assess frequency and characteristics of anginal attacks periodically throughout therapy.
- **Vascular Headache Prophylaxis:** Assess frequency, severity, characteristics, and location of vascular headaches periodically throughout therapy.
- ***Lab Test Considerations:*** May cause increased BUN, serum lipoprotein, potassium, triglyceride, and uric acid levels.
  - May cause increased ANA titers.
  - May cause decrease or increase in blood glucose levels. In labile diabetics, hypoglycemia may be accompanied by precipitous elevation of blood pressure.
- ***Toxicity and Overdose:*** Monitor patients receiving beta-adrenergic blocking agents for signs of overdose (bradycardia, severe dizziness or fainting, severe drowsiness, dyspnea, bluish fingernails or palms, seizures). Notify physician or other health care professional immediately if these signs occur.
  - Hypotension may be treated with Trendelenburg position and IV fluids unless contraindicated. Vasopressors (epinephrine, norepinephrine, dopamine, dobutamine) may also be used. Hypotension does not respond to $beta_2$ agonists.
  - Glucagon has been used to treat bradycardia and hypotension.

POTENTIAL NURSING DIAGNOSES

- Cardiac output, decreased (Side Effects).
- Knowledge deficit, related to medication regimen (Patient/Family Teaching).
- Noncompliance, related to medication regimen (Patient/Family Teaching).

IMPLEMENTATION

- **General Info:** Oral and parenteral doses of *propranolol* are not interchangeable. Check dose carefully. IV dose is 1/10 the oral dose and may be a temporary alternative if patient is NPO.
- **PO:** Take apical pulse prior to administering. If <50 bpm or if arrhythmia occurs, withhold medication and notify physician or other health care professional.

- Administer with meals or directly after eating to enhance absorption.
- Extended-release capsules should be swallowed whole; do not crush, open, or chew. *Propranolol tablets* may be crushed and mixed with food.
- Mix propranolol oral solution with liquid or semisolid food (water, juices, soda, applesauce, puddings). Make sure entire dose is taken. Rinse glass with more liquid to ensure all medication is taken. Do not store after mixing.

Propranolol

- **Direct IV:** Administer undiluted or dilute each 1 mg in 10 ml of D5W for injection.
- ***Rate:*** Administer over at least 1 min.
- **Intermittent Infusion:** May also be diluted for infusion in 50 ml of 0.9% NaCl, D5W, D5/0.45% NaCl, D5/0.9% NaCl, or lactated Ringer's injection.
- ***Rate:*** Infuse over 10–15 min.
- **Syringe Compatibility:** ▪ amrinone ▪ milrinone.
- **Y-Site Compatibility:** ▪ alteplase ▪ amrinone ▪ heparin ▪ hydrocortisone sodium succinate ▪ meperidine ▪ milrinone ▪ morphine ▪ potassium chloride ▪ tacrolimus ▪ vitamin B complex with vitamin C.
- **Y-Site Incompatibility:** ▪ diazoxide.

PATIENT/FAMILY TEACHING

- **General Info:** Instruct patient to take medication exactly as directed, at the same time each day, even if feeling well; do not skip or double up on missed doses. If a dose is missed, it should be taken as soon as possible up to 4 hr before next dose (8 hr with extended-release propranolol). Abrupt withdrawal may precipitate life-threatening arrhythmias, hypertension, or myocardial ischemia.
- Advise patient to make sure enough medication is available for weekends, holidays, and vacations. A written prescription may be kept in wallet in case of emergency.
- Teach patient and family how to check pulse and blood pressure. Instruct them to check pulse daily and blood pressure biweekly. Advise patient to hold dose and contact health care professional if pulse is <50 bpm or blood pressure changes significantly.
- May cause drowsiness or dizziness. Caution patients to avoid driving or other activities that require alertness until response to the drug is known.
- Advise patients to change positions slowly to minimize orthostatic hypotension, especially during initiation of therapy or when dose is increased.
- Caution patient that this medication may increase sensitivity to cold.
- Instruct patient to consult health care professional before taking any OTC medications, especially cold preparations, concurrently with this medication.
- Diabetics should closely monitor blood sugar, especially if weakness, malaise, irritability, or fatigue occurs. May mask tachycardia and increased blood pressure as signs of hypoglycemia, but dizziness and sweating may still occur.
- Advise patient to notify health care professional if slow pulse, difficulty breathing, wheezing, cold hands and feet, dizziness, lightheadedness, confusion, depression, rash, fever, sore throat, unusual bleeding, or bruising occurs.
- Instruct patient to inform health care professional of medication regimen prior to treatment or surgery.
- Advise patient to carry identification describing disease process and medication regimen at all times.
- **Hypertension:** Reinforce the need to continue additional therapies for hypertension (weight loss, sodium restriction, stress reduction, regular exercise, moderation of alcohol consumption, and smoking cessation). Medication controls but does not cure hypertension.
- **Angina:** Caution patient to avoid overexertion with decrease in chest pain.
- **Vascular Headache Prophylaxis:** Caution patient that sharing this medication may be dangerous.

EVALUATION

Effectiveness of therapy can be demonstrated by: ▪ Decrease in blood pressure ▪ Control of arrhythmias without appearance of detrimental side effects ▪ Reduction in frequency of anginal attacks ▫ Increase in activity tolerance ▪ Prevention of myocardial infarction ▪ Prevention of vascular headaches ▪ Management of thyrotoxicosis ▪ Management of pheochromocytoma ▪ Decrease in tremors ▪ Management of hypertrophic cardiomyopathy.

PROPYLTHIOURACIL
(proe-pill-thye-oh-**yoor**-a-sill)
{Propyl-Thyracil}, PTU

CLASSIFICATION(S):
Antithyroid agent

Pregnancy Category D

INDICATIONS
▪ Palliative treatment of hyperthyroidism ▪ Adjunct in the control of hyperthyroidism in preparation for thyroidectomy or radioactive iodine therapy.

ACTION
▪ Inhibits the synthesis of thyroid hormones. **Therapeutic Effects:** ▪ Decreased signs and symptoms of hyperthyroidism.

PHARMACOKINETICS
Absorption: Rapidly absorbed from the GI tract.
Distribution: Concentrates in the thyroid gland; crosses the placenta and enters breast milk in low concentrations.
Metabolism and Excretion: Metabolized by the liver.
Half-life: 1–2 hr.

CONTRAINDICATIONS AND PRECAUTIONS
Contraindicated in: ▪ Hypersensitivity.
Use Cautiously in: ▪ Decreased bone marrow reserve ▪ Pregnancy (may be used safely; however, fetus may develop thyroid problems) ▪ Lactation (safety not established).

ADVERSE REACTIONS AND SIDE EFFECTS*
CNS: drowsiness, headache, vertigo.
GI: nausea, vomiting, diarrhea, drug-induced hepatitis, loss of taste.
Derm: rash, skin discoloration, urticaria.
Endo: hypothyroidism.
Hemat: AGRANULOCYTOSIS, leukopenia, thrombocytopenia.
MS: arthralgia.
Misc: fever, lymphadenopathy, parotitis.

INTERACTIONS
Drug-Drug: ▪ Additive bone marrow depression with **antineoplastic agents** or **radiation therapy** ▪ Additive antithyroid effects with **lithium, potassium iodide,** or **sodium iodide** ▪ Increased risk of agranulocytosis with **phenothiazines.**

ROUTE AND DOSAGE
- **PO (Adults):** *Thyrotoxic crisis*—200–400 mg q 4 hr during the first 24 hr. *Hyperthyroidism*—300–900 mg once daily or in 2–4 divided doses initially (up to 1.2 g/day); maintenance dose 50–600 mg/day once daily or in 2–4 divided doses.
- **PO (Children >10 yr):** 50–300 mg/day given once daily or in 2–4 divided doses.
- **PO (Children 6–10 yr):** 50–150 mg/day given once daily or in 2–4 divided doses.
- **PO (Neonates):** 10 mg/kg/day in divided doses.

AVAILABILITY
▪ ***Tablets:*** 50 mg[Rx], {100 mg[Rx]}.

TIME/ACTION PROFILE (effects on clinical thyroid status)

	ONSET	PEAK	DURATION
PO	10–21 days†	6–10 wk	wks

†Effects on serum thyroid hormone concentration may occur within 60 min of a single dose.

NURSING IMPLICATIONS

ASSESSMENT
- ☐ Monitor response of symptoms of hyperthyroidism or thyrotoxicosis (tachycardia, palpitations, nervousness, insomnia, fever, diaphoresis, heat intolerance, tremors, weight loss, diarrhea).
- ☐ Assess patient for development of hypothyroidism (intolerance to cold, constipation, dry skin, headache, listlessness, tiredness, or weakness). Dosage adjustment may be required.

{} = Available in Canada only.
*CAPITALS indicate life-threatening; underlines indicate most frequent.

□ Assess patient for skin rash or swelling of cervical lymph nodes. Treatment may be discontinued if this occurs.

■ ***Lab Test Considerations:*** Thyroid function studies should be monitored prior to therapy, monthly during initial therapy, and every 2–3 mo throughout therapy.

□ WBC and differential counts should be monitored periodically throughout course of therapy. Agranulocytosis may develop rapidly and usually occurs during first 2 mo. This necessitates discontinuation of therapy.

□ May cause increased AST, ALT, LDH, alkaline phosphatase, serum bilirubin, and prothrombin time.

POTENTIAL NURSING DIAGNOSES

■ Knowledge deficit, related to medication regimen (Patient/Family Teaching).

■ Noncompliance (Patient/Family Teaching).

IMPLEMENTATION

■ **General Info:** Can be compounded by pharmacist into enema or suppository.

■ **PO:** Administer at same time in relation to meals every day. Food may either increase or decrease absorption.

PATIENT/FAMILY TEACHING

□ Instruct patient to take medication exactly as directed, around the clock. If a dose is missed, take as soon as remembered; take both doses together if almost time for next dose; check with health care professional if more than 1 dose is missed. Consult health care professional prior to discontinuing medication.

□ Instruct patient to monitor weight 2–3 times weekly. Report significant changes.

□ May cause drowsiness. Caution patient to avoid driving or other activities requiring alertness until response to medication is known.

□ Advise patient to consult health care professional regarding dietary sources of iodine (iodized salt, shellfish).

□ Advise patient to report sore throat, fever, chills, headache, malaise, weakness, yellowing of eyes or skin, unusual bleeding or bruising, symptoms of hyperthyroidism or hypothyroidism, or rash to health care professional promptly.

□ Instruct patient to consult health care professional before taking any OTC medications containing iodine concurrently with this medication.

□ Advise patient to carry identification describing medication regimen at all times and to notify health care professional of medication regimen prior to treatment or surgery.

□ Emphasize the importance of routine exams to monitor progress and to check for side effects.

EVALUATION

Effectiveness of therapy can be demonstrated by: ■ Decrease in severity of symptoms of hyperthyroidism (lowered pulse rate and weight gain) ■ Return of thyroid function studies to normal ■ May be used as short-term adjunctive therapy to prepare patient for thyroidectomy or radiation therapy or may be used in treatment of hyperthyroidism. Treatment of 6 mo to several years may be necessary, usually averaging 1 yr.

PROTAMINE SULFATE

(**proe**-ta-meen)

CLASSIFICATION(S):
Antidote (antiheparin agent)

Pregnancy Category C

INDICATIONS

■ Acute management of severe heparin overdosage ■ Used to neutralize heparin received during dialysis, cardiopulmonary bypass, and other procedures. **Unlabeled Uses:** ■ Management of overdosage of: □ Dalteparin □ Enoxaparin.

ACTION

■ A strong base that forms a complex with heparin (an acid). **Therapeutic Effects:** ■ Inactivation of heparin.

PHARMACOKINETICS

Absorption: Administered IV only, resulting in complete bioavailability.
Distribution: UK.
Metabolism and Excretion: Metabolic fate not known. Protamine-heparin complex eventually degrades.
Half-life: UK.

CONTRAINDICATIONS AND PRECAUTIONS

Contraindicated in: ▪ Hypersensitivity to protamine or fish ▪ Avoid reconstitution with diluents containing benzyl alcohol if used in neonates.
Use Cautiously in: ▪ Patients who have received previous protamine-containing insulin or vasectomized men (increased risk of hypersensitivity reactions) ▪ Pregnancy, lactation, and children (safety not established).

ADVERSE REACTIONS AND SIDE EFFECTS*

Resp: dyspnea.
CV: bradycardia, hypertension, hypotension, pulmonary hypertension.
GI: nausea, vomiting.
Derm: flushing, warmth.
Hemat: bleeding.
MS: back pain.
Misc: hypersensitivity reactions, including ANAPHYLAXIS, ANGIOEDEMA, and PULMONARY EDEMA.

INTERACTIONS

Drug-Drug: ▪ None significant.

ROUTE AND DOSAGE

- **IV (Adults and Children):** *Heparin overdosage*—1 mg/100 units of heparin. If given >30 min after heparin, give 0.5 mg/100 units of heparin (not to exceed 100 mg/2 hr). Further doses should be determined by coagulation tests. *Enoxaparin overdose*—1 mg/each mg of enoxaparin to be neutralized (unlabeled). *Dalteparin overdose*—1 mg/100 anti-Xa IU of dalteparin. If required, a 2nd dose of 0.5 mg/100 anti-Xa IU of dalteparin may be given 2–4 hr later if laboratory assessment indicates need (unlabeled).

AVAILABILITY

▪ ***Injection:*** 10 mg/ml in 5- and 25-ml ampules and 5-, 10-, and 25-ml vials[Rx].

TIME/ACTION PROFILE (reversal of heparin effect)

	ONSET	PEAK	DURATION
IV	30 sec–1 min	UK	2 hr†

†Depends on body temperature.

NURSING IMPLICATIONS

ASSESSMENT

- ▫ Assess for bleeding and hemorrhage throughout therapy. Hemorrhage may recur 8–9 hr after therapy because of rebound effects of heparin. Rebound may occur as late as 18 hr after therapy in patients heparinized for cardiopulmonary bypass.
- ▫ Assess for allergy to fish (salmon), previous reaction to or use of protamine insulin or protamine sulfate. Vasectomized and infertile men also have higher risk of hypersensitivity reaction.
- ▫ Observe patient for signs and symptoms of hypersensitivity reaction (hives, edema, coughing, wheezing). Keep epinephrine, an antihistamine, and resuscitative equipment close by in the event of anaphylaxis.
- ▫ Assess for hypovolemia prior to initiation of therapy. Failure to correct hypovolemia may result in cardiovascular collapse from peripheral vasodilating effects of protamine sulfate.
- ▪ ***Lab Test Considerations:*** Monitor clotting factors, activated clotting time (ACT), activated partial thromboplastin time (aPTT), and thrombin time (TT) 5–15 min after therapy and again as necessary.

POTENTIAL NURSING DIAGNOSES

- ▪ Injury, risk for (Indications).
- ▪ Tissue perfusion, altered (Indications).

IMPLEMENTATION

- ▪ **General Info:** Discontinue heparin infusion. In milder cases, overdosage may be treated by heparin withdrawal alone.
- ▫ In severe cases, fresh frozen plasma or whole blood may also be required to control bleeding.
- ▫ Dosage varies with type of heparin, route of heparin therapy, and amount of time elapsed since discontinuation of heparin.
- ▫ Do not administer >100 mg in 2 hr without rechecking clotting studies, as protamine sulfate has its own anticoagulant properties.
- ▪ **IV:** Reconstitute 50-mg vial with 5 ml and 250-mg vial with 25 ml of sterile water for injection or bacteriostatic water for injection for a concentration of 10 mg/ml. Shake vigorously. Solution reconstituted with sterile water for in-

*CAPITALS indicate life-threatening; underlines indicate most frequent.

jection should be discarded after dose is withdrawn. Solution reconstituted with bacteriostatic water is stable for 24 hr when refrigerated.

- **Direct IV:** May be administered undiluted.
- ***Rate:*** May be administered slow IV push over 1–3 min.
- **Intermittent Infusion:** May be diluted in D5W or 0.9% NaCl.
- ***Rate:*** Infuse no faster than 50 mg over 10 min. Rapid infusion rate may result in hypotension, bradycardia, flushing, or feeling of warmth. If these symptoms occur, stop infusion and notify physician.

PATIENT/FAMILY TEACHING

- Explain purpose of the medication to patient. Instruct patient to report recurrent bleeding immediately.
- Advise patient to avoid activities that may result in bleeding (shaving, brushing teeth, receiving injections or rectal temperatures, or ambulating) until risk of hemorrhage has passed.

EVALUATION

Effectiveness of therapy can be demonstrated by: ▪ Control of bleeding ▪ Normalization of clotting factors in heparinized patients.

PSEUDOEPHEDRINE

(soo-doe-e-**fed**-rin)

{Balminil Decongestant Syrup}, {Benylin Decongestant}, {Cenafed}, Decofed, Dorcol Children's Decongestant liquid, Drixoral Non-Drowsy Formula, Efidac/24, {Eltor 120}, Genafed, Halofed, Myfedrine, Novafed, PediaCare Infants' Oral Decongestant Drops, Pseudo, Pseudogest, {Robidrine}, Sudafed, Sudafed 12 Hour, Sufedrin

CLASSIFICATION(S):

Decongestant

Pregnancy Category B

INDICATIONS

▪ Symptomatic management of nasal congestion associated with acute viral upper respiratory tract infections ▪ Used in combination with antihistamines in the management of allergic conditions ▪ Used to open obstructed eustachian tubes in chronic otic inflammation or infection.

ACTION

▪ Stimulates alpha- and beta-adrenergic receptors ▪ Produces vasoconstriction in the respiratory tract mucosa (alpha-adrenergic stimulation) and possibly bronchodilation ($beta_2$-adrenergic stimulation). **Therapeutic Effects:** ▪ Reduction of nasal congestion, hyperemia, and swelling in nasal passages.

PHARMACOKINETICS

Absorption: Well absorbed following oral administration.

Distribution: Appears to enter the CSF; probably crosses the placenta and enters breast milk.

Metabolism and Excretion: Partially metabolized by the liver. 55–75% excreted unchanged by the kidneys (depends on urine pH).

Half-life: 7 hr (depends on urine pH).

CONTRAINDICATIONS AND PRECAUTIONS

Contraindicated in: ▪ Hypersensitivity to sympathomimetic amines ▪ Hypertension, severe coronary artery disease ▪ Concurrent MAO inhibitor therapy ▪ Known alcohol intolerance (some liquid products).

Use Cautiously in: ▪ Hyperthyroidism ▪ Diabetes mellitus ▪ Prostatic hypertrophy ▪ Ischemic heart disease ▪ Glaucoma ▪ Pregnancy or lactation (safety not established).

ADVERSE REACTIONS AND SIDE EFFECTS*

CNS: SEIZURES, anxiety, nervousness, dizziness, drowsiness, excitability, fear, hallucinations, headache, insomnia, restlessness, weakness.

Resp: respiratory difficulty.

CV: CARDIOVASCULAR COLLAPSE, palpitations, hypertension, tachycardia.

{} = Available in Canada only.
***CAPITALS indicate life-threatening; underlines indicate most frequent.**

GI: anorexia, dry mouth.
GU: dysuria.

INTERACTIONS

Drug-Drug: ▪ Concurrent use with **MAO inhibitors** may cause hypertensive crisis ▪ Additive sympathomimetic effects with other **sympathomimetic agents** ▪ Concurrent use with **beta-adrenergic blockers** may result in hypertension or bradycardia ▪ **Drugs that acidify the urine** may decrease effectiveness ▪ **Drugs that alkalinize the urine (sodium bicarbonate, high-dose antacid therapy)** may intensify effectiveness.

Drug-Food: ▪ **Foods that acidify the urine** may decrease effectiveness ▪ **Foods that alkalinize the urine** may intensify effectiveness (see lists in Appendix K).

ROUTE AND DOSAGE

- **PO (Adults and Children >12 yr):** 60 mg q 4–6 hr as needed (not to exceed 240 mg/day) or 120 mg of extended-release preparation q 12 hr or 240 mg extended-release preparation q 24 hr.
- **PO (Children 6–12 yr):** 30 mg q 4–6 hr as needed (not to exceed 120 mg/day) *or* 4 mg/kg/day (125 mg/m²/day) in 4 divided doses.
- **PO (Children 2–6 yr):** 15 mg q 4–6 hr (not to exceed 60 mg/day) *or* 4 mg/kg/day (125 mg/m²/day) in 4 divided doses.
- **PO (Children 1–2 yr):** 7 drops (of 7.5 mg/0.8 ml solution)/kg q 4–6 hr (not to exceed 4 doses/24 hr).
- **PO (Children 3–12 mo):** 3 drops (of 7.5 mg/0.8 ml solution)/kg q 4–6 hr (not to exceed 4 doses/24 hr).

AVAILABILITY

▪ ***Tablets:*** 30 mg^OTC, 60 mg^OTC ▪ ***Extended-release tablets:*** 120 mg^OTC, 240 mg^OTC ▪ ***Capsules:*** {60 mg^OTC} ▪ ***Extended-release capsules:*** 120 mg^Rx, {240 mg^OTC} ▪ ***Syrup:*** 30 mg/5 ml^OTC ▪ ***Oral solution:*** 15 mg/5 ml^OTC, 30 mg/5 ml^OTC ▪ ***Drops:*** 7.5 mg/0.8 ml (0.8 ml = 1 dropperful)^OTC ▪ ***In combination with:*** antihistamines, acetaminophen, cough suppressants, and expectorants^OTC. See Appendix A.

TIME/ACTION PROFILE (decongestant effects)

	ONSET	PEAK	DURATION
PO	30 min	UK	4–8 hr
PO-ER	60 min	UK	12 hr

P

NURSING IMPLICATIONS

ASSESSMENT

- ☐ Assess congestion (nasal, sinus, eustachian tube) prior to and periodically throughout therapy.
- ☐ Monitor pulse and blood pressure before beginning therapy and periodically throughout therapy.
- ☐ Assess lung sounds and character of bronchial secretions. Maintain fluid intake of 1500–2000 ml/day to decrease viscosity of secretions.

POTENTIAL NURSING DIAGNOSES

- Airway clearance, ineffective (Indications).
- Knowledge deficit, related to medication regimen (Patient/Family Teaching).

IMPLEMENTATION

- **General Info:** Administer pseudoephedrine at least 2 hr before bedtime to minimize insomnia.
- **PO:** Extended-release tablets and capsules should be swallowed whole; do not crush, break, or chew. Contents of the capsule can be mixed with jam or jelly and swallowed without chewing for patients with difficulty swallowing.

PATIENT/FAMILY TEACHING

- ☐ Instruct patient to take medication exactly as directed and not to take more than recommended. If a dose is missed, take within 1 hr; if remembered later, omit. Do not double doses.
- ☐ Instruct patient to notify health care professional if nervousness, slow or fast heart rate, breathing difficulties, hallucinations, or seizures occur, as these symptoms may indicate overdosage.
- ☐ Instruct patient to contact health care professional if symptoms do not improve within 7 days or if fever is present.

EVALUATION

Effectiveness of therapy can be demonstrated by: ▪ Decreased nasal, sinus, or eustachian tube congestion.

PSYLLIUM

(**sill**-i-yum)

Alramucil, Cillium, Effer-Syllium, Fiberall, Fibrepur, Genfiber, Hydrocil, {Karacil}, Konsyl, Metamucil, Modane Bulk, Muci-Lax, Mylanta Natural Fiber Supplement, Naturacil Caramels, {Natural Source Fibre Laxative}, Perdiem, {Prodiem}, Pro-Lax, Reguloid Natural, Serutan, Siblin, Syllact, UniLaxative, Vitalax, V-Lax

CLASSIFICATION(S):

Laxative (bulk-forming agent)

Pregnancy Category UK

INDICATIONS

▪ Management of simple or chronic constipation, particularly if associated with a low-fiber diet ▪ Useful in situations in which straining should be avoided (after myocardial infarction, rectal surgery, prolonged bed rest) ▪ Used in the management of chronic watery diarrhea.

ACTION

▪ Combines with water in the intestinal contents to form an emollient gel or viscous solution that promotes peristalsis and reduces transit time. **Therapeutic Effects:** ▪ Relief and prevention of constipation.

PHARMACOKINETICS

Absorption: Not absorbed from the GI tract.
Distribution: No distribution occurs.
Metabolism and Excretion: Excreted in feces.
Half-life: UK.

CONTRAINDICATIONS AND PRECAUTIONS

Contraindicated in: ▪ Hypersensitivity ▪ Abdominal pain, nausea, or vomiting (especially when associated with fever) ▪ Serious adhesions ▪ Dysphagia.
Use Cautiously in: ▪ Some dosage forms contain sugar, aspartame, or excessive sodium and should be avoided in patients on restricted diets ▪ Pregnancy and lactation (has been used safely).

ADVERSE REACTIONS AND SIDE EFFECTS

Resp: bronchospasm.
GI: cramps, intestinal or esophageal obstruction, nausea, vomiting.

INTERACTIONS

Drug-Drug: ▪ May decrease the absorption of **warfarin, salicylates,** or **digitalis glycosides.**

ROUTE AND DOSAGE

- **PO (Adults):** 1–2 tsp/packet/wafer (3–6 g psyllium) in or with a full glass of liquid 2–3 times daily. Up to 30 g daily in divided doses.
- **PO (Children >6 yr):** 1 tsp/packet/wafer (1.5–3 g psyllium) in or with ½–1 glass of liquid 2–3 times daily. Up to 15 g daily in divided doses.

AVAILABILITY

▪ ***Powder:*** 3.3–3.5 g/dose or packet^OTC ▪ ***Effervescent powder:*** 3–3.5 g/dose or packet^OTC ▪ ***Granules:*** 2.5 g/dose ▪ ***Wafers:*** 3.4 g/dose^OTC.

TIME/ACTION PROFILE (laxative effect)

	ONSET	PEAK	DURATION
PO	12–24 hr	2–3 days	UK

NURSING IMPLICATIONS

ASSESSMENT

- ☐ Assess patient for abdominal distention, presence of bowel sounds, and usual pattern of bowel function.
- ☐ Assess color, consistency, and amount of stool produced.
- ▪ ***Lab Test Considerations:*** May cause elevated blood glucose levels with prolonged use of preparations containing sugar.

POTENTIAL NURSING DIAGNOSES

- Constipation (Indications).
- Knowledge deficit, related to medication regimen (Patient/Family Teaching).

IMPLEMENTATION

- **General Info:** Packets are not standardized for volume, but each contains 3–3.5 g of psyllium.
- **PO:** Administer with a full glass of water or juice, followed by an additional glass of liquid. Solution should be taken immediately after mixing, as it will congeal. Do not administer without sufficient fluid and do not chew granules.

PATIENT/FAMILY TEACHING

- Encourage patient to use other forms of bowel regulation, such as increasing bulk in the diet, increasing fluid intake, and increasing mobility. Normal bowel habits are individualized and may vary from 3 times/day to 3 times/wk.
- May be used for long-term management of chronic constipation.
- Instruct patients with cardiac disease to avoid straining during bowel movements (Valsalva maneuver).
- Advise patient not to use laxatives when abdominal pain, nausea, vomiting, or fever is present.

EVALUATION

Effectiveness of therapy can be demonstrated by: ▪ A soft, formed bowel movement, usually within 12–24 hr. May require 3 days of therapy for results.

PYRIDOSTIGMINE

(peer-id-oh-**stig**-meen)
Mestinon, {Mestinon SR}, Mestinon Timespan, Regonol

CLASSIFICATION(S):
Antimyasthenic, Cholinergic (anticholinesterase)

Pregnancy Category C

INDICATIONS

▪ Used to increase muscle strength in the symptomatic treatment of myasthenia gravis ▪ Reversal of nondepolarizing neuromuscular blockers.

ACTION

▪ Inhibits the breakdown of acetylcholine and prolongs its effects ▪ Effects include: □ Miosis □ Increased intestinal and skeletal muscle tone □ Bronchial and ureteral constriction □ Bradycardia □ Increased salivation □ Lacrimation □ Sweating. **Therapeutic Effects:** ▪ Improved muscular function in patients with myasthenia gravis ▪ Reversal of paralysis from nondepolarizing neuromuscular blocking agents.

PHARMACOKINETICS

Absorption: Poorly absorbed following oral administration, necessitating large oral doses as compared with parenteral doses.
Distribution: Appears to cross the placenta.
Metabolism and Excretion: Metabolized by plasma cholinesterases and the liver.
Half-life: *PO:* 3.7 hr; *IV:* 1.9 hr.

CONTRAINDICATIONS AND PRECAUTIONS

Contraindicated in: ▪ Hypersensitivity to pyridostigmine or bromides ▪ Mechanical obstruction of the GI or GU tract ▪ Known alcohol intolerance (syrup only).
Use Cautiously in: ▪ History of asthma ▪ Ulcer disease ▪ Cardiovascular disease ▪ Epilepsy ▪ Hyperthyroidism ▪ Pregnancy or lactation (may cause uterine irritability following IV administration near term; 20% of newborns display transient muscle weakness).

ADVERSE REACTIONS AND SIDE EFFECTS*

CNS: SEIZURES, dizziness, weakness.
EENT: lacrimation, miosis.
Resp: bronchospasm, excessive secretions.
CV: bradycardia, hypotension.
GI: abdominal cramps, diarrhea, excessive salivation, nausea, vomiting.
Derm: sweating, rashes.

{} = Available in Canada only.
***CAPITALS indicate life-threatening; underlines indicate most frequent.**

INTERACTIONS

Drug-Drug: ▪ Cholinergic effects may be antagonized by other **drugs possessing anticholinergic properties**, including **antihistamines, antidepressants, atropine, haloperidol, phenothiazines, procainamide, quinidine,** or **disopyramide** ▪ Prolongs the action of **depolarizing muscle-relaxing agents (succinylcholine, decamethonium)** ▪ Additive toxicity with other **cholinesterase inhibitors,** including **demecarium, echothiophate,** and **isoflurophate** ▪ Antimyasthenic effects may be decreased by concurrent **guanadrel, guanethidine,** or **trimethophan.**

ROUTE AND DOSAGE

❑ Myasthenia Gravis

- **PO (Adults):** *Tablets/syrup*—30–60 mg q 3–4 hr initially; then adjusted as required; usual maintenance dose is 600 mg/day in divided doses (range 60–1500 mg/day). *Extended-release tablets*—180–540 mg 1–2 times daily (dosing interval should be at least 6 hr; may be associated with increased risk of cholinergic crisis; concurrent immediate-release products may be required).
- **PO (Children):** 7 mg/kg (200 mg/m^2)/day in 5–6 divided doses.
- **IM, IV (Adults):** 2 mg (1/30 of oral dose); may be repeated q 2–3 hr. *During labor/delivery*—1 mg before 2nd stage of labor is complete.
- **IM (Neonates Born to Myasthenic Mothers):** 50–150 mcg/kg q 4–6 hr.

❑ Antidote for Nondepolarizing Neuromuscular Blockers

- **IV (Adults):** 10–20 mg; pretreat with 0.6–1.2 mg atropine IV.

AVAILABILITY

▪ ***Tablets:*** 60 mg[Rx] ▪ ***Extended-release tablets:*** 180 mg[Rx] ▪ ***Syrup:*** 60 mg/5 ml[Rx] ▪ ***Injection:*** 5 mg/ml in 2-ml ampules and 5-ml vials[Rx].

TIME/ACTION PROFILE (cholinergic effects)

	ONSET	PEAK	DURATION
PO	30–35 min	UK	3–6 hr
PO-SR	30–60 min	UK	6–12 hr
IM	15 min	UK	2–4 hr
IV	2–5 min	UK	2–3 hr

NURSING IMPLICATIONS

ASSESSMENT

- **General Info:** Assess pulse, respiratory rate, and blood pressure prior to administration. Report significant changes in heart rate.
- **Myasthenia Gravis:** Assess neuromuscular status, including vital capacity, ptosis, diplopia, chewing, swallowing, hand grasp, and gait prior to administering and at peak effect. Patients with myasthenia gravis may be advised to keep a daily record of their condition and the effects of this medication.
  - ❑ Assess patient for overdosage and underdosage or resistance. Both have similar symptoms (muscle weakness, dyspnea, dysphagia), but symptoms of overdosage usually occur within 1 hr of administration, while symptoms of underdosage occur ≥3 hr after administration. Overdosage (cholinergic crisis) symptoms may also include increased respiratory secretions and saliva, bradycardia, nausea, vomiting, cramping, diarrhea, and diaphoresis. A Tensilon test (edrophonium chloride) may be used to differentiate between overdosage and underdosage.
- **Antidote to Nondepolarizing Neuromuscular Blocking Agents:** Monitor reversal of effect of neuromuscular blocking agents with a peripheral nerve stimulator. Recovery usually occurs consecutively in the following muscles: diaphragm, intercostal muscles, muscles of the glottis, abdominal muscles, limb muscles, muscles of mastication, and levator muscles of eyelids. Closely observe patient for residual muscle weakness and respiratory distress throughout the recovery period. Maintain airway patency and ventilation until recovery of normal respirations occurs.
- ***Toxicity and Overdose:*** Atropine is the antidote.

POTENTIAL NURSING DIAGNOSES

- Physical mobility, impaired (Indications).
- Breathing pattern, ineffective (Indications).
- Knowledge deficit, related to medication regimen (Patient/Family Teaching).

IMPLEMENTATION

- **General Info:** For patients who have difficulty chewing, pyridostigmine may be administered 30 min before meals.

□ Oral dose is not interchangeable with IV dose. Parenteral form is 30 times more potent.
□ When used as an antidote to nondepolarizing neuromuscular blocking agents, atropine may be ordered prior to or currently with large doses of pyridostigmine to prevent or to treat bradycardia and other side effects.
■ **PO:** Administer with food or milk to minimize side effects. Extended-release tablets should be swallowed whole; do not crush, break, or chew. Regular tablets or syrup may be administered with extended-release tablets for optimum control of symptoms. Mottled appearance of sustained-release tablet does not affect potency.
■ **Direct IV:** Administer undiluted. Do not add to IV solutions. May be given through Y-site of infusion of D5W, 0.9% NaCl, lactated Ringer's solution, D5/Ringer's solution, or D5/LR.
■ ***Rate:*** For myasthenia gravis, administer each 0.5 mg over 1 min. For reversal of nondepolarizing neuromuscular blocking agents, administer each 5 mg over 1 min.
■ **Syringe Compatibility:** ■ glycopyrrolate.
■ **Y-Site Compatibility:** ■ heparin ■ hydrocortisone sodium succinate ■ potassium chloride ■ vitamin B complex with C.

PATIENT/FAMILY TEACHING

□ Instruct patient to take medication exactly as directed. Do not skip or double up on missed doses. Patients with a history of dysphagia should have a nonelectric or battery-operated back-up alarm clock to remind them of exact dose time. Patients with dysphagia may not be able to swallow medication if the dose is not taken exactly on time. Taking dose late may result in myasthenic crisis. Taking dose early may result in cholinergic crisis. Patients with myasthenia gravis must continue this regimen as a lifelong therapy.
□ Advise patient to carry identification describing disease and medication regimen at all times.
□ Instruct patient to space activities to avoid fatigue.

EVALUATION

Effectiveness of therapy can be demonstrated by: ■ Relief of ptosis and diplopia; improved chewing, swallowing, extremity strength, and breathing without the appearance of cholinergic symptoms ■ Reversal of nondepolarizing neuromuscular blocking agents in general anesthesia.

PYRIDOXINE

(peer-i-**dox**-een)
Beesix, Doxine, Nestrex, Pyri, Rodex, Vitabee 6, vitamin B_6

CLASSIFICATION(S):
Vitamin (water-soluble)

Pregnancy Category A

INDICATIONS

■ Treatment and prevention of pyridoxine deficiency (may be associated with poor nutritional status or chronic debilitating illnesses) ■ Treatment and prevention of neuropathy, which may develop from isoniazid, penicillamine, or hydralazine therapy ■ Management of isoniazid overdose $>$10 g.

ACTION

■ Required for amino acid, carbohydrate, and lipid metabolism ■ Used in the transport of amino acids, formation of neurotransmitters, and synthesis of heme. **Therapeutic Effects:** ■ Prevention of pyridoxine deficiency ■ Prevention or reversal of neuropathy associated with hydralazine, penicillamine, or isoniazid therapy.

PHARMACOKINETICS

Absorption: Well absorbed from the GI tract.
Distribution: Stored in liver, muscle, and brain. Crosses the placenta and enters breast milk.
Metabolism and Excretion: Converted in RBCs to pyridoxal phosphate and another active metabolite. Amounts in excess of requirements are excreted unchanged by the kidneys.
Half-life: 15–20 days.

CONTRAINDICATIONS AND PRECAUTIONS

Contraindicated in: ■ No known contraindications.
Use Cautiously in: ■ Parkinson's disease (treatment with levodopa only) ■ Pregnancy (chronic ingestion of large doses may produce pyridoxine-dependency syndrome in newborn).

ADVERSE REACTIONS AND SIDE EFFECTS

Adverse reactions listed are seen with excessive doses only.
Neuro: sensory neuropathy.
Misc: pyridoxine-dependency syndrome.

INTERACTIONS

Drug-Drug: ▪ Interferes with the therapeutic response to **levodopa** ▪ Requirements are increased by **isoniazid, hydralazine, chloramphenicol, penicillamine, estrogens,** and **immunosuppressants.**

ROUTE AND DOSAGE

❑ **Prevention of Deficiency**

- **PO (Adults and Children >10 yr):** 1.4–2.2 mg/day (larger doses required with cycloserine, ethionamide, hydralazine, immunosuppressants, isoniazid, penicillamine, and estrogen-containing oral contraceptives).
- **PO (Children 4–10 yr):** 1.1–1.4 mg/day (larger doses required with cycloserine, ethionamide, hydralazine, immunosuppressants, isoniazid, and penicillamine).
- **PO (Children birth–3 yr):** 0.3–1 mg/day (larger doses required with cycloserine, ethionamide, hydralazine, immunosuppressants, isoniazid, and penicillamine).

❑ **Treatment of Deficiency**

- **PO, IM, IV (Adults and Children):** Must be individualized.

❑ **Pyridoxine-Dependency Syndrome**

- **IM, IV (Adults and Children):** 30–600 mg/day.

❑ **Isoniazid Overdose (>10 g)**

- **IM, IV (Adults):** Amount in mg equal to amount of isoniazid ingested given as 4 g IV, then 1 g IM q 30 min.

AVAILABILITY

▪ ***Tablets:*** 10 mg^OTC^, 25 mg^OTC^, 50 mg^OTC^, 100 mg^OTC^, 200 mg^OTC^, 250 mg^OTC^, 500 mg^OTC^ ▪ ***Extended-release tablets:*** 100 mg^OTC^, 200 mg^OTC^, 500 mg^OTC^ ▪ ***Extended-release capsules:*** 150 mg^OTC^ ▪ ***Injection:*** 100 mg/ml in 10- and 30-ml vials^Rx^ ▪ ***In combination with:*** vitamins, minerals, and trace elements in a variety of multivitamin preparations^OTC^.

TIME/ACTION PROFILE

	ONSET	PEAK	DURATION
PO, IM, IV	UK	UK	UK

NURSING IMPLICATIONS

ASSESSMENT

❑ Assess patient for signs of vitamin B_6 deficiency (anemia, dermatitis, cheilosis, irritability, seizures, nausea, and vomiting) prior to and periodically throughout therapy. Institute seizure precautions in pyridoxine-dependent infants.

▪ ***Lab Test Considerations:*** May cause false elevations in urobilinogen concentrations.

POTENTIAL NURSING DIAGNOSES

- Nutrition, altered, less than body requirements (Indications).
- Knowledge deficit, related to medication regimen (Patient/Family Teaching).

IMPLEMENTATION

▪ **General Info:** Because of infrequency of single B-vitamin deficiencies, combinations are commonly administered.

❑ Administration of parenteral vitamin B_6 is limited to patients who are NPO or who have nausea and vomiting or malabsorption syndromes.

❑ Protect parenteral solution from light, as decomposition will occur.

▪ **PO:** Extended-release capsules and tablets should be swallowed whole, without crushing, breaking, or chewing. For patients unable to swallow capsule, contents of capsules may be mixed with jam or jelly.

▪ **SC, IM:** Rotate sites; burning or stinging at site may occur.

▪ **IV:** May be administered direct IV or as infusion in standard IV solutions.

❑ B_6-dependent seizures should cease within 2–3 min of IV administration of pyridoxine.

▪ ***Rate:*** Infusion rates of 15–30 min and up to 3 hr have been used.

▪ **Additive Incompatibility:** ▪ alkaline solutions ▪ riboflavin.

PATIENT/FAMILY TEACHING

❑ Instruct patient to take medication as directed. If a dose is missed, it may be omitted, as an extended period of time is required to become deficient in vitamin B_6.

- Encourage patient to comply with diet recommended by health care professional. Explain that the best source of vitamins is a well-balanced diet with foods from the four basic food groups. Foods high in vitamin B_6 include bananas, whole-grain cereals, potatoes, lima beans, and meats.
- Patients self-medicating with vitamin supplements should be cautioned not to exceed RDA (see Appendix L). The effectiveness of megadoses for treatment of various medical conditions is unproved and may cause side effects, such as unsteady gait, numbness in feet, and difficulty with hand coordination.
- Emphasize the importance of follow-up exams to evaluate progress.

EVALUATION

Effectiveness of therapy can be demonstrated by: ▪ Decrease in the symptoms of vitamin B_6 deficiency.

PYRIMETHAMINE

(peer-i-**meth**-a-meen)
Daraprim

CLASSIFICATION(S):
Antimalarial, Antiprotozoal
Pregnancy Category C

INDICATIONS

▪ Used in combination with other antimalarials in the treatment of chloroquine-resistant malaria ▪ Used in combination with a sulfonamide in the treatment of toxoplasmosis. **Unlabeled Uses:** ▪ Used in combination with other agents (sulfonamides, dapsone) in the treatment of *Pneumocystis carinii* pneumonia.

ACTION

▪ Binds to an enzyme in the protozoa, which results in depletion of folic acid. **Therapeutic Effects:** ▪ Death and arrested growth of susceptible organisms (protozoa).

PHARMACOKINETICS

Absorption: Well absorbed following oral administration.
Distribution: Widely distributed with high concentrations achieved in blood cells, kidneys, lungs, liver, and spleen. Some enters CSF (13–26% of serum levels). Crosses the placenta and enters breast milk.
Metabolism and Excretion: Mostly metabolized by the liver. 20–30% excreted unchanged by the kidneys.
Half-life: 4 days (shortened in patients with AIDS).

CONTRAINDICATIONS AND PRECAUTIONS

Contraindicated in: ▪ Hypersensitivity ▪ First 14–16 wk of pregnancy ▪ Megaloblastic anemia due to folate deficiency ▪ Concurrent folate antagonist therapy (because of risk of megaloblastic anemia).
Use Cautiously in: ▪ History of seizures (high doses) ▪ Underlying anemia or bone marrow depression ▪ Impaired liver function ▪ Lactation (large doses to mother may cause folic acid deficiency in infant) ▪ G6PD deficiency ▪ Pregnancy >16 wk (may require concurrent leucovorin).

ADVERSE REACTIONS AND SIDE EFFECTS*

CNS: SEIZURES (high doses), headache, insomnia, light-headedness, malaise, mental depression.
Resp: dry throat, pulmonary eosinophilia.
CV: ARRHYTHMIAS (large doses).
GI: atrophic glossitis (high doses), anorexia, diarrhea, nausea.
GU: hematuria.
Derm: abnormal pigmentation, dermatitis.
Hemat: megaloblastic anemia (high doses), pancytopenia, thrombocytopenia.
Misc: fever.

INTERACTIONS

Drug-Drug: ▪ Increased risk of bone marrow depression with other **bone marrow depressants**, including **antineoplastic agents** or **radiation therapy** ▪ Increased risk of megaloblastic anemia with **folate antagonists**

***CAPITALS indicate life-threatening; underlines indicate most frequent.**

(methotrexate); concurrent use should be avoided.

ROUTE AND DOSAGE

❑ Treatment of Malaria

- **PO (Adults):** 75 mg single dose in combination with other agents.
- **PO (Children):** 1.25 mg/kg single dose in combination with other agents.

❑ Toxoplasmosis

- **PO (Adults):** 50–200 mg/day for 1–2 days, followed by 25–50 mg/day for 2–6 wk; given with a sulfonamide.
- **PO (Children):** 1 mg/kg/day for 1–3 days, then 0.5 mg/kg/day for 4–6 wk; given with a sulfonamide.

❑ Toxoplasmosis in AIDS Patients

- **PO (Adults):** 100–200 mg/day for 1–2 days, followed by 50–100 mg/day for 3–6 wk, then 25–50 mg/day for life; given with clindamycin or sulfadiazine.

AVAILABILITY

▪ ***Tablets:*** 25 mg[Rx] ▪ ***In combination with:*** sulfadoxine (Fansidar)[Rx]. See Appendix A.

TIME/ACTION PROFILE (blood levels)

	ONSET	PEAK	DURATION
PO	UK	3 hr	2 wk*

*Suppressive levels.

NURSING IMPLICATIONS

ASSESSMENT

- ❑ Assess patient for improvement in signs and symptoms of infection daily throughout therapy.
- ▪ ***Lab Test Considerations:*** Monitor CBC and platelet count periodically throughout therapy; semi-weekly in patients with toxoplasmosis. May cause decreased WBC and platelet counts.

POTENTIAL NURSING DIAGNOSES

- Infection, risk for (Indications).
- Knowledge deficit, related to medication regimen (Patient/Family Teaching).

IMPLEMENTATION

- **General Info:** Leucovorin may be administered concurrently to prevent folic acid deficiency and restore normal hematopoiesis.
- **PO:** Administer with milk or meals to minimize GI distress.
- ❑ Tablets may be crushed and mixed with saline or with other vehicles by pharmacist for patients with difficulty swallowing.

PATIENT/FAMILY TEACHING

- ❑ Instruct patient to take medication exactly as directed on a regular schedule and continue full course of therapy, even if feeling better. If a dose is missed, take as soon as possible unless almost time for next dose; do not double doses.
- ❑ Advise patient to notify health care professional promptly if sore throat, pallor, purpura, or glossitis occurs. Instruct patient to stop taking pyrimethamine and notify health care professional immediately at the first sign of a skin rash or if no improvement is seen within a few days.
- ❑ Emphasize the importance of lab tests at scheduled intervals, especially in patients taking high doses. Tests should not be delayed or missed.

EVALUATION

Effectiveness of therapy can be demonstrated by: ▪ Improvement in the signs and symptoms of malaria ▪ Improvement in signs and symptoms of toxoplasmosis.

QUETIAPINE

(kwet-**eye**-a-peen)
Seroquel

CLASSIFICATION(S):
Antipsychotic agent

Pregnancy Category C

INDICATIONS

▪ Management of the symptoms of psychotic disorders (including schizophrenia).

ACTION

▪ Probably acts by serving as an antagonist of dopamine and serotonin ▪ Also antagonizes histamine H_1 receptors and $alpha_1$-adrenergic receptors. **Therapeutic Effects:** ▪ Decreased manifestations of psychoses.

PHARMACOKINETICS

Absorption: Well absorbed following oral administration.
Distribution: Widely distributed.
Metabolism and Excretion: Extensively metabolized by the liver; <1% excreted unchanged in the urine.
Half-life: 6 hr.

CONTRAINDICATIONS AND PRECAUTIONS

Contraindicated in: ▪ Hypersensitivity ▪ Lactation.
Use Cautiously in: ▪ Cardiovascular disease, cerebrovascular disease, dehydration or hypovolemia (increased risk of hypotension) ▪ History of seizures, Alzheimer's dementia, or age ≥65 yr ▪ Hepatic impairment (dosage reduction may be necessary) ▪ Hypothyroidism (may be exacerbated) ▪ History of suicide attempt ▪ Pregnancy or children (safety not established).

ADVERSE REACTIONS AND SIDE EFFECTS*

CNS: NEUROLEPTIC MALIGNANT SYNDROME, SEIZURES, dizziness, cognitive impairment, extrapyramidal symptoms, sedation, tardive dyskinesia.
EENT: ear pain, rhinitis.
Resp: cough, dyspnea, pharyngitis.
CV: palpitations, peripheral edema, postural hypotension.
GI: anorexia, constipation, dry mouth, dyspepsia.
Derm: sweating.
Hemat: leukopenia.
Metab: weight gain.
Misc: flu-like syndrome.

INTERACTIONS

Drug-Drug: ▪ Additive CNS depression may occur with **alcohol, antihistamines, opioids,** and **sedative/hypnotics** ▪ Increased risk of hypotension with acute ingestion of **alcohol** or **antihypertensive agents** ▪ **Phenytoin** and **thioridazine** increase clearance and decrease effectiveness of quetiapine (dosage adjustment may be necessary); similar effects may occur with **carbamazepine, barbiturates, rifampin,** or **glucocorticoids** ▪ Effects may be increased by **ketoconazole, itraconazole, fluconazole,** or **erythromycin.**

ROUTE AND DOSAGE

▪ **PO (Adults):** 25 mg twice daily initially, increased by 25–50 mg 2–3 times daily over 3 days, up to 300–400 mg/day in 2–3 divided doses by the 4th day.

AVAILABILITY

▪ ***Tablets:*** 25 mg [Rx], 100 mg[Rx], 200 mg[Rx].

TIME/ACTION PROFILE (antipsychotic effects)

	ONSET	PEAK	DURATION
PO	UK	UK	8–12 hr

NURSING IMPLICATIONS

ASSESSMENT

- ☐ Monitor patient's mental status (delusions, hallucinations, and behavior) prior to and periodically throughout therapy.
- ☐ Monitor mood changes. Assess for suicidal tendencies, especially during early therapy. Restrict amount of drug available to patient.
- ☐ Monitor blood pressure (sitting, standing, lying) and pulse prior to and frequently during initial dosage titration. If hypotension occurs during dose titration, return to the previous dose.
- ☐ Observe patient carefully when administering medication to ensure medication is actually swallowed and not hoarded.
- ☐ Monitor patient for onset of extrapyramidal side effects (*akathisia*—restlessness; *dystonia*—muscle spasms and twisting motions; or *pseudoparkinsonism*—mask facies, rigidity, tremors, drooling, shuffling gait, dysphagia). Report these symptoms; reduction of dosage or discontinuation of medication may be necessary. Trihexyphenidyl or diphenhydramine may be used to control these symptoms.
- ☐ Monitor for tardive dyskinesia (involuntary rhythmic movement of mouth, face, and extremities). Report immediately; may be irreversible.

***CAPITALS indicate life-threatening; underlines indicate most frequent.**

- □ Monitor for development of neuroleptic malignant syndrome (fever, respiratory distress, tachycardia, convulsions, diaphoresis, hypertension or hypotension, pallor, tiredness). Notify physician or other health care professional immediately if these symptoms occur.
- ▪ ***Lab Test Considerations:*** May cause asymptomatic increases in AST and ALT.
- □ May also cause anemia, thrombocytopenia, leukocytosis, and leukopenia.
- □ May cause increased total cholesterol and triglycerides.

POTENTIAL NURSING DIAGNOSES

- ▪ Violence, risk for, directed at others (Indications).
- ▪ Thought processes, altered, related to panic anxiety (Indications).
- ▪ Injury, risk for (Side Effects).

IMPLEMENTATION

- ▪ **General Info:** If therapy is reinstituted after an interval of ≥1 wk off, follow initial titration schedule.
- ▪ **PO:** May be administered without regard to food.

PATIENT/FAMILY TEACHING

- □ Instruct patient to take medication exactly as directed.
- □ Inform patient of the possibility of extrapyramidal symptoms. Instruct patient to report these symptoms immediately to health care professional.
- □ Advise patient to change positions slowly to minimize orthostatic hypotension.
- □ May cause drowsiness. Caution patient to avoid driving or other activities requiring alertness until response to medication is known.
- □ Advise patient that extremes in temperature should be avoided, as this drug impairs body temperature regulation.
- □ Caution patient to avoid concurrent use of alcohol, other CNS depressants, and OTC medications without consulting health care professional.
- □ Advise female patients to notify health care professional if pregnancy is planned or suspected or if they are breast-feeding or planning to breast-feed.
- □ Advise patient to notify health care professional of medication regimen prior to treatment or surgery.
- □ Instruct patient to notify health care professional promptly of sore throat, fever, unusual bleeding or bruising, or rash.
- □ Emphasize the need for continued follow-up for psychotherapy and monitoring for side effects. Ophthalmologic exams should be performed prior to and every 6 mo during therapy.

EVALUATION

Effectiveness of therapy can be demonstrated by: ▪ Decrease in excited, paranoic, or withdrawn behavior.

QUINIDINE

(**kwin**-i-deen)

quinidine gluconate

Duraquin, Quinaglute Dura-Tabs, Quinalan, {Quinate}

quinidine polygalacturonate

Cardioquin

quinidine sulfate

{Apo-Quinidine}, Cin-Quin, {Novoquinidin}, Quinidex Extentabs, Quinora

CLASSIFICATION(S):

Antiarrhythmic (group IA)

Pregnancy Category C

INDICATIONS

▪ Management of a wide variety of atrial and ventricular arrhythmias, including: □ Atrial premature contractions □ Premature ventricular contractions □ Ventricular tachycardia □ Paroxysmal atrial tachycardia □ Maintenance of normal sinus rhythm after conversion from atrial fibrillation or flutter. **Unlabeled Uses:** ▪ Treatment of malaria (IV gluconate only).

ACTION

▪ Decrease myocardial excitability ▪ Slow conduction velocity. **Therapeutic Effects:** ▪ Suppression of arrhythmias.

{} = Available in Canada only.

PHARMACOKINETICS

Absorption: Well absorbed from the GI tract and IM sites. Extended-release quinidine sulfate (Quinidex Extentabs) or gluconate (Duraquin, Quinaglute, Quinalan) oral preparations and polygalacturonate salt are absorbed more slowly following oral administration.
Distribution: Widely distributed. Cross the placenta; enter breast milk.
Metabolism and Excretion: Metabolized by the liver; 10–30% excreted unchanged by the kidneys.
Half-life: 6–8 hr (increased in congestive heart failure [CHF] or severe liver impairment).

CONTRAINDICATIONS AND PRECAUTIONS

Contraindicated in: ▪ Hypersensitivity ▪ Conduction defects ▪ Digitalis glycoside toxicity.
Use Cautiously in: ▪ CHF or severe liver disease (dosage reduction recommended) ▪ Pregnancy, lactation, or children (safety not established; extended-release preparations should not be used in children).

ADVERSE REACTIONS AND SIDE EFFECTS*

CNS: dizziness, headache, syncope.
EENT: blurred vision, diplopia, mydriasis, photophobia, tinnitus.
CV: HYPOTENSION, arrhythmias, tachycardia.
GI: <u>anorexia</u>, <u>cramping</u>, <u>diarrhea</u>, <u>nausea</u>, bitter taste, drug-induced hepatitis.
Derm: rashes.
Hemat: hemolytic anemia, thrombocytopenia.
Misc: fever.

INTERACTIONS

Drug-Drug: ▪ Increases serum **digoxin** levels and may cause toxicity (dosage reduction recommended) ▪ **Amiodarone** increases quinidine levels and risk of toxicity ▪ **Phenytoin, phenobarbital,** or **rifampin** may increase metabolism and decrease effectiveness ▪ **Cimetidine** and **verapamil** decrease metabolism and may increase blood levels ▪ Potentiates **neuromuscular blocking agents** and **warfarin** ▪ Additive hypotension with **antihypertensives, nitrates,** and acute ingestion of **alcohol** ▪ May increase **procainamide, propafenone,** or **tricyclic antidepressant** levels and risk of toxicity ▪ May antagonize **anticholinesterase therapy** in patients with myasthenia gravis ▪ **Drugs that alkalinize the urine,** including high-dose **antacid** therapy or **sodium bicarbonate,** increase blood levels and the risk of toxicity ▪ Additive anticholinergic effects may occur with **agents having anticholinergic properties (antihistamines, tricyclic antidepressants)** ▪ Increased risk of arrhythmias with **pimozide.**
Drug-Food: ▪ **Foods that alkalinize the urine** (see Appendix K) may increase serum quinidine levels and the risk of toxicity.

ROUTE AND DOSAGE

❑ Quinidine Gluconate (62% Quinidine)

- **PO (Adults):** 324–660 mg q 6–12 hr as extended-release tablets (325–650 mg q 6 hr if not extended release).
- **IM (Adults):** 600 mg initially, followed by 400 mg as often as q 2 hr.
- **IV (Adults):** *Antiarrhythmic*—Infuse at 16 mg/min until arrhythmia is suppressed, QRS complex widens, bradycardia or hypotension occurs.

❑ Quinidine Polygalacturonate (60% Quinidine)

- **PO (Adults):** 275–825 mg q 3–4 hr for 3–4 doses, then may increase by 137.5–275 mg every 3rd or 4th dose until arrhythmia is controlled. Usual maintenance dose is 275 mg q 8–12 hr.
- **PO (Children):** 8.25 mg/kg (247.5 mg/m^2) 5 times daily.

❑ Quinidine Sulfate (83% Quinidine)

- **PO (Adults):** *Paroxysmal supraventricular tachycardia*—400–600 mg q 2–3 hr until arrhythmia is terminated. *Conversion of atrial fibrillation*—200 mg q 2–3 hr for 5–8 doses; dosage may be increased at daily intervals if necessary. *Premature atrial/ventricular contractions*—200–300 mg q 6–8 hr or 300–600 mg of extended-release preparation every 8–12 hr maintenance (not to exceed 4 g/day).
- **PO (Children):** 6 mg/kg or 180 mg/m^2 5 times daily.

*CAPITALS indicate life-threatening; <u>underlines</u> indicate most frequent.

AVAILABILITY

❑ **Quinidine Gluconate**

▪ ***Tablets:*** {325 mg[Rx]} ▪ ***Extended-release tablets:*** 324 mg[Rx], 330 mg[Rx] ▪ ***Injection:*** 80 mg/ml in 10-ml vials[Rx].

❑ **Quinidine Polygalacturonate**

▪ ***Tablets:*** 275 mg[Rx].

❑ **Quinidine Sulfate**

▪ ***Tablets:*** 100 mg[Rx], 200 mg[Rx], 300 mg[Rx] ▪ ***Extended-release tablets:*** 300 mg[Rx] ▪ ***Capsules:*** 200 mg[Rx], 300 mg[Rx].

TIME/ACTION PROFILE (antiarrhythmic effects)

	ONSET	PEAK	DURATION
PO (sulfate)	30 min	1–1.5 hr	6–8 hr
PO (sulfate-ER)	UK	4 hr	8–12 hr
PO (gluconate)	UK	3–4 hr	6–8 hr
PO (polygalacturonate)	UK	6 hr	8–12 hr
IM	30 min	30–90 min	6–8 hr
IV	1–5 min	rapid	6–8 hr

NURSING IMPLICATIONS

ASSESSMENT

- Monitor ECG, pulse, and blood pressure continuously throughout IV administration and periodically during oral administration. IV administration is usually discontinued if any of the following occur: arrhythmia is resolved, QRS complex widens by 50%, PR or QT intervals are prolonged, frequent ventricular ectopic beats or tachycardia develops. Patient should remain supine throughout IV administration to minimize hypotension.
- ***Lab Test Considerations:*** Hepatic and renal function, CBC, and serum potassium levels should be periodically monitored during prolonged therapy.
- ***Toxicity and Overdose:*** Serum quinidine levels may be monitored periodically during dosage adjustment. Therapeutic serum concentrations are 2–6 mcg/ml. Toxic effects usually occur at concentrations >8 mcg/ml.
- Signs and symptoms of toxicity or cinchonism include tinnitus, hearing loss, visual disturbances, headache, nausea, and dizziness. These may occur after a single dose.
- Cardiac signs of toxicity include QRS widening, cardiac asystole, ventricular ectopic beats, idioventricular rhythms (ventricular tachycardia, ventricular fibrillation), paradoxical tachycardia, and arterial embolism.

POTENTIAL NURSING DIAGNOSES

- Cardiac output, decreased (Indications).
- Knowledge deficit, related to medication regimen (Patient/Family Teaching).

IMPLEMENTATION

- **General Info:** A test dose of a single 200-mg quinidine sulfate tablet or 200 mg IM quinidine gluconate may be administered prior to quinidine therapy to check for intolerance.
- Higher doses may be required to correct atrial arrhythmias than are required for ventricular arrhythmias.
- **PO:** Administer with a full glass of water on an empty stomach either 1 hr before or 2 hr after meals for faster absorption. If GI irritation becomes a problem, may be administered with or immediately after meals. Extended-release preparations (Quinaglute Dura-Tabs, Quinidex Extentabs, Quinalan) should be swallowed whole; do not break, crush, or chew.
- **IV:** Use only clear, colorless solution.
- **Intermittent Infusion:** Dilute 800 mg of quinidine gluconate (10 ml) in 50 ml of D5W for injection for a concentration of 16 mg/ml. Solution is stable for 24 hr at room temperature.
- ***Rate:*** Administer quinidine gluconate at a rate not to exceed 1 ml/min. Administer via infusion pump to ensure accurate dose. Rapid administration may cause hypotension.
- **Y-Site Compatibility:** ▪ diazepam ▪ milrinone.
- **Y-Site Incompatibility:** ▪ furosemide.

PATIENT/FAMILY TEACHING

- Instruct patient to take medication around the clock, exactly as directed, even if feeling well. If a dose is missed, take as soon as remembered if within 2 hr; if remembered later, omit. Do not double doses.
- Instruct patient or family member on how to take pulse. Advise patient to report changes in pulse rate or rhythm to health care professional.
- May cause dizziness or blurred vision. Caution patient to avoid driving or other activities re-

quiring alertness until response to medication is known.

- Inform patient that quinidine may cause increased sensitivity to light. Dark glasses may minimize this effect.
- Advise patient to inform health care professional of medication regimen prior to treatment or surgery.
- Instruct patient not to take OTC medications with quinidine without consulting health care professional.
- Advise patient to consult health care professional if symptoms of cinchonism, rash, or dyspnea occur or if diarrhea is severe or persistent.
- Advise patient to carry identification describing disease process and medication regimen at all times.
- Emphasize the importance of routine follow-up exams to monitor progress.

EVALUATION

Effectiveness of therapy can be demonstrated by: ▪ Resolution of cardiac arrhythmias without detrimental side effects.

RALOXIFENE

(ra-**lox**-i-feen)
Evista

CLASSIFICATION(S):
Selective estrogen receptor modulator

Pregnancy Category X

INDICATIONS

▪ Prevention of osteoporosis in postmenopausal women.

ACTION

▪ Binds to estrogen receptors, producing estrogen-like effects on bone, resulting in reduced resorption of bone and decreased bone turnover. **Therapeutic Effects:** ▪ Prevention of osteoporosis in patients at risk.

PHARMACOKINETICS

Absorption: Although well absorbed (>60%) following oral administration, extensive first-pass metabolism results in 2% bioavailability.

Distribution: Highly bound to plasma proteins, remainder of distribution UK.

Metabolism and Excretion: Extensively metabolized by the liver; undergoes enterohepatic cycling; excreted primarily in feces.

Half-life: 27.7 hr.

CONTRAINDICATIONS AND PRECAUTIONS

Contraindicated in: ▪ Hypersensitivity ▪ Pregnancy, lactation, or children ▪ Childbearing potential ▪ History of thromboembolic events.

Use Cautiously in: ▪ Potential immobilization (increased risk of thromboembolic events).

ADVERSE REACTIONS AND SIDE EFFECTS*

MS: leg cramps.
Misc: hot flashes.

INTERACTIONS

Drug-Drug: ▪ **Cholestyramine** decreases absorption (avoid concurrent use) ▪ May alter effects of **warfarin** and other **highly protein bound drugs** ▪ Concurrent systemic **estrogen** therapy is not recommended.

ROUTE AND DOSAGE

▪ **PO (Adults):** 60 mg once daily.

AVAILABILITY

▪ ***Tablets:*** 60 mg[Rx].

TIME/ACTION PROFILE (effects on bone turnover)

	ONSET	PEAK	DURATION
PO	UK	3 mo	UK

NURSING IMPLICATIONS

ASSESSMENT

- Assess patient for bone mineral density with x ray and serum and urine bone turnover markers (bone-specific alkaline phosphatase, osteocalcin, and collagen breakdown products) prior to and periodically during therapy.
- ***Lab Test Considerations:*** May cause increased apolipoprotein A-I and reduced serum total cholesterol, LDL cholesterol, fibrinogen, apolipoprotein B, and lipoprotein.
- May cause increased hormone-binding glob-

*CAPITALS indicate life-threatening; underlines indicate most frequent.

ulin (sex steroid–binding globulin, thyroxine-binding globulin, corticosteroid-binding globulin) with increases in total hormone concentrations.
- □ May cause small decreases in serum total calcium, inorganic phosphate, total protein, and albumin.
- □ May also cause slight decrease in platelet count.

POTENTIAL NURSING DIAGNOSES
- ■ Injury, risk for (Indications).
- ■ Knowledge deficit, related to medication regimen (Patient/Family Teaching).

IMPLEMENTATION
- ■ May be administered without regard to meals.
- □ Calcium supplementation should be added to diet if daily intake is inadequate.

PATIENT/FAMILY TEACHING
- □ Instruct patient to take raloxifene as directed. Discuss the importance of adequate calcium and vitamin D intake or supplementation. Advise patient to discontinue smoking and alcohol consumption.
- □ Emphasize the importance of regular weight-bearing exercise. Advise patient that raloxifene should be discontinued at least 72 hr prior to and during prolonged immobilization (recovery from surgery, prolonged bed rest). Instruct patient to avoid prolonged restrictions of movement during travel because of the increased risk of venous thrombosis.
- □ Advise patient that raloxifene will not reduce hot flashes or flushes associated with estrogen deficiency and may cause hot flashes.
- □ Advise patient that raloxifene may have teratogenic effects. Instruct patient to notify health care provider immediately if pregnancy is planned or suspected.
- □ Instruct patient to read the patient package insert when initiating therapy and again with each prescription refill.

EVALUATION
Effectiveness of therapy can be demonstrated by: ■ Prevention of osteoporosis in postmenopausal women.

Rh_0(D) IMMUNE GLOBULIN
(arr aych oh dee im-**yoon glob**-yoo-lin)

Rh_0(D) IMMUNE GLOBULIN STANDARD DOSE IM
Gamulin Rh, HypRho-D, Rhesonativ, RhoGAM

Rh_0(D) GLOBULIN MICRODOSE IM
HypRho-D Mini-Dose, MICRhoGAM, Mini-Gamulin R

Rh_0(D) GLOBULIN IV
WinRho SD, WinRho SDF

CLASSIFICATION(S):
Immune globulins

Pregnancy Category C

INDICATIONS
■ **IM, IV:** Administered to Rh_0(D)-negative patients who have been exposed to Rh_0(D)-positive blood by: □ Delivering an Rh_0(D)-positive infant □ Miscarrying or aborting an Rh_0(D)-positive fetus □ Having amniocentesis or intra-abdominal trauma while carrying an Rh_0(D)-positive fetus □ Following accidental transfusion of Rh_0(D)-positive blood to an Rh_0(D)-negative patient ■ **IV:** Management of immune thrombocytopenic purpura (ITP).

ACTION
■ Prevent production of anti-Rh_0(D) antibodies in Rh_0(D)-negative patients who were exposed to Rh_0(D)-positive blood ■ Increase platelet counts in patients with ITP. **Therapeutic Effects:** ■ Prevention of antibody response and hemolytic disease of the newborn (erythroblastosis fetalis) in future pregnancies of women who have conceived an Rh_0(D)-positive fetus ■ Prevention of Rh_0(D) sensitization following transfusion accident ■ Decreased bleeding in patients with ITP.

PHARMACOKINETICS
Absorption: Well absorbed from IM sites.
Distribution: UK.
Metabolism and Excretion: UK.
Half-life: *IM*—30 days; *IV*—24 days.

CONTRAINDICATIONS AND PRECAUTIONS

Contraindicated in: ▪ Rh_o(D)- or D^u-positive patients ▪ Patients previously sensitized to Rh_o(D) or D^u.
Use Cautiously in: ▪ Patients with previous hypersensitivity reactions to immune globulins or thimerosal (IM product) ▪ ITP patients with preexisting anemia (decreased dose if Hgb <10 g/dl).

ADVERSE REACTIONS AND SIDE EFFECTS*

Hemat: anemia (when used for ITP).
Local: pain at IM site.
Misc: fever.

INTERACTIONS

Drug-Drug: ▪ May decrease antibody response to some **live virus vaccines (measles, mumps, rubella).**

ROUTE AND DOSAGE

❑ **Rh_o (D) Immune Globulin (for IM use only)**

❑ ***Following Delivery***

- **IM (Adults):** 1 vial standard dose (300 mcg) within 72 hr of delivery.

❑ ***Before Delivery***

- **IM (Adults):** 1 vial standard dose (300 mcg) at 26–28 wk.

❑ ***Termination of Pregnancy (<13 wk Gestation)***

- **IM (Adults):** 1 vial of microdose (50 mcg) within 72 hr.

❑ ***Termination of Pregnancy (>13 wk Gestation)***

- **IM (Adults):** 1 vial standard dose (300 mcg) within 72 hr.

❑ ***Large Fetal-Maternal Hemorrhage***

- **IM (Adults):** Packed red blood cell volume of hemorrhage/15 = number of vials of standard dose (300 mcg) preparation (round to next whole number of vials).

❑ ***Transfusion Accident***

- **IM (Adults):** (Volume of Rh-positive blood administered × Hct of donor blood)/15 = number of vials of standard dose (300 mcg) preparation (round to next whole number of vials).

❑ **Rh_o (D) Immune Globulin IV (for IM or IV Use)**

❑ ***Following Delivery***

- **IM, IV (Adults):** 600 IU (120 mcg) within 72 hr of delivery.

❑ ***Prior to Delivery***

- **IV, IM (Adults):** 1500 IU (300 mcg) of Rh_o (D) immune globulin IV at 28 wk; if initiated earlier in pregnancy, repeat q 12 wk.

❑ ***Following Abortion, Amniocentesis, or Other Manipulation >34 wk Gestation***

- **IM, IV (Adults):** 600 IU (120 mcg) within 72 hr.

❑ ***Following Amniocentesis <34 wk or Chorionic Villus Sampling***

- **IM, IV (Adults):** 1500 IU (300 mcg) within 72 hr; repeat q 12 wk during pregnancy.

❑ ***Large Fetal-Maternal Hemorrhage/ Transfusion Accident***

- **IM (Adults):** 6000 IU (1200 mcg) q 12 hr until total dose is given (total dose determined by amount of blood loss/hemorrhage).
- **IV (Adults):** 3000 IU (600 mcg) q 8 hr until total dose is given (total dose determined by amount of blood loss/hemorrhage).

❑ ***Immune Thrombocytopenic Purpura (ITP)***

- **IV (Adults):** 250 IU (50 mcg)/kg initially (if Hgb <10g/dl, decrease dose to 125–200 IU [25–40 mcg]/kg); further dosing/frequency determined by clinical response (range 125–300 IU [25–60 mcg]). Each dose may be given as a single dose or in 2 divided doses on separate days.

AVAILABILITY

❑ **Rh_o (D) Immune Globulin (for IM Use)**

▪ ***Injection:*** 50 mcg/vial (microdose)[Rx], 300 mcg/vial (standard dose)[Rx].

❑ **Rh_o (D) Immune Globulin Intravenous (for IM or IV Use)**

▪ ***Injection:*** 600 IU (120 mcg)/vial[Rx], 1500 IU (300 mcg)/vial[Rx], 5000 IU (1000 mcg)/vial[Rx].

***CAPITALS indicate life-threatening; underlines indicate most frequent.**

TIME/ACTION PROFILE (blood levels)

	ONSET	PEAK	DURATION
IM	rapid	5–10 days	UK
IV*	UK	2 hr	UK

*When given for ITP, platelet counts start to rise in 1–2 days, peak after 5–7 days, and last for 30 days.

NURSING IMPLICATIONS

ASSESSMENT

- **IV:** Assess vital signs periodically during therapy in patients receiving Rh_o (D) IG IV.
- ***Lab Test Considerations:*** *Pregnancy:* Type and crossmatch of mother and newborn's cord blood must be performed to determine need for medication. Mother must be Rh_o(D)-negative and D^u-negative. Infant must be Rh_o(D)-positive. If there is doubt regarding infant's blood type or if father is Rh_o(D)-positive, medication should be given.
  - An infant born to a woman treated with Rh_o(D) immune globulin antepartum may have a weakly positive direct Coombs' test result on cord or infant blood.
  - *ITP:* Monitor platelet counts, RBC counts, hemoglobin, and reticulocyte levels to determine effectiveness of therapy.

POTENTIAL NURSING DIAGNOSES

- Knowledge deficit, related to medication regimen (Patient/Family Teaching).

IMPLEMENTATION

- **General Info:** Do not give to infant, to Rh_o(D)-positive individual, or to Rh_o(D)-negative individual previously sensitized to the Rh_o(D) antigen. However, there is no more risk than when given to a woman who is not sensitized. When in doubt, administer Rh_o (D) immune globulin.
- **IM:** Reconstitute Rh_o (D) immune globulin IV for IM use immediately before use with 1.25 ml of 0.9% NaCl. Inject diluent onto inside wall of vial and wet pellet by gently swirling until dissolved. Do not shake.
  - Administer into the deltoid muscle. Dose should be given within 3 hr but may be given up to 72 hr after delivery, miscarriage, abortion, or transfusion.
  - Do not administer *Rh_o(D) immune globulin* or *Rh_o(D) immune globulin microdose* intravenously.
- **Direct IV:** Reconstitute Rh_o (D) immune globulin IV for IV administration immediately before use with 2.5 ml of 0.9% NaCl. Inject diluent onto inside wall of vial and wet pellet by gently swirling until dissolved. Do not shake.
- ***Rate:*** Administer over 3–5 min.

PATIENT/FAMILY TEACHING

- **Pregnancy:** Explain to patient that the purpose of this medication is to protect future Rh_o(D)-positive infants.
- **ITP:** Explain purpose of medication to patient.

EVALUATION

Effectiveness of therapy can be demonstrated by: ▪ Prevention of erythroblastosis fetalis in future Rh_o(D)-positive infants ▪ Prevention of Rh_o(D) sensitization following transfusion accident ▪ Decreased bleeding episodes in patients with ITP.

RIBAVIRIN

(rye-ba-**vye**-rin)
Virazole

CLASSIFICATION(S):
Antiviral

Pregnancy Category X

INDICATIONS

▪ Treatment of severe lower respiratory tract infections caused by the respiratory syncytial virus (RSV) in infants and young children. **Unlabeled Uses:** ▪ Early (within 24 hr of symptoms) secondary treatment of influenza A or B in young adults.

ACTION

▪ Inhibits viral DNA and RNA synthesis and subsequent replication ▪ Must be phosphorylated intracellularly to be active. **Therapeutic Effects:** ▪ Virustatic action.

PHARMACOKINETICS

Absorption: Systemic absorption occurs following nasal and oral inhalation.
Distribution: 70% of inhaled drug is deposited in the respiratory tract. Appears to concentrate in the respiratory tract and red blood cells. Enters breast milk.

Metabolism and Excretion: Eliminated from the respiratory tract by distribution across membranes, macrophages, and ciliary motion. Metabolized primarily by the liver.
Half-life: 9.5 hr (40 days in red blood cells).

CONTRAINDICATIONS AND PRECAUTIONS

Contraindicated in: ▪ Hypersensitivity ▪ Women with childbearing potential ▪ Patients receiving mechanically assisted ventilation.
Use Cautiously in: ▪ Underlying anemia ▪ Adults (safety not established).

ADVERSE REACTIONS AND SIDE EFFECTS*

CNS: dizziness, faintness.
EENT: blurred vision, conjunctivitis, erythema of the eyelids, ocular irritation, photosensitivity.
CV: CARDIAC ARREST, hypotension.
Derm: rash.
Hemat: reticulocytosis.

INTERACTIONS

Drug-Drug: ▪ May antagonize the antiviral action of **zidovudine** ▪ May potentiate the hematologic toxicity of **zidovudine.**

ROUTE AND DOSAGE

- **Inhalation (Infants and Young Children):** 300 ml of 20 mg/ml solution delivered via mist for 12–18 hr/day.

AVAILABILITY

▪ ***Powder for reconstitution for aerosol use:*** 6 g/vial[Rx].

TIME/ACTION PROFILE (blood levels)

	ONSET	PEAK	DURATION
Inhaln	UK	end of inhaln	UK

NURSING IMPLICATIONS

ASSESSMENT

- □ Assess patient for infection (vital signs, sputum, WBC) at beginning of and throughout therapy.
- □ Obtain specimens for culture and sensitivity prior to initiating therapy. First dose may be given before receiving results.
- □ Assess respiratory (lung sounds, quality and rate of respirations) and fluid status prior to and frequently throughout therapy.

POTENTIAL NURSING DIAGNOSES

- Infection, risk for (Indications, Side Effects).
- Gas exchange, impaired (Indications).
- Knowledge deficit, related to medication regimen (Patient/Family Teaching).

IMPLEMENTATION

- **General Info:** Infants requiring assisted ventilation should be suctioned every 1–2 hr and pulmonary pressures monitored every 2–4 hr.
- □ Ribavirin treatment should begin within the first 3 days of RSV infection to be effective.
- **Inhalation:** Ribavirin aerosol should be administered using the Viratek SPAG model SPAG-2 only. Do not administer via other aerosol-generating devices. Usually administered using an infant oxygen hood attached to the SPAG-2 aerosol generator. Administration by face mask may be used if the oxygen hood cannot be used.
- □ Reconstitute ribavirin 6-g vial with preservative-free sterile water for injection or inhalation. Transfer to clean, sterilized Erlenmeyer flask of the SPAG-2 reservoir and dilute to a final volume of 300 ml. This recommended concentration (20 mg/ml) in the reservoir provides a concentration of aerosol ribavirin of 190 mcg/liter of air over a 12-hr period. Solution should be discarded and replaced every 24 hr.
- □ Aerosol treatments should be administered continuously 12–18 hr/day for 3–7 days.

PATIENT/FAMILY TEACHING

- □ Explain the purpose and route of treatment to the patient and parents.
- □ Inform patient and parents that ribavirin may cause blurred vision and photosensitivity.
- □ Emphasize the importance of receiving ribavirin for the full course of therapy and on a regular or continuous schedule.

EVALUATION

Clinical response to therapy can be evaluated by: ▪ Resolution of the signs and symptoms of RSV.

***CAPITALS indicate life-threatening; underlines indicate most frequent.**

R

RIBOFLAVIN

(**rye**-boe-flay-vin)
vitamin B_2

CLASSIFICATION(S):
Vitamin (water-soluble)

Pregnancy Category A

INDICATIONS

▪ Treatment and prevention of riboflavin deficiency, which may be associated with poor nutritional status or chronic debilitating illnesses.

ACTION

▪ Active metabolites serve as coenzymes for metabolic reactions involving transfer of hydrogen ions, including tissue respiration ▪ Necessary for normal red blood cell function. **Therapeutic Effects:** ▪ Replacement in or prevention of deficiency.

PHARMACOKINETICS

Absorption: Well absorbed from the upper GI tract by an active transport process.
Distribution: Widely distributed. Crosses the placenta and enters breast milk.
Metabolism and Excretion: Converted to flavin mononucleotide (FMN) and flavin adenine dinucleotide (FAD), which are the active coenzymes. Amounts in excess of requirements are excreted unchanged by the kidneys.
Half-life: 66–84 min.

CONTRAINDICATIONS AND PRECAUTIONS

Contraindicated in: ▪ No known contraindications.
Use Cautiously in: ▪ No known precautions.

ADVERSE REACTIONS AND SIDE EFFECTS

GU: yellow discoloration of urine (large doses only).

INTERACTIONS

Drug-Drug: ▪ **Phenothiazines, tricyclic antidepressants, probenecid,** and chronic ingestion of **alcohol** increase riboflavin requirements.

ROUTE AND DOSAGE

❑ **Prevention of Deficiency**

▪ **PO (Adults and Children):** Must be individualized.

AVAILABILITY

▪ ***Tablets:*** {5 mg^{OTC}}, 10 mg^{OTC}, 25 mg^{OTC}, 50 mg^{OTC}, 100 mg^{OTC}, 250 mg^{OTC}.

TIME/ACTION PROFILE

	ONSET	PEAK	DURATION
PO	UK	UK	UK

NURSING IMPLICATIONS

ASSESSMENT

- Assess patient for signs of vitamin B_2 deficiency (dermatoses, stomatitis, ocular inflammation and irritation, photophobia, and cheilosis) prior to and periodically throughout therapy.
- ***Lab Test Considerations:*** May cause false elevations in urobilinogen and urinary catecholamine measurements.

POTENTIAL NURSING DIAGNOSES

- Nutrition, altered, less than body requirements (Indications).
- Knowledge deficit, related to medication regimen (Patient/Family Teaching).

IMPLEMENTATION

- **General Info:** Because of infrequency of single B-vitamin deficiencies, combinations are commonly administered.

PATIENT/FAMILY TEACHING

- Instruct patient to take as directed. If a dose is missed, it may be omitted, as an extended period of time is required to become deficient in riboflavin.
- Encourage patient to comply with diet recommendations of health care professional. Explain that the best source of vitamins is a well-balanced diet with foods from the four basic food groups. Foods high in riboflavin include dairy products; enriched flour; nuts; meats; fish; and green, leafy vegetables; little is lost from cooking.
- Patients self-medicating with vitamin supplements should be cautioned not to exceed RDA

(see Appendix L). The effectiveness of megadoses for treatment of various medical conditions is unproved and may cause side effects.

- Advise patient to avoid alcoholic beverages; alcohol impairs the absorption of riboflavin.
- Explain to patient that medically insignificant increase in yellow coloration of urine may occur.
- Emphasize the importance of follow-up exams to evaluate progress.

EVALUATION

Effectiveness of therapy can be demonstrated by: ▪ Prevention of or decrease in the symptoms of riboflavin deficiency.

RIFABUTIN
(riff-a-**byoo**-tin)
Mycobutin

CLASSIFICATION(S):
Antimycobacterial

Pregnancy Category B

INDICATIONS

▪ Prevention of disseminated *Mycobacterium avium* complex (MAC) disease in patients with advanced HIV infection.

ACTION

▪ Appears to inhibit DNA-dependent RNA polymerase in susceptible organisms. **Therapeutic Effects:** ▪ Antimycobacterial action against susceptible organisms **Spectrum:** ▪ Active against *M. avium* and most strains of *Mycobacterium tuberculosis*.

PHARMACOKINETICS

Absorption: Well absorbed following oral administration (50–85%). Absorption is decreased in HIV-positive patients (20%).
Distribution: Widely distributed to body tissues and fluids.
Metabolism and Excretion: Mostly metabolized by the liver; <5% excreted unchanged by the kidneys.
Half-life: 45 hr.

CONTRAINDICATIONS AND PRECAUTIONS

Contraindicated in: ▪ Hypersensitivity. Cross-sensitivity with other rifamycins (rifampin) may occur ▪ Active tuberculosis ▪ Concurrent ritonavir.
Use Cautiously in: ▪ Pregnancy, lactation, or children (safety not established).

ADVERSE REACTIONS AND SIDE EFFECTS*

EENT: brown-orange discoloration of tears, ocular disturbances.
Resp: dyspnea.
CV: chest pain, chest pressure.
GI: brown-orange discoloration of saliva, altered taste, drug-induced hepatitis.
GU: brown-orange discoloration of urine.
Derm: rash, skin discoloration.
Hemat: hemolysis, neutropenia, thrombocytopenia.
MS: arthralgia, myositis.
Misc: brown-orange discoloration of body fluids, flu-like syndrome.

INTERACTIONS

Drug-Drug: ▪ Increases metabolism and may decrease the effectiveness of other drugs, including **glucocorticoids, disopyramide, quinidine, opioids, oral hypoglycemic agents, warfarin, estrogens, oral contraceptives** (estrogen-containing), **phenytoin, verapamil, fluconazole, quinidine, tocainide, theophylline, zidovudine,** and **chloramphenicol** ▪ **Ritonavir** increases blood levels of rifabutin (concurrent use is contraindicated).

ROUTE AND DOSAGE

- **PO (Adults):** 300 mg once daily. If GI upset occurs, may give as 150 mg twice daily with food.

AVAILABILITY

▪ ***Capsules:*** 150 mg[Rx].

TIME/ACTION PROFILE (blood levels)

	ONSET	PEAK	DURATION
PO	rapid	2–4 hr	24 hr

***CAPITALS indicate life-threatening; underlines indicate most frequent.**

NURSING IMPLICATIONS

ASSESSMENT

- □ Monitor patient for signs of active tuberculosis (purified protein derivative [PPD], chest x ray, sputum culture, blood culture, urine culture, biopsy of suspicious lymph nodes) prior to and throughout therapy. Rifabutin must not be administered to patients with active tuberculosis.
- ■ ***Lab Test Considerations:*** Monitor CBC periodically throughout therapy. May cause neutropenia and thrombocytopenia.

POTENTIAL NURSING DIAGNOSES

- ■ Infection, risk for (Indications).
- ■ Knowledge deficit, related to medication regimen (Patient/Family Teaching).
- ■ Noncompliance (Patient/Family Teaching).

IMPLEMENTATION

- ■ **PO:** May be administered without regard to meals. High-fat meals slow rate but not extent of absorption. May be mixed with foods such as applesauce. If GI upset occurs, administer with food.

PATIENT/FAMILY TEACHING

- □ Advise patient to take medication exactly as directed. Do not skip doses or double up on missed doses. Emphasize the importance of continuing therapy even if asymptomatic.
- □ Advise patient to notify health care professional promptly if signs and symptoms of neutropenia (sore throat, fever, signs of infection), thrombocytopenia (unusual bleeding or bruising), or hepatitis (yellow eyes and skin, nausea, vomiting, anorexia, unusual tiredness, weakness) occur.
- □ Caution patient to avoid the use of alcohol during this therapy, as this may increase the risk of hepatotoxicity.
- □ Instruct patient to report symptoms of myositis (myalgia, arthralgia) or uveitis (intraocular inflammation) to health care professional promptly.
- □ Inform patient that saliva, sputum, sweat, tears, urine, and feces may become red-orange to red-brown and that soft contact lenses may become permanently discolored.
- □ Advise patient that this medication has teratogenic properties and may decrease the effectiveness of oral contraceptives. Counsel patient to use a nonhormonal form of contraception throughout therapy.
- □ Emphasize the importance of regular follow-up exams to monitor progress and to check for side effects.

EVALUATION

Effectiveness of therapy can be demonstrated by: ■ Prevention of disseminated MAC in patients with advanced HIV infection.

RIFAMPIN

(rif-**am**-pin)

Rifadin, Rimactane, {Rofact}

CLASSIFICATION(S):

Antitubercular

Pregnancy Category C

INDICATIONS

■ Management of active tuberculosis (in combination with other agents) ■ Elimination of the carrier state of meningococcal disease. **Unlabeled Uses:** ■ Prevention of disease caused by *Haemophilus influenzae* type B in close contacts.

ACTION

■ Inhibits RNA synthesis by blocking RNA transcription in susceptible organisms. **Therapeutic Effects:** ■ Bactericidal action against susceptible organisms. **Spectrum:** ■ Broad spectrum notable for activity against: □ *Mycobacterium* spp. □ *Staphylococcus aureus* □ *H. influenzae* □ *Legionella pneumophila* □ *Neisseria meningitidis*.

PHARMACOKINETICS

Absorption: Well absorbed following oral administration.

Distribution: Widely distributed into many body tissues and fluids, including CSF. Crosses the placenta; enters breast milk.

Metabolism and Excretion: Mostly metabolized by the liver; 60% eliminated in the feces via biliary elimination.

Half-life: 3 hr.

CONTRAINDICATIONS AND PRECAUTIONS

Contraindicated in: ▪ Hypersensitivity. ▪ Concurrent indinavir, nelfinavir, or saquinavir.
Use Cautiously in: ▪ History of liver disease ▪ Concurrent use of other hepatotoxic agents ▪ Pregnancy or lactation.

ADVERSE REACTIONS AND SIDE EFFECTS*

CNS: ataxia, confusion, drowsiness, fatigue, headache, weakness.
EENT: red discoloration of tears.
GI: abdominal pain, diarrhea, flatulence, heartburn, nausea, vomiting, drug-induced hepatitis, red discoloration of saliva.
GU: red discoloration of urine.
Hemat: hemolytic anemia, thrombocytopenia.
MS: arthralgia, myalgia.
Misc: red discoloration of all body fluids, flu-like syndrome.

INTERACTIONS

Drug-Drug: ▪ Rifampin stimulates liver enzymes, which may increase metabolism and decrease the effectiveness of other drugs, including **glucocorticoids, disopyramide, quinidine, opioid analgesics, oral hypoglycemic agents, warfarin, estrogens, phenytoin, verapamil, fluconazole, quinidine, tocainide, theophylline, chloramphenicol,** and **oral contraceptive agents** ▪ Increased risk of hepatotoxicity with other **hepatotoxic agents,** including **alcohol, isoniazid, ketoconazole,** and **miconazole** ▪ Rifampin significantly decreases blood levels of **indinavir, nelfinavir,** and **saquinavir;** concurrent use is contraindicated.

ROUTE AND DOSAGE

❑ Tuberculosis

- **PO, IV (Adults):** 600 mg/day or 10 mg/kg/day (up to 600 mg/day) single dose; may also be given 2–3 times weekly.
- **PO, IV (Children):** 10–20 mg/kg/day single dose (not to exceed 600 mg/day); may also be given 2–3 times weekly.

❑ Asymptomatic Carriers of Meningococcus

- **PO, IV (Adults):** 600 mg q 12 hr for 2 days.
- **PO, IV (Children ≥1 mo):** 10 mg/kg q 12 hr for 2 days.
- **PO (Infants <1 mo):** 5 mg/kg q 12 hr for 2 days.

❑ Prevention of *Haemophilus influenzae* Type B Infection

- **PO (Adults):** 600 mg/day for 4 days.
- **PO (Children):** 20 mg/kg/day for 4 days.

AVAILABILITY

▪ ***Capsules:*** 150 mg[Rx], 300 mg[Rx] ▪ ***Powder for injection:*** 600 mg/vial[Rx] ▪ ***In combination with:*** isoniazid (Rifamate)[Rx]; isoniazid and pyrazinamide (Rifater)[Rx]. See Appendix A.

TIME/ACTION PROFILE (blood levels)

	ONSET	PEAK	DURATION
PO	rapid	2–4 hr	12–24 hr
IV	rapid	end of infusion	12–24 hr

NURSING IMPLICATIONS

ASSESSMENT

- ❑ Mycobacterial studies and susceptibility tests should be performed prior to and periodically throughout therapy to detect possible resistance.
- ❑ Assess lung sounds and character and amount of sputum periodically throughout therapy.
- ▪ ***Lab Test Considerations:*** Renal function, CBC, and urinalysis should be evaluated periodically and throughout course of therapy.
- ❑ Monitor hepatic function at least monthly during therapy. May cause increased BUN, AST, ALT, and serum alkaline phosphatase, bilirubin, and uric acid concentrations.
- ❑ May cause false-positive direct Coombs' test results. May interfere with folic acid and vitamin B_{12} assays.
- ❑ May interfere with dexamethasone suppression test results; discontinue rifampin 15 days prior to test.
- ❑ May interfere with methods for determining serum folate and vitamin B_{12} levels and with urine tests based on color reaction.

***CAPITALS indicate life-threatening; underlines indicate most frequent.**

- ☐ May delay hepatic uptake and excretion of SBP during sulfobromophthalein (SBP) uptake and excretion tests; perform test prior to daily dose of rifampin.

POTENTIAL NURSING DIAGNOSES

- ▪ Infection, risk for (Indications).
- ▪ Knowledge deficit, related to medication regimen (Patient/Family Teaching).
- ▪ Noncompliance (Patient/Family Teaching).

IMPLEMENTATION

- ▪ **PO:** Administer medication on an empty stomach at least 1 hr before or 2 hr after meals with a full glass (240 ml) of water. If GI irritation becomes a problem, may be administered with food. Antacids may also be taken 1 hr prior to administration. Capsules may be opened and contents mixed with applesauce or jelly for patients with difficulty swallowing.
- ☐ Pharmacist can compound a syrup for patients unable to swallow solids.
- ▪ **Intermittent Infusion:** Reconstitute 600-mg vial with 10 ml of sterile water for injection and swirl gently to dissolve completely. Dilute further in 500 ml or 100 ml of D5W or 0.9% NaCl. Solution is stable for 24 hr at room temperature; however, manufacturer recommends administration within 4 hr to prevent precipitation.
- ▪ ***Rate:*** Administer solutions diluted in 500 ml over 3 hr and solutions diluted in 100 ml over 30 min.
- ▪ **Additive Incompatibility:** ▪ Do not admix with other solutions or medications.

PATIENT/FAMILY TEACHING

- ☐ Advise patient to take medication once daily (unless biweekly regimens are used), exactly as directed, and not to skip doses or double up on missed doses. Emphasize the importance of continuing therapy even after symptoms have subsided. Length of therapy for tuberculosis depends on regimen being used and underlying disease states. Patients on short-term prophylactic therapy should also be advised of the importance of compliance with therapy.
- ☐ Advise patient to notify health care professional promptly if signs and symptoms of hepatitis (yellow eyes and skin, nausea, vomiting, anorexia, unusual tiredness, weakness) or of thrombocytopenia (unusual bleeding or bruising) occur.
- ☐ Caution patient to avoid the use of alcohol during this therapy, as this may increase the risk of hepatotoxicity.
- ☐ Instruct patient to report the occurrence of flu-like symptoms (fever, chills, myalgia, headache) promptly.
- ☐ Rifampin may occasionally cause drowsiness. Caution patient to avoid driving or other activities requiring alertness until response to medication is known.
- ☐ Inform patient that saliva, sputum, sweat, tears, urine, and feces may become red-orange to red-brown and that soft contact lenses may become permanently discolored.
- ☐ Advise patient that this medication has teratogenic properties and may decrease the effectiveness of oral contraceptives. Counsel patient to use a nonhormonal form of contraception throughout therapy.
- ☐ Emphasize the importance of regular follow-up exams to monitor progress and to check for side effects.

EVALUATION

Effectiveness of therapy can be demonstrated by: ▪ Decreased fever and night sweats ☐ Diminished cough and sputum production ☐ Negative sputum cultures ☐ Increased appetite ☐ Weight gain ☐ Reduced fatigue ☐ Sense of well-being in patients with tuberculosis ▪ Prevention of meningococcal meningitis ▪ Prevention of *H. influenzae* type B infection. Prophylactic course is usually short-term.

RISPERIDONE

(riss-**per**-i-done)

Risperdal

CLASSIFICATION(S):

Antipsychotic agent (miscellaneous)

Pregnancy Category C

INDICATIONS

- ▪ Management of psychoses.

ACTION

▪ May act by antagonizing dopamine and serotonin in the CNS. **Therapeutic Effects:** ▪ Decreased symptoms of psychoses.

PHARMACOKINETICS

Absorption: Well absorbed (70%) following oral administration.
Distribution: UK.
Metabolism and Excretion: Extensively metabolized by the liver. Metabolism is genetically determined; extensive metabolizers (most patients) convert risperidone to 9-hydroxyrisperidone rapidly. Poor metabolizers (6–8% of whites) convert it more slowly. The 9-hydroxyrisperidone is an antipsychotic compound. Risperidone and its active metabolite are renally eliminated.
Half-life: *Extensive metabolizers*—3 hr for risperidone, 21 hr for 9-hydroxyrisperidone. *Poor metabolizers*—20 hr for risperidone and 30 hr for 9-hydroxyrisperidone.

CONTRAINDICATIONS AND PRECAUTIONS

Contraindicated in: ▪ Hypersensitivity.
Use Cautiously in: ▪ Geriatric or debilitated patients, patients with renal or hepatic impairment (initial dosage reduction recommended) ▪ Underlying cardiovascular disease (may be more prone to arrhythmias and hypotension) ▪ History of seizures ▪ History of suicide attempt or drug abuse ▪ Pregnancy, lactation, or children (safety not established).

ADVERSE REACTIONS AND SIDE EFFECTS*

CNS: NEUROLEPTIC MALIGNANT SYNDROME, aggressive behavior, dizziness, extrapyramidal reactions, headache, increased dreams, increased sleep duration, insomnia, sedation, fatigue, impaired temperature regulation, nervousness, tardive dyskinesia.
EENT: pharyngitis, rhinitis, visual disturbances.
Resp: cough, dyspnea, rhinitis.
CV: arrhythmias, orthostatic hypotension, tachycardia.
GI: constipation, diarrhea, dry mouth, nausea, abdominal pain, anorexia, dyspepsia, increased salivation, vomiting.
GU: decreased libido, dysmenorrhea/menorrhagia, difficulty urinating, polyuria.
Derm: itching/skin rash, dry skin, increased pigmentation, increased sweating, photosensitivity, seborrhea.
Endo: galactorrhea.
MS: arthralgia, back pain.
Misc: weight gain, weight loss, polydipsia.

INTERACTIONS

Drug-Drug: ▪ May decrease the antiparkinsonian effects of **levodopa** or other **dopamine agonists** ▪ **Carbamazepine** increases metabolism and may decrease effectiveness ▪ **Clozapine** decreases metabolism and may increase the effects of risperidone ▪ Additive CNS depression may occur with other **CNS depressants,** including **alcohol, antihistamines, sedative/hypnotics,** or **opioids.**

ROUTE AND DOSAGE

- **PO (Adults):** 1 mg twice daily, increased by 3rd day to 3 mg twice daily. Further increments may be made at weekly intervals by 1 mg twice daily (usual range, 4–6 mg/day; not to exceed 16 mg/day). *Geriatric or debilitated patients, patients prone to hypotension, or patients with impaired renal or hepatic function*—Start with 0.5 mg twice daily; increase by 0.5 mg twice daily, up to 1.5 mg twice daily; then increase at weekly intervals if necessary. May also be given as a single daily dose following initial titration.

AVAILABILITY

- ***Tablets:*** 1 mg^{Rx}, 2 mg^{Rx}, 3 mg^{Rx}, 4 mg^{Rx}.

TIME/ACTION PROFILE (clinical effects)

	ONSET	PEAK	DURATION
PO	1–2 wk	UK	up to 6 wk†

†Following discontinuation.

NURSING IMPLICATIONS

ASSESSMENT

- ▫ Monitor patient's mental status (delusions, hallucinations, and behavior) prior to and periodically throughout therapy.
- ▫ Monitor mood changes. Assess for suicidal tendencies, especially during early therapy. Restrict amount of drug available to patient.
- ▫ Monitor blood pressure (sitting, standing, lying) and pulse prior to and frequently during initial dosage titration. May cause prolonged QT interval, tachycardia, and orthostatic hy-

*CAPITALS indicate life-threatening; underlines indicate most frequent.

potension. If hypotension occurs, dose may need to be decreased.

- □ Observe patient carefully when administering medication to ensure medication is actually swallowed and not hoarded.
- □ Monitor patient for onset of extrapyramidal side effects (*akathisia*—restlessness; *dystonia*—muscle spasms and twisting motions; or *pseudoparkinsonism*—mask facies, rigidity, tremors, drooling, shuffling gait, dysphagia). Report these symptoms; reduction of dosage or discontinuation of medication may be necessary. Trihexyphenidyl or diphenhydramine may be used to control these symptoms.
- □ Monitor for tardive dyskinesia (involuntary rhythmic movement of mouth, face, and extremities). Report immediately; may be irreversible.
- □ Monitor for development of neuroleptic malignant syndrome (fever, respiratory distress, tachycardia, convulsions, diaphoresis, hypertension or hypotension, pallor, tiredness). Notify physician or other health care professional immediately if these symptoms occur.
- ▪ ***Lab Test Considerations:*** May cause increased serum prolactin levels.
- □ May cause increased AST and ALT.
- □ May also cause anemia, thrombocytopenia, leukocytosis, and leukopenia.

POTENTIAL NURSING DIAGNOSES

- ▪ Violence, risk for, directed at others (Indications).
- ▪ Thought processes, altered, related to panic anxiety (Indications).
- ▪ Injury, risk for (Side Effects).

IMPLEMENTATION

- ▪ **General Info:** When switching from other antipsychotics, discontinue previous agents when starting risperidone and minimize the period of overlapping antipsychotic agents.
- □ If therapy is reinstituted after an interval off risperidone, follow initial 3-day titration schedule.

PATIENT/FAMILY TEACHING

- □ Instruct patient to take medication exactly as directed.
- □ Inform patient of the possibility of extrapyramidal symptoms. Instruct patient to report these symptoms immediately to health care professional.
- □ Advise patient to change positions slowly to minimize orthostatic hypotension.
- □ May cause drowsiness. Caution patient to avoid driving or other activities requiring alertness until response to medication is known.
- □ Advise patient to use sunscreen and protective clothing when exposed to the sun to prevent photosensitivity reactions. Extremes in temperature should also be avoided, as this drug impairs body temperature regulation.
- □ Caution patient to avoid concurrent use of alcohol, other CNS depressants, and OTC medications without consulting health care professional.
- □ Advise female patients to notify health care professional if pregnancy is planned or suspected or if they are breast-feeding or planning to breast-feed.
- □ Advise patient to notify health care professional of medication regimen prior to treatment or surgery.
- □ Instruct patient to notify health care professional promptly if sore throat, fever, unusual bleeding or bruising, rash, or tremors occur.
- □ Emphasize the need for continued follow-up for psychotherapy and monitoring for side effects.

EVALUATION

Effectiveness of therapy can be demonstrated by: ▪ Decrease in excited, paranoic, or withdrawn behavior.

RITONAVIR

(ri-**toe**-na-veer)
Norvir

CLASSIFICATION(S):
Antiretroviral (protease inhibitor)

Pregnancy Category B

INDICATIONS

▪ Management of HIV infection in combination with other antiretrovirals (may be used alone in patients who are intolerant to combination regimens).

ACTION

▪ Inhibits the action of HIV protease and prevents the cleavage of viral polyproteins. **Therapeutic Effects:** ▪ Increased CD4 cell counts and decreased viral load with subsequent slowed progression of HIV infection and its sequelae.

PHARMACOKINETICS

Absorption: Appears to be well absorbed following oral administration.
Distribution: Poor CNS penetration.
Metabolism and Excretion: Highly metabolized by the liver; one metabolite has antiretroviral activity; 3.5% excreted unchanged in urine.
Half-life: 3–5 hr.

CONTRAINDICATIONS AND PRECAUTIONS

Contraindicated in: ▪ Hypersensitivity ▪ Concurrent use of alprazolam, amiodarone, bepridil, bupropion, cisapride, clorazepate, clozapine, diazepam, dihydroergotamine, encainide, ergotamine, estazolam, flecainide, flurazepam, meperidine, midazolam, pimozide, piroxicam, propafenone, propoxyphene, quinidine, rifabutin, triazolam, or zolpidem ▪ Hypersensitivity or intolerance to alcohol or castor oil (present in capsules and liquid).
Use Cautiously in: ▪ Impaired hepatic function, history of hepatitis ▪ Diabetes mellitus ▪ Hemophilia (increased risk of bleeding) ▪ Pregnancy, lactation, or children <12 yr (safety not established; breast-feeding not recommended in HIV-infected patients).

ADVERSE REACTIONS AND SIDE EFFECTS*

CNS: SEIZURES, abnormal thinking, weakness, dizziness, headache, malaise, somnolence, syncope.
EENT: pharyngitis, throat irritation.
Resp: ANGIOEDEMA, bronchospasm.
CV: orthostatic hypotension, vasodilation.
GI: abdominal pain, altered taste, anorexia, diarrhea, nausea, vomiting, constipation, dyspepsia, flatulence.
GU: renal insufficiency.
Derm: rash, skin eruptions, sweating, urticaria.
Endo: hyperglycemia.
F and E: dehydration.
Metab: hyperlipidemia.
MS: ↑ creatine phosphokinase, myalgia.
Neuro: circumoral paresthesia, peripheral paresthesia.
Misc: hypersensitivity reactions including STEVENS-JOHNSON SYNDROME and ANAPHYLAXIS, fever.

INTERACTIONS

Drug-Drug: ▪ Produces large increases in blood levels and effects of **amiodarone, astemizole, bepridil, bupropion, cisapride, clozapine, encainide, flecainide, meperidine, piroxicam, propafenone, propoxyphene, quinidine,** and **rifabutin**; because of the increased risk of serious arrhythmias, hematologic toxicity, or seizures, these agents should not be used with ritonavir ▪ Ergot toxicity may occur with concurrent use of **ergotamine** or **dihydroergotamine;** concurrent use should be avoided ▪ Should not be used with **pimozide** ▪ Increases blood levels and the risk of excessive sedation and/or respiratory depression from **alprazolam, clorazepate, diazepam, estazolam, flurazepam, midazolam, triazolam,** and **zolpidem;** concurrent use should be avoided ▪ May also increase blood levels and effects of **some opioid analgesics (alfentanil, fentanyl, hydrocodone, oxycodone, tramadol), some NSAIDs (diclofenac, ibuprofen, indomethacin), some antiarrhythmics (disopyramide, lidocaine, mexiletine), some anti-infectives (clarithromycin, erythromycin), many antidepressants (amitriptyline, clomipramine, desipramine, imipramine, maprotiline, nortriptyline, nefazodone, sertraline, trazodone, fluoxetine, paroxetine, venlafaxine), some antiemetics (dronabinol, ondansetron), some beta blockers (metoprolol, pindolol, propranolol, timolol), many calcium channel blockers (amlodipine, diltiazem, felodipine, isradipine, nicardipine, nifedipine, nimodipine, nisoldipine, verapamil), some antineoplastic agents (etoposide, paclitaxel, tamoxifen, vinblastine, vincristine), some glucocorticoids (dexamethasone, prednisone), some lipid-lowering agents (lovastatin, pravastatin), some immunosuppresants (cyclosporine, tacrolimus), some antipsychotics (chlorpromazine, haloperidol, perphenazine, risperidone,**

***CAPITALS indicate life-threatening; underlines indicate most frequent.**

thioridazine), as well as **quinidine, saquinavir, methamphetamine,** and **warfarin.** Dosage reduction may be necessary ▪ Decreases blood levels and effects of **oral contraceptives, zidovudine, sulfamethoxazole,** and **theophylline**; dosage alteration or alternative therapy may be necessary ▪ Levels may be increased by **clarithromycin** or **fluoxetine.**
Drug-Food: ▪ Food promotes absorption.

ROUTE AND DOSAGE

- **PO (Adults):** 300 mg twice daily for 1 day, then 400 mg twice daily for 3 days, then 500 mg twice daily for 1 day, then 600 mg twice daily as maintenance.
- **PO (Children):** 250 mg/m² twice daily initially; increase by 50 mg/m² twice daily q 2–3 days up to 400 mg/m² twice daily (if unable to get up to 400 mg/m² twice daily, additional antiretroviral therapy is required).

AVAILABILITY

▪ ***Capsules:*** 100 mg^Rx ▪ ***Oral solution:*** 600 mg/7.5 ml (80 mg/ml) in 240-ml bottles^Rx.

TIME/ACTION PROFILE (blood levels)

	ONSET	PEAK	DURATION
PO	rapid	4 hr*	12 hr

*Nonfasting.

NURSING IMPLICATIONS

ASSESSMENT

- □ Assess patient for change in severity of HIV symptoms and for symptoms of opportunistic infections throughout therapy.
- ▪ ***Lab Test Considerations:*** Monitor viral load and CD4 counts regularly during therapy.
- □ May cause hyperglycemia.
- □ May cause elevated serum AST, ALT, GGT, total bilirubin, CPK, triglycerides, and uric acid concentrations.

POTENTIAL NURSING DIAGNOSES

- Infection, risk for (Indications).
- Knowledge deficit, related to disease process and medication regimen (Patient/Family Teaching).
- Noncompliance (Patient/Family Teaching).

IMPLEMENTATION

- ▪ **General Info:** Do not confuse with Retrovir (zidovudine).
- ▪ **PO:** Administer with a meal or light snack.
- □ Oral powder may be mixed with chocolate milk, Ensure, or Advera within 1 hr of dosing to improve taste. Capsules should be stored in the refrigerator and protected from light. Use calibrated oral dosing syringe for oral solution. Oral solution does not require refrigeration if used within 30 days and stored below 77°F in the original container. Keep cap tightly closed.
- □ If nausea occurs on dose of 600 mg twice daily, may titrate by 300 mg twice daily for 1 day, then 400 mg twice daily for 2 days, then 500 mg twice daily for 1 day, then 600 mg twice daily thereafter.
- □ Patients initiating concurrent therapy with nucleoside analogues may have less GI intolerance by initiating ritonavir for 2 wk and then adding the nucleoside analogue.

PATIENT/FAMILY TEACHING

- □ Emphasize the importance of taking ritonavir exactly as directed, at evenly spaced times throughout day. Do not take more than prescribed amount and do not stop taking without consulting health care professional. If a dose is missed, take as soon as remembered; do not double doses.
- □ Instruct patient that ritonavir should not be shared with others.
- □ Advise patient to avoid taking other medications, prescription or OTC, without consulting health care professional.
- □ Inform patient that ritonavir does not cure AIDS or prevent associated or opportunistic infections. Ritonavir does not reduce the risk of transmission of HIV to others through sexual contact or blood contamination. Caution patient to use a condom during sexual contact and to avoid sharing needles or donating blood to prevent spreading the AIDS virus to others. Advise patient that the long-term effects of ritonavir are unknown at this time.
- □ Inform patient that ritonavir may cause hyperglycemia. Advise patient to notify health care professional if increased thirst or hunger; unexplained weight loss; increased urination; fatigue; or dry, itchy skin occurs.
- □ Advise patients taking oral contraceptives to

use a nonhormonal method of birth control during ritonavir therapy.

- Emphasize the importance of regular follow-up exams and blood counts to determine progress and monitor for side effects.

EVALUATION

Effectiveness of therapy can be demonstrated by: ▪ Delayed progression of AIDS and decreased opportunistic infections in patients with HIV ▪ Decrease in viral load and improvement in CD4 cell counts.

RITUXIMAB

(ri-**tux**-i-mab)

Rituxan

CLASSIFICATION(S):
Antineoplastic (monoclonal antibody)

Pregnancy Category C

INDICATIONS

▪ Treatment of low-grade or follicular, CD20-positive, B-cell non-Hodgkin's lymphoma that has relapsed during or has become refractory to other therapies.

ACTION

▪ Binds to the CD20 antigen on the surface of lymphoma cells, preventing the activation process for cell cycle initiation and differentiation. **Therapeutic Effects:** ▪ Death of lymphoma cells.

PHARMACOKINETICS

Absorption: IV administration results in complete bioavailability.
Distribution: Binds specifically to CD20 binding sites on lymphoma cells.
Metabolism and Excretion: UK.
Half-life: 59.8–174 hr (depends on tumor burden).

CONTRAINDICATIONS AND PRECAUTIONS

Contraindicated in: ▪ Hypersensitivity to murine (mouse) proteins ▪ Pregnancy or lactation.
Use Cautiously in: ▪ Pre-existing bone marrow depression ▪ Children (safety not established).

ADVERSE REACTIONS AND SIDE EFFECTS*

CNS: headache.
Resp: bronchospasm, cough, dyspnea.
CV: ARRHYTHMIAS, hypotension, peripheral edema.
GI: abdominal pain, altered taste, dyspepsia.
Derm: flushing, urticaria.
Endo: hyperglycemia.
F and E: hypocalcemia.
Hemat: ANEMIA, NEUTROPENIA, THROMBOCYTOPENIA, B-cell depletion (with decreased immunoglobulins).
MS: arthralgia, back pain.
Misc: allergic reactions including ANAPHYLAXIS and ANGIOEDEMA, fever/chills/rigors (infusion related).

INTERACTIONS

Drug-Drug: ▪ None known.

ROUTE AND DOSAGE

▪ **IV (Adults):** 375 mg/m² once weekly for 4 doses.

AVAILABILITY

▪ ***Solution for injection (requires dilution):*** 10 mg/ml in 100-mg and 500-mg vials[Rx].

TIME/ACTION PROFILE (B-cell depletion)

	ONSET	PEAK	DURATION
IV	within 14 days	3–4 wk	6–9 mo†

†Duration of depletion following 4 wk of treatment.

NURSING IMPLICATIONS

ASSESSMENT

- Monitor patient for fever, chills/rigors, nausea, urticaria, fatigue, headache, pruritus, bronchospasm, dyspnea, sensation of tongue or throat swelling, rhinitis, vomiting, hypotension, flushing, and pain at disease sites. These infusion-related events occur frequently within 30 min–2 hr of beginning first infusion and may resolve with slowing or discontinuing infusion and treatment with IV saline, diphen-

*CAPITALS indicate life-threatening; underlines indicate most frequent.

hydramine, and acetaminophen. Incidence decreases with subsequent infusions.

- □ Assess patient for hypersensitivity reactions (hypotension, bronchospasm, angioedema) during administration. May respond to decrease in infusion rate. Premedication with diphenhydramine and acetaminophen is recommended. Treatment includes diphenhydramine, acetaminophen, bronchodilators, or IV saline as indicated. Epinephrine, antihistamines, and glucocorticoids should be readily available in the event of a severe reaction. If severe reactions occur, discontinue infusion; may be resumed at 50% of the rate when symptoms have resolved completely.
- □ Monitor ECG during and immediately post infusion in patients with pre-existing cardiac conditions (arrhythmias, angina) or patients who have developed arrhythmias during previous infusions of rituximab. Life-threatening arrhythmias may occur.
- ▪ ***Lab Test Considerations:*** Monitor CBC and platelet count regularly during therapy and frequently in patients with blood dyscrasias. May cause anemia, thrombocytopenia, or neutropenia.

POTENTIAL NURSING DIAGNOSES

- ▪ Infection, risk for (Side Effects).
- ▪ Knowledge deficit, related to medication regimen (Patient/Family Teaching).

IMPLEMENTATION

- ▪ **General Info:** Transient hypotension may occur during infusion; antihypertensive medications may be held for 12 hr prior to infusion.
- ▪ **Intermittent Infusion:** Dilute to a concentration of 1–4 mg/ml with 0.9% NaCl or D5W. Gently invert bag to mix. Solution is clear and colorless; do not administer solutions that are discolored or contain particulate matter. Discard unused portion remaining in vial. Solution is stable for 12 hr at room temperature and for 24 hr if refrigerated.
- ▪ ***Rate:*** Do not administer as an IV push or bolus.
- □ *First infusion:* Administer at an initial rate of 50 mg/hr. If hypersensitivity or infusion-related events do not occur, rate may be escalated in 50-mg/hr increments every 30 min to a maximum of 400 mg/hr.
- □ ***Subsequent infusions:*** May be administered at an initial rate of 100 mg/hr and increased by 100-mg/hr increments at 30 min intervals to a maximum of 400 mg/hr.
- ▪ **Additive Incompatibility:** ▪ Do not admix with other medications.

PATIENT/FAMILY TEACHING

- □ Inform patient of the purpose of the medication.
- □ Advise patient to report infusion-related events or symptoms of hypersensitivity reactions immediately.
- □ Instruct patient to notify health care professional promptly if fever; chills; cough; hoarseness; sore throat; signs of infection; lower back or side pain; painful or difficult urination; bleeding gums; bruising; petechiae; blood in stools, urine, or emesis; increased fatigue; dyspnea; or orthostatic hypotension occurs. Caution patient to avoid crowds and persons with known infections. Instruct patient to use soft toothbrush and electric razor and to avoid falls. Caution patient not to drink alcoholic beverages or take medication containing aspirin or NSAIDs; may precipitate gastric bleeding.
- □ Instruct patient to use contraception throughout therapy.

EVALUATION

Effectiveness of therapy can be demonstrated by: ▪ Decrease in spread of malignancy.

ROPINIROLE

(roe-**pin**-i-role)
Requip

CLASSIFICATION(S):
Anti-Parkinson agent (dopamine agonist)

Pregnancy Category C

INDICATIONS

▪ Management of signs and symptoms of idiopathic Parkinson's disease.

ACTION

▪ Stimulates dopamine receptors in the brain. **Therapeutic Effects:** ▪ Decreased tremor and rigidity in Parkinson's disease.

PHARMACOKINETICS

Absorption: 55% absorbed following oral administration.
Distribution: Widely distributed.
Metabolism and Excretion: Extensively metabolized by the liver; <10% excreted unchanged in urine.
Half-life: 6 hr.

CONTRAINDICATIONS AND PRECAUTIONS

Contraindicated in: ▪ Hypersensitivity.
Use Cautiously in: ▪ Geriatric patients (increased risk of hallucinations in patients >65 yr) ▪ Hepatic impairment (slower titration may be required) ▪ Severe cardiovascular disease ▪ Pregnancy, lactation, or children (safety not established; may inhibit lactation).

ADVERSE REACTIONS AND SIDE EFFECTS*

CNS: dizziness, syncope, confusion, drowsiness, fatigue, hallucinations, headache, increased dyskinesia, weakness.
EENT: abnormal vision.
CV: orthostatic hypotension, peripheral edema.
GI: constipation, dry mouth, dyspepsia, nausea, vomiting.
Derm: increased sweating.

INTERACTIONS

Drug-Drug: ▪ **Drugs that alter the activity of certain drug-metabolizing enzymes** may affect the activity or ropinirole ▪ Effects may be increased by **estrogens** ▪ Effects may be decreased by **phenothiazines, butyrophenones, thioxanthenes,** or **metoclopramide.**

ROUTE AND DOSAGE

- **PO (Adults):** 0.25 mg 3 times daily for 1 wk, then 0.5 mg 3 times daily for 1 wk, then 0.75 mg 3 times daily for 1 wk, then 1 mg 3 times daily for 1 wk; then may increase by 1.5 mg/day every wk, up to 9 mg/day; then may increase by up to 3 mg/day every wk up to 24 mg/day.

AVAILABILITY

▪ ***Tablets:*** 0.25 mg[Rx], 0.5 mg[Rx], 1 mg[Rx], 2 mg[Rx], 5 mg[Rx].

TIME/ACTION PROFILE

	ONSET	PEAK	DURATION
PO	UK	UK	8 hr

NURSING IMPLICATIONS

ASSESSMENT

- □ Assess patient for signs and symptoms of Parkinson's disease (tremor, muscle weakness and rigidity, ataxic gait) prior to and throughout therapy.
- □ Assess blood pressure periodically throughout therapy.
- ▪ ***Lab Test Considerations:*** May cause elevated BUN.

POTENTIAL NURSING DIAGNOSES

- Physical mobility, impaired (Indications).
- Injury, risk for (Indications, Side Effects).
- Knowledge deficit, related to medication regimen (Patient/Family Teaching).

IMPLEMENTATION

- **PO:** May be administered with or without food. Administration with food may decrease nausea.

PATIENT/FAMILY TEACHING

- □ Instruct patient to take medication exactly as directed. Missed doses should be taken as soon as possible, but not if almost time for next dose. Do not double doses.
- □ Caution patient to change positions slowly to minimize orthostatic hypotension.
- □ May cause drowsiness. Caution patient to avoid driving or other activities requiring alertness until effects of medication are known.
- □ Advise patient to avoid alcohol and other CNS depressants concurrently with ropinirole.
- □ Advise patient that increasing fluids, sugarless gum or candy, ice, or saliva substitutes may help minimize dry mouth. Consult health care professional if dry mouth continues for >2 wk.

EVALUATION

Effectiveness of therapy can be demonstrated by: ▪ Decreased tremor and rigidity in Parkinson's disease.

***CAPITALS indicate life-threatening; underlines indicate most frequent.**

SALICYLATES

aspirin

(**as**-pir-in)

acetylsalicylic acid, Acuprin, {Apo-ASA}, {Apo-ASEN}, {Arthrinol}, {Arthrisin}, {Artria S.R.}, ASA, Aspergum, Aspir-Low, Aspirtab, {Astrin}, Bayer Aspirin, Bayer Timed-Release Arthritic Pain Formula, {Coryphen}, Easprin, Ecotrin, 8-Hour Bayer Timed-Release, Empirin, {Entrophen}, Halfprin, {Headache Tablets}, Healthprin, Norwich Aspirin, {Novasen}, {PMS-ASA}, Sloprin, St. Joseph Adult Chewable Aspirin, Therapy Bayer, ZORprin

choline salicylate

(**koe**-leen sal-**i**-sil-ate)

Arthropan

choline and magnesium salicylates

(**koe**-leen mag-**neez**-ee-um sal-**i**-sil-ates)

CMT, Tricosal, Trilisate

magnesium salicylate

(mag-**neez**-ee-um sal-**i**-sil-ate)

{Doan's Backache Pills}, Doan's Regular Strength Tablets, Magan, Mobidin

salsalate

(**sal**-sa-late)

Amigesic, Anaflex, Dilsalcid, Marthritic, Mono-Gesic, Salflex, Salgesic, Salsitab

sodium salicylate

(**soe**-dee-yum sal-**i**-sil-ate)

{Dodd's Extra Strength}, {Dodd's Pills}, {Gin Pain Pills}

CLASSIFICATION(S):

Antiplatelet agent (aspirin only), Antipyretics, Nonopioid analgesics/Nonsteroidal anti-inflammatory agents (NSAIDs)

Pregnancy Category D

INDICATIONS

▪ Inflammatory disorders including: ▫ Rheumatoid arthritis ▫ Osteoarthritis ▪ Mild to moderate pain ▪ Fever ▪ **Aspirin:** Prophylaxis of transient ischemic attacks and myocardial infarction.

ACTION

▪ Produce analgesia and reduce inflammation and fever by inhibiting the production of prostaglandins ▪ **Aspirin Only:** Decreases platelet aggregation. **Therapeutic Effects:** ▪ Analgesia ▪ Reduction of inflammation ▪ Reduction of fever ▪ **Aspirin:** Decreased incidence of transient ischemic attacks and myocardial infarction.

PHARMACOKINETICS

Absorption: *Aspirin*—Well absorbed from the upper small intestine; absorption from enteric-coated preparations may be unreliable; rectal absorption is slow and variable. *Choline and magnesium salicylates*—Well absorbed following oral administration. *Salsalate*—Splits into 2 molecules of salicylic acid following oral administration; absorbed in the small intestine.

Distribution: All salicylates are rapidly and widely distributed; cross the placenta and enter breast milk.

Metabolism and Excretion: Extensively metabolized by the liver; inactive metabolites excreted by the kidneys. Amount excreted unchanged by the kidneys depends on urine pH; as pH increases, amount excreted unchanged increases from 2–3% up to 80%.

Half-life: 2–3 hr for low doses; up to 15–30 hr with larger doses because of saturation of liver metabolism.

CONTRAINDICATIONS AND PRECAUTIONS

Contraindicated in: ▪ Hypersensitivity to aspirin, tartrazine (FDC yellow dye #5), or other salicylates ▪ Cross-sensitivity with other NSAIDs may exist (less with nonaspirin salicylates) ▪ Bleeding disorders or thrombocytopenia (more important with aspirin).

Use Cautiously in: ▪ History of GI bleeding or ulcer disease ▪ Chronic alcohol use/abuse ▪ Severe renal disease (magnesium toxicity may occur with magnesium salicylate) ▪ Severe hepatic disease ▪ Children or adolescents with viral infections (may increase the risk of Reye's syndrome) ▪ Geriatric patients (increased risk of adverse reactions; more sensitive to toxic levels) ▪ Pregnancy (may have adverse effects on fetus and mother; avoid use in 3rd trimester) ▪ Lactation (safety not established).

ADVERSE REACTIONS AND SIDE EFFECTS*

EENT: hearing loss, tinnitus.

GI: GI BLEEDING, dyspepsia, epigastric distress, heartburn, nausea, abdominal pain, anorexia, hepatotoxicity, vomiting.

Hemat: *aspirin*—anemia, hemolysis, increased bleeding time.

Misc: allergic reactions including ANAPHYLAXIS and LARYNGEAL EDEMA, noncardiogenic pulmonary edema.

INTERACTIONS

Drug-Drug: ▪ **Aspirin:** May potentiate **warfarin, heparin,** or **thrombolytic agents** ▪ **Aspirin:** May increase the risk of bleeding with **cefamandole, cefoperazone, cefotetan, valproic acid,** or **plicamycin** ▪ **All salicylates:** May enhance the activity of **penicillins, phenytoin, methotrexate, valproic acid, oral hypoglycemic agents,** and **sulfonamides** ▪ May antagonize the beneficial effects of **probenecid** or **sulfinpyrazone** ▪ **Glucocorticoids** may decrease serum salicylate levels ▪ **Urinary acidification** enhances reabsorption and may increase serum salicylate levels ▪ **Alkalinization of the urine** or the ingestion of large amounts of **antacids** promotes excretion and decreases serum salicylate levels ▪ May blunt the therapeutic response to **diuretics, antihypertensives,** or some **NSAIDs** ▪ Increased risk of gastrointestinal irritation with **NSAIDs** ▪ Increased risk of ototoxicity with **vancomycin.**

Drug-Food: ▪ **Foods capable of acidifying the urine** (see Appendix K) may increase serum salicylate levels.

ROUTE AND DOSAGE

❑ **Aspirin**

❑ ***Pain/Fever***

- **PO, Rect (Adults):** 325–500 mg q 3 hr or 325–650 mg q 4 hr or 650–1000 mg q 6 hr (not to exceed 4 g/day). *Extended-release tablets*—650 mg q 8 hr or 800 mg q 12 hr.
- **PO, Rect (Children 2–11 yr):** 65 mg/kg/day (1.5 g/m^2/day) in 4–6 divided doses.

❑ ***Inflammation***

- **PO (Adults):** 2.4 g/day initially; increased to maintenance dose of 3.6–5.4 g/day in divided doses (up to 7.8 g/day for acute rheumatic fever).
- **PO (Children):** 80–100 mg/kg/day in divided doses (up to 130 mg/kg/day for acute rheumatic fever).

❑ ***Prevention of Transient Ischemic Attacks***

- **PO (Adults):** 1–1.3 g daily in 2–4 divided doses (doses as low as 325 mg/day may be used in patients who are intolerant of the higher dose).

❑ ***Prevention of Myocardial Infarction***

- **PO (Adults):** 300–325 mg/day (doses as low as 80 mg/day may be effective).

❑ ***Kawasaki Disease***

- **PO (Children):** 80–120 mg/kg/day in 4 divided doses initially; may be followed by maintenance dose of 3–8 mg/kg/day as a single dose for up to 8 wk.

❑ **Choline Salicylate**

435 mg of choline salicylate is equivalent to 325 mg of aspirin.

- **PO (Adults):** *Analgesic/antipyretic*—435–669 mg (½–¾ tsp) q 3 hr or 425–870 mg (½–1 tsp) q 4 hr or 870–1305 mg (1–1½ tsp) q 6 hr as needed. *Anti-inflammatory*—4.8–7.2 g/day in divided doses.
- **PO (Children):** *Pain/fever*—2 g/m^2/day in 4–6 divided doses. *Inflammation*—107–133 mg/kg/day in 4–6 divided doses (up to 174 mg/kg).

❑ **Magnesium Salicylate**

- **PO (Adults):** 303.7 mg q 6 hr or 467 mg q 8 hr.

❑ **Choline and Magnesium Salicylates**

5 ml of liquid equivalent to 500 mg salicylate or 650 mg of aspirin. Tablet strength expressed in mg of salicylate: 500-mg tablet equivalent to 650 mg of aspirin, 750-mg tablet equivalent to 975

*CAPITALS indicate life-threatening; underlines indicate most frequent.

mg of aspirin, 1000-mg tablet equivalent to 1.3 g of aspirin.

- **PO (Adults):** *Analgesic/antipyretic*—2–3 g of salicylate/day in 2–3 divided doses. *Anti-inflammatory*—3 g/day at bedtime or in 2–3 divided doses.
- **PO (Children >37 kg):** 2.2 g of salicylate/day in 2 divided doses.
- **PO (Children <37 kg):** 50 mg of salicylate/kg/day in 2 divided doses.

❑ **Salsalate**

- **PO (Adults):** 1 g 3 times daily initially; further titration may be required.

❑ **Sodium Salicylate**

- **PO (Adults):** *Pain/fever*—325–650 mg q 4 hr. *Inflammation*—3.6–5.4 g/day in divided doses.
- **PO (Children):** *Pain/fever*—1.5 g/m²/day in 4–6 divided doses. *Inflammation*—80–100 mg/kg/day in 4–6 divided doses.

AVAILABILITY

❑ **Aspirin**

▪ ***Tablets:*** 81 mg^OTC^, 162.5 mg^OTC^, 325 mg^OTC^, 500 mg^OTC^, 650 mg^OTC^, {975 mg^OTC^} ▪ ***Chewable tablets:*** {80 mg^OTC^}, 81 mg^OTC^ ▪ ***Chewing gum:*** 227 mg^OTC^ ▪ {***Dispersible tablets:*** 325 mg^OTC^, 500 mg^OTC^} ▪ ***Enteric-coated (delayed-release) tablets:*** 80 mg^OTC^, 165 mg^OTC^, {300 mg^OTC^}, 325 mg^OTC^, 500 mg^OTC^, {600 mg^OTC^}, 650 mg^OTC^, 975 mg^OTC^ ▪ ***Extended-release tablets:*** {325 mg^OTC^}, 650 mg^OTC^, 800 mg^Rx^ ▪ {***Delayed-release capsules:*** 325 mg^OTC^, 500 mg^OTC^} ▪ ***Suppositories:*** 60 mg^OTC^, 120 mg^OTC^, 125 mg^OTC^, 130 mg^OTC^, {150 mg^OTC^}, {160 mg^OTC^}, 195 mg^OTC^, 200 mg^OTC^, 300 mg^OTC^, {320 mg^OTC^}, 325 mg^OTC^, 600 mg^OTC^, {640 mg^OTC^}, 650 mg^OTC^, 1.2 g^OTC^ ▪ ***In combination with:*** antihistamines, decongestants, cough suppressants^OTC^, and opioids^Rx^. See Appendix A.

❑ **Choline Salicylate**

▪ ***Oral solution:*** 870 mg/5 ml^OTC^.

❑ **Magnesium Salicylate**

▪ ***Tablets:*** 325 mg^OTC^, 500 mg^OTC^, 545 mg^Rx^, 600 mg^Rx^.

❑ **Choline and Magnesium Salicylates (listed as salicylate content)**

▪ ***Tablets:*** 500 mg^Rx^, 750 mg^Rx^, 1000 mg^Rx^ ▪ ***Liquid:*** 500 mg/5 ml^Rx^.

❑ **Salsalate**

▪ ***Tablets:*** 500 mg^Rx^, 750 mg^Rx^ ▪ ***Capsules:*** 500 mg^Rx^.

❑ **Sodium Salicylate**

▪ ***Tablets:*** 325 mg^OTC^, 650 mg^OTC^ ▪ ***Delayed-release tablets:*** 324 mg^OTC^, 325 mg^OTC^, 650 mg^OTC^.

TIME/ACTION PROFILE (analgesia/fever reduction*)

	ONSET	PEAK	DURATION
Aspirin–PO	5–30 min	1–3 hr	3–6 hr
Aspirin–PO-ER	5–30 min	2–4 hr	8–12 hr
Aspirin–Rect	1–2 hr	4–5 hr	7 hr
All other salicylates–PO	5–30 min	1–3 hr	3–6 hr

*Antirheumatic effect may take 2–3 wk of chronic dosing.

NURSING IMPLICATIONS

ASSESSMENT

- **General Info:** Patients who have asthma, allergies, and nasal polyps or who are allergic to tartrazine are at an increased risk for developing hypersensitivity reactions.
- **Pain:** Assess pain and limitation of movement; note type, location, and intensity prior to and at the peak (see Time/Action Profile) following administration.
- **Fever:** Assess fever and note associated signs (diaphoresis, tachycardia, malaise, chills).
- ***Lab Test Considerations:*** Monitor hepatic function prior to antirheumatic therapy and if symptoms of hepatotoxicity occur; more likely in patients, especially children, with rheumatic fever, systemic lupus erythematosus, juvenile arthritis, or pre-existing hepatic disease. May cause elevated serum AST, ALT, and alkaline phosphatase, especially when plasma concentrations exceed 25 mg/100 ml. May return to normal despite continued use or dose reduction. If severe abnormalities or active liver disease occurs, discontinue and use with caution in future.
  - ❑ Monitor serum salicylate levels periodically with prolonged high-dose therapy to determine dose, safety, and efficacy, especially in children with Kawasaki disease.
  - ❑ May alter results of serum uric acid, urine vanillylmandelic acid (VMA), protirelin-induced thyroid-stimulating hormone (TSH), urine hydroxyindoleacetic acid (5-HIAA) de-

terminations, and radionuclide thyroid imaging.

- May cause decreased serum potassium and cholesterol concentrations.
- *Aspirin:* In addition to the above lab tests, aspirin prolongs bleeding time for 4–7 days and, in large doses, may cause prolonged prothrombin time. Monitor hematocrit periodically in prolonged high-dose therapy to assess for GI blood loss.
- ***Toxicity and Overdose:*** Monitor patient for the onset of tinnitus, headache, hyperventilation, agitation, mental confusion, lethargy, diarrhea, and sweating. If these symptoms appear, withhold medication and notify physician or other health care professional immediately.

POTENTIAL NURSING DIAGNOSES

- Pain (Indications).
- Physical mobility, impaired (Indications).
- Knowledge deficit, related to medication regimen (Patient/Family Teaching).

IMPLEMENTATION

- **PO:** Administer after meals or with food or an antacid to minimize gastric irritation. Food slows but will not alter the total amount absorbed.
- Do not crush or chew enteric-coated tablets. Do not take antacids within 1–2 hr of enteric-coated tablets. Chewable tablets may be chewed, dissolved in liquid, or swallowed whole. Some extended-release tablets may be broken or crumbled but must not be ground up before swallowing. See manufacturer's prescribing information for individual products.

PATIENT/FAMILY TEACHING

- **General Info:** Instruct patient to take salicylates with a full glass of water and to remain in an upright position for 15–30 min after administration.
- Advise patient to report tinnitus; unusual bleeding of gums; bruising; black, tarry stools; or fever lasting longer than 3 days.
- Caution patient to avoid concurrent use of alcohol with this medication to minimize possible gastric irritation; 3 or more glasses of alcohol per day may increase the risk of GI bleeding. Caution patient to avoid taking concurrently with acetaminophen or NSAIDs for more than a few days, unless directed by health care professional to prevent analgesic nephropathy.
- Teach patients on a sodium-restricted diet to avoid effervescent tablets or buffered-aspirin preparations.
- Tablets with an acetic (vinegar-like) odor should be discarded.
- Advise patients on long-term therapy to inform health care professional of medication regimen prior to surgery. Aspirin may need to be withheld for 1 wk prior to surgery.
- Centers for Disease Control and Prevention warns against giving aspirin to children or adolescents with varicella (chickenpox) or influenza-like or viral illnesses because of a possible association with Reye's syndrome.
- **Transient Ischemic Attacks or Myocardial Infarction:** Advise patients receiving aspirin prophylactically to take only prescribed dosage. Increasing the dosage has not been found to provide additional benefits.

EVALUATION

Effectiveness of therapy can be demonstrated by: ▪ Relief of mild to moderate discomfort ▪ Increased ease of joint movement. May take 2–3 wk for maximum effectiveness ▪ Reduction of fever ▪ Prevention of transient ischemic attacks ▪ Prevention of myocardial infarction.

S

SALMETEROL

(sal-**me**-te-role)
Serevent

CLASSIFICATION(S):
Bronchodilator (beta-adrenergic agonist)

Pregnancy Category C

INDICATIONS

▪ Used as a long-acting bronchodilator in the long-term control of reversible airway obstruction due to asthma ▪ Prevention of exercise-induced asthma.

ACTION

▪ Produces accumulation of cyclic adenosine monophosphate (cAMP) at beta-adrenergic receptors ▪ Relatively specific for $beta_2$ (pulmonary) receptors. **Therapeutic Effects:** ▪ Bronchodilation.

PHARMACOKINETICS

Absorption: Minimal systemic absorption follows inhalation.
Distribution: Action is primarily local.
Metabolism and Excretion: UK.
Half-life: UK.

CONTRAINDICATIONS AND PRECAUTIONS

Contraindicated in: ▪ Hypersensitivity ▪ Acute attack of asthma (onset of action is delayed).
Use Cautiously in: ▪ Cardiovascular disease (including angina and hypertension) ▪ Diabetes ▪ Glaucoma ▪ Hyperthyroidism ▪ Pheochromocytoma ▪ Excessive use (may lead to tolerance and paradoxical bronchospasm) ▪ Pregnancy, lactation, or children <12 yr (safety not established).

ADVERSE REACTIONS AND SIDE EFFECTS*

CNS: headache, nervousness.
CV: palpitations, tachycardia.
GI: abdominal pain, diarrhea, nausea.
MS: muscle cramps/soreness.
Neuro: trembling.

INTERACTIONS

Drug-Drug: ▪ **Beta-adrenergic blocking agents** may decrease the therapeutic effects of salmeterol.

ROUTE AND DOSAGE

▪ **Inhalation (Adults and Children ≥12 yr):** 50 mcg (2 inhalations) twice daily (approximately 12 hr apart); *exercise-induced bronchospasm*—50 mcg (2 inhalations) 30–60 min prior to exercise.

AVAILABILITY

▪ ***Aerosol for inhalation:*** 25 mcg/spray in 6.5-g (60 spray) or 13-g (120 spray) canisters[Rx] ▪ {***Powder for inhalation:*** 50 mcg/blister}.

TIME/ACTION PROFILE (bronchodilation)

	ONSET	PEAK	DURATION
Inhalation	10–25 min	3–4 hr	12 hr

NURSING IMPLICATIONS

ASSESSMENT

- Assess lung sounds, pulse, and blood pressure before administration and periodically during therapy.
- Monitor pulmonary function tests before initiating therapy and periodically throughout course to determine effectiveness of medication.
- Observe for paradoxical bronchospasm (wheezing, dyspnea, tightness in chest) and hypersensitivity reaction (rash; urticaria; swelling of the face, lips, or eyelids). If condition occurs, withhold medication and notify physician or other health care professional immediately.

▪ ***Lab Test Considerations:*** May cause increased serum glucose concentrations; occurs rarely with recommended doses and is more pronounced with frequent use of high doses.

- May cause decreased serum potassium concentrations, which are usually transient and dose related; rarely occurs at recommended doses and is more pronounced with frequent use of high doses.

▪ ***Toxicity and Overdose:*** Symptoms of overdose include persistent agitation, chest pain or discomfort, decreased blood pressure, dizziness, hyperglycemia, hypokalemia, seizures, tachyarrhythmias, persistent trembling, and vomiting.

- Treatment includes discontinuing salmeterol and other beta-adrenergic agonists and providing symptomatic, supportive therapy. Cardioselective beta-adrenergic blocking agents are used cautiously, as they may induce bronchospasm.

POTENTIAL NURSING DIAGNOSES

▪ Airway clearance, ineffective (Indications).
▪ Knowledge deficit, related to medication regimen (Patient/Family Teaching).

IMPLEMENTATION

▪ **Inhalation:** See Appendix D for instructions in the use of metered-dose inhalers.

- Salmeterol metered-dose inhaler should be primed or tested prior to 1st use.
- Do not use a spacer with powder for inhalation.

*CAPITALS indicate life-threatening; underlines indicate most frequent.

PATIENT/FAMILY TEACHING

- Instruct patient on proper technique for use of metered-dose inhaler or powder for inhalation and advise patient to take salmeterol exactly as directed. Do not use more than the prescribed dose. If a regularly scheduled dose is missed, use as soon as possible and resume regular schedule. Do not double doses. If symptoms occur before next dose is due, use a rapid-acting inhaled bronchodilator.
- Instruct patient using *powder for inhalation* to never exhale into discus device and to always hold device in a level horizontal position. Mouthpiece should be kept dry; never wash.
- Caution patient not to use salmeterol to treat acute symptoms. A rapid-acting inhaled beta-adrenergic bronchodilator should be used for relief of acute asthma attacks.
- Do not spray inhaler near eyes.
- Instruct patient to save inhaler; refill canisters may be available.
- Advise patients on chronic therapy not to use additional salmeterol to prevent exercise-induced bronchospasm. Patients using salmeterol for prevention of exercise-induced bronchospasm should not use additional doses of salmeterol for 12 hr after prophylactic administration.
- Advise patient to notify health care professional immediately if difficulty in breathing persists after use of salmeterol, if condition worsens, if more inhalations of rapid-acting bronchodilator than usual are needed to relieve an acute attack, or if using 4 or more inhalations of a rapid-acting bronchodilator for 2 or more consecutive days or more than 1 canister in an 8-wk period.
- Advise patients using inhalation or systemic glucocorticoids to consult health care professional prior to stopping or reducing therapy.
- Emphasize the importance of regular follow-up exams to determine progress during therapy.

EVALUATION

Effectiveness of therapy can be demonstrated by: ▪ Prevention of bronchospasm or reduction of frequency of acute asthma attacks in patients with chronic asthma ▪ Prevention of exercise-induced asthma.

SAQUINAVIR
(sa-**kwin**-a-vir)
Fortovase, Invirase

CLASSIFICATION(S):
Antiretroviral (protease inhibitor)

Pregnancy Category B

INDICATIONS

▪ Management of HIV infection in combination with other antiretroviral agents.

ACTION

▪ Inhibits the action of HIV protease and prevents the cleavage of viral polyproteins. **Therapeutic Effects:** ▪ Slowing of the progression of HIV infection and its sequelae ▪ Increased CD4 cell counts and decreased viral load.

PHARMACOKINETICS

Absorption: Incompletely absorbed following oral administration; rapidly undergoes extensive first-pass hepatic metabolism. Absorption of Invirase and Fortovase is not the same; products are not interchangeable.
Distribution: Distributes into tissues, but CNS penetration is poor.
Metabolism and Excretion: Mostly metabolized by the liver. <1% excreted unchanged in urine.
Half-life: 13 hr.

CONTRAINDICATIONS AND PRECAUTIONS

Contraindicated in: ▪ Hypersensitivity ▪ Lactation ▪ Concurrent astemizole, dihydroergotamine, cisapride, midazolam, rifabutin, rifampin, and triazolam.
Use Cautiously in: ▪ Pregnancy or children <16 yr (safety not established) ▪ Diabetes mellitus (may exacerbate hyperglycemia) ▪ Hemophilia (increased risk of bleeding) ▪ Hepatic impairment.

ADVERSE REACTIONS AND SIDE EFFECTS*

CNS: SEIZURES, confusion, headache, mental depression, psychic disorders, weakness.

*CAPITALS indicate life-threatening; underlines indicate most frequent.

CV: thrombophlebitis.
GI: abdominal discomfort, diarrhea, increased liver enzymes, jaundice, nausea.
Derm: photosensitivity, severe cutaneous reactions.
Endo: hyperglycemia.
Hemat: acute myeloblastic leukemia, hemolytic anemia, thrombocytopenia.
Neuro: ataxia.
Misc: STEVENS-JOHNSON SYNDROME.

INTERACTIONS

Drug-Drug: ▪ **Rifampin** and **rifabutin** significantly decrease saquinavir levels; concurrent use is contraindicated ▪ Saquinavir increases blood levels of **astemizole** and **cisapride** (increased risk of arrhythmias); **dihydroergotamine** and **ergotamine** (increased risk of vasoconstriction); **midazolam** and **triazolam** (excessive CNS depression); concurrent use is contraindicated ▪ Coadministration with **clarithromycin** significantly increases saquinavir levels and decreases clarithromycin levels ▪ Saquinavir levels are also significantly increased by **indinavir, nelfinavir, ritonavir, delavirdine,** and **ketoconazole** (dosage adjustments may be necessary) ▪ **Carbamazepine, phenobarbital, phenytoin, nevirapine,** and **dexamethasone** may decrease saquinavir levels.
Drug-Food: ▪ Food significantly increases the absorption of saquinavir.

ROUTE AND DOSAGE

□ **Invirase**
- **PO (Adults):** 600 mg 3 times daily within 2 hr of a meal.

□ **Fortovase**
- **PO (Adults):** 1200 mg 3 times daily within 2 hr of a meal.

AVAILABILITY

□ **Invirase**
- ***Capsules:*** 200 mg[Rx].

□ **Fortovase**
- ***Soft gelatin capsules:*** 200 mg[Rx].

TIME/ACTION PROFILE (blood levels)

	ONSET	PEAK	DURATION
PO	UK	UK	8 hr

NURSING IMPLICATIONS

ASSESSMENT

□ Assess patient for change in severity of symptoms of HIV and for symptoms of opportunistic infections throughout therapy.
▪ ***Lab Test Considerations:*** Monitor viral load and CD4 count regularly during therapy.
□ May cause hyperglycemia.
□ Monitor hematologic and hepatic function prior to and periodically during therapy. May cause anemia, thrombocytopenia, and elevated liver enzymes.

POTENTIAL NURSING DIAGNOSES

- Infection, risk for (Indications, Side Effects).
- Knowledge deficit, related to medication regimen (Patient/Family Teaching).

IMPLEMENTATION

▪ **PO:** Administer within 2 hr after a full meal to increase effectiveness. Taking without food causes decreased blood concentrations and may result in no antiviral activity.
□ Capsules are stable until expiration date if refrigerated or for 3 mo when brought to room temperature.

PATIENT/FAMILY TEACHING

□ Instruct patient to take saquinavir exactly as directed at the same time each day, within 2 hr after a full meal. Missed doses should be taken as soon as possible if not almost time for next dose; do not double doses. Do not discontinue without consulting health care professional. Changes from Invirase to Fortovase should be made under supervision of health care professional.
□ Instruct patient that saquinavir should not be shared with others.
□ Inform patient that saquinavir does not cure HIV or prevent associated or opportunistic infections. Saquinavir does not reduce the risk of transmission of HIV to others through sexual contact or blood contamination. Caution patient to use a condom during sexual contact and to avoid sharing needles or donating blood to prevent spreading HIV to others. Advise patient that the long-term effects of saquinavir are unknown at this time.
□ Advise patient not to take other medications,

prescription or OTC, concurrently without consulting health care professional.
- Inform patient that saquinavir may cause hyperglycemia. Advise patient to notify health care professional if increased thirst or hunger; unexplained weight loss; increased urination; fatigue; or dry, itchy skin occurs.
- Inform patient that long-term effects of saquinavir are unknown at this time.
- Emphasize the importance of regular follow-up exams and blood tests to determine progress and monitor for side effects.

EVALUATION

Effectiveness of therapy can be demonstrated by: ▪ Slowing of the progression of HIV infection and its sequelae ▪ Decrease in viral load and improvement in CD4 cell counts.

SARGRAMOSTIM

(sar-**gram**-oh-stim)

Leukine, (recombinant human granulocyte/macrophage colony-stimulating factor), rHu GM-CSF

CLASSIFICATION(S):

Colony-stimulating factor

Pregnancy Category C

INDICATIONS

▪ Acceleration of bone marrow recovery following: ▫ Autologous bone marrow transplantation in patients with non-Hodgkin's lymphoma, acute lymphoblastic leukemia, or Hodgkin's disease ▫ Allogenic bone marrow transplantation from HLA-matched donors ▪ Management of bone marrow transplant failure or engraftment delay ▪ Following induction chemotherapy for acute myelogenous leukemia (AML) in patients ≥55 yr ▪ Mobilization and following transplant of autologous peripheral blood progenitor cells (PBPCs); increases harvest by leukapheresis.

ACTION

▪ Consists of a glycoprotein produced by recombinant DNA technique that is capable of binding to and stimulating the production, division, differentiation, and activation of granulocytes and macrophages. **Therapeutic Effects:** ▪ Accelerated recovery of bone marrow following autologous bone marrow transplantation, resulting in decreased risk of infection and other complications.

PHARMACOKINETICS

Absorption: Following IV administration, absorption is essentially complete. Well absorbed following SC administration.
Distribution: UK.
Metabolism and Excretion: UK.
Half-life: UK.

CONTRAINDICATIONS AND PRECAUTIONS

Contraindicated in: ▪ Presence of ≥10% leukemic myeloid blast cells in bone marrow or peripheral blood ▪ Hypersensitivity to GM-CSF, yeast products, or additives (mannitol, tromethamine, or sucrose) ▪ Products containing benzyl alcohol should not be used in newborns.
Use Cautiously in: ▪ Pre-existing fluid retention, congestive heart failure, or pulmonary infiltrates ▪ Pre-existing cardiac disease ▪ Myeloid malignancies ▪ Previous extensive radiation or chemotherapy (response may be limited) ▪ Pregnancy (use only if clearly needed) ▪ Lactation or children (safety not established).

ADVERSE REACTIONS AND SIDE EFFECTS*

CNS: headache, malaise, weakness.
Resp: dyspnea.
CV: pericardial effusion, peripheral edema, transient supraventricular tachycardia.
GI: diarrhea.
Derm: itching, rash.
MS: arthralgia, bone pain, myalgia.
Misc: chills, fever, first-dose reaction.

INTERACTIONS

Drug-Drug: ▪ **Lithium** or **glucocorticoids** may potentiate myeloproliferative effects of sargramostim (concurrent use should be undertaken cautiously).

ROUTE AND DOSAGE

▫ **Following Bone Marrow Transplantation**

▪ **IV (Adults):** 250 mcg/m²/day for 21 days.

*CAPITALS indicate life-threatening; underlines indicate most frequent.

❑ **Failure/Delay of Engraftment following Bone Marrow Transplantation**

- **IV (Adults):** 250 mcg/m²/day for 14 days; may be repeated after a 7-day rest between courses; if results are inadequate, a 3rd course at 500 mcg/m²/day for 14 days may be given following a 7-day rest.

❑ **Following Chemotherapy for AML**

- **IV (Adults):** 250 mcg/m²/day started around day 11 or 4 days following induction if day 10 bone marrow is hypoplastic with <5% blast cells and continued until absolute neutrophil count (ANC) >1500 cells/mm³ for 3 consecutive days (not to exceed 42 days); if adverse reactions occur, decrease dose by 50% or temporarily discontinue.

❑ **Mobilization of PBPCs**

- **IV, SC (Adults):** 250 mcg/m²/day continued throughout collection of PBPCs.

❑ **Following PBPC Transplantation**

- **IV, SC (Adults):** 250 mcg/m²/day continued until ANC >1500 cells/mm³ for 3 consecutive days.

AVAILABILITY

- ***Powder for injection:*** 250 mcg/vial^Rx^, 500 mcg/vial^Rx^.

TIME/ACTION PROFILE (noted as effects on blood counts)

	ONSET	PEAK	DURATION
SC, IV	rapid	UK	3–7 days

NURSING IMPLICATIONS

ASSESSMENT

- Monitor heart rate, blood pressure, and respiratory status during and immediately following infusion. If dyspnea develops, slow infusion rate by half. Reassess; medication may need to be discontinued. Assess for peripheral edema daily throughout therapy. Capillary leak syndrome (swelling of feet or lower legs, sudden weight gain, dyspnea) and pleural or pericardial effusion may occur, usually at doses >32 mcg/kg/day.
- Monitor for first-dose reaction (flushing, hypotension, syncope, weakness). Does not recur with first dose of each course but may occur with first dose of more than 1 course.
- Assess patient for fever daily during therapy. Usually mild and dose related and resolves with discontinuation or administration of antipyretics.
- Assess patient for arthralgias and myalgias, usually in lower extremities, which tend to occur when granulocyte counts are returning to normal. May also cause mild to moderate bone pain, possibly due to bone marrow expansion. Usually occurs over a 1–3-day period before myeloid recovery and occurs in the sternum, spine, pelvis, and long bones. Treat with analgesics.
- ***Lab Test Considerations:*** Obtain a CBC with differential and platelet count prior to chemotherapy and twice weekly during therapy to avoid leukocytosis. Monitor ANC; may increase rapidly. If ANC >20,000/mm³ or 10,000/mm³ after the nadir has occurred or if platelet count >500,000/mm³, interrupt administration and reduce dose by half or discontinue. Excessive blood levels usually return to baseline 3–7 days following discontinuation of therapy. If blast cells appear, sargramostim should be discontinued.
- Monitor renal and hepatic function prior to and biweekly throughout therapy in patients with renal or hepatic dysfunction. May cause increased BUN, creatinine, and hepatic enzymes.
- May cause decreased serum albumin concentrations.

POTENTIAL NURSING DIAGNOSES

- Infection, risk for (Indications).
- Knowledge deficit, related to medication regimen (Patient/Family Teaching).

IMPLEMENTATION

- **General Info:** Administer 2–4 hr after bone marrow transplant and no earlier than 24 hr following cytotoxic chemotherapy or 12 hr after last dose of radiotherapy.
- Refrigerate but do not freeze powder, reconstituted solution, or diluted solution. Reconstitute with 1 ml of sterile water without preservatives injected toward side of vial. Swirl gently to avoid foaming. Do not shake. Solution should be clear and colorless. Discard if

left at room temperature for >6 hr. Vial is for 1-time use only.
- **SC:** Administer reconstituted solution without further dilution.
- **Intermittent Infusion:**
- □ Dilute in 0.9% NaCl. If final concentration is <10 mcg/ml, add a final concentration of 0.1% human albumin to 0.9% NaCl prior to addition of sargramostim to prevent absorption of the components of the drug delivery system. Do not administer with an in-line filter.
- ***Rate:*** Usually infused over 2–4 hr. Has been administered over 30–60 min, over 5–12 hr, and as a continuous infusion over 24 hr.
- □ *Following bone marrow transplantation or failure of engraftment:* Administer over 2 hr.
- □ *Chemotherapy for AML:* Administer over 4 hr.
- □ *Mobilization of PBPCs or PBPC transplant:* Administer as a continuous infusion over 24 hr.
- **Y-Site Compatibility:** ▪ amikacin ▪ aminophylline ▪ aztreonam ▪ bleomycin ▪ butorphanol ▪ calcium gluconate ▪ carboplatin ▪ carmustine ▪ cefazolin ▪ cefepime ▪ cefotaxime ▪ cefotetan ▪ ceftizoxime ▪ ceftriaxone ▪ cefuroxime ▪ cimetidine ▪ cisplatin ▪ clindamycin ▪ cyclophosphamide ▪ cyclosporine ▪ cytarabine ▪ dacarbazine ▪ dactinomycin ▪ dexamethasone sodium phosphate ▪ diphenhydramine ▪ dopamine ▪ doxorubicin ▪ doxycycline ▪ droperidol ▪ etoposide ▪ famotidine ▪ fentanyl ▪ floxuridine ▪ fluconazole ▪ fluorouracil ▪ furosemide ▪ gentamicin ▪ heparin ▪ idarubicin ▪ ifosfamide ▪ immune globulin ▪ magnesium sulfate ▪ mannitol ▪ mechlorethamine ▪ meperidine ▪ mesna ▪ methotrexate ▪ metoclopramide ▪ metronidazole ▪ mezlocillin ▪ miconazole ▪ minocycline ▪ mitoxantrone ▪ netilmicin ▪ pentostatin ▪ piperacillin/tazobactam ▪ potassium chloride ▪ prochlorperazine ▪ promethazine ▪ ranitidine ▪ teniposide ▪ ticarcillin ▪ ticarcillin/clavulanate ▪ trimethoprim/sulfamethoxazole ▪ vinblastine ▪ vincristine ▪ zidovudine.
- **Y-Site Incompatibility:** ▪ acyclovir ▪ ampicillin ▪ ampicillin/sulbactam ▪ cefonicid ▪ cefoperazone ▪ chlorpromazine ▪ ganciclovir ▪ haloperidol ▪ hydrocortisone ▪ hydromorphone ▪ imipenem/cilastatin ▪ lorazepam ▪ methylprednisolone sodium succinate ▪ mitomycin ▪ morphine ▪ nalbuphine ▪ ondansetron ▪ piperacillin ▪ sodium bicarbonate ▪ tobramycin.
- **Additive Incompatibility:** ▪ Do not admix with other medications.

PATIENT/FAMILY TEACHING

- □ Instruct patient to notify nurse or physician if dyspnea or palpitations occur.

EVALUATION

Effectiveness of therapy can be demonstrated by: ▪ Acceleration of bone marrow recovery and decreased incidence of infection in patients following autologous and allogenic bone marrow transplantation, bone marrow transplant failure or engraftment delay, chemotherapy for AML, and PBPC transplantation.

S

SCOPOLAMINE

(scoe-**pol**-a-meen)
Isopto Hyoscine, Transderm-Scōp, {Transderm-V}

CLASSIFICATION(S):
Anticholinergic, Antiemetic

Pregnancy Category C

INDICATIONS

▪ **Transdermal:** Prevention of motion sickness ▪ Management of nausea and vomiting associated with opioid analgesia or general anesthesia ▪ **IM, IV, SC:** Preoperatively to produce amnesia and to decrease salivation and excessive respiratory secretions.

ACTION

▪ Inhibits the muscarinic activity of acetylcholine ▪ Corrects the imbalance of acetylcholine and norepinephrine in the CNS, which may be responsible for motion sickness. **Therapeutic Effects:** ▪ Reduction of nausea and vomiting ▪ Preoperative amnesia and decreased secretions.

PHARMACOKINETICS

Absorption: Well absorbed following IM, SC, and transdermal administration.
Distribution: Crosses the placenta and blood-brain barrier.

{} = Available in Canada only.

Metabolism and Excretion: Mostly metabolized by the liver.
Half-life: 8 hr.

CONTRAINDICATIONS AND PRECAUTIONS

Contraindicated in: ▪ Hypersensitivity ▪ Hypersensitivity to bromides (injection only) ▪ Narrow-angle glaucoma ▪ Acute hemorrhage ▪ Tachycardia secondary to cardiac insufficiency or thyrotoxicosis.
Use Cautiously in: ▪ Geriatric patients, infants, and children (increased risk of adverse reactions) ▪ Possible intestinal obstruction ▪ Prostatic hypertrophy ▪ Chronic renal, hepatic, pulmonary, or cardiac disease ▪ Pregnancy or lactation (safety not established).

ADVERSE REACTIONS AND SIDE EFFECTS*

CNS: drowsiness, confusion.
EENT: blurred vision, mydriasis, photophobia.
CV: tachycardia, palpitations.
GI: dry mouth, constipation.
GU: urinary hesitancy, urinary retention.
Derm: decreased sweating.

INTERACTIONS

Drug-Drug: ▪ Additive anticholinergic effects with **antihistamines, antidepressants, quinidine**, or **disopyramide** ▪ Additive CNS depression with **alcohol, antidepressants, antihistamines, opioid analgesics**, or **sedative/hypnotics** ▪ May alter the absorption of other **orally administered drugs** by slowing motility of the GI tract ▪ May increase GI mucosal lesions in patients taking oral **wax-matrix potassium chloride preparations.**

ROUTE AND DOSAGE

- **Transdermal (Adults):** —1.5 mg Transderm-Scōp system delivers 1 mg over 72 hr; for motion sickness, apply 4 hr prior to travel (US product).
- **IM, IV, SC (Adults):** *Antiemetic/anticholinergic*—0.3–0.65 mg; *antisecretory effect*—0.2–0.6 mg; *amnestic effect*—0.32–0.65 mg; *sedation*—0.6 mg 3–4 times daily.
- **IM, IV, SC (Children):** *Antiemetic/anticholinergic*—6 mcg/kg or 0.2 mg/m².
- **IM (Children 8–12 yr):** *Antisecretory*—0.3 mg.
- **IM (Children 3–8 yr):** *Antisecretory*—0.2 mg.
- **IM (Children 7 mo–3 yr):** *Antisecretory*—0.15 mg.
- **IM (Children 4–7 mo):** *Antisecretory*—0.1 mg.

AVAILABILITY

▪ ***Transdermal therapeutic system:*** *Transderm-Scōp*—1.5 mg scopolamine/patch releases 0.5 mg scopolamine over 3 days in packs of 4 units[Rx], {*Transderm-V*—1.5 mg scopolamine/patch releases 1 mg scopolamine over 3 days[Rx]} ▪ ***Injection:*** 0.3 mg/ml in 1-ml vials[Rx], 0.4 mg/ml in 0.5-ml ampules and 1-ml vials[Rx], 0.86 mg/ml in 0.5-ml ampules[Rx], 1 mg/ml in 1-ml vials[Rx].

TIME/ACTION PROFILE (antiemetic, sedative properties)

	ONSET	PEAK	DURATION
PO, IM, SC	30 min	1 hr	4–6 hr
IV	10 min	1 hr	2–4 hr
Transdermal	4 hr	UK	72 hr

NURSING IMPLICATIONS

ASSESSMENT

- **General Info:** Assess patient for signs of urinary retention periodically throughout therapy.
  - Monitor heart rate periodically throughout parenteral therapy.
  - Assess patient for pain prior to administration. Scopolamine may act as a stimulant in the presence of pain, producing delirium if used without morphine or meperidine.
- **Antiemetic:** Assess patient for nausea and vomiting periodically during therapy.

POTENTIAL NURSING DIAGNOSES

- Oral mucous membrane, altered (Indications, Side Effects).
- Injury, risk for (Side Effects).
- Knowledge deficit, related to medication regimen (Patient/Family Teaching).

*CAPITALS indicate life-threatening; underlines indicate most frequent.

IMPLEMENTATION

- **Direct IV:** Scopolamine should be diluted with sterile water for injection prior to IV administration. Inject slowly.
- **Syringe Compatibility:** ▪ benzquinamide ▪ butorphanol ▪ chlorpromazine ▪ cimetidine ▪ diphenhydramine ▪ droperidol ▪ fentanyl ▪ hydromorphone ▪ meperidine ▪ metoclopramide ▪ midazolam ▪ morphine ▪ nalbuphine ▪ pentazocine ▪ pentobarbital ▪ perphenazine ▪ prochlorperazine ▪ promazine ▪ promethazine ▪ ranitidine ▪ sufentanil ▪ thiopental.
- **Y-Site Compatibility:** ▪ heparin ▪ hydrocortisone sodium succinate ▪ potassium chloride ▪ sufentanil ▪ vitamin B complex with C.

PATIENT/FAMILY TEACHING

- **General Info:** Instruct patient to take medication exactly as directed. If a dose is missed, take as soon as remembered. Do not double doses.
- □ Medication may cause drowsiness or blurred vision. Caution patient to avoid driving or other activities requiring alertness until response to medication is known.
- □ Patient should use caution when exercising and in hot weather; overheating may result in heatstroke.
- □ Advise patient to avoid concurrent use of alcohol and other CNS depressants with this medication.
- □ Inform patient that frequent mouth rinses, good oral hygiene, and sugarless gum or candy may minimize dry mouth.
- **Transdermal:** Instruct patient on application of transdermal patches. Apply at least 4 hr (US product) before exposure to travel to prevent motion sickness. Wash hands and dry thoroughly before and after application. Apply to hairless, clean, dry area behind ear; avoid areas with cuts or irritation. Apply pressure over system to ensure contact with skin. System is effective for 3 days. If system becomes dislodged, replace with a new system on another site behind the ear. System is waterproof and not affected by bathing or showering.
- □ Instruct patient to remove patch and notify health care professional immediately if symptoms of acute narrow-angle glaucoma (pain or reddening of the eyes with pupil dilation) occur.
- □ Caution patients engaging in underwater sports of potentially distorting effects of scopolamine.

EVALUATION

Effectiveness of therapy can be demonstrated by: ▪ Decrease in salivation and respiratory secretion preoperatively ▪ Postoperative amnesia ▪ Prevention of motion sickness ▪ Prevention and treatment of opioid- or anesthesia-induced nausea and vomiting.

SELEGILINE

(se-**le**-ji-leen)

Carbex, Eldepryl, {Novo-selegiline}, SD-Deprenyl

CLASSIFICATION(S):

Anti-Parkinson agent (monoamine oxidase type B inhibitor)

Pregnancy Category C

INDICATIONS

▪ Management of Parkinson's disease (with levodopa or levodopa/carbidopa) in patients who fail to respond to levodopa/carbidopa alone.

ACTION

▪ Following conversion by monoamine oxidase to its active form, selegiline inactivates monoamine oxidase by irreversibly binding to it at type B (brain) sites ▪ Inactivation of monoamine oxidase leads to increased amounts of dopamine available in the CNS. **Therapeutic Effects:** ▪ Increased response to levodopa/dopamine therapy in Parkinson's disease.

PHARMACOKINETICS

Absorption: Appears to be well absorbed following oral administration.

Distribution: Widely distributed.

Metabolism and Excretion: Metabolism involves some conversion to amphetamine and methamphetamine. 45% excreted in urine as metabolites.

Half-life: UK.

S

{} = Available in Canada only.

CONTRAINDICATIONS AND PRECAUTIONS

Contraindicated in: ▪ Hypersensitivity ▪ Concurrent meperidine or opioid analgesic therapy (possible fatal reactions) ▪ Concurrent use of SSRIs or tricyclic antidepressants.
Use Cautiously in: ▪ Doses >10 mg/day (increased risk of hypertensive reactions with tyramine-containing foods and some medications) ▪ History of peptic ulcer disease.

ADVERSE REACTIONS AND SIDE EFFECTS*

CNS: confusion, dizziness, fainting, hallucinations, insomnia, vivid dreams.
GI: nausea, abdominal pain, dry mouth.

INTERACTIONS

Drug-Drug: ▪ Concurrent use with **meperidine** or other **opioids** may possibly result in a potentially fatal reaction (excitation, sweating, rigidity, and hypertension; or hypotension and coma) ▪ Serotonin syndrome (confusion, agitation, hyperpyrexia, hypertension, seizures) may occur with concurrent use of **SSRI antidepressants** (fluoxetine should be discontinued 5 wk prior to selegiline), venlafaxine should be discontinued 7 days before selegiline, other agents should be discontinued 2 wk before selegiline). Selegiline should be discontinued 2 wk before SSRI's are initiated ▪ Concurrent use with **tricyclic antidepressants** may result in asystole, diaphoresis, hypertension, syncope, behavioral changes, altered consciousness, hyperpyrexia, tremors, muscle rigidity, and seizures (avoid concurrent use; discontinue selegiline 2 wk before initiating tricyclic antidepressant therapy) ▪ May initially increase risk of side effects of **levodopa/carbidopa** (dosage of levodopa/carbidopa may need to be decreased by 10–30%).
Drug-Food: ▪ Doses >10 mg/day may produce hypertensive reactions with **tyramine-containing foods** (see list in Appendix K).

ROUTE AND DOSAGE

- **PO (Adults):** 5 mg bid, with breakfast and lunch (some patients may require further dividing of doses—2.5 mg 4 times daily).

AVAILABILITY

▪ ***Capsules:*** 5 mg[Rx] ▪ ***Tablets:*** 5 mg[Rx].

TIME/ACTION PROFILE (onset of beneficial effects in Parkinson's disease)

	ONSET	PEAK	DURATION
PO	2–3 days	UK	UK

NURSING IMPLICATIONS

ASSESSMENT

- □ Assess patient for signs and symptoms of Parkinson's disease (tremor, muscle weakness and rigidity, ataxic gait) prior to and throughout therapy.
- □ Assess blood pressure periodically throughout therapy.

POTENTIAL NURSING DIAGNOSES

- Physical mobility, impaired (Indications).
- Injury, risk for (Indications, Side Effects).
- Knowledge deficit, related to medication regimen (Patient/Family Teaching).

IMPLEMENTATION

- **General Info:** An attempt to reduce the dose of levodopa/carbidopa by 10–30% may be made after 2–3 days of selegiline therapy.
- **PO:** Administer 5-mg tablet with breakfast and lunch.

PATIENT/FAMILY TEACHING

- □ Instruct patient to take medication exactly as directed. Missed doses should be taken as soon as possible, but not if late afternoon or evening or almost time for next dose. Do not double doses. Caution patient that taking more than the prescribed dose may increase side effects and place patient at risk for hypertensive crisis if foods containing tyramine are consumed (see Appendix K).
- □ Advise patients taking selegiline ≥20 mg/day to avoid large amounts of tyramine-containing foods (see Appendix K), alcoholic beverages, large quantities of caffeine-containing beverages, or OTC cough or cold medications.
- □ Inform patient and family of the signs and symptoms of MAO inhibitor–induced hypertensive crisis (severe headache, chest pain,

*CAPITALS indicate life-threatening; underlines indicate most frequent.

nausea, vomiting, photosensitivity, enlarged pupils). Advise patient to notify health care professional immediately if severe headache or any other unusual symptom occurs.

- Caution patient to change positions slowly to minimize orthostatic hypotension.
- Advise patient that increasing fluids, sugarless gum or candy, ice, or saliva substitutes may help minimize dry mouth. Consult health care professional if dry mouth continues for >2 wk.

EVALUATION

Effectiveness of therapy can be demonstrated by: ▪ Improved response to levodopa/carbidopa in patients with Parkinson's disease.

SENNA, SENNOSIDES

(**se**-na, **sen**-oh-sides)

Black-Draught, Dosaflext, Dr. Caldwell Senna Laxative, Ex-Lax Gentle Nature Laxative Pills, Fletchers' Castoria, Sena-Gen, Senexon, Senna-tural, Senna X-Prep Liquid, Senokot, Senokot Syrup, SenokotXTRA, Senolax

CLASSIFICATION(S):
Laxative (stimulant)

Pregnancy Category C

INDICATIONS

▪ Treatment of constipation, particularly when associated with: ▫ Slow transit time ▫ Constipating drugs ▫ Irritable or spastic bowel syndrome ▫ Neurologic constipation.

ACTION

▪ Active components of senna (sennosides) alter water and electrolyte transport in the large intestine, resulting in accumulation of water and increased peristalsis. **Therapeutic Effects:** ▪ Laxative action.

PHARMACOKINETICS

Absorption: Minimally absorbed following oral administration.
Distribution: UK.
Metabolism and Excretion: UK.
Half-life: UK.

CONTRAINDICATIONS AND PRECAUTIONS

Contraindicated in: ▪ Hypersensitivity ▪ Abdominal pain of unknown cause, especially if associated with fever ▪ Rectal fissures ▪ Ulcerated hemorrhoids ▪ Known alcohol intolerance (some liquid products).
Use Cautiously in: ▪ Chronic use (may lead to laxative dependence) ▪ Possible intestinal obstruction ▪ Pregnancy or lactation (safety not established; may be used safely during breast-feeding).

ADVERSE REACTIONS AND SIDE EFFECTS*

GI: <u>cramping</u>, <u>diarrhea</u>, nausea.
GU: pink-red or brown-black discoloration of urine.
F and E: electrolyte abnormalities (chronic use or dependence).
Misc: laxative dependence.

INTERACTIONS

Drug-Drug: ▪ May decrease absorption of other **orally administered drugs** because of decreased transit time.

ROUTE AND DOSAGE

Larger doses have been used to treat/prevent opioid-induced constipation.

- **PO (Adults and Children >12 yr):** *Senna*—0.5–2 g; *sennosides*—12–50 mg 1–2 times daily; *evacuation of the bowel prior to colonic radiographic examination*—105–157.5 mg sennosides 12–14 hr prior to exam (in addition to other laxatives).
- **PO (Children 6–11 yr):** 50% of the adult dose.
- **PO (Children 1–5 yr):** 33% of the adult dose.
- **Rect (Adults and Children ≥12 yr):** 30 mg 1–2 times daily.

AVAILABILITY

▫ **Senna Leaf Powder**
▪ ***Tablets:*** 600 mg senna[OTC].

***CAPITALS indicate life-threatening; <u>underlines</u> indicate most frequent.**

❑ **Senna Concentrate**

▪ ***Granules:*** 15 mg sennosides/3g^{OTC} ▪ ***Tablets:*** 8.6 mg sennosides^{OTC}, 17 mg sennosides^{OTC}, 20 mg sennosides^{OTC} ▪ ***Suppositories:*** 30 mg sennosides^{OTC}.

❑ **Senna Fluidextract**

▪ ***Oral solution:*** 3 mg sennosides/ml^{OTC}.

❑ **Senna Fruit Extract**

▪ ***Oral solution:*** 3.25 mg sennosides/5 ml^{OTC}, 8.8 mg/5 ml^{OTC} ▪ ***In combination with:*** psyllium and docusate^{OTC}. See Appendix A.

TIME/ACTION PROFILE (laxative effect)

	ONSET	PEAK	DURATION
PO	6–12 hr*	UK	3–4 days
Rectal	½–2 hr	UK	UK

*May take as long as 24 hr.

NURSING IMPLICATIONS

ASSESSMENT

- Assess patient for abdominal distention, presence of bowel sounds, and usual pattern of bowel function.
- Assess color, consistency, and amount of stool produced.

POTENTIAL NURSING DIAGNOSES

- Constipation (Indications).
- Diarrhea (Side Effects).
- Knowledge deficit, related to medication regimen (Patient/Family Teaching).

IMPLEMENTATION

- **PO:** Take with a full glass of water. Administer at bedtime for evacuation 6–12 hr later. Administer on an empty stomach for more rapid results.
- Shake oral solution well before administering.
- Granules should be dissolved or mixed in water or other liquid before administration.

PATIENT/FAMILY TEACHING

- Advise patient that laxatives should be used only for short-term therapy. Long-term therapy may cause electrolyte imbalance and dependence.
- Encourage patient to use other forms of bowel regulation, such as increasing bulk in the diet, increasing fluid intake, and increasing mobility. Normal bowel habits are individualized and may vary from 3 times/day to 3 times/wk.
- Inform patient that this medication may cause a change in urine color to pink, red, violet, yellow, or brown.
- Instruct patients with cardiac disease to avoid straining during bowel movements (Valsalva maneuver).
- Advise patient not to use laxatives when abdominal pain, nausea, vomiting, or fever is present.

EVALUATION

Effectiveness of therapy can be demonstrated by: ▪ A soft, formed bowel movement.

SERTRALINE

(**ser**-tra-leen)

Zoloft

CLASSIFICATION(S):

Antidepressant (selective serotonin reuptake inhibitor)

Pregnancy Category B

INDICATIONS

▪ Management of the following (in conjunction with psychotherapy): ❑ Depression ❑ Panic disorder ❑ Obsessive-compulsive disorder (OCD).

ACTION

▪ Inhibits neuronal uptake of serotonin in the CNS, thus potentiating the activity of serotonin. Has little effect on norepinephrine or dopamine. **Therapeutic Effects:** ▪ Antidepressant action ▪ Decreased incidence of pain attacks ▪ Decreased obsessive and compulsive behavior.

PHARMACOKINETICS

Absorption: Appears to be well absorbed following oral administration.

Distribution: Extensively distributed throughout body tissues.

Metabolism and Excretion: Extensively metabolized by the liver; 14% excreted unchanged in feces.

Half-life: 26 hr.

CONTRAINDICATIONS AND PRECAUTIONS

Contraindicated in: ▪ Hypersensitivity ▪ Concurrent MAO inhibitor therapy (may result in serious, potentially fatal reactions).

Use Cautiously in: ▪ Severe hepatic or renal impairment ▪ Patients with a history of mania ▪ Children (increased incidence of adverse CNS reactions) ▪ Patients at risk of suicide ▪ Pregnancy or lactation.

ADVERSE REACTIONS AND SIDE EFFECTS*

CNS: dizziness, drowsiness, fatigue, headache, insomnia, agitation, anxiety, confusion, emotional lability, impaired concentration, manic reaction, nervousness, weakness, yawning.
EENT: pharyngitis, rhinitis, tinnitus, visual abnormalities.
CV: chest pain, palpitations.
GI: diarrhea, dry mouth, nausea, abdominal pain, altered taste, anorexia, constipation, dyspepsia, flatulence, increased appetite, vomiting.
GU: sexual dysfunction, menstrual disorders, urinary disorders, urinary frequency.
Derm: increased sweating, hot flashes, rash.
MS: back pain, myalgia.
Neuro: tremor, hypertonia, hypoesthesia, paresthesia, twitching.
Misc: fever, thirst.

INTERACTIONS

Drug-Drug: ▪ Serious, potentially fatal reactions (hyperthermia, rigidity, myoclonus, autonomic instability, with fluctuating vital signs and extreme agitation, which may proceed to delirium and coma) may occur with concurrent **MAO inhibitor** therapy. MAO inhibitors should be stopped at least 14 days prior to sertraline therapy. Sertraline should be stopped at least 14 days prior to MAO inhibitor therapy ▪ Concurrent use with **alcohol** is not recommended ▪ May increase the effect of **warfarin.**

ROUTE AND DOSAGE

❑ Depression/Obsessive-Compulsive Disorder

- **PO (Adults):** 50 mg/day as a single dose in the morning or evening initially; after several weeks may be increased at weekly intervals up to 200 mg/day, depending on response.
- **PO (Children 13–17 yr):** *Obsessive-compulsive disorder*—50 mg once daily.
- **PO (Children 6–12 yr):** *Obsessive-compulsive disorder*—25 mg once daily.

❑ Panic Disorder

- **PO (Adults):** 25 mg/day initially, may increase after 1 wk to 50 mg/day.

AVAILABILITY

▪ ***Tablets:*** 50 mg[Rx], 100 mg[Rx] ▪ ***Capsules:*** {50 mg[Rx]}, {100 mg[Rx]}.

TIME/ACTION PROFILE (antidepressant effect)

	ONSET	PEAK	DURATION
PO	within 2–4 wk	UK	UK

NURSING IMPLICATIONS

ASSESSMENT

- **General Info:** Monitor appetite and nutritional intake. Weigh weekly. Notify physician or other health care professional of continued weight loss. Adjust diet as tolerated to support nutritional status.
- **Depression:** Monitor mood changes. Inform physician or other health care professional if patient demonstrates significant increase in anxiety, nervousness, or insomnia.
- □ Assess for suicidal tendencies, especially during early therapy. Restrict amount of drug available to patient.
- **Obsessive-Compulsive Disorder:** Assess patient for frequency of obsessive-compulsive behaviors. Note degree to which these thoughts and behaviors interfere with daily functioning.
- **Panic Attacks:** Assess frequency and severity of panic attacks.

POTENTIAL NURSING DIAGNOSES

- Coping, ineffective individual (Indications).
- Injury, risk for (Side Effects).
- Knowledge deficit, related to medication regimen (Patient/Family Teaching).

*CAPITALS indicate life-threatening; underlines indicate most frequent.

IMPLEMENTATION

- **General Info:** Periodically reassess dose and continued need for therapy.
- **PO:** Administer as a single dose in the morning or evening.

PATIENT/FAMILY TEACHING

- Instruct patient to take sertraline exactly as directed. If a dose is missed, take as soon as possible and return to regular dosing schedule. Do not double doses.
- May cause drowsiness or dizziness. Caution patient to avoid driving and other activities requiring alertness until response to the drug is known.
- Advise patient to avoid alcohol or other CNS-depressant drugs during therapy and to consult with health care professional before taking other medications with sertraline.
- Inform patient that frequent mouth rinses, good oral hygiene, and sugarless gum or candy may minimize dry mouth. If dry mouth persists for more than 2 wk, consult health care professional regarding use of saliva substitute.
- Advise patient to wear sunscreen and protective clothing to prevent photosensitivity reactions.
- Instruct female patient to inform health care professional if pregnancy is planned or suspected or if she is breast-feeding.
- Advise patient to notify health care professional if headache, weakness, nausea, anorexia, anxiety, or insomnia persists.
- Emphasize the importance of follow-up exams to monitor progress. Encourage patient participation in psychotherapy.

EVALUATION

Effectiveness of therapy can be demonstrated by: ▪ Increased sense of well-being ▫ Renewed interest in surroundings. May require 1–4 wk of therapy to obtain antidepressant effects ▪ Decrease in obsessive-compulsive behaviors ▪ Decrease in frequency and severity of panic attacks.

SIBUTRAMINE

(si-**byoo**-tra-meen)
Meridia

CLASSIFICATION(S):
Appetite suppressant

Schedule IV
Pregnancy Category C

INDICATIONS

▪ Treatment of obesity in patients with body mass index ≥ 30 kg/m^2 (or ≥ 27 kg/m^2 in patients with diabetes, hypertension, or other risk factors) in conjunction with other interventions (dietary restriction, exercise); used to produce and maintain weight loss.

ACTION

▪ Acts as an inhibitor of the reuptake of serotonin, norepinephrine, and dopamine; increases the satiety-producing effects of serotonin. **Therapeutic Effects:** ▪ Decreased hunger with resultant weight loss in obese patients.

PHARMACOKINETICS

Absorption: 77% absorbed, then rapidly undergoes extensive first-pass hepatic metabolism to 2 active metabolites (M_1 and M_2).
Distribution: Widely and rapidly distributed; high concentrations in liver and kidneys.
Metabolism and Excretion: Active metabolites are extensively metabolized to inactive metabolites that are mostly excreted by the kidneys.
Half-life: *M_1 metabolite*—14 hr; *M_2 metabolite*—16 hr.

CONTRAINDICATIONS AND PRECAUTIONS

Contraindicated in: ▪ Hypersensitivity ▪ Anorexia nervosa ▪ Concurrent use of other centrally acting appetite suppressants, MAO inhibitors, SSRIs, sumatriptan, naratriptan, zolmitriptan, dihydroergotamine, dextromethorphan, meperidine, pentazocine, fentanyl, lithium, or tryptophan ▪ Organic causes of obesity (untreated hypothyroidism) ▪ Severe hepatic/renal impairment ▪ Uncontrolled/poorly controlled hypertension ▪ History of coronary artery disease, CHF, arrhythmias, or stroke ▪ Excessive consumption of alcohol ▪ Pregnancy or lactation.
Use Cautiously in: ▪ History of seizures ▪ Narrow-angle glaucoma ▪ Geriatric patients ▪ Children <16 yr (safety not established).

ADVERSE REACTIONS AND SIDE EFFECTS*

CNS: SEIZURES, headache, insomnia, CNS stimulation, dizziness, drowsiness, emotional lability, nervousness.
EENT: laryngitis/pharyngitis, rhinitis, sinusitis.
CV: hypertension, palpitations, tachycardia, vasodilation.
GI: anorexia, constipation, dry mouth, altered taste, dyspepsia, increased appetite, nausea.
GU: dysmenorrhea.
Derm: increased sweating, rash.

INTERACTIONS

Drug-Drug: ▪ Concurrent use of **other centrally acting appetite suppressants, MAO inhibitors, SSRIs, naratriptan, zolmitriptan, sumatriptan, dihydroergotamine, dextromethorphan, meperidine, pentazocine, fentanyl, lithium,** or **tryptophan** may result in potentially fatal "serotinin syndrome" (avoid concurrent use; allow 2 wk between use of MAO inhibitors and sibutramine) ▪ Concurrent use of **decongestants** may increase the risk of hypertension ▪ **Ketoconazole** may increase blood levels and effects.

ROUTE AND DOSAGE

- **PO (Adults):** 10 mg once daily; may be increased to 15 mg/day after 4 wk. Patients who do not tolerate an initial dose of 10 mg/day may be started on 5 mg/day.

AVAILABILITY

- ***Capsules:*** 5 mg[Rx], 10 mg[Rx], 15 mg[Rx].

TIME/ACTION PROFILE (appetite suppression/weight loss)

	ONSET	PEAK	DURATION
PO	days	4 wk	UK

NURSING IMPLICATIONS

ASSESSMENT

- □ Monitor patients for weight loss and adjust concurrent medications (antihypertensives, antidiabetic agents, lipid-lowering agents) as needed.
- □ Monitor blood pressure and heart rate regularly during therapy. Increases in blood pressure or heart rate, especially during early therapy, may require decrease in dose or discontinuation of sibutramine.

POTENTIAL NURSING DIAGNOSES

- Body image disturbance (Indications).
- Nutrition, altered, more than body requirements (Indications).
- Knowledge deficit, related to diet and medication regimen (Patient/Family Teaching).

IMPLEMENTATION

- **PO:** Capsules should be taken once daily without regard to meals.

PATIENT/FAMILY TEACHING

- □ Instruct patient to take medication as directed and not to exceed dose recommended. Medication may need to be discontinued gradually.
- □ Caution patient to avoid using other CNS depressants or excessive amounts of alcohol with this medication.

EVALUATION

Effectiveness of therapy can be demonstrated by: ▪ Slow, consistent weight loss when combined with a reduced-calorie diet. If this does not occur, therapy should be re-evaluated. Loss of at least 10% of initial body weight should occur within 1 yr.

SIMETHICONE

(si-**meth**-i-kone)

Extra Strength Gas-X, Extra Strength Maalox Anti-Gas, {Extra Strength Maalox GRF Gas Relief Formula}, Flatulex, Gas Relief, Gas-X, Genasyme, Maalox Anti-Gas, {Maalox GRF Gas Relief Formula}, Maximum Strength Gas Relief, Maximum Strength Mylanta Gas Relief, Maximum Strength Phazyme, Mylanta Gas, Mylanta Gas Relief, Mylicon Drops, {Ovol}, {Ovol-40}, Phazyme Drops, Phazyme-95, {Phazyme 125}

CLASSIFICATION(S):
Antiflatulent

Pregnancy Category UK

*CAPITALS indicate life-threatening; underlines indicate most frequent.
{} = Available in Canada only.

INDICATIONS

■ Relief of painful symptoms of excess gas in the GI tract that may occur postoperatively or as a consequence of: □ Air swallowing □ Dyspepsia □ Peptic ulcer □ Diverticulitis.

ACTION

■ Causes the coalescence of gas bubbles ■ Does not prevent the formation of gas. **Therapeutic Effects:** ■ Passage of gas through the GI tract by belching or passing flatus.

PHARMACOKINETICS

Absorption: No systemic absorption occurs.
Distribution: Not systemically distributed.
Metabolism and Excretion: Excreted unchanged in the feces.
Half-life: UK.

CONTRAINDICATIONS AND PRECAUTIONS

Contraindicated in: ■ Not recommended for infant colic.
Use Cautiously in: ■ Abdominal pain of unknown cause, especially when accompanied by fever ■ Has been used safely during pregnancy and lactation.

ADVERSE REACTIONS AND SIDE EFFECTS

None significant.

INTERACTIONS

Drug-Drug: ■ None significant.

ROUTE AND DOSAGE

- **PO (Adults):** 40–125 mg qid, after meals and at bedtime (up to 500 mg/day).
- **PO (Children 2–12 yr):** 40 mg 4 times daily.
- **PO (Children <2 yr):** 20 mg 4 times daily (up to 240 mg/day).

AVAILABILITY

■ ***Chewable tablets:*** 40 mg^{OTC}, 80 mg^{OTC}, 125 mg^{OTC}, 150 mg^{OTC} ■ ***Tablets:*** 60 mg^{OTC}, 80 mg^{OTC}, 95 mg^{OTC} ■ ***Capsules:*** {95 mg^{OTC}}, 125 mg^{OTC} ■ ***Drops:*** 40 mg/0.6 ml^{OTC}, {40 mg/1 ml^{OTC}}, {95 mg/1.425 ml^{OTC}} ■ ***In combination with:*** antacids^{OTC}. See Appendix A.

TIME/ACTION PROFILE (antiflatulent effect)

	ONSET	PEAK	DURATION
PO	immediate	UK	3 hr

NURSING IMPLICATIONS

ASSESSMENT

- □ Assess patient for abdominal pain, distention, and bowel sounds prior to and periodically throughout course of therapy. Frequency of belching and passage of flatus should also be assessed.

POTENTIAL NURSING DIAGNOSES

- ■ Pain (Indications).
- ■ Knowledge deficit, related to medication regimen (Patient/Family Teaching).

IMPLEMENTATION

- ■ **PO:** Administer after meals and at bedtime for best results. Shake liquid preparations well prior to administration. Chewable tablets should be chewed thoroughly before swallowing, for faster and more complete results.
- □ Drops can be mixed with 30 ml of cool water, infant formula, or other liquid as directed. Shake well before using.

PATIENT/FAMILY TEACHING

- □ Explain to patient the importance of diet and exercise in the prevention of gas. Also explain that this medication does not prevent the formation of gas.
- □ Advise patient to notify health care professional if symptoms are persistent.

EVALUATION

Effectiveness of therapy can be demonstrated by: ■ Decrease in abdominal distention and discomfort.

SODIUM BICARBONATE

(**soe**-dee-um bye-**kar**-boe-nate)
Baking Soda, Bell-Ans, Citrocarbonate, Neut, Soda Mint

CLASSIFICATION(S):
Antacid, Electrolyte modifier (alkalinizing agent)

Pregnancy Category C

INDICATIONS

■ **PO, IV:** Management of metabolic acidosis ■ **PO, IV:** Used to alkalinize urine and promote excretion of certain drugs in overdosage situations (phenobarbital, aspirin) ■ **PO:** Antacid.

ACTION

■ Acts as an alkalinizing agent by releasing bicarbonate ions ■ Following oral administration, releases bicarbonate, which is capable of neutralizing gastric acid. **Therapeutic Effects:** ■ Alkalinization ■ Neutralization of gastric acid.

PHARMACOKINETICS

Absorption: Following oral administration, excess bicarbonate is absorbed and results in metabolic alkalosis and alkaline urine.
Distribution: Widely distributed into extracellular fluid.
Metabolism and Excretion: Sodium and bicarbonate are excreted by the kidneys.
Half-life: UK.

CONTRAINDICATIONS AND PRECAUTIONS

Contraindicated in: ■ Metabolic or respiratory alkalosis ■ Hypocalcemia ■ Excessive chloride loss ■ As an antidote following ingestion of strong mineral acids ■ Patients on sodium-restricted diets (oral use as an antacid only) ■ Renal failure (oral use as an antacid only) ■ Severe abdominal pain of unknown cause, especially if associated with fever (oral use as an antacid only).
Use Cautiously in: ■ Congestive heart failure ■ Renal insufficiency ■ Concurrent glucocorticoid therapy ■ Chronic use as an antacid (may cause metabolic alkalosis and possible sodium overload).

ADVERSE REACTIONS AND SIDE EFFECTS*

CV: edema.
GI: *PO*—flatulence, gastric distention.
F and E: metabolic alkalosis, hypernatremia, hypocalcemia, hypokalemia, sodium and water retention.
Local: irritation at IV site.
Neuro: tetany.

INTERACTIONS

Drug-Drug: ■ Following oral administration, may decrease the absorption of **ketoconazole** ■ Concurrent use with **calcium-containing antacids** may lead to milk-alkali syndrome ■ Urinary alkalinization may result in decreased **salicylate** or **barbiturate** blood levels; increased blood levels of **quinidine, mexiletine, flecainide,** or **amphetamines;** increased risk of crystalluria from **fluoroquinolones;** decreased effectiveness of **methenamine** ■ May negate the protective effects of enteric-coated products (do not administer within 1–2 hr of each other).

ROUTE AND DOSAGE

Contains 12 mEq of sodium/g.

❑ Alkalinization of Urine

- **PO (Adults):** 48 mEq (4 g) initially. Then 12–24 mEq (1–2 g) q 4 hr (up to 48 mEq q 4 hr) or 1 tsp of powder q 4 hr as needed.
- **PO (Children):** 1–10 mEq/kg (12–120 mg/kg) per day in divided doses.
- **IV (Adults and Children):** 2–5 mEq/kg as a 4–8 hr infusion.

❑ Antacid

- **PO (Adults):** *Tablets/powder*—325 mg–2 g 1–4 times daily or ½ tsp q 2 hr as needed. *Effervescent powder*—3.9–10 g in water after meals; patients >60 yr should receive 1.9–3.9 g after meals.
- **PO (Children 6–12 yr):** 520 mg; may repeat in 30 min.

❑ Systemic Alkalinization/Cardiac Arrest

- **IV (Adults and Children):** *Cardiac arrest/urgent situations*—1 mEq/kg; may repeat 0.5 mEq/kg q 10 min. *Less urgent situations*—2–5 mEq/kg as a 4–8 hr infusion.

AVAILABILITY

■ ***Oral powder:*** (20.9 mEq Na/½ tsp) in 120-, 240-, 480-, and 2400-g containers^OTC ■ ***Tablets*** **:** 325 mg (3.9 mEq Na/tablet)^OTC, {500 mg (6.0 mEq Na/tablet^OTC}, 520 mg (6.2 mEq Na/tablet)^OTC, 650 mg (7.7 mEq Na/tablet)^OTC ■ ***Solution for injection:*** 4.2% (0.5 mEq/ml) in 2.5-, 5-, and 10-ml prefilled syringes^Rx, 5% (0.6 mEq/ml) in 500-ml

***CAPITALS indicate life-threatening; underlines indicate most frequent.**

containers^Rx, 7.5% (0.9 mEq/ml) in 50-ml vials and prefilled syringes and 200-ml vials^Rx, 8.4% (1 mEq/ml) in 10- and 50-ml vials and prefilled syringes^Rx ▪ ***Neutralizing additive solution for injection:*** 4% (0.48 mEq/ml) in 5-ml vials^Rx, 4.2% (0.5 mEq/ml) in 6-ml vials^Rx.

TIME/ACTION PROFILE (PO = antacid effect; IV = alkalinization)

	ONSET	PEAK	DURATION
PO	immediate	30 min	1–3 hr
IV	immediate	rapid	UK

NURSING IMPLICATIONS

ASSESSMENT

▪ **IV:** Assess fluid balance (intake and output, daily weight, edema, lung sounds) throughout therapy. Report symptoms of fluid overload (hypertension, edema, dyspnea, rales/crackles, frothy sputum) if they occur.

□ Assess patient for signs of acidosis (disorientation, headache, weakness, dyspnea, hyperventilation), alkalosis (confusion, irritability, paresthesia, tetany, altered breathing pattern), hypernatremia (edema, weight gain, hypertension, tachycardia, fever, flushed skin, mental irritability), or hypokalemia (weakness, fatigue, U wave on ECG, arrhythmias, polyuria, polydipsia) throughout therapy.

□ Observe IV site closely. Avoid extravasation, as tissue irritation or cellulitis may occur. If infiltration occurs, confer with physician or other health care professional regarding warm compresses and infiltration of site with lidocaine or hyaluronidase.

▪ **Antacid:** Assess patient for epigastric or abdominal pain and frank or occult blood in the stool, emesis, or gastric aspirate.

▪ ***Lab Test Considerations:*** Monitor serum sodium, potassium, calcium, bicarbonate concentrations, serum osmolarity, acid-base balance, and renal function prior to and periodically throughout therapy.

□ Arterial blood gases (ABGs) should be obtained frequently in emergency situations and during parenteral therapy.

□ Monitor urine pH frequently when used for urinary alkalinization.

□ Antagonizes effects of pentagastrin and histamine during gastric acid secretion test. Avoid administration during the 24 hr preceding the test.

POTENTIAL NURSING DIAGNOSES

▪ Gas exchange, impaired (Indications).

▪ Fluid volume excess (Side Effects).

▪ Knowledge deficit, related to medication regimen (Patient/Family Teaching).

IMPLEMENTATION

▪ **General Info:** This medication may cause premature dissolution of enteric-coated tablets in the stomach.

▪ **PO:** Tablets must be taken with a full glass of water.

□ When used in treatment of peptic ulcers, may be administered 1 and 3 hr after meals and at bedtime.

▪ **Direct IV:** Administer direct IV push in arrest situation. Use premeasured ampules or prefilled syringes to ensure accurate dosage. Doses should be based on ABG results. Dose may be repeated every 10 min.

▪ ***Rate:*** May be administered by rapid bolus.

□ Flush IV line before and after administration to prevent incompatible medications used in arrest management from precipitating.

▪ **Continuous Infusion:** May be diluted in dextrose, saline, and dextrose/saline combinations.

▪ ***Rate:*** May be administered over 4–8 hr.

▪ **Y-Site Compatibility:** ▪ acyclovir ▪ amifostine ▪ asparaginase ▪ aztreonam ▪ cefepime ▪ ceftriaxone ▪ cyclophosphamide ▪ cytarabine ▪ daunorubicin ▪ dexamethasone ▪ doxorubicin ▪ etoposide ▪ famotidine ▪ filgrastim ▪ fludarabine ▪ gallium nitrate ▪ granisetron ▪ heparin ▪ ifosfamide ▪ indomethacin ▪ insulin ▪ melphalan ▪ mesna ▪ morphine ▪ paclitaxel ▪ piperacillin/tazobactam ▪ potassium chloride ▪ tacrolimus ▪ teniposide ▪ thiotepa ▪ tolazoline ▪ vancomycin ▪ vitamin B complex with C.

▪ **Y-Site Incompatibility:** ▪ amiodarone ▪ amrinone ▪ calcium chloride ▪ idarubicin ▪ imipenem/cilastatin ▪ leucovorin calcium ▪ midazolam ▪ nalbuphine ▪ ondansetron ▪ oxacillin ▪ sargramostim ▪ verapamil ▪ vincristine ▪ vinorelbine.

▪ **Solution Incompatibility:** ▪ Do not add to Ringer's solution, lactated Ringer's solution, or Ionosol products, as compatibility varies with concentration.

PATIENT/FAMILY TEACHING

- **General Info:** Instruct patient to take medication as directed. A missed dose should be taken as soon as remembered unless almost time for next dose.
- □ Review symptoms of electrolyte imbalance with patients on chronic therapy; instruct patient to notify health care professional if these symptoms occur.
- □ Advise patient not to take milk products concurrently with this medication. Renal calculi or hypercalcemia (milk-alkali syndrome) may result.
- □ Emphasize the importance of regular follow-up examinations to monitor serum electrolyte levels and acid-base balance and to monitor progress.
- **Antacid:** Advise patient to avoid routine use of sodium bicarbonate for indigestion. Dyspepsia that persists >2 wk should be evaluated by a health care professional.
- □ Advise patient on sodium-restricted diet to avoid use of baking soda as a home remedy for indigestion.
- □ Instruct patient to notify health care professional if indigestion is accompanied by chest pain, difficulty breathing, or diaphoresis or if stools become dark and tarry.

EVALUATION

Effectiveness of therapy can be demonstrated by: ▪ Increase in urinary pH ▪ Clinical improvement of acidosis ▪ Enhanced excretion of selected overdoses and poisonings ▪ Decreased gastric discomfort.

SODIUM CHLORIDE

(**soe**-dee-um **klor**-ide)

intravenous

oral

Slo-Salt

CLASSIFICATION(S):

Electrolyte (replacement solution)

Pregnancy Category C

INDICATIONS

▪ **IV:** Hydration and provision of sodium chloride in deficiency states ▪ Maintenance of fluid and electrolyte status in situations in which losses may be excessive (excess diuresis or severe salt restriction) ▪ 0.45% ("half-normal saline") solution is most commonly used for hydration and the treatment of hyperosmolar diabetes ▪ 0.9% ("normal saline") solution is used for: □ Replacement □ Treatment of metabolic alkalosis □ A priming fluid for hemodialysis □ To begin and end blood transfusions ▪ Small volumes of 0.9% sodium chloride (preservative-free or bacteriostatic) are used to reconstitute or dilute other medications ▪ Hypertonic solution (3%, 5%) may be required in situations in which rapid replacement of sodium is necessary: □ Hyponatremia □ Hypochloremia □ Renal failure □ Heart failure ▪ **PO:** Prevention of or management of volume depletion due to salt restriction or heat prostration when excessive sweating occurs during exposures to high temperatures ▪ **Irrigating Solutions:** 0.9% and 0.45% may be used as irrigating solutions.

ACTION

▪ Sodium is a major cation in extracellular fluid and helps maintain water distribution, fluid and electrolyte balance, acid-base equilibrium, and osmotic pressure ▪ Chloride is the major anion in extracellular fluid and is involved in maintaining acid-base balance. Solutions of sodium chloride resemble extracellular fluid ▪ Reduces corneal edema by an osmotic effect. **Therapeutic Effects:** ▪ **IV, PO:** Replacement in deficiency states and maintenance of homeostasis.

PHARMACOKINETICS

Absorption: Well absorbed following oral administration. Replacement solutions of sodium chloride are administered IV only.
Distribution: Rapidly and widely distributed.
Metabolism and Excretion: Excreted primarily by the kidneys.
Half-life: UK.

CONTRAINDICATIONS AND PRECAUTIONS

Contraindicated in: ▪ **IV solution:** □ Hypertonic (3%, 5%) solutions should not be used in patients with elevated, slightly decreased, or normal serum sodium □ Fluid retention or hypernatremia.
Use Cautiously in: ▪ **IV:** Patients prone to metabolic, acid-base, or fluid and electrolyte

S

abnormalities, including: □ Geriatric patients □ Those with nasogastric suctioning □ Vomiting □ Diarrhea □ Diuretic therapy □ Glucocorticoid therapy □ Fistulas □ Congestive heart failure □ Severe renal failure □ Severe liver diseases (additional electrolytes may be required) ▪ Sodium chloride preserved with benzyl alcohol should not be used in neonates ▪ **PO:** Inadequate hydration (water and other electrolytes must be replaced).

ADVERSE REACTIONS AND SIDE EFFECTS*

Seen primarily during PO and IV use.

CV: CONGESTIVE HEART FAILURE, PULMONARY EDEMA, edema.

F and E: hypernatremia, hypervolemia, hypokalemia.

Local: *IV*—extravasation, irritation at IV site.

INTERACTIONS

Drug-Drug: ▪ Excessive amounts of sodium chloride may partially antagonize the effects of **antihypertensive medications** ▪ Use with **glucocorticoids** may result in excess sodium retention.

ROUTE AND DOSAGE

- **IV (Adults):** *0.9% sodium chloride (isotonic)*—1 liter (contains 150 mEq sodium per liter) rate and amount determined by condition being treated. *0.45% sodium chloride (hypotonic)*—1–2 liter (contains 75 mEq sodium per liter), rate and amount determined by condition being treated. *3%, 5% sodium chloride (hypertonic)*—100 ml over 1 hr (3% contains 50 mEq sodium per 100 ml; 5% contains 83.3 mEq sodium per 100 ml).
- **PO (Adults):** 1–2 g 3 times daily.

AVAILABILITY

▪ ***IV solutions:*** 0.45%^Rx^, 0.9%^Rx^, 3%^Rx^, 5%^Rx^ ▪ ***Diluents:*** 0.9%^Rx^ ▪ ***Concentrate for dilution:*** 14.6%^Rx^, 23.4%^Rx^ ▪ ***Tablets:*** 650 mg^OTC^ ▪ ***In combination with:*** dextrose, electrolytes^Rx^.

TIME/ACTION PROFILE (various clinical effects†)

	ONSET	PEAK	DURATION
PO	UK	UK	UK
IV	rapid (min)	end of infusion	UK

†PO, IV = electrolyte effects.

NURSING IMPLICATIONS

ASSESSMENT

- □ Assess fluid balance (intake and output, daily weight, edema, lung sounds) throughout therapy.
- □ Assess patient for symptoms of hyponatremia (headache, tachycardia, lassitude, dry mucous membranes, nausea, vomiting, muscle cramps) or hypernatremia (edema, weight gain, hypertension, tachycardia, fever, flushed skin, mental irritability) throughout therapy. Sodium is measured in relation to its concentration to fluid in the body, and symptoms may change based on patient's hydration status.
- ▪ ***Lab Test Considerations:*** Monitor serum sodium, potassium, bicarbonate, and chloride concentrations and acid-base balance periodically for patients receiving prolonged therapy with sodium chloride.
- □ Monitor serum osmolarity in patients receiving hypertonic saline solutions.

POTENTIAL NURSING DIAGNOSES

- ▪ Fluid volume deficit (Indications).
- ▪ Fluid volume excess (Side Effects).

IMPLEMENTATION

- ▪ **General Info:** Dosage of sodium chloride depends on patient's age, weight, condition, fluid and electrolyte balance, and acid-base balance.
- □ Do not administer bacteriostatic sodium chloride containing benzyl alcohol as a preservative to neonates. This should not be used to reconstitute or to dilute solutions or to flush intravascular catheters in neonates.
- □ Infusion of 0.45% NaCl is hypotonic, 0.9% NaCl is isotonic, and 3% and 5% NaCl are hypertonic.
- ▪ **Intermittent Infusion:** Administer 3% or 5% NaCl via a large vein and prevent infiltration. After the first 100 ml, sodium, chloride, and bicarbonate concentrations should be re-

***CAPITALS indicate life-threatening; underlines indicate most frequent.**

evaluated to determine the need for further administration.

- ***Rate:*** Rate of hypertonic sodium chloride solutions should not exceed 100 ml/hr.
- **Solution Compatibility:** ▪ D5W ▪ D10W ▪ Ringer's and lactated Ringer's injection ▪ dextrose/Ringer's solution combinations ▪ dextrose/lactated Ringer's solution combinations ▪ dextrose/saline combinations ▪ ⅙ M sodium lactate.

PATIENT/FAMILY TEACHING

- ☐ Explain to patient the purpose of the infusion.
- ☐ Advise patients at risk for dehydration due to exposure to extreme temperatures when and how to take sodium chloride tablets.

EVALUATION

Effectiveness of therapy can be demonstrated by: ▪ Prevention or correction of dehydration ▪ Normalization of serum sodium and chloride levels ▪ Prevention of heat prostration during exposure to high temperatures.

SODIUM CITRATE AND CITRIC ACID

(**soe**-dee-um **sye**-trate and **sit**-rik **as**-id)

Bicitra, Oracit, {PMS-Dicitrate}, Shohl's Solution modified

CLASSIFICATION(S):

Antiurolithic, Electrolyte modifier (alkalinizing agent)

Pregnancy Category C

INDICATIONS

▪ Management of chronic metabolic acidosis associated with chronic renal insufficiency or renal tubular acidosis ▪ Alkalinization of urine ▪ Prevention of cystine and urate urinary calculi ▪ Prevention of aspiration pneumonitis during surgical procedures.

ACTION

▪ Converted to bicarbonate in the body, resulting in increased blood pH ▪ As bicarbonate is renally excreted, urine is also alkalinized, increasing the solubility of cystine and uric acid ▪ Neutralizes gastric acid. **Therapeutic Effects:** ▪ Provision of bicarbonate in metabolic acidosis ▪ Alkalinization of the urine ▪ Prevention of cystine and urate urinary calculi ▪ Prevention of aspiration pneumonitis.

PHARMACOKINETICS

Absorption: Well absorbed following oral administration.

Distribution: Rapidly and widely distributed.

Metabolism and Excretion: Rapidly oxidized to bicarbonate, which is excreted primarily by the kidneys. Small amounts (<5%) excreted unchanged by the lungs.

Half-life: UK.

CONTRAINDICATIONS AND PRECAUTIONS

Contraindicated in: ▪ Severe renal insufficiency ▪ Severe sodium restriction ▪ Congestive heart failure, untreated hypertension, edema, or toxemia of pregnancy.

Use Cautiously in: ▪ Pregnancy or lactation (safety not established).

ADVERSE REACTIONS AND SIDE EFFECTS

GI: diarrhea.

F and E: fluid overload, hypernatremia (severe renal impairment), hypocalcemia, metabolic alkalosis (large doses only).

MS: tetany.

INTERACTIONS

Drug-Drug: ▪ May partially antagonize the effects of **antihypertensives** ▪ Urinary alkalinization may result in decreased **salicylate** or **barbiturate** blood levels or increased blood levels of **quinidine, flecainide,** or **amphetamines.**

ROUTE AND DOSAGE

Adjust dosage according to urine pH. Contains 1 mEq sodium and 1 mEq bicarbonate/ml solution.

☐ Alkalinizer

- **PO (Adults):** 10–30 ml solution diluted in water qid.
- **PO (Children):** 5–15 ml solution diluted in water qid.

S

❑ **Antiurolithic**

- **PO (Adults):** 10–30 ml solution diluted in water qid.

❑ **Neutralization of Gastric Acid**

- **PO (Adults):** 15 ml solution diluted in 15 ml of water.

AVAILABILITY

- ***Oral solution:*** 500 mg sodium citrate/334 mg citric acid/5 ml (Bicitra, PMS-Dicitrate)[Rx], 490 mg sodium citrate/640 mg citric acid/5 ml (Oracit)[Rx].

TIME/ACTION PROFILE (effects on serum pH)

	ONSET	PEAK	DURATION
PO	rapid (min–hr)	UK	4–6 hr

NURSING IMPLICATIONS

ASSESSMENT

- Assess patient for signs of alkalosis (confusion, irritability, paresthesia, tetany, altered breathing pattern) or hypernatremia (edema, weight gain, hypertension, tachycardia, fever, flushed skin, mental irritability) throughout therapy.
- Monitor patients with renal dysfunction for fluid overload (discrepancy in intake and output, weight gain, edema, rales/crackles, and hypertension).
- ***Lab Test Considerations:*** Prior to and every 4 mo throughout chronic therapy, monitor hematocrit, hemoglobin, electrolytes, pH, creatinine, urinalysis, and 24-hr urine for citrate.
- Monitor urine pH if used to alkalinize urine.

POTENTIAL NURSING DIAGNOSES

- Knowledge deficit, related to medication regimen (Patient/Family Teaching).

IMPLEMENTATION

- **PO:** Solution is more palatable if chilled. Administer with 30–90 ml of chilled water. Administer 30 min after meals or as bedtime snack to minimize saline laxative effect.
- When used as preanesthetic, administer 15–30 ml of sodium citrate with 15–30 ml of chilled water.

PATIENT/FAMILY TEACHING

- Instruct patient to take as directed. Missed doses should be taken within 2 hr. Do not double doses.
- Instruct patients receiving chronic sodium citrate on correct method of monitoring urine pH, maintenance of alkaline urine, and the need to increase fluid intake to 3000 ml/day. When treatment is discontinued, pH begins to fall toward pretreatment levels.
- Advise patients receiving long-term therapy on need to avoid salty foods.

EVALUATION

Effectiveness of therapy can be demonstrated by: ▪ Correction of metabolic acidosis ▪ Maintenance of alkaline urine with resulting decreased stone formation ▪ Buffering the pH of gastric secretions, thereby preventing aspiration pneumonitis associated with intubation and anesthesia.

SODIUM PHOSPHATE

(**soe**-dee-um **foss**-fate)

CLASSIFICATION(S):
Electrolyte (phosphate supplement)

Pregnancy Category C

INDICATIONS

- Treatment and prevention of phosphate depletion in patients who are unable to ingest adequate dietary phosphates.

ACTION

- Phosphate is present in bone and is involved in energy transfer and carbohydrate metabolism ▪ Serves as a buffer for the excretion of hydrogen ions by the kidney. **Therapeutic Effects:** ▪ Replacement of phosphorus in deficiency states.

PHARMACOKINETICS

Absorption: Administered IV only, resulting in complete bioavailability.
Distribution: Phosphates enter extracellular fluids and are then actively transported to sites of action.
Metabolism and Excretion: Excreted mainly (>90%) by the kidneys.
Half-life: UK.

CONTRAINDICATIONS AND PRECAUTIONS

Contraindicated in: ▪ Hyperphosphatemia ▪ Hypocalcemia ▪ Severe renal impairment.
Use Cautiously in: ▪ Hyperparathyroidism ▪ Cardiac disease ▪ Hypernatremia ▪ Hypertension.

ADVERSE REACTIONS AND SIDE EFFECTS*

Related to hyperphosphatemia, unless otherwise indicated.
CNS: confusion, listlessness, weakness.
Resp: *hypernatremia*—shortness of breath.
CV: ARRHYTHMIAS, CARDIAC ARREST, ECG changes (absent P waves, widening of the QRS complex with biphasic curve), hypotension; *hypernatremia*—edema.
GI: diarrhea, abdominal pain, nausea, vomiting.
F and E: hyperkalemia, hypernatremia, hyperphosphatemia, hypocalcemia, hypomagnesemia.
Local: irritation at IV site, phlebitis.
MS: *hypocalcemia*—tremors.
Neuro: flaccid paralysis, heaviness of legs, paresthesias of extremities.

INTERACTIONS

Drug-Drug: ▪ Concurrent use of **glucocorticoids** with sodium phosphate may result in hypernatremia.

ROUTE AND DOSAGE

- **IV (Adults):** 12–15 mM phosphorus/liter of parenteral nutrition.
- **IV (Neonates):** 1.5–2 mM/kg/day (infused as part of parenteral nutrition).

AVAILABILITY

▪ ***IV injection for dilution:*** 3 mM phosphate and 4 mEq sodium/ml in 10-, 15-, 30-, and 50-ml vials[Rx].

TIME/ACTION PROFILE (effects on serum phosphate levels)

	ONSET	PEAK	DURATION
IV	rapid (min–hr)	end of infusion	UK

NURSING IMPLICATIONS

ASSESSMENT

- □ Assess patient for signs and symptoms of hypophosphatemia (anorexia, weakness, decreased reflexes, bone pain, confusion, blood dyscrasias) throughout therapy.
- □ Monitor intake and output ratios and daily weight. Report significant discrepancies.
- ▪ ***Lab Test Considerations:*** Monitor serum phosphate, potassium, sodium, and calcium levels prior to and periodically throughout therapy. Increased phosphate may cause hypocalcemia.
- □ Monitor renal function studies prior to and periodically throughout therapy.
- ▪ ***Toxicity and Overdose:*** Symptoms of toxicity are those of hyperphosphatemia or hypocalcemia (paresthesia, muscle twitching, laryngospasm, colic, cardiac arrhythmias, Chvostek's or Trousseau's signs) or hypernatremia (thirst; dry, flushed skin; fever; tachycardia; hypotension; irritability; decreased urine output).

POTENTIAL NURSING DIAGNOSES

- ▪ Nutrition, altered, less than body requirements (Indications).
- ▪ Knowledge deficit, related to medication regimen (Patient/Family Teaching).

IMPLEMENTATION

- ▪ **General Info:** Available in oral form in combination with potassium phosphate to acidify urine and to prevent formation of renal calculi (see potassium and sodium phosphates monograph on p. 828).
- ▪ **IV:** Administer IV only in dilute concentrations and infuse slowly.
- ▪ **Additive Incompatibility:** ▪ calcium ▪ magnesium.

PATIENT/FAMILY TEACHING

- □ Explain purpose of the medication to patient.

EVALUATION

Effectiveness of therapy can be demonstrated by: ▪ Prevention and correction of serum phosphate deficiency.

***CAPITALS indicate life-threatening; underlines indicate most frequent.**

SODIUM POLYSTYRENE SULFONATE

(**soe**-dee-um po-lee-**stye**-reen **sul**-fon-ate)

Kayexalate, {K-Exit}, Kionex, {PMS-Sodium Polystyrene Sulfonate}, SPS

CLASSIFICATION(S):
Electrolyte modifier (cation exchange resin)

Pregnancy Category C

INDICATIONS

▪ Mild to moderate hyperkalemia (if severe, more immediate measures such as sodium bicarbonate IV, calcium, or glucose/insulin infusion should be instituted).

ACTION

▪ Exchanges sodium ions for potassium ions in the intestine (each 1 g is exchanged for 0.5–1 mEq potassium). **Therapeutic Effects:** ▪ Reduction of serum potassium levels.

PHARMACOKINETICS

Absorption: Distributed throughout the intestine but is nonabsorbable.
Distribution: Not distributed.
Metabolism and Excretion: Eliminated in the feces.
Half-life: UK.

CONTRAINDICATIONS AND PRECAUTIONS

Contraindicated in: ▪ Life-threatening hyperkalemia (other, more immediate measures should be instituted) ▪ Hypersensitivity to saccharin or parabens (some products) ▪ Ileus ▪ Known alcohol intolerance (suspension only).
Use Cautiously in: ▪ Geriatric patients ▪ Congestive heart failure, hypertension, edema ▪ Sodium restriction ▪ Constipation.

ADVERSE REACTIONS AND SIDE EFFECTS*

GI: constipation, fecal impaction, anorexia, gastric irritation, nausea, vomiting.
F and E: hypocalcemia, hypokalemia, sodium retention.

INTERACTIONS

Drug-Drug: ▪ Administration with **calcium** or **magnesium-containing antacids** may decrease resin-exchanging ability and increase risk of systemic alkalosis ▪ Hypokalemia may enhance **digitalis glycoside** toxicity.

ROUTE AND DOSAGE

4 level tsp = 15 g (4.1 mEq sodium/g).
- **PO (Adults):** 15 g 1–4 times daily in water or sorbitol (up to 40 g 4 times daily).
- **Rect (Adults):** 25–100 g as a retention enema; repeat as needed.
- **PO, Rect (Children):** 1 g/kg/dose.

AVAILABILITY

▪ ***Suspension:*** 15 g sodium polystyrene sulfonate with 20 g sorbitol/60 ml[Rx], 15 g sodium polystyrene sulfonate with 14.1 g sorbitol/60 ml[Rx] ▪ ***Powder:*** 15 g/4 level tsp[Rx].

TIME/ACTION PROFILE (decrease in serum potassium)

	ONSET	PEAK	DURATION
PO	2–12 hr	UK	6–24 hr
Rect	2–12 hr	UK	4–6 hr

NURSING IMPLICATIONS

ASSESSMENT

- ☐ Monitor response of symptoms of hyperkalemia (fatigue, muscle weakness, paresthesia, confusion, dyspnea, peaked T waves, depressed ST segments, prolonged QT segments, widened QRS complexes, loss of P waves, and cardiac arrhythmias). Assess for development of hypokalemia (weakness, fatigue, arrhythmias, flat or inverted T waves, prominent U waves).
- ☐ Monitor intake and output ratios and daily weight. Assess for symptoms of fluid overload (dyspnea, rales/crackles, jugular venous distention, peripheral edema). Concurrent low-sodium diet may be ordered for patients with congestive heart failure (see Appendix K for foods included).

{} = Available in Canada only.
***CAPITALS indicate life-threatening; underlines indicate most frequent.**

- □ In patients receiving concurrent cardiac glycosides, assess for symptoms of digitalis toxicity (anorexia, nausea, vomiting, visual disturbances, arrhythmias).
- □ Assess abdomen and note character and frequency of stools. Concurrent sorbitol or laxatives may be ordered to prevent constipation or impaction. Some products contain sorbitol to prevent constipation. Patient should ideally have 1–2 watery stools each day during course of therapy.
- ▪ ***Lab Test Considerations:*** Monitor serum potassium daily during therapy. Notify physician or other health care professional when potassium decreases to 4–5 mEq/liter.
- □ Monitor renal function and electrolytes (especially sodium, calcium, bicarbonate, and magnesium) prior to and periodically throughout therapy.

POTENTIAL NURSING DIAGNOSES

- ▪ Constipation (Side Effects).
- ▪ Knowledge deficit, related to medication regimen (Patient/Family Teaching).

IMPLEMENTATION

- ▪ **General Info:** Solution is stable for 24 hr when refrigerated.
- □ Consult physician or other health care professional regarding discontinuation of medications that may increase serum potassium (ACE inhibitors, potassium-sparing diuretics, potassium supplements, salt substitutes).
- ▪ **PO:** An osmotic laxative (sorbitol) is usually administered concurrently to prevent constipation.
- □ For oral administration, add prescribed amount of powder to 3–4 ml water/g of powder. Shake well. Syrup may be ordered to improve palatability. Resin cookie or candy recipes are available; discuss with pharmacist or dietitian.
- ▪ **Retention Enema:** Precede retention enema with cleansing enema. Administer solution via rectal tube or 28 French Foley catheter with 30-ml balloon. Insert tube at least 20 cm and tape in place.
- □ For retention enema, add powder to 100 ml of prescribed solution (usually sorbitol or 20% dextrose in water). Shake well to dissolve powder thoroughly; should be of liquid consistency. Position patient on left side and elevate hips on pillow if solution begins to leak. Follow administration of medication with additional 50–100 ml of diluent to ensure administration of complete dose. Encourage patient to retain enema as long as possible, at least 30–60 min.
- □ After retention period, irrigate colon with 1–2 liters of non–sodium-containing solution. Y-connector with tubing may be attached to Foley or rectal tube; cleansing solution is administered through one port of the Y and allowed to drain by gravity through the other port.

PATIENT/FAMILY TEACHING

- □ Explain purpose and method of administration of medication to patient.
- □ Inform patient of need for frequent lab tests to monitor effectiveness.

EVALUATION

Effectiveness of therapy can be demonstrated by: ▪ Normalization of serum potassium levels.

SOTALOL

(**soe**-ta-lole)
Betapace, {Sotacor}

CLASSIFICATION(S):
Antiarrhythmic (group II), Beta-adrenergic blocking agent (nonselective)

Pregnancy Category B

INDICATIONS

▪ Management of life-threatening ventricular arrhythmias.

ACTION

▪ Blocks stimulation of $beta_1$ (myocardial) and $beta_2$ (pulmonary, vascular, and uterine) -adrenergic receptor sites. **Therapeutic Effects:** ▪ Suppression of arrhythmias.

PHARMACOKINETICS

Absorption: Well absorbed following oral administration.

Distribution: Crosses the placenta; enters breast milk.
Metabolism and Excretion: Elimination is mostly renal.
Half-life: 12 hr (increased in renal impairment).

CONTRAINDICATIONS AND PRECAUTIONS

Contraindicated in: ▪ Uncompensated congestive heart failure ▪ Pulmonary edema ▪ Cardiogenic shock ▪ Bradycardia or heart block.
Use Cautiously in: ▪ Renal impairment (increased dosing interval recommended if CCr ≤60 ml/min) ▪ Hepatic impairment ▪ Geriatric patients (increased sensitivity to beta-adrenergic blockers; initial dosage reduction recommended) ▪ Pulmonary disease (including asthma) ▪ Diabetes mellitus (may mask signs of hypoglycemia) ▪ Thyrotoxicosis (may mask symptoms) ▪ Patients with a history of severe allergic reactions (intensity of reactions may be increased) ▪ Pregnancy, lactation, or children (safety not established; may cause fetal/neonatal bradycardia, hypotension, hypoglycemia, or respiratory depression).

ADVERSE REACTIONS AND SIDE EFFECTS*

CNS: fatigue, weakness, anxiety, dizziness, drowsiness, insomnia, memory loss, mental depression, mental status changes, nervousness, nightmares.
EENT: blurred vision, dry eyes, nasal stuffiness.
Resp: bronchospasm, wheezing.
CV: ARRHYTHMIAS, BRADYCARDIA, CONGESTIVE HEART FAILURE, PULMONARY EDEMA, orthostatic hypotension, peripheral vasoconstriction.
GI: constipation, diarrhea, nausea.
GU: impotence, decreased libido.
Derm: itching, rashes.
Endo: hyperglycemia, hypoglycemia.
MS: arthralgia, back pain, muscle cramps.
Neuro: paresthesia.

INTERACTIONS

Drug-Drug: ▪ **General anesthesia, IV phenytoin,** and **verapamil** may cause additive myocardial depression ▪ Additive bradycardia may occur with **digitalis glycosides** ▪ Additive hypotension may occur with other **antihypertensives,** acute ingestion of **alcohol,** or **nitrates** ▪ Concurrent use with **amphetamines, cocaine, ephedrine, epinephrine, norepinephrine, phenylephrine,** or **pseudoephedrine** may result in unopposed alpha-adrenergic stimulation (excessive hypertension, bradycardia) ▪ Concurrent **thyroid** administration may decrease effectiveness ▪ May alter the effectiveness of **insulin** or **oral hypoglycemic agents** (dosage adjustments may be necessary) ▪ May decrease the effectiveness of **beta-adrenergic bronchodilators** and **theophylline** ▪ May decrease the beneficial $beta_1$ cardiovascular effects of **dopamine** or **dobutamine** ▪ Use cautiously within 14 days of **MAO inhibitor** therapy (may result in hypertension).

ROUTE AND DOSAGE

- **PO (Adults):** 80 mg twice daily; may be gradually increased (usual maintenance dose is 160–320 mg/day in 2–3 divided doses; up to 480–640 mg/day).

AVAILABILITY

- ***Tablets:*** 80 mg[Rx], 120 mg[Rx], 160 mg[Rx], 240 mg[Rx].

TIME/ACTION PROFILE (antiarrhythmic effects)

	ONSET	PEAK	DURATION
PO	hrs	2–3 days	8–12 hr

NURSING IMPLICATIONS

ASSESSMENT

- **General Info:** Monitor blood pressure and pulse frequently during dosage adjustment period and periodically throughout therapy. Assess for orthostatic hypotension when assisting patient up from supine position.
- Monitor intake and output ratios and daily weight. Assess patient routinely for evidence of fluid overload (peripheral edema, dyspnea, rales/crackles, fatigue, weight gain, jugular venous distention).
- ***Lab Test Considerations:*** May cause increased BUN, serum lipoprotein, potassium, triglyceride, and uric acid levels.
- May cause increased ANA titers.

*CAPITALS indicate life-threatening; underlines indicate most frequent.

- May cause increase in blood glucose levels.
- ***Toxicity and Overdose:*** Monitor patients receiving beta-adrenergic blocking agents for signs of overdose (bradycardia, severe dizziness or fainting, severe drowsiness, dyspnea, bluish fingernails or palms, seizures). Notify physician or other health care professional immediately if these signs occur.
- Glucagon has been used to treat bradycardia and hypotension.

POTENTIAL NURSING DIAGNOSES

- Cardiac output, decreased (Side Effects).
- Knowledge deficit, related to medication regimen (Patient/Family Teaching).
- Noncompliance, related to medication regimen (Patient/Family Teaching).

IMPLEMENTATION

- **PO:** Take apical pulse prior to administering. If <50 bpm or if arrhythmia occurs, withhold medication and notify physician or other health care professional.
- Administer on an empty stomach, 1 hr before or 2 hr after meals. Administration with food, especially milk or milk products, reduces absorption by approximately 20%.

PATIENT/FAMILY TEACHING

- **General Info:** Instruct patient to take medication exactly as directed, at the same time each day, even if feeling well; do not skip or double up on missed doses. If a dose is missed, it should be taken as soon as possible up to 8 hr before next dose. Abrupt withdrawal may precipitate life-threatening arrhythmias, hypertension, or myocardial ischemia.
- Advise patient to make sure enough medication is available for weekends, holidays, and vacations. A written prescription may be kept in wallet in case of emergency.
- Teach patient and family how to check pulse and blood pressure. Instruct them to check pulse daily and blood pressure biweekly. Advise patient to hold dose and contact physician or other health care professional if pulse is <50 bpm or if blood pressure changes significantly.
- May cause drowsiness or dizziness. Caution patients to avoid driving or other activities that require alertness until response to the drug is known.
- Advise patients to change positions slowly to minimize orthostatic hypotension, especially during initiation of therapy or when dose is increased.
- Caution patient that this medication may increase sensitivity to cold.
- Instruct patient to consult health care professional before taking any OTC medications, especially cold preparations, concurrently with this medication.
- Diabetics should closely monitor blood sugar, especially if weakness, malaise, irritability, or fatigue occurs. Medication may mask tachycardia and increased blood pressure as signs of hypoglycemia, but dizziness and sweating may still occur.
- Advise patient to notify health care professional if slow pulse, difficulty breathing, wheezing, cold hands and feet, dizziness, confusion, depression, rash, fever, sore throat, unusual bleeding, or bruising occurs.
- Instruct patient to inform health care professional of medication regimen prior to treatment or surgery.
- Advise patient to carry identification describing disease process and medication regimen at all times.

EVALUATION

Effectiveness of therapy can be demonstrated by: ▪ Control of arrhythmias without appearance of detrimental side effects.

SPECTINOMYCIN

(spek-tin-oh-**mye**-sin)

Trobicin

CLASSIFICATION(S):

Anti-infective (miscellaneous)

Pregnancy Category B

INDICATIONS

▪ Second-line treatment of gonorrhea and gonococcal urethritis, cervicitis, or proctitis in patients who are infected with penicillin-resistant strains of *Neisseria gonorrhoeae*. ▪ Treatment of gonorrhea and gonococcal urethritis, cervicitis, or proctitis in patients allergic to beta-lactam anti-infectives (including ceftriaxone).

ACTION

▪ Inhibits bacterial protein synthesis at the level of the 30S ribosome. **Therapeutic Effects:** ▪ Bactericidal action against susceptible organisms. **Spectrum:** ▪ Most notable for activity against *N. gonorrhoeae,* including penicillinase-producing strains (PPNG) ▪ Not active against *Treponema pallidum* or *Chlamydia trachomatis*.

PHARMACOKINETICS

Absorption: Rapidly absorbed from IM sites.
Distribution: Concentrates in urine; poor distribution into saliva.
Metabolism and Excretion: Excreted primarily by the kidneys.
Half-life: 1.2–2.8 hr.

CONTRAINDICATIONS AND PRECAUTIONS

Contraindicated in: ▪ Hypersensitivity ▪ Neonates (diluent contains benzyl alcohol).
Use Cautiously in: ▪ Concurrent infection with other sexually transmitted disease (additional anti-infectives may be required) ▪ Pregnancy, lactation, or children (safety not established; has been used).

ADVERSE REACTIONS AND SIDE EFFECTS*

CNS: dizziness, headache, insomnia, nervousness.
GI: nausea, vomiting.
Derm: pruritus, transient rashes, urticaria.
Local: <u>pain</u> at IM site.
Misc: hypersensitivity reactions, including ANAPHYLAXIS, chills, fever.

INTERACTIONS

Drug-Drug: ▪ None significant.

ROUTE AND DOSAGE

- **IM (Adults and Children >45 kg):** 2 g single dose (2 g q 12 hr for 3 days for disseminated gonorrhea).
- **IM (Infants and Children <45 kg):** 40 mg/kg single dose.

AVAILABILITY

▪ ***Powder for injection:*** 2-g vial[Rx], 4-g vial[Rx].

TIME/ACTION PROFILE (blood levels)

	ONSET	PEAK	DURATION
IM	rapid	1 hr	N/A

NURSING IMPLICATIONS

ASSESSMENT

- □ Assess patient for gonorrheal infection (dysuria, urethral discharge, vaginal discharge, perianal discomfort).
- □ Obtain gram-stain smear and specimens for culture and sensitivity prior to initiating therapy. Dose may be given before receiving results.
- □ Monitor patients with history of allergies for hypersensitivity reactions (urticaria, wheezing).
- ▪ ***Lab Test Considerations:*** Additional serologic testing for syphilis should be conducted at the time of therapy and again 3 mo later. Spectinomycin does not cure syphilis, but it may mask symptom development.
- □ When multiple doses are given, increased ALT, BUN, and alkaline phosphatase and decreased hemoglobin, hematocrit, and CCr may occur. Urine output often decreases, but this is not associated with renal toxicity.

POTENTIAL NURSING DIAGNOSES

- ▪ Infection, risk for (Indications).
- ▪ Knowledge deficit, related to safe sex practices (Patient/Family Teaching).

IMPLEMENTATION

- ▪ **IM:** Reconstitute 2-g vial with 3.2 ml provided diluent (bacteriostatic water with 0.9% benzyl alcohol for injection) and 4-g vial with 6.2 ml diluent. Administer deep into well-developed muscle of dorsogluteal site. The 2-g vial yields 5 ml, which can be injected slowly into one site. The 4-g vial yields 10 ml, which should be divided into two 5-ml injections and administered at separate sites. Suspension is stable for 24 hr.
- □ Most patients are concurrently infected with chlamydia and should be treated with tetracycline, erythromycin, or doxycycline.

***CAPITALS indicate life-threatening; <u>underlines</u> indicate most frequent.**

PATIENT/FAMILY TEACHING

□ Discuss need for all sexual contacts to receive treatment. Patient should abstain from sex until repeat tests confirm resolution of infection. Patient should not share washcloths, towels, or underclothes. Review safe sex practices to prevent reinfection.
□ Inform patient that temporary soreness at injection site, nausea, fever, chills, dizziness, and insomnia may occur.
□ Explain need for repeat smears or culture and sensitivity tests 1 wk after treatment to ensure effectiveness of treatment.

EVALUATION

Clinical response to therapy can be evaluated by: ▪ Resolution of the signs and symptoms of gonorrheal urethritis □ Recurrence of symptoms is usually indicative of re-exposure, not treatment failure.

STAVUDINE
(**stav**-yoo-deen)
d4T, Zerit
CLASSIFICATION(S):
Antiretroviral
Pregnancy Category C

INDICATIONS

▪ Treatment of HIV infection in patients who do not respond to or who cannot tolerate conventional therapy.

ACTION

▪ Converted intracellularly to stavudine triphosphate, which inhibits viral DNA synthesis and replication. **Therapeutic Effects:** ▪ Virustatic action against HIV ▪ Decreased viral load and increased cell count ▪ Not curative, but may slow progression of HIV infection and decrease the incidence and severity of its sequelae.

PHARMACOKINETICS

Absorption: Well absorbed following oral administration (78–80% bioavailability).
Distribution: Crosses the blood-brain barrier; enters RBCs and plasma equally.
Metabolism and Excretion: Converted intracellularly to stavudine triphosphate, which is the active drug; 40% excreted unchanged in urine; 50% nonrenally eliminated.
Half-life: *Adults*—1–1.6 hr; *children*—0.9–1.1 hr; *adults with renal impairment*—4.8 hr; *intracellular half-life*—3.5 hr.

CONTRAINDICATIONS AND PRECAUTIONS

Contraindicated in: ▪ Hypersensitivity.
Use Cautiously in: ▪ Patients with a history of alcohol abuse ▪ Patients with a history of liver disease or hepatic impairment ▪ Renal impairment (dosage reduction and/or increased dosing interval recommended if CCr <50 ml/min) ▪ History of peripheral neuropathy ▪ Pregnancy, lactation, or children (safety not established; breast-feeding should be avoided by HIV-infected mothers due to transmission of the virus in breast milk).

ADVERSE REACTIONS AND SIDE EFFECTS*

CNS: headache, insomnia, weakness.
GI: anorexia, diarrhea, pancreatitis.
Hemat: anemia.
MS: arthralgia, myalgia.
Neuro: <u>peripheral neuropathy</u>.

INTERACTIONS

Drug-Drug: ▪ Use cautiously with **drugs causing peripheral neuropathy (chloramphenicol, cisplatin, dapsone, didanosine, ethambutol, ethionamide, hydralazine, isoniazid, lithium, metronidazole, nitrofurantoin, phenytoin, vincristine,** or **zalcitabine**) ▪ Concurrent use with **zidovudine** is not recommended due to possible antiviral antagonism.

ROUTE AND DOSAGE

- **PO (Adults ≥60 kg):** 40 mg q 12 hr.
- **PO (Adults <60 kg):** 30 mg q 12 hr.
- **PO (Children):** 1 mg/kg every 12 hr (not to exceed 40 mg q 12 hr; unlabeled).

AVAILABILITY

▪ ***Capsules:*** 15 mg^{Rx}, 20 mg^{Rx}, 30 mg^{Rx}, 40 mg^{Rx}.

*CAPITALS indicate life-threatening; <u>underlines</u> indicate most frequent.

TIME/ACTION PROFILE (blood levels)

	ONSET	PEAK	DURATION
PO	UK	0.5–1.5 hr	12 hr

NURSING IMPLICATIONS

ASSESSMENT

- Assess patient for change in severity of symptoms of HIV infection and for symptoms of opportunistic infection throughout therapy.
- Monitor patient for signs and symptoms of peripheral neuropathy (tingling, burning, numbness, or pain in hands or feet); may be difficult to differentiate from peripheral neuropathy of severe HIV disease. May resolve if stavudine therapy is discontinued promptly or may temporarily worsen after discontinuation of therapy. If symptoms resolve completely, stavudine therapy may resume at 50% of the regular dose.
- Assess patient for signs of pancreatitis (nausea, vomiting, abdominal pain) periodically throughout therapy. Occurs rarely, but may require discontinuation of therapy.
- ***Lab Test Considerations:*** Monitor viral load CD4 counts prior to and regularly throughout therapy.
- Monitor liver function. May cause elevated levels of AST, ALT, and alkaline phosphatase, which usually resolve following interruption of therapy.
- May cause elevated serum amylase and lipase levels.

POTENTIAL NURSING DIAGNOSES

- Infection, risk for (Indications).
- Knowledge deficit, related to medication regimen (Patient/Family Teaching).

IMPLEMENTATION

- **PO:** May be administered without regard to food.
- Shake solution vigorously prior to administration. Keep refrigerated; discard unused portion after 30 days.

PATIENT/FAMILY TEACHING

- Instruct patient to take stavudine exactly as directed every 12 hr. Emphasize the importance of compliance with full course of therapy, not taking more than the prescribed amount, and not discontinuing without consulting health care professional. If a dose is missed, take as soon as possible unless almost time for next dose. Do not double doses. Caution patient not to share medication with others.
- Inform patient that stavudine does not cure HIV disease and does not reduce the risk of transmission of HIV to others through sexual contact or blood contamination. Caution patient to avoid sexual contact, to use a condom, and to avoid sharing needles or donating blood to prevent spreading HIV to others.
- Instruct patient to notify health care professional promptly if signs of peripheral neuropathy or pancreatitis occur.
- Advise patient not to take other OTC or prescription medications without consulting health care professional.
- Emphasize the importance of regular follow-up exams and blood tests to determine progress and monitor for side effects.

EVALUATION

Effectiveness of therapy can be demonstrated by: ▪ Decrease in viral load and improvement in CD4 counts in patients with advanced HIV infection.

SUCCIMER

(**sux**-i-mer)

Chemet

CLASSIFICATION(S):

Antidote (lead chelator)

Pregnancy Category C

INDICATIONS

▪ Treatment of lead poisoning in children with blood lead levels >45 mcg/dl.

ACTION

▪ Forms a water-soluble compound with lead, allowing urinary elimination of excessive amounts of lead. **Therapeutic Effects:** ▪ Decreased blood lead levels and decreased target organ damage in lead poisoning.

PHARMACOKINETICS

Absorption: Rapidly but variably absorbed following oral administration.

Distribution: UK.
Metabolism and Excretion: Extensively metabolized; 10% excreted unchanged by the kidneys.
Half-life: 2 days.

CONTRAINDICATIONS AND PRECAUTIONS

Contraindicated in: ▪ Hypersensitivity or allergy to succimer ▪ Lactation (should be discouraged during succimer therapy).
Use Cautiously in: ▪ Renal failure (chelates are not dialyzable) ▪ Pregnancy or children <1 yr (safety not established).

ADVERSE REACTIONS AND SIDE EFFECTS*

CNS: dizziness, drowsiness, headache.
EENT: cloudy film in eye, otitis media, plugged ears, watery eyes.
Resp: cough, nasal congestion, rhinorrhea, sore throat.
CV: arrhythmias.
GI: nausea, vomiting, abdominal cramps, anorexia, diarrhea, elevated liver function tests, hemorrhoidal symptoms, metallic taste.
GU: oliguria, proteinuria, voiding difficulty.
Derm: mucocutaneous eruptions, pruritus, rashes.
Hemat: eosinophilia, thrombocytosis.
MS: back, rib, flank pain; leg pain.
Neuro: paresthesia, sensorimotor neuropathy.
Misc: chills, fever, flu-like syndrome, moniliasis.

INTERACTIONS

Drug-Drug: ▪ Not recommended for use with other **chelating agents.**

ROUTE AND DOSAGE

- **PO (Adults and Children):** 10 mg/kg (350 mg/m²) q 8 hr for 5 days, then reduce to 10 mg/kg (350 mg/m²) q 12 hr for 2 more wk. Repeated courses should follow a 2-wk rest period.

AVAILABILITY

- ***Capsules:*** 100 mg[Rx].

TIME/ACTION PROFILE (urinary lead excretion)

	ONSET	PEAK	DURATION
PO	within 2 hr	2–4 hr	8–12 hr

NURSING IMPLICATIONS

ASSESSMENT

- Assess patient and family members for evidence of lead poisoning prior to and frequently throughout therapy. Acute lead poisoning is characterized by a metallic taste, colicky abdominal pain, vomiting, diarrhea, oliguria, and coma. Symptoms of chronic poisoning vary with severity and include anorexia, a blue-black line along the gums, intermittent vomiting, paresthesia, encephalopathy, seizures, and coma.
- Monitor strict intake and output and daily weight. Notify physician or other health care professional of any discrepancies. Patients undergoing succimer therapy should be adequately hydrated.
- Monitor neurologic status closely (level of consciousness, pupil response, movement). Notify physician or other health care professional immediately of any changes.
- Monitor patient for signs of allergic or other mucocutaneous reactions, especially during repeated courses of succimer therapy.
- ***Lab Test Considerations:*** Monitor blood and urine lead levels prior to and periodically throughout therapy. After therapy, monitor patients for rebound of blood levels at least once weekly until stable. Succimer is indicated for treatment of blood lead levels of >45 mcg/dl.
- May cause elevated serum transaminases, alkaline phosphatase, and cholesterol; monitor prior to and at least weekly during therapy.
- May interfere with serum and urine lab tests.

POTENTIAL NURSING DIAGNOSES

- Injury, risk for, poisoning (Indications, Patient/Family Teaching).
- Home maintenance management, impaired (Indications).
- Knowledge deficit, related to medication regimen (Patient/Family Teaching).

S

*CAPITALS indicate life-threatening; underlines indicate most frequent.

IMPLEMENTATION

- **General Info:** Coadministration of succimer with other chelation agents is not recommended. Patients who have received ethylenediamine tetraacetic acid (EDTA) or dimercaprol (BAL) may receive subsequent therapy with succimer after 4 wk.
- □ Course of treatment lasts 19 days. Doses are administered every 8 hr for 5 days and then every 12 hr for 14 days. Unless blood levels indicate prompt treatment is needed, a minimum of 2 wk between courses is recommended.
- **PO:** If patient is unable to swallow the capsule, open capsule and sprinkle medicated beads on a small amount of soft food or place in a spoon and follow with a fruit drink.

PATIENT/FAMILY TEACHING

- □ Discuss need for follow-up appointments to monitor lead levels. Additional treatments may be necessary.
- □ Instruct patient to drink adequate fluids throughout therapy.
- □ Advise patient to notify health care professional if rash occurs.
- □ Consult public health department regarding potential sources of lead poisoning in the home, workplace, and recreational areas. Chelation therapy cannot be used as prophylaxis for lead poisoning.

EVALUATION

Effectiveness of therapy can be demonstrated by: ▪ Decrease in symptoms of lead poisoning □ Decrease in blood lead levels to below 45 mcg/dl, although the normal upper limit is 29 mcg/dl.

SUCCINYLCHOLINE

(sux-sin-il-**koe**-leen)

Anectine, Quelicin, Sucostrin

CLASSIFICATION(S):

Neuromuscular blocking agent (depolarizing)

Pregnancy Category UK

INDICATIONS

▪ Used after induction of anesthesia in surgical procedures to produce skeletal muscle paralysis.

ACTION

▪ Prevents neuromuscular transmission by blocking the effect of acetylcholine at the myoneural junction ▪ Has agonist activity initially, producing fasciculation ▪ Causes the release of histamine ▪ Has no analgesic or anxiolytic effects. **Therapeutic Effects:** ▪ Skeletal muscle paralysis.

PHARMACOKINETICS

Absorption: Well absorbed following deep IM administration.

Distribution: Widely distributed into extracellular fluid. Crosses the placenta in small amounts.

Metabolism and Excretion: 90% metabolized by pseudocholinesterase in plasma. 10% excreted unchanged by the kidneys.

Half-life: UK.

CONTRAINDICATIONS AND PRECAUTIONS

Contraindicated in: ▪ Hypersensitivity to succinylcholine or parabens ▪ Plasma pseudocholinesterase deficiency ▪ Children and neonates (continuous infusions).

Use Cautiously in: ▪ History of malignant hyperthermia ▪ History of pulmonary disease, renal or liver impairment ▪ Geriatric or debilitated patients ▪ Major trauma, burns, or underlying myopathy (increased risk of rhabdomyolysis and hyperkalemia, especially in children or adolescents) ▪ Glaucoma ▪ Electrolyte disturbances ▪ Patients receiving digitalis glycosides ▪ Fractures or muscular spasm ▪ Myasthenia gravis or myasthenic syndromes ▪ Has been used in pregnant women undergoing cesarean section ▪ Neonates and children (increased risk of malignant hyperthermia).

ADVERSE REACTIONS AND SIDE EFFECTS*

Most adverse reactions to succinylcholine are extensions of pharmacologic effects.

Resp: APNEA, bronchospasm.

CV: arrhythmias, bradycardia, hypotension.

***CAPITALS indicate life-threatening; underlines indicate most frequent.**

F and E: HYPERKALEMIA.
MS: RHABDOMYOLYSIS, muscle fasciculation.
Misc: MALIGNANT HYPERTHERMIA, myoglobinemia (↑ in children), myoglobinuria (↑ in children), tachyphylaxis.

INTERACTIONS

Drug-Drug: ▪ Concurrent administration of **cholinesterase inhibitors (echothiophate, isofluorophate, demecarium eyedrops)** reduces pseudocholinesterase activity and intensifies paralysis ▪ Intensity and/or duration of paralysis may be prolonged by pretreatment with **general anesthesia, aminoglycoside anti-infectives, polymyxin B, colistin, clindamycin, lidocaine, quinidine, procainamide, beta-adrenergic blocking agents, lithium, cyclophosphamide, phenelzine, potassium-losing diuretics,** and **magnesium** ▪ Increased risk of adverse cardiovascular reactions with **opioids** or **digitalis glycosides.**

ROUTE AND DOSAGE

IV route is preferred, but deep IM injection may be used in children and patients without vascular access.

❑ Test Dose

- **IV (Adults):** 5–10 mg (0.1 mg/kg), then assess respiratory function.

❑ Short Procedures

- **IV (Adults):** 0.6 mg/kg (range 0.3–1.1 mg/kg); additional doses depend on response.
- **IV (Children):** 1–2 mg/kg; additional doses depend on response (continuous infusion not recommended in children or neonates).

❑ Prolonged Procedures

- **IV (Adults):** 2.5 mg/min infusion (range 0.5–10 mg/min) or 0.6 mg/kg (range 0.3–1.1 mg/kg) initially, then 0.04–0.07 mg/kg as necessary (continuous infusion preferred in adults).

❑ Intramuscular Dosing

- **IM (Adults):** 2.5–4 mg/kg (total dose not to exceed 150 mg).
- **IM (Children):** *Endotracheal intubation*—up to 2.5 mg/kg (total dose not to exceed 150 mg).

❑ Electroshock Therapy

- **IV (Adults):** 10–30 mg 1 min prior to shock (further individualization of dose may be required).
- **IM (Adults):** Up to 2.5 mg/kg (not to exceed 150 mg).

AVAILABILITY

▪ ***Injection:*** 20 mg/ml in 10-ml vials[Rx], 50 mg/ml in 10-ml vials[Rx], 100 mg/ml in 10- and 20-ml vials[Rx] ▪ ***Powder for injection:*** 100 mg/vial[Rx] ▪ ***Powder for infusion:*** 500 mg/vial[Rx], 1 g/vial[Rx].

TIME/ACTION PROFILE (skeletal muscle paralysis)

	ONSET	PEAK	DURATION
IM	up to 3 min	UK	10–30 min
IV	0.5–1 min	1–2 min	4–10 min

NURSING IMPLICATIONS

ASSESSMENT

- ❑ Assess respiratory status continuously throughout use of succinylcholine. Succinylcholine should be used only by individuals experienced in endotracheal intubation, and equipment for this procedure should be immediately available.
- ❑ Monitor neuromuscular response to succinylcholine with a peripheral nerve stimulator intraoperatively. Paralysis is initially selective and usually occurs consecutively in the following muscles: levator muscles of eyelids, muscles of mastication, limb muscles, abdominal muscles, muscles of the glottis, intercostal muscles, and the diaphragm.
- ❑ Monitor ECG, heart rate, and blood pressure throughout use of succinylcholine.
- ❑ Assess patient for history of malignant hyperthermia prior to administration. Monitor for signs of malignant hyperthermia (tachycardia, tachypnea, hypercarbia, jaw muscle spasm, lack of laryngeal relaxation, hyperthermia) throughout administration.
- ❑ Observe patient for residual muscle weakness and respiratory distress during the recovery period.
- ▪ ***Lab Test Considerations:*** May cause hyperkalemia, especially in patients with severe trauma, burns, or neurologic disorders.
- ▪ ***Toxicity and Overdose:*** If overdose occurs, use peripheral nerve stimulator to determine degree of neuromuscular blockade.

S

Maintain airway patency and ventilation until recovery of normal respirations occurs.

POTENTIAL NURSING DIAGNOSES

- Breathing pattern, ineffective (Indications).
- Communication, impaired verbal (Side Effects).

IMPLEMENTATION

- **General Info:** Succinylcholine has no effect on consciousness or the pain threshold. Adequate anesthesia should *always* be used when succinylcholine is used as an adjunct to surgical procedures or when painful procedures are performed. Benzodiazepines and/or analgesics should be administered concurrently when prolonged succinylcholine therapy is used for ventilator patients, as patient is awake and able to feel all sensations.
- □ If eyes remain open throughout prolonged administration, protect corneas with artificial tears.
- □ To prevent excessive salivation, patients may be premedicated with atropine or scopolamine.
- □ A small dose of a nondepolarizing agent may be used prior to succinylcholine to decrease the severity of muscle fasciculations.
- **IM:** If IM route is used, administer deep into the deltoid muscle.
- **IV:** A test dose of 5–10 mg or 0.1 mg/kg may be administered to determine patient's sensitivity and recovery time.
- **Direct IV:** May be administered undiluted.
- ***Rate:*** Usual adult dose is administered over 10–30 sec. Dose is titrated to patient response.
- **Continuous Infusion:** Dilute as a 0.1–0.2% solution (1–2 mg/ml) in dextrose/Ringer's or lactated Ringer's combinations, dextrose/saline combinations, 0.45% NaCl, 0.9% NaCl, D5W, D10W, Ringer's or lactated Ringer's injection. Solution is stable for 24 hr at room temperature. Administer only clear solutions. Discard any unused solution.
- ***Rate:*** Administer at a rate of 0.5–10 mg/min; usual rate is 2.5–4.3 mg/min. Titrate dose to patient response and degree of paralysis required.
- **Y-Site Compatibility:** ▪ etomidate ▪ potassium chloride ▪ vitamin B complex with C.
- **Y-Site Incompatibility:** ▪ thiopental.

PATIENT/FAMILY TEACHING

- □ Explain all procedures to patient receiving succinylcholine therapy without anesthesia, as consciousness is not affected by succinylcholine alone. Provide emotional support.
- □ Reassure patient that communication abilities will return as the medication wears off.

EVALUATION

Effectiveness of therapy can be demonstrated by: ▪ Adequate suppression of the twitch response when tested with peripheral nerve stimulation, with subsequent muscle paralysis.

SUCRALFATE

(soo-**kral**-fate)
Carafate, {Sulcrate}

CLASSIFICATION(S):
Antiulcer agent (protectant)

Pregnancy Category B

INDICATIONS

▪ Short-term management of duodenal ulcers ▪ Maintenance (preventive) therapy of duodenal ulcers. **Unlabeled Uses:** ▪ Management of gastric ulcer or gastroesophageal reflux ▪ Prevention of gastric mucosal injury due to high-dose aspirin or NSAIDs in patients with rheumatoid arthritis or in high-stress situations (ICU). **Suspension:** Mucositis/stomatitis/oral ulceration due to various etiologies.

ACTION

▪ Reacts with gastric acid to form a thick paste, which selectively adheres to the ulcer surface. **Therapeutic Effects:** ▪ Protection of ulcers, with subsequent healing.

PHARMACOKINETICS

Absorption: Systemic absorption is minimal (<5%).
Distribution: UK.
Metabolism and Excretion: >90% is eliminated in the feces.
Half-life: 6–20 hr.

CONTRAINDICATIONS AND PRECAUTIONS

Contraindicated in: ▪ Hypersensitivity.
Use Cautiously in: ▪ Children (safety not established).

ADVERSE REACTIONS AND SIDE EFFECTS*

CNS: dizziness, drowsiness.
GI: constipation, diarrhea, dry mouth, gastric discomfort, indigestion, nausea.
Derm: pruritus, rashes.

INTERACTIONS

Drug-Drug: ▪ May decrease the absorption of **phenytoin, fat-soluble vitamins,** or **tetracycline** ▪ Concurrent **antacids** decrease the effectiveness of sucralfate ▪ Decreases absorption of **fluoroquinolones** (do not administer within 1 hr of each other).

ROUTE AND DOSAGE

❑ **Treatment of Ulcers**

- **PO (Adults):** 1 g qid, 1 hr before meals and at bedtime; or 2 g twice daily, on waking and at bedtime.

❑ **Prevention of Ulcers**

- **PO (Adults):** 1 g twice daily, 1 hr before a meal.

❑ **Gastroesophageal Reflux**

- **PO (Adults):** 1 g qid, 1 hr before meals and at bedtime (unlabeled).
- **PO (Children):** 500 mg–1 g qid, 1 hr before meals and at bedtime (unlabeled).

AVAILABILITY

▪ ***Tablets:*** 1 g[Rx] ▪ ***Oral suspension:*** 500 mg/5 ml[Rx].

TIME/ACTION PROFILE (mucosal protectant effect)

	ONSET	PEAK	DURATION
PO	30 min	UK	5 hr

NURSING IMPLICATIONS

ASSESSMENT

❑ Assess patient routinely for abdominal pain and frank or occult blood in the stool.

POTENTIAL NURSING DIAGNOSES

- Pain (Indications).
- Constipation (Side Effects).
- Knowledge deficit, related to medication regimen (Patient/Family Teaching).

IMPLEMENTATION

- **PO:** Administer on an empty stomach, 1 hr before meals and at bedtime. Do not crush or chew tablets. Shake suspension well prior to administration.

❑ If nasogastric administration is required, consult pharmacist, as protein-binding properties of sucralfate have resulted in formation of a bezoar when administered with enteral feedings and other medications.
❑ If antacids are also required for pain, administer 30 min before or after sucralfate dosage.

PATIENT/FAMILY TEACHING

❑ Advise patient to continue with course of therapy for 4–8 wk, even if feeling better, to ensure ulcer healing. If a dose is missed, take as soon as remembered unless almost time for next dose; do not double doses.
❑ Advise patient that increase in fluid intake, dietary bulk, and exercise may prevent drug-induced constipation.
❑ Emphasize the importance of routine examinations to monitor progress.

EVALUATION

Effectiveness of therapy can be demonstrated by: ▪ Decrease in abdominal pain ❑ Healing of duodenal ulcers, seen by x-ray examination and endoscopy.

SULFAMETHOXAZOLE

(sul-fa-meth-**ox**-a-zole)
{Apo-Sulfamethoxazole}, Gantanol, Urobak

CLASSIFICATION(S):
Anti-infective (sulfonamide)

Pregnancy Category C

S

*CAPITALS indicate life-threatening; underlines indicate most frequent.
{} = Available in Canada only.

INDICATIONS

▪ Treatment of: ▫ Urinary tract infections ▫ Nocardiosis ▫ Toxoplasmosis and malaria (in combination with other anti-infectives).

ACTION

▪ Interferes with bacterial folic acid synthesis. **Therapeutic Effects:** ▪ Bacteriostatic action against susceptible bacteria. **Spectrum:** ▪ Notable for activity against some gram-positive pathogens, including: ▫ Streptococci and staphylococci ▫ *Clostridium perfringens* ▫ *Clostridium tetani* ▫ *Nocardia asteroides* ▪ Active against some gram-negative pathogens, including: ▫ *Enterobacter* ▫ *Escherichia coli* ▫ *Klebsiella* ▫ *Proteus mirabilis* ▫ *Proteus vulgaris* ▫ *Salmonella* ▫ *Shigella*.

PHARMACOKINETICS

Absorption: Well absorbed following oral administration.
Distribution: Widely distributed; crosses the placenta and enters breast milk.
Metabolism and Excretion: Mostly metabolized by the liver (some metabolites may contribute to toxic effects); 20% excreted unchanged by the kidneys.
Half-life: 7–12 hr.

CONTRAINDICATIONS AND PRECAUTIONS

Contraindicated in: ▪ Hypersensitivity ▪ Glucose-6-phosphate dehydrogenase (G6PD) deficiency ▪ Porphyria ▪ Pregnancy or lactation ▪ Infants <2 mo (unless treating congenital toxoplasmosis).
Use Cautiously in: ▪ Geriatric patients (increased risk of adverse reactions) ▪ Severe renal or hepatic impairment.

ADVERSE REACTIONS AND SIDE EFFECTS*

CNS: ataxia, confusion, dizziness, drowsiness, mental depression, psychosis, restlessness.
GI: nausea, anorexia, drug-induced hepatitis, vomiting.
GU: crystalluria.
Derm: rashes, exfoliative dermatitis, photosensitivity.
Hemat: AGRANULOCYTOSIS, APLASTIC ANEMIA, eosinophilia, thrombocytopenia.
Neuro: peripheral neuropathy.
Misc: hypersensitivity reactions including STEVENS-JOHNSON SYNDROME and SERUM SICKNESS, fever, superinfection.

INTERACTIONS

Drug-Drug: ▪ May enhance the action of and increase the risk of toxicity from **oral hypoglycemic agents, phenytoin, methotrexate, warfarin**, or **zidovudine** ▪ Concurrent use with **methenamine** may increase the risk of crystalluria ▪ Increased risk of drug-induced hepatitis with other **hepatotoxic agents.**

ROUTE AND DOSAGE

- **PO (Adults):** 2 g initially, then 1 g q 8–12 hr.
- **PO (Children >2 mo):** 50–60 mg/kg initially (not to exceed 2 g), then 25–30 mg/kg q 12 hr (not to exceed 75 mg/kg/day).

AVAILABILITY

▪ ***Tablets:*** 500 mg[Rx] ▪ ***Oral suspension:*** 500 mg/5 ml[Rx] ▪ ***In combination with:*** trimethoprim (see trimethoprim/sulfamethoxazole monograph on page 1011)[Rx].

TIME/ACTION PROFILE (blood levels)

	ONSET	PEAK	DURATION
PO	1 hr	2 hr	12 hr

NURSING IMPLICATIONS

ASSESSMENT

- ▫ Assess patient for infection (vital signs; appearance of wound, sputum, urine, and stool; WBC) at beginning of and throughout therapy.
- ▫ Obtain specimens for culture and sensitivity prior to initiating therapy. First dose may be given before receiving results.
- ▫ Assess patient for allergy to sulfonamides.
- ▫ Monitor intake and output ratios. Fluid intake should be sufficient to maintain a urine output of at least 1200–1500 ml daily to prevent crystalluria and stone formation.
- ▪ ***Lab Test Considerations:*** Monitor CBC and urinalysis periodically throughout therapy.

*CAPITALS indicate life-threatening; underlines indicate most frequent.

□ May produce elevated serum bilirubin, creatinine, and alkaline phosphatase concentrations.

POTENTIAL NURSING DIAGNOSES

- Infection, risk for (Indications, Side Effects).
- Knowledge deficit, related to medication regimen (Patient/Family Teaching).
- Noncompliance, related to medication regimen (Patient/Family Teaching).

IMPLEMENTATION

- **PO:** Administer around the clock with a full glass of water. Tablets may be crushed and taken with fluid of patient's choice for patients with difficulty swallowing. Use calibrated measuring device for liquid preparations.

PATIENT/FAMILY TEACHING

□ Instruct patient to take medication around the clock and to finish the drug completely as directed, even if feeling better. If a dose is missed, it should be taken as soon as remembered. Advise patient that sharing of this medication may be dangerous.

□ May cause dizziness. Caution patient to avoid driving or other activities requiring alertness until response to medication is known.

□ Caution patient to use sunscreen and protective clothing to prevent photosensitivity reactions.

□ Advise patient to notify health care professional if skin rash, sore throat, fever, mouth sores, or unusual bleeding or bruising occurs.

□ Instruct patient to notify health care professional if symptoms do not improve within a few days. Emphasize the importance of follow-up exams to monitor progress and side effects.

EVALUATION

Clinical response to therapy can be evaluated by: ■ Resolution of the signs and symptoms of infection. Length of time for complete resolution depends on the organism and site of infection.

SULFISOXAZOLE

(sul-fi-**sox**-a-zole)

Apo-Sulfisoxazole, Gantrisin, {Novo-Soxazole}, {Sulfizole}

CLASSIFICATION(S):

Anti-infective (sulfonamide)

Pregnancy Category C

INDICATIONS

■ **PO:** Treatment of urinary tract infections, nocardiosis, and, in combination with other anti-infectives, malaria and pelvic inflammatory disease in prepubertal adolescents. **Unlabeled Uses:** ■ Prevention of recurrent otitis media.

ACTION

■ Interferes with bacterial folic acid synthesis. **Therapeutic Effects:** ■ Bacteriostatic action against susceptible bacteria. **Spectrum:** ■ Notable for activity against some gram-positive pathogens, including: □ Streptococci and staphylococci □ *Clostridium perfringens* □ *Clostridium tetani* □ *Nocardia asteroides* ■ Active against some gram-negative pathogens, including: □ *Enterobacter* □ *Escherichia coli* □ *Klebsiella* □ *Proteus mirabilis* □ *Proteus vulgaris* □ *Salmonella* □ *Shigella*.

PHARMACOKINETICS

Absorption: Well absorbed following oral administration.

Distribution: Widely distributed. Crosses the placenta; enters breast milk.

Metabolism and Excretion: Mostly metabolized by the liver.

Half-life: 5–8 hr.

CONTRAINDICATIONS AND PRECAUTIONS

Contraindicated in: ■ Hypersensitivity to sulfonamides ■ Cross-sensitivity with furosemide, thiazides, sulfonylurea oral hypoglycemic agents, or carbonic anhydrase inhibitors may exist ■ Porphyria ■ Pregnancy or lactation ■ Glucose-6-phosphate dehydrogenase (G6PD) deficiency ■ Known alcohol intolerance (oral suspension

only) ▪ Infants <2 mo (unless with pyrimethamine for congenital toxoplasmosis).
Use Cautiously in: ▪ Severe renal or hepatic impairment.

ADVERSE REACTIONS AND SIDE EFFECTS*

CNS: ataxia, confusion, dizziness, drowsiness, mental depression, psychosis, restlessness.
GI: nausea, anorexia, drug-induced hepatitis, vomiting.
GU: crystalluria.
Derm: rashes, exfoliative dermatitis, photosensitivity.
Hemat: AGRANULOCYTOSIS, APLASTIC ANEMIA, eosinophilia, thrombocytopenia.
Neuro: peripheral neuropathy.
Misc: hypersensitivity reactions including SERUM SICKNESS and STEVENS-JOHNSON SYNDROME, fever, superinfection.

INTERACTIONS

Drug-Drug: ▪ May enhance the action and increase the risk of toxicity from **oral hypoglycemic agents, methotrexate, phenytoin, zidovudine,** or **warfarin** ▪ Increased risk of crystalluria with **methenamine** ▪ Increased risk of drug-induced hepatitis with other **hepatotoxic agents.**

ROUTE AND DOSAGE

- **PO (Adults):** 2–4 g initially, then 750 mg–1.5 g q 4 hr or 1–2 g q 6 hr (not to exceed 12 g/day).
- **PO (Children >2 mo):** 75 mg/kg (2 g/m^2) initially, then 25 mg (667 mg/m^2) q 4 hr or 37.5 mg/kg (1g/m^2) q 6 hr (not to exceed 6 g/day).

AVAILABILITY

▪ ***Tablets:*** 500 mg[Rx] ▪ ***Oral suspension:*** 500 mg/5 ml[Rx].

TIME/ACTION PROFILE (blood levels)

	ONSET	PEAK	DURATION
PO	1 hr	2–4 hr	4–6 hr

NURSING IMPLICATIONS

ASSESSMENT

- Assess patient for infection (vital signs; appearance of wound, sputum, urine, and stool; WBC; earache) at beginning of and throughout therapy.
- Obtain specimens for culture and sensitivity prior to initiating therapy. First dose may be given before receiving results.
- Assess patient for allergy to sulfonamides.
- Monitor intake and output ratios. Fluid intake should be sufficient to maintain a urine output of at least 1200–1500 ml daily to prevent crystalluria and stone formation.
- ***Lab Test Considerations:*** Monitor CBC prior to and monthly during prolonged therapy. Therapy should be discontinued if blood dyscrasias occur.
- Monitor urinalysis prior to and periodically throughout therapy for crystalluria and formation of urinary calculi.

POTENTIAL NURSING DIAGNOSES

- Infection, risk for (Indications, Side Effects).
- Knowledge deficit, related to medication regimen (Patient/Family Teaching).
- Noncompliance, related to medication regimen (Patient/Family Teaching).

IMPLEMENTATION

- **PO:** Administer around the clock with a full glass of water. Tablets may be crushed and taken with liquids for patients with difficulty swallowing. Use calibrated measuring device for liquid preparations.

PATIENT/FAMILY TEACHING

- Instruct patient to take medication around the clock and to finish the drug completely as directed, even if feeling better. If a dose is missed, it should be taken as soon as remembered unless almost time for next dose. Advise patient that sharing of this medication may be dangerous.
- May cause dizziness. Caution patient to avoid driving and other activities requiring alertness until response to medication is known.
- Caution patient to use sunscreen and protec-

***CAPITALS indicate life-threatening; underlines indicate most frequent.**

tive clothing to prevent photosensitivity reactions.

- Advise patient to notify health care professional if skin rash, sore throat, fever, mouth sores, or unusual bleeding or bruising occurs.
- Instruct patient to notify health care professional if symptoms do not improve within a few days. Emphasize the importance of follow-up exams to monitor blood counts.

EVALUATION

Clinical response to therapy can be evaluated by: ▪ Resolution of the signs and symptoms of infection. Length of time for complete resolution depends on the organism and site of infection.

SULINDAC

(**soo**-lin-dak)

{Apo-Sulin}, Clinoril, {Novo-Sundac}

CLASSIFICATION(S):

Nonsteroidal anti-inflammatory agent

Pregnancy Category B (first trimester)

INDICATIONS

▪ Management of inflammatory disorders, including: ▫ Rheumatoid arthritis ▫ Osteoarthritis ▫ Acute gouty arthritis ▫ Bursitis.

ACTION

▪ Inhibits prostaglandin synthesis. **Therapeutic Effects:** ▪ Suppression of pain and inflammation.

PHARMACOKINETICS

Absorption: Well absorbed from the GI tract following oral administration.
Distribution: UK. Enters breast milk in small amounts.
Metabolism and Excretion: Converted by the liver to active drug. Minimal amounts excreted unchanged by the kidneys.
Half-life: 7.8 hr (16.4 hr for active metabolite).

CONTRAINDICATIONS AND PRECAUTIONS

Contraindicated in: ▪ Hypersensitivity ▪ Cross-sensitivity may occur with other NSAIDs, including aspirin ▪ Active GI bleeding or ulcer disease.
Use Cautiously in: ▪ Severe cardiovascular, renal, or hepatic disease (dosage modification recommended) ▪ History of ulcer disease ▪ Pregnancy, lactation, or children (safety not established; avoid use during 2nd half of pregnancy).

ADVERSE REACTIONS AND SIDE EFFECTS*

CNS: dizziness, headache, drowsiness.
EENT: blurred vision, tinnitus.
CV: edema.
GI: GI BLEEDING, DRUG-INDUCED HEPATITIS, constipation, diarrhea, discomfort, dyspepsia, nausea, vomiting, anorexia, flatulence, pancreatitis.
GU: renal failure.
Derm: rashes, photosensitivity.
Hemat: blood dyscrasias, prolonged bleeding time.
Misc: allergic reactions including ANAPHYLAXIS and HYPERSENSITIVITY SYNDROME.

INTERACTIONS

Drug-Drug: ▪ Concurrent use of **aspirin** may decrease effectiveness ▪ Increased risk of bleeding with **anticoagulants, thrombolytic agents, cefamandole, cefoperazone, cefotetan, valproic acid,** or **plicamycin** ▪ Additive adverse GI side effects with **aspirin, glucocorticoids,** and other **NSAIDs** ▪ May decrease response to **antihypertensives** or **diuretics** ▪ May increase serum levels and risk of toxicity from **lithium** ▪ May increase the risk of hematologic toxicity from **antineoplastic agents** or **radiation therapy** ▪ Increased risk of adverse renal effects with **gold compounds, cyclosporine,** or chronic use of **acetaminophen** ▪ **Antacids** decrease blood levels and decrease effectiveness of sulindac ▪ Increased risk of photosensitivity reactions with other **photosensitizing medications** ▪ Increased risk of hypoglycemia with **insulin** or **oral hypoglycemic agents.**

{} = Available in Canada only.
***CAPITALS indicate life-threatening; underlines indicate most frequent.**

ROUTE AND DOSAGE

- **PO (Adults):** 150–200 mg bid (not to exceed 400 mg/day).

AVAILABILITY

- ***Tablets:*** 150 mg[Rx], 200 mg[Rx].

TIME/ACTION PROFILE

	ONSET	PEAK	DURATION
PO (analgesic)	1–2 days	UK	12 hr
PO (anti-inflammatory)	few days–1 wk	2 wk or more	UK

NURSING IMPLICATIONS

ASSESSMENT

- Patients who have asthma, aspirin-induced allergy, and nasal polyps are at increased risk for developing hypersensitivity reactions. Monitor for rhinitis, asthma, and urticaria.
- Assess pain and range of movement prior to and after 1–2 wk of therapy.
- ***Lab Test Considerations:*** BUN, serum creatinine, CBC, and liver function tests should be evaluated periodically in patients receiving prolonged therapy.
- Serum potassium, glucose, alkaline phosphatase, AST, and ALT may show increased levels.
- Bleeding time may be prolonged for 1 day following discontinuation of therapy.

POTENTIAL NURSING DIAGNOSES

- Pain (Indications).
- Physical mobility, impaired (Indications).
- Knowledge deficit, related to medication regimen (Patient/Family Teaching).

IMPLEMENTATION

- **General Info:** Administration in higher than recommended doses does not provide increased effectiveness but may cause increased side effects.
- **PO:** May be administered with food, milk, or antacids to decrease GI irritation. Food slows but does not reduce the extent of absorption. Tablets may be crushed and mixed with fluids or food.

PATIENT/FAMILY TEACHING

- Advise patient to take this medication with a full glass of water and to remain in an upright position for 15–30 min after administration.
- Instruct patient to take medication exactly as directed. If a dose is missed, it should be taken as soon as remembered but not if almost time for the next dose. Do not double doses.
- May cause dizziness. Advise patient to avoid driving or other activities requiring alertness until response to the medication is known.
- Caution patient to avoid the concurrent use of alcohol, aspirin, NSAIDs, acetaminophen, or other OTC medications without consulting health care professional.
- Advise patient to inform health care professional of medication regimen prior to treatment or surgery.
- Advise patient to use sunscreen and protective clothing to prevent photosensitivity reactions.
- Advise patient to consult health care professional if rash, itching, visual disturbances, tinnitus, weight gain, edema, black stools, persistent headache, or influenza-like syndrome (chills, fever, muscle aches, pain) occurs.

EVALUATION

Effectiveness of therapy can be demonstrated by: ▪ Decreased pain and improved joint mobility. Partial arthritic relief may be seen within 7 days, but maximum effectiveness may require 2–3 wk of continuous therapy. Patients who do not respond to one NSAID may respond to another.

SUMATRIPTAN

(soo-ma-**trip**-tan)
Imitrex

CLASSIFICATION(S):
Vascular headache suppressant

Pregnancy Category C

INDICATIONS

▪ Acute treatment of migraine attacks ▪ **SC:** Acute treatment of cluster headache episodes.

ACTION

▪ Acts as a selective agonist at specific vascular serotonin receptor sites, causing vasoconstriction in large intracranial arteries. **Therapeutic Effects:** ▪ Relief of acute attacks of migraine.

PHARMACOKINETICS

Absorption: Well absorbed (97%) following SC administration. Absorption following oral administration is incomplete and significant amounts undergo substantial hepatic metabolism, resulting in poor bioavailability (14%). Well absorbed following intranasal administration.
Distribution: Does not cross the blood-brain barrier. Remainder of distribution not known.
Metabolism and Excretion: Mostly metabolized (80%) by the liver.
Half-life: 2 hr.

CONTRAINDICATIONS AND PRECAUTIONS

Contraindicated in: ▪ Hypersensitivity ▪ Patients with ischemic heart disease or signs and symptoms of ischemic heart disease, Prinzmetal's angina, or uncontrolled hypertension.
Use Cautiously in: ▪ Patients with any history of cardiovascular disease ▪ Patients with childbearing potential ▪ Pregnancy, lactation, or children <18 yr (safety not established).

ADVERSE REACTIONS AND SIDE EFFECTS*

All adverse reactions are less common following oral administration.
CNS: dizziness, vertigo, anxiety, drowsiness, fatigue, feeling of heaviness, feeling of tightness, headache, malaise, strange feeling, tight feeling in head, weakness.
EENT: alterations in vision, nasal sinus discomfort, throat discomfort.
CV: MYOCARDIAL INFARCTION, angina, chest pressure, chest tightness, coronary vasospasm, ECG changes, transient hypertension.
GI: abdominal discomfort, dysphagia.
Derm: tingling, warm sensation, burning sensation, cool sensation, flushing.
Local: injection site reaction.
MS: jaw discomfort, muscle cramps, myalgia, neck pain, neck stiffness.
Neuro: numbness.

INTERACTIONS

Drug-Drug: ▪ The risk of vasospastic reactions may be increased by concurrent use of **ergotamine** (avoid use of ergotamine and sumatriptan within 24 hr of each other) ▪ Concurrent use with **lithium, MAO inhibitors,** or **selective serotonin reuptake inhibitor antidepressants** should be avoided because the combined effects with sumatriptan are unknown.

ROUTE AND DOSAGE

- **PO (Adults):** 25 mg initially; if response is inadequate at 2 hr, up to 100 mg may be given. If headache recurs, doses may be repeated q 2 hr (not to exceed 300 mg/day). If PO therapy is to follow SC injection, additional PO sumatriptan may be taken q 2 hr (not to exceed 200 mg/day).
- **SC (Adults):** 6 mg; may repeat after 1 hr (not to exceed 12 mg in 24 hr).
- **Nasal (Adults):** Single dose of 5, 10, or 20 mg in one nostril; may be repeated in 2 hr, not to exceed 40 mg/24 hr or treatment of >5 episodes/mo.

AVAILABILITY

▪ ***Tablets:*** 25 mg[Rx], 50 mg[Rx], {100 mg[Rx]} ▪ ***Injection:*** 6 mg/0.5-ml prefilled syringes[Rx], 0.6 mg/0.5-ml vials[Rx], SELFdose injection kit (containing 2 prefilled syringes and instructions)[Rx] ▪ ***Nasal spray:*** 5 mg in 100 mcl-unit dose spray device (package of 6)[Rx], 20 mg in 100 mcl-unit dose spray device (package of 6)[Rx].

TIME/ACTION PROFILE (relief of migraine)

	ONSET	PEAK	DURATION
PO	within 30 min	2–4 hr	up to 24 hr
SC	30 min	up to 2 hr	up to 24 hr
Nasal	within 60 min	2 hr	UK

NURSING IMPLICATIONS

ASSESSMENT

- Assess pain location, intensity, duration, and associated symptoms (photophobia, phonophobia, nausea, vomiting) during migraine attack.
- Give initial SC under observation to patients with potential for coronary artery disease (CAD) (postmenopausal women, men over 40 years, patients with risk factors for CAD—[hypertension], hypercholesterolemia, obesity, diabetes, smoking, family history). Monitor blood pressure prior to and for 1 hr fol-

*CAPITALS indicate life-threatening; underlines indicate most frequent.

lowing initial injection. If angina occurs, monitor ECG for ischemic changes.

POTENTIAL NURSING DIAGNOSES

- Pain (Indications).
- Knowledge deficit, related to medication regimen (Patient/Family Teaching).

IMPLEMENTATION

- **PO:** Tablets should be swallowed whole; do not crush, break, or chew. Tablets are film-coated to prevent contact with tablet contents, which have an unpleasant taste and may cause nausea and vomiting.
- **SC:** Administer as a single injection just below the skin.
- **Intranasal:** 10-mg dose may be administered as 2 sprays of 5 mg in one nostril or 1 spray in each nostril.

PATIENT/FAMILY TEACHING

- **General Info:** Inform patient that sumatriptan should be used only during a migraine attack. It is meant to be used for relief of migraine attacks but not to prevent or reduce the number of attacks.
- □ Instruct patient to administer sumatriptan as soon as symptoms of a migraine attack appear, but it may be administered at any time during an attack. If migraine symptoms return, a 2nd injection may be used. Allow at least 1 hr between doses, and do not use more than 2 injections in any 24-hr period.
- □ Advise patient that lying down in a darkened room following sumatriptan administration may further help relieve headache.
- □ Caution patient not to use sumatriptan if she is pregnant, suspects she is pregnant, or plans to become pregnant. Adequate contraception should be used during therapy.
- □ Advise patient to notify health care professional prior to next dose of sumatriptan if pain or tightness in the chest occurs during use. If pain is severe or does not subside, notify health care professional immediately. If wheezing; heart throbbing; swelling of eyelids, face, or lips; skin rash; skin lumps; or hives occur, notify health care professional immediately and do not take more sumatriptan without approval of health care professional. Additional sumatriptan doses are not likely to be effective and alternative medications, as previously discussed with health care professional, may be used. If usual dose fails to relieve 3 consecutive headaches or if frequency and/or severity increases, notify health care professional. If feelings of tingling, heat, flushing, heaviness, pressure, drowsiness, dizziness, tiredness, or sickness develop, discuss with health care professional at next visit.
- □ Sumatriptan may cause dizziness or drowsiness. Caution patient to avoid driving or other activities requiring alertness until response to medication is known.
- □ Advise patient to avoid alcohol, which aggravates headaches, during sumatriptan use.
- **SC:** Instruct patient on the proper technique for loading, administering, and discarding the auto-injector. Patient information pamphlet is provided. Instructional video is available from the manufacturer.
- □ Inform patient that pain or redness at the injection site usually lasts less than 1 hr.
- **Intranasal:** Instruct patient in proper technique for intranasal administration. Usual dose is a single spray in one nostril. If headache returns, a 2nd dose may be administered in $\geq$2 hr. Do not administer 2nd dose if no relief was provided by 1st dose without consulting health care professional.

EVALUATION

Effectiveness of therapy can be demonstrated by: ▪ Relief of migraine attack.

TACRINE

(**tak**-rin)

Cognex

CLASSIFICATION(S):

Cholinesterase inhibitor (reversible)

Pregnancy Category C

INDICATIONS

▪ Mild to moderate dementia associated with Alzheimer's disease.

ACTION

▪ Increases levels of acetylcholine in the CNS by inhibiting its breakdown. **Therapeutic Effects:** ▪ Improved cognitive function in patients with mild to moderate Alzheimer's disease. Does not affect the course of the disease.

PHARMACOKINETICS

Absorption: Rapidly absorbed following oral administration, although bioavailability is low (17%).
Distribution: UK.
Metabolism and Excretion: Highly metabolized by the liver.
Half-life: 2–4 hr.

CONTRAINDICATIONS AND PRECAUTIONS

Contraindicated in: ▪ Hypersensitivity to tacrine or other acridines ▪ Jaundice associated with previous courses of tacrine therapy.
Use Cautiously in: ▪ Patients with a history or risk of GI bleeding, including current therapy with NSAIDs.

ADVERSE REACTIONS AND SIDE EFFECTS

CNS: dizziness, headache.
CV: bradycardia.
GI: GI BLEEDING, anorexia, diarrhea, drug-induced hepatitis, dyspepsia, nausea, vomiting.

INTERACTIONS

Drug-Drug: ▪ Increases **theophylline** levels and risk of toxicity (blood level monitoring recommended; dosage reduction may be required) ▪ Potentiates the effects of **succinylcholine** (increases neuromuscular blockade) during anesthesia ▪ May potentiate the action of **cholinergic agents** (bethanechol) ▪ **Cigarette smoking** decreases blood levels of tacrine ▪ **Cimetidine** increases tacrine levels ▪ May interfere with the action of **anticholinergic agents** ▪ Concurrent use of **NSAIDs** may increase the risk of GI bleeding.
Drug-Food: ▪ Food decreases absorption of tacrine by 30–40%.

ROUTE AND DOSAGE

- **PO (Adults):** 10 mg 4 times daily for 4 wk. If ALT remains unchanged, increase dose to 20 mg 4 times daily. Further increments may be made at 4-wk intervals as tolerated, up to 160 mg/day.

AVAILABILITY

- ***Capsules:*** 10 mg^{Rx}, 20 mg^{Rx}, 30 mg^{Rx}, 40 mg^{Rx}.

TIME/ACTION PROFILE (improvement in cognitive function)

	ONSET	PEAK	DURATION
PO	within 6 wk	18–24 wk	UK

NURSING IMPLICATIONS

ASSESSMENT

- □ Assess cognitive function (memory, attention, reasoning, language, ability to perform simple tasks) periodically throughout therapy.
- □ Monitor heart rate periodically during therapy. May cause bradycardia.
- ▪ ***Lab Test Considerations:*** May cause ALT elevations; monitor levels every other wk for the first 16 wk of therapy, monthly for 2 mo, and then every 3 mo throughout therapy. Biweekly monitoring should be resumed for at least 6 wk after any dose increase. If ALT levels are <3 times the upper limit of normal, continue dose titration; if levels are >3 to <5 times the upper limit of normal, decrease the dose of tacrine by 40 mg/day and resume dose titration when ALT returns to normal. Tacrine should be discontinued if ALT levels are >5 times the upper limit of normal. Levels usually return to normal 4–6 wk after discontinuation of therapy.
- □ Tacrine should be permanently discontinued and a new trial should not be attempted in patients with clinical jaundice and a total bilirubin >3 mg/dl.

POTENTIAL NURSING DIAGNOSES

- ▪ Thought processes, altered (Indications).
- ▪ Injury, risk for (Indications).
- ▪ Knowledge deficit, related to medication regimen (Patient/Family Teaching).

IMPLEMENTATION

- ▪ **PO:** Administer at regular intervals between meals on an empty stomach. If GI upset occurs, may be administered with meals; however, plasma levels may be reduced by 30–40%.
- □ Tacrine capsules may be dissolved in any aqueous solution for patients with difficulty swallowing (orange juice best masks the bitter taste). Place intact capsule in liquid to avoid loss of medication by spillage.

T

PATIENT/FAMILY TEACHING

- Emphasize the importance of taking tacrine at regular intervals as directed. If a dose is missed, take as soon as possible unless within 2 hr of next dose; do not double doses or discontinue without consulting health care professional. Abrupt discontinuation of doses >80 mg/day may cause a decline in cognitive function and behavioral disturbances.
- Caution patient and caregiver that tacrine may cause dizziness, unsteadiness, and clumsiness.
- Advise patient and caregiver to notify health care professional if nausea, vomiting, diarrhea, rash, jaundice, or changes in the color of the stool occur or if new symptoms occur or previously noted symptoms increase in severity.
- Advise patient to notify health care professional of medication regimen prior to treatment or surgery.

EVALUATION

Clinical response to therapy can be evaluated by: ▪ Improvement in cognitive function (memory, attention, reasoning, language, ability to perform simple tasks) in patients with Alzheimer's disease.

TACROLIMUS
(tak-roe-**lye**-mus)

CLASSIFICATION(S):
Immunosuppressant

Pregnancy Category C

INDICATIONS

▪ Prevention of organ rejection in patients who have undergone allogenic liver transplantation (used concurrently with glucocorticoids). **Unlabeled Uses:** ▪ Prevention of rejection of other types of organ transplantation ▪ Autoimmune diseases ▪ Severe recalcitrant psoriasis.

ACTION

▪ Inhibits T-lymphocyte activation. **Therapeutic Effects:** ▪ Prevention of transplanted organ rejection.

PHARMACOKINETICS

Absorption: Absorption following oral administration is variable (bioavailability ranges from 14.4–21.8%).
Distribution: Crosses the placenta and enters breast milk.
Metabolism and Excretion: 99% metabolized by the liver.
Half-life: *Liver transplant patients*—11.7 hr; *healthy volunteers*—21.2 hr.

CONTRAINDICATIONS AND PRECAUTIONS

Contraindicated in: ▪ Hypersensitivity to tacrolimus or to castor oil (a component in the injection) ▪ Concurrent use with cyclosporine should be avoided ▪ Breast-feeding should be avoided.
Use Cautiously in: ▪ Renal or hepatic impairment (dosage reduction may be required; if oliguria occurs, wait 48 hr before initiating tacrolimus) ▪ Children (higher end of dosing range required to maintain adequate blood levels) ▪ Pregnancy (hyperkalemia and renal impairment may occur in the newborn; use only if benefit to mother justifies risk to the fetus).

ADVERSE REACTIONS AND SIDE EFFECTS*

CNS: SEIZURES, <u>headache</u>, <u>insomnia</u>, <u>tremor</u>, abnormal dreams, agitation, anxiety, confusion, dizziness, emotional lability, mental depression, hallucinations, psychoses, somnolence.
EENT: abnormal vision, amblyopia, rhinitis, sinusitis, tinnitus, voice change.
Resp: asthma, bronchitis, cough, pharyngitis, pneumonia, pulmonary edema.
CV: <u>ascites</u>, <u>hypertension</u>, <u>peripheral edema</u>.
GI: GI BLEEDING, <u>abdominal pain</u>, <u>anorexia</u>, <u>diarrhea</u>, <u>nausea</u>, <u>vomiting</u>, cholangitis, cholestatic jaundice, dyspepsia, dysphagia, flatulence, increased appetite, increased liver function studies, oral thrush, peritonitis.
GU: <u>nephrotoxicity</u>, <u>urinary tract infection</u>.
Derm: <u>pruritus</u>, <u>rash</u>, alopecia, herpes simplex, hirsutism, photosensitivity, sweating.
Endo: <u>hyperglycemia</u>.
F and E: <u>hyperkalemia</u>, <u>hypomagnesemia</u>, acidosis, alkalosis, hyperlipidemia, hyperphospha-

***CAPITALS indicate life-threatening; <u>underlines</u> indicate most frequent.**

temia, hyperuricemia, hypocalcemia, hypokalemia, hyponatremia, hypophosphatemia.
Hemat: anemia, lymphocytosis, thrombocytopenia, coagulation defects, leukopenia.
MS: arthralgia, hypertonia, leg cramps, muscle spasm, myalgia, myasthenia, osteoporosis.
Neuro: paresthesia, neuropathy.
Misc: allergic reactions including ANAPHYLAXIS, generalized pain, abnormal healing, chills, fever, increased risk of lymphoma.

INTERACTIONS

Drug-Drug: ▪ Risk of nephrotoxicity is increased by concurrent use of **aminoglycoside anti-infectives, amphotericin B, cisplatin,** or **cyclosporine** (allow 24 hr to pass after stopping cyclosporine before starting tacrolimus) ▪ Concurrent use of **potassium-sparing diuretics** or **angiotensin-converting enzyme (ACE) inhibitors** increases the risk of hyperkalemia ▪ The following drugs increase tacrolimus blood levels: **antifungals, bromocriptine, calcium channel blockers, cimetidine, clarithromycin, cyclosporine, danazol, erythromycin, methylprednisolone,** and **metoclopramide** ▪ **Phenobarbital, phenytoin, carbamazepine,** and **rifamycins** may decrease tacrolimus blood levels ▪ **Vaccinations** may be less effective if given concurrently with tacrolimus (avoid use of live vaccines).
Drug-Food: ▪ Food decreases the rate and extent of GI absorption ▪ **Grapefruit juice** increases absorption.

ROUTE AND DOSAGE

- **PO (Adults):** 0.075–0.15 mg/kg q 12 hr.
- **PO (Children):** Start therapy at 0.15 mg/kg q 12 hr.
- **IV (Adults):** 0.05–0.1 mg/kg/day as a continuous infusion.
- **IV (Children):** 0.1 mg/kg/day as a continuous infusion.

AVAILABILITY

▪ ***Capsules:*** 1 mg[Rx], 5 mg[Rx] ▪ ***Injection:*** 5 mg/ml in 1-ml ampules[Rx].

TIME/ACTION PROFILE (immunosuppression)

	ONSET	PEAK	DURATION
PO	rapid	1.3–3.2 hr*	12 hr
IV	rapid	UK	8–12 hr

*Blood level.

NURSING IMPLICATIONS

ASSESSMENT

- Monitor blood pressure closely during therapy. Hypertension is a common complication of tacrolimus therapy and should be treated.
- Observe patients receiving IV tacrolimus for the development of anaphylaxis (rash, pruritus, laryngeal edema, wheezing) for at least 30 min and frequently thereafter. If signs develop, stop infusion and initiate treatment.
- ***Lab Test Considerations:*** Tacrolimus blood level monitoring may be helpful in the evaluation of rejection and toxicity, dose adjustments, and assessment of compliance. Tacrolimus whole blood concentrations measured with ELISA were the most variable during the 1st wk post-transplantation. After the 1st wk, median trough blood concentrations ranged from 9.8–19.4 ng/ml.
- Monitor serum creatinine, potassium, and glucose closely. Elevated serum creatinine and decreased urine output may indicate nephrotoxicity. May cause hyperglycemia; may require insulin therapy.
- May also cause hyperuricemia, hypokalemia, hypomagnesemia, acidosis, alkalosis, hyperlipidemia, hyperphosphatemia, hypophosphatemia, hypocalcemia, and hyponatremia.
- Monitor CBC and platelet count. May cause anemia, lymphocytosis, and thrombocytopenia.
- ***Toxicity and Overdose:*** Tremor and headache have been associated with high whole blood concentrations of tacrolimus and may respond to dose adjustment.

POTENTIAL NURSING DIAGNOSES

- Infection, risk for (Adverse Reactions).
- Knowledge deficit, related to medication regimen (Patient/Family Teaching).

IMPLEMENTATION

- **General Info:** Therapy with tacrolimus should be started no sooner than 6 hr posttransplant. Concurrent therapy with glucocorticoids is recommended in the early postoperative period.
- Oral therapy is preferred because of the risk of anaphylactic reactions with intravenous tacrolimus. Intravenous therapy should be replaced with oral therapy as soon as possible.

T

- □ Adults should be started at the lower end of the dose range; children require and tolerate higher doses and should be started at upper end of dosing range.
- ▪ **PO:** Oral doses can be initiated 8–12 hr after discontinuation of IV doses.
- ▪ **Continuous Infusion:** Dilute in 0.9% NaCl or D5W for a concentration of 0.004–0.02 mg/ml prior to use. May be stored in polyethylene or glass containers for 24 hr following dilution. Do not store in PVC containers.
- ▪ ***Rate:*** Administer daily dose as a continuous infusion over 24 hr.
- ▪ **Y-Site Compatibility:** ▪ acyclovir ▪ aminophylline ▪ amphotericin B ▪ ampicillin ▪ ampicillin/sulbactam ▪ benztropine ▪ calcium gluconate ▪ cefazolin ▪ cefotetan ▪ ceftazidime ▪ ceftriaxone ▪ cefuroxime ▪ chloramphenicol ▪ cimetidine ▪ ciprofloxacin ▪ clindamycin ▪ dexamethasone ▪ digoxin ▪ diphenhydramine ▪ dobutamine ▪ dopamine ▪ doxycycline ▪ erythromycin lactobionate ▪ esmolol ▪ fluconazole ▪ furosemide ▪ ganciclovir ▪ gentamicin ▪ haloperidol ▪ heparin ▪ hydrocortisone sodium succinate ▪ imipenem/cilastatin ▪ insulin ▪ isoproterenol ▪ leucovorin ▪ lorazepam ▪ methylprednisolone ▪ metoclopramide ▪ metronidazole ▪ mezlocillin ▪ multivitamins ▪ nitroglycerin ▪ oxacillin ▪ penicillin G potassium ▪ perphenazine ▪ phenytoin ▪ piperacillin ▪ potassium ▪ propranolol ▪ ranitidine ▪ sodium bicarbonate ▪ tobramycin ▪ trimethoprim/sulfamethoxazole ▪ vancomycin.

PATIENT/FAMILY TEACHING

- □ Instruct patient to take tacrolimus at the same time each day, as directed. Do not skip or double up on missed doses. Do not discontinue medication without advice of health care professional.
- □ Reinforce the need for lifelong therapy to prevent transplant rejection. Review symptoms of rejection for transplanted organ and stress need to notify health care professional immediately if they occur.
- □ Emphasize the importance of repeated lab tests during tacrolimus therapy.
- □ Advise patient of the risk of taking tacrolimus during pregnancy.
- □ Inform patient of the risk of lymphoma with tacrolimus therapy.

EVALUATION

Effectiveness of therapy can be demonstrated by: ▪ Prevention of transplanted liver rejection.

TAMOXIFEN

(ta-**mox**-i-fen)
{Alpha-Tamoxifen}, {Med Tamoxifen}, Nolvadex, {Nolvadex-D}, {Novo-Tamoxifen}, {Tamofen}, {Tamone}, {Tamoplex}

CLASSIFICATION(S):
Antineoplastic (estrogen blocker)

Pregnancy Category D

INDICATIONS

▪ Adjuvant therapy of breast cancer following surgery and radiation (delays recurrence) ▪ Palliative or adjunctive treatment of advanced breast cancer.

ACTION

▪ Competes with estrogen for binding sites in breast and other tissues ▪ Reduces DNA synthesis and estrogen response. **Therapeutic Effects:** ▪ Suppression of tumor growth.

PHARMACOKINETICS

Absorption: Absorbed following oral administration.
Distribution: Widely distributed.
Metabolism and Excretion: Mostly metabolized by the liver. Slowly eliminated in the feces. Minimal amounts excreted in the urine.
Half-life: 7 days.

CONTRAINDICATIONS AND PRECAUTIONS

Contraindicated in: ▪ Hypersensitivity ▪ Pregnancy or lactation.
Use Cautiously in: ▪ Women with childbearing potential ▪ Decreased bone marrow reserve.

ADVERSE REACTIONS AND SIDE EFFECTS*

CNS: confusion, depression, headache, weakness.
EENT: blurred vision.
CV: edema.
GI: nausea, vomiting.
GU: endometrial carcinoma, vaginal bleeding.
F and E: hypercalcemia.
Hemat: leukopenia, thrombocytopenia.
Metab: hot flashes.
MS: bone pain.
Misc: tumor flare.

INTERACTIONS

Drug-Drug: ▪ **Estrogens** and **aminoglutethimide** may decrease the effectiveness of concurrently administered tamoxifen ▪ Blood levels are increased by **bromocriptine** ▪ May increase the anticoagulant effect of **warfarin** ▪ Risk of thromboembolic events is increased by concurrent use of other **antineoplastic agents.**

ROUTE AND DOSAGE

▪ **PO (Adults):** 10–20 mg twice daily; doses of 20 mg/day may be taken as a single dose.

AVAILABILITY

▪ ***Tablets:*** 10 mg^Rx^, 20 mg^Rx^ ▪ ***Enteric-coated tablets:*** {20 mg^Rx^}.

TIME/ACTION PROFILE (tumor response)

	ONSET	PEAK	DURATION
PO	4–10 wk	several mo	several wk

NURSING IMPLICATIONS

ASSESSMENT

□ Assess for an increase in bone or tumor pain. Confer with physician or other health care professional regarding analgesics. This transient pain usually resolves despite continued therapy.

▪ ***Lab Test Considerations:*** Monitor CBC, platelets, and calcium levels prior to and throughout therapy. May cause transient hypercalcemia in patients with metastases to the bone. An estrogen receptor assay should be assessed prior to initiation of therapy.

□ Monitor serum cholesterol and triglyceride concentrations in patients with pre-existing hyperlipidemia. May cause increased concentrations.

□ Monitor hepatic function tests and thyroxine (T_4) periodically during therapy. May cause elevated serum hepatic enzyme and thyroxine concentrations.

□ Gynecologic examinations should be performed regularly; may cause variations in PAP and vaginal smears.

POTENTIAL NURSING DIAGNOSES

▪ Knowledge deficit, related to medication regimen (Patient/Family Teaching).

IMPLEMENTATION

▪ **PO:** Administer with food or fluids if GI irritation becomes a problem. Consult physician or other health care professional if patient vomits shortly after administration of medication to determine need for repeat dose.

□ Do not crush, break, chew, or administer an antacid within 1–2 hr of enteric-coated tablet.

PATIENT/FAMILY TEACHING

□ Instruct patient to take medication exactly as directed. If a dose is missed, it should be omitted.

□ If skin lesions are present, inform patient that lesions may temporarily increase in size and number and may have increased erythema.

□ Advise patient to report bone pain to health care professional promptly. This pain may be severe. Inform patient that this may be an indication of the drug's effectiveness and will resolve over time. Analgesics should be ordered to control pain.

□ Instruct patient to monitor weight weekly. Weight gain or peripheral edema should be reported to health care professional.

□ This medication may induce ovulation and may have teratogenic properties. Advise patient to use a nonhormonal method of contraception during and for 1 mo after the course of therapy.

□ Advise patient that medication may cause hot flashes. Notify health care professional if these become bothersome.

□ Instruct patient to notify health care professional promptly if pain or swelling of legs,

***CAPITALS indicate life-threatening; underlines indicate most frequent.**

T

shortness of breath, weakness, sleepiness, confusion, nausea, vomiting, weight gain, dizziness, headache, loss of appetite, or blurred vision occurs. Patient should also report menstrual irregularities, vaginal bleeding, pelvic pain or pressure.

EVALUATION

Effectiveness of therapy can be demonstrated by: ▪ Decrease in the size or spread of breast cancer. Observable effects of therapy may not be seen for 4–10 wk after initiation.

TAMSULOSIN
(tam-**soo**-loe-sin)
Flomax

CLASSIFICATION(S):
Antiadrenergic (peripherally acting)

Pregnancy Category B

INDICATIONS

▪ Management of outflow obstruction in male patients with prostatic hyperplasia.

ACTION

▪ Decreases contractions in smooth muscle of the prostatic capsule by preferentially binding to $alpha_1$-adrenergic receptors. **Therapeutic Effects:** ▪ Decreased symptoms of prostatic hyperplasia (urinary urgency, hesitancy, nocturia).

PHARMACOKINETICS

Absorption: Slowly absorbed following oral administration.
Distribution: Widely distributed.
Metabolism and Excretion: Extensively metabolized by the liver; <10% excreted unchanged in urine.
Half-life: 14 hr.

CONTRAINDICATIONS AND PRECAUTIONS

Contraindicated in: ▪ Hypersensitivity.
Use Cautiously in: ▪ Patients at risk for prostate carcinoma (symptoms may be similar).

ADVERSE REACTIONS AND SIDE EFFECTS*

CNS: dizziness, headache.
EENT: rhinitis.
CV: orthostatic hypotension.
GU: retrograde/diminished ejaculation.

INTERACTIONS

Drug-Drug: ▪ **Cimetidine** may increase blood levels and the risk of toxicity ▪ Increased risk of hypotension with other **peripherally acting antiadrenergics** (doxazosin, prazosin, terazosin); concurrent use should be avoided.

ROUTE AND DOSAGE

▪ **PO (Adults):** 0.4 mg once daily following a meal; may be increased after 2–4 wk to 0.8 mg/day.

AVAILABILITY

▪ ***Capsules:*** 0.4 mg[Rx].

TIME/ACTION PROFILE (increase in urine flow)

	ONSET	PEAK	DURATION
PO	UK	2 wk	UK

NURSING IMPLICATIONS

ASSESSMENT

□ Assess patient for symptoms of prostatic hyperplasia (urinary hesitancy, feeling of incomplete bladder emptying, interruption of urinary stream, impairment of size and force of urinary stream, terminal urinary dribbling, straining to start flow, dysuria, urgency) prior to and periodically throughout therapy.
□ Assess patient for first-dose orthostatic hypotension and syncope. Incidence may be dose related. Observe patient closely during this period and take precautions to prevent injury.
□ Monitor intake and output ratios and daily weight, and assess for edema daily, especially at beginning of therapy. Report weight gain or edema.

POTENTIAL NURSING DIAGNOSES

▪ Injury, risk for (Side Effects).
▪ Urinary elimination, altered patterns of (Indications).

*CAPITALS indicate life-threatening; underlines indicate most frequent.

- Knowledge deficit, related to medication regimen (Patient/Family Teaching).

IMPLEMENTATION

- **PO:** Administer daily dose 30 min following the same meal each day.
  - If dose is interrupted for several days at either the 0.4-mg or 0.8-mg dose, restart therapy with the 0.4-mg/day dose.

PATIENT/FAMILY TEACHING

- **General Info:** Emphasize the importance of continuing to take this medication, even if feeling well. Instruct patient to take medication at the same time each day. If a dose is missed, take as soon as remembered unless almost time for next dose. Do not double doses.
  - May cause dizziness. Advise patient to avoid driving or other activities requiring alertness until response to medication is known.
  - Caution patient to change positions slowly to minimize orthostatic hypotension.
  - Advise patient to consult health care professional before taking any cough, cold, or allergy remedies.
  - Emphasize the importance of follow-up visits to determine effectiveness of therapy.

EVALUATION

Effectiveness of therapy can be demonstrated by: ▪ Decrease in urinary symptoms of benign prostatic hyperplasia.

TEMAZEPAM
(tem-**az**-a-pam)
Restoril

CLASSIFICATION(S):
Sedative/hypnotic (benzodiazepine)

Schedule IV
Pregnancy Category X

INDICATIONS

▪ Short-term management of insomnia.

ACTION

▪ Acts at many levels in the CNS, producing generalized depression ▪ Effects may be mediated by gamma-aminobutyric acid (GABA), an inhibitory neurotransmitter. **Therapeutic Effects:** ▪ Relief of insomnia.

PHARMACOKINETICS

Absorption: Well absorbed following oral administration.
Distribution: Widely distributed, crosses blood-brain barrier. Probably crosses the placenta and enters breast milk. Accumulation of drug occurs with chronic dosing.
Metabolism and Excretion: Metabolized by the liver.
Half-life: 10–20 hr.

CONTRAINDICATIONS AND PRECAUTIONS

Contraindicated in: ▪ Hypersensitivity ▪ Cross-sensitivity with other benzodiazepines may exist ▪ Pre-existing CNS depression ▪ Severe uncontrolled pain ▪ Narrow-angle glaucoma ▪ Pregnancy or lactation.
Use Cautiously in: ▪ Pre-existing hepatic dysfunction ▪ History of suicide attempt or drug addiction ▪ Geriatric or debilitated patients (dosage reduction recommended).

ADVERSE REACTIONS AND SIDE EFFECTS*

CNS: <u>hangover</u>, dizziness, drowsiness, lethargy, paradoxical excitation.
EENT: blurred vision.
GI: constipation, diarrhea, nausea, vomiting.
Derm: rashes.
Misc: physical dependence, psychological dependence, tolerance.

INTERACTIONS

Drug-Drug: ▪ Additive CNS depression with **alcohol, antidepressants, antihistamines, opioids**, and other **sedative/hypnotics** ▪ May decrease efficacy of **levodopa** ▪ **Rifampin** or **smoking** increases metabolism and may decrease effectiveness of temazepam ▪ **Probenecid** may prolong the effects of temazepam ▪ Sedative effects may be antagonized by **theophylline.**

ROUTE AND DOSAGE

- **PO (Adults):** 15–30 mg at bedtime initially; some patients may require only 7.5 mg.

***CAPITALS** indicate life-threatening; <u>underlines</u> indicate most frequent.**

- **PO (Geriatric Patients or Debilitated Patients):** 7.5 mg at bedtime.

AVAILABILITY

- ***Tablets:*** 15 mg^{Rx}, 30 mg^{Rx} - ***Capsules:*** 7.5 mg^{Rx}, 15 mg^{Rx}, 30 mg^{Rx}.

TIME/ACTION PROFILE (sedation)

	ONSET	PEAK	DURATION
PO	30 min	2–3 hr	6–8 hr

NURSING IMPLICATIONS

ASSESSMENT

- Assess sleep patterns prior to and periodically throughout course of therapy.
- Prolonged high-dose therapy may lead to psychological or physical dependence. Restrict amount of drug available to patient, especially if patient is depressed or suicidal or has a history of addiction.

POTENTIAL NURSING DIAGNOSES

- Sleep pattern disturbance (Indications).
- Injury, risk for (Side Effects).
- Knowledge deficit, related to medication regimen (Patient/Family Teaching).

IMPLEMENTATION

- **General Info:** Supervise ambulation and transfer of patients following administration. Remove cigarettes. Side rails should be raised and call bell within reach at all times.
- **PO:** Administer with food if GI irritation becomes a problem.

PATIENT/FAMILY TEACHING

- Instruct patient to take temazepam exactly as directed. Discuss the importance of preparing environment for sleep (dark room, quiet, avoidance of nicotine and caffeine). If less effective after a few weeks, consult health care professional; do not increase dose.
- May cause daytime drowsiness or dizziness. Caution patient to avoid driving or other activities requiring alertness until response to medication is known.
- Advise patient to avoid the use of alcohol and other CNS depressants and to consult health care professional prior to the use of OTC preparations that contain antihistamines or alcohol.
- Advise patient to inform health care professional if pregnancy is planned or suspected.
- Emphasize the importance of follow-up appointments to monitor progress.

EVALUATION

Effectiveness of therapy can be demonstrated by: - Improvement in sleep habits, which may not be noticeable until the 3rd day of therapy.

TERAZOSIN

(ter-**ay**-zoe-sin)
Hytrin

CLASSIFICATION(S):
Antihypertensive agent (peripherally acting antiadrenergic)

Pregnancy Category C

INDICATIONS

- Treatment of mild to moderate hypertension (alone or with other agents, such as diuretics) - Management of outflow obstruction in patients with prostatic hyperplasia.

ACTION

- Dilates both arteries and veins by blocking postsynaptic alpha$_1$-adrenergic receptors - Decreases contractions in smooth muscle of the prostatic capsule. **Therapeutic Effects:** - Lowering of blood pressure - Decreased symptoms of prostatic hyperplasia (urinary urgency, hesitancy, nocturia).

PHARMACOKINETICS

Absorption: Well absorbed following oral administration.
Distribution: UK.
Metabolism and Excretion: 50% metabolized by the liver. 10% excreted unchanged by the kidneys. 20% excreted unchanged in feces. 40% eliminated in bile.
Half-life: 12 hr.

CONTRAINDICATIONS AND PRECAUTIONS

Contraindicated in: - Hypersensitivity.
Use Cautiously in: - Deyhdration, volume or sodium depletion, increased risk of hypotension

- Pregnancy, lactation, or children (safety not established).

ADVERSE REACTIONS AND SIDE EFFECTS*

CNS: dizziness, headache, weakness, drowsiness, nervousness.
EENT: nasal congestion, blurred vision, conjunctivitis, sinusitis.
Resp: dyspnea.
CV: first-dose orthostatic hypotension, arrhythmias, chest pain, palpitations, peripheral edema, tachycardia.
GI: nausea, abdominal pain, diarrhea, dry mouth, vomiting.
GU: impotence, urinary frequency.
Derm: pruritus.
Metab: weight gain.
MS: arthralgia, back pain, extremity pain.
Neuro: paresthesia.
Misc: fever.

INTERACTIONS

Drug-Drug: ▪ Additive hypotension with other **antihypertensive agents**, acute ingestion of **alcohol**, or **nitrates** ▪ **NSAIDs, sympathomimetics**, or **estrogens** may decrease the effects of antihypertensive therapy.

ROUTE AND DOSAGE

The first dose should be taken at bedtime.

❑ Hypertension

- **PO (Adults):** 1 mg initially, then slowly increase up to 5 mg/day (usual range 1–5 mg/day); may be given as single dose or in 2 divided doses (not to exceed 20 mg/day).

❑ Benign Prostatic Hyperplasia

- **PO (Adults):** 1 mg at bedtime; gradually may be increased up to 5–10 mg/day.

AVAILABILITY

- ***Tablets:*** 1 mg[Rx], 2 mg[Rx], 5 mg[Rx], 10 mg[Rx].

TIME/ACTION PROFILE

	ONSET†	PEAK‡	DURATION†
PO-hypertension	15 min	6–8 wk	24 hr
PO-prostatic hyperplasia	2–6 wk	UK	UK

†After single dose.
‡After multiple oral dosing.

NURSING IMPLICATIONS

ASSESSMENT

- **General Info:** Monitor blood pressure (lying and standing) and pulse frequently during initial dosage adjustment and periodically throughout therapy. Notify physician or other health care professional of significant changes.
- □ Assess patient for first-dose orthostatic reaction and syncope. May occur 30 min–2 hr following initial dose and occasionally thereafter. Incidence may be dose related. Volume-depleted or sodium-restricted patients may be more sensitive to this effect.
- □ Monitor intake and output ratios and daily weight; assess for edema daily, especially at beginning of therapy.
- **Benign Prostatic Hyperplasia:** Assess patient for symptoms of prostatic hyperplasia (urinary hesitancy, feeling of incomplete bladder emptying, interruption of urinary stream, impairment of size and force of urinary stream, terminal urinary dribbling, straining to start flow, dysuria, urgency) prior to and periodically throughout therapy.
- □ Rule out prostatic carcinoma prior to therapy; symptoms are similar.

POTENTIAL NURSING DIAGNOSES

- Injury, risk for (Side Effects).
- Knowledge deficit, related to medication regimen (Patient/Family Teaching).
- Noncompliance (Patient/Family Teaching).

IMPLEMENTATION

- **General Info:** May be used in combination with diuretic or beta-adrenergic blocker to minimize sodium and water retention. If these are added to terazosin therapy, reduce dose of terazosin initially and titrate to effect.
- **PO:** Administer daily dose at bedtime. If necessary, dosage may be increased to twice daily.

PATIENT/FAMILY TEACHING

- **General Info:** Instruct patient to take medication at the same time each day. If a dose is missed, take as soon as remembered. If not remembered until next day, omit; do not double doses.

***CAPITALS indicate life-threatening; underlines indicate most frequent.**

- □ Advise patient to weigh self twice weekly and assess feet and ankles for fluid retention.
- □ May cause dizziness or drowsiness. Advise patient to avoid driving or other activities requiring alertness until response to the medication is known.
- □ Caution patient to avoid sudden changes in position to decrease orthostatic hypotension. Alcohol, CNS depressants, standing for long periods, hot showers, and exercising in hot weather should be avoided because of enhanced orthostatic effects.
- □ Advise patient to consult health care professional before taking any cough, cold, or allergy remedies.
- □ Instruct patient to notify health care professional of medication regimen prior to any surgery.
- □ Advise patient to notify health care professional if frequent dizziness, fainting, or swelling of feet or lower legs occurs.
- □ Emphasize the importance of follow-up exams to evaluate effectiveness of medication.
- ■ **Hypertension:** Emphasize the importance of continuing to take this medication as directed, even if feeling well. Medication controls but does not cure hypertension.
- □ Encourage patient to comply with additional interventions for hypertension (weight reduction, low-sodium diet, smoking cessation, moderation of alcohol consumption, regular exercise, and stress management).
- □ Instruct patient and family on proper technique for blood pressure monitoring. Advise them to check blood pressure at least weekly and to report significant changes.

EVALUATION

Effectiveness of therapy can be demonstrated by: ■ Decrease in blood pressure without appearance of side effects ■ Decreased symptoms of prostatic hyperplasia. May require 2–6 wk of therapy before effects are noticeable.

TERBINAFINE†

(ter-**bi**-na-feen)
Lamisal

CLASSIFICATION(S):
Antifungal (systemic)

Pregnancy Category B

†For topical use, refer to antifungals, topical, monograph on page 69.

INDICATIONS

■ Onychomycosis (fungal nail infection).

ACTION

■ Interferes with fungal cell wall synthesis by inhibiting the enzyme squalene epoxidase. **Therapeutic Effects:** ■ Fungal cell death. **Spectrum:** ■ Active against dermatophytes and other fungi.

PHARMACOKINETICS

Absorption: 70–80% absorbed following oral administration.
Distribution: Extensively distributed; penetrates dermis and epidermis; concentrates in stratum corneum, hair, scalp, and nails. Enters breast milk.
Metabolism and Excretion: Extensively metabolized by the liver.
Half-life: *Plasma*—22 days; longer from skin and nails.

CONTRAINDICATIONS AND PRECAUTIONS

Contraindicated in: ■ Hypersensitivity.
Use Cautiously in: ■ History of alcoholism ■ Renal/hepatic impairment (dosage reduction recommended for stable chronic liver impairment or CCr <50 ml/min) ■ Pregnancy, lactation, or children (safety not established).

ADVERSE REACTIONS AND SIDE EFFECTS*

GI: anorexia, diarrhea, nausea, stomach pain, vomiting, altered taste, drug-induced hepatitis.
Derm: TOXIC EPIDERMAL NECROLYSIS, itching, rash.
Hemat: neutropenia, pancytopenia.
Misc: STEVENS-JOHNSON SYNDROME.

INTERACTIONS

Drug-Drug: ■ **Alcohol** or other **hepatotoxic agents** may increase the risk of hepatotoxicity

*CAPITALS indicate life-threatening; underlines indicate most frequent.

■ **Rifampin** and other **drugs that induce hepatic drug-metabolizing enzymes** may decrease effectiveness ■ **Cimetidine** and other **drugs that inhibit hepatic drug-metabolizing enzymes** may increase effectiveness.

ROUTE AND DOSAGE

- **PO (Adults):** 250 mg once daily for 6 wk for fingernail infection or 12 wk for toenail infection.

AVAILABILITY

- ***Tablets:*** 250 mg[Rx].

TIME/ACTION PROFILE (antifungal tissue levels)

	ONSET	PEAK	DURATION
PO	several days	days–wks	several wk

NURSING IMPLICATIONS

ASSESSMENT

- □ Assess patient for signs and symptoms of infection (nail beds) prior to and periodically throughout therapy.
- □ Specimens for culture should be taken prior to instituting therapy. Therapy may be started before results are obtained.
- ■ ***Lab Test Considerations:*** CBC and hepatic function tests should be monitored in patients receiving therapy for >6 wk. Discontinue if abnormal values occur.
- □ If signs of secondary infection occur, monitor neutrophil count. If <1000/mm³, discontinue treatment.
- □ May cause decrease in absolute lymphocyte count.
- □ Monitor serum potassium. May cause hypokalemia.

POTENTIAL NURSING DIAGNOSES

- Infection, risk for (Indications).
- Knowledge deficit, related to medication regimen (Patient/Family Teaching).
- Noncompliance, related to medication regimen (Patient/Family Teaching).

IMPLEMENTATION

- **PO:** May be administered without regard to food.

PATIENT/FAMILY TEACHING

- □ Instruct patient to take medication exactly as directed, for the full course of therapy, even if feeling better. Doses should be taken at the same time each day.
- □ Instruct patient to notify health care professional if signs and symptoms of liver dysfunction (unusual fatigue, anorexia, nausea, vomiting, jaundice, dark urine, or pale stools) occur.
- □ Advise patient to consult health care professional prior to taking any Rx or OTC medications concurrently with terbinafine.

EVALUATION

Effectiveness of therapy can be demonstrated by: ■ Resolution of clinical and laboratory indications of fungal nail infections. Inadequate period of treatment may lead to recurrence of active infection.

TERBUTALINE

(ter-**byoo**-ta-leen)
Brethaire, Bricanyl

CLASSIFICATION(S):
Bronchodilator (adrenergic agonist)

Pregnancy Category B

INDICATIONS

■ Management of reversible airway disease due to asthma or COPD; inhalation and SC used for short-term control and oral agent as long-term control. **Unlabeled Uses:** ■ Management of preterm labor (tocolytic).

ACTION

■ Results in the accumulation of cyclic adenosine monophosphate (cAMP) at beta-adrenergic receptors ■ Produces bronchodilation ■ Inhibits the release of mediators of immediate hypersensitivity reactions from mast cells ■ Relatively selective for $beta_2$ (pulmonary) -adrenergic receptor sites, with less effect on $beta_1$ (cardiac) -adrenergic receptors. **Therapeutic Effects:** ■ Bronchodilation.

PHARMACOKINETICS

Absorption: 35–50% absorbed following oral administration but rapidly undergoes first-pass metabolism. Well absorbed following SC admin-

istration. Minimal absorption occurs following inhalation.
Distribution: Enters breast milk.
Metabolism and Excretion: Partially metabolized by the liver; 60% excreted unchanged by the kidneys following SC administration.
Half-life: UK.

CONTRAINDICATIONS AND PRECAUTIONS

Contraindicated in: ▪ Hypersensitivity to adrenergic amines ▪ Known hypersensitivity or intolerance to fluorocarbons (inhalation only).
Use Cautiously in: ▪ Cardiac disease ▪ Hypertension ▪ Hyperthyroidism ▪ Diabetes ▪ Glaucoma ▪ Geriatric patients (more susceptible to adverse reactions; may require dosage reduction) ▪ Excessive use may lead to tolerance and paradoxical bronchospasm (inhaler) ▪ Pregnancy (near term), lactation, and children <2 yr (safety not established).

ADVERSE REACTIONS AND SIDE EFFECTS*

CNS: nervousness, restlessness, tremor, headache, insomnia.
Resp: PARADOXICAL BRONCHOSPASM (excessive use of inhalers).
CV: angina, arrhythmias, hypertension, tachycardia.
GI: nausea, vomiting.
Endo: hyperglycemia.

INTERACTIONS

Drug-Drug: ▪ Concurrent use with other **adrenergic (sympathomimetic) agents** will have additive adrenergic side effects ▪ Use with **MAO inhibitors** may lead to hypertensive crisis ▪ **Beta-adrenergic blockers** may negate therapeutic effect.

ROUTE AND DOSAGE

- **PO (Adults and Children >15 yr):** *Bronchodilation*—2.5–5 mg 3 times daily, given q 6 hr (not to exceed 15 mg/24 hr). *Tocolysis*—2.5 mg q 4–6 hr until delivery (unlabeled).
- **PO (Children 12–15 yr):** 2.5 mg 3 times daily (given q 6 hr).
- **Inhalation (Adults and Children ≥12 yr):** 2 inhalations (200 mcg/spray) q 4–6 hr.
- **SC (Adults):** *Bronchodilation*—250 mcg; may repeat in 15–30 min (not to exceed 500 mcg/4 hr). *Tocolysis*—250 mcg q 1 hr until contractions stop (unlabeled).
- **IV (Adults):** *Tocolysis*—10 mcg/min infusion; increase by 5 mcg/min q 10 min until contractions stop (not to exceed 80 mcg/min). After contractions have stopped for 30 min, decrease infusion rate to lowest effective amount and maintain for 4–8 hr (unlabeled).

AVAILABILITY

▪ ***Tablets:*** 2.5 mg[Rx], 5 mg[Rx] ▪ ***Injection:*** 1 mg/ml[Rx] ▪ ***Inhalation aerosol:*** 200 mcg/spray (≥300 inhalations/10.5-g canister)[Rx], {500 mcg/spray[Rx]}.

TIME/ACTION PROFILE (bronchodilation)

	ONSET	PEAK	DURATION
PO	within 60–120 min	within 2–3 hr	4–8 hr
Inhaln	5–30 min	1–2 hr	3–6 hr
SC	within 15 min	within 0.5–1 hr	1.5–4 hr

NURSING IMPLICATIONS

ASSESSMENT

- **Bronchodilator:** Assess lung sounds, respiratory pattern, pulse, and blood pressure before administration and during peak of medication. Note amount, color, and character of sputum produced, and notify physician or other health care professional of abnormal findings.
  - Monitor pulmonary function tests before initiating therapy and periodically throughout course to determine effectiveness of medication.
  - Observe for paradoxical bronchospasm (wheezing). If condition occurs, withhold medication and notify physician or other health care professional immediately.
  - Observe patient for drug tolerance and rebound bronchospasm. Patients requiring more than 3 inhalation treatments in 24 hr should be under close supervision. If minimal or no relief is seen after 3–5 inhalation treat-

*CAPITALS indicate life-threatening; underlines indicate most frequent.

ments within 6–12 hr, further treatment with aerosol alone is not recommended.

- **Preterm Labor:** Monitor maternal pulse and blood pressure, frequency and duration of contractions, and fetal heart rate. Notify physician or other health care professional if contractions persist or increase in frequency or duration or if symptoms of maternal or fetal distress occur. Maternal side effects include tachycardia, palpitations, tremor, anxiety, and headache.
- □ Assess maternal respiratory status for symptoms of pulmonary edema (increased rate, dyspnea, rales/crackles, frothy sputum).
- □ Monitor mother and neonate for symptoms of hypoglycemia (anxiety; chills; cold sweats; confusion; cool, pale skin; difficulty in concentration; drowsiness; excessive hunger; headache; irritability; nausea; nervousness; rapid pulse; shakiness; unusual tiredness; or weakness) and mother for hypokalemia (weakness, fatigue, U wave on ECG, arrhythmias).
- ***Lab Test Considerations:*** May cause transient decrease in serum potassium concentrations with higher than recommended doses.
- □ Monitor maternal serum glucose and electrolytes. May cause hypokalemia and hypoglycemia. Monitor neonate's serum glucose, as hypoglycemia may also occur in neonates.
- ***Toxicity and Overdose:*** Symptoms of overdose include persistent agitation, chest pain or discomfort, decreased blood pressure, dizziness, hyperglycemia, hypokalemia, seizures, tachyarrhythmias, persistent trembling, and vomiting.
- □ Treatment includes discontinuing beta-adrenergic agonists and symptomatic, supportive therapy. Cardioselective beta-adrenergic blocking agents are used cautiously, as they may induce bronchospasm.

POTENTIAL NURSING DIAGNOSES

- Airway clearance, ineffective (Indications).
- Knowledge deficit, related to medication regimen (Patient/Family Teaching).

IMPLEMENTATION

- **PO:** Administer with meals to minimize gastric irritation.
- □ Tablet may be crushed and mixed with food or fluids for patients with difficulty swallowing.
- **SC:** Administer SC injections in lateral deltoid area. Do not use solution if discolored.
- **Continuous Infusion:** May be diluted in D5W, 0.9% NaCl, or 0.45% NaCl.
- ***Rate:*** Use infusion pump to ensure accurate dosage. Begin infusion at 10 mcg/min. Increase dosage by 5 mcg every 10 min until contractions cease. Maximum dose is 80 mcg/min. Begin to taper dose in 5-mcg decrements after a 30–60 min contraction-free period is attained. Switch to oral dosage form after patient is contraction-free 4–8 hr on the lowest effective dose.
- **Y-Site Compatibility:** ▪ insulin.

PATIENT/FAMILY TEACHING

- **General Info:** Instruct patient to take medication exactly as directed. If on a scheduled dosing regimen, take a missed dose as soon as possible; space remaining doses at regular intervals. Do not double doses. Caution patient not to exceed recommended dose; may cause adverse effects, paradoxical bronchospasm, or loss of effectiveness of medication.
- □ Instruct patient to contact health care professional immediately if shortness of breath is not relieved by medication or is accompanied by diaphoresis, dizziness, palpitations, or chest pain.
- □ Advise patient to consult health care professional before taking any OTC medications or alcoholic beverages concurrently with this therapy. Caution patient also to avoid smoking and other respiratory irritants.
- **Inhalation:** Review correct administration technique with patient. See Appendix H for administration with metered-dose inhaler. Wait 1–5 min before administering next dose. Mouthpiece should be washed after each use.
- □ Do not spray inhaler near eyes.
- □ Instruct patient to save inhaler; refill canisters may be available.
- □ Advise patients to use bronchodilator first if using other inhalation medications, and allow 15 min to elapse before administering other inhalant medications, unless otherwise directed.
- □ Advise patient to rinse mouth with water after each inhalation dose to minimize dry mouth.
- □ Advise patient to maintain adequate fluid intake (2000–3000 ml/day) to help liquefy tenacious secretions.

- Advise patient to consult health care professional if respiratory symptoms are not relieved or worsen after treatment or if chest pain, headache, severe dizziness, palpitations, nervousness, or weakness occurs.
- Instruct patient to notify health care professional if contents of one canister are used up in less than 2 wk.

- **Preterm Labor:** Health care professional should be notified immediately if labor resumes or if significant side effects occur.

EVALUATION

Effectiveness of therapy can be demonstrated by: ▪ Prevention or relief of bronchospasm ▪ Increase in ease of breathing ▪ Control of preterm labor in a fetus of 20–36 wk gestational age.

TESTOSTERONE
(tess-**toss**-te-rone)

testosterone base
Andro, Histerone, {Malogen}, Testamone, Testaqua, Testoject

testosterone cypionate
Andro-Cyp, Andronate, depAndro, Depotest, Depo-Testosterone, Duratest, T-Cypionate, Testa-C, Testred, Testoject-LA, Virilon IM

testosterone enanthate
Andro LA, Andropository, Andryl, Delatest, Delatestryl, Everone, {Malogex}, Testone LA, Testrin-PA

testosterone propionate
{Malogen}, Testex

testosterone transdermal
Androderm, Testoderm

CLASSIFICATION(S):
Hormone (androgen)

Schedule III
Pregnancy Category X

INDICATIONS

▪ Treatment of hypogonadism in androgen-deficient men ▪ Treatment of delayed puberty in men ▪ Palliative treatment of androgen-responsive breast cancer.

ACTION

▪ Responsible for the normal growth and development of male sex organs ▪ Maintenance of male secondary sex characteristics: □ Growth and maturation of the prostate, seminal vesicles, penis, scrotum □ Development of male hair distribution □ Vocal cord thickening □ Alterations in body musculature and fat distribution. **Therapeutic Effects:** ▪ Correction of hormone deficiency in male hypogonadism □ Initiation of male puberty ▪ Suppression of tumor growth in some forms of breast cancer.

PHARMACOKINETICS

Absorption: Well absorbed from IM sites. Cypionate, propionate, and enanthate salts are absorbed slowly. Well absorbed through skin (scrotal skin is 5–30 times more permeable than other sites).
Distribution: Probably cross the placenta and enter breast milk.
Metabolism and Excretion: Metabolized by the liver.
Half-life: *Base*—10–100 min; *cypionate*—8 days.

CONTRAINDICATIONS AND PRECAUTIONS

Contraindicated in: ▪ Hypersensitivity ▪ Pregnancy and lactation ▪ Male patients with breast or prostate cancer ▪ Hypercalcemia ▪ Severe liver, renal, or cardiac disease ▪ Some products contain tartrazine and should be avoided in patients with known hypersensitivity.
Use Cautiously in: ▪ Diabetes mellitus ▪ Coronary artery disease ▪ History of liver disease ▪ Prepubertal males.

ADVERSE REACTIONS AND SIDE EFFECTS*

EENT: deepening of voice.
CV: edema.

{} = Available in Canada only.
*CAPITALS indicate life-threatening; underlines indicate most frequent.

GI: changes in appetite, drug-induced hepatitis, nausea, vomiting.
GU: bladder irritability, menstrual irregularities, prostatic enlargement.
Endo: *women*—change in libido, clitoral enlargement, decreased breast size; *men*—acne, facial hair, gynecomastia, impotence, oligospermia, priapism.
F and E: hypercalcemia.
Local: local reactions to transdermal systems, pain at injection site.

INTERACTIONS

Drug-Drug: ▪ Decrease metabolism and may enhance the action of **warfarin, oral hypoglycemic agents,** and **glucocorticoids** ▪ May also enhance the effect of **insulin** ▪ Additive hepatotoxicity with other **hepatotoxic agents.**

ROUTE AND DOSAGE

❑ **Replacement Therapy**

- **IM (Adults):** 25–50 mg 2–3 times/wk (base or propionate) or 50–400 mg q 2–4 wk (enanthate or cypionate).
- **Transdermal (Adults):** *Testoderm*—4–6 mg applied q 22–24 hr. *Androderm*—5 mg applied q 24 hr.

❑ **Delayed Male Puberty**

- **IM (Children >12 yr):** Up to 100 mg/mo for up to 6 mo.

❑ **Palliative Management of Breast Cancer**

- **IM (Adults):** 50–100 mg 3 times/wk (propionate or base) or 200–400 mg q 2–4 wk (cypionate or enanthate).

AVAILABILITY

▪ ***Sterile testosterone suspension for injection (base):*** 25 mg/ml in 10-ml vials[Rx], 50 mg/ml in 10- and 30-ml vials[Rx], 100 mg/ml in 10-ml vials[Rx] ▪ ***Testosterone cypionate injection (in oil):*** 100 mg/ml in 10-ml vials[Rx], 200 mg/ml in 1- and 10-ml vials[Rx] ▪ ***Testosterone enanthate injection (in oil):*** 100 mg/ml in 10-ml vials[Rx], 200 mg/ml in 5- and 10-ml vials and 1-ml prefilled syringes[Rx] ▪ ***Testosterone propionate injection (in oil):*** 100 mg/ml in 10-ml vials[Rx] ▪ ***Testosterone transdermal patches:*** *Testoderm*—4 mg/day in packages of 30[Rx], 6 mg/day in packages of 30[Rx]; *Androderm*—2.5 mg/day in packages of 60[Rx], 5 mg/day in packages of 60[Rx] ▪ ***In combination with:*** estradiol[Rx]. See Appendix A.

TIME/ACTION PROFILE (androgenic effects*)

	ONSET	PEAK	DURATION
IM—base	UK	UK	1–3 days
IM—cypionate, enanthate	UK	UK	2–4 wk
IM—propionate	UK	UK	1–3 days
Transdermal	UK	2–4 hr †	2 hr‡

*Response is highly variable among individuals; may take months.

†Plasma testosterone levels following applications of patch (plateaus after 3–4 wk).

‡Following patch removal.

NURSING IMPLICATIONS

ASSESSMENT

- **General Info:** Monitor intake and output ratios, weigh patient twice weekly, and assess patient for edema. Report significant changes indicative of fluid retention.
- **Men:** Monitor for precocious puberty in boys (acne, darkening of skin, development of male secondary sex characteristics—increase in penis size, frequent erections, growth of body hair). Bone age determinations should be measured every 6 mo to determine rate of bone maturation and effects on epiphyseal closure.
  - ❑ Monitor for breast enlargement, persistent erections, and increased urge to urinate in men. Monitor for difficulty urinating in elderly men, as prostate enlargement may occur.
- **Women:** Assess for virilism (deepening of voice, unusual hair growth or loss, clitoral enlargement, acne, menstrual irregularity).
  - ❑ In women with metastatic breast cancer, monitor for symptoms of hypercalcemia (nausea, vomiting, constipation, lethargy, loss of muscle tone, thirst, polyuria).
- ***Lab Test Considerations:*** Monitor hemoglobin and hematocrit periodically throughout therapy; may cause polycythemia.
  - ❑ Monitor hepatic function tests and serum cholesterol levels periodically throughout course of therapy. May cause increased serum AST

T

and bilirubin, increased or decreased cholesterol levels, and suppression of clotting factors II, V, VII, and X.

- Monitor serum and urine calcium levels and serum alkaline phosphatase concentrations in metastatic cancer.
- May alter results of fasting blood sugar, glucose tolerance tests, thyroid function tests, and metyrapone tests. Increased creatine and CCr may last up to 2 wk following discontinuation of therapy. Serum chloride, potassium, phosphate, and sodium levels may be increased.
- May cause increased levels in 24-hr urine tests for 17-ketosteroid concentrations.
- May cause decreased corticosteroid-binding globulin and sex steroid–binding globulin; free hormone concentrations remain unchanged. May also cause reduced folicle-stimulating hormone (FSH), luteinizing hormone (LH), spermatozoa count, and hamster ova penetration test (HOPT).
- *Transdermal:* Monitor prostatic acid phosphatase and prostatic specific antigen at regular intervals during therapy with transdermal patch. Serum testosterone determinations should be measured 2–4 hr after patch application, after 3–4 wk use.
- Luteinizing hormone and serum ALT should be measured every 6 mo during gender change androgen therapy to monitor success and side effects.

POTENTIAL NURSING DIAGNOSES

- Sexual dysfunction (Indications, Side Effects).
- Knowledge deficit, related to medication regimen (Patient/Family Teaching).

IMPLEMENTATION

- **General Info:** Range-of-motion exercises should be done with all bedridden patients to prevent mobilization of calcium from the bone.
- **IM:** Administer IM deep into gluteal muscle. Crystals may form at low temperatures; warming and shaking vial will redissolve crystals. Use of a wet syringe or needle will cause a cloudy solution but will not affect potency.
- **Transdermal:** Apply patch(es) to clean, dry, hairless skin. Skin may be dry-shaved; do not use chemical depilatories. May be reapplied after bathing, showering, or swimming. *Testoderm* is applied to skin of scrotum. *Androderm* is applied to skin of back, abdomen, upper arms, or thighs.

PATIENT/FAMILY TEACHING

- **General Info:** Advise patient to report the following signs and symptoms promptly: in male patients, priapism (sustained and often painful erections) or gynecomastia; in female patients, virilism (which may be reversible if medication is stopped as soon as changes are noticed), hypercalcemia (nausea, vomiting, constipation, and weakness), edema (unexpected weight gain, swelling of feet), hepatitis (yellowing of skin or eyes and abdominal pain), or unusual bleeding or bruising.
- Explain rationale for prohibition of use for increasing athletic performance. Testosterone is neither safe nor effective for this use and has a potential risk of serious side effects.
- Instruct patient to notify health care professional immediately if pregnancy is planned or suspected.
- Advise diabetic patients to monitor blood or urine closely for alterations in blood sugar concentrations.
- Emphasize the importance of regular follow-up physical exams, lab tests, and x-ray exams to monitor progress.
- Radiologic bone age determinations should be evaluated every 6 mo in prepubertal children to determine rate of bone maturation and effects on epiphyseal centers.
- **Transdermal:** Advise patient to notify health care professional if female sexual partner develops mild virilization.

EVALUATION

Effectiveness of therapy can be demonstrated by: ▪ Resolution of the signs of androgen deficiency without side effects. Therapy is usually limited to 3–6 mo followed by bone growth or maturation determinations ▪ Decrease in the size and spread of breast malignancy in postmenopausal women. In antineoplastic therapy, response may require 3 mo of therapy; if signs of disease progression appear, therapy should be discontinued.

TETRACYCLINES

doxycycline

(dox-i-**sye**-kleen)

{Apo-Doxy}, Doryx, Doxy, Doxy-Caps, {Doxycin}, Monodox, {Novo-doxylin}, Vibramycin, Vibra-Tabs

minocycline

(min-oh-**sye**-kleen)

Minocin

tetracycline

(te-tra-**sye**-kleen)

Achromycin, {Apo-Tetra}, {Novotetra}, {Nu-Tetra}, Panmycin, Robitet, Sumycin, Tetracyn

CLASSIFICATION(S):

Anti-infectives

Pregnancy Category UK

INDICATIONS

▪ Treatment of various infections due to unusual organisms, including: ▫ *Mycoplasma* ▫ *Chlamydia* ▫ *Rickettsia* ▫ *Borrelia burgorferi* ▪ Treatment of gonorrhea and syphilis in penicillin-allergic patients ▪ Prevention of exacerbations of chronic bronchitis ▪ Treatment of acne. **Unlabeled Uses:** ▪ **Doxycycline:** Treatment of Lyme disease.

ACTION

▪ Inhibit bacterial protein synthesis at the level of the 30S bacterial ribosome. **Therapeutic Effects:** ▪ Bacteriostatic action against susceptible bacteria. **Spectrum:** ▪ Include activity against some gram-positive pathogens: ▫ *Bacillus anthracis* ▫ *Clostridium perfringens* ▫ *Clostridium tetani* ▫ *Listeria monocytogenes* ▫ *Nocardia* ▫ *Propionibacterium acnes* ▫ *Actinomyces israelii* ▪ Active against some gram-negative pathogens: ▫ *Haemophilus influenzae* ▫ *Legionella pneumophila* ▫ *Yersinia entercolitica* ▫ *Yersinia pestis* ▫ *Neisseria gonorrhoeae* ▫ *Neisseria meningitidis* ▪ Also active against several other pathogens, including: ▫ *Mycoplasma* ▫ *Treponema pallidum* ▫ *Chlamydia* ▫ *Rickettsia* ▫ *B. burgdorferi*.

PHARMACOKINETICS

Absorption: *Tetracycline*—60–80% absorbed following oral administration. *Doxycycline, minocycline*—Well absorbed from the GI tract.

Distribution: Widely distributed, some penetration into CSF; cross the placenta and enter breast milk.

Metabolism and Excretion: *Doxycycline*—20–40% excreted unchanged by the urine; some inactivation in the intestine and some enterohepatic circulation with excretion in bile and feces. *Minocycline*—5–20% excreted unchanged by the urine; some metabolism by the liver with enterohepatic circulation and excretion in bile and feces. *Tetracycline*—Excreted mostly unchanged by the kidneys.

Half-life: *Doxycycline*—14–17 hr (increased in severe renal impairment). *Minocycline*—11–26 hr. *Tetracycline*—6–12 hr.

CONTRAINDICATIONS AND PRECAUTIONS

Contraindicated in: ▪ Hypersensitivity ▪ Some products contain alcohol or bisulfites and should be avoided in patients with known hypersensitivity or intolerance ▪ Children <8 yr (permanent staining of teeth) ▪ Pregnancy (risk of permanent staining of teeth in infant if used during last half of pregnancy) ▪ Lactation.

Use Cautiously in: ▪ Cachectic or debilitated patients ▪ Renal disease ▪ Hepatic impairment (doxycycline, minocycline) ▪ Nephrogenic diabetes insipidus.

ADVERSE REACTIONS AND SIDE EFFECTS*

CNS: benign intracranial hypertension (↑ in children); *minocycline*—dizziness.

EENT: *minocycline*—vestibular reactions.

GI: diarrhea, nausea, vomiting, esophagitis, hepatotoxicity, pancreatitis.

Derm: photosensitivity, rashes; *minocycline*—pigmentation of skin and mucous membranes.

Hemat: blood dyscrasias.

Local: *doxycycline, minocycline*—phlebitis at IV site.

Misc: hypersensitivity reactions, superinfection.

{} = Available in Canada only.

***CAPITALS indicate life-threatening; underlines indicate most frequent.**

T

INTERACTIONS

Drug-Drug: ▪ May enhance the effect of **warfarin** ▪ May decrease the effectiveness of **estrogen-containing oral contraceptives** ▪ **Antacids, calcium, iron**, and **magnesium** form insoluble compounds (chelates) and decrease absorption of tetracyclines; effect is least with doxycycline ▪ **Sucralfate** may bind to tetracycline and prevent its absorption from the GI tract ▪ **Cholestyramine** or **colestipol** decrease oral absorption of tetracyclines ▪ **Adsorbent antidiarrheals** may decrease absorption ▪ **Barbiturates, phenytoin**, or **carbamazepine** may decrease the activity of doxycycline.

Drug-Food: ▪ **Calcium** in foods or **dairy products** decreases absorption by forming insoluble compounds (chelates).

ROUTE AND DOSAGE

❑ Doxycycline

- **PO (Adults and Children >45 kg):** *Most infections*—100 mg q 12 hr on the 1st day, then 100–200 mg once daily or 50–100 mg q 12 hr. *Gonorrhea*—100 mg q 12 hr for 7 days or 300 mg followed 1 hr later by another 300-mg dose. *Malaria prophylaxis*—100 mg once daily. *Lyme disease*—100 mg twice daily.
- **PO (Children ≤45 kg):** 2.2 mg/kg q 12 hr on the 1st day, then 2.2–4.4 mg/kg/day given once daily or 1.1–2.2 mg/kg q 12 hr.
- **IV (Adults and Children >45 kg):** 200 mg once daily or 100 mg q 12 hr on the 1st day, then 100–200 mg once daily or 50–100 mg q 12 hr.
- **IV (Children ≤45 kg):** 4.4 mg/kg once daily or 2.2 mg/kg q 12 hr on the 1st day, then 2.2–4.4 mg/kg/day given once daily or 1.1–2.2 mg/kg q 12 hr.

❑ Minocycline

- **PO (Adults):** 100–200 mg initially, then 100 mg q 12 hr or 50 mg q 6 hr.
- **PO (Children ≥8 yr):** 4 mg/kg initially, then 2 mg/kg q 12 hr.
- **IV (Adults):** 200 mg initially, then 100 mg q 12 hr (up to 400 mg/day).
- **IV (Children ≥8 yr):** 4 mg/kg initially, then 2 mg/kg q 12 hr.

❑ Tetracycline

- **PO (Adults):** 250–500 mg q 6 hr or 500 mg–1 g q 12 hr. *Chronic treatment of acne*—500 mg–2 g/day for 3 wk, then decreased to 125 mg–1 g/day.
- **PO (Children ≥8 yr):** 6.25–12.5 mg/kg q 6 hr or 12.5–25 mg/kg q 12 hr.

AVAILABILITY

❑ Doxycycline

▪ ***Tablets:*** 100 mg[Rx] ▪ ***Capsules:*** 50 mg[Rx], 100 mg[Rx] ▪ ***Delayed-release capsules:*** 100 mg[Rx] ▪ ***Oral suspension:*** 25 mg/5 ml[Rx], 50 mg/5 ml[Rx] ▪ ***Powder for injection:*** 100 mg[Rx], 200 mg[Rx].

❑ Minocycline

▪ ***Capsules:*** 50 mg[Rx], 100 mg[Rx] ▪ ***Tablets:*** 50 mg[Rx], 100 mg[Rx] ▪ ***Oral suspension:*** 50 mg/5 ml[Rx] ▪ ***Powder for injection:*** 100 mg[Rx].

❑ Tetracycline

▪ ***Tablets:*** 250 mg[Rx], 500 mg[Rx] ▪ ***Capsules:*** 250 mg[Rx], 500 mg[Rx] ▪ ***Oral suspension:*** 125 mg/5 ml[Rx].

TIME/ACTION PROFILE (blood levels)

	ONSET	PEAK	DURATION
Doxycycline—PO	1–2 hr	1.5–4 hr	12 hr
Doxycycline—IV	rapid	end of infusion	12 hr
Minocycline—PO	rapid	2–3 hr	6–12 hr
Minocycline—IV	rapid	end of infusion	6–12 hr
Tetracycline—PO	1–2 hr	2–4 hr	6–12 hr

NURSING IMPLICATIONS

ASSESSMENT

- **Infection:** Assess patient for infection (vital signs; appearance of wound, sputum, urine, and stool; WBC) at beginning of and throughout therapy.
- ▫ Obtain specimens for culture and sensitivity prior to initiating therapy. First dose may be given before receiving results.
- **IV:** Assess IV site frequently; may cause thrombophlebitis.
- ***Lab Test Considerations:*** Renal and hepatic functions and CBC should be monitored periodically during long-term therapy.
- ▫ May cause increased AST, ALT, serum alkaline phosphatase, bilirubin, and amylase concen-

trations. Tetracyclines, except doxycycline, may cause elevated serum BUN.
- May cause false elevations in urinary catecholamine levels.

POTENTIAL NURSING DIAGNOSES

- Infection, risk for (Indications, Side Effects).
- Knowledge deficit, related to medication regimen (Patient/Family Teaching).
- Noncompliance, related to medication regimen (Patient/Family Teaching).

IMPLEMENTATION

- **General Info:** May cause yellow-brown discoloration and softening of teeth and bones if administered prenatally or during early childhood. Not recommended for children under 8 yr of age or during pregnancy or lactation.
- **PO:** Administer around the clock. Administer at least 1 hr before or 2 hr after meals. *Doxycycline and minocycline* may be taken with food or milk if GI irritation occurs. Administer with a full glass of liquid at least 1 hr before going to bed to avoid esophageal ulceration. Use calibrated measuring device for liquid preparations. Shake liquid preparations well. Do not administer within 1–3 hr of other medications.
- Avoid administration of calcium, antacids, magnesium-containing medications, sodium bicarbonate, or iron supplements within 1–3 hr of oral tetracyclines.

Doxycycline

- **Intermittent Infusion:** Dilute each 100 mg with 10 ml of sterile water or 0.9% NaCl for injection. Dilute further in 100–1000 ml of 0.9% NaCl, D5W, D5/LR, Ringer's or lactated Ringer's solution. Solution is stable for 12 hr at room temperature and 72 hr if refrigerated. If diluted with D5/LR or lactated Ringer's solution, administer within 6 hr. Protect solution from direct sunlight. Concentrations of less than 1 mcg/ml or greater than 1 mg/ml are not recommended.
- ***Rate:*** Administer over a minimum of 1–4 hr. Avoid rapid administration. Avoid extravasation.
- **Y-Site Compatibility:** ▪ acyclovir ▪ amifostine ▪ amiodarone ▪ aztreonam ▪ cyclophosphamide ▪ diltiazem ▪ filgrastim ▪ fludarabine ▪ hydromorphone ▪ magnesium sulfate ▪ melphalan ▪ meperidine ▪ morphine ▪ ondansetron ▪ perphenazine ▪ sargramostim ▪ tacrolimus ▪ teniposide ▪ thiotepa ▪ vinorelbine.
- **Y-Site Incompatibility:** ▪ heparin ▪ piperacillin/tazobactam.

Minocycline

- **Intermittent Infusion:** Dilute each 100 mg with 5–10 ml of sterile water for injection. Dilute further in 500–1000 ml of 0.9% NaCl, D5W, D5/0.9% NaCl, Ringer's or lactated Ringer's solution. Solution is stable for 24 hr at room temperature.
- ***Rate:*** Administer over 6 hr immediately following dilution. Avoid rapid infusions. May cause thrombophlebitis; avoid extravasation.
- **Y-Site Compatibility:** ▪ aztreonam ▪ cyclophosphamide ▪ filgrastim ▪ fludarabine ▪ heparin ▪ hydrocortisone sodium succinate ▪ magnesium sulfate ▪ melphalan ▪ perphenazine ▪ potassium chloride ▪ sargramostim ▪ teniposide ▪ vinorelbine ▪ vitamin B complex with C.
- **Y-Site Incompatibility:** ▪ amifostine ▪ hydromorphone ▪ meperidine ▪ morphine ▪ piperacillin/tazobactam ▪ thiotepa.

PATIENT/FAMILY TEACHING

- **General Info:** Instruct patient to take medication around the clock and to finish the drug completely, as directed, even if feeling better. If a dose is missed, take as soon as possible unless almost time for next dose; do not double doses. Advise patient that sharing of this medication may be dangerous.
- Advise patient to avoid taking milk or other dairy products concurrently with *tetracycline.* Also avoid taking antacids, calcium, magnesium-containing medications, sodium bicarbonate, and iron supplements within 1–3 hr of oral tetracyclines.
- Advise female patients to use a nonhormonal method of contraception while taking tetracyclines and until next menstrual period.
- *Minocycline* commonly causes dizziness or unsteadiness. Caution patient to avoid driving or other activities requiring alertness until response to medication is known. Notify health care professional if these symptoms occur.
- Caution patient to use sunscreen and protective clothing to prevent photosensitivity reactions.
- Advise patient to report the signs of superinfection (black, furry overgrowth on the

tongue; vaginal itching or discharge; loose or foul-smelling stools). Skin rash, pruritus, and urticaria should also be reported.

- Instruct patient to notify health care professional of medication regimen prior to treatment or surgery.
- Instruct patient to notify health care professional if symptoms do not improve within a few days for systemic preparations.
- Caution patient to discard outdated or decomposed tetracyclines; they may be toxic.

EVALUATION

Clinical response to therapy can be evaluated by: ▪ Resolution of the signs and symptoms of infection. Length of time for complete resolution depends on the organism and site of infection ▪ Decrease in acne lesions.

THIAMINE

(**thye**-a-min)

{Betaxin}, {Bewon}, Biamine, vitamin B_1

CLASSIFICATION(S):

Vitamin (water-soluble)

Pregnancy Category A

INDICATIONS

- Treatment of thiamine deficiencies (beriberi)
- Prevention of Wernicke's encephalopathy
- Dietary supplement in patients with GI disease, alcoholism, or cirrhosis.

ACTION

▪ Required for carbohydrate metabolism. **Therapeutic Effects:** ▪ Replacement in deficiency states.

PHARMACOKINETICS

Absorption: Well absorbed from the GI tract by an active process. Excessive amounts are not absorbed completely. Also well absorbed from IM sites.

Distribution: Widely distributed. Enters breast milk.

Metabolism and Excretion: Metabolized by the liver. Excess amounts are excreted unchanged by the kidneys.

Half-life: UK.

CONTRAINDICATIONS AND PRECAUTIONS

Contraindicated in: ▪ Hypersensitivity ▪ Known alcohol intolerance or bisulfite hypersensitivity (elixir only).

Use Cautiously in: ▪ Wernicke's encephalopathy (condition may be worsened unless thiamine is administered before glucose).

ADVERSE REACTIONS AND SIDE EFFECTS*

Adverse reactions and side effects are extremely rare and are usually associated with IV administration or extremely large doses.

CNS: restlessness, weakness.

EENT: tightness of the throat.

Resp: pulmonary edema, respiratory distress.

CV: VASCULAR COLLAPSE, hypotension, vasodilation.

GI: GI bleeding, nausea.

Derm: cyanosis, pruritus, sweating, tingling, urticaria, warmth.

Misc: angioedema.

INTERACTIONS

Drug-Drug: ▪ May enhance **neuromuscular blocking agents.**

ROUTE AND DOSAGE

Thiamine Deficiency (Beriberi)

- **PO (Adults):** 5–10 mg 3 times daily.
- **PO (Children):** 10–50 mg/day in divided doses.
- **IM, IV (Adults):** 5–100 mg tid.
- **IM, IV (Children):** 10–25 mg/day.

Dietary Supplement

- **PO (Adults):** 1–1.6 mg/day.
- **PO (Children 4–10 yr):** 0.9–1 mg/day.
- **PO (Children birth–3 yr):** 0.3–0.7 mg/day.

AVAILABILITY

▪ ***Tablets:*** 5 mg^{OTC}, 10 mg^{OTC}, 25 mg^{OTC}, 50 mg^{OTC}, 100 mg^{OTC}, 250 mg^{OTC}, 500 mg^{OTC} ▪ {***Elixir:*** 250 mcg/5 ml^{OTC}} ▪ ***Injection:*** 100

{} = Available in Canada only.

***CAPITALS indicate life-threatening; underlines indicate most frequent.**

mg/ml in 1-ml ampules and prefilled syringes and 1-, 2-, 10-, and 30-ml vials[Rx] ▪ ***In combination with:*** other vitamins, minerals, and trace elements in multi-vitamin preparations[OTC].

TIME/ACTION PROFILE (time for symptoms of deficiency—edema and heart failure—to resolve*)

	ONSET	PEAK	DURATION
PO, IM, IV	hr	days	days–wks

*Confusion and psychosis take longer to respond.

NURSING IMPLICATIONS

ASSESSMENT

- ▫ Assess patient for signs and symptoms of thiamine deficiency (anorexia, GI distress, irritability, palpitations, tachycardia, edema, paresthesia, muscle weakness and pain, depression, memory loss, confusion, psychosis, visual disturbances, elevated serum pyruvic acid levels).
- ▫ Assess patient's nutritional status (diet, weight) prior to and throughout therapy.
- ▫ Monitor patients receiving IV thiamine for anaphylaxis (wheezing, urticaria, edema).
- ▪ ***Lab Test Considerations:*** May interfere with certain methods of testing serum theophylline, uric acid, and urobilinogen concentrations.

POTENTIAL NURSING DIAGNOSES

- ▪ Nutrition, altered, less than body requirements (Indications).
- ▪ Knowledge deficit, related to diet and medication regimen (Patient/Family Teaching).

IMPLEMENTATION

- ▪ **General Info:** Because of infrequency of single B-vitamin deficiencies, combinations are commonly administered.
- ▪ **IM, IV:** Parenteral administration is reserved for patients in whom oral administration is not feasible.
- ▪ **IM:** Administration may cause tenderness and induration at injection site. Cool compresses may decrease discomfort.
- ▪ **IV:** Sensitivity reactions and deaths have occurred from IV administration. An intradermal test dose is recommended in patients with suspected sensitivity. Monitor site for erythema and induration.
- ▪ **Direct IV:** Administer undiluted.
- ▪ ***Rate:*** Administer at a rate of 100 mg over 5 min.
- ▪ **Continuous Infusion:** May be diluted in dextrose/Ringer's or lactated Ringer's combinations, dextrose/saline combinations, D5W, D10W, Ringer's and lactated Ringer's injection, 0.9% NaCl, or 0.45% NaCl and is usually administered with other vitamins.
- ▪ **Y-Site Compatibility:** ▪ famotidine.
- ▪ **Additive Incompatibility:** ▪ solutions with neutral or alkaline pH, such as carbonates, bicarbonates, citrates, and acetates.

PATIENT/FAMILY TEACHING

- ▫ Encourage patient to comply with dietary recommendations of health care professional. Explain that the best source of vitamins is a well-balanced diet with foods from the four basic food groups.
- ▫ Teach patient that foods high in thiamine include cereals (whole grain and enriched), meats (especially pork), and fresh vegetables; loss is variable during cooking.
- ▫ Caution patients self-medicating with vitamin supplements not to exceed RDA (see Appendix L). The effectiveness of megadoses of vitamins for treatment of various medical conditions is unproved and may cause side effects.

EVALUATION

Effectiveness of therapy can be demonstrated by: ▪ Prevention of or decrease in the signs and symptoms of vitamin B_1 deficiency ▫ Decrease in the symptoms of neuritis, ocular signs, ataxia, edema, and heart failure may be seen within hours of administration and may disappear within a few days ▫ Confusion and psychosis may take longer to respond and may persist if nerve damage has occurred.

THIETHYLPERAZINE

(thye-eth-il-**per**-a-zeen)
Norzine, Torecan

CLASSIFICATION(S):
Antiemetic (phenothiazine)

Pregnancy Category UK

INDICATIONS

- ▪ Management of nausea and vomiting.

ACTION

▪ Alters the effects of dopamine in the CNS ▪ Depresses the chemoreceptive trigger zone (CTZ) and vomiting center in the CNS. **Therapeutic Effects:** ▪ Diminished nausea and vomiting.

PHARMACOKINETICS

Absorption: Well absorbed following oral, rectal, or IM administration.
Distribution: Widely distributed, high concentrations in the CNS. Crosses the placenta and probably enters breast milk.
Metabolism and Excretion: Highly metabolized by the liver and GI mucosa.
Half-life: UK.

CONTRAINDICATIONS AND PRECAUTIONS

Contraindicated in: ▪ Hypersensitivity ▪ Hypersensitivity to bisulfites (IM) ▪ Hypersensitivity to aspirin or tartrazine (tablets) ▪ Cross-sensitivity with other phenothiazines may occur ▪ Narrow-angle glaucoma ▪ Bone marrow depression ▪ Severe liver or cardiovascular disease ▪ Pregnancy.
Use Cautiously in: ▪ Geriatric or debilitated patients (dosage reduction recommended) ▪ Diabetes mellitus ▪ Respiratory disease ▪ Prostatic hypertrophy ▪ CNS tumors ▪ Epilepsy ▪ Intestinal obstruction ▪ Children <12 yr or lactation (safety not established).

ADVERSE REACTIONS AND SIDE EFFECTS*

CNS: NEUROLEPTIC MALIGNANT SYNDROME, sedation, cerebral vascular spasm, extrapyramidal reactions, headache, restlessness, tardive dyskinesia.
EENT: dry eyes, blurred vision, lens opacities, tinnitus.
CV: hypotension (following IM use), peripheral edema.
GI: constipation, dry mouth, altered taste, anorexia, drug-induced hepatitis, ileus.
GU: urinary retention.
Derm: photosensitivity, pigment changes, rashes.
Endo: galactorrhea.
Hemat: AGRANULOCYTOSIS, leukopenia.
Metab: hyperthermia.
Neuro: trigeminal neuralgia.
Misc: allergic reactions.

INTERACTIONS

Drug-Drug: ▪ Additive hypotension with **antihypertensive agents**, acute ingestion of **alcohol**, or **nitrates** ▪ Additive CNS depression with other **CNS depressants**, including **alcohol, antihistamines, opioids, sedative/hypnotics**, or **general anesthetics** ▪ Additive anticholinergic effects with other **drugs possessing anticholinergic properties**, including **antihistamines, antidepressants, atropine, disopyramide, haloperidol**, and other **phenothiazines** ▪ May decrease the beneficial effects of **levodopa** ▪ May block alpha-adrenergic effects of **epinephrine**, resulting in severe hypotension and tachycardia.

ROUTE AND DOSAGE

▪ **PO, IM (Adults):** 10 mg 1–3 times daily.

AVAILABILITY

▪ ***Tablets:*** 10 mg[Rx] ▪ ***Injection:*** 5 mg/ml in 2-ml ampules[Rx].

TIME/ACTION PROFILE (antiemetic effect)

	ONSET	PEAK	DURATION
PO	30 min	UK	4 hr
IM	UK	UK	UK

NURSING IMPLICATIONS

ASSESSMENT

- □ Assess patient for nausea and vomiting prior to and 30–60 min following administration.
- □ Monitor blood pressure (sitting, standing, lying), pulse, and respiratory rate prior to and frequently during initial therapy.
- □ Assess patient for level of sedation following administration.
- □ Monitor patient for onset of akathisia (restlessness or desire to keep moving) and extrapyramidal side effects (*parkinsonian*—difficulty speaking or swallowing, loss of balance control, pill rolling, mask-like face, shuffling gait, rigidity, tremors; and *dystonic*—muscle spasms, twisting motions, twitching, inability to move eyes, weakness of arms or legs) every

***CAPITALS indicate life-threatening; underlines indicate most frequent.**

2 mo during therapy and 8–12 wk after therapy has been discontinued. Report these symptoms; reduction in dosage or discontinuation of medication may be necessary. Trihexyphenidyl or diphenhydramine may be used to control these symptoms.
- Monitor for tardive dyskinesia (uncontrolled rhythmic movement of mouth, face, and extremities; lip smacking or puckering; puffing of cheeks; uncontrolled chewing; rapid or worm-like movements of tongue). Report immediately; may be irreversible.
- Monitor for development of neuroleptic malignant syndrome (fever, respiratory distress, tachycardia, convulsions, diaphoresis, hypertension or hypotension, pallor, tiredness, severe muscle stiffness, loss of bladder control). Notify physician or other health care professional immediately if these symptoms occur.
- ***Lab Test Considerations:*** CBC and liver function tests should be evaluated periodically throughout course of prolonged therapy.
- May cause false-positive or false-negative pregnancy tests.
- May cause increased serum prolactin levels, thereby interfering with gonadorelin test results.

POTENTIAL NURSING DIAGNOSES

- Fluid volume deficit (Indications).
- Injury, risk for (Side Effects).
- Knowledge deficit, related to medication regimen (Patient/Family Teaching).

IMPLEMENTATION

- **IM:** Inject slowly into deep, well-developed muscle. Administer only clear, colorless solution. Keep patient recumbent for at least 60 min following injection to minimize hypotensive effects.
- Do not administer IV; may cause severe hypotension.
- **Syringe Compatibility:** ▪ butorphanol ▪ hydromorphone ▪ midazolam ▪ ranitidine.
- **Syringe Incompatibility:** ▪ ketorolac.

PATIENT/FAMILY TEACHING

- Instruct patient to take medication exactly as directed. Do not take within 2 hr of antacids or antidiarrheal agents.
- Advise patient to change positions slowly to minimize orthostatic hypotension.
- May cause drowsiness. Caution patient to avoid driving or other activities requiring alertness until response to medication is known.
- Caution patient to avoid taking alcohol or other CNS depressants concurrently with this medication.
- Inform patient of possibility of extrapyramidal symptoms and tardive dyskinesia. Caution patient to report these symptoms immediately to health care professional.
- Advise patient to use sunscreen and protective clothing when exposed to the sun to prevent photosensitivity reactions. Extremes in temperature should also be avoided, as this drug impairs body temperature regulation.
- Instruct patient to use frequent mouth rinses, good oral hygiene, and sugarless gum or candy to minimize dry mouth. Consult health care professional if dry mouth continues for >2 wk.
- Advise patient that increasing bulk and fluids in the diet and exercise may help minimize the constipating effects of this medication.
- Instruct patient to notify health care professional promptly if sore throat, fever, unusual bleeding or bruising, skin rashes, weakness, tremors, visual disturbances, dark-colored urine, or clay-colored stools are noted.
- Patients on prolonged therapy should have periodic lab tests and ocular exams.

EVALUATION

Effectiveness of therapy can be demonstrated by: ▪ Relief of nausea and vomiting.

T

THIORIDAZINE

(thye-oh-**rid**-a-zeen)
{Apo-Thioridazine}, Mellaril, Mellaril-S, {Novo-Ridazine}, {PMS Thioridazine}

CLASSIFICATION(S):
Antipsychotic agent (phenothiazine)

Pregnancy Category C

INDICATIONS

▪ Acute and chronic psychoses ▪ Management of depression/anxiety in geriatric patients ▪ Severe behavioral problems in children.

ACTION

▪ Alters the effects of dopamine in the CNS ▪ Possesses significant anticholinergic and alpha-adrenergic blocking activity. **Therapeutic Effects:** ▪ Diminished signs and symptoms of psychoses.

PHARMACOKINETICS

Absorption: Absorption from tablets is variable; may be better with oral liquid formulations.
Distribution: Widely distributed, high concentrations in the CNS. Crosses the placenta and enters breast milk.
Metabolism and Excretion: Highly metabolized by the liver and GI mucosa.
Half-life: 21–24 hr.

CONTRAINDICATIONS AND PRECAUTIONS

Contraindicated in: ▪ Hypersensitivity ▪ Cross-sensitivity with other phenothiazines may exist ▪ Narrow-angle glaucoma ▪ Bone marrow depression ▪ Severe liver or cardiovascular disease □ Known alcohol intolerance (concentrate only).
Use Cautiously in: ▪ Geriatric or debilitated patients ▪ Diabetes mellitus ▪ Respiratory disease ▪ Prostatic hypertrophy ▪ CNS tumors ▪ Epilepsy ▪ Intestinal obstruction ▪ Pregnancy or lactation (safety not established).

ADVERSE REACTIONS AND SIDE EFFECTS*

CNS: NEUROLEPTIC MALIGNANT SYNDROME, sedation, extrapyramidal reactions, tardive dyskinesia.
EENT: blurred vision, dry eyes, lens opacities, pigmentary retinopathy (high doses).
CV: hypotension, tachycardia.
GI: constipation, dry mouth, anorexia, drug-induced hepatitis, ileus.
GU: urinary retention.
Derm: photosensitivity, pigment changes, rashes.
Endo: galactorrhea.
Hemat: AGRANULOCYTOSIS, leukopenia.
Metab: hyperthermia.
Misc: allergic reactions.

INTERACTIONS

Drug-Drug: ▪ Additive hypotension with other **antihypertensive agents, nitrates,** and acute ingestion of **alcohol** ▪ Additive CNS depression with other **CNS depressants,** including **alcohol, antihistamines, opioids, sedative/hypnotics,** and **general anesthetics** ▪ Additive anticholinergic effects with other **drugs possessing anticholinergic properties,** including **antihistamines, antidepressants, atropine, haloperidol,** other **phenothiazines,** and **disopyramide** ▪ **Lithium** decreases blood levels of thioridazine ▪ Thioridazine may mask early signs of **lithium** toxicity and increase the risk of extrapyramidal reactions ▪ Increased risk of agranulocytosis with **antithyroid agents** ▪ Concurrent use with **epinephrine** may result in severe hypotension and tachycardia ▪ May decrease the effectiveness of **levodopa.**

ROUTE AND DOSAGE

- **PO (Adults and Children >12 yr):** 25–100 mg tid initially; maintenance 10–200 mg 2–4 times daily up to 800 mg/day.
- **PO (Children >2 yr):** 0.25–3 mg/kg (7.5 mg/m^2) 4 times daily or 10–25 mg 2–3 times daily.

AVAILABILITY

▪ ***Tablets:*** 10 mg[Rx], 15 mg[Rx], 25 mg[Rx], 50 mg[Rx], 100 mg[Rx], 150 mg[Rx], 200 mg[Rx] ▪ ***Oral suspension:*** {10 mg/5 ml[Rx]}, 25 mg/5 ml[Rx], 100 mg/5 ml[Rx] ▪ ***Concentrated oral solution:*** 30 mg/ml[Rx], 100 mg/ml[Rx].

TIME/ACTION PROFILE (antipsychotic effects)

	ONSET	PEAK	DURATION
PO	UK	UK	8–12 hr

NURSING IMPLICATIONS

ASSESSMENT

□ Assess mental status (orientation, mood, behavior) and degree of anxiety prior to and periodically throughout therapy.
□ Monitor blood pressure (sitting, standing, lying), ECG, pulse, and respiratory rate prior to

*CAPITALS indicate life-threatening; underlines indicate most frequent.

and frequently during the period of dosage adjustment. May cause Q-wave and T-wave changes in ECG.

- Observe patient carefully when administering medication to ensure that medication is actually taken and not hoarded.
- Assess patient for level of sedation following administration.
- Monitor intake and output ratios and daily weight. Report significant discrepancies.
- Monitor patient for onset of akathisia (restlessness or desire to keep moving) and extrapyramidal side effects (*parkinsonian*—difficulty speaking or swallowing, loss of balance control, pill rolling, mask-like face, shuffling gait, rigidity, tremors; and *dystonic*—muscle spasms, twisting motions, twitching, inability to move eyes, weakness of arms or legs) every 2 mo during therapy and 8–12 wk after therapy has been discontinued. Report these symptoms; reduction in dosage or discontinuation of medication may be necessary. Trihexyphenidyl or diphenhydramine may be used to control these symptoms.
- Monitor for tardive dyskinesia (uncontrolled rhythmic movement of mouth, face, and extremities; lip smacking or puckering; puffing of cheeks; uncontrolled chewing; rapid or worm-like movements of tongue). Report immediately; may be irreversible.
- Monitor for development of neuroleptic malignant syndrome (fever, respiratory distress, tachycardia, convulsions, diaphoresis, hypertension or hypotension, pallor, tiredness, severe muscle stiffness, loss of bladder control). Notify physician or other health care professional immediately if these symptoms occur.

- ***Lab Test Considerations:*** CBC, liver function tests, and ocular examinations should be evaluated periodically throughout therapy. May cause decreased hematocrit, hemoglobin, leukocytes, granulocytes, platelets. May cause elevated bilirubin, AST, ALT, and alkaline phosphatase. Agranulocytosis occurs between 4–10 wk of therapy with recovery 1–2 wk following discontinuation. May recur if medication is restarted. Liver function abnormalities may require discontinuation of therapy.
  - May cause false-positive or false-negative pregnancy tests and false-positive urine bilirubin test results.
  - May cause increased serum prolactin levels, thereby interfering with gonadorelin test results.

POTENTIAL NURSING DIAGNOSES

- Coping, ineffective individual (Indications).
- Thought processes, altered (Indications).
- Knowledge deficit, related to medication regimen (Patient/Family Teaching).

IMPLEMENTATION

- **General Info:** To prevent contact dermatitis, avoid getting liquid preparations on hands, and wash hands thoroughly if spillage occurs.
  - Phenothiazines should be discontinued 48 hr before and not resumed for 24 hr following myelography, as they lower the seizure threshold.
- **PO:** Administer with food, milk, or full glass of water to minimize gastric irritation.
  - Dilute concentrate in 120 ml of distilled or acidified tap water or fruit juice just prior to administration.

PATIENT/FAMILY TEACHING

- Advise patient to take medication exactly as directed and not to skip doses or double up on missed doses. If a dose is missed, it should be taken as soon as remembered unless almost time for the next dose. If more than 2 doses a day are ordered, the missed dose should be taken within 1 hr of the scheduled time or omitted. Abrupt withdrawal may lead to gastritis, nausea, vomiting, dizziness, headache, tachycardia, and insomnia.
- Inform patient of possibility of extrapyramidal symptoms and tardive dyskinesia. Instruct patient to report these symptoms immediately to health care professional.
- Advise patient to change positions slowly to minimize orthostatic hypotension.
- May cause drowsiness. Caution patient to avoid driving or other activities requiring alertness until response to medication is known.
- Advise patient to use sunscreen and protective clothing when exposed to the sun. Exposed surfaces may develop a blue-gray pigmentation, which may fade following discontinuation of the medication. Extremes in temperature should also be avoided, as this drug impairs body temperature regulation.
- Instruct patient to use frequent mouth rinses, good oral hygiene, and sugarless gum or

candy to minimize dry mouth. Consult health care professional if dry mouth continues for >2 wk.

- □ Advise patient that increasing activity and bulk and fluids in the diet helps minimize the constipating effects of this medication.
- □ Caution patient to avoid taking alcohol or other CNS depressants concurrently with this medication.
- □ Advise patient not to take thioridazine within 2 hr of antacids or antidiarrheal medication.
- □ Inform patient that this medication may turn urine pink to reddish brown.
- □ Advise patient to notify health care professional of medication regimen prior to treatment or surgery.
- □ Instruct patient to notify health care professional promptly if sore throat, fever, unusual bleeding or bruising, rash, weakness, tremors, visual disturbances, dark-colored urine, or clay-colored stools occur.
- □ Emphasize the importance of routine follow-up exams to monitor response to medication and to detect side effects. Periodic ocular exams are indicated. Encourage continued participation in psychotherapy.

EVALUATION

Effectiveness of therapy can be demonstrated by: ▪ Decrease in excitable, paranoic, or withdrawn behavior ▪ Decrease in anxiety associated with depression ▪ Improvement in severe behavioral problems in children.

THROMBOLYTIC AGENTS

alteplase
(**al**-te-plase)
Activase, {Activase rt-PA}, {Lysatec rt-PA}, tissue plasminogen activator, t-PA

anistreplase
(an-**eye**-strep-lase)
anisoylated plasminogen–streptokinase activator complex, APSAC, Eminase

reteplase
(**re**-te-plase)
Retavase

streptokinase
(strep-toe-**kye**-nase)
Kabbikinase, Streptase

urokinase
(yoor-oh-**kye**-nase)
Abbokinase, Abbokinase Open-Cath

CLASSIFICATION(S):
Thrombolytic agents (plasminogen activators)

Pregnancy Category B (urokinase), C (alteplase, anistreplase, reteplase, streptokinase)

INDICATIONS

▪ Acute management of coronary thrombosis (myocardial infarction) ▪ **Streptokinase, urokinase:** Management of massive pulmonary emboli ▪ **Alteplase:** Management of acute ischemic stroke ▪ **Streptokinase, urokinase:** □ Management of deep vein thrombosis or arterial thromboembolism □ Management of occluded cannulae/catheters (streptokinase unlabeled for this indication).

ACTION

▪ Convert plasminogen to plasmin, which is then able to degrade fibrin present in clots. Alteplase, reteplase, and urokinase directly activate plasminogen. Anistreplase and streptokinase combine with plasminogen to form activator complexes, which then convert plasminogen to plasmin. **Therapeutic Effects:** ▪ Lysis of thrombi in coronary arteries, with preservation of ventricular function ▪ Lysis of pulmonary emboli or deep vein thrombosis ▪ Decreased neurologic sequelae of stroke ▪ Clearing of clots in cannulae/catheters.

PHARMACOKINETICS

Absorption: Following IV administration, absorption is essentially complete. Intracoronary administration or administration into occluded catheters or cannulae has a more localized effect.

Distribution: Streptokinase appears to minimally, if at all, cross the placenta. Remainder of distribution for streptokinase or other agents is not known.

{} = Available in Canada only.

Metabolism and Excretion: *Alteplase*—Rapidly metabolized by the liver. *Anistreplase*—Inactivated by binding to plasmin inactivators. *Reteplase*—Cleared primarily by the liver and kidneys. *Streptokinase*—Rapidly cleared from circulation.

Half-life: *Alteplase*—35 min; *anistreplase*—70–120 min; *reteplase*—13–16 min; *streptokinase activator complex*—23 min; *urokinase*—up to 20 min.

CONTRAINDICATIONS AND PRECAUTIONS

Contraindicated in: ▪ Active internal bleeding ▪ History of cerebrovascular accident, recent CNS trauma or surgery, neoplasm, or arteriovenous malformation ▪ Severe uncontrolled hypertension ▪ Known bleeding tendencies ▪ Hypersensitivity; cross-sensitivity with anistreplase and streptokinase may occur.

Use Cautiously in: ▪ Recent (within 10 days) major surgery, trauma, GI or GU bleeding ▪ Left heart thrombus ▪ Severe hepatic or renal disease ▪ Hemorrhagic ophthalmic conditions ▪ Septic phlebitis ▪ Previous puncture of a noncompressible vessel ▪ Geriatric patients (>75 yr) ▪ Subacute bacterial endocarditis or acute pericarditis ▪ Recent streptococcal infection or previous therapy with anistreplase or streptokinase (from 5 days–6 mo); may produce resistance due to antibody formation; increased dosage requirements may be encountered (anistreplase and streptokinase only) ▪ Pregnancy, lactation, or children (safety not established).

Exercise Extreme Caution in: ▪ Early postpartum period (10 days) ▪ Patients receiving warfarin therapy.

ADVERSE REACTIONS AND SIDE EFFECTS*

CNS: INTRACRANIAL HEMORRHAGE, headache.
EENT: epistaxis, gingival bleeding; *streptokinase*—periorbital edema.
Resp: bronchospasm, hemoptysis.
CV: <u>reperfusion arrhythmias</u>, hypotension.
GI: GI BLEEDING, RETROPERITONEAL BLEEDING.
GU: GU TRACT BLEEDING.
Derm: ecchymoses, flushing, urticaria.
Hemat: <u>BLEEDING</u>.
Local: hemorrhage at injection sites, phlebitis at IV site.
MS: musculoskeletal pain.
Misc: allergic reactions including ANAPHYLAXIS, fever.

INTERACTIONS

Drug-Drug: ▪ **Aspirin, NSAIDs, warfarin, heparins, abciximab, ticlopidine,** or **dipyridamole**—concurrent use may increase the risk of bleeding, although these agents are frequently used together or in sequence ▪ Risk of bleeding may be increased by concurrent use of **cefamandole, cefotetan, cefoperazone, plicamycin, ticlopidine,** or **valproic acid.**

ROUTE AND DOSAGE

❑ **Alteplase**

❑ ***Myocardial Infarction (Accelerated or Front-Loading Regimen)***

- **IV (Adults):** 15 mg initially, then 0.75 mg/kg (up to 50 mg) over 30 min, then 0.5 mg/kg (up to 35 mg) over next 60 min; usually accompanied by heparin therapy.

❑ ***Myocardial Infarction (Standard Regimen)***

- **IV (Adults >65 kg):** 60 mg over 1st hr (6–10 mg given as a bolus over first 1–2 min), 20 mg over the 2nd hr, and 20 mg over the 3rd hr for a total dose of 100 mg.
- **IV (Adults <65 kg):** 0.75 mg/kg over 1st hr (0.075–0.125 mg/kg given as a bolus over first 1–2 min), 0.25 mg/kg over the 2nd hr, and 0.25 mg/kg over the 3rd hr for a total dose of 1.25 mg/kg (not to exceed 100 mg total).

❑ ***Pulmonary Embolism***

- **IV (Adults):** 100 mg over 2 hr; follow with heparin.

❑ ***Acute Ischemic Stroke***

- **IV (Adults):** 0.9 mg/kg (not to exceed 90 mg), given as an infusion over 1 hr, with 10% of the dose given as a bolus over the 1st min.

❑ **Anistreplase**

- **IV (Adults):** 30 units over 2–5 min.

***CAPITALS indicate life-threatening; <u>underlines</u> indicate most frequent.**

❑ **Reteplase**

- **IV (Adults):** 10 units, followed 30 min later by an additional 10 units.

❑ **Streptokinase**

❑ ***Myocardial Infarction***

- **IV (Adults):** 1.5 million IU.
- **Intracoronary (Adults):** 20,000 IU bolus followed by 2000 IU/min infusion for 60 min (140,000 IU total dose).

❑ ***Deep Vein Thrombosis, Pulmonary Emboli, Arterial Emboli, or Thromboses***

- **IV (Adults):** 250,000 IU loading dose, followed by 100,000 IU/hr for 24 hr for pulmonary emboli, 72 hr for recurrent pulmonary emboli or deep vein thrombosis.

❑ ***AV Cannula Occlusion***

- **Into Cannula (Adults):** 100,000 IU–250,000 IU; clamp for 2 hr, then aspirate (unlabeled).

❑ **Urokinase**

❑ ***Myocardial Infarction***

- **Intracoronary (Adults):** 6000 IU/min for up to 2 hr, preceded by 2500–10,000 units of heparin IV.

❑ ***Pulmonary Emboli***

- **IV (Adults):** 4400 IU/kg loading dose, followed by 4400 IU/kg/hr for 12 hr.

❑ ***Occluded IV Catheters***

- **IV (Adults):** 1–1.8 ml of 5000 IU/ml solution injected into catheter, then aspirated. May repeat q 5 min for 30 min; if no result, may cap and leave in catheter for 30–60 min, then aspirate.
- **IV (Children):** Fill catheter with solution containing 5000 IU/ml or infuse 150 IU/kg/hr for 8 hr.

❑ ***Arterial Thrombi***

- **IA (Adults):** 60,000–240,000 units/hr infused directly into affected artery as guided by radiologic exam.

AVAILABILITY

❑ **Alteplase**

- ***Powder for injection:*** 20 mg/vial^{Rx}, 50 mg/vial^{Rx}.

❑ **Anistreplase**

- ***Powder for injection:*** 30 units/vial^{Rx}.

❑ **Reteplase**

- ***Powder for injection:*** 10.8 units (18.8 mg)/vial^{Rx}.

❑ **Streptokinase**

- ***Powder for injection:*** 250,000 IU/vial^{Rx}, 600,000 IU/vial^{Rx}, 750,000 IU/vial^{Rx}, 1,500,000 IU/vial^{Rx}.

❑ **Urokinase**

- ***Powder for injection:*** 5000 IU/vial^{Rx}, 250,000 IU/vial^{Rx}.

TIME/ACTION PROFILE (fibrinolysis)

	ONSET	PEAK	DURATION
Alteplase IV	UK	20 min–2 hr (45 min avg)	UK
Anistreplase IV	UK	45 min	6 hr*
Reteplase IV	rapid	within 2 hr	48 hr
Streptokinase IV	immediate	rapid	4 hr (up to 12 hr)
Urokinase IV	immediate	rapid	up to 12 hr

*Systemic hyperfibrinolytic state may persist for 2 days.

NURSING IMPLICATIONS

ASSESSMENT

- **General Info:** Begin therapy as soon as possible after the onset of symptoms.
  - ▫ Monitor vital signs, including temperature, continuously for coronary thrombosis and at least every 4 hr during therapy for other indications. Do not use lower extremities to monitor blood pressure.
  - ▫ Assess patient carefully for bleeding every 15 min during the 1st hr of therapy, every 15–30 min during the next 8 hr, and at least every 4 hr for the duration of therapy. Frank bleeding may occur from sites of invasive procedures or from body orifices. Internal bleeding may also occur (decreased neurologic status; abdominal pain with coffee-ground emesis or black, tarry stools; hematuria; joint pain). If uncontrolled bleeding occurs, stop medication and notify physician immediately.
  - ▫ Inquire about previous reaction to anistreplase or streptokinase therapy. Assess patient for hypersensitivity reaction (rash, dyspnea, fever, changes in facial color, swelling around the eyes, wheezing). If these occur, inform physician promptly. Keep epinephrine, an antihistamine, and resuscitation equipment close by in the event of an anaphylactic reaction.
  - ▫ Inquire about recent streptococcal infection.

Anistreplase and *streptokinase* may be less effective if administered between 5 days and 6 mo of a streptococcal infection.

- Assess neurologic status throughout therapy. Altered sensorium or neurologic changes may be indicative of intracranial bleeding.
- **Coronary Thrombosis:** Monitor ECG continuously. Notify physician if significant arrhythmias occur. IV lidocaine or procainamide (Pronestyl) may be ordered prophylactically. Cardiac enzymes should be monitored. Radionuclide myocardial scanning and/or coronary angiography may be ordered 7–10 days following therapy to monitor effectiveness of therapy.
- Assess intensity, character, location, and radiation of chest pain. Note presence of associated symptoms (nausea, vomiting, diaphoresis). Administer analgesics as directed. Notify physician if chest pain is unrelieved or recurs.
- Monitor heart sounds and breath sounds frequently. Inform physician if signs of congestive heart failure occur (rales/crackles, dyspnea, S_3 heart sound, jugular venous distention, relieved CVP).
- **Pulmonary Embolism:** Monitor pulse, blood pressure, hemodynamics, and respiratory status (rate, degree of dyspnea, ABGs).
- **Deep Vein Thrombosis/Acute Arterial Occlusion:** Observe extremities and palpate pulses of affected extremities every hour. Notify physician immediately if circulatory impairment occurs. Computerized tomography, impedance plethysmography, quantitative Doppler effect determination, and/or angiography or venography may be used to determine restoration of blood flow and duration of therapy; however, repeated venograms are not recommended.
- **Cannula/Catheter Occlusion:** Monitor ability to aspirate blood as indicator of patency. Ensure that patient exhales and holds breath when connecting and disconnecting IV syringe to prevent air embolism.
- **Acute Ischemic Stroke:** Assess neurologic status. Determine time of onset of stroke symptoms. Alteplase must be administered within 3 hr of onset.
- ***Lab Test Considerations:*** Hematocrit, hemoglobin, platelet count, fibrin/fibrin degradation product (FDP/fdp) titer, fibrinogen concentration, prothrombin time, thrombin time, and activated partial thromboplastin time may be evaluated prior to and frequently throughout therapy. Bleeding time may be assessed prior to therapy if patient has received platelet aggregation inhibitors.
- Obtain type and crossmatch and have blood available at all times in case of hemorrhage.
- Stools should be tested for occult blood loss and urine for hematuria periodically during therapy.
- ***Toxicity and Overdose:*** If local bleeding occurs, apply pressure to site. If severe or internal bleeding occurs, discontinue infusion. Clotting factors and/or blood volume may be restored through infusions of whole blood, packed RBCs, fresh frozen plasma, or cryoprecipitate. Do not administer dextran, as it has antiplatelet activity. Aminocaproic acid (Amicar) may be used as an antidote.

POTENTIAL NURSING DIAGNOSES

- Tissue perfusion, altered (Indications).
- Injury, risk for (Side Effects).
- Knowledge deficit, related to medication regimen (Patient/Family Teaching).

IMPLEMENTATION

- **General Info:** This medication should be used only in settings in which hematologic function and clinical response can be adequately monitored.
- Starting two IV lines prior to therapy is recommended: one for the thrombolytic agent, the other for any additional infusions.
- Avoid invasive procedures, such as IM injections or arterial punctures, with this therapy. If such procedures must be performed, apply pressure to all arterial and venous puncture sites for at least 30 min. Avoid venipunctures at noncompressible sites (jugular vein, subclavian site).
- Systemic anticoagulation with heparin is usually begun several hours after the completion of thrombolytic therapy.
- Acetaminophen may be ordered to control fever.

Alteplase

- **Intermittent Infusion:** Vials are packaged with sterile water for injection (without pre-

T

servatives) to be used as diluent. Do not use bacteriostatic water for injection. Reconstitute 20-mg vials with 20 ml and 50-mg vials with 50 ml using an 18-gauge needle. Avoid excess agitation during dilution; swirl or invert gently to mix. Solution may foam upon reconstitution. Bubbles will resolve upon standing a few min. Solution will be clear to pale yellow. Stable for 8 hr at room temperature. May be administered as reconstituted (1 mg/ml) or may be further diluted immediately prior to use in an equal amount of 0.9% NaCl or D5W.

- ***Rate:*** See infusion rate table in Appendix D. Flush line with 20–30 ml of saline at completion of infusion to ensure entire dose is received.
  - Standard dose for *myocardial infarction* is administered over 3 hr.
  - For *pulmonary embolism,* administer over 2 hr.
  - For *acute ischemic stroke,* administer 10% of total dose IV bolus over 1 min, with the remaining dose infused over 60 min.
- **Y-Site Compatibility:** ▪ lidocaine ▪ metoprolol ▪ propranolol.
- **Y-Site Incompatibility:** ▪ dobutamine ▪ dopamine ▪ heparin ▪ nitroglycerin.

❑ Anistreplase

- **Direct IV:** Reconstitute with 5 ml of sterile water for injection (direct to sides of vial) and swirl gently; do not shake, to minimize foaming. Do not dilute further. Use reconstituted solution within 30 min of preparation.
- ***Rate:*** Administer via IV line or vein over 2–5 min.
- **Y-Site/Additive Incompatibility:** Do not admix or administer via Y-site injection with any other medications.

❑ Reteplase

- **Direct IV:** Reconstitute using diluent, needle, syringe, and dispensing pin provided. Reconstitute only with sterile water for injection without preservatives. Solution is colorless. Do not administer solutions that are discolored or contain a precipitate. Slight foaming may occur; allow vial to stand undisturbed for several min to dissipate bubbles. Reconstitute immediately prior to use. Stable for 4 hr at room temperature.
- ***Rate:*** Administer each bolus over 2 min into an IV line containing D5W; flush line prior to and following bolus.
- **Y-Site Incompatibility:** ▪ heparin ▪ No other medication should be infused or injected into line used for reteplase.

❑ Streptokinase

- **Intracoronary:** Dilute 250,000 IU vial to a total volume of 125 ml with 0.9% NaCl or D5W. Administer 20,000 IU (10 ml) via bolus injection.
- ***Rate:*** Intracoronary bolus is administered over 15 sec–2 min.
- **Intermittent Infusion:** Reconstitute with 5 ml of 0.9% NaCl or D5W (direct to sides of vial) and swirl gently; do not shake. Dilute further with 0.9% NaCl for a total volume of 45–500 ml (45 ml for MI, 90 ml for deep vein thrombosis or pulmonary embolism). Solution is slightly yellow in color. Administer through 0.8-micron pore–size filter. Use reconstituted solution within 24 hr.
- ***Rate:*** Administer dose for MI within 60 min.
  - Intracoronary bolus should be followed by an intracoronary maintenance infusion of 2000 IU/min for 60 min.
  - Loading dose for *deep vein thrombosis* or *pulmonary embolism* is administered over 30 min, followed by an infusion of 100,000 IU/hr.
  - Use infusion pump to ensure accurate dose.
- **Y-Site Compatibility:** ▪ dobutamine ▪ dopamine ▪ heparin ▪ lidocaine ▪ nitroglycerin.
- **Additive Incompatibility:** ▪ Do not admix with any other medication.
- **Cannula/Catheter Clearance:** Dilute 250,000 IU in 2 ml of 0.9% NaCl or D5W.
- ***Rate:*** Administer slowly, over 25–35 min, into each occluded limb of cannula, and then clamp for at least 2 hr. Aspirate contents carefully and flush lines with 0.9% NaCl.

❑ Urokinase

- **Intermittent Infusion:** Reconstitute each 250,000 IU vial with 5 ml of sterile water for injection without preservatives (direct to sides of vial) and swirl gently; do not shake. Solution is light straw–colored. Do not administer solutions that are discolored or contain a precipitate. Use reconstituted solution immediately after preparation. Infuse through a 0.45-micron filter.

- For *intracoronary infusion,* add the contents of 3 reconstituted 250,000 IU vials to 500 ml of D5W or 0.9% NaCl for a solution containing 1,500 IU/ml.
- For *pulmonary embolism,* dilute the reconstituted solution further with 190 ml of 0.9% NaCl or D5W for treatment of pulmonary embolism.
- ***Rate:*** For *intracoronary infusion,* administer at a rate of 6000 IU (4 ml)/min until the artery is maximally opened, up to 2 hr.
- For *pulmonary embolism,* administer loading dose over 10 min and follow with infusion of 4400 IU/kg/hr for 12 hr.
- Administer via infusion pump to ensure accurate dosage.
- **Cannula/Catheter Clearance:** Add 1 ml of the previously reconstituted drug to 9 ml of sterile water for injection without preservatives. Available in a dual-chamber vial, which reconstitutes to 5000 IU/ml concentration for clearance of occluded cannulae and catheters.
- ***Rate:*** Inject 1 ml slowly and gently into occluded cannula, and then clamp for 5 min. Aspirate contents carefully to remove clot. If unsuccessful, reclamp for 5 min. Repeat aspiration every 5 min until clot clears or for 30 min. If still unsuccessful, clamp for 30–60 min and attempt to aspirate again. A 2nd dose of urokinase may be needed. Once catheter is patent, aspirate 4–5 ml of blood, then irrigate catheter with 10 ml of 0.9% NaCl from a separate syringe.

PATIENT/FAMILY TEACHING

- Explain purpose of medication and the need for close monitoring to patient and family. Instruct patient to report hypersensitivity reactions (rash, dyspnea) and bleeding or bruising.
- Explain need for bed rest and minimal handling during therapy to avoid injury. Avoid all unnecessary procedures such as shaving and vigorous tooth brushing.

EVALUATION

Effectiveness of therapy can be demonstrated by: ▪ Lysis of thrombi and restoration of blood flow ▪ Prevention of neurologic sequelae in acute ischemic stroke ▪ Cannula or catheter patency.

THYROID PREPARATIONS

levothyroxine

(lee-voe-thye-**rox**-een)

{Eltroxin}, Levo-T, Levothroid, Levoxyl, {PMS-Levothyroxine Sodium}, Synthroid, T_4

liothyronine

(lye-oh-**thye**-roe-neen)

Cytomel, L-triiodothyronine, T_3, Triostat

liotrix

(**lye**-oh-trix)

T_3/T_4, Thyrolar

thyroid

(**thye**-royd)

Armour thyroid, Thyrar, Thyroid Strong, Westhroid

CLASSIFICATION(S):
Hormones (thyroid)

Pregnancy Category A

INDICATIONS

▪ Replacement or substitution therapy in diminished or absent thyroid function of many causes ▪ Treatment of some types of thyroid cancer.

ACTION

▪ Principal effect is increasing metabolic rate of body tissues: ▫ Promote gluconeogenesis ▫ Increase utilization and mobilization of glycogen stores ▫ Stimulate protein synthesis ▫ Promote cell growth and differentiation ▫ Aid in the development of the brain and CNS ▪ Contain T_3 (triiodothyronine) and T_4 (thyroxine) activity. **Therapeutic Effects:** ▪ Replacement in deficiency states with restoration of normal hormonal balance ▪ Suppression of thyrotropin-dependent thyroid cancers.

PHARMACOKINETICS

Absorption: Levothyroxine is variably (50–80%) absorbed from the GI tract. Liothyronine and thyroid hormone are well absorbed.
Distribution: Distributed into most body tis-

T

sues. Thyroid hormones do not readily cross the placenta; minimal amounts enter breast milk.
Metabolism and Excretion: Metabolized by the liver and other tissues. Thyroid hormone undergoes enterohepatic recirculation and is excreted in the feces via the bile.
Half-life: T_3 *(liothyronine)*—1–2 days; T_4 *(thyroxine)*—6–7 days.

CONTRAINDICATIONS AND PRECAUTIONS

Contraindicated in: ▪ Hypersensitivity ▪ Recent myocardial infarction ▪ Thyrotoxicosis ▪ Known alcohol intolerance (liothyronine injection only) ▪ Hypersensitivity to beef (Thyrar product).
Use Cautiously in: ▪ Cardiovascular disease (initiate therapy with lower doses) ▪ Severe renal insufficiency ▪ Uncorrected adrenocortical disorders ▪ Geriatric and myxedematous patients (extremely sensitive to thyroid hormones—initial dosage should be markedly reduced).

ADVERSE REACTIONS AND SIDE EFFECTS*

Seen mostly with excessive doses.
CNS: insomnia, irritability, nervousness, headache.
CV: CARDIOVASCULAR COLLAPSE, arrhythmias, tachycardia, angina pectoris, hypotension, increased BP, increased cardiac output.
GI: cramps, diarrhea, vomiting.
Derm: hair loss (in children), increased sweating.
Endo: hyperthyroidism, menstrual irregularities.
Metab: weight loss, heat intolerance.
MS: accelerated bone maturation in children.

INTERACTIONS

Drug-Drug: ▪ **Cholestyramine** or **colestipol** decreases absorption of orally administered thyroid preparations ▪ May alter the effectiveness of **warfarin** ▪ May cause an increase in the requirement for **insulin** or **oral hypoglycemic agents** in diabetics ▪ Additive cardiovascular effects with **adrenergic agents (sympathomimetics)** ▪ May decrease response to **beta-adrenergic blockers.**

ROUTE AND DOSAGE

Each 1 gr = 60 mg and is equivalent to 100 mcg or less of levothyroxine (T_4) or 25 mcg of liothyronine (T_3).

❑ Levothyroxine

- **PO (Adults):** *Hypothyroidism*—50 mcg as a single dose initially; may be increased q 2–3 wk; usual maintenance dose is 75–125 mcg/day (1.5 mcg/kg/day). *Severe hypothyroidism*—12.5–25 mcg/day; may increase q 2–3 wk by 25 mcg/day; usual maintenance dose is 75–125 mcg/day (1.5 mcg/kg/day).
- **PO (Geriatric Patients and Patients with Increased Sensitivity to Thyroid Hormones):** 12.5–25 mcg as a single dose initially; may be increased q 3–4 wk; usual maintenance dose is 75 mcg/day.
- **PO (Children >10 yr):** 2–3 mcg/kg/day (up to 150–200 mcg/day).
- **PO (Children 6–10 yr):** 4–5 mcg/kg/day (100–150 mcg/day).
- **PO (Children 1–5 yr):** 3–5 mcg/kg/day (75–100 mcg/day).
- **PO (Children 6–12 mo):** 5–6 mcg/kg/day (50–75 mcg/day).
- **PO (Infants <6 mo):** 5–6 mcg/kg/day (25–50 mcg/day).
- **PO (Infants <2000 g or Infants at Risk for Cardiac Failure):** 25 mcg/day; may be increased after 4–6 wk to 50 mcg.
- **IM, IV (Adults):** *Hypothyroidism*—50–100 mcg/day as a single dose. *Myxedema coma/stupor*—200–500 mcg IV; additional 100–300 mcg may be given on 2nd day, followed by daily administration of smaller doses.
- **IM, IV (Children):** *Hypothyroidism*—75% of the calculated oral dose.

❑ Liothyronine

- **PO (Adults):** *Mild hypothyroidism*–25 mcg once daily; may increase by 12.5–25 mcg/day q 1–2 wk intervals; usual maintenance dose is 25–50 mcg/day. *Myxedema*—2.5–5 mcg once daily initially; increase by 5–10 mcg/day q 1–2 wk up to 25 mcg/day, then increase by 12.5–25 mcg/day; usual maintenance dose is 25–50 mcg/day. *Simple goiter*—5 mcg once daily initially; increase by 5–10 mcg/day

*CAPITALS indicate life-threatening; underlines indicate most frequent.

q 1–2 wk up to 25 mcg/day, then increase by 12.5–25 mcg/day q wk until desired effect is obtained; usual maintenance dose is 50–100 mcg/day. *T_3 suppression test*—75–100 mcg daily for 7 days. Radioactive ^{131}I is administered before and after 7-day course.

- **PO (Geriatric Patients or Patients with Cardiovascular Disease):** 5 mcg /day initially; increase by not more than 5 mcg/day q 2 wk.
- **IV (Adults):** *Myxedema coma/precoma*—25–50 mcg initially (if cardiovascular disease is present, initial dose should be 10–20 mcg). Additional doses may be given, to a total of at least 65 mcg/day (not to exceed 100 mcg/day). Doses should be at least 4 hr but not more than 12 hr apart.

❑ Liotrix

Contains T_4 and T_3 in a ratio of 4:1.

- **PO (Adults):** *Hypothyroidism*—Start with 50 mcg levothyroxine/12.5 mg liothyronine; increase by 50 mcg levothyroxine/12.5 mcg liothyronine q mo until desired effect is obtained; usual maintenance dose is 50–100 mcg levothyroxine/12.5–25 mcg liothyronine daily. *Myxedema/hypothyroidism with cardiovascular disease*—12.5 mcg levothyroxine/3.1 mcg liothyronine/day; increase by 12.5 mcg levothyroxine/3.1 mcg liothyronine q 2–3 wk until desired effect is obtained.
- **PO (Geriatric Patients):** 12.5–25 mcg levothyroxine/3.1–6.2 mcg liothyronine/day; increase by 12.5–25 mcg levothyroxine/3.1–6.2 mcg liothyronine q 6–8 wk until desired effect is obtained.

❑ Thyroid

- **PO (Adults and Children):** *Hypothyroidism*–60 mg/day; increase q mo by 30 mg; usual maintenance dose is 60–120 mg/day. *Myxedema/hypothyroidism with cardiovascular disease*—15 mg/day initially; increase by 30 mg/day q 2 wk, then may increase by 30–60 mg q 2 wk; usual maintenance dose is 60–120 mg/day.
- **PO (Geriatric Patients):** 7.5–15 mg/day initially; may double dose q 6–8 wk until desired effect is obtained.

AVAILABILITY

❑ Levothyroxine

- ***Tablets:*** 25 mcg^{Rx}, 50 mcg^{Rx}, 75 mcg^{Rx}, 88 mcg^{Rx}, 100 mcg^{Rx}, 112 mcg^{Rx}, 125 mcg^{Rx}, 137 mcg^{Rx}, 150 mcg^{Rx}, 175 mcg^{Rx}, 200 mcg^{Rx}, 300 mcg^{Rx} ▪ ***Powder for injection:*** 200 mcg/vial in 6- and 10-ml vials^{Rx}, 500 mcg/vial in 6- and 10-ml vials^{Rx}.

❑ Liothyronine

- ***Tablets:*** 5 mcg^{Rx}, 25 mcg^{Rx}, 50 mcg^{Rx}
- ***Injection:*** 10 mcg/ml in 1-ml vials^{Rx}.

❑ Liotrix

- ***Tablets:*** 12.5 mcg levothyroxine/3.1 mcg liothyronine^{Rx}, 25 mcg levothyroxine/6.25 mcg liothyronine^{Rx}, 50 mcg levothyroxine/12.5 mcg liothyronine^{Rx}, 100 mcg levothyroxine/25 mcg liothyronine^{Rx}, 150 mcg levothyroxine/37.5 mcg liothyronine^{Rx}.

❑ Thyroid

- ***Tablets (regular):*** 15 mg^{Rx}, 30 mg^{Rx}, 60 mg^{Rx}, 90 mg^{Rx}, 120 mg^{Rx}, 180 mg^{Rx}, 240 mg^{Rx}, 300 mg^{Rx} ▪ ***Tablets (bovine):*** 30 mg^{Rx}, 60 mg^{Rx}, 120 mg^{Rx} ▪ ***Tablets (strong) 0.3% Iodine:*** 30 mg^{Rx}, 60 mg^{Rx}, 90 mg^{Rx}, 120 mg^{Rx}, {125 mg^{Rx}}, 180 mg^{Rx}.

TIME/ACTION PROFILE (effects on thyroid function tests)

	ONSET	PEAK	DURATION
Levothyroxine PO	UK	1–3 wk	1–3 wk
Levothyroxine IV	6–8 hr	24 hr	UK
Liothyronine PO	UK	24–72 hr	72 hr
Liothyronine IV	UK	UK	UK
Thyroid PO	days–wks	1–3 wk	days–wks

NURSING IMPLICATIONS

ASSESSMENT

- **General Info:** Assess apical pulse and blood pressure prior to and periodically during therapy. Assess for tachyarrhythmias and chest pain.
- **Children:** Monitor height, weight, and psychomotor development.
- ***Lab Test Considerations:*** Thyroid function studies should be monitored prior to and throughout therapy.
- ❑ Monitor blood and urine glucose in diabetic patients. Insulin or oral hypoglycemic dose may need to be increased.
- ***Toxicity and Overdose:*** Overdose is man-

ifested as hyperthyroidism (tachycardia, chest pain, nervousness, insomnia, diaphoresis, tremors, weight loss). Usual treatment is to withhold dose for 2–6 days. Acute overdose is treated by induction of emesis or gastric lavage, followed by activated charcoal. Sympathetic overstimulation may be controlled by antiadrenergic drugs (beta blockers), such as propranolol. Oxygen and supportive measures to control symptoms such as fever are also used.

POTENTIAL NURSING DIAGNOSES

- Knowledge deficit, related to medication regimen (Patient/Family Teaching).

IMPLEMENTATION

- **General Info:** Administer as a single dose, preferably before breakfast to prevent insomnia.
  - Initial dose is low, especially in geriatric and cardiac patients. Dosage is increased gradually, based on thyroid function tests. Side effects occur more rapidly with liothyronine because of its rapid onset of effect.

❑ Levothyroxine

- **Direct IV:** Dilute the 200-mcg and 500-mcg vials with 2 or 5 ml, respectively, of 0.9% NaCl without preservatives (diluent usually provided), for a concentration of 100 mcg/ml. Shake well to dissolve completely. Administer solution immediately after preparation; discard unused portion.
- ***Rate:*** Administer at a rate of 100 mcg over 1 min. Do not add to IV infusions; may be administered through Y-tubing.

❑ Liothyronine

- **IV:** Liothyronine injection is for IV use only. Do not give IM or SC. Administer doses at least 4 hr and not more than 12 hr apart. Base doses on continuous monitoring of patient and response to therapy.
  - Resume PO therapy as soon as patient is stable and able to take PO medication. When switching to PO therapy, discontinue IV liothyronine and initiate PO at low dose, increasing gradually according to patient's response.
- **Direct IV:** May be administered undiluted.
- ***Rate:*** Administer as a bolus.

PATIENT/FAMILY TEACHING

- **General Info:** Instruct patient to take medication exactly as directed at the same time each day. If a dose is missed, take as soon as remembered unless almost time for next dose. If more than 2–3 doses are missed, notify health care professional. Do not discontinue without consulting health care professional.
  - Instruct patient and family on correct technique for checking pulse. Dose should be withheld and health care professional notified if resting pulse >100 bpm.
  - Explain to patient that medication does not cure hypothyroidism; it provides a thyroid hormone. Therapy is lifelong.
  - Caution patient not to change brands of thyroid preparations, as this may affect drug bioavailability.
  - Advise patient to notify health care professional if headache, nervousness, diarrhea, excessive sweating, heat intolerance, chest pain, increased pulse rate, palpitations, weight loss >2 lb/wk, or any unusual symptoms occur.
  - Caution patient to avoid taking other medications concurrently with thyroid preparations unless instructed by health care professional.
  - Instruct patient to inform health care professional of thyroid therapy.
  - Emphasize importance of follow-up exams to monitor effectiveness of therapy. Thyroid function tests are performed at least yearly.
- **Children:** Discuss with parents the need for routine follow-up studies to ensure correct development. Inform patient that partial hair loss may be experienced by children on thyroid therapy. This is usually temporary.

EVALUATION

Clinical response to therapy can be evaluated by: ▪ Resolution of symptoms of hypothyroidism. Response includes: ▫ Diuresis ▫ Weight loss ▫ Increased sense of well-being ▫ Increased energy, pulse rate, appetite, psychomotor activity ▫ Normalization of skin texture and hair ▫ Correction of constipation ▫ Increased T_3 and T_4 levels ▪ In children, effectiveness of therapy is determined by: ▫ Appropriate physical and psychomotor development.

TIAGABINE
(tye-a-ga-been)
Gabatril

CLASSIFICATION(S):
Anticonvulsant (miscellaneous)

Pregnancy Category C

INDICATIONS
- Adjunctive treatment of partial seizures.

ACTION
- Enhances the activity of gamma-aminobutyric acid, an inhibitory neurotransmitter. **Therapeutic Effects:** - Decreased frequency of seizures.

PHARMACOKINETICS
Absorption: 90% absorbed following oral administration.
Distribution: UK.
Metabolism and Excretion: Mostly metabolized by the liver; 2% excreted unchanged in urine.
Half-life: *Without enzyme-inducing antiepileptic drugs*—7–9 hr; *with enzyme-inducing antiepileptic drugs*—4–7 hr.

CONTRAINDICATIONS AND PRECAUTIONS
Contraindicated in: - Hypersensitivity.
Use Cautiously in: - Hepatic impairment (decreased dose/increased interval may be necessary) - Patients receiving concurrent non–enzyme-inducing antiepileptic drug therapy such as valproates (may require lower doses and/or slower titration) - Pregnancy, lactation, or children <12 yr (safety not established).

ADVERSE REACTIONS AND SIDE EFFECTS*
CNS: DIZZINESS, drowsiness, nervousness, weakness, confusion, difficulty concentrating, hallucinations, headache, mental depression, personality disorder.
EENT: abnormal vision, ear pain, tinnitus.
Resp: dyspnea, epistaxis.
CV: chest pain, edema, hypertension, palpitations, syncope, tachycardia.
GI: abdominal pain, gingivitis, nausea, stomatitis.
GU: dysmenorrhea, dysuria, metrorrhagia, urinary incontinence.
Derm: alopecia, dry skin, rash, sweating.
Metab: weight gain, weight loss.
MS: arthralgia, neck pain.
Neuro: ataxia, tremors.
Misc: allergic reactions, chills, lymphadenopathy.

INTERACTIONS
Drug-Drug: - **Carbamazepine, phenytoin, primidone,** and **phenobarbital** induce metabolism and decrease blood levels; although concurrent therapy is usually necessary, adjustments may be required when altering regimens.

ROUTE AND DOSAGE
- **PO (Adults >18 yr):** 4 mg once daily initially for 1 wk; may increase by 4–8/day at weekly intervals, up to 56 mg/day in 2–4 divided doses.
- **PO (Children 12–18 yr):** 4 mg once daily initially for 1 wk; may increase by 4/day for 1 wk, then may increase by 4–8/day at weekly intervals, up to 32 mg/day in 2–4 divided doses.

AVAILABILITY
- ***Tablets:*** 4 mg[Rx], 12 mg[Rx], 16 mg[Rx], 20 mg[Rx].

TIME/ACTION PROFILE (blood levels)

	ONSET	PEAK	DURATION
PO	UK	45 min	UK

NURSING IMPLICATIONS

ASSESSMENT
- Assess location, duration, and characteristics of seizure activity.
- ***Toxicity and Overdose:*** Therapeutic serum levels have not been determined. However, levels may be monitored prior to and following changes in the therapeutic regimen.

POTENTIAL NURSING DIAGNOSES
- Injury, risk for (Side Effects).
- Knowledge deficit, related to medication regimen (Patient/Family Teaching).

***CAPITALS indicate life-threatening; underlines indicate most frequent.**

IMPLEMENTATION

- **PO:** Administer with food.
- Tiagabine should be discontinued gradually. Abrupt discontinuation may cause increase in seizure frequency.

PATIENT/FAMILY TEACHING

- Instruct patient to take medication exactly as directed. If a dose is missed, take as soon as possible unless almost time for next dose. Do not double doses. Do not discontinue abruptly; may cause increase in frequency of seizures.
- Advise patient to notify health care professional immediately if frequency of seizures increases.
- May cause dizziness. Caution patient to avoid driving or activities requiring alertness until response to medication is known. Do not resume driving until physician gives clearance based on control of seizure disorder.
- Advise patient to notify health care professional if pregnancy is planned or suspected or if patient intends to breast-feed or is breast-feeding.
- Instruct patient to notify health care professional of medication regimen prior to treatment or surgery.
- Advise patient to carry identification describing disease process and medication regimen at all times.

EVALUATION

Effectiveness of therapy can be demonstrated by: ▪ Decrease in the frequency or cessation of seizures.

TICARCILLIN
(tye-kar-**sil**-in)
Ticar

TICARCILLIN/CLAVULANATE
(tye-kar-**sil**-in/klav-yoo-**la**-nate)
Timentin

CLASSIFICATION(S):
Anti-infective (extended-spectrum penicillin)

Pregnancy Category B

INDICATIONS

▪ Treatment of : ▫ Skin and skin structure infections ▫ Bone and joint infections ▫ Septicemia ▫ Respiratory tract infections ▫ Intra-abdominal, gynecologic, and urinary tract infections.

ACTION

▪ Binds to bacterial cell wall membrane, causing cell death ▪ Addition of clavulanate enhances resistance to beta-lactamase, an enzyme that can inactivate penicillins. **Therapeutic Effects:** ▪ Bactericidal action. **Spectrum:** ▪ Similar to penicillin but extended to include several gram-negative aerobic pathogens, notably: ▫ *Pseudomonas aeruginosa* ▫ *Escherichia coli* ▫ *Proteus mirabilis* ▫ *Providencia rettgeri* ▪ Active against some anaerobic bacteria, including bacteroides.

PHARMACOKINETICS

Absorption: Ticarcillin is well absorbed following IM administration.
Distribution: Widely distributed. Enters CSF well when meninges are inflamed. Crosses the placenta; enters breast milk in low concentrations.
Metabolism and Excretion: 10% of ticarcillin is metabolized by the liver; 90% excreted unchanged by the kidneys. Clavulanate is metabolized by the liver.
Half-life: *Ticarcillin*—0.9–1.3 hr (increased in renal impairment); *clavulanate*—1.1–1.5 hr.

CONTRAINDICATIONS AND PRECAUTIONS

Contraindicated in: ▪ Hypersensitivity to penicillins (cross-sensitivity with cephalosporins may occur).
Use Cautiously in: ▪ Renal impairment (dosage reduction and/or increased interval required if CCr <60 ml/min) ▪ Pregnancy and lactation (safety not established) ▪ Severe liver disease.

ADVERSE REACTIONS AND SIDE EFFECTS*

CNS: SEIZURES (high doses), confusion, lethargy.
CV: CONGESTIVE HEART FAILURE, arrhythmias.
GI: PSEUDOMEMBRANOUS COLITIS, <u>diarrhea</u>, nausea.
GU: hematuria (children only).

***CAPITALS indicate life-threatening; <u>underlines</u> indicate most frequent.**

Derm: rashes, urticaria.
F and E: hypokalemia, hypernatremia.
Hemat: bleeding, blood dyscrasias, increased bleeding time.
Local: phlebitis.
Metab: metabolic alkalosis.
Misc: hypersensitivity reactions including ANAPHYLAXIS, superinfection.

INTERACTIONS

Drug-Drug: ▪ **Probenecid** decreases renal excretion and increases blood levels ▪ May alter excretion of **lithium** ▪ **Diuretics, amphotericin B,** or **glucocorticoids** may increase the risk of hypokalemia ▪ Hypokalemia increases the risk of **digitalis glycoside** toxicity.

ROUTE AND DOSAGE

Ticarcillin contains 5.2 mEq sodium/g; ticarcillin/clavulanate contains 4.75–6.2 mEq sodium/g ticarcillin and 0.15 mEq potassium/100 mg clavulanate.

❑ Ticarcillin

- **IV (Adults and Children >40 kg):** *Most infections*—3 g q 4 hr or 4 g q 6 hr (150–300 mg/kg/day in divided doses; not to exceed 24 g/day). *Bacterial meningitis*—75 mg/kg q 6 hr IV. *Complicated urinary tract infections*—3 g q 6 hr IV. *Uncomplicated urinary tract infections*—1 g q 6 hr IM/IV.
- **IV (Children <40 kg):** *Most infections*—33.3–50 mg/kg q 4 hr or 50–75 mg/kg q 6 hr IV. *Complicated urinary tract infections*—25–33.3 mg/kg q 4 hr or 37.5–50 mg/kg q 6 hr IV. *Uncomplicated urinary tract infections*—12.5 –25 mg/kg q 6 hr or 16.7–33.3 mg/kg q 8 hr IM/IV.
- **IM, IV (Neonates ≥2 kg):** 75 mg/kg q 8 hr for the first 7 days of life, then 75 mg/kg q 6 hr.
- **IM, IV (Neonates <2 kg):** 75 mg/kg q 12 hr for the first 7 days of life, then 75 mg/kg q 8 hr.

❑ Ticarcillin/Clavulanate

3 g ticarcillin plus 100 mg clavulanate labeled as 3.1 g combined potency.

- **IV (Adults ≥60 kg):** 3.1 g q 4–6 hr.
- **IV (Adults <60 kg):** 33.3–50 mg/kg ticarcillin plus 1.1–1.7 mg/kg clavulanate q 4 hr or 50–75 mg/kg ticarcillin plus 1.7–2.5 mg clavulanate q 6 hr.
- **IV (Children ≥3 mo–<60 kg):** 50 mg ticarcillin/kg plus 1.7 mg clavulanate/kg q 4–6 hr. *Children with cystic fibrosis*—up to 350–450 mg ticarcillin/kg plus 11.7–17 mg clavulanate/kg daily in divided doses.

AVAILABILITY

❑ Ticarcillin

▪ ***Powder for injection:*** 1 g/vial[Rx], 3 g/vial[Rx], 6 g/vial[Rx], 20 g/vial[Rx], 30 g/vial[Rx].

❑ Ticarcillin/Clavulanate

▪ ***Powder for injection:*** 3.1 g/vials and piggyback bottles[Rx] ▪ ***Solution for injection:*** 3.1 g premixed 100-ml bottles[Rx].

TIME/ACTION PROFILE (blood levels)

	ONSET	PEAK	DURATION
IM	rapid	30–75 min	4–6 hr
IV	rapid	end of infusion	4–6 hr

T

NURSING IMPLICATIONS

ASSESSMENT

- ❑ Assess patient for infection (vital signs; appearance of wound, sputum, urine, and stool; WBC) at beginning of and throughout therapy.
- ❑ Obtain a history before initiating therapy to determine use of and reactions to penicillins or cephalosporins. Persons with a negative history of penicillin sensitivity may still have an allergic response.
- ❑ Obtain specimens for culture and sensitivity before initiating therapy. First dose may be given before receiving results.
- ❑ Observe patient for signs and symptoms of anaphylaxis (rash, pruritus, laryngeal edema, wheezing). Discontinue drug and notify physician immediately if these problems occur. Keep epinephrine, an antihistamine, and resuscitation equipment close by in case of anaphylactic reaction.
- ▪ ***Lab Test Considerations:*** Renal and hepatic function, CBC, serum potassium, and bleeding times should be evaluated prior to and routinely throughout therapy.
- ❑ May cause false-positive urine protein testing and increased BUN, creatinine, AST, ALT, serum bilirubin, alkaline phosphatase, LDH, and uric acid levels. May also cause increased bleeding time.

- May cause hypernatremia and hypokalemia with high doses.

POTENTIAL NURSING DIAGNOSES

- Infection, risk for (Indications, Side Effects).
- Knowledge deficit, related to medication regimen (Patient/Family Teaching).

IMPLEMENTATION

- **IM:** Reconstitute with 2 ml of sterile or bacteriostatic water for injection or 1% lidocaine hydrochloride injection (without epinephrine) to each 1-g vial for a concentration of 1 g/2.5 ml.
- Inject deep into a well-muscled mass to minimize discomfort, and massage well. IM injections should not exceed 2 g at each site. Do not administer ticarcillin/clavulanate IM.
- **IV:** Change IV sites every 48 hr to prevent phlebitis.

Ticarcillin

- **Direct IV:** Add at least 4 ml of sterile water for injection to each 1-g vial. Further dilute to at least 20 ml with 0.9% NaCl, D5W, Ringer's or lactated Ringer's solution. Solution is stable for 48 hr at room temperature, 14 days if refrigerated.
- ***Rate:*** Administer as slowly as possible to minimize vein irritation. Do not administer concentrations >50 mg/ml.
- **Intermittent Infusion:** Dilute further for a concentration of 10–100 mg/ml.
- ***Rate:*** Administer over 30 min–2 hr, 10–20 min in neonates.
- **Y-Site Compatibility:** ▪ acyclovir ▪ amifostine ▪ aztreonam ▪ cyclophosphamide ▪ diltiazem ▪ famotidine ▪ filgrastim ▪ fludarabine ▪ hydromorphone ▪ insulin ▪ magnesium sulfate ▪ melphalan ▪ meperidine ▪ morphine ▪ ondansetron ▪ perphenazine ▪ sargramostim ▪ teniposide ▪ theophylline ▪ thiotepa ▪ verapamil ▪ vinorelbine.
- **Y-Site Incompatibility:** ▪ fluconazole. If aminoglycosides and penicillins must be administered concurrently, administer in separate sites at least 1 hr apart.

Ticarcillin/Clavulanate

- **Intermittent Infusion:** Add 13 ml of sterile water or 0.9% NaCl for injection to each 3.1-g vial, to provide a concentration of ticarcillin 200 mg/ml and clavulanic acid 6.7 mg/ml. Further dilute in 0.9% NaCl, D5W, or Ringer's or lactated Ringer's solution. Stable for 6 hr at room temperature, 72 hr if refrigerated.
- ***Rate:*** Administer over 30 min via Y-site or direct IV.
- **Y-Site Compatibility:** ▪ amifostine ▪ aztreonam ▪ cefepime ▪ cyclophosphamide ▪ diltiazem ▪ famotidine ▪ filgrastim ▪ fludarabine ▪ foscarnet ▪ gallium nitrate ▪ granisetron ▪ heparin ▪ insulin ▪ melphalan ▪ meperidine ▪ morphine ▪ ondansetron ▪ perphenazine ▪ sargramostim ▪ teniposide ▪ theophylline ▪ thiotepa ▪ vinorelbine.
- **Y-Site Incompatibility:** ▪ If aminoglycosides and penicillins must be administered concurrently, administer in separate sites at least 1 hr apart.

PATIENT/FAMILY TEACHING

- Advise patient to report signs of superinfection (black, furry overgrowth on the tongue; vaginal itching or discharge; loose or foul-smelling stools) and allergy.

EVALUATION

Clinical response to therapy can be evaluated by: ▪ Resolution of the signs and symptoms of infection. Length of time for complete resolution depends on the organism and site of infection.

TICLOPIDINE

(tye-**cloe**-pi-deen)
Ticlid

CLASSIFICATION(S):
Platelet aggregation inhibitor

Pregnancy Category B

INDICATIONS

▪ Prevention of stroke in patients who have had a completed thrombotic stroke or precursors to stroke and are unable to tolerate aspirin. **Unlabeled Uses:** ▪ Prevention of early restenosis in intracoronary stents.

ACTION

▪ Inhibits platelet aggregation by altering the function of platelet membranes ▪ Prolongs bleeding time. **Therapeutic Effects:** ▪ Decreased incidence of stroke in high-risk patients.

PHARMACOKINETICS

Absorption: >80% absorbed following oral administration.
Distribution: UK.
Metabolism and Excretion: Extensively metabolized by the liver; minimal excretion of unchanged drug by the kidneys.
Half-life: *Single dose*—12.6 hr; *multiple dosing*—4–5 days.

CONTRAINDICATIONS AND PRECAUTIONS

Contraindicated in: ▪ Hypersensitivity ▪ Bleeding disorders ▪ Active bleeding ▪ Severe liver disease.
Use Cautiously in: ▪ Risk of bleeding (trauma, surgery, history of ulcer disease) ▪ Renal or hepatic impairment (dosage adjustments may be necessary) ▪ Geriatric patients (increased sensitivity) ▪ Pregnancy, lactation, or children <18 yr (safety not established).

ADVERSE REACTIONS AND SIDE EFFECTS*

CNS: dizziness, headache, weakness.
EENT: epistaxis, tinnitus.
GI: diarrhea, abnormal liver function tests, anorexia, GI fullness, GI pain, nausea, vomiting.
GU: hematuria.
Derm: rashes, ecchymoses, pruritus, urticaria.
Hemat: AGRANULOCYTOSIS, INTRACEREBRAL BLEEDING, NEUTROPENIA, bleeding, thrombocytopenia.
Metab: hypercholesterolemia, hypertriglyceridemia.

INTERACTIONS

Drug-Drug: ▪ **Aspirin** potentiates the effect of ticlopidine on platelets (concurrent use not recommended) ▪ Increased risk of bleeding with **heparins, warfarin,** or **thrombolytic agents** ▪ **Cimetidine** decreases metabolism of ticlopidine and may increase the risk of toxicity ▪ Ticlopidine decreases metabolism of **theophylline** and increases the risk of toxicity.
Drug-Food: ▪ Absorption of ticlopidine is increased by taking with **food.**

ROUTE AND DOSAGE

- **PO (Adults):** 250 mg bid with food.

AVAILABILITY

- ***Tablets:*** 250 mg[Rx].

TIME/ACTION PROFILE (effect on platelet function)

	ONSET	PEAK	DURATION
PO	within 4 days	8–11 days	2 wk

NURSING IMPLICATIONS

ASSESSMENT

- Assess patient for symptoms of stroke periodically throughout therapy.
- ***Lab Test Considerations:*** Monitor bleeding time throughout therapy. Prolonged bleeding time (2–5 times the normal limit), which is time- and dose-dependent, is expected.
- Monitor CBC with differential and platelet count every 2 wk from the 2nd wk to the end of the 3rd mo of therapy; more frequently if absolute neutrophil count (ANC) is declining or <30% of baseline. If neutropenia occurs, ticlopidine should be discontinued. Neutrophil counts usually return to normal within 1–3 wk of discontinuation of therapy. After the first 3 mo of therapy, CBCs need to be obtained only for patients with signs and symptoms of infection.
- May cause thrombocytopenia, usually within 3–12 wk of initiation of therapy. If platelet count is <80,000/mm³, discontinue ticlopidine.
- May cause increased serum total cholesterol and triglyceride levels. Levels usually increase 8–10% within the first mo and persist at that level.
- May cause elevated alkaline phosphatase, bilirubin, AST, and ALT levels during the first 4 mo of therapy.
- ***Toxicity and Overdose:*** Prolonged bleeding time is normalized within 2 hr after administration of IV methylprednisolone. May also use platelet transfusions to reverse effects of ticlopidine on bleeding time.

POTENTIAL NURSING DIAGNOSES

- Injury, risk for (Indications, Side Effects).
- Knowledge deficit, related to medication regimen (Patient/Family Teaching).

*CAPITALS indicate life-threatening; underlines indicate most frequent.

IMPLEMENTATION

- **PO:** Administer with food or immediately after eating to minimize GI discomfort and increase absorption.

PATIENT/FAMILY TEACHING

- Instruct patient to take medication exactly as directed. Missed doses should be taken as soon as possible unless almost time for next dose; do not double doses.
- Advise patient to notify health care professional promptly if fever, chills, sore throat, unusual bleeding or bruising, severe or persistent diarrhea, skin rash, jaundice, dark-colored urine, or light-colored stools occur.
- Advise patient to notify health care professional of medication regimen prior to treatment or surgery. Medication may need to be discontinued 10–14 days prior to surgery.
- Emphasize the importance of routine lab tests during the first 3 mo of therapy to monitor for side effects.

EVALUATION

Effectiveness of therapy can be demonstrated by: ▪ Prevention of stroke.

TILUDRONATE

(tye-**loo**-droe-nate)
Skelid

CLASSIFICATION(S):
Bone resorption inhibitor (biphosphonate)

Pregnancy Category C

INDICATIONS

▪ Management of Paget's disease of the bone in patients with: ▫ Serum alkaline phosphatase ≥2 times the upper limit of normal ▫ Symptoms ▫ Risk for complications.

ACTION

▪ Inhibits resorption of bone by inhibiting osteoclast activity. **Therapeutic Effects:** ▪ Decreased progression of Paget's disease.

PHARMACOKINETICS

Absorption: Rapidly but poorly absorbed following oral administration (6% bioavailability).
Distribution: Distributes to bone and soft tissue; subsequently is slowly released from bone.
Metabolism and Excretion: Excreted mostly in urine.
Half-life: 150 hr.

CONTRAINDICATIONS AND PRECAUTIONS

Contraindicated in: ▪ Hypersensitivity ▪ Severe renal impairment (CCr <30 ml/min).
Use Cautiously in: ▪ Pregnancy, lactation, or children <18 yr (safety not established).

ADVERSE REACTIONS AND SIDE EFFECTS

CNS: anxiety, drowsiness, fatigue, insomnia, nervousness, syncope, vertigo, weakness.
EENT: cataracts, conjunctivitis, glaucoma, pharyngitis, rhinitis, sinusitis.
Resp: bronchitis.
CV: chest pain, dependent edema, hypertension, peripheral edema.
GI: abdominal pain, anorexia, constipation, diarrhea, dry mouth, dysphagia, esophageal ulcer, esophagitis, flatulence, gastric ulcer, gastritis, nausea, tooth disorder, vomiting.
GU: urinary tract infection.
Derm: flushing, increased sweating, pruritus, rash, skin disorder.
Endo: hyperparathyroidism.
F and E: hypocalcemia.
MS: arthrosis, involuntary muscle contractions, pathological fractures.
Neuro: paresthesia.
Misc: infection.

INTERACTIONS

Drug-Drug: ▪ Absorption is decreased by concurrent administration of **calcium supplements**, **aspirin**, or **aluminum-** or **magnesium-containing antacids** ▪ Bioavailability is increased by concurrent administration of **indomethacin.**
Drug-Food: ▪ **Food** decreases absorption.

ROUTE AND DOSAGE

- **PO (Adults):** 400 mg/day taken with 8 oz of plain water only, for 3 mo.

AVAILABILITY

- ***Tablets:*** 400 mg[Rx].

TIME/ACTION PROFILE (blood levels)

	ONSET	PEAK	DURATION
PO	UK	within 2 hr	UK

NURSING IMPLICATIONS

ASSESSMENT

- **Paget's Disease:** Assess for symptoms of Paget's disease (bone pain, headache, decreased visual and auditory acuity, increased skull size).
- ***Lab Test Considerations:*** Monitor alkaline phosphatase prior to and periodically during therapy. Tiluronate is indicated for patients with alkaline phosphatase 2 times the upper limit of normal.

POTENTIAL NURSING DIAGNOSES

- Injury, risk for (Indications).
- Knowledge deficit, related to diet and medication regimen (Patient/Family Teaching).

IMPLEMENTATION

- **PO:** Administer first thing in the morning with 6–8 oz plain water 30 min prior to other medications, beverages, or food.
- □ Calcium supplements, aspirin, or indomethacin should not be taken for 2 hr before or 2 hr after tiludronate; antacids should not be taken for at least 2 hr following tiludronate.

PATIENT/FAMILY TEACHING

- □ Instruct patient on the importance of taking exactly as directed, first thing in the morning, 30 min prior to other medications, beverages, or food. Waiting longer than 30 min will improve absorption. Tiluronate should be taken with 6–8 oz plain water (mineral water, orange juice, coffee, and other beverages decrease absorption). If a dose is missed, skip dose and resume the next morning; do not double doses or take later in the day. Do not discontinue without consulting health care professional.
- □ Caution patients to remain upright for 30 min following dose to facilitate passage to stomach and minimize risk of esophageal irritation.
- □ Advise patient to eat a balanced diet and consult health care professional about the need for supplemental calcium and vitamin D.
- □ Encourage patient to participate in regular exercise and to modify behaviors that increase the risk of osteoporosis (stop smoking, reduce alcohol consumption).
- □ Advise female patient to notify health care professional if pregnancy is planned or suspected or if she is nursing.

EVALUATION

Effectiveness of therapy can be demonstrated by: ▪ Decrease in the progression of Paget's disease.

TIMOLOL*

(**tim**-oh-lole)

{Apo-Timol}, Blocadren, {Novo-Timol}

CLASSIFICATION(S):

Antihypertensive agent, Beta-adrenergic blocking agent (nonselective)

Pregnancy Category C

*For ophthalmic use, see Appendix O.

INDICATIONS

▪ Management of hypertension ▪ Prevention of myocardial infarction ▪ Prevention of migraine headaches. **Unlabeled Uses:** ▪ Ventricular arrhythmias ▪ Essential tremor ▪ Anxiety.

ACTION

▪ Blocks stimulation of $beta_1$ (myocardial) and $beta_2$ (pulmonary, vascular, and uterine) -adrenergic receptor sites. **Therapeutic Effects:** ▪ Decreased heart rate and blood pressure ▪ Prevention of myocardial infarction ▪ Decreased frequency of migraine headache.

PHARMACOKINETICS

Absorption: Well absorbed following oral administration.

Distribution: Enters breast milk.

Metabolism and Excretion: Extensively metabolized by the liver.
Half-life: 3–4 hr.

CONTRAINDICATIONS AND PRECAUTIONS

Contraindicated in: ▪ Uncompensated congestive heart failure ▪ Pulmonary edema ▪ Cardiogenic shock ▪ Bradycardia or heart block.
Use Cautiously in: ▪ Renal impairment ▪ Hepatic impairment ▪ Geriatric patients (increased sensitivity to beta-adrenergic blockers; initial dosage reduction recommended) ▪ Pulmonary disease (including asthma) ▪ Diabetes mellitus (may mask signs of hypoglycemia) ▪ Thyrotoxicosis (may mask symptoms) ▪ Patients with a history of severe allergic reactions (intensity of reactions may be increased) ▪ Pregnancy, lactation, or children (safety not established; all agents cross the placenta and may cause fetal/neonatal bradycardia, hypotension, hypoglycemia, or respiratory depression).

ADVERSE REACTIONS AND SIDE EFFECTS*

CNS: fatigue, weakness, anxiety, depression, dizziness, drowsiness, insomnia, memory loss, mental status changes, nervousness, nightmares.
EENT: blurred vision, dry eyes, nasal stuffiness.
Resp: bronchospasm, wheezing.
CV: ARRHYTHMIAS, BRADYCARDIA, CONGESTIVE HEART FAILURE, PULMONARY EDEMA, orthostatic hypotension, peripheral vasoconstriction.
GI: constipation, diarrhea, nausea.
GU: impotence, decreased libido.
Derm: itching, rashes.
Endo: hyperglycemia, hypoglycemia.
MS: arthralgia, back pain, muscle cramps.
Neuro: paresthesia.

INTERACTIONS

Drug-Drug: ▪ **General anesthesia, IV phenytoin,** and **verapamil** may cause additive myocardial depression ▪ Additive bradycardia may occur with **digitalis glycosides** ▪ Additive hypotension may occur with other **antihypertensives,** acute ingestion of **alcohol,** or **nitrates** ▪ Concurrent use with **amphetamines, cocaine, ephedrine, epinephrine, norepinephrine, phenylephrine,** or **pseudoephedrine** may result in unopposed alpha-adrenergic stimulation (excessive hypertension, bradycardia) ▪ Concurrent **thyroid** administration may decrease effectiveness ▪ May alter the effectiveness of **insulin** or **oral hypoglycemic agents** (dosage adjustments may be necessary) ▪ May decrease the effectiveness of **beta-adrenergic bronchodilators** and **theophylline** ▪ May decrease the beneficial $beta_1$ cardiovascular effects of **dopamine** or **dobutamine** ▪ Use cautiously within 14 days of **MAO inhibitor** therapy (may result in hypertension) ▪ **Cimetidine** may increase toxicity ▪ Concurrent **NSAIDs** may decrease antihypertensive action.

ROUTE AND DOSAGE

- **PO (Adults):** *Antihypertensive*—10 mg twice daily initially, may be increased q 7 days as needed (usual maintenance dose is 10–20 mg twice daily; up to 60 mg/day). *Prevention of myocardial infarction*—10 mg twice daily, starting 1–4 wk after myocardial infarction. *Prevention of vascular headache*—10 mg twice daily initially, may be given as a single daily dose; may be increased up to 10 mg in the morning and 20 mg in the evening.

AVAILABILITY

- ***Tablets:*** 5 g[Rx], 10 mg[Rx], 20 mg[Rx].

TIME/ACTION PROFILE (cardiovascular effects)

	ONSET	PEAK	DURATION
PO	UK	1–2 hr†	12–24 hr

†Following single dose, full effect not seen until several weeks of therapy.

NURSING IMPLICATIONS

ASSESSMENT

- **General Info:** Monitor blood pressure and pulse frequently during dosage adjustment period and periodically throughout therapy. Assess for orthostatic hypotension when assisting patient up from supine position.
- □ Monitor intake and output ratios and daily weight. Assess patient routinely for evidence of fluid overload (peripheral edema, dyspnea,

*CAPITALS indicate life-threatening; underlines indicate most frequent.

rales/crackles, fatigue, weight gain, jugular venous distention).

- **Vascular Headache Prophylaxis:** Assess frequency, severity, characteristics, and location of vascular headaches periodically throughout therapy.
- ***Lab Test Considerations:*** May cause increased BUN, serum lipoprotein, potassium, triglyceride, and uric acid levels.
  - May cause increased ANA titers.
  - May cause increase in blood glucose levels.
- ***Toxicity and Overdose:*** Monitor patients receiving beta-adrenergic blocking agents for signs of overdose (bradycardia, severe dizziness or fainting, severe drowsiness, dyspnea, bluish fingernails or palms, seizures). Notify physician or other health care provider immediately if these signs occur.
  - Glucagon has been used to treat bradycardia and hypotension.

POTENTIAL NURSING DIAGNOSES

- Cardiac output, decreased (Side Effects).
- Knowledge deficit, related to medication regimen (Patient/Family Teaching).
- Noncompliance, related to medication regimen (Patient/Family Teaching).

IMPLEMENTATION

- **PO:** Take apical pulse prior to administering. If <50 bpm or if arrhythmia occurs, withhold medication and notify physician or other health care professional.
  - May be administered with food or on an empty stomach.
  - Tablets may be crushed and mixed with food.

PATIENT/FAMILY TEACHING

- **General Info:** Instruct patient to take medication exactly as directed, at the same time each day, even if feeling well; do not skip or double up on missed doses. If a dose is missed, it should be taken as soon as possible up to 4 hr before next dose. Abrupt withdrawal may precipitate life-threatening arrhythmias, hypertension, or myocardial ischemia.
  - Advise patient to make sure enough medication is available for weekends, holidays, and vacations. A written prescription may be kept in wallet in case of emergency.
  - Teach patient and family how to check pulse and blood pressure. Instruct them to check pulse daily and blood pressure biweekly. Advise patient to hold dose and contact health care professional if pulse is <50 bpm or blood pressure changes significantly.
  - May cause drowsiness or dizziness. Caution patients to avoid driving or other activities that require alertness until response to the drug is known.
  - Advise patients to change positions slowly to minimize orthostatic hypotension, especially during initiation of therapy or when dose is increased.
  - Caution patient that this medication may increase sensitivity to cold.
  - Instruct patient to consult health care professional before taking any OTC medications, especially cold preparations, concurrently with this medication.
  - Diabetics should closely monitor blood sugar, especially if weakness, malaise, irritability, or fatigue occurs. Medication may mask tachycardia and increased blood pressure as signs of hypoglycemia, but dizziness and sweating may still occur.
  - Advise patient to notify health care professional if slow pulse, difficulty breathing, wheezing, cold hands and feet, dizziness, confusion, depression, rash, fever, sore throat, unusual bleeding, or bruising occurs.
  - Instruct patient to inform health care professional of medication regimen prior to treatment or surgery.
  - Advise patient to carry identification describing disease process and medication regimen at all times.
- **Hypertension:** Reinforce the need to continue additional therapies for hypertension (weight loss, sodium restriction, stress reduction, regular exercise, moderation of alcohol consumption, and smoking cessation). Medication controls but does not cure hypertension.
- **Vascular Headache Prophylaxis:** Caution patient that sharing this medication may be dangerous.

EVALUATION

Effectiveness of therapy can be demonstrated by: ▪ Decrease in blood pressure ▪ Prevention of myocardial infarction ▪ Prevention of vascular headaches.

T

TIZANIDINE
(tye-**zan**-i-deen)
Zanaflex

CLASSIFICATION(S):
Alpha-adrenergic agonist (centrally acting)

Pregnancy Category C

INDICATIONS

▪ Management of increased muscle tone associated with spasticity in patients with multiple sclerosis or spinal cord injury.

ACTION

▪ Acts as an agonist at central alpha-adrenergic receptor sites ▪ Reduces spasticity by increasing presynaptic inhibition of motor neurons. **Therapeutic Effects:** ▪ Decreased spasticity, allowing better function.

PHARMACOKINETICS

Absorption: Completely absorbed following oral administration but rapidly metabolized, resulting in 40% bioavailability.
Distribution: Widely distributed.
Metabolism and Excretion: 95% metabolized by the liver.
Half-life: 2.5 hr.

CONTRAINDICATIONS AND PRECAUTIONS

Contraindicated in: ▪ Hypersensitivity.
Use Cautiously in: ▪ Renal impairment ▪ Geriatric patients ▪ Concurrent antihypertensive therapy ▪ Pregnancy, lactation, or children (safety not established).
Exercise Extreme Caution in: ▪ Impaired hepatic function.

ADVERSE REACTIONS AND SIDE EFFECTS*

CNS: anxiety, depression, dizziness, sedation, weakness, dyskinesia, hallucinations, nervousness.
EENT: blurred vision, pharyngitis, rhinitis.
CV: hypotension, bradycardia.
GI: abdominal pain, diarrhea, dry mouth, dyspepsia, constipation, hepatocellular injury, increased liver enzymes, vomiting.
GU: urinary frequency.
Derm: rash, skin ulcers, sweating.
MS: back pain, myasthenia, paresthesia.
Misc: fever, speech disorder.

INTERACTIONS

Drug-Drug: ▪ Blood levels and effects may be increased by concurrent use of **oral contraceptives** and **alcohol** ▪ Additive CNS depression may occur with **alcohol** and other **CNS depressants** including some **antidepressants, sedative/hypnotics, antihistamines,** and **opioids.**

ROUTE AND DOSAGE

▪ **PO (Adults):** 4 mg q 6–8 hr initially (no more than 3 doses/24 hr); increase by 2–4 mg/dose up to 8 mg/dose or 24 mg/day (not to exceed 36 mg/day).

AVAILABILITY

▪ ***Tablets:*** 4 mg[Rx].

TIME/ACTION PROFILE (reduced muscle tone)

	ONSET	PEAK	DURATION
PO	UK	1–2 hr	3–6 hr

NURSING IMPLICATIONS

ASSESSMENT

□ Assess muscle spasticity prior to and periodically throughout therapy.
□ Monitor blood pressure and pulse, especially during dose titration. May cause orthostatic hypotension, bradycardia, dizziness, and, rarely, syncope. Effects are usually dose related.
□ Observe patient for drowsiness, dizziness, and asthenia. A change in dose may alleviate these problems.
▪ ***Lab Test Considerations:*** Monitor liver function tests prior to and at 1, 3, and 6 mo of therapy. May cause increase in serum glucose, alkaline phosphatase, AST, and ALT levels.

*CAPITALS indicate life-threatening; underlines indicate most frequent.

POTENTIAL NURSING DIAGNOSES

- Physical mobility, impaired (Indications).
- Injury, risk for (Adverse Reactions).
- Knowledge deficit, related to medication regimen (Patient/Family Teaching).

IMPLEMENTATION

- **General Info:** Doses should be titrated carefully to prevent side effects.
- **PO:** May be taken without regard to meals.

PATIENT/FAMILY TEACHING

- Instruct patient to take tizanidine as directed. Tizanidine may need to be discontinued gradually.
- May cause dizziness and drowsiness. Advise patient to avoid driving or other activities requiring alertness until response to drug is known.
- Instruct patient to change positions slowly to minimize orthostatic hypotension.
- Advise patient to avoid concurrent use of alcohol or other CNS depressants while taking this medication.

EVALUATION

Effectiveness of therapy can be demonstrated by: ▪ Decrease in muscle spasticity with an increased ability to perform activities of daily living.

TOCAINIDE

(toe-**kay**-nide)
Tonocard

CLASSIFICATION(S):
Antiarrhythmic (group IB)

Pregnancy Category C

INDICATIONS

- Life-threatening ventricular arrhythmias, including multifocal and unifocal premature ventricular contractions and ventricular tachycardia.

ACTION

▪ Suppresses automaticity of conduction tissue and spontaneous depolarization of the ventricles during diastole ▪ Has little or no effect on heart rate. **Therapeutic Effects:** ▪ Suppression of arrhythmias.

PHARMACOKINETICS

Absorption: Well absorbed following oral administration.
Distribution: Widely distributed; crosses the blood-brain barrier.
Metabolism and Excretion: Partially metabolized by the liver. 30–50% excreted unchanged by the kidneys.
Half-life: 11–23 hr.

CONTRAINDICATIONS AND PRECAUTIONS

Contraindicated in: ▪ Hypersensitivity ▪ Advanced heart block.
Use Cautiously in: ▪ Congestive heart failure ▪ Hepatic or renal impairment (dosage reduction recommended) ▪ Pregnancy, lactation, or children (safety not established).

ADVERSE REACTIONS AND SIDE EFFECTS*

CNS: SEIZURES, changes in mood, drowsiness, hallucinations, headache, restlessness, tremor, coma, dizziness, mental depression, paranoia.
EENT: blurred vision, thirst, tinnitus.
Resp: PULMONARY FIBROSIS, pneumonia.
CV: SINUS ARREST, CONGESTIVE HEART FAILURE, arrhythmias, bradycardia, hypotension, palpitations, tachycardia, angina, conduction disturbances, hypertension.
GI: anorexia, diarrhea, nausea, vomiting, abdominal discomfort, constipation, drug-induced hepatitis, dyspepsia, dysphagia.
GU: urinary retention.
Derm: alopecia, flushing, rashes, sweating.
Hemat: AGRANULOCYTOSIS, leukopenia, neutropenia, thrombocytopenia.
MS: arthralgia, myalgia.
Neuro: myasthenia gravis, numbness.

INTERACTIONS

Drug-Drug: ▪ Additive cardiac effects with other **antiarrhythmics** ▪ Concurrent use with **beta-adrenergic blocking agents** may precipitate congestive heart failure ▪ **Cimetidine** or **rifampin** may decrease blood levels of tocainide.

***CAPITALS indicate life-threatening; underlines indicate most frequent.**

T

ROUTE AND DOSAGE

- **PO (Adults):** 400 mg q 8 hr initially; usual maintenance dose 1.2–1.8 g/day in divided doses q 8–12 hr.

AVAILABILITY

- ***Tablets:*** 400 mg^{Rx}, 600 mg^{Rx}.

TIME/ACTION PROFILE (antiarrhythmic effects)

	ONSET	PEAK	DURATION
PO	30–60 min	0.5–2 hr	8–12 hr

NURSING IMPLICATIONS

ASSESSMENT

- ECG, pulse, and blood pressure should be monitored prior to and periodically throughout therapy.
- Assess lungs periodically throughout therapy. Notify physician or other health care professional if cough, wheezing, or shortness of breath occurs. Pulmonary side effects usually occur after 3–18 wk of therapy and may be fatal. Chest x rays should also be evaluated if signs of pulmonary complications occur.
- ***Lab Test Considerations:*** CBC and WBC with differential and platelet counts should be monitored weekly during the first 3 mo of therapy and frequently thereafter. Blood counts should be performed promptly if patient develops signs of infection (fever, chills, sore throat, stomatitis), bleeding, or bruising. Leukopenia, agranulocytosis, and thrombocytopenia usually occur after 2–12 wk of therapy and return to normal 1 mo after discontinuation.

POTENTIAL NURSING DIAGNOSES

- Cardiac output, decreased (Indications).
- Knowledge deficit, related to medication regimen (Patient/Family Teaching).

IMPLEMENTATION

- **PO:** Administer with food or milk to minimize GI irritation.

PATIENT/FAMILY TEACHING

- Instruct patient to take medication around the clock, exactly as directed, even if feeling well. If a dose is missed, take as soon as remembered if within 4 hr; do not take if remembered later. Do not double doses. Consult health care professional prior to discontinuing medication, as gradual reduction in dosage may be needed to prevent worsening of condition.
- Instruct patient or family member on how to take pulse. Advise patient to report changes in pulse rate or rhythm.
- May cause dizziness. Caution patient to avoid driving or other activities requiring alertness until response to medication is known.
- Advise patient to inform health care professional of medication regimen prior to treatment or surgery.
- Advise patient to carry identification describing disease process and medication regimen at all times.
- Instruct patient to notify health care professional if trembling, shaking, fever, chills, sore throat, ulcers in the mouth, unusual bleeding or bruising, dyspnea, cough, wheezing, or palpitations occur. The occurrence of tremor may be used as an indication that maximum dose has been reached. Health care professional should also be notified if nausea, vomiting, or diarrhea becomes severe. Tocainide may be discontinued if pulmonary fibrosis, bone marrow depression, or severe skin reaction occurs.
- Emphasize the importance of routine follow-up exams to monitor progress.

EVALUATION

Effectiveness of therapy can be demonstrated by: ▪ Resolution of ventricular arrhythmias without detrimental side effects.

TOLMETIN

(**tole**-met-in)

Tolectin, Tolectin DS, {Novo-Tolmetin}

CLASSIFICATION(S):
Nonsteroidal anti-inflammatory agent

Pregnancy Category C (first trimester)

INDICATIONS

▪ Management of inflammatory disorders including: ▫ Rheumatoid arthritis ▫ Juvenile rheumatoid arthritis ▫ Osteoarthritis.

ACTION

▪ Inhibits prostaglandin synthesis. **Therapeutic Effects:** ▪ Suppression of pain and inflammation.

PHARMACOKINETICS

Absorption: Well absorbed from the GI tract following oral administration.
Distribution: UK.
Metabolism and Excretion: Mostly metabolized by the liver; 20% excreted unchanged by the kidneys.
Half-life: 1 hr.

CONTRAINDICATIONS AND PRECAUTIONS

Contraindicated in: ▪ Hypersensitivity ▪ Cross-sensitivity may exist with other NSAIDs, including aspirin ▪ Active GI bleeding or ulcer disease.
Use Cautiously in: ▪ Severe cardiovascular, renal, or hepatic disease ▪ History of ulcer disease ▪ Severe hepatic or renal impairment (dosage reduction recommended) ▪ Pregnancy and lactation (safety not established; avoid use during 2nd half of pregnancy).

ADVERSE REACTIONS AND SIDE EFFECTS*

CNS: dizziness, headache, drowsiness, mental depression, sleep disturbances.
EENT: tinnitus, visual disturbances.
CV: edema, hypertension.
GI: DRUG-INDUCED HEPATITIS, GI BLEEDING, diarrhea, discomfort, dyspepsia, nausea, vomiting, constipation, flatulence.
GU: renal failure.
Derm: rashes.
Hemat: prolonged bleeding time.
MS: muscle weakness.
Misc: allergic reactions including ANAPHYLAXIS.

INTERACTIONS

Drug-Drug: ▪ Increased risk of bleeding with **anticoagulants, cefamandole, cefoperazone, cefotetan, thrombolytic agents, clopidogrel,** or **plicamycin** ▪ Additive adverse GI side effects with **aspirin, glucocorticoids,** and other **NSAIDs** ▪ May decrease response to **antihypertensives** or **diuretics** ▪ May increase serum levels and risk of toxicity from **lithium** ▪ May increase the risk of hematologic toxicity from **antineoplastic agents** or **radiation therapy** ▪ Increased risk of adverse renal effects with **gold compounds, cyclosporine,** or chronic use of **acetaminophen** ▪ May increase the risk of hypoglycemia from **insulin** or **oral hypoglycemic agents.**

ROUTE AND DOSAGE

- **PO (Adults):** 400 mg 3 times daily initially, followed by maintenance dose of 600–1800 mg/day in 3–4 divided doses (not to exceed 2000 mg/day).
- **PO (Children >2 yr):** 20 mg/kg/day in 3–4 divided doses initially, followed by maintenance dose of 15–30 mg/kg/day in 3–4 divided doses.

AVAILABILITY

▪ ***Tablets:*** 200 mg[Rx], 600 mg[Rx] ▪ ***Capsules:*** 400 mg[Rx].

TIME/ACTION PROFILE (anti-inflammatory effects)

	ONSET	PEAK	DURATION
PO	within 7 days	1–2 wk	UK

NURSING IMPLICATIONS

ASSESSMENT

▫ Patients who have asthma, aspirin-induced allergy, and nasal polyps are at increased risk for developing hypersensitivity reactions. Monitor for rhinitis, asthma, and urticaria.
▫ Assess pain and range of motion prior to and weekly during therapy.
▪ ***Lab Test Considerations:*** BUN, serum creatinine, CBC, and liver function tests should be evaluated periodically in patients receiving prolonged courses of therapy.
▫ Serum potassium, BUN, AST, and ALT may show increased levels.
▫ Hemoglobin and hematocrit may be decreased. Bleeding time may be prolonged for up to 2 days after discontinuation.
▫ May cause false-positive results for urinary protein.

T

*CAPITALS indicate life-threatening; underlines indicate most frequent.

POTENTIAL NURSING DIAGNOSES

- Pain (Indications).
- Physical mobility, impaired (Indications).
- Knowledge deficit, related to medication regimen (Patient/Family Teaching).

IMPLEMENTATION

- **General Info:** Administration in higher than recommended doses does not provide increased effectiveness but may cause increased side effects.
- **PO:** May be administered with food, milk, or antacids to decrease GI irritation. Tablets may be crushed and capsules opened and mixed with fluids or food.

PATIENT/FAMILY TEACHING

- □ Advise patient to take this medication with a full glass of water and to remain in an upright position for 15–30 min after administration.
- □ Instruct patient to take medication exactly as directed. If a dose is missed, it should be taken as soon as remembered but not if almost time for the next dose. Do not double doses.
- □ May cause drowsiness or dizziness. Advise patient to avoid driving or other activities requiring alertness until response to medication is known.
- □ Caution patient to avoid the concurrent use of alcohol, aspirin, NSAIDs, acetaminophen, or other OTC medications without consulting health care professional.
- □ Advise patient to use sunscreen and protective clothing to prevent photosensitivity reactions.
- □ Advise patient to inform health care professional of medication regimen prior to treatment or surgery.
- □ Advise patient to consult health care professional if rash, itching, visual disturbances, tinnitus, weight gain, edema, black stools, persistent headache, or influenza-like syndrome (chills, fever, muscle aches, pain) occurs.

EVALUATION

Effectiveness of therapy can be demonstrated by: ▪ Decrease in pain ▪ Improved joint mobility. Partial arthritic relief is usually seen within 7 days, but maximum effectiveness may require 1–2 wk of continuous therapy. Patients who do not respond to one NSAID may respond to another.

TOPIRAMATE

(toe-**peer**-i-mate)
Topamax

CLASSIFICATION(S):
Anticonvulsant (sulfamate-substituted monosaccharide)

Pregnancy Category C

INDICATIONS

▪ Adjunctive therapy of partial-onset seizures in adults.

ACTION

▪ Action may be due to: □ Blockade of sodium channels in neurons □ Enhancement of gamma-aminobutyrate, an inhibitory neurotransmitter □ Prevention of activation of excitatory receptors.
Therapeutic Effects: ▪ Decreased incidence of seizures.

PHARMACOKINETICS

Absorption: Well absorbed (80%) following oral administration.
Distribution: UK.
Metabolism and Excretion: 70% excreted unchanged in urine.
Half-life: 21 hr.

CONTRAINDICATIONS AND PRECAUTIONS

Contraindicated in: ▪ Hypersensitivity.
Use Cautiously in: ▪ Renal impairment (dosage reduction recommended if CCr <70 ml/min/1.73 m^2) ▪ Hepatic impairment ▪ Dehydration ▪ Pregnancy, lactation, or children (safety not established).

ADVERSE REACTIONS AND SIDE EFFECTS*

CNS: INCREASED SEIZURES, <u>dizziness</u>, <u>drowsiness</u>, <u>fatigue</u>, <u>impaired concentration/memory</u>, <u>nervousness</u>, <u>psychomotor slowing</u>, <u>speech problems</u>, aggressive reaction, agitation, anxiety, confusion, depression, malaise, mood problems.
EENT: <u>abnormal vision</u>, <u>diplopia</u>, <u>nystagmus</u>.

***CAPITALS indicate life-threatening; <u>underlines</u> indicate most frequent.**

GI: nausea, abdominal pain, anorexia, constipation, dry mouth.
GU: kidney stones.
Hemat: leukopenia.
Metab: weight loss.
Neuro: ataxia, paresthesia, tremor.
Misc: SUICIDE ATTEMPT, fever.

INTERACTIONS

Drug-Drug: ▪ Blood levels and effects may be decreased by concurrent **phenytoin, carbamazepine,** or **valproic acid** ▪ May increase blood levels and effects of **phenytoin** ▪ May decrease blood levels and effects of **oral contraceptives** or **valproic acid** ▪ Increased risk of CNS depression with **alcohol** or other **CNS depressants** ▪ Concurrent use with **carbonic anhydrase inhibitors (acetazolamide)** may increase the risk of kidney stones.

ROUTE AND DOSAGE

- **PO (Adults):** 50 mg/day initially, gradually increased to 200 mg twice daily (not to exceed 1600 mg/day).

AVAILABILITY

- ***Tablets:*** 25 mg[Rx], 100 mg[Rx], 200 mg[Rx].

TIME/ACTION PROFILE (blood levels*)

	ONSET	PEAK	DURATION
PO	UK	2 hr	12 hr

*Following single dose.

NURSING IMPLICATIONS

ASSESSMENT

- Assess location, duration, and characteristics of seizure activity.
- ***Lab Test Considerations:*** Monitor CBC with differential and platelet count prior to therapy to determine baseline levels and periodically during therapy. Frequently causes anemia.
- Hepatic function should be monitored periodically throughout therapy. May cause elevated AST and ALT levels.

POTENTIAL NURSING DIAGNOSES

- Injury, risk for (Indications, Side Effects).
- Knowledge deficit, related to medication regimen (Patient/Family Teaching).

IMPLEMENTATION

- **General Info:** Implement seizure precautions.
- **PO:** May be administered without regard to meals.
- Do not break tablets because of bitter taste.

PATIENT/FAMILY TEACHING

- Instruct patient to take topiramate exactly as directed. If a dose is missed, take as soon as possible but not just before next dose; do not double doses. Notify health care professional if more than 1 dose is missed. Medication should be gradually discontinued to prevent seizures and status epilepticus.
- May cause dizziness, drowsiness, confusion, and difficulty concentrating. Caution patients to avoid driving or other activities requiring alertness until response to medication is known.
- Advise patient to maintain a fluid intake of 2000–3000 ml of fluid/day to prevent the formation of kidney stones.
- Caution patient to make position changes slowly to minimize orthostatic hypotension.
- Advise patient not to take alcohol or other CNS depressants concurrently with this medication.
- Advise patient to use a nonhormonal form of contraception while taking topiramate.
- Instruct patient to notify health care professional of medication regimen prior to treatment or surgery.
- Advise patient to use sunscreen and wear protective clothing to prevent photosensitivity reactions.
- Advise patient to carry identification describing disease and medication regimen at all times.

EVALUATION

Clinical response to therapy can be evaluated by: ▪ Absence or reduction of seizure activity.

TOPOTECAN

(toe-poe-**tee**-kan)
Hycamtin

CLASSIFICATION(S):
Antineoplastic (enzyme inhibitor)

Pregnancy Category D

T

INDICATIONS

■ Treatment of metastatic ovarian cancer that has not responded to previous chemotherapy.

ACTION

■ Interferes with DNA synthesis by inhibiting the enzyme topoisomerase. **Therapeutic Effects:** ■ Death of rapidly replicating cells, particularly malignant ones.

PHARMACOKINETICS

Absorption: IV administration results in complete bioavailability.
Distribution: UK.
Metabolism and Excretion: 30% excreted in urine; small amounts metabolized by the liver.
Half-life: 2–3 hr.

CONTRAINDICATIONS AND PRECAUTIONS

Contraindicated in: ■ Hypersensitivity ■ Pregnancy or lactation ■ Pre-existing severe myelosuppression.
Use Cautiously in: ■ Impaired renal function (dosage reduction recommended if CCR $<$40 ml/min) ■ Patients with childbearing potential.

ADVERSE REACTIONS AND SIDE EFFECTS*

CNS: headache, fatigue, weakness.
Resp: dyspnea.
GI: abdominal pain, diarrhea, nausea, vomiting, anorexia, constipation, increased liver enzymes, stomatitis.
Derm: alopecia.
Hemat: anemia, leukopenia, thrombocytopenia.
MS: arthralgia.

INTERACTIONS

Drug-Drug: ■ Neutropenia is prolonged by concurrent use of **G-CSF** (do not use until day 6; 24 hr following completion of topotecan) ■ Additive myelosuppression with other **antineoplastic agents** (especially **cisplatin**) or **radiation therapy.**

ROUTE AND DOSAGE

■ **IV (Adults):** 1.5 mg/m²/day for 5 days starting on day 1 of a 21-day course.

TIME/ACTION PROFILE (effects on WBC counts)

	ONSET	PEAK	DURATION
IV	within days	11 days	7 days

NURSING IMPLICATIONS

ASSESSMENT

□ Monitor vital signs frequently during administration.
□ Monitor for bone marrow depression. Assess for bleeding (bleeding gums, bruising, petechiae, guaiac stools, urine, and emesis) and avoid IM injections and rectal temperatures if platelet count is low. Apply pressure to venipuncture sites for 10 min. Assess for signs of infection during neutropenia. Anemia may occur. Monitor for increased fatigue, dyspnea, and orthostatic hypotension.
□ Nausea and vomiting are common. Pretreatment with antiemetics should be considered.
□ Assess IV site frequently for extravasation, which causes mild local erythema and bruising.
■ ***Lab Test Considerations:*** Monitor CBC with differential and platelet count prior to administration and frequently during therapy. Baseline neutrophil count of $\geq$1500 cells/mm³ and platelet count of $\geq$100,000 cells/mm³ are required before first dose. The nadir of neutropenia occurs in 11 days, with a duration of 7 days. The nadir of thrombocytopenia occurs in 15 days, with a duration of 5 days. The nadir of anemia occurs in 15 days. Subsequent doses should not be administered until neutrophils recover to $>$1000 cells/mm³, platelets recover to $>$100,000 cells/mm³, and hemoglobin levels recover to 9.0 mg/dl. If severe neutropenia occurs during any course, subsequent doses should be reduced by 0.25 mg/m² or filgrastim may be administered following the subsequent course of therapy starting on day 6, 24 hr after the completion of topotecan.
□ Monitor liver function. May cause transient in-

*CAPITALS indicate life-threatening; underlines indicate most frequent.

creases in AST, ALT, and bilirubin concentrations.

POTENTIAL NURSING DIAGNOSES

- Infection, risk for (Adverse Reactions).
- Knowledge deficit, related to medication regimen (Patient/Family Teaching).

IMPLEMENTATION

- **General Info:** Solution should be prepared in a biologic cabinet. Wear gloves, gown, and mask while handling IV medication. Discard IV equipment in specially designated containers.
- **Intermittent Infusion:** Reconstitute each vial with 4 ml of sterile water for injection. Dilute further in 0.9% NaCl or D5W. Use solution immediately after preparing. Solution is yellow to yellow-green. Solution is stable for 24 hr at room temperature.
- ***Rate:*** Administer dose over 30 min.
- **Additive Incompatibility:** ▪ Information unavailable. Do not admix with other solutions or medications.

PATIENT/FAMILY TEACHING

- □ Instruct patient to notify health care professional if fever; chills; sore throat; signs of infection; bleeding gums; bruising; petechiae; blood in urine, stool, or emesis occurs. Caution patient to avoid crowds and persons with known infections. Instruct patient to use soft toothbrush and electric razor. Patient should be cautioned not to drink alcoholic beverages or take products containing aspirin or NSAIDs.
- □ Discuss with patient the possibility of hair loss. Explore methods of coping.
- □ Advise patient that this medication may have teratogenic effects. Contraception should be used during therapy.
- □ Instruct patient not to receive any vaccinations without advice of health care professional.
- □ Emphasize the need for periodic lab tests to monitor for side effects.

EVALUATION

Effectiveness of therapy can be demonstrated by: ▪ Decrease in size and and spread of malignancy.

TORSEMIDE

(**tore**-se-mide)
Demedex

CLASSIFICATION(S):
Diuretic (loop)

Pregnancy Category B

INDICATIONS

▪ Management of edema associated with: □ Congestive heart failure □ Renal disease □ Hepatic disease ▪ Management of hypertension.

ACTION

▪ Acts in the lumen of the thick ascending limb of the loop of Henle, where it increases the renal excretion of water, sodium, chloride, magnesium, hydrogen, and calcium ▪ Also possesses vasodilatory activity that reduces cardiac preload and afterload ▪ Effectiveness persists in impaired renal function. **Therapeutic Effects:** ▪ Induction of diuresis with subsequent mobilization of excess fluid (ascites, pleural effusions, edema) ▪ Lowers blood pressure.

PHARMACOKINETICS

Absorption: 80% absorbed following oral administration.
Distribution: UK.
Metabolism and Excretion: 80% metabolized by the liver; 20% excreted in urine.
Half-life: 210 min.

CONTRAINDICATIONS AND PRECAUTIONS

Contraindicated in: ▪ Hypersensitivity ▪ Cross-sensitivity with thiazides and sulfonamides may occur ▪ Pre-existing uncorrected electrolyte imbalance, hepatic coma, or anuria.
Use Cautiously in: ▪ Patients with hepatic disease accompanied by cirrhosis or ascites (may precipitate hepatic coma; concurrent use with aldosterone antagonists or potassium-sparing diuretics is recommended) ▪ Geriatric patients (difficult to assess hearing status; more prone to hypotension) ▪ Patients with electrolyte depletion, diabetes mellitus, or increasing azotemia ▪ Pregnancy, lactation, or children (safety not established).

T

ADVERSE REACTIONS AND SIDE EFFECTS*

CNS: dizziness, headache, insomnia, nervousness, weakness.
EENT: ototoxicity (↑ doses).
Resp: increased cough, rhinitis, sore throat.
CV: chest pain, ECG abnormalities, hypotension.
GI: constipation, stomach upset, dyspepsia, nausea.
GU: excessive urination.
Derm: photosensitivity.
F and E: hypokalemia, hypomagnesemia.
MS: arthralgia, myalgia.

INTERACTIONS

Drug-Drug: ▪ Additive hypokalemia may occur with concurrent use of **mezlocillin, piperacillin, amphotericin B,** and **glucocorticoids** ▪ Hypokalemia increases the risk of **cardiac glycoside** toxicity ▪ Additive hypotension may occur with other **antihypertensives** or **nitrates** ▪ Concurrent use of other **ototoxic drugs (aminoglycoside anti-infectives, cisplatin)** increases the risk of ototoxicity ▪ May increase the risk of salicylate toxicity in patient on high doses of **salicylates** ▪ Risk of renal dysfunction may be increased by concurrent use of **NSAIDs** ▪ Concurrent use with **indomethacin** in sodium-restricted patients may decrease the effectiveness of torsemide ▪ Diuretic activity may be decreased by **probenecid** ▪ May decrease **lithium** excretion and increase the risk of lithium toxicity.

ROUTE AND DOSAGE

- **PO, IV (Adults):** *Congestive heart failure*—10–20 mg once daily. *Chronic renal failure*—20 mg once daily; dose may be doubled until desired effect is obtained. *Hepatic cirrhosis*—5–10 mg once daily (with aldosterone antagonist or potassium-sparing diuretic); dose may be doubled until desired effect is obtained. *Hypertension*—5 mg once daily; may be increased to 10 mg once daily after 4–6 wk (if still not effective, add another agent).

AVAILABILITY

▪ ***Tablets:*** 5 mg[Rx], 10 mg[Rx], 20 mg[Rx], 100 mg[Rx] ▪ ***Injection:*** 10 mg/ml in 2- and 5-ml ampules[Rx].

TIME/ACTION PROFILE (diuresis)

	ONSET	PEAK	DURATION
PO	within 60 min	60–120 min	6–8 hr
IV	within 10 min	within 60 min	6–8 hr

NURSING IMPLICATIONS

ASSESSMENT

- Assess fluid status throughout therapy. Monitor daily weight, intake and output ratios, amount and location of edema, lung sounds, skin turgor, and mucous membranes. Notify physician or other health care professional if dry mouth, lethargy, weakness, hypotension, or oliguria occurs.
- Monitor blood pressure and pulse before and periodically during therapy.
- Assess patients receiving cardiac glycosides for anorexia, nausea, vomiting, muscle cramps, paresthesia, and confusion. Patients taking cardiac glycosides are at increased risk of digitalis toxicity because of the potassium-depleting effect of the diuretic.
- Assess patient for tinnitus and hearing loss. Audiometry is recommended for patients receiving prolonged therapy. Hearing loss is most common following rapid or high-dose IV administration in patients with decreased renal function or in those taking other ototoxic drugs.
- Assess for allergy to sulfonamides. Cross-sensitivity may occur.
- ***Lab Test Considerations:*** Monitor electrolytes, renal and hepatic function, serum glucose and uric acid levels prior to and periodically throughout therapy. Torsemide may cause decreased serum potassium, calcium, and magnesium concentrations. May also cause increased BUN, serum glucose, creatinine, and uric acid levels.
- Torsemide may cause increases in total plasma cholesterol and lipids during initial therapy. Those elevations usually return to normal with chronic therapy.

POTENTIAL NURSING DIAGNOSES

- Fluid volume excess (Indications).
- Fluid volume deficit (Adverse Reactions).
- Knowledge deficit, related to medication regimen (Patient/Family Teaching).

***CAPITALS indicate life-threatening; underlines indicate most frequent.**

IMPLEMENTATION

- **General Info:** Administer torsemide in the morning to prevent disruption of the sleep cycle.
- □ Doses for IV and oral routes are the same.
- **PO:** May be administered without regard to meals.
- **Direct IV:** Administer undiluted. Do not administer if solution is discolored or contains particulate matter.
- ***Rate:*** Administer slowly over 2 min.
- **Syringe Incompatibility:** ▪ Information unavailable. Do not mix with other drugs or solutions.

PATIENT/FAMILY TEACHING

- **General Info:** Instruct patient to take torsemide exactly as directed at the same time each day. If a dose is missed, take as soon as possible unless almost time for next dose; do not double doses.
- □ Caution patient to make position changes slowly to minimize orthostatic hypotension. Caution patient that use of alcohol, exercise during hot weather, or standing for long periods during therapy may enhance orthostatic hypotension.
- □ Instruct patient to consult health care professional regarding a diet high in potassium (see Appendix K).
- □ Caution patient to use sunscreen and wear protective clothing to prevent photosensitivity reactions.
- □ Advise patient to consult health care professional before taking OTC medications concurrently with this therapy.
- □ Advise diabetic patients to monitor blood sugar closely, as torsemide may cause increased blood sugar levels.
- □ Instruct patient to notify health care professional of medication regimen prior to treatment or surgery.
- □ Advise patient to contact health care professional immediately if muscle weakness, cramps, nausea, dizziness, numbness or tingling of extremities, ringing in ears, loss of hearing, or rash occurs.
- □ Emphasize the importance of routine follow-up exams.
- **Hypertension:** Advise patients on antihypertensive regimen to continue taking medication even if feeling better. Torsemide controls but does not cure hypertension.
- □ Reinforce the need to continue additional therapies for hypertension (weight loss, restricted sodium intake, stress reduction, regular exercise, moderation of alcohol consumption, cessation of smoking).

EVALUATION

Effectiveness of therapy can be demonstrated by: ▪ Increase in urinary output □ Decrease in edema ▪ Decrease in blood pressure.

TRACE METAL COMBINATION ADDITIVE

Concentrated Multiple Trace Element, ConTE-PAK-4, M.T.E.-4, M.T.E.-4 Concentrated, M.T.E.-5, M.T.E.-5 Concentrated, M.T.E.-6, M.T.E.-6 Concentrated, M.T.E.-7, MulTE-PAK-4, MulTE-PAK-5, Multiple Trace Element, Multiple Trace Element Neonatal, Multiple Trace Element Pediatric, Neotrace 4, PedTE-PAK-4, Pedtrace-4, P.T.E.-4, P.T.E.-5

CLASSIFICATION(S):
Nutritional supplement

Pregnancy Category C

INDICATIONS

▪ Administered as a component in total parenteral nutrition (TPN, parenteral hyperalimentation) ▪ May contain any or all of the following: □ Chromium □ Copper □ Iodine □ Manganese □ Molybdenum □ Selenium □ Zinc.

ACTION

▪ Trace metals serve as cofactors or catalysts for numerous diverse homeostatic processes. **Therapeutic Effects:** ▪ Replacement in deficiency states when oral ingestion is not feasible.

PHARMACOKINETICS

Absorption: Administered IV only, resulting in complete bioavailability.
Distribution: Widely distributed.

Metabolism and Excretion: Excretion depends on individual trace element.
Half-life: UK.

CONTRAINDICATIONS AND PRECAUTIONS

Contraindicated in: ▪ Hypersensitivity to iodine (iodine-containing products only).
Use Cautiously in: ▪ Pregnancy or lactation ▪ Nasogastric suction, fistula drainage, prolonged vomiting or diarrhea (may increase requirements) ▪ Renal impairment or biliary obstruction (may increase risk of toxicity) ▪ Isolated trace element deficiency (other additives may be excessive—use only those required).

ADVERSE REACTIONS AND SIDE EFFECTS*

Listed for individual trace metals—usually associated with toxicity.
Misc: *Chromium*—COMA, SEIZURES, GI ulceration, hepatic damage, nausea, renal damage, vomiting. *Copper*—behavioral changes, diarrhea, peripheral edema, photophobia, progressive marasmus, weakness. *Iodine*—acneiform skin lesions, headache, increased salivation, metallic taste, parotitis, runny nose, sneezing, sore mouth, swelling of eyelids. *Manganese*—anorexia, apathy, gait disturbances, headache, impotence, irritability, speech difficulties. *Molybdenum*—gout-like syndrome. *Selenium*—garlic-like breath, garlic-like sweat, GI discomfort, hair loss, mental depression, metallic taste, nervousness, vomiting, weak nails. *Zinc*—blurred vision, hypotension, jaundice, loss of consciousness, oliguria, pulmonary edema, tachycardia, toxicity poorly defined but may include hypothermia, vomiting.

INTERACTIONS

Drug-Drug: ▪ None significant in replacement doses.

ROUTE AND DOSAGE

- **IV (Adults and Children):** Amount necessary to maintain normal trace element levels.

AVAILABILITY

All must be diluted in large-volume parenterals prior to use.

▪ ***Injection:*** Each ml contains 0.85–4 mcg chromium, 0.1–0.4 mg copper, 0.025–0.16 mg manganese, and 0.5–1.5 mg zinc. Some products also contain iodide, selenium, and molybdenum[Rx] ▪ ***Concentrated injection:*** Each ml contains 10 mcg chromium, 1 mg copper, 0.5 mg manganese, and 5 mg zinc. Some products also contain iodide and selenium[Rx].

TIME/ACTION PROFILE (replacement)

	ONSET	PEAK	DURATION
IV	rapid	UK	UK

NURSING IMPLICATIONS

ASSESSMENT

- Assess nutritional status by 24-hr recall prior to therapy.
- Monitor patient for signs and symptoms of trace metal deficiencies prior to and throughout therapy, as follows:
- *Chromium:* glucose intolerance, ataxia, peripheral neuropathy, confusion.
- *Copper:* leukopenia, neutropenia, anemia, iron deficiency, skeletal abnormalities, defective tissue formation.
- *Iodine:* impaired thyroid function, goiter, cretinism.
- *Manganese:* nausea, vomiting, weight loss, dermatitis, changes in hair.
- *Molybdenum:* tachycardia, tachypnea, headache, night blindness, nausea, vomiting, edema, lethargy, disorientation, coma, hypouricemia, hypouricosuria.
- *Selenium:* cardiomyopathy, muscle pain, kwashiorkor, Keshan disease.
- *Zinc:* diarrhea, apathy, depression, anorexia, hypogonadism, growth retardation, anemia, hepatosplenomegaly, impaired wound healing, decreased sense of taste and smell.

▪ ***Lab Test Considerations:*** Serum trace metal concentrations should be monitored periodically throughout TPN therapy.

POTENTIAL NURSING DIAGNOSES

- Nutrition, altered, less than body requirements (Indications).
- Knowledge deficit, related to medication regimen (Patient/Family Teaching).

*CAPITALS indicate life-threatening; underlines indicate most frequent.

IMPLEMENTATION

- **IV:** Solution usually does not contain preservatives; discard unused portion.
- **Continuous Infusion:** Must be diluted prior to administration. Dilute each dose in at least 1 liter of IV solution.
- Administer at prescribed rate for TPN infusion.
- **Additive Compatibility:** ▪ Usually compatible with other trace metals, electrolytes, and dextrose/amino acid combinations used for TPN.

PATIENT/FAMILY TEACHING

- Explain purpose of infusion of TPN and components to patient.

EVALUATION

Effectiveness of therapy can be demonstrated by: ▪ Prevention or treatment of trace metal deficiencies.

TRAMADOL

(**tra**-ma-dol)
Ultram

CLASSIFICATION(S):
Analgesic (centrally acting)

Pregnancy Category C

INDICATIONS

▪ Treatment of moderate to moderately severe pain.

ACTION

▪ Binds to mu-opioid receptors ▪ Inhibits reuptake of serotonin and norepinephrine in the CNS. **Therapeutic Effects:** ▪ Decreased pain.

PHARMACOKINETICS

Absorption: 75% absorbed following oral administration.
Distribution: Crosses the placenta; enters breast milk.
Metabolism and Excretion: Mostly metabolized by the liver; one metabolite has analgesic activity; 30% is excreted unchanged in urine.
Half-life: *Tramadol*—5–9 hr; *active metabolite*—5–9 hr (both are increased in renal or hepatic impairment).

CONTRAINDICATIONS AND PRECAUTIONS

Contraindicated in: ▪ Hypersensitivity ▪ Cross-sensitivity with opioids may occur ▪ Patients who are acutely intoxicated with alcohol, sedative/hypnotics, centrally acting analgesics, opioid analgesics, or psychotropic agents ▪ Patients who are physically dependent on opioids (may precipitate withdrawal) ▪ Not recommended for use during pregnancy or lactation.
Use Cautiously in: ▪ Geriatric patients (not to exceed 300 mg/day in patients >75 yr) ▪ Patients with a history of epilepsy or risk factors for seizures ▪ Renal impairment (increased dosing interval recommended if CCr >30 ml/min) ▪ Hepatic impairment (increased interval recommended in patients with cirrhosis) ▪ Patients receiving MAO inhibitors or CNS depressants ▪ Increased intracranial pressure or head trauma ▪ Acute abdomen (may preclude accurate clinical assessment) ▪ Patients with a history of opioid dependence or who have recently received large doses of opioids ▪ Children <16 yr (safety not established).

ADVERSE REACTIONS AND SIDE EFFECTS*

CNS: SEIZURES, dizziness, headache, somnolence, anxiety, CNS stimulation, confusion, coordination disturbance, euphoria, malaise, nervousness, sleep disorder, weakness.
EENT: visual disturbances.
CV: vasodilation.
GI: constipation, nausea, abdominal pain, anorexia, diarrhea, dry mouth, dyspepsia, flatulence, vomiting.
GU: menopausal symptoms, urinary retention/frequency.
Derm: pruritus, sweating.
Neuro: hypertonia.
Misc: physical dependence, psychological dependence, tolerance.

INTERACTIONS

Drug-Drug: ▪ Increased risk of CNS depression when used concurrently with other **CNS depressants**, including **alcohol, antihistamines, sedative/hypnotics, opioids, anesthetics**, or **psychotropic agents** ▪ Increased risk of seizures with high doses of **penicillins**

*CAPITALS indicate life-threatening; underlines indicate most frequent.

or **cephalosporins, phenothiazines, antidepressants,** or **MAO inhibitors** ▪ **Carbamazepine** increases the metabolism and decreases the effectiveness of tramadol (increased doses may be required) ▪ Use cautiously in patients who are receiving **MAO inhibitors** (increased risk of adverse reactions) ▪ Effectiveness may be altered by concurrent **quinidine.**

ROUTE AND DOSAGE

- **PO (Adults):** 50–100 mg q 4–6 hr (not to exceed 400 mg/day or 300 mg in patients >75 yr).

AVAILABILITY

- ***Tablets:*** 50 mg^Rx^.

TIME/ACTION PROFILE (analgesia)

	ONSET	PEAK	DURATION
PO	1 hr	2–3 hr	4–6 hr

NURSING IMPLICATIONS

ASSESSMENT

- Assess type, location, and intensity of pain prior to and 2–3 hr (peak) following administration.
- Assess blood pressure and respiratory rate before and periodically during administration. Respiratory depression has not occurred with recommended doses.
- Assess bowel function routinely. Prevention of constipation should be instituted with increased intake of fluids and bulk and with laxatives to minimize constipating effects.
- Assess prior analgesic history. Tramadol is not recommended for patients dependent on opioids or who have previously received opioids for more than 1 wk; may cause opioid withdrawal symptoms.
- Prolonged use may lead to physical and psychological dependence and tolerance, although these may be milder than with opioids. This should not prevent patient from receiving adequate analgesia. Most patients who receive tramadol for pain do not develop psychological dependence. If tolerance develops, changing to an opioid agonist may be required to relieve pain.
- ***Lab Test Considerations:*** May cause increased serum creatinine, elevated liver enzymes, decreased hemoglobin, and proteinuria.
- ***Toxicity and Overdose:*** Overdose may cause respiratory depression and seizures. Naloxone (Narcan) may reverse some, but not all, of the symptoms of overdose. Treatment should be symptomatic and supportive. Maintain adequate respiratory exchange. Hemodialysis is not helpful, as it removes only a small portion of administered dose. Seizures may be managed with barbiturates or benzodiazepines; naloxone increases seizures.

POTENTIAL NURSING DIAGNOSES

- Pain (Indications).
- Injury, risk for (Side Effects).
- Knowledge deficit, related to medication regimen (Patient/Family Teaching).

IMPLEMENTATION

- **General Info:** Tramadol is considered to provide more analgesia than codeine 60 mg but less than aspirin 650 mg/codeine 60 mg for acute postoperative pain.
- For chronic pain, daily doses of 250 mg of tramadol provide pain relief similar to that of 5 doses/day of acetaminophen 300 mg/codeine 30 mg, 5 doses/day of aspirin 325 mg/codeine 30 mg, or 2–3 doses/day of acetaminophen 500 mg/oxycodone 5 mg.
- Explain therapeutic value of medication prior to administration to enhance the analgesic effect.
- Regularly administered doses may be more effective than prn administration. Analgesic is more effective if given before pain becomes severe.
- Tramadol should be discontinued gradually after long-term use to prevent withdrawal symptoms.
- **PO:** Tramadol may be administered without regard to meals.

PATIENT/FAMILY TEACHING

- Instruct patient on how and when to ask for pain medication.
- May cause dizziness and drowsiness. Caution patient to avoid driving or other activities requiring alertness until response to medication is known.
- Advise patient to change positions slowly to minimize orthostatic hypotension.

- Caution patient to avoid concurrent use of alcohol or other CNS depressants with this medication.
- Encourage patient to turn, cough, and breathe deeply every 2 hr to prevent atelectasis.

EVALUATION

Effectiveness of therapy can be demonstrated by: ▪ Decrease in severity of pain without a significant alteration in level of consciousness or respiratory status.

TRAZODONE

(**traz**-oh-done)

Desyrel, Trazon, Trialodine

CLASSIFICATION(S):

Antidepressant (miscellaneous)

Pregnancy Category C

INDICATIONS

▪ Treatment of major depression often in conjunction with psychotherapy. **Unlabeled Uses:** ▪ Management of chronic pain syndromes, including diabetic neuropathy.

ACTION

▪ Alters the effects of serotonin in the CNS. **Therapeutic Effects:** ▪ Antidepressant action, which may develop only over several weeks.

PHARMACOKINETICS

Absorption: Well absorbed following oral administration.

Distribution: Widely distributed.

Metabolism and Excretion: Extensively metabolized by the liver; minimal excretion of unchanged drug by the kidneys.

Half-life: 5–9 hr.

CONTRAINDICATIONS AND PRECAUTIONS

Contraindicated in: ▪ Hypersensitivity ▪ Recovery period following myocardial infarction ▪ Concurrent electroconvulsive therapy.

Use Cautiously in: ▪ Cardiovascular disease ▪ Suicidal behavior ▪ Severe hepatic or renal disease (dosage reduction recommended) ▪ Geriatric patients (initial dosage reduction recommended) ▪ Pregnancy, lactation, or children (safety not established).

ADVERSE REACTIONS AND SIDE EFFECTS*

CNS: drowsiness, confusion, dizziness, fatigue, hallucinations, headache, insomnia, nightmares, slurred speech, syncope, weakness.

EENT: blurred vision, tinnitus.

CV: hypotension, arrhythmias, chest pain, hypertension, palpitations, tachycardia.

GI: dry mouth, altered taste, constipation, diarrhea, excess salivation, flatulence, nausea, vomiting.

GU: hematuria, impotence, priapism, urinary frequency.

Derm: rashes.

Hemat: anemia, leukopenia.

MS: myalgia.

Neuro: tremor.

INTERACTIONS

Drug-Drug: ▪ May increase **digoxin** or **phenytoin** serum levels ▪ Additive CNS depression with other **CNS depressants,** including **alcohol, antihistamines, opioids,** and **sedative/hypnotics** ▪ Additive hypotension with **antihypertensive agents,** acute ingestion of **alcohol,** or **nitrates** ▪ Concurrent use with **fluoxetine** increases levels and risk of toxicity from trazodone.

ROUTE AND DOSAGE

- **PO (Adults):** 150 mg/day in 3 divided doses; increase by 50 mg/day q 3–4 days until desired response (not to exceed 400 mg/day in outpatients or 600 mg/day in hospitalized patients).
- **PO (Geriatric Patients):** 75 mg/day in divided doses initially; may be increased q 3–4 days.
- **PO (Children 6–18 yr):** 1.5–2 mg/kg/day in divided doses. May be increased q 3–4 days up to 6 mg/kg/day.

AVAILABILITY

▪ ***Tablets:*** 50 mg[Rx], 100 mg[Rx], 150 mg[Rx], 300 mg[Rx].

*CAPITALS indicate life-threatening; underlines indicate most frequent.

T

TIME/ACTION PROFILE (antidepressant effect)

	ONSET	PEAK	DURATION
PO	1–2 wk	2–4 wk	wks

NURSING IMPLICATIONS

ASSESSMENT

- **General Info:** Monitor blood pressure and pulse rate prior to and during initial therapy. Patients with pre-existing cardiac disease should have ECGs monitored prior to and periodically during therapy to detect arrhythmias.
- **Depression:** Assess mental status and mood changes frequently. Assess for suicidal tendencies, especially during early therapy. Restrict amount of drug available to patient.
- **Pain:** Assess location, duration, intensity, and characteristics of pain prior to and periodically during therapy.
- ***Lab Test Considerations:*** Assess CBC and renal and hepatic function prior to and periodically during therapy. Slight, clinically insignificant decrease in leukocyte and neutrophil counts may occur.

POTENTIAL NURSING DIAGNOSES

- Coping, ineffective individual (Indications).
- Knowledge deficit, related to medication regimen (Patient/Family Teaching).

IMPLEMENTATION

- **PO:** Administer with or immediately after meals to minimize side effects (nausea, dizziness) and allow maximum absorption of trazodone. A larger portion of the total daily dose may be given at bedtime to decrease daytime drowsiness and dizziness.

PATIENT/FAMILY TEACHING

- Instruct patient to take medication exactly as directed. If a dose is missed, take as soon as remembered. Do not take if within 4 hr of next scheduled dose; do not double doses. Consult health care professional prior to discontinuing medication; gradual dosage reduction is necessary to prevent aggravation of condition.
- May cause drowsiness and blurred vision. Caution patient to avoid driving and other activities requiring alertness until response to drug is known.
- Caution patient to change positions slowly to minimize orthostatic hypotension.
- Advise patient to avoid concurrent use of alcohol or other CNS depressant drugs.
- Inform patient that frequent rinses, good oral hygiene, and sugarless candy or gum may diminish dry mouth. Health care professional should be notified if this persists >2 wk. An increase in fluid intake, fiber, and exercise may prevent constipation.
- Advise patient to notify health care professional of medication regimen prior to treatment or surgery.
- Instruct patient to notify health care professional if priapism, irregular heartbeat, fainting, confusion, skin rash, or tremors occur or if dry mouth, nausea and vomiting, dizziness, headache, muscle aches, constipation, or diarrhea becomes pronounced.
- Emphasize the importance of follow-up exams to evaluate progress.

EVALUATION

Effectiveness of therapy can be demonstrated by: ▪ Resolution of depression ▫ Increased sense of well-being ▫ Renewed interest in surroundings ▫ Increased appetite ▫ Improved energy level ▫ Improved sleep ▪ Decrease in severity of pain in chronic pain syndromes. Therapeutic effects are usually seen within 1 wk, although 4 wk may be required to obtain significant therapeutic results.

TRIAZOLAM

(trye-**az**-oh-lam)

{Apo-Triazo}, {Gen-Triazolam}, Halcion, {Novo-Triolam}, {Nu-Triazo}

CLASSIFICATION(S):
Sedative/hypnotic (benzodiazepine)

Schedule IV
Pregnancy Category X

INDICATIONS

- Short-term management of insomnia.

{} = Available in Canada only.

ACTION

▪ Acts at many levels in the CNS, producing generalized depression ▪ Effects may be mediated by gamma-aminobutyric acid (GABA), an inhibitory neurotransmitter. **Therapeutic Effects:** ▪ Relief of insomnia.

PHARMACOKINETICS

Absorption: Well absorbed following oral administration.
Distribution: Widely distributed, crosses blood-brain barrier. Probably crosses the placenta and enters breast milk.
Metabolism and Excretion: Metabolized by the liver.
Half-life: 1.6–5.4 hr.

CONTRAINDICATIONS AND PRECAUTIONS

Contraindicated in: ▪ Hypersensitivity ▪ Cross-sensitivity with other benzodiazepines may occur ▪ Pre-existing CNS depression ▪ Uncontrolled severe pain ▪ Pregnancy, lactation, or children.
Use Cautiously in: ▪ Pre-existing hepatic dysfunction (dosage reduction recommended) ▪ History of suicide attempt or drug addiction ▪ Geriatric or debilitated patients (initial dosage reduction recommended).

ADVERSE REACTIONS AND SIDE EFFECTS*

CNS: dizziness, excessive sedation, hangover, headache, anterograde amnesia, confusion, lethargy, mental depression, paradoxical excitation.
EENT: blurred vision.
GI: constipation, diarrhea, nausea, vomiting.
Derm: rashes.
Misc: physical dependence, psychological dependence, tolerance.

INTERACTIONS

Drug-Drug: ▪ **Cimetidine**, **erythromycin**, **fluconazole**, **itraconazole**, **ketoconazole**, **indinavir**, **nelfinavir**, **ritonavir**, or **saquinavir** may decrease metabolism and enhance actions of triazolam; combination should be avoided ▪ Additive CNS depression with **alcohol, antidepressants, antihistamines,** and **opioids** ▪ May decrease effectiveness of **levodopa** ▪ May increase toxicity of **zidovudine** ▪ **Isoniazid** may decrease excretion and increase effects of triazolam ▪ Sedative effects may be decreased by **theophylline.**
Drug-Food: ▪ **Grapefruit juice** increases absorption.

ROUTE AND DOSAGE

▪ **PO (Adults):** 125–250 mcg (up to 500 mcg) at bedtime.
▪ **PO (Geriatric Patients or Debilitated Patients):** 125 mcg at bedtime initially; may be increased as needed.

AVAILABILITY

▪ ***Tablets:*** 125 mcg[Rx], 250 mcg[Rx].

TIME/ACTION PROFILE (sedation)

	ONSET	PEAK	DURATION
PO	15–30 min	6–8 hr	UK

NURSING IMPLICATIONS

ASSESSMENT

- Assess sleep patterns prior to and periodically throughout therapy.
- Prolonged high-dose therapy may lead to psychological or physical dependence. Restrict the amount of drug available to patient, especially if patient is depressed, suicidal, or has a history of addiction.

POTENTIAL NURSING DIAGNOSES

▪ Sleep pattern disturbance (Indications).
▪ Injury, risk for (Side Effects).
▪ Knowledge deficit, related to medication regimen (Patient/Family Teaching).

IMPLEMENTATION

▪ **General Info:** Supervise ambulation and transfer of patients following administration. Remove cigarettes. Side rails should be raised and call bell within reach at all times.
▪ **PO:** Administer with food if GI irritation becomes a problem.

PATIENT/FAMILY TEACHING

- Instruct patient to take triazolam exactly as directed. Discuss the importance of preparing environment for sleep (dark room, quiet, avoidance of nicotine and caffeine). If less ef-

*CAPITALS indicate life-threatening; underlines indicate most frequent.

T

fective after a few weeks, consult health care professional; do not increase dose.

- May cause daytime drowsiness or dizziness. Caution patient to avoid driving or other activities requiring alertness until response to medication is known.
- Advise patient to avoid the use of alcohol and other CNS depressants and to consult health care professional prior to using OTC preparations that contain antihistamines or alcohol.
- Advise patient to inform health care professional if pregnancy is planned or suspected or if confusion, depression, or persistent headaches occur. Instruct family or caregiver to notify health care professional if personality changes occur.
- Instruct patient to notify health care professional if an increase in daytime anxiety occurs. May occur after as few as 10 days of therapy. May require discontinuation of triazolam.
- Emphasize the importance of follow-up appointments to monitor progress.

EVALUATION

Effectiveness of therapy can be demonstrated by: ▪ Improvement in sleep patterns, which may not be noticeable until the 3rd day of therapy.

TRIFLUOPERAZINE

(trye-floo-oh-**pair**-a-zeen)
{Apo-Trifluoperazine}, {Novo-Flurazine}, {PMS-Trifluoperazine}, {Solazine}, Stelazine, {Terfluzine}

CLASSIFICATION(S):
Antipsychotic agent (phenothiazine)

Pregnancy Category C

INDICATIONS

▪ Treatment of acute and chronic psychoses ▪ Adjunct in the management of anxiety when safer agents are contraindicated.

ACTION

▪ Alters the effects of dopamine in the CNS ▪ Possesses significant anticholinergic and alpha-adrenergic blocking activity. **Therapeutic Effects:** ▪ Diminished signs and symptoms of psychoses.

PHARMACOKINETICS

Absorption: Absorption from tablets is variable; may be better with oral liquid formulations. Well absorbed following IM administration.
Distribution: Widely distributed, high concentrations in the CNS. Crosses the placenta and enters breast milk.
Protein Binding: ≥90%.
Metabolism and Excretion: Highly metabolized by the liver.
Half-life: UK.

CONTRAINDICATIONS AND PRECAUTIONS

Contraindicated in: ▪ Hypersensitivity ▪ Cross-sensitivity with other phenothiazines may exist ▪ Hypersensitivity to bisulfites (oral concentrate only) ▪ Narrow-angle glaucoma ▪ Bone marrow depression ▪ Severe liver or cardiovascular disease.
Use Cautiously in: ▪ Geriatric or debilitated patients (dosage reduction recommended) ▪ Pregnancy or lactation (safety not established; may cause adverse effects in the newborn) ▪ Diabetes mellitus ▪ Respiratory disease ▪ Prostatic hypertrophy ▪ CNS tumors ▪ Epilepsy ▪ Intestinal obstruction ▪ Pregnancy or lactation (safety not established; may cause adverse effects in the newborn).

ADVERSE REACTIONS AND SIDE EFFECTS*

CNS: NEUROLEPTIC MALIGNANT SYNDROME, extrapyramidal reactions, sedation, tardive dyskinesia.
EENT: dry eyes, blurred vision, lens opacities.
CV: hypotension, tachycardia.
GI: constipation, anorexia, dry mouth, hepatitis, ileus.
GU: urinary retention.
Derm: photosensitivity, pigment changes, rashes.
Endo: galactorrhea.
Hemat: AGRANULOCYTOSIS, leukopenia.
Metab: hyperthermia.
Misc: allergic reactions.

{} = Available in Canada only.
***CAPITALS indicate life-threatening; underlines indicate most frequent.**

INTERACTIONS

Drug-Drug: ▪ Additive hypotension with **antihypertensive agents**, acute ingestion of **alcohol,** or **nitrates** ▪ Additive CNS depression with other **CNS depressants**, including **alcohol, antihistamines, opioids, sedative/hypnotics,** and **general anesthetics** ▪ Additive anticholinergic effects with other **drugs having anticholinergic properties**, including **antihistamines, antidepressants,** other **phenothiazines, quinidine,** and **disopyramide** ▪ Acute encephalopathy may occur with **lithium** ▪ May decrease the effectiveness of **levodopa** ▪ Increased risk of agranulocytosis with **antithyroid drugs** ▪ **Lithium** decreases absorption and may increase risk of extrapyramidal reactions.

ROUTE AND DOSAGE

- **PO (Adults):** *Psychoses*—2–5 mg bid (up to 40 mg/day). *Anxiety*—1–2 mg bid (not to exceed 6 mg/day or more than 12 mg/wk).
- **PO (Children 6–12 yr):** 1 mg once or twice daily (up to 15 mg/day).
- **IM (Adults):** 1–2 mg q 4–6 hr (up to 10 mg/day).
- **IM (Children):** 1 mg once or twice daily.

AVAILABILITY

▪ ***Tablets:*** 1 mg[Rx], 2 mg[Rx], 5 mg[Rx], 10 mg[Rx], {20 mg[Rx]} ▪ ***Syrup:*** {1 mg/ml[Rx]}, {10 mg/ml[Rx]} ▪ ***Oral solution:*** 10 mg/ml in 60-ml bottles[Rx] ▪ ***Injection:*** 2 mg/ml in 10-ml vials[Rx].

TIME/ACTION PROFILE (antipsychotic effects)

	ONSET	PEAK	DURATION
PO	UK	UK	12–24 hr
IM	UK	UK	4–6 hr

NURSING IMPLICATIONS

ASSESSMENT

- □ Assess mental status (orientation, mood, behavior) and degree of anxiety prior to and periodically throughout therapy.
- □ Monitor blood pressure (sitting, standing, lying), ECG, pulse, and respiratory rate prior to and frequently during the period of dosage adjustment. May cause Q-wave and T-wave changes in ECG.
- □ Observe patient carefully when administering medication to ensure that medication is actually taken and not hoarded.
- □ Assess patient for level of sedation following administration.
- □ Monitor intake and output ratios and daily weight. Notify physician or other health care provider if significant discrepancies occur.
- □ Monitor patient for onset of akathisia (restlessness or desire to keep moving) and extrapyramidal side effects (*parkinsonian*—difficulty speaking or swallowing, loss of balance control, pill rolling, mask-like face, shuffling gait, rigidity, tremors; and *dystonic*—muscle spasms, twisting motions, twitching, inability to move eyes, weakness of arms or legs) every 2 mo during therapy and 8–12 wk after therapy has been discontinued. Notify physician or other health care professional if these symptoms occur, as reduction in dosage or discontinuation of medication may be necessary. Trihexyphenidyl or diphenhydramine may be used to control these symptoms.
- □ Monitor for tardive dyskinesia (uncontrolled rhythmic movement of mouth, face, and extremities; lip smacking or puckering; puffing of cheeks; uncontrolled chewing; rapid or worm-like movements of tongue). Notify physician or other health care professional immediately if these symptoms occur, as they may be irreversible.
- □ Monitor for development of neuroleptic malignant syndrome (fever, respiratory distress, tachycardia, convulsions, diaphoresis, hypertension or hypotension, pallor, tiredness, severe muscle stiffness, loss of bladder control). Notify physician or other health care professional immediately if these symptoms occur.
- ▪ ***Lab Test Considerations:*** CBC, liver function tests, and ocular examinations should be evaluated periodically throughout course of therapy. May cause decreased hematocrit, hemoglobin, leukocytes, granulocytes, platelets. May cause elevated bilirubin, AST, ALT, and alkaline phosphatase. Agranulocytosis occurs at 4–10 wk of therapy, with recovery 1–2 wk following discontinuation. May recur if medication is restarted. Liver function abnormalities may require discontinuation of therapy.
- □ May cause false-positive or false-negative pregnancy tests and false-positive urine bilirubin test results.
- □ May cause increased serum prolactin levels,

thereby interfering with gonadorelin test results.

POTENTIAL NURSING DIAGNOSES

- Coping, ineffective individual (Indications).
- Thought processes, altered (Indications).
- Knowledge deficit, related to medication regimen (Patient/Family Teaching).

IMPLEMENTATION

- **General Info:** To prevent contact dermatitis, avoid getting liquid preparations on hands, and wash hands thoroughly if spillage occurs.
- □ Phenothiazines should be discontinued 48 hr before and not resumed for 24 hr following myelography, as they lower the seizure threshold.
- □ Solution may be slightly yellow. Do not use if solution is brown or contains a precipitate. Protect from light.
- **PO:** Administer oral doses with food, water, or milk to minimize GI irritation. Tablets may be crushed and mixed with food or fluids for patients with difficulty swallowing.
- □ Dilute concentrate just prior to administration, in at least 120 ml of tomato or fruit juice, milk, carbonated beverage, coffee, tea, or water. Semisolid foods (soups, puddings) may also be used.
- **IM:** Administer deep into well-developed muscle. SC administration may cause tissue necrosis. Keep patient recumbent for at least 30 min following injection to minimize hypotensive effects.

PATIENT/FAMILY TEACHING

- □ Advise patient to take medication exactly as directed and not to skip doses or double up on missed doses. If a dose is missed, it should be taken as soon as remembered unless almost time for the next dose. If more than 2 doses a day are ordered, the missed dose should be taken within 1 hr of the scheduled time or omitted. Abrupt withdrawal may lead to gastritis, nausea, vomiting, dizziness, headache, tachycardia, and insomnia.
- □ Inform patient of possibility of extrapyramidal symptoms and tardive dyskinesia. Instruct patient to report these symptoms immediately to physician or other health care provider.
- □ May cause drowsiness. Caution patient to avoid driving or other activities requiring alertness until response to medication is known.
- □ Advise patient to make position changes slowly to minimize orthostatic hypotension.
- □ Advise patient to use sunscreen and protective clothing when exposed to the sun to prevent photosensitivity reactions. Extremes in temperature should also be avoided, as this drug impairs body temperature regulation.
- □ Caution patient to avoid taking alcohol or other CNS depressants concurrently with this medication.
- □ Instruct patient to use frequent mouth rinses, good oral hygiene, and sugarless gum or candy to minimize dry mouth. Consult health care professional if dry mouth continues for >2 wk.
- □ Advise patient that increasing activity and bulk and fluids in the diet helps minimize the constipating effects of this medication.
- □ Inform patient that this medication may turn urine pink to reddish brown.
- □ Advise patient to notify health care professional of medication regimen prior to treatment or surgery.
- □ Instruct patient to notify health care professional promptly if sore throat, fever, unusual bleeding or bruising, rash, weakness, tremors, visual disturbances, dark-colored urine, or clay-colored stools occur.
- □ Emphasize the importance of routine follow-up examinations to monitor response to medication and detect side effects. Periodic ocular examinations are indicated. Encourage continued participation in psychotherapy.

EVALUATION

Effectiveness of therapy can be demonstrated by: ▪ Decrease in excitable, paranoic, or withdrawn behavior ▪ Decrease in anxiety associated with depression. Therapeutic effects of oral doses may not be seen for 2–3 wk.

TRIHEXYPHENIDYL

(trye-hex-ee-**fen**-i-dill)
{Apo-Trihex}, Artane, {PMS-Trihexyphenidyl}, Trihexane, Trihexy

{} = Available in Canada only.

CLASSIFICATION(S):
Anti-Parkinson agent (anticholinergic)
Pregnancy Category C

INDICATIONS

▪ Adjunct in the management of parkinsonian syndrome due to many causes, including drug-induced parkinsonism.

ACTION

▪ Inhibits the action of acetylcholine, resulting in: ▫ Decreased sweating and salivation ▫ Mydriasis (pupillary dilation) ▫ Increased heart rate ▪ Also has spasmolytic action on smooth muscle ▪ Inhibits cerebral motor centers and blocks efferent impulses. **Therapeutic Effects:** ▪ Diminished signs and symptoms of parkinsonian syndrome (tremors, rigidity).

PHARMACOKINETICS

Absorption: Well absorbed following oral administration.
Distribution: UK.
Metabolism and Excretion: Excreted mostly in urine.
Half-life: 3.7 hr.

CONTRAINDICATIONS AND PRECAUTIONS

Contraindicated in: ▪ Hypersensitivity ▪ Narrow-angle glaucoma ▪ Acute hemorrhage ▪ Tachycardia secondary to cardiac insufficiency ▪ Thyrotoxicosis ▪ Known alcohol intolerance (elixir only).
Use Cautiously in: ▪ Geriatric and very young patients (increased risk of adverse reactions) ▪ Intestinal obstruction or infection ▪ Prostatic hypertrophy ▪ Chronic renal, hepatic, pulmonary, or cardiac disease ▪ Pregnancy, lactation, or childen (safety not established).

ADVERSE REACTIONS AND SIDE EFFECTS*

CNS: dizziness, nervousness, confusion, drowsiness, headache, psychoses, weakness.
EENT: blurred vision, mydriasis.
CV: orthostatic hypotension, tachycardia.
GI: dry mouth, nausea, constipation, vomiting.
GU: urinary hesitancy, urinary retention.
Derm: decreased sweating.

INTERACTIONS

Drug-Drug: ▪ Additive anticholinergic effects with other **drugs having anticholinergic properties**, including **phenothiazines, tricyclic antidepressants, quinidine**, and **disopyramide** ▪ May increase the efficacy of **levodopa** but may increase the risk of psychoses ▪ Additive CNS depression with other **CNS depressants**, including **alcohol, antihistamines, opioids**, and **sedative/hypnotics** ▪ Anticholinergics may alter the absorption of other **orally administered drugs** by slowing motility of the GI tract ▪ **Antacids** may decrease absorption ▪ May increase GI mucosal lesions in patients taking oral **wax-matrix potassium chloride preparations.**

ROUTE AND DOSAGE

▪ **PO (Adults):** 1–2 mg/day initially; increase by 2 mg q 3–5 days. Usual maintenance dose is 5–15 mg/day in 3 divided doses. Extended-release (Artane Sequels) preparations may be given q 12 hr after daily dose has been determined using conventional tablets or liquid.

AVAILABILITY

▪ ***Tablets:*** 2 mg[Rx], 5 mg[Rx] ▪ ***Elixir:*** 2 mg/5 ml[Rx] ▪ ***Extended-release capsules:*** 5 mg[Rx].

TIME/ACTION PROFILE (antiparkinson effects)

	ONSET	PEAK	DURATION
PO	1 hr	2–3 hr	6–12 hr
PO-ER	UK	UK	12–24 hr

NURSING IMPLICATIONS

ASSESSMENT

▫ Assess parkinsonian and extrapyramidal symptoms (restlessness or desire to keep moving, rigidity, tremors, pill rolling, mask-like face, shuffling gait, muscle spasms, twisting motions, difficulty speaking or swallowing, loss of balance control) prior to and throughout therapy.

▫ Monitor intake and output ratios and assess patient for urinary retention (dysuria, dis-

*CAPITALS indicate life-threatening; underlines indicate most frequent.

tended abdomen, infrequent voiding of small amounts, overflow incontinence).

- Patients with mental illness are at risk of developing exaggerated symptoms of their disorder during early therapy with this medication. Withhold drug and report significant behavioral changes.

POTENTIAL NURSING DIAGNOSES

- Physical mobility, impaired (Indications).
- Injury, risk for (Indications).
- Knowledge deficit, related to medication regimen (Patient/Family Teaching).

IMPLEMENTATION

- **General Info:** Extended-release capsules are not used until dosage is established with shorter-acting forms.
- **PO:** Usually administered after meals. May be administered before meals if patient suffers from dry mouth or with meals if gastric distress is a problem. Extended-release capsules should be swallowed whole; do not break, crush, or chew. Use calibrated measuring device to ensure accurate dosage of elixir.

PATIENT/FAMILY TEACHING

- Instruct patient to take this drug exactly as directed. If a dose is missed, take as soon as remembered, unless next scheduled dose is within 2 hr; do not double doses.
- Medication should be tapered gradually when discontinuing or a withdrawal reaction may occur (anxiety, tachycardia, insomnia, return of parkinsonian or extrapyramidal symptoms).
- May cause drowsiness or dizziness. Advise patient to avoid driving or other activities that require alertness until response to medication is known.
- Caution patient to change positions slowly to minimize orthostatic hypotension.
- Instruct patient that frequent rinsing of mouth, good oral hygiene, and sugarless gum or candy may decrease dry mouth. Patient should notify health care professional if dryness persists (saliva substitutes may be used). Also, notify the dentist if dryness interferes with use of dentures.
- Advise patient to confer with health care professional prior to taking OTC medications, especially cold remedies, or drinking alcoholic beverages.
- Caution patient that this medication decreases perspiration. Overheating may occur during hot weather. Patient should remain indoors, in an air-conditioned environment, during hot weather.
- Advise patient to increase activity and bulk and fluid in diet to minimize constipating effects of medication.
- Advise patient to avoid taking antacids or antidiarrheals within 1–2 hr of this medication.
- Advise patient to notify health care professional if confusion, rash, urinary retention, severe constipation, or visual changes occur.
- Emphasize the importance of routine follow-up exams.

EVALUATION

Effectiveness of therapy can be demonstrated by: ▪ Decrease in tremors and rigidity and an improvement in gait and balance. Therapeutic effects are usually seen 2–3 days after the initiation of therapy ▪ Resolution of drug-induced extrapyramidal symptoms.

TRIMETHOBENZAMIDE

(trye-meth-oh-**ben**-za-mide)

Arrestin, Benzacot, Brogan, Stemetic, Tebamide, Tegamide, T-Gen, Ticon, Tigan, Tiject-20, Triban, Tribenzagan, Trimazide

CLASSIFICATION(S):
Antiemetic (miscellaneous)

Pregnancy Category C

INDICATIONS

▪ Management of mild to moderate nausea and vomiting.

ACTION

▪ Inhibits emetic stimulation of the chemoreceptor trigger zone in the medulla. **Therapeutic Effects:** ▪ Decreased nausea and vomiting.

PHARMACOKINETICS

Absorption: Absorption following oral, IM, and rectal administration.
Distribution: UK.

Metabolism and Excretion: UK. Appears to be mostly metabolized by the liver.
Half-life: UK.

CONTRAINDICATIONS AND PRECAUTIONS

Contraindicated in: ▪ Hypersensitivity ▪ Hypersensitivity to benzocaine (suppositories only) ▪ Premature or newborn infants.
Use Cautiously in: ▪ Children who may have a viral illness (may increase risk of Reye's syndrome) ▪ Pregnancy or lactation (safety not established).

ADVERSE REACTIONS AND SIDE EFFECTS*

CNS: COMA, SEIZURES, drowsiness, depression, extrapyramidal reactions.
CV: hypotension.
GI: diarrhea, hepatitis.
Derm: rashes.
Hemat: blood dyscrasias.
Local: pain, rectal irritation (suppositories), burning at IM injection site, redness at IM injection site, stinging at IM injection site.

INTERACTIONS

Drug-Drug: ▪ Additive CNS depression with other **CNS depressants**, including **alcohol, antidepressants, antihistamines, opioids,** and **sedative/hypnotics.**

ROUTE AND DOSAGE

- **PO (Adults):** 250 mg 3–4 times daily.
- **PO (Children 15–45 kg):** 100–200 mg 3–4 times daily as needed or 15 mg/kg/day in 3–4 divided doses.
- **IM, Rect (Adults):** 200 mg 3–4 times daily as needed.
- **Rect (Children 15–45 kg):** 100–200 mg 3–4 times daily as needed.
- **Rect (Children <15 kg):** 100 mg 3–4 times daily as needed.

AVAILABILITY

▪ ***Capsules:*** 100 mg[Rx], 250 mg[Rx] ▪ ***Suppositories:*** 100 mg[Rx], 200 mg[Rx] ▪ ***Injection:*** 100 mg/ml in 2-ml ampules and prefilled syringes and in 20-ml vials[Rx].

TIME/ACTION PROFILE (antiemetic effect)

	ONSET	PEAK	DURATION
PO	10–40 min	UK	3–4 hr
IM	15–35 min	UK	2–3 hr
Rect	10–40 min	UK	3–4 hr

NURSING IMPLICATIONS

ASSESSMENT

- ▫ Assess patient for nausea and vomiting prior to and 30–60 min following administration.
- ▫ Assess blood pressure for hypotension following parenteral administration.

POTENTIAL NURSING DIAGNOSES

- Fluid volume deficit (Indications).
- Injury, risk for (Side Effects).
- Knowledge deficit, related to medication regimen (Patient/Family Teaching).

IMPLEMENTATION

- **PO:** Capsules can be opened and contents mixed with food or fluids for patients with difficulty swallowing.
- **IM:** Inject deep into well-developed muscle mass to minimize tissue irritation.
- **Syringe Compatibility:** ▪ glycopyrrolate ▪ hydromorphone ▪ midazolam ▪ nalbuphine.
- **Y-Site Compatibility:** ▪ heparin ▪ hydrocortisone sodium succinate ▪ potassium chloride ▪ vitamin B complex with C.

PATIENT/FAMILY TEACHING

- ▫ Instruct patient to take medication exactly as directed. Missed doses should be taken as soon as remembered unless almost time for next dose; do not double doses.
- ▫ Advise patient to make position changes slowly to minimize orthostatic hypotension following parenteral doses.
- ▫ May cause drowsiness. Caution patient to avoid driving or other activities requiring alertness until response to medication is known.
- ▫ Caution patient to avoid taking alcohol or other CNS depressants concurrently with this medication.
- ▫ Instruct patient to notify health care professional promptly if sore throat, fever, unusual weakness or tiredness, tremors, or yellowing of the skin and eyes occurs.

T

*CAPITALS indicate life-threatening; underlines indicate most frequent.

EVALUATION

Effectiveness of therapy can be demonstrated by: ▪ Prevention and relief of nausea and vomiting.

TRIMETHOPRIM
(trye-**meth**-oh-prim)
Primsol, Proloprim, Trimpex
CLASSIFICATION(S):
Anti-infective (miscellaneous)
Pregnancy Category C

INDICATIONS

▪ Treatment of uncomplicated urinary tract infections. **Unlabeled Uses:** ▪ Prophylaxis of chronic recurrent urinary tract infections ▪ With dapsone in the management of mild to moderate *Pneumocystis carinii* pneumonia (PCP).

ACTION

▪ Interferes with bacterial folic acid synthesis. **Therapeutic Effects:** ▪ Bactericidal action against susceptible organisms. **Spectrum:** ▪ Some gram-positive pathogens, including: ▫ *Streptococcus pneumoniae* ▫ Group A beta-hemolytic streptococci ▫ Some staphylococci and *Enterococcus* ▪ Gram-negative spectrum includes the following Enterobacteriaceae: ▫ *Acinetobacter* ▫ *Citrobacter* ▫ *Enterobacter* ▫ *Escherichia coli* ▫ *Klebsiella pneumoniae* ▫ *Proteus mirabilis* ▫ *Salmonella* ▫ *Shigella* ▪ Other strains of *Proteus*, some *Providencia*, some *Serratia*, and *P. carinii* are also susceptible.

PHARMACOKINETICS

Absorption: Well absorbed following oral administration.
Distribution: Widely distributed. Crosses the placenta and is distributed into breast milk in high concentrations.
Metabolism and Excretion: 80% excreted unchanged in the urine; 20% metabolized by the liver.
Half-life: 8–11 hr (increased in renal impairment).

CONTRAINDICATIONS AND PRECAUTIONS

Contraindicated in: ▪ Hypersensitivity ▪ Megaloblastic anemia secondary to folate deficiency.
Use Cautiously in: ▪ Renal impairment (dosage reduction required if CCr ≤30 ml/min) ▪ Debilitated patients ▪ Severe hepatic impairment ▪ Folate deficiency ▪ Pregnancy, lactation, or children <12 yr (safety as a single agent not established).

ADVERSE REACTIONS AND SIDE EFFECTS*

GI: altered taste, epigastric discomfort, glossitis, nausea, vomiting, drug-induced hepatitis.
Derm: pruritus, rash.
Hemat: megaloblastic anemia, neutropenia, thrombocytopenia.
Misc: fever.

INTERACTIONS

Drug-Drug: ▪ Increased risk of folate deficiency when used with **phenytoin** or **methotrexate** ▪ Increased risk of bone marrow depression when used with **antineoplastic agents** or **radiation therapy** ▪ **Rifampin** may decrease effectiveness by increasing elimination.

ROUTE AND DOSAGE

▫ Treatment of Urinary Tract Infections

▪ **PO (Adults and Children ≥12 yr):** 100 mg q 12 hr or 200 mg as a single daily dose.

▫ Prophylaxis of Chronic Urinary Tract Infections

▪ **PO (Adults):** 100 mg/day as a single dose (unlabeled).

▫ *Pneumocystis Carinii* Pneumonia

▪ **PO (Adults):** 20 mg/kg/day with 100 mg dapsone daily for 21 days (unlabeled).

AVAILABILITY

▪ ***Tablets:*** 100 mg[Rx], 200 mg[Rx] ▪ ***In combination with:*** sulfamethoxazole[Rx]. See trimethoprim/sulfamethoxazole monograph on page 1011.

*CAPITALS indicate life-threatening; underlines indicate most frequent.

TIME/ACTION PROFILE (blood levels)

	ONSET	PEAK	DURATION
PO	rapid	1–4 hr	12–24 hr

NURSING IMPLICATIONS

ASSESSMENT

- Assess patient for urinary tract infection (fever, cloudy urine, frequency, urgency, pain and burning on urination) or other signs of infection at beginning of and throughout therapy.
- Obtain specimens for culture and sensitivity prior to initiating therapy. First dose may be given before receiving results.
- Monitor intake and output ratios. Fluid intake should be sufficient to maintain urine output of at least 1200–1500 ml daily.
- ***Lab Test Considerations:*** May produce elevated serum bilirubin, creatinine, BUN, AST, and ALT.
- Monitor CBC and urinalysis periodically throughout therapy. Therapy should be discontinued if blood dyscrasias occur.

POTENTIAL NURSING DIAGNOSES

- Infection, risk for (Indications, Side Effects).
- Knowledge deficit, related to medication regimen (Patient/Family Teaching).

IMPLEMENTATION

- **PO:** Administer on an empty stomach, at least 1 hr before or 2 hr after meals, with a full glass of water. May be administered with food if GI irritation occurs.

PATIENT/FAMILY TEACHING

- Instruct patient to take medication and to finish medication completely as directed, even if feeling better. If a dose is missed, it should be taken as soon as remembered, with subsequent doses spaced evenly apart. Advise patient that sharing of this medication may be dangerous.
- Advise patient to notify health care professional if skin rash, sore throat, fever, mouth sores, or unusual bleeding or bruising occurs. Leucovorin (folinic acid) may be administered if folic acid deficiency occurs.
- Instruct patient to notify health care professional if symptoms do not improve.
- Emphasize the importance of routine follow-up exams to evaluate progress.

EVALUATION

Clinical response to therapy can be evaluated by: ▪ Resolution of the signs and symptoms of infection. Therapy is usually required for 10–14 days for resolution of urinary tract infection ▪ Decreased incidence of urinary tract infections during prophylactic therapy.

TRIMETHOPRIM/ SULFAMETHOXAZOLE

(trye-**meth**-oh-prim/sul-fa-meth-**ox**-a-zole)

{Apo-Sulfatrim}, {Apo-Sulfatrim DS}, Bactrim, Bactrim DS, Cofatrim, Cotrim, Cotrim DS, {Novo-Trimel}, {Novo-Trimel DS}, {Nu-Cotrimox}, {Nu-Cotrimox DS}, {Roubac}, Septra, Septra DS, SMZ/TMP, Sulfatrim, Sulfatrim DS, TMP/SMX, TMP/SMZ

CLASSIFICATION(S):
Anti-infective (sulfonamide)

Pregnancy Category C

INDICATIONS

▪ Treatment of: ▫ Bronchitis ▫ *Shigella* enteritis ▫ Otitis media ▫ *Pneumocystis carinii* pneumonia ▫ Urinary tract infections ▫ Traveler's diarrhea ▪ Prevention of *Pneumocystis carinii* pneumonia in HIV-positive patients. **Unlabeled Uses:** ▪ Biliary tract infections, osteomyelitis, burn and wound infections, chlamydial infections, endocarditis, gonorrhea, intra-abdominal infections, nocardiosis, rheumatic fever prophylaxis, sinusitis, eradication of meningococcal carriers, prophylaxis of urinary tract infections, and an alternative agent in the treatment of chancroid ▪ Prevention of bacterial infections in immunosuppressed patients.

ACTION

▪ Combination inhibits the metabolism of folic acid in bacteria at two different points. **Therapeutic Effects:** ▪ Bactericidal action against sus-

T

ceptible bacteria. **Spectrum:** ▪ Active against many strains of gram-positive aerobic pathogens including: ▫ *Streptococcus pneumoniae* ▫ *Staphylococcus aureus* ▫ Group A beta-hemolytic streptococci ▫ *Nocardia* ▫ *Enterococcus* ▪ Has activity against many aerobic gram-negative pathogens, such as: ▫ *Acinetobacter* ▫ *Enterobacter* ▫ *Klebsiella pneumoniae* ▫ *Escherichia coli* ▫ *Proteus mirabilis* ▫ *Shigella* ▫ *Haemophilus influenzae*, including ampicillin-resistant strains ▪ *Pneumocystis carinii* (a protozoa) ▪ Not active against *Pseudomonas aeruginosa*.

PHARMACOKINETICS

Absorption: Well absorbed from the GI tract.
Distribution: Widely distributed. Crosses the blood-brain barrier and placenta and enters breast milk.
Metabolism and Excretion: Some metabolism by the liver (20%); remainder excreted unchanged by the kidneys.
Half-life: *Trimethoprim*—8–11 hr; *sulfamethoxazole*—7–12 hr.

CONTRAINDICATIONS AND PRECAUTIONS

Contraindicated in: ▪ Hypersensitivity to sulfonamides or trimethoprim ▪ Megaloblastic anemia secondary to folate deficiency ▪ Pregnancy, lactation, or children <2 mo ▪ Severe renal impairment.
Use Cautiously in: ▪ Impaired hepatic or renal function (dosage reduction required if CCr <30 ml/min) ▪ HIV-positive patients (increased incidence of adverse reactions).

ADVERSE REACTIONS AND SIDE EFFECTS*

CNS: fatigue, hallucinations, headache, insomnia, mental depression.
GI: HEPATIC NECROSIS, nausea, vomiting, diarrhea, stomatitis.
GU: crystalluria.
Derm: TOXIC EPIDERMAL NECROLYSIS, rashes, photosensitivity.
Hemat: AGRANULOCYTOSIS, APLASTIC ANEMIA, hemolytic anemia, leukopenia, megaloblastic anemia, thrombocytopenia.
Local: phlebitis at IV site.
Misc: allergic reactions including ERYTHEMA MULTIFORME, STEVENS-JOHNSON SYNDROME, fever.

INTERACTIONS

Drug-Drug: ▪ May increase half-life, decrease clearance, and exaggerate folic acid deficiency caused by **phenytoin** ▪ May enhance the effects of **oral hypoglycemic agents** and **warfarin** ▪ May increase the toxicity of **methotrexate** ▪ Increases the risk of thrombocytopenia from **thiazide diuretics** (↑ geriatric patients) ▪ Decreases efficacy of **cyclosporine** and increases risk of nephrotoxicity.

ROUTE AND DOSAGE

(TMP = trimethoprim, SMZ = sulfamethoxazole)

▫ Bacterial Infections

- **PO (Adults and Children ≥40 kg):** 160 mg TMP/800 mg SMZ q 12 hr.
- **PO (Children >2 mo):** 4–6 mg/kg TMP/20–30 mg/kg SMZ q 12 hr.
- **IV (Adults and Children >2 mo):** 2–2.5 mg/kg TMP/10–12.5 mg/kg SMZ q 6 hr *or* 2.7–3.3 mg/kg TMP/13.3–16.7 mg/kg SMZ q 8 hr *or* 4–5 mg/kg TMP/20–25 mg/kg SMZ q 12 hr.

▫ *Pneumocystis Carinii* Pneumonia (Treatment)

- **PO (Adults and Children >2 mo):** 3.75–5 mg/kg TMP/18.75–25 mg SMZ q 6 hr.
- **IV (Adults and Children >2 mo):** 3.75–5 mg/kg TMP/18.75–25 mg SMZ q 6 hr *or* 5–6.7 mg/kg TMP/25–33.3 mg SMZ q 8 hr.

▫ *Pneumocystis Carinii* Pneumonia (Prevention)

- **PO (Adults):** 160 mg TMP/800 mg SMZ daily (may also be given 3 times weekly).
- **PO (Children >1 mo):** 75 mg/m² TMP/325 mg/m² SMZ q 12 hr on 3 consecutive days/wk (not to exceed 320 mg TMP/1600 mg SMZ per day).

AVAILABILITY

▪ ***Tablets:*** {20 mg TMP/100 mg SMZ^Rx}, 80 mg TMP/400 mg SMZ^Rx, 160 mg TMP/800 mg SMZ^Rx
▪ ***Suspension:*** 40 mg TMP/200 mg SMZ per 5

*CAPITALS indicate life-threatening; underlines indicate most frequent.

ml[Rx] ▪ ***Injection:*** 80 mg TMP/400 mg SMZ per 5 ml in 5-, 10-, 20-, and 30-ml vials[Rx].

TIME/ACTION PROFILE (blood levels)

	ONSET	PEAK	DURATION
PO	rapid	2–4 hr	6–12 hr
IV	rapid	end of infusion	6–12 hr

NURSING IMPLICATIONS

ASSESSMENT

□ Assess patient for infection (vital signs; appearance of wound, sputum, urine, and stool; WBC) at beginning of and throughout therapy.
□ Obtain specimens for culture and sensitivity prior to initiating therapy. First dose may be given before receiving results.
□ Inspect IV site frequently. Phlebitis is common.
□ Assess patient for allergy to sulfonamides.
□ Monitor intake and output ratios. Fluid intake should be sufficient to maintain a urine output of at least 1200–1500 ml daily to prevent crystalluria and stone formation.
▪ ***Lab Test Considerations:*** Monitor CBC and urinalysis periodically throughout therapy.
□ May produce elevated serum bilirubin, creatinine, and alkaline phosphatase.

POTENTIAL NURSING DIAGNOSES

▪ Infection, risk for (Indications, Side Effects).
▪ Knowledge deficit, related to medication regimen (Patient/Family Teaching).
▪ Noncompliance, related to medication regimen (Patient/Family Teaching).

IMPLEMENTATION

▪ **General Info:** Do not administer medication IM.
▪ **PO:** Administer around the clock with a full glass of water. Use calibrated measuring device for liquid preparations.
▪ **Intermittent Infusion:** Dilute each 5-ml ampule with 100–125 ml of D5W. May reduce diluent to 75 ml if fluid restriction required. Do not use if solution is cloudy or contains a precipitate. Solution is stable for 6 hr in standard dilution and 2 hr in fluid-restricted dilution at room temperature. Do not refrigerate.
▪ ***Rate:*** Infuse over 60–90 min. Do not administer rapidly or by bolus injection.
▪ **Y-Site Compatibility:** ▪ acyclovir ▪ aldesleukin ▪ amifostine ▪ atracurium ▪ aztreonam ▪ cefepime ▪ cyclophosphamide ▪ diltiazem ▪ enalaprilat ▪ esmolol ▪ filgrastim ▪ fludarabine ▪ gallium nitrate ▪ hydromorphone ▪ labetalol ▪ lorazepam ▪ magnesium sulfate ▪ melphalan ▪ meperidine ▪ morphine ▪ pancuronium ▪ perphenazine ▪ piperacillin/tazobactam ▪ sargramostim ▪ tacrolimus ▪ teniposide ▪ thiotepa ▪ vecuronium ▪ zidovudine.
▪ **Y-Site Incompatibility:** ▪ fluconazole ▪ midazolam ▪ vinorelbine.
▪ **Additive Incompatibility:** ▪ Manufacturer recommends that no other medication or solution be admixed with trimethoprim/sulfamethoxazole.

PATIENT/FAMILY TEACHING

□ Instruct patient to take medication around the clock and to finish drug completely as directed, even if feeling well. If a dose is missed, it should be taken as soon as remembered unless almost time for next dose. Advise patient that sharing of this medication may be dangerous.
□ Caution patient to use sunscreen and protective clothing to prevent photosensitivity reactions.
□ Advise patient to notify health care professional if skin rash, sore throat, fever, mouth sores, or unusual bleeding or bruising occurs.
□ Instruct patient to notify health care professional if symptoms do not improve within a few days.
□ Emphasize importance of regular follow-up exams to monitor blood counts in patients on prolonged therapy.
▪ **Home Care Issues:** Instruct family or caregiver on dilution, rate, and administration of drug and proper care of IV equipment.

EVALUATION

Clinical response to therapy can be evaluated by: ▪ Resolution of the signs and symptoms of infection. Length of time for complete resolution depends on organism and site of infection ▪ Resolution of symptoms of traveler's diarrhea ▪ Prevention of *Pneumocystis carinii* pneumonia in patients with HIV.

TRIMETREXATE

(trye-me-**trex**-ate)
NeuTrexin

CLASSIFICATION(S):
Antiprotozoal

Pregnancy Category D

INDICATIONS

▪ Treatment of moderate to severe *Pneumocystis carinii* pneumonia (PCP) in immunocompromised patients who are unable to tolerate therapy with trimethoprim/sulfamethoxazole.

ACTION

▪ Inhibits dihydrofolate reductase, thereby acting as a folic acid antagonist. Must be given concurrently with leucovorin, which prevents bone marrow depression from trimetrexate while allowing its antiprotozoal action against *P. carinii* to continue. **Therapeutic Effects:** ▪ Antiprotozoal action.

PHARMACOKINETICS

Absorption: IV administration results in complete bioavailability.
Distribution: UK.
Metabolism and Excretion: Metabolized by the liver; some metabolites have antiprotozoal activity. 10–30% excreted unchanged by the kidneys.
Half-life: 11 hr.

CONTRAINDICATIONS AND PRECAUTIONS

Contraindicated in: ▪ Hypersensitivity to trimetrexate, methotrexate, or leucovorin ▪ Pregnant or lactating patients should not receive trimetrexate.
Use Cautiously in: ▪ Underlying renal disease (temporarily discontinue if serum creatinine levels are >2.5 mg/dl during trimetrexate therapy) ▪ Underlying liver disease (temporarily discontinue if transaminases or alkaline phosphatase increases to more than 5 times normal) ▪ Patients with bone marrow depression (dosage reduction of trimetrexate and/or increased leucovorin recommended if neutrophils are <1000/mm³ or platelets are less than 75,000/mm³) ▪ Patients with childbearing potential ▪ Children <18 yr (safety not established).

ADVERSE REACTIONS AND SIDE EFFECTS*

CNS: confusion, fatigue.
GI: increased AST/ALT, increased alkaline phosphatase, increased bilirubin, nausea, vomiting.
GU: increased serum creatinine.
Derm: pruritus, rash.
F and E: hypocalcemia, hyponatremia.
Hemat: neutropenia, thrombocytopenia, anemia.
Misc: fever.

INTERACTIONS

Drug-Drug: ▪ The concurrent use of the following medications may alter blood levels and effectiveness of trimetrexate: **acetaminophen, erythromycin, rifampin, rifabutin, ketoconazole,** or **fluconazole** ▪ Toxicity of trimetrexate may be increased by concurrent **cimetidine, clotrimazole, ketoconazole,** or **miconazole** ▪ Leucovorin administered concurrently with trimetrexate may decrease the anticonvulsant effectiveness of **phenobarbital, phenytoin, primidone** ▪ Increased risk of hematologic toxicity when used concurrently with **antineoplastic agents** or **radiation therapy** ▪ Increased risk of nephrotoxicity when used concurrently with other **nephrotoxic drugs.**

ROUTE AND DOSAGE

▪ **IV (Adults):** *Trimetrexate* — 45 mg/m² (1.2 mg/kg) once daily for 21 days. *Concurrent leucovorin* — 20 mg/m² PO or IV every 6 hr for 24 days with the 1st dose given IV prior to 1st dose of trimetrexate.

AVAILABILITY

▪ ***Injection:*** 25 mg/5 ml vial[Rx].

TIME/ACTION PROFILE (blood levels)

	ONSET	PEAK	DURATION
IV	rapid	end of infusion	N/A

***CAPITALS indicate life-threatening; underlines indicate most frequent.**

NURSING IMPLICATIONS

ASSESSMENT

- □ Monitor IV site frequently for signs of infection.
- □ Monitor temperature daily. If patient becomes febrile, an antipyretic may be administered. Assess for fever, chills, sore throat, and signs of infection. Assess bleeding (bleeding gums; bruising; petechiae; guaiac test stools, urine, and emesis). Avoid giving IM injection and taking rectal temperatures. Apply pressure to venipuncture sites for 10 min. Initiate bleeding precautions for platelet counts $<50,000/mm^3$ and infection control measures for absolute neutrophil counts (ANC) $\leq 1000/mm^3$ (see Patient/Family Teaching). Dosage reduction is required for neutrophils $<1000/mm^3$ or platelets $<75,000/mm^3$.
- ■ ***Lab Test Considerations:*** Monitor hematologic, renal, and hepatic functions twice weekly during therapy. May cause decreased ANC and platelet counts. May cause increased serum creatinine, BUN, AST, ALT, and alkaline phosphatase.

POTENTIAL NURSING DIAGNOSES

- ■ Infection, risk for (Indications).
- ■ Knowledge deficit, related to medication regimen (Patient/Family Teaching).

IMPLEMENTATION

- ■ **General Info:** Concurrent leucovorin (leucovorin protection) must be administered during and for 72 hr after the last dose of trimetrexate to prevent life-threatening toxicity.
- □ Solution should be prepared in a biologic cabinet. Wear gloves, gown, and mask while handling medication. Discard IV equipment in specially designated containers (see Appendix I).
- ■ **Intermittent Infusion:** Reconstitute each vial of trimetrexate with 2 ml of D5W or sterile water for injection for a concentration of 12.5 mg/ml. Filter the solution with a 0.22-micron filter prior to further dilution. Dilute further with D5W for a final concentration of 0.25 mg/ml to 2 mg/ml. Solution is stable for 24 hr at room temperature.
- ■ ***Rate:*** Administer over 60 min.
- ■ **Y-Site Incompatibility/Additive Incompatibilty:** ■ 0.9% NaCl ■ leucovorin ■ sodium chloride. Administer trimetrexate and leucovorin separately. Flush IV lines with at least 10 ml of D5W between infusions.

PATIENT/FAMILY TEACHING

- □ Instruct patient about the purpose of trimetrexate and leucovorin and the importance of complying with the full course of therapy.
- □ Instruct the patient to take his or her temperature at least once daily and more frequently if fever is suspected.
- □ Advise patient with ANC $<1000/mm^3$ to practice infection control measures (rigorous handwashing, coverage of IV site during showers or bathing, thorough washing of fresh fruit, avoidance of raw or undercooked meat and vegetables, elimination of fresh flowers and house plants, and avoidance of crowds and persons with known infections).
- □ Instruct patients with a platelet count of $<50,000/mm^3$ to practice bleeding precautions (use soft toothbrush and electric razor; be especially careful to avoid falls; avoid alcoholic beverages and medications containing aspirin or NSAIDs, as these may precipitate gastric bleeding).
- □ Instruct patient to report promptly to health care professional a fever of >101°F; rash; flu-like symptoms; numbness or tingling in the extremities; nausea or vomiting; abdominal pain; mouth sores; increased bruising or bleeding; or black, tarry stools.
- □ Emphasize the importance of frequent lab tests to monitor side effects.

EVALUATION

Effectiveness of therapy can be demonstrated by: ■ Decrease in the symptoms of *P. carinii* pneumonia in immunocompromised patients.

T

TRIPROLIDINE

(trye-**proe**-li-deen)
Myidyl

CLASSIFICATION(S):
Antihistamine

Pregnancy Category B

INDICATIONS

▪ Symptomatic relief of allergic symptoms caused by histamine release ▪ Most useful in management of nasal allergies and allergic dermatoses.

ACTION

▪ Antagonizes the effects of histamine at peripheral histamine-1 (H_1) receptors, including pruritus and urticaria ▪ Also has a drying effect on the nasal mucosa. **Therapeutic Effects:** ▪ Relief of symptoms associated with histamine excess usually seen in allergic conditions.

PHARMACOKINETICS

Absorption: Well absorbed following oral administration.
Distribution: Widely distributed. Minimal amounts excreted in breast milk. Crosses the blood-brain barrier.
Metabolism and Excretion: Extensively metabolized by the liver.
Half-life: 3–3.3 hr.

CONTRAINDICATIONS AND PRECAUTIONS

Contraindicated in: ▪ Hypersensitivity ▪ Acute attacks of asthma ▪ Lactation ▪ Known alcohol intolerance (some liquids).
Use Cautiously in: ▪ Geriatric patients (increased risk of adverse reactions) ▪ Narrow-angle glaucoma ▪ Liver disease ▪ Prostatic hypertrophy ▪ Pregnancy (safety not established).

ADVERSE REACTIONS AND SIDE EFFECTS*

CNS: drowsiness, dizziness, excitation (↑ in children).
EENT: blurred vision.
CV: arrhythmias, hypertension, hypotension, palpitations.
GI: dry mouth, constipation.
GU: urinary hesitancy, urinary retention.

INTERACTIONS

Drug-Drug: ▪ Additive CNS depression with other **CNS depressants,** including **alcohol, opioids,** and **sedative/hypnotics** ▪ Additive anticholinergic effects with other **drugs possessing anticholinergic properties,** including **antidepressants, atropine, haloperidol, phenothiazines, quinidine,** and **disopyramide** ▪ **MAO inhibitors** intensify and prolong anticholinergic effects of antihistamines.

ROUTE AND DOSAGE

- **PO (Adults):** 2.5 mg q 4–6 hr (not to exceed 10 mg/24 hr).
- **PO (Children 6–12 yr):** 1.25 mg q 6–8 hr (not to exceed 5 mg/24 hr).
- **PO (Children 4–6 yr):** 937 mcg q 6–8 hr (not to exceed 3.75 mg/24 hr).
- **PO (Children 2–4 yr):** 625 mcg q 6–8 hr (not to exceed 2.5 mg/24 hr).
- **PO (Children 4 mo–2 yr):** 312 mcg q 6–8 hr (not to exceed 1.25 mg/24 hr).

AVAILABILITY

▪ ***Syrup:*** 1.25 mg/5 ml[Rx] ▪ ***In combination with:*** pseudoephedrine[OTC]. See Appendix A.

TIME/ACTION PROFILE (antihistaminic effects)

	ONSET	PEAK	DURATION
PO	15–60 min	1–2 hr	4–8 hr

NURSING IMPLICATIONS

ASSESSMENT

- □ Assess allergy symptoms (rhinitis, conjunctivitis, hives) prior to and periodically throughout therapy.
- □ Assess lung sounds and character of bronchial secretions. Maintain fluid intake of 1500–2000 ml/day to decrease viscosity of secretions.
- ▪ ***Lab Test Considerations:*** May cause false-negative reactions on allergy skin tests; discontinue 3 days prior to testing.

POTENTIAL NURSING DIAGNOSES

- Airway clearance, ineffective (Indications).
- Injury, risk for (Adverse Reactions).
- Knowledge deficit, related to medication regimen (Patient/Family Teaching).

IMPLEMENTATION

- **PO:** Administer oral doses with food or milk to decrease GI irritation. Use calibrated measuring device to ensure accurate dose of syrup.

PATIENT/FAMILY TEACHING

- Instruct patient to take as directed. If a dose is missed, it should be taken as soon as remembered unless almost time for next dose.
- Instruct patient to contact health care professional if symptoms persist.
- May cause drowsiness. Caution patient to avoid driving or other activities requiring alertness until response to drug is known.
- Caution patient against using alcohol or other CNS depressants concurrently with this drug.
- Advise patient that good oral hygiene, frequent mouth rinses, and sugarless gum or candy may help relieve mouth dryness. Health care professional should be notified if mouth dryness persists >2 wk.

EVALUATION

Effectiveness of therapy can be demonstrated by: ▪ Decrease in allergic symptoms.

TROGLITAZONE

(troe-**glit**-a-zone)
Rezulin

CLASSIFICATION(S):
Oral hypoglycemic agent (thiazolidinedione)

Pregnancy Category B

INDICATIONS

▪ Management of type II diabetes (non–insulin-dependent diabetes mellitus [NIDDM]), especially in patients whose blood sugar is poorly controlled with >30 units of insulin/day; can be used with insulin, with sulfonylurea oral hypoglycemic agents, or as monotherapy.

ACTION

▪ Improves sensitivity to insulin in muscle and in adipose tissue ▪ Inhibits hepatic gluconeogenesis ▪ Requires insulin for activity. **Therapeutic Effects:** ▪ Decreased insulin resistance with improved control of blood sugar in diabetic patients.

PHARMACOKINETICS

Absorption: Rapidly absorbed following oral administration.
Distribution: Partitions into red blood cells.
Metabolism and Excretion: Highly metabolized by the liver; negligible renal excretion.
Half-life: 16–34 hr.

CONTRAINDICATIONS AND PRECAUTIONS

Contraindicated in: ▪ Hypersensitivity ▪ Type I (insulin-dependent) diabetes mellitus ▪ Diabetic ketoacidosis ▪ Concurrent use of cholestyramine.
Use Cautiously in: ▪ Premenopausal anovulatory patients (ovulation may be restored with resultant pregnancy) ▪ Congestive heart failure ▪ Hepatic impairment or chronic alcohol ingestion ▪ Pregnancy, lactation, or children (safety not established; not recommended for use during pregnancy or lactation).

ADVERSE REACTIONS AND SIDE EFFECTS*

CNS: headache, dizziness, weakness.
EENT: pharyngitis, rhinitis.
CV: peripheral edema.
GI: HEPATOCELLULAR INJURY, diarrhea, nausea, reversible increase in liver enzymes.
Hemat: ↓ hemoglobin.
MS: back pain.
Misc: infection, pain.

INTERACTIONS

Drug-Drug: ▪ **Cholestyramine** significantly decreases absorption; concurrent use should be avoided ▪ Decreases blood levels and may decrease effectiveness of **oral contraceptives;** similar effects may occur with **cyclosporine, tacrolimus,** and some **HMG-CoA reductase inhibitors.**
Drug-Food: ▪ **Food** significantly improves absorption.

ROUTE AND DOSAGE

- **PO (Adults):** *Monotherapy*—400–600 mg/day initially; if starting dose is 400 mg/day, may increase to 600 mg/day after 6–8 wk. *If currently receiving sulfonylurea oral hypo-*

***CAPITALS indicate life-threatening; underlines indicate most frequent.**

glycemic agent—200 mg once daily initially; after 2–4 wk may be increased to 400 mg (not to exceed 600 mg/day).

AVAILABILITY

▪ ***Tablets:*** 200 mg^{Rx}, 400 mg^{Rx}.

TIME/ACTION PROFILE (blood levels)

	ONSET	PEAK	DURATION
PO	UK	2–3 hr	UK

NURSING IMPLICATIONS

ASSESSMENT

□ Observe patient taking current insulin for signs and symptoms of hypoglycemic reactions (sweating, hunger, weakness, dizziness, tremor, tachycardia, anxiety).

▪ ***Lab Test Considerations:*** Serum glucose and glycosylated hemoglobin should be monitored periodically throughout therapy to evaluate effectiveness of treatment.

□ Monitor CBC with differential periodically throughout therapy. May cause decrease in hemoglobin, hematocrit, and neutrophil counts, usually during the first 4–8 wk of therapy; then levels stabilize.

□ Monitor AST and ALT monthly during the first 6 mo of therapy and then every other month during the next 6 mo of troglitazone therapy and periodically thereafter or if jaundice or symptoms of hepatic dysfunction occur. May cause irreversible elevations in AST and ALT, serum bilirubin, and alkaline phosphatase concentrations or hepatic failure (rare). Discontinue troglitazone if ALT is >3 times normal.

POTENTIAL NURSING DIAGNOSES

▪ Nutrition, altered, more than body requirements (Indications).

▪ Knowledge deficit, related to medication regimen (Patient/Family Teaching).

▪ Noncompliance (Patient/Family Teaching).

IMPLEMENTATION

▪ **General Info:** Patients stabilized on a diabetic regimen who are exposed to stress, fever, trauma, infection, or surgery may require administration of insulin.

▪ **PO:** Administer with a meal.

PATIENT/FAMILY TEACHING

□ Instruct patient to take medication with a meal. If a dose is missed at the usual meal, take at the next meal. If dose for 1 day is missed, do not double dose the next day.

□ Explain to patient that this medication controls hyperglycemia but does not cure diabetes. Therapy is long-term.

□ Review signs of hypoglycemia and hyperglycemia with patient, especially those on combined therapy with insulin. If hypoglycemia occurs, advise patient to take a glass of orange juice or 2–3 tsp of sugar, honey, or corn syrup dissolved in water and notify health care professional.

□ Encourage patient to follow prescribed diet, medication, and exercise regimen to prevent hypoglycemic or hyperglycemic episodes.

□ Instruct patient in proper testing of serum glucose and ketones. These tests should be closely monitored during periods of stress or illness and health care professional notified if significant changes occur.

□ Advise patient to notify health care professional immediately if signs of hepatic dysfunction (nausea, vomiting, abdominal pain, fatigue, anorexia, dark urine, jaundice) occur.

□ Insulin is the preferred method of controlling blood sugar during pregnancy. Counsel female patients that higher doses of oral contraceptives or a form of contraception other than oral contraceptives may be required and to notify health care professional promptly if pregnancy is planned or suspected.

□ Advise patient to inform health care professional of medication regimen prior to treatment or surgery.

□ Advise patient to carry a form of sugar (sugar packets, candy) and identification describing disease process and medication regimen at all times.

□ Emphasize the importance of routine follow-up exams.

EVALUATION

Effectiveness of therapy can be demonstrated by: ▪ Control of blood glucose levels without the appearance of hypoglycemic or hyperglycemic episodes. □ Reduction in insulin requirements in patients taking concurrent insulin therapy.

VALACYCLOVIR
(val-a-**sye**-kloe-vir)
Valtrex

CLASSIFICATION(S):
Antiviral

Pregnancy Category B

INDICATIONS

▪ Treatment of herpes zoster in patients who are not immunosuppressed ▪ Initial treatment and suppression of recurrent genital herpes in patients who are not immunosuppressed.

ACTION

▪ Rapidly converted to acyclovir. Acyclovir interferes with viral DNA synthesis. **Therapeutic Effects:** ▪ Inhibited viral replication, decreased viral shedding, and reduced time to healing of lesions.

PHARMACOKINETICS

Absorption: 54% bioavailable as acyclovir following oral administration of valacyclovir.
Distribution: CSF concentrations of acyclovir are 50% of plasma concentrations. Acyclovir crosses the placenta and enters breast milk.
Metabolism and Excretion: Rapidly converted to acyclovir via intestinal/hepatic metabolism.
Half-life: 2.5–3.3 hr; up to 14 hr in renal impairment (acyclovir).

CONTRAINDICATIONS AND PRECAUTIONS

Contraindicated in: ▪ Hypersensitivity to valacyclovir or acyclovir.
Use Cautiously in: ▪ Renal impairment (dosage reduction/increased dosing interval recommended if CCr <50 ml/min) ▪ Geriatric patients (dosage reduction may be necessary) ▪ Pregnancy, lactation, or children (safety not established).

ADVERSE REACTIONS AND SIDE EFFECTS*

CNS: headache, dizziness, weakness.
GI: nausea, abdominal pain, anorexia, constipation, diarrhea.

INTERACTIONS

Drug-Drug: ▪ **Probenecid** and **cimetidine** increase blood levels of acyclovir during valacyclovir therapy.

ROUTE AND DOSAGE

❑ Herpes Zoster

▪ **PO (Adults):** 1 g 3 times daily for 7 days.

❑ Genital Herpes

▪ **PO (Adults):** *Initial treatment*—1 g twice daily for 10 days. *Suppression of recurrence*—1 g once daily or 500 mg once daily in patients experiencing fewer than 10 recurrences/yr.

AVAILABILITY

▪ ***Tablets:*** 500 mg[Rx].

TIME/ACTION PROFILE (blood levels†)

	ONSET	PEAK	DURATION
PO	UK	1.5–2.5 hr	8–24 hr

†Acyclovir.

NURSING IMPLICATIONS

ASSESSMENT

❑ Assess lesions prior to and daily during therapy.

POTENTIAL NURSING DIAGNOSES

▪ Skin integrity, impaired (Indications).
▪ Infection transmission, risk for (Indications, Patient/Family Teaching).
▪ Knowledge deficit, related to disease process and medication regimen (Patient/Family Teaching).

IMPLEMENTATION

▪ **PO:** May be administered without regard to meals.
▪ **Herpes Zoster:** Valacyclovir should be implemented as soon as possible following the onset of signs or symptoms of herpes zoster and is most effective if started within 48 hr of the onset of zoster rash. Efficacy of treatment started >72 hr after rash onset is unknown.
▪ **Genital Herpes:** Implement treatment for gential herpes as soon as possible following onset of symptoms.

***CAPITALS indicate life-threatening; underlines indicate most frequent.**

V

PATIENT/FAMILY TEACHING

- **General Info:** Instruct patient to take valacyclovir exactly as directed for the full course of therapy. If a dose is missed, take as soon as remembered if not just before next dose.
- **Herpes Zoster:** Inform patient that valacyclovir does not prevent the spread of infection to others. Precautions should be taken around others who have not had chickenpox or varicella vaccine, or are immunosuppressed until all lesions have crusted.
- **Genital Herpes:** Inform patient that valacyclovir does not prevent the spread of infection to others. Advise patient to avoid contact with lesions and to avoid intercourse while lesions or symptoms are present.

EVALUATION

Effectiveness of therapy can be demonstrated by: ▪ Decrease in time to full crusting, loss of vesicles, loss of ulcers, and development of crusts in patients with acute herpes zoster (shingles) ▪ Decrease in time to full crusting, loss of vesicles, loss of ulcers, and development of crusts in patients with genital herpes ▪ Decrease in frequency of outbreaks in patients with genital herpes.

VALPROATES

divalproex sodium
(dye-val-**proe**-ex **soe**-dee-um)
Depakote, {Epival}

valproate sodium
(val-**proe**-ate **soe**-dee-um)
Depacon

valproic acid
(val-**proe**-ik **as**-id)
Depakene, Myproic Acid

CLASSIFICATION(S):
Anticonvulsants

Pregnancy Category D

INDICATIONS

▪ Simple and complex absence seizures ▪ Partial seizures with complex symptomatology ▪ **Divalproex only:** □ Manic episodes associated with bipolar disorder (manic-depressive illness) □ Prevention of migraine headache.

ACTION

▪ Increase levels of gamma-aminobutyric acid (GABA), an inhibitory neurotransmitter in the CNS. **Therapeutic Effects:** ▪ Suppression of absence seizures ▪ Decreased manic behavior ▪ Decreased frequency of migraine headaches.

PHARMACOKINETICS

Absorption: Well absorbed following oral administration; divalproex is enteric-coated, and absorption is delayed. IV administration results in complete bioavailability.
Distribution: Rapidly distributed into plasma and extracellular water. Cross blood-brain barrier and placenta; enter breast milk.
Metabolism and Excretion: Mostly metabolized by the liver; minimal amounts excreted unchanged in urine.
Half-life: 5–20 hr.

CONTRAINDICATIONS AND PRECAUTIONS

Contraindicated in: ▪ Hypersensitivity ▪ Hepatic impairment ▪ Some products contain tartrazine; avoid in patients with known hypersensitivity.
Use Cautiously in: ▪ Bleeding disorders ▪ History of liver disease ▪ Organic brain disease ▪ Bone marrow depression ▪ Renal impairment ▪ Children (increased risk of hepatotoxicity) ▪ Pregnancy and lactation (safety not established).

ADVERSE REACTIONS AND SIDE EFFECTS*

CNS: confusion, dizziness, headache, sedation.
EENT: visual disturbances.
GI: HEPATOTOXICITY, indigestion, nausea, vomiting, anorexia, constipation, diarrhea, hypersalivation, increased appetite, pancreatitis.
Derm: rashes.
Hemat: leukopenia, prolonged bleeding time, thrombocytopenia.
Metab: hyperammonemia.
Neuro: ataxia, paresthesia.

{} = Available in Canada only.
***CAPITALS indicate life-threatening; underlines indicate most frequent.**

INTERACTIONS

Drug-Drug: ▪ Increased risk of bleeding with **antiplatelet agents** (including **aspirin** and **NSAIDs**), **cefamandole, cefoperazone, cefotetan, heparin, thrombolytic agents,** or **warfarin** ▪ Decreases metabolism of **barbiturates** and **primidone,** increasing risk of toxicity ▪ Blood levels and toxicity may be increased by **carbamazepine, cimetidine, erythromycin,** or **felbamate.** ▪ Additive CNS depression with other **CNS depressants,** including **alcohol, antihistamines, antidepressants, opioids, MAO inhibitors,** and **sedative/hypnotics** ▪ Large doses of **salicylates** (in children) increase the effects of valproic acid ▪ May increase or decrease effects and toxicity of **phenytoin** ▪ **MAO inhibitors** and other **antidepressants** may lower seizure threshold and decrease effectiveness of valproates ▪ **Carbamazepine, rifampin,** or **lamotrigine** may decrease valproic acid blood levels ▪ Valproic acid may increase toxicity of **carbamazepine, ethosuximide, lamotrigine,** or **zidovudine.**

ROUTE AND DOSAGE

Doses expressed in mg of valproic acid.

❑ Anticonvulsant

- **PO (Adults):** *Single-agent therapy*—Initial dose of 5–15 mg/kg/day; increase by 5–10 mg/kg/day weekly until therapeutic levels are reached (not to exceed 60 mg/kg/day); when daily dosage exceeds 250 mg, give in 2 divided doses. *Polytherapy*—Initial dose of 10–30 mg/kg/day; increase by 5–10 mg/kg/day weekly until therapeutic levels are reached (not to exceed 60 mg/kg/day); when daily dosage exceeds 250 mg, give in 2 divided doses.
- **PO (Children):** *Single-agent therapy*—Initial dose of 15–45 mg/kg/day; increase by 5–10 mg/kg/day weekly until therapeutic levels are reached. *Polytherapy*—Initial dose of 30–100 mg/kg/day.
- **IV (Adults and Children):** Give same daily dose as was given orally; if daily dose >250 mg, give in divided doses q 6 hr.

❑ Antimanic

- **PO (Adults):** *Divalproex*—750 mg/day in divided doses initially, titrated rapidly to desired clinical effect or trough plasma levels of 50–125 mcg/ml (not to exceed 60 mg/kg/day).

❑ Migraine Prevention

- **PO (Adults):** 250 mg twice daily (up to 1000 mg/day).

AVAILABILITY

❑ Valproic Acid

▪ ***Capsules:*** 250 mg[Rx], {500 mg[Rx]} ▪ ***Syrup:*** 250 mg/5 ml[Rx].

❑ Valproate Sodium

▪ ***Injection:*** 100mg/ml in 5-ml vials[Rx].

❑ Divalproex Sodium

▪ ***Delayed-release tablets:*** 125 mg[Rx], 250 mg[Rx], 500 mg[Rx] ▪ ***Delayed-release capsules (sprinkle):*** 125 mg[Rx].

TIME/ACTION PROFILE (onset = anticonvulsant effect; peak = blood levels)

	ONSET	PEAK	DURATION
PO—liquid	2–4 days	15–120 min	6–24 hr
PO—capsules	2–4 days	1–4 hr	6–24 hr
PO—delayed-release products	2–4 days	3–5 hr	12–24 hr
IV	2–4 days	end of infusion	6–24 hr

NURSING IMPLICATIONS

ASSESSMENT

- **Seizures:** Assess location, duration, and characteristics of seizure activity. Institute seizure precautions.
- **Bipolar Disorder:** Assess mood, ideation, and behavior frequently.
- **Migraine Prophylaxis:** Monitor frequency of migraine headaches.
- ***Lab Test Considerations:*** Monitor CBC, platelet count, and bleeding time prior to and periodically throughout therapy. May cause leukopenia and thrombocytopenia.
- ❑ Monitor hepatic function (LDH, AST, ALT, and bilirubin) and serum ammonia concentrations prior to and periodically throughout therapy. May cause hepatotoxicity; monitor closely, especially during initial 6 mo of therapy; fatalities have occurred. Therapy should be discontinued if hyperammonemia occurs.
- ❑ May interfere with accuracy of thyroid function tests and decrease response to metyrapone tests.

V

- May cause false-positive results in urine ketone tests.
- ***Toxicity and Overdose:*** Therapeutic serum levels range from 50–100 mcg/ml. Doses are gradually increased until a predose serum concentration of at least 50 mcg/ml is reached. However, a good correlation among daily dose, serum level, and therapeutic effects has not been established. Patients receiving near the maximum recommended 60 mg/kg/day should be monitored for toxicity.

POTENTIAL NURSING DIAGNOSES

- Injury, risk for (Indications).
- Knowledge deficit, related to medication regimen (Patient/Family Teaching).

IMPLEMENTATION

- **General Info:** Single daily doses are usually administered at bedtime because of sedation.
- **PO:** Administer with or immediately after meals to minimize GI irritation. Tell patient to swallow capsules and enteric-coated tablets whole, not to break or chew them, as this will cause irritation of the mouth or throat. Do not administer tablets with milk, to prevent premature dissolution. Delayed-release divalproex sodium may cause less GI irritation than valproic acid capsules.
- Shake liquid preparations well before pouring. Use calibrated measuring device to ensure accurate dosage. Syrup may be mixed with food or other liquids to improve taste.
- Sprinkle capsules may be swallowed whole or opened and entire capsule contents sprinkled on a teaspoonful of soft, cool food (applesauce, pudding). Tell patient to swallow drug/food mixture immediately, not to chew it. Do not store for future use.
- To convert from valproic acid to divalproex sodium, initiate divalproex sodium at same total daily dose and dosing schedule as valproic acid. Once patient is stabilized on divalproex sodium, attempt administration 2–3 times daily.
- **Intermittent Infusion:** May be diluted in D5W, 0.9% NaCl, or LR. Solution is stable for 24 hr at room temperature.
- ***Rate:*** Infuse over 60 min (≤20 mg/min). Rapid infusion may cause increased side effects.

PATIENT/FAMILY TEACHING

- Instruct patient to take medication exactly as directed. If a dose is missed on a once-a-day schedule, it should be taken as soon as remembered that day. If on a multiple-dose schedule, patient should take it within 6 hr of the scheduled time, then space remaining doses throughout the remainder of the day. Abrupt withdrawal may lead to status epilepticus.
- May cause drowsiness or dizziness. Caution patient to avoid driving or other activities requiring alertness until effects of medication are known. Tell patient not to resume driving until physician gives clearance based on control of seizure disorder.
- Caution patient to avoid taking alcohol, CNS depressants, or OTC medications concurrently with valproates without consulting health care professional.
- Instruct patient to notify health care professional of medication regimen prior to treatment or surgery.
- Advise patient to carry identification describing medication regimen at all times.
- Advise patient to notify health care professional if anorexia, severe nausea and vomiting, yellow skin or eyes, fever, sore throat, malaise, weakness, facial edema, lethargy, unusual bleeding or bruising, pregnancy, or loss of seizure control occurs. Children <2 yr of age are especially at risk for fatal hepatotoxicity.
- Emphasize the importance of routine exams to monitor progress.

EVALUATION

Effectiveness of therapy can be demonstrated by: ▪ Decrease in or cessation of seizures without excessive sedation ▪ Decreased incidence of mood swings in patients with bipolar disorders ▪ Decreased frequency of migraine headaches.

VANCOMYCIN

(van-koe-**mye**-sin)

Lyphocin, Vancocin, Vancoled

CLASSIFICATION(S):

Anti-infective (miscellaneous)

Pregnancy Category C

INDICATIONS

▪ **IV:** Treatment of potentially life-threatening infections when less toxic anti-infectives are contraindicated. Particularly useful in staphylococcal infections, including: ▫ Endocarditis ▫ Osteomyelitis ▫ Pneumonia ▫ Septicemia ▫ Soft-tissue infections in patients who have allergies to penicillin or its derivatives or when sensitivity testing demonstrates resistance to methicillin ▪ **PO:** Treatment of pseudomembranous colitis due to *Clostridium difficile* ▪ **IV:** Part of endocarditis prophylaxis in high-risk patients who are allergic to penicillin (see Appendix N).

ACTION

▪ Binds to bacterial cell wall, resulting in cell death. **Therapeutic Effects:** ▪ Bactericidal action against susceptible organisms. **Spectrum:** ▪ Active against gram-positive pathogens, including: ▫ Staphylococci (including methicillin-resistant strains of *Staphylococcus aureus*) ▫ Group A beta-hemolytic streptococci ▫ *Streptococcus pneumoniae* ▫ *Corynebacterium* ▫ *Clostridium* ▫ *Enterococcus faecalis* ▫ *Enterococcus faecium*.

PHARMACOKINETICS

Absorption: Poorly absorbed from the GI tract.
Distribution: Widely distributed. Some penetration (20–30%) of CSF; crosses placenta.
Metabolism and Excretion: Oral doses excreted primarily in the feces; IV vancomycin eliminated almost entirely by the kidneys.
Half-life: 6 hr (increased in renal impairment).

CONTRAINDICATIONS AND PRECAUTIONS

Contraindicated in: ▪ Hypersensitivity.
Use Cautiously in: ▪ Renal impairment (dosage reduction required if CCr ≤80 ml/min) ▪ Hearing impairment ▪ Intestinal obstruction or inflammation (increased systemic absorption when given orally) ▪ Pregnancy and lactation (safety not established).

ADVERSE REACTIONS AND SIDE EFFECTS*

Mainly associated with IV administration.
EENT: ototoxicity.
CV: hypotension.
GI: nausea, vomiting.
GU: <u>nephrotoxicity</u>.
Derm: rashes.
Hemat: eosinophilia, leukopenia.
Local: <u>phlebitis</u>.
MS: back and neck pain.
Misc: hypersensitivity reactions including ANAPHYLAXIS, chills, fever, red man syndrome, superinfection.

INTERACTIONS

Drug-Drug: ▪ May cause additive ototoxicity and nephrotoxicity with other **ototoxic** and **nephrotoxic drugs (aspirin, aminoglycosides, cyclosporine, cisplatin, loop diuretics)** ▪ May enhance neuromuscular blockade from **nondepolarizing neuromuscular blockers** ▪ Increased risk of histamine flush when used with **anesthetics** in children.

ROUTE AND DOSAGE

▫ Serious Systemic Infections

- **IV (Adults):** 500 mg (7.5 mg/kg) q 6 hr *or* 1 g (15 mg/kg) q 12 hr (up to 3–4 g/day).
- **IV (Children >1 mo):** 10 mg/kg q 6 hr *or* 20 mg/kg q 12 hr.
- **IV (Neonates 1 wk–1 mo):** 15 mg/kg initially, then 10 mg/kg q 8 hr.
- **IV (Neonates <1 wk):** 15 mg/kg initially, then 10 mg/kg q 12 hr.

▫ Endocarditis Prophylaxis in Penicillin-Allergic Patients

- **IV (Adults and Adolescents):** 1 g single dose 1 hr preprocedure.
- **IV (Children):** 20 mg/kg single dose 1 hr preprocedure.

▫ Pseudomembranous Colitis

- **PO (Adults):** 125–500 mg q 6 hr.
- **PO (Children):** 10 mg/kg q 6 hr (up to 125 mg/dose; not to exceed 2 g/day).

AVAILABILITY

▪ ***Capsules:*** 125 mg[Rx], 250 mg[Rx] ▪ ***Oral solution:*** 250 mg/5 ml[Rx], 500 mg/6 ml[Rx] ▪ ***Injection:*** 500-mg, 1-, 5-, 10-g vials[Rx].

TIME/ACTION PROFILE (blood levels)

	ONSET	PEAK	DURATION
IV	rapid	end of infusion	12–24 hr

***CAPITALS** indicate life-threatening; <u>**underlines**</u> **indicate most frequent.**

V

NURSING IMPLICATIONS

ASSESSMENT

- Assess patient for infection (vital signs; appearance of wound, sputum, urine, and stool; WBC) at beginning of and throughout therapy.
- Obtain specimens for culture and sensitivity prior to initiating therapy. First dose may be given before receiving results.
- Monitor IV site closely. Vancomycin is irritating to tissues and causes necrosis and severe pain with extravasation. Rotate infusion site.
- Monitor blood pressure throughout IV infusion.
- Evaluate eighth cranial nerve function by audiometry and serum vancomycin levels prior to and throughout therapy in patients with borderline renal function or those >60 yr of age. Prompt recognition and intervention are essential in preventing permanent damage.
- Monitor intake and output ratios and daily weight. Cloudy or pink urine may be a sign of nephrotoxicity.
- Assess patient for signs of superinfection (black, furry overgrowth on tongue; vaginal itching or discharge; loose or foul-smelling stools). Report occurrence.
- **Pseudomembranous Colitis:** Assess bowel status (bowel sounds, frequency and consistency of stools, presence of blood in stools) throughout therapy.
- ***Lab Test Considerations:*** Monitor for casts, albumin, or cells in the urine or decreased specific gravity, CBC, and renal function periodically throughout course of therapy.
- May cause increased BUN levels.
- ***Toxicity and Overdose:*** Peak serum vancomycin levels should not exceed 25 mcg/ml. Trough concentrations should not exceed 5–10 mcg/ml.

POTENTIAL NURSING DIAGNOSES

- Infection, risk for (Indications).
- Sensory-perceptual alterations: auditory (Side Effects).
- Knowledge deficit, related to medication regimen (Patient/Family Teaching).

IMPLEMENTATION

- **PO:** Use calibrated measuring device for liquid preparations. IV dosage form may be diluted in 30 ml of water for oral or nasogastric tube administration. Resulting solution has bitter, unpleasant taste. Stable for 14 days if refrigerated.
- **Intermittent Infusion:** Dilute each 500-mg vial with 10 ml of sterile water for injection. Dilute further with 100–200 ml of 0.9% NaCl, D5W, D10W, or lactated Ringer's solution. Solution is stable for 14 days after initial reconstitution if refrigerated. After further dilution, solution is stable for 96 hr if refrigerated.
- ***Rate:*** Administer over at least 60 min. Do not administer rapidly or as a bolus to minimize risk of thrombophlebitis, hypotension, and red man or red neck syndrome (sudden, severe hypotension; flushing and/or maculopapular rash of face, neck, chest, and upper extremities). Thrombophlebitis can be minimized by using dilute solutions of 2.5–5 mg/ml and rotating sites.
- **Continuous Infusion:** Should be used only if intermittent infusion is not feasible.
- ***Rate:*** May also be prepared with 1–2 g in sufficient volume to infuse over 24 hr.
- **Y-Site Compatibility:** ▪ acyclovir ▪ amifostine ▪ amiodarone ▪ atracurium ▪ cyclophosphamide ▪ diltiazem ▪ enalaprilat ▪ esmolol ▪ filgrastim ▪ fluconazole ▪ fludarabine ▪ gallium nitrate ▪ hydromorphone ▪ insulin ▪ labetalol ▪ lorazepam ▪ magnesium sulfate ▪ melphalan ▪ meperidine ▪ midazolam ▪ morphine ▪ ondansetron ▪ paclitaxel ▪ pancuronium ▪ perphenazine ▪ sodium bicarbonate ▪ tacrolimus ▪ teniposide ▪ theophylline ▪ thiotepa ▪ tolazoline ▪ vecuronium ▪ vinorelbine ▪ zidovudine.
- **Y-Site Incompatibility:** ▪ albumin ▪ cefepime ▪ heparin ▪ idarubicin ▪ piperacillin/tazobactam.

PATIENT/FAMILY TEACHING

- Advise patients on oral vancomycin to take exactly as directed. Tell patients that missed doses should be taken as soon as remembered unless almost time for next dose; do not double dose.
- Instruct patient to report signs of hypersensitivity, tinnitus, vertigo, or hearing loss.
- Advise patient to notify health care professional if no improvement is seen in a few days.
- Patients with a history of rheumatic heart disease or valve replacement need to be taught importance of using antimicrobial prophylaxis

prior to invasive dental or medical procedures.

EVALUATION

Clinical response to therapy can be evaluated by: ▪ Resolution of signs and symptoms of infection. Length of time for complete resolution depends on organism and site of infection ▪ Endocarditis prophylaxis.

VENLAFAXINE

(ven-la-**fax**-een)
Effexor, Effexor XR

CLASSIFICATION(S):
Antidepressant (miscellaneous)

Pregnancy Category C

INDICATIONS

▪ Treatment of major depressive illness, often in conjunction with psychotherapy.

ACTION

▪ Inhibits the reuptake of serotonin and norepinephrine in the CNS. **Therapeutic Effects:** ▪ Decrease in depressive symptomatology.

PHARMACOKINETICS

Absorption: Well absorbed (92–100%) following oral administration.
Distribution: Extensive distribution into body tissues.
Metabolism and Excretion: Extensively metabolized on 1st pass through the liver. One metabolite, O-desmethylvenlafaxine (ODV), has antidepressant activity; 5% of venlafaxine is excreted unchanged in urine; 30% of the active metabolite is excreted in urine.
Half-life: *Venlafaxine*—3–5 hr; *ODV*—9–11 hr (both are increased in hepatic/renal impairment).

CONTRAINDICATIONS AND PRECAUTIONS

Contraindicated in: ▪ Hypersensitivity ▪ Concurrent MAO inhibitor therapy.
Use Cautiously in: ▪ Cardiovascular disease, including hypertension ▪ Hepatic impairment (decrease dose by 50% or more if impairment is moderate to severe) ▪ Impaired renal function (decrease dose by 25% in mild impairment; 50% if CCr <50 ml/min) ▪ History of seizures or neurologic impairment ▪ History of mania ▪ History of drug abuse ▪ Pregnancy, lactation, or children <18 yr (use only if clearly required during pregnancy; safety not established).

ADVERSE REACTIONS AND SIDE EFFECTS*

CNS: SEIZURES, abnormal dreams, anxiety, dizziness, headache, nervousness, weakness, abnormal thinking, agitation, confusion, depersonalization, drowsiness, emotional lability, worsening depression.
EENT: rhinitis, visual disturbances, tinnitus.
CV: chest pain, hypertension, palpitations, tachycardia.
GI: abdominal pain, altered taste, anorexia, constipation, diarrhea, dry mouth, dyspepsia, nausea, vomiting, weight loss.
GU: sexual dysfunction, urinary frequency, urinary retention.
Derm: itching, photosensitivity, skin rash.
Neuro: paresthesia, twitching.
Misc: chills, yawning.

INTERACTIONS

Drug-Drug: ▪ Concurrent use with **MAO inhibitors** may result in serious, potentially fatal reactions (wait at least 2 wk after stopping MAO inhibitor before initiating venlafaxine; wait at least 1 wk after stopping venlafaxine before starting MAO inhibitors) ▪ Concurrent use with **alcohol** or other **CNS depressants,** including **sedative/hypnotics, antihistamines,** and **opioid analgesics,** in depressed patients is not recommended ▪ **Lithium** may have additive serotonergic effects with venlafaxine; use cautiously in patients receiving venlafaxine ▪ **Cimetidine** may increase the effects of venlafaxine (may be more pronounced in elderly patients, those with hepatic or renal impairment, or those with preexisting hypertension).

ROUTE AND DOSAGE

▪ **PO (Adults):** 75 mg/day in 2–3 divided doses; may increase by up to 75 mg/day every 4 or more days, up to 225 mg/day (not to

*CAPITALS indicate life-threatening; underlines indicate most frequent.

V

exceed 375 mg/day in 3 divided doses); extended-release (XR) formulation can be given as a single daily dose.

AVAILABILITY

▪ ***Tablets:*** 25 mg[Rx], 37.5 mg[Rx], 50 mg[Rx], 75 mg[Rx], 100 mg[Rx] ▪ ***Extended-release tablets:*** 37.5 mg[Rx], 75 mg[Rx], 150 mg[Rx].

TIME/ACTION PROFILE (antidepressant action)

	ONSET	PEAK	DURATION
PO	within 2 wk	2–4 wk	UK

NURSING IMPLICATIONS

ASSESSMENT

□ Assess mental status and mood changes. Inform physician or other health care professional if patient demonstrates significant increase in anxiety, nervousness, or insomnia.
□ Assess suicidal tendencies, especially in early therapy. Restrict amount of drug available to patient.
□ Monitor blood pressure prior to and periodically throughout therapy. Sustained hypertension may be dose related; decrease dose or discontinue therapy if this occurs.
□ Monitor appetite and nutritional intake. Weigh weekly. Report continued weight loss. Adjust diet as tolerated to support nutritional status.
▪ ***Lab Test Considerations:*** Monitor CBC with differential and platelet count periodically during therapy. May cause anemia, leukocytosis, leukopenia, thrombocytopenia, basophilia, and eosinophilia.
□ May cause an increase in serum alkaline phosphatase, bilirubin, AST, ALT, BUN, and creatinine.
□ May also cause increased serum cholesterol.
□ May cause electrolyte abnormalities (hyperglycemia or hypoglycemia, hyperkalemia or hypokalemia, hyperuricemia, hyperphosphatemia or hypophosphatemia, and hyponatremia.

POTENTIAL NURSING DIAGNOSES

▪ Coping, ineffective individual (Indications).
▪ Injury, risk for (Side Effects).
▪ Knowledge deficit, related to medication regimen (Patient/Family Teaching).

IMPLEMENTATION

▪ **PO:** Administer venlafaxine with food.
□ Extended-release tablets should be swallowed whole; do not crush, break, or chew.

PATIENT/FAMILY TEACHING

□ Instruct patient to take medication exactly as directed. If a dose is missed, take as soon as possible unless almost time for next dose. Do not double doses or discontinue abruptly. Patients taking venlafaxine for >6 wk should have dose gradually decreased prior to discontinuation.
□ May cause drowsiness or dizziness. Caution patient to avoid driving or other activities requiring alertness until response to the drug is known.
□ Caution patient to avoid taking alcohol or other CNS-depressant drugs during therapy and not to take other prescription or OTC medications without consulting health care professional.
□ Instruct female patients to inform health care professional if pregnancy is planned or suspected or if breast-feeding.
□ Instruct patient to notify health care professional if signs of allergy (rash, hives) occur.
□ Emphasize the importance of follow-up exams to monitor progress. Encourage patient participation in psychotherapy.

EVALUATION

Effectiveness of therapy can be demonstrated by: ▪ Increased sense of well-being □ Renewed interest in surroundings. Need for therapy should be periodically reassessed. Therapy is usually continued for several mo.

VERAPAMIL

(ver-**ap**-a-mil)
Apo-Verap, Calan, Calan SR, Covera-HS, Isoptin, Isoptin SR, {Novo-Veramil}, {Nu-Verap}, Verelan

{} = Available in Canada only.

CLASSIFICATION(S):
Antianginals, Antiarrhythmic, Antihypertensive agent, Calcium channel blockers, Vascular headache suppressant

Pregnancy Category C

INDICATIONS

▪ Management of hypertension, angina pectoris, and/or vasospastic (Prinzmetal's) angina ▪ Management of supraventricular arrhythmias and rapid ventricular rates in atrial flutter or fibrillation. **Unlabeled Uses:** ▪ Prevention of migraine headache ▪ Management of cardiomyopathy.

ACTION

▪ Inhibits the transport of calcium into myocardial and vascular smooth muscle cells, resulting in inhibition of excitation-contraction coupling and subsequent contraction ▪ Decreases SA and AV conduction and prolongs AV node refractory period in conduction tissue. **Therapeutic Effects:** ▪ Systemic vasodilation resulting in decreased blood pressure ▪ Coronary vasodilation resulting in decreased frequency and severity of attacks of angina ▪ Suppression of ventricular tachyarrhythmias.

PHARMACOKINETICS

Absorption: 90% absorbed following oral administration, but much is rapidly metabolized, resulting in bioavailability of 20–25%.
Distribution: Small amounts enter breast milk.
Metabolism and Excretion: Mostly metabolized by the liver.
Half-life: 4.5–12 hr.

CONTRAINDICATIONS AND PRECAUTIONS

Contraindicated in: ▪ Hypersensitivity ▪ Sick sinus syndrome ▪ 2nd- or 3rd-degree AV block (unless an artificial pacemaker is in place) ▪ Blood pressure <90 mm Hg ▪ Congestive heart failure (CHF), severe ventricular dysfunction, or cardiogenic shock, unless associated with supraventricular tachyarrhythmias ▪ Concurrent IV beta-adrenergic blocker therapy.
Use Cautiously in: ▪ Severe hepatic impairment (dosage reduction recommended for most agents) ▪ Geriatric patients (dosage reduction/slower IV infusion rates recommended for most agents; increased risk of hypotension) ▪ History of serious ventricular arrhythmias or CHF ▪ Pregnancy or lactation (safety not established; verapamil is approved for use in children).

ADVERSE REACTIONS AND SIDE EFFECTS*

CNS: abnormal dreams, anxiety, confusion, dizziness/light-headedness, drowsiness, headache, jitteriness, nervousness, psychiatric disturbances, weakness.
EENT: blurred vision, disturbed equilibrium, epistaxis, tinnitus.
Resp: cough, dyspnea, shortness of breath.
CV: ARRHYTHMIAS, CHF, bradycardia, chest pain, hypotension, palpitations, peripheral edema, syncope, tachycardia.
GI: abnormal liver function studies, anorexia, constipation, diarrhea, dry mouth, dysgeusia, dyspepsia, nausea, vomiting.
GU: dysuria, nocturia, polyuria, sexual dysfunction, urinary frequency.
Derm: dermatitis, erythema multiforme, flushing, increased sweating, photosensitivity, pruritus/urticaria, rash.
Endo: gynecomastia, hyperglycemia.
Hemat: anemia, leukopenia, thrombocytopenia.
Metab: weight gain.
MS: joint stiffness, muscle cramps.
Neuro: paresthesia, tremor.
Misc: STEVENS-JOHNSON SYNDROME, gingival hyperplasia.

INTERACTIONS

Drug-Drug: ▪ Additive hypotension may occur when used concurrently with **fentanyl**, other **antihypertensives, nitrates**, acute ingestion of **alcohol**, or **quinidine** ▪ Antihypertensive effects may be decreased by concurrent use of **NSAIDs** ▪ Serum **digoxin** levels may be increased ▪ Concurrent use with **beta-adrenergic blockers, digoxin, disopyramide**, or **phenytoin** may result in bradycardia, conduction defects, or CHF ▪ May decrease the metabolism of and increase the risk of toxicity from **cyclosporine, prazosin, quinidine**, or **carbamazepine** ▪ May decrease the effectiveness of **rifampin** ▪ Increases the muscle-paralyzing effects

***CAPITALS indicate life-threatening; underlines indicate most frequent.**

V

of **nondepolarizing neuromuscular-blocking agents** ▪ Effectiveness may be decreased by coadministration with **vitamin D** and **calcium** ▪ May alter serum **lithium** levels.

ROUTE AND DOSAGE

- **PO (Adults):** 80–120 mg 3 times daily, increased as needed. *Patients with poor ventricular function, hepatic impairment, or geriatric patients*—40 mg 3 times daily initially. *Extended-release preparations*—120–240 mg/day as a single dose; may be increased as needed (range 240–480 mg/day).
- **PO (Children up to 15 yr):** 4–8 mg/kg/day in divided doses.
- **IV (Adults):** 5–10 mg (75–150 mcg/kg); may repeat with 10 mg (150 mcg/kg) after 15–30 min.
- **IV (Children 1–15 yr):** 2–5 mg (100–300 mcg/kg); may repeat after 30 min (initial dose not to exceed 5 mg; repeat dose not to exceed 10 mg).
- **IV (Children <1 yr):** 0.75–2 mg (100–200 mcg/kg); may repeat after 30 min.

AVAILABILITY

▪ ***Tablets:*** 40 mg[Rx], 80 mg[Rx], 120 mg[Rx] ▪ ***Extended-release tablets:*** 120 mg[Rx], 180 mg[Rx], 240 mg[Rx] ▪ ***Extended-release capsules:*** 120 mg[Rx], 180 mg[Rx], 240 mg[Rx], 360 mg[Rx] ▪ ***Injection:*** 2.5 mg/ml[Rx] in 2- and 4-ml vials, ampules, and syringes ▪ ***In combination with:*** trandolapril (Tarka[Rx]; see Appendix A).

TIME/ACTION PROFILE (cardiovascular effects)

	ONSET	PEAK	DURATION
PO	1–2 hr	30–90 min*	3–7 hr
PO-ER	UK	5–7 hr	24 hr
IV	1–5 min†	3–5 min	2 hr†

*Single dose; effects from multiple doses may not be evident for 24–48 hr.

†Antiarrhythmic effects; hemodynamic effects begin 3–5 min following injection and persist for 10–20 min.

NURSING IMPLICATIONS

ASSESSMENT

- **General Info:** Monitor blood pressure and pulse prior to therapy, during dosage titration, and periodically throughout therapy. Monitor ECG periodically during prolonged therapy. Verapamil may cause prolonged PR interval.
  - □ Monitor intake and output ratios and daily weight. Assess for signs of CHF (peripheral edema, rales/crackles, dyspnea, weight gain, jugular venous distention).
  - □ Patients receiving digitalis glycosides concurrently with calcium channel blockers should have routine serum digitalis glycoside levels and be monitored for signs and symptoms of digitalis glycoside toxicity.
- **Angina:** Assess location, duration, intensity, and precipitating factors of patient's anginal pain.
- **Arrhythmias:** Monitor ECG continuously during administration. Notify physician promptly if bradycardia or prolonged hypotension occurs. Emergency equipment and medication should be available. Monitor blood pressure and pulse before and frequently during administration.
- ***Lab Test Considerations:*** Total serum calcium concentrations are not affected by calcium channel blockers.
  - □ Monitor serum potassium periodically. Hypokalemia increases the risk of arrhythmias and should be corrected.
  - □ Monitor renal and hepatic functions periodically during long-term therapy. May cause increase in hepatic enzymes after several days of therapy, which return to normal on discontinuation of therapy.

POTENTIAL NURSING DIAGNOSES

- Cardiac output, decreased (Indications).
- Pain (Indications).
- Knowledge deficit, related to medication regimen (Patient/Family Teaching).

IMPLEMENTATION

- **PO:** Administer verapamil with meals or milk to minimize gastric irritation.
  - □ Do not open, crush, break, or chew sustained-release capsules or tablets. Empty tablets that appear in stool are not significant.
- **IV:** Patients should remain recumbent for at least 1 hr following IV administration to minimize hypotensive effects.
- **Direct IV:** Administer IV undiluted through Y-site over 2 min for each single dose. Administer over 3 min in elderly patients.
- **Syringe Compatibility:** ▪ amrinone ▪ heparin ▪ milrinone.
- **Y-Site Compatibility:** ▪ amrinone ▪ cipro-

floxacin ▪ dobutamine ▪ dopamine ▪ famotidine ▪ hydralazine ▪ meperidine ▪ methicillin ▪ milrinone ▪ penicillin G potassium ▪ piperacillin ▪ ticarcillin.

▪ **Y-Site Incompatibility:** ▪ albumin ▪ ampicillin ▪ mezlocillin ▪ nafcillin ▪ oxacillin ▪ sodium bicarbonate.

PATIENT/FAMILY TEACHING

- **General Info:** Advise patient to take medication exactly as directed, even if feeling well. If a dose is missed, take as soon as possible unless almost time for next dose; do not double doses. May need to be discontinued gradually.
- □ Instruct patient on correct technique for monitoring pulse. Instruct patient to contact health care professional if heart rate is <50 bpm.
- □ Caution patient to change positions slowly to minimize orthostatic hypotension.
- □ May cause drowsiness or dizziness. Advise patient to avoid driving or other activities requiring alertness until response to the medication is known.
- □ Instruct patient on importance of maintaining good dental hygiene and seeing dentist frequently for teeth cleaning to prevent tenderness, bleeding, and gingival hyperplasia (gum enlargement).
- □ Instruct patient to avoid concurrent use of alcohol or OTC medications, especially cold preparations, without consulting health care professional.
- □ Advise patient to notify health care professional if irregular heartbeats, dyspnea, swelling of hands and feet, pronounced dizziness, nausea, constipation, or hypotension occurs or if headache is severe or persistent.
- □ Caution patient to wear protective clothing and use sunscreen to prevent photosensitivity reactions.
- **Angina:** Instruct patient on concurrent nitrate or beta-blocker therapy to continue taking both medications as directed and use SL nitroglycerin as needed for anginal attacks.
- □ Advise patient to contact health care professional if chest pain does not improve, worsens after therapy, or occurs with diaphoresis; if shortness of breath occurs; or if severe, persistent headache occurs.
- □ Caution patient to discuss exercise restrictions with health care professional prior to exertion.
- **Hypertension:** Encourage patient to comply with other interventions for hypertension (weight reduction, low-sodium diet, smoking cessation, moderation of alcohol consumption, regular exercise, and stress management). Medication controls but does not cure hypertension.
- □ Instruct patient and family in proper technique for monitoring blood pressure. Advise patient to take blood pressure weekly and to report significant changes to health care professional.

EVALUATION

Effectiveness of therapy can be demonstrated by: ▪ Decrease in blood pressure ▪ Decrease in frequency and severity of anginal attacks □ Decrease in need for nitrate therapy □ Increase in activity tolerance and sense of well-being ▪ Suppression and prevention of atrial tachyarrhythmias.

VINBLASTINE

(vin-**blass**-teen)

Velban, {Velbe}, Velsar

CLASSIFICATION(S):

Antineoplastic (vinca alkaloid)

Pregnancy Category D

INDICATIONS

▪ Combination chemotherapy of: □ Lymphomas □ Nonseminomatous testicular carcinoma □ Advanced breast cancer □ Other tumors.

ACTION

▪ Binds to proteins of mitotic spindle, causing metaphase arrest. Cell replication is stopped as a result (cell cycle–specific for M phase). **Therapeutic Effects:** ▪ Death of rapidly replicating cells, particularly malignant ones ▪ Has immunosuppressive properties.

PHARMACOKINETICS

Absorption: Administered IV only, resulting in complete bioavailability.

V

Distribution: Does not cross the blood-brain barrier well.
Metabolism and Excretion: Converted by the liver to an active antineoplastic compound; excreted in the feces via biliary excretion, some renal elimination.
Half-life: 24 hr.

CONTRAINDICATIONS AND PRECAUTIONS

Contraindicated in: ▪ Hypersensitivity ▪ Pregnancy or lactation.
Use Cautiously in: ▪ Patients with childbearing potential ▪ Infections ▪ Decreased bone marrow reserve ▪ Other chronic debilitating illnesses ▪ Patients with impaired hepatic function (decrease dose by 50% if serum bilirubin >3 mg/dl).

ADVERSE REACTIONS AND SIDE EFFECTS*

CNS: SEIZURES, mental depression, neurotoxicity, weakness.
Resp: BRONCHOSPASM.
GI: nausea, vomiting, anorexia, constipation, diarrhea, stomatitis.
GU: gonadal suppression.
Derm: alopecia, dermatitis, vesiculation.
Endo: syndrome of inappropriate antidiuretic hormone (SIADH).
Hemat: anemia, leukopenia, thrombocytopenia.
Local: phlebitis at IV site.
Metab: hyperuricemia.
Neuro: neuritis, paresthesia, peripheral neuropathy.

INTERACTIONS

Drug-Drug: ▪ Additive bone marrow depression with other **antineoplastic agents** or **radiation therapy** ▪ Bronchospasm may occur in patients who have been previously treated with **mitomycin** ▪ May decrease antibody response to **live virus vaccines** and increase the risk of adverse reactions ▪ May decrease serum **phenytoin** levels.

ROUTE AND DOSAGE

Doses may vary greatly, depending on tumor, schedule, condition of patient, and blood counts.

- **IV (Adults):** *Initial*—3.7 mg/m^2 (100 mcg/kg), single dose; increase weekly as tolerated by 1.8 mg/m^2 (50 mcg/kg) to maximum of 18.5 mg/m^2 (usual dose is 5.5–7.4 mg/m^2). *Maintenance*—10 mg 1–2 times/mo or 1 increment less than last dose q 7–14 days.
- **IV (Children):** *Initial*—2.5 mg/m^2, single dose; increase weekly as tolerated by 1.25 mg/m^2 to maximum of 7.5 mg/m^2. *Maintenance*—1 increment less than last dose q 7–14 days.

AVAILABILITY

▪ ***Solution for injection:*** 1 mg/ml in 10-ml vials[Rx] ▪ ***Powder for injection:*** 10 mg/vial[Rx].

TIME/ACTION PROFILE (effects on white blood cell counts)

	ONSET	PEAK	DURATION
IV	5–7 days	10 days	7–14 days

NURSING IMPLICATIONS

ASSESSMENT

- Monitor blood pressure, pulse, and respiratory rate during course of therapy. Notify physician immediately if respiratory distress occurs. Bronchospasm can be life-threatening and may occur at time of infusion or several hours to weeks later.
- Monitor for bone marrow depression. Assess for bleeding (bleeding gums, bruising, petechiae, guaiac stools, urine, and emesis) and avoid IM injections and rectal temperatures if platelet count is low. Apply pressure to venipuncture sites for 10 min. Assess for signs of infection during neutropenia. Anemia may occur. Monitor for increased fatigue, dyspnea, and orthostatic hypotension.
- May cause nausea and vomiting. Monitor intake and output, appetite, and nutritional intake. Prophylactic antiemetics may be used. Adjust diet as tolerated.
- Assess injection site frequently for redness, irritation, or inflammation. If extravasation occurs, infusion must be stopped and restarted elsewhere to avoid damage to SC tissue. Standard treatment includes infiltration with hyaluronidase and application of heat.

***CAPITALS indicate life-threatening; underlines indicate most frequent.**

- Monitor for symptoms of gout (increased uric acid, joint pain, edema). Encourage patient to drink at least 2 liters of fluid per day. Allopurinol or alkalinization of urine may be used to decrease uric acid levels.
- ***Lab Test Considerations:*** Monitor CBC prior to and routinely throughout therapy. If WBC <2000, subsequent doses are usually withheld until WBC is at least 4000. The nadir of leukopenia occurs in 5–10 days and recovery usually occurs 7–14 days later. Thrombocytopenia may also occur in patients who have received radiation or other chemotherapy agents.
- Monitor liver function studies (AST, ALT, LDH, bilirubin) and renal function studies (BUN, creatinine) prior to and periodically throughout therapy.
- May cause increased uric acid. Monitor periodically during therapy.

POTENTIAL NURSING DIAGNOSES

- Infection, risk for (Adverse Reactions).
- Nutrition, altered, less than body requirements (Adverse Reactions).
- Knowledge deficit, related to medication regimen (Patient/Family Teaching).

IMPLEMENTATION

- **General Info:** Solution should be prepared in a biologic cabinet. Wear gloves, gown, and mask while handling medication. Discard IV equipment in specially designated containers (see Appendix I).
- Do not administer SC, IM, or IT. Intrathecal administration is fatal. Vinblastine must be dispensed in an overwrap stating, "For IV use only." Overwrap should remain in place until immediately before administration.
- Do not inject into extremities with impaired circulation; may cause thrombophlebitis.
- **Direct IV:** Dilute each 10 mg with 10 ml of 0.9% NaCl for injection with phenol or benzyl alcohol for a concentration of 1 mg/ml. Solution is clear. Reconstituted medication is stable for 28 days if refrigerated.
- ***Rate:*** Administer each single dose over 1 min through Y-site injection of a free-flowing infusion of 0.9% NaCl or D5W.
- **Intermittent Infusion:** Dilution in large volumes (100–250 ml) or prolonged infusion (≥30 min) increases chance of vein irritation and extravasation.
- **Syringe Compatibility:** ▪ bleomycin ▪ cisplatin ▪ cyclophosphamide ▪ droperidol ▪ fluorouracil ▪ leucovorin calcium ▪ methotrexate ▪ metoclopramide ▪ mitomycin ▪ vincristine.
- **Y-Site Compatibility:** ▪ amifostine ▪ aztreonam ▪ bleomycin ▪ cefepime ▪ cisplatin ▪ cyclophosphamide ▪ doxorubicin ▪ droperidol ▪ filgrastim ▪ fludarabine ▪ fluorouracil ▪ heparin ▪ leucovorin calcium ▪ melphalan ▪ methotrexate ▪ metoclopramide ▪ mitomycin ▪ ondansetron ▪ paclitaxel ▪ piperacillin/tazobactam ▪ sargramostim ▪ teniposide ▪ thiotepa ▪ vincristine ▪ vinorelbine.
- **Y-Site Incompatibility:** ▪ furosemide.

PATIENT/FAMILY TEACHING

- Advise patient to notify health care professional if fever; chills; sore throat; signs of infection; bleeding gums; bruising; petechiae; or blood in urine, stool, or emesis occurs. Caution patient to avoid crowds and persons with known infections. Instruct patient to use soft toothbrush and electric razor. Caution patient not to drink alcoholic beverages or take products containing aspirin or NSAIDs.
- Instruct patient to inspect oral mucosa for redness and ulceration. Advise patient that, if ulceration occurs, to avoid spicy foods, use sponge brush, and rinse mouth with water after eating and drinking. Topical agents may be used if mouth pain interferes with eating. Stomatitis pain may require treatment with opioid analgesics.
- Instruct patient to report symptoms of neurotoxicity (paresthesia, pain, difficulty walking, persistent constipation).
- Advise patient that jaw pain, pain in organs containing tumor tissue, nausea, and vomiting may occur. Avoid constipation and report other adverse reactions.
- Advise patient that this medication may have teratogenic effects. Contraception should be used during and for at least 2 mo after therapy is concluded.
- Discuss with patient the possibility of hair loss. Explore coping strategies.
- Instruct patient not to receive any vaccinations without advice of health care professional.

□ Emphasize need for periodic lab tests to monitor for side effects.

EVALUATION

Effectiveness of therapy can be demonstrated by: ▪ Regression of malignancy without the appearance of detrimental side effects.

VINCRISTINE
(vin-**kriss**-teen)
Oncovin, Vincasar PFS, Vincrex

CLASSIFICATION(S):
Antineoplastic (vinca alkaloid)

Pregnancy Category D

INDICATIONS

▪ Used alone and in combination with other treatment modalities (antineoplastic agents, surgery, or radiation therapy) in treatment of: □ Hodgkin's disease □ Leukemias □ Neuroblastoma □ Malignant lymphomas □ Rhabdomyosarcoma □ Wilms' tumor □ Other tumors.

ACTION

▪ Binds to proteins of mitotic spindle, causing metaphase arrest ▪ Cell replication is stopped as a result (cell cycle–specific for M phase) ▪ Has little or no effect on bone marrow. **Therapeutic Effects:** ▪ Death of rapidly replicating cells, particularly malignant ones ▪ Has immunosuppressive properties.

PHARMACOKINETICS

Absorption: Administered IV only, resulting in complete bioavailability.
Distribution: Rapidly and widely distributed.
Metabolism and Excretion: Metabolized by the liver and eliminated in the feces via biliary excretion.
Half-life: 10.5–37.5 hr.

CONTRAINDICATIONS AND PRECAUTIONS

Contraindicated in: ▪ Hypersensitivity ▪ Pregnancy or lactation.
Use Cautiously in: ▪ Patients with childbearing potential ▪ Infections ▪ Decreased bone marrow reserve ▪ Other chronic debilitating illnesses ▪ Hepatic impairment (dosage reduction recommended if serum bilirubin >3 mg/dl).

ADVERSE REACTIONS AND SIDE EFFECTS*

CNS: agitation, insomnia, mental depression, mental status changes.
EENT: cortical blindness, diplopia.
Resp: bronchospasm.
GI: <u>nausea</u>, <u>vomiting</u>, abdominal cramps, anorexia, constipation, ileus, stomatitis.
GU: gonadal suppression, nocturia, oliguria, urinary retention.
Derm: <u>alopecia</u>.
Endo: syndrome of inappropriate antidiuretic hormone (SIADH).
Hemat: anemia, leukopenia, thrombocytopenia (mild and brief).
Local: <u>phlebitis</u> at IV site, tissue necrosis (from extravasation).
Metab: hyperuricemia.
Neuro: <u>ascending peripheral neuropathy</u>.

INTERACTIONS

Drug-Drug: ▪ Bronchospasm may occur in patients who have been previously treated with **mitomycin** ▪ **L-asparaginase** may decrease hepatic metabolism of vincristine (give vincristine 12–24 hr prior to asparaginase) ▪ May decrease antibody response to **live virus vaccines** and increase the risk of adverse reactions.

ROUTE AND DOSAGE

Many other protocols are used.

- **IV (Adults):** 10–30 mcg/kg (0.4–1.4 mg/m^2); may repeat weekly (not to exceed 2 mg/dose).
- **IV (Children >10 kg):** 1.5–2 mg/m^2 single dose; may repeat weekly.
- **IV (Children <10 kg):** 50 mcg/kg single dose; may repeat weekly.

AVAILABILITY

▪ ***Solution for injection:*** 1 mg/ml in 1-, 2-, 5-ml vials[Rx] ▪ ***Powder for injection:*** 5 mg/vial[Rx].

***CAPITALS indicate life-threatening; <u>underlines</u> indicate most frequent.**

TIME/ACTION PROFILE (effects on blood counts*)

	ONSET	PEAK	DURATION
IV	UK	4 days	7 days

*Usually mild.

NURSING IMPLICATIONS

ASSESSMENT

- Monitor blood pressure, pulse, and respiratory rate during course of therapy. Report significant changes.
- Monitor neurologic status. Assess for paresthesia (numbness, tingling, pain), loss of deep tendon reflexes (Achilles reflex is usually first involved), weakness (wrist drop or footdrop, gait disturbances), cranial nerve palsies (jaw pain, hoarseness, ptosis, visual changes), autonomic dysfunction (ileus, difficulty voiding, orthostatic hypotension, impaired sweating), and CNS dysfunction (decreased level of consciousness, agitation, hallucinations). Notify physician if these symptoms develop, as they may persist for months.
- Monitor intake and output ratios and daily weight; report significant discrepancies. Decreased urine output with concurrent hyponatremia may indicate SIADH, which usually responds to fluid restriction.
- Assess infusion site frequently for redness, irritation, or inflammation. If extravasation occurs, infusion must be stopped and restarted elsewhere to avoid damage to SC tissue. Cellulitis and discomfort may be minimized by infiltration with hyaluronidase and application of moderate heat or by application of cold compresses.
- Assess nutritional status. An antiemetic may be used to minimize nausea and vomiting.
- Monitor for symptoms of gout (increased uric acid, joint pain, edema). Encourage patient to drink at least 2 liters of fluid per day. Allopurinol or alkalinization of urine may be used to decrease uric acid levels.
- ***Lab Test Considerations:*** Monitor CBC prior to and periodically throughout therapy. May cause slight leukopenia 4 days after therapy, which resolves within 7 days. Platelet count may increase or decrease.
- Monitor liver function studies (AST, ALT, LDH, bilirubin) and renal function studies (BUN, creatinine) prior to and periodically throughout therapy.
- May cause increased uric acid. Monitor periodically during therapy.

POTENTIAL NURSING DIAGNOSES

- Injury, risk for (Adverse Reactions).
- Nutrition, altered, less than body requirements (Adverse Reactions).
- Knowledge deficit, related to medication regimen (Patient/Family Teaching).

IMPLEMENTATION

- **General Info:** Solution should be prepared in a biologic cabinet. Wear gloves, gown, and mask while handling medication. Discard IV equipment in specially designated containers (see Appendix I).
- Do not administer SC, IM, or IT. Intrathecal administration is fatal. Vincristine must be dispensed in an overwrap stating, "For IV use only." Overwrap should remain in place until immediately before administration.
- **Direct IV:** Reconstitute by adding 5 ml of sterile water for injection to each vial for a concentration of 1 mg/ml. Administer undiluted.
- ***Rate:*** Administer each dose direct IV push over 1 min through Y-site injection of a free-flowing infusion of 0.9% NaCl or D5W.
- **Syringe Compatibility:** ▪ bleomycin ▪ cisplatin ▪ cyclophosphamide ▪ doxapram ▪ doxorubicin ▪ droperidol ▪ fluorouracil ▪ heparin ▪ leucovorin calcium ▪ methotrexate ▪ metoclopramide ▪ mitomycin ▪ vinblastine.
- **Syringe Incompatibility:** ▪ furosemide.
- **Y-Site Compatibility:** ▪ allopurinol sodium ▪ amifostine ▪ aztreonam ▪ bleomycin ▪ cisplatin ▪ cyclophosphamide ▪ doxorubicin ▪ droperidol ▪ filgrastim ▪ fludarabine ▪ fluorouracil ▪ granisetron ▪ heparin ▪ leucovorin calcium ▪ melphalan ▪ methotrexate ▪ metoclopramide ▪ mitomycin ▪ ondansetron ▪ paclitaxel ▪ piperacillin/tazobactam ▪ sargramostim ▪ teniposide ▪ thiotepa ▪ vinblastine ▪ vinorelbine.
- **Y-Site Incompatibility:** ▪ cefepime ▪ furosemide ▪ idarubicin ▪ sodium bicarbonate.

PATIENT/FAMILY TEACHING

- Instruct patient to notify health care professional immediately if redness, swelling, or pain at injection site occurs.
- Instruct patient to report symptoms of neu-

rotoxicity (paresthesia, pain, difficulty walking, persistent constipation). Inform patient that increased fluid intake, dietary fiber, and exercise may minimize constipation. Stool softeners or laxatives may be used. Patient should inform health care professional if severe constipation or abdominal discomfort occurs, as this may be a sign of neuropathy.

- Advise patient to notify health care professional if fever; chills; sore throat; signs of infection; bleeding gums; bruising; petechiae; blood in urine, stool, or emesis; or mouth sores occur. Caution patient to avoid crowds and persons with known infections.
- Advise patient that this medication may have teratogenic effects. Contraception should be used during and for at least 2 mo after therapy is concluded.
- Discuss with patient the possibility of hair loss. Explore coping strategies.
- Instruct patient not to receive any vaccinations without advice of health care professional.
- Emphasize need for periodic lab tests to monitor for side effects.

EVALUATION

Effectiveness of therapy can be demonstrated by: ▪ Regression of malignancy without the appearance of detrimental side effects.

VINORELBINE

(vine-oh-**rel**-been)

Navelbine

CLASSIFICATION(S):

Antineoplastic (vinca alkaloid)

Pregnancy Category D

INDICATIONS

▪ Used alone or in combination with cisplatin in the treatment of ambulatory patients with inoperable non–small-cell cancer of the lung.

ACTION

▪ Binds to a protein (tubulin) of cellular microtubules, where it interferes with microtubule assembly. Cell replication is stopped as a result (cell cycle–specific for M phase). **Therapeutic Effects:** ▪ Death of rapidly replicating cells, particularly malignant ones.

PHARMACOKINETICS

Absorption: IV administration results in complete bioavailability.

Distribution: Highly bound to platelets and lymphocytes.

Metabolism and Excretion: Mostly metabolized by the liver. At least one metabolite is active. Large amounts eliminated in feces; 11% excreted unchanged by the kidneys.

Half-life: 28–44 hr.

CONTRAINDICATIONS AND PRECAUTIONS

Contraindicated in: ▪ Hypersensitivity ▪ Pregnancy or lactation ▪ Active infections ▪ Decreased bone marrow reserve ▪ Other chronic debilitating illnesses.

Use Cautiously in: ▪ Childbearing potential ▪ Impaired hepatic function (dosage reduction recommended if total bilirubin >2 mg/dl) ▪ Granulocytopenic patients (temporarily discontinue or reduce dose) ▪ Children (safe use not established).

ADVERSE REACTIONS AND SIDE EFFECTS*

CNS: fatigue.

Resp: shortness of breath.

CV: chest pain.

GI: constipation, nausea, anorexia, diarrhea, transient ↑ in liver enzymes, vomiting.

Derm: alopecia, rashes.

Hemat: anemia, neutropenia, thrombocytopenia.

Local: irritation at IV site, skin reactions, phlebitis.

MS: arthralgia, jaw pain, myalgia.

Neuro: neurotoxicity.

INTERACTIONS

Drug-Drug: ▪ Additive bone marrow depression with other **antineoplastic agents** or **radiation therapy** ▪ Concurrent use with **cisplatin** increases the risk and severity of bone marrow depression ▪ Concurrent use with **mitomycin** or **chest radiation** increases the risk of acute pulmonary reactions.

***CAPITALS indicate life-threatening; underlines indicate most frequent.**

ROUTE AND DOSAGE

- **IV (Adults):** 30 mg/m^2 once weekly.

AVAILABILITY

- ***Injection:*** 10 mg/ml[Rx].

TIME/ACTION PROFILE (effect on WBC counts)

	ONSET	PEAK	DURATION
IV	UK	7–10 days	7–15 days

NURSING IMPLICATIONS

ASSESSMENT

- Monitor blood pressure, pulse, and respiratory rate during course of therapy. Note significant changes. Acute shortness of breath and severe bronchospasm may occur infrequently shortly after administration. Treatment with corticosteroids, bronchodilators, and supplemental oxygen may be required, especially in patients with a history of pulmonary disease.
- Assess frequently for signs of infection (sore throat, temperature, cough, mental status changes), especially when nadir of granulocytopenia is expected.
- Monitor neurologic status. Assess for paresthesia (numbness, tingling, pain), loss of deep tendon reflexes (Achilles reflex is usually first involved), weakness (wrist drop or footdrop, gait disturbances), cranial nerve palsies (jaw pain, hoarseness, ptosis, visual changes), autonomic dysfunction (constipation, ileus, difficulty voiding, orthostatic hypotension, impaired sweating), and CNS dysfunction (decreased level of consciousness, agitation, hallucinations). These symptoms may persist for months. The incidence of neurotoxicity associated with vinorelbine is less than that of other vinca alkaloids.
- Monitor intake and output and daily weight for significant discrepancies.
- Assess nutritional status. Mild to moderate nausea is common. An antiemetic may be used to minimize nausea and vomiting.
- Monitor for symptoms of gout (increased uric acid, joint pain, edema). Encourage patient to drink at least 2 liters of fluid/day. Allopurinol and alkalinization of urine may decrease uric acid levels.
- ***Lab Test Considerations:*** Monitor CBC prior to each dose and routinely throughout therapy. The nadir of granulocytopenia usually occurs 7–10 days after vinorelbine administration and recovery usually follows within 7–15 days. If granulocyte count is <1500/mm^3, dosage reduction or temporary interruption of vinorelbine may be warranted. If repeated episodes of fever and/or sepsis occur during granulocytopenia, future dosage of vinorelbine should be modified. May also cause mild to moderate anemia. Thrombocytopenia rarely occurs.
- Monitor liver function studies (AST, ALT, LDH, bilirubin) and renal function studies (BUN, creatinine) prior to and periodically throughout therapy. May cause increased uric acid; monitor periodically during therapy.

POTENTIAL NURSING DIAGNOSES

- Injury, risk for (Adverse Reactions).
- Infection, risk for (Adverse Reactions).
- Knowledge deficit, related to medication regimen (Patient/Family Teaching).

IMPLEMENTATION

- **General Info:** Solution should be prepared in a biologic cabinet. Wear gloves, gown, and mask while handling medication. Discard IV equipment in specially designated containers (see Appendix I).
- Assess infusion site frequently for redness, irritation, or inflammation. Vinorelbine is a vesicant. If extravasation occurs, infusion must be stopped and restarted elsewhere to avoid damage to SC tissue. Treatment of extravasation includes application of warm compresses applied over the area immediately for 30–60 min, then alternating on/off every 15 min for 1 day to increase systemic absorption of the drug. Hyaluronidase 150 U diluted in 1–2 ml of 0.9% NaCl, 1 ml for each ml extravasated, should be injected through existing IV cannula or SC if the needle has been removed to enhance absorption and dispersion of the extravasated drug.
- **Direct IV:** Dilute vinorelbine to a concentration of 1.5–3 mg/ml with 0.9% NaCl or D5W.
- ***Rate:*** Infuse over 6–10 min into Y-site closest to bag of a free-flowing IV or into a central line.
- Flush vein with at least 75–125 ml of 0.9% NaCl or D5W administered over 10 min or more following administration of vinorelbine.

V

- **Intermittent Infusion:** Dilute vinorelbine to a concentration of 0.5–2 mg/ml with 0.9% NaCl, D5W, 0.45% NaCl, D5/0.45% NaCl, Ringer's or lactated Ringer's injection. Solution should be colorless to pale yellow. Do not administer solutions that are discolored or contain particulate matter. Diluted solution is stable for 24 hr at room temperature.
- ***Rate:*** Infuse over 6–10 min into Y-site closest to bag of a free-flowing IV or into a central line.
- □ Flush vein with at least 75–125 ml of 0.9% NaCl or D5W administered over 10 min or more following administration of vinorelbine.
- **Y-Site Compatibility:** ▪ amikacin ▪ aztreonam ▪ bleomycin ▪ bumetanide ▪ buprenorphine ▪ butorphanol ▪ calcium gluconate ▪ carboplatin ▪ carmustine ▪ cefotaxime ▪ ceftazidime ▪ ceftizoxime ▪ ceftriaxone ▪ chlorpromazine ▪ cimetidine ▪ cisplatin ▪ clindamycin ▪ cyclophosphamide ▪ cytarabine ▪ dacarbazine ▪ dactinomycin ▪ daunorubicin ▪ dexamethasone sodium phosphate ▪ diphenhydramine ▪ doxorubicin ▪ doxycycline ▪ droperidol ▪ enalaprilat ▪ etoposide ▪ famotidine ▪ floxuridine ▪ fluconazole ▪ fludarabine ▪ gallium nitrate ▪ gentamicin ▪ haloperidol ▪ heparin ▪ hydrocortisone ▪ hydromorphone ▪ idarubicin ▪ ifosfamide ▪ imipenem/cilastatin ▪ lorazepam ▪ mannitol ▪ mechlorethamine ▪ melphalan ▪ meperidine ▪ mesna ▪ methotrexate ▪ metoclopramide ▪ metronidazole ▪ miconazole ▪ minocycline ▪ mitoxantrone ▪ morphine ▪ nalbuphine ▪ netilmicin ▪ ondansetron ▪ plicamycin ▪ streptozocin ▪ teniposide ▪ ticarcillin ▪ ticarcillin/clavulanate ▪ tobramycin ▪ vancomycin ▪ vinblastine ▪ vincristine ▪ zidovudine.
- **Y-Site Incompatibility:** ▪ acyclovir ▪ aminophylline ▪ amphotericin B ▪ ampicillin ▪ cefazolin ▪ cefoperazone ▪ ceforanide ▪ cefotetan ▪ ceftriaxone ▪ cefuroxime ▪ fluorouracil ▪ furosemide ▪ ganciclovir ▪ methylprednisolone ▪ mitomycin ▪ piperacillin ▪ sodium bicarbonate ▪ thiotepa ▪ trimethoprim/sulfamethoxazole.

PATIENT/FAMILY TEACHING

- □ Instruct patient to report symptoms of neurotoxicity (paresthesia, pain, difficulty walking, persistent constipation).
- □ Inform patient that increased fluid intake, dietary fiber, and exercise may minimize constipation. Stool softeners or laxatives may be necessary. Patient should be advised to report severe constipation or abdominal discomfort, as this may be a sign of ileus, which may occur as a consequence of neuropathy.
- □ Advise patient to notify health care professional if fever; chills; sore throat; signs of infection; bleeding gums; bruising; petechiae; blood in urine, stool, or emesis; or mouth sores occur.
- □ Caution patient to avoid crowds and persons with known infections.
- □ Advise patient that this medication may have teratogenic effects. Contraception should be used during and for at least 2 mo after therapy is concluded.
- □ Discuss with patient the possibility of hair loss and explore coping strategies.
- □ Instruct patient not to receive any vaccinations without advice of health care professional.
- □ Emphasize the need for periodic lab tests to monitor for side effects.

EVALUATION

Effectiveness of therapy can be demonstrated by: ▪ Decrease in the size or spread of malignancy without detrimental side effects.

VITAMIN A

(**vye**-ta-min A)

Aquasol A

CLASSIFICATION(S):

Vitamin (fat-soluble)

Pregnancy Category A (oral), X (parenteral, or doses > RDA)

INDICATIONS

▪ Treatment and prevention of deficiency states ▪ Prevention of vitamin A deficiency in patients who have fat malabsorption or are taking bile acid sequestrants.

ACTION

▪ Serves as a cofactor in many biochemical processes ▪ Necessary for growth, bone development, vision, reproduction, integrity of mucosal and epithelial surfaces, and formation of visual pigment. **Therapeutic Effects:** ▪ Resolution of deficiency signs ▪ Prevention of deficiency.

PHARMACOKINETICS

Absorption: GI absorption requires bile acids, fat, lipase, and protein. Aqueous preparations are absorbed more readily than emulsions.
Distribution: Stored primarily in the liver (2-yr supply); small amounts stored in kidneys and lungs. Does not cross the placenta but enters breast milk.
Metabolism and Excretion: Mostly metabolized by the liver.
Half-life: UK.

CONTRAINDICATIONS AND PRECAUTIONS

Contraindicated in: ▪ Hypervitaminosis A ▪ Malabsorption (oral products) ▪ Hypersensitivity to ingredients in preparations (chlorobutanol, polysorbate 80, butylated hydroxyanisole, butylated hydroxytoluene).
Use Cautiously in: ▪ Lactation (supplements to infant necessary) ▪ Pregnancy (avoid amounts greater than RDA; see Appendix L) ▪ Severely impaired renal function.

ADVERSE REACTIONS AND SIDE EFFECTS

Misc: hypervitaminosis A syndrome.

INTERACTIONS

Drug-Drug: ▪ **Cholestyramine, colestipol,** and **mineral oil** decrease absorption of vitamin A ▪ **Oral contraceptives** increase plasma levels of vitamin A.

ROUTE AND DOSAGE

RE = retinol equivalents. Doses should be individualized on the basis of degree of deficiency.

- **PO (Adults):** *Deficiency*—If xerophthalmia is present, 7500–15,000 RE (25,000–50,000 units)/day.
- **PO (Children ≥1 yr):** *Measles*—60,000 RE (200,000 units) single dose. *Xerophthalmia*—60,000 RE (200,000 units) daily for 2 days; repeat at 4 wk.
- **PO (Children 6 mo–1 yr):** *Measles*—30,000 RE (100,000 units) single dose. *Xerophthalmia*—30,000 RE (100,000 units) daily for 2 days; repeat at 4 wk.
- **IM (Adults and Children ≥8 yr):** 15,000–30,000 RE (50,000–100,000 units)/day for 3 days; then 15,000 RE (50,000 units)/day for 2 wk.
- **IM (Children 1–8 yr):** 5000–35,000 units/day for 10 days.
- **IM (Children <1 yr):** 1500–4500 RE (5000–15,000 units)/day for 10 days.
- **IV (Adults and Children):** Infused as part of TPN in amounts required to meet nutritional needs (in parenteral multivitamin preparations).

AVAILABILITY

▪ ***Capsules:*** 3000 RE (10,000 units)[Rx,OTC], 7500 RE (25,000 units)[Rx], 15,000 RE (50,000 units)[Rx] ▪ ***Tablets:*** 3000 RE (10,000 units)[Rx,OTC], 7500 RE (25,000 units)[Rx,OTC], 15,000 RE (50,000 units)[Rx] ▪ ***Oral solution:*** 1500 RE (5000 units)/0.1 ml in 30-ml containers[Rx] ▪ ***Injection:*** 50,000 units/ml in 2-ml vials[Rx] ▪ ***In combination with:*** other vitamins and minerals (see multiple vitamins on p. 683).

TIME/ACTION PROFILE

	ONSET	PEAK	DURATION
PO	UK	UK	UK
IM	UK	UK	UK

V

NURSING IMPLICATIONS

ASSESSMENT

- □ Assess patient for signs of vitamin A deficiency (night blindness; frequent eye, ear, sinus, and GU infections; dry mucous membranes; rough, scaly skin with goose pimple–like lesions; photophobia; and dry eyes) prior to and periodically throughout therapy.
- □ Assess nutritional status through 24-hr diet recall. Determine frequency of consumption of vitamin A–rich foods.
- ▪ ***Lab Test Considerations:*** Chronic toxicity may cause increased blood glucose, calcium, BUN, cholesterol, and triglyceride levels.
- □ Plasma vitamin A and carotene levels may be evaluated prior to therapy to determine vitamin A deficiency.
- □ With high doses, erythrocyte and leukocyte counts may be decreased, and erythrocyte sedimentation rate (ESR) and prothrombin time (PT) may be increased.

POTENTIAL NURSING DIAGNOSES

- ▪ Nutrition, altered, less than body requirements (Indications).

- Knowledge deficit, related to medication regimen (Patient/Family Teaching).

IMPLEMENTATION

- **PO:** Administer with or after meals.
- Solution may be dropped directly into mouth or mixed with cereal, fruit juice, or other food. Use calibrated dropper supplied by manufacturer to measure solution accurately.
- **IM:** Parenteral administration is indicated only when oral administration is not possible (because of malabsorption, NPO status, vomiting, or severe ocular damage).
- Do not administer vitamin A intravenously because of the risk of anaphylactic shock and death.

PATIENT/FAMILY TEACHING

- Instruct patient to take medication as directed. If a dose is missed, it should be omitted, as fat-soluble vitamins are stored in the body for long periods.
- Encourage patient to comply with diet recommendations of health care professional. Explain that the best source of vitamins is a well-balanced diet with foods from the four basic food groups.
- Foods high in vitamin A include liver, fish liver oils, egg yolks, yellow-orange fruits and vegetables, dark green leafy vegetables, whole milk, vitamin A–fortified skim milk, butter, and margarine. Ordinary cooking does not destroy vitamin A, but frozen foods lose 5–10% during storage for 12 mo.
- Patients self-medicating with vitamin supplements should be cautioned not to exceed RDA (see Appendix L). The effectiveness of megadoses for treatment of various medical conditions is unproved, and this may cause side effects and toxicity.
- Review symptoms of hypervitaminosis A syndrome (headaches, bulging fontanelles in infants, irritability, yellow-orange discoloration of skin, drying and desquamation of skin and lips, hair loss, anorexia, vomiting, joint and bone pain). Instruct patient to report these symptoms promptly to health care professional.
- Advise patient that mineral oil may interfere with the absorption of fat-soluble vitamins and should not be used concurrently.
- Emphasize the importance of follow-up exams to evaluate progress. Ophthalmologic exams may be required prior to and periodically throughout therapy.

EVALUATION

Effectiveness of therapy can be demonstrated by: ▪ Prevention of or decrease in the symptoms of vitamin A deficiency.

VITAMIN B COMPLEX WITH VITAMIN C

Oral

Albee-T, Albee with C, Arcobee with C, B-Complex/Vitamin C, Beminal, Econo B & C, Enviro-Stress, Farbee with Vitamin C, Gen-bee with C, High Potency N-Vites, Nion B Plus C, Probec-T, Sublingual B Total Liquid, Surbex T, Surbu-Gen-T, Surplex-T, Therapeutic B Complex with C, ThexForte, T-Vites, Vicon-C, Viogen-C, Vita-Bee with C

Parenteral

Key Plex, Neurodep, Vicam

CLASSIFICATION(S):

Vitamin (water-soluble)

Pregnancy Category UK

INDICATIONS

- Treatment and prevention of vitamin deficiencies.

ACTION

- Contain most or all of the B-complex vitamins (B_1, B_2, B_3, B_5, B_6, B_{12}) and vitamin C, a diverse group of compounds necessary for normal growth and development that act as coenzymes or catalysts in numerous metabolic processes. **Therapeutic Effects:** ▪ Replacement of vitamins in patients who are deficient or at risk for deficiency.

PHARMACOKINETICS

Absorption: Well absorbed following oral administration. Some absorptive processes require cofactors (B_{12}).

Distribution: Widely distributed; crosses the placenta and enters breast milk.
Metabolism and Excretion: Used in various biologic processes. Excess amounts are excreted unchanged by the kidneys.
Half-life: UK.

CONTRAINDICATIONS AND PRECAUTIONS

Contraindicated in: ▪ Hypersensitivity to ingredients in preparations (benzyl alcohol, parabens, bisulfites, tartrazine).
Use Cautiously in: ▪ Undiagnosed anemias.

ADVERSE REACTIONS AND SIDE EFFECTS*

In recommended doses, adverse reactions are extremely rare.
Misc: ANAPHYLAXIS (vitamin B_1-thiamine), allergic reactions to preservatives.

INTERACTIONS

Drug-Drug: ▪ Large amounts of vitamin B_6 may interfere with the beneficial effect of **levodopa.**

ROUTE AND DOSAGE

- **PO, IV (Adults and Children):** Amount sufficient to meet RDA for age group (see table in Appendix L).

AVAILABILITY

▪ ***Tablets, capsules, sublingual liquid:*** contain vitamins B_1 (6–50 mg); B_2 (5–50 mg); B_3 (20–150 mg); B_5 (10–50 mg); B_6 (4–50 mg); vitamin B_{12} (0–1000 mcg); and vitamin C (50–600 mg) per tablet, capsule, or ml[OTC] ▪ ***In combination with:*** folic acid, biotin, chromium, soy protein, brewers yeast, potassium, manganese, and zinc in multivitamin/mineral products[Rx,OTC] ▪ ***Injection:*** contains vitamin B_1 (50 mg), B_2 (5 mg), B_3 (125 mg), B_5 (6 mg), B_{12} (1000 mcg), and vitamin C (50 mg/ml)[Rx].

TIME/ACTION PROFILE

	ONSET	PEAK	DURATION
PO	UK	UK	UK

NURSING IMPLICATIONS

ASSESSMENT

- Assess patient for signs of vitamin deficiency prior to and periodically throughout therapy. Assess nutritional status through 24-hr diet recall. Determine frequency of consumption of vitamin-rich foods. Therapy is limited to periods of high physiologic stress when patient is not able to ingest adequate vitamins orally.
- Monitor patient for anaphylaxis (wheezing, urticaria, edema); contains thiamine.

POTENTIAL NURSING DIAGNOSES

- Nutrition, altered, less than body requirements (Indications).
- Knowledge deficit, related to medication regimen (Patient/Family Teaching).

IMPLEMENTATION

- **Continuous Infusion:** Usually administered as part of a large-volume parenteral admixture.

PATIENT/FAMILY TEACHING

- Encourage patient to comply with diet recommendations of health care professional. Explain that the best source of vitamins is a well-balanced diet with foods from the four basic food groups.

EVALUATION

Effectiveness of therapy can be demonstrated by: ▪ Prevention of or decrease in the symptoms of vitamin deficiencies.

VITAMIN B_{12} PREPARATIONS

cyanocobalamin

(sye-an-oh-koe-**bal**-a-min)
{Anacobin}, {Bedoz}, Cobex, Cobolin-M, Crystamine, Crysti-1000, Cyanoject, Cyomin, Ener-B, Neuroforte-R, Primabalt, Rubesol-1000, Rubramin PC, Shovite, Vibal, Vitabee-12

*CAPITALS indicate life-threatening; underlines indicate most frequent.
{} = Available in Canada only.

hydroxocobalamin
(hye-drox-oh-koe-**bal**-a-min)
Alphamin, Hydrobexan, Hydro Cobex, Hydro-Crysti-12, Hydroxy-Cobal, LA-12, Vibal LA, vitamin B_{12}

CLASSIFICATION(S):
Antianemic, Vitamin (water-soluble)

Pregnancy Category C

INDICATIONS

▪ Treatment and prevention of vitamin B_{12} deficiency ▪ Treatment of pernicious anemia ▪ Used diagnostically as part of the Schilling test.

ACTION

▪ A necessary coenzyme for many metabolic processes, including fat and carbohydrate metabolism and protein synthesis ▪ Required for the formation of red blood cells. **Therapeutic Effects:** ▪ Correction of manifestations of pernicious anemia (megaloblastic indices, GI lesions, and neurologic damage) ▪ Prevention of vitamin B_{12} deficiency.

PHARMACOKINETICS

Absorption: Absorption from the GI tract requires intrinsic factor and calcium (only 5 mcg/day may be absorbed); well absorbed following IM and SC administration. 89% absorbed from nasal mucosa.
Distribution: Stored in the liver; crosses the placenta and enters breast milk.
Metabolism and Excretion: Excess amounts are eliminated unchanged in the urine.
Half-life: 6 days (400 days in liver).

CONTRAINDICATIONS AND PRECAUTIONS

Contraindicated in: ▪ Hypersensitivity ▪ Hereditary optic nerve atrophy (accelerates nerve damage) ▪ Avoid using benzyl alcohol–containing preparations in premature infants (associated with fatal "gasping syndrome").
Use Cautiously in: ▪ Cardiac disease ▪ Uremia, folic acid deficiency, concurrent infection, iron deficiency (response to B_{12} will be impaired).

ADVERSE REACTIONS AND SIDE EFFECTS*

CV: peripheral vascular thrombosis.
GI: diarrhea.
Derm: itching, swelling of the body, urticaria.
F and E: hypokalemia.
Local: pain at IM site.
Misc: hypersensitivity reactions including ANAPHYLAXIS.

INTERACTIONS

Drug-Drug: ▪ **Chloramphenicol** and **antineoplastic agents** may decrease the hematologic response to vitamin B_{12} ▪ **Aminoglycosides, colchicine, extended-release potassium supplements, aminosalicylic acid, anticonvulsants, cimetidine,** excess intake of **alcohol,** or **vitamin C** may decrease oral absorption/effectiveness of vitamin B_{12}.

ROUTE AND DOSAGE

❑ Cyanocobalamin Deficiency

- **PO (Adults and Children):** Amount depends on degree of deficiency; up to 1000 mcg/day.
- **IM, SC (Adults):** 30–100 mcg/day for 6–7 days; then 100–200 mcg/month. (Doses up to 1000 mcg have been used.) "Flushing" dose for Schilling test is 1000 mcg.
- **IM, SC (Children):** 30–50 mcg/day for 14 or more days; then 100 mcg/month. (Doses up to 1000 mcg have been used.) "Flushing" dose for Schilling test is 1000 mcg.
- **Intranasal:** 500 mcg (one spray in one nostril) once weekly.

❑ Hydroxocobalamin Deficiency

- **IM, SC (Adults):** 30–50 mcg/day for 5–10 days; then 100–200 mcg monthly. "Flushing" dose for Schilling test is 1000 mcg.
- **IM, SC (Children):** 30–50 mcg/day for 5–10 days; then 100 mcg monthly.

AVAILABILITY

❑ Cyanocobalamin

▪ ***Tablets:*** {25 mcg^{OTC}}, {50 mcg^{OTC}}, {100 mcg^{OTC}}, {250 mcg^{OTC}}, 500 mcg^{OTC}, 1000 mcg^{OTC} ▪ ***Extended-release tablets:*** {100 mcg^{OTC}}, {200 mcg^{OTC}}, 500 mcg^{OTC}, 1000

*CAPITALS indicate life-threatening; underlines indicate most frequent.

mcg[OTC] ▪ ***Nasal gel:*** 500 mcg/spray (8 sprays/bottle) ▪ ***Injection:*** 100 mcg/ml in 30-ml vials[Rx], 1000 mcg/ml in 10- and 30-ml vials[Rx].

□ **Hydroxocobalamin**

▪ ***Injection:*** 1000 mcg/ml in 30-ml vials[Rx].

TIME/ACTION PROFILE (reticulocytosis)

	ONSET	PEAK	DURATION
Cyanocobalamin IM, SC, nasal	UK	3–10 days	UK
Hydroxocobalamin IM, SC	UK	3–10 days	UK

NURSING IMPLICATIONS

ASSESSMENT

□ Assess patient for signs of vitamin B_{12} deficiency (pallor; neuropathy; psychosis; red, inflamed tongue) prior to and periodically throughout therapy.

▪ ***Lab Test Considerations:*** Monitor plasma folic acid levels, reticulocyte count, and plasma vitamin B_{12} levels prior to and between the 5th and 7th day of therapy. Patients receiving vitamin B_{12} for megaloblastic anemia should have serum potassium level evaluated for hypokalemia during the first 48 hr of treatment. Patients with pernicious anemia should be monitored every 5–6 mo.

POTENTIAL NURSING DIAGNOSES

▪ Nutrition, altered, less than body requirements (Indications).

▪ Activity intolerance (Indications).

▪ Knowledge deficit, related to medication regimen (Patient/Family Teaching).

IMPLEMENTATION

▪ **General Info:** Usually administered in combination with other vitamins, as solitary vitamin B deficiencies are rare.

□ Administration of vitamin B_{12} by the oral route is useful only for nutritional deficiencies. Patients with small bowel disease, malabsorption syndrome, or gastric or ileal resections require parenteral administration.

▪ **PO:** Administer with meals to increase absorption.

□ May be mixed with fruit juices. Administer immediately after mixing, as ascorbic acid alters stability.

▪ **IV:** IV route is not recommended; however, small amounts of cyanocobalamin may be admixed in TPN solutions.

▪ **Y-Site Compatibility:** ▪ heparin ▪ hydrocortisone sodium succinate ▪ potassium chloride ▪ vitamin B complex with C.

▪ **Additive/Solution Compatibility:** ▪ dextrose/Ringer's or lactated Ringer's combinations ▪ dextrose/saline combinations ▪ D5W ▪ D10W ▪ 0.45% NaCl ▪ 0.9% NaCl ▪ Ringer's or lactated Ringer's solution ▪ ascorbic acid ▪ vitamin B complex with C.

▪ **Intranasal:** Dose should not be administered within 1 hr of hot food or fluids.

PATIENT/FAMILY TEACHING

▪ **General Info:** Encourage patient to comply with diet recommendations of health care professional. Explain that the best source of vitamins is a well-balanced diet with foods from the four basic food groups.

□ Foods high in vitamin B_{12} include meats, seafood, egg yolk, and fermented cheeses; few vitamins are lost with ordinary cooking.

□ Patients self-medicating with vitamin supplements should be cautioned not to exceed RDA (see Appendix L). Effectiveness of megadoses for treatment of various medical conditions is unproved and may cause side effects.

□ Inform patients of the lifelong need for vitamin B_{12} replacement following gastrectomy or ileal resection.

□ Emphasize the importance of follow-up exams to evaluate progress.

▪ **Intranasal:** Instruct patient in proper administration technique. Unit must be primed with 3 strokes if not used for 18 hr or longer. Advise patient to clear nose, then place tip approximately 1 in. into nostril and press pump once, firmly and quickly. After dose, remove unit from nose and massage dosed nostril gently for a few seconds. Vial delivers 8 doses.

EVALUATION

Effectiveness of therapy can be demonstrated by: ▪ Resolution of the symptoms of vitamin B_{12} deficiency □ Increase in reticulocyte count ▪ Improvement in manifestations of pernicious anemia.

VITAMIN D COMPOUNDS

calcitriol
(kal-si-**trye**-ole)
1,25-dihydroxycholecalciferol, Calcijex, Rocaltrol, vitamin D_3

dihydrotachysterol
(dye-hye-droh-tak-**iss**-ter-ole)
DHT, Hytakerol

ergocalciferol
(er-goe-kal-**sif**-e-role)
Calciferol, Deltalin, Drisdol, {Ostoforte}, {Radiostol}, vitamin D_2

CLASSIFICATION(S):
Vitamins (fat-soluble)

Pregnancy Category C

INDICATIONS

▪ **Calcitriol:** Management of hypocalcemia in chronic renal failure patients ▪ Treatment of hypoparathyroidism or pseudohypoparathyroidism ▪ **Dihydrotachysterol:** Treatment of hypophosphatemia ▪ Treatment of hypocalcemia ▪ Prevention and treatment of rickets ▪ Prevention and treatment of vitamin D deficiency ▪ Prevention and treatment of postoperative and idiopathic tetany ▪ **Ergocalciferol:** Prophylaxis and treatment of vitamin D deficiency ▪ Treatment of hypophosphatemia or hypocalcemia ▪ Treatment of osteodystrophy ▪ Treatment of osteomalacia secondary to chronic anticonvulsant therapy ▪ Treatment of rickets.

ACTION

▪ Dihydrotachysterol and ergocalciferol are inactive forms of vitamin D; activation occurs in the liver and kidneys. Calcitriol is the active form ▪ Vitamin D ▫ Promotes the absorption of calcium and phosphorus ▫ Regulates calcium homeostasis in conjunction with parathyroid hormone and calcitonin. **Therapeutic Effects:** ▪ Treatment and prevention of deficiency states, particularly bone manifestations.

PHARMACOKINETICS

Absorption: *Calcitriol*—Well absorbed following oral administration. *Dihydrotachysterol, ergocalciferol*—Well absorbed in an inactive form.
Distribution: Stored in the liver and other fatty tissues; calcitriol crosses the placenta.
Metabolism and Excretion: *Calcitriol*—Undergoes enterohepatic recycling and is excreted mostly in bile. *Dihydrotachysterol, ergocalciferol*—Converted to active form by sunlight, the liver, and the kidneys.
Half-life: *Calcitriol*—3–8 hr.

CONTRAINDICATIONS AND PRECAUTIONS

Contraindicated in: ▪ Hypersensitivity ▪ Hypercalcemia ▪ Vitamin D toxicity ▪ Lactation (large doses).
Use Cautiously in: ▪ Sarcoidosis ▪ Hyperparathyroidism ▪ Patients receiving digitalis glycosides ▪ Pregnancy (larger doses; safety not established).

ADVERSE REACTIONS AND SIDE EFFECTS

Seen primarily as manifestations of toxicity (hypercalcemia).
CNS: headache, somnolence, weakness.
EENT: conjunctivitis, photophobia, rhinorrhea.
CV: arrhythmias, hypertension.
GI: anorexia, constipation, dry mouth, metallic taste, nausea, polydipsia, vomiting, weight loss.
GU: albuminuria, decreased libido, nocturia, polyuria.
Derm: pruritus.
F and E: hypercalcemia.
Metab: hyperthermia.
MS: bone pain, muscle pain.

INTERACTIONS

Drug-Drug: ▪ **Cholestyramine, colestipol,** or **mineral oil** decreases absorption of vitamin D analogues ▪ Use with **thiazide diuretics** in patients with hypoparathyroidism may result in hypercalcemia ▪ **Glucocorticoids** decrease the effectiveness of vitamin D analogues ▪ Use with **digitalis glycosides** increases the risk of arrhythmias ▪ Vitamin D requirements are increased by **phenytoin** and other **hydantoin anticonvulsants, sucralfate, barbiturates,** and **primidone** ▪ Use with caution in patients

receiving **magnesium-containing antacids** or **calcium-containing drugs.**
Drug-Food: ▪ Ingestion of **foods high in calcium content** (see Appendix K) may lead to hypercalcemia.

ROUTE AND DOSAGE

❑ Calcitriol

- **PO (Adults):** *Hypocalcemia during chronic dialysis*—0.5–3 mcg/day (larger doses have been used). *Hypoparathyroidism*—0.25–2.7 mcg/day. *Renal osteodystrophy*—0.25 mcg every other day–3 mcg/day (larger doses have been used).
- **PO (Children):** *Hypocalcemia during chronic dialysis*—0.25–2 mcg/day. *Hypoparathyroidism*—0.04–0.08 mcg/kg/day. *Renal osteodystrophy*—0.014–0.041 mcg/kg/day. Children with liver disease may require larger initial doses.
- **IV (Adults):** *Initial*—0.5 mcg (0.01 mcg/kg) 3 times weekly. May be increased by 0.25–0.5 mcg/dose at 2- to 4-wk intervals. *Maintenance*—0.5–3.0 mcg 3 times weekly (0.01–0.05 mcg/kg 3 times weekly).

❑ Dihydrotachysterol

- **PO (Adults):** *Hypocalcemic tetany*—0.75–2.5 mg/day for 3 days initially; then 0.25/week–1 mg/day. *Hypoparathyroidism/pseudohypoparathyroidism*—0.75–2.5 mg/day initially for several days; then 0.2–1 mg/day (up to 1.5 mg/day). *Renal osteodystrophy*—0.1–0.25 mg/day initially; then 0.2–1 mg/day.
- **PO (Children):** *Hypoparathyroidism/pseudohypoparathyroidism*—1–5 mg/day for 4 days; then 0.5–1.5 mg/day.

❑ Ergocalciferol

- **PO (Adults):** *Vitamin D deficiency*—Depends on degree of deficiency. *Vitamin D–resistant rickets*—12,000–150,000 units/day. *Vitamin D–dependent rickets*—10,000–60,000 units/day (up to 150,000 units/day). *Familial hypophosphatemia*—50,000–100,000 units/day. *Osteomalacia from anticonvulsants*—1000–4000 units/day. *Hypoparathyroidism*—50,000–150,000 units/day.
- **PO (Children):** *Vitamin D deficiency*—Depends on degree of deficiency. *Vitamin D–dependent rickets*—3000–10,000 units/day (up to 50,000 units/day). *Osteomalacia from anticonvulsants*—1000 units/day. *Hypoparathyroidism*—50,000–200,000 units/day.
- **IM (Adults and Children):** *Malabsorption*—10,000 units/day.
- **IV (Adults and Children):** As part of TPN, amount determined by need on an individual basis.

AVAILABILITY

❑ Calcitriol

▪ ***Capsules:*** 0.25 mcg^Rx^, 0.5 mcg^Rx^ ▪ ***Injection:*** 1 mcg/ml in 1-ml ampules^Rx^, 2 mcg/ml in 1-ml ampules^Rx^.

❑ Dihydrotachysterol

▪ ***Tablets:*** 0.125 mg^Rx^, 0.2 mg^Rx^, 0.4 mg^Rx^ ▪ ***Capsules:*** 0.125 mg^Rx^ ▪ ***Oral solution:*** 0.2 mg/ml in 30-ml bottles^Rx^.

❑ Ergocalciferol

▪ ***Liquid:*** 8000 units/ml in 60-ml bottles^Rx,OTC^ ▪ ***Capsules:*** 50,000 units^Rx^ ▪ ***Tablets:*** 50,000 units^Rx^ ▪ ***Injection:*** 500,000 units/ml in 1-ml ampules^Rx^.

V

TIME/ACTION PROFILE (effects on serum calcium)

	ONSET	PEAK	DURATION
Calcitriol-PO	2–6 hr	2–6 hr	3–5 days
Calcitriol-IV	UK	UK	UK
Dihydrotachysterol-PO	several hr	1–2 wk	2 wk
Ergocalciferol-PO	12–24 hr*	UK	up to 6 mo

*Therapeutic effect may take 10–14 days.

NURSING IMPLICATIONS

ASSESSMENT

- ❑ Assess for symptoms of vitamin deficiency prior to and periodically throughout therapy.
- ❑ Assess patient for bone pain and weakness prior to and throughout therapy.
- ❑ Observe patient carefully for evidence of hypocalcemia (paresthesia, muscle twitching, laryngospasm, colic, cardiac arrhythmias, and Chvostek's or Trousseau's sign). Protect symptomatic patient by raising and padding side rails; keep bed in low position.
- ▪ **Children:** Monitor height and weight; growth arrest may occur in prolonged high-dose therapy.

- **Ricketts/Osteomalacia:** Assess patient for bone pain and weakness prior to and throughout therapy.
- ***Lab Test Considerations:*** Serum ionized calcium concentrations should be drawn weekly during initial therapy.
- □ Monitor BUN, serum creatinine, alkaline phosphatase, parathyroid hormone levels, urinary calcium/creatinine ratio, 24-hr urinary calcium periodically.
- □ Monitor serum phosphorus levels prior to and periodically throughout course of therapy. Serum phosphorus must be controlled prior to initiating calcitriol. Aluminum carbonate or aluminum hydroxide is used for this purpose in dialysis patients.
- □ A fall in alkaline phosphatase levels may signal onset of hypercalcemia. Overdosage is associated with a serum calcium times phosphate ($Ca \times P$) level of >70 and elevated BUN, AST, and ALT.
- □ May cause false elevated cholesterol levels.
- ***Toxicity and Overdose:*** Toxicity is manifested as hypercalcemia, hypercalciuria, and hyperphosphatemia. Assess patient for appearance of nausea, vomiting, anorexia, weakness, constipation, headache, bone pain, and metallic taste. Later symptoms include polyuria, polydipsia, photophobia, rhinorrhea, pruritus, and cardiac arrhythmias. Notify physician or other health care professional immediately if these signs of hypervitaminosis D occur. Treatment usually consists of discontinuation of calcitriol, a low-calcium diet, use of low-calcium dialysate in peritoneal dialysis patients, and administration of a laxative. IV hydration and loop diuretics may be ordered to increase urinary excretion of calcium. Hemodialysis may also be used.

POTENTIAL NURSING DIAGNOSES

- Nutrition, altered, less than body requirements (Indications).
- Knowledge deficit, related to medication regimen (Patient/Family Teaching).

IMPLEMENTATION

- **General Info:** Because solitary vitamin deficiencies are rare, combinations are commonly administered.
- **PO:** May be administered without regard to meals. Measure solution accurately with calibrated dropper provided by manufacturer. May be mixed with juice, cereal, or food, or dropped directly into mouth.
- **IM:** *Ergocalciferol* injection is oil-based; avoid IV administration.
- **Direct IV:** Administer *calcitriol* by rapid injection through the catheter at the end of a hemodialysis period.

PATIENT/FAMILY TEACHING

- □ Advise patient to take medication exactly as directed. If a dose is missed, tell patient to take as soon as remembered that day, unless almost time for next dose; do not double up on doses.
- □ Review diet modifications with patient. See Appendix K for foods high in calcium and vitamin D. Renal patients must still consider renal failure diet in food selection. Health care professional may order concurrent calcium supplement.
- □ Encourage patient to comply with diet recommendations of health care professional. Explain that the best source of vitamins is a well-balanced diet with foods from the four basic food groups and the importance of sunlight exposure. See Appendix K for foods high in vitamin D.
- □ Patients self-medicating with vitamin supplements should be cautioned not to exceed RDA (see Appendix L). The effectiveness of megadoses for treatment of various medical conditions is unproved and may cause side effects.
- □ Advise patient to avoid concurrent use of antacids containing magnesium.
- □ Review symptoms of overdosage and instruct patient to report these promptly to health care professional.
- □ Emphasize the importance of follow-up exams to evaluate progress.

EVALUATION

Effectiveness of therapy can be demonstrated by: ▪ Normalization of serum calcium and parathyroid hormone levels ▪ Decreased bone pain and weakness in patients with renal osteodystrophy ▪ Improvement in symptoms of vitamin D–resistant rickets.

VITAMIN E

(**vye**-ta-min E)
alpha tocopherol, Amino-Opti-E, Aquasol E, E-200, E-400, E-1000, E-Complex-600, E-Vitamin, Liqui-E, Pheryl-E, Vita Plus E, {Webber Vitamin E}

CLASSIFICATION(S):
Vitamin (fat-soluble)

Pregnancy Category A (doses within RDA), C (doses > RDA)

INDICATIONS

▪ **PO:** Used as a dietary supplement ▪ Used in low-birth-weight infants to prevent and treat hemolysis due to vitamin E deficiency ▪ **Topical:** Treatment of irritated, chapped, or dry skin. **Unlabeled Uses:** ▪ Prevention of coronary artery disease.

ACTION

▪ Prevents the oxidation (antioxidant) of other substances ▪ Protects red blood cell membranes against hemolysis, especially in low-birth-weight neonates. **Therapeutic Effects:** ▪ Prevention and treatment of deficiency in high-risk patients.

PHARMACOKINETICS

Absorption: 20–80% absorbed following oral administration. Absorption requires fat and bile salts.
Distribution: Widely distributed, stored in adipose tissue (4-yr supply).
Metabolism and Excretion: Metabolized by the liver, excreted in bile.
Half-life: UK.

CONTRAINDICATIONS AND PRECAUTIONS

Contraindicated in: ▪ Hypersensitivity to ingredients in preparations (parabens, propylene, glycol).
Use Cautiously in: ▪ Anemia due to iron deficiency ▪ Low-birth-weight infants (oral administration may cause necrotizing enterocolitis) ▪ Vitamin K deficiency (may increase risk of bleeding).

ADVERSE REACTIONS AND SIDE EFFECTS*

Seen primarily with large doses over long periods of time.
CNS: fatigue, headache, weakness.
EENT: blurred vision.
GI: NECROTIZING ENTEROCOLITIS (oral administration in low-birth-weight infants), cramps, diarrhea, nausea.
Derm: rash.
Endo: gonadal dysfunction.

INTERACTIONS

Drug-Drug: ▪ **Cholestyramine, colestipol, mineral oil,** and **sucralfate** decrease absorption ▪ May decrease hematologic response to **iron supplements** ▪ May increase the risk of bleeding with **warfarin.**

ROUTE AND DOSAGE

Other dosing regimens may be used.
- **PO (Adults and Children):** Determined by nutritional intake or degree of deficiency.
- **Topical (Adults and Children):** Apply to affected areas as needed.

AVAILABILITY

▪ ***Capsules:*** 100 units^OTC^, 200 units^OTC^, 400 units^OTC^, 600 units^OTC^, {800 units^OTC^}, 1000 units^OTC^ ▪ ***Oral solution:*** 26.6 units/ml^OTC^, 50 units/ml^OTC^, 77 units/ml^OTC^ ▪ ***Tablets:*** 100 units^OTC^, 200 units^OTC^, 400 units^OTC^, 500 units^OTC^, 800 units^OTC^ ▪ ***Chewable tablets:*** 400 units^OTC^ ▪ ***Ointment:*** ^OTC^ ▪ ***Cream:*** ^OTC^ ▪ ***Lotion:*** ^OTC^ ▪ ***Oil:*** ^OTC^.

TIME/ACTION PROFILE

	ONSET	PEAK	DURATION
PO	UK	UK	UK

NURSING IMPLICATIONS

ASSESSMENT

☐ Assess patient for signs of vitamin E deficiency (*neonates*—irritability, edema, hemolytic

{} = Available in Canada only.
*CAPITALS indicate life-threatening; underlines indicate most frequent.

anemia, creatinuria; *adults/children [rare]*—muscle weakness, ceroid deposits, anemia, creatinuria) prior to and periodically throughout therapy.
- □ Assess nutritional status through 24-hr diet recall. Determine frequency of consumption of vitamin E–rich foods.
- ▪ ***Lab Test Considerations:*** Large doses may increase cholesterol, triglyceride, and CPK levels.

POTENTIAL NURSING DIAGNOSES

- ▪ Nutrition, altered, less than body requirements (Indications).
- ▪ Knowledge deficit, related to medication regimen (Patient/Family Teaching).

IMPLEMENTATION

- ▪ **PO:** Administer with or after meals.
- □ Chewable tablets should be chewed well or crushed before swallowing. Solution may be dropped directly into mouth or mixed with cereal, fruit juice, or other food. Use calibrated dropper supplied by manufacturer to measure solution accurately.

PATIENT/FAMILY TEACHING

- □ Instruct patient to take medication as directed. If a dose is missed, it should be omitted, as fat-soluble vitamins are stored in the body for long periods.
- □ Encourage patient to comply with diet recommendations of health care professional. Explain that the best source of vitamins is a well-balanced diet with foods from the four basic food groups.
- □ Foods high in vitamin E include vegetable oils, wheat germ, whole-grain cereals, egg yolk, and liver. Vitamin E content is not markedly affected by cooking.
- □ Patients self-medicating with vitamin supplements should be cautioned not to exceed RDA (see Appendix L). The effectiveness of megadoses for treatment of various medical conditions is unproved, and this may cause side effects and toxicity.
- □ Review symptoms of overdosage (blurred vision, flu-like symptoms, headache, breast enlargement). Instruct patient to report these promptly to health care professional.
- □ Mineral oil may interfere with the absorption of fat-soluble vitamins and should not be used concurrently.

EVALUATION

Effectiveness of therapy can be demonstrated by: ▪ Prevention of or decrease in the symptoms of vitamin E deficiency ▪ Control of dry or chapped skin.

WARFARIN

(war-fa-rin)

Coumadin, {Warfilone}

CLASSIFICATION(S):

Anticoagulant

Pregnancy Category UK

INDICATIONS

▪ Prophylaxis and treatment of: □ Venous thrombosis □ Pulmonary embolism □ Atrial fibrillation with embolization ▪ Management of myocardial infarction to: □ Decrease risk of death □ Decrease risk of subsequent myocardial infarction □ Decrease risk of future thromboembolic events ▪ Prevention of thrombus formation and embolization after prosthetic valve placement.

ACTION

▪ Interferes with hepatic synthesis of vitamin K–dependent clotting factors (II, VII, IX, and X). **Therapeutic Effects:** ▪ Prevention of thromboembolic events.

PHARMACOKINETICS

Absorption: Well absorbed from the GI tract following oral administration.
Distribution: Crosses the placenta but does not enter breast milk.
Metabolism and Excretion: Metabolized by the liver.
Half-life: 0.5–3 days.

CONTRAINDICATIONS AND PRECAUTIONS

Contraindicated in: ▪ Pregnancy ▪ Uncontrolled bleeding ▪ Open wounds ▪ Active ulcer disease ▪ Recent brain, eye, or spinal cord injury or surgery ▪ Severe liver disease ▪ Uncontrolled hypertension.

Use Cautiously in: ▪ Malignancy ▪ Patients with history of ulcer or liver disease ▪ History of poor compliance ▪ Women with childbearing potential.

ADVERSE REACTIONS AND SIDE EFFECTS*

GI: cramps, nausea.
Derm: dermal necrosis.
Hemat: BLEEDING.
Misc: fever.

INTERACTIONS

Drug-Drug: ▪ **Abciximab, androgens, cefamandole, cefoperazone, cefotetan, chloral hydrate, chloramphenicol, clopidogrel, disulfiram, fluconazole, fluoroquinolones, itraconazole, metronidazole, plicamycin, thrombolytic agents, ticlopidine, sulfonamides, quinidine, NSAIDs, valproates,** and **aspirin** may increase the response to warfarin and increase the risk of bleeding ▪ **Alcohol, barbiturates,** and **oral contraceptives containing estrogen** may decrease the anticoagulant response to warfarin ▪ Many **other drugs** may affect the activity of warfarin.
Drug-Food: ▪ Ingestion of large quantities of **foods high in vitamin K content** (see list in Appendix K) may antagonize the anticoagulant effect of warfarin.

ROUTE AND DOSAGE

- **PO, IV (Adults):** 2.5–10 mg/day for 2–4 days; then adjust daily dose by results of prothrombin time or INR. Initiate therapy with lower doses in elderly or debilitated patients (usual range 2–10 mg/day).

AVAILABILITY

▪ ***Tablets:*** 1 mg[Rx], 2 mg[Rx], 2.5 mg[Rx], 3 mg[Rx], 4 mg[Rx], 5 mg[Rx], 6 mg[Rx], 7.5 mg[Rx], 10 mg[Rx] ▪ ***Injection:*** 5 mg/vial[Rx].

TIME/ACTION PROFILE (effects on coagulation tests)

	ONSET	PEAK	DURATION
PO, IV	several hr	0.5–3 days	2–5 days

NURSING IMPLICATIONS

ASSESSMENT

- Assess patient for signs of bleeding and hemorrhage (bleeding gums; nosebleed; unusual bruising; tarry, black stools; hematuria; fall in hematocrit or blood pressure; guaiac-positive stools, urine, or nasogastric aspirate).
- Assess patient for evidence of additional or increased thrombosis. Symptoms will depend on area of involvement.
- ***Lab Test Considerations:*** Prothrombin time (PT) and other clotting factors should be monitored frequently during therapy. Therapeutic PT ranges from 1.3–1.5 times greater than control. May also be reported as INR, a standardized system that provides a common basis for communicating and interpreting PT results. PT values of 1.3–1.5 times the control are equivalent to INR values of 2–3 times the control value. PT of 1.5–2 or INR of 3–4.5 may be used for patients with high risk of embolization.
- Hepatic function and CBC should be monitored prior to and periodically throughout therapy.
- Stool and urine should be monitored for occult blood prior to and periodically throughout therapy.
- ***Toxicity and Overdose:*** Withholding 1 or more doses of medication is usually sufficient if PT is excessively prolonged or if minor bleeding occurs. If overdose occurs or anticoagulation needs to be immediately reversed, the antidote is vitamin K (phytonadione, AquaMEPHYTON). Administration of whole blood or plasma also may be required in severe bleeding because of the delayed onset of vitamin K.

POTENTIAL NURSING DIAGNOSES

- Tissue perfusion, altered (Indications).
- Injury, risk for (Side Effects).
- Knowledge deficit, related to medication regimen (Patient/Family Teaching).

IMPLEMENTATION

- **General Info:** Administer medication at same time each day.
- **PO:** Medication requires 3–5 days to reach

W

*CAPITALS indicate life-threatening; underlines indicate most frequent.

effective levels. It is usually begun while patient is still on IV heparin.

- □ Do not interchange brands; potencies may not be equivalent.
- ■ **Direct IV:** Reconstitute with 2.7 ml of sterile water for injection. Do not use solutions that are discolored or contain particulate matter. Stable for 4 hr at room temperature.
- ■ ***Rate:*** Administer as low bolus injection over 1–2 min into a peripheral vein.

PATIENT/FAMILY TEACHING

- □ Instruct patient to take medication exactly as directed. If a dose is missed, tell patient to take it as soon as remembered that day. Patient should not double doses. Health care professional should be informed of missed doses at time of checkup or lab tests.
- □ Review foods high in vitamin K (see Appendix K). Patient should have consistent limited intake of these foods, as vitamin K is the antidote for warfarin, and alternating intake of these foods will cause PT levels to fluctuate.
- □ Caution patient to avoid IM injections and activities leading to injury. Instruct patient to use a soft toothbrush, not to floss, and to shave with an electric razor during warfarin therapy. Advise patient that venipunctures and injection sites require application of pressure to prevent bleeding or hematoma formation.
- □ Advise patient to report any symptoms of unusual bleeding or bruising (bleeding gums; nosebleed; black, tarry stools; hematuria; excessive menstrual flow). Notify health care professional if these occur.
- □ Instruct patient not to drink alcohol or take OTC medications, especially those containing aspirin or NSAIDs, without advice of health care professional.
- □ Emphasize the importance of frequent lab tests to monitor coagulation factors.
- □ Instruct patient to carry identification describing medication regimen at all times and to inform all health care personnel caring for patient on anticoagulant therapy prior to lab tests, treatment, or surgery.

EVALUATION

Clinical response to therapy can be evaluated by: ■ Prolonged PT (1.3–2.0 times the control; may vary with indication) or INR of 2–4.5 without signs of hemorrhage.

ZAFIRLUKAST

(za-**feer**-loo-kast)

Accolate

CLASSIFICATION(S):

Bronchodilator (leukotriene receptor antagonist)

Pregnancy Category B

INDICATIONS

■ Long-term control agent in the management of asthma.

ACTION

■ Antagonizes the effects of leukotrienes, which are components of slow-reacting substance of anaphylaxis (SRSA) ■ These substances mediate the following: □ Airway edema □ Smooth muscle constriction □ Altered cellular activity ■ Result is decreased inflammatory process that is part of asthma. **Therapeutic Effects:** ■ Decreased frequency and severity of asthma.

PHARMACOKINETICS

Absorption: Rapidly absorbed following oral administration.

Distribution: Enters breast milk.

Metabolism and Excretion: Mostly metabolized by the liver; 10% excreted unchanged by the kidneys.

Half-life: 10 hr.

CONTRAINDICATIONS AND PRECAUTIONS

Contraindicated in: ■ Hypersensitivity ■ Lactation.

Use Cautiously in: ■ Acute attacks of asthma ■ Patients $>$55 yr (increased risk of infection) ■ Geriatric patients $\geq$65 yr or patients with hepatic impairment (may need lower doses) ■ Pregnancy or children $<$12 yr (safety not established).

ADVERSE REACTIONS AND SIDE EFFECTS*

CNS: headache, dizziness, weakness.
GI: abdominal pain, diarrhea, dyspepsia, ↑ liver enzymes, nausea, vomiting.
MS: back pain, myalgia.
Misc: CHURG-STRAUSS SYNDROME, fever, infection, pain.

INTERACTIONS

Drug-Drug: ▪ Blood levels are increased by **aspirin** ▪ Blood levels are decreased by **erythromycin** and **theophylline** ▪ Increases effects and risk of bleeding with **warfarin.**
Drug-Food: ▪ **Food** decreases absorption.

ROUTE AND DOSAGE

- **PO (Adults and Children ≥12 yr):** 20 mg twice daily.

AVAILABILITY

- ***Tablets:*** 20 mg[Rx].

TIME/ACTION PROFILE (improved symptoms of asthma)

	ONSET	PEAK	DURATION
PO	UK	1 wk	UK

NURSING IMPLICATIONS

ASSESSMENT

- □ Assess lung sounds and respiratory function prior to and periodically throughout therapy.
- ▪ ***Lab Test Considerations:*** Monitor liver function periodically during therapy. May cause elevated ALT concentrations.

POTENTIAL NURSING DIAGNOSES

- Airway clearance, ineffective (Indications).
- Knowledge deficit, related to medication regimen (Patient/Family Teaching).

IMPLEMENTATION

- **PO:** Administer at regular intervals on an empty stomach, 1 hr before or 2 hr after meals.

PATIENT/FAMILY TEACHING

- □ Instruct patient to take medication on an empty stomach as directed, at evenly spaced intervals, even if not experiencing symptoms of asthma. If a dose is missed, take as soon as remembered unless almost time for next dose. Do not double doses. Do not discontinue therapy without consulting health care professional.
- □ Instruct patient not to discontinue or reduce other asthma medications without consulting health care professional.
- □ Advise patient that zafirlukast is not used to treat acute asthma attacks but may be continued during an acute exacerbation.
- □ Advise patient to notify health care professional if symptoms of Churg-Strauss syndrome (generalized flu-like syndrome, fever, muscle aches and pain, weight loss, worsening respiratory symptoms) occur. Occurs rarely but may be life-threatening. More likely to occur when weaning from systemic glucocorticoids.

EVALUATION

Effectiveness of therapy can be demonstrated by: ▪ Prevention of and reduction in symptoms of asthma.

ZALCITABINE

(zal-**site**-a-been)
ddC, dideoxycitidine, HIVID

CLASSIFICATION(S):
Antiretroviral (nucleoside reverse transcriptase inhibitor)

Pregnancy Category C

INDICATIONS

▪ Management of HIV infection in combination with other antiretrovirals ▪ Has also been used as a single agent in patients who are intolerant of or who progress on other regimens.

ACTION

▪ Following intracellular conversion to its active form, it inhibits viral DNA synthesis and subsequent viral replication. **Therapeutic Effects:** ▪ Slowed progression and decreased sequelae of

*CAPITALS indicate life-threatening; underlines indicate most frequent.

Z

HIV infection ▪ Decreased viral load and increased CD4 cell count.

PHARMACOKINETICS

Absorption: Well absorbed following oral administration (80%).
Distribution: Distributes into intracellular fluid. Crosses the blood-brain barrier. Remainder of distribution not known.
Metabolism and Excretion: 70% excreted by the kidneys.
Half-life: 2 hr.

CONTRAINDICATIONS AND PRECAUTIONS

Contraindicated in: ▪ Hypersensitivity.
Use Cautiously in: ▪ Patients with renal impairment (dosage modification recommended if CCr is <40 ml/min) ▪ Patients with any signs of peripheral neuropathy (zalcitabine should be briefly discontinued and restarted at 50% of the previous dose if improvement occurs) ▪ Pre-existing liver disease or history of alcohol abuse (increased risk of liver function abnormalities) ▪ History of pancreatitis or hypertriglyceridemia ▪ Safe use in pregnancy, lactation, or children has not been established.

ADVERSE REACTIONS AND SIDE EFFECTS*

CNS: confusion, dizziness, fatigue, headache, impaired concentration.
EENT: pharyngitis.
CV: CARDIOMYOPATHY, CONGESTIVE HEART FAILURE, chest pain.
GI: PANCREATITIS, oral ulcers, abdominal pain, anorexia, diarrhea, dysphagia, esophageal ulcerations, ↑ liver enzymes, nausea, vomiting.
Derm: dermatitis, pruritus, rash.
Hemat: leukopenia, neutropenia.
MS: arthralgia, myalgia.
Neuro: peripheral neuropathy.
Misc: hypersensitivity reactions, weight loss.

INTERACTIONS

Drug-Drug: ▪ Risk of neuropathy is increased by concurrent use of other **drugs causing neuropathy** (chloramphenicol, cisplatin, disulfiram, ethionamide, glutethimide, gold, hydralazine, iodoquinol, isoniazid, metronidazole, nitrofurantoin, phenytoin, ribavirin, vincristine) ▪ Concurrent use with **didanosine** is not recommended ▪ Risk of pancreatitis is increased by concurrent use of other **drugs causing pancreatitis** (alcohol, asparaginase, azathioprine, estrogens, furosemide, methyldopa, nitrofurantoin, pentamidine, sulfonamides, tetracyclines, thiazide diuretics, valproic acid) ▪ **Aminoglycoside anti-infectives, amphotericin B, cimetidine, probenicid,** and **foscarnet** may increase the risk of toxicity from zalcitabine by decreasing its elimination.
Drug-Food: ▪ **Food** decreases absorption.

ROUTE AND DOSAGE

▪ **PO (Adults):** 0.75 mg zalcitabine q 8 hr.

AVAILABILITY

▪ ***Tablets:*** 0.375 mg[Rx], 0.75 mg[Rx].

TIME/ACTION PROFILE (blood levels)

	ONSET	PEAK	DURATION
PO	rapid	1–2 hr	8 hr

NURSING IMPLICATIONS

ASSESSMENT

- ☐ Assess patient for change in severity of symptoms of AIDS and for symptoms of opportunistic infections throughout therapy.
- ☐ Monitor patient for signs and symptoms of peripheral neuropathy. Zalcitabine should be discontinued when moderate discomfort from numbness, tingling, burning, or pain of the extremities; loss of an Achilles tendon reflex; or any related symptoms occur, especially if symptoms last longer than 3 days and are bilateral. If zalcitabine is not stopped promptly, peripheral neuropathy may progress to severe pain and may be potentially irreversible. Neuropathy may progress despite discontinuation of zalcitabine but usually is slowly reversible with prompt discontinuation. If peripheral neuropathy improves to very mild symptoms, zalcitabine may be reintroduced at 50% of the regular dose.
- ☐ Monitor patients for symptoms of pancreatitis (nausea, vomiting, abdominal pain) throughout therapy. If these symptoms or associated

*CAPITALS indicate life-threatening; underlines indicate most frequent.

lab test signs occur, discontinue zalcitabine, as fatalities have occurred.

- ***Lab Test Considerations:*** Monitor viral load and CD4 levels prior to and periodically throughout therapy.
- Monitor serum amylase, lipase, triglyceride, and calcium throughout therapy. Rising serum amylase, lipase, and triglyceride and decreasing calcium levels may indicate pancreatitis. Assess baseline in patients with prior history of pancreatitis or increased amylase, those on parenteral nutrition, or those with history of alcohol abuse. Zalcitabine should be discontinued if serum amylase is elevated by 1.5–2 times the normal limits.
- Monitor CBC and liver function studies prior to and periodically during therapy. May cause leukopenia and anemia and increase in AST, ALT, and alkaline phosphatase levels.

POTENTIAL NURSING DIAGNOSES

- Infection, risk for (Indications, Side Effects).
- Knowledge deficit, related to medication regimen (Patient/Family Teaching).

IMPLEMENTATION

- **PO:** Administer on an empty stomach, 1 hr before or 2 hr after meals for maximum absorption. Administer every 8 hr around the clock.
- Antacids should not be administered concurrently with zalcitabine.

PATIENT/FAMILY TEACHING

- Instruct patient to take zalcitabine exactly as directed, around the clock. Emphasize the importance of compliance with therapy, not taking more than the prescribed amount, and not discontinuing without consulting health care professional. Missed doses should be taken as soon as remembered, unless almost time for next dose; patient should not double doses.
- Inform patient that zalcitabine does not cure AIDS and does not reduce the risk of transmission of HIV to others through sexual contact or blood contamination. Caution patient to use a condom during sexual contact and avoid sharing needles or donating blood to prevent spreading the AIDS virus to others.
- Instruct patient to notify health care professional promptly if signs of peripheral neuropathy or pancreatitis occur.
- Advise women with childbearing potential to use a nonhormonal method of contraception throughout therapy.
- Advise patient not to take other medications, including antacids, without consulting health care professional.
- Emphasize the importance of regular follow-up exams and blood tests to determine progress and monitor for side effects.

EVALUATION

Effectiveness of therapy can be demonstrated by: ▪ Decrease in viral load and improvement in CD4 levels in patients with advanced HIV infection.

ZIDOVUDINE

(zye-**doe**-vue-deen)
{Apo-Zidovudine}, azidothymidine, AZT, {Novo-AZT}, Retrovir

CLASSIFICATION(S):
Antiretroviral (nucleoside reverse transcriptase inhibitor)

Pregnancy Category C

INDICATIONS

▪ Management of HIV infection in combination with other antiretrovirals ▪ Reduction of maternal/fetal transmission of HIV.

ACTION

▪ Following intracellular conversion to its active form, inhibits viral RNA synthesis by inhibiting the enzyme DNA polymerase (reverse transcriptase) ▪ Prevents viral replication. **Therapeutic Effects:** ▪ Virustatic action against selected retroviruses ▪ Slowed progression and decreased sequelae of HIV infection ▪ Decreased viral load and improved CD4 cell counts ▪ Decreased transmission of HIV to infants born to HIV-infected mothers.

PHARMACOKINETICS

Absorption: Well absorbed following oral administration.

Z

Distribution: Widely distributed; enters the CNS. Crosses the placenta.
Metabolism and Excretion: Mostly (75%) metabolized by the liver. 15–20% excreted unchanged by the kidneys.
Half-life: 1 hr.

CONTRAINDICATIONS AND PRECAUTIONS

Contraindicated in: ▪ Hypersensitivity ▪ Lactation.
Use Cautiously in: ▪ Decreased bone marrow reserve (dosage reduction required for anemia or granulocytopenia) ▪ Severe hepatic or renal disease (dosage modification may be required).

ADVERSE REACTIONS AND SIDE EFFECTS*

CNS: SEIZURES, headache, weakness, anxiety, confusion, decreased mental acuity, dizziness, insomnia, mental depression, restlessness, syncope.
GI: abdominal pain, diarrhea, nausea, anorexia, drug-induced hepatitis, dyspepsia, vomiting.
Derm: nail pigmentation.
Hemat: anemia, granulocytopenia, thrombocytosis.
MS: back pain, myopathy.
Neuro: tremor.

INTERACTIONS

Drug-Drug: ▪ Additive bone marrow depression with other **agents having bone marrow–depressing properties, antineoplastic agents, radiation therapy**, or **ganciclovir** ▪ Additive neurotoxicity may occur with **acyclovir** ▪ Toxicity may be increased by concurrent administration of **probenecid** or **fluconazole** ▪ Zidovudine levels are decreased by **clarithromycin.**

ROUTE AND DOSAGE

❑ Management of HIV Infection

- **PO (Adults and Children >13 yr):** 100 mg q 4 hr while awake or 200 mg 3 times daily or 300 mg twice daily (depends on combination and clinical situation).
- **PO (Children 3 mo–12 yr):** 90–180 mg/m^2 every 6 hr (not to exceed 200 mg q 6 hr).
- **IV (Adults and Children >12 yr):** 1 mg/kg infused over 1 hr q 4 hr. Change to oral therapy as soon as possible.
- **IV (Children):** 120 mg/m^2 q 6 hr (not to exceed 160 mg/dose).

❑ Prevention of Maternal/Fetal Transmission of HIV Infection

- **PO (Adults >14 wk Pregnant):** 100 mg 5 times daily until onset of labor.
- **IV (Adults during Labor and Delivery):** 2 mg/kg over 1 hr; then continuous infusion of 1 mg/kg/hr until umbilical cord is clamped.
- **IV (Infants):** 1.5 mg/kg q 6 hr until able to take PO.
- **PO (Infants):** 2 mg/kg q 6 hr started within 12 hr of birth and continued for 6 wk.

AVAILABILITY

▪ ***Capsules:*** 100 mg[Rx], 300 mg[Rx] ▪ ***Oral syrup:*** 50 mg/5 ml[Rx] ▪ ***Injection:*** 200 mg/20 ml[Rx] ▪ ***In combination with:*** lamivudine (Combivir[Rx]; see Appendix A).

TIME/ACTION PROFILE (blood levels)

	ONSET	PEAK	DURATION
PO	UK	0.5–1.5 hr	4 hr
IV	rapid	end of infusion	4 hr

NURSING IMPLICATIONS

ASSESSMENT

- ❑ Assess patient for change in severity of symptoms of HIV and for symptoms of opportunistic infections throughout therapy.
- ▪ ***Lab Test Considerations:*** Monitor viral load and CD4 counts prior to and periodically during therapy.
- ❑ Monitor CBC every 2 wk during the first 8 wk of therapy in patients with advanced HIV disease, and decrease to every 4 wk after the first 2 mo if zidovudine is well tolerated or monthly during the first 3 mo and every 3 mo thereafter unless indicated in patients who are asymptomatic or have early symptoms. Commonly causes granulocytopenia and anemia. Anemia may occur 2–4 wk after initiation of therapy. Anemia may respond to epoetin administration (see monograph on p. 332). Granulocytopenia usually occurs after 6–8 wk of therapy. Dosage reduction, discontinuation of therapy, or blood transfusions should be

*CAPITALS indicate life-threatening; underlines indicate most frequent.

considered if hemoglobin is <7.5 g/dl or reduction of >25% from baseline and/or granulocyte count is <750/mm^3 or reduction of >50% from baseline. Treatment with sargramostim may be necessary (see sargramostim monograph on p. 907). Therapy may be gradually resumed when bone marrow recovery is evident.

POTENTIAL NURSING DIAGNOSES

- Infection, risk for (Indications, Side Effects).
- Knowledge deficit, related to medication regimen (Patient/Family Teaching).

IMPLEMENTATION

- **General Info:** Administer doses around the clock.
- **IV:** Patient should receive the IV infusion only until oral therapy can be administered.
- **Intermittent Infusion:** Remove the calculated dose from the vial and dilute with D5W or 0.9% NaCl for concentration of <4 mg/ml. Do not use solutions that are discolored. Stable for 8 hr at room temperature or 24 hr if refrigerated.
- ***Rate:*** Infuse at a constant rate over 1 hr. Avoid rapid infusion or bolus injection.
- **Y-Site Compatibility:** ▪ acyclovir ▪ amifostine ▪ amikacin ▪ amphotericin B ▪ aztreonam ▪ cefepime ▪ ceftazidine ▪ ceftriaxone ▪ cimetidine ▪ clindamycin ▪ dexamethasone ▪ dobutamine ▪ dopamine ▪ erythromycin lactobionate ▪ filgrastim ▪ fluconazole ▪ fludarabine ▪ gentamicin ▪ heparin ▪ imipenem/cilastatin ▪ lorazepam ▪ melphalan ▪ metoclopramide ▪ morphine ▪ nafcillin ▪ ondansetron ▪ oxacillin ▪ paclitaxel ▪ pentamidine ▪ phenylephrine ▪ piperacillin ▪ piperacillin/tazobactam ▪ potassium chloride ▪ ranitidine ▪ sargramostim ▪ teniposide ▪ thiotepa ▪ tobramycin ▪ trimethoprim/sulfamethoxazole ▪ trimetrexate ▪ vancomycin ▪ vinorelbine.
- **Additive Incompatibility:** ▪ blood products or protein solutions.

PATIENT/FAMILY TEACHING

- □ Instruct patient to take zidovudine exactly as directed, around the clock, even if sleep is interrupted. Emphasize the importance of compliance with therapy, not taking more than prescribed amount, and not discontinuing without consulting health care professional. Missed doses should be taken as soon as remembered unless almost time for next dose; patient should not double doses. Inform patient that long-term effects of zidovudine are unknown at this time.
- □ Instruct patient that zidovudine should not be shared with others.
- □ Zidovudine may cause dizziness or fainting. Caution patient to avoid driving or other activities requiring alertness until response to medication is known.
- □ Inform patient that zidovudine does not cure HIV and does not reduce the risk of transmission of HIV to others through sexual contact or blood contamination. Caution patient to use a condom during sexual contact and avoid sharing needles or donating blood to prevent spreading the AIDS virus to others.
- □ Instruct patient to notify health care professional promptly if fever, sore throat, or signs of infection occur. Caution patient to avoid crowds and persons with known infections. Instruct patient to use soft toothbrush, to use caution when using toothpicks or dental floss, and to have dental work done prior to therapy or deferred until blood counts return to normal. Patient should also notify health care professional if shortness of breath, muscle aches, symptoms of hepatitis or pancreatitis, or other unexpected reactions occur.
- □ Advise patient to avoid taking any Rx or OTC medications without consulting health care professional.
- □ Emphasize the importance of regular follow-up exams and blood counts to determine progress and monitor for side effects.

EVALUATION

Effectiveness of therapy can be demonstrated by: ▪ Decrease in viral load and increase in CD4 counts in patients with HIV ▪ Delayed progression of AIDS and decreased opportunistic infections in patients with HIV.

ZILEUTON

(zye-**loo**-ton)
Zyflo

CLASSIFICATION(S):
Bronchodilator (enzyme inhibitor)

Pregnancy Category C

INDICATIONS

▪ Long-term control agent in the management of asthma.

ACTION

▪ Inhibits the enzyme 5-lipoxygenase that catalyzes to formation of leukotrienes. Leukotrienes are components of slow-reacting substance of anaphylaxis (SRSA) and mediate the following: □ Airway edema □ Smooth muscle constriction □ Altered cellular activity ▪ Result is decreased inflammatory process that is part of asthma. **Therapeutic Effects:** ▪ Decreased incidence and severity of asthma.

PHARMACOKINETICS

Absorption: Rapidly absorbed following oral administration.
Distribution: UK.
Metabolism and Excretion: Mostly metabolized by the liver.
Half-life: 2.5 hr.

CONTRAINDICATIONS AND PRECAUTIONS

Contraindicated in: ▪ Hypersensitivity ▪ Active liver disease or transaminases ≥3 times upper limit of normal.
Use Cautiously in: ▪ Acute attacks of asthma ▪ History of liver disease or alcohol consumption ▪ Pregnancy, lactation, or children <12 yr (safety not established).

ADVERSE REACTIONS AND SIDE EFFECTS*

CNS: headache, dizziness, insomnia, malaise, nervousness, somnolence, weakness.
EENT: conjunctivitis.
CV: chest pain.
GI: abdominal pain, constipation, dyspepsia, flatulence, increased liver enzymes, nausea, vomiting.
GU: urinary tract infection, vaginitis.
Derm: pruritus.
MS: arthralgia, myalgia, neck pain.
Neuro: hypertonia.
Misc: fever, lymphadenopathy.

INTERACTIONS

Drug-Drug: ▪ Increases blood levels and effects of **theophylline, propranolol, terfenadine,** and **warfarin.**
Drug-Food: ▪ **Food** slows but does not alter extent of absorption.

ROUTE AND DOSAGE

▪ **PO (Adults and Children ≥12 yr):** 600 mg 4 times daily.

AVAILABILITY

▪ ***Tablets:*** 600 mg[Rx].

TIME/ACTION PROFILE (improvement in pulmonary function)

	ONSET	PEAK	DURATION
PO	UK	1.7 hr	UK

NURSING IMPLICATIONS

ASSESSMENT

□ Assess lung sounds and respiratory function prior to and periodically throughout therapy.
▪ ***Lab Test Considerations:*** Monitor ALT prior to therapy, monthly for the first 3 mo, every 2 mo for the 1st yr of therapy, and periodically thereafter. May cause elevated ALT concentrations. If ALT ≥5 times the upper limit of normal or the patient is symptomatic, zileuton therapy should be discontinued.
□ May occasionally cause transient low WBC.

POTENTIAL NURSING DIAGNOSES

▪ Airway clearance, ineffective (Indications).
▪ Knowledge deficit, related to medication regimen (Patient/Family Teaching).

IMPLEMENTATION

▪ **PO:** Administer 4 times daily, with meals and at bedtime.

PATIENT/FAMILY TEACHING

□ Instruct patient to take medication as directed, at evenly spaced intervals, even if not experiencing symptoms of asthma. If a dose is missed, take as soon as remembered unless almost time for next dose. Do not double

*CAPITALS indicate life-threatening; underlines indicate most frequent.

doses. Do not discontinue therapy without consulting health care professional.

- Instruct patient not to discontinue or reduce other asthma medications without consulting health care professional. Health care professional should be notified if more short-acting bronchodilators than usual or more than the maximum number for 24 hr of inhalations of short-acting bronchodilator are needed.
- Advise patient that zileuton is not used to treat acute asthma attacks but may be continued during an acute exacerbation.
- Advise patient to consult health care professional before starting or stopping other medications, including OTC drugs, while taking zileuton.
- Instruct patient to notify health care professional immediately if upper right quadrant pain, nausea, fatigue, lethargy, pruritus, jaundice, or flu-like symptoms occur.

EVALUATION

Effectiveness of therapy can be demonstrated by: ▪ Reduction in symptoms of asthma.

ZINC SULFATE

(zink **sul**-fate)

Orazinc, {PMS Egozinc}, Verazinc, Zinc 220, Zincate, Zinkaps

CLASSIFICATION(S):

Nutritional supplement (trace metal)

Pregnancy Category C (parenteral)

INDICATIONS

▪ Replacement and supplementation therapy in patients who are at risk for zinc deficiency, including patients on long-term parenteral nutrition. **Unlabeled Uses:** ▪ Management of impaired wound healing due to zinc deficiency.

ACTION

▪ Serves as a cofactor for many enzymatic reactions ▪ Required for normal growth and tissue repair, wound healing, and senses of taste and smell. **Therapeutic Effects:** ▪ Replacement in deficiency states.

PHARMACOKINETICS

Absorption: Poorly absorbed from the GI tract (20–30%).

Distribution: Widely distributed. Concentrates in muscle, bone, skin, kidney, liver, pancreas, retina, prostate, red blood cells, and white blood cells.

Metabolism and Excretion: 90% excreted in feces, remainder lost in urine and sweat.

Half-life: UK.

CONTRAINDICATIONS AND PRECAUTIONS

Contraindicated in: ▪ Hypersensitivity or allergy to any components in formulation ▪ Pregnancy or lactation (supplemental amounts >RDA for pregnant or lactating patients; see list in Appendix L) ▪ Preparations containing benzyl alcohol should not be used in neonates.

Use Cautiously in: ▪ Renal failure.

ADVERSE REACTIONS AND SIDE EFFECTS

GI: gastric irritation (oral use only), nausea, vomiting.

INTERACTIONS

Drug-Drug: ▪ Oral zinc may decrease the absorption of **tetracyclines** or **fluoroquinolones.**

Drug-Food: ▪ **Caffeine**, **dairy products**, and **bran** may decrease the absorption of orally administered zinc.

ROUTE AND DOSAGE

RDA = 15 mg. Doses expressed in mg of elemental zinc unless otherwise noted. Zinc sulfate contains 23% zinc.

Deficiency

- **PO (Adults):** *Prevention of deficiency*—15–19 mg/day; *treatment of deficiency*—must be individualized; based on degree of deficiency.

IV Nutritional Supplementation—Metabolically Stable Patients

- **IV (Adults):** 2.5–4 mg/day; up to 12 mg/day in patients with excessive losses.

Z

- **IV (Infants and Children ≤5 yr):** 100 mcg/kg/day.
- **IV (Infants up to 3 kg):** 300 mcg/kg/day.

AVAILABILITY

- ***Tablets:*** 66 mg[OTC], 110 mg[OTC] ▪ ***Capsules:*** 220 mg[Rx,OTC] ▪ ***Injection:*** 1 mg/ml in 10- and 30-ml vials[Rx], 5 mg/ml in 5- and 10-ml vials[Rx].

TIME/ACTION PROFILE (blood levels)

	ONSET	PEAK	DURATION
PO	UK	2 hr	UK
IV	UK	UK	UK

NURSING IMPLICATIONS

ASSESSMENT

- □ Monitor progression of zinc deficiency symptoms (impaired wound healing, growth retardation, decreased sense of taste, decreased sense of smell) throughout therapy.
- ***Lab Test Considerations:*** Serum zinc levels may not accurately reflect zinc deficiency.
- □ Long-term high-dose zinc therapy may cause reduced serum copper concentrations.
- □ Monitor serum alkaline phosphatase concentrations monthly; may increase with zinc therapy.
- □ Monitor high-density lipoprotein (HDL) concentrations monthly in patients on long-term high-dose zinc therapy. Serum concentrations may be decreased.

POTENTIAL NURSING DIAGNOSES

- Nutrition, altered, less than body requirements (Indications).
- Knowledge deficit, related to medication regimen (Patient/Family Teaching).

IMPLEMENTATION

- **PO:** Administer oral doses with food to decrease gastric irritation. Administration with caffeine, dairy products, or bran may impair absorption.
- **IV:** Zinc is often included as a trace mineral in total parenteral nutrition solution prepared by pharmacist.

PATIENT/FAMILY TEACHING

- □ Encourage patient to comply with diet recommendations of health care professional. Explain that the best source of vitamins is a well-balanced diet with foods from the four basic food groups. Foods high in zinc include seafood, organ meats, and wheat germ.
- □ Patients self-medicating with vitamin supplements should be cautioned not to exceed RDA (see Appendix L). The effectiveness of megadoses for treatment of various medical conditions is unproved and may cause side effects.
- □ Instruct patients receiving oral zinc to notify health care professional if severe nausea or vomiting, abdominal pain, or tarry stools occur.
- □ Emphasize the importance of follow-up exams to evaluate progress.

EVALUATION

Effectiveness of therapy can be demonstrated by: ▪ Improved wound healing □ Improved senses of taste or smell. 6–8 wk of therapy may be required before full effect is seen.

ZOLPIDEM

(**zole**-pi-dem)
Ambien

CLASSIFICATION(S):
Hypnotic (nonbenzodiazepine)

Schedule IV
Pregnancy Category B

INDICATIONS

- Short-term treatment of insomnia.

ACTION

- Produces CNS depression by binding to gamma-aminobutyric acid (GABA) receptors ▪ Has no analgesic properties. **Therapeutic Effects:** ▪ Sedation and induction of sleep.

PHARMACOKINETICS

Absorption: Rapidly absorbed following oral administration.
Distribution: Minimal amounts enter breast milk; remainder of distribution not known.
Metabolism and Excretion: Converted to inactive metabolites, which are excreted by the kidneys.
Half-life: 2.5–2.6 hr (increased in geriatric patients and patients with hepatic impairment).

ZOLMITRIPTAN
(zole-mi-**trip**-tan)
Zomig

CLASSIFICATION(S):
Vascular headache suppressant (5-hydroxytryptamine agonist)

Pregnancy Category C

INDICATIONS
▪ Acute treatment of migraine headache.

ACTION
▪ Acts as an agonist at specific 5-hydroxytryptamine receptor sites in intracranial blood vessels and sensory trigeminal nerves. **Therapeutic Effects:** ▪ Cranial vessel vasoconstriction with resultant decrease in migraine headache.

PHARMACOKINETICS
Absorption: Well absorbed (40%) following oral administration.
Distribution: UK.
Metabolism and Excretion: Mostly metabolized by the liver; some conversion to metabolites that are more active than zolmitriptan. 8% excreted unchanged in urine.
Half-life: 3 hr (for zolmitriptan and active metabolite).

CONTRAINDICATIONS AND PRECAUTIONS
Contraindicated in: ▪ Hypersensitivity ▪ Significant underlying heart disease (including ischemic heart disease, history of myocardial infarction, coronary artery vasospasm, uncontrolled hypertension) ▪ Concurrent (or within 24 hr) use of other 5-HT agonists, ergotamine, or ergot-type medications ▪ Concurrent (or within 2 wk) use of MAO inhibitors ▪ Hemiplegic or basilar migraine ▪ Symptomatic Wolff-Parkinson-White syndrome or other arrhythmias.
Use Cautiously in: ▪ Cardiovascular risk factors (hypertension, hypercholesterolemia, cigarette smoking, obesity, diabetes, strong family history, menopausal females or males >40 yr (use only if cardiovascular status has been evaluated and determined to be safe and first dose is administered under supervision) ▪ Hepatic impairment (use lower doses) ▪ Pregnancy, lactation, or children (safety not established).

ADVERSE REACTIONS AND SIDE EFFECTS
CNS: dizziness, drowsiness, vertigo, weakness.
EENT: throat pain/tightness/pressure.
CV: chest pain/pressure/tightness/heaviness, hypertension, palpitations.
GI: dry mouth, dyspepsia, dysphagia, nausea.
Derm: sweating, warm/cold sensation.
MS: myalgia, myasthenia.
Neuro: hypesthesia, paresthesia.
Misc: feeling of heaviness, pain.

INTERACTIONS
Drug-Drug: ▪ Because of increased risk of cerebral vasospasm, avoid concurrent use of other **5-HT agonists (naratriptan** and **sumatriptan)** or **ergot-type preparations** ▪ Concurrent use of **MAO inhibitors** increases blood level and risk of toxicity (avoid use within 2 wk of MAO inhibitors) ▪ Blood levels may be increased by **oral contraceptives** ▪ May increase the risk of adverse reactions with SSRIs ▪ **Cimetidine** increases half-life of zolmitriptan and its active metabolite.

ROUTE AND DOSAGE
- **PO (Adults):** 2.5 mg or less initially; if headache returns, dose may be repeated after 2 hr (not to exceed 10 mg/24 hr).

AVAILABILITY
▪ ***Tablets:*** 2.5 mg[Rx], 5 mg[Rx].

TIME/ACTION PROFILE (relief of headache)

	ONSET	PEAK	DURATION
PO	UK	2 hr	UK

NURSING IMPLICATIONS

ASSESSMENT
□ Assess pain location, intensity, duration, and associated symptoms (photophobia, phonophobia, nausea, vomiting) during migraine attack.

POTENTIAL NURSING DIAGNOSES

- Pain (Indications).
- Knowledge deficit, related to medication regimen (Patient/Family Teaching).

IMPLEMENTATION

- **PO:** Initial dose is 2.5 mg. Lower doses can be achieved by breaking 2.5-mg tablet.

PATIENT/FAMILY TEACHING

- **General Info:** Inform patient that zolmitriptan should be used only during a migraine attack. It is meant to be used to relieve migraine attack but not to prevent or reduce the number of attacks.
- □ Instruct patient to administer zolmitriptan as soon as symptoms appear, but it may be administered any time during an attack. If migraine symptoms return, a second dose may be used. Allow at least 2 hr between doses, and do not use more than 10 mg in any 24-hr period.
- □ If dose does not relieve headache, additional zolmitriptan doses are not likely to be effective; notify health care professional.
- □ Advise patient that lying down in a darkened room following zolmitriptan administration may further help relieve headache.
- □ Caution patient not to use zolmitriptan if she is pregnant, suspects she is pregnant, plans to become pregnant, or is breast-feeding. Adequate contraception should be used during therapy.
- □ Advise patient to notify health care professional prior to next dose of zolmitriptan if pain or tightness in the chest occurs during use. If pain is severe or does not subside, notify health care professional immediately. If wheezing; heart throbbing; swelling of eyelids, face, or lips; skin rash; skin lumps; or hives occur, notify health care professional immediately and do not take more zolmitriptan without approval of health care professional. If feelings of tingling, heat, flushing, heaviness, pressure, drowsiness, dizziness, tiredness, or sickness develop, discuss with health care professional at next visit.
- □ May cause dizziness or drowsiness. Caution patient to avoid driving or other activities requiring alertness until response to medication is known.
- □ Advise patient to avoid alcohol, which aggravates headaches, during zolmitriptan use.

EVALUATION

Effectiveness of therapy can be demonstrated by: ▪ Relief of migraine attack.

CONTRAINDICATIONS AND PRECAUTIONS

Contraindicated in: ▪ Hypersensitivity ▪ Sleep apnea.

Use Cautiously in: ▪ History of previous psychiatric illness, suicide attempt, drug or alcohol abuse ▪ Geriatric patients and patients with impaired hepatic function (initial dosage reduction recommended) ▪ Patients with pulmonary disease ▪ Pregnancy, lactation, or children (safety not established).

ADVERSE REACTIONS AND SIDE EFFECTS

CNS: amnesia, daytime drowsiness, dizziness, "drugged" feeling.

GI: diarrhea, nausea, vomiting.

Misc: hypersensitivity reactions, physical dependence, psychological dependence, tolerance.

INTERACTIONS

Drug-Drug: ▪ Additive CNS depression may occur with concurrent use of other **sedative/hypnotics, tricyclic antidepressants, opioids,** or **antihistamines.**

Drug-Food: ▪ Food decreases and delays absorption.

ROUTE AND DOSAGE

- **PO (Adults):** 10 mg at bedtime; may be increased to 20 mg.
- **PO (Geriatric Patients, Debilitated Patients, or Patients with Hepatic Impairment):** 5 mg at bedtime initially; may be increased to 10 mg.

AVAILABILITY

- ***Tablets:*** 5 mg[Rx], 10 mg[Rx].

TIME/ACTION PROFILE (sedation)

	ONSET	PEAK	DURATION
PO	rapid	30 min–2 hr	6–8 hr

NURSING IMPLICATIONS

ASSESSMENT

- □ Assess mental status, sleep patterns, and potential for abuse prior to administering this medication. Prolonged use of >7–10 days may lead to physical and psychological dependence. Limit amount of drug available to the patient.
- □ Assess alertness at time of peak effect. Notify physician or other health care professional if desired sedation does not occur.
- □ Assess patient for pain. Medicate as needed. Untreated pain decreases sedative effects.

POTENTIAL NURSING DIAGNOSES

- Sleep pattern disturbance (Indications).
- Injury, risk for (Side Effects).
- Knowledge deficit, related to medication regimen (Patient/Family Teaching).

IMPLEMENTATION

- **General Info:** Before administering, reduce external stimuli and provide comfort measures to increase effectiveness of medication.
- □ Protect patient from injury. Raise bed side rails. Assist with ambulation. Take patient's cigarettes.
- **PO:** Tablets should be swallowed whole with full glass of water. For faster onset of sleep, do not administer with or immediately after a meal.

PATIENT/FAMILY TEACHING

- □ Instruct patient to take zolpidem exactly as directed. Do not take more than the amount prescribed because of the habit-forming potential. Not recommended for use longer than 7–10 days. If used for 2 wk or longer, abrupt withdrawal may result in fatigue, nausea, flushing, light-headedness, uncontrolled crying, vomiting, GI upset, panic attack, or nervousness.
- □ Because of rapid onset, advise patient to go to bed immediately after taking zolpidem.
- □ May cause daytime drowsiness or dizziness. Advise patient to avoid driving or other activities requiring alertness until response to this medication is known.
- □ Caution patient to avoid concurrent use of alcohol or other CNS depressants.

EVALUATION

Effectiveness of therapy can be demonstrated by: ▪ Relief of insomnia.

APPENDIX CONTENTS

APPENDIX A

Commonly Used Combination Drugs

Note: The drugs listed in this section are in alphabetical order according to trade names. If the trade name does not specify dosage form, the dosage form is either a tablet or capsule. Following each trade name are the generic names and doses of the active ingredients contained in each preparation. For information on these drugs, look up each generic name in the combination, listed separately in the *Drug Guide*. For inert ingredients, see drug label. **Rx** signifies that a physician's prescription is required. **Otc** signifies "over the counter" or nonprescription medication.

A-200 Shampoo—0.33% pyrethrins/4% piperonyl butoxide **(otc)**
Acid-X—acetaminophen 500 mg/calcium carbonate 250 mg **(otc)**
Actifed—pseudoephedrine 60 mg/triprolidine 2.5 mg **(otc)**
Actifed Allergy, Nighttime—pseudoephedrine 30 mg/diphenhydramine 25 mg **(otc)**
Actifed Plus—pseudoephedrine 30 mg/triprolidine 1.25 mg/acetaminophen 500 mg **(otc)**
Actifed Sinus Daytime—pseudoephedrine 30 mg/acetaminophen 500 mg **(otc)**
Actifed Sinus Nighttime—pseudoephedrine 30 mg/diphenhydramine 25 mg/acetaminophen 500 mg **(otc)**
Advil Cold & Sinus—pseudoephedrine 30 mg/ibuprofen 200 mg **(otc)**
AK-Cide Ophthalmic Suspension/Ointment—0.5% prednisolone acetate/10% sulfacetamide sodium **(Rx)**
Aldactazide 25/25—hydrochlorothiazide 25 mg/spironolactone 25 mg **(Rx)**
Aldactazide 50/50—hydrochlorothiazide 50 mg/spironolactone 50 mg **(Rx)**
Aldoclor-150—methyldopa 250 mg/chlorothiazide 150 mg **(Rx)**
Aldoclor-250—methyldopa 250 mg/chlorothiazide 250 mg **(Rx)**
Aldoril-15—hydrochlorothiazide 15 mg/methyldopa 250 mg **(Rx)**
Aldoril-25—hydrochlorothiazide 25 mg/methyldopa 250 mg **(Rx)**
Alka-Seltzer Effervescent, Original—citric acid 1000 mg/sodium bicarbonate 1916 mg/aspirin 325 mg **(otc)**
Alka-Seltzer Plus Allergy Liqui-Gels—pseudoephedrine 30 mg/chlorpheniramine 2 mg/acetaminophen 325 mg **(otc)**
Alka-Seltzer Plus Cold & Cough—phenylpropanolamine 20 mg/chlorpheniramine 2 mg/dextromethorphan 10 mg/aspirin 325 mg **(otc)**
Alka-Seltzer Plus Cold & Cough Liqui-Gels—dextromethorphan 10 mg/pseudoephedrine 30 mg/chlorpheniramine 2 mg/acetaminophen 250 mg **(otc)**
Alka-Seltzer Plus Cold Liqui-Gels—pseudoephedrine 30 mg/chlorpheniramine 2 mg/acetaminophen 250 mg **(otc)**
Alka-Seltzer Plus Cold Medicine—chlorpheniramine 2 mg/phenylpropanolamine 20 mg/aspirin 325 mg **(otc)**
Alka-Seltzer Plus Flu & Body Aches Non-Drowsy Liqui-Gels—pseudoephedrine 30 mg/dextromethorphan 10 mg/acetaminophen 250 mg **(otc)**
Alka-Seltzer Plus Night-Time Cold—phenylpropanolamine 20 mg/doxylamine 6.25 mg/dextromethorphan 15 mg/aspirin 500 mg **(otc)**
Alka-Seltzer Plus Night-Time Cold Liqui-Gels—doxylamine 6.25 mg/dextromethorphan 10 mg/pseudoephedrine 30 mg/acetaminophen 250 mg **(otc)**
Alka-Seltzer Plus Sinus—phenylpropanolamine 20 mg/aspirin 325 mg **(otc)**
Allerest Headache Strength Advanced Formula—pseudoephedrine 30 mg/chlorpheniramine 2 mg/acetaminophen 325 mg **(otc)**
Allerest Maximum Strength—pseudoephedrine 30 mg/chlorpheniramine 2 mg **(otc)**

Allerest Maximum Strength 12 Hour—phenylpropanolamine 75 mg/chlorpheniramine 12 mg **(Rx)**
Allerest No-Drowsiness—pseudoephedrine 30 mg/acetaminophen 325 mg **(otc)**
Allerest Sinus Pain Formula—pseudoephedrine 30 mg/chlorpheniramine 2 mg/acetaminophen 500 mg **(otc)**
All-Nite Cold Formula Liquid—(per 5 ml) pseudoephedrine 10 mg/doxylamine 1.25 mg/dextromethorphan 5 mg/acetaminophen 167 mg **(otc)**
Alor 5/500—hydrocodone 5 mg/aspirin 500 mg **(Rx)**
Amaphen—acetaminophen 325 mg/butalbital 50 mg/caffeine 40 mg **(Rx)**
Ambenyl Cough Syrup—(per 5 ml) codeine 10 mg/bromodiphenhydramine 12.5 mg/5% alcohol **(Rx)**
Anacin—aspirin 400 mg/caffeine 32 mg **(otc)**
Anacin Maximum Strength—aspirin 500 mg/caffeine 32 mg **(otc)**
Anacin PM (Aspirin Free)—diphenhydramine 25 mg/acetaminophen 500 mg **(otc)**
Anaplex HD Syrup—(per 5 ml) hydrocodone 1.7 mg/phenylephrine 5 mg/chlorpheniramine 2 mg **(Rx)**
Anaplex Liquid—(per 5 ml) chlorpheniramine 2 mg/pseudoephedrine 30 mg **(Rx)**
Anatuss—guaifenesin 100 mg/dextromethorphan 15 mg/phenylpropanolamine 25 mg/acetaminophen 325 mg **(Rx)**
Anatuss DM—guaifenesin 400 mg/pseudoephedrine 60 mg/dextromethorphan 20 mg **(otc)**
Anatuss DM Syrup—(per 5 ml) guaifenesin 100 mg/pseudoephedrine 30 mg/dextromethorphan 10 mg **(otc)**
Anatuss LA—pseudoephedrine 120 mg/guaifenesin 400 mg **(Rx)**
Anatuss Syrup—(per 5 ml) guaifenesin 100 mg/dextromethorphan 15 mg/phenylpropanolamine 25 mg **(otc)**
Anexsia 5/500—hydrocodone 5 mg/acetaminophen 500 mg **(Rx)**
Anexsia 7.5/650—hydrocodone 7.5 mg/acetaminophen 650 mg **(Rx)**
Anexsia 10/660—hydrocodone 10 mg/acetaminophen 660 mg **(Rx)**
Antihist-D—clemastine 1.34 mg/phenylpropanolamine 75 mg **(otc)**
Antrocol Elixir—(per 5 ml) atropine 0.195 mg/phenobarbital 16 mg/alcohol 20% **(Rx)**
Apresazide 25/25—hydralazine 25 mg/hydrochlorothiazide 25 mg **(Rx)**
Aprodine Syrup—(per 5 ml) pseudoephedrine 30 mg/triprolidine 1.25 mg **(otc)**
Aprodine w/Codeine Syrup—(per 5 ml) pseudoephedrine 30 mg/triprolidine 1.25 mg/codeine 10 mg **(Rx)**
A.R.M.—phenylpropanolamine 25 mg/chlorpheniramine 4 mg **(otc)**
Arthritis Pain Formula—aspirin 500 mg/aluminum hydroxide 27 mg/magnesium hydroxide 100 mg **(otc)**
Arthrotec—diclofenac 50 or 75 mg/misoprostol 200 mcg **(Rx)**
Ascriptin A/D—aspirin 325 mg/aluminum hydroxide 75 mg/magnesium hydroxide 75 mg/calcium carbonate 75 mg **(otc)**
Aspirin Free Bayer Select Allergy Sinus—pseudoephedrine 30 mg/chlorpheniramine 2 mg/acetaminophen 500 mg **(otc)**
Aspirin Free Bayer Select Head & Chest Cold—pseudoephedrine 30 mg/guaifenesin 100 mg/dextromethorphan 10 mg/acetaminophen 325 mg **(otc)**
Aspirin Free Excedrin—acetaminophen 500 mg/caffeine 65 mg **(otc)**
Aspirin Free Excedrin Dual—acetaminophen 500 mg/calcium carbonate 111 mg/magnesium carbonate 64 mg/magnesium oxide 30 mg **(otc)**
Arthotec—diclofenac 50 or 75 mg/misoprostol 200 mcg **(Rx)**
Augmentin 250—amoxicillin 250 mg/clavulanic acid 125 mg **(Rx)**
Augmentin 500—amoxicillin 500 mg/clavulanic acid 125 mg **(Rx)**
Augmentin 875—amoxicillin 875 mg/clavulanic acid 125 mg **(Rx)**
Augmentin 125 Chewable—amoxicillin 125 mg/clavulanic acid 31.25 mg **(Rx)**
Augmentin 250 Chewable—amoxicillin 250 mg/clavulanic acid 62.5 mg **(Rx)**

Augmentin 125 mg/5 ml Suspension—(per 5 ml) amoxicillin 125 mg/clavulanic acid 31.25 mg **(Rx)**
Augmentin 250 mg/5 ml Suspension—(per 5 ml) amoxicillin 250 mg/clavulanic acid 62.5 mg **(Rx)**
Auralgan Otic Solution—5.4% antipyrine/1.4% benzocaine **(Rx)**
B & O Supprettes No. 15A Supps—belladonna extract 15 mg/opium 30 mg **(Rx)**
B & O Supprettes No. 16A Supps—belladonna extract 16.2 mg/opium 60 mg **(Rx)**
Bactrim—trimethoprim 80 mg/sulfamethoxazole 400 mg **(Rx)**
Bactrim DS—trimethoprim 160 mg/sulfamethoxazole 800 mg **(Rx)**
Bactrim I.V. For Injection—(per 5 ml) trimethoprim 80 mg/sulfamethoxazole 400 mg **(Rx)**
Bancap HC—acetaminophen 500 mg/hydrocodone 5 mg **(Rx)**
Bayer Plus, Extra Strength—aspirin 500 mg buffered with: calcium carbonate/magnesium carbonate, magnesium oxide **(otc)**
Bayer Select Chest Cold—dextromethorphan 15 mg/acetaminophen 500 mg **(otc)**
Bayer Select Flu Relief—acetaminophen 500 mg/pseudoephedrine 30 mg/dextromethorphan 15 mg/chlorpheniramine 2 mg **(otc)**
Bayer Select Head & Chest Cold, Apirin Free Caplets—pseudoephedrine 30 mg/dextromethorphan 10 mg/guaifenesin 100 mg/acetaminophen 325 mg **(otc)**
Bayer Select Head Cold—pseudoephedrine 30 mg/acetaminophen 500 mg **(otc)**
Bayer Select Maximum Strength Headache—acetaminophen 500 mg/caffeine 65 mg **(otc)**
Bayer Select Maximum Strength Menstrual—acetaminophen 500 mg/pamabrom 25 mg **(otc)**
Bayer Select Maximum Strength Night Time Pain Relief—acetaminophen 500 mg/diphenhydramine 25 mg **(otc)**
Bayer Select Maximum Strength Sinus Pain Relief—acetaminophen 500 mg/pseudoephedrine 30 mg **(otc)**
Bayer Select Night Time Cold—acetaminophen 500 mg/pseudoephedrine 30 mg/dextromethorphan 15 mg/triprolidine 1.25 mg **(otc)**
Bellatal—phenobarbital 16.2 mg/hyoscyamine sulfate 0.1037 mg/atropine sulfate 0.0194 mg/scopolamine hydrobromide 0.0065 mg **(Rx)**
Bellergal-S—ergotamine 0.6 mg/phenobarbital 40 mg/l-alkaloids of belladonna 0.2 mg **(Rx)**
Bel-Phen-Ergot-SR—phenobarbital 40 mg/ergotamine tartrate 0.6 mg/l-alkaloids of belladonna 0.2 mg **(Rx)**
Benadryl Allergy Decongestant Liquid—(per 5 ml) diphenhydramine 12.5 mg/pseudoephedrine 30 mg **(otc)**
Benadryl Allergy/Sinus Headache Caplets—diphenhydramine 12.5 mg/pseudoephedrine 30 mg/acetaminophen 500 mg **(otc)**
Benadryl Decongestant Allergy—pseudoephedrine 60 mg/diphenhydramine 25 mg **(otc)**
Benylin Expectorant Liquid—(per 5 ml) guaifenesin 100 mg/dextromethorphan 5 mg/5% alcohol **(otc)**
Benylin Multi-Symptom Liquid—(per 5 ml) dextromethorphan 5 mg/pseudoephedrine 15 mg/guaifenesin 100 mg **(otc)**
Betoptic-Pilo—0.25% betaxolol/1.75% pilocarpine **(Rx)**
Bicitra Solution—(per 5 ml) sodium citrate 500 mg/citric acid 334 mg **(Rx)**
Bion Tears Ophthalmic Solution—0.1% dextran 70/0.3% hydroxypropyl methylcellulose 2910 **(otc)**
Blephamide Ophthalmic Suspension/Ointment—0.2% prednisolone/10% sodium sulfacetamide **(Rx)**
Bromfed Capsules—brompheniramine 12 mg/pseudoephedrine 120 mg **(Rx)**
Bromfed Tablets—pseudoephedrine 60 mg/brompheniramine 4 mg **(Rx)**
Bromfenex—brompheniramine 12 mg/pseudoephedrine 120 mg **(Rx)**
Bromfenex PD—brompheniramine 6 mg/pseudoephedrine 60 mg **(Rx)**

Bromo Seltzer—(effervescent granules) sodium bicarbonate 2781 mg/acetaminophen 325 mg/citric acid 2224 mg **(otc)**

Bromophen T.D.—brompheniramine 12 mg/phenylephrine 15 mg/phenylpropanolamine 15 mg **(Rx)**

Bronkaid Dual Action—ephedrine 25 mg/guaifenesin 400 mg **(otc)**

Brontex—codeine 10 mg/guaifenesin 300 mg **(Rx)**

Bufferin—aspirin 325 mg/calcium carbonate 158 mg/magnesium oxide 63 mg/magnesium carbonate 34 mg **(otc)**

Bufferin AF Nite Time—acetaminophen 500 mg/diphenhydramine 38 mg **(otc)**

Butibel—belladonna extract 15 mg/butabarbital 15 mg **(Rx)**

Cafatine PB—ergotamine 1 mg/caffeine 100 mg/l-alkaloids of belladonna 0.125 mg/sodium pentobarbital 30 mg **(Rx)**

Cafergot—ergotamine 1 mg/caffeine 100 mg **(Rx)**

Cafergot Supps—ergotamine 2 mg/caffeine 100 mg **(Rx)**

Caladryl Lotion—8% calamine and camphor/2.2% alcohol/1% pramoxine/diazolidinyl urea **(otc)**

Calcet—elemental calcium 152.8 mg/vitamin D 100 IU **(otc)**

Calcidrine Syrup—(per 5 ml) codeine 8.4 mg/calcium iodide 152 mg **(Rx)**

Caltrate 600+D—vitamin D 200 IU/calcium 600 mg **(otc)**

Cama Arthritis Pain Reliever—aspirin 500 mg/magnesium oxide 150 mg/aluminum hydroxide 125 mg **(otc)**

Capozide 25/15—captopril 25 mg/hydrochlorothiazide 15 mg **(Rx)**

Capozide 25/25—captopril 25 mg/hydrochlorothiazide 25 mg **(Rx)**

Capozide 50/15—captopril 50 mg/hydrochlorothiazide 15 mg **(Rx)**

Capozide 50/25—captopril 50 mg/hydrochlorothiazide 25 mg **(Rx)**

Cardec DM Syrup—(per 5 ml) pseudoephedrine 60 mg/carbinoxamine 4 mg/dextromethorphan 15 mg **(Rx)**

Cetacaine Topical—14% benzocaine/2% tetracaine/0.5% benzalkonium chloride/0.005% cetyl dimethyl ethyl ammonium bromide **(Rx)**

Ceta Plus—hydrocodone 5 mg/acetaminophen 500 mg **(Rx)**

Cetapred Ophthalmic Ointment—0.25% prednisolone/10% sodium sulfacetamide **(Rx)**

Cheracol Cough Syrup—(per 5 ml) codeine 10 mg/guaifenesin 100 mg **(Rx)**

Cheracol Plus Liquid—(per 5 ml) phenylpropanolamine 8.3 mg/chlorpheniramine 1.3 mg/dextromethorphan 6.7 mg/8% alcohol **(otc)**

Children's Cepacol Liquid—(per 5 ml) acetaminophen 160 mg/pseudoephedrine 15 mg **(otc)**

Chlor-Trimeton Allergy-Sinus Caplets—phenylpropanolamine 12.5 mg/chlorpheniramine 2 mg/acetaminophen 500 mg **(otc)**

Chlor-Trimeton 4 Hour Relief—pseudoephedrine 60 mg/chlorpheniramine 4 mg **(otc)**

Chlor-Trimeton 12 Hour Relief—pseudoephedrine 120 mg/chlorpheniramine 8 mg **(otc)**

Chromagen—ferrous fumarate 66 mg/vitamin B_{12} 10 mcg/vitamin C 250 mg/intrinsic factor 100 mg **(Rx)**

Claritin-D—loratadine 5 mg/pseudoephedrine 120 mg **(Rx)**

Claritin-D 24-Hour—loratadine 10 mg/pseudoephedrine 240 mg **(Rx)**

Clindex—chlordiazepoxide 5 mg/clidinium 2.5 mg **(Rx)**

Clomycin Ointment—bacitracin 500 units/neomycin sulfate (equiv. to 3.5 g neomycin base)/polymyxin B sulfate 500 units/lidocaine 40 mg **(otc)**

Co-Apap—pseudoephedrine 30 mg/chlorpheniramine 2 mg/dextromethorphan 15 mg/acetaminophen 325 mg **(otc)**

Co-Gesic—acetaminophen 500 mg/hydrocodone 5 mg **(Rx)**

Codamine Syrup—(per 5 ml) hydrocodone 5 mg/phenylpropanolamine 25 mg **(Rx)**

Codehist DH Elixir—(per 5 ml) pseudoephedrine 30 mg/chlorpheniramine 2 mg/codeine 10 mg **(Rx)**

Codiclear DH Syrup—(per 5 ml) hydrocodone 5 mg/guaifenesin 100 mg **(Rx)**

Codimal—pseudoephedrine 30 mg/chlorpheniramine 2 mg/acetaminophen 500 mg **(otc)**
Codimal DH Syrup—(per 5 ml) hydrocodone 1.66 mg/phenylephrine 5 mg/pyrilamine 8.33 mg **(Rx)**
Codimal DM Syrup—(per 5 ml) phenylephrine 5 mg/pyrilamine 8.33 mg/dextromethorphan 10 mg **(otc)**
Codimal-L.A.—chlorpheniramine 8 mg/pseudoephedrine 120 mg **(Rx)**
Codimal PH Syrup—(per 5 ml) codeine 10 mg/phenylephrine 5 mg/pyrilamine 8.33 mg **(Rx)**
ColBenemid—colchicine 0.5 mg/probenecid 500 mg **(Rx)**
Coldrine—pseudoephedrine 30 mg/acetaminophen 500 mg **(otc)**
Col-Probenecid—probenecid 500 mg/colchicine 0.5 mg **(Rx)**
Coly-Mycin S Otic Suspension—1% hydrocortisone/neomycin base 3.3 mg/ml/colistin 3 mg/ml /0.05% thonzonium bromide **(Rx)**
Combipres 0.1—chlorthalidone 15 mg/clonidine 0.1 mg **(Rx)**
Combipres 0.2—chlorthalidone 15 mg/clonidine 0.2 mg **(Rx)**
Combipres 0.3—chlorthalidone 15 mg/clonidine 0.3 mg **(Rx)**
Combivent—(per actuation) ipratropium bromide 18 mcg/albuterol 103 mcg **(Rx)**
Combivir—lamivudine 150 mg/zidovudine 300 mg **(Rx)**
Combist—phenylephrine 10 mg/chlorpheniramine 2 mg/phenyltoloxamine 25 mg **(Rx)**
Combist LA—phenylephrine 20 mg/chlorpheniramine 4 mg/phenyltoloxamine 50 mg **(Rx)**
Comtrex Allergy-Sinus—chlorpheniramine 2 mg/acetaminophen 500 mg/pseudoephedrine 30 mg **(otc)**
Comtrex Liquid—(per 5 ml) chlorpheniramine 0.67 mg/acetaminophen 108.3 mg/dextromethorphan 3.3 mg/pseudoephedrine 10 mg **(otc)**
Comtrex Liqui-Gels—acetaminophen 325 mg/phenylpropanolamine 12.5 mg/chlorpheniramine 2 mg/dextromethorphan 10 mg **(otc)**
Comtrex Maximum Strength Caplets—acetaminophen 500 mg/pseudoephedrine 30 mg/chlorpheniramine 2 mg/dextromethorphan 15 mg **(otc)**
Comtrex Maximum Strength Liqui-Gels—acetaminophen 500 mg/phenylpropanolamine 12.5 mg/chlorpheniramine 2 mg/dextromethorphan 15 mg **(otc)**
Comtrex Maximum Strength Multi-Symptom Cold & Flu Relief—pseudoephedrine 30 mg/dextromethorphan 15 mg/chlorpheniramine 2 mg/acetaminophen 500 mg **(otc)**
Comtrex Maximum Strength Multi-Symptom Cold & Flu Relief Liqui-Gels—acetaminophen 500 mg/phenylpropanolamine 12.5 mg/chlorpheniramine 2 mg/dextromethorphan 15 mg **(otc)**
Comtrex Maximum Strength Non-Drowsy Caplets—acetaminophen 500 mg/pseudoephedrine 30 mg/dextromethorphan 15 mg **(otc)**
Congess SR—guaifenesin 250 mg/pseudoephedrine 120 mg **(Rx)**
Congestac—guaifenesin 400 mg/pseudoephedrine 60 mg **(otc)**
Contac Cough & Chest Cold Liquid—(per 5 ml) pseudoephedrine 15 mg/dextromethorphan 5 mg/guaifenesin 50 mg/acetaminophen 125 mg **(otc)**
Contac Cough & Sore Throat Liquid—(per 5 ml) dextromethorphan 5 mg/acetaminophen 125 mg **(otc)**
Contac Day Allergy/Sinus—pseudoephedrine 60 mg/acetaminophen 650 mg **(otc)**
Contac Day Cold and Flu—pseudoephedrine 60 mg/dextromethorphan 30 mg/acetaminophen 650 mg **(otc)**
Contac 12 Hour—phenylpropanolamine 75 mg/chlorpheniramine 8 mg **(otc)**
Contac Maximum Strength 12 Hour—phenylpropanolamine 75 mg/chlorpheniramine 12 mg **(Rx)**
Contac Night Allergy Sinus—pseudoephedrine 60 mg/diphenhydramine 50 mg/acetaminophen 650 mg **(otc)**
Contac Night Cold and Flu Caplets—pseudoephedrine 60 mg/diphenhydramine 50 mg/acetaminophen 650 mg **(otc)**

Contac Severe Cold & Flu Nighttime Liquid—(per 5 ml) pseudoephedrine 10 mg/chlorpheniramine 0.67 mg/dextromethorphan 5 mg/acetaminophen 167 mg/18.5% alcohol **(otc)**
Contuss Liquid—(per 5 ml) phenylpropanolamine 20 mg/phenylephrine 5 mg/guaifenesin 100 mg **(Rx)**
Coricidin—chlorpheniramine 2 mg/acetaminophen 325 mg **(otc)**
Coricidin D—phenylpropanolamine 12.5 mg/chlorpheniramine 2 mg/acetaminophen 325 mg **(otc)**
Coricidin Maximum Strength Sinus Headache Caplets—phenylpropanolamine 12.5 mg/chlorpheniramine 2 mg/acetaminophen 500 mg **(otc)**
Cortisporin Ophthalmic (Suspension)/Otic (Solution/Suspension)—0.35% neomycin base/polymyxin B 10,000 units/ml/1% hydrocortisone **(Rx)**
Cortisporin Ophthalmic Ointment—(per g) 0.35% neomycin base/bacitracin 400 units/polymyxin B 10,000 units/hydrocortisone 1% **(Rx)**
Cortisporin Topical Cream—0.5% neomycin sulfate/polymyxin B 10,000 units/0.5% hydrocortisone **(Rx)**
Cortisporin Topical Ointment—0.5% neomycin sulfate/bacitracin 400 units/polymyxin B 5000 units/1% hydrocortisone **(Rx)**
Corzide 40/5—nadolol 40 mg/bendroflumethiazide 5 mg **(Rx)**
Cough-X—dextromethorphan 5 mg/benzocaine 2 mg **(otc)**
Creon—lipase 8000 units/amylase 30,000 units/protease 13,000 units/pancreatin 300 mg **(Rx)**
Cyclomydril Ophthalmic Solution—0.2% cyclopentolate/1% phenylephrine **(Rx)**
Dallergy Caplets—chlorpheniramine 8 mg/phenylephrine 20 mg/methscopolamine 2.5 mg **(Rx)**
Dallergy Syrup—(per 5 ml) chlorpheniramine 2 mg/phenylephrine 10 mg/methscopolamine 0.625 mg **(Rx)**
Dallergy Tablets—chlorpheniramine 4 mg/phenylephrine 10 mg/methscopolamine 1.25 mg **(Rx)**
Dallergy-D Syrup—(per 5 ml) phenylephrine 5 mg/chlorpheniramine 2 mg **(otc)**
Damason-P—hydrocodone 5 mg/aspirin 500 mg **(Rx)**
Darvocet-N 100—propoxyphene-N 100 mg/acetaminophen 650 mg **(Rx)**
Darvon Compound-65—propoxyphene 65 mg/aspirin 389 mg/caffeine 32.4 mg **(Rx)**
Deconamine—pseudoephedrine 60 mg/chlorpheniramine 4 mg **(Rx)**
Deconamine CX—hydrocodone 5 mg/pseudoephedrine 30 mg/guaifenesin 300 mg **(Rx)**
Deconamine SR—pseudoephedrine 120 mg/chlorpheniramine 8 mg **(Rx)**
Deconamine Syrup—(per 5 ml) pseudoephedrine 30 mg/chlorpheniramine 2 mg **(Rx)**
Defen-LA—pseudoephedrine 60 mg/guaifenesin 600 mg **(Rx)**
Demazin—phenylpropanolamine 25 mg/chlorpheniramine 4 mg **(otc)**
Demi-Regroton—chlorthalidone 25 mg/reserpine 0.125 mg **(Rx)**
Demulen 1/50—ethinyl estradiol 50 mcg/ethynodiol diacetate 1 mg **(Rx)**
Dexacidin Ophthalmic Ointment/Suspension—(per g/per ml) 0.1% dexamethasone/0.35% neomycin base/polymyxin B 10,000 units **(Rx)**
Dexasporin Ophthalmic Ointment—(per g) 0.1% dexamethasone/0.35% neomycin base/polymyxin B 10,000 units **(Rx)**
DHC Plus—dihydrocodeine 16 mg/acetaminophen 356.4 mg/caffeine 30 mg **(Rx)**
Dialose Plus—docusate sodium 100 mg/yellow phenolphthalein 65 mg **(otc)**
Di-Gel, Advanced Formula—magnesium hydroxide 128 mg/calcium carbonate 280 mg/simethicone 20 mg **(otc)**
Di-Gel Liquid—(per 5 ml) aluminum hydroxide 200 mg/magnesium hydroxide 200 mg/simethicone 20 mg **(otc)**
Dieutrim T.D.—benzocaine 9 mg/phenylpropanolamine 75 mg/carboxymethylcellulose 75 mg **(otc)**
Dibistine DH Liquid—(per 5 ml) pseudoephedrine 30 mg/chlorpheniramine 2 mg/codeine 10 mg **(Rx)**
Dilaudid Cough Syrup—(per 5 ml) guaifenesin 100 mg/hydromorphone 1 mg/5% alcohol **(Rx)**

Dilor-G—dyphylline 200 mg/guaifenesin 200 mg **(Rx)**
Dimetane Decongestant—brompheniramine 4 mg/phenylephrine 10 mg **(otc)**
Dimetane-DC Cough Syrup—(per 5 ml) brompheniramine 2 mg/phenylpropanolamine 12.5 mg/codeine 10 mg **(Rx)**
Dimetane-DX Cough Syrup—(per 5 ml) brompheniramine 2 mg/pseudoephedrine 30 mg/dextromethorphan 10 mg **(Rx)**
Dimetapp—brompheniramine 4 mg/phenylpropanolamine 25 mg **(otc)**
Dimetapp Cold & Allergy Chewable—phenylpropanolamine 6.25 mg/brompheniramine 1 mg **(otc)**
Dimetapp Cold & Flu—phenylpropanolamine 12.5 mg/brompheniramine 2 mg/acetaminophen 500 mg **(otc)**
Dimetapp DM Elixir—(per 5 ml) phenylpropanolamine 12.5 mg/brompheniramine 2 mg/dextromethorphan 10 mg **(otc)**
Dimetapp Elixir—(per 5 ml) phenylpropanolamine 12.5 mg/brompheniramine 2 mg **(otc)**
Dimetapp Extentabs—phenylpropanolamine 75 mg/brompheniramine 12 mg **(otc)**
Dimetapp Sinus—pseudoephedrine 30 mg/ibuprofen 200 mg **(otc)**
Diutensin-R—methyclothiazide 2.5 mg/reserpine 0.1 mg **(Rx)**
Doan's PM Extra Strength—magnesium salicylate 500 mg/diphenhydramine 25 mg **(otc)**
Dolacet—hydrocodone 5 mg/acetaminophen 500 mg **(Rx)**
Donnatal—phenobarbital 16.2 mg/hyoscyamine 0.1037 mg/atropine 0.0194 mg/scopolamine 0.0065 mg **(Rx)**
Donnatal Elixir—(per 5 ml) phenobarbital 16.2 mg/hyoscyamine 0.1037 mg/atropine 0.0194 mg/scopolamine 0.0065 mg/23% alcohol **(Rx)**
Donnatal Extentabs—phenobarbital 48.6 mg/hyoscyamine 0.3111 mg/atropine 0.0582 mg/scopolamine 0.0195 mg **(Rx)**
Donnazyme—pancreatin 500 mg/lipase 1000 units/protease 12,500 units/amylase 12,500 units **(Rx)**
Dorcol Children's Cold Formula Liquid—(per 5 ml) pseudoephedrine 15 mg/chlorpheniramine 1 mg **(otc)**
Doxidan—docusate calcium 60 mg/phenolphthalein 65 mg **(otc)**
Dristan Cold—pseudoephedrine 30 mg/acetaminophen 500 mg **(otc)**
Dristan Cold Maximum Strength Caplets—pseudoephedrine 30 mg/brompheniramine 2 mg/acetaminophen 500 mg **(otc)**
Dristan Cold Multi-Symptom Formula—acetaminophen 325 mg/phenylephrine 5 mg/chlorpheniramine 2 mg **(otc)**
Dristan Sinus—pseudoephedrine 30 mg/ibuprofen 200 mg **(otc)**
Drixoral Allergy Sinus—pseudoephedrine 60 mg/dexbrompheniramine 3 mg/acetaminophen 500 mg **(otc)**
Drixoral Cold & Allergy—pseudoephedrine 120 mg/dexbrompheniramine 6 mg **(otc)**
Drixoral Cold & Flu—pseudoephedrine 60 mg/dexbrompheniramine 3 mg/acetaminophen 500 mg **(otc)**
Drixoral Cough & Congestion Liquid Caps—pseudoephedrine 60 mg/dextromethorphan 30 mg **(otc)**
Drixoral Cough & Sore Throat Liquid Caps—dextromethorphan 15 mg/acetaminophen 325 mg **(otc)**
Drixoral Plus—pseudoephedrine 60 mg/dexbrompheniramine 3 mg/acetaminophen 500 mg **(otc)**
DT Vaccine—(per 0.5-ml dose) diphtheria toxoid 2 Lf units/tetanus toxoid 5 Lf units **(Rx)**
DTP Vaccine—(per 0.5-ml dose) (by Connaught®) diphtheria toxoid 6.5 Lf units/tetanus toxoid 5 LF units/pertussis 4 Lf units **(Rx)**
Dura-Vent—phenylpropanolamine 75 mg/guaifenesin 600 mg **(Rx)**
Dura-Vent/A—phenylpropanolamine 75 mg/chlorpheniramine 10 mg **(Rx)**
Dura-Vent/DA—phenylephrine 20 mg/chlorpheniramine 8 mg/methscopolamine 2.5 mg **(Rx)**

Dyazide—hydrochlorothiazide 25 mg/triamterene 37.5 mg **(Rx)**
Dynafed Asthma Relief—ephedrine 25 mg/guaifenesin 200 mg **(otc)**
Dynafed Plus Maximum Strength—pseudoephedrine 30 mg/acetaminophen 500 mg **(otc)**
Dyphylline-GG Elixir—(per 5 ml) dyphylline 100 mg/guaifenesin 100 mg **(Rx)**
Elase-Chloromycetin Ointment—(per g) fibrinolysin 1 unit/desoxyribonuclease 666.6 units/chloramphenicol 10 mg **(Rx)**
Elase Ointment—(per g) fibrinolysin 1 unit/desoxyribonuclease 666.6 units **(Rx)**
Elixophyllin-GG Liquid—(per 5 ml) guaifenesin 100 mg/theophylline 100 mg **(Rx)**
EMLA Cream—lidocaine 2.5 mg/prilocaine 2.5 mg **(Rx)**
Empirin w/Codeine No. 3—aspirin 325 mg/codeine phosphate 30 mg **(Rx)**
Empirin w/Codeine No. 4—aspirin 325 mg/codeine phosphate 60 mg **(Rx)**
Enduronyl—methyclothiazide 5 mg/deserpidine 0.25 mg **(Rx)**
Entex—phenylephrine 5 mg/phenylpropanolamine 45 mg/guaifenesin 200 mg **(Rx)**
Entex LA—phenylpropanolamine 75 mg/guaifenesin 400 mg **(Rx)**
Entex PSE—pseudoephedrine 120 mg/guaifenesin 600 mg **(Rx)**
Epifoam Aerosol Foam—1% hydrocortisone/1% pramoxine **(Rx)**
E-Pilo-1 Ophthalmic Solution—1% epinephrine bitartrate/1% pilocarpine **(Rx)**
E-Pilo-2 Ophthalmic Solution—1% epinephrine bitartrate/2% pilocarpine **(Rx)**
E-Pilo-4 Ophthalmic Solution—1% epinephrine bitartrate/4% pilocarpine **(Rx)**
Esgic-Plus—butalbital 50 mg/acetaminophen 500 mg/caffeine 40 mg **(Rx)**
Esimil—guanethidine 10 mg/hydrochlorothiazide 25 mg **(Rx)**
Estratest—esterified estrogens 1.25 mg/methyltestosterone 2.5 mg **(Rx)**
Etrafon—perphenazine 2 mg/amitriptyline 25 mg **(Rx)**
Etrafon-Forte—perphenazine 4 mg/amitriptyline 25 mg **(Rx)**
Excedrin Migraine—aspirin 250 mg/acetaminophen 250 mg/caffeine 65 mg **(otc)**
Excedrin P.M.—acetaminophen 500 mg/diphenhydramine citrate 38 mg **(otc)**
Excedrin P.M. Liquid—(per 30 ml) acetaminophen 1000 mg/diphenhydramine 50 mg **(otc)**
Excedrin P.M. Liquigels—acetaminophen 500 mg/diphenhydramine 25 mg **(otc)**
Excedrin Sinus Extra Strength—pseudoephedrine 30 mg/acetaminophen 500 mg **(otc)**
Fansidar—sulfidoxine 500 mg/pyrimethamine 25 mg **(Rx)**
Fedahist—pseudoephedrine 60 mg/chlorpheniramine 4 mg **(otc)**
Fedahist Expectorant Syrup—(per 5 ml) guaifenesin 200 mg/pseudoephedrine 20 mg **(otc)**
Fedahist Gyrocaps—pseudoephedrine 65 mg/chlorpheniramine 10 mg **(Rx)**
Fedahist Timecaps—pseudoephedrine 120 mg/chlorpheniramine 8 mg **(Rx)**
Feen-A-Mint Pills—docusate sodium 100 mg/phenolphthalein 65 mg **(otc)**
Fem-1—acetaminophen 500 mg/pamabrom 25 mg **(otc)**
Ferro-Sequels—docusate sodium 100 mg/ferrous fumarate 150 mg **(otc)**
Fioricet—acetaminophen 325 mg/caffeine 40 mg/butalbital 50 mg **(Rx)**
Fioricet w/Codeine—acetaminophen 325 mg/caffeine 40 mg/butalbital 50 mg/codeine 30 mg **(Rx)**
Fiorinal—aspirin 325 mg/caffeine 40 mg/butalbital 50 mg **(Rx)**
Fiorinal w/Codeine—aspirin 325 mg/caffeine 40 mg/butalbital 50 mg/codeine 30 mg **(Rx)**
FML-S Ophthalmic Suspension—0.1% fluorometholone/10% sulfacetamide **(Rx)**
Gas-Ban—calcium carbonate 500 mg/simethicone 40 mg **(otc)**
Gas-Ban DS Liquid—(per 5 ml) aluminum hydroxide 400 mg/magnesium hydroxide 400 mg/simethicone 40 mg **(otc)**
Gaviscon—magnesium trisilicate 20 mg/aluminum hydroxide 80 mg **(otc)**
Gaviscon Liquid—(per 5 ml) aluminum hydroxide 31.7 mg/magnesium carbonate 119.3 mg **(otc)**
Gelpirin—acetaminophen 125 mg/aspirin 240 mg/caffeine 32 mg **(otc)**
Gelusil—aluminum hydroxide 200 mg/magnesium hydroxide 200 mg/simethicone 25 mg **(otc)**
Genatuss DM Syrup—(per 5 ml) guaifenesin 100 mg/dextromethorphan 10 mg **(otc)**
Granulex Aerosol—(per 0.82 ml) trypsin 0.1 mg/Balsam Peru 72.5 mg/castor oil 650 mg **(Rx)**

Guaifenex PPA 75—guiafenesin 600 mg/phenylpropanolamine 75 mg **(Rx)**
Guaifenex PSE 60—pseudoephedrine 60 mg/guaifenesin 600 mg **(Rx)**
Guaifenex PSE 120—pseudoephedrine 120 mg/guaifenesin 600 mg **(Rx)**
Haley's M-O Liquid—(per 15 ml) magnesium hydroxide 900 mg/mineral oil 3.75 ml **(otc)**
Halotussin-DM Sugar Free Liquid—(per 5 ml) guaifenesin 100 mg/dextromethorphan 10 mg **(otc)**
Helidac—bismuth subsalicylate 262.4-mg tablets plus metronidazole 250-mg tablets plus tetracycline 500-mg capsules in a compliance package **(Rx)**
Humibid DM Sprinkle Caps—dextromethorphan 15 mg/guaifenesin 300 mg **(Rx)**
Humibid DM Tablets—dextromethorphan 30 mg/guaifenesin 600 mg **(Rx)**
Hycodan—hydrocodone 5 mg/homatropine 1.5 mg **(Rx)**
Hycodan Syrup—(per 5 ml) hydrocodone 5 mg/homatropine 1.5 mg **(otc)**
Hycomine Compound—chlorpheniramine 2 mg/acetaminophen 250 mg/phenylephrine 10 mg/hydrocodone 5 mg/caffeine 30 mg **(Rx)**
Hycomine Syrup—(per 5 ml) hydrocodone 5 mg/phenylpropanolamine 25 mg **(Rx)**
Hycotuss Expectorant—(per 5 ml) guaifenesin 100 mg/hydrocodone 5 mg/10% alcohol **(Rx)**
Hydrocet—hydrocodone 5 mg/acetaminophen 500 mg **(Rx)**
Hydrogesic—hydrocodone 5 mg/acetaminophen 500 mg **(Rx)**
Hydropres-50—hydrochlorothiazide 50 mg/reserpine 0.125 mg **(Rx)**
Hydro-Serp—hydrochlorothiazide 50 mg/reserpine 0.125 mg **(Rx)**
Hydroserpine #1—hydrochlorothiazide 25 mg/reserpine 0.125 mg **(Rx)**
Hyzaar—losartan potassium 50 mg/hydrochlorothiazide 12.5 mg/potassium 4.24 mg **(Rx)**
Iberet Filmtab—ferrous sulfate 105 mg/ascorbic acid 150 mg/B-complex vitamins **(otc)**
Iberet Liquid—(per 5 ml) ferrous sulfate 78.75 mg/ascorbic acid 112.5 mg/B-complex vitamins **(otc)**
Imodium Advanced—loperamide 2 mg/simethicone 125 mg **(otc)**
Inderide 40/25—propranolol 40 mg/hydrochlorothiazide 25 mg **(Rx)**
Innovar—(per 1 ml) 2.5 mg droperidol/0.05 mg fentanyl **(Rx)**
Iofed—brompheniramine 12 mg/pseudoephedrine 120 mg **(Rx)**
Iofed PD—brompheniramine 6 mg/pseudoephedrine 60 mg **(Rx)**
Iophen-C Liquid—(per 5 ml) iodinated glycerol 30 mg/codeine 10 mg **(Rx)**
Iophen-DM Liquid—(per 5 ml) iodinated glycerol 30 mg/dextromethorphan 10 mg **(Rx)**
Kondremul w/Phenolphthalein—(per 15 ml) phenolphthalein 150 mg/55% mineral oil/Irish Moss **(otc)**
Lactinex—mixed culture of *Lactobacillus acidophilus* and *Lactobacillus bulgaricus* **(otc)**
Levsin PB Drops—(per ml) hyoscyamine 0.125 mg/phenobarbital 15 mg/5% alcohol **(Rx)**
Levsin w/Phenobarbital—hyoscyamine 0.125 mg/phenobarbital 15 mg **(Rx)**
Lexxel—enalapril 5 mg/felodipine 5 mg **(Rx)**
Librax—chlordiazepoxide 5 mg/clidinium 2.5 mg **(Rx)**
Lida-Mantle-HC Cream—0.5% hydrocortisone/3% lidocaine **(Rx)**
Limbitrol DS 10-25—chlordiazepoxide 10 mg/amitriptyline 25 mg **(Rx)**
Lobac—salicylamide 200 mg/phenyltoloxamine 20 mg/acetaminophen 300 mg **(Rx)**
Loestrin Fe 1.5/30—norethindrone acetate 1.5 mg/ethinyl estradiol 30 mcg **(Rx)**
Lomotil—diphenoxylate 2.5 mg/atropine 0.025 mg **(Rx)**
Lomotil Liquid—(per 5 ml) diphenoxylate 2.5 mg/atropine 0.025 mg **(Rx)**
Lo/Ovral—ethinyl estradiol 30 mcg/norgestrel 0.3 mg **(Rx)**
Lopressor HCT 50/25—metoprolol 50 mg/hydrochlorothiazide 25 mg **(Rx)**
Lopressor HCT 100/25—metoprolol 100 mg/hydrochlorothiazide 25 mg **(Rx)**
Lopressor HCT 100/50—metoprolol 100 mg/hydrochlorothiazide 50 mg **(Rx)**
Lorcet 10/650—acetaminophen 650 mg/hydrocodone 10 mg **(Rx)**
Lortab 2.5/500—hydrocodone 2.5 mg/acetaminophen 500 mg **(Rx)**
Lortab 5/500—hydrocodone 5 mg/acetaminophen 500 mg **(Rx)**
Lortab 7.5/500—hydrocodone 7.5 mg/acetaminophen 500 mg **(Rx)**

Lortab 10/500—hydrocodone 10 mg/acetaminophen 500 mg **(Rx)**
Lortab ASA—aspirin 500 mg/hydrocodone 5 mg **(Rx)**
Lortab Elixir—(per 5 ml) hydrocodone 2.5 mg/acetaminophen 167 mg **(Rx)**
Lotensin HCT 5/6.25—benazepril 5 mg/hydrochlorothiazide 6.25 mg **(Rx)**
Lotensin HCT 10/12.5—benazepril 10 mg/hydrochlorothiazide 12.5 mg **(Rx)**
Lotensin HCT 20/12.5—benazepril 20 mg/hydrochlorothiazide 12.5 mg **(Rx)**
Lotensin HCT 20/25—benazepril 20 mg/hydrochlorothiazide 25 mg **(Rx)**
Lotrel 2.5/10—amlodipine 2.5 mg/benazepril 10 mg **(Rx)**
Lotrel 5/10—amlodipine 5 mg/benazepril 10 mg **(Rx)**
Lotrel 5/20—amlodipine 5 mg/benazepril 20 mg **(Rx)**
Lotrisone Topical—0.05% betamethasone/1% clotrimazole **(Rx)**
Lufyllin-EPG Elixir—(per 5 ml) ephedrine 24 mg/dyphylline 150 mg/guaifenesin 300 mg/ phenobarbital 24 mg **(Rx)**
Lufyllin-GG—dyphylline 200 mg/guaifenesin 200 mg **(Rx)**
M-M-R II—mixture of 3 viruses: measles/mumps/rubella **(Rx)**
M-R-Vax II—mixture of 2 viruses: measles/rubella **(Rx)**
Maalox—aluminum hydroxide 200 mg/magnesium hydroxide 200 mg **(otc)**
Maalox Plus—aluminum hydroxide 200 mg/magnesium hydroxide 200 mg/simethicone 25 mg **(otc)**
Maalox Plus Extra Strength Suspension—(per 5 ml) aluminum hydroxide 500 mg/magnesium hydroxide 450 mg/simethicone 40 mg **(otc)**
Maalox Suspension—(per 5 ml) aluminum hydroxide 225 mg/magnesium hydroxide 200 mg **(otc)**
Mapap Cold Formula—acetaminophen 325 mg/chlorpheniramine 2 mg/pseudoephedrine 30 mg/dextromethorphan 15 mg **(otc)**
Marax—ephedrine 25 mg/theophylline 130 mg/hydroxyzine 10 mg **(Rx)**
Maxitrol Ophthalmic Suspension/Ointment—0.35% neomycin base/0.1% dexamethasone/ polymyxin B 10,000 U/ml **(Rx)**
Maxzide—hydrochlorothiazide 50 mg/triamterene 75 mg **(Rx)**
Maxzide-25MG—hydrochlorothiazide 25 mg/triamterene 37.5 mg **(Rx)**
Medi-Flu-Liquid—(per 5 ml) pseudoephedrine 10 mg/chlorpheniramine 0.67 mg/dextromethorphan 5 mg/acetaminophen 167 mg/18.5% alcohol **(otc)**
Mepergan Fortis—meperidine 50 mg/promethazine 25 mg **(Rx)**
Metimyd Ophthalmic Suspension/Ointment—0.5% prednisolone/10% sodium sulfacetamide **(Rx)**
Midol Maximum Strength Multi-Symptom Menstrual Gelcaps—acetaminophen 500 mg/ pyrilamine 15 mg/caffeine 60 mg **(otc)**
Midol PM—acetaminophen 500 mg/diphenhydramine 25 mg **(otc)**
Midol PMS Maximum Strength Caplets—acetaminophen 500 mg/pyrilamine 15 mg/pamabrom 25 mg **(otc)**
Midol, Teen—acetaminophen 400 mg/pamabrom 25 mg **(otc)**
Midrin—isometheptene 65 mg/acetaminophen 325 mg/dichloralphenazone 100 mg **(Rx)**
Minizide 1—prazosin 1 mg/polythiazide 0.5 mg **(Rx)**
Minizide 2—prazosin 2 mg/polythiazide 0.5 mg **(Rx)**
Minizide 5—prazosin 5 mg/polythiazide 0.5 mg **(Rx)**
Modane Plus—docusate sodium 100 mg/phenolphthalein 65 mg **(otc)**
Moduretic—hydrochlorothiazide 50 mg/amiloride 5 mg **(Rx)**
Motrin IB Sinus—pseudoephedrine 30 mg/ibuprofen 200 mg **(otc)**
Murocoll-2 Ophthalmic Drops—0.3% scopolamine/10% phenylephrine **(Rx)**
Mycolog II Topical—0.1% triamcinolone acetonide/nystatin 100,000 units/g **(Rx)**
Mylanta—aluminum hydroxide 200 mg/magnesium hydroxide 200 mg/simethicone 20 mg **(otc)**
Mylanta Double Strength Liquid—(per 5 ml) aluminum hydroxide 400 mg/magnesium hydroxide 400 mg/simethicone 40 mg **(otc)**

Mylanta Gelcaps—calcium carbonate 311 mg/magnesium carbonate 232 mg **(otc)**
Naldecon—phenylpropanolamine 40 mg/chlorpheniramine 5 mg/phenyltoloxamine 5 mg **(Rx)**
Naldecon Syrup—(per 5 ml) chlorpheniramine 2.5 mg/phenylephrine 5 mg/phenylpropanolamine 20 mg/phenyltoloxamine 7.5 mg **(Rx)**
Naldecon CX Adult Liquid—(per 5 ml) guaifenesin 200 mg/phenylpropanolamine 12.5 mg/codeine 10 mg **(Rx)**
Naldecon DX Adult Liquid—(per 5 ml) guaifenesin 200 mg/dextromethorphan 10 mg/phenylpropanolamine 12.5 mg **(otc)**
Naldecon DX Children's Syrup—(per 5 ml) phenylpropanolamine 6.25 mg/dextromethorphan 5 mg/guaifenesin 100 mg **(otc)**
Naldecon DX Pediatric Drops—(per 1 ml) phenylpropanolamine 6.25 mg/dextromethorphan 5 mg/guaifenesin 50 mg **(otc)**
Naldecon EX Children's Syrup—(per 5 ml) guaifenesin 100 mg/phenylpropanolamine 6.25 mg **(otc)**
Naldecon EX Pediatric Drops—(per 1 ml) phenylpropanolamine 6.25 mg/guaifenesin 50 mg **(otc)**
Naldecon Pediatric Drops—(per 1 ml) phenylpropanolamine 5 mg/phenylephrine 1.25 mg/chlorpheniramine 0.5 mg/phenyltoloxamine 2 mg **(Rx)**
Naldecon Pediatric Syrup—(per 5 ml) phenylpropanolamine 5 mg/phenylephrine 1.25 mg/chlorpheniramine 0.5 mg/phenyltoloxamine 2 mg **(Rx)**
Naldecon Senior DX Liquid—(per 5 ml) dextromethorphan 10 mg/guiafenesin 200 mg **(otc)**
Naphcon-A Ophthalmic Solution—0.25% naphazoline/0.3% pheniramine **(otc)**
Nasatab LA—guaifenesin 500 mg/pseudoephedrine 120 mg **(Rx)**
NeoDecadron Ophthalmic Ointment—0.35% neomycin/0.05% dexamethasone **(Rx)**
NeoDecadron Ophthalmic Solution—0.35% neomycin/0.1% dexamethasone **(Rx)**
NeoDecadron Topical—0.5% neomycin sulfate/0.1% dexamethasone **(Rx)**
Neosporin Cream—(per g) polymyxin B 10,000 units/neomycin 3.5 mg **(otc)**
Neosporin G.U. Irrigant—(per ml) neomycin 40 mg/polymyxin B 200,000 units **(Rx)**
Neosporin Ophthalmic Ointment—(per g) polymyxin B 10,000 units/neomycin 3.5 mg/bacitracin 400 units **(Rx)**
Neosporin Ophthalmic Solution—(per ml) polymyxin B 10,000 units/neomycin 1.75 mg/gramicidin 0.025 mg **(Rx)**
Neosporin Plus Cream—(per g) polymyxin B 10,000 units/neomycin 3.5 mg/lidocaine 40 mg **(otc)**
Neosporin Topical Ointment—(per g) neomycin 3.5 mg/bacitracin zinc 400 units/polymyxin B 5000 units **(otc)**
Niferex-150 Forte—ferrous sulfate 150 mg/vitamin B_{12} 25 mcg/folic acid 1 mg **(Rx)**
Norgesic—orphenadrine 25 mg/caffeine 30 mg/aspirin 385 mg **(Rx)**
Norgesic Forte—orphenadrine 50 mg/caffeine 60 mg/aspirin 770 mg **(Rx)**
Novacet Lotion—10% sodium sulfacetamide/5% sulfur **(Rx)**
Novafed A—chlorpheniramine 8 mg/pseudoephedrine 120 mg **(Rx)**
NuLytely—PEG 3350 420 g/sodium bicarbonate 5.72 g/sodium chloride 11.2 g/potassium chloride 1.48 g **(Rx)**
Nyquil Hot Therapy—(per packet) acetaminophen 1000 mg/pseudoephedrine 60 mg/dextromethorphan 30 mg/doxylamine 12.5 mg **(otc)**
NyQuil Nighttime Cold/Flu Medicine Liquid—(per 5 ml) pseudoephedrine 10 mg/doxylamine 1.25 mg/dextromethorphan 5 mg/acetaminophen 167 mg/25% alcohol (may contain tartrazine) **(otc)**
Octicair Otic Suspension—1% hydrocortisone/neomycin 5 mg/ml/polymyxin B 10,000 units/ml **(Rx)**
Opcon-A Ophthalmic Solution—0.027% naphazoline/0.315% pheniramine **(otc)**
Ornade—phenylpropanolamine 75 mg/chlorpheniramine 12 mg **(Rx)**
Ornex—pseudoephedrine 30 mg/acetaminophen 500 mg **(otc)**

Ornex No Drowsiness—pseudoephedrine 30 mg/acetaminophen 325 mg **(otc)**
Ortho-cept—ethinyl estradiol 30 mcg/desogestrel 0.15 mg **(Rx)**
Ortho-Novum 7/7/7:
Phase I—norethindrone 0.5 mg/ethinyl estradiol 35 mcg **(Rx)**
Phase II—norethindrone 0.75 mg/ethinyl estradiol 35 mcg **(Rx)**
Phase III—norethindrone 1 mg/ethinyl estradiol 35 mcg **(Rx)**
Otocort Otic Suspension—1% hydrocortisone/neomycin 5 mg/ml/polymyxin B 10,000 units/ml **(Rx)**
P-V-Tussin—guaifenesin 200 mg/hydrocodone 5 mg/phenindamine 25 mg **(Rx)**
Pain-X Topical—0.05% capsaicin/5% menthol/4% camphor **(otc)**
Pamprin Maximum Pain Relief—acetaminophen 250 mg/pamabrom 25 mg/magnesium salicylate 250 mg **(otc)**
Pamprin Multi-Symptom—acetaminophen 500 mg/pamabrom 25 mg/pyrilamine 15 mg **(otc)**
Panacet 5/500—hydrocodone 5 mg/acetaminophen 500 mg **(Rx)**
Panasal 5/500—hydrocodone 5 mg/aspirin 500 mg **(Rx)**
Pancrease—lipase 4500 units/amylase 20,000 units/protease 25,000 units **(Rx)**
Pedia Care Cold-Allergy Chewable—pseudoephedrine 15 mg/chlorpheniramine 1 mg **(otc)**
Pedia Care Cough-Cold Liquid—(per 5 ml) pseudoephedrine 15 mg/chlorpheniramine 1 mg/dextromethorphan 5 mg **(otc)**
Pedia Care NightRest Cough-Cold Liquid—(per 5 ml) pseudoephedrine 15 mg/chlorpheniramine 1 mg/dextromethorphan 7.5 mg **(otc)**
Pediacof Syrup—(per 5 ml) codeine 5 mg/phenylephrine 2.5 mg/chlorpheniramine 0.75 mg/potassium iodide 75 mg/5% alcohol **(Rx)**
Pediacon DX Children's Syrup—(per 5 ml) phenylpropanolamine 6.25 mg/guaifenesin 100 mg/dextromethorphan 5 mg **(otc)**
Pediacon DX Pediatric Drops—(per 1 ml) phenylpropanolamine 6.25 mg/guaifenesin 50 mg/dextromethorphan 5 mg **(otc)**
Pediacon EX Drops—(per 1 ml) phenylpropanolamine 6.25 mg/guaifenesin 50 mg **(otc)**
Pediazole Suspension—(per 5 ml) erythromycin 200 mg/sulfisoxazole 600 mg **(Rx)**
Percocet—oxycodone 5 mg/acetaminophen 325 mg **(Rx)**
Percodan—oxycodone 4.88 mg/aspirin 325 mg **(Rx)**
Percogesic—phenyltoloxamine 30 mg/acetaminophen 325 mg **(otc)**
Perdiem Granules—(per teaspoonful) senna 0.74 g/psyllium 3.25 g/sodium 1.8 mg/potassium 35.5 mg **(otc)**
Peri-Colace—docusate sodium 100 mg/casanthranol 30 mg **(otc)**
Peri-Colace Syrup—(per 15 ml) docusate sodium 60 mg/casanthranol 30 mg **(otc)**
Phenerbel-S—phenobarbital 40 mg/ergotamine tartrate 0.6 mg/l-alkaloids of belladonna 0.2 mg **(Rx)**
Phenergan VC Syrup—(per 5 ml) phenylephrine 5 mg/promethazine 6.25 mg **(Rx)**
Phenergan VC w/Codeine Syrup—(per 5 ml) phenylephrine 5 mg/promethazine 6.25 mg/codeine 10 mg **(Rx)**
Phenergan w/Codeine Syrup—(per 5 ml) promethazine 6.25 mg/codeine 10 mg **(Rx)**
Phenylfenesin LA—phenylpropanolamine 75 mg/guaifenesin 400 mg **(Rx)**
Pherazine DM Syrup—(per 5 ml) dextromethorphan 15 mg/promethazine 6.25 mg/7% alcohol **(Rx)**
Phillips' Laxative Gelcaps—docusate sodium 83 mg/phenolphthalein 90 mg **(otc)**
PMB 400—conjugated estrogens 0.45 mg/meprobamate 400 mg **(Rx)**
Polaramine Expectorant Liquid—(per 5 ml) guaifenesin 100 mg/dexchlorpheniramine 2 mg/pseudoephedrine 20 mg/7.5% alcohol **(Rx)**
Polycillin-PRB Oral Suspension—(single dose) ampicillin 3.5 g/probenecid 1 g **(Rx)**
Polycitra Syrup—(per 5 ml) potassium citrate 550 mg/sodium citrate 500 mg/citric acid 334 mg **(Rx)**

Poly-Histine CS Syrup—(per 5 ml) phenylpropanolamine 12.5 mg/brompheniramine 2 mg/codeine 10 mg **(Rx)**
Poly-Histine DM Syrup—(per 5 ml) brompheniramine 2 mg/phenylpropanolamine 12.5 mg/dextromethorphan 10 mg **(Rx)**
Poly-Histine Elixir—(per 5 ml) pheniramine 4 mg/pyrilamine 4 mg/phenyltoloxamine 4 mg/4% alcohol **(Rx)**
Poly-Pred Ophthalmic Suspension—(per ml) 0.5% prednisolone acetate/0.35% neomycin/polymyxin B 10,000 units **(Rx)**
Polysporin Ophthalmic Ointment—(per g) polymyxin B 10,000 units/bacitracin 500 units **(Rx)**
Polysporin Topical Ointment—(per g) polymyxin B 10,000 units/bacitracin 500 units **(otc)**
Polytrim Ophthalmic Solution—(per ml) polymyxin B 10,000 units/trimethoprim 1 mg **(Rx)**
Premphase—conjugated estrogens 0.625 mg/medroxyprogesterone 5 mg plus conjugated estrogens 0.625 mg in a compliance package **(Rx)**
Prempro—conjugated estrogens 0.625 mg/medroxyprogesterone 2.5 mg in a compliance package **(Rx)**
Premsyn PMS—acetaminophen 500 mg/pamabrom 25 mg/pyrilamine 15 mg **(otc)**
Prevpac—amoxicillin 500 mg capsules/clarithromycin 500 mg tablets/lansoprazole 30 mg capsules in a compliance package **(Rx)**
Primatene—theophylline 130 mg/ephedrine 24 mg/phenobarbital 7.5 mg **(otc)**
Primatene Dual Action—theophylline 60 mg/ephedrine 12.5 mg/guaifenesin 100 mg **(otc)**
Primaxin 250 mg I.V. For Injection—imipenem 250 mg/cilastatin sodium 250 mg **(Rx)**
Primaxin 500 mg I.V. For Injection—imipenem 500 mg/cilastatin sodium 500 mg **(Rx)**
Prinzide 10-12.5—lisinopril 10 mg/hydrochlorothiazide 12.5 mg **(Rx)**
Prinzide 20-12.5—lisinopril 20 mg/hydrochlorothiazide 12.5 mg **(Rx)**
Prinzide 20-25—lisinopril 20 mg/hydrochlorothiazide 25 mg **(Rx)**
Probampacin Oral Suspension—(single dose) ampicillin 3.5 g/probenecid 1 g **(Rx)**
Proben-C—colchicine 0.5 mg/probenecid 500 mg **(Rx)**
Proctofoam-HC Aerosol Foam—1% hydrocortisone/1% pramoxine **(Rx)**
Propacet 100—propoxyphene-N 100 mg/acetaminophen 650 mg **(Rx)**
Pseudo-Chlor—pseudoephedrine 120 mg/chlorpheniramine 8 mg **(Rx)**
Pseudo-Gest Plus—pseudoephedrine 60 mg/chlorpheniramine 4 mg **(otc)**
Quadrinal—ephedrine 24 mg/theophylline 65 mg/potassium iodide 320 mg/phenobarbital 24 mg **(Rx)**
Quelidrine Cough Syrup—(per 5 ml) dextromethorphan 10 mg/phenylephrine 5 mg/ephedrine 5 mg/chlorpheniramine 2 mg/ammonium chloride 40 mg/ipecac 0.005 ml **(otc)**
Quibron-300—guaifenesin 180 mg/theophylline 300 mg **(Rx)**
R&C Shampoo—0.3% pyrethrins/3% piperonyl butoxide **(otc)**
Rauzide—bendroflumethiazide 4 mg/powdered rauwolfia serpentina 50 mg **(Rx)**
Regroton—chlorthalidone 50 mg/reserpine 0.25 mg **(Rx)**
Regulace—docusate sodium 100 mg/casanthranol 30 mg **(otc)**
Renese-R—polythiazide 2 mg/reserpine 0.25 mg **(Rx)**
Respahist—pseudoephedrine 60 mg/brompheniramine 6 mg **(Rx)**
Respaire-60—guaifenesin 200 mg/pseudoephedrine 60 mg **(Rx)**
RID Shampoo—0.3% pyrethrins/3% piperonyl butoxide **(otc)**
Rifamate—isoniazid 150 mg/rifampin 300 mg **(Rx)**
Rifater—rifampin 120 mg/isoniazid 50 mg/pyrazinamide 300 mg **(Rx)**
Riopan Plus Suspension—(per 5 ml) magaldrate 540 mg/simethicone 40 mg **(otc)**
Robaxisal—aspirin 325 mg/methocarbamol 400 mg **(Rx)**
Robitussin A-C Syrup—(per 5 ml) codeine 10 mg/guaifenesin 100 mg/3.5% alcohol **(Rx)**
Robitussin-CF Liquid—(per 5 ml) guaifenesin 100 mg/dextromethorphan 10 mg/phenylpropanolamine 12.5 mg/4.75% alcohol **(otc)**

Robitussin Cold & Cough Liqui-Gels—pseudoephedrine 30 mg/guaifenesin 200 mg/dextromethorphan 10 mg **(otc)**
Robitussin-DAC Syrup—(per 5 ml) codeine 10 mg/guaifenesin 100 mg/pseudoephedrine 30 mg/1.4% alcohol **(Rx)**
Robitussin-DM Liquid—(per 5 ml) guaifenesin 100 mg/dextromethorphan 10 mg **(otc)**
Robitussin Maximum Strength Cough and Cold Liquid—dextromethorphan 15 mg/pseudoephedrine 30 mg **(otc)**
Robitussin Night Relief Liquid—dextromethorphan 5 mg/pyrilamine 8.3 mg/pseudoephedrine 10 mg/acetaminophen 108.3 mg **(otc)**
Robitussin Pediatric Cough & Cold Liquid—(per 5 ml) pseudoephedrine 15 mg/dextromethorphan 7.5 mg **(otc)**
Robitussin-PE Syrup—guaifenesin 100 mg/pseudoephedrine 30 mg/1.4% alcohol **(otc)**
Robitussin Severe Congestion Liqui-Gels—guaifenesin 200 mg/pseudoephedrine 30 mg **(otc)**
Rolaids Calcium Rich—magnesium hydroxide 80 mg/calcium carbonate 412 mg **(otc)**
Rondec—pseudoephedrine 60 mg/carbinoxamine 4 mg **(Rx)**
Rondec DM Drops—(per 1 ml) pseudoephedrine 25 mg/carbinoxamine 2 mg/dextromethorphan 4 mg **(Rx)**
Rondec DM Syrup—(per 5 ml) pseudoephedrine 60 mg/carbinoxamine 4 mg/dextromethorphan 15 mg **(Rx)**
Rondec Oral Drops—(per 1 ml) pseudoephedrine 25 mg/carbinoxamine 2 mg **(Rx)**
Roxicet—oxycodone 5 mg/acetaminophen 325 mg **(Rx)**
Roxicet 5/500—oxycodone 5 mg/acetaminophen 500 mg **(Rx)**
Ru-Tuss—phenylephrine 25 mg/phenylpropanolamine 50 mg/chlorpheniramine 8 mg/hyoscyamine 0.19 mg/atropine 0.04 mg/scopolamine 0.01 mg **(Rx)**
Ru-Tuss DE—pseudoephedrine 120 mg/guaifenesin 600 mg **(Rx)**
Ru-Tuss Expectorant Liquid—(per 5 ml) guaifenesin 100 mg/pseudoephedrine 30 mg/dextromethorphan 10 mg/10% alcohol **(otc)**
Ru-Tuss w/Hydrocodone Liquid—(per 5 ml) hydrocodone 1.7 mg/phenylephrine 5 mg/pyrilamine 3.3 mg/pheniramine 3.3 mg/phenylpropanolamine 3.3 mg/5% alcohol **(Rx)**
Ryna-C Liquid—(per 5 ml) pseudoephedrine 30 mg/chlorpheniramine 2 mg/codeine 10 mg **(Rx)**
Ryna Liquid—(per 5 ml) pseudoephedrine 30 mg/chlorpheniramine 2 mg **(otc)**
Rynatan—phenylephrine 25 mg/chlorpheniramine 8 mg/pyrilamine 25 mg **(Rx)**
Rynatan Pediatric Suspension—(per 5 ml) phenylephrine 5 mg/chlorpheniramine 2 mg/pyrilamine 12.5 mg **(Rx)**
Rynatuss—ephedrine 10 mg/carbetapentane 60 mg/chlorpheniramine 5 mg/phenylephrine 10 mg **(Rx)**
Salutensin—reserpine 0.125 mg/hydroflumethiazide 50 mg **(Rx)**
Salutensin-Demi—reserpine 0.125 mg/hydroflumethiazide 25 mg **(Rx)**
Scot-Tussin DM Liquid—(per 5 ml) chlorpheniramine 2 mg/dextromethorphan 15 mg **(otc)**
Scot-Tussin Original 5-Action Liquid—phenylephrine 4.2 mg/pheniramine 13.3 mg/sodium citrate 83.3 mg/sodium salicylate 83.3 mg/caffeine citrate 25 mg **(otc)**
Scot-Tussin Senior Clear Liquid—(per 5 ml) guaifenesin 200 mg/dextromethorphan 15 mg **(otc)**
Sedapap-10—acetaminophen 650 mg/butalbital 50 mg **(Rx)**
Semprex-D—acrivastine 8 mg/pseudoephedrine 60 mg **(Rx)**
Senokot-S—standardized senna concentrate 187 mg/docusate sodium 50 mg **(otc)**
Septra—trimethoprim 80 mg/sulfamethoxazole 400 mg **(Rx)**
Septra DS—trimethoprim 160 mg/sulfamethoxazole 800 mg **(Rx)**
Septra I.V. For Injection—(per 5 ml) trimethoprim 80 mg/sulfamethoxazole 400 mg **(Rx)**
Septra Suspension—(per 5 ml) trimethoprim 40 mg/sulfamethoxazole 200 mg **(Rx)**
Ser-Ap-Es—hydralazine 25 mg/hydrochlorothiazide 15 mg/reserpine 0.1 mg **(Rx)**

Silafed Syrup—(per 5 ml) pseudoephedrine 30 mg/triprolidine 1.25 mg **(otc)**
Silaminic Cold Syrup—(per 5 ml) phenylpropanolamine 12.5 mg/chlorpheniramine 2 mg **(otc)**
Silaminic Expectorant Liquid—(per 5 ml) phenylpropanolamine 12.5 mg/guaifenesin 100 mg **(otc)**
Sinarest Extra Strength—pseudoephedrine 30 mg/chlorpheniramine 2 mg/acetaminophen 500 mg **(otc)**
Sinarest No Drowsiness—pseudoephedrine 30 mg/acetaminophen 500 mg **(otc)**
Sinarest Sinus—pseudoephedrine 30 mg/chlorpheniramine 2 mg/acetaminophen 325 mg **(otc)**
Sine-Aid IB—pseudoephedrine 30 mg/ibuprofen 200 mg **(otc)**
Sine-Aid Maximum Strength—pseudoephedrine 30 mg/acetaminophen 500 mg **(otc)**
Sinemet 10/100—carbidopa 10 mg/levodopa 100 mg **(Rx)**
Sinemet 25/100—carbidopa 25 mg/levodopa 100 mg **(Rx)**
Sinemet 25/250—carbidopa 25 mg/levodopa 250 mg **(Rx)**
Sinemet CR 25-100—carbidopa 25 mg/levodopa 100 mg **(Rx)**
Sinemet CR 50-200—carbidopa 50 mg/levodopa 200 mg **(Rx)**
Sine-Off Maximum Strength No Drowsiness Formula Caplets—pseudoephedrine 30 mg/acetaminophen 500 mg **(otc)**
Sine-Off Sinus Medicine—pseudoephedrine 30 mg/chlorpheniramine 2 mg/acetaminophen 500 mg **(otc)**
Sinutab Maximum Strength Sinus Allergy—acetaminophen 500 mg/chlorpheniramine 2 mg/pseudoephedrine 30 mg **(otc)**
Sinutab Maximum Strength Without Drowsiness—pseudoephedrine 30 mg/acetaminophen 500 mg **(otc)**
Sinutab Non-Drying—pseudoephedrine 30 mg/guaifenesin 200 mg **(otc)**
Slo-Phyllin GG—guaifenesin 90 mg/theophylline 150 mg **(Rx)**
Soma Compound—aspirin 325 mg/carisoprodol 200 mg **(Rx)**
Spec-T Lozenge—dextromethorphan 10 mg/benzocaine 10 mg **(otc)**
St. Joseph Cold Tablets For Children—phenylpropanolamine 3.125 mg/acetaminophen 80 mg **(otc)**
Sudafed Cold & Cough Liquicaps—pseudoephedrine 30 mg/dextromethorphan 10 mg/guaifenesin 100 mg/acetaminophen 250 mg **(otc)**
Sudafed Plus—pseudoephedrine 60 mg/chlorpheniramine 4 mg **(otc)**
Sudafed Severe Cold—pseudoephedrine 30 mg/dextromethorphan 15 mg **(otc)**
Sudafed Sinus Maximum Strength—pseudoephedrine 30 mg/acetaminophen 500 mg **(otc)**
Sudal 60/500—pseudoephedrine 60 mg/guaifenesin 500 mg **(Rx)**
Sudal 120/600—pseudoephedrine 120 mg/guaifenesin 600 mg **(Rx)**
Sultrin Triple Sulfa Vaginal Cream—3.42% sulfathiazole/2.86% sulfacetamide/3.7% sulfabenzamide **(Rx)**
Sultrin Triple Sulfa Vaginal Tablets—sulfathiazole 172.5 mg/sulfacetamide 143.75 mg/sulfabenzamide 184 mg/urea **(Rx)**
Synalgos-DC—aspirin 356.4 mg/caffeine 30 mg/dihydrocodeine 16 mg **(Rx)**
Talacen—acetaminophen 650 mg/pentazocine 25 mg **(Rx)**
Talwin Compound—aspirin 325 mg/pentazocine 12.5 mg **(Rx)**
Talwin NX—pentazocine 50 mg/naloxone 0.5 mg **(Rx)**
Tarka 182—trandolapril 2 mg (immediate release)/verapamil 180 mg (sustained release) **(Rx)**
Tarka 241—trandolapril 1 mg (immediate release)/verapamil 240 mg (sustained release) **(Rx)**
Tarka 242—trandolapril 2 mg (immediate release)/verapamil 240 mg (sustained release) **(Rx)**
Tarka 244—trandolapril 4 mg (immediate release)/verapamil 240 mg (sustained release) **(Rx)**
Tavist-D—clemastine 1.34 mg/phenylpropanolamine 75 mg **(otc)**
Tavist Sinus—acetaminophen 500 mg/pseudoephedrine 30 mg **(otc)**
Teczem—enalapril 5 mg (extended release)/diltiazem 180 mg (extended release) **(Rx)**
Tedrigen—ephedrine 22.5 mg/theophylline 120 mg/phenobarbital 7.5 mg **(Rx)**
Teen Midol—see ***Midol, Teen***

Tegrin-LT Shampoo—0.33% pyrethrins/3.15% piperonyl butoxide **(otc)**
Tenoretic 50—chlorthalidone 25 mg/atenolol 50 mg **(Rx)**
Tenoretic 100—chlorthalidone 25 mg/atenolol 100 mg **(Rx)**
Terra-Cortril Ophthalmic Suspension—1.5% hydrocortisone acetate/0.5% oxytetracycline **(Rx)**
Terramycin with Polymyxin B Sulfate Ophthalmic Ointment—(per g) polymyxin B 10,000 units/oxytetracycline 5 mg **(Rx)**
T-Gesic—hydrocodone 5 mg/acetaminophen 500 mg **(Rx)**
Theodrine—ephedrine 22.5 mg/theophylline 120 mg **(otc)**
Thera-Flu, Flu & Cold Medicine Powder—(per packet) pseudoephedrine 60 mg/chlorpheniramine 4 mg/acetaminophen 650 mg **(otc)**
Thera-Flu, Flu, Cold & Cough Powder—(per pack) pseudoephedrine 60 mg/chlorpheniramine 4 mg/dextromethorphan 20 mg/acetaminophen 650 mg **(otc)**
Thera-Flu NightTime Powder—(per pack) pseudoephedrine 60 mg/chlorpheniramine 4 mg/dextromethorphan 30 mg/acetaminophen 1000 mg **(otc)**
Thera-Flu Non-Drowsy Flu, Cold & Cough Maximum Strength Powder—(per pack) pseudoephedrine 60 mg/dextromethorphan 30 mg/acetaminophen 1000 mg **(otc)**
Thera-Flu Non-Drowsy Formula Maximum Strength Caplets—pseudoephedrine 30 mg/dextromethorphan 15 mg/acetaminophen 500 mg **(otc)**
Timentin For Injection—(3.1-g vials) ticarcillin 3 g/clavulanic acid 0.1 g **(Rx)**
Timolide 10-25—timolol 10 mg/hydrochlorothiazide 25 mg **(Rx)**
Titralac Plus—calcium carbonate 420 mg/simethicone 21 mg **(otc)**
TobraDex Ophthalmic Suspension/Ointment—0.1% dexamethasone/0.3% tobramycin **(Rx)**
Triacin-C Cough Syrup—(per 5 ml) codeine 10 mg/pseudoephedrine 30 mg/triprolidine 1.25 mg **(Rx)**
Tri-Hydroserpine—hydralazine 25 mg/hydrochlorothiazide 15 mg/reserpine 0.1 mg **(Rx)**
Tri-Levlen:
- ***Phase I***—levonorgestrel 0.05 mg/ethinyl estradiol 30 mcg **(Rx)**
- ***Phase II***—levonorgestrel 0.075 mg/ethinyl estradiol 40 mcg **(Rx)**
- ***Phase III***—levonorgestrel 0.125 mg/ethinyl estradiol 30 mcg **(Rx)**

Triaminic Allergy—phenylpropanolamine 25 mg/chlorpheniramine 4 mg **(otc)**
Triaminic AM Cough & Decongestant Formula Liquid—(per 5 ml) pseudoephedrine 15 mg/dextromethorphan 7.5 mg **(otc)**
Triaminic Cold—phenylpropanolamine 12.5 mg/chlorpheniramine 2 mg **(otc)**
Triaminic-DM Syrup—(per 5 ml) dextromethorphan 5 mg/phenylpropanolamine 6.25 mg **(otc)**
Triaminic Expectorant Liquid—(per 5 ml) guaifenesin 50 mg/phenylpropanolamine 6.25 mg **(otc)**
Triaminic Expectorant DH Liquid—(per 5 ml) guaifenesin 100 mg/hydrocodone 1.67 mg/phenylpropanolamine 12.5 mg/pheniramine 6.25 mg/pyrilamine 6.25 mg/5% alcohol **(Rx)**
Triaminic Expectorant w/Codeine Liquid—(per 5 ml) phenylpropanolamine 12.5 mg/codeine 10 mg/guaifenesin 100 mg **(Rx)**
Triaminic Nite Light Liquid—(per 5 ml) pseudoephedrine 15 mg/chlorpheniramine 1 mg/dextromethorphan 7.5 mg **(otc)**
Triaminic Oral Infant Drops—(per 1 ml) phenylpropanolamine 20 mg/pyrilamine 10 mg/pheniramine 10 mg **(Rx)**
Triaminic Sore Throat Formula Liquid—(per 5 ml) pseudoephedrine 15 mg/dextromethorphan 7.5 mg/acetaminophen 160 mg **(otc)**
Triaminic Syrup—(per 5 ml) phenylpropanolamine 6.25 mg/chlorpheniramine 1 mg **(otc)**
Triaminicin Cold, Allergy, Sinus—phenylpropanolamine 25 mg/chlorpheniramine 4 mg/acetaminophen 650 mg **(otc)**
Triaminicol Multi-Symptom Cough and Cold—phenylpropanolamine 12.5 mg/chlorpheniramine 2 mg/dextromethorphan 10 mg **(otc)**

Triaminicol Multi-Symptom Relief Liquid—(per 5 ml) phenylpropanolamine 12.5 mg/chlorpheniramine 2 mg/dextromethorphan 10 mg **(otc)**
Triavil 2-10—perphenazine 2 mg/amitriptyline 10 mg **(Rx)**
Triavil 2-25—perphenazine 2 mg/amitriptyline 25 mg **(Rx)**
Triavil 4-10—perphenazine 4 mg/amitriptyline 10 mg **(Rx)**
Triminol Cough Syrup—(per 5 ml) dextromethorphan 10 mg/chlorpheniramine 2 mg/phenylpropanolamine 12.5 mg **(otc)**
Trinalin Repetabs—azatadine maleate 1 mg/pseudoephedrine 120 mg **(Rx)**
Triphasil:
Phase I—levonorgestrel 0.05 mg/ethinyl estradiol 30 mcg **(Rx)**
Phase II—levonorgestrel 0.075 mg/ethinyl estradiol 40 mcg **(Rx)**
Phase III—levonorgestrel 0.125 mg/ethinyl estradiol 30 mcg **(Rx)**
Triple Antibiotic Ophthalmic Ointment—(per g) polymyxin B 10,000 units/neomycin 3.5 mg/bacitracin 400 units **(Rx)**
Tuinal 100 mg—amobarbital 50 mg/secobarbital 50 mg **(Rx)**
Tuinal 200 mg—amobarbital 100 mg/secobarbital 100 mg **(Rx)**
Tusibron-DM Syrup—(per 5 ml) guaifenesin 100 mg/dextromethorphan 15 mg **(otc)**
Tussionex Pennkinetic Suspension—(per 5 ml) chlorpheniramine 8 mg/hydrocodone 10 mg (as polistirex) **(Rx)**
Tussi-Organidin NR Liquid—(per 5 ml) codeine 10 mg/guaifenesin 100 mg **(Rx)**
Tussi-Organidin DM NR Liquid—(per 5 ml) guaifenesin 100 mg/dextromethorphan 10 mg **(Rx)**
Tylenol Allergy Sinus, Maximum Strength Gelcaps—acetaminophen 500 mg/chlorpheniramine 2 mg/pseudoephedrine 30 mg **(otc)**
Tylenol Children's Cold—acetaminophen 80 mg/chlorpheniramine 0.5 mg/pseudoephedrine 7.5 mg **(otc)**
Tylenol Children's Cold Liquid—(per 5 ml) acetaminophen 160 mg/chlorpheniramine 1 mg/pseudoephedrine 15 mg **(otc)**
Tylenol Children's Cold Multi-Symptom Plus Cough Liquid—(per 5 ml) acetaminophen 160 mg/dextromethorphan 5 mg/chlorpheniramine 1 mg/pseudoephedrine 15 mg **(otc)**
Tylenol Children's Cold Plus Cough Chewable—acetaminophen 80 mg/pseudoephedrine 7.5 mg/dextromethorphan 2.5 mg/chlorpheniramine 0.5 mg **(otc)**
Tylenol Cold Multi-Symptom—acetaminophen 325 mg/chlorpheniramine 2 mg/pseudoephedrine 30 mg/dextromethorphan 15 mg **(otc)**
Tylenol Cold No Drowsiness—acetaminophen 325 mg/pseudoephedrine 30 mg/dextromethorphan 15 mg **(otc)**
Tylenol Flu Maximum Strength Gelcaps—dextromethorphan 15 mg/pseudoephedrine 30 mg/acetaminophen 500 mg **(otc)**
Tylenol Flu NightTime Maximum Strength Gelcaps—pseudoephedrine 30 mg/chlorpheniramine 2 mg/acetaminophen 500 mg **(otc)**
Tylenol Flu NightTime Maximum Strength Powder—pseudoephedrine 60 mg/diphenhydramine 50 mg/acetaminophen 1000 mg **(otc)**
Tylenol Headache Plus, Extra Strength—acetaminophen 500 mg/calcium carbonate 250 mg **(otc)**
Tylenol Multi-Symptom Cough Liquid—(per 5 ml) dextromethorphan 10 mg/acetaminophen 216.7 mg/5% alcohol **(otc)**
Tylenol Multi-Symptom Cough w/Decongestant Liquid—(per 5 ml) dextromethorphan 10 mg/acetaminophen 200 mg/pseudoephedrine 20 mg **(otc)**
Tylenol Multi-Symptom Hot Medication—(per pack) acetaminophen 650 mg/chlorpheniramine 4 mg/pseudoephedrine 60 mg/dextromethorphan 30 mg **(otc)**
Tylenol PM, Extra Strength—acetaminophen 500 mg/diphenhydramine 25 mg **(otc)**
Tylenol Severe Allergy—diphenhydramine 12.5 mg/acetaminophen 500 mg **(otc)**
Tylenol Sinus Maximum Strength—pseudoephedrine 30 mg/acetaminophen 500 mg **(otc)**

Tylenol w/Codeine Elixir—(per 5 ml) codeine 12 mg/acetaminophen 120 mg **(Rx)**
Tylenol w/Codeine No. 2—acetaminophen 300 mg/codeine 15 mg **(Rx)**
Tylenol w/Codeine No. 3—acetaminophen 300 mg/codeine 30 mg **(Rx)**
Tylenol w/Codeine No. 4—acetaminophen 300 mg/codeine 60 mg **(Rx)**
Tylox—oxycodone 5 mg/acetaminophen 500 mg **(Rx)**
Tyrodone Liquid—(per 5 ml) hydrocodone 5 mg/pseudoephedrine 60 mg/5% alcohol **(Rx)**
Unasyn For Injection 1.5 g—ampicillin 1 g/sulbactam 0.5 g **(Rx)**
Unasyn For Injection 3 g—ampicillin 2 g/sulbactam 1 g **(Rx)**
Uniretic—moexipril 7.5 mg/hydrochlorothiazide 12.5 mg or moexipril 15 mg/hydrochlorothiazide 25 mg **(Rx)**
Unituss HC Syrup—(per 5 ml) hydrocodone 2.5 mg/phenylephrine 5 mg/chlorpheniramine 2 mg **(Rx)**
Urised—methenamine 40.8 mg/phenyl salicylate 18.1 mg/atropine 0.03 mg/hyoscyamine 0.3 mg/benzoic acid 4.5 mg/methylene blue 5.4 mg **(Rx)**
Ursinus Inlay—pseudoephedrine 30 mg/aspirin 325 mg **(otc)**
Vanquish—aspirin 227 mg/acetaminophen 194 mg/caffeine 33 mg **(otc)**
Vaseretic 10-25—enalapril 10 mg/hydrochlorothiazide 25 mg **(Rx)**
Vasocidin Ophthalmic Ointment—0.5% prednisolone/10% sulfacetamide **(Rx)**
Vasocidin Ophthalmic Solution—0.25% prednisolone/10% sulfacetamide **(Rx)**
Vasocon-A Ophthalmic Solution—0.05% naphazoline/0.5% antazoline **(Rx)**
Vicks 44D Cough & Head Congestion Liquid—(per 5 ml) dextromethorphan 10 mg/pseudoephedrine 20 mg **(otc)**
Vicks 44E Liquid—(per 5 ml) dextromethorphan 6.7 mg/guaifenesin 66.7 mg **(otc)**
Vicks 44M Cold, Flu,& Cough LiquiCaps—dextromethorphan 10 mg/pseudoephedrine 30 mg/chlorpheniramine 2 mg/acetaminophen 250 mg **(otc)**
Vicks 44 Non-Drowsy Cold & Cough LiquiCaps—dextromethorphan 30 mg/pseudoephedrine 60 mg **(otc)**
Vicks Children's NyQuil Nighttime Cough/Cold Liquid—(per 5 ml) pseudoephedrine 10 mg/chlorpheniramine 0.67 mg/dextromethorphan 5 mg **(otc)**
Vicks Cough Silencers—dextromethorphan 2.5 mg/benzocaine 1 mg **(otc)**
Vicks DayQuil Allergy Relief 4 Hour—phenylpropanolamine 25 mg/brompheniramine 4 mg **(otc)**
Vicks DayQuil Allergy Relief 12 Hour ER—phenylpropanolamine 75 mg/brompheniramine 12 mg **(otc)**
Vicks DayQuil Liquid—(per 5 ml) dextromethorphan 3.3 mg/pseudoephedrine 10 mg/acetaminophen 108.3 mg/guaifenesin 33.3 mg **(otc)**
Vicks DayQuil Sinus Pressure & Pain Relief—pseudoephedrine 30 mg/acetaminophen 500 mg **(otc)**
Vicks NyQuil Liquicaps—pseudoephedrine 30 mg/doxylamine 6.25 mg/dextromethorphan 10 mg/acetaminophen 250 mg **(otc)**
Vicks NyQuil Multi-Symptom Cold Flu Relief Liquid—(per 5 ml) pseudoephedrine 10 mg/doxylamine 2.1 mg/dextromethorphan 5 mg/acetaminophen 167 mg **(otc)**
Vicks Pediatric Formula 44e Liquid—(per 5 ml) dextromethorphan 3.3 mg/guaifenesin 33.3 mg **(otc)**
Vicks Pediatric Formula 44m Multi-Symptom Cough & Cold Liquid—(per 5 ml) pseudoephedrine 10 mg/chlorpheniramine 0.67 mg/dextromethorphan 5 mg **(otc)**
Vicodin—acetaminophen 500 mg/hydrocodone 5 mg **(Rx)**
Vicodin ES—hydrocodone 7.5 mg/acetaminophen 750 mg **(Rx)**
Vicodin HP—hydrocodone 10 mg/acetaminophen 660 mg **(Rx)**
VicodinTuss—(per 5 ml) hydrocodone 5 mg/guaifenesin 100 mg **(Rx, C-III)**
Vicoprofen—hydrocodone 7.5 mg/ibuprofen 200 mg **(Rx)**
Wigraine Supps—ergotamine 2 mg/caffeine 100 mg **(Rx)**
Zestoretic 10/12.5—lisinopril 10 mg/hydrochlorothiazide 12.5 mg **(Rx)**

Zestoretic 20/12.5—lisinopril 20 mg/hydrochlorothiazide 12.5 mg **(Rx)**
Zestoretic 20/25—lisinopril 20 mg/hydrochlorothiazide 25 mg **(Rx)**
Ziac 2.5 mg—bisoprolol 2.5 mg/hydrochlorothiazide 6.25 mg **(Rx)**
Ziac 5 mg—bisoprolol 5 mg/hydrochlorothiazide 6.25 mg **(Rx)**
Ziac 10 mg—bisoprolol 10 mg/hydrochlorothiazide 6.25 mg **(Rx)**
Zydone—hydrocodone 5 mg/acetaminophen 500 mg **(Rx)**

APPENDIX B

Equianalgesic Tables

DOSING DATA FOR OPIOID ANALGESICS*

DRUG	APPROXIMATE EQUIANALGESIC DOSE		RECOMMENDED STARTING DOSE (adults >50 kg body weight)		RECOMMENDED STARTING DOSE (children and adults <50 kg body weight)[1]	
	ORAL	PARENTERAL	ORAL	PARENTERAL	ORAL	PARENTERAL
Opioid Agonist						
Morphine[2]	30 mg q 3–4 hr (around-the-clock dosing) 60 mg q 3–4 hr (single dose or intermittent dosing)	10 mg q 3–4 hr	30 mg q 3–4 hr	10 mg q 3–4 hr	0.3 mg/kg q 3–4 hr	0.1 mg/kg q 3–4 hr
Codeine[3]	180–200 mg q 3–4 hr	130 mg q 3–4 hr	60 mg q 3–4 hr	60 mg q 2 hr (intramuscular/subcutaneous)	1 mg/kg q 3–4 hr[4]	Not recommended
Hydrocodone (in Lorcet, Lortab, Vicodin, others)	30 mg q 3–4 hr	Not available	10 mg q 3–4 hr	Not available	0.2 mg/kg q 3–4 hr[4]	Not available
Hydromorphone[2] (Dilaudid)	7.5 mg q 3–4 hr	1.5 mg q 3–4 hr	6 mg q 3–4 hr	1.5 mg q 3–4 hr	0.06 mg/kg q 3–4 hr	0.015 mg/kg q 3–4 hr
Levorphanol (Levo-Dromoran)	4 mg q 6–8 hr	2 mg q 6–8 hr	4 mg q 6–8 hr	2 mg q 6–8 hr	0.04 mg/kg q 6–8 hr	0.02 mg/kg q 6–8 hr
Meperidine (Demerol)	300 mg q 2–3 hr	100 mg q 3 hr	Not recommended	100 mg q 3 hr	Not recommended	0.75 mg/kg q 2–3 hr
Methadone (Dolophine, others)	20 mg q 6–8 hr	10 mg q 6–8 hr	20 mg q 6–8 hr	10 mg q 6–8 hr	0.2 mg/kg q 6–8 hr	0.1 mg/kg q 6–8 hr
Oxycodone (Roxicodone, also in Percocet, Percodan, Tylox, others)	30 mg q 3–4 hr	Not available	10 mg q 3–4 hr	Not available	0.2 mg/kg q 3–4 hr[4]	Not available
Oxymorphone[2] (Numorphan)	Not available	1 mg q 3–4 hr	Not available	1 mg q 3–4 hr	Not recommended	Not recommended

Opioid Agonist-Antagonist and Partial Agonist						
Buprenorphine (Buprenex)	Not available	0.3–0.4 mg q 6–8 hr	Not available	0.4 mg q 6–8 hr	Not available	0.004 mg/kg q 6–8 hr
Butorphanol (Stadol)	Not available	2 mg q 3–4 hr	Not available	2 mg q 3–4 hr	Not available	Not recommended
Dezocine (Dalgan)	Not available	10 mg q 3–4 hr	Not available	10 mg q 3–4 hr	Not available	Not recommended
Nalbuphine (Nubain)	Not available	10 mg q 3–4 hr	Not available	10 mg q 3–4 hr	Not available	0.1 mg/kg q 3–4 hr
Pentazocine (Talwin, others)	150 mg q 3–4 hr	60 mg q 3–4 hr	50 mg q 4–6 hr	Not recommended	Not recommended	Not recommended

Note: Published tables vary in the suggested doses that are equianalgesic to morphine. Clinical response is the criterion that must be applied for each patient; titration to clinical response is necessary. Because there is not complete cross-tolerance among these drugs, it is usually necessary to use a lower than equianalgesic dose when changing drugs and to retitrate to response.

Caution: Recommended doses do not apply to patients with renal or hepatic insufficiency or other conditions affecting drug metabolism and kinetics.

[1]**Caution:** Doses listed for patients with body weight less than 50 kg cannot be used as initial starting doses in babies less than 6 mo of age.

[2]For morphine, hydromorphone, and oxymorphone, rectal administration is an alternate route for patients unable to take oral medications, but equianalgesic doses may differ from oral and parenteral doses because of pharmacokinetic differences.

[3]**Caution:** Codeine doses above 65 mg often are not appropriate because of diminishing incremental analgesia with increasing doses but continually increasing constipation and other side effects. Oral doses refer to combination with aspirin or acetaminophen.

[4]**Caution:** Doses of aspirin and acetaminophen in combination opioid/NSAID preparations must also be adjusted to the patient's body weight.

*Adapted from Acute Pain Management Guideline Panel: *Acute Pain Management in Adults: Operative Procedures. Quick Reference Guide for Clinicians.* Agency for Health Care Policy and Research, Public Health and Human Services, Rockville, MD. AHCPR Publication No. 92-0019.

FENTANYL TRANSDERMAL DOSE BASED ON DAILY MORPHINE DOSE*

ORAL 24-HR MORPHINE (mg/day)	IM 24-HR MORPHINE (mg/day)	FENTANYL TRANSDERMAL (mcg/hr)
45–134	8–22	25
135–224	23–37	50
225–314	38–52	75
315–404	53–67	100
405–494	68–82	125
495–584	83–97	150
585–674	98–112	175
675–764	113–127	200
765–854	128–142	225
855–944	143–157	250
945–1034	158–172	275
1035–1124	173–187	300

*A 10-mg IM or 60-mg oral dose of morphine every 4 hr for 24 hr (total of 60 mg/day IM or 360 mg/day oral) was considered approximately equivalent to fentanyl transdermal 100 mcg/hr.

OPIOID ANALGESICS COMMONLY USED FOR MILD TO MODERATE PAIN

NAME	STARTING DOSE* ADULTS (mg)	CHILDREN (mg/kg)	COMMENTS	PRECAUTIONS AND CONTRAINDICATIONS
Morphine-like Agonists				
Codeine	30–60	0.5–1	Many preparations include combination with nonopioid analgesics.†	Caution in patients with impaired ventilation, bronchial asthma, increased intracranial pressure, liver failure.
Hydrocodone (in Lorcet, Lortab, Vicodin, Zydone, others)	5–10	0.2	Preparations include acetaminophen, which limits daily dose.	Same as codeine.
Meperidine (Demerol)	NR‡	NR‡	Shorter acting; biotransformed to normeperidine, a toxic metabolite.	Normeperidine accumulates with repetitive dosing, causing CNS excitation; avoid in patients with impaired renal function or who are receiving monoamine oxidase inhibitors; avoid any chronic use.
Oxycodone	5–10	0.1	Shorter acting; many preparations include acetaminophen, which limits dose to 12 tabs/day.†	Same as for codeine.
Propoxyphene (Darvon)	65–130	NR‡	Weak analgesic; many preparations include nonopioid analgesics; biotransformed to potentially toxic metabolite (norpropoxyphene).	Propoxyphene and metabolite accumulate with repetitive dosing; overdose complicated by convulsions.
Mixed Agonist-Antagonist				
Pentazocine (Talwin)	50	NR‡	Some preparations include naloxone to discourage parenteral abuse.	May cause psychotomimetic effects; may precipitate withdrawal in opioid-dependent patients.

*Starting doses are approximately equianalgesic to aspirin 650 mg (adults) or 10–15 mg/kg (children). The optimal dose for each patient is determined by titration.
†In children, opioid-acetaminophen formulations must not exceed the maximum safe dose of acetaminophen, 90 mg/kg/day.
‡NR = not recommended.
Adapted from American Pain Society: *Principles of Analgesic Use in the Treatment of Acute Pain and Cancer Pain*, ed 3, 1992.

APPENDIX C

Schedules of Controlled Substances

Classes or schedules are determined by the Drug Enforcement Agency (DEA), an arm of the United States Justice Department, and are based on the potential for abuse and dependence liability (physical and psychological) of the medication. Some states may have stricter prescription regulations. Physicians, dentists, podiatrists, and veterinarians may prescribe controlled substances. Nurse practitioners and physician's assistants may prescribe controlled substances with certain limitations.

Schedule I (C-I):

Potential for abuse is so high as to be unacceptable. May be used for research with appropriate limitations. Examples are LSD and heroin.

Schedule II (C-II):

High potential for abuse and extreme liability for physical and psychological dependence (amphetamines, opioid analgesics, dronabinol, certain barbiturates). Outpatient prescriptions must be in writing. In emergencies, telephone orders may be acceptable if a written prescription is provided within 72 hr. No refills are allowed.

Schedule II Drugs Included in *Davis's Drug Guide for Nurses*

afentanil
alfentanil
amphetamine
codeine (single entity; solid dosage form or injectable)
dronabinol
fentanyl
fentanyl transmucosal
hydromorphone
levorphanol
meperidine
methadone
methylphenidate
morphine
oxycodone (alone and in combination with nonopioid analgesics)
oxymorphone
pentobarbital (oral and parenteral)
remifentanil
sufentanil

Schedule III (C-III):

Intermediate potential for abuse (less than C-II) and intermediate liability for physical and psychological dependence (certain nonbarbiturate sedatives, certain nonamphetamine CNS stimulants, and limited dosages of certain opioid analgesics). Outpatient prescriptions can be refilled 5 times within 6 mo from date of issue if authorized by prescriber. Telephone orders are acceptable.

Schedule III Drugs Included in *Davis's Drug Guide for Nurses*

anabolic steroids (testosterone)
butalbital compound (in combination with nonopioid analgesics)
codeine (in combination with nonopioid analgesics; solid oral dosage forms)
hydrocodone (in combination with nonopioid analgesics)
pentobarbital (rectal)
thiopental

Schedule IV (C-IV):

Less abuse potential than Schedule III with minimal liability for physical or psychological dependence (certain sedative/hypnotics, certain antianxiety agents, some barbiturates, benzodiazepines, chloral hydrate, pentazocine, and propoxyphene). Outpatient prescriptions can be refilled 6 times within 6 mo from date of issue if authorized by prescriber. Telephone orders are acceptable.

Schedule IV Drugs Included in *Davis's Drug Guide for Nurses*

alprazolam
butorphanol
chloral hydrate
chlordiazepoxide
clonazepam
clorazepate
codeine (elixir or oral suspension with acetaminophen)
diazepam
difenoxin/atropine
flurazepam
lorazepam
methohexital
midazolam
oxazepam
pemoline
pentazocine
phenobarbital
phentermine
propoxyphene
quazepam
temazepam
triazolam
zolpidem

Schedule V (C-V):

Minimal abuse potential. Number of outpatient refills determined by prescriber. Some products (cough suppressants with small amounts of codeine, antidiarrheals containing paregoric) may be available without prescription to patients >18 yr of age.

Schedule V Drugs Included in *Davis's Drug Guide for Nurses*

buprenorphine
codeine (in cough preparations; ≤ 10 mg/5 ml or dosage unit)
diphenoxylate/atropine

APPENDIX D

Infusion Rate Tables

ALTEPLASE (Activase) Accelerated Infusion for Acute Myocardial Infarction*

Dilution: 50-mg vial with 50-ml diluent, or 100-mg vial with 100-ml diluent = 1 mg/ml.

Alteplase	dose (vol) bolus	dose (vol) next 30 min	dose (vol) next 60 min
pt >67 kg	15 mg (15 ml)	50 mg (50 ml)	35 mg (35 ml)
pt ≤67 kg	15 mg (15 ml)	0.75 mg/kg (0.75 ml/kg)	0.5 mg/kg (0.5 ml/kg)

*Total dose should not exceed 100 mg.

ALTEPLASE (Activase) 3-hr Infusion for Acute Myocardial Infarction

Dilution: 50-mg vial with 50-ml diluent or 100-mg vial with 100-ml diluent = 1 mg/ml.

Alteplase	**dose (vol)**	**dose (vol)**	**dose (vol)**
1 mg/ml	*first hr**	*second hr*	*third hr*
pt ≥65 kg	60 mg (60 ml)	20 mg (20 ml)	20 mg (20 ml)
Alteplase	**dose (vol)**	**dose (vol)**	**dose (vol)**
1 mg/ml	*first hr*†	*second hr*	*third hr*
pt <65 kg	0.75 mg/kg (0.75 ml/kg)	0.25 mg/kg (0.25 ml/kg)	0.25 mg/kg (0.25 ml/kg)

*Give 6–10 mg (6–10 ml) as a bolus over first 1–2 min.
†0.075–0.125 mg/kg of this given as a bolus over the first 1–2 min.

ALTEPLASE (Activase) for Acute Ischemic Stroke

Dilution: 50-mg vial with 50-ml diluent or 100-mg vial with 100-ml diluent = 1 mg/ml.

	Patient Weight					
Alteplase dose	**50 kg**	**60 kg**	**70 kg**	**80 kg**	**90 kg**	**100 kg**
Total dose over 60 min (0.9 mg/kg)*	45 mg (45 ml)	54 mg (54 ml)	63 mg (63 ml)	72 mg (72 ml)	81 mg (81 ml)	90 mg (90 ml)
Bolus dose over first min	4.5 mg (4.5 ml)	5.4 mg (5.4 ml)	6.3 mg (6.3 ml)	7.2 mg (7.2 ml)	8.1 mg (8.1 ml)	9 mg (9 ml)
Remaining dose over next 59 min	40.5 mg (40.5 ml)	48.6 mg (48.6 ml)	56.7 mg (56.7 ml)	64.8 mg (64.8 ml)	72.9 mg (72.9 ml)	81 mg (81 ml)
Rate over remaining 59 min	0.69 mg/min (0.69 ml/min)	0.82 mg/min (0.82 ml/min)	0.96 mg/min (0.96 ml/min)	1.1 mg/min (1.1 ml/min)	1.24 mg/min (1.24 ml/min)	1.37 mg/min (1.37 ml/min)

*Total dose should not exceed 90 mg.

AMINOPHYLLINE

Dilution: 250 mg in 250 ml or 500 mg in 500 ml or 1000 mg in 1000 ml = 1 mg/ml.
Loading dose in patients who have not received aminophylline in preceding 24 hr = 5.6 mg/kg (5.6 ml/kg) of above dilution administered over 20 min. Aminophylline is approximately 85% theophylline.

Aminophylline Infusion Rates (ml/hr)
Concentration = 1 mg/ml
Patient Weight

Dose	**50 kg**	**60 kg**	**70 kg**	**80 kg**	**90 kg**	**100 kg**
loading dose (mg)*	**280 mg**	**336 mg**	**392 mg**	**448 mg**	**504 mg**	**560 mg**
0.9 mg/kg/hr	45 ml/hr	54 ml/hr	63 ml/hr	72 ml/hr	81 ml/hr	90 ml/hr
0.8 mg/kg/hr	40 ml/hr	48 ml/hr	56 ml/hr	64 ml/hr	72 ml/hr	80 ml/hr
0.7 mg/kg/hr	35 ml/hr	42 ml/hr	49 hl/hr	56 ml/hr	63 ml/hr	70 ml/hr
0.6 mg/kg/hr	30 ml/hr	36 ml/hr	42 ml/hr	48 ml/hr	54 ml/hr	60 ml/hr
0.5 mg/kg/hr	25 ml/hr	30 ml/hr	35 ml/hr	40 ml/hr	45 ml/hr	50 ml/hr
0.4 mg/kg/hr	20 ml/hr	24 ml/hr	28 ml/hr	32 ml/hr	36 ml/hr	40 ml/hr
0.3 mg/kg/hr	15 ml/hr	18 ml/hr	21 ml/hr	24 ml/hr	27 ml/hr	30 ml/hr
0.2 mg/kg/hr	10 ml/hr	12 ml/hr	14 ml/hr	16 ml/hr	18 ml/hr	20 ml/hr
0.1 mg/kg/hr	5 ml/hr	6 ml/hr	7 ml/hr	8 ml/hr	9 ml/hr	10 ml/hr

*Loading dose administered over 20 min.

AMIODARONE (Cordarone)

Type of Infusion	**Dose (rate)**	**Dilution (concentration)**
First rapid loading infusion	150 mg over 10 min (15 mg/min)	150 mg in 100 ml D5W (1.5 mg/ml)
Second slow loading infusion	360 mg over next 6 hr (1 mg/min)	900 mg in 500 ml D5W (1.8 mg/ml)
Maintenance infusion	540 mg over next 18 hr (0.5 mg/min)*	900 mg in 500 ml D5W (1.8 mg/ml)

*Infusion may be continued at 0.5 mg/min after first 24 hr using a concentration of 1–6 mg/ml (if concentration >2 mg/ml, use a central line). Breakthrough arrhythmias may be treated with additional doses of 150 mg mixed in 100 ml D5W and infused over 10 min. A subsequent increase in infusion rate may be required.

AMRINONE (Inocor)

Dilution: 100 mg/100 ml = 1 mg/ml.
Dilute with 0.45% or 0.9% sodium chloride.
Loading dose: 0.75 mg/kg (0.75 ml/kg) over 2–3 min.
To calculate infusion rate (ml/min), multiply patient's weight (kg) by dose in ml/kg/min.
To calculate infusion rate (ml/hr), multiply patient's weight (kg) by dose in mg/kg/min × 60.

Amrinone Infusion Rates (ml/hr)
Concentration = 1 mg/ml
Patient Weight

Dose	**50 kg**	**60 kg**	**70 kg**	**80 kg**	**90 kg**	**100 kg**
loading dose (mg)*	**37.5 mg**	**45 mg**	**52.5 mg**	**60 mg**	**67.5 mg**	**75 mg**
5 mcg/kg/min	15 ml/hr	18 ml/hr	21 ml/hr	24 ml/hr	27 ml/hr	30 ml/hr
6 mcg/kg/min	18 ml/hr	21.6 ml/hr	25.5 ml/hr	28.8 ml/hr	32.4 ml/hr	36 ml/hr
7 mcg/kg/min	21 ml/hr	25.2 ml/hr	29.4 ml/hr	33.6 ml/hr	37.8 ml/hr	47 ml/hr
8 mcg/kg/min	24 ml/hr	28.8 ml/hr	33.6 ml/hr	38.4 ml/hr	43.2 ml/hr	48 ml/hr
9 mcg/kg/min	27 ml/hr	32.4 ml/hr	37.8 ml/hr	43.2 ml/hr	48.6 ml/hr	54 ml/hr
10 mcg/kg/min	30 ml/hr	36 ml/hr	42 ml/hr	48 ml/hr	54 ml/hr	60 ml/hr

*Given over 2–3 min.

BRETYLIUM (Bretylol)

A. For life-threatening ventricular arrhythmias: (Ventricular fibrillation or hemodynamically unstable ventricular tachycardia.) Administer 5 mg/kg (0.1 ml/kg) of *undiluted* drug by rapid IV injection. *Undiluted* drug concentration = 50 mg/1 ml.

Rapid IV Injection of Undiluted Bretylium
Doses given in volume of undiluted bretylium injection
>50 mg/1 ml

	Patient Weight					
Dose	**50 kg**	**60 kg**	**70 kg**	**80 kg**	**90 kg**	**100 kg**
5 mg/kg	5 ml	6 ml	7 ml	8 ml	9 ml	10 ml

B. For other ventricular arrhythmias: Dilution: 2 g/500 ml = 4 mg/ml. Administer as 5–10 mg/kg (1.25–2.5 ml/kg) IV over 10–30 min; may be repeated q 6 hr or adminstered as a continuous infusion at 1–2 mg/min.

Bretylium Intermittent Infusion Rates
Volume of diluted bretylium
to infuse over 10–30 min
Concentration = 4 mg/ml

	Patient Weight					
Dose	**50 kg**	**60 kg**	**70 kg**	**80 kg**	**90 kg**	**100 kg**
5 mg/kg	62.5 ml	75 ml	87.5 ml	100 ml	112.5 ml	125 ml
6 mg/kg	75 ml	90 ml	105 ml	120 ml	135 ml	150 ml
7 mg/kg	87.5 ml	105 ml	122.5 ml	140 ml	157.5 ml	175 ml
8 mg/kg	100 ml	120 ml	140 ml	160 ml	180 ml	200 ml
9 mg/kg	112.5 ml	135 ml	157.5 ml	180 ml	202.5 ml	225 ml
10 mg/kg	125 ml	150 ml	175 ml	200 ml	225 ml	250 ml

Bretylium Continuous Infusion Rates
Concentration = 4 mg/ml

Dose (mg/min)	Dose (ml/hr)
1.0 mg/min	15 ml/hr
1.5 mg/min	23 ml/hr
2.0 mg/min	30 ml/hr

DOBUTAMINE (Dobutrex)

Dilution: May be prepared as 250 mg/1000 ml = 250 mcg/ml.
500 mg/1000 ml = 500 mcg/ml.
1000 mg/1000 ml = 1000 mcg/ml.
To calculate infusion rate (ml/min), multiply patient's weight (kg) by dose in ml/kg/min.
To calculate infusion rate (ml/hr), multiply patient's weight (kg) by dose in ml/kg/min × 60.

Dobutamine Infusion Rates

	Infusion rates (ml/kg/min) at various concentrations		
Dose (mcg/kg/min)	**250 mcg/ml concentration**	**500 mcg/ml concentration**	**1000 mcg/ml concentration**
2.5 mcg/kg/min	0.01 ml/kg/min	0.005 ml/kg/min	0.0025 ml/kg/min
5 mcg/kg/min	0.02 ml/kg/min	0.01 ml/kg/min	0.005 ml/kg/min
7.5 mcg/kg/min	0.03 ml/kg/min	0.015 ml/kg/min	0.0075 ml/kg/min
10 mcg/kg/min	0.04 ml/kg/min	0.02 ml/kg/min	0.01 ml/kg/min
12.5 mcg/kg/min	0.05 ml/kg/min	0.025 ml/kg/min	0.0125 ml/kg/min
15 mcg/kg/min	0.06 ml/kg/min	0.03 ml/kg/min	0.015 ml/kg/min

DOPAMINE (Intropin)

Dilution: May be prepared as 200 mg/500 ml = 400 mcg/ml.
400 mg/500 ml = 800 mcg/ml.
800 mg/500 ml = 1600 mcg/ml.
To calculate infusion rate (ml/min), multiply patient's weight (kg) by dose in ml/kg/min.
To calculate infusion rate (ml/hr), multiply patient's weight (kg) by dose in ml/kg/min × 60.

Dopamine Infusion Rates

	Infusion rates (ml/kg/min) at various concentrations		
Dose (mcg/kg/min)	**400 mcg/ml concentration**	**800 mcg/ml concentration**	**1600 mcg/ml concentration***
2 mcg/kg/min	0.005 ml/kg/min	0.0025 ml/kg/min	0.000125 ml/kg/min
5 mcg/kg/min	0.0125 ml/kg/min	0.00625 ml/kg/min	0.003125 ml/kg/min
10 mcg/kg/min	0.025 ml/kg/min	0.0125 ml/kg/min	0.00625 ml/kg/min
20 mcg/kg/min	0.05 ml/kg/min	0.025 ml/kg/min	0.0125 ml/kg/min
30 mcg/kg/min	0.075 ml/kg/min	0.0375 ml/kg/min	0.01875 ml/kg/min
40 mcg/kg/min	0.1 ml/kg/min	0.05 ml/kg/min	0.025 ml/kg/min
50 mcg/kg/min	0.125 ml/kg/min	0.0625 ml/kg/min	0.03125 ml/kg/min

*Appropriate concentration for patients with restricted fluid intake.

ESMOLOL (Brevibloc)

Dilution: 5 g/500 ml = 10 mg/ml.
Loading regimen = 500 mcg/kg (0.05 ml/kg) loading dose over 1 min followed by 50 mcg/kg/min (0.005 ml/kg/min) infusion over 4 min. If no response, repeat loading dose over 1 min and increase infusion rate to 100 mcg/kg/min for 4–10 min. If no response, loading may be repeated before increasing infusion rates in 50 mcg/kg/min increments.

Esmolol Infusion Rates
Concentration = 10 mg/ml
Patient Weight

Dose	**50 kg**	**60 kg**	**70 kg**	**80 kg**	**90 kg**	**100 kg**
loading dose (ml)*	**2.5 ml**	**3 ml**	**3.5 ml**	**4 ml**	**4.5 ml**	**5 ml**
50 mcg/kg/min	15 ml/hr	18 ml/hr	21 ml/hr	24 ml/hr	27 ml/hr	30 ml/hr
75 mcg/kg/min	22.5 ml/hr	27 ml/hr	31.5 ml/hr	36 ml/hr	40.5 ml/hr	45 ml/hr
100 mcg/kg/min	30 ml/hr	36 ml/hr	42 ml/hr	48 ml/hr	54 ml/hr	60 ml/hr
125 mcg/kg/min	37.5 ml/hr	45 ml/hr	52.5 ml/hr	60 ml/hr	67.5 ml/hr	75 ml/hr
150 mcg/kg/min	38 ml/hr	54 ml/hr	63 ml/hr	72 ml/hr	81 ml/hr	90 ml/hr
175 mcg/kg/min	52.5 ml/hr	63 ml/hr	73.5 ml/hr	84 ml/hr	94.5 ml/hr	105 ml/hr
200 mcg/kg/min	60 ml/hr	72 ml/hr	84 ml/hr	96 ml/hr	108 ml/hr	120 ml/hr

*Loading dose given over 1 min.

HEPARIN

Dilution: 20,000 units/1000 ml = 20 units/ml.
Loading dose: 1000–2000 units as a bolus.

Heparin Infusion Rates (ml/hr)
Concentration = 20 units/ml

Dose (units/hr)	**Dose (ml/hr)**
500 units/hr	25 ml/hr
750 units/hr	37.5 ml/hr
1000 units/hr	50 ml/hr
1250 units/hr	62.5 ml/hr
1500 units/hr	75 ml/hr
1750 units/hr	87.5 ml/hr
2000 units/hr	100 ml/hr

LIDOCAINE (Xylocaine)

Dilution: May be prepared as 1 g/1000 ml = 1 mg/ml.
2 g/1000 ml = 2 mg/ml.
4 g/1000 ml = 4 mg/ml.
8 g/1000 ml = 8 mg/ml.
Loading dose: 50–100 mg at 25–50 mg/min.

Lidocaine Infusion Rates (ml/hr)

Dose (mg/min)	1 mg/ml concentration	2 mg/ml concentration	4 mg/ml concentration	8 mg/ml concentration
1 mg/min	60 ml/hr	30 ml/hr	15 ml/hr	7.5 ml/hr
2 mg/min	120 ml/hr	60 ml/hr	30 ml/hr	15 ml/hr
3 mg/min	180 ml/hr	90 ml/hr	45 ml/hr	22.5 ml/hr
4 mg/min	240 ml/hr	120 ml/hr	60 ml/hr	30 ml/hr

MILRINONE (Primacor)

Loading dose: 50 mcg/kg given over 10 min.

Milrinone Infusion Rates (ml/hr)
Patient Weight

Dose	50 kg	60 kg	70 kg	80 kg	90 kg	100 kg
loading dose (mg)	2.5 mg	3.0 mg	3.5 mg	4.0 mg	4.5 mg	5.0 mg

Milrinone Infusion Rates

Dose (mcg/kg/min)	Infusion rates (ml/kg/min) at various concentrations		
	100 mcg/ml concentration	150 mcg/ml concentration	200 mcg/ml concentration
0.375 mcg/kg/min	0.00375 ml/kg/min	0.0025 ml/kg/min	0.001875 ml/kg/min
0.400 mcg/kg/min	0.004 ml/kg/min	0.00267 ml/kg/min	0.002 ml/kg/min
0.500 mcg/kg/min	0.005 ml/kg/min	0.0033 ml/kg/min	0.0025 ml/kg/min
0.600 mcg/kg/min	0.006 ml/kg/min	0.004 ml/kg/min	0.003 ml/kg/min
0.700 mcg/kg/min	0.007 ml/kg/min	0.00467 ml/kg/min	0.0035 ml/kg/min
0.750 mcg/kg/min	0.0075 ml/kg/min	0.005 ml/kg/min	0.00375 ml/kg/min

NITROGLYCERIN (Nitro-Bid, Nitrol, Nitrostat, Tridil)

Dilution: May be prepared as 5 mg/100 ml (25 mg/500 ml, 50 mg/1000 ml) = 50 mcg/ml.
25 mg/250 ml (50 mg/500 ml, 100 mg/1000 ml) = 100 mcg/ml.
50 mg/250 ml (100 mg/500 ml, 200 mg/1000 ml) = 200 mcg/ml.
Note that different products are available in different concentrated solutions and should be used with appropriate infusion tubing. Changes in tubing may result in altered response to a given dose.

Nitroglycerin Infusion Rates (ml/hr)

Dose (mcg/min)	50 mcg/ml concentration	100 mcg/ml concentration	200 mcg/ml concentration
2.5 mcg/min	3 ml/hr	1.5 ml/hr	0.75 ml/hr
5 mcg/min	6 ml/hr	3 ml/hr	1.5 ml/hr
10 mcg/min	12 ml/hr	6 ml/hr	3 ml/hr
15 mcg/min	18 ml/hr	9 ml/hr	4.5 ml/hr
20 mcg/min	24 ml/hr	12 ml/hr	6 ml/hr
30 mcg/min	36 ml/hr	18 ml/hr	9 ml/hr
40 mcg/min	48 ml/hr	24 ml/hr	12 ml/hr
50 mcg/min	60 ml/hr	30 ml/hr	15 ml/hr
60 mcg/min	72 ml/hr	36 ml/hr	18 ml/hr

NITROPRUSSIDE (Nipride, Nitropress)

Dilution: May be prepared as 50 mg/1000 ml = 50 mcg/ml.
100 mg/1000 ml = 100 mcg/ml.
200 mg/1000 ml = 200 mcg/ml.
To calculate infusion rate (ml/min), multiply patient's weight (kg) by dose in ml/kg/min.
To calculate infusion rate (ml/hr), multiply patient's weight (kg) by dose in ml/kg/min × 60.
Dosing range: 0.3 mcg/kg/min–10 mcg/kg/min.

	Nitroprusside Infusion Rates (ml/kg/min)		
Dose (mcg/kg/min)	**50 mcg/ml concentration**	**100 mcg/ml concentration**	**200 mcg/ml concentration**
0.3 mcg/kg/min	0.006 ml/kg/min	—	—
0.5 mcg/kg/min	0.01 ml/kg/min	—	—
1 mcg/kg/min	0.02 ml/kg/min	0.01 ml/kg/min	—
2 mcg/kg/min	0.04 ml/kg/min	0.02 ml/kg/min	0.01 ml/kg/min
3 mcg/kg/min	0.06 ml/kg/min	0.03 ml/kg/min	0.015 ml/kg/min
4 mcg/kg/min	0.08 ml/kg/min	0.04 ml/kg/min	0.02 ml/kg/min
5 mcg/kg/min	0.1 ml/kg/min	0.05 ml/kg/min	0.025 ml/kg/min
6 mcg/kg/min	0.12 ml/kg/min	0.06 ml/kg/min	0.03 ml/kg/min
7 mcg/kg/min	0.14 ml/kg/min	0.07 ml/kg/min	0.035 ml/kg/min
8 mcg/kg/min	0.16 ml/kg/min	0.08 ml/kg/min	0.04 ml/kg/min
9 mcg/kg/min	0.18 ml/kg/min	0.09 ml/kg/min	0.045 ml/kg/min
10 mcg/kg/min	0.2 ml/kg/min	0.1 ml/kg/min	0.05 ml/kg/min

PROCAINAMIDE (Pronestyl)

Dilution: May be prepared as 1000 mg/500 ml = 2 mg/ml.
Loading dose: 50–100 mg q 5 min until arrhythmia is controlled, adverse reaction occurs, or 500 mg have been given; or 500–600 mg as a loading infusion over 25–30 min.

Procainamide Infusion Rates (ml/hr)

Concentration = 2 mg/ml	
Dose (mg/min)	**Dose (ml/hr)**
1 mg/min	30 ml/hr
2 mg/min	60 ml/hr
3 mg/min	90 ml/hr
4 mg/min	120 ml/hr
5 mg/min	150 ml/hr
6 mg/min	180 ml/hr

APPENDIX E

Food and Drug Administration Pregnancy Categories

Category A

As demonstrated by studies that are adequate and well controlled, no risk to the fetus has been shown in the first trimester. In addition, there does not appear to be risk in the second or third trimester. Fetal harm is probably remote.

Category B

Studies in animals may or may not have shown risk. If risk has been shown in animals, no risk has been shown in human studies. If risk has not been seen in animals, there are insufficient data in pregnant women.

Category C

Adverse effects have been demonstrated in animals, but there are insufficient data in pregnant women. In certain clinical situations, the benefits of the medication could outweigh possible risks.

Category D

Based on information collected in clinical investigations or postmarketing surveillance, human fetal risk has been demonstrated. In certain clinical situations, the benefits of the medication could outweigh possible risks.

Category X

Human fetal risk has been clearly documented in human studies, animal studies, clinical investigation, or postmarketing surveillance. Possible risks to the fetus outweigh potential benefits to the pregnant woman. Avoid using in patients who are pregnant or who may become pregnant.

APPENDIX F

Formulas Helpful for Calculating Doses

Ratio and Proportion

A ratio is the same as a fraction and can be expressed as a fraction (1/2) or in the algebraic form (1:2). This relationship is stated as *one is to two.*

A proportion is an equation of equal fractions or ratios.

$$\frac{1}{2} = \frac{4}{8}$$

To calculate doses, begin each proportion with the two known values, for example, 15 grains = 1 gram (known equivalent) or 10 milligrams = 2 milliliters (dosage available) on one side of the equation. Next, make certain that the units of measure on the opposite side of the equation are the same as the units of the known values and are placed on the same level of the equation.

Problem A:

$$\frac{15 \text{ gr}}{1 \text{ g}} = \frac{10 \text{ gr}}{x \text{ g}}$$

Problem B:

$$\frac{10 \text{ mg}}{2 \text{ ml}} = \frac{5 \text{ mg}}{x \text{ ml}}$$

Once the proportion is set up correctly, cross-multiply the opposing values of the proportion.

Problem A:

$$\frac{15 \text{ gr}}{1 \text{ gr}} \times \frac{10 \text{ gr}}{x \text{ g}}$$

$$15x = 10$$

Problem B:

$$\frac{10 \text{ mg}}{2 \text{ ml}} \times \frac{5 \text{ mg}}{x \text{ ml}}$$

$$10x = 10$$

Next, divide each side of the equation by the number with the x to determine the answer. Then, add the unit of measure corresponding to x in the original equation.

Problem A:

$$\frac{15x}{15} = \frac{10}{15}$$

$$x = \frac{2}{3} \text{ or } 0.6 \text{ g}$$

Problem B:

$$\frac{10x}{10} = \frac{10}{10}$$

$$x = 1 \text{ ml}$$

Calculation of IV Drip Rate

To calculate the drip rate for an intravenous infusion, 3 values are needed:

I. The amount of solution and corresponding time for infusion. May be ordered as:

1000 ml over 8 hr

or

125 ml/hr

II. The equivalent in time to convert hours to minutes.

$$1 \text{ hr} = 60 \text{ min}$$

III. The drop factor or number of drops that equal 1 ml of fluid. (This information can be found on the IV tubing box.)

$$10 \text{ gtt} = 1 \text{ ml}$$

Set up the problem by placing each of the 3 values in a proportion.

$$\frac{125 \text{ ml}}{1 \text{ hr}} \times \frac{1 \text{ hr}}{60 \text{ min}} \times \frac{10 \text{ gtt}}{1 \text{ ml}}$$

Numbers and units of measure can be canceled out from the upper and lower levels of this equation.

The numbers cancel, leaving:

$$\frac{125 \text{ ml}}{1 \text{ hr}} \times \frac{1 \text{ hr}}{\underset{6}{\cancel{60}} \text{ min}} \times \frac{\overset{1}{\cancel{10}} \text{ gtt}}{1 \text{ ml}}$$

The units cancel, leaving:

$$\frac{125 \cancel{\text{ml}}}{1 \cancel{\text{hr}}} \times \frac{1 \cancel{\text{hr}}}{6 \text{ min}} \times \frac{1 \text{ gtt}}{1 \cancel{\text{ml}}}$$

Next, multiply each level across and divide the numerator by the denominator for the answer.

$$\frac{125 \cancel{\text{ml}}}{1 \cancel{\text{hr}}} \times \frac{1 \cancel{\text{hr}}}{6 \text{ min}} \times \frac{1 \text{ gtt}}{1 \cancel{\text{ml}}} = \frac{125 \text{ gtt}}{6 \text{ min}}$$

$$125 \div 6 = 20.8 \text{ or } 21 \text{ gtt/min}$$

Calculation of Creatinine Clearance (CCr) in Adults from Serum Creatinine

$$\text{Men: CCr} = \frac{\text{weight (kg)} \times (140 - \text{age})}{72 \times \text{serum creatinine (mg/dl)}}$$

$$\text{Women: CCr} = 0.85 \times \text{calculation for men}$$

Calculation of Ideal Body Weight (kg) in Adults

$$\text{Men} = 50 \text{ kg} + 2.3 \text{ kg (each inch} > 5 \text{ ft)}$$

$$\text{Women} = 45.5 \text{ kg} + 2.3 \text{ kg (each inch} > 5 \text{ ft)}$$

Calculation of Body Surface Area (BSA) in Adults and Children

Dubois method:

$$SA\ (cm^2) = wt\ (kg)^{0.425} \times ht\ (cm)^{0.725} \times 71.84$$

$$SA\ (m^2)\ K \times \sqrt[3]{wt^2\ (kg)}$$ (common K value 0.1 for toddlers, 0.103 for neonates)

Simplified method:

$$BSA\ (m^2) = \sqrt{\frac{ht\ (cm) \times wt\ (kg)}{3600}}$$

Body Mass Index

$$BMI = wt\ (kg) \div ht\ (m^2)$$

APPENDIX G

Body Surface Area Nomograms

ESTIMATING BODY SURFACE AREA IN CHILDREN

For pediatric patients of average size, body surface area may be estimated with the scale on the left. Match weight to corresponding surface area. For other pediatric patients, use the scale on the right. Lay a straightedge on the correct height and weight points for your patient, and observe the point where it intersects on the surface area scale at center.

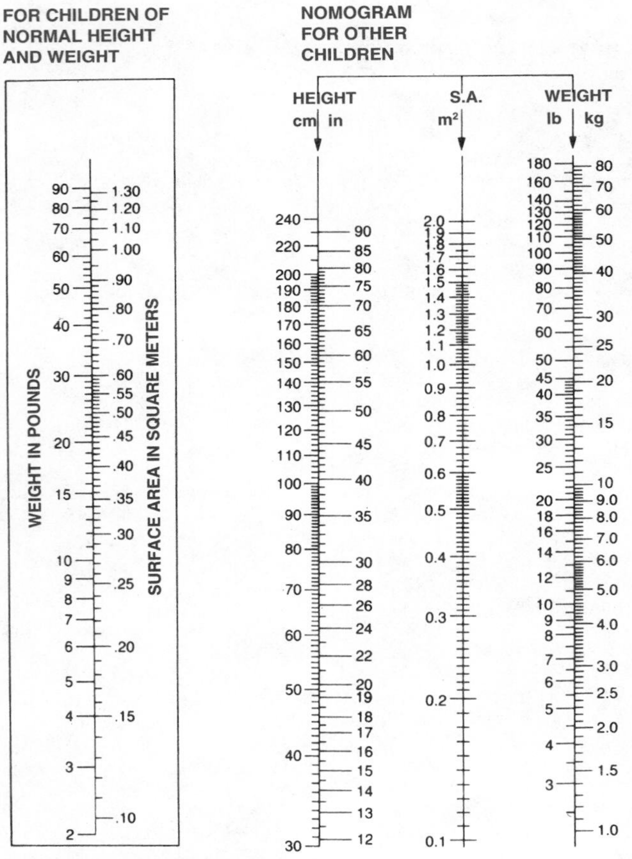

Reproduced from *Nelson Textbook of Pediatrics*, 13th edition. Courtesy W.B. Saunders Co., Philadelphia, Pa.

ESTIMATING BODY SURFACE AREA IN ADULTS

Use a straightedge to connect the patient's height in the left-hand column to weight in the right-hand column. The intersection of this line with the center scale estimates the body surface area.

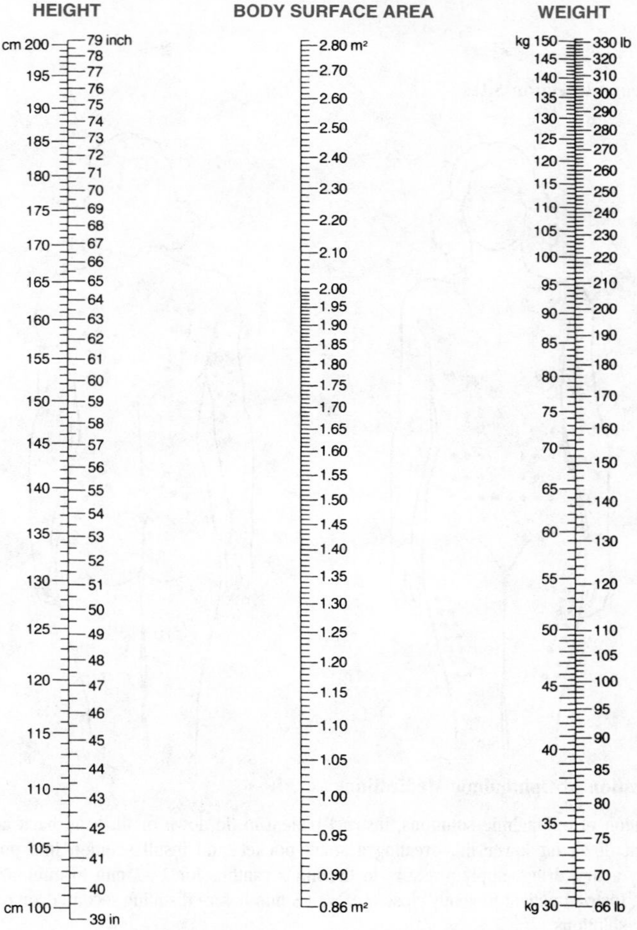

Reproduced from Lenter, C. (ed.), *Geigy Scientific Tables*, 8th edition. Courtesy CIBA-GEIGY, Basel, Switzerland.

APPENDIX H

Administration Techniques

Subcutaneous Injection Sites

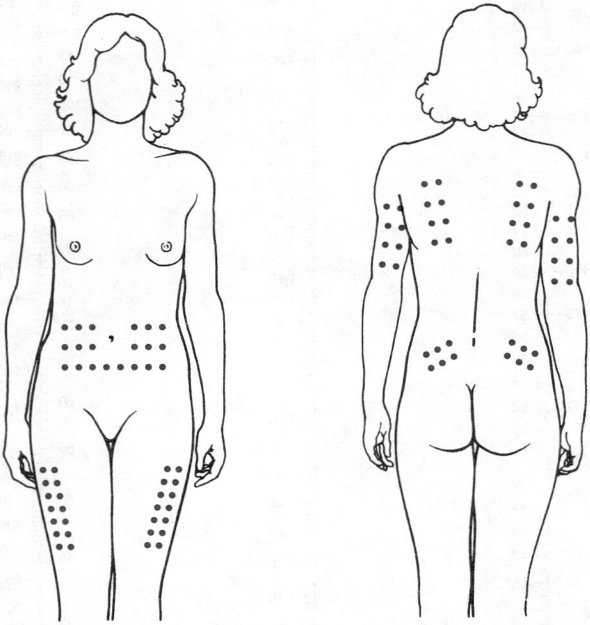

Administration of Ophthalmic Medications

For instillation of ophthalmic solutions, instruct patient to lie down or tilt head back and look at ceiling. Pull down on lower lid, creating a small pocket, and instill solution into pocket. With systemically acting drugs, apply pressure to the inner canthus for 1–2 min to minimize systemic absorption. Instruct patient to gently close eye. Wait 5 min before instilling second drop or any other ophthalmic solutions.

For instillation of ophthalmic ointment, instruct patient to hold tube in hand for several minutes to warm. Squeeze a small amount of ointment (¼–½ in.) inside lower lid. Instruct patient to close eye gently and roll eyeball around in all directions with eye closed. Wait 10 min before instilling any other ophthalmic ointments.

Do not touch cap or tip of container to eye, fingers, or any surface.

Administration of Medications with Metered-Dose Inhalers

Instruct patient on the proper use of the metered-dose inhaler. There are 3 methods of using a metered-dose inhaler. Shake inhaler well. (1) Take a drink of water to moisten the throat; place the inhaler mouthpiece 2 finger-widths away from mouth; tilt head back slightly. While activating the inhaler, take a slow, deep breath for 3–5 sec; hold the breath for 10 sec; and breathe out slowly.

(2) Exhale and close lips firmly around mouthpiece. Administer during second half of inhalation, and hold breath for as long as possible to ensure deep instillation of medication. (3) Use of spacer. Consult health care professional to determine method desired prior to instruction. Allow 1–2 min between inhalations. Rinse mouth with water or mouthwash after each use to minimize dry mouth and hoarseness. Wash inhalation assembly at least daily in warm running water.

For use of dry powder inhalers, turn head away from inhaler and exhale (do not blow into inhaler). Do not shake. Close mouth tightly around the mouthpiece of the inhaler and inhale rapidly. (See inside of back cover for diagrams.)

STEPS FOR USING YOUR INHALER

Please demonstrate your inhaler technique at every visit.

1. Remove the cap and hold inhaler upright.
2. Shake the inhaler.
3. Tilt your head back slightly and breathe out slowly.
4. Position the inhaler in one of the following ways (A or B is optimal, but C is acceptable for those who have difficulty with A or B. C is required for breath-activated inhalers):

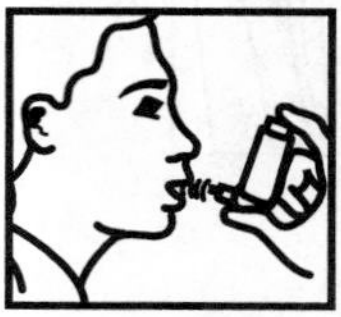

A. Open mouth with inhaler 1 to 2 inches away.

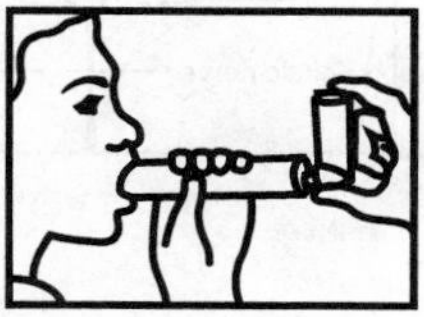

B. Use spacer/holding chamber (that is recommended especially for young children and for people using corticosteroids).

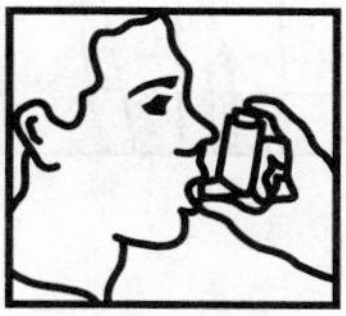

C. In the mouth. Do not use for corticosteroids.

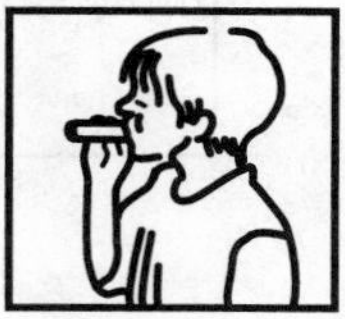

D. NOTE: Inhaled dry powder capsules require a different inhalation technique. To use a dry powder inhaler, it is important to close the mouth tightly around the mouthpiece of the inhaler and to inhale rapidly.

5. Press down on the inhaler to release medication as you start to breathe in slowly.
6. Breathe in slowly (3 to 5 seconds).
7. Hold your breath for 10 seconds to allow the medicine to reach deeply into your lungs.
8. Repeat puff as directed. Waiting 1 minute between puffs may permit second puff to penetrate your lungs better.
9. Spacers/holding chambers are useful for all patients. They are particularly recommended for young children and older adults and for use with inhaled corticosteroids.

Avoid common inhaler mistakes. Follow these inhaler tips:

- Breathe out *before* pressing your inhaler.
- Inhale *slowly.*
- Breathe in through your mouth, not your nose.
- Press down on your inhaler at the *start* of inhalation (or within the first second of inhalation).
- Keep inhaling as you press down on inhaler.
- Press your inhaler only *once* while you are inhaling (one breath for each puff).
- Make sure you breathe in evenly and deeply.

NOTE: Other inhalers are becoming available in addition to those illustrated above. Different types of inhalers may require different techniques.

Source: *Expert Panel Report 2: Guidelines for the Diagnosis and Management of Asthma.* National Asthma Education and Prevention Program, National Heart, Lung, and Blood Institute, 1997.

Administration of Nasal Sprays

Clear nasal passages of secretions prior to use. If nasal passages are blocked, use a decongestant immediately prior to use to ensure adequate penetration of the spray. Keep head upright. Breathe in through nose during administration. Sniff hard for a few minutes after adminstration.

Intramuscular Injection Sites

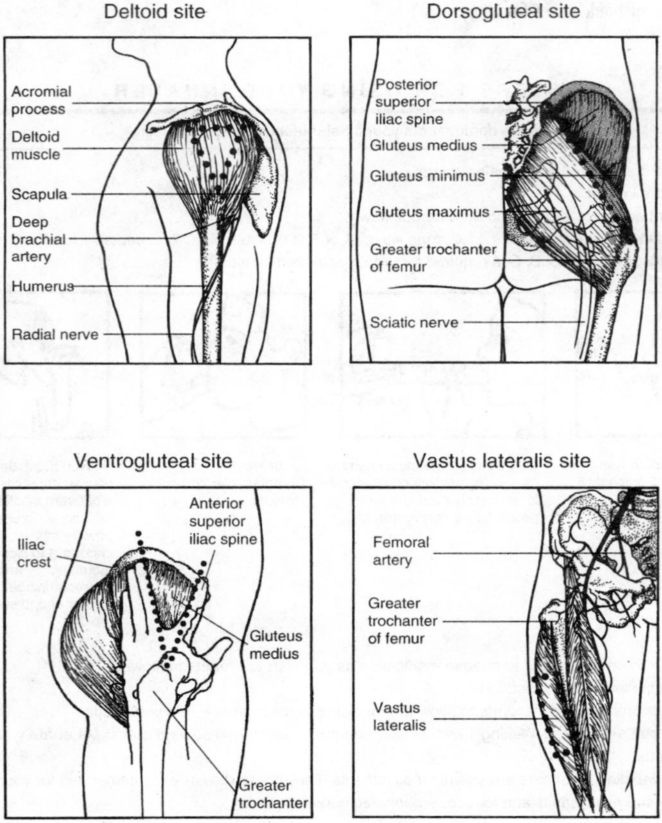

APPENDIX I

Recommendations for the Safe Handling of Hazardous Drugs*

INTRODUCTION/CATEGORIZATION

This is a summary of the revised Occupational Safety and Health Administration Guidelines for the Safe Handling of Hazardous Drugs. Previous guidelines referred to Safe Handling of *Cytotoxic* Drugs. The revised guidelines use the term *Hazardous* Drugs (HDs) in order to include other drugs (such as some antivirals, hormones) that also display toxic, carcinogenic, mutagenic, and/or teratogenic potential. These agents may also cause irritation to the skin, eyes, and mucous membranes and ulceration and necrosis of tissue. The toxicity of HDs dictates that the exposure of health care personnel to these drugs in any setting should be minimized. At the same time, the requirement for maintenance of aseptic conditions for most agents must be satisfied.

HDs AS OCCUPATIONAL RISKS

Exposure to HDs should be minimized because they bind to genetic material and may affect cellular protein synthesis. HDs also may not be able to differentiate between cancerous and normal cells. These risks have been documented in animal and human studies.

The primary potential routes of exposure during preparation and administration are via inhalation of dusts or aerosols, dermal absorption, and ingestion. Potential exposure to hazardous drugs may occur at many points in the handling of these agents. These sources of exposure have been documented by studies demonstrating the presence of HDs or their metabolites in the blood or urine of workers who handle them, in overt toxicity to organ systems in these workers, or in reproductive abnormalities. Deleterious effects may be increased if workers also smoke cigarettes.

Preparation Areas

In large specialized institutions, HDs are usually prepared in the pharmacy. However, in many small hospitals, clinics, and physicians' offices, HDs are routinely prepared in uncontrolled settings. The risk of exposure is greatest for nurses who work in outpatient settings. During the preparation of HDs for administration, even when great care is taken, splattering, spraying, and aerosolization may occur during needle withdrawal from vials, during drug transfer, during opening of ampules, and during expulsion of air from syringes. Although horizontal-airflow workbenches provide an aseptic area for preparation of HDs, they increase exposure to HDs by personnel in the work area. As a result, horizontal Biologic Safety Cabinets (BSCs) should not be used in preparation areas. Risk of exposure is also increased by smoking, drinking, applying cosmetics, or eating in areas where HDs are prepared, stored, or administered.

Other activities that increase exposure during administration should also be prohibited. These include clipping needles and crushing syringes. Excreta from patients receiving HDs may contain potentially damaging concentrations of HDs and/or their metabolites; unprotected handling should be avoided. When materials contaminated in any way with HDs are to be handled, the use of properly labeled, sealed, and covered containers by trained personnel is required. Additional procedures are required where contamination with blood or body fluids has occurred.

*Controlling occupational exposure to hazardous drugs. *Am J Health Syst Pharm* 1996;53:1669–1685.

PREVENTION OF EMPLOYEE EXPOSURE

Each setting should have a written HD safety and health plan. This plan should be easily accessible and include the following:

- Procedures that safeguard safety and health of workers exposed to HDs
- Criteria for measures designed to reduce HD exposure
- Presence of ventilation equipment and its maintenance
- Provision of information and training
- Procedures for handling investigational HDs
- Provision of medical care for employees exposed to HDs
- Designation of specific employees responsible for implementation of the HD safety and health plan

Preparation of HDs

Where allowable, specified HD-handling areas should be designated in a restricted, centralized location. Activities known to increase exposure should be prohibited in this area. The posting in the work area of guidelines for handling spills and emergencies is recommended. Under optimum conditions, preparation of HDs should take place in a Class II, Type B, or Class III BSC (with venting to the outside) that undergoes routine maintenance and decontamination. If a BSC is not available, personnel preparing HDs should wear a respirator with a high-efficiency filter until a BSC is available. Full face coverage or partial face coverage with splash goggles should be used with the respirator.

Personnel handling HDs should wear personal protective equipment (PPE). Double latex gloving is generally recommended. Gloves should be changed hourly or more frequently if damaged or contaminated. Protective gowns should also be worn and should be tucked into gloves at the wrist (inner glove under cuff, outer glove over cuff). Employees should be trained in the proper removal of PPE. Chemical-barrier face and eye protection should be used near splashes, sprays, or aerosols. Eyewash facilities should be available. All PPEs should be disposed of properly or, when appropriate, cleaned for reuse.

When working with HDs, a disposable plastic-backed paper liner should be placed in the BCS and changed routinely. Syringes and IV sets with Luer-Lok fittings should be used for preparation of HDs. Syringe size should be compatible with volume required. Excess solution should be discarded in a covered disposable container; a covered "sharps" container should also be available. All HDs and materials should be disposed of in clearly labeled bags.

Aseptic technique should be used in a manner consistent with working in a BSC. PPEs should be donned prior to work and necessary equipment placed in the BSC. All syringes and IV bags must be labeled with a distinctive warning label in addition to standard labeling. Needles must be disposed of in "sharps" containers (crushing, clipping, or capping is prohibited). Extremes in pressure generated in vials should be avoided. Multi-use dispensing pins or venting devices may be preferable to needles alone for this purpose. The remainder of the procedure involving vials or ampules should be performed to minimize spraying or dripping. Once prepared, bags or bottles should be wiped with moist gauze; entry ports should be swabbed with alcohol and capped. The entire unit should be packaged in a sealed plastic bag placed inside a secure container. Nonliquid doses should be counted, compounded, or handled inside a BSC using equipment designated for that purpose only.

Administration of HDs

The same PPEs should be worn as for preparation (gown, gloves, splash goggles). A respirator should be worn while administering aerosolized drugs. In addition to PPE the following equipment may be packaged for use during administration: gauze for cleanup, alcohol wipes, disposable plastic-backed absorbent liner, puncture-resistant container (for needles/syringes), resealable plastic bag with warning label and other accessory warning labels.

The following work practices should be employed:

- Hands should be washed before donning gloves and after gloves are removed. Contaminated equipment should be replaced immediately and disposed of properly.

- All infusion pumps and IV sets should have Luer-Lok fittings and be inspected frequently for leakage. Disposable plastic-backed absorbent liner should be placed under tubing; sterile gauze should cover IV push sites and connection sites should be taped.
- Priming/air expelling should take place in the BSC; if not, priming should be done with a nondrug solution or a backflow closed system should be used. Vented systems should not be used.
- Syringes, IV bottles, bags, and pumps should be wiped clean with gauze. Needles and syringes should be placed in a puncture-resistant container and then into an HD disposal bag. Administration sets should be disposed of intact. Waste bags should follow HD disposal requirements and unused drugs should be returned to the pharmacy. PPE should be properly disposed of and reusable materials washed for future use.
- Spill and emergency skin and eye decontamination kits and other materials should be readily available in areas where HDs are administered.
- If splashing is a possibility, PPE should be used during administration of oral HDs.
- Investigational HDs should be administered only by experienced personnel.

These procedures should be observed as closely as possible in the home care environment. Patients and caregivers should have ready access to providers and emergency protocols.

Aerosolized drugs require controls to prevent exposure to individuals in the vicinity of drug administration. Specific isolation and ventilation techniques may be used.

Caring for Patients Receiving HDs

Universal precautions should be observed to prevent contact with any potentially infectious/hazardous materials. Gowns and gloves should be worn by personnel for 48 hr following administration and replaced if contamination occurs. If splashing is possible, eye protection should be worn. Contaminated linens should be bagged separately and prewashed before being washed with other laundry. Laundry personnel should wear gowns/gloves when handling contaminated linens. Reusable items should be washed twice with detergent by personnel wearing gowns and double gloves.

Disposed equipment must be specially bagged and labeled. Needles/syringes/breakable items contaminated with blood or other potentially infectious materials must be disposed of in a "sharps" container. Such disposal containers should be readily available in patient care areas and sealed and replaced routinely. Care should be taken to avoid exterior contamination of all waste containers; if this occurs, the contaminated container should be placed inside another uncontaminated container. HD waste must be disposed of separately from other waste in accordance with applicable regulations.

Spills should be cleaned up by properly protected personnel, using the facility's procedure. The area of spill should be identified and reported.

If contamination of personnel occurs, the following should be performed:

- Immediately remove gloves/gown.
- Immediately cleanse the affected skin with soap and water.
- Flood affected eye at eyewash fountain or flush with water or isotonic eyewash for at least 15 min.
- Obtain medical attention and follow protocols for specific exposure.
- Document exposure.

Small spills (less than 5 ml or 5 g) should be cleaned up by personnel in gowns, gloves, splash protectors, and a respirator, if necessary. Liquids may be mopped up with absorbent gauze, solids with damp gauze, followed by three washings of the area with detergent followed by water. Broken fragments should be picked up with a scoop and properly disposed of.

Large spill areas should be isolated. Absorbent sheets or spill-control pads should be used. Damp cloths should be used if a powder is spilled. Spills greater than 150 ml (or 1 vial) in a BSC necessitate decontamination of the BSC. If the filter of the BSC is contaminated, the unit should be sealed until maintenance can be performed by experienced personnel.

Spill kits should be readily available in areas where HDs are handled. The kit should include splash goggles, 2 pairs of gloves, utility gloves, gown, 2 sheets of absorbent material, spill-control pillows (2 sizes), "sharps" container, and 2 large HD disposal bags.

MEDICAL SURVEILLANCE

Personnel who work with HDs should be routinely monitored to prevent occupational injury and disease. This should include examination before employment, routinely during employment, following acute exposure, and upon termination of employment. Special consideration should be given to reproductive issues. Employers must develop and maintain hazard communication programs and provide information about HDs. Employees must be informed of the risks of working with HDs. Training must be provided to minimize exposure. Records of such programs must be maintained by the institution.

APPENDIX J

Normal Values of Common Laboratory Tests

SERUM TESTS

HEMATOLOGIC	MEN		WOMEN
Hemoglobin	13.5–18 g/dl		12–16 g/dl
Hematocrit	40–54%		38–47%
Red blood cells (RBC)	4.6–6.2 million/mm^3		4.2–5.4 million/mm^3
Mean corpuscular volume (MCV)		76–100 (micrometer)^3	
Mean corpuscular hemoglobin (MCH)		27–33 picogram	
Mean corpuscular hemoglobin concentration (MCHC)		33–37 g/dl	
Erythrocyte sedimentation rate (ESR)	≤20 mm/hr		≤30 mm/hr
Leukocytes (WBC)		5000–10,000/mm^3	
Neutrophils		54–75% (3000–7500/mm^3)	
Bands		3–8% (150–700/mm^3)	
Eosinophils		1–4% (50–400/mm^3)	
Basophils		0–1% (25–100/mm^3)	
Monocytes		2–8% (100–500/mm^3)	
Lymphocytes		25–40% (1500–4500/mm^3)	
T lymphocytes		60–80% of lymphocytes	
B lymphocytes		10–20% of lymphocytes	
Platelets		150,000–450,000/mm^3	
Prothrombin time (PT)	9.6–11.8 sec		9.5–11.3 sec
Partial thromboplastin time (PTT)	30–45 sec		
Bleeding time (duke)	1–3 min		
(ivy)	3–6 min		
(template)	3–6 min		
Clotting time (Lee-White)	4–8 min		

CHEMISTRY	MEN AND WOMEN
Sodium	135–145 mEq/L
Potassium	3.5–5.0 mEq/L
Chloride	95–105 mEq/L
Bicarbonate (HCO_3)	19–25 mEq/L
Total calcium	9–11 mg/dl or 4.5–5.5 mEq/L
Ionized calcium	4.2–5.4 mg/dl or 2.1–2.6 mEq/L
Phosphorus/phosphate	2.4–4.7 mg/dl
Magnesium	1.8–3.0 mg/dl or 1.5–2.5 mEq/L
Glucose	70–110 mg/dl
Osmolality	285–310 mOsm/kg
Ammonia (NH_3)	10–80 mcg/dl
Amylase	≤130 U/L
Creatine phosphokinase total (CK, CPK)	<150 U/L
Creatine kinase isoenzymes, MB fraction	>5% in MI
Lactic dehydrogenase (LDH)	50–150 U/L
Protein, total	6–8 g/dl
Albumin	4–6 g/dl

HEPATIC	MEN		WOMEN
AST	8–46 U/L		7–34 U/L
ALT		10–30 IU/ml	
Total bilirubin		0.3–1.2 mg/dl	
Conjugated bilirubin		0.0–0.2 mg/dl	
Unconjugated (indirect) bilirubin		0.2–0.8 mg/dl	
Alkaline phosphatase		20–90 U/L	

RENAL	MEN	WOMEN
BUN	6–20 mg/dl	
Creatinine	0.6–1.3 mg/dl	0.5–1.0 mg/dl
Uric acid	4.0–8.5 mg/dl	2.7–7.3 mg/dl

ARTERIAL BLOOD GASES	MEN AND WOMEN
pH	7.35–7.45
Po_2	80–100 mm Hg
Pco_2	35–45 mm Hg
O_2 saturation	95–97%
Base excess	+2–(−2)
Bicarbonate (HCO_3^-)	22–26 mEq/L

URINE TESTS

URINE	MEN AND WOMEN
pH	4.5–8.0
Specific gravity	1.010–1.025

APPENDIX K

Dietary Guidelines for Food Sources

Potassium-Rich Foods

avocados	grapefruit	oranges	rhubarb
bananas	lima beans	peaches	spinach
broccoli	navy beans	potatoes	sunflower seeds
cantaloupe	nuts	prunes	tomatoes
dried fruits			

Sodium-Rich Foods

baking mixes (pancakes, muffins)	canned soups	Parmesan cheese
	canned spaghetti sauce	pickles
barbecue sauce	cured meats	potato salad
butter/margarine	dry onion soup mix	pretzels, potato chips
buttermilk	"fast" foods	sauerkraut
canned chili	macaroni and cheese	tomato ketchup
canned seafood	microwave dinners	TV dinners

Calcium-Rich Foods

bok choy	cream soups	oysters
broccoli	milk and dairy products	spinach
canned salmon/sardines	molasses (blackstrap)	tofu
clams		

Vitamin K–Rich Foods

asparagus	cabbage	fish	rice
beans	cauliflower	milk	spinach
broccoli	cheeses	mustard greens	turnips
brussel sprouts	collards	pork	yogurt

Low-Sodium Foods

baked or broiled poultry	grits (not instant)	potatoes
canned pumpkin	honey	puffed wheat and rice
cooked turnips	jams and jellies	red kidney and lima beans
egg yolk	lean meats	sherbet
fresh vegetables	low-calorie mayonnaise	unsalted nuts
fruit	macaroons	whiskey

Foods That Acidify Urine

cheeses	fish	meats	poultry
cranberries	grains (breads and cereals)	plums	prunes
eggs			

Foods That Alkalinize Urine

all fruits except cranberries, prunes, plums	all vegetables	milk

Foods Containing Tyramine

aged cheeses (blue, Boursault, brick, Brie, Camembert, cheddar, Emmenthaler, Gruyère, mozzarella, Parmesan, Romano, Roquefort, Stilton, Swiss)
American processed cheese
avocados (especially over-ripe)
bananas
bean curd
beer and ale
caffeine-containing beverages (coffee, tea, colas)
caviar
chocolate
distilled spirits
fermented sausage (bologna, salami, pepperoni, summer sausage)
liver
meats prepared with tenderizer
miso soup
over-ripe fruit
raisins
red wine (especially Chianti)
sauerkraut
sherry
shrimp paste
smoked or pickled fish
soy sauce
vermouth
yeasts
yogurt

Iron-Rich Foods

cereals
dried beans and peas
dried fruit
leafy green vegetables
lean red meats
organ meats

Vitamin D–Rich Foods

breads
cereals
fish
fish liver oils
fortified milk

APPENDIX L

Recommended Dietary Allowances (RDAs),* Revised 1989

	WEIGHT†		HEIGHT†			FAT-SOLUBLE VITAMINS			
AGE (yr) AND SEX GROUP	kg	lb	cm	in	PROTEIN	VITAMIN A	VITAMIN D	VITAMIN E	VITAMIN K
					gm	μg RE‡	μg§	mg α-TE¶	μg
Infants									
0.0–0.5	6	13	60	24	13	375	7.5	3	5
0.5–1.0	9	20	71	28	14	375	10	4	10
Children									
1–3	13	29	90	35	16	400	10	6	15
4–6	20	44	112	44	24	500	10	7	20
7–10	28	62	132	52	28	700	10	7	30
Men									
11–14	45	99	157	62	45	1000	10	10	45
15–18	66	145	176	69	59	1000	10	10	65
19–24	72	160	177	70	58	1000	10	10	70
25–50	79	174	176	70	63	1000	5	10	80
51+	77	170	173	68	63	1000	5	10	80
Women									
11–14	46	101	157	62	46	800	10	8	45
15–18	55	120	163	64	44	800	10	8	55
19–24	58	128	164	65	46	800	10	8	60
25–50	63	138	163	64	50	800	5	8	65
51+	65	143	160	63	50	800	5	8	65
Pregnant					60	800	10	10	65
Lactating									
first 6 mo					65	1300	10	12	65
second 6 mo					62	1200	10	11	65

RECOMMENDED DIETARY ALLOWANCES (RDAS),* REVISED 1989 (CONTINUED)

AGE (yr) AND SEX GROUP	WATER-SOLUBLE VITAMINS							MINERALS						
	VITAMIN C	THIAMIN	RIBOFLAVIN	NIACIN	VITAMIN B_6	FOLATE	VITAMIN B_{12}	CALCIUM	PHOSPHORUS	MAGNESIUM	IRON	ZINC	IODINE	SELENIUM
	mg			mg NE**	mg	μg		mg					μg	
Infants														
0.0–0.5	30	0.3	0.4	5	0.3	25	0.3	400	300	40	6	5	40	10
0.5–1.0	35	0.4	0.5	6	0.6	35	0.5	600	500	60	10	5	50	15
Children														
1–3	40	0.7	0.8	9	1.0	50	0.7	800	800	80	10	10	70	20
4–6	45	0.9	1.1	12	1.1	75	1.0	800	800	120	10	10	90	20
7–10	45	1.0	1.2	13	1.4	100	1.4	800	800	170	10	10	120	30
Men														
11–14	50	1.3	1.5	17	1.7	150	2.0	1200	1200	270	12	15	150	40
15–18	60	1.5	1.8	20	2.0	200	2.0	1200	1200	400	12	15	150	50
19–24	60	1.5	1.7	19	2.0	200	2.0	1200	1200	350	10	15	150	70
25–50	60	1.5	1.7	19	2.0	200	2.0	800	800	350	10	15	150	70
51+	60	1.2	1.4	15	2.0	200	2.0	800	800	350	10	15	150	70
Women														
11–14	50	1.1	1.3	15	1.4	150	2.0	1200	1200	280	15	12	150	45
15–18	60	1.1	1.3	15	1.5	180	2.0	1200	1200	300	15	12	150	50
19–24	60	1.1	1.3	15	1.6	180	2.0	1200	1200	280	15	12	150	55
25–50	60	1.1	1.3	15	1.6	180	2.0	800	800	280	15	12	150	55
51+	60	1.0	1.2	13	1.6	180	2.0	800	800	280	10	12	150	55
Pregnant	70	1.5	1.6	17	2.2	400	2.2	1200	1200	320	30	15	175	65
Lactating														
first 6 mo	95	1.6	1.8	20	2.1	280	2.6	1200	1200	355	15	19	200	75
second 6 mo	90	1.6	1.7	20	2.1	260	2.6	1200	1200	340	15	16	200	75

* The allowances, expressed as average daily intakes over time, are intended to provide for individual variations among most normal persons as they live in the United States under usual environmental stresses. Diets should be based on a variety of common foods in order to provide other nutrients for which human requirements have been less well defined. See text for detailed discussion of allowances and nutrients not tabulated.

† Weights and heights of Reference Adults are actual medians for the US population of the designated age, as reported by NHANES II. The median weights and heights of those under 19 yr of age were taken from Hamill, PVV, Drizd, TA, Johnson, CL, Reed, RB, Roche, AF, and Moore, WM: Physical growth. National Center for Health Statistics Percentiles. *Am J Clin Nutr* 1979;32:607. The use of these figures does not imply that the height-to-weight ratios are ideal.

‡ Retinol equivalents. 1 retinol equivalent = 1 μg retinol or 6 μg β-carotene. See text for calculation of vitamin A activity of diets as retinol equivalents.

§ As cholecalciferol. 10 μg cholecalciferol = 400 IU of vitamin D.

¶ α-Tocopherol equivalents. 1 mg d-α tocopherol = 1 α-TE. See text for variation in allowances and calculation of vitamin E activity of the diet as α-tocopherol equivalents.

** NE (niacin equivalent) is equal to 1 mg of niacin or 60 mg of dietary tryptophan.

APPENDIX M

Routine Pediatric and Adult Immunizations

ROUTINE PEDIATRIC IMMUNIZATIONS

GENERIC NAME (BRAND NAMES)	ROUTE AND DOSAGE	CONTRAINDICATIONS AND PRECAUTIONS	ADVERSE REACTIONS/ SIDE EFFECTS	NOTES
DTaP diphtheria toxoid, tetanus toxoid, and acellular pertussis vaccine (Acel-Imune, Tripedia)*	0.5 ml IM at 2, 4, 6, and 15–18 mo; booster at 4–6 yr (either product).	Acute infection, immunosuppressive therapy, previous CNS damage or convulsions.	Redness, tenderness, induration at site; fever; malaise; myalgia; urticaria; hypotension; neurologic reactions; allergic reactions (all less than with DTwP).	Individual components may be given as separate injections if unusual reactions occur. Tetanus and diphtheria toxoids absorbed (Td) should be repeated every 10 yr.
Polio vaccine, oral trivalent (Orimune, OPV)	0.5 ml PO at 2 mo, 4 mo, 6–18 mo, and booster at 4–6 yr.	Vomiting, diarrhea, allergy to streptomycin or neomycin, acute illness, immunosuppression.	Vaccine-associated paralysis.	May also be given as IPV at 2 and 4 mo, then OPV at 12–18 mo with a booster at 4–6 yr.
Polio vaccine, inactivated (IPV, IPOL, Poliovax)	0.5 ml SC at 2, 4, and 12–18 mo with a booster at 4–6 yr.	Hypersensitivity to neomycin, streptomycin, or polymyxin B; acute febrile illness.	Erythema, induration, pain at injection site; fever.	May also be given as IPV at 2 and 4 mo, then OPV at 12–18 mo with a booster at 4–6 yr. Only IPV should be used in immunocompromised patients and their household contacts.
Measles, mumps, and rubella vaccines (M-M-R II)	Single dose 0.5 ml SC at 12–15 mo with a booster at 4–6 yr or 11–12 yr (at least 1 mo should elapse between doses).	Allergy to egg or neomycin; active infection; immunosuppression.	Burning, stinging, pain at injection site; arthritis/arthralgia (40%); fever; encephalitis; allergic reactions.	If unusual reactions occur, individual components may be given as separate injections.
Hemophilus b conjugate vaccine (Hib-TITER, Pedvax-HIB, ProHIBit)*	0.5 ml IM at 2, 4, and 6 mo (6 mo dose not needed for Pedvax HIB), with a booster at 12–18 mo.	Allergy to diphtheria toxoid or thimerosal.	Induration, erythema, tenderness at injection site; fever.	
Hepatitis B vaccine (Engerix-B, Recombivax HB)†	10 mcg IM Engerix-B or 2.5 mcg IM Recombivax HB 1st dose at 0–2 mo, 2nd dose at 1–4 mo, and 3rd dose at 6–18 mo (1st and 2nd dose about 1 mo apart).	Hypersensitivity to thimerosal (Recombivax) or yeast (both products).	Local soreness.	Children who have not been vaccinated as infants should complete the series by 12 yr.

ROUTINE PEDIATRIC IMMUNIZATIONS (CONTINUED)

GENERIC (BRAND NAMES)	ROUTE AND DOSAGE	CONTRAINDICATIONS AND PRECAUTIONS	ADVERSE REACTIONS/ SIDE EFFECTS	NOTES
	Infants born to HBsAg-positive mothers: 1st dose of 5 mcg Recombivax HB or 10 mcg of Engerix-B preceded by hepatitis B immune globulin, 2nd dose at 1–2 mo, 3rd dose at 6 mo. *Children up to 10 yr:* 2.5 mcg Recombivax HB or 10 mcg Engerix-B as 3-dose series; 2nd dose 1 mo after 1st dose, 3rd dose 4 mo after 1st dose and 2 mo after 2nd dose. *Children up to 11–19 yr:* 5 mcg Recombivax HB or 10 mcg Engerix-B as 3-dose series; 2nd dose 1 mo after 1st dose, 3rd dose 4 mo after 1st dose and 2 mo after 2nd dose.			
Varicella vaccine (Varivax)	0.5 ml IM single dose given any time after 1st birthday; those without a reliable history should be vaccinated at the 11–12 yr visit; children around age 13 yr should receive 2 doses 1 mo apart.	Allergy to gelatin or neomycin; active infection; immunosuppression, including HIV.	Local soreness, fever.	Given to children who have not been vaccinated or have not had chickenpox. Salicylates should be avoided for 6 wk following vaccination.
Hepatitis A vaccine (Havrix, Vaqta)	*Children 2–18 yr:* 0.5 ml IM (pediatric formulation), repeated 6–12 mo later (pediatric dose form).	Acute febrile illness.	Local reactions, headache.	For high-risk groups including travelers to endemic areas and patients with clotting disorders.

*DTaP is preferred to DTwP for all vaccinations in the series; combination injections DTwP-HIB = diphtheria and tetanus toxoids and whole-cell pertussis and hemophilus b conjugate vaccine (Tetramune).
†Available in varying concentrations.

Nursing Implications:

Assessment
- Assess previous immunization history and history of hypersensitivity.

Potential Nursing Diagnoses
- Infection, risk for (Indications).
- Knowledge deficit, related to medication regimen (Patient/Family Teaching).

Implementation
- Measles, mumps, and rubella vaccine; trivalent oral poliovirus vaccine; and diphtheria toxoid, tetanus toxoid, and pertussis vaccine may be given concomitantly.
- Administer each immunization by appropriate route: ▪ **PO:** Polio (Orimune) ▪ **SC:** measles, mumps, rubella, polio (IPOL, Poliovax) ▪ **IM:** diphtheria, tetanus toxoid, pertussis.

Patient/Family Teaching
- Inform parent of potential and reportable side effects of immunization. Physician should be notified if patient develops fever higher than 39.4°C (103°F); difficulty breathing; hives; itching; swelling of eyes, face, or inside of nose; sudden, severe tiredness or weakness; or convulsions.
- Review next scheduled immunization with parent.

Evaluation
Effectiveness of therapy can be demonstrated by: ▪ Prevention of diseases through active immunity.

ROUTINE ADULT IMMUNIZATIONS

GENERIC NAME (BRAND NAMES)	INDICATIONS	DOSAGE/ROUTE	CONTRAINDICATIONS	ADVERSE REACTIONS/SIDE EFFECTS
Hepatitis A vaccine (Havrix, Vaqta)	High-risk patients, some health care workers, persons who are food handlers in the food service industry, patients with clotting disorders, travelers to endemic areas, patients with chronic liver disease.	1 ml IM, followed by 1 ml IM 6–12 mo later (adult dose form).	Concurrent febrile illness.	Local soreness, headache.
Hepatitis B vaccine (Engerix-B, Recombivax HB, Recombivax HB dialysis formulation)	High-risk patients, health care workers.	3 doses of 0.5 ml IM, given at 0, 1, and 6 mo. Dialysis patients should receive special formulation (40 mcg surface antigen/ml).	Hypersensitivity to thimerosal (Recombivax) or yeast.	Local sorenesss.
Influenza vaccine (Flu-Imune, Fluogen, Fluzone, influenza virus vaccine [trivalent])	General population, especially patients >65 yr, health care workers, teenagers receiving chronic salicylate therapy, patients with chronic illnesses including HIV, international travelers.	0.5 ml IM every year (new strain developed yearly).	Allergy to eggs, egg protein, chickens, bisulfites, or thimerosal.	Fever, chills, myalgia, malaise.
Pneumococcal vaccine, polyvalent (Pneumovax 23, Pnu-Imune 23)	Everyone >65 yr, high-risk patients with chronic illnesses including HIV.	0.5 ml IM, high-risk patients (asplenics) should have a booster after 6 yr.	Hypersensitivity to phenol or thimerosal.	Local soreness.
Tetanus-diphtheria (Adult Td)	Unimmunized.	2 doses 0.5 ml IM 1–2 mo apart, then a 3rd dose 6–12 mo later.	Hypersensitivity to previous dose or to thimerosal; previous neurologic reaction.	Local pain and swelling.
	Everyone.	Booster every 10 yr.		
Varicella vaccine (Varivax)	Any adult without a history of chickenpox or herpes zoster.	0.5 ml SC; repeated 4–8 wk later.	Allergy to gelatin or neomycin; active infection; immunosuppression including HIV.	Salicylates should be avoided for 6 wk following vaccination.

SOURCE: Adapted from Update: Influenza Activity–United States, 1995–1996 season. *Morbidity and Mortality Weekly Report* 1996; 44:937–939. *Recommended Childhood Immunization Schedule–United States*, Jan–Dec 1997. [Online] Available http://aap.org/family/parents/immunize.htm, Nov 17,1997.

APPENDIX N

Prevention of Bacterial Endocarditis

Many physicians believe that antimicrobial prophylaxis before procedures that may cause transient bacteremia can prevent endocarditis in patients with valvular heart disease, prosthetic heart valves, or other cardiac abnormalities, although the effectiveness of this common practice has never been established by controlled trials. The drugs and dosages in the table are identical to those recommended recently by the American Heart Association (Dajani, AS, et al, JAMA 277:1794, June 11, 1997).

ENDOCARDITIS PROPHYLAXIS[1]

	Dosage for Adults	Dosage for Children*
	DENTAL AND UPPER RESPIRATORY PROCEDURES[2]	
Oral		
Amoxicillin[3] (*Amoxil* and others)	2 g 1 hr before procedure	50 mg/kg 1 hr before procedure
Penicillin allergy:		
Clindamycin (*Cleocin* and others)	600 mg 1 hr before procedure	20 mg/kg 1 hr before procedure
or		
Cephalexin† (*Keflex* and others) or cefadroxil† (*Duricef* and others)	2 g 1 hr before procedure	50 mg/kg 1 hr before procedure
or		
Azithromycin (*Zithromax*) or clarithromycin (*Biaxin*)	500 mg 1 hr before procedure	15 mg/kg 1 hr before procedure
Parenteral		
Ampicillin (*Polycillin* and others)	2 g IM or IV 30 min before procedure	50 mg/kg IM or IV 30 min before procedure
Penicillin allergy:		
Clindamycin	600 mg IV within 30 min before procedure	20 mg/kg IV 30 min before procedure
or		
Cefazolin† (*Ancef* and others)	1 g IM or IV within 30 min before procedure	25 mg/kg IM or IV within 30 min before procedure
	GASTROINTESTINAL AND GENITOURINARY PROCEDURES[2]	
Oral		
Amoxicillin[3]	2 g 1 hr before procedure	50 mg/kg 1 hr before procedure
Parenteral[4]		
Ampicillin	2 g IM or IV within 30 min before procedure	50 mg/kg IM or IV 30 min before procedure
± Gentamicin (*Garamycin* and others)	1.5 mg/kg (120 mg max) IM or IV 30 min before procedure	2 mg/kg IM or IV 30 min before procedure
Penicillin allergy:[4]		
Vancomycin (*Vancocin* and others)	1 g IV infused *slowly over 1 hr* beginning 1 hr before procedure	20 mg/kg IV infused *slowly over 1 hr* beginning 1 hr before procedure
± Gentamicin	1.5 mg/kg (120 mg max) IM or IV 30 min before procedure	2 mg/kg IM or IV 30 min before procedure

* Should not exceed adult dosage.

† Not recommended for patients with history of immediate-type (urticaria, angioedema, anaphylaxis) allergy to penicillin.

1. The risk of endocarditis is considered high in patients with previous endocarditis, prosthetic heart valves, complex cyanotic congenital heart disease such as tetralogy of Fallot or surgically constructed systemic pulmonary shunts or conduits. The risk is considered moderate in patients with other forms of congenital heart disease (but not uncomplicated secundum atrial septal defect), acquired (such as rheumatic) valvular disease, hypertrophic cardiomyopathy, and mitral valve prolapse with regurgitation or thickened leaflets. *Streptococcus viridans* is the most common cause of endocarditis after dental or upper respiratory procedures; enterococci are the most common cause after gastrointestinal or genitourinary procedures.

2. For a review of the risk of bacteremia and endocarditis with various procedures, see Dajani, AS, et al, JAMA, 277:1794, June 11, 1997.
3. Amoxicillin is recommended because of its excellent bioavailability and good activity against streptococci and enterococci.
4. Gentamicin should be added for patients with a high risk of endocarditis (see footnote 1. High-risk patients given parenteral ampicillin before the procedure should receive a dose of ampicillin 1 g IM or IV or a dose of amoxicillin 1 g orally 6 hr afterward.

(From: Prevention of Bacterial Endocarditis. *The Medical Letter,* vol. 39, October 24, 1997, with permission.)

APPENDIX O

Ophthalmic Medications

General Info: See Appendix H for administration techniques for ophthalmic agents.
Consult health care professional regarding:
Concurrent use of contact lenses (medication or additives may be absorbed by the lens).
Concurrent administration of other ophthalmic agents (order and spacing may be important).

Alpha-Adrenergic Blocker
Uses: Reverses mydriasis from phenylephrine or tropicamide.
Cautions: Avoid using in conditions in which miosis is undesirable; not to be used more than once weekly.

Generic Name (Brand Name) {Canadian Brand Name}	Dose	Notes
dapiprazole (Rev-Eyes)	Adults: 1 drop followed after 5 min by another drop	■ Administer immediately following retinal exam ■ ADRs*: blurred vision, irritation, corneal edema, punctate keratitis

Anesthetics
Uses: Provide brief local anesthesia to allow measurement of intraocular pressure, removal of foreign bodies, or other superficial procedures.
Cautions: Repeated use may result in increased risk of CNS and cardiovascular toxicity; cross-sensitivity with some local anesthetics may occur.

Generic Name (Brand Name) {Canadian Brand Name}	Dose	Notes
proparacaine (AK-Taine, Alcaine, Ocu-Caine, Ophthaine, Ophthetic, Spectro-Caine), {Diocane}	Adults and children: 1–2 drops of 0.5% solution (single dose)	■ Does not interact with ophthalmic cholinesterase inhibitors ■ ADRs: *ophthalmic*—irritation; *systemic*—irregular heartbeat, CNS depression, CNS stimulation
tetracaine (Pontocaine), {Minims Tetracaine}	Adults: 1–2 drops of 0.5–1% solution (single dose)	■ May interact with ophthalmic cholinesterase inhibitors, resulting in increased duration of action and risk of toxicity ■ ADRs: *ophthalmic*—irritation; *systemic*—irregular heartbeat, CNS depression, CNS stimulation

Antihistamines
Uses: Various forms of allergic conjunctivitis.

Generic Name (Brand Name) {Canadian Brand Name}	Dose	Notes
emedastine (Emadine)	Adults: 1 drop in affected eye up to 4 times daily	■ ADRs: headache, drowsiness, malaise, local irritation
levocabastine (Livostin)	Adults: 1 drop of 0.05% solution 4 times daily	■ ADRs: mild transient stinging, burning, headache, lid edema, drowsiness, dry mouth, nausea
olopatadine (Patanol)	Adults and children >3 yr: 1–2 drops of 0.1% solution twice daily (given 6–8 hr apart)	■ Small amounts are absorbed; excreted in urine ■ ADRs: headache, conjunctival irritation

Anti-infectives/Antifungals/Antivirals
Uses: Localized superficial ophthalmic infections.
Cautions: Small amounts may be absorbed and result in hypersensitivity reactions.

Generic Name (Brand Name) {Canadian Brand Name}	Dose	Notes
chloramphenicol (AK-Chlor, Chlorofair, Chloroptic, Clorachol, Econochlor, I-Chlor, Ocu-Chlor, Ophthochlor, Spectro-Chlor), {Fenicol}, {Ophtho-Chloram}, {Pentamycetin}	Adults and children: 1 drop of solution or thin strip of ointment q 1–4 hr	■ May rarely cause systemic hematologic toxicity if used chronically and in excessive doses
ciprofloxacin (Ciloxan)	Adult: *bacterial conjunctivitis*—1 drop in each eye q 2 hr while awake for 48 hr, then q 4 hr while awake for 5 days; *corneal ulcers*—1 drop in affected eye q 15 min for 6 hr, then q 30 min while awake for rest of day, then q 1 hr while awake for next 24 hr, then q 4 hr while awake until re-epithelialization occurs	■ May cause harmless white crystalline precipitate that resolves over time ■ ADRs: altered taste, systemic allergic reactions, photophobia
erythromycin (Ilotycin)	Adults and children: *treatment of infections*—thin strip up to 6 times daily Infants: *prophylaxis of ophthalmia neonatorum*—thin strip in each eye as a single dose	■ ADRs: irritation
norfloxacin (Chibroxin)	Adults and children ≥1 yr: 1 drop 4 times daily while awake (up to q 2 hr while awake)	■ ADRs: altered taste, systemic allergic reactions, photophobia
gentamicin (Garamycin, Genoptic, Gentacidin, Gentafair, Gentak, Gentrasul, Ocu-Mycin, Spectro-Genta), {Alcomicin}	Adults and children: 1 drop of solution q 1–4 hr or thin strip of ointment q 8–12 hr	■ ADRs: irritation, burning, stinging, blurred vision (ointment)

OPHTHALMIC MEDICATIONS (CONTINUED)

Generic Name (Brand Name) {Canadian Brand Name}	Dose	Notes
ofloxacin (Ocuflox)	Adults and children $\geq$1 yr: 1 drop q 2–4 hr while awake for 2 days, then 4 times daily for up to 5 more days	■ ADRs: altered taste, systemic allergic reactions, photophobia
sulfacetamide (AK-Sulf, Bleph, Isopto Cetamide, I-Sulfacet, Ocu-Sul, Ocusulf, Sodium Sulamyd, Spectro-Sulf, Sulf, Sulfair, Sulfamide, Sulten), {Sulfex}	Adults: 1 drop of solution q 1–3 hr while awake (less frequently at night) or thin strip of ointment 4 times daily and at bedtime	■ Cross-sensitivity with other sulfonamides (including thiazides) may occur ■ ADRs: local irritation
tobramycin (Tobrex)	Adults and children: 1 drop of solution q 1–4 hr depending on severity of infection or thin strip of ointment q 8–12 hr	■ ADRs: irritation, burning, stinging, blurred vision (ointment)

Antifungal

Generic Name (Brand Name) {Canadian Brand Name}	Dose	Notes
natamycin (Natacyn)	Adults: 1 drop q 1–6 hr, depending on severity of infection	■ ADRs: irritation, swelling, chemosis

Antivirals

Generic Name (Brand Name) {Canadian Brand Name}	Dose	Notes
trifluridine (Viroptic)	Adults and children $\geq$6 yr: 1 drop q 2 hr (up to 9 drops/day) while awake until cornea re-epithelializes, then 1 drop q 4 hr (at least 5 times daily) for up to 7 days	■ ADRs: burning, stinging; keratopathy rarely
vidarabine (Vira-A)	Adults and children: thin strip of ointment q 3 hr (5 times daily) until cornea is re-epithelialized, then twice daily for up to 7 days	■ ADRs: irritation, hypersensitivity

Artificial Tears/Ocular Lubricants (sterile buffered isotonic solutions/ointments)

Uses: *Artificial tears*—keep the eyes moist with isotonic solutions and wetting agents in the management of dry eyes due to lack of tears; also provide lubrication for artificial eyes. *Ocular lubricants*—provide lubrication and protection in a variety of conditions including exposure keratitis, decreased corneal sensitivity, corneal erosions, keratitis sicca, during/following ocular surgery or removal of a foreign body.

Generic Name (Brand Name) {Canadian Brand Name}	Dose	Notes
(Adsorbotear, Akwa Tears, Aquasite, Artifical Tears Plus, Cellufresh, Celluvisc, Comfort Tears, Dakrina, Dry Eye Therapy, Dry Eyes Duratears Naturale, Dwelle, Eye-Lube-A, HypoTears, HypoTears PF, Isopto Alkaline, Isopto Plain, Just Tears, Lacril, Lacri-Lube NP, Lacri-Lube S.O.P., Lacrisert, Liquifilm Forte, Liquifilm Tears, LubriTears, Moisture Drops, Murine Solution, Murocel, Nature's Tears, Nu-Tears, Nu-Tears II, Nutra Tear, Paralube, Refresh, Refresh PM, Tear Drop, TearGard, Teargen, Tearisol, Tears Naturale, Tears Naturale Free, Tears Naturale II, Tears Plus, Tears Renewed, Ultra Tears, Vit-A-Drops, Viva-Drops)	*Artificial tears* Adults and children: 1–2 drops 3–4 times daily or 1 insert (Lacrisert) 1–2 times daily *Ocular lubricants* Adults and children: small amount instilled into conjunctiva several times daily	■ May alter effects of other concurrently administered ophthalmic medications ■ ADRs: photophobia, lid edema stinging (insert only), temporarily blurred vision, eye discomfort

Beta-Adrenergic Blockers

Uses: Management of chronic open-angle glaucoma and other forms of ocular hypertension (decreases the formation of aqueous humor).

Cautions: Systemic absorption is minimal but may occur. Systemic absorption may result in additive adverse cardiovascular effects (bradycardia, hypotension), especially when used with other cardiovascular agents (antihypertensives, antiarrhythmics). Other systemic adverse reactions may occur, including bronchospasm or delirium (geriatric patients). Concurrent use with ophthalmic epinephrine may decrease effectiveness.

Generic Name (Brand Name) {Canadian Brand Name}	Dose	Notes
betaxolol (Betoptic, Betoptic S)	Adults: 1 drop of 0.5% solution twice daily or 1 drop of 0.25% suspension twice daily	■ ADRs: conjunctivitis, decreased visual acuity, ocular burning, rashes (may be less likely than others to cause bronchospasm if systemically absorbed)
carteolol (Ocupress)	Adults: 1 drop of 1% solution twice daily	■ ADRs: bronchospasm, conjunctivitis, decreased visual acuity, ocular burning, rashes (may be less likely than others to cause bradycardia if systemically absorbed)
levobunolol (AKBeta, Betagan)	Adults: 1 drop of 0.25% solution 1–2 times daily or 1 drop of 0.5% solution once daily	■ ADRs: conjunctivitis, decreased visual acuity, ocular burning, rashes
metipranolol (OptiPranolol)	Adults: 1 drop of 0.3% solution twice daily	■ ADRs: conjunctivitis, decreased visual acuity, ocular burning, rashes ■ Lasts up to 24 hr
timolol (Betimol, Timoptic), {Apo-Timop}	Adults and children ≥10 yr: *0.25% or 0.5% solution*—1 drop 1–2 times daily; *0.25% or 0.5% gel*—1 drop once daily Children <10 yr: 1 drop 0.25% solution 1–2 times daily	■ ADRs: conjunctivitis, decreased visual acuity, ocular burning, rashes ■ Lasts up to 24 hr

OPHTHALMIC MEDICATIONS (CONTINUED)

Carbonic Anhydrase Inhibitor

Uses: Management of open-angle glaucoma or other forms of ocular hypertension (decreases formation of aqueous humor).

Cautions: May exacerbate kidney stones; should not be used in patients with CCr <30 ml/min.

Generic Name (Brand Name) {Canadian Brand Name}	Dose	Notes
dorzolamide (Trusopt)	Adults: 1 drop 3 times daily	■ ADRs: bitter taste, cross-sensitivity with sulfonamides, ocular irritation or allergy

Cholinergic Agents (direct-acting)

Uses: Treatment of open-angle glaucoma (facilitates the outflow of aqueous humor); also used to facilitate miosis after ophthalmic surgery or before examination (to counteract mydriatics).

Cautions: Conditions in which pupillary constriction should be avoided. If significant systemic absorption occurs, bronchospasm, sweating, increased urination and salivation may occur.

Generic Name (Brand Name) {Canadian Brand Name}	Dose	Notes
carbachol (Carboptic, Isopto Carbachol)	Adults and children: 1 drop of 0.75–3% solution 1–3 times daily	■ ADRs: blurred vision, altered vision, stinging, eye pain
pilocarpine (Adsorbocarpine, Akarpine, Isopto Carpine, Ocu-Carpine, Ocusert Pilo, Pilocar, Pilopine, Piloptic, Pilostat), {Miocarpine}, {Spersacarpine}	Adults and children: *glaucoma*—1 drop of 1–4% solution 2–4 times daily (may be given more frequently for acute angle-closure glaucoma) or 1 ocular insert weekly or ½-in. strip of 4% gel at bedtime; *counteracting mydriatic sympathomimetics*—1 drop of 1% solution (may be repeated prior to surgery)	■ Use 1% or less solution in infants ■ ADRs: blurred vision, altered vision, stinging, eye pain, headache, browache

Cholinergic Agents (cholinesterase inhibitors)

Uses: Management of glaucoma not controlled with short-acting miotics or other agents; also used in varying doses for accommodative esotropia (diagnosis and treatment).

Cautions: Enhance neuromuscular blockade from succinylcholine; intensify the actions of cocaine and some other local anesthetics; additive toxicity with antimyasthenics, anticholinergics, and cholinesterase inhibitors (including some pesticides). Use cautiously in patients with history or risk of retinal detachment.

Generic Name (Brand Name) {Canadian Brand Name}	Dose	Notes
demecarium (Humorsol)	Adults: 1 drop 1–2 times daily	■ Avoid use during pregnancy ■ ADRs: blurred vision, change in vision, browache, miosis, eyelid twitching, watering eyes
echothiophate (Phospholine Iodide)	Adults: 1 drop 1–2 times daily	■ May cause hyperactivity in patients with Down syndrome ■ ADRs: blurred vision, change in vision, browache, miosis, eyelid twitching, watering eyes ■ Irreversible cholinesterase inhibitor

isoflurophate (Floropryl)	Adults: thin strip of ointment once every 3 days, 3 times daily	■ Avoid use during pregnancy ■ ADRs: blurred vision, change in vision, browache, miosis, eyelid twitching, watering eyes
physostigmine (Eserine Salicylate, Isopto Eserin)	Adults and children: 1 drop of 0.25–0.5% solution up to 4 times daily or 1 cm of 0.25% ointment 1–3 times daily	■ ADRs: blurred vision (ointment), change in vision, browache, miosis, eyelid twitching, watering eyes

Cycloplegic Mydriatics

Uses: Preparation for cycloplegic refraction; management of uveitis (not tropicamide).

Cautions: Use cautiously in patients with a history of glaucoma; systemic absorption may cause anticholinergic effects such as confusion, unusual behavior, flushing, hallucinations, slurred speech, drowsiness, swollen stomach (infants), tachycardia, dry mouth.

Generic Name (Brand Name) {Canadian Brand Name}	Dose	Notes
atropine (Atropair, Atropisol, Atrosulf, Isopto Atropine, I-Tropine, Ocu-Tropine)	Children: *cycloplegic refraction (solution)*—1 drop twice daily for 1–3 days prior to refraction (use 0.125% solution in children <1 yr, 0.25% solution for children 1–5 yr, 0.25% solution for children >5 yr with blue irides, 0.5–1% for children >5 yr with dark irides; *cycloplegic refraction (ointment)*—0.3 cm of 0.5% ointment in children <2 yr with blue irides, 1% ointment in children <2 yr with dark irides or children >2 yr 3 times daily for 1–3 days prior to refraction; *uveitis*—1 drop of 0.125–1% solution 1–3 times daily Adults: *uveitis*—1 drop of 1% solution 1–2 times daily (up to 4 times daily) or 0.3–0.5 cm of 1% ointment 1–2 times daily	■ Cycloplegic refraction in children only (too long-acting to use in adults); treatment of uveitis ■ Avoid using in children who have had a prior serious reaction to atropine ■ Effects on accommodation may last 6 days; mydriasis may last 12 days ■ ADRs: irritation, blurred vision, photophobia
cyclopentolate (AK-Pentolate, Cyclogyl, I-Pentolate, Cyclopentolate, Ocu-Pentolate, Pentolair, Spectro-Pentolate), {Minims}	Adults: 1 drop of 0.5–2% solution; may repeat in 5–10 min Children: 1 drop of 0.5–2% solution; may be followed 5–10 min later by 1 drop of 0.5–1% solution Premature and small infants: 1 drop of 0.5% solution single dose	■ Peak of cycloplegia is within 25–75 min and lasts 6–24 hr ■ Peak of mydriasis is within 30–60 min and may last several days ■ ADRs: irritation, blurred vision, photophobia
homatropine (Isopto Homatropine, Spectro-Homatropine), {Minims Homatropine}	Adults and children: *cycloplegic refraction*—1 drop of 2–5% solution, may repeat in 5–10 min for 2–3 more doses; *uveitis*—1 drop of 2–5% solution 2–3 times daily (up to q 3–4 hr in adults)	■ Cycloplegia and mydriasis may persist for 24–72 hr ■ ADRs: irritation, blurred vision, photophobia
scopolamine (Isopto Hyoscine)	Adults and children: *cycloplegic refraction*—1 drop of 0.25% solution (repeat twice daily for 2 days in children); *uveitis*—1 drop of 0.25% solution up to 4 times daily	■ Shorter duration than atropine, but mydriasis and cycloplegia may persist for 3–7 days ■ ADRs: irritation, blurred vision, photophobia

OPTHALMIC MEDICATIONS (CONTINUED)

Generic Name (Brand Name) {Canadian Brand Name}	Dose	Notes
tropicamide (Mydriacyl, Mydriafair, Ocu-Tropic, Opticyl, Spectro-Cyl, Tropicacyl), {Minims Tropicamide}	Adults and children: 1 drop of 0.5–1% solution	■ Stronger solution/repeated dosing may be required in patients with dark irides ■ Peak effect occurs in 20–40 min ■ Cycloplegia lasts 2–6 hr; mydriasis lasts up to 7 hr ■ ADRs: irritation, blurred vision, photophobia

Glucocorticoids

Uses: Management of inflammatory eye conditions including allergic conjunctivitis, nonspecific superficial keratitis, infectious conjunctivitis (with anti-infectives); management of corneal injury; suppression of graft rejection following keratoplasty.

Cautions: Infectious ocular processes (avoid in herpes simplex keratitis), especially fungal and viral ocular infections (may mask symptoms); diabetes; glaucoma.

Generic Name (Brand Name) {Canadian Brand Name}	Dose	Notes
dexamethasone (AK-Dex, Decadron, Maxidex), {Diodex}, {PMS Dexamethasone}, {RO-Dexasone}, {Spersadex}	Adults and children: 1–2 drops of solution 4–6 times daily (up to q 1 hr) or thin strip of ointment 3–4 times daily initially	■ As condition improves, decrease frequency of administration ■ ADRs: blurred vision (ointment), corneal thinning, increased intraocular pressure, irritation
fluorometholone (FML, Flarex, Fluor-Op)	1–2 drops 4 times daily (up to 1–2 drops q 1 hr) as suspension or thin strip of ointment 1–3 times daily (up to q 4 hr) initially	■ As condition improves, decrease frequency of administration ■ ADRs: blurred vision (ointment), corneal thinning, increased intraocular pressure, irritation
medrysone (HMS)	Adults and children: 1 drop of 1% suspension up to q 4 hr initially	■ As condition improves, decrease frequency of administration ■ ADRs: corneal thinning, increased intraocular pressure, irritation
prednisolone (AK-Pred, Econopred, Inflamase, Pred Mild)	Adults and children: 1–2 drops of 0.12–1% solution/suspension 2–6 times daily (up to q 1 hr) initially	■ As condition improves, decrease frequency of administration ■ ADRs: corneal thinning, increased intraocular pressure, irritation
rimexolone (Vexol)	Adults and children: 1–2 drops of 1% suspension q 6 hr (up to q 1 hr) initially	■ As condition improves, decrease frequency of administration ■ ADRs: corneal thinning, increased intraocular pressure, irritation

Mast Cell Stabilizers

Uses: Vernal keratoconjunctivitis.

Cautions: Require several days of treatment before effects are seen.

Generic Name (Brand Name) {Canadian Brand Name}	Dose	Notes
cromolyn (Crolom), {Opticrom}	Adults and children ≥4 yr: 1 drop of 4% solution 4–6 times daily	■ ADRs: chemosis, irritation
lodoxamide (Alomide)	Adults and children ≥2 yr: 1 drop of 0.1% solution 4 times daily	■ ADRs: blurred vision, foreign body sensation, irritation

Nonsteroidal Anti-inflammatory Agents

Uses: Management of inflammation following cataract surgery (diclofenac), allergic conjunctivitis (ketorolac), inhibition of perioperative miosis (flurbiprofen, suprofen).

Cautions: Cross-sensitivity with systemic NSAIDs may occur; concurrent use of anticoagulants, other NSAIDs, thrombolytics, some cephalosporins, and valproates may increase the risk of bleeding.

Generic Name (Brand Name) {Canadian Brand Name}	Dose	Notes
diclofenac (Voltaren)	Adults: 1 drop of 0.1% solution 4 times daily for up to 6 wk	■ Do not wear hydrocel contact lenses concurrently ■ ADRs: irritation, allergic reactions
flurbiprofen (Ocufen)	Adults: 1 drop of 0.03% solution q 30 min, beginning 2 hr prior to surgery (4 drops total)	■ ADRs: irritation, allergic reactions
ketorolac (Acular)	Adults: 1 drop of 0.5% solution 4 times daily	■ ADRs: irritation, allergic reactions
suprofen (Profenal)	Adults: 2 drops of 1% solution given 3 hr, 2 hr, and 1 hr before surgery or 2 drops q 4 hr while awake on day prior to surgery	■ ADRs: irritation, allergic reactions

Ocular Decongestants/Vasoconstrictors

Uses: Decrease ocular congestion due to irritation by vasoconstricting conjunctival blood vessels; stronger solutions have mydriatic effects.

Cautions: Systemic absorption may result in adverse cardiovascular effects; excessive/prolonged use may produce rebound hyperemia; use caution in patients at risk for acute angle-closure glaucoma; cardiovascular effects may be exaggerated by MAO inhibitors and dose adjustment may be required within 21 days of MAO inhibitors; increased risk of arrhythmias with inhalation anesthetics.

Generic Name (Brand Name) {Canadian Brand Name}	Dose	Notes
naphazoline (Albalon, Allerest, Allergy Drops, Clear Eyes Lubricating Eye Redness Reliever, Comfort Eye Drops, Degest 2, Estivin II, Nafazair, Naphcon, Ocu-Zoline, VasoClear, Vasocon), {AK-Con}	Adults: 1 drop of 0.012% solution 4 times daily as needed or 1 drop of 0.1% solution q 3–4 hr as needed	■ ADRs: *ophthalmic*—rebound hyperemia; *systemic*—dizziness, headache, nausea, sweating, weakness
oxymetazoline (OcuClear, Visine LR)	Adults and children >6 yr: 1 drop of 0.025% solution q 6 hr as needed	■ ADRs: *ophthalmic*—rebound hyperemia; *systemic*—headache, insomnia, nervousness, tachycardia
phenylephrine (AK-Dilate, AK-Nefrin, Dilatair, I-Phrine, Isopto Frin, Mydfrin, Ocu-Phrin, Prefrin), {Minims Phenylephrine}, {Spersaphrine}	Adults: *decongestant*—1 drop of 0.12% solution q 3–4 hr as needed; *mydriasis*—2.5 or 10% solution up to 3 times daily Children: *mydriasis*—2.5% solution up to 3 times daily	■ ADRs: *ophthalmic*—blurred vision, browache, irritation; *systemic*—dizziness, tachycardia, hypertension, paleness, sweating, trembling

OPHTHALMIC MEDICATIONS (CONTINUED)

Generic Name (Brand Name) {Canadian Brand Name}	Dose	Notes
tetrahydrozoline (Collyrium Fresh, Eyesine, Geneye, Mallazine, Murine Plus, Optigene 3, Tetrazine, Visine)	Adults: 1–2 drops of 0.05% solution up to 4 times daily	■ ADRs: *ophthalmic*—irritation; *systemic*—tachycardia, hypertension

Osmotic Agent
Uses: Decreases superficial edema of the cornea prior to examination.

Generic Name (Brand Name) {Canadian Brand Name}	Dose	Notes
glycerin (Ophthalgan)	Adults: 1–2 drops prior to exam	■ Avoid using in patients with hypersensitivity to chlorobutanol

Prostaglandin Agonist
Uses: Management of glaucoma or lowering of intraocular pressure (increases outflow of aqueous humor).
Cautions: May change eye color to brown; will form precipitate with thimerosal-containing products; can be used with other agents to lower intraocular pressure.

Generic Name (Brand Name) {Canadian Brand Name}	Dose	Notes
latanoprost (Xalatan)	Adults: 1 drop once daily	■ ADRs: local irritation, foreign body sensation

Sympathomimetics
Uses: Management of glaucoma (lowers intraocular pressure by decreasing formation of aqueous humor).
Cautions: Systemic absorption may result in adverse cardiovascular and CNS reactions (especially in patients with cardiovascular disease); avoid use in patients predisposed to acute angle-closure glaucoma.

Generic Name (Brand Name) {Canadian Brand Name}	Dose	Notes
apraclonidine (Iopidine)	Adults: *glaucoma*—1–2 drops of 0.5% solution 3 times daily; *preoperative use*—1 drop of 1% solution 1 hr prior to surgery	■ A selective alpha-adrenergic agonist ■ ADRs: *ophthalmic*—irritation, mydriasis; *systemic*—allergic reactions, arrhythmias, bradycardia, drowsiness, dry nose, fainting, headache, nervousness, weakness ■ Monitor pulse and blood pressure ■ Avoid concurrent use with MAO inhibitors

brimonidine (Alphagan)	Adults: 1 drop 3 times daily (8 hr apart)	■ A selective alpha-adrenergic agonist ■ ADRs: *ophthalmic*—irritation; *systemic*—drowsiness, dizziness, dry mouth, headache, weakness, muscular pain ■ Avoid concurrent use with MAO inhibitors ■ Tricyclic antidepressants may decrease effectiveness; additive CNS depression may occur with other CNS depressants, additive adverse cardiovascular effects with other cardiovascular agents
dipivefrin (Propine)	Adults: 1 drop q 12 hr	■ Converted to epinephrine in the eye ■ ADRs: *ophthalmic*—local irritation, macular edema (aphakic patients); *systemic*—arrhythmias, hypertension ■ Wait 15 min before inserting soft contact lenses
epinephrine (Epifrin, Epinal, Eppy/N, Glaucon)	Adults: 1 drop of 1–2% solution 1–2 times daily	■ Increased risk of arrhythmias with inhalation anesthetics ■ ADRs: headache, local irritation ■ Cardiovascular effects may be exaggerated by MAO inhibitors; dose adjustment may be required within 21 days of MAO inhibitors

*ADRs = adverse reactions.

APPENDIX P

Recent Drug Release Update

Generic Name (Brand Name) Rx/OTC	Classification(s)	Use(s)	Dose	Notes
acetretin (Soriatane) Rx	Retinoid	Severe psoriasis unresponsive to other therapies	PO (Adults): 25 or 50 mg once daily with main meal until lesions resolve	Will replace etretinate (Tegison) ADRs*: cheilitis, hair loss, dry skin, desquamation, increased liver enzymes, increased vitamin A toxicity, decreased effectiveness of progestin contraceptives, increased risk of pseudotumor cerebri with tetracycline Pregnancy category X
amlexanox (Aphthasol) Rx	Mast cell stabilizer	Management of aphthous ulcers in patients with intact immune systems	Top (Adults): Apply a dab (0.5 cm) of 5% paste to each ulcer 4 times daily	ADRs: transient pain, stinging, burning at site of application
arbutamine (GenESA) Rx	Diagnostic agent (synthetic catecholamine)	Part of a diagnostic system that mimics exercise in patients who cannot exercise adequately	IV (Adults): 0.1 mcg/kg/min initially; automated system calculates further doses up to 0.8 mcg/kg/min (up to a total dose of 10 mcg/kg) To be given only with specific infusion device	Should not be used in patients receiving digitalis glycosides, tricyclic antidepressants or atropine, or Group I antiarrhythmics or in patients with idiopathic hypertrophic subaortic stenosis, severe CHF, or recurrent sustained VT
azelastine (Astelin) Rx	Antihistamine	Treatment of seasonal allergic rhinitis	Intranasal (Adults and Children): 2 sprays/nostril twice daily (137 mcg/spray)	ADRs: nasal irritation
becaplermin (Regranex) Rx	Platelet-derived growth factor	Treatment of lower extremity diabetic neuropathic ulcers that extend into subcutaneous tissue or beyond and have an adequate blood supply	Top (Adults): Apply once daily, cover with moist gauze for 12 hr, remove	Should not be applied to neoplasms ADRs: erythematous rash

cefdinir (Omnicef) Rx	Anti-infective (cephalosporin)	Treatment of respiratory tract infections, skin and skin structure infections, and otitis media	PO (Adults and Adolescents): 300 mg q 12 hr or 600 mg q 24 hr PO (Children 6 mo–12 yr): 7 mg/kg q 12 hr or 14 mg/kg q 24 hr	Do not take concurrently (within 2 hr) of antacids or iron supplements Dosage reduction required if CCr <30 ml/min
citric acid (Citrol Oral Spray) OTC	Smoking cessation deterrent	Decreases craving for cigarettes	Oral Spray (Adults): Spray as needed	When sprayed in back of throat, mimics the sensation of smoking a cigarette
daclizumab (Zenapax) Roche Rx	Immunosuppressant (monoclonal antibody)	Prevention of acute organ rejection in renal transplant patients (with cyclosporine and glucocorticoids)	IV (Adults): 1 mg/kg for 5 doses; 1st dose no more than 24 hr before transplant, then q 14 days for 4 more doses	ADRs: bleeding, changes in blood pressure, dizziness, edema, gastrointestinal symptoms, insomnia, tremor
fomepizole (Antizol) Rx	Antidote	Antidote to antifreeze (ethylene glycol) poisoning	IV (Adults): 15 mg/kg loading dose, then 10 mg/kg q 12 hr for 4 doses, then 15 mg/kg q 12 hr until ethylene glycol level is <20 mg/dl (give q 4 hr during hemodialysis)	ADRs: dizziness, headache, nausea All doses given as a slow infusion over 30 min
glatiramer (Copaxone) Rx	Immune modifier	Management of relapsing-remitting multiple sclerosis	SC (Adults): 20 mg/day	ADRs: allergic reactions, anxiety, chest pain, coughing, injection site reactions, weight gain May be refrigerated (no longer requires freezing)
halofantrine (Halfan) Rx	Antimalarial	Mild to moderate malaria	PO (Adults): 500 mg q 6 hr for 3 doses; may need to repeat in 7 days	Take 1 hr before or 2 hr after food
hylan G-F 20 (Synvisc) Rx	Synovial fluid viscosity agent	Management of the symptoms of osteoarthritis of the knee	Intra-articular (Adults): 5 injections/treatment cycle	ADRs: injection site reactions, headache Contraindicated in patients with avian allergies
imiquimod (Aldara) Rx	Immune modifier	Management of genital and perianal warts	Top (Adults): Apply 5% cream 3 times weekly prior to sleep; leave on for 6–10 hr, then remove with mild soap and water	ADRs: local skin irritation
interferon alfacon-1 (Infergen) Rx	Immune modifier	Management of chronic hepatitis C infection	SC (Adults): 9 mcg 3 times weekly for 24 wk (at least 48 hr between injections)	ADRs: depression, flu-like symptoms, hypertension, palpitations, tachycardia
ivermectin (Stromectol) Rx	Antihelmintic	Treatment of strongyloidiasis and onchocerciasis	PO (Adults and Children >15 kg): *Strongyloidiasis*—200 mcg/kg single dose; *onchocerciasis*—150 mcg/kg single dose (re-treatment may be necessary)	ADRs: reactions related to killing of filaria (Manzotti reaction)

RECENT DRUG RELEASE UPDATE (CONTINUED)

Generic Name (Brand Name) Rx/OTC	Classification(s)	Use(s)	Dose	Notes
midodrine (ProAmatine) Rx	Vasopressor ($alpha_1$-adrenergic agonist)	Management of symptomatic orthostatic hypotension	PO (Adults): 10 mg 3 times daily at least 3–4 hr apart; last dose taken no less than 4 hr before bedtime	ADRs: dysuria, paresthesias, piloerection Increased risk of adverse cardiovascular reactions with other cardioactive agents
samarium SM 153 lexidronam (Quadramet) Rx	Radiopharmaceutical	Management of pain due to osteoblastic metastatic cancer	IV (Adults): 1 mCi/kg	ADRs: transient increase in bone pain Radioactivity excreted in urine; take appropriate precautions Additive bone marrow depression with antineoplastic agents
sodium hyaluronate (Hyalagan) Rx	Synovial fluid viscosity agent	Management of the symptoms of osteoarthritis of the knee	Intra-articular (Adults): 3 injections/treatment cycle	ADRs: local swelling Contraindicated in patients with avian allergies
talc aerosol (Sclerosol) Rx	Sclerosing agent	Prevention of recurrence of pleural effusions	Intrapleurally (Adults): 4–8 g	ADRs: pain, fever
tazarotene (Tazorac) Rx	Antipsoriatic agent (receptor-selective retinoid)	Management of stable-plaque psoriasis <20% of BSA Mild to moderately severe facial acne vulgaris	Top (Adults): *Psoriasis*—apply as thin film once daily to dry skin (not to exceed 20% of body surface area)	Available as 0.05 and 0.1% gel Small amounts are absorbed Converted in skin to active metabolite Irritation, stinging, burning, pruritus, erythema (more common with 0.1%)
tolcapone (Tasmar) Rx	Anti-Parkinson agent (catechol-*O*-methyltransferase inhibitor	Management of Parkinson's disease with levodopa/carbidopa	PO (Adults): 100–200 mg 3 times daily with levodopa/carbidopa	ADRs: diarrhea, headache, muscle cramps, nausea, sleep disorders
toremifene (Fareston) Rx	Antineoplastic (antiestrogen)	Treatment of postmenopausal metastatic breast cancer in patients who are estrogen receptor–positive or unknown	PO (Adults): 60 mg once daily	May cause hypercalcemia and tumor flare Increases effects of warfarin
NEW INDICATIONS				
cefepime (Maxipime) Rx	Anti-infective (3rd generation cephalosporin)	Treatment of **intra-abdominal infections** (with metronidazole)	IM (Adults): 0.5–1 g q 12 hr IV (Adults): 1–2 g q 12 hr up to 2 g q 8 hr	ADRs: allergic reactions Dosage reduction/increased interval recommended if CCr ≤60 ml/mm
enoxaparin (Lovenox) Rx	Anticoagulant (heparin-like)	Prevention of deep vein thrombosis following hip replacment	SC (Adults): 40 mg once daily	Approved **for at home use** for ≤3 wk as a **once-daily** dose

propafenone (Rythmol) Rx	Antiarrhythmic	Management of **paroxysmal supraventricular tachyarrhythmias**	PO (Adults): 150 mg q 8 hr; may be gradually increased at 3–4 day intervals as required, up to 300 mg q 8–12 hr	ADRs: arrhythmias, dizziness, GI complaints Increases serum digoxin levels
salmeterol (Serevent) Rx	Bronchodilator (adrenergic)	Long-term maintenance treatment of bronchospasm due to **COPD**	Inhalation (Adults): 50 mcg (as 2 inhalations or 1 blister) q 12 hr	Should not be used to treat acute bronchospasm
NEW DOSAGE FORMS				
carbamazepine **extended-release capsules** (Carbatrol) Rx	Anticonvulsant	Prevention of seizures; management of trigeminal neuralgia	PO (Adults): 300 mg twice daily PO (Children): 200 mg twice daily	Capsules can be opened and sprinkled over food
etodolac (Lodine XL) **500 mg extended-release tablet** Rx	Nonsteroidal anti-inflammatory agent	Management of osteoarthritis/rheumatoid arthritis	PO (Adults): 400–1000 mg once daily	ADRs: gastrointestinal complaints, GI bleeding
niacin **extended-release tablets** (Niaspan) Rx	Lipid-lowering agent	Part of a comprehensive program to lower lipids (including cholesterol and triglycerides)	PO (Adults): 375 mg at bedtime initially; increased weekly up to 1 g	Should be taken with a low-fat snack
ofloxacin otic solution (Floxin Otic) Rx	Anti-infective (fluoroquinolone)	Otitis externa in adults and children ≥1 yr, otitis media in children ≥1 yr with tympanostomy tubes, chronic suppurative otitis media in adolescents ≥ 12 yr, and adults with chronic perforations of the tympanic membrane	Adults and Children >12 yr: 10 drops (0.5 ml) in each ear twice daily for 10–14 days Children 1–12 yr: 5 drops (0.25 ml) in each ear twice daily for 10–14 days	ADRs: application site reactions, dizziness, earache, pruritus, vertigo
tobramycin inhalation solution (TOBI) Rx	Anti-infective (aminoglycoside)	Bronchopulmonary infections due to *Pseudomonas aeruginosa* in patients with cystic fibrosis	Inhalation: (Adults and Children): 300mg/5 ml inhaled over 10–15 min twice daily for 28 days, then off for 28 days	ADRs: irritation, resistant organisms

DISCONTINUED DRUGS

Generic Name (Brand Name) {Canadian Brand Name} Rx/OTC	Reason for Discontinuation
dexfenfluramine (Redux) Rx	Risk of valvular heart disease
etretinate (Tegison) Rx	Will be replaced by acetretin (Soriatane); see acetretin entry at beginning of table; better safety profile

RECENT DRUG RELEASE UPDATE (CONTINUED)

Generic Name (Brand Name) {Canadian Brand Name} Rx/OTC	Reason for Discontinuation
fenfluramine (Pondimin) Rx	Risk of valvular heart disease
prazepam (Centrax) Rx	Removed from market; many other choices available
terfenadine (Seldane) Rx	Removed from market because of risk of serious interactions

*ADRs = adverse reactions.
†Boldface in Dose column and New Indications section = change in dose or usage.

APPENDIX Q

Infrequently Used Drugs

Generic Name (Brand Name) {Canadian Brand Name} Rx/OTC Controlled Substance	Classification(s)	Use(s)	Route/Dosage	Notes
abciximab (ReoPro) Rx	Platelet aggregation inhibitor	With heparin and/or aspirin to decrease/prevent cardiac ischemic complications before or after percutaneous coronary intervention (PCI)	IV (Adults): 0.25 mg/kg bolus 10–60 min before PCI, followed by 0.125 mcg/kg/min (up to 10 mcg/min) for 12 hr following PCI; *or* 0.25 mg/kg bolus followed by 0.125 mcg/kg/min (up to 10 mcg/min) for 18–24 hr ending 1 hr after PCI	ADRs*: hypersensitivity reactions, increased risk of bleeding
albendazole (Albenza) Rx	Antihelmintic	Neurocysticercosis, hydatid disease	PO (Adults and Children >6 yr): 400 mg twice daily in patients ≥60 kg, 7.5 mg/kg twice daily in patients <60 kg (*neurocysticercosis*—treat for 8–30 days; *hydatid disease*—treat for 28 days, off for 14 days, for 3 cycles)	ADRs: neutropenia Avoid use in pregnancy
alpha$_1$-proteinase inhibitor (alpha$_1$-antitrypsin, Prolastin) Rx	Enzyme inhibitor	Replacement therapy (chronic) in patients with panacinar emphysema due to alpha$_1$-antitrypsin deficiency	IV (Adults): 60 mg/kg once weekly; has also been given as 240 mg/kg once monthly (unlabeled)	ADRs: delayed fever, dizziness, light-headedness, transient leukocytosis
alprostadil intracavernosal (Caverject, Edex, Muse) Rx	Prostaglandin	Diagnosis and treatment of erectile dysfunction	Intracavernosal (Adults): 1.25—2.5 mg initially, increased until optimal response is obtained Intraurethral (Adults): 125–1000 mcg	ADRs: ecchymoses, edema, penile fibrosis (intracavernosal), priapism Should be used only once/24 hr no more than 3 times weekly
amantadine (Symadine, Symmetrel) Rx	Anti-Parkinson agent Antiviral	Management of Parkinson's disease Prophylaxis and treatment of influenza A infection	PO (Adults): *Parkinson's disease*—100 mg 1–2 times daily; *influenza A*—200 mg daily as a single dose or 100 mg twice daily (100 mg/day in geriatric patients) PO (Children 9–12 yr): *Influenza A*—100 mg q 12 hr PO (Children 1–9 yr): *Influenza A*—1.5–3 mg/kg q 12 hr or 2.2–4.4 mg/kg q 12 hr (not >150 mg/day)	ADRs: ataxia, dizziness, hypotension, insomnia, mottling Additive anticholinergic effects, increased risk of adverse CNS effects with alcohol or CNS stimulants

Generic Name (Brand Name) {Canadian Brand Name} Rx/OTC Controlled Substance	Classification(s)	Use(s)	Route/Dosage	Notes
aminocaproic acid (Amicar) Rx	Hemostatic	Management of hemorrhage due to fibrinolysis *Unlabeled*—prevention of recurrent subarachnoid hemorrhage; prevention of bleeding following oral surgery in hemophiliacs; management of hemorrhage due to thrombolytic agents	PO (Adults): *Bleeding due to increased fibrinolysis*—5 g 1st hr, followed by 1–1.25 g q hr for 8 hr or until bleeding stops or 6 g/24 hr after prostate surgery; *subarachnoid hemorrhage*—(following IV) 3 g q 2 hr (36 g/day). If no surgery is performed, continue for 21 days, then taper dose over several days; *management of bleeding following oral surgery in hemophiliacs*—6 g immediately after procedure, then q 6 hr for 9–10 days; or 2 g 30–60 min before procedure, then 2 g 3–4 times daily for 3–7 days IV (Adults): *Bleeding due to increased fibrinolysis*—4–5 g over 1st hr, followed by 1 g/hr for 8 hr or until bleeding stops or 6 g/24 hr after prostate surgery (not >30 g/day) PO, IV (Children): 100 mg/kg or 3 g/m^2 over 1st hr, followed by continuous infusion of 33.3 mg/kg/hr or 1 $g/m^2/hr$ (not >18 $g/m^2/24$ hr)	ADRs: anorexia, arrhythmias, bloating, cramping, diarrhea, diuresis, hypotension (IV only), myopathy, nasal stuffiness, nausea, renal failure, tinnitus
ammonium chloride Rx	Electrolyte modifier	Acidifying agent	PO (Adults): 1 g 3 times daily for up to 6 days IV (Adults): Administer by infusion at concentration not to exceed 2% at a rate not to exceed 5 ml/min	ADRs: acidosis, nausea, vomiting Avoid using in patients with hepatic impairment
amphetamine Rx C-II	CNS stimulant	Narcolepsy ADHD (unlabeled)	PO (Adults): 5–20 mg 1–3 times daily PO (Children 6–12 yr): *Narcolepsy*—2.5 mg twice daily initially, increased weekly until desired effect or adult dose; *ADHD*—5 mg 1–2 times daily, increased weekly as needed PO (Children 3–6 yr): *ADHD*—2.5 mg once daily, increased weekly as needed	ADRs: insomnia, hypertension, tachycardia Avoid use in patients with hypertension, diabetes
amyl nitrite Rx	Antianginal Antidote (cyanide poisoning)	Acute treatment of angina pectoris Acute management of cyanide poisoning	Inhalation (Adults): *Angina*—1 ampule crushed and vapors inhaled, may be repeated in 3–5 min (1–6 inhalations); *cyanide poisoning*—inhale vapors for 15–30 sec of each minute until sodium nitrite is prepared or inhale vapors for 30–60 sec q 5 min until patient is conscious, then repeat at longer intervals for 24 hr	ADRs: headache, hypotension, tachycardia

anagralide (Agrylin) Rx	Platelet reduction agent	Essential thrombocythemia	PO (Adults): 0.5 mg 4 times daily or 1 mg twice daily for at least 7 days, then adjust dose to maintain platelet count <600,000/mcl (not to exceed 10 mg/day or 2.5 mg/dose)	ADRs: abdominal pain, diarrhea, nausea, palpitations Platelet count should respond in 7–14 days Use cautiously in patients with hepatic, cardiovascular, or renal disease
aprotinin (Trasylol) Rx	Hemostatic agent (protein-ase inhibitor)	Reduces bleeding and need for transfusions following coronary artery bypass grafting in high-risk patients	IV (Adults): *Test dose*—1 ml (1.4 mg or 10,000 kallikrein inhibitor units [KIU]) given 10 min prior to loading dose; if no reaction occurs, give loading dose; *loading dose*—200 ml (280 mg or 2 million KIU) followed by continuous infusion; *continuous infusion*—50 ml/hr (70 mg/hr) or 500,000 KIU/hr; *pump prime dose*—200 ml (280 mg or 2 million KIU) may be added to priming fluid of cardiopulmonary bypass circuit (other regimens are used)	ADRs: hypersensitivity reactions, phlebitis, renal tubular necrosis Incidence of hypersensitivity reactions increases with repeat exposure, especially within first 6 mo
attapulgite (Diar-Aid, Diasorb, Kaopectate, Kaopectate Advanced Formula, Kaopectate Maximum Strength, K-Pek, Parepectolin, Rheaban), {Fowler's Diarrhea Tablets} OTC	Antidiarrheal (adsorbent)	Adjunct symptomatic management of mild-to-moderate acute diarrhea	PO (Adults): 1.2–1.5 g after each loose stool (not >9 g/24 hr) PO (Children 6–12 yr): 600 mg after each loose stool (not >4.2 g/24 hr) PO (Children 3–6 yr): 300 mg after each loose stool (not >2.1 g/24 hr)	ADRs: constipation Attapulgite is hydrated magnesium aluminum silicate
BCG-Connaught Strain (ImmuCyst, TheraCys) Rx	Antineoplastic	Transitional cell carcinoma of the bladder	Intracavitary (Adults): 81 mg instilled and retained for 1–2 hr q wk for 6 wk, then at 3, 6, 12, 18, and 24 mo	ADRS: bladder irritation, flu-like symptoms, nausea Connaught Strain and Tice Strain products are not interchangeable
BCG-Tice Strain (TICE BCG) Rx	Antineoplastic	Transitional cell carcinoma of the bladder	Intracavitary (Adults): 1–8 × 10^8 CFU instilled and retained for 1–2 hr q wk for 6–12 wk, then monthly for 6–12 mo	ARDs: bladder irritation, flu-like symptoms, nausea Connaught Strain and Tice Strain products are not interchangeable
bacitracin (Baci-IM) Rx	Anti-infective	Infants with pneumonia/empyema due to susceptible staphylococci	IM (Infants >2.5 kg): 1000 U/kg/day in 2–3 divided doses IM (Infants <2.5 kg): 900 U/kg/day in 2–3 divided doses	ADRs: renal failure Largely replaced by less toxic agents
benzonatate (Tessalon) Rx	Antitussive (locally acting)	Management of nonproductive cough	PO (Adults and Children ≥10 yr): 100 mg 3 times daily (up to 600 mg/day)	ADRs: dizziness, headache, hypersensitivity reactions, sedation

INFREQUENTLY USED DRUGS (CONTINUED)

Generic Name (Brand Name) {Canadian Brand Name} Rx/OTC Controlled Substance	Classification(s)	Use(s)	Route/Dosage	Notes
benzquinamide (Emete-Con) Rx	Antiemetic	Prevention/treatment of nausea and vomiting associated with anesthesia and surgery	IM (Adults): 50 mg (0.5–1 mg/kg); may repeat in 1 hr, then q 3–4 hr as needed IV (Adults): 25 mg (0.2–0.4 mg/kg)	ADRs: drowsiness Use lower doses in geriatric patients Additive CNS depression with other CNS depressants May cause hypertension with vasopressors or epinephrine
beractant (Survanta) Rx	Pulmonary surfactant	Treatment/prevention of RDS in premature infants	Intratracheal (Infants): 100 mg/kg; may be repeated 4 times, at least 6 hr apart, during first 2 days of life	Each dose is given as 4 aliquots (25 mg/kg) using specific technique
botulinum toxin type A (Botox) Rx	Ophthalmic (neuromuscular blocking agent)	Treatment of blepharospasm or strabismus	IM (Adults and Children >12 yr): 1.25–5 U/muscle	Injected into ophthalmic muscles
cabergoline (Dostinex) Rx	Dopamine agonist	Management of hyperprolactinemia	PO (Adults): 0.25 mg twice weekly (up to 1 mg twice weekly)	ADRs: dizziness, headache, hypotension, nausea Dopamine antagonists (phenothiazines, metoclopramide) may decrease effectiveness
calcipotriene (Dovonex) Rx	Antipsoriatic (local)	Management of moderate-plaque psoriasis	Topical (Adults): Apply twice daily	ADRs: burning, itching, and skin irritation
carboprost (Hemabate) Rx	Oxytocic Prostaglandin Abortifacient	Induction of abortion Control of postpartum bleeding	IM (Adults): *Abortion*—250 mcg, may repeat q 1.5–3.5 hr (dosage may be increased to 500 mcg but should not exceed a cumulative dose of 12 mg or more than 2 days of continuous use). *Control of bleeding*—250 mcg; may repeat q 15–90 min (not to exceed 2 mg total or 8 doses)	ADRs: diarrhea, nausea, vomiting 100-mcg test dose may be used before inducing abortion
chlorpropamide (Diabinese) {Apo-Chlorpropamide}, {Novo-Propamide} Rx	Oral hypoglycemic agent	Management of type II (non–insulin-dependent) diabetes mellitus	PO (Adults): 250–500 mg/day in 1–2 divided doses (range 100–750 mg/day)	ADRs: allergic reactions, hypoglycemia, photosensitivity, SIADH

chlorzoxazone (EZE-DS, Paraflex, Parafon Forte DSC, Relaxazone, Remular, Strifon Forte DCS) Rx	Skeletal muscle relaxant (centrally acting)	Acute painful musculoskeletal conditions	PO (Adults): 250–750 mg 3–4 times daily PO (Children): 20 mg/kg (600 mg/m^2)/day in 3–4 divided doses	ADRs: hepatotoxicity
cladribine (Leustatin) Rx	Antineoplastic (antimetabolite)	Management of refractory hairy cell leukemia	IV (Adults): 0.09–0.1 mg/kg/day for 7 days	ADRs: bone marrow depression, diarrhea, flu-like syndrome, injection site reactions, nausea, vomiting, tumor lysis syndrome
colfosceril (Exosurf Neonatal) Rx	Pulmonary surfactant	Treatment/prevention of RDS in premature infants	Intratracheal (Infants): *Prophylaxis*—67.5 mg/kg, repeated 12 and 24 hr later; *treatment*—67.5 mg/kg, repeated 12 hr later	Each dose is given as 2 aliquots (33.75 mg/kg) using specific technique
corticotropin (ACTH, Acthar) Rx	Hormone (adrenocorticotropic)	Diagnosis of adrenocortical disorders	IV (Adults): 10–25 U infused over 8 hr	ADRs: minimal, because of single-dose use
cosyntropin (Cortrosyn) Rx	Hormone (adrenocorticotropic)	Diagnosis of adrenocortical disorders	SC, IM, IV (Adults and Children $>$2 yr): 0.25 mg IM (Children $<$2 yr): 0.125 mg	ADRs: hypersensitivity reactions
cyclizine (Marezine), {Marzine} Rx	Antiemetic	Motion sickness	PO (Adults): 50 mg q 3–4 hr as needed PO (Children): 1 mg/kg (33 mg/m^2) 3 times daily or 25 mg q 6–8 hr as needed	ADRs: dizziness, drowsiness, dry mouth Give initial dose 30 min before travel
cromolyn, oral (Gastrocrom), {Nalcrom} Rx	Mast cell stabilizer	Treatment of mastocytosis	PO (Adults): 200 mg 4 times daily PO (Children 2–12 yr): 100 mg 4 times daily PO (Children up to 2 yr): 20 mg/kg/day in 4 divided doses (up to 30 mg/kg/day)	ADRs: abdominal pain, diarrhea, myalgia, irritability
cytomegalovirus immune globulin (CMVIG, CytoGam) Rx	Immune globulin	Suppression of cytomegalovirus (CMV) disease in CMV-negative recipients of transplanted CMV-positive kidneys	IV (Adults): 150 mg/kg within 72 hr of transplantation, then 100 mg/kg at 2, 4, 6, and 8 wk, then 50 mg/kg at 12 and 16 wk	ADRs: allergic reactions, hypotension
dapsone (Avlosulfon) Rx	Antifungal Anti-infective Antiprotozoal	Leprosy, dermatitis herpetiformis *Unlabeled uses:* prophylaxis of malaria, treatment and prevention of *Pneumocystis carinii* pneumonia	PO (Adults): 50–100 mg once daily	ADRs: blood dyscrasias, hemolytic anemia, peripheral motor weakness, liver damage Concurrent use with didanosine may decrease dapsone levels

Generic Name (Brand Name) {Canadian Brand Name} Rx/OTC Controlled Substance	Classification(s)	Use(s)	Route/Dosage	Notes
delavirdine (Rescriptor) Rx	Antiretroviral (non-nucleoside reverse transcriptase inhibitor)	Management of HIV infection with other antiretrovirals	PO (Adults): 400 mg 3 times daily	ADRs: nausea, neutropenia, rash Interacts with many other drugs: antacids decrease absorption; levels increased by clarithromycin, fluoxetine, ketoconazole; delavirdine increases indinavir levels; didanosine, some anticonvulsants, and rifampin decrease delavirdine levels; delaviridine decreases didanosine levels
demeclocycline (Declomycin) Rx	Anti-infective (tetracycline)	Treatment of infections Management of syndrome of inappropriate diuretic hormone (SIADH; unlabeled)	PO (Adults): *Infections*—150 mg q 6 hr or 300 mg q 12 hr; *SIADH*—3.25–3.75 mg/kg q 6 hr	ADRs: photosensitivity, allergic reactions, diabetes insipidus Concurrent ingestion of antacids, calcium or iron supplements, or dairy products decreases absorption
desipramine (Norpramin) Rx	Antidepressant (tricyclic)	Treatment of depression *Unlabeled uses:* chronic neurogenic pain, panic disorder, vascular headache prophylaxis	PO (Adults): 100–200 mg/day as a single dose or in divided doses PO (Adolescents): 25–50 mg/day in divided doses (up to 100 mg/day) PO (Children 6–12 yr): 10–30 mg (1–5 mg/kg)/day in divided doses	ADRs: arrhythmias, blurred vision, constipation, dry mouth, hypotension
dicyclomine (Antispas, A-Spas, Bentyl, Dibent, Di-Spaz, Spasmoject), {Bentylol}, {Formulex}, {Lomine}, {Neoquess}, {Or-Tyl}, {Spasmoban}, Rx	Anticholinergic (antispasmodic)	Management of irritable bowel syndrome in patients who do not respond to standard interventions	PO (Adults): 10–20 mg 3–4 times daily (up to 160 mg/day; 30-mg ER tablets may be given twice daily) PO (Children ≥2 yr): 10 mg 3–4 times daily PO (Children 6 mo–2 yr): 5–10 mg 3–4 times daily IM (Adults): 20 mg q 4–6 hr	ADRs: blurred vision, constipation, dry eyes, dry mouth
dienestrol (Ortho Dienestrol) Rx	Hormone (estrogen)	Symptomatic management of atrophic vaginitis in postmenopausal women	Vag (Adults): 1 applicatorful 1–2 times daily for 1–2 wk, then 1/2 dose for 1–2 wk. *Maintenance dose*—1 applicatorful 1–3 times wk for 3 wk, then 1 wk off	ADRs: breakthrough bleeding, breast tenderness, edema, headache

dimercaprol (BAL in Oil) Rx	Antidote (heavy metal antagonist)	Treatment of heavy metal poisoning (mercury, gold, arsenic, lead)	IM (Adults): *Severe lead poisoning*—4 mg/kg q 4 hr for 2–7 days; regimen may repeat for 5 days after 2-day rest. *Mild lead poisoning*—4 mg/kg initially, then 3 mg/kg q 4 hr. *Severe arsenic/gold poisoning*—3 mg/kg q 4 hr for 2 days, then 4 times daily on the 3rd day, then twice daily for 10 days or until recovered (other doses used). *Mild arsenic/gold poisoning*—2.5 mg/kg q 6 hr for 2 days, then twice daily on the 3rd day, then once daily for 10 days or until recovered IM (Children): *Lead poisoning*—50–75 mg/m^2 q 4 hr for 5 days; may repeat after 2-day rest	ADRs: abscesses/pain at IM sites, hypertension, unpleasant breath Used with other agents in lead poisoning
dirithromycin (Dynabac) Rx	Anti-infective (macrolide)	Treatment of infections	PO (Adults): 500 mg once daily; some infections require only 5 days of treatment	ADRs: GI complaints
disulfiram (Antabuse) Rx	Alcohol abuse deterrent	Prevention of alcohol abuse in predisposed patients	PO (Adults): 125–500 mg/day	ADRs: drowsiness (give as a single bedtime dose)
dornase alfa (Pulmozyme) Rx	Enzyme	Adjunct management of cystic fibrosis	Inhalation (Adults and Children >5 yr): 2.5 mg 1–2 times daily	ADRs: dysphonia, pharyngitis
edetate calcium disodium (Calcium Disodium Versenate, calcium EDTA, edathamil calcium disodium, sodium calcium edetate) Rx	Antidote (lead chelator)	Management of acute or chronic lead poisoning	IM, IV (Adults): 15–25 mg/kg (0.5–0.75 g/m^2) q 12 hr for 3–5 days (not >2 g/day); may repeat after 2-day rest IM, IV (Children): 1–1.5 g/m^2/day in 6 divided doses for 5 days; may repeat after 2-day rest	ADRs: nephrotoxicity, pain at IM site
epoprostenol (Flolan, prostacyclin) Rx	Prostaglandin (vasodilator)	Management of primary pulmonary hypertension in selected patients	IV (Adults): *Acute dose ranging*—2 ng/kg/min; may increase by 2 ng/kg/min q 15 min or more until dose-limiting effects are noted; *chronic dosing*—begin with 4 ng/kg/min less than maximum tolerated rate determined during acute dose ranging. If initial maximum tolerated rate was <5 ng/kg/min, initiate therapy at 50% of maximum tolerated rate. Further adjustments may be made; increments of 1–2 ng/kg/min may be made at intervals of at least 15 min; decrements of 2 ng/kg/min may be made at intervals of at least 15 min (avoid abrupt discontinuation)	ADRs: anxiety, headache, flu-like symptoms, hypotension, nausea, paresthesia, tachycardia, vomiting

INFREQUENTLY USED DRUGS (CONTINUED)

Generic Name (Brand Name) {Canadian Brand Name} Rx/OTC Controlled Substance	Classification(s)	Use(s)	Route/Dosage	Notes
estramustine (Emcyt) Rx	Antineoplastic (hormone/alkylating agent)	Palliative treatment of metastatic prostate cancer	PO (Adults): 600 mg/m²/day in 3 divided doses *or* 14 mg/kg/day in 3–4 divided doses (range 10–16 mg/kg/day)	ADRs: edema, gynecomastia, nausea, decreased libido, diarrhea
ethosuximide (Zarontin) Rx	Anticonvulsant	Management of absence seizures	PO (Adults and Children >6 yr): 15–30 mg/kg/day in 2 divided doses; may be increased up to 1.5 g/day in divided doses PO (Children <6 yr): 15–40 mg/kg/day; may be increased up to 1 g/day (usual dose is 20 mg/kg/day)	ADRs: anorexia, gastric upset
felbamate (Felbatol) Rx	Anticonvulsant	Alone or with other agents in the management of partial seizures unresponsive to other agents Adjunct in the management of Lennox-Gastaut syndrome	PO (Adults): 1200 mg/day in 3–4 divided doses initially; may be increased up to 3600 mg/day PO (Children 2–14 yr): 15 mg/kg/day in 3–4 divided doses; may be increased up to 45 mg/kg/day or 3600 mg	ADRs: acute hepatic damage, blood dyscrasias Dosage adjustments are necessary when used with other anticonvulsants
fentanyl transmucosal (Oralet) Rx C-II	Opioid analgesic	Anesthetic premedication Induction of conscious sedation	Transmucosal (Adults and Children): 5 mcg/kg (not >5 mcg/kg in adults; children <40 kg may require 10–15 mcg/kg; no dose >400 mcg) Transmucosal (Geriatric Patients): 2.5–5 mcg/kg	ADRs: euphoria, excessive sedation, hallucinations
fibrinolysin/ deoxyribonuclease (Elase) Rx	Enzyme	Debriding agent for wounds, burns, cervicitis, vaginitis	Topical (Adults): Apply ointment and dress wound, repeat 2–3 times daily or soak dressings in prepared solution, pack into wound, and allow to dry for 6–8 hr; remove and repeat 3–4 times daily for 2 days Intravaginal (Adults): 5 g as ointment nightly for 5 nights or 10 ml of solution followed by tampon insertion, removed next morning	ADRs: hypersensitivity reactions
floxuridine (FUDR) Rx	Antineoplastic (antimetabolite)	Treatment of hepatic and gastric carcinoma	Intra-arterial (Adults): 100–600 mcg/kg/day as a continuous infusion for 14–21 days, followed by a 2-wk rest	Bone marrow depression and gastrointestinal adverse reactions are common
fludarabine (Fludara) Rx	Antineoplastic (antimetabolite)	Treatment of B-cell chronic lymphocytic leukemia unresponsive to standard therapy Treatment of non-Hodgkin's lymphoma	IV (Adults): 25 mg/m²/day for 5 days; repeat cycle q 28 days	ADRs: bone marrow depression, diarrhea, nausea, neurotoxicity, pulmonary hypersensitivity, vomiting

gonadotropin, chorionic (A.P.P., Pregnyl, Profasi, Profasi HP) Rx	Hormone (gonadotropin)	Treatment of cryptorchidism, management of infertility	IM (Adults): *Male infertility*—500–4000 U 2–3 times weekly; *induction of ovulation*—5000–10,000 U 1 day after menotropins or urofollitropin or 5–9 days after clomiphene IM (Children): 500–4000 U 2–3 times weekly for up to 6 wk	ADRs: when used to induce ovulation, observe for ovarian hyperstimulation syndrome (abdominal/gastrointestinal symptoms, peripheral edema)
hepatitis B immune globulin (H-BIG, Hep-B-Gammagee, HyperHep) Rx	Immune globulin	Acute management of exposure to hepatitis B, provides passive immunity	IM (Adults): 0.06 ml/kg (3–5 ml) IM (Neonates): 0.5 ml	ADRs: allergic reactions, pain at IM site
histrelin (Supprelin) Rx	Hormone (gonadotropin-releasing)	Management of central precocious puberty	SC (Children): 10 mcg/kg/day	ADRs: GI complaints, hypersensitivity reactions, vasodilation
hyoscyamine (Cystospaz, Cystospaz-M, Levsinex) Rx	Anticholinergic/antispasmodic	Management of irritable bowel syndrome; GU tract spasm	PO (Adults): 0.125–0.5 mg 3–4 times daily or 0.375 mg twice daily as extended-release product	ADRs: constipation, blurred vision, dry eyes, dry mouth
imiglucerase (Cerezyme) Rx	Replacement enzyme	Treatment of symptomatic type 1 Gaucher's disease	IV (Adults and Children): 15–60 U/kg q 2 wk	ADRs: hypersensitivity reactions Some patients may require dosing several times weekly
interferon gamma-1b (Actimmune) Rx	Immune modulator	Treatment of chronic granulomatous disease	SC (Children BSA >0.5 m^2): 50 mcg/m^2 3 times weekly SC (Children BSA ≤ 0.5 m^2): 1.5 mcg/kg 3 times weekly	ADRs: flu-like symptoms, leukopenia Use deltoids and anterior thighs as injection sites
isoproterenol (Isuprel) Rx	Bronchodilator (adrenergic) Vasopressor	Management of reversible airway disease Management of shock, some arrhythmias	Inhalation (Adults and Children): 1–2 inhalations 4–6 times daily or up to 8 times daily as a nebulization treatment IV (Adults): *Bronchodilator*—1–20 mcg; *antiarrhythmic*—20–60 mcg initially, may follow with 10–200 mcg boluses or 5 mcg/min infusion; *vasopressor*—0.5–5 mcg/min infusion	ADRs: angina, hypertension, nervousness, paradoxical bronchospasm, restlessness, tachycardia, tremor
isotretinoin (Accutane) Rx	Antiacne agent	Management of cystic acne unresponsive to conventional therapy	PO (Adults): 0.5–1 mg/kg/day in 2 divided doses (up to 2 mg/kg) for 15–20 wk	ADRs: skin irritation, mental depression Pregnancy testing recommended prior to use in female patients Pregnancy category X
ketamine (Ketalar) Rx	General anesthetic	Anesthesia for short procedures, induction of anesthesia, supplemental anesthesia	IV (Adults and Children): *Induction*—1–2 mg/kg as a single dose or as an infusion at 0.5 mg/kg/min; *maintenance*—0.01–0.05 mg/kg by continuous infusion at 1–2 mg/min IM (Adults and Children): 5–10 mg/kg	ADRs: emergence (benzodiazepines may minimize)

Generic Name (Brand Name) {Canadian Brand Name} Rx/OTC Controlled Substance	Classification(s)	Use(s)	Route/Dosage	Notes
levomethadyl (Orlaam) Rx	Opioid agonist	Heroin addiction	PO (Adults): 60–90 mg 3 times weekly (maintenance)	May be dispensed only through approved programs
masoprocol (Actinex) Rx	Antineoplastic (topical)	Multiple actinic keratoses	Top (Adults): Apply 10% cream twice daily for 28 days	ADRs: contact dermatitis
menotropins (Pergonal) Rx	Hormone (gonadotropin)	Management of infertility	IM (Adults): *Induction of ovulation*—75 units FSH/75 units LH once daily for 7 days or more followed by chorionic gonadotropin (dosage may be increased up to 450 units FSH/450 units LH); *male infertility*—3 times weekly concurrently with and following pretreatment with chorionic gonadotropin for at least 4 mo (dosage may be increased up to 150 units FSH/150 units LH)	ADRs: ovarian hyperstimulation syndrome (abdominal/gastrointestinal symptoms, peripheral edema)
mercaptopurine (Purinethol) Rx	Antineoplastic (antimetabolite)	Combination treatment of leukemias	PO (Adults): 2.5 mg/kg (80–100 mg/m^2) day; may increase to 5 mg/kg after 4 wk (round dose to nearest 25 mg) PO (Children): 2.5 mg/kg (75 mg/m^2) day	ADRs: bone marrow depression, hepatotoxicity
methohexital (Brevital), {Brietal} Rx C-IV	Anesthetic (general) Barbiturate (ultra–short acting)	Induction of general anesthesia Sole anesthesia in short (<15 min), minimally painful procedures Supplement with other anesthetic agents To produce unconsciousness during balanced anesthesia	IV (Adults): *Induction*—1–2 mg/kg; *maintenance*—0.25–1 mg/kg as needed or continuous infusion of 0.2% solution, usually at rate of 3 ml/min (6 mg/min), with additional doses of 20–40 mg q 4–7 min as needed	ADRs: emergence delirium, hypotension, laryngospasm, seizures, shivering
methyclothiazide (Aquatensen, Enduron) Rx	Antihypertensive agent Diuretic (thiazide)	Management of hypertension and/or edema	PO (Adults): 2.5–10 mg/day	ADRs: hypokalemia, photosensitivity
minoxidil topical (Rogaine for Men, Rogaine Extra Strength for Men, Rogaine for Women) {Apo-Gain} {Gen-Minoxidil} {Minoxigaine} {Rogaine} OTC	Hair growth stimulant	Management of androgenetic alopecia (male pattern baldness)	Topical (Adults): Apply 2 or 5% solution twice daily	ADRs: local irritation; if absorption occurs, fluid retention and hypotension may result Extra-strength product may allow more and faster hair regrowth At least 4 mo of regular therapy is required for benefit

mitotane (Lysodren, o, p′-DDD) Rx	Antineoplastic	Treatment of carcinoma of the adrenal cortex *Unlabeled*—treatment of Cushing's syndrome due to pituitary disorders	PO (Adults): *Adrenocortical carcinoma*—8–10 g/day in 3–4 divided doses; may be increased as tolerated (range 2–16 g/day); *Cushing's syndrome*—3–6 g/day in 3–4 divided doses initially, decreased to maintenance dose of 500 mg twice weekly to 2 g/day.	ADRs: GI complaints, lethargy, rash, somnolence
norepinephrine (Levarterenol, Levophed) Rx	Vasopressor	Management of shock	IV (Adults): 0.5–1 mcg/min initially (range 2–12 mcg/min, depending on blood pressure) IV (Children): 0.1 mcg/kg/min (up to 1 mcg/kg/min depending on blood pressure)	ADRs: angina, hypertension, tachycardia Fluid replacement should be initiated prior to norepinephrine
orphenadrine (Norflex), {Disipal} Rx	Skeletal muscle relaxant (centrally acting)	Acute painful musculoskeletal conditions	PO (Adults): 50 mg 3 times daily or 100 mg twice daily as extended-release product	ADRs: blurred vision, constipation, dry eyes, dry mouth, tachycardia Elderly patients may be more sensitive to the effects of orphenadrine
papaverine (Cerespan, Genabid, Pavabid, Pavabid HP, Pavacot, Pavagen, Pavarine, Pavased, Pavatine, Pavatym, Paverolan) Rx	Vasodilator	Cerebral and peripheral ischemia	PO (Adults): 100–300 mg 3–5 times daily or 150 mg q 8–12 hr as extended-release product or 300 mg q 12 hr as extended-release product	FDA notes that papaverine has not been shown to be effective for cerebral and peripheral ischemia
paromomycin (Humatin) Rx	Anti-infective	Amebiasis; hepatic coma; cryptosporidiosis in HIV-infected patients	PO (Adults): *Amebiasis*—25–35 mg/kg/day in 3 divided doses; *hepatic coma*—4 g/day in 2–4 divided doses; *cryptosporidiosis in HIV-infected patients*—1.5–3 g/day in divided doses	Minimal systemic absorption follows oral administration
pentostatin (Nipent) Rx	Antineoplastic (enzyme inhibitor)	Hairy-cell leukemia	IV (Adults): 4 mg/m^2 every other week	ADRs: CNS, hepatic, pulmonary, and renal toxicity; myelosuppression; GI complaints; headache
phenoxybenzamine (Dibenzyline) Rx	Antihypertensive agent (alpha-adrenergic blocking agent)	Management of adrenergic excess (pheochromocytoma)	PO (Adults): 10 mg twice daily initially; may be increased (range 20–40 mg 2–3 times daily) PO (Children): 0.2 mg/kg /day; may be increased (range 0.4–1.2 mg/kg/day in 3–4 divided doses)	ADRs: orthostatic hypotension
phentermine (Adipex-P, Fastin, Obe-Nix, OBY-CAP, Phentercot, Phentride, T-Diet, Teramine, Zantryl) Rx C-IV	Appetite suppressant	Short-term management of exogenous obesity in conjunction with a program that includes caloric restriction, exercise, and behavior modification	PO (Adults): 15–37.5 mg once daily	ADRs: CNS stimulation, hypertension, insomnia, tachycardia Avoid use in patients with hypertension, diabetes

Generic Name (Brand Name) {Canadian Brand Name} Rx/OTC Controlled Substance	Classification(s)	Use(s)	Route/Dosage	Notes
physostigmine (Antilirium) Rx	Cholinergic (anticholinesterase agent)	Reversal of CNS effects due to overdose of drugs capable of causing the anticholinergic syndrome, including belladonna or other plant alkaloids, phenothiazines, tricyclic antidepressants, or antihistamines	IM, IV (Adults): *Anticholinergic toxicity*—2 mg initially, may be repeated as symptoms recur. *Postanesthesia*—0.5–1 mg; may be repeated q 10–30 min IM, IV (Children): 20 mcg/kg; may repeat every 5–10 min as needed (up to 2-mg total dose)	ADRs: bradycardia, bronchospasm, GI complaints, restlessness, seizures
pimozide (Orap) Rx	Antipsychotic agent	Treatment of Gilles de la Tourette's syndrome	PO (Adults): 1–2 mg/day in divided doses initially, titrated as needed up to 300 mcg/kg/day or 20 mg/day	ADRs: arrhythmias, blurred vision, dry eyes, dry mouth, extrapyramidal reactions, tardive dyskinesia Increased risk of arrhythmias with azithromycin, clarithromycin, dirithromycin, erythromycin, azole antifungals, or cardioactive agents
podofilox (Condylox) Rx	Antimitotic agent	Treatment of anogenital warts	Topical (Adults): Apply 0.5% gel or solution twice daily for 3 days, then off for 4 days; may continue for up to 4 cycles	ADRs: local irritation
porfimer (Photofrin) Rx	Antineoplastic (photosensitize)	Palliative treatment of esophageal cancer	IV (Adults): 2 mg/kg followed 40–50 hr later by laser light therapy; 2nd session of laser therapy may be given 96–120 hr after porfimer	ADRs: photosensitivity Avoid concurrent use of photosensitizing agents
pralidoxime (Protopam) Rx	Antidote (anticholinesterase poisoning)	Early treatment of organophosphate anticholinesterase insecticide poisoning Management of overdose of anticholinesterase agents (neostigmine, pyridostigmine)	IV (Adults): 1–2 g; additional doses may be given as needed IV (Children): 20–40 mg/kg	ADRs: blurred vision, dizziness, hypertension, tachycardia Atropine should be given after ventilation is established
primaquine Rx	Antimalarial	Treatment of malaria *Unlabeled*—combination treatment of *Pneumocystis carinii* pneumonia (PCP)	PO (Adults): *Malaria*—26.3 mg/day for 14 days; *PCP*—26.3–52.6 mg/day for 21 days	ADRs: hemolytic anemia Used only for PCP when TMP/SMX and pentamidine cannot be used
progesterone IM (Gestrol), {PMS-Progesterone} Rx	Hormone (progestin)	Amenorrhea, dysfunctional uterine bleeding	IM (Adults): *Amenorrhea*—5–10 mg/day for 6–10 days or 100–150-mg single dose; *dysfunctional uterine bleeding*—5–10 mg/day for 6 days	ADRs: abdominal pain, edema, mood changes, nervousness When used for amenorrhea, withdrawal bleeding should start 48–72 hr after last injection; for dysfunctional bleeding, bleeding should stop within 6 days

progesterone gel 8% (Crinone) Rx	Hormone (progestin)	Progesterone supplementation during Assisted Reproductive Technology (ART) treatment	Vag (Adults): 90 mg 1–2 times daily for up to 12 wk	ADRs: breast enlargement, drowsiness, GI complaints, headache
progesterone intrauterine system (Progestasert) Rx	Hormone (progestin)	Intrauterine contraceptive	Intrauterine (Adults): 38 mg once yearly	ADRs: bleeding, cramps
protirelin (Relefact TRH) Rx	Diagnostic aid	Tests thyroid and pituitary function	IV (Adults): 0.5 mg IV (Children 6–16 yr): 7 mcg (0.007 mg)/kg (up to 0.5 mg)	ADRs: flushing, headache, nausea, unpleasant taste sensation Discontinue thyroid supplements before testing.
pyrazinamide {PMS Pyrazinamide}, {Tebrazid} Rx	Antitubercular	Part of combination treatment for tuberculosis *Unlabeled use:* initial management of *Mycobacterium avium* complex (MAC) infection	PO (Adults): *Tuberculosis*—15–30 mg/kg/day	ADRs: arthralgia Used only for MAC until cultures are back; never use for prevention
quazepam (Doral) Rx C-IV	Sedative/hypnotic (benzodiazepine)	Hypnotic (short-term use)	PO (Adults): 7.5–15 mg at bedtime	ADRs: excessive sedation, hangover Due to accumulation, may give larger dose for 1–2 nights, then decrease
riluzole (Rilutek) Rx	Antiglutamate	Treatment of amyotrophic lateral sclerosis	PO (Adults): 50 mg q 12 hr	ADRs: GI complaints, worsening of symptoms
rimantadine (Flumadine) Rx	Antiviral	Prevention/treatment of influenza viral A infection	PO (Adults and Children >10 yr): 100 mg twice daily (once daily in geriatric patients) PO (Children <10 yr): 5 mg/kg/day (not >150 mg/day)	ADRs: GI complaints, seizures
ritodrine (Yutopar) Rx	Tocolytic	Premature labor	IV (Adults): 50–100 mcg/min; increase by 50 mcg/min to maintenance of 150–350 mcg/min PO (Adults): 10 mg q 2 hr for 24 hr, then 10–20 mg q 4–6 hr	ADRs: angina, arrhythmias, pulmonary edema, tachycardia Continue IV for 12–24 hr after contractions cease; begin PO 30 min before IV is stopped
saliva substitutes (Entertainers' Secret, MouthKote, Optimoist, Salivart, Salix) OTC	Electrolyte solution/thickening agent	Management of dry mouth or throat, which may occur as a consequence of medications (tricyclic antidepressants, antihistamines, anticholinergics), radiation therapy, other illnesses, emotional factors	PO (Adults): Spray/apply to oral mucosa as needed	ADRs: excess absorption of electrolytes

INFREQUENTLY USED DRUGS (CONTINUED)

Generic Name (Brand Name) {Canadian Brand Name} Rx/OTC Controlled Substance	Classification(s)	Use(s)	Route/Dosage	Notes
silver sulfadiazine (Flint SSD, Sildimac, Silvadene, Thermazene), {Flamazine} Rx	Anti-infective (topical)	Prevention/treatment of infections in burns or skin	Topical (Adults and Children >1 mo): Apply 1% cream 1–2 times daily in layer 1.5 mm thick	ADRs: crystalluria, leukopenia, local reactions
sodium nitrite Rx	Antidote (cyanide)	Cyanide poisoning	IV (Adults): 300 mg (4–6 mg/kg); may repeat with 50% of initial dose in 2 hr IV (Children): 180–240 mg/m² (4–6 mg/kg, not to exceed 300 mg); may repeat with 50% of initial dose in 2 hr	Administer amyl nitrite (see amyl nitrite entry) by inhalation while sodium nitrite is prepared. Follow sodium nitrite with sodium thiosulfate (see sodium thiosulfate entry)
sodium thiosulfate Rx	Antidote (cyanide)	Cyanide poisoning	IV (Adults and Children): 12.5 g (50 ml of 25% solution over 10 min)	Sodium nitrite is administered first (see previous entry)
streptozocin (Zanosar) Rx	Antineoplastic (antitumor antibiotic)	Management of metastatic islet cell carcinoma of the pancreas	IV (Adults): 500 mg/m²/day for 5 days q 4–6 wk or 1 g/m²/wk for 2 wk; then may be increased up to 1.5 g/m² weekly for 4–6 doses	ADRs: bone marrow depression, hepatotoxicity, hypoglycemia, nephrotoxicity, phlebitis at IV site
strontium-89 chloride (Metastron) Rx	Radiopharmaceutical	Management of bone pain in patients with painful skeletal metastases	IV (Adults): 148 megabecquerels (4 millicuries) or 1.5–2.2 megabecquerels/kg (40–60 microcuries/kg), not to be repeated any sooner than 90 days	ADRs: bone marrow depression, transient increase in bone pain
teniposide (VM-26, Vumon) Rx	Antineoplastic (podophyllotoxin derivative)	Induction therapy for refractory acute lymphoblastic leukemia in children (in combination with other agents)	Several regimens have been used; these are examples: IV (Children): Teniposide 165 mg/m² in combination with cytarabine 300 mg/m² twice weekly for 8–9 doses. Another regimen uses teniposide 250 mg/m² in combination with vincristine 1.5 mg/m² weekly for 4–8 wk with prednisone 40 mg/m²/day for 28 days	ADRs: allergic reactions, bone marrow depression, GI complaints
thioguanine {Lanvis} Rx	Antineoplastic (antimetabolite)	Used to induce remission in acute myelogenous leukemia (with other agents) Used in the treatment of acute lymphocytic leukemia and chronic myelogenous leukemia (with other agents)	Many protocols are used PO (Adults and Children): *Induction*—2 mg/kg (75–100 mg/m²) per day, rounded off to nearest 20 mg given as single dose; after 4 wk may increase to 3 mg/kg; *maintenance*—2–3 mg/kg (100 mg/m²) per day	ADRs: bone marrow depression, hepatotoxicity

thiopental (Pentothal) Rx C-III	Anesthetic (barbiturate)	Induction and maintenance of general anesthesia	IV (Adults): 50–100 mg (3–5 mg/kg), followed by 50–100 mg as needed	ADRs: excessive sedation Test dose may be given to determine unusual sensitivity
thiotepa (Thioplex) Rx	Antineoplastic (alkylating agent)	Management or prophylaxis of superficial tumors of the bladder following local resection (local instillation) Palliative treatment for breast and ovarian cancer (IV) Prevention of recurrent malignant effusions in pleura, pericardium, or peritoneum (intracavitary)	Intravesical (Adults): 30–60 mg retained in the bladder for 2 hr weekly for 4 wk, then monthly IV (Adults): 300–400 mcg/kg q 1–4 wk or 200 mcg/kg daily for 4–5 days q 2–4 wk Intracavitary (Adults): 600–800 mcg/kg q 1–4 wk (range 70–800 mcg/kg)	ADRs: bone marrow depression, local irritation
thiothixene (Navane) Rx	Antipsychotic agent	Management of psychoses	PO (Adults): 2 mg 3 times daily initially, may be increased up to 60 mg/day IM (Adults): 4 mg 2–4 times daily, may be increased up to 30 mg/day	ADRs: blurred vision, constipation, dry mouth, extrapyramidal reactions, hypotension, tardive dyskinesia are more common
tolazamide (Tolamide, Tolinase) Rx	Oral hypoglycemic agent	Management of type II (non–insulin-dependent) diabetes mellitus	PO (Adults): 100–250 mg/day (range 100–1000 mg/day; doses >500 mg/day should be given as divided doses)	ADRs: allergic reactions, hypoglycemia, photosensitivity
tolbutamide (Orinase, Tol-Tab) {Apo-Tolbutamide}, {Mobenol}, {Novobutamide} Rx	Oral hypoglycemic agent	Management of type II (non–insulin-dependent) diabetes mellitus	PO (Adults): 500–2000 mg/day in divided doses (range 250–3000 mg/day)	ADRs: allergic reactions, hypoglycemia, photosensitivity
tranexamic acid (Cyklokapron) Rx	Hemostatic agent (plasminogen activator) Antifibrinolytic agent	Prevention of hemorrhage following dental surgery in hemophiliacs	PO (Adults and Children): 25 mg/kg 3–4 times daily beginning the day before surgery, then 3–4 times daily for 2–8 days postop IV (Adults and Children): 10 mg/kg just prior to surgery, then 3–4 times daily for 2–8 days	ADRs: dizziness, GI complaints, hypotension, thromboembolism
tretinoin (topical) (Avita, Renova, Retin-A, Retin-A Micro, vitamin A acid, Vitinoin), {Stieva-A} Rx	Antiacne agent (retinoid)	Management of acne vulgaris Palliation of fine wrinkles, mottled hyperpigmentation, and tactile roughness in patients who cannot achieve this through good skin care and sun avoidance	Topical (Adults and Adolescents): Apply once daily at bedtime	ADRs: local irritation

Generic Name (Brand Name) {Canadian Brand Name} Rx/OTC Controlled Substance	Classification(s)	Use(s)	Route/Dosage	Notes
tretinoin (oral) (Vesanoid) Rx	Antineoplastic (retinoid)	Induction of remission in acute promyelocytic leukemia in patients who have not responded to or cannot tolerate anthracyclines	PO (Adults): 45 $mg/m^2/day$ in 2 divided doses; treatment should be continued for 30 days after a complete remission has been achieved or for a total of 90 days, whichever is first	ADRs: bone marrow depression, CNS reactions, edema, GI complaints, hypertension
trichlormethiazide (Metahydrin, Naqua) Rx	Antihypertensive agent Diuretic (thiazide)	Management of hypertension and/or edema	PO (Adults): 1–4 mg/day	ADRs: hypokalemia, photosensitivity
ursodiol, ursodeoxycholic acid (Actigall, URSO) Rx	Anticholelithic	Gallstone dissolution Treatment of primary biliary cirrhosis	PO: 8–10 mg/kg/day in 1–3 doses	ADRs: diarrhea Avoid concurrent use with bile acid sequestrants, aluminum-containing antacids, estrogens, oral contraceptives, clofibrate
vasopressin (Pitressin), {Pressyn} Rx	Hormone (antidiuretic)	Treatment of central diabetes insipidus due to deficient antidiuretic hormone Treatment of severe, refractory GI bleeding (IA, IV; unlabeled)	IM, SC (Adults): 5–10 units 2–3 times daily IM, SC (Children): 2.5–10 units 3–4 times daily IA, IV (Adults): *GI bleeding*—0.2–0.4 units/hr (unlabeled)	ADRs: abdominal cramps, angina, myocardial infarction
vidarabine (Vira-A) Rx	Ophthalmic antiviral	Treatment of acute keratoconjunctivitis, recurrent epithelial keratitis, or superficial keratitis due to herpes simplex virus	Ophth (Adults): 0.5 in. into lower conjunctival sac 5 times daily (q 3 hr) for 7–21 days; give less frequently for 7 more days following re-epithelialization	ADRs: local irritation If improvement does not occur in 7 days or re-epithelialization after 21 days, consider alternative agents

*ADRs = adverse reactions.

Sample FDA Medication Error and Adverse Reaction Reporting Forms

MEDWATCH

THE FDA MEDICAL PRODUCTS REPORTING PROGRAM F. A. DAVIS

A. Patient information

1. Patient identifier	2. Age at time of event:	3. Sex	4. Weight
In confidence	or ______ Date of birth:	☐ female ☐ male	____ lbs or ____ kgs

B. Adverse event or product problem

1. ☐ **Adverse event** and/or ☐ **Product problem** (e.g., defects/malfunctions)

2. **Outcomes attributed to adverse event** (check all that apply)

- ☐ death ______ (mo/day/yr)
- ☐ life-threatening
- ☐ hospitalization – initial or prolonged
- ☐ disability
- ☐ congenital anomaly
- ☐ required intervention to prevent permanent impairment/damage
- ☐ other: ______

3. Date of event (mo/day/yr)	4. Date of this report (mo/day/yr)

5. **Describe event or problem**

SAMPLE

6. **Relevant tests/laboratory data,** including dates

7. **Other relevant history, including preexisting medical conditions** (e.g., allergies, race, pregnancy, smoking and alcohol use, hepatic/renal dysfunction, etc.)

PLEASE TYPE OR USE BLACK INK

FDA **Mail to:** MEDWATCH 5600 Fishers Lane Rockville, MD 20852-9787 *or* **FAX to:** 1-800-FDA-0178

FDA Form 3500 (6/93)

MEDWATCH

THE FDA MEDICAL PRODUCTS REPORTING PROGRAM **F. A. DAVIS**

C. Suspect medication(s)

1. **Name** (give labeled strength & mfr/labeler, if known)
#1 ______
#2 ______

2. **Dose, frequency & route used**
#1 ______
#2 ______

3. **Therapy dates** (if unknown, give duration) from/to (or best estimate)
#1 ______
#2 ______

4. **Diagnosis for use** (indication)
#1 ______
#2 ______

5. **Event abated after use stopped or dose reduced**
#1 ☐ yes ☐ no ☐ doesn't apply
#2 ☐ yes ☐ no ☐ doesn't apply

6. **Lot #** (if known)
#1 ______
#2 ______

7. **Exp. date** (if known)
#1 ______
#2 ______

8. **Event reappeared after reintroduction**
#1 ☐ yes ☐ no ☐ doesn't apply
#2 ☐ yes ☐ no ☐ doesn't apply

9. **NDC #** (for product problems only)
– –

10. **Concomitant medical products** and therapy dates (exclude treatment of event)

D. Suspect medical device

1. **Brand name**

2. **Type of device**

3. **Manufacturer name & address**

4. **Operator of device**
☐ health professional
☐ lay user/patient
☐ other: ______

5. **Expiration date** (mo/day/yr)

6.
model # ______
catalog # ______
serial # ______
lot # ______
other #

7. **If implanted, give date** (mo/day/yr)

8. **If explanted, give date** (mo/day/yr)

9. **Device available for evaluation?** (Do not send to FDA)
☐ yes ☐ no ☐ returned to manufacturer on ______ (mo/day/yr)

10. **Concomitant medical products** and therapy dates (exclude treatment of event)

E. Reporter (see confidentiality section on back)

1. **Name, address & phone #**

2. **Health professional?**
☐ yes ☐ no

3. **Occupation**

4. **Also reported to**
☐ manufacturer
☐ user facility
☐ distributor

5. **If you do NOT want your identity disclosed to the manufacturer, place an " X " in this box.** ☐

FDA

Mail to: MEDWATCH
5600 Fishers Lane
Rockville, MD 20852-9787

or **FAX to:**
1-800-FDA-0178

FDA Form 3500 (6/93)

USP MEDICATION ERRORS REPORTING PROGRAM

Presented in cooperation with the Institute for Safe Medication Practices

The USP Practitioners' Reporting Network℠ is an FDA MEDWATCH partner

❑ ACTUAL ERROR ❑ POTENTIAL ERROR

Please describe the error. Include sequence of events, personnel involved, and work environment (e.g., code situation, change of shift, short staffing, no 24-hr. pharmacy, floor stock). If more space is needed, please attach separate page.

Was the medication administered to or used by the patient? ❑ No ❑ Yes

Date and time of event: ______

What type of staff or health care practitioner made the initial error? ______

Describe outcome (e.g., death, type of injury, adverse reaction). ______

If the medication did not reach the patient, describe the intervention.

Who discovered the error? ______

When and how was error discovered? ______

Where did the error occur (e.g., hospital, outpatient or retail pharmacy, nursing home, patient's home)? ______

Was another practitioner involved in the error ? ❑ No ❑ Yes

If yes, what type of practitioner? ______

Was patient counseling provided? ❑ No ❑ Yes

If yes, before or after error was discovered? ______

If a product was involved, please complete the following:

	Product #1	Product #2
Brand name of product involved		
Generic name		
Manufacturer		
Labeler (if different from mfr.)		
Dosage form		
Strength/concentration		
Type and size of container		
NDC number		

If available, please provide relevant patient information (age, gender, diagnosis, etc.). Patient identification not required.

Reports are most useful when relevant materials such as product label, copy of prescription/order, etc. can be reviewed. Can these materials be provided?

❑ No ❑ Yes If yes, please specify. ______________________

Suggest any recommendations you have to prevent recurrence of this error or describe policies or procedures you have instituted to prevent future similar errors.

A copy of this report is routinely sent to the Institute for Safe Medication Practices (ISMP), to the manufacturer/labeler, and to the Food and Drug Administration (FDA).

USP may release my identity to: (check boxes that apply)

❑ ISMP ❑ The manufacturer and/or labeler as listed above ❑ FDA

❑ Other persons requesting a copy of this report ❑ Anonymous to all

Your name and title | Telephone number (include area code)

Your facility name, address, and ZIP

Signature | Date

Date Received by USP:	File Access Number:

DAVIS3/96

Return to the attention of:
Diane D. Cousins, R.Ph.
USP PRN
12601 Twinbrook Parkway
Rockville, MD 20852-1790

Call Toll Free: **800-23-ERROR** (800-233-7767) or FAX 301-816-8532

Electronic reporting forms are available. Please call for additional information and/or your free diskette.

Additional forms can be found in the USP DI Vol. I and Vol. III and in all monthly Updates.

C212-G

APPENDIX S

NANDA Nursing Diagnoses from the 12th Conference

ACTIVITY/REST

Activity intolerance
Activity intolerance, risk for
Disuse syndrome, risk for
Diversional activity deficit
Fatigue
Sleep pattern disturbance

CIRCULATION

Adaptive capacity: intracranial, decreased
Cardiac output, decreased
Dysreflexia
Tissue perfusion, altered (specify): cerebral, cardiopulmonary, renal, gastrointestinal, peripheral

EGO INTEGRITY

Adjustment, impaired
Anxiety (specify level)
Body image disturbance
Coping, defensive
Coping, ineffective individual
Decisional conflict (specify)
Denial, ineffective
Energy field disturbance
Fear
Grieving, anticipatory
Grieving, dysfunctional
Hopelessness
Personal identity disturbance
Post-trauma response
Powerlessness
Rape-trauma syndrome
Rape-trauma syndrome: compound reaction
Rape-trauma syndrome: silent reaction
Self-esteem, chronic low
Self-esteem disturbance
Self-esteem, situational low
Spiritual distress
Spiritual well-being, potential for enhanced

ELIMINATION

Bowel incontinence
Constipation
Constipation, colonic
Constipation, perceived
Diarrhea
Incontinence, functional
Incontinence, reflex
Incontinence, stress
Incontinence, total
Incontinence, urge
Urinary elimination, altered
Urinary retention (acute/chronic)

FOOD/FLUID

Breastfeeding, effective
Breastfeeding, ineffective
Breastfeeding, interrupted
Fluid volume deficit (active loss)
Fluid volume deficit (regulatory failure)
Fluid volume deficit, risk for
Fluid volume excess
Infant feeding pattern, ineffective
Nutrition, altered: less than body requirements
Nutrition, altered: more than body requirements
Nutrition, altered: risk for more than body requirements
Oral mucous membrane, altered
Swallowing, impaired

HYGIENE

Self-care deficit (specify): feeding, bathing/hygiene, dressing/grooming, toileting

NEUROSENSORY

Confusion, acute
Confusion, chronic
Infant behavior, disorganized
Infant behavior, disorganized, risk for

Infant behavior, organized, potential for enhanced
Memory, impaired
Peripheral neurovascular dysfunction, risk for
Sensory/perceptual alterations (specify): visual, auditory, kinesthetic, gustatory, tactile, olfactory
Thought processes, altered
Unilateral neglect

PAIN/COMFORT

Pain (acute)
Pain, chronic

RESPIRATION

Airway clearance, ineffective
Aspiration, risk for
Breathing pattern, ineffective
Gas exchange, impaired
Spontaneous ventilation: inability to sustain
Ventilatory weaning response, dysfunctional (DVWR)

SAFETY

Body temperature, altered, risk for
Environmental interpretation syndrome, impaired
Health maintenance, altered
Home maintenance management, impaired
Hyperthermia
Hypothermia
Infection, risk for
Injury, risk for
Perioperative positioning injury, risk for
Physical mobility, impaired
Poisoning, risk for
Protection, altered
Self-mutilation, risk for
Skin integrity, impaired
Skin integrity, impaired, risk for
Suffocation, risk for
Thermoregulation, ineffective
Tissue integrity, impaired
Trauma, risk for
Violence, risk for, directed at self/others

SEXUALITY (COMPONENT OF EGO INTEGRITY AND SOCIAL INTERACTION)

Sexual dysfunction
Sexuality patterns, altered

SOCIAL INTERACTION

Caregiver role strain
Caregiver role strain, risk for
Communication, impaired verbal
Community coping, ineffective
Community coping, potential for enhanced
Family coping, ineffective, compromised
Family coping, ineffective, disabling
Family coping, potential for growth
Family processes, altered
Family process, altered: alcoholism
Loneliness, risk for
Parent/infant/child attachment, altered, risk for
Parental role conflict
Parenting, altered
Parenting, altered, risk for
Relocation stress syndrome
Role performance, altered
Social interaction, impaired
Social isolation

TEACHING/LEARNING

Growth and development, altered
Health-seeking behaviors (specify)
Knowledge deficit (learning need) (specify)
Noncompliance (compliance, altered) (specify)
Therapeutic regimen: community, ineffective management
Therapeutic regimen: families, ineffective management
Therapeutic regimen: individual, effective management
Therapeutic regimen (individuals), ineffective management

BIBLIOGRAPHY

Acute Pain Management Guideline Panel: Acute Pain Management in Adults: Operative Procedures. Quick Reference Guide for Clinicians. Agency for Health Care Policy and Research, Public Health Service, US Department of Health and Human Services, Rockville, MD, 1992.

American Hospital Formulary Service: Drug Information 97. American Society of Hospital Pharmacists, Bethesda, 1997.

American Pain Society: Principles of Analgesic Use in the Treatment of Acute Pain and Cancer Pain, ed 3. American Pain Society, Skokie, IL, 1992.

Briggs, GG, Freeman, RK, and Yaffee, SJ: Drugs in Pregnancy and Lactation: A Reference Guide to Fetal and Neonatal Risks, ed 4. Williams & Wilkins, Baltimore, 1994.

Cancer Chemotherapy Guidelines. Recommendations for the Management of Vesicant Extravasation, Hypersensitivity, and Anaphylaxis. Oncology Nursing Society, Pittsburgh, PA, 1996.

Expert Panel Report 2: Guidelines for the Diagnosis and Management of Asthma. National Asthma Education and Prevention Program, National Heart, Lung, and Blood Institute, 1997.

Facts and Comparisons. JB Lippincott, Philadelphia, 1998.

Koda-Kimble, MA, Young, LY, Kradjian, WA, and Guglielmo, BJ: Handbook of Applied Therapeutics, ed 2. Applied Therapeutics, Vancouver, WA, 1992.

Koda-Kimble, MA, and Young, LY (eds): Applied Therapeutics: The Clinical Use of Drugs, ed 5. Applied Therapeutics, Vancouver, WA, 1992.

Lutz, CA, and Przytulski, KR: Nutrition and Diet Therapy, ed 2. FA Davis, Philadelphia, 1997.

McCaffery, M, and Pasero, C: Pain: Clinical Manual. St Louis, Mosby-Yearbook, 1998.

Phelps, SJ, and Cochran, EB: Guidelines for Administration of Intravenous Medications to Pediatric Patients, ed 4. American Society of Hospital Pharmacists, Bethesda, 1993.

Physicians' Desk Reference (PDR). Medical Economics Company, Oradell, NJ, 1998.

Semla, TP, Beizer, J, and Higbee, MD: Geriatric Dosage Handbook. LexiComp, Cleveland, 1993.

Trissel, LA: Supplement to Handbook on Injectable Drugs, ed 9. American Society of Hospital Pharmacists, Bethesda, 1997.

Trissel, LA: Handbook on Injectable Drugs, ed 9. American Society of Hospital Pharmacists, Bethesda, 1996.

USP Dispensing Information (USP-DI): Drug Information for the Health Care Professional, Volume I. United States Pharmacopeial Convention, Rockville, MD, 1998.

USP Dispensing Information (USP-DI): Advice for the Patient, Volume II, ed 17. United States Pharmacopeial Convention, Rockville, MD, 1998.

Watson, J, and Jaffe, MS: Nurse's Manual of Laboratory and Diagnostic Tests, ed 2. FA Davis, Philadelphia, 1995.

COMPREHENSIVE INDEX*

generic / Trade / *classification*

*Entries for **generic** names appear in **boldface type,** trade names appear in regular type, **CLASSIFICATIONS** appear in **BOLDFACE SMALL CAPS,** and Combination Drugs appear in *italics.* A **"C"** and a **boldface** page number following a generic name identify the page in the "Classification" section on which that drug is listed.

*Entries for **generic** names appear in **boldface type,** trade names appear in regular type, **CLASSIFICATIONS** appear in **BOLDFACE SMALL CAPS,** and Combination Drugs appear in *italics.* A **"C"** and a **boldface** page number following a generic name identify the page in the "Classification" section on which that drug is listed.

*Entries for **generic** names appear in **boldface type,** trade names appear in regular type, **CLASSIFICATIONS** appear in **BOLDFACE SMALL CAPS,** and Combination Drugs appear in *italics.* A **"C"** and a **boldface** page number following a generic name identify the page in the "Classification" section on which that drug is listed.

*Entries for **generic** names appear in **boldface type,** trade names appear in regular type, **CLASSIFICATIONS** appear in **BOLDFACE SMALL CAPS,** and Combination Drugs appear in *italics.* A **"C"** and a **boldface** page number following a generic name identify the page in the "Classification" section on which that drug is listed.

*Entries for **generic** names appear in **boldface type,** trade names appear in regular type, **CLASSIFICATIONS** appear in **BOLDFACE SMALL CAPS,** and Combination Drugs appear in *italics.* A **"C"** and a **boldface** page number following a generic name identify the page in the "Classification" section on which that drug is listed.

*Entries for **generic** names appear in **boldface type,** trade names appear in regular type, **CLASSIFICATIONS** appear in **BOLDFACE SMALL CAPS,** and Combination Drugs appear in *italics.* A **"C"** and a **boldface** page number following a generic name identify the page in the "Classification" section on which that drug is listed.

*Entries for **generic** names appear in **boldface type**, trade names appear in regular type, **CLASSIFICATIONS** appear in **BOLDFACE SMALL CAPS**, and Combination Drugs appear in *italics*. A **"C"** and a **boldface** page number following a generic name identify the page in the "Classification" section on which that drug is listed.

C

*Entries for **generic** names appear in **boldface type**, trade names appear in regular type, **CLASSIFICATIONS** appear in **BOLDFACE SMALL CAPS**, and Combination Drugs appear in *italics.* A **"C"** and a **boldface** page number following a generic name identify the page in the "Classification" section on which that drug is listed.

*Entries for **generic** names appear in **boldface type,** trade names appear in regular type, **CLASSIFICATIONS** appear in **BOLDFACE SMALL CAPS,** and Combination Drugs appear in *italics.* A **"C"** and a **boldface** page number following a generic name identify the page in the "Classification" section on which that drug is listed.

*Entries for **generic** names appear in **boldface type,** trade names appear in regular type, **CLASSIFICATIONS** appear in **BOLDFACE SMALL CAPS,** and Combination Drugs appear in *italics.* A **"C"** and a **boldface** page number following a generic name identify the page in the "Classification" section on which that drug is listed.

*Entries for **generic** names appear in **boldface type,** trade names appear in regular type, **CLASSIFICATIONS** appear in **BOLDFACE SMALL CAPS,** and Combination Drugs appear in *italics.* A **"C"** and a **boldface** page number following a generic name identify the page in the "Classification" section on which that drug is listed.

*Entries for **generic** names appear in **boldface type,** trade names appear in regular type, **CLASSIFICATIONS** appear in **BOLDFACE SMALL CAPS,** and Combination Drugs appear in *italics.* A **"C"** and a **boldface** page number following a generic name identify the page in the "Classification" section on which that drug is listed.

*Entries for **generic** names appear in **boldface type**, trade names appear in regular type, **CLASSIFICATIONS** appear in **BOLDFACE SMALL CAPS**, and Combination Drugs appear in *italics*. A **"C"** and a **boldface** page number following a generic name identify the page in the "Classification" section on which that drug is listed.

*Entries for **generic** names appear in **boldface type**, trade names appear in regular type, **CLASSIFICATIONS** appear in **BOLDFACE SMALL CAPS**, and Combination Drugs appear in *italics*. A **"C"** and a **boldface** page number following a generic name identify the page in the "Classification" section on which that drug is listed.

*Entries for **generic** names appear in **boldface type**, trade names appear in regular type, **CLASSIFICATIONS** appear in **BOLDFACE SMALL CAPS**, and Combination Drugs appear in *italics*. A **"C"** and a **boldface** page number following a generic name identify the page in the "Classification" section on which that drug is listed.

E

*Entries for **generic** names appear in **boldface type,** trade names appear in regular type, **CLASSIFICATIONS** appear in **BOLDFACE SMALL CAPS,** and Combination Drugs appear in *italics.* A **"C"** and a **boldface** page number following a generic name identify the page in the "Classification" section on which that drug is listed.

*Entries for **generic** names appear in **boldface type**, trade names appear in regular type, **CLASSIFICATIONS** appear in **BOLDFACE SMALL CAPS**, and Combination Drugs appear in *italics*. A **"C"** and a **boldface** page number following a generic name identify the page in the "Classification" section on which that drug is listed.

F

*Entries for **generic** names appear in **boldface type,** trade names appear in regular type, **CLASSIFICATIONS** appear in **BOLDFACE SMALL CAPS,** and Combination Drugs appear in *italics.* A **"C"** and a **boldface** page number following a generic name identify the page in the "Classification" section on which that drug is listed.

*Entries for **generic** names appear in **boldface type**, trade names appear in regular type, **CLASSIFICATIONS** appear in **BOLDFACE SMALL CAPS**, and Combination Drugs appear in *italics*. A **"C"** and a **boldface** page number following a generic name identify the page in the "Classification" section on which that drug is listed.

G

*Entries for **generic** names appear in **boldface type**, trade names appear in regular type, **CLASSIFICATIONS** appear in **BOLDFACE SMALL CAPS**, and Combination Drugs appear in *italics*. A **"C"** and a **boldface** page number following a generic name identify the page in the "Classification" section on which that drug is listed.

*Entries for **generic** names appear in **boldface type**, trade names appear in regular type, **CLASSIFICATIONS** appear in **BOLDFACE SMALL CAPS**, and Combination Drugs appear in *italics*. A **"C"** and a **boldface** page number following a generic name identify the page in the "Classification" section on which that drug is listed.

*Entries for **generic** names appear in **boldface type**, trade names appear in regular type, **CLASSIFICATIONS** appear in **BOLDFACE SMALL CAPS**, and Combination Drugs appear in *italics*. A **"C"** and a **boldface** page number following a generic name identify the page in the "Classification" section on which that drug is listed.

*Entries for **generic** names appear in **boldface type,** trade names appear in regular type, **CLASSIFICATIONS** appear in **BOLDFACE SMALL CAPS,** and Combination Drugs appear in *italics.* A **"C"** and a **boldface** page number following a generic name identify the page in the "Classification" section on which that drug is listed.

*Entries for **generic** names appear in **boldface type,** trade names appear in regular type, **CLASSIFICATIONS** appear in **BOLDFACE SMALL CAPS,** and Combination Drugs appear in *italics.* A **"C"** and a **boldface** page number following a generic name identify the page in the "Classification" section on which that drug is listed.

*Entries for **generic** names appear in **boldface type,** trade names appear in regular type, CLASSIFICATIONS appear in **BOLDFACE SMALL CAPS,** and Combination Drugs appear in *italics.* A **"C"** and a **boldface** page number following a generic name identify the page in the "Classification" section on which that drug is listed.

*Entries for **generic** names appear in **boldface type,** trade names appear in regular type, **CLASSIFICATIONS** appear in **BOLDFACE SMALL CAPS,** and Combination Drugs appear in *italics.* A **"C"** and a **boldface** page number following a generic name identify the page in the "Classification" section on which that drug is listed.

M

*Entries for **generic** names appear in **boldface type,** trade names appear in regular type, **CLASSIFICATIONS** appear in **BOLDFACE SMALL CAPS,** and Combination Drugs appear in *italics.* A **"C"** and a **boldface** page number following a generic name identify the page in the "Classification" section on which that drug is listed.

*Entries for **generic** names appear in **boldface type,** trade names appear in regular type, **CLASSIFICATIONS** appear in **BOLDFACE SMALL CAPS,** and Combination Drugs appear in *italics.* A **"C"** and a **boldface** page number following a generic name identify the page in the "Classification" section on which that drug is listed.

*Entries for **generic** names appear in **boldface type,** trade names appear in regular type, **CLASSIFICATIONS** appear in **BOLDFACE SMALL CAPS,** and Combination Drugs appear in *italics.* A **"C"** and a **boldface** page number following a generic name identify the page in the "Classification" section on which that drug is listed.

*Entries for **generic** names appear in **boldface type,** trade names appear in regular type, **CLASSIFICATIONS** appear in **BOLDFACE SMALL CAPS,** and Combination Drugs appear in *italics.* A **"C"** and a **boldface** page number following a generic name identify the page in the "Classification" section on which that drug is listed.

*Entries for **generic** names appear in **boldface type,** trade names appear in regular type, **CLASSIFICATIONS** appear in **BOLDFACE SMALL CAPS,** and Combination Drugs appear in *italics.* A **"C"** and a **boldface** page number following a generic name identify the page in the "Classification" section on which that drug is listed.

*Entries for **generic** names appear in **boldface type**, trade names appear in regular type, **CLASSIFICATIONS** appear in **BOLDFACE SMALL CAPS**, and Combination Drugs appear in *italics*. A "**C**" and a **boldface** page number following a generic name identify the page in the "Classification" section on which that drug is listed.

*Entries for **generic** names appear in **boldface type**, trade names appear in regular type, **CLASSIFICATIONS** appear in **BOLDFACE SMALL CAPS**, and Combination Drugs appear in *italics.* A **"C"** and a **boldface** page number following a generic name identify the page in the "Classification" section on which that drug is listed.

O

*Entries for **generic** names appear in **boldface type,** trade names appear in regular type, **CLASSIFICATIONS** appear in **BOLDFACE SMALL CAPS,** and Combination Drugs appear in *italics.* A **"C"** and a **boldface** page number following a generic name identify the page in the "Classification" section on which that drug is listed.

*Entries for **generic** names appear in **boldface type,** trade names appear in regular type, **CLASSIFICATIONS** appear in **BOLDFACE SMALL CAPS,** and Combination Drugs appear in *italics.* A **"C"** and a **boldface** page number following a generic name identify the page in the "Classification" section on which that drug is listed.

*Entries for **generic** names appear in **boldface type,** trade names appear in regular type, **CLASSIFICATIONS** appear in **BOLDFACE SMALL CAPS,** and Combination Drugs appear in *italics.* A **"C"** and a **boldface** page number following a generic name identify the page in the "Classification" section on which that drug is listed.

*Entries for **generic** names appear in **boldface type,** trade names appear in regular type, **CLASSIFICATIONS** appear in **BOLDFACE SMALL CAPS,** and Combination Drugs appear in *italics.* A **"C"** and a **boldface** page number following a generic name identify the page in the "Classification" section on which that drug is listed.

*Entries for **generic** names appear in **boldface type**, trade names appear in regular type, **CLASSIFICATIONS** appear in **BOLDFACE SMALL CAPS**, and Combination Drugs appear in *italics*. A **"C"** and a **boldface** page number following a generic name identify the page in the "Classification" section on which that drug is listed.

*Entries for **generic** names appear in **boldface type**, trade names appear in regular type, CLASSIFICATIONS appear in **BOLDFACE SMALL CAPS**, and Combination Drugs appear in *italics*. A **"C"** and a **boldface** page number following a generic name identify the page in the "Classification" section on which that drug is listed.

Q

*Entries for **generic** names appear in **boldface type,** trade names appear in regular type, **CLASSIFICATIONS** appear in **BOLDFACE SMALL CAPS,** and Combination Drugs appear in *italics.* A **"C"** and a **boldface** page number following a generic name identify the page in the "Classification" section on which that drug is listed.

R

*Entries for **generic** names appear in **boldface type**, trade names appear in regular type, **CLASSIFICATIONS** appear in **BOLDFACE SMALL CAPS**, and Combination Drugs appear in *italics*. A **"C"** and a **boldface** page number following a generic name identify the page in the "Classification" section on which that drug is listed.

*Entries for **generic** names appear in **boldface type,** trade names appear in regular type, **CLASSIFICATIONS** appear in **BOLDFACE SMALL CAPS,** and Combination Drugs appear in *italics.* A **"C"** and a **boldface** page number following a generic name identify the page in the "Classification" section on which that drug is listed.

*Entries for **generic** names appear in **boldface type,** trade names appear in regular type, **CLASSIFICATIONS** appear in **BOLDFACE SMALL CAPS,** and Combination Drugs appear in *italics.* A "**C**" and a **boldface** page number following a generic name identify the page in the "Classification" section on which that drug is listed.

*Entries for **generic** names appear in **boldface type,** trade names appear in regular type, **CLASSIFICATIONS** appear in **BOLDFACE SMALL CAPS,** and Combination Drugs appear in *italics.* A **"C"** and a **boldface** page number following a generic name identify the page in the "Classification" section on which that drug is listed.

T

*Entries for **generic** names appear in **boldface type,** trade names appear in regular type, **CLASSIFICATIONS** appear in **BOLDFACE SMALL CAPS,** and Combination Drugs appear in *italics.* A **"C"** and a **boldface** page number following a generic name identify the page in the "Classification" section on which that drug is listed.

*Entries for **generic** names appear in **boldface type**, trade names appear in regular type, **CLASSIFICATIONS** appear in **BOLDFACE SMALL CAPS**, and Combination Drugs appear in *italics*. A **"C"** and a **boldface** page number following a generic name identify the page in the "Classification" section on which that drug is listed.

*Entries for **generic** names appear in **boldface type,** trade names appear in regular type, **CLASSIFICATIONS** appear in **BOLDFACE SMALL CAPS,** and Combination Drugs appear in *italics.* A **"C"** and a **boldface** page number following a generic name identify the page in the "Classification" section on which that drug is listed.

*Entries for **generic** names appear in **boldface type**, trade names appear in regular type, **CLASSIFICATIONS** appear in **BOLDFACE SMALL CAPS,** and Combination Drugs appear in *italics.* A **"C"** and a **boldface** page number following a generic name identify the page in the "Classification" section on which that drug is listed.

*Entries for **generic** names appear in **boldface type,** trade names appear in regular type, **CLASSIFICATIONS** appear in **BOLDFACE SMALL CAPS,** and Combination Drugs appear in *italics.* A **"C"** and a **boldface** page number following a generic name identify the page in the "Classification" section on which that drug is listed.

*Entries for **generic** names appear in **boldface type**, trade names appear in regular type, **CLASSIFICATIONS** appear in **BOLDFACE SMALL CAPS**, and Combination Drugs appear in *italics*. A **"C"** and a **boldface** page number following a generic name identify the page in the "Classification" section on which that drug is listed.

W

X

Y

Z

*Entries for **generic** names appear in **boldface type,** trade names appear in regular type, **CLASSIFICATIONS** appear in **BOLDFACE SMALL CAPS,** and Combination Drugs appear in *italics.* A **"C"** and a **boldface** page number following a generic name identify the page in the "Classification" section on which that drug is listed.

*Entries for **generic** names appear in **boldface type,** trade names appear in regular type, **CLASSIFICATIONS** appear in **BOLDFACE SMALL CAPS,** and Combination Drugs appear in *italics.* A **"C"** and a **boldface** page number following a generic name identify the page in the "Classification" section on which that drug is listed.

Deltoid site

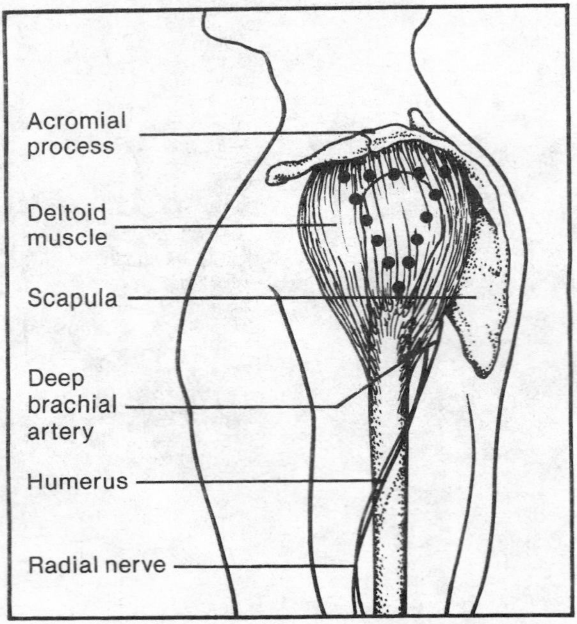

Dorsogluteal site

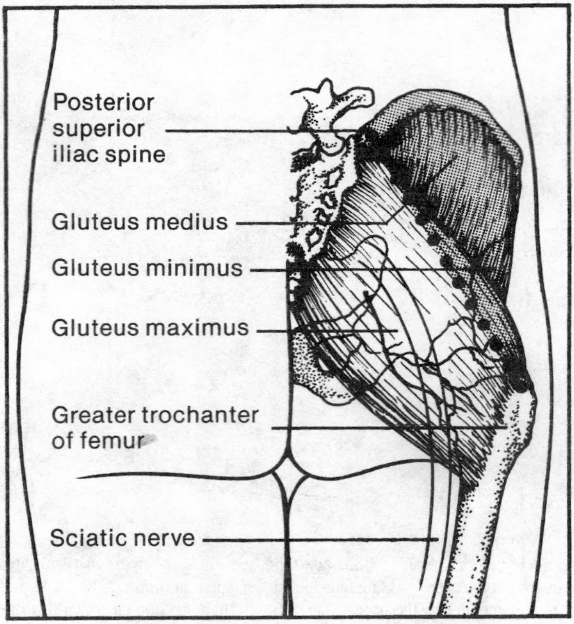

Ventrogluteal site

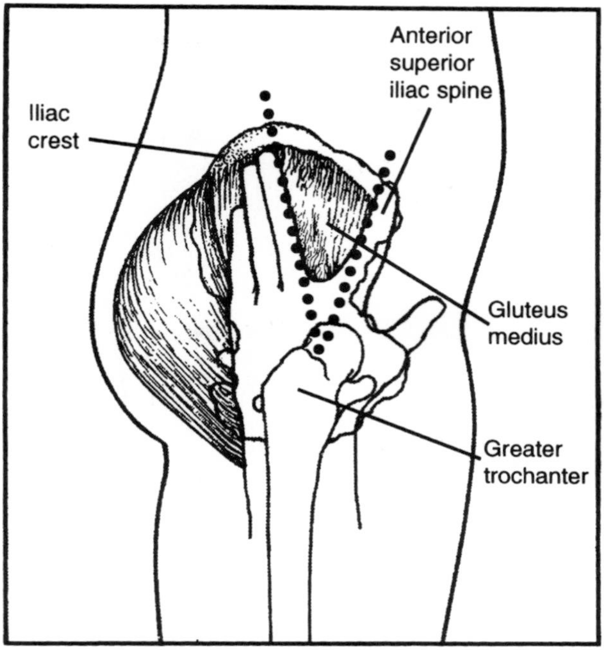

Vastus lateralis site

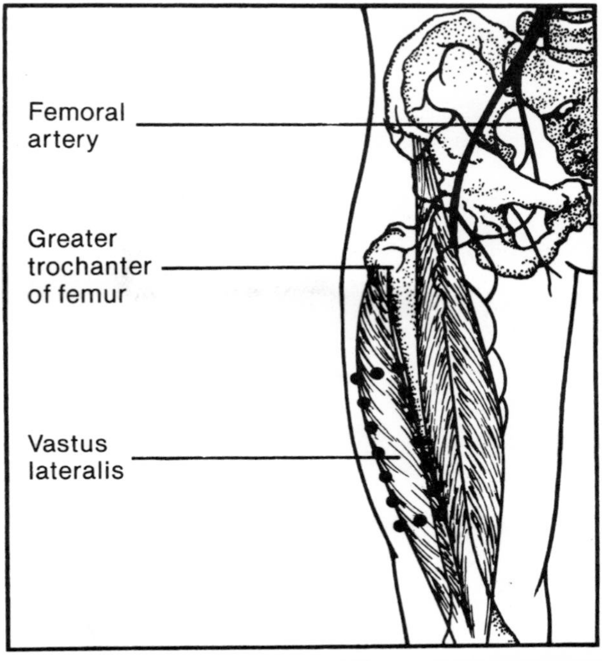